BARRY

Gastrointestinal Disease

Volume 2

Pathophysiology
Diagnosis
Management

FOURTH EDITION

MARVIN H. SLEISENGER, M.D.

Professor of Medicine
Vice Chairman for Academic Affairs
Department of Medicine
Director, Clinical Training Program in Gastroenterology
University of California, San Francisco
Attending Physician, Moffitt-Long Hospital
San Francisco, California

JOHN S. FORDTRAN, M.D.

Professor of Medicine,
Chief, Department of Internal Medicine,
Baylor University Medical Center,
Dallas, Texas

with a foreword by

THOMAS P. ALMY, M.D.

1989

W.B. SAUNDERS COMPANY

Harcourt Brace Jovanovich, Inc.

Philadelphia London Toronto Montreal Sydney Tokyo

Gastrointestinal Disease

Volume 2

Pathophysiology
Diagnosis
Management

FOURTH EDITION

W. B. SAUNDERS COMPANY
Harcourt Brace Jovanovich, Inc.

The Curtis Center
Independence Square West
Philadelphia, PA 19106

Library of Congress Cataloging-in-Publication Data

Gastrointestinal disease: pathophysiology, diagnosis, management/ [edited by] Marvin Sleisenger, John S. Fordtran; with a foreword by Thomas P. Almy.—4th ed.
p. cm.

Includes bibliographical references and index.

ISBN 0–7216–2298–4 (set)

1. Gastrointestinal system—Diseases. I. Sleisenger, Marvin H. II. Fordtran, John S.

RC801.G384 1989

616.3′3—dc19 88–15668

Listed here is the latest translated edition of this book together with the language of the translation and the publisher.

Italian *(3rd Edition)*—Piccin Nuova Libraria S.P.A., Padova, Italy.
Spanish *(3rd Edition)*—Panamericana, Buenos Aires, Argentina.
Portuguese *(2nd Edition)*—Editora Guanabara Koogan S.A., Rio de Janeiro, Brazil.

Editor: Edward Wickland
Developmental Editor: David Kilmer
Designer: W. B. Saunders Staff
Production Manager: Bob Butler
Manuscript Editor: Mark Coyle
Illustration Coordinator: Peg Shaw
Indexer: Helene Taylor

Gastrointestinal Disease

Single Volume ISBN 0–7216–2078–7
Volume I ISBN 0–7216–2079–5
Volume II ISBN 0–7216–2080–9
Set ISBN 0–7216–2298–4

Last digit is the print number: 9 8 7 6 5 4 3 2 1

CONTRIBUTORS

THOMAS P. ALMY, M.D.

Professor of Medicine and Community and Family Medicine, Emeritus, Dartmouth Medical School; Staff Member, Mary Hitchcock Memorial Hospital, Hanover, New Hampshire, and Veterans Administration Hospital, White River Junction, Vermont
Diverticular Disease of the Colon

DAVID H. ALPERS, M.D.

Professor of Medicine and Chief, Gastroenterology Division, Washington University School of Medicine; Physician, Barnes Hospital, St. Louis, Missouri
Absorption of Vitamins and Divalent Minerals; Eating Behavior and Nutrient Requirements; Nutritional Deficiency in Gastrointestinal Disease; Dietary Management and Vitamin-Mineral Replacement Therapy

DAVID F. ALTMAN, M.D.

Associate Dean of Student and Curricular Affairs, University of California, San Francisco, School of Medicine; Director, Gastroenterology Clinic, University of California Medical Center, San Francisco, California
The Effect of Age on Gastrointestinal Function; Neoplasms of the Gallbladder and Bile Ducts

MARVIN E. AMENT, M.D.

Professor of Pediatrics, University of California, Los Angeles, School of Medicine; Chief, Division of Pediatric Gastroenterology and Nutrition, and Chief, Hospital Parenteral and Enteral Nutritional Support Service, UCLA Medical Center, Los Angeles, California
The Stomach and Duodenum: Anatomy, Embryology, and Developmental Anomalies

JAMES L. AUSTIN, M.D.

Assistant Professor of Surgery, University of Missouri School of Medicine; Staff Surgeon, Truman Veterans Administration Hospital, Columbia, Missouri
Abdominal Abscesses and Gastrointestinal Fistulas

JOHN G. BARTLETT, M.D.

Professor of Medicine, Johns Hopkins University School of Medicine; Chief of Infectious Diseases Division, Johns Hopkins Hospital, Baltimore, Maryland
The Pseudomembranous Enterocolitides

THEODORE M. BAYLESS, M.D.

Professor of Medicine, Johns Hopkins University School of Medicine; Medical Director, Meyerhoff Digestive Disease–Inflammatory Bowel Disease Center, Johns Hopkins Hospital, Baltimore, Maryland
Small Intestinal Ulcers and Strictures: Isolated and Diffuse

MICHAEL D. BENDER, M.D.

Associate Clinical Professor of Medicine and Family and Community Medicine, University of California, San Francisco, School of Medicine, San Francisco, California; Chief of Medicine and Director of Medical Education, Peninsula Hospital, Burlingame, California
Ascites; Diseases of the Peritoneum, Mesentery, and Diaphragm

JEFFREY A. BILLER, M.D.

Assistant Clinical Professor of Pediatrics, Tufts University School of Medicine; Pediatric Gastroenterologist, Division of Pediatric Gastroenterology and Nutrition, The Floating Hospital, New England Medical Center, Boston, Massachusetts
Pancreatic Disorders in Childhood

HENRY J. BINDER, M.D.

Professor of Medicine and Director, Gastrointestinal Research Training Program, Yale University School of Medicine; Director, General Clinical Research Center, Yale–New Haven Medical Center, New Haven, Connecticut
Absorption and Secretion of Water and Electrolytes by Small and Large Intestine

C. RICHARD BOLAND, M.D.

Associate Professor of Medicine, University of Michigan Medical School; Chief of Gastroenterology, Ann Arbor Veterans Administration Medical Center, Ann Arbor, Michigan
Colonic Polyps and the Gastrointestinal Polyposis Syndromes

GEORGE W. BO-LINN, M.D.

St. John's Mercy Medical Center, St. Louis, Missouri
Obesity, Anorexia Nervosa, Bulimia, and Other Eating Disorders

JOHN H. BOND, M.D.

Professor of Medicine, University of Minnesota; Chief, Gastroenterology Section, Veterans Administration Medical Center, Minneapolis, Minnesota
Intestinal Gas

H. WORTH BOYCE, JR., M.S., M.D.

Professor of Medicine; Director, Division of Digestive Diseases and Nutrition; Director, The Center for Swallowing Disorders, University of South Florida College of Medicine, Tampa, Florida
Tumors of the Esophagus

ROBERT S. BRESALIER, M.D.

Assistant Professor of Medicine, University of California, San Francisco, School of Medicine; Attending Physician, Veterans Administration Medical Center, San Francisco, California
Malignant Neoplasms of the Large and Small Intestine

JOHN P. CELLO, M.D.

Associate Professor of Medicine, University of California, San Francisco, School of Medicine; Chief of Gastroenterology, San Francisco General Hospital, San Francisco, California
Ulcerative Colitis; Chronic Pancreatitis; Carcinoma of the Pancreas

RAY E. CLOUSE, M.D.

Assistant Professor of Medicine, Washington University School of Medicine; Assistant Physician, Barnes Hospital, St. Louis, Missouri
Motor Disorders of the Esophagus; Intensive Nutritional Support

SIDNEY COHEN, M.D.

Professor, Temple University School of Medicine; Chairman, Department of Medicine, Temple University Hospital, Philadelphia, Pennsylvania
Movement of the Small and Large Intestine

JEFFREY CONKLIN, M.D.

Assistant Professor, Division of Gastroenterology, Department of Internal Medicine, University of Iowa Hospitals and Clinics, Iowa City, Iowa
Gastrointestinal Smooth Muscle

JEFFREY R. CRIST, M.D.
Instructor in Medicine, Harvard Medical School; Assistant in Medicine, Gastroenterology Division, Beth Israel Hospital, Boston, Massachusetts
Neurology of the Gut

GLENN R. DAVIS, M.D.
Assistant Clinical Professor, University of Arkansas for Medical Science; Staff Physician, St. Vincent Infirmary, Little Rock, Arkansas
Neoplasms of the Stomach

JOHN DELVALLE, M.D.
Instructor of Internal Medicine, Division of Gastroenterology, University of Michigan Medical School, Ann Arbor, Michigan
Secretory Tumors of the Pancreas

GHISLAIN DEVROEDE, M.D.
Professor of Surgery and Physiology, Université de Sherbrooke; Attending Physician, Centre Hospitalier Universitaire, Sherbrooke, Québec, Canada
Constipation

NICHOLAS E. DIAMANT, M.D., F.R.C.P.(C)
Professor of Medicine and Physiology, University of Toronto; Head, Division of Gastroenterology, Toronto Western Hospital, Toronto, Ontario, Canada
Physiology of the Esophagus

WYLIE J. DODDS, M.D.
Professor of Radiology and Medicine, Medical College of Wisconsin; Staff Radiologist, Milwaukee County Medical Center and Froedtert Memorial Lutheran Hospital, Milwaukee, Wisconsin
Gastroesophageal Reflux Disease (Reflux Esophagitis)

ROBERT M. DONALDSON, JR., M.D.
David Paige Smith Professor of Medicine, Yale University School of Medicine; Attending Physician, Yale–New Haven Hospital, New Haven, Connecticut
The Relation of Enteric Bacterial Populations to Gastrointestinal Function and Disease; The Blind Loop Syndrome; Crohn's Disease

DOUGLAS A. DROSSMAN, M.D.
Associate Professor of Medicine and Psychiatry, Division of Digestive Diseases, University of North Carolina School of Medicine; Associate Attending, North Carolina Memorial Hospital, Chapel Hill, North Carolina
The Physician and the Patient: Review of the Psychosocial Gastrointestinal Literature with an Integrated Approach to the Patient

DAVID L. EARNEST, M.D.
Professor of Medicine, University of Arizona College of Medicine; Attending Physician, Gastroenterology Section, University of Arizona Health Sciences Center, Tucson, Arizona
Radiation Enteritis and Colitis; Other Diseases of the Colon and Rectum

ABRAM M. EISENSTEIN, M.D.
Clinical Professor of Medicine, University of Texas Southwestern Medical School at Dallas; Chief of Gastroenterology, Presbyterian Hospital of Dallas; Attending Physician, Parkland Memorial Hospital, Dallas, Texas
Caustic Injury to the Upper Gastrointestinal Tract

THOMAS H. ERMAK, Ph.D.
Assistant Research Cell Biologist, Department of Medicine, University of California, San Francisco, School of Medicine; Attending Staff, Cell Biology and Aging Section, Veterans Administration Medical Center, San Francisco, California
The Pancreas: Anatomy, Histology, Embryology, and Developmental Anomalies

ANTHONY S. FAUCI, M.D.
Director, National Institute of Allergy and Infectious Diseases, National Institutes of Health, Bethesda, Maryland
Acquired Immunodeficiency Syndrome (AIDS)

MARK FELDMAN, M.D.
Professor of Internal Medicine, University of Texas Southwestern Medical School at Dallas; Associate Chief of Staff for Research and Development, Dallas Veterans Administration Medical Center, Dallas, Texas
Nausea and Vomiting; Gastric Secretion in Health and Disease

KENNETH D. FINE, M.D.
Resident in Internal Medicine, Baylor University Medical Center, Dallas, Texas
Diarrhea

JOHN S. FORDTRAN, M.D.
Professor of Medicine and Chief, Department of Internal Medicine, Baylor University Medical Center, Dallas, Texas
Diarrhea

SCOTT L. FRIEDMAN, M.D.
Assistant Professor of Medicine, University of California, San Francisco, School of Medicine; Attending Physician, San Francisco General Hospital, San Francisco, California
Gastrointestinal Manifestations of AIDS and Other Sexually Transmissible Diseases

SHERWOOD L. GORBACH, M.D.
Professor of Community Health and Medicine, Tufts University School of Medicine, Boston, Massachusetts
Infectious Diarrhea

RAJ K. GOYAL, M.D.
Charlotte F. and Irving W. Rabb Professor of Medicine, Harvard Medical School; Chief, Gastroenterology Division, Beth Israel Hospital, Boston, Massachusetts
Neurology of the Gut; Gastrointestinal Smooth Muscle

DAVID Y. GRAHAM, M.D.
Professor of Medicine and Virology, Baylor College of Medicine; Chief of Digestive Disease Division, Veterans Administration Medical Center, Houston, Texas
Complications of Peptic Ulcer Disease and Indications for Surgery

RICHARD J. GRAND, M.D.
Professor of Pediatrics, Tufts University School of Medicine; Chief, Division of Pediatric Gastroenterology and Nutrition, The Floating Hospital, New England Medical Center, Boston, Massachusetts
Pancreatic Disorders in Childhood

JAMES H. GRENDELL, M.D.
Assistant Professor of Medicine and Physiology, University of California, San Francisco, School of Medicine; Attending Physician, San Francisco General Hospital, San Francisco, California
The Pancreas: Anatomy, Histology, and Developmental Anomalies; Chronic Pancreatitis; Vascular Diseases of the Bowel

J. KENT HAMILTON, M.D.
Clinical Instructor of Medicine, University of Texas Southwestern Medical School at Dallas; Attending Physician, Baylor University Medical Center, Dallas, Texas
Foreign Bodies in the Gut

MELVIN B. HEYMAN, M.D., M.P.H.
Assistant Professor, Department of Pediatrics, University of California, San Francisco, School of Medicine; Associate Director, Division of Pediatric Gastroenterology and Nutrition, University of California Children's Medical Center, San Francisco, California
Food Sensitivity and Eosinophilic Gastroenteropathies

MARTIN F. HEYWORTH, M.D., M.R.C.P.

Associate Professor of Medicine, University of California, San Francisco, School of Medicine; Staff Physician, Veterans Administration Medical Center, San Francisco, California
Maldigestion and Malabsorption

ALAN F. HOFMANN, M.D., Ph.D.

Professor of Medicine in Gastroenterology, University of California, San Diego, School of Medicine; Professor of Medicine, University of California, San Diego, Medical Center
The Enterohepatic Circulation of Bile Acids in Health and Disease

WALTER J. HOGAN, M.D.

Professor of Medicine, Medical College of Wisconsin; Chief, Gastrointestinal Diagnostic Laboratory, Froedtert Memorial Lutheran Hospital, Milwaukee, Wisconsin
Gastroesophageal Reflux Disease (Reflux Esophagitis)

R. THOMAS HOLZBACH, M.D.

Head, Gastrointestinal Research Unit, Research Institute, and Department of Gastroenterology, Cleveland Clinic Foundation, Cleveland, Ohio
Pathogenesis and Medical Treatment of Gallstones

STEVEN H. ITZKOWITZ, M.D.

Assistant Professor of Medicine, University of California, San Francisco, School of Medicine; Research Associate, Veterans Administration Medical Center, San Francisco, California
Chronic Polyps and the Gastrointestinal Polyposis Syndromes

GRAHAM H. JEFFRIES, M.S., Ch.B. (N.Z.), D. Phil. (Oxon), F.A.C.P.

Professor and Chairman, Department of Medicine, Pennsylvania State University College of Medicine, Hershey, Pennsylvania
Protein-Losing Gastroenteropathy

R. SCOTT JONES, M.D.

Stephen H. Watts Professor and Chairman, Department of Surgery, University of Virginia; Surgeon-in-Chief, University of Virginia Medical Center, Charlottesville, Virginia
Intestinal Obstruction, Pseudo-Obstruction, and Ileus

PAUL H. JORDAN, JR., M.D.

Professor of Surgery, Baylor College of Medicine; Senior Attending Surgeon, The Methodist Hospital, Houston, Texas
Operations for Peptic Ulcer Disease and Early Postoperative Complications

MARTIN F. KAGNOFF, M.D.

Professor of Medicine, University of California, San Diego, School of Medicine; Attending Physician, University of California, San Diego, Medical Center, San Diego, California
Immunology and Disease of the Gastrointestinal Tract

GORDON L. KAUFFMAN, JR., M.D.

Professor of Surgery and Physiology, and Chief, Division of General Surgery, The Milton S. Hershey Medical Center, Pennsylvania State University, Hershey, Pennsylvania
Stress Ulcers, Erosions, and Gastric Mucosal Injury

YOUNG S. KIM, M.D.

Professor of Medicine and Pathology, University of California, San Francisco, School of Medicine; Director, Gastrointestinal Research Laboratory, Veterans Administration Medical Center, San Francisco, California
Colonic Polyps and the Gastrointestinal Polyposis Syndromes; Malignant Neoplasms of the Large and Small Intestine

FREDERICK A. KLIPSTEIN, M.D.

Professor of Medicine, University of Rochester; Attending Physician, Strong Memorial Hospital, Rochester, New York
Tropical Sprue

O. DHODANAND KOWLESSAR, M.D.

Professor of Medicine and Associate Chairman, Department of Medicine, Jefferson Medical College of Thomas Jefferson University, Philadelphia, Pennsylvania
The Carcinoid Syndrome

GUENTER J. KREJS, M.D.

Professor and Chairman, Department of Internal Medicine, Karl Franzens University, Graz, Austria
Diarrhea

MICHAEL D. LEVITT, M.D.

Professor of Medicine, University of Minnesota; Associate Chief of Staff for Research, Veterans Administration Medical Center, Minneapolis, Minnesota
Intestinal Gas

MARVIN LIPSKY, M.D.

Research Fellow in Medicine, Harvard Medical School; Research/Clinical Fellow in Medicine, Brigham and Women's Hospital, Boston, Massachusetts
The Short Bowel Syndrome

PETER M. LOEB, M.D.

Clinical Professor of Medicine, University of Texas Southwestern Medical School at Dallas; Gastroenterologist, Presbyterian Hospital; Attending Gastroenterologist, Parkland Memorial Hospital and Veterans Administration Medical Center, Dallas, Texas
Caustic Injury to the Upper Gastrointestinal Tract

TIMOTHY P. MARONEY, M.D.

Assistant Professor of Radiology, University of California, San Francisco, School of Medicine; Attending Physician, University of California Medical Center, San Francisco, California
Endoscopic/Radiologic Treatment of Biliary Tract Diseases

HENRY MASUR, M.D.

Deputy Chief, Critical Care Medicine Department, Clinical Center, National Institutes of Health, Bethesda, Maryland; Clinical Professor of Medicine, George Washington University School of Medicine, Washington, D.C.
Acquired Immunodeficiency Syndrome (AIDS)

RICHARD W. McCALLUM, M.D., F.A.C.P., F.R.A.C.P. (Aust.), F.A.C.S.

Paul Janssen Professor of Medicine, University of Virginia School of Medicine; Chief, Division of Gastroenterology, University of Virginia Medical Center, Charlottesville, Virginia; Director of Gastrointestinal Fellowship Program at University of Virginia and Salem Veterans Administration Center, Salem, Virginia
Motor Function of the Stomach in Health and Disease

GEORGE B. McDONALD, M.D.

Professor of Medicine, University of Washington School of Medicine; Attending Physician, Veterans Administration Medical Center, Fred Hutchinson Cancer Research Center, University Hospital, Harborview Medical Center, and Pacific Medical Center, Seattle, Washington
Esophageal Diseases Caused by Infection, Systemic Illness, and Trauma

JAMES E. McGUIGAN, M.D.

Professor and Chairman, Department of Medicine, University of Florida College of Medicine; Physician-in-Chief, Shands Hospital, Gainesville, Florida
Anatomy, Embryology, and Developmental Anomalies; The Zollinger-Ellison Syndrome

JAMES H. MEYER, M.D.

Chief of Gastroenterology, Veterans Administration Medical Center, Sepulveda, California
Chronic Morbidity after Ulcer Surgery; Pancreatic Physiology

ARTHUR NAITOVE, M.D.

Professor of Surgery, Dartmouth Medical School; Attending Physician, Mary Hitchcock Memorial Hospital, Hanover, New Hampshire; Attending Physician, Veterans Administration Medical Center, White River Junction, Vermont
Diverticular Disease of the Colon

THOMAS F. O'BRIEN, JR., M.D.

Professor of Medicine, East Carolina University School of Medicine, Greenville, North Carolina
Benign Neoplasms and Vascular Malformations of the Large and Small Intestine

ROBERT K. OCKNER, M.D.

Professor of Medicine, University of California, San Francisco, School of Medicine; Chief, Division of Gastroenterology, Moffitt-Long Hospitals; Attending Physician, San Francisco General Hospital and Veterans Administration Medical Center; Consultant, Letterman Army Medical Center, San Francisco, California
Ascites; Vascular Diseases of the Bowel

ROBERT L. OWEN, M.D.

Professor of Medicine, Epidemiology, and International Health, University of California, San Francisco, School of Medicine; Staff Physician, Veterans Administration Medical Center, San Francisco, California
Parasitic Diseases; Gastrointestinal Manifestations of AIDS and Other Sexually Transmissible Diseases

WALTER L. PETERSON, M.D.

Associate Professor of Internal Medicine, University of Texas Southwestern Medical School at Dallas; Chief, Gastroenterology Section, Dallas Veterans Administration Medical Center, Dallas, Texas
Gastrointestinal Bleeding

SIDNEY F. PHILLIPS, M.D.

Professor of Medicine, Mayo Medical School; Director, Gastroenterology Unit, Mayo Clinic, Rochester, Minnesota
Megacolon: Congenital and Acquired; Conventional and Alternative Ileostomies

DANIEL E. POLTER, M.D.

Clinical Professor of Medicine, University of Texas Southwestern Medical School at Dallas; Attending Staff, Baylor University Medical Center, Dallas, Texas
Foreign Bodies in the Gut

CHARLES E. POPE, II, M.D.

Professor of Medicine, University of Washington School of Medicine; Chief, Gastroenterology, Veterans Administration Medical Center, Seattle, Washington
Heartburn, Dysphagia, and Other Esophageal Symptoms; The Esophagus: Anatomy and Developmental Anomalies; Rings and Webs; Diverticula

STEVEN B. RAFFIN, M.D., F.A.C.P.

Associate Clinical Professor of Medicine, University of California, San Francisco, School of Medicine, San Francisco, California; Attending Physician, Peninsula Hospital and Medical Center, Burlingame, California
The Stomach and Duodenum: Diverticula, Rupture, and Volvulus; Bezoars

HOWARD A. REBER, M.D.

Professor of Surgery and Vice Chairman, Department of Surgery, University of California, Los Angeles, School of Medicine, Los Angeles, California; Chief, Surgical Service, Sepulveda Veterans Administration Hospital, Sepulveda, California
Abdominal Abscesses and Gastrointestinal Fistulas

CHARLES T. RICHARDSON, M.D.

Patterson Professor of Medicine, University of Texas Southwestern Medical Center at Dallas; Chief of Staff, Dallas Veterans Administration Medical Center, Dallas, Texas
Gastric Ulcer

ERNEST J. RING, M.D.

Professor of Radiology and Chief of Interventional Radiology, University of California, San Francisco, School of Medicine
Endoscopic/Radiologic Treatment of Biliary Tract Diseases

ANDRÉ ROBERT, M.D., Ph.D.

Senior Scientist, Drug Metabolism Research, The Upjohn Company, Kalamazoo, Michigan
Stress Ulcers, Erosions, and Gastric Mucosal Injury

IRWIN H. ROSENBERG, M.D.

Professor of Medicine and Nutrition, and Director of USDA Human Nutrition Research Center on Aging, Tufts University; Attending Physician, New England Medical Center, Boston, Massachusetts
Eating Behavior and Nutrient Requirements; Nutritional Deficiency in Gastrointestinal Disease; Intensive Nutritional Support

TODD L. SACK, M.D.

Assistant Professor of Medicine in Residence, University of California, San Francisco, School of Medicine; Attending Physician, University of California Medical Center and Veterans Administration Medical Center, San Francisco, California
Effects of Systemic and Extraintestinal Disease on the Gut; Oral Diseases and Cutaneous Manifestations of Gastrointestinal Disease

BRUCE F. SCHARSCHMIDT, M.D.

Professor of Medicine, University of California, San Francisco, School of Medicine; Attending Physician, University of California, San Francisco, Affiliated Hospitals, San Francisco, California
Jaundice; Bile Formation and Gallbladder and Bile Duct Function

LAWRENCE R. SCHILLER, M.D.

Clinical Assistant Professor of Internal Medicine, University of Texas Southwestern Medical School at Dallas; Associate Attending Physician and Director, Gastroenterology Physiology Laboratory, Baylor University Medical Center, Dallas, Texas
Fecal Incontinence

BRUCE D. SCHIRMER, M.D.

Assistant Professor of Surgery, University of Virginia Medical Center, Charlottesville, Virginia
Intestinal Obstruction, Pseudo-Obstruction, and Ileus

DAVID J. SCHNEIDERMAN, M.D.

Assistant Professor of Medicine, University of Arizona School of Medicine; Director, Gastrointestinal Endoscopy Unit, Arizona Health Sciences Center, Tucson, Arizona
Ulcerative Colitis; Other Diseases of the Colon and Rectum

THEODORE SCHROCK, M.D.

Professor of Surgery, University of California, San Francisco, School of Medicine, San Francisco, California
Complications of Gastrointestinal Endoscopy; Acute Appendicitis; Examination of the Anorectum, Rigid Sigmoidoscopy, Flexible Sigmoidoscopy, and Diseases of the Anorectum

MARVIN M. SCHUSTER, M.D., F.A.C.P., F.A.P.A.

Professor of Medicine with Joint Appointment in Psychiatry, Johns Hopkins University School of Medicine; Director, Division of Digestive Diseases, Francis Scott Key Medical Center, Baltimore, Maryland
Irritable Bowel Syndrome

HOWARD A. SHAPIRO, M.D.

Clinical Professor of Medicine, University of California, San Francisco, School of Medicine; Attending Physician, University of California, Medical Center, San Francisco, California
Endoscopic/Radiologic Treatment of Biliary Tract Diseases

JAMES SHOREY, M.D.

Chief, Hepatology Section, Medical Service, Dallas Veterans Administration Medical Center, Dallas, Texas
Evaluation of Mass Lesions in the Liver

SOL SILVERMAN, JR., M.A., D.D.S.

Professor and Chairman, Division of Oral Medicine, University of California, San Francisco, School of Dentistry; Attending Dentist, Moffitt-Long Hospital, San Francisco, California
Oral Diseases and Cutaneous Manifestations of Gastrointestinal Disease

DENNIS R. SINAR, M.D.

Associate Professor of Medicine, East Carolina University School of Medicine; Chairman, Laser Committee, Pitt County Memorial Hospital, Greenville, North Carolina
Benign Neoplasms and Vascular Malformations of the Large and Small Intestine

MARVIN H. SLEISENGER, M.D.

Professor of Medicine and Vice Chairman for Academic Affairs, Department of Medicine; Director, Clinical Training Program in Gastroenterology, University of California, San Francisco, School of Medicine; Attending Physician, Moffitt-Long Hospital, San Francisco, California
Effects of Systemic and Extraintestinal Disease on the Gut; Cholelithiasis; Chronic and Acute Cholecystitis; Biliary Obstruction, Cholangitis, and Choledocholithiasis; Postoperative Syndromes

WILLIAM J. SNAPE, JR.

Professor of Medicine, University of California, Los Angeles, School of Medicine; Chief of Gastroenterology, Harbor-UCLA Medical Center, Los Angeles, California
Movement of the Small and Large Intestine

KONRAD H. SOERGEL, M.D.

Professor of Medicine and Chief, Division of Gastroenterology, Medical College of Wisconsin; Chief, Gastroenterology Service, Froedtert Memorial Lutheran Hospital and Milwaukee County Medical Complex, Milwaukee, Wisconsin
Acute Pancreatitis

ANDREW H. SOLL, M.D.

Professor of Medicine, University of California, Los Angeles, School of Medicine; Key Investigator, Center for Ulcer Research and Education, Wadsworth Veterans Administration Medical Center, Los Angeles, California
Duodenal Ulcer and Drug Therapy

M. MICHAEL THALER, M.D.

Professor of Pediatrics and Director, Pediatric Gastroenterology and Nutrition, University of California, San Francisco, School of Medicine; Attending Physician, University of California Medical Center, San Francisco, California
The Biliary Tract: Embryology and Anatomy; Biliary Disease in Infancy and Childhood

RICHARD C. THIRLBY, M.D.

Staff Surgeon, The Virginia Mason Clinic, Seattle, Washington
Postoperative Recurrent Ulcer

PHILLIP P. TOSKES, M.D.

Professor of Medicine and Director, Division of Gastroenterology, Hepatology and Nutrition, University of Florida College of Medicine and Gainesville Veterans Administration Medical Center; Attending Physician, Shands Hospital of the University of Florida, Gainesville, Florida
The Relation of Enteric Bacterial Populations to Gastrointestinal Function and Disease; The Blind Loop Syndrome

ROGER B. TRAYCOFF, M.D.

Associate Professor of Medicine and Anesthesiology, Department of Medicine, Section of Algology, Southern Illinois University School of Medicine, Springfield, Illinois
The Management of Abdominal Pain

JERRY S. TRIER, M.D.

Professor of Medicine, Harvard Medical School; Co-Director, Gastroenterology Division, and Senior Physician, Brigham and Women's Hospital, Boston, Massachusetts
Anatomy, Embryology, and Developmental Abnormalities of the Small and Large Intestine and Colon; The Short Bowel Syndrome; Celiac Sprue; Whipple's Disease; Radiation Enteritis and Colitis

REBECCA W. VAN DYKE, M.D.

Assistant Professor of Medicine, University of California, San Francisco, School of Medicine; Attending Physician, Moffitt-Long Hospital, University of California Medical Center, San Francisco, California
Mechanisms of Digestion and Absorption of Food

JOHN H. WALSH, M.D.

Professor of Medicine, Division of Gastroenterology, University of California, Los Angeles, School of Medicine; Director, Center for Ulcer Research and Education, Wadsworth Veterans Administration Medical Center, Los Angeles, California
Gastrointestinal Peptide Hormones

LAWRENCE W. WAY, M.D.

Professor of Surgery, University of California, San Francisco, School of Medicine; Attending Surgeon, University of California Medical Center; Chief, Surgical Service, Veterans Administration Medical Center, San Francisco, California
Abdominal Pain; Cholelithiasis; Chronic and Acute Cholecystitis; Biliary Obstruction, Cholangitis, and Choledocholithiasis; Postoperative Syndromes; Neoplasms of the Gallbladder and Bile Ducts

WILFRED M. WEINSTEIN, M.D.

Professor of Medicine, Division of Gastroenterology, University of California, Los Angeles, School of Medicine; Attending Physician, UCLA Medical Center, Los Angeles, California
Gastritis

HARLAND S. WINTER, M.D.

Assistant Professor of Pediatrics, Harvard Medical School; Associate in Gastroenterology, The Children's Hospital; Associate Pediatrician, Massachusetts General Hospital, Boston, Massachusetts
Anatomy, Embryology, and Developmental Abnormalities of the Small Intestine and Colon

TERESA L. WRIGHT, B.M., B.S., M.D.

Assistant Professor of Medicine, University of California, San Francisco, School of Medicine; Attending Staff, Veterans Administration Medical Center, San Francisco, California
Maldigestion and Malabsorption

TADATAKA YAMADA, M.D.

Professor of Internal Medicine and Chief of Division of Gastroenterology, University of Michigan Medical School, Ann Arbor, Michigan
Secretory Tumors of the Pancreas

FOREWORD

Since its first publication in 1973, the appearance of a new edition of this widely acclaimed text has served as a milestone in the progress of our knowledge of digestive disease. For twenty years the Editors, themselves deeply involved in the logarithmic growth of fundamental research and in the rising standards of clinical training and education, have enlisted more than one hundred of the major North American participants in that progress as contributors to this trusted resource for learning and for patient care.

Like its predecessors, the Fourth Edition affords the reader a sound orientation to current concepts of biology, human behavior, pathophysiology, pharmacology, and nutrition essential for understanding the broad spectrum of manifestations of digestive illness; yet its chief emphasis is on the rational and effective management of the principal gastrointestinal diseases and disorders encountered in developed Western countries. As before, the Editors have excluded from the scope of the book only the diseases of the liver, some conditions common in children, and most specific infections of the gut, in view of excellent coverage of those fields by other texts.

The veteran reader of this work will find extensive revisions, incorporating new advances in the basic and clinical aspects of our field and bringing into play the insights of thirteen new authors or coauthors. Eight wholly new chapters present important fresh perspectives on, among other things, the acquired immunodeficiency syndrome (AIDS), the gastrointestinal effects of aging, the management of intrahepatic masses disclosed by modern methods of imaging, and the endoscopic treatment of biliary tract disease. The material on cytoprotection of the gut mucosa, on the pathogenesis of gallstones, on premalignant conditions in the digestive tract, and on psychological interactions between physician and patient has been thoroughly updated. The section on nutritional management has been revised to reflect recent advances in basic nutritional concepts and to provide authoritative guidance on the benefits and limitations of enteral and parenteral feedings for functionally impaired patients. The coverage of new diagnostic procedures is no less extensive than in the previous edition but will be found, suitably indexed, in the chapters that describe their most important clinical applications. This change should facilitate the most appropriate, timely, and cost-effective use of these rapidly evolving and expensive resources.

The Editors are to be congratulated on their conspicuous success in keeping their far-flung readership abreast of the current rapid advances in digestive disease. Their Fourth Edition is a volume of large but still manageable proportions, whose weight will be measured not in pounds but by its continuing impact on the modern practice of gastroenterology.

THOMAS P. ALMY

ACKNOWLEDGMENTS

The Editors are grateful to the many authors of this book who have written wisely and well. Numerous colleagues have aided us by their constant encouragment and support; among them we would like especially to thank Dick Root, Holly Smith, Bob Ockner, John Cello, Bruce Scharschmidt, and Young Kim; and Boone Powell, Jr., Don Seldin, Dan Foster, Floyd Rector, Carol Santa Ana, and Lawrence Schiller. The Editors have also benefited from the continuing advice and support of the veteran contributors who helped to plan the First Edition: Bob Donaldson, Chuck Pope, Jerry Trier, and Larry Way, and Dave Alpers and Irv Rosenberg for their efforts in behalf of the section on Nutrition. For excellent secretarial assistance we thank Eva Fruit, Connie Van, Janie Francis, Marcia Horvitz, and Sharon Michael. We also happily acknowledge the fine efforts of the professionals at the W. B. Saunders Company: Lew Reines, Ed Wickland, Bob Butler, Dave Kilmer, Mark Coyle, Peg Shaw, and Helene Taylor.

We are especially proud to acknowledge the encouragement of our wives, Lenore Sleisenger and Jewel Fordtran; and of our children and grandchildren, Tom Sleisenger; Bill, Micki, Joey, and Amy Fordtran; and Bess, Bryan, Emily and Sarah Stone.

Again, we cannot fail to mention the influence of the late Mort Grossman and the late Franz Ingelfinger, and the continuing encouragement of Tom Almy. Directly and indirectly they all influenced this work. We hope we have justified their efforts and confidence.

PREFACE

In the five years since the Third Edition, the avalanche of information has been greater than during the intervals between preceding editions. Once again we have found it impossible to eliminate enough of the older material in making way for the newer to maintain constant the size of the work. So, the Fourth Edition is a bit bigger. Fortunately, availability of thinner and lighter paper has allowed this to be done with little increase in the book's weight. The bibliography remains rather complete, reflecting our belief that all important statements require documentation.

Many chapters have been completely rewritten, and all the others were thoroughly updated. In Part I, Some Psychologic and Biologic Aspects of Gastrointestinal Disease, we have a new chapter, The Effect of Age on Gastrointestinal Function. New additions to Part II, Major Symptoms and Syndromes, include chapters on Complications of Gastrointestinal Endoscopy, Fecal Incontinence, and Evaluation of Mass Lesions in the Liver. We have also given greater emphasis to the oral and cutaneous manifestations of gastrointestinal disease by discussing these important clinical findings in a separate chapter. In Part V, The Small and Large Intestine, there is a new chapter on Acquired Immunodeficiency Syndrome, and several chapters have been expanded considerably (including those on Colon Cancer and Food Sensitivity and Eosinophilic Gastroenteropathies. Part VI, The Biliary Tract: Anatomy, Physiology, and Disease, contains a new chapter on Endoscopic and Radiologic Treatment. Finally, much new information on nutrition will be found in Part IX, particularly on the biomedical effects of alcohol, on vitamin and mineral deficiencies, and on enteral nutrition therapy.

We have deleted the section in the Third Edition entitled Special Diagnostic Procedures. Indications for endoscopy of the upper intestinal tract, biliary tract, pancreas, and colon and for the various scanning techniques will be found in the chapters devoted to the diseases of the various organ systems.

Although we have tried our best to control it, we are still guilty of some repetition. We hope it will be looked upon as educational reinforcement rather than poor editing. We hope this Fourth Edition will be found both helpful and stimulating for all who are interested in the theory and practice of gastroenterology.

CONTENTS

PART I

SOME PSYCHOLOGIC AND BIOLOGIC ASPECTS OF GASTROINTESTINAL FUNCTIONS AND DISEASES

PART II

MAJOR SYMPTOMS AND SYNDROMES: PATHOPHYSIOLOGY, DIAGNOSIS, AND MANAGEMENT

PART III

THE ESOPHAGUS: ANATOMY, PHYSIOLOGY, AND DISEASE

PART IV

THE STOMACH AND DUODENUM: ANATOMY, PHYSIOLOGY, AND DISEASE

PART V
THE SMALL AND LARGE INTESTINE: ANATOMY, PHYSIOLOGY, AND DISEASE

PART VI

THE BILIARY TRACT: ANATOMY, PHYSIOLOGY, AND DISEASE

PART VII

THE PANCREAS: ANATOMY, PHYSIOLOGY, AND DISEASE

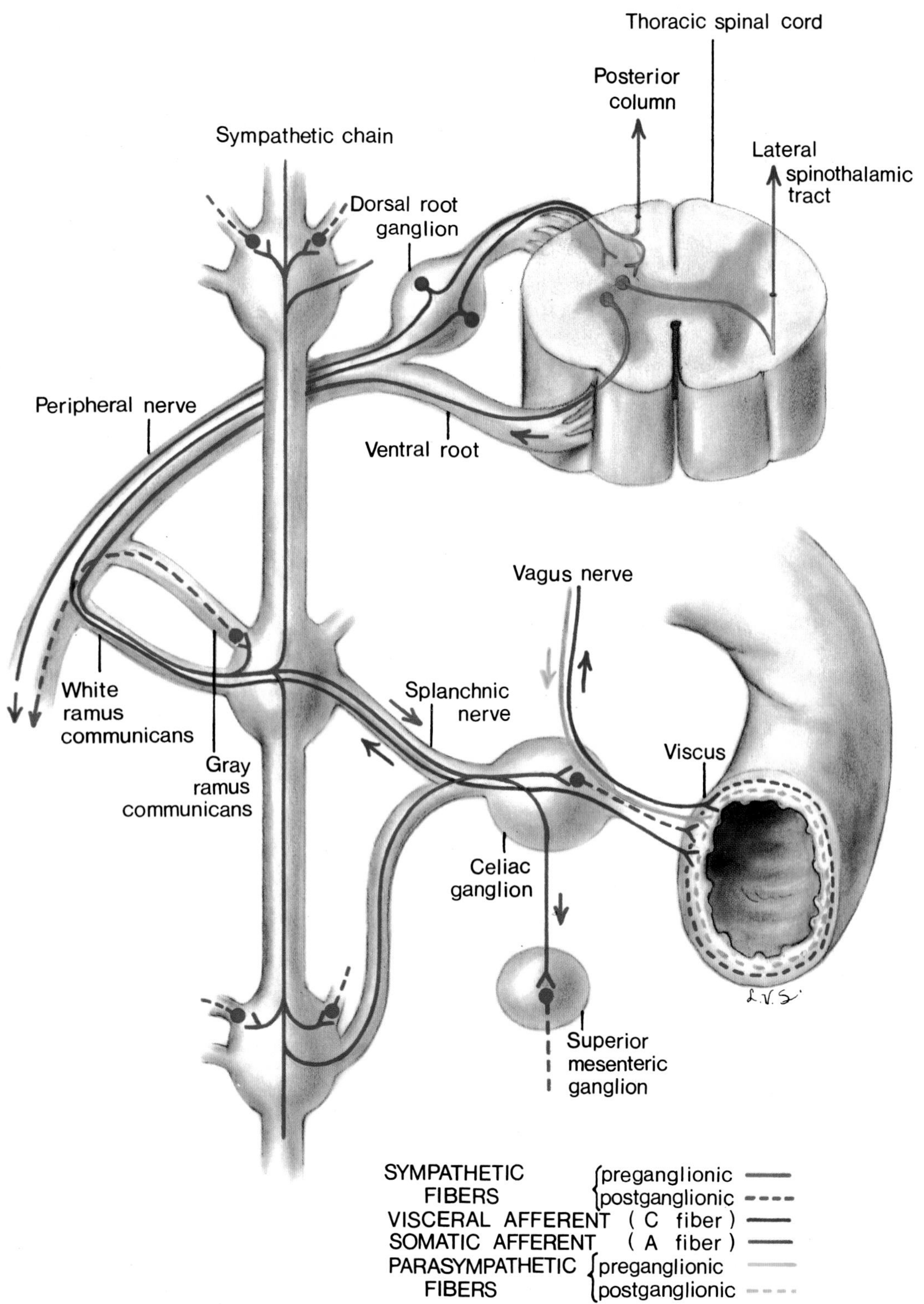

Figure 15–2. Relationship of visceral afferent fibers that transmit pain impulses to autonomic and somatic afferent fibers. The visceral afferents for pain pass through the splanchnic ganglia, reach the sympathetic chain in the splanchnic nerves, and enter the dorsal root via the white ramus communicans. They synapse with cell bodies in the dorsal horn that send impulses toward the brain in the lateral spinothalamic tract. These relays may be inhibited by sensory impulses that enter in large afferents from the periphery (A fibers). The connections undoubtedly are much more complex than shown here. (Adapted from Netter.)

PART VIII

DISEASES OF THE INTRA-ABDOMINAL VASCULATURE AND SUPPORTIVE STRUCTURES

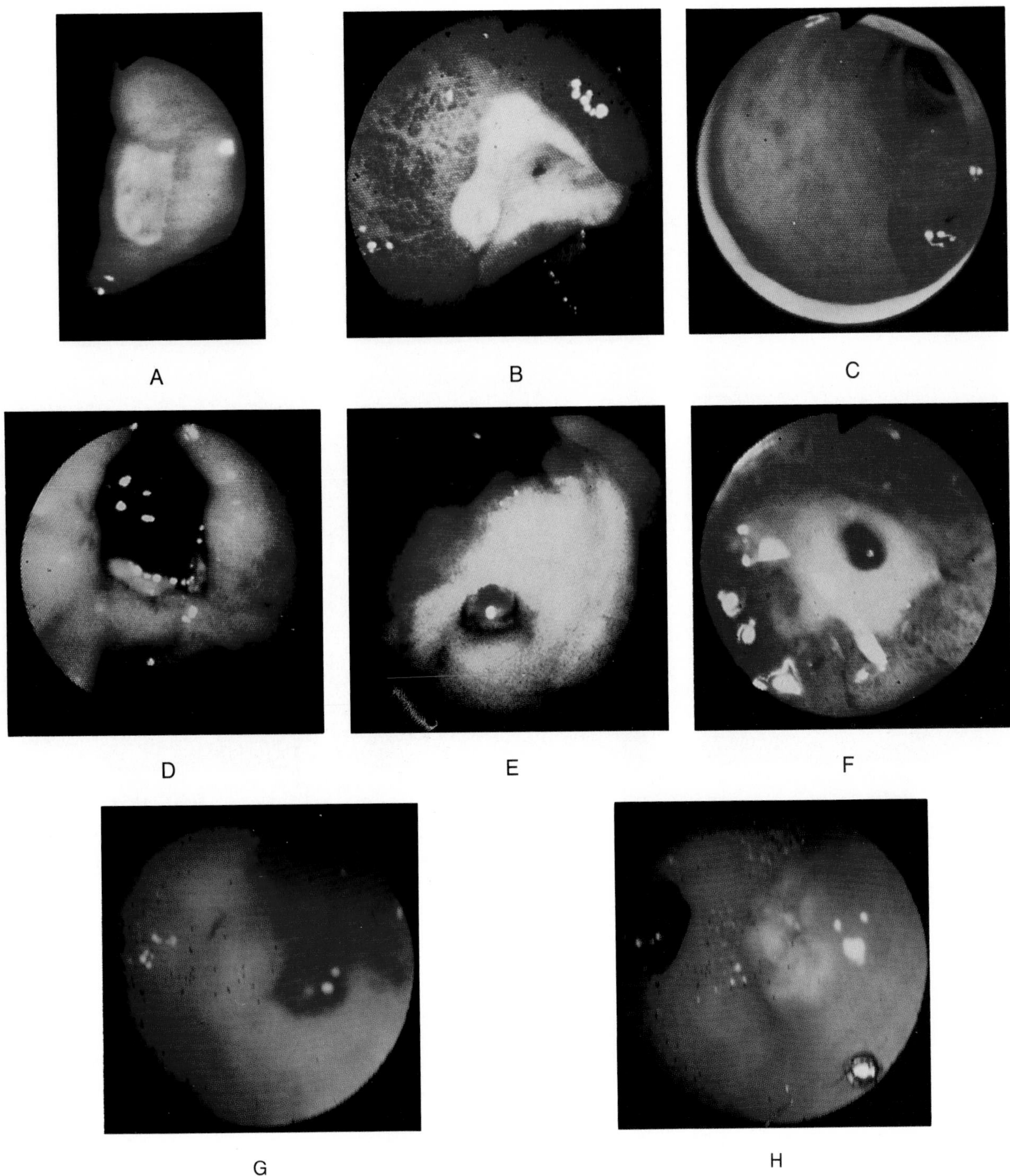

Figure 25–4. Bleeding peptic ulcers. *A,* Clean base. *B,* Central spot. *C,* Fresh clot. *D,* Black clot. *E* and *F,* Visible vessels (sentinel clots). *G,* Active bleeding. *H,* After electrocoagulation. (Photos courtesy of D. Fleischer, M.D. [C]; H. Parker, M.D. [D and E]; and J. Morrissey, M.D. [G, H].)

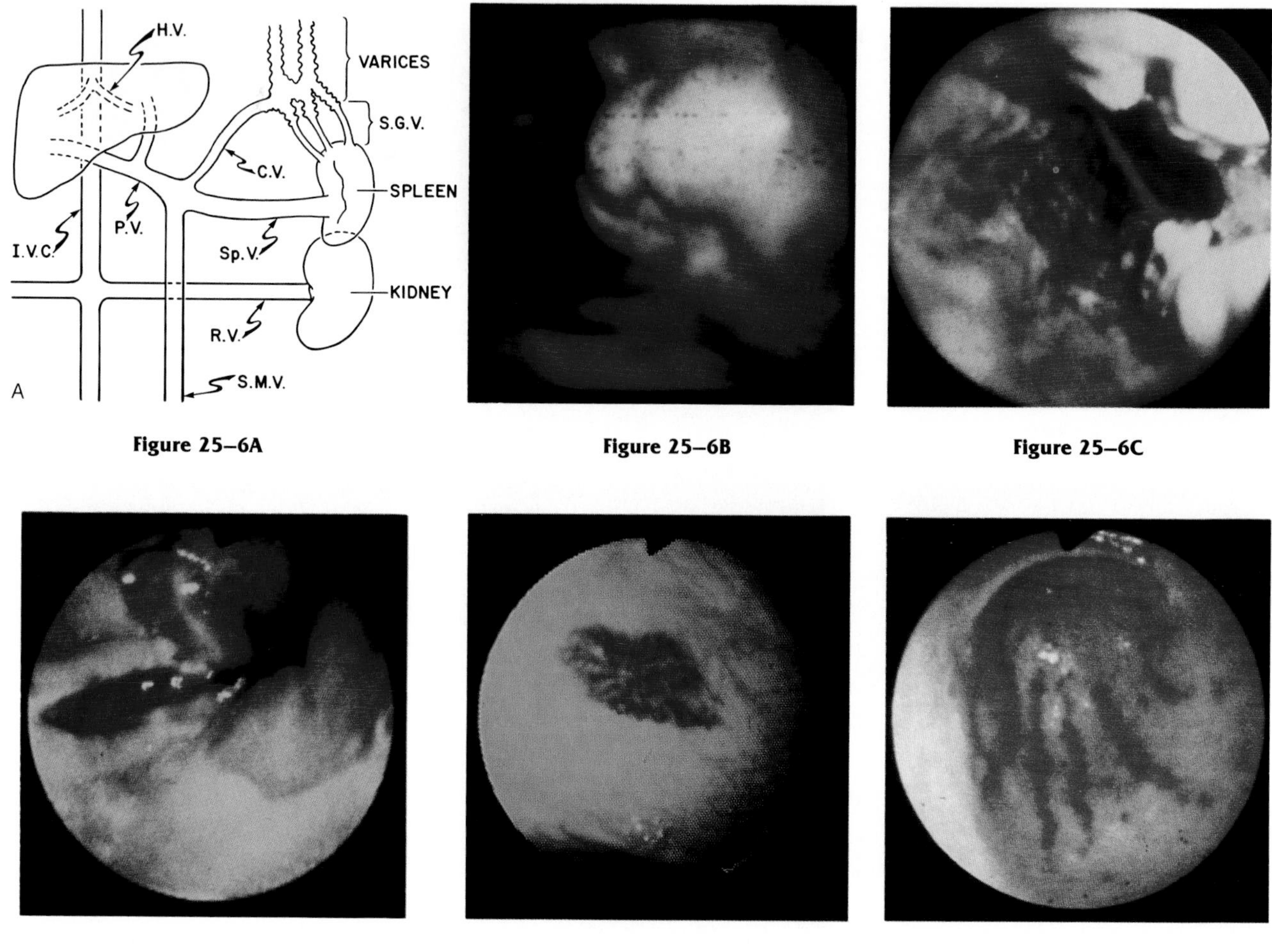

Figure 25–6A **Figure 25–6B** **Figure 25–6C**

Figure 25–10 **Figure 25–14A** **Figure 25–14B**

Figure 25–6. *A,* Diagrammatic representation of the portal circulation showing esophagogastric varices. H.V., hepatic vein; I.V.C., inferior vena cava; P.V., portal vein; C.V., coronary vein; Sp.V., splenic vein; R.V., renal vein; S.M.V., superior mesenteric vein; S.G.V., short gastric veins. *B,* Large, nonbleeding varices. *C,* Actively bleeding esophageal varix. (Courtesy of J. Morrissey, M.D.)

Figure 25–10. Mallory-Weiss tear at gastroesophageal junction. (Courtesy of J. Noble, M.D.)

Figure 25–14. *A,* Cecal vascular ectasia. (Courtesy of H. Parker, M.D.). *B,* Antral vascular ectasia. (Reprinted with permission from: Gastric antral vascular ectasia: The watermelon stomach, by Jabbari, M., Cherry, R., Lough, J. O., et al. Gastroenterology *87:*1165. Copyright 1984 by The American Gastroenterological Association.)

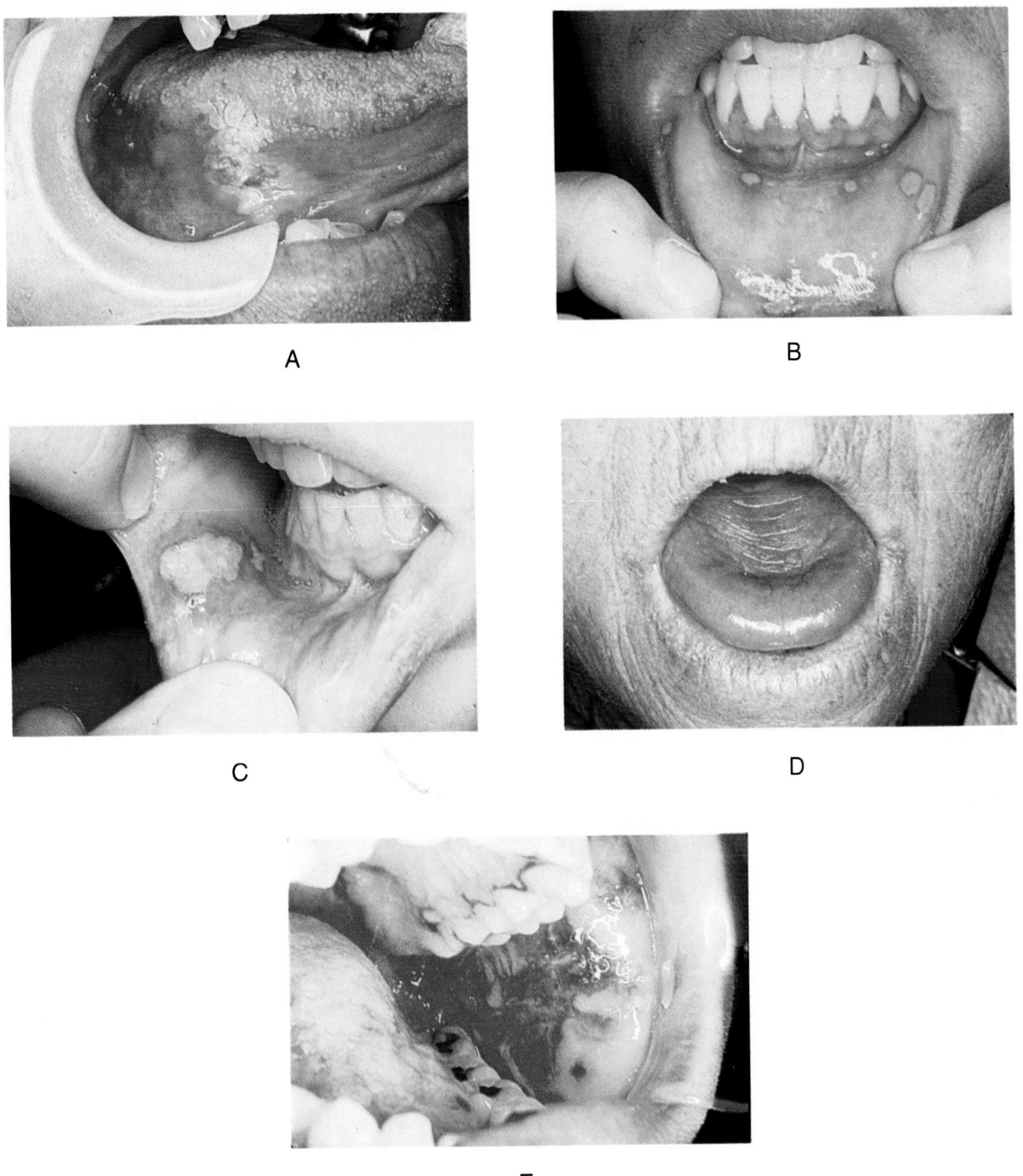

Figure 30–2. Oral lesions associated with gastrointestinal disorders. *A*, Oral leukoplakia and associated squamous carcinoma. *B*, Multiple minor aphthous ulcers. *C*, Major aphthous ulcer. *D*, Glossitis in a patient with diabetes and malabsorption. The tongue is smooth (depapillation) and red; angular cheilitis is present. *E*, Marked erythema and ulceration associated with erythema multiforme. This patient had Stevens-Johnson syndrome.

Illustration continued on following page

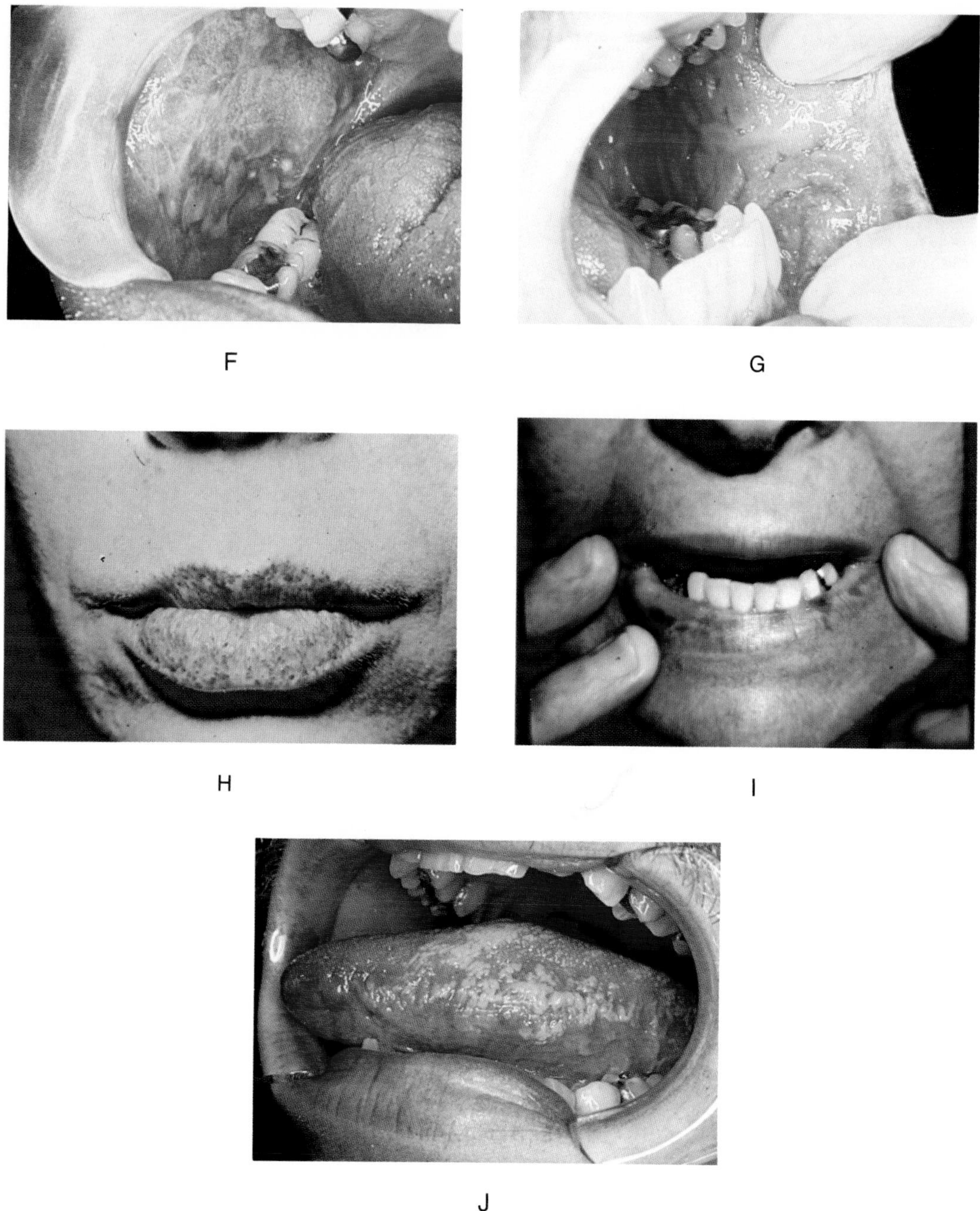

Figure 30–2 *Continued F*, The erosive form of oral lichen planus involving the buccal mucosa. Note lace-like keratoses, erythema, and ulceration. *G*, Pyostomatitis vegetans in a patient with ulcerative colitis. Biopsy revealed micro-abscesses. *H*, Hereditary hemorrhagic telangiectasia (Osler-Weber-Rendu disease). *I*, Mucocutaneous pigmentation of Peutz-Jeghers syndrome. *J*, Hairy leukoplakia in a patient with AIDS. (Courtesy of Sol Silverman Jr., D.D.S., and Victor Newcomer, M.D.)

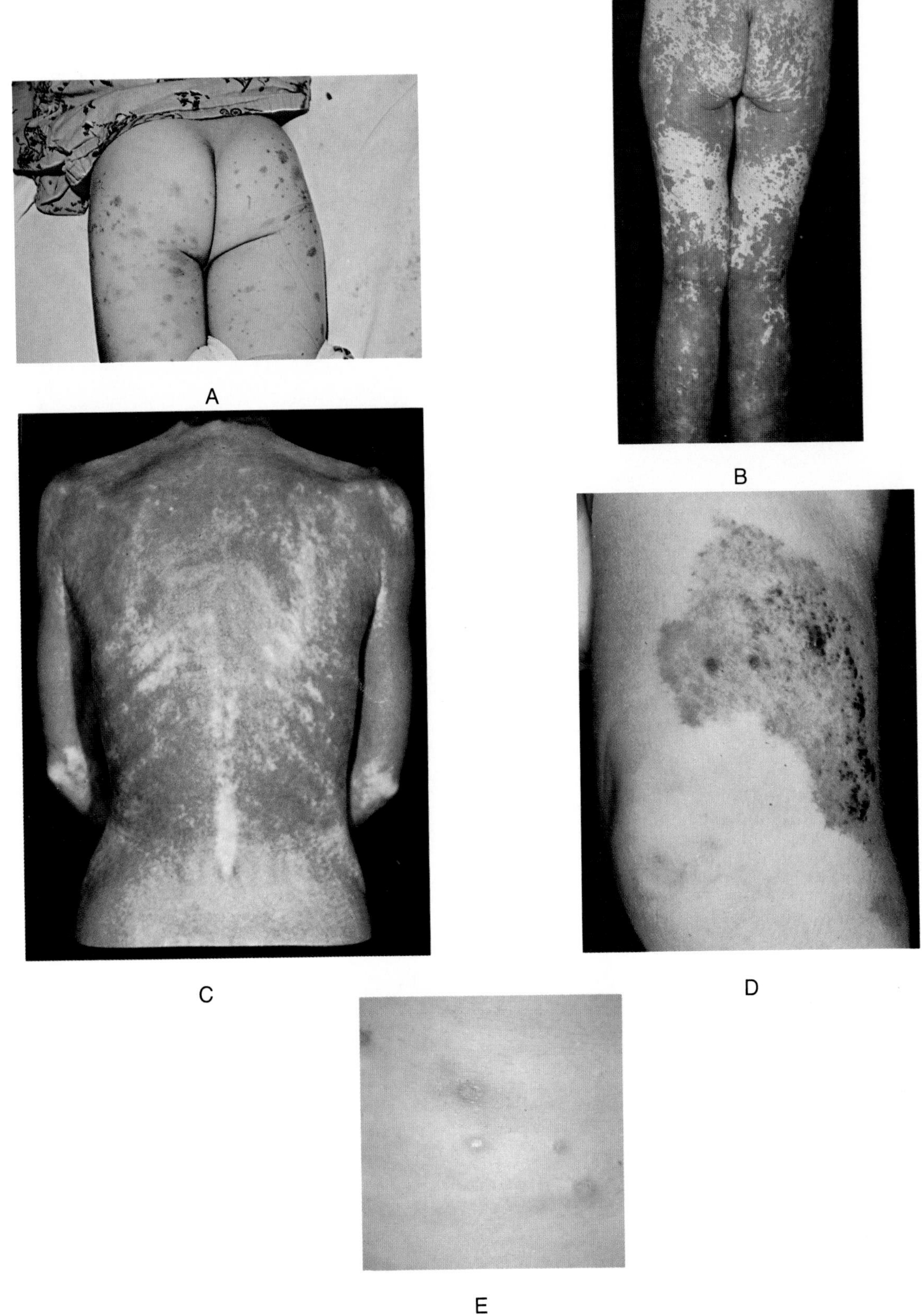

Figure 30–3. Cutaneous lesions associated with gastrointestinal disorders. *A*, Henoch-Schönlein purpura. *B*, Cryoglobulinemia with drug eruption. *C*, Urticaria pigmentosa in a patient with systemic mastocytosis. *D*, Cutaneous vascular hemangioma associated with intestinal hemorrhage. *E*, Degos' disease, with vasculitic lesions of different stages.

Illustration continued on following page

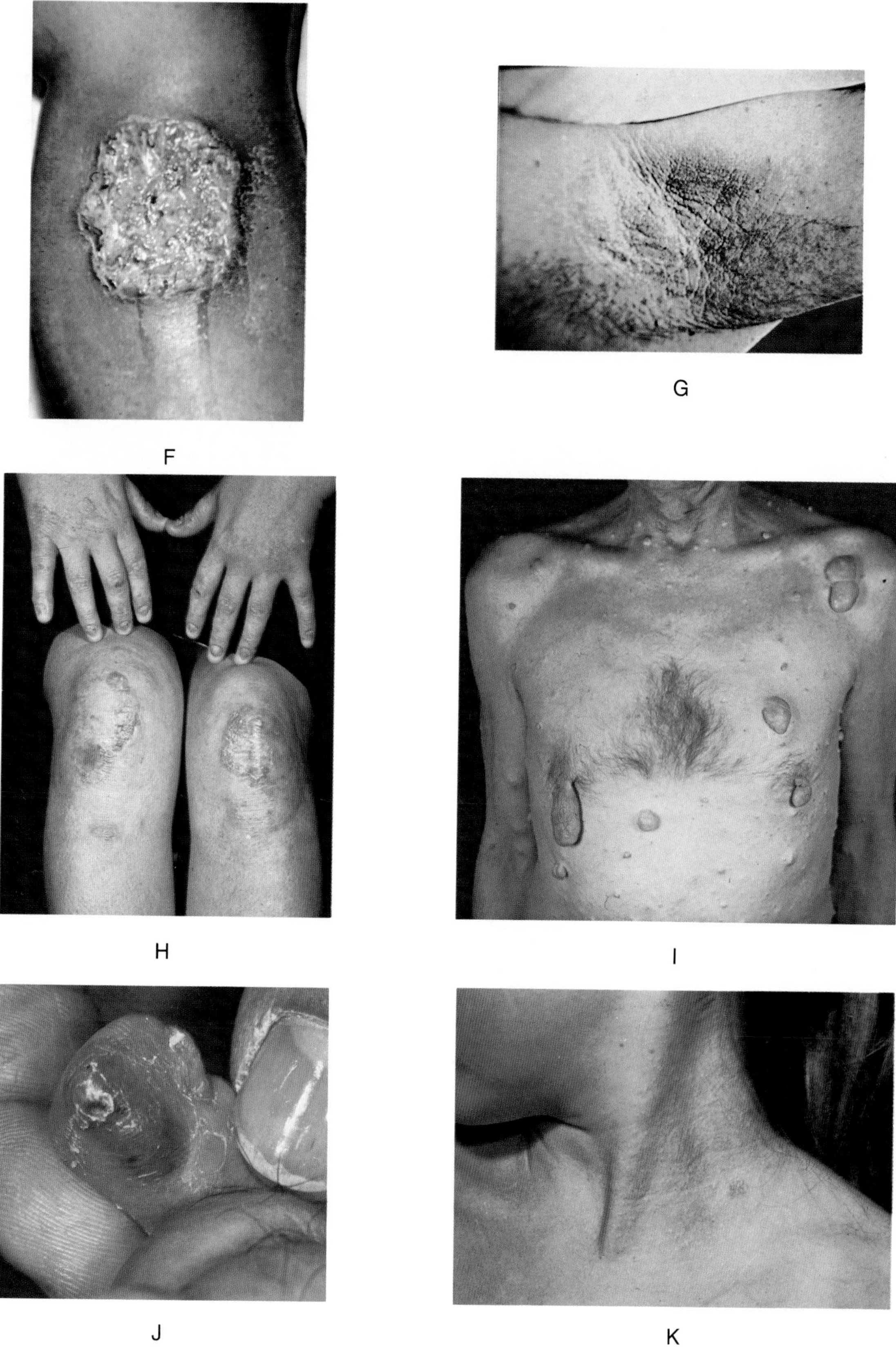

Figure 30–3 *Continued F*, Pyoderma gangrenosum associated with ulcerative colitis. *G*, Acanthosis nigricans. *H*, Skin fragility in epidermolysis bullosa dystrophica. *I*, Neurofibromatosis. *J*, Finger tip lesion in blue rubber bleb nevus syndrome. *K*, Pseudoxanthoma elasticum. (Courtesy of Victor Newcomer, M.D.)

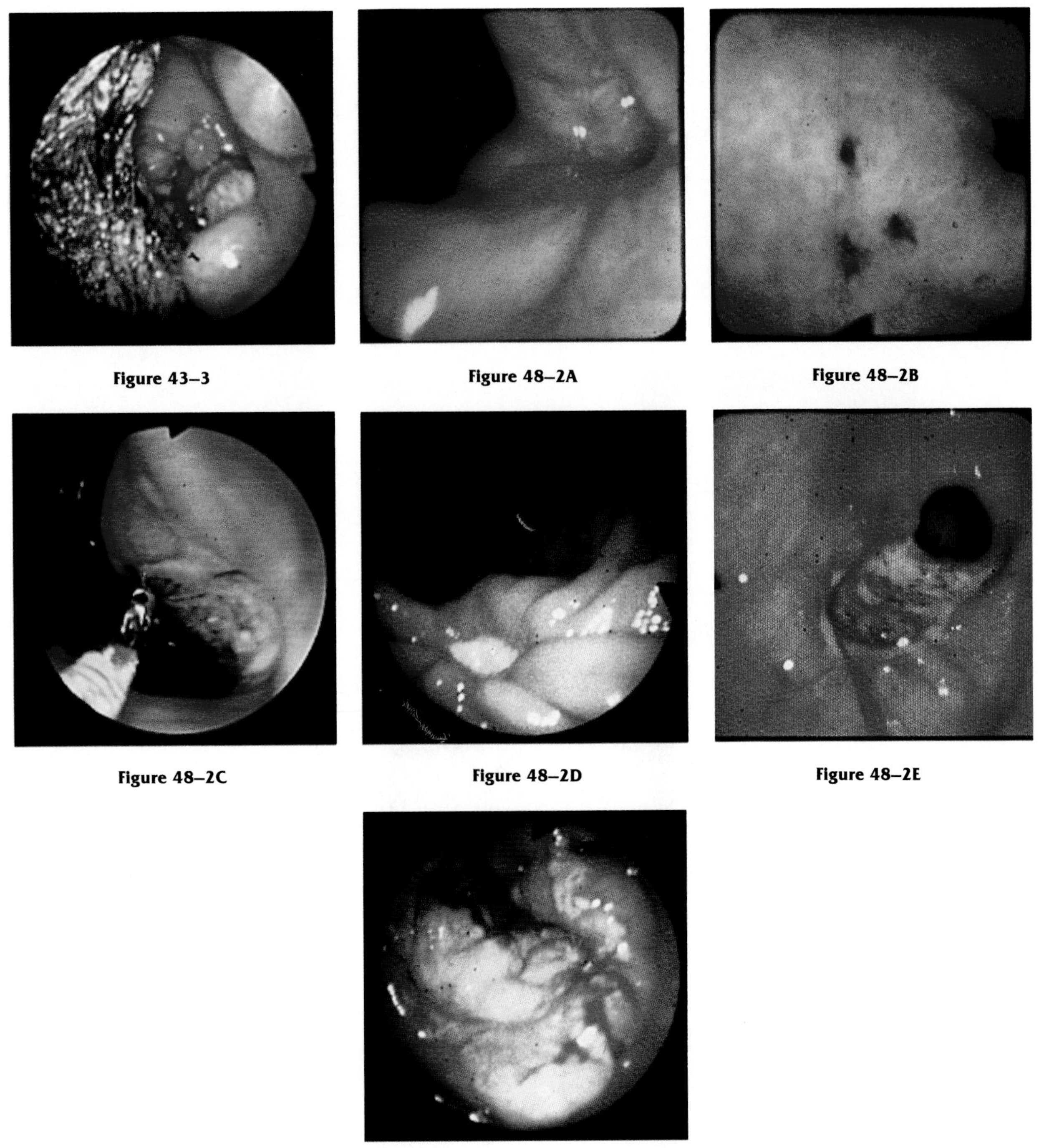

Figure 43–3

Figure 48–2A

Figure 48–2B

Figure 48–2C

Figure 48–2D

Figure 48–2E

Figure 48–2F

Figure 43–3. Endoscopic view of trichobezoar adjacent to an area of nodular gastritis. (Courtesy of Emmet B. Keefe, M.D.)

Figure 48–2. *A*, Endoscopic picture of a relatively deep, benign-appearing gastric ulcer. Folds radiate to the ulcer margin. *B*, Endoscopic picture illustrating blood-tinged, superficial erosions. In this patient the erosions resulted from therapy with indomethacin. (Courtesy of Frank Lanza, M.D.) *C*, Endoscopic picture illustrating gastric ulcer. Biopsy forceps can be seen obtaining tissue from edge of the ulcer crater. (Courtesy of Doug Thurman, M.D.) *D*, Endoscopic picture demonstrating folds radiating to a benign-appearing gastric ulcer. The edges of the crater are regular but slightly indurated. *E*, Oval or somewhat linear gastric ulcer. The pylorus is seen in the background. *F*, Malignant-appearing gastric ulcer.

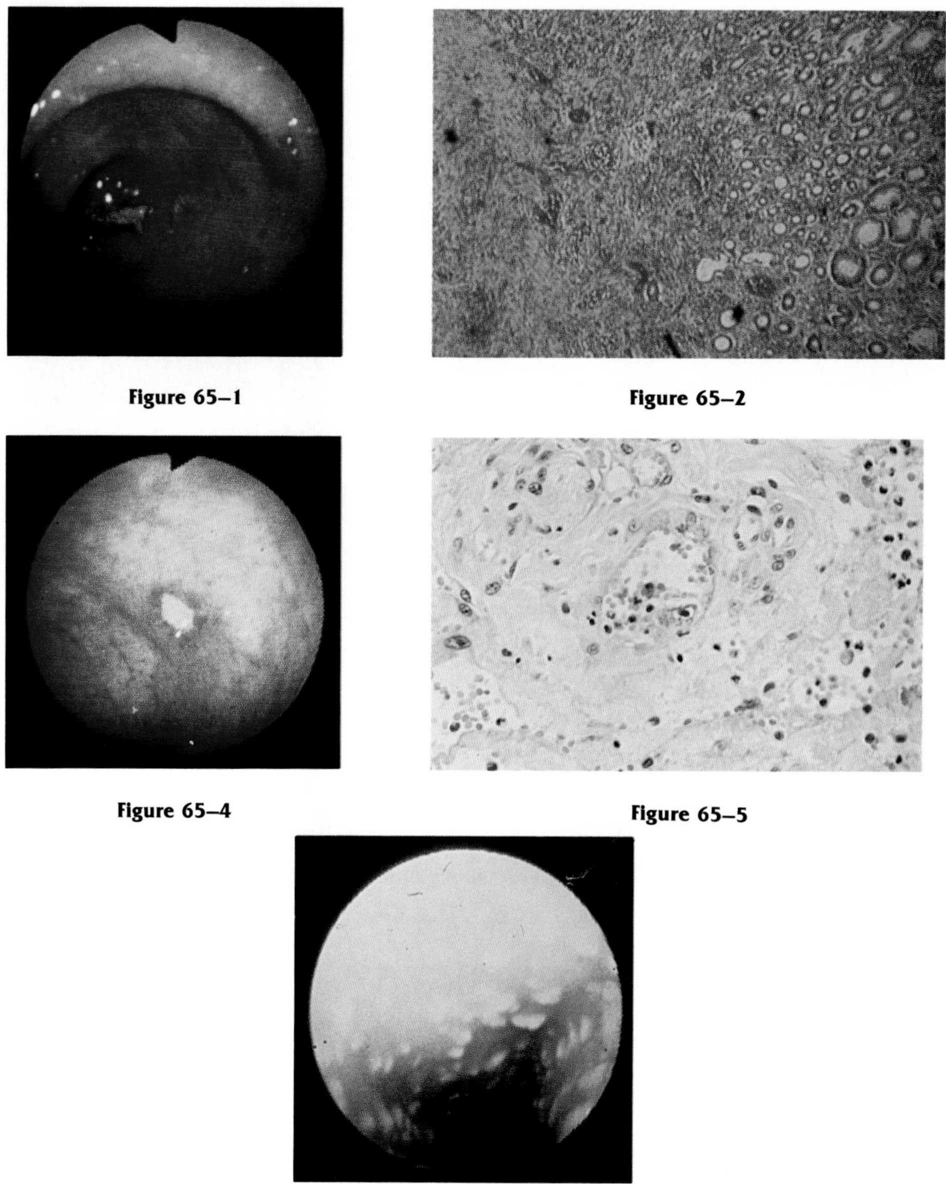

Figure 65–1

Figure 65–2

Figure 65–4

Figure 65–5

Figure 65–6

Figure 65–1. Endoscopic view of Kaposi's sarcoma involving the gastric antrum. There is a nodular lesion along the incisura angularis, as well as submucosal hemorrhage in the prepyloric region. (Courtesy of D. F. Altman, M.D.)

Figure 65–2. Endoscopic biopsy specimen of Kaposi's sarcoma of the sigmoid colon. There is hemorrhage and infiltration of the submucosa and lamina propria by numerous spindle-shaped cells. Hematoxylin and eosin stain, ×50. (Reprinted with permission from: Gastrointestinal Kaposi's sarcoma in patients with acquired immunodeficiency syndrome: endoscopic and autopsy findings, by Freidman, S. L., Wright, T. L., and Altman, D. F. Gastroenterology *89*:102–108. Copyright 1985 by The American Gastroenterological Association.)

Figure 65–4. Endoscopic view of a focal colonic mucosal ulcer due to cytomegalovirus. (Courtesy of J. P. Cello, M.D.)

Figure 65–5. Endoscopic biopsy specimen of cytomegalovirus infection of the colon, demonstrating characteristic CMV inclusion in a capillary endothelial cell. Hematoxylin and eosin stain, ×50. (Courtesy of D. F. Altman, M.D.)

Figure 65–6. Endoscopic appearance of *Candida* eosphagitis, demonstrating focal mucosal exudates and erythema. (From Blackstone, M. O. Endoscopic Interpretation: Normal and Pathologic Appearances of the Gastrointestinal Tract, 1984. Used by permission of Raven Press, New York).

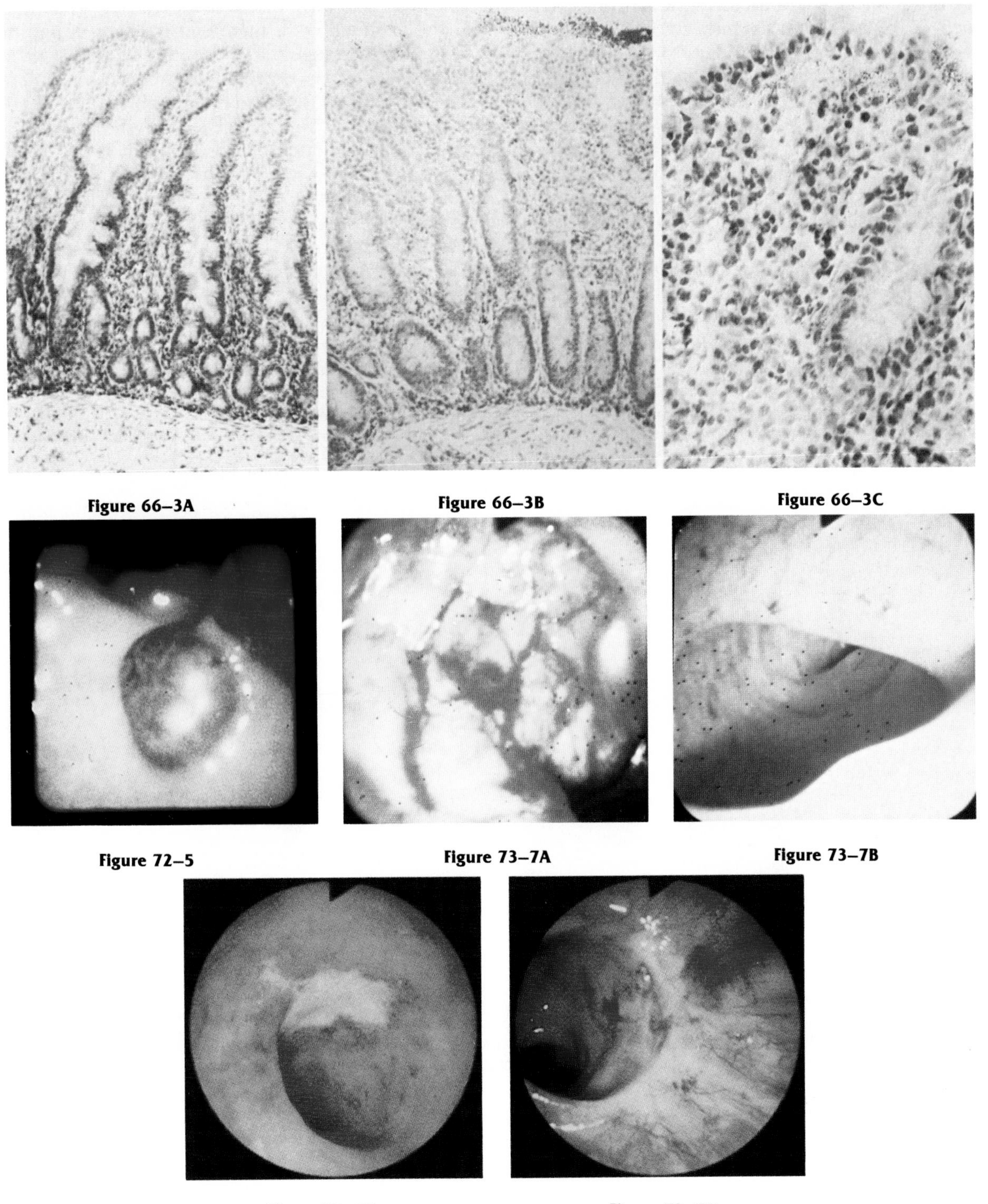

Figure 66–3. Lipid distribution in jejunal biopsies stained with oil-red-O. *A*, Normal control (× 84). Lipid (stained red) is present within the basal portion of the lamina propria. *B*, Celiac disease (× 84). Lipid is present within the surface epithelium. *C*, Tropical sprue (× 210). Lipid is located principally subjacent to the surface epithelium.

Figure 72–5. Kaposi's sarcoma of the sigmoid colon. Although malignant histologically, such tumors of gut behave biologically in a benign fashion. (Courtesy of Dr. M. H. Sleisenger.)

Figure 73–7. Endoscopic changes in colorectal mucosa induced by radiation therapy. *A*, Acute radiation proctitis with mucosal hemorrhage may appear much the same as acute idiopathic inflammatory bowel disease. *B*, Small telangiectatic vessels on pale, opaque mucosa may be all that is seen in a later stage. (*A* and *B* courtesy of Jerome D. Waye, M.D.) *C*, Radiation-induced ulceration with surrounding telangiectasia located at rectosigmoid junction. *D*, Healing of an indolent radiation-induced rectal ulcer may lead to scar formation, retraction, and ultimately a stricture. (*C* and *D* from Silverstein, F. E., and Tytgat, G. N. J. Atlas of Gastrointestinal Endoscopy. London, Gower Medical Publishing, and Philadelphia, W. B. Saunders Co., 1987. Used by permission.)

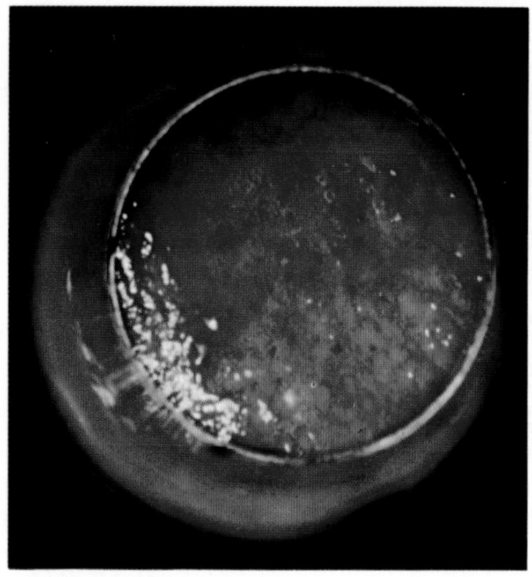

Figure 78–3A

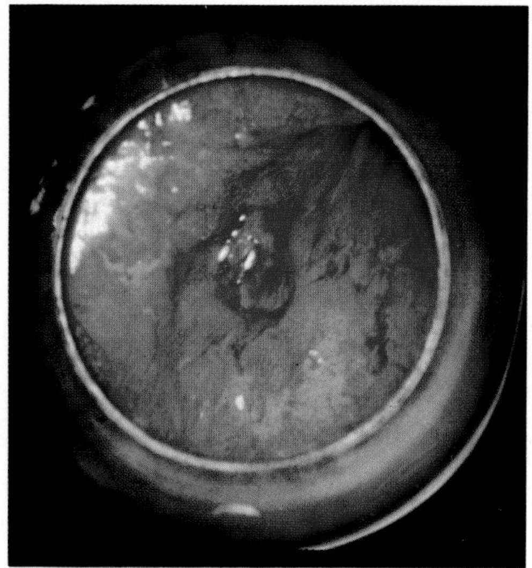

Figure 78–3B

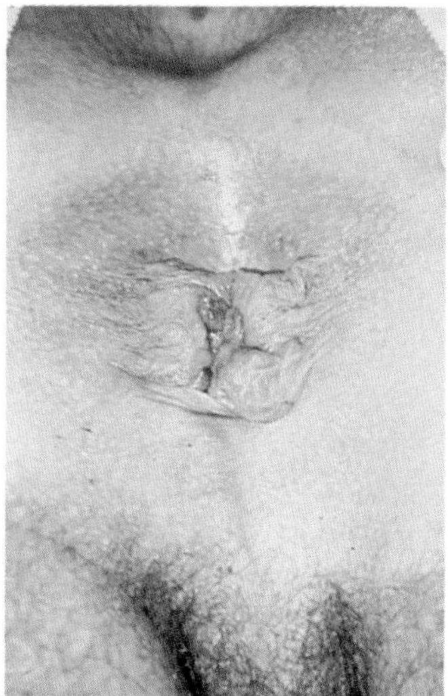

Figure 83–6

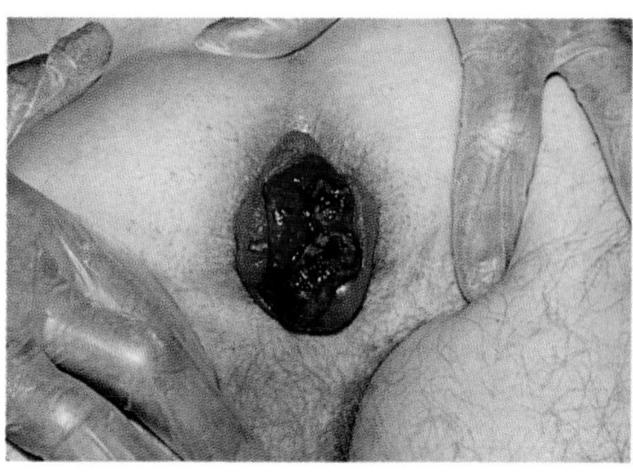

Figure 83–7

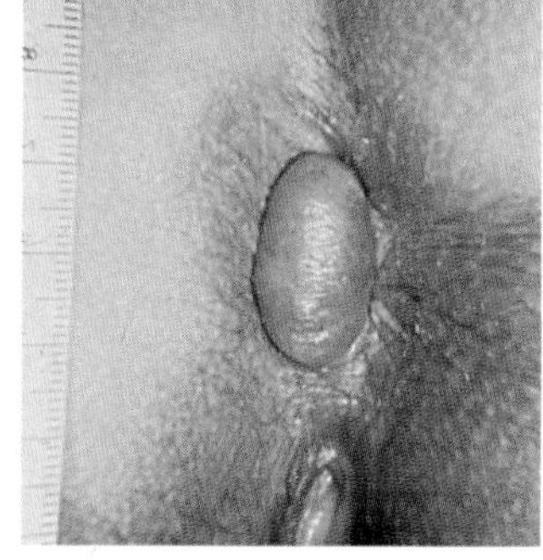

Figure 83–8

Figure 78–3. Proctoscopic views of colonic mucosa in two patients with ulcerative colitis. *A*, Granularity and minute bleeding mucosal ulcerations. *B*, Minimal granularity, but mucosa is friable and a pseudopolyp can be seen. (Courtesy of M. H. Sleisenger, M.D.)

Figure 83–6. Typical prolapsing mixed internal and external hemorrhoids. The patient is prone. Note hemorrhoidal masses in the three primary locations: left lateral, right posterior, and right anterior. Radial grooves are prominent between adjacent hemorrhoids.

Figure 83–7. Acute prolapsed, thrombosed internal hemorrhoids. Note congestion and edema of the external components below the pectinate line. Mucosal ulceration has developed.

Figure 83–8. Thrombosed external hemorrhoid. The mass is entirely covered by skin.

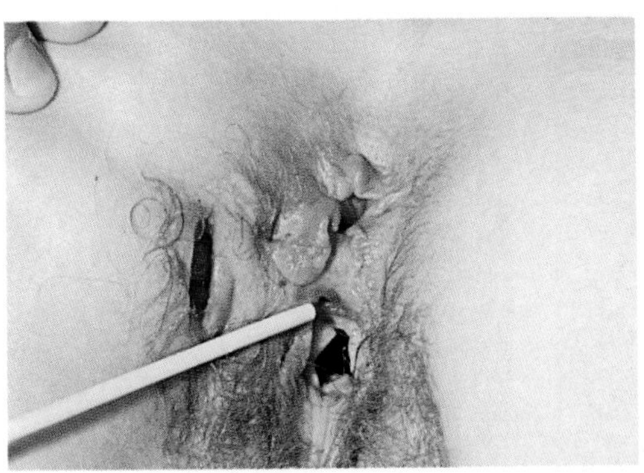

Figure 83–12

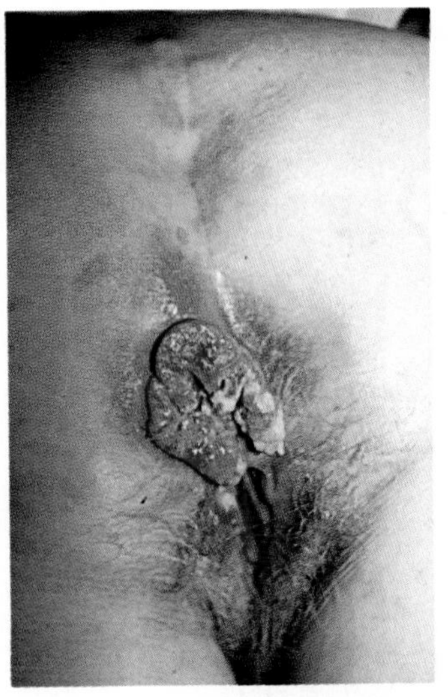

Figure 83–13

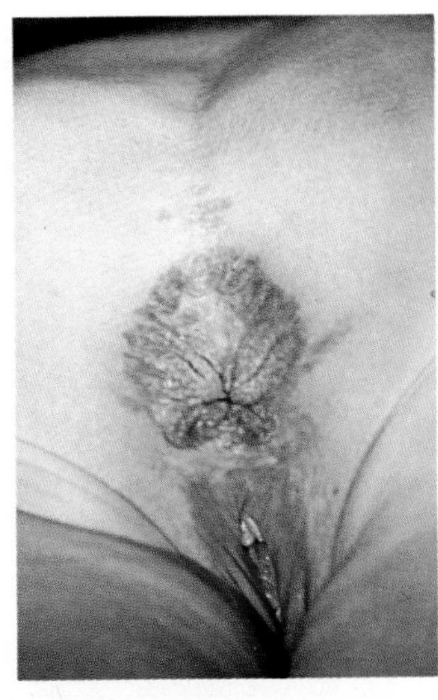

Figure 83–14

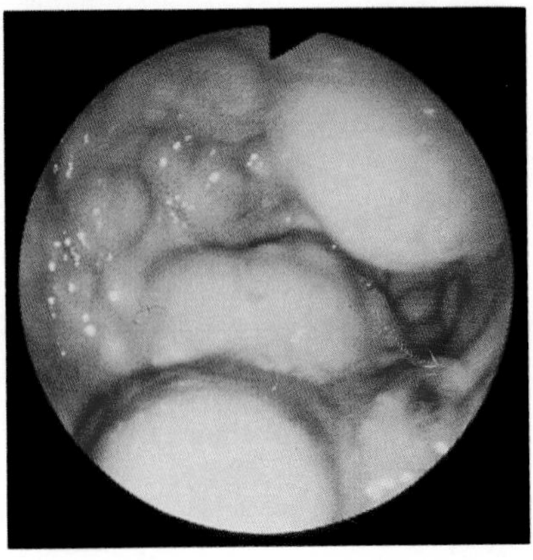

Figure 84–5

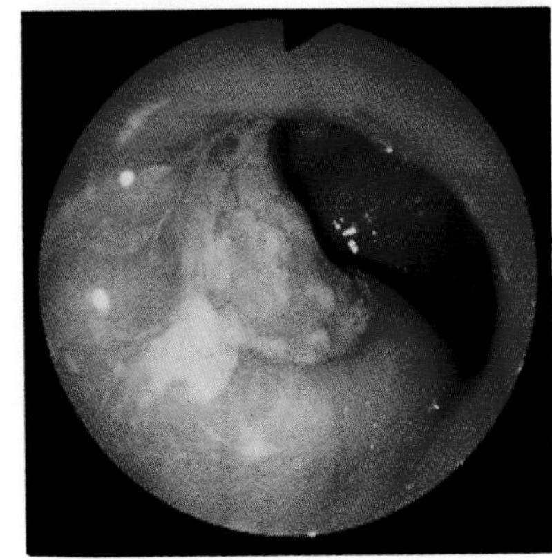

Figure 84–9

Figure 83–12. Complex anorectal fistulas due to Crohn's disease in a young woman. Pointer indicates rectovaginal fistula. The anus is edematous and deformed. A large secondary fistula orifice gapes open on the left.

Figure 83–13. Large epidermoid carcinoma involving much of the circumference at the anal verge.

Figure 83–14. Perianal Bowen's disease.

Figure 84–5. Pneumatosis coli as seen by fiberoptic colonoscopy. The tense air cysts are often mistaken for sessile polyps but collapse with a popping sound when biopsy samples are taken. (From Silverstein, F. E., and Tytgat, G. N. J. Atlas of Gastrointestinal Endoscopy. London, Gower Medical Publishing, and Philadelphia, W. B. Saunders Co., 1987. Used by permission.)

Figure 84–9. Solitary rectal ulcer. Sharply demarcated ulceration is present in the anterior wall of the rectum. The ulcer size can vary from several millimeters to 5 centimeters and may have an irregular outline or be linear in shape. The ulcer edge is often flat but clearly demarcated from normal mucosa by a thin line of hyperemia. The surrounding mucosa may have a nodular appearance. (From Silverstein, F. E., and Tytgat, G. N. J: Atlas of Gastrointestinal Endoscopy. London, Gower Medical Publishing, and Philadelphia, W. B. Saunders Co., 1987. Used by permission.)

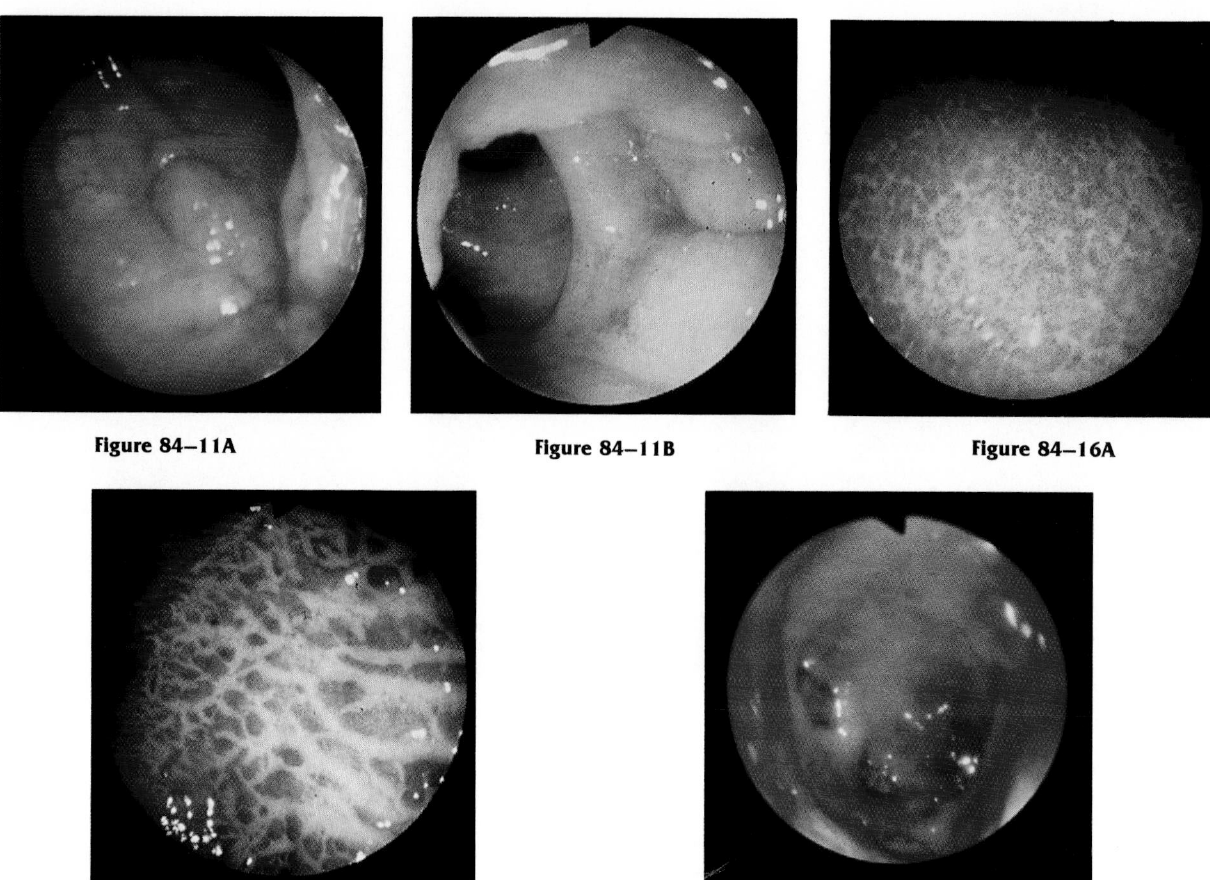

Figure 84–11A **Figure 84–11B** **Figure 84–16A**

Figure 84–16B **Figure 84–20**

Figure 84–11. Two endoscopic photographs of colitis cystica profunda in the rectum. The cysts are covered by normal-appearing mucosa and appear as submucosal wounds or plaques. In some cases, the mucosa may be edematous, hyperemic or even ulcerated similar to that shown in Figure 84–9. (From Silverstein, F. E., and Tytgat, G. N. J. Atlas of Gastrointestinal Endoscopy. London, Gower Medical Publishing, and Philadelphia, W. B. Saunders Co., 1987. Used by permission.)

Figure 84–16. *A*, Endoscopic photograph of rectal mucosa showing melanosis coli. *B*, Close-up view showing that darker areas are divided in a polyhedral design by lighter areas of less pigmentation. The gross appearance of the mucosa may vary from light brown to black coloration.

Figure 84–20. Endoscopic photograph of rectal mucosa in an elderly woman with acute colitis following a hydrogen peroxide enema. There is marked mucosal hyperemia, areas of bullous-like edema and necrotic ulceration. (Courtesy of P. Bryan Hudson, Ph.D., M.D.)

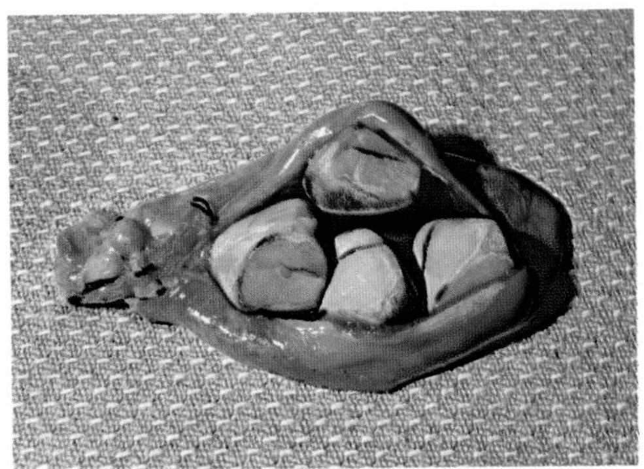

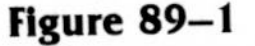

Figure 89–1

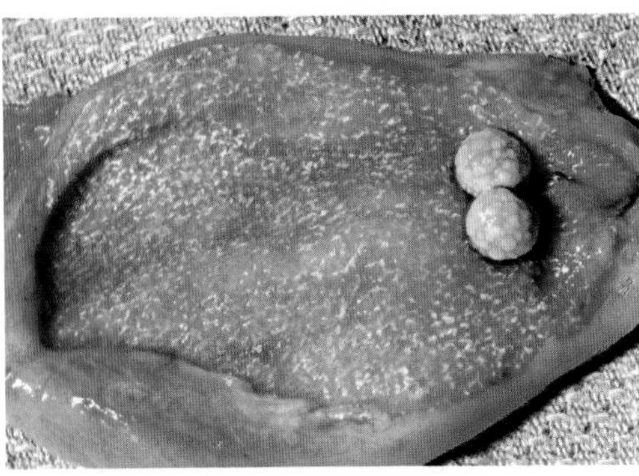

Figure 89–2

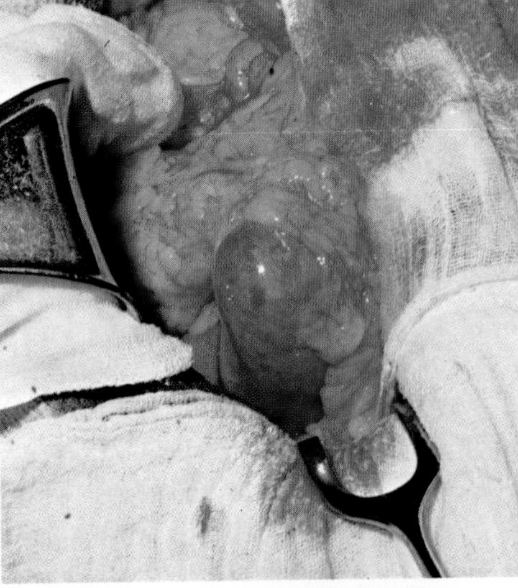

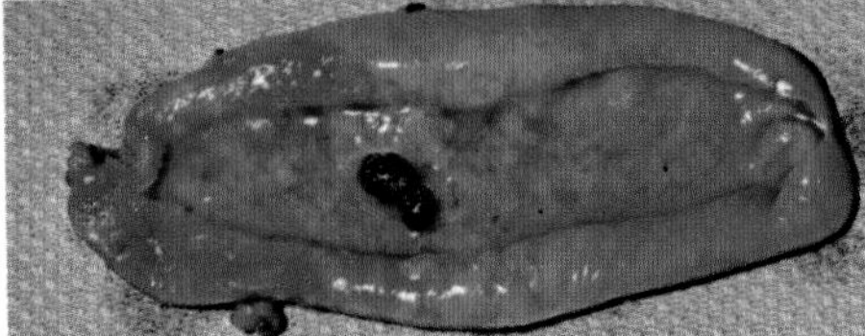

Figure 89–3

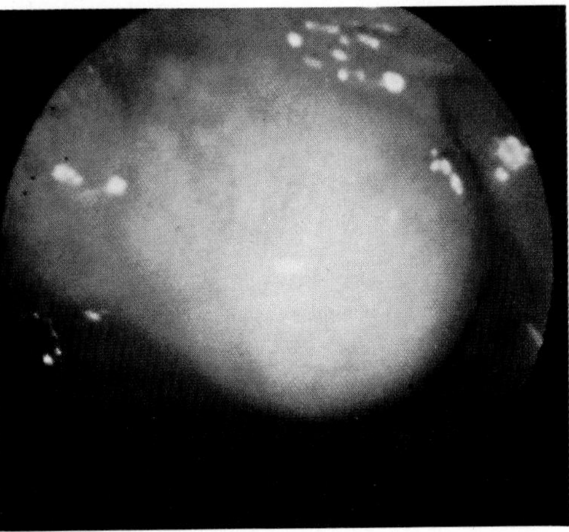

Figure 97–14

Figure 89–1. Gallbladder removed for episodic biliary colic. There is moderate thickening of the gallbladder wall from chronic inflammation and collagen deposition. The stones are typical faceted mixed-cholesterol gallstones.

Figure 89–2. Gallbladder showing prominent cholesterolosis of the mucosal surface. Operation was performed for episodic colic. The gallbladder had opacified on the preoperative oral cholecystogram. The gallstones are "mulberry stones," which are almost pure cholesterol.

Figure 89–3. The gallbladder as seen at laparotomy in a case of early acute cholecystitis. Onset of the attack was less than 48 hours before operation. The gallbladder is inflamed and edematous and surrounded by adherent omentum. The open specimen *(inset)* shows two bilirubin pigment stones as well as mucosal inflammation and minor submucosal hemorrhages. At the start of the operation, one stone had been lodged in the infundibulum, obstructing the gallbladder.

Figure 97–14. Endoscopic appearance of a *choledochocele.* An enlarged, hemispherical structure is seen protruding into the duodenal lumen after injection of contrast material into the common bile duct. The duodenoscope and cannulation catheter have been withdrawn. The orifice of the papilla of Vater is not visible; it is eccentrically placed, behind and slightly inferior to the protruding choledochocele. Same patient as in Figure 97–15, page 1837.

V

THE SMALL AND LARGE INTESTINE: ANATOMY, PHYSIOLOGY, AND DISEASE

Anatomy, Embryology, and Developmental Abnormalities of the Small Intestine and Colon

54

JERRY S. TRIER
HARLAND S. WINTER

Remarkable structural specifications greatly facilitate the digestive and absorptive functions of the small and large intestine.[1,2] The clinician should be familiar with these morphologic features, because their alteration in disease results in defective intestinal function as well as in significant and often predictable clinical symptoms.[3]

GROSS MORPHOLOGY OF THE SMALL INTESTINE

The small intestine is efficiently designed. Its many redundant loops allow it to occupy limited space within the abdominal cavity.[4,5] The adult human small intestine is an elongated tube 12 to 22 feet long, its length depending on both the tone of the muscular wall and the way in which it is measured. The small intestine lies in the peritoneal cavity and is mobile except for the duodenum, which, except for the first inch, is retroperitoneal and hence immobile. The anatomic relationship of the duodenum to other viscera is important, because disease of the duodenum may extend into these adjacent organs and vice versa (Fig. 54–1). The duodenum is molded around the head of the pancreas in a horseshoe fashion. In view of this intimate contact between the pancreas and all portions of the duodenum, disease of the pancreas may distort or invade adjacent duodenal tissue. On the other hand, duodenal disease, especially peptic ulceration, may penetrate into and involve pancreatic tissue. Disease of the duodenum in the region of the ampulla of Vater may obstruct the distal portion of the common bile duct and the main pancreatic duct, thus interfering with normal delivery of bile and pancreatic secretions into the duodenum.

Because both the liver and the gallbladder are in immediate contact with the anterosuperior aspect of the proximal or first portion of the duodenum (Fig. 54–1), disease of one of these organs may involve the other and result in complications such as cholecystoduodenal fistulas or penetration of peptic duodenal ulcerations into either the quadrate or right lobe of the liver. Less often, the common bile duct, which passes behind the proximal duodenum en route to its entry into the descending duodenum, may be jointly involved with the proximal duodenum by disease. Carcinoma of the transverse colon may extend into and involve the descending or the second portion of the duodenum, because the transverse colon normally crosses it anteriorly (Fig. 54–1). The superior mesenteric artery and vein cross the transverse or third portion of the duodenum near the midline as they emerge from the root of the mesentery of the small intestine. Rarely, these vessels may produce functional obstruction of the third portion of the duodenum by compressing it as it crosses the spine, especially in thin individuals. The descending aorta passes directly behind the duodenum, and aneurysms or prosthethic grafts of this major vessel may erode through the wall and rupture into the lumen of the duodenum, causing catastrophic gastrointestinal bleeding (see pp. 1919–1921).

Unlike the fixed retroperitoneal duodenum, the jejunum and the ileum are suspended by an extensive mesentery and have considerable mobility within the abdominal cavity. Usually, the jejunal loops lie over the duodenum, pancreas, and left kidney in the upper abdomen and thus may be affected by disease of those organs. For example, the radiolucent "sentinel" loop seen by X-ray in patients with acute pancreatitis results from ileus localized to a loop of jejunum overlying the pancreas (see p. 1827). The ileum generally occupies the lower abdomen and a portion of the pelvis. The distal few inches are the least mobile, because the cecum is affixed to the posterior abdominal wall.

No specific anatomic structure marks the end of the jejunum and the beginning of the ileum; instead the proximal two fifths of the mobile small intestine are arbitrarily considered jejunum and the distal three fifths are designated ileum. However, significant differences in the structure of the proximal jejunum and

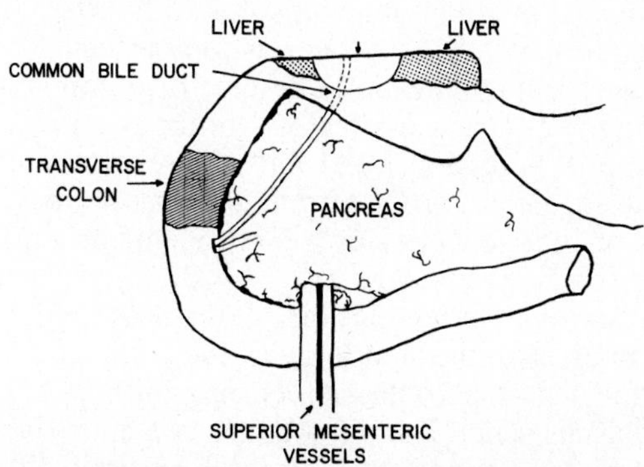

Figure 54–1. Diagram showing relationship of the duodenum to adjacent viscera.

the distal ileum facilitate their identification by the radiologist and surgeon.

The diameter of the proximal jejunum is almost twice that of the distal ileum, and its wall is considerably thicker. The circumferential, spiral, or circular folds, the *plicae circulares*, which consist of a fold of submucosa covered by a full thickness of mucosa, are most abundant and well developed (up to 1 cm in height) in the distal duodenum and proximal jejunum. These folds gradually become sparser and often may disappear entirely in the distal third of the ileum. Elliptical aggregates of lymphoid follicles (Peyer's patches) up to 1 inch or more in length are present along the antimesenteric border in the distal half of the ileum; smaller aggregates of lymphoid follicles are seen in the more proximal small intestine and isolated follicles are present throughout the alimentary canal. Peyer's patches are most prominent in young individuals; they atrophy toward middle age and may be difficult to identify in old age. The amount of fat in the mesentery adjacent to the jejunum is very small; hence the mesentery appears translucent. In contrast, the mesentery adjacent to the ileum contains much fat and appears opaque—another difference that helps the surgeon identify the level of a specific segment of small intestine.

HISTOLOGY OF THE SMALL INTESTINE

The wall of the small intestine consists of four layers; the serosa, the muscularis, the submucosa, and the mucosa (Fig. 54–2).

The *serosa*, or outermost layer, is an extension of the peritoneum. It encircles the jejunum and ileum but covers only a part of the anterior portion of the retroperitoneal duodenum. Like the peritoneum, the serosa consists of a single layer of flattened mesothelial cells overlying some loose connective tissue.

The *muscularis* consists of two layers of smooth muscle, an outer or longitudinal layer in which the long axis of the individual smooth muscle cells parallels the long axis of the intestine, and an inner or circular layer in which the individual muscle cells tend to encircle the bowel (Fig. 54–2). This arrangement of muscle cells facilitates efficient propulsion of intraluminal contents of the gut. Specialized junctional complexes, the gap junctions found in the plasma membranes of adjacent smooth muscle cells, permit cell-to-cell communication and electrical coupling, facilitating the muscularis' ability to act as an electrical syncytium. Ganglion cells and nerve fibers of the myenteric plexus are interposed between these two layers of muscle, and small nerve elements ramify in the muscle fibers.

The *submucosa* consists largely of dense connective tissue sparsely infiltrated by cells, including fibroblasts, lymphocytes, macrophages, eosinophils, mast cells, and plasma cells. The submucosa contains elaborate lymphatic and venous plexuses, which drain the lymphatic and venous capillaries of the lamina propria of the mucosa. It also contains an extensive network of arterioles and the ganglion cells and nerve fibers that form the autonomic submucosal plexus. Although the submucosal (Meissner's) and myenteric (Auerbach's) plexuses are generally considered as separate entities, they are interconnected by nerve fibrils. Moreover, the nerve fibrils of the mucosa are continuous with the submucosal plexus. Thus, the autonomic nerve elements of all layers of the bowel are interconnected, a fact that has significant physiologic implications.

Elaborately branched acinar glands, Brunner's glands, which contain both mucous and serous secretory cells, fill much of the submucosal space of the duodenal cap and the proximal half of the descending duodenum. Small islands of Brunner's glands are regularly present in the submucosa of the distal duodenum, and isolated islets may extend well into the jejunum. The secretion elaborated by Brunner's glands, which is rich in both mucus and bicarbonate, may help protect the proximal duodenum from acid-peptic digestion. Moreover, these glands are of additional clinical importance in that they regularly penetrate and extend into the lamina propria of the mucosa of the proximal duodenum (Fig. 54–3). This often results in marked distortion of the so-called normal villous pattern in this segment of the small intestine. Failure to appreciate this normal variant in *proximal* duodenal tissue may result in serious misinterpretation of peroral biopsies obtained from this region, including incorrect diagnosis of primary mucosal disease in individuals whose biopsy specimens from the *distal* duodenum or proximal jejunum would be normal.[6] In addition, Brunner's glands hypertrophy in some patients with cystic fibrosis. The clinical significance of this observation is unknown, but failure to recognize this finding may result in unnecessary endoscopic procedures, or the erroneous diagnosis of duodenal ulceration.

The numerous villi that greatly amplify the absorptive and digestive surface, which is in contact with the intraluminal intestinal contents, are a striking structural feature of the innermost layer of the small intestine, the *mucosa*. Although the villi are often described as finger-like structures 0.5 to 1 mm in height, their appearance in humans may vary in relation to their location in the small intestine and from individual to individual. The villi are normally broad and ridge-shaped in the proximal duodenum, where the lamina is infiltrated with Brunner's glands and, especially in young individuals, with lymphoid follicles. Sectioned biopsies in this area often fail to show discrete villi and may resemble, to some degree, the flattened mucosa found in the more distal bowel in patients with celiac sprue.[6] In the more distal duodenum and proximal jejunum, the villi are often leaf-shaped, but may be finger-shaped. In the distal jejunum and ileum, finger-shaped villi are the rule. The villi are tallest in the distal duodenum and proximal jejunum and progressively become shorter toward the ileocecal valve.

The villous architecture of the small intestine varies significantly among normal inhabitants of different

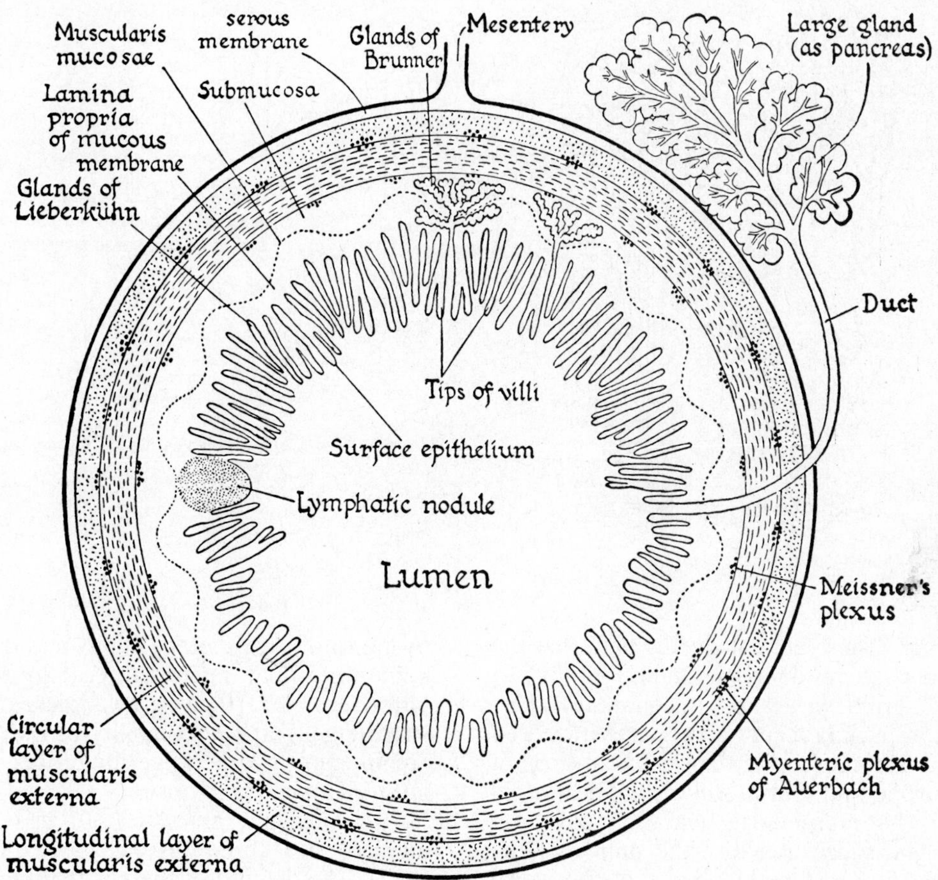

Figure 54–2. Schematic diagram of a cross section of the intestinal tract. (From Bloom, W. N., and Fawcett, D. W. A Textbook of Histology. Philadelphia, W. B. Saunders Company, 1968.)

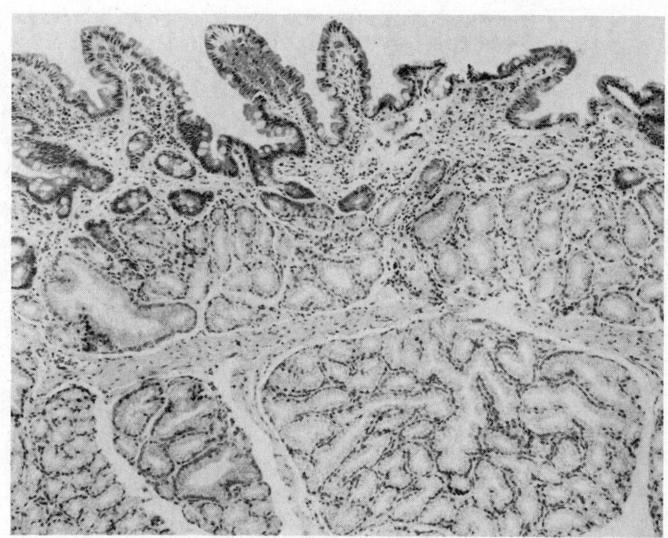

Figure 54–3. Normal human duodenal mucosa. Brunner's glands are infiltrating the submucosa and the lamina propria. As a result, the villous architecture appears distorted. Hematoxyin and eosin stain, approximately ×70. (From Brandborg, L. L., Rubin, G. E., and Quinton, W. E.: A multipurpose instrument for suction biopsy of the esophagus, stomach, and small bowel. Gastroenterology *37*:1–16. © by Williams & Wilkins, 1959.)

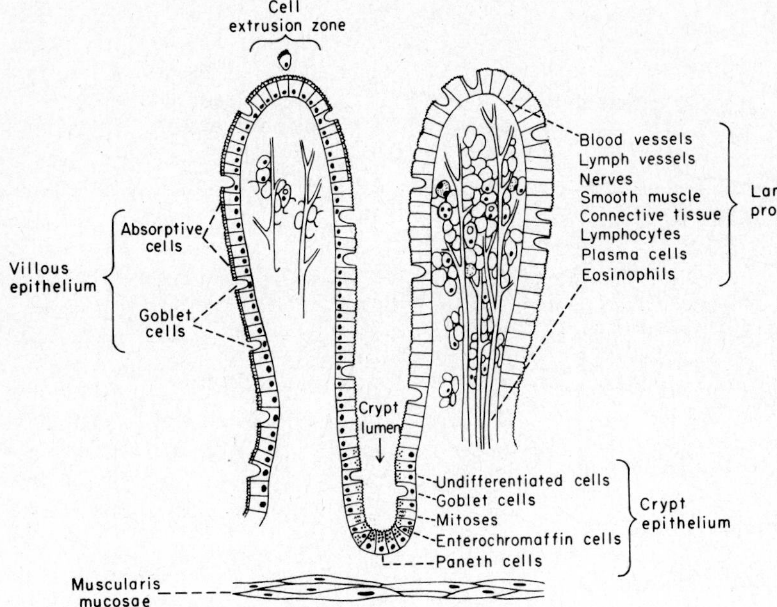

Figure 54–4. Schematic diagram of two sectioned villi and a crypt to illustrate the histologic organization of the small intestinal mucosa.

parts of the world. There are convincing data that the intestinal mucosa of residents of India,[7] Southeast Asia,[8] and the Caribbean islands[9] is commonly characterized by shorter villi, deeper crypts, and increased cellularity in the lamina propria than is the mucosa of residents of Europe and North America. The factors responsible for this morphologic variation have not been defined. The suggestion that the milieu of the intestinal lumen differs in various parts of the world owing to diverse dietary habits and distinctive intraluminal intestinal microbial ecology is attractive but unproved. Nevertheless, awareness of this sometimes striking geographic variability of the "normal" villous architecture is imperative for proper interpretation of intestinal mucosal biopsies.

The intestinal mucosa itself can be conveniently divided into three distinct layers (Figs. 54–4 and 54–5). The deepest of these is the *muscularis mucosae,*

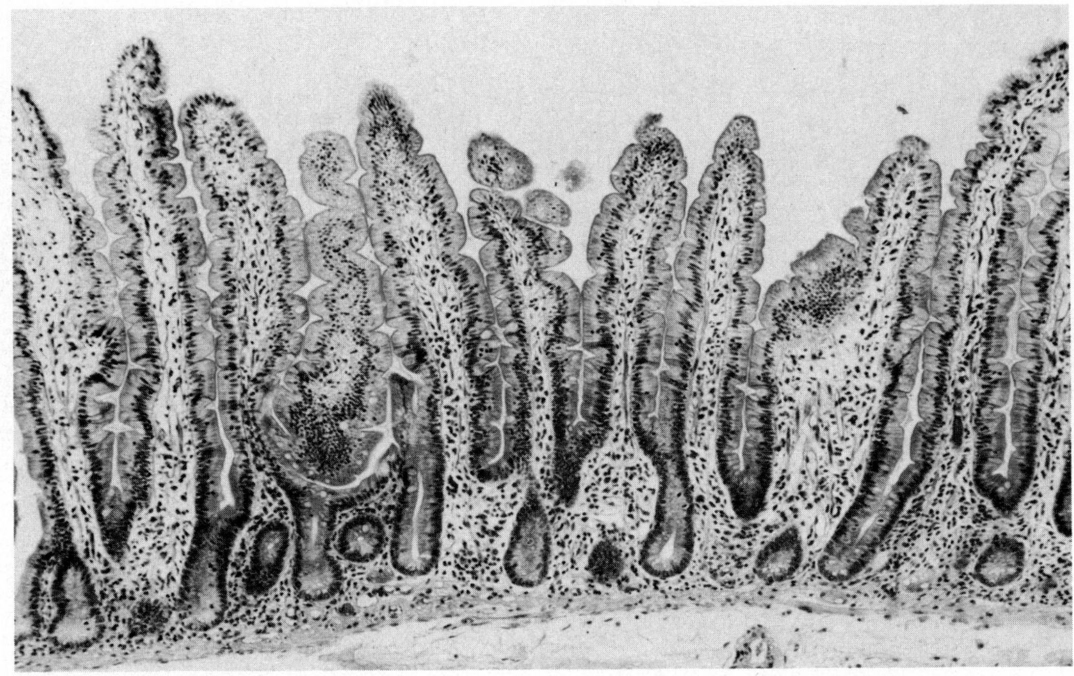

Figure 54–5. Light micrograph of a section of mucosa obtained by peroral biopsy from the proximal jejunum of a normal man. Hematoxylin and eosin stain, approximately ×93.

a thin sheet of smooth muscle, three to ten cells thick, that separates the mucosa from the submucosa.

The middle layer, the *lamina propria,* is a continuous connective tissue space bounded below by the muscularis mucosae and above by the intestinal epithelium. The lamina forms the connective tissue core of the numerous villi and surrounds the pitlike crypts that encircle villi around their base. The lamina propria normally contains many types of cells, including plasma cells, lymphocytes, mast cells, eosinophils, macrophages, smooth muscle cells, fibroblasts, and noncellular connective tissue elements (collagen, reticular, and elastin fibers).

There is increasing evidence that the lamina propria serves important protective functions by combating microorganisms and other foreign substances that may penetrate the overlying epithelial barrier. The lamina contains macrophages capable of phagocytosis along with numerous plasma cells, helper-inducer T lymphocytes, and other T lymphocyte subtypes. Thus, this area is well suited immunologically to be an active site of immunoglobulin synthesis.[10, 11] Indeed, significant intestinal dysfunction is often seen in patients in whom the plasma cell population and immunoglobin synthesis of the lamina propria are deficient (see pp. 114–144).

The lamina propria also provides important structural support, not only for the overlying epithelium but also for the many small vascular channels that nourish the mucosa and that carry away absorbed materials to the systemic circulation. These blood and lymphatic capillaries differ structurally from one another. The blood capillaries are surrounded by a closely applied continuous basal lamina and have thin endothelial walls with many tiny (0.05 to 0.1 μm) diaphragm-covered fenestrations (Fig. 54–6). These pores have a greater permeability to large molecules and particulate material than does the pore-free portion of the capillary wall.[12] In contrast, the walls of the lymphatic capillaries contain no such discrete fenestrations, and the basal lamina on the external surface is discontinuous. The lamina propria also contains small unmyelinated nerve fibers.

The inner layer of the mucosa consists of a continuous sheet of a single layer of *columnar epithelial cells,* which lines both the crypts and the villi. The base of each epithelial cell rests on a thin basal lamina that separates the epithelium from the underlying lamina propria. The main known functions of the crypt epithelium are cell renewal and exocrine, endocrine, water, and ion secretion; the main function of the villous epithelium is absorption. The crypt epithelium is composed of at least four distinct cell types: the Paneth, goblet, undifferentiated, and endocrine cells (Figs. 54–4 and 54–7).

Morphologically, *Paneth cells* strongly resemble zymogenic cells, such as the pancreatic and salivary gland acinar cells that are known to secrete large amounts of protein-rich materials. The Paneth cells are readily identified by their location in the base of the crypts, by their strongly basophilic cytoplasm, and by their large eosinophilic secretory granules.

The *goblet cells* of the crypts are located on the lateral walls of the crypts, and their morphology resembles that of goblet cells elsewhere in the gastrointestinal tract, including the villous epithelium. They are shaped like a brandy goblet, and the bulk of their cytoplasm

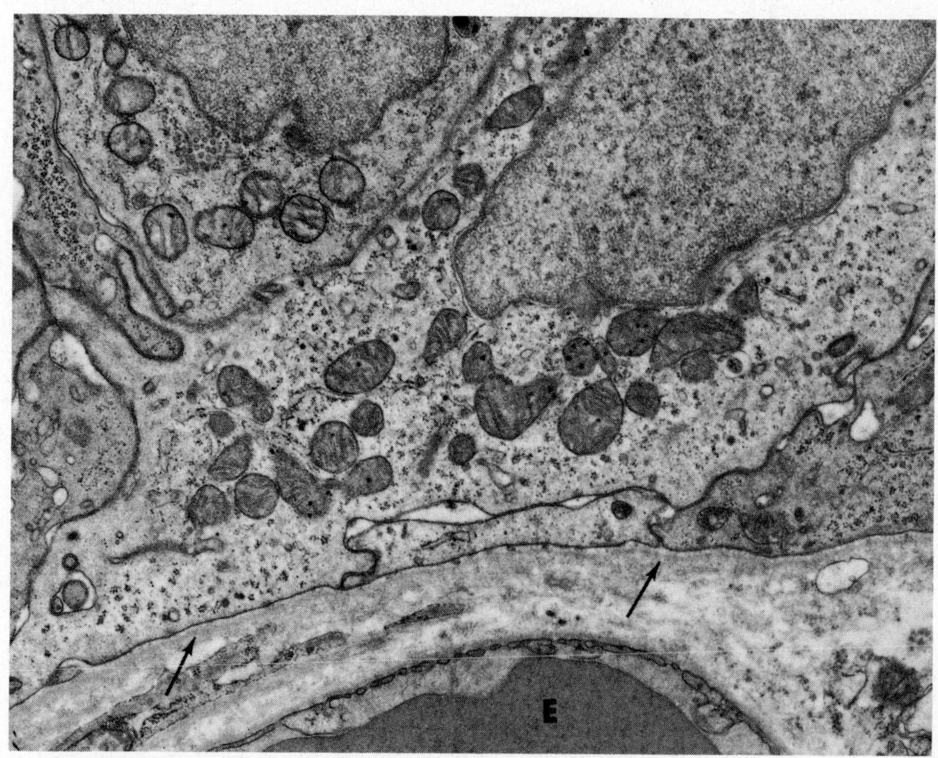

Figure 54–6. Basal portion of several jejunal absorptive cells from a normal man. Note the continuous basal lamina *(arrows),* which is closely applied to the basal cell membrane of absorptive cells. Part of a capillary containing an erythrocyte (E) within its lumen is seen in the underlying lamina propria. Approximately × 12,000. (From Trier, J. S. *In* Code, C. [ed.]. Handbook of Physiology: Vol. 3, Alimentary Canal. Washington, D.C., American Physiological Society, 1968.)

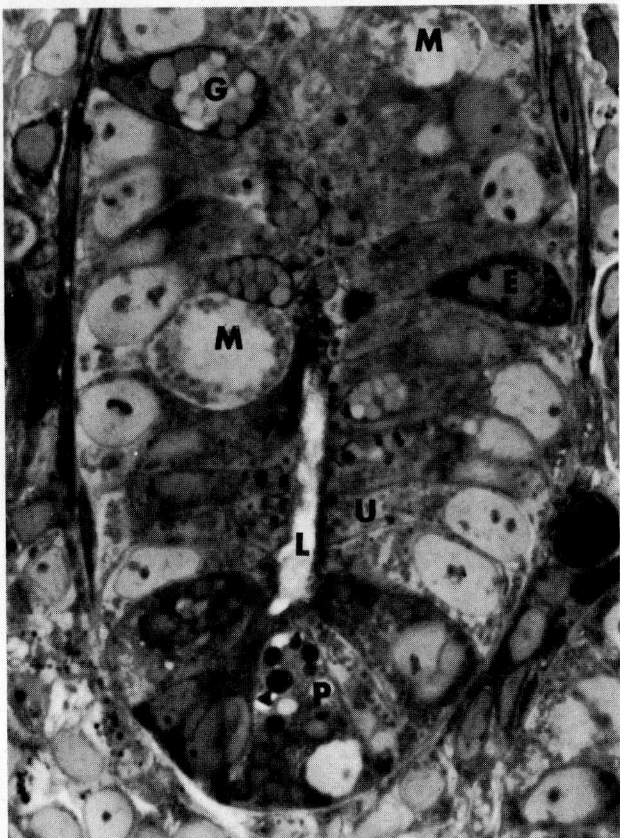

Figure 54–7. High magnification light micrograph of a jejunal crypt from a biopsy from a normal volunteer. Paneth cells (P) help form the base of the crypt. Undifferentiated cells (U), goblet cells (G), and an endocrine cell (E) are seen along the lateral wall of the crypt. Two of the undifferentiated cells are undergoing mitosis (M). The crypt lumen (L) is sectioned tangentially. Toluidine blue stain of resin-embedded section, approximately ×1400. (From Trier, J. S. *In* Code, C. [ed.]. Handbook of Physiology: Vol. 3, Alimentary Canal. Washington, D.C., American Physiological Society, 1968.)

between the basally located nucleus and the apical brush border is packed with many mucous granules.

The most abundant cells in the crypts are the *undifferentiated cells* that form the lateral walls of the crypts and are also interspersed in the crypt base between Paneth cells. Their cytoplasm contains many secretory granules. These granules are quite small and not obvious in routine histologic preparations, but they are easily seen in the apical cytoplasm near the crypt lumen when sections are stained for glycoprotein with the periodic acid–Schiff (PAS) technique.

The *endocrine cells* (often called enterochromaffin, argentaffin, or basal granular cells in the older literature) are characterized by their "inverted" appearance compared with other crypt cells, in that their small secretory granules are distributed in the basal cytoplasm between the nucleus and the cell base (Figs. 54–4 and 54–7). This basal location suggests that the endocrine cells secrete their granules along the basolateral membrane into the lamina propria. This is in contrast to the other crypt epithelial cells, which are exocrine cells in that they secrete their granules along their apical surface into the gastrointestinal lumen via the crypt lumen. The endocrine cell granules do not stain with hematoxylin or eosin after routine formalin fixation and hence cannot be identified in routinely processed tissue sections. Rather, special fixation and staining methods that utilize the strong reducing potential of some endocrine cell granules or immunocytochemical techniques must be employed. There are more than ten distinct populations of small endocrine intestinal cells that can be distinguished from one another immunocytochemically, histochemically, or by subtle morphologic criteria at the electron microscopic level. This heterogeneity of the endocrine cell structure reflects their diverse secretory products.

It is established that the four epithelial cell types that form the crypts are active secretory cells. The goblet cells constantly secrete mucus into the intestinal lumen. Although this mucus is said to protect and lubricate the intestinal mucosa, firm experimental data on this role are surprisingly limited. The endocrine cells are the site of production of gastrointestinal hormones and peptides including gastrin, secretin, cholecystokinin, somatostatin, enteroglucagon, motilin, neurotensin, gastric inhibitory peptide, and vasoactive intestinal peptide as well as serotonin.[13] Clearly these cells, by virtue of their secretory products, play a major role in the regulation of diverse physiologic processes in the digestive organs. The potential significance of excessive secretion by endocrine cell tumors, as, for example, in patients with gastrinomas and carcinoid syndrome, is well known.

Less is known about the function of Paneth and undifferentiated cell exocrine secretions.[2] One might expect that these actively secreting cells would contribute important digestive enzymes, such as proteases and lipases, to the intraluminal contents. However, available data indicate that such enzymes are not produced in the crypts. Indeed, the only major digestive enzymes found in cell-free filtrates of intestinal juice are amylase and enterokinase. Thus the significance of Paneth and undifferentiated cell secretion is simply not known. Human Paneth cells contain lysozyme,[14] IgA, and IgG.[15] Paneth cells in rat small intestine are able to phagocytose selected protozoa and bacteria,[16] but the physiologic implications of these findings are not yet clear. There is increasing evidence based on morphologic and electrophysiologic studies that undifferentiated crypt cells contribute in a major fashion to intestinal water and ion secretion.[2, 17]

Like other alimentary epithelia, the epithelium of the small intestine is a rapidly proliferating tissue. A major function of the undifferentiated crypt cells is the constant renewal of the intestinal epithelium;[18, 19] hence mitoses are abundant in these cells.

The epithelium that covers intestinal villi is composed of absorptive cells, goblet cells, a few endocrine cells, and tuft or caveolated cells. The morphology of the villous goblet and endocrine cells closely resembles that of crypt goblet and endocrine cells. Tuft or caveolated cells, characterized by broad, long apical microvilli and an intracytoplasmic system of tubules and vesicles, are uncommon (1 per cent or less of villous epithelial cells) and their function is not known.[2] Intraepithelial lymphocytes are located in many of the intercellular spaces between villous epithelial cells. In contrast to the lamina propria in which helper-inducer T lymphocytes predominate, the majority of intraepithelial lymphocytes are cytotoxic-suppressor T lymphocytes and a small percentage exhibit natural killing activity after viral challenge.[11] Although the functions of intraepithelial lymphocytes are not fully understood, they likely contribute in a substantive fashion to host defenses at the interface between the mucosal surface and luminal contents. Since the major known functions of the villi are digestion and absorption and the absorptive cells play a major role in these processes, their highly specialized structure will now be considered in some detail.

The absorptive cells are tall, columnar cells with basally located nuclei (Figs. 54–8 and 54–9). The surface they present to the intraluminal intestinal contents is amplified about 30-fold by the numerous finger-like microvilli that form the brush border of their luminal surface. The plasma membrane covering the microvilli is in direct contact with the contents of the bowel lumen and is both morphologically and biochemically distinctive. It is appreciably wider, is richer in protein, and contains more cholesterol and glycolipids than the plasma membrane lining the basolateral borders of absorptive cells.[20, 21]

A continuous filamentous-appearing glycoprotein coat, the glycocalyx, is applied directly to the outer surface of the microvillous membrane (Figs. 54–10 and 54–11). This surface coat is well developed in humans and is produced by the absorptive cells on which it is found. It is firmly anchored in the membrane and cannot be removed entirely with proteolytic agents as long as the cells remain viable, although pancreatic elastase removes some components of the glycocalyx.[22, 23] Hence this glycoprotein fuzzy coat must be considered an integral part of the microvillous membrane of the cells.

The microvillous membrane, together with its surface coat, does more than provide an immense surface area to facilitate absorption of nutrients previously digested within the gut lumen. Rather, the microvilli participate in absorptive and digestive phenomena in several ways. Disaccharidases and peptidases have been localized to the microvillous membrane–surface coat portion of intestinal absorptive cells and isolated microvillous membranes covered with their surface coat effectively hydrolyze disaccharides and polypeptides to monosaccharides, amino acids, and di- and tripeptides.[24] Thus digestion of carbohydrates and peptides occurs at the level of the microvillous membrane–surface coat complex prior to monosaccharide, amino acid, and small peptide absorption by cells.[25] Moreover, there is evidence that specific receptors are located on the microvillous membrane surface coat complex. These receptors selectively bind substances prior to their absorption and may explain the selective absorption of certain nutrients at specific sites along the small intestine. For example, the receptor for intrinsic factor—cobalamin—is selectively located in the apical membrane of the distal small intestine,[26] and in dog ileum has been localized by immunocytochemistry to small pits between microvilli of absorptive

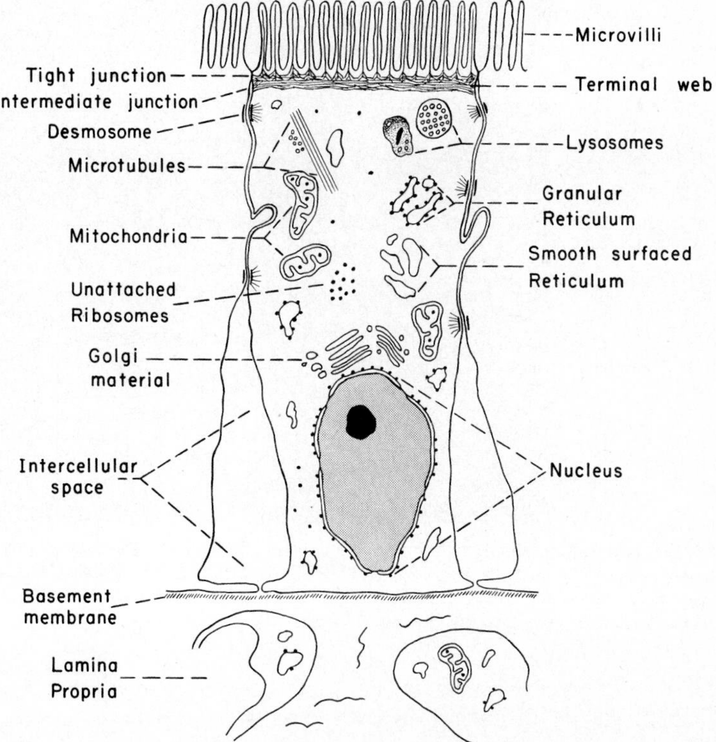

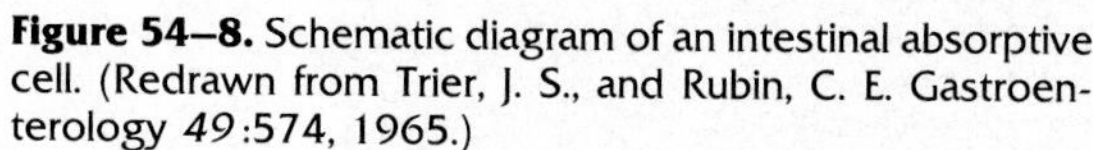
Figure 54–8. Schematic diagram of an intestinal absorptive cell. (Redrawn from Trier, J. S., and Rubin, C. E. Gastroenterology *49*:574, 1965.)

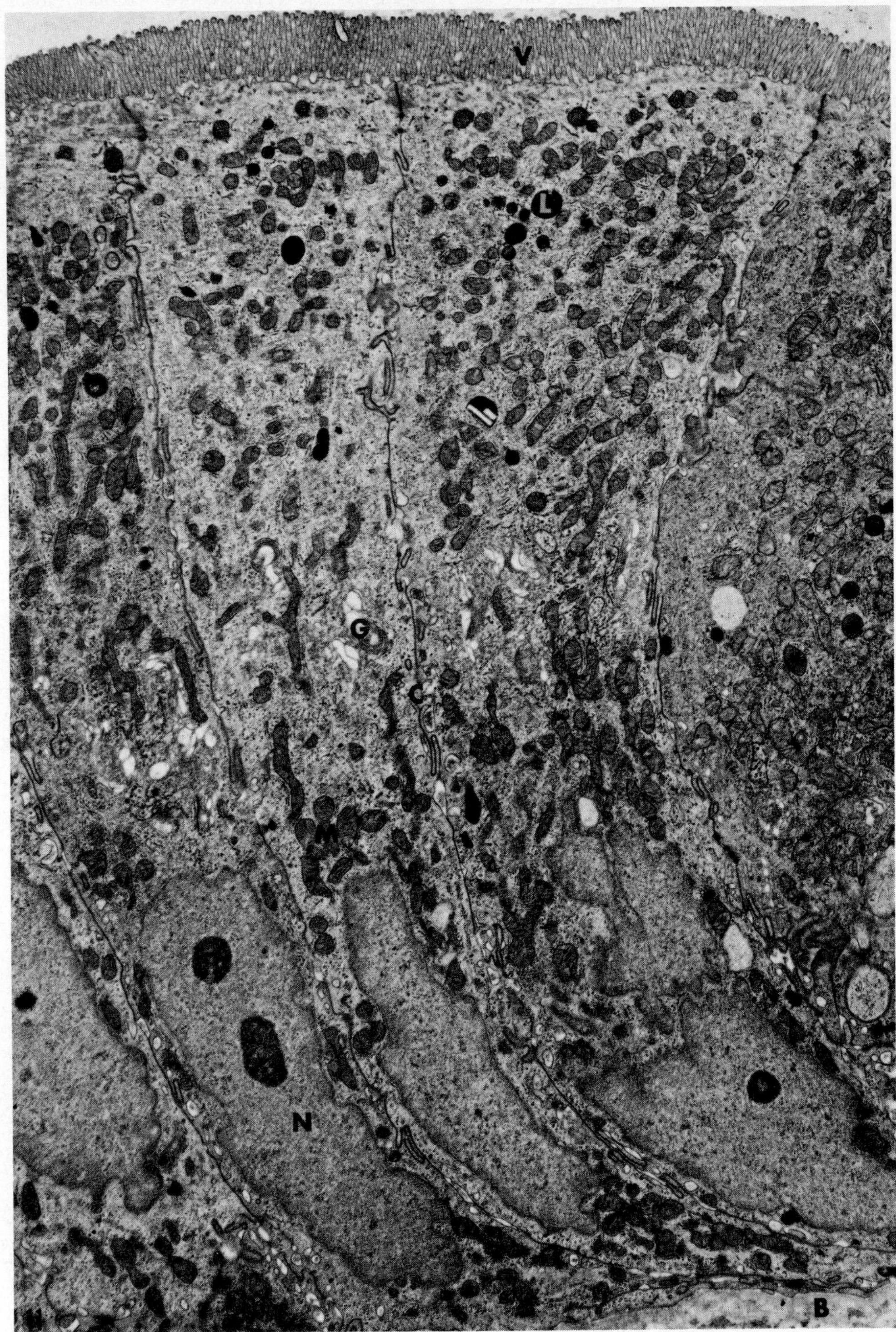

Figure 54–9. Low magnification electron micrograph of intestinal absorptive cells from the middle third of a jejunal villus from a normal man. Basal lamina (B) is seen in the lower right corner. (V) microvilli; (N) nucleus; (G) Golgi material; (L) lysosomes; (M) mitochondria; (C) lateral cell membrane. Approximately ×450. (From Trier, J. S. *In* Code, C. [ed.]. Handbook of Physiology: Vol. 3, Alimentary Canal. Washington, D.C., American Physiological Society, 1968.)

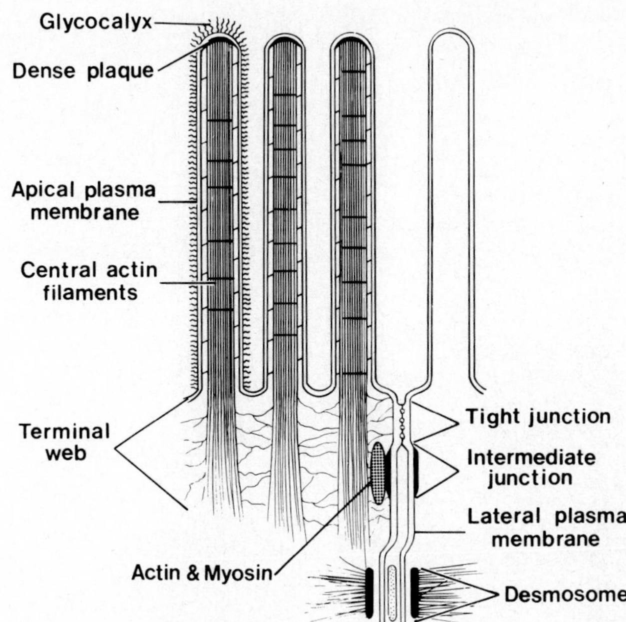

Figure 54–10. Schematic illustration of the specializations of the apical cytoplasm of the plasma membrane of intestinal absorptive cells.

cells.[27] This helps explain why absorption of cobalamin is greatest in the ileum. Receptors may also play a role in the preferential absorption of conjugated bile salts in the distal intestine and food iron and calcium in the proximal intestine. In addition, transport proteins that cotransport Na^+ and D-glucose and Na^+ and amino acids have been localized to the microvillous membranes of absorptive cells.[28]

An important morphologic specialization is seen at the upper part of the lateral plasma membrane. Here, the outer leaflets of adjacent plasma membranes appear to fuse to form a "tight junction" (Figs. 54–10 and 54–11).[29] Actually, electron microscopic freeze fracture studies have revealed that these tight junctions (also termed zonula occludens) consist of a series of linear epithelial cells,[30] suggesting that true fusion of adjacent membranes is focal along the tight junction. The tight junctions of intestinal epitheleum have important implications with regard to transport phenomena. They completely encircle the upper part of adjacent epithelial cells and, in most instances, appear to be impermeable to macromolecular tracers. On the other hand, in the intestine they do permit passive transport of small molecules such as water and small ions by the paracellular route. It has been noted that the depths of the tight junctions and the number of strands that constitute the junctions are greater between adjacent absorptive cells than between adjacent undifferentiated crypt cells (Fig. 54–12).[31] Junctions that involve goblet cells also vary in depth and strand count.[32] Thus, the permeability of this barrier between the intestinal lumen and the paracellular space appears to vary focally with cell type in the intestinal epithelium with leaky junctions in the crypts and relatively tight junctions on villi.[33] Such partitioning of paracellular

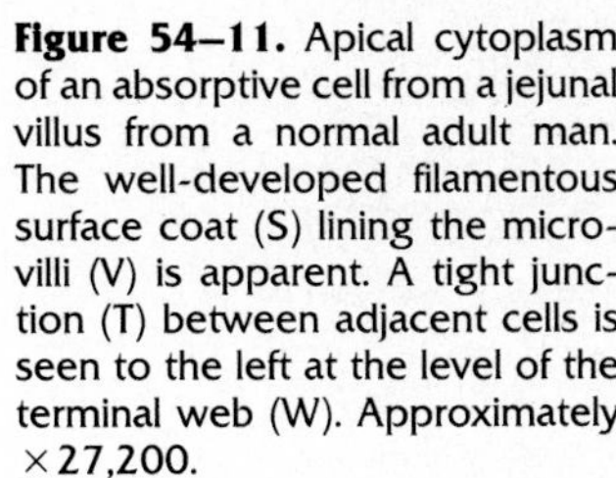

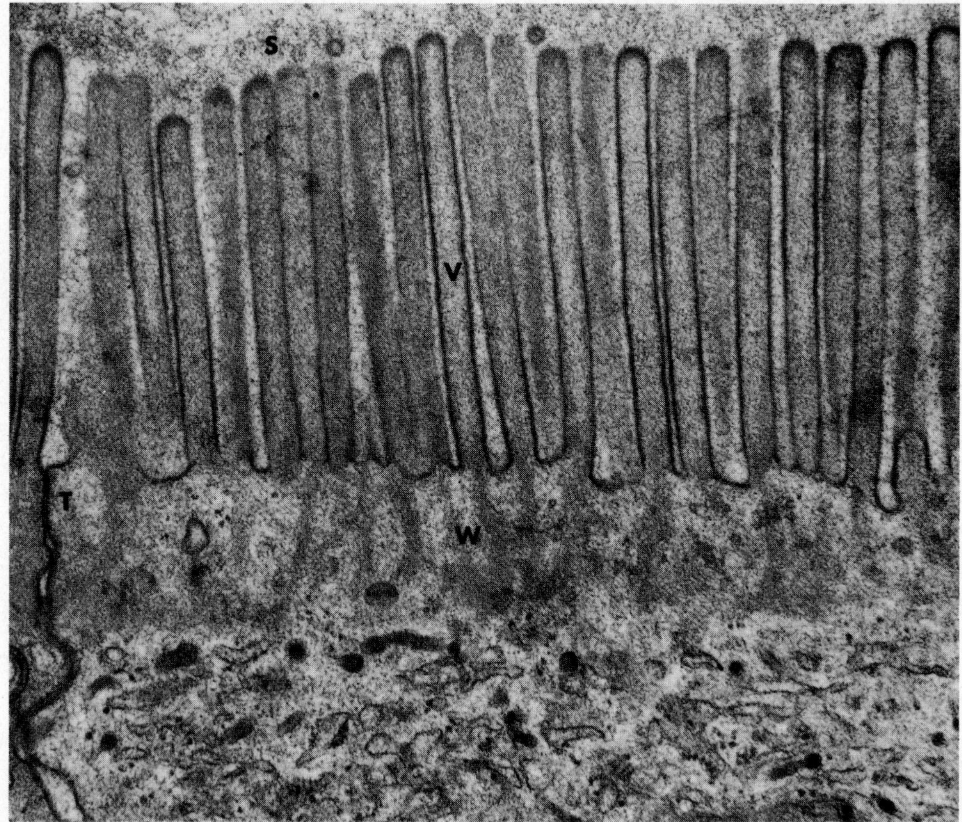

Figure 54–11. Apical cytoplasm of an absorptive cell from a jejunal villus from a normal adult man. The well-developed filamentous surface coat (S) lining the microvilli (V) is apparent. A tight junction (T) between adjacent cells is seen to the left at the level of the terminal web (W). Approximately ×27,200.

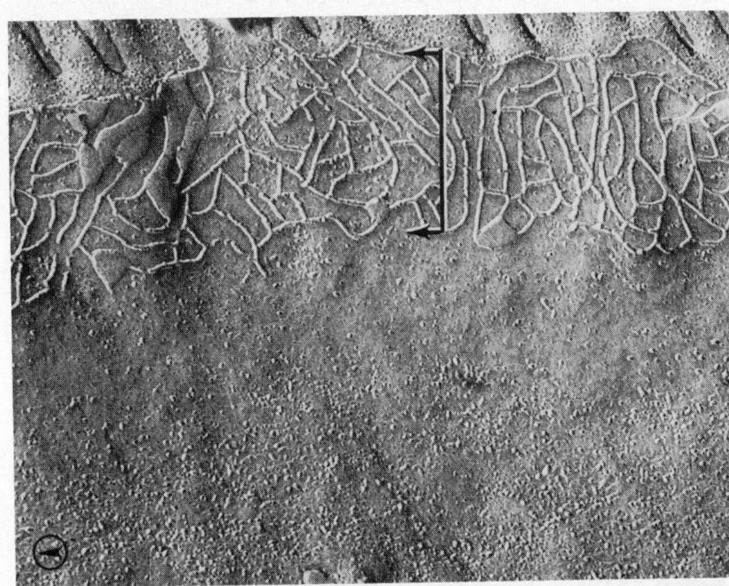

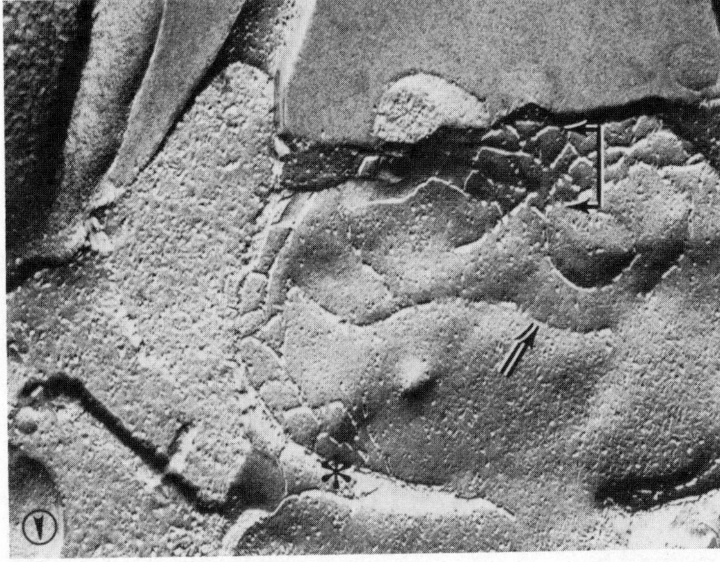

Figure 54–12. Freeze-fracture replicas of tight junctions of villus (top) and crypt cells (bottom). Tight junctions of villus absorptive cells have greater depth *(brackets)* and are more uniformly organized than those of crypt cells. Unconnected lateral aberrant strands *(double arrow)* are common in the crypt but rare on the villus. Cells in both crypts and villi show ladder-like specializations at three-cell junctions *(asterisk)*. Approximately ×56,100. Reprinted with permission from: Structural changes in the plasma membrane accompanying differentiation of epithelial cells in human and monkey small intestine, by Madara, J. L., Trier, J. S., and Neutra, M. R. Gastroenterology *78*[5 pt. 2]:963–975. Copyright 1980 by The American Gastroenterological Association.)

conductance between crypts and villi fits well with current models of intestinal water and electrolyte absorption and secretion. However, because of the barrier provided by these junctions, most dietary nutrients that are considerably larger than water and selected ions must cross at least the microvillous membrane, the apical cytoplasm, and the lateral plasma membrane of the absorptive cells in order to gain access to the intercellular space between epithelial cells during absorption from the gut lumen (Fig. 54–10). As in other epithelia, the tight junction also plays a key role in maintaining the polarity of the plasma membrane of the absorptive cells.

The intercellular space between adjacent absorptive cells may vary considerably in width from a small fraction of a micron between absorptive cells at the base of the villi to a micron or more between absorptive cells near the tip of the villus. The intermediate junction (zonula adherens) is located just below the tight junction, and spot desmosomes are located along the lateral membrane and serve to anchor adjacent cells to each other. The intercellular space widens during active fluid absorption; hence its greater width near the tip of the villi is not surprising.

The rim of cytoplasm immediately beneath the microvilli consists of numerous filaments and is known as the terminal web region (Figs. 54–8, 54–10, and 54–11). The filaments that form the cores of the microvilli extend as rootlets into and associate with the filaments of the web (Fig. 54–11). It has been established that the core filaments consist of actin, and there is now evidence that the brush border and web region of intestinal absorptive cells contains other muscle-associated proteins, including myosin, which is most prominently associated with actin in a peripheral ring adjacent to the intermediate junction (Fig. 54–10).[34] Recent observations suggest that these contractile proteins might form the basis for microvillar motion.[34] Thus the terminal web and cores of the microvilli could cause stirring of the intraluminal contents in addition to providing structural support for the microvillous absorptive surface, although it remains to be shown that contraction of absorptive cell microvilli occurs *in vivo*.

Various organelles are distributed in the cytoplasm beneath the terminal web. These include many mitochondria, a variable number of lysosomes, granular and smooth-surfaced endoplasmic reticulum, a well-defined supranuclear Golgi complex, microtubules, and a moderate number of unattached ribosomes. Although all the specific functions of each of these organelles in absorptive processes have not been defined precisely, some information is available. The mitochondria, as in other cells, participate in oxidative reactions that provide energy needed for metabolic processes. The lysosomes, as in other cells, are sites of intracellular digestion where both endogenous and exogenous substances that might damage the cell can be degraded.

The endoplasmic reticulum plays an important role in intracellular transport and synthetic processes. For example, during fat absorption, the endoplasmic reticulum resynthesizes triglyceride from absorbed monoglyceride and fatty acid (see pp. 1068–1075). There is also evidence that, at least in part, the liprotein coat that surrounds chlomicrons is synthesized by the endoplasmic reticulum and applied to the triglyceride droplets as they travel through channels of the endoplasmic reticulum. The endoplasmic reticulum is also the site for synthesis of the peptide core of digestive enzymes, such as peptidases and disacchardidases and other membrane proteins found in absorptive cells.

The Golgi material is regularly located in the cytoplasm above or alongside the nucleus (Figs. 54–8 and 54–9) Available data indicate that the Golgi material segregates and chemically modifies material absorbed and synthesized by cells and plays a key role in the sorting process that ultimately targets these products to their final destination.[35]

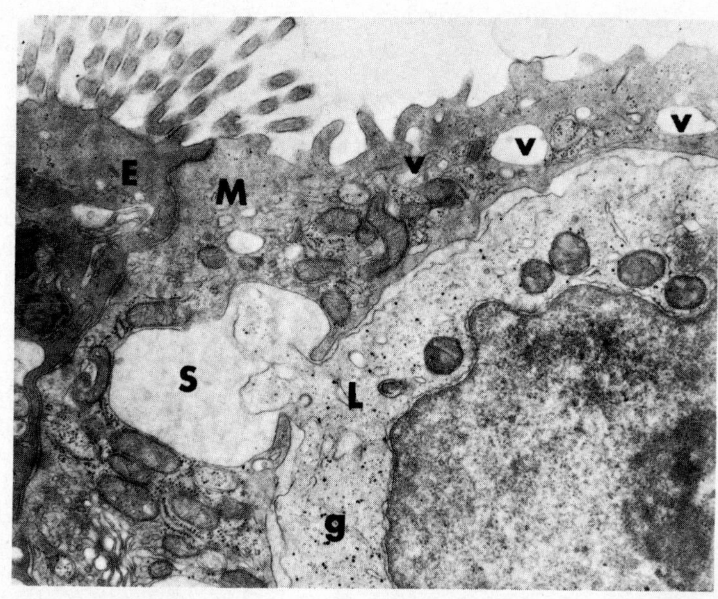

Figure 54–13. Transmission electron micrograph showing the apical junction and subsurface desmosomes between an M cell (M) and an epithelial cell (E) on its left. The attenuated cytoplasm, containing mitochondria, rough endoplasmic reticulum, vesicles (v) of various sizes, and Golgi apparatus, is only as thick as five of the overhanging microvilli, which are each approximately 0.1 μm wide. The microfolds lack the thick coat of glycocalyx material adherent to microvilli on the adjacent cell. Flocculent material fills the space (S) separating the underlying lymphoid cell (L) and the internal cell membrane of the M cell The lymphoid cell contains vesicles, mitochondria, free ribosomes, and glycogen (g) but lacks a well-developed endoplasmic reticulum. A pseudopod of the lymphoid cell (L) is seen projecting into an M cell cavity. Along the lymphoid cell surface are vesicles in continuity with the material within the intercellular space. Approximately × 18,500. (From Owen, R. L., and Jones, A. L. Epithelial cell specialization with human Peyer's patches. An ultrastructural study of intestinal lymphoid follicles. Gastroenterology *66*:189–203. © by Williams & Wilkins, 1974.)

The thin basal lamina is closely applied to the basal plasma membrane of the absorptive cells and bridges the gap between adjacent lateral plasma membranes (Figs. 54–6 and 54–8). The capillaries and lymphatics in the lamina propria may lie in close proximity to the basal surface of absorptive cells (Fig. 54–6), but absorbed material must cross the epithelial basal lamina to gain access to these vascular channels. Thus, in the process of nutrient absorption, material first cotacts the glycoprotein surface coat of the microvilli, where terminal digestion of the nutrients may occur. The products of digestion then penetrate the microvillous membrane and traverse the terminal web region and a variable amount of cytoplasmic matrix. The absorbed material then either may enter the intercellular space between absorptive cells by crossing the lateral plasma membrane, or may enter the intracellular channels of the endolasmic reticulum. In the reticulum, the material may be biochemically modified and travel to the Golgi material, where it may be further modified and directed to its final destination in the cell. Eventually most abosorbed material leaves the cell by crossing either the lateral or the basal plasma membrane. Finally, the absorbed material penetrtes the epithelial cell basal lamina to enter the lamina propria, in which it traverses the lymphatic or capillary wall to gain access to the lymph or the blood.

An important specialized epithelial cell has been described relatively recently overlying lymphoid follicles in Peyer's patches in the ileum.[36] These cells have been termed "M" cells. Their cytoplasm is indented centrally by macrophages and lymphocytes, hence only a thin bridge of M cell cytolasm separates intraluminal contents from the underlying immunocompetent cells (Fig. 54–13). M cells are capable of endocytosing macromolecules and selected micro-organisms such as reovirus and cholera vibrios.[37–39] M cells appear to provide a specific route for antigen uptake into the intestinal lymphoid system and may play a key role in the intestinal immune response.[37–39] Moreover, they may serve as a site for penetration of the intestinal mucosal barrier by pathogens[38] (see pp. 114–144).

GROSS MORPHOLOGY OF THE COLON

The colon is concerned primarily with absorption of water and electrolytes (see pp. 1022–1045) and storage and propulsion of its intraluminal contents (see pp. 1093–1102). The colon also can absorb volatile fatty acids that are formed by intraluminal bacteria from unabsorbed carbohydrates. This may be nutritionally significant in young infants. The proximal colon is derived from the embryonal midgut and is nourished by the superior mesenteric artery. The distal colon springs from the hindgut and receives the greater part of its blood supply from the inferior mesenteric artery and its branches.

The length of the colon of the average adult is 4 to 5 feet. The diameter of the colon diminishes from cecum to anus. The colon is characterized grossly by some tortuosity and redundancy of the sigmoid and by two sharp angulations, the splenic and hepatic flexures, the former situated superior to the latter (Fig. 54–14).

The wall of the colon, like that of the small intestine, contains an outer longitudinal and inner circular muscle coat, but in the colon the longitudinal muscle forms three separate bands, the teniae coli, about 0.6 to 1.0 cm in width, which run from the tip of the cecum to the rectum and converge at the base of the appendix. Between the teniae are outpouchings, which are called haustra, separated by folds. The size and shape of the haustra are determined by the state of contraction of the smooth and longitudinal muscle layers. Covering the serosal surface of the colon are the appendices epiploicae, which are fatty structures attached to the peritoneum. Unlike the jejunum and the ileum, the colon does not have a mesentery for its entire length, containing a structure of this sort only along the transverse colon and the sigmoid.[4] Thus, the cecum, ascending and descending colon, and rectum are "fixed" and not as freely movable as those segments with a mesentery.

On plain films of the abdomen, the colon is frequently seen to contain some gas, more than is normally seen in the small intestine. The course of the colon can often be traced by identification of haustra, the relatively high position of the splenic flexure, and the often partially gas-filled rectum and rectosigmoid (Fig. 54–15). In contrast, the small intestine, overlying or underlying the colon in many areas, normally appears only as radiolucent spots scattered about the abdomen.

Although the mucosa of the colon is flat, it is thrown into some irregular folds, the *plicae semilunares* (Fig. 54–14), by contraction of the underlying muscle coats. The crypts of Lieberkühn open into the colonic lumen all along the flat mucosal surface.

Segmental Characteristics of the Colon

The most proximal segment of the colon is the cecum. The terminal segment of ileum enters the cecum at its posterior medial aspect in a horizontal and often slightly downward directed fashion. The distal aspect of the cecal lumen is defined by the ileocecal valve (Figs. 54–16 and 54–17).

Ileocecal Valve. Studies have indicated that the ileocecal valve behaves like a sphincter.[40] Anatomically, it is composed of an upper and a lower lip; at their corners of fusion they taper to form transverse folds that are part of the cecal wall (Fig. 54–16). In man, the resting pressure of the sphincter is about 20 mm Hg above colonic pressure and the length of the zone is approximately 4 cm. Splanchnic and vagal nerve stimulation as well as cecal distention increase sphincteric pressure. In contrast, distention of the terminal ileum causes relaxation of the ileocecal valve and facilitates movement of chyme into the colon. Together with the normal propulsive activity of the small intestine, the ileocecal sphincter serves to regulate delivery

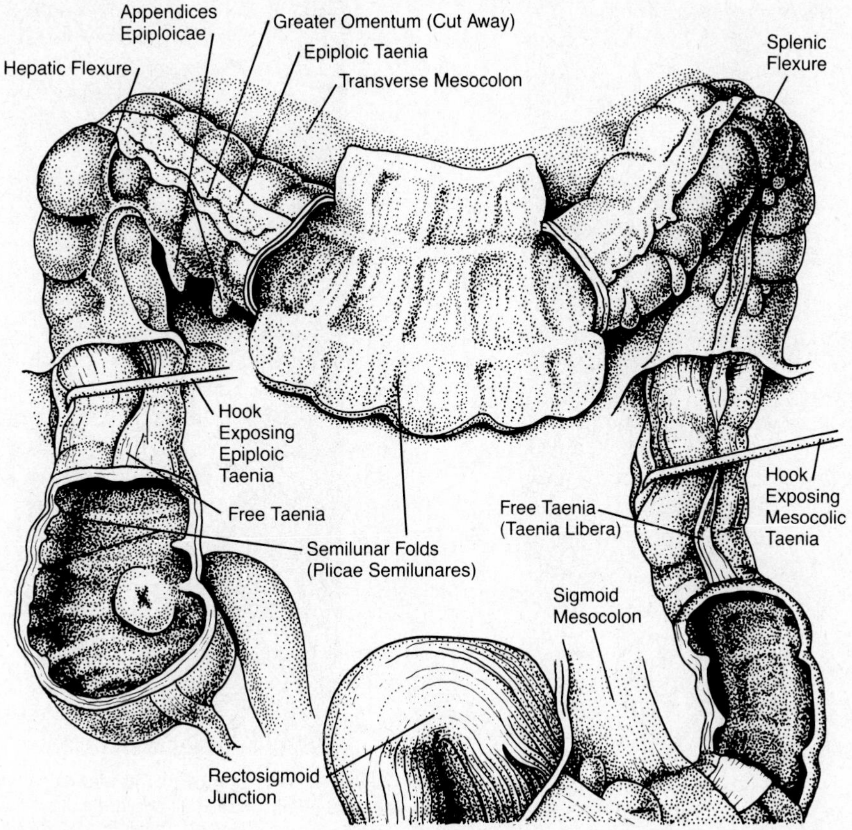

Figure 54–14. Contour and gross anatomy of the colon. Note the ileocecal junction, which is not labeled. (From Netter, F., Ciba Collection of Medical Illustrations. Volume 3, Section X.)

of ileal contents into the proximal colon and minimize reflux of cecal contents into the ileum. If sufficient pressure is exerted, as, for example, during a barium enema X-ray examination, colonic contents may reflux into the terminal ileum (Fig. 54–17). Although the anatomy of the ileocecal valve is not exactly the same in all individuals, certain features are rather constant: the terminal ileum is directed horizontally and slightly downward and forms a slotlike orifice in the cecum; the lips of the valves are often thicker in children because of the presence of more lymphoid tissue; and the last few centimeters of ileum are usually fixed either by fusion to the cecal wall or by Lane's membrane to the posterior parietal peritoneum.

Cecum. The cecum is the most proximal and widest segment of the colon, occupying the right iliac fossa by virtue of rotation of the intestine during a later embryonic stage. Occasionally it may be located a bit more toward the midline, particularly in an individual whose colon is somewhat long and redundant. When intestinal rotation has been incomplete, the cecum may be found in the right upper quadrant and in extreme instances in the midline or in the left side of the abdominal cavity. This abnormality is clinically important because it is the basis for cecal volvulus (see pp. 372–373). The cecum possesses no mesentery, because it is an outpouching of the antimesenteric border of the gut and is "fixed" posteriorly in only a small percentage of individuals; therefore it has a certain degree of mobility and in extreme instances may actually become twisted. When fully matured, the cecum is somewhat eccentric in shape because of the greater growth of the lateral than the medial sacculation.

Attached to the cecum is the *vermiform appendix*; originally it is found at the apex of the cecum, but with full development it is attached to the medial aspect. It is located below the ileocecal junction where the teniae converge, ranges from a little over 2 cm to over 20 cm in length, and averages about 0.8 cm in diameter. It may be located behind the cecum (over 50 per cent of dissections); downward and to the right of the cecum; pointed over the brim of the pelvis; or anterior or posterior to the ileum (less than 1 per cent of dissections). The appendix is attached to the posterior parietal wall by a triangular fold of mesoappendix. Frequently, however, when the appendix is located behind the cecum, this fold is not present, and the appendix adheres to the colon or to the posterior abdominal wall.

Ascending Colon. An approximately 20-cm segment distal to the cecum between it and the lower pole of the right kidney, is known as the ascending colon. This is located below the undersurface of the right lobe of the liver, at which point it turns toward the midline and downward rather sharply, forming the hepatic flexure. It is usually fixed to the posterior peritoneum.

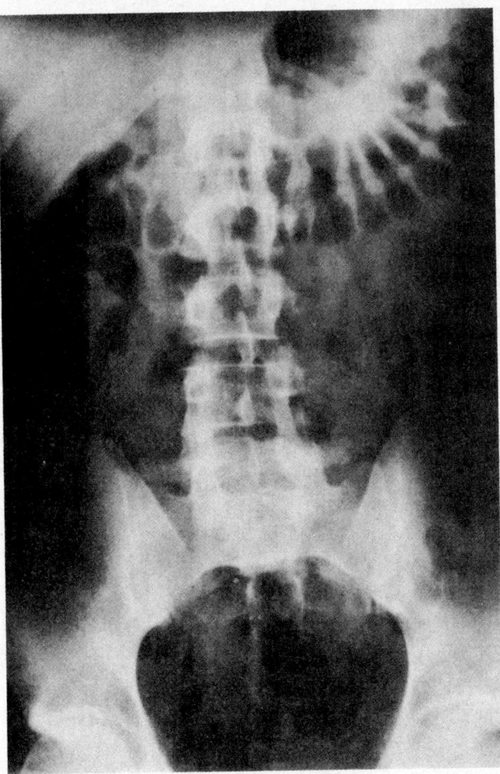

Figure 54–15. Plain film of the abdomen. Air outlines haustra of transverse colon particularly. Normally, only scattered pockets of air in small bowel are noted.

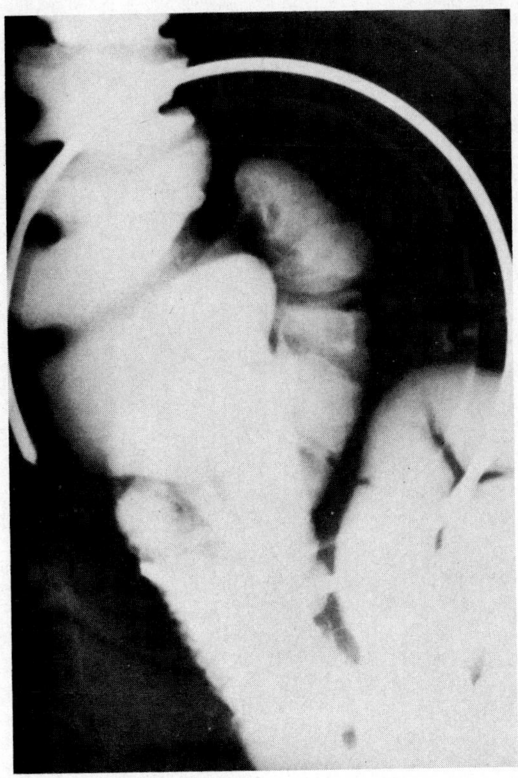

Figure 54–17. Contour of the ileocecal junction as seen on X-ray. Note the "bird beak" appearance.

Occasionally, the hepatic flexure containing gas may be interposed between the liver and the diaphragm, obscuring liver dullness on physical examination. Thus, it is not a fixed segment of colon, although it is sometimes supported by a fold extending from the hepatorenal ligament.

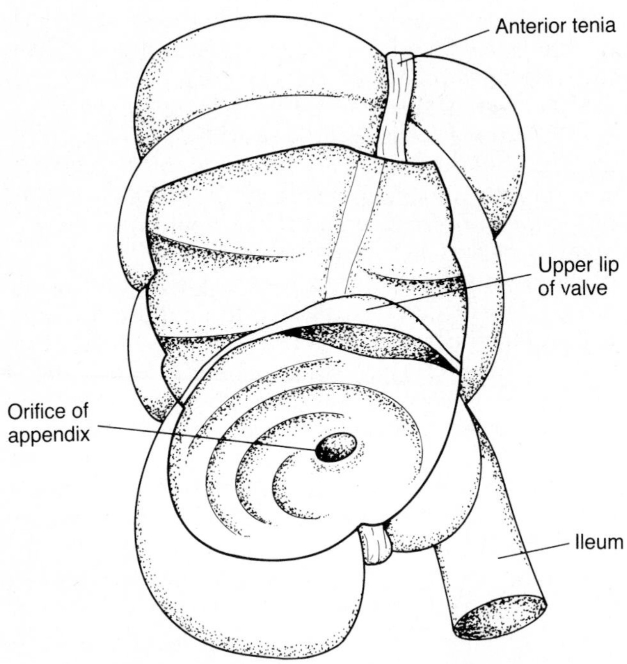

Figure 54–16. Diagram of ileocecal junction.

Transverse Colon. The transverse colon lies between the hepatic flexure and the splenic flexure, traversing the abdomen from right to left; it is quite mobile, often descending into the pelvis in individuals in the upright position. It is located anteriorly and is suspended by the transverse mesocolon that originates from the posterior peritoneum. The transverse mesocolon is a fold; its upper part is continuous posteriorly with the lesser peritoneal sac, and its lower portion forms a part of the wall of the greater omentum.

The splenic flexure marks the junction between the transverse and descending colon, and it is attached to the diaphragm at about the level of the tenth to eleventh ribs by phrenicocolic ligaments. At the flexure, the colon is directed posteriorly so that the distal transverse colon lies in front of the proximal descending colon when viewed laterally. The splenic flexure is located higher than the hepatic flexure. The location and configuration plus fixation of the splenic flexure may contribute to the discomfort noted in some patients with the irritable colon syndrome; a special entity known as the "splenic flexure syndrome" may occur in an occasional patient who complains of upper abdominal and even anterior thoracic pain due to an inordinate amount of gas trapped at this juncture.

Descending Colon. The descending colon descends inferiorly between the psoas and quadratus lumborum muscles and is joined to the sigmoid colon at the pelvic brim; it is only partially peritonealized and usually has no mesentery. Although this segment of the colon is capable of absorbing water, electrolytes, and glucose, the degree of this function is normally less than in the more promixal colon. Its main purposes are temporary storage and, presumably, mucous secretion.

Sigmoid Colon. From the pelvic brim to the rectum, which begins at the peritoneal reflection, lies the sigmoid colon, a redundant loop of large bowel with the characteristic sigma shape. Its length varies considerably; the longer ones are coiled to variable degrees. In most individuals it has a mesentery, which explains much of its mobility and winding course. Because of its twists and curves, adjacent loops are superimposed on each other in anteroposterior projections. This is especially relevant during barium contrast radiologic examinations in individuals suspected of having tumors in the "blind alleys" of the rectosigmoid curve as well as in more superior segments, which are partly obscured by the turns of this portion of the colon as it courses superiorly to join the descending colon. Therefore special maneuvers are essential to visualize the loops in lateral or oblique projections. The sharpest angulation is at the rectosigmoid junction, the point at which the bowel becomes peritonealized, which is approximately 15 cm from the anus in adults. In children the location of the rectosigmoid junction varies with age; this becomes clinically important when an internal examination is necessary. In the first three months of life, the anal canal is approximately 2 cm in length and the rectosigmoid junction is 9 cm from the anus. In infants less than two years of age, the anal canal has elongated to 2.5 cm and the rectosigmoid junction is approximately 12 cm from the anus. By age 10 years, the distance between the rectosigmoid junction and the anal orifice is approximately the same as in adults (15 cm).

Rectum and Anal Canal. From above downward the rectum begins at the termination of the pelvic mesocolon. At the rectosigmoid junction, the mucosa changes in appearance, being smoother in the rectum. The rectum follows the curve of the sacrum and, although not firmly fixed, does not have a great degree of mobility. Anteriorly, it may be impinged upon by the uterus or the cervix uteri in women. In infants, the rectum does not follow the curve of the sacrum as closely as it will when the child becomes older. Thus, there often is a much straighter course to follow when negotiating an examination of the rectosigmoid region in a young child.

From below upward, the rectum rapidly becomes capacious, and the enlarged, fusiform-shaped segment is known as the ampulla; it begins a few centimeters beyond the pectinate line (Fig. 54–18); its upper portion gradually merges into the segment that is the upper rectum, which in turn joins the sigmoid at the peritoneal reflection. The rectal mucosa has three shelflike folds termed valves of Houston—two on the left and one on the right.

The terminal 3 cm of rectum and anal canal is marked by longitudinal folds called the columns of Morgagni, which terminate in the anal papillae. These papillae may be quite accentuated in some individuals; they appear whitish and are sometimes sufficiently thickened to look polypoid. The anal canal terminates at the mucocutaneous junction where the lining of the canal changes from columnar epithelium to the stratified squamous epithelium of skin. The transition is not sudden but is a rather gradual blending; an intermediate cuboidal epithelium is frequently noted. Several plexuses of veins may be found in the anus—the internal hemorrhoidal plexus in the submucosal space at the level of the columns of Morgagni and the anal papillae, and the external hemorrhoidal plexus in the subcutaneous space near the anal verge (Fig. 54–18).

On page 1100, a full description is given of the muscular pelvic diaphragm and its function with regard to the defecation reflex and the function of the sphincters. Components of the levator ani muscles—puborectalis, pubococcygeus, and ileococcygeus—make up this pelvic diaphragm, which is joined in its most posterior portion by the small coccygeus muscle. The fibers of the levator ani form a puborectal sling within which the lower rectum turns posteriorly. Contraction of the levator ani raises the pelvic diaphragm, the rectum, and the anus and narrows the anal-rectal angle, contributing to anal continence, which is maintained principally by the contraction of the external sphincter (Fig. 54–19).

The internal sphincter of the anal canal is the distal portion of the circular smooth muscle of the rectum (Fig. 54–18). It extends from the distal tip of the rectum to within 1 cm of the anal orifice. The external sphincter circumscribes the anal canal and is separated from the internal sphincter by a thin layer of elastic fibers and longitudinal muscle coat of the rectum. Superiorly, its fibers blend with those of the levator ani muscle; it is attached posteriorly to the coccyx and anteriorly to the perineal body (Fig. 54–19). Distally, the external sphincter ends subcutaneously at the anal margin.

Examination of the Rectum. Examination of the rectum is extremely important and is an integral part of every physical examination. It must be done with the greatest of care, particularly in patients in whom one has reason to believe a tumor exists in the lower bowel, or in whom other evidence suggests the possibility of tumor with possible extension into the pelvis. The perianal area should first be examined carefully for evidence of fistulas, fissures, rash, ulcerations, and external hemorrhoids. The examining finger can detect much; for example, the tone of the sphincter (internal sphincter), the feel of the mucosa, and the presence or absence of strictures, mucosal tumors, or metastatic tumors impinging on the anterior wall of the rectum, which may form a firm, indurated, ridgelike deformity known as Blumer's shelf. In men, the prostate and retrovesical and retroprostatic spaces may be palpated as well as the seminal vesicles. In women, anteriorly one may feel the cervix of the uterus and the posterior vaginal wall. Laterally, the examiner may palpate the ischiorectal space on each side, an important area for abscess formation (see pp. 1573–1574).

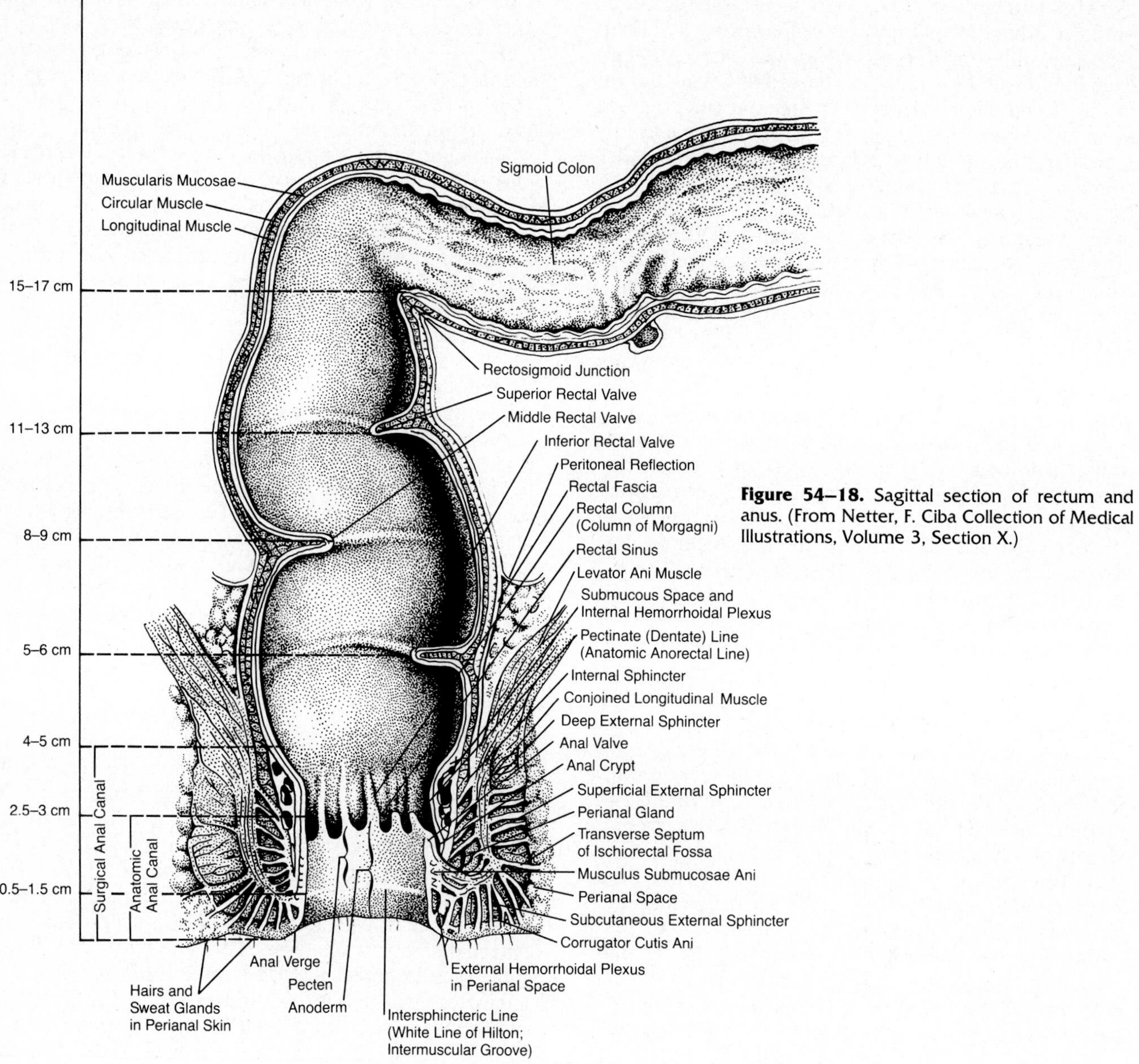

Figure 54–18. Sagittal section of rectum and anus. (From Netter, F. Ciba Collection of Medical Illustrations, Volume 3, Section X.)

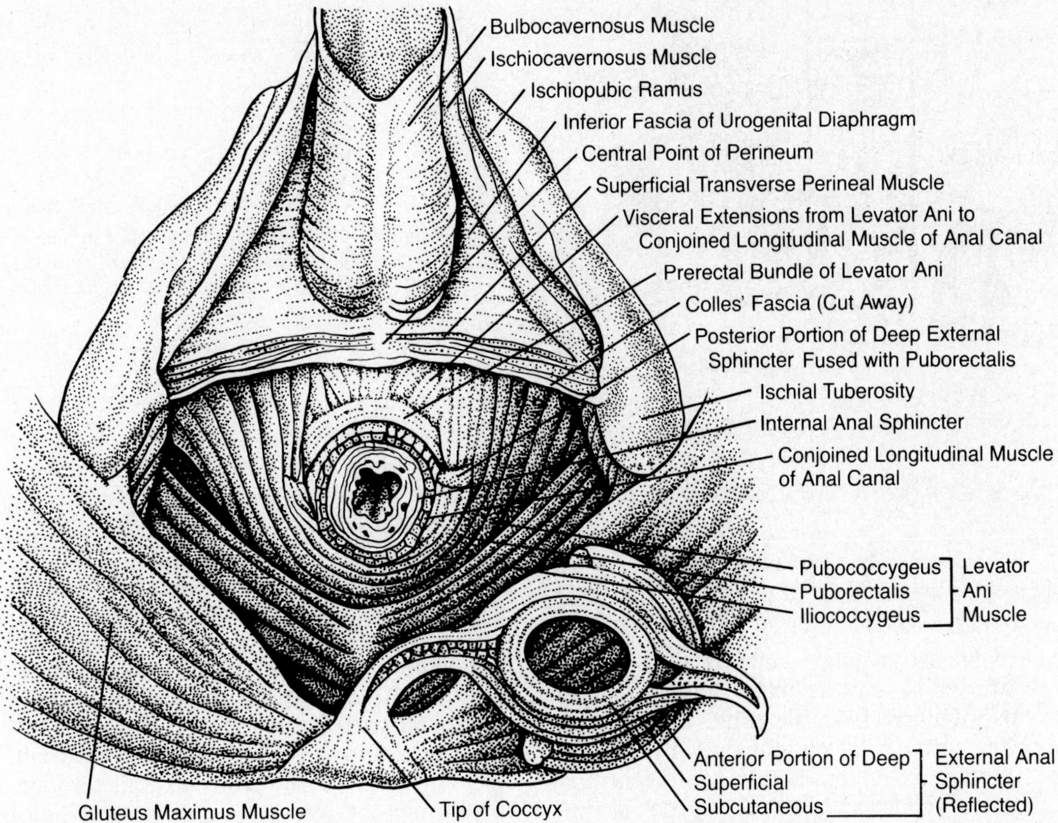

Figure 54–19. The muscular pelvic diaphragm, its anatomic relationship to the rectum and anus. (From Netter, F. Ciba Collection of Medical Illustrations, Volume 3, Section X.)

HISTOLOGY OF THE COLON

The wall of the large intestine, like that of the small intestine, consists of four distinct layers (Fig. 54–2).[1] The outermost layer, the serosa, is composed of mesothelial cells to which are attached fatty appendices' epiploicae, which are extensions of peritoneal fat. The serosa covers only the portions of the large bowel that lie within the peritoneal cavity; thus it is not found in the rectum.

The muscle coat, found immediately beneath the serosa, is composed of an inner circular muscular layer forming a tight spiral circumferentially along the course of the colon and an incomplete outer longitudinal muscle layer composed of three separate longitudinal strips (teniae coli) which run from the rectum to the cecum. The ganglion cells of the myenteric plexus of Auerbach may be found between the circular and longitudinal muscle layers, with the majority being located along the external surface of the circular muscle coat. Unmyelinated postganglionic fibers are also found in the circular muscle layer and communicate with the submucosal (Meissner's) plexus.

The submucosa of the colon resembles the submucosa of the other tubular digestive organs. It contains many blood and lymph vessels, dense connective tissue sparsely infiltrated by cells (fibroblasts, lymphocytes, plasma cells, mast cells, macrophages, and eosinophils), and the unmyelinated nerve fibers and ganglion cells that form the submucosal plexus.

The innermost layer of the mucosa is separated from the submucosa by the muscularis mucosae, a layer of smooth muscle cells roughly 8 to 12 cells thick. The mucosa of the large intestine differs from that of the small intestine in that villi are absent; instead, the absorptive surface is flat. However, numerous straight tubular crypts up to 0.7 mm in length are normally present and extend from the muscularis mucosae to the flat absorptive surface (Fig. 54–20).[1, 41] The crypts and the absorptive surface are lined by a continuous sheet of columnar epithelial cells, which are separated from mesenchymal tissue of the lamina propria by a well-defined, continuous basal lamina applied to the basal plasma membrane of the epithelial cells.

The epithelium in the lower half of the crypts is composed of proliferating undifferentiated columnar cells, mucus-secreting goblet cells, and at least six types of endocrine epithelial cells.[13] The epithelium of the upper half of the crypts consists of differentiating columnar cells, goblet cells, and a few endocrine cells. Young goblet cells are capable of cell proliferation. The flat absorptive surface is lined by many columnar cells as well as a moderate number of goblet cells, most of which are largely depleted of their mucous

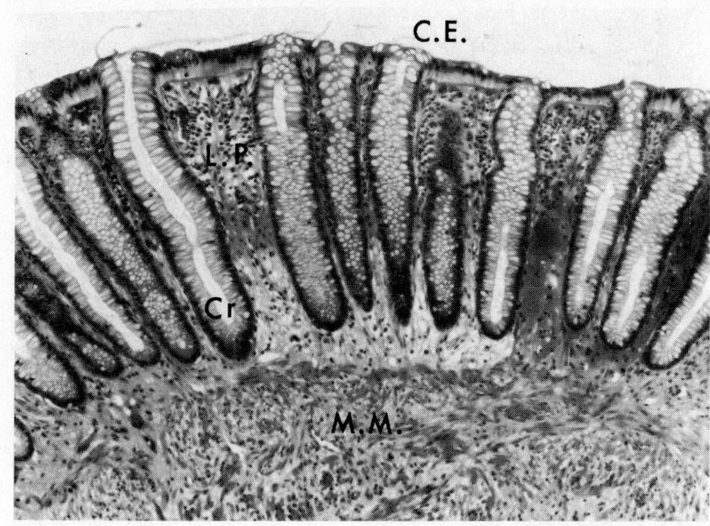

Figure 54–20. Biopsy of normal adult human rectum, showing rectal mucosa. C.E., columnar epithelium; L.P., lamina propria; Cr, crypt; M.M., muscularis mucosae. × 100.

granules. The decrease in goblet cells on the surface epithelium of the colon may be more apparent than real owing to loss of mucus from the goblet cells during their ascent to the surface. Intraepithelial lymphocytes are scattered throughout the epithelium, and as in the small intestine, the predominant T cell subset is the cytotoxic-suppressor type. In contrast with the epithelium of the small intestine, the intraepithelial lymphocytes in the colon are more numerous in the crypt than in the surface epithelium.

The morphology of the columnar cells of the large intestine differs significantly from that of absorptive cells in the small intestine. Although the absorptive surface of both cell types is line by microvilli, the microvilli on the colonic columnar cells are less abundant (Fig. 54–21). However, as in the small intestine, an elaborate fibrillar glycoprotein surface coat is applied directly to the apical plasma membrane that delineates the microvilli (Fig. 54–21). Numerous membrane-bounded glycoprotein-containing vesicles 0.1 to 1 μm in diameter are present in the apical cytoplasm of colonic and rectal columnar cells (Fig. 54–21). Although their function is unknown, these vesicles are distinctive, are not found in the cytoplasm of absorptive cells of the small intestine, and suggest that colonic columnar cells may secrete glycoproteins as well as absorb water and electrolytes. The morphology of the goblet and endocrine cells of the large intestine resembles that of goblet and some endocrine cells in the small intestine.

The cellular elements of the lamina propria of the large intestine resemble closely those seen in the small intestine and include lymphocytes, many plasma cells, mast cells, macrophages, eosinophils, and fibroblasts. Occasional macrophage-like cells, muciphages, which contain glycoprotein and stain positively with PAS, are found in otherwise normal colonic biopsies and are considered a normal variant. It is postulated that they phagocytose goblet cell mucus.[42] In addition, there are blood and lymph vessels and unmyelinated nerve fibers in the lamina. Large lymph follicles with typical B cell germinal centers are often seen in the lamina propria of the colon and the rectum, especially in young persons. These frequently extend through the muscalaris mucosae into the submucosa. When present, the follicles may markedly distort mucosal architecture and thus make interpretation of the results of biopsy difficult (Fig. 54–22).

Lymphatic Drainage

The small intestine and colon are drained by a vast network of lymphatics that begin in the intramural lymph capillaries associated with lymph follicles. Applied to the surface of the intestine are the "epi-" group of lymph nodes (e.g., epicolic), which drain through the mesentery to another group of nodes identified as the "para-" group (e.g., paracolic) along the marginal artery. These drain proximally to nodes along the mesenteric and colic arteries. In those areas of the intestine in which there is no mesentery, lymphatic flow is retroperitoneal. The smaller and larger lymph channels merge and drain into the three groups of pre-aortic nodes—inferior mesenteric, superior mesenteric, and celiac. All the lymph eventually flows into the cisterna chyli, a sac between the aorta and the right crus of the diaphragm. Here lymphatic vessels from other viscera, the abdominal wall, and the lower extremities join before the thoracic duct ascends through the diaphragm to empty into the left subclavian vein at the jugulosubclavian angle.

The importance of the colonic lymphatics lies in their involvement in both inflammatory—particularly granulomatous—and neoplastic disease of the colon and rectum. Further discussion of the lymphatics in these diseases of the colon will be found on pages 1328 to 1331 and 1533 to 1546.

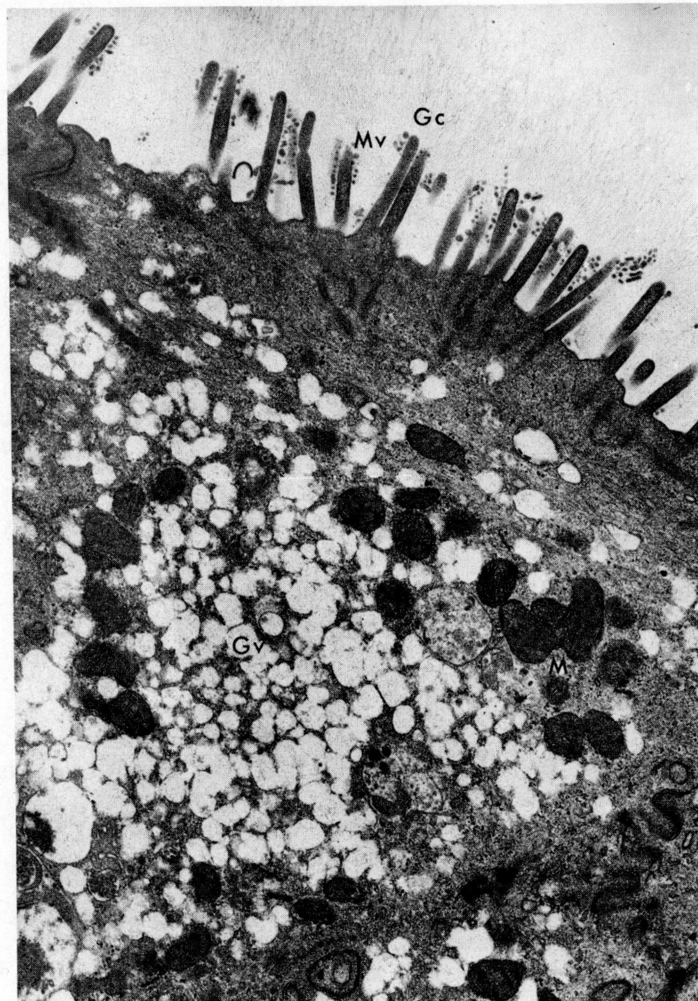

Figure 54–21. Electron micrograph of a normal human rectal absorptive cell. Cc, glycocalyx; Mv, microvilli; Gv, glycoprotein vesicles; M, mitochondria. ×20,000. (Courtesy of Gregory Eastwood, M.D.)

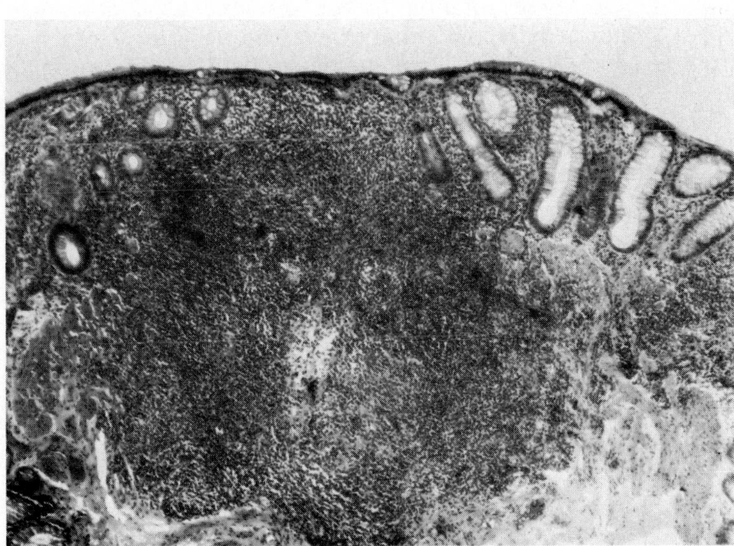

Figure 54–22. Large lymph follicle of lamina propria of normal human rectum. ×75.

VASCULATURE OF THE SMALL INTESTINE, COLON, AND RECTUM

The arterial blood supply and venous drainage of the small intestine, colon, and rectum are described in detail on pages 1903 to 1932.

INNERVATION OF THE SMALL INTESTINE, COLON, AND RECTUM

The innervation of the small intestine, colon, and rectum, both efferent and afferent, is described in detail on pages 21 to 52.

CELL RENEWAL IN THE SMALL AND LARGE INTESTINE

Cell proliferation in the epithelium of the intestine is confined to the intestinal crypts; mitoses are not normally seen on the villi or on the colonic absorptive surface. Within the crypts, the undifferentiated cells divide most actively, although young goblet cells are also capable of proliferating. As new cells are formed within the crypts, cells migrate up the wall of the crypts and onto the base of the villi in the small intestine and onto the flat absorptive surface in the colon. In the upper crypt of the small intestine, the cells begin to differentiate into absorptive cells; they lose their capacity for proliferation and secretion but begin to develop the specialized features that characterize absorptive cells. Differentiation continues as the cells migrate up the villus until they reach its upper third, where their absorptive capacity reaches its peak and they are fully differentiated cells. When the absorptive cells reach the extreme villous tip, they degenerate, lose their absorptive capacity, and eventually slough off onto the intestinal lumen.[18, 19] In the large intestine, substantial differentiation occurs in the upper half of the crypts as well as on the absorptive surface; mitoses are normally confined to the lower half of the crypts, whereas senescent cells exfoliate into the lumen from the flat absorptive surface between crypts.

In human beings, the entire process of cell migration and maturation from cell birth in the crypts to cell loss from the villous tips or colonic absorptive surface normally takes place in only five to seven days in the duodenum and jejunum, four to five days in the ileum, and four to six days in the large intestine.[18, 19] Thus, the epithelium lining the absorptive surface of the small and large intestine is normally replaced completely every four to seven days. The rapid cell renewal of this epithelium may at times protect its integrity and, under other circumstances, increase its vulnerability to noxious substances. A continuous intestinal epithelial lining could not be maintained in patients with celiac sprue were it not for its rapid renewal rate. In this disease, absorptive cells are being damaged by gluten and are rapidly sloughed into the gut lumen[43, 44] (see p. 1136). Moreover, the rapid repair and healing seen in the small intestine of celiac sprue patients after removal of gluten from the diet is a reflection of the tremendous regenerative potential of the intestinal epithelium. More rapid than normal epithelial cell proliferation has been demonstrated in the rectum in acute ulcerative colitis[45] and probably occurs in most infectious colitides. On the other hand, because of its great proliferative activity, the intestinal epithelium is particularly susceptible to damage by mitotic inhibitors that interfere with normal cell proliferation. Thus significant damage to the intestinal and rectal epithelium may be seen in patients receiving abdominal irradiation or cancer chemotherapeutic agents that inhibit cell renewal.[46]

In any case, the dynamic nature of this epithelium with its constant and rapid renewal rate must always be considered when one interprets its morphology in normal or pathologic conditions.

EMBRYOLOGY OF THE SMALL INTESTINE AND COLON

The human intestinal tract can be recognized at four weeks of embryonic development as a simple tube stretching from the stomach to the cloaca, joined ventrally to the yolk stalk, and evenly divided into cephalic and caudal limbs supported by a dorsal mesentery. Beginning in the fifth week, the tube elongates, forming a hairpin-shaped primary intestinal loop, extending ventrally into the belly stalk and joined at its apex to the yolk sac by the vitelline or omphalomesenteric duct. The cephalic limb develops into the distal duodenum to proximal ileum; the caudal limb becomes the distal ileum to proximal two thirds of the transverse colon. The embryonic junction of the cephalic and caudal limbs in the adult can be recognized only if a portion of the vitelline duct persists as a Meckel's diverticulum. Further elongation of the primary loop results in temporary umbilical herniation and counterclockwise rotation of the intestine around an axis formed by the superior mesenteric artery, which is located in the dorsal mesentery between the two limbs of the loop.

Although rotation is a continuous process, it is convenient to divide it into three stages (Fig. 54–23). The first, from the fifth to tenth week of embryonic life, includes umbilical herniation, 90-degree counterclockwise rotation, and return of the intestine to the abdominal cavity. The proximal jejunum is the first to re-enter the abdomen, and it comes to lie on the left side. Subsequent returning loops settle more and more to the right. The cecal swelling is the last part of the gut to re-enter the abdominal cavity, temporarily located in the right upper quadrant, directly below the right lobe of the liver. During the second stage, between 10 and 12 weeks, the cephalic and caudal loops rotate an additional 180 degrees as the gut re-enters the abdomen, completing a full 270 degrees with respect to the starting point. The third stage, from the twelfth week to the fifth month, includes further de-

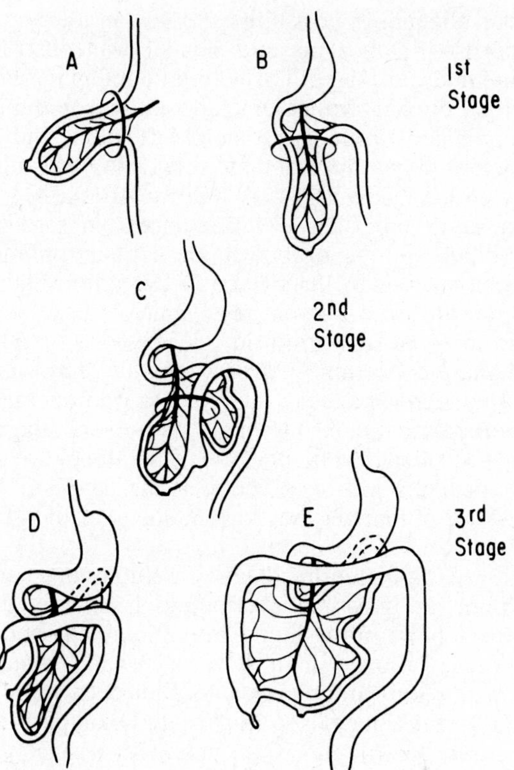

Figure 54–23. Rotation of the intestine. *A*, At 6 weeks gestational age, the superior mesenteric artery is the central axis around which the duodenojejunal loop rotates 270 degrees counterclockwise. *B*, Eight weeks gestational age, incomplete rotation. *C*, Nine weeks gestational age, incomplete rotation. *D*, Eleven weeks gestational age. *E*, Twelve weeks gestational age. (From Filston, H. C., and Kirk, D. R. J. Pediatr. Surg. *16*:614, 1981. Adapted from Snyder, W. H., Jr., and Chaffin, L. Ann. Surg. *140*:368, 1954. Used by permission.)

scent of the cecum to its normal position at the level of the iliac crest and fixation to the posterior abdominal wall of the cecum, the ascending and descending colon, and the entire mesentery of the small intestine from the ligament of Treitz to the ileocecal junction.

Histogenesis. The human digestive tract is formed from an entodermal tube, producing the epithelial cells and glands, and an encasing layer of mesoderm that ultimately forms connective tissue, muscle, and peritoneum. Circular muscle appears by the seventh week, longitudinal by the twelfth. Simple columnar epithelium first lines the entire gastrointestinal tract. Between the sixth and seventh weeks, the epithelial lining of the duodenum proliferates, forming a stratified epithelium that may occlude the lumen. Formation of coalescing vacuoles eventually restores the patency of the lumen. This process may occur to a greater or lesser extent in the entire small and large intestine. Villi begin to develop during the ninth to tenth week in the duodenum. Villus formation proceeds in a cranial-caudal fashion, and by the twelfth week the entire small intestine and colon are lined by villi. Differentiated crypt cells such as enteroendocrine, goblet, and Paneth cells appear between the ninth and twentieth weeks of gestation.[47] In the duodenum, Brunner's glands appear by the fifteenth week. During the third month, outgrowths of epithelium at the base of the villi form the intestinal glands of Lieberkühn. This dynamic developmental process continues in the small intestine, with glands and villi increasing in number throughout childhood. In the large intestine, the villi found during early gestation gradually begin to disappear toward the end of the second trimester; by term, flat mucosa with well-developed deep crypts of Lieberkühn comparable to that of the adult is seen. Teniae and haustra appear late in the first trimester.

Sucrase activity has been found in the human fetus as early as eight weeks. By the tenth to the eleventh week, sucrase, maltase, and isomaltase activity are already at the level found in mature intestine.[48] Lactase activity is low before 24 weeks of gestation, when it begins to increase, rising, at term, to two to four times the values found in normal infants 2 to 11 weeks of age.[48] Activity of disaccharidases is generally greatest in the proximal jejunum and decreases toward the distal ileum. Peptidases are also present early in gestation in the mucosa of the small intestine, and levels of the dipeptidases remain constant between the eleventh and the twenty-third week, with the exception of leucine aminopeptidase, which rises with increasing gestational age.

Spontaneous rhythmic activity of the small and large intestine is seen by the ninth week of gestation when nervous elements in Auerbach's plexus are first found. Peristaltic movements of the small intestine develop at approximately the fourth to fifth months, and the fetus begins to swallow amniotic fluid at this time. Beginning with the fourth month, an increasing amount of material accumulates in the intestine. This material, meconium, consists of a mixture of desquamated epithelial cells, lanugo hairs, and sebaceous secretion. The intestinal contents are sterile until postpartum oral feeding begins, at which time a bacterial flora first forms.

DEVELOPMENTAL ABNORMALITIES OF THE SMALL INTESTINE

The major developmental anomalies of the small intestine include: (1) atresia and stenosis; (2) duplication; (3) persistence of vestigial structures; (4) errors of rotation and defective fixation; and (5) defective innervation. Symptomatic disorders resulting from congenital anomalies of the intestine frequently appear during infancy and childhood, although the presence of a congenital defect may be discovered for the first time in the adult.

Jejunoileal Atresia and Stenosis

Duodenal obstructions have been considered in an earlier chapter (see p. 666), and only jejunoileal lesions will be considered in this section. *Jejunoileal atresia* refers to a congenitally acquired complete obstruction of the lumen of the intestine; stenosis is defined as a partial intestinal obstruction. In the small intestine, 40 per cent of atresias occur in the duodenum, 35 per cent in the ileum and 25 per cent in the jejunum. The distribution for small intestinal stenoses is somewhat different in that 75 per cent occur in the duodenum and only 20 per cent and 5 per cent occur in the ileum and jejunum, respectively. Atresias are the most common of the obstructive anomalies, responsible for 95 per cent of all the occlusions. Thus, in obstruction of the jejunum and ileum a stenosis is identified as the cause in only 5 per cent of affected children.

The reported incidence of jejunoileal atresia in the United States ranges from 1 in 330 to 1 in 1500 live births. The ratio of boys to girls appears to be equal. In contrast to duodenal atresia or stenosis, in which approximately one third of the children have Down's syndrome, the incidence of trisomy 21 in infants with jejunoileal obstruction is low. However, a significant number will be low-birth-weight infants.

Two mechanisms of pathogenesis have been proposed: a primary developmental defect caused by persistence or failure of resolution of the epithelial proliferative phase during the fifth through eighth weeks of development, or an acquired defect caused later by vascular insufficiency.[49] Arrest in growth at the solid stage may result in atresia of the duodenum, but there is considerable evidence that this is not the cause of atresia in the jejunum and ileum. Observations at surgery and autopsy reveal evidence of vascular insufficiency at the atretic or stenotic segment of bowel. Experimentally, *in utero* ligation of mesenteric vessels in unborn puppies and lambs leads to intestinal atresia, whereas incomplete vascular occlusion leads to stenosis.[50] Because the bowel distal to the site of atresia frequently contains bile (secreted after the eleventh week), squamous cells (shed by the fetal skin and swallowed during the third month), and lanugo (present after the sixth month), jejunoileal atresia must occur relatively late in the course of fetal development. Whether the association of intrauterine volvulus or intussusception with atretic lesions is causative remains unknown.[51] Additionally, there are isolated case reports associating jejunal atresia with maternal Cafergot use during pregnancy,[52] congenital rubella,[53] and genetic factors.[54]

The most common clinical manifestations of jejunoileal atresia are polyhydramnios, bilious emesis, abdominal distention, failure to pass meconium, and jaundice. Jaundice (primarily elevated indirect bilirubin) and polyhydramnios are more common in an atresia involving the proximal jejunum than in a more distal obstruction. Bilious vomiting occurs in over 80 per cent of children with any small bowel obstruction, but abdominal distention is more severe and generalized with a more distal obstruction. The passage of meconium does not eliminate the possibility of an atresia; approximately one third of children with atresia will expel meconium presumably formed prior to development of the obstruction. Atresias may be single or multiple.

Other diagnostic possibilities to be considered in the newborn with distal or mid small bowel obstruction include malrotation with or without a midgut volvulus, intestinal duplication, colonic atresia, meconium ileus, adynamic ileus from sepsis, small left colon syndrome, meconium plug syndrome, and total colonic aganglionosis (see pp. 1389–1402). A bubbly, ground-glass appearance in the right lower quadrant in association with dilated loops of bowel on a plain radiograph suggests meconium ileus (Fig. 54–24) and a diagnosis of *cystic fibrosis.* A sweat test, which is usually diagnostic, may be inaccurate in the newborn because of inadequate collection of sweat. For this reason and to avoid unnecessary delay, a hyperosmotic enema may be therapeutic and also strongly support the diagnosis. A sweat test should be performed on all children with jejunoileal obstructions; if possible the sample of sweat should be obtained when the infant is stable (see p. 1790).

Prior to implementing diagnostic studies in a neonate in whom an intestinal obstruction is suspected, the infant's temperature should be maintained, and orogastric aspiration with a 10 French tube should be initiated. Fluids and electrolytes should be monitored carefully when diagnostic studies are being performed. If organic obstruction is documented, surgical intervention is mandatory immediately following the decompression of the proximal gastrointestinal tract and the restoration of fluid and electrolyte balance.

The diagnosis of jejunoileal atresia must be suspected clinically and supported radiologically by recumbent and upright abdominal films. Proximal atresias will demonstrate only few air-fluid levels and a lack of intestinal gas beyond the point of putative

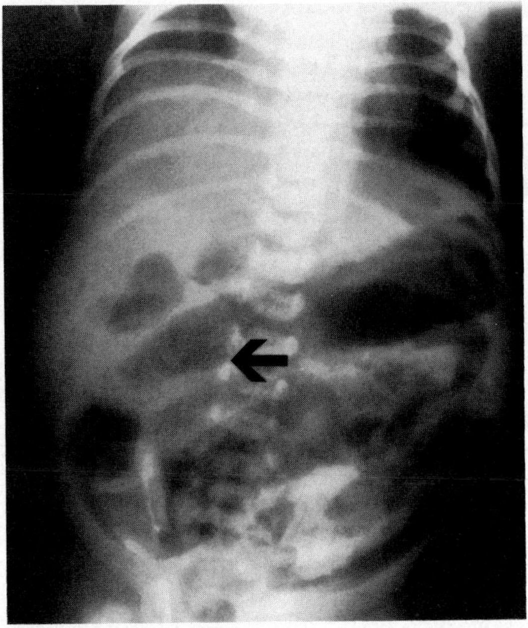

Figure 54–24. Plain radiograph of an infant with meconium ileus. Small bubbles of air are mixed with the meconium to produce a "soap bubble" appearance in the right side of the abdomen *(arrow)*. The small bowel is dilated proximally.

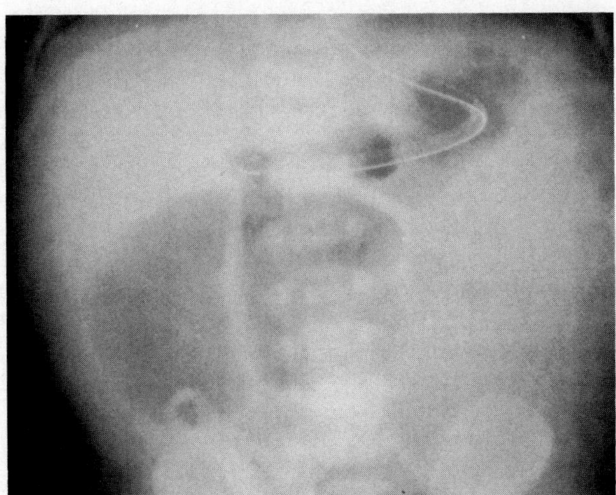

Figure 54–25. Jejunal atresia in an infant with bilious emesis. Marked dilatation of the proximal intestine is evident without gas distally.

obstruction (Fig. 54–25). The more distal the obstruction, the more distended loops of small bowel and air-fluid levels become evident. Peritoneal calcification is an unusual finding, but when present denotes an intrauterine bowel perforation with resultant meconium peritonitis. Because haustral markings are frequently not visible on a plain abdominal radiograph in the newborn, precise localization of the obstruction is not possible. For this reason, a barium enema should be performed in all children with suspected intestinal obstruction. Individuals experienced in performing barium enemas in neonates should be consulted as the procedure is not without risk.[55] The presence of a microcolon suggests that the colon has not had intestinal contents passing through it during gestation (Fig. 54–26). Most infants with a low jejunoileal atresia will

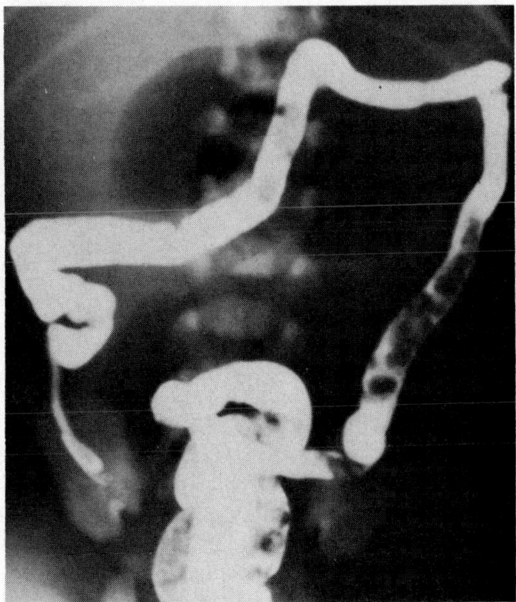

Figure 54–26. Microcolon in a newborn with distal small bowel obstruction because of ileal atresia. (Courtesy of C. A. Gooding, M.D.)

have a microcolon. The barium enema will determine if the obstruction is in the small or large bowel and if the cecum is in the correct position. Although malrotations are associated with jejunoileal atresia in approximately 10 per cent of patients, the position of the cecum is not the most reliable criterion with which to establish this diagnosis. Determining the position of the ligament of Treitz is the only way to establish with certainty whether or not a malrotation coexists.

The dilated, often atonic small intestine proximal to the atresia may fail to function following primary anastomosis. Postoperative obstruction results when insufficient intestine proximal to the atresia is resected. An end-to-end small bowel anastomosis is preferred, because of the possible development of the blind loop syndrome following side-to-side anastomoses. In jejunal atresia adequate resection of the dilated proximal bowel may not be possible or may result in unacceptable loss of absorptive surface. In these situations, a tapering jejunoplasty with end-to-end jejunojejunostomy permits conservation of bowel while promoting effective peristalsis.

Thirty-five years ago, the mortality rate in infants with intestinal atresia was over 90 per cent. The most common cause of death resulted from infection, which was related to nutritional compromise, pneumonia, peritonitis, or generalized sepsis. Prognosis was poorest when the atresia was proximal, multiple, or associated with other congenital anomalies. Recent improvements in the nutritional and pulmonary care of neonates has resulted in an improved survival. In a more recent series extending from 1965 to 1978, overall mortality had decreased to 22 per cent.[56] In those infants who survive, long-term follow-up of growth and development is essential. Malabsorption, poor motility with stasis, and bacterial overgrowth may persist for many years following initial correction (see pp. 263–282 and 1289–1297). However, most children who survive with this disorder grow normally and are without chronic gastrointestinal problems.

Duplications

An *intestinal duplication* is a spherical or tubular cyst intimately attached to a portion of the gastrointestinal tract. The term has been used to describe a wide range of rare lesions, but such cysts are only infrequently true intestinal duplications and might more properly be termed enterogenous cysts. In contrast to Meckel's diverticula, intestinal duplications are located on the mesenteric side of the gut, usually between the leaves of the mesentery. The pathogenesis remains unknown. For classification as a true duplication, there must be intimate adherence of the cystic structure to the gut, a smooth wall, and a gastrointestinal type mucosal lining. The duplication may or may not communicate with the intestinal lumen. Most duplications are seen in the ileum (Fig. 54–27), although they may occasionally be found in the jejunum.[57]

There are three basic types of duplications: large single, long tubular, and smaller intramural cysts. The

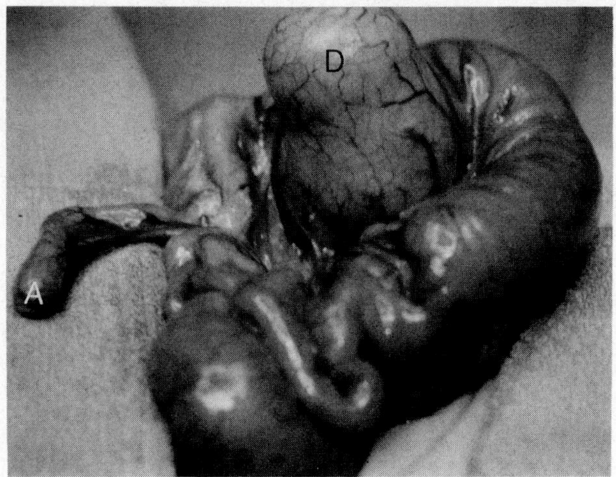

Figure 54–27. Spherical, cystic type of ileal duplication (D). The appendix (A) is on the towel.

large single cyst may cause obstructive symptoms because of compression of the attached bowel, or it may present as a visible or palpable mass on examination. Although the large spherical cysts generally do not communicate with the bowel, the *long tubular duplications* commonly do. Communicating duplications are generally lined by gastric mucosa, whereas spherical cysts are often lined by intestinal mucosa. If the duplication contains ectopic gastric mucosa, peptic ulceration of the adjacent bowel or of the duplication itself may occur and result in gastrointestinal hemorrhage and/or perforation. The *smaller intramural cysts* are most common at or near the ileocecal valve and may cause intestinal obstruction by compression of the ileum at the entrance to the cecum or, more commonly, by causing intussusception (see p. 371). Therefore, intestinal duplications primarily present with symptoms of obstruction, but may cause gastrointestinal hemorrhage or perforation. Mild manifestations in childhood may delay diagnosis until adulthood. Duplication should be considered in the patient who presents with the combination of hematochezia and obstruction. Many duplications can be identified with ultrasound[58] (Fig. 54–28). Because a significant number of duplications contain gastric mucosa, a technetium scan also may identify the anomaly.[59]

Surgical resection is the treatment of choice for these lesions. In adults, malignancies have been reported to arise in the mucosa lining the duplication. Large enterogenous cysts may be readily removed at surgery, but the long tubular duplications may require resection of both the duplication and the adjacent segment of the main channel, because frequently blood supply and muscle layers are intimately shared.

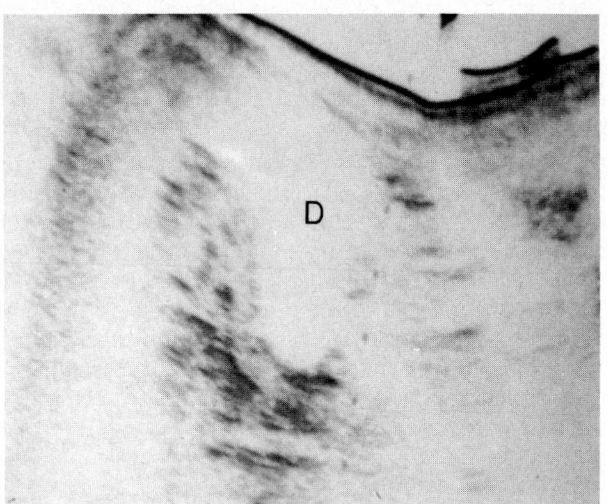

Figure 54–28. Ultrasonographic appearance of a cystic type (D) of ileal duplication. (Courtesy of Dr. Rita Teele.)

Meckel's Diverticulum

Although Fredericus Ruysch described an ileal diverticulum in 1757, this anomaly is known as *Meckel's diverticulum* following Johann Friedrich Meckel the Younger's report in 1809. Meckel's diverticulum is the most frequent congenital anomaly of the intestinal tract, having an incidence of 0.3 to 3.0 per cent in autopsy reports; it most commonly remains asymptomatic throughout life.[60] Of the patients presenting with complications, 60 per cent are under two years of age and more than one third are less than one year of age. At birth the vitelline duct normally is completely obliterated, the closure proceeding from the umbilicus inward. With incomplete obliteration, the intestinal end of the duct persists as a sac. Occasionally, the blind end is joined to the umbilicus by a fibrous band, and rarely the vitelline duct persists intact, maintaining a patent communication between ileum and the umbilicus from which intestinal contents may escape. The diverticulum arises from the antimesenteric border of the ileum, usually within 100 cm of the ileocecal valve (the average being between 80 and 85 cm), is approximately 5 cm in length, and ends blindly. It contains all the layers of the intestinal tract. The mouth of the sac is wide, often being equal to the width of the intestinal lumen itself. About 45 per cent of resected diverticula contain only normal ileal mucosa. Gastric mucosa is present in 80 to 85 per cent of the other 55 per cent, but duodenal, colonic, pancreatic, and endometrial ectopic mucosae have occasionally been described adjacent to the mouth of the diverticulum. Blood is supplied through a terminal branch of the superior mesenteric artery, which is carried to the diverticulum by a separate mesentery.

Complications of Meckel's diverticulum include hemorrhage, intestinal obstruction, diverticulitis, umbilical discharge, intussusception, and perforation with peritonitis. Rarely, the diverticulum may become incarcerated in an indirect inguinal (Littre's) hernia. Prolapse of a short segment of ileum through a patent vitelline duct may produce a complicated form of intussusception. Rarely, foreign bodies may be impacted in Meckel's diverticulum, or a neoplasm may develop within the wall.

Bleeding is the most common complication, resulting from ulceration of ileal mucosa adjacent to ectopic

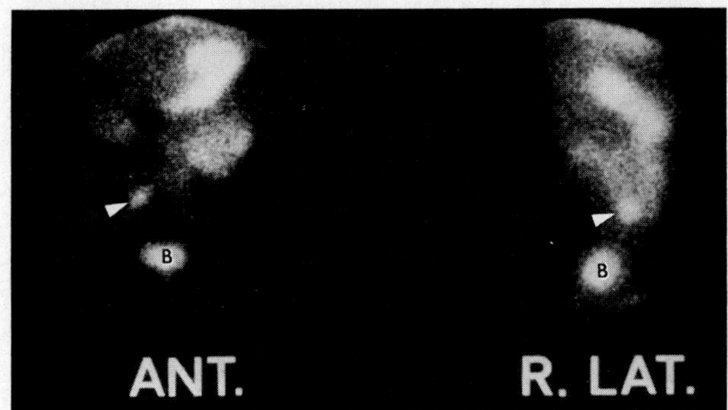

Figure 54–29. Technetium-99m scan of Meckel's diverticulum demonstrating ectopic uptake *(arrowheads)* in an area superior to the bladder (B) in the anterior projection and in the right lateral projection.

gastric mucosa; it is often painless and is usually encountered in children less than two years of age. Tarry stools suggest a small amount of bleeding with a slow transit time, but more commonly, the blood is dark red in color, and may become more like "currant jelly" as the hemorrhage persists. Meckel's diverticulum accounts for nearly half of all significant lower gastrointestinal bleeding in children. Only infrequently can a diagnosis be made in children by X-ray study; however, enteroclysis in adults has been shown to be of diagnostic benefit.[61] Gas filling the pouch or a large opaque stone may occasionally be recognized on plain film of the abdomen. Less commonly, barium may fill the diverticulum. If a Meckel's diverticulum is suspected, the technetium-99m scan must be done prior to any barium studies. Abdominal scanning after administration of radioactive technetium, which is concentrated by parietal cell–containing gastric mucosa, is the diagnostic study of choice (Fig. 54–29), but both false-negative and false-positive results have been reported. The use of pentagastrin to stimulate technetium-99m uptake in the diverticulum may decrease the number of false negative studies[62] (see pp. 412–413).

The principal mechanisms causing *intestinal obstruction* are intussusception, with the diverticulum as lead point, and herniation through, or volvulus around, a persistent fibrous cord remnant of the vitelline duct, which may extend to the abdominal wall, base of mesentery, or an adjacent segment of bowel. Early surgical intervention is mandatory for survival (see pp. 369–381).

Diverticulitis may produce a clinical picture indistinguishable from acute appendicitis. Failure to find an inflamed appendix necessitates making a search for a Meckel's diverticulum. *Perforation* may occur, associated with thrombosis of the blood supply to the diverticulum. In addition, the peptic ulceration may cause postprandial abdominal pain. Rarely, it may result in obstruction. Drainage from the umbilicus should alert the clinician that, in addition, the patient may have a persistent vitelline duct remnant.

Although it was taught for many years that local excision of a Meckel's diverticulum was indicated even when the anomaly was found incidentally, this concept has now been challenged. The morbidity from such incidental removal of asymptomatic diverticula may well exceed the risk of complications if they are left alone.[60]

Anomalies of Rotation and Fixation

Aberrations of intestinal rotation and fixation result in anomalous positioning of the small intestine and colon, predisposing to internal herniation and volvulus. These anomalies can be classified according to the stage of development in which they occur. By the third week of gestation, the intestine of the fetus can be divided into three regions—foregut, midgut, and hindgut. At the fifth week, the intestine has grown so rapidly that it cannot be contained within the abdominal cavity and extrudes into the base of the umbilical cord. Rotational movements occur in the next six weeks which permit the intestine to return to the abdominal cavity by the eleventh week (see p. 1010 and Fig. 54–23). Between weeks 12 and 20, the cecum takes its place in the right lower quadrant, signifying completion of the rotation of the colon. Fixation of the cecum, the ascending colon and the descending colon to the posterior abdominal wall begins at this time and continues even after birth. Therefore, anomalies of rotation can be classified in a broad sense into three main categories—failure to return to the abdominal cavity, aberrant rotational movements (malpositions), and failures of fixation. Omphalocele and gastroschisis represent failure of the intestine to return to the abdominal cavity; malposition of the ligament of Treitz and/or the colon results in a variety of clinical entities depending upon when in the complex series of rotations the aberrant twist occurred; failure of fixation results in free mobility of the duodenum, the distal ileum, and/or the cecum.

An *omphalocele* is the persistent herniation of abdominal viscera into a sac lined by peritoneum and amniotic membrane through a defect in the umbilical and supraumbilical portions of the abdominal wall (Fig. 54–30*A*). If the defect is less than 4 cm it is called a hernia of the umbilical cord. Because the bowel is protected in the sac, the intestinal wall is usually not thickened from intrauterine exposure to amniotic fluid. In contrast, *gastroschisis* is caused by an extraumbilical abdominal wall defect, usually to the right of the umbilicus, in which the viscera are not enclosed in a membranous sac (Fig. 54–30*B*). Presumably, the chronic exposure to amniotic fluid results in a serositis and a markedly thickened intestinal wall.

Malformations associated with omphalocele and gastroschisis include vesicointestinal fistula, imperforate anus, colonic agenesis, bladder exstrophy, and defects in the sternum, diaphragm, pericardium, and heart. These are more frequent in patients with omphalocele than in infants with either gastroschisis or hernia of the umbilical cord. As many as 25 per cent of infants with omphalocele have cardiovascular malformations, with tetralogy of Fallot being the most common.

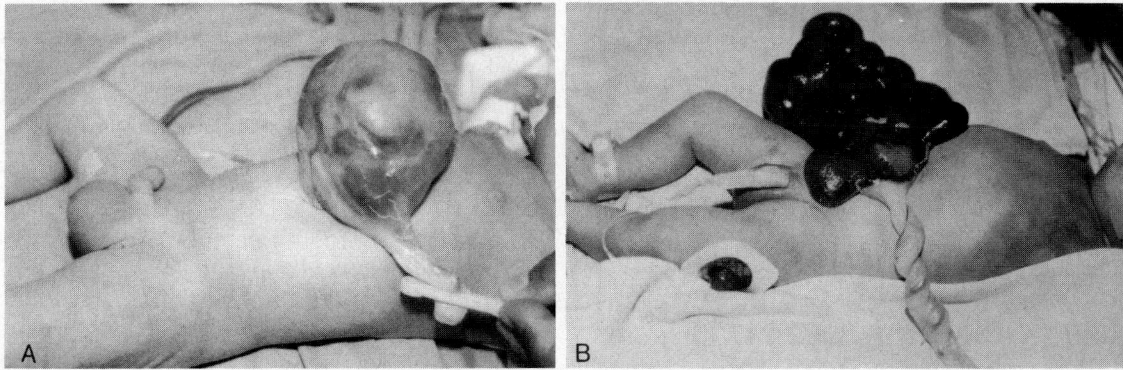

Figure 54–30. *A,* Infant with an omphalocele. Note how abdominal contents are enclosed in a sac-like structure that is related to the umbilical cord. *B,* Infant with a gastroschisis. Note the thickened abdominal viscera and the position of the umbilical cord. Courtesy of Robert Shamberger.

Surgical repair of these abdominal wall defects is complex and requires expert surgical technique. Concomitant careful nutritional and metabolic management are crucial. If the contents of the abdomen cannot be returned, staged closure using prosthetic materials is performed allowing the infant and the abdominal cavity to grow. Because of the edema and thickening of the bowel in infants with gastroschisis, normal function of the intestine returns more slowly than in infants with omphalocele. Even though these children have some degree of malrotation, late intestinal obstruction is not a major problem. Other sequelae, such as mental retardation and growth failure, seem to be related to length of hospital stay and level of prematurity.

Four types of anomalies may occur from faulty rotation during the second stage: nonrotation, malrotation, reversed rotation, and mesocolic hernia. When the midgut fails to rotate, this anomaly is referred to as *nonrotation*. The duodenum descends straight downward to the right of the superior mesenteric artery and is in direct continuity with the jejunum, which is located in the right half of the abdominal cavity. The colon lies entirely on the left, and the terminal ileum enters the cecum by crossing the midline from the right (Fig. 54–31). The patient is usually asymptomatic.

Malrotation is the most common of the anomalies in this group.[63] The midgut fails to complete the process of rotation and instead becomes arrested at some point. Therefore, the ligament of Treitz is never in its normal

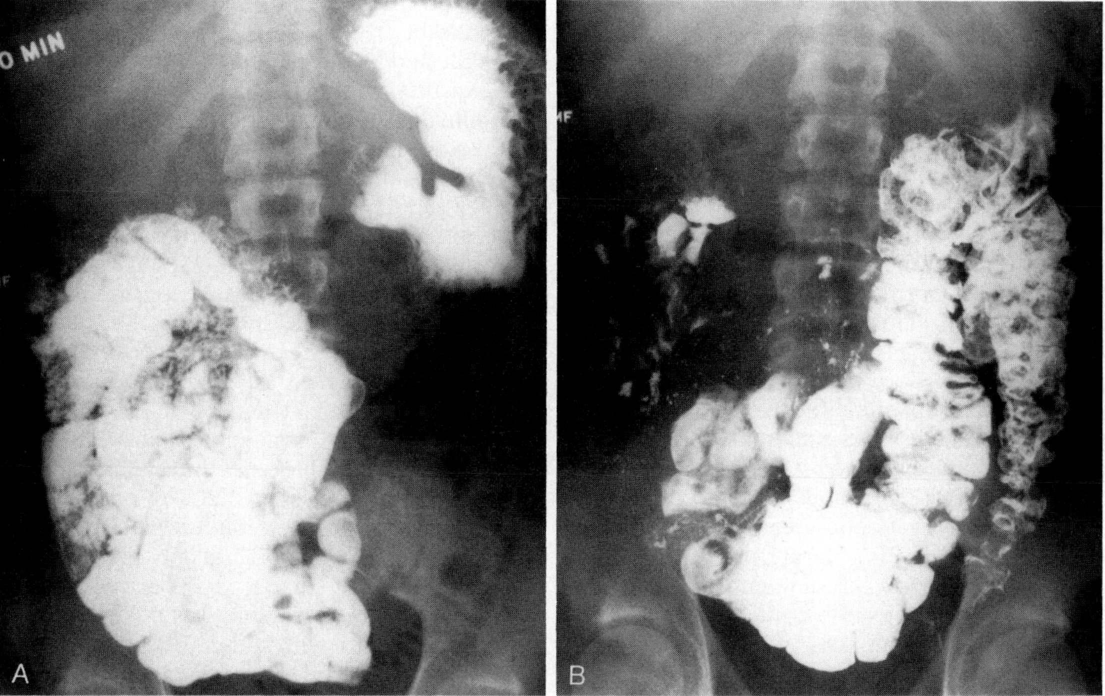

Figure 54–31. In nonrotation of the bowel, the small bowel lies to the right of the spine *(A)* and the entire colon lies to the left of the spine *(B).*

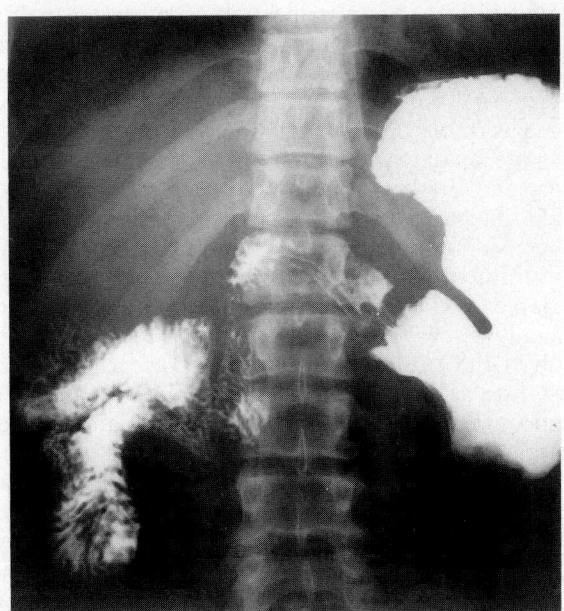

Figure 54–32. Upper gastrointestinal examination in a patient with malrotation reveals malposition of the ligament of Treitz.

position (Fig. 54–32). The cecum may be found at the splenic level, in front of the superior mesenteric vessels, or, most frequently, below the liver. Two major clinical problems are associated with malrotation—volvulus and duodenal obstruction. Because in malrotation the mesentery is narrow and not fixed to the retroperitoneum by a broad-based attachment, there is a greater propensity for the midgut to rotate on itself and cause a volvulus. Although 75 to 80 per cent of patients with malrotation will develop a midgut volvulus in the first month of life,[63] it may occur in adults without warning and, if not promptly recognized, cause substantial morbidity or mortality. Volvulus due to malrotation is not always associated with a catastrophic event, and some individuals will have subacute clinical presentations. Recurrent torsion may result in chronic abdominal pain and malabsorption related to intermittent partial obstruction of lymphatics and venules.[63] This process may cause a radiographic image of the small bowel similar to that observed in celiac disease.[64] Partial obstruction of the duodenum by peritoneal bands (Ladd's bands), may cause bilious vomiting, poor weight gain, and intermittent, crampy abdominal pain.

Reversed rotation is a rare abnormality in which the duodenum and the jejunum are anterior to the superior mesenteric vessels and the transverse colon is posterior to these vessels. This results in passage of the transverse colon through a defect in the mesentery and clinically results in obstruction of the colon. Individuals with this anomaly usually present in adulthood.

Mesocolic hernias (formerly called paraduodenal hernias) may occur on the right or the left side of the abdomen. In both conditions small intestine is trapped within the mesentery of the colon, which has failed to become properly fixed. With a right mesocolic hernia, small intestine that is in the hernial sac lies posterior to the right colon on the right side of the abdomen. The cecum is in the right upper quadrant, and Ladd's bands are present from the cecum to the duodenum. With a left mesocolic hernia, the rotation of the small intestine is normal, but the herniated portion is enclosed in a hernial sac formed from the left mesocolon. The inferior mesenteric vein demarcates the right margin of the sac. The most common clinical manifestations are colicky abdominal pain, vomiting, and occasional constipation. With incarceration, persistent obstruction necessitating urgent surgery may occur.

Conditions that are caused by failures in fixation usually involve the cecum and/or the ascending colon. However, in some patients the distal duodenum may be free. Depending upon the degree of malfixation, these individuals may be asymptomatic and not require any surgical intervention.

Surgical therapy is predicated upon the development of obstruction from volvulus, Ladd's bands, or an incarcerated hernia. Those patients who have a narrow mesentery are particularly at risk for developing volvulus. Occasionally adults may present with symptoms of chronic, partial, or intermittent obstruction. Although there is disagreement about whether or not to recommend surgery for the asymptomatic patient who has a malrotation identified coincidentally, most physicians would urge exploration to avert such a potentially life-threatening complication as volvulus. During laparotomy, bands are lysed, the volvulus (if present) is reduced, and the bowel is positioned to prevent twisting. It is not clear if adhesions play a more important role in the prevention of volvulus than does the repositioning of the bowel. In uncomplicated cases, the prognosis is excellent and recurrent problems are unusual.

Miscellaneous Abnormalities

A number of rather rare congenital abnormalities of the small intestine have been described. Isolated *heterotopic gastric mucosa* has been found in the small intestine[65] and the rectum. In the rectum it may appear as a tumorous, polypoid, nodular, or rugose mass as large as 3 to 12 cm in size.[66] Lesions have resulted in intussusception or bleeding, or, in the absence of associated symptoms, have been recognized as polyps on X-ray study.

A very rare disorder of segmental absence of intestinal musculature has been encountered in neonates presenting with intestinal obstruction caused by intussusception. Segments of ileum entirely lack muscle layers and contain only mucosa and serosa.[67] *Hirschsprung's disease* may involve the entire colon as well as distal small intestine. Plain film of the abdomen reveals small intestinal obstruction of a distal type, as in ileal atresia. However, gas may be seen in the rectum, and barium enema may reveal a small but yet "used" colon (see p. 1393).

DEVELOPMENTAL ABNORMALITIES OF THE LARGE INTESTINE

Clinically, congenital anomalies of the colon consist principally of malrotations as described earlier in this chapter, megacolon caused by aganglionosis, and a group of anorectal anomalies. Congenital aganglionosis (Hirschsprung's disease) is discussed on pages 1390 to 1395.

Incidence and Etiology

Malformations of the anus and rectum are among the most common congenital abnormalities found in infants.[68] They occur with a frequency ranging from 1:3500 to 1:9630 live births.[69] Embryologically, these anomalies result from arrests or abnormalities in the development of the fetal caudal region between the first and sixth months of intrauterine life. A family history is uncommon, and there is no racial predilection; however, a slight preponderance of affected males is reported.[70]

Classification

There is considerable confusion and lack of uniformity in the various published classifications.[71] Most are modifications of the classification of anorectal malformations described by Ladd and Gross in 1934,[72] which still provides a clear basis for understanding the lesions. The International Classification, although detailed, has gained wide acceptance.[71] Essentially, 90 per cent of cases are of the two major types, the *low* or translevator, and the *high* or supralevator (see Figs. 54–33 and 54–34 and Table 54–1). Anal agenesis and stenosis are considered *intermediate* types, whereas the rare imperforate anal membrane and cloacal exstrophy are relegated to a *miscellaneous* group. Fistula formation is mainly associated with the high and low lesions and involves the urethra, bladder, vagina, or perineum. Most fistulas in females communicate with the perineum or vagina, and rarely with the urinary tract. In contrast, three fourths of the fistulas in males communicate with the urinary tract. These "fistulas" actually represent ectopic openings of the distal bowel, which develop with a migration arrest of the normal orifice. The high rectal atresia is considered by some investigators to result from gestational vascular ischemia.[73]

As a rule, those infants in whom the terminal portion of the colon passes through the puborectalis muscle sling of the levator ani (translevator) demonstrate less morbidity and fewer associated anomalies and have a much better prognosis than those in whom the colonic tip ends proximally (supralevator). Abnormalities of the lumbosacral spine, such as sacral agenesis, hemi-

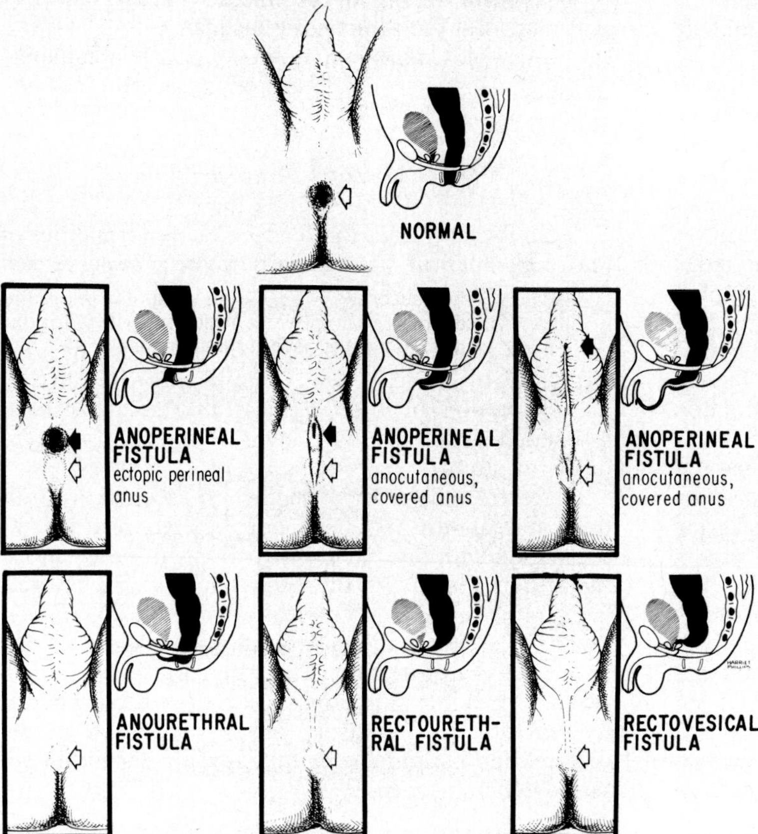

Figure 54–33. Anorectal anomalies in the male with fistula formation. Note relationship of the rectum to the puborectalis sling of the levator ani muscle. Anoperineal fistulas may be located anywhere between the perineoscrotal junction and the anal dimple. In the ectopic perineal anus, the opening resembles a normal anus. In the anocutaneous fistula or covered anus, the orifice is usually small and is anterior to a thickened median band. Anourethral fistulas are rare and open into the bulbar or membranous urethra. The common rectourethral and the rare rectovesical fistulas represent high anomalies in which the bowel has not traversed the sling. (From Santulli, T. V., Kiesewetter, W. B., and Bill, A. H., Jr. J. Pediatr. Surg. 5:281, 1970. Used by permission.)

agenesis, or errors in lumbar segmentation, occur in 50 per cent of the high lesions. Seventy per cent of the patients with vertebral abnormalities additionally demonstrate urologic anomalies, particularly hydronephrosis or a double collecting system.

At least one third of patients with any type of anorectal anomaly have developmental malformations involving areas other than the vertebral column and urinary tract.[73] The most significant of these are congenital heart disease and esophageal atresia. Less commonly one may find small and large intestinal atresias, annular pancreas, intestinal malrotation and duplication, bicornuate uterus, vaginal atresia, septate vagina, absence of the rectus abdominis muscle, Down's syndrome, anomalies of the fingers and hands, omphalocele, and exstrophy of the bladder and ileocecal area of the intestine.

Diagnosis

A careful perineal inspection of the infant with problems of micturition or defecation or unusual external perineal structures will often reveal the anomaly. Anorectal stenoses and anal membranes have orifices in normal locations and can be diagnosed by digital examination. In the supralevator anomalies, the normal orifice, although imperforate, can usually be detected as a pigmented depression (anal dimple) or elevation of thickened skin. Puckering may be noted at this site when the sphincter is stimulated to contract. Occasionally the ectopic perineal anus may be adequate for stool evacuation, and the definitive anomaly may be overlooked for many months or years.

Roentgenographic studies to outline the distal intestinal pouch are adequately achieved by cinefluoroscopy or radiocontrast studies. Adding indigo carmine as a marker will demonstrate rectourinary communications. The traditional plain film with the baby held in an upside down position is now known to be inaccurate.[74]

Treatment

Anal stenosis is easily treated with daily dilations, using bougies or a finger. The parents should subsequently be taught the procedure in order to continue treatment for a total period of three to six months. The thin, bulging anorectal membrane is easily excised or incised with subsequent dilations as in anal stenosis.

In lower lesions with fistulous formation, the orifice may be enlarged by a simple "cutback" procedure in the newborn period and continence is invariably uncompromised. A daily digital dilation program is necessary during follow-up.

In high lesions, a more extensive surgical procedure is indicated. A preliminary divided sigmoid colostomy is recommended to decompress the bowel, followed by

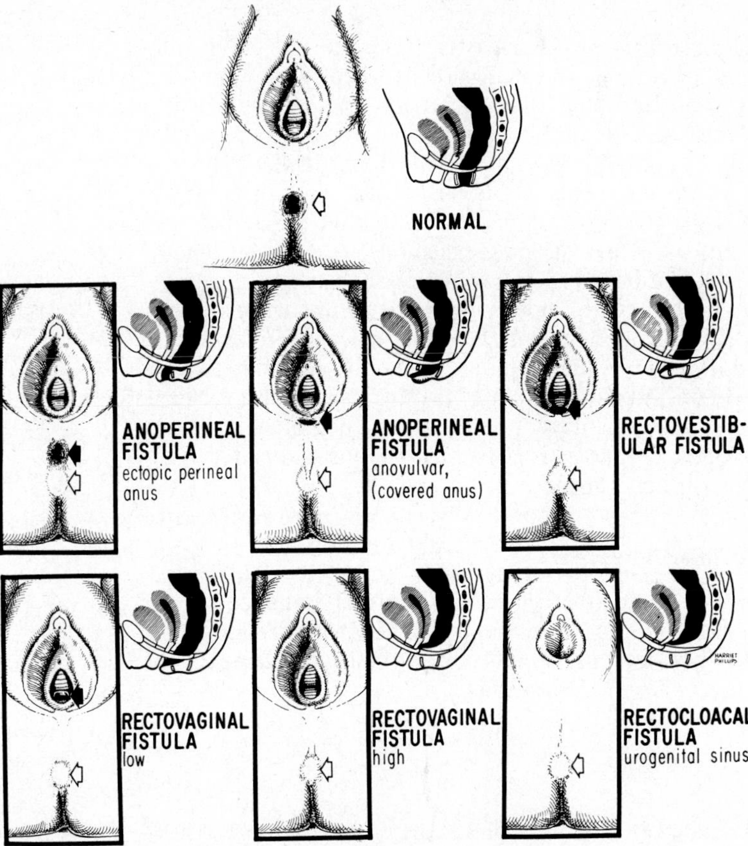

Figure 54–34. Anorectal anomalies in the female with anoperineal fistulas, which may be either an ectopic perineal anus or an anovulvar fistula, which is in the fourchette. The rectovestibular fistula lies within the vestibule of the vagina and courses cephalad, paralleling the posterior vaginal wall. The anovulvar fistula is directed posteriorly and is relatively superficial to the skin. Rectovaginal fistulas are usually low but may be located high in the posterior vaginal wall. The rectocloacal fistula occurs as a high-communication in a urogenital sinus. The bowel traverses the sling in all but the last two malformations. (From Santulli, T. V., Kiesewetter, W. B., and Bill, A. H., Jr. J. Pediatr. Surg. *5*:281, 1970. Used by permission.)

Table 54–1. ANORECTAL ANOMALIES: A SUGGESTED INTERNATIONAL CLASSIFICATION

Male	Female
A. Low (translevator)	
1. At normal anal site	1. Same
a. Anal stenosis	a. Same
b. Covered anus—complete	b. Same
2. At perineal site	2. Same
a. Anocutaneous fistula (covered anus—incomplete)	a. Same
b. Anterior perineal anus	b. Same
	3. At vulvar site
	a. Anovular fistula
	b. Anovestibular fistula
	c. Vestibular anus
B. Intermediate	
1. Anal agenesis	1. Same
a. Without fistula	a. Without fistula
b. With fistula	b. With fistula
Rectobular	(1) Rectovestibular
	(2) Rectovaginal—low
2. Anorectal stenosis	2. Same
C. High (supralevator)	
1. Anorectal agenesis	1. Same
a. Without fistula	a. Without fistula
b. With fistula	b. With fistula
(1) Rectourethral	(1) Rectovaginal—high
(2) Rectovesical	(2) Rectocloacal
	(3) Rectovesical
2. Rectal atresia	2. Same
D. Miscellaneous	
Imperforate and membrane	
Cloacal exstrophy	
Others	

From Santulli, T. V., Kiesewetter, W. B., and Bill, A. H., Jr.: J. Pediatr. Surg. 5:281, 1970. Used by permission.

an appropriate reconstructive operation at about one year of age. In selected cases, the colostomy may be avoided and dilation or cutback of the fistula may suffice as a temporizing measure. For the rectal atresias, a preliminary sigmoid colostomy in the newborn is performed. This is followed at one year of age by a pull-through procedure similar to that utilized in patients with aganglionic megacolon.

All patients are followed closely for many years, because they are more vulnerable to impactions, strictures, rectal dysfunction, and anal incontinence. In addition, a cystic fistulous tract, missed at first, may be detected at a later date. In general, the best surgical results are achieved with lower anomalies and the poorest prognosis is with high lesions associated with severe sacral agenesis.

Acknowledgment

We would like to thank Robert Shamberger, M.D. of the Department of Surgery, The Children's Hospital, Boston, for his review of the surgical aspects of congenital malformations.

References

1. Bloom, W., and Fawcett, D. W. Intestines. *In* A Textbook of Histology. 10th ed. Philadelphia, W. B. Saunders Co., 1975, pp. 658–687.
2. Madara, J. L., and Trier, J. S. Functional morphology of the mucosa of the small intestine. *In* Johnson, L. R. (ed.). Physiology of the Gastrointestinal Tract. 2nd ed. New York, Raven Press, 1987, pp. 1209–1249.
3. Trier, J. S. Structure of the mucosa of the small intestine as it relates to intestinal function. Fed. Proc. *26*:1391, 1967.
4. Clemente, C. D. The digestive system. *In* Clemente, C. D. (ed.). Gray's Anatomy of the Human Body. Philadelphia, Lea & Febiger, 1985, pp. 1402–1514.
5. Basmajian, J. V. Abdominopelvic cavity. *In* Grant's Method of Anatomy. Baltimore, Williams & Wilkins, 1975, pp. 190–211.
6. Perera, D. R., Weinstein, W. M., and Rubin, C. E. Small intestinal biopsy. Hum. Pathol. *6*:157, 1975.
7. Baker, S. J., Ignatius, M., Mathan, V. I., Vaish, S. K., and Chacko, C. C. Intestinal biopsy in tropical sprue. *In* Wolstenholme, G. E. W., Cameron, M. P. (eds.). Intestinal Biopsy. Boston, Little, Brown & Co., 1962, pp. 84–101.
8. Sprinz, H., Sribhibhadh, R., Gangrosa, E. J., Benyajati, C., Kundel, D., and Halstead, S. Biopsy of the small bowel of Thai people. Am. J. Clin. Pathol. *38*:43, 1962.
9. Brunser, O., Eidelman, S., and Klipstein, F. A. Intestinal morphology of rural Haitians. A comparison between overt tropical sprue and asymptomatic subjects. Gastroenterology *58*:655, 1970.
10. Crabbé, P. A., Carbonara, A. O., Heremans, J. F. The normal human intestinal mucosa as a major source of plasma cells containing gamma-A-immunoglobulin. Lab. Invest. *14*:235, 1965.
11. Elson, C. O., Kagnoff, M. F., Fiocchi, C., Befus, A. D., and Targan, S. Intestinal immunity and inflammation: recent progress. Gastroenterology *91*:746, 1986.
12. Clementi, F., Palade, G. E. Intestinal capillaries. I. Permeability to peroxidase and ferritin. J. Cell Biol. *41*:33, 1969.
13. Solicia, E., Capella, C., Buffa, R., Usellini, L., Fiocca, R., and Sessa, F. Endocrine cells of the digestive system. *In* Johnson, L. R., Christensen, J., Grossman, M. I., Jacobson, E. D., and Schultz, S. G. (eds.). Physiology of the Gastrointestinal Tract. New York, Raven Press, 1981, pp. 39–58.
14. Erlandsen, S. L., Parsons, J. A., and Taylor, T. D. Ultrastructural immunocytochemical localization of lysozyme on the Paneth cells of man. J. Histochem. Cytochem. *22*:401, 1974.
15. Rodning, C. B., Wilson, I. D., and Erlandsen, S. L. Immunoglobulins within human small intestinal Paneth cells. Lancet *1*:984, 1976.
16. Erlandsen, S. L., Chase, D. G. Paneth cell function: phagocytosis and intracellular digestion of intestinal microorganism. II. Spiral microorganism. J. Ultrastruct. Res. *41*:319, 1972.
17. Field, M. Secretion by the small intestine. *In* Johnson, L. R., Christensen, J., Grossman, M. I., Jacobson, E. D., and Schultz, S. G. (eds.). Physiology of the Gastrointestinal Tract. New York, Raven Press, 1981, pp. 983–990.
18. Lipkin, M., Sherlock, P., and Bell, B. Cell renewal in stomach, ileum, colon, and rectum. Gastroenterology *45*:721, 1963.
19. MacDonald, W. C., Trier, J. S., and Everett, N. B. Cell proliferation and migration in the stomach, duodenum, and rectum of man: radioautographic studies. Gastroenterology *46*:405, 1964.
20. Douglas, A. P., Kerley, R., and Isselbacher, K. J. Preparation and characterization of the lateral and basal plasma membranes of the rat intestinal epithelial cell. Biochem. J. *128*:1329, 1972.
21. Glickman, R. M., and Bouhours, J. F. Characterization, distribution and biosynthesis of the major ganglioside of rat intestinal mucosa. Biochim. Biophys. Acta *424*:17, 1976.
22. Ito, S. The enteric surface coat on cat intestinal microvilli. J. Cell Biol. *27*:475, 1965.
23. Alpers, D. H., and Tedesco, F. J. The possible role of pancreatic proteases in the turnover of intestinal brush border proteins. Biochim. Biophys. Acta *401*:28, 1975.
24. Crane, R. K. A digestive-absorptive surface as illustrated by the intestinal cell brush border. Trans. Am. Microsc. Soc. *94*:529, 1975.
25. Alpers, D. H., and Seetharam, B. Pathophysiology of diseases involving intestinal brush-border proteins. N. Engl. J. Med. *296*:1047, 1977.
26. Mackenzie, I. L., and Donaldson, R. M. Vitamin B_{12} absorption and the intestinal surface. Fed. Proc. *28*:41, 1969.

27. Levine, J. S., Allen, R. H., Alpers, D. H., and Seetharam, B. Immunocytochemical localization of the intrinsic factor–cobalamin receptor in dog-ileum: distribution of intracellular receptor during cell maturation. J. Cell Biol. *98*:111, 1984.
28. Hopfer, U. Isolated membrane vesicles as tools for analysis of epithelial transport. Am. J. Physiol. *233*:E445, 1977.
29. Farquhar, M. G., Palade, G. E. Junctional complexes in various epithelia. J. Cell Biol. *17*:375, 1963.
30. Claude, P., and Goodenough, D. A. Fracture faces of zonulae occludentes from "tight" and "leaky" epithelia. J. Cell Biol. *58*:390, 1973.
31. Madara, J. L., Trier, J. S., and Neutra, M. R. Structural changes in the plasma membrane accompanying differentiation of epithelial cells in human and monkey small intestine. Gastroenterology *78*:963, 1980.
32. Madara, J. L., and Trier, J. S. Structure and permeability of goblet cell tight junctions in rat small intestine. J. Membr. Biol. *66*:145, 1982.
33. Marcial, M. A., Carlson, S. L., and Madara, J. L. Partitioning of paracellular conductance along the crypt-villus axis: a hypothesis based on structural analysis with detailed consideration of tight junction structure-function relationships. J. Membr. Biol. *80*:59, 1984.
34. Hirokawa, N., Keller, T. C. S., Chasan, R., and Mooseker, M. S. Mechanism of brush border contractility studied in the quick-freeze, deep-etch method. J. Cell Biol. *96*:1325, 1983.
35. Farquhar, M. G. Progress in unraveling pathways of Golgi traffic. Ann. Rev. Cell Biol. *1*:447, 1985.
36. Owen, R. L., Jones, A. L. Epithelial cell specialization within human Peyer's patches: an ultrastructural study of intestinal lymphoid follicles. Gastroenterology *66*:189, 1974.
37. Owen, R. L. Sequential uptake of horseradish peroxidase by lymphoid follicle epithelium of Peyer's patches in the normal unobstructed mouse intestine: an ultrastructural study. Gastroenterology *72*:440, 1977.
38. Wolf, J. L., and Bye, W. A. The membranous epithelial (M) cell and the mucosal immune system. Ann. Rev. Med. *35*:95, 1984.
39. Owen, R. L., Pierce, N. F., Apple, R. T., and Cray, W. C. J. M cell transport of *Vibrio cholerae* from the intestinal lumen into Peyer's patches: a mechanism for antigen sampling and for microbial transmigration. J. Infect. Dis. *153*:1108, 1986.
40. Cohen, S., Harris, L. D., and Levitan, R. Manometric characteristics of human ileocecal juntional zone. Gastroenterology *54*:72, 1968.
41. Goldman, H., and Antonioli, D. A. Mucosal biopsy of the rectum, colon, and distal ileum. Hum. Pathol. *13*:981, 1982.
42. Azzopardi, J. G., and Evans, D. J. Mucoprotein-containing histiocytes (muciphages) in the rectum. J. Clin. Pathol. *19*:368, 1966.
43. Padykula, H. A., Strauss, E. W., Ladman, A. J., and Gardner, F. H. A morphologic and histochemical analysis of the human jejunal epithelium in non-tropical sprue. Gastroenterology *40*:735, 1961.
44. Trier, J. S., and Browning, T. H. Epithelial cell renewal in cultured duodenal biopsies in celiac sprue. N. Engl. J. Med. *283*:1245, 1970.
45. Eastwood, G. L., and Trier, J. S. Epithelial cell renewal in cultured rectal biopsies in ulcerative colitis. Gastroenterology *64*:383, 1973.
46. Trier, J. S., and Browning, T. H. Morphologic response of the mucosa of human small intestine to X-ray exposure. J. Clin. Invest. *45*:194, 1966.
47. Trier, J. S., and Moxey, P. C. Morphogenesis of the small intestine during fetal development. *In* Development of Mammalian Absorptive Processes, Ciba Foundation Series 70 (new series). New York, Excerpta Medica, 1979, pp. 3–29.
48. Grand, R. J., Watkins, J. B., and Torti, F. M. Development of the human gastrointestinal tract: a review. Gastroenterology *70*:790, 1976.
49. Nixon, H. H., and Tawes, R. Etiology and treatment of small intestinal atresia: analysis of a series of 127 jejunoileal atresias and comparison with 62 duodenal atresias. Surgery *69*:41, 1971.
50. Abrams, J. S. Experimental intestinal atresia. Surgery *64*:185, 1968.
51. Grosfeld, J. L., and Clatworthy, H. W., Jr. The nature of ileal atresia due to intrauterine intussusception. Arch. Surg. *100*:714, 1970.
52. Graham, J. M., Marin-Padilla, M., and Hoefnagel, D. Jejunal atresia associated with Cafergot ingestion during pregnancy. Clin. Pediatr. *22*:226, 1983.
53. Esterly, J. R., and Talbert, J. L. Jejunal atresia in twins with presumed congenital rubella. Lancet *1*:1028, 1969.
54. Al-Awadi, S. A., Naguib, K., Farag, T. I., and Cuschieri, A. Familial jejunal atresia with "apple-peel" variant. J. R. Soc. Med. *74*:499, 1981.
55. Wolfson, J. J., and Williams, H. A hazard of barium enema studies in infants with small bowel atresia. Radiology *95*:341, 1970.
56. Miller, R. C. Complicated intestinal atresias. Ann. Surg. *189*:606, 1979.
57. Chavez, C. M., and Timmis, H. H. Duplication cysts of the gastrointestinal tract. Am. J. Surg. *110*:960, 1965.
58. Lamont, A. C., Strainsky, R., and Cremin, B. J. Ultrasonic diagnosis of duplication cysts in children. Br. J. Radiol. *57*:463, 1984.
59. Curran, J. P., Behbahane, M., Kim, B. H., and Palamis, N. Ectopic gastric duplication cyst in an infant. Clin. Pediatr. *23*:50, 1984.
60. Soltero, M. J., and Bill, A. H. The natural history of Meckel's diverticulum and its relation to incidental removal. Am. J. Surg. *132*:168, 1976.
61. Maglinte, D. D. T., Hall, R., Miller, R. E., Chernish, S. M., Rosenak, B., Elmore, M., and Burney, B. T. Detection of surgical lesions of the small bowel by enteroclysis. Am. J. Surg. *147*:225, 1984.
62. Treves, S., Grand, R. J., Eraklis, A. J. Pentagastrin stimulation of technetium-99m uptake by ectopic gastric mucosa in a Meckel's diverticulum. Radiology *128*:711, 1978.
63. Andrassy, R. J., and Mahour, G. H. Malrotation of the midgut in infants and children: a 25-year review. Arch. Surg. *116*:158, 1981.
64. Nussbaum, A., and Kirkpatrick, J. A. Malrotation of the midgut in infants and children. Contemp. Diagn. Radiol. *6*:1, 1983.
65. Lee, S. M., Mosenthal, W. T., and Weisman, R. E. Tumorous heterotopic gastric mucosa in the small intestine. Arch. Surg. *100*:619, 1970.
66. Pistioa, M. A., Guardani, S., Ventura, T., Pistioa, F., and Carboni, M. Gastric heterotopia of the rectum. Endoscopy *18*:34, 1986.
67. Steiner, D. H., Maxwell, J. G., Rasmussen, B. L., and Jones, R. Segmental absence of intestinal musculature. An unusual cause of intestinal obstruction in the neonate. Am. J. Surg. *118*:963, 1969.
68. Walpole, I. R., and Hockey, A. Syndrome of imperforate anus, abnormalities of hands and feet, satyr ears, and sensorineural deafness. J. Pediatr. *100*:250, 1982.
69. Kiesewetter, W. B. Malformations of the rectum and anus. *In* Ravitch, M. M., Welch, K. J., Benson, C. D., Aberdeen, E., and Randolph, J. G. (eds.). Pediatric Surgery. 3rd ed. Chicago, Year Book Medical Publishers, 1979, pp. 1059–1072.
70. Weinstein, E. D. Sex-linked imperforate anus. Pediatrics *35*:715, 1965.
71. Santulli, T. V., Kiesewetter, W. B., and Bill, A. H., Jr. Anorectal anomalies: a suggested international classification. J. Pediatr. Surg. *5*:281, 1970.
72. Ladd, W. E., Gross, E. D. Congenital malformations of the anus and rectum: report of 162 cases. Am. J. Surg. *23*:167, 1934.
73. Santulli, T. V., and Blanc, W. A. Congenital malformation of the rectum and anus: 11 associated anomalies encountered in a series of 120 cases. Surg. Gynecol. Obstet. *95*:281, 1952.
74. Berdon, W. E., and Baker, D. H. The inherent errors in measurements of inverted films in patients with imperforate anus. Ann. Radiol. *10*:235, 1967.

55 Absorption and Secretion of Water and Electrolytes by Small and Large Intestine

HENRY J. BINDER

The small intestine and colon possess specialized function to regulate fluid and electrolyte movement. Although there are significant differences in the details of specific transport processes in these two organs, the absorptive and secretory processes of the small and large intestine are sufficiently similar to permit a unified discussion of their normal physiology and their alteration in various diarrheal disorders (see pp. 290–316).

In normal healthy persons, the small intestine absorbs large quantities of water and electrolytes. Although dietary intake is only 1000 to 1500 ml/day, the fluid load to the small intestine is considerably greater. Figure 55–1 shows that the fluid volume presented to the entire small intestine is approximately 7 to 9 L daily and represents the sum of salivary, gastric, biliary, and pancreatic secretions, in addition to the fluid contained in the diet. Although there is undoubtedly fluid secretion that originates in the intestine under normal conditions, present methodology precludes a reliable estimate of the volume of intestinal secretion. The small intestine is relatively efficient in that it absorbs approximately 75 to 80 per cent of this load. This estimate is based on a few studies in normal subjects in whom ileocecal flow has been measured and has been found to be approximately 1.5 to 2.0 L/day.[1] It is important to note that this estimate of ileocecal flow is considerably greater than "normal" ileostomy output.[2] The difference probably reflects adaptation (i.e., increased fluid and electrolyte absorption) by the small intestine following colectomy, probably the result of chronic salt depletion and secondary aldosteronism.[3] In addition to absorbing water, the small intestine absorbs significant quantities of sodium, chloride, and potassium while secreting bicarbonate. The maximal absorptive capacity of the small intestine is unknown but may be at least 12 L/day. The fluid absorbed by the small intestine is approximately isotonic; in contrast to the colon, the small intestine, especially the jejunum, has a limited capacity to conserve sodium (that is, to absorb sodium against a chemical concentration gradient). Luminal glucose markedly stimulates water absorption in the small intestine but not in the colon.

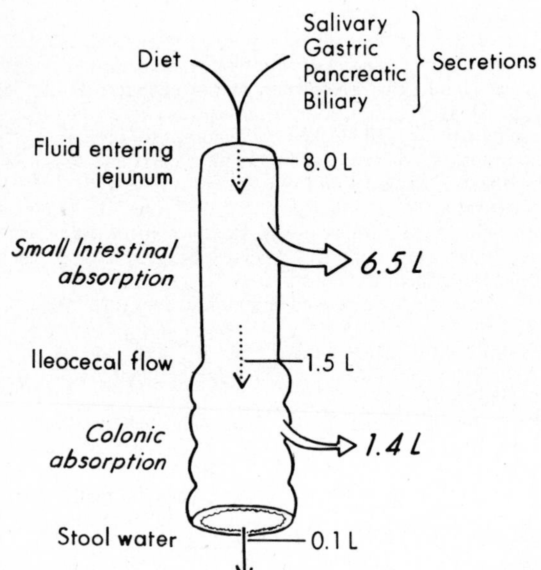

Figure 55–1. Diagram showing the approximate values for both the volume of fluid entering the small intestine and colon, and the small intestinal and colonic water absorption each day in healthy adults.

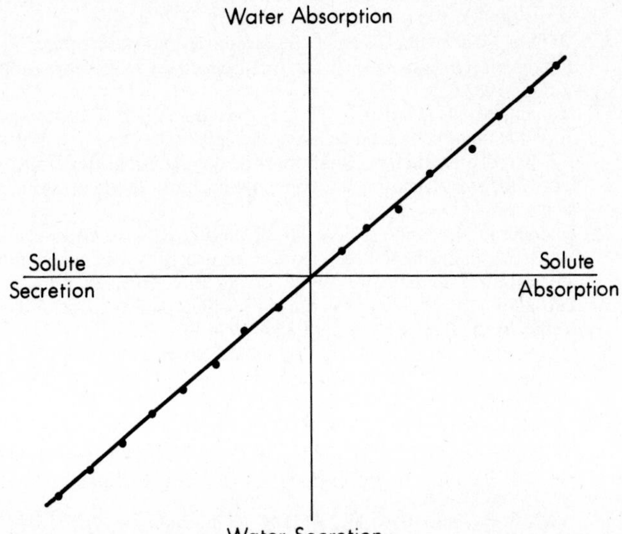

Figure 55–2. Solute and water movements are parallel. Solute movement is the driving force for water movement in the small and large intestine. The composition of the absorbed fluid in the jejunum (shown in this figure) is isotonic, but it is slightly hypertonic in more distal intestinal segments.

Compared with the small intestine, the colon absorbs a smaller quantity of fluid but does so much more efficiently.[4] Of the approximate 1500 to 2000 ml presented to the colon each day, the large intestine absorbs all but 100 to 200 ml (an efficiency of more than 90 per cent). The colon can absorb sodium even though the luminal concentration of sodium may be as low as

30 mEq/L; thus, the colon has a significant capacity to conserve sodium. Of greater importance is the maximal fluid absorptive capacity of the colon, which is approximately 5 L/day.[5] Diarrhea secondary to small intestinal disease occurs when the fluid load to the large intestine exceeds this maximal fluid absorptive capacity. Sodium and chloride are absorbed while bicarbonate and potassium are secreted by the colon.

This discussion of overall fluid absorption by the small and large intestine, as well as a subsequent one regarding the development of diarrhea, emphasizes water movement. As there is no evidence suggesting the presence of an active transport process for water, it is accepted that fluid movement (both absorption and secretion) is secondary to solute (either electrolyte or nonelectrolyte) movement (Fig. 55–2). Therefore, an understanding of fluid absorption and secretion requires knowledge of electrolyte transport and its coupling to fluid movement.

COUPLING OF WATER MOVEMENT TO SOLUTE TRANSPORT

How are solute absorption and water absorption coupled? Curran and MacIntosh proposed the so-called three compartment–double membrane hypothesis to explain it.[6] This model proposed that the intestinal (and other) epithelial cells and their surrounding structures could be represented as three separate compartments that are separated by two membranes with different permeabilities (Fig. 55–3). Although over the past two decades this model has been modified and considerable controversy has developed over how fluid and solute flow coupled, the major features of this hypothesis remain the most likely explanation of the linking of fluid absorption to solute absorption.[7] This model, initially proposed to explain the observation that water absorption does not cease during perfusion of the intestine with hyperosmolar (that is, up to approximately 340 mOsm/kg water) solutions, explains the movement of water against a concentration gradient and provides a mechanism to couple fluid absorption to solute absorption (Fig. 55–3).

This model proposes that three compartments are separated by two semipermeable membranes of different porosities. If membrane α were less permeable than membrane β, a solution in compartment B with a higher osmolarity than that in compartment A or C would provide a driving force for fluid to move from compartment A to compartment B. The resulting increase in hydrostatic pressure in compartment B would cause fluid to move from compartment B to compartment C. Figure 55–3 also presents a possible structural analogy of this model to the intestine (or any other epithelium). Sodium is extruded across the basolateral membrane (membrane α) of the epithelial cell (compartment A) into the intercellular space (compartment B). Thus, it is proposed that the cell interior and the intercellular space represent compartments A and B, respectively. The basolateral cell membrane is thought

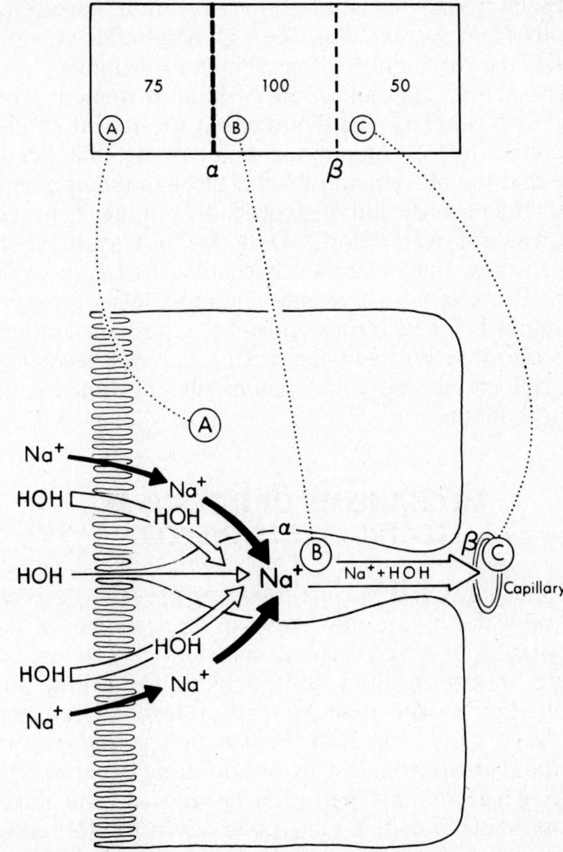

Figure 55–3. Proposed model to explain coupling of fluid absorption to solute absorption. The top panel depicts a double-membrane model that can result in fluid moving from compartment A to compartment C against an apparent concentration gradient (see text). The bottom panel provides proposed anatomic sites of the double-membrane model in epithelia. As discussed in the text, the exact route of water movement is not known but probably is predominately through the epithelial cell. According to this proposal, the basolateral membrane would function as the α membrane and the basement membrane–capillary membrane as the β membrane of the double-membrane model.

to represent the relatively tight membrane α, whereas membrane β would be the basement or capillary membrane. Confirmation of the exact location of the critical middle compartment for this model (i.e., compartment B) is lacking.

Recent studies of the hydraulic conductivity of the opposing membranes of epithelial cells have yielded relatively high estimates for this value. If these measurements are correct, very small increments in osmolarity could provide a sufficient driving force for isotonic fluid movement. Thus, it might not be technically feasible to demonstrate such a small increase in the osmolarity in compartment B even if it were possible to place micropipettes into the intercellular space. At present, there are few or no data that substantially contradict this hypothesis, and sodium extrusion across the basolateral membrane by the so-called sodium pump, with the maintenance of an increased intercellular sodium concentration, is central to most active transport processes present in the intestine. It should be noted that in the jejunum, a relatively "leaky" epithelium, a significant fraction of sodium absorption results from *solvent drag* (i.e., glucose-induced water flow is the driving force for sodium absorption).[8]

The actual anatomic route of fluid movement from lumen to capillary is unknown, but the recent studies that measure cell membrane water permeability indicate that the movement of water through the epithelial cell is the primary, although probably not the exclusive, pathway for water flow.[9] Data are not available to explain how fluid secretion is coupled to solute secretion. There is no convincing anatomic locus for compartment B for secretory processes. One speculation is that the area between the unstirred water layer and the cell membrane could potentially function as this compartment.

MECHANISMS OF INTESTINAL ELECTROLYTE TRANSPORT

Both *active* and *passive transport* processes are responsible for solute movement in all segments of the intestine, but their relative contributions to overall solute transport differ in the jejunum, ileum, and colon. During the past 20 years, intestinal transport has been studied in both human beings and experimental animals primarily by two different experimental approaches: luminal perfusion *in vivo* and ion fluxes across short-circuited mucosa *in vitro*.[10–12] In recent years membrane vesicles have also been employed to identify and characterize transport processes across isolated apical and basolateral cell membranes.[13] Unfortunately, considerable confusion has arisen when *in vivo* and *in vitro* studies of intestinal transport are compared. *In vitro* experiments in which unidirectional fluxes are determined under voltage clamp conditions measure primarily active transport processes as a result of eliminating motility, hydrostatic pressure, and blood flow, including the role of countercurrent mechanism[14] (Fig. 55–4). Furthermore, this methodologic approach minimizes those factors that promote passive processes, including the effects of water flow. In contrast, *in vivo* studies provide knowledge of the role of both active and passive processes and water flow–induced processes but may not allow precise determination of active transport events. Thus, understanding of overall intestinal fluid and electrolyte movement requires integration of the results of both *in vivo* and *in vitro* studies and the contributions of both active and passive transport processes.

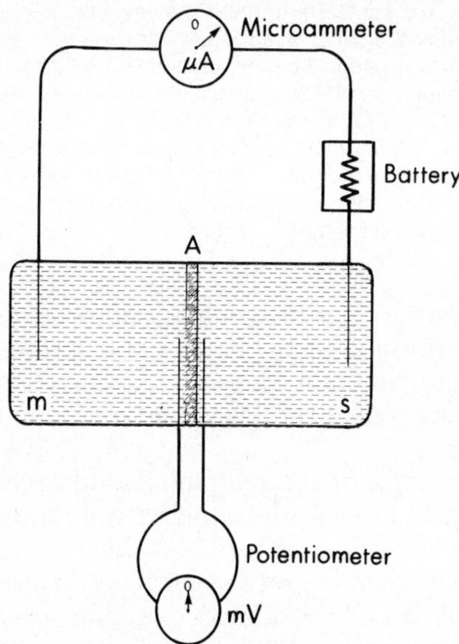

Figure 55–4. This diagram illustrates the general design of experiments in which unidirectional fluxes are determined from both mucosa to serosa solution and serosa to mucosa solution across intestinal tissue (A) under short-circuit conditions (i.e., in the absence of a spontaneous potential difference). The short-circuit current represents the current (generated by a battery) necessary to nullify the spontaneous potential difference (measured by a potentiometer) and is a measure of the total ion movement across the tissue. Under these circumstances, in which there is no electrochemical, hydrostatic, or osmotic concentration difference, the demonstration of net movement by radiolabeled isotopes provides excellent evidence of *active transport.*

Net solute movement represents the sum of several transport events. In addition to the contributions of both active and passive processes, absorptive and secretory processes are also operative simultaneously. At present, it is generally believed that active absorptive processes are located in the villous epithelial cells, whereas active secretory processes are present in crypt epithelium (see Fig. 55–16).[15] Thus, net electrolyte absorption (or secretion) represents the sum of oppositely directed active and passive transport processes.

Three different mechanisms are responsible for electrolyte movement across intestinal mucosa: *passive diffusion, convection,* and *carrier-mediated active transport.* A comprehensive presentation of membrane physiology of electrolyte transport processes is beyond the scope of this chapter and the interested reader is referred to several recent discussions.[16, 17]

Passive Diffusion. Electrolyte movement secondary to passive diffusion accounts for a considerable component of overall electrolyte absorption and reflects the relatively low resistance ("leakiness") of the intestinal epithelium (jejunum $<$ ileum $<$ colon). Leaky epithelia are characterized by low electrical resistances, low transepithelial potential differences, high water permeabilities, and an inability to absorb sodium against significant concentration gradients. Some of the characteristics of intestinal transport that are manifestations of the varying degrees of permeability in the jejunum, ileum, and colon are compared in Table 55–1. Electrolyte movement across the tight junctions (shunt pathway) is often called "paracellular" transport and always is secondary to passive driving forces. The presence of fixed negative charges in aqueous channels of the tight junction results in higher rates of cation than anion movement through the tight junction (permselectivity). In contrast, electrolyte transport through epithelial cells (transcellular movement) may be either active or passive.

The forces responsible for generating passive ion movement are either chemical concentration gradients or electrical potential concentration (PD) gradients: It

Table 55–1. TRANSPORT CHARACTERISTICS THAT REFLECT VARYING PERMEABILITY OF JEJUNUM, ILEUM, AND COLON

	Jejunum	Ileum	Colon
Spontaneous transepithelial potential difference (lumen negative) (approximate values)	−3mV	−6mV	−20mV
Mucosal resistance	Low	Moderate	High
Apparent pore size (mean radius)	700 nm	300 nm	230 nm
Passive NaCl movement	High	Low	Minimal
Equilibrium concentration for net Na absorption	133 mEq/L	~75 mEq/L	~30 mEq/L

is possible to determine whether net ion movement can be explained by existing electrochemical concentration gradients by the use of either the Nernst equation or the Ussing flux equation or by the measurement of ion fluxes under short-circuit conditions (Fig. 55–4).

Convection. An additional form of passive ion transport is that of *convective,* or *solvent drag.* Convective flow is solute movement that is secondary to water flow. In the jejunum, a large component of total sodium movement is secondary to water flow and is another manifestation of the relatively high permeability and low resistance of the jejunal mucosa compared with ileum and colon.[4, 18] Most *in vitro* studies are *not* designed to provide quantitative detail of this transport process.

Active Transport. Considerable effort has been directed during the past quarter century toward the study of active, carrier-mediated transport processes in the small and large intestine. Active transport is an energy-dependent process that results in net movement against or in the absence of an electrochemical concentration gradient. Additional characteristics of active transport processes include the presence of *saturation kinetics* and *competitive inhibition.* Saturation kinetics is the phenomenon that, as the concentration of the transported substance increases, the rate of transport increases up to a maximal (or "saturated") rate. Active transport processes can be described in terms of their Vmax (maximal transport rate) and Km (the concentration at which transport is one half of that at Vmax). Substances that are transported by the same transport process will inhibit each other's transport by "competing" for the transport process. Competitive inhibition is the observation that the transport rate of substance A decreases as the concentration of substance B increases, but when the concentration of substance A increases the inhibition of its transport by substance B decreases.

Sodium absorption, probably in all intestinal segments but definitely in the ileum and colon, is secondary to active transport. Sodium transport appears central to most intestinal transport processes. It is generally accepted that sodium extrusion from the cell across the basolateral membrane by Na-K-ATPase (the so-called *sodium pump*) results in the maintenance of a *low* intracellular sodium concentration and electro-

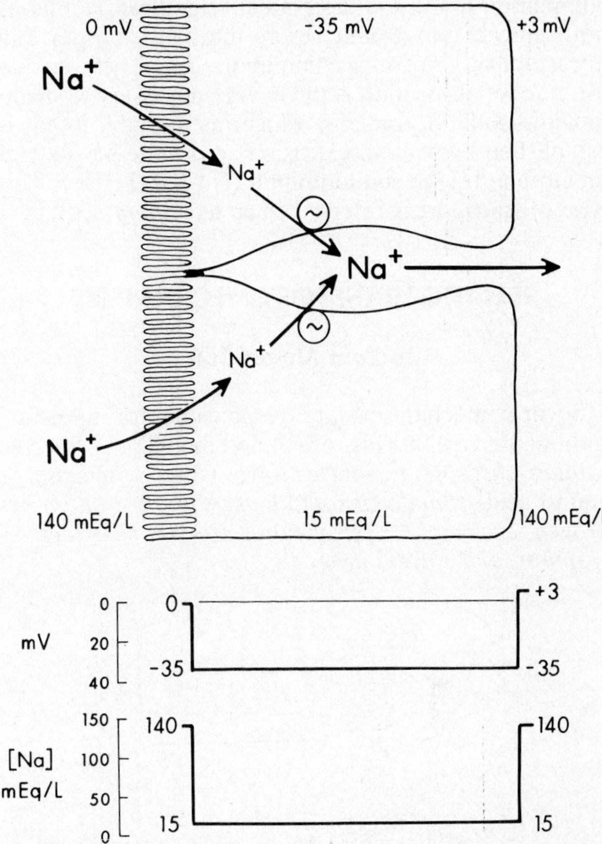

Figure 55–5. This figure emphasizes that transcellular sodium movement is a two-step process. The basolateral sodium pump (Na-K-ATPase) is the driving force for sodium extrusion from the epithelial cell. Intracellular sodium activity is approximately 15 mEq/L, and the potential difference across the luminal membane is approximately 35 mV. Although transcellular sodium movement is against an electrochemical concentration gradient, sodium movement into the epithelial cell is down an electrochemical concentration gradient, as emphasized by the two bottom panels.

negativity of the cell interior (Fig. 55–5). As a result, a considerable PD as well as a sodium concentration gradient exists across the mucosal membrane of the cell. Thus, sodium movement across the brush border into the cell is driven by the resulting electrochemical concentration gradient. The permeability of sodium across the apical membrane (especially that of the colon) is regulated in part by several factors, including the intraluminal and intracellular concentration of sodium, which contribute to the maintenance of a stable intracellular Na concentration.[19] The mechanism of absorption of several nonelectrolytes (e.g., glucose, amino acids, and so on) is active (that is, movement against a concentration gradient) and is sodium-dependent. The movement of these substances across the brush border that results in their intracellular accumulation, however, is not linked directly to an energy source but rather is coupled indirectly to an energy process by the so-called *sodium gradient* (Fig. 55–6*c*).[20] Mucosal accumulation of glucose (i.e., "uphill" movement) depends on the existence of a sodium gradient. Metabolic inhibitors do not impair glucose entry into the mucosal cell if the sodium gradient is maintained;

elimination of the sodium gradient significantly inhibits both glucose movement across the brush border and intracellular glucose accumulation. Thus, the energy for glucose absorption is the energy necessary to maintain the sodium gradient, which, as already noted, is established by sodium extrusion across the basolateral membrane by the sodium pump (Na-K-ATPase). This type of transport is referred to as *secondary active.*[21]

SPECIFIC TRANSPORT MECHANISMS

Sodium Absorption

Several mechanisms are responsible for intestinal sodium absorption (Fig. 55–6) and include *electrogenic sodium absorption, nonelectrolyte* (that is, glucose or amino acid)*-stimulated sodium absorption, sodium-hydrogen exchange, electroneutral sodium-chloride absorption, and solvent drag.*

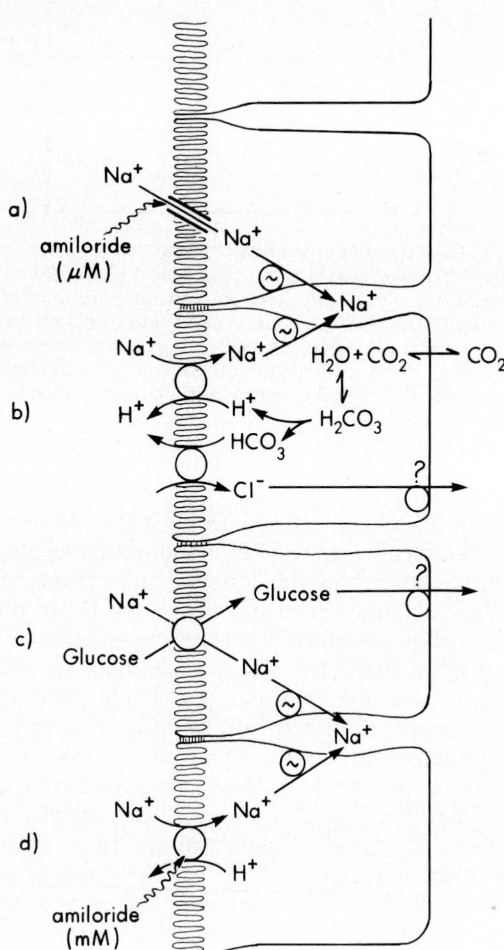

Figure 55–6. Modes of active intestinal sodium absorption. There are at least four mechanisms by which sodium can be absorbed. Electrogenic sodium absorption *(a)* is usually inhibited by micromolar concentrations of amiloride in the distal colon. Parallel ion exchanges *(b)* appear the primary process in the ileum and proximal colon, whereas glucose-stimulated (c) and bicarbonate-dependent *(d)* sodium absorption is the predominant mechanism of sodium absorption in the jeunum.

Electrogenic Sodium Absorption. This is the simplest form of active sodium transport and is associated with the development of a potential difference.[8] This process, which is probably present in all segments of the intestine, is the predominant mechanism of sodium transport in the colon and is similar to sodium transport in several other epithelia (Fig. 55–6). Electrogenic sodium absorption in the distal colon is chloride-independent and in the distal large intestine is inhibited by micromolar concentrations of the diuretic amiloride.[22] Net sodium absorption ceases in the jejunum when the luminal sodium concentration falls below 133 mEq/L; in contrast, it persists in the colon despite luminal sodium concentrations as low as 30 mEq/L.[4, 8] It is likely that the apparent differences in the efficiency of sodium transport in the jejunum, ileum, and colon reflect not the electrogenic sodium absorptive process but rather the different permeability characteristics of the intestine. The increased permeability in the jejunum (reflected by the lowered PD) causes a greater plasma-to-lumen movement ("back-leak") of sodium, resulting in an apparent diminished ability of the jejunum to absorb sodium against a concentration gradient.

Glucose (or Amino Acid)-Stimulated Sodium Absorption. This refers to the increased entry of sodium that is associated with glucose or amino acid movement across the mucosal brush border.[23] This process, which is present in the small intestine but not in the colon, is depicted in Figure 55–6*c*. The increase in sodium absorption stimulated by actively transported nonelectrolytes is associated with an increase in PD. The colon does not possess active absorptive processes for glucose or amino acids, and thus glucose- and amino acid–stimulated sodium absorption is not present in the large intestine. The coupling of glucose and sodium transport is well demonstrated in *in vitro* studies with intact tissue under short-circuited conditions (in which the PD is nullified by external current) and with apical membrane vesicles.[23, 24] In the human ileum, *in vivo* glucose increases the PD but not sodium absorption.[8] It has been suggested that glucose increases lumen-to-plasma sodium movement, but the increased PD results in an increase in plasma-to-lumen sodium movement, producing no net change in sodium transport.

Sodium-Hydrogen Exchange. Sodium absorption of the human jejunum is significantly increased by luminal bicarbonate.[8] Turnberg and associates provided compelling evidence that a sodium-hydrogen exchange is responsible for this bicarbonate stimulation of sodium absorption.[25] *In vitro* studies employing vesicles prepared from both small and large intestinal brush border membranes of experimental animals and humans have demonstrated the existence of a sodium-hydrogen exchange[26–29] (Fig. 55–6*d*). This process results in a 1:1 exchange of sodium for hydrogen ion and is inhibited by millimolar concentrations of the diuretic amiloride. The extrusion of protons across the brush border membrane energizes the movement of sodium into the epithelial cell. Sodium-hydrogen exchanges are ubiquitous and have been associated with transepithelial sodium movement, regulation of intracellular volume, and modulation of cell growth.[30]

Electroneutral (or Coupled) Sodium-Chloride Absorption. This form of transport is not associated with the development of a PD and has been identified in ileal, colonic, and gall bladder mucosa.[31] Overall electroneutral sodium-chloride absorption can occur as a result of one of three different transport processes (Fig. 55–7): Sodium-chloride (Na-Cl) cotransport; sodium-potassium-chloride (Na-K-2Cl) cotransport; and the coupling of parallel ion (sodium-hydrogen and chloride-bicarbonate or chloride-hydroxyl) exchanges. All three processes produce the same overall event: sodium-chloride absorption. Electroneutral sodium-chloride absorption is inhibited by increased mucosal cyclic adenosine monophosphate (cAMP), by changes in the concentration of cytosolic calcium, and by activation of protein kinase C.[31–33]

Turnberg and associates provided the initial evidence that, in the human ileum, sodium-chloride absorption could be a result of dual ion exchange processes: sodium-hydrogen and chloride-bicarbonate[34] (Fig. 55–6*b*). Recent studies with brush border membrane vesicles have established that these two ion exchange processes are coupled by intracellular pH and by carbonic anhydrase in that sodium and chloride absorption was inhibited either by millimolar concentrations of amiloride or by acetazolamide, an inhibitor of carbonic anhydrase.[35] It appears likely that electroneutral sodium-chloride absorption is primarily a result of these two ion exchange processes in the apical membrane of intestinal epithelial cells. It should be noted that the model of active chloride secretion in the intestine (see p. 1028) also requires the presence of electroneutral sodium-chloride uptake across the basolateral membrane. However, studies of this process indicate the involvement of a Na-K-2Cl cotransport mechanism[36] (see Fig. 55–9). Whether the Na-Cl cotransport process is at all present in intestinal epithelial cells is not as yet established.

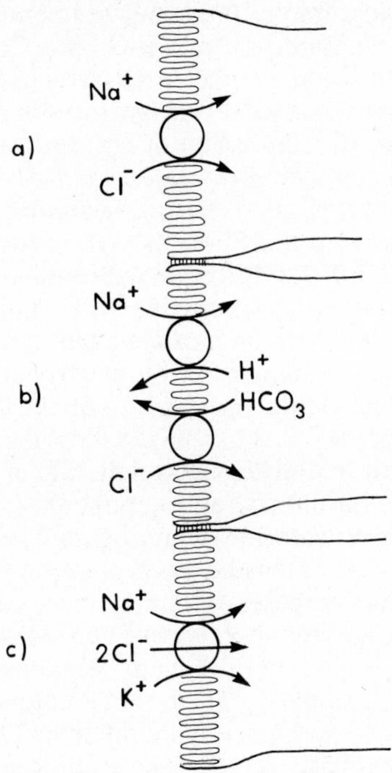

Figure 55–7. Models of electroneutral sodium-chloride transport. Three different models can explain overall electroneutral (i.e., without the development of an electrical potential difference) sodium-chloride absorption. These models can best be distinguished by the use of several inhibitors (diuretics) and by apical membrane vesicle studies.[13] Parallel ion (Na-H and Cl-HCO_3) exchanges *(b)* are now thought to explain electroneutral sodium-chloride in the mammalian small and large intestine. NA-K-2Cl cotransport *(c)* is likely responsible for sodium-chloride uptake across the basolateral membrane (See Fig. 55–9).

Almost all secretagogues inhibit electroneutral sodium-chloride absorption (together with stimulation of active chloride secretion). It is likely that inhibition of this absorptive process is primarily responsible for the observed net fluid and electrolyte secretion observed in most diarrheal disorders (see p. 1033 for full discussion).

Solvent Drag. Although there is no doubt that glucose stimulates sodium absorption in the small intestine, but not in the colon, there is controversy regarding the mechanism of this stimulation. *In vitro* studies have emphasized glucose-sodium cotransport (Fig. 55–6), which is likely present in the jejunum and ileum, including that of humans.[37, 38] In contrast, Fordtran has clearly provided evidence that as much as 85 per cent of glucose stimulation of sodium absorption in the human jejunum is secondary to solvent drag.[39] Water flow–dependent solute movement does not occur in the distal small intestine, probably because of the higher mucosal resistance of the ileum.

Sodium Secretion

In contrast to sodium absorptive processes, sodium secretion is primarily passive; the increased lumen-negative PD that is produced by several secretagogues is the driving force for sodium secretion in several diarrheal disorders. Whether there is an active sodium secretory process regulating basal transport, similar to that described in the guinea pig ileum, is unknown.[40]

Chloride Absorption

Both active and passive transport processes mediate the significant amounts of chloride that are absorbed daily from the small and large intestine. The mechanism of chloride absorption includes potential-sensitive and concentration-dependent passive processes as well as electroneutral sodium-chloride absorption and chloride-bicarbonate exchange (Fig. 55–8).

Passive Chloride Transport. Potential-sensitive chloride absorption is responsible for a major fraction of net chloride absorption in the intestine (Fig. 55–8*a*). Since the PD across the intestinal mucosa is oriented in such a way that the lumen is electronegative, the magnitude of the PD will influence chloride absorption quantitatively. Thus, glucose stimulation of sodium

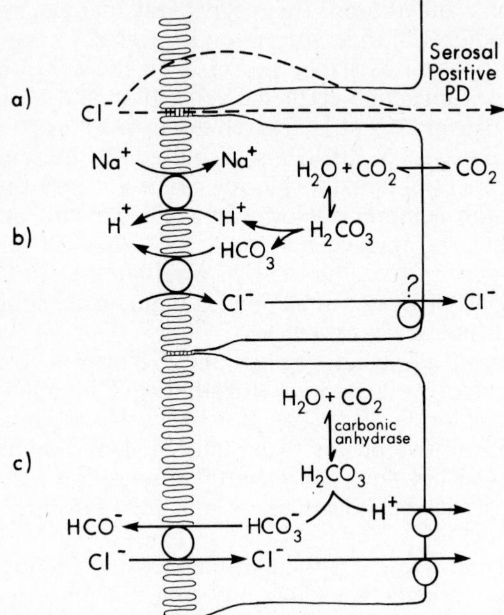

Figure 55–8. Modes of intestinal chloride absorption. There are three predominant mechanisms by which chloride can be absorbed. Potential-dependent chloride absorption *(a)* is probably the primary mechanism of chloride absorption. A bicarbonate-chloride exchange *(c)* results in the active absorption of chloride and the active secretion of bicarbonate. Inhibition of this process by acetazolamide is consistent with the proposed model. Carbon dioxide is derived from metabolic activity and plasma CO_2.

absorption results in increased chloride absorption *in vivo,* primarily by increasing the PD.[39] The route of potential-sensitive chloride absorption is probably paracellular, but a transcellular pathway has not been completely excluded.

It should also be noted that the absorption of chloride during perfusion of an intestinal segment with a solution containing a chloride concentration greater than 100 mEq/L will be mediated in part by the chloride concentration gradient from lumen to plasma.

Bicarbonate-Dependent Chloride Absorption. Chloride absorption and bicarbonate secretion* are closely linked in both ileum and colon and can result in the movement of these two anions against their concentration gradients. Both *in vivo* and *in vitro* experimental evidence indicate that a chloride-bicarbonate exchange process accounts for the observed chloride absorption and bicarbonate secretion.[41, 42] In contrast to other chloride absorptive secretory processes that are sodium-dependent, this chloride-bicarbonate exchange is not affected by the absence of sodium and is inhibited by stilbene derivatives that alter anion exchange processes in several other tissues.[22] The model represented in Figure 55–8*c* is consistent with present observations, including the inhibition of this transport process by acetazolamide, a carbonic anhydrase inhibitor.

*It is important to recognize that bicarbonate secretion may not necessarily represent HCO_3 secretion; hydroxyl ion secretion or hydrogen ion absorption can also result in apparent "bicarbonate" secretion.

In *congenital chloridorrhea,* deletion of this chloride-bicarbonate exchange in ileum and colon is responsible for the significant elevation of fecal chloride concentrations.[43, 44]

Electroneutral Sodium-Chloride Absorption. As described in the discussion of sodium absorption on page 1026 and as depicted in Figures 55–6*b* and 55–8*b*, it is most likely that electroneutral sodium-dependent chloride absorption is the result of the coupling of sodium-hydrogen and chloride-bicarbonate exchanges by intracellular pH.[34, 35]

Chloride Secretion

A large experimental literature exists regarding secretory processes in various diarrheal disorders, especially cyclic nucleotide–stimulated active electrogenic chloride secretion[2] in the small and large intestine.[45, 46] Little information, however, is available that characterizes basal intestinal secretion. Recently, evidence has been provided that demonstrates active chloride secretion in the jejunum in normal human subjects.[47] The relationship of this basal chloride secretory process to cAMP-mediated chloride secretion is unknown, and it is possible that the cellular regulation of these two processes differs. Electroneutral sodium-anion secretion has been documented in the guinea pig ileum and explains the fluid secretion observed in the basal state in this perhaps unique intestinal segment.[40] Also unknown are whether a similar or parallel secretory process is the driving force for basal secretion in the human intestine and what role hydrostatic pressure has in the genesis and regulation of basal secretion.

Secretagogues whose action is mediated by cAMP primarily produce active chloride secretion *in vitro* but active bicarbonate secretion *in vivo.* Little is known about why there should be a significant difference in anion secretion *in vivo* and *in vitro,* and, although considerable information and speculation are available regarding the details of active electrogenic chloride secretion, much less is known about the bicarbonate secretory process.

Electrogenic Chloride Secretion. Several bacterial enterotoxins, hormones, and detergents (see p. 1037) stimulate active chloride secretion *in vitro.*[45, 46] This secretory process is located in crypt epithelial cells and is initiated by increases either in mucosal cAMP or cyclic guanosine monophosphate (cGMP) or in the cytosolic concentration of calcium. An attractive model based on initial experiments in rabbit colon by Heintze and colleagues[48] and recently modified by Dharmsathaphorn and co-workers[36, 49, 50] in studies with the T_{84} colon cancer cell line is presented in Figure 55–9.

This model proposes that normally sodium, potassium, and chloride enter the epithelial cell across the basolateral border via the Na-K-2Cl transport process (step *a*).[36] A sodium concentration gradient, which is maintained by sodium extrusion across the basolateral membrane by Na-K-ATPase (step *b*), is the driving force for coupled Na-K-2Cl entry across the basolateral

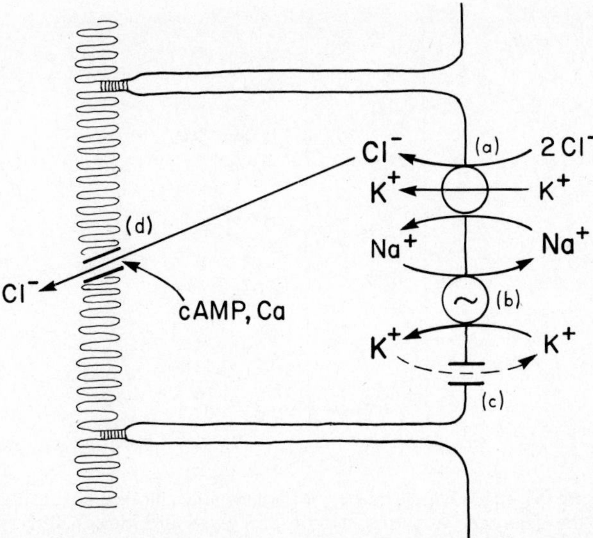

Figure 55–9. Cellular model of electrogenic chloride secretion. In this proposed model, chloride enters the cell via the Na-K-2Cl cotransport process across the basolateral membrane *(a)*, driven by a sodium gradient that would result in chloride activity above its electrochemical concentration gradient. The sodium gradient is maintained by the sodium pump *(b)*. Normally, the luminal membrane is relatively impermeable to chloride; increases in intracellular calcium concentrations and cyclic adenosine monophosphate (cAMP) (possibly by mobilizing intracellular calcium) result in active chloride secretion by increasing the permeability of the basolateral membrane to potassium *(c)* and the luminal membrane to chloride *(d)*. Specific chloride channel blocker can inhibit chloride secretion.[51] See text for additional details.

membrane. This model predicts that the intracellular concentration of chloride is above its equilibrium concentration but that chloride movement across the mucosal border does not occur because this membrane is relatively impermeable to chloride. It is proposed that cAMP, cGMP, or changes in the intracellular concentration of calcium induce potassium channels in the basolateral membrane (step *c*), resulting in an increase in the electrical potential difference across the luminal membrane. Cyclic AMP and calcium activate different potassium channels.[49] Chloride movement across the apical membrane is stimulated both by the presence of chloride channels (step *d*) in the apical membrane that are activated (or inserted) by increased mucosal cAMP, cGMP, or increased intracellular calcium (whether calcium "opens" apical chloride channels has recently been questioned[49, 50]) and by the increase in potential difference across the apical membrane. These several cellular events—*Na-K-ATPase, Na-K-2Cl cotransport* processes in the basolateral membrane, *K channel* in the basolateral membrane, and *chloride channel* in the apical membrane—act in concert to produce active chloride secretion. Considerable experimental evidence consistent with this model has been presented.[36, 49, 50] It is not known how changes in the cytosolic concentration of cyclic nucleotides or calcium might result in active chloride secretion; see page 1035 for further discussion of the effect of intracellular mediators on ion transport.

Potassium Transport

Until recently there has been considerable controversy regarding the mechanism of potassium transport in the intestine. It is generally agreed that potassium movement in the small intestine is passive, altered by changes in water flow, and can be explained solely by existing electrochemical concentration gradients.[52] In the colon, significant rates of net potassium secretion are a constant finding. Because the potential difference across the colon is approximately 20 to 30 mV (lumen-negative), potential-dependent potassium secretion explains a considerable portion of overall net potassium secretion (Fig. 55–10). There is now substantial evidence that both active potassium absorption and active potassium secretion are also present in the colon.[46, 53, 54] An active electrogenic potassium secretory process is present throughout the colon, whereas an active electroneutral, sodium-independent potassium absorptive process has been identified in the distal colon of experimental animals[53, 55, 56]; it is not known whether a similar potassium absorptive process is present in the human colon. This absorptive process is likely the result of a potassium-hydrogen exchange mechanism that is located in the luminal membrane and that may be similar to the exchange process responsible for gastric acid secretion by the parietal cell (see pp. 715–716). Whether similar K-ATPases energize both transport processes is not known.[57]

Both aldosterone and cAMP stimulate active colonic potassium secretion.[53, 58] This cAMP-induced potassium

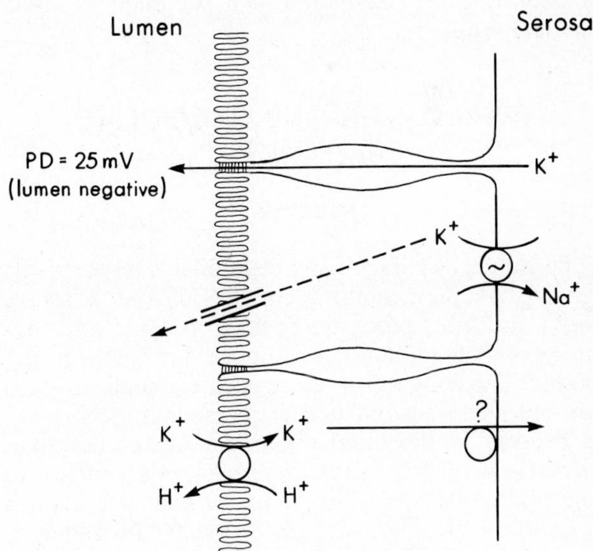

Figure 55–10. Mechanisms of potassium transport in the distal colon. Net potassium secretion in the colon occurs in the large part as a result of potential-dependent potassium movement across the tight junction. Also present are active electrogenic potassium secretion (also identified in the proximal colon) and electroneutral sodium-independent potassium absorption, which is likely secondary to a potassium-hydrogen exchange in the luminal membrane. This absorptive process is not present in the proximal colon. It is not known whether the two active transport processes are located in the same or in different cells.

secretion probably accounts for the increased stool potassium losses seen in many diarrheal disorders. Because increases in dietary potassium induce potassium secretion whereas potassium depletion stimulates active potassium absorption (or decreases net potassium secretion) in the distal colon, these potassium transport processes may function as an auxilliary modulator of overall potassium homeostasis working in concert with the renal tubule.[56] Thus, overall net potassium movement is the result of both passive (potential-dependent secretion) and active (absorptive and secretory) processes.

Short-Chain Fatty Acid Absorption

Short-chain fatty acids, predominantly acetate, butyrate, and propionate, are produced in the colon by enteric bacteria by fermentation of unabsorbed carbohydrate. Luminal bicarbonate neutralizes a significant fraction of the acid load generated by these volatile short-chain fatty acids, resulting in the production of carbon dioxide and water. The human large intestine absorbs significant quantities of short-chain fatty acids by a non–active transport process—primarily nonionic diffusion.[59] In contrast to long-chain fatty acids (with carbon chain lengths greater than 12), which stimulate fluid and electrolyte secretion, these short-chain fatty acids increase fluid and electrolyte absorption. Colonic absorption of these catabolic products of unabsorbed carbohydrates results in significant energy conservation[60] and may play a critical role in compensating for small intestinal secretion in some diarrheal disorders.

OVERALL FLUID AND ELECTROLYTE MOVEMENT

Jejunum

The primary characteristic of jejunal transport is its high passive permeability (Fig. 55–11). As a result, passive transport processes provide a major contribution to overall sodium and chloride movement in the jejunum. Although both electrogenic sodium absorption and glucose-stimulated active sodium absorption are present in the human jejunum, water flow–mediated (solvent drag) sodium absorption secondary to monosaccharide absorption is the primary mechanism of sodium absorption in this segment. In addition, bicarbonate-stimulated sodium absorption (via a sodium-hydrogen exchange) is also an important process. Chloride is absorbed primarily via potential- and concentration-dependent processes; it is also actively secreted in human jejunum in the basal state.

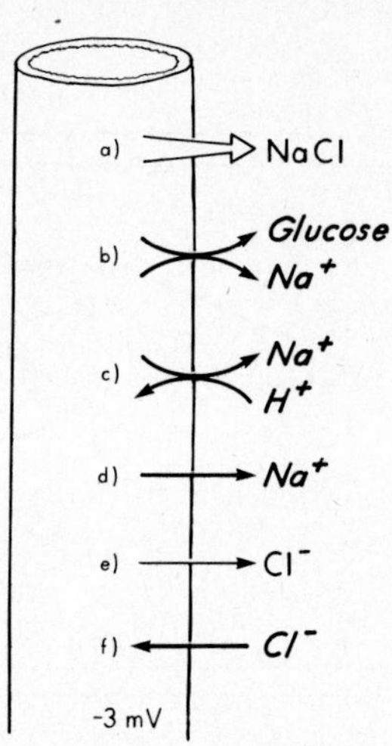

Figure 55–11. Overall model of sodium and chloride absorption in the jejunum. Active transport processes are designated by boldface italics, passive processes by roman type. Although there is evidence for active (electrogenic) sodium absorption *(d)*, glucose-stimulated sodium absorption *(b)*, and sodium-hydrogen exchange *(c)*, the majority of sodium absorption in the human jejunum is secondary to water flow *(a)*, which is induced by monosaccharide absorption. Details are provided in the text.

Ileum

Electroneutral sodium-chloride absorption results from parallel ion exchanges (Na-H and Cl-HCO_3) and is the predominant mechanism of sodium absorption in the ileum (Fig. 55–12). Although sodium is absorbed electrogenically in the ileum, little sodium is absorbed secondary to solvent drag (i.e., associated with glucose transport). Although such glucose-coupled sodium absorption is readily demonstrated *in vitro,* the greater mucosal resistance of the ileum than of the jejunum is probably the explanation for the failure of glucose to stimulate sodium absorption *in vivo.*

Colon

Both similarities and differences exist in the characteristics of colonic (compared with small intestinal)

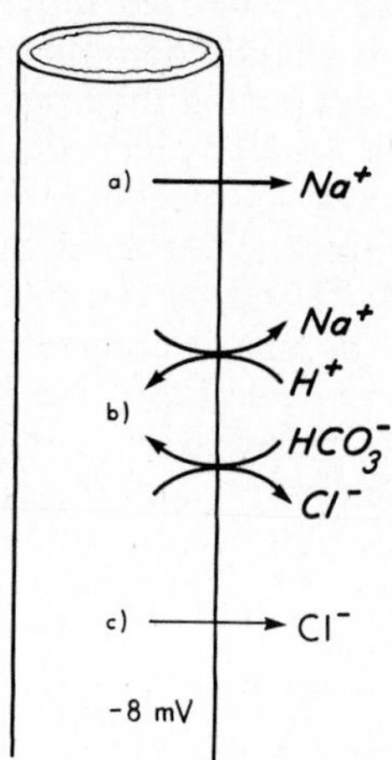

Figure 55–12. Overall model of sodium-chloride absorption in the ileum. As noted in the text and in Figure 55–6, recent studies establish that electroneutral sodium-chloride absorption is secondary to dual ion exchanges. Electrogenic sodium absorption and potential-dependent chloride absorption also occur in the ileum.

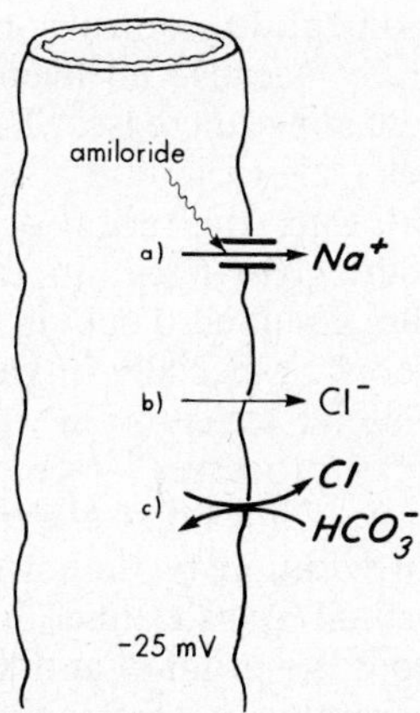

Figure 55–13. Overall model of sodium-chloride absorption in the distal colon. Electrogenic sodium absorption inhibited by micromolar concentration of amiloride is the major process for sodium absorption in rabbit and human; in the rat, electroneutral sodium-chloride absorption is present. Sodium-independent chloride-bicarbonate exchange is also present in the large intestine. In the more proximal colon, amiloride-sensitive sodium transport is less dominant, and characteristics of sodium and chloride transport resemble more those in small bowel than in distal colon.

electrolyte transport (Fig. 55–13). Colonic transport differs from that of the small intestine in several significant ways: (1) The large intestine is characterized by relatively high mucosal resistance (compared with jejunum and ileum), which is reflected by a high PD and low permeability (see Table 55–1); (2) glucose (and other nonelectrolytes) do not stimulate sodium and water absorption; (3) active nutrient absorptive processes are absent in the colon; and (4) mineralocorticoids have significant effect on colonic, but not small intestinal, electrolyte transport.

Most studies of fluid and electrolyte absorption in the large intestine have tacitly assumed that electrolyte transport processes are uniform throughout the colon. Thus, *in vivo* luminal perfusion studies have frequently been performed without regard for the possibility that electrolyte movement may differ in one or more segments, and *in vitro* studies have been performed primarily in the distal portion of the colon. More recent studies provide compelling evidence that these assumptions are not correct and that there are significant differences in function between different colonic segments of both experimental animals and humans.[22, 61–65] The traditional description of colonic ion transport—amiloride-sensitive, electrogenic sodium absorption and electroneutral bicarbonate-dependent chloride absorption—is probably present only in the most distal segment of the colon. Electroneutral sodium-chloride absorption (i.e., Na-H and Cl-HCO_3 exchanges) has been identified in the colon of some species[66] and amiloride-insensitive sodium absorption is present in the more proximal portions of the large intestine of humans.[62] In addition to chloride-bicarbonate exchange, chloride absorption is also the result of potential-dependent mechanism.

The following segmental differences of colonic electrolyte transport can be characterized: Sodium-chloride transport in the more proximal portions of the large intestine, as in the small intestine, has a high capacity but relatively low efficiency, an observation that may explain why diarrhea is greater following resection of the ascending colon than after removal of the descending colon. In addition, the rate of sodium-chloride transport in the distal colon is lower but more efficient (i.e., there is significant sodium conservation or movement against large electrochemical concentration gradients).

REGULATION OF ELECTROLYTE TRANSPORT

Intestinal electrolyte transport is influenced by multiple factors, including neural and hormonal. Evidence of neural regulation of intestinal electrolyte transport has only recently been provided and involves participation of both the *enteric* and *central nervous systems.* Hubel and Cooke and their collaborators have demonstrated that electrical field stimulation of isolated sheets of mucosa (small and large intestine of both humans and experimental animals) stimulates active chloride secretion, which is blocked by tetrodotoxin, an inhibitor of neurotransmission.[67–70] These results indicate that the intrinsic nerves of the enteric nervous system can release one or more substances that alter electrolyte transport. It is likely that acetylcholine (and perhaps vasoactive intestine peptide), as well as other unidentified neurotransmitters, are responsible for these changes in intestinal electrolyte transport. It is probable that cholinergic agonists also exert a basal secretory tone.

The enteric nervous system may also participate in the stimulation of electrolyte secretion by secretagogues (e.g., cholera enterotoxin) that have traditionally been believed to act solely at the level of the enterocyte.[71, 72]

Despite the common assumption that stress affects intestinal function (i.e., is responsible for "functional" diarrhea), evidence for an association between central nervous system and intestinal electrolyte transport has been minimal. It has been reported that intraventricular injection of peptides, including enkephalins, and of prostaglandins can alter gastric acid secretion, intestinal motility, and fluid and electrolyte movement.[73–77] Thus, central administration of minute amounts of prostaglandins and enkephalins stimulates small intestinal fluid and water absorption.[76, 77]

Hormones and neurotransmitters also affect intestinal electrolyte transport. These regulators of intestinal transport function as *endocrine hormones,* as so-called *paracrine mediators,* and as *neurotransmitters.* Peptides, bioactive amines, and corticosteroids may produce either increases or decreases in fluid and electrolyte movement. Although potent effects of these agents are observed in both *in vivo* studies (usually observations following intravenous infusion of agonists) and *in vitro* experiments (addition of the agonist to isolated mucosa), it is often uncertain whether the observed changes represent *physiologic* and not *pharmacologic* actions, especially because, in some experiments, extremely high concentrations are employed.

Many hormones and neurotransmitters are found in the intestine and may exert a direct effect on epithelial function ("paracrine" mediator).[78] *Paracrine* control is the regulation of intestinal function by agonists present in intestinal endocrine cells that are released from these cells and alter the function of adjacent epithelial cells but do not necessarily enter the systemic circulation. Enkephalin, somatostatin, substance P, and serotonin are such paracrine mediators[79]; (see also pp. 21–52 and 78–107).

Aldosterone. Similar to its effects on electrolyte transport in the kidney, increased plasma aldosterone increases sodium absorption and potassium secretion in the colon.[55, 80, 81] Adrenalectomy decreases sodium absorption. Mineralocorticoids have no effects on ion transport in the jejunum and minimal action in the ileum. Because sodium depletion is a major stimulant for aldosterone secretion, the response of the colon to aldosterone represents an important compensatory mechanism to dehydration. A patient with an ileostomy is at increased risk when dehydrated owing to the loss of aldosterone-responsive colonic mucosa (see p. 1478).

Evidence exists for hormonal regulation of fluid balance by the small intestine during volume depletion and dehydration,[82] although aldosterone does not have potent effects on sodium absorption in the small intestine. In this situation, circulating angiotensin II is increased, stimulating fluid and electrolyte absorption more in the small intestine than in the colon and complementing the role of aldosterone in the colon during periods of volume depletion.[82]

Glucocorticoids. Glucocorticoids not only regulate small intestinal maturation significantly but also help regulate both small intestinal and colonic fluid and electrolyte transport.[81, 83, 84] Dexamethasone and methylprednisolone in experimental animals increase water, sodium, and chloride absorption and potassium secretion.[83, 84] Although glucocorticoids interact with the aldosterone receptor, recent studies establish that there are glucocorticoid receptors in small and large intestinal epithelial cells and that the effect of glucocorticoids on electrolyte transport is glucocorticoid-specific and cannot be explained completely by cross-over binding to the aldosterone receptor.[85, 86] Intravenous hydrocortisone increases sodium and water absorption acutely in the rectum of normal subjects and patients with ulcerative colitis.[87] In this way, glucocorticoids augment their anti-inflammatory action in ameliorating symptoms in patients with diarrhea. It is likely that basal colonic electrolyte transport is also mediated to some extent by glucocorticoids.

Opiates and Opioid Peptides. *In vitro* studies have demonstrated that synthetic enkephalins and morphine stimulate active sodium and chloride absorption in the ileum.[88, 89] Opioid peptides affect ion transport not by directly interacting with the intestinal epithelial cell but by inducing the release of an unidentified neurotransmitter (e.g., norepinephrine) that stimulates active sodium-chloride absorption.[90] Opioid peptides also help to regulate basal electrolyte movement as their antagonists decrease basal water and electrolyte absorption.[91] Opioid peptides control some intestinal fluid absorption centrally because intraventricular administration of enkephalins increases fluid absorption.[92] Opioid peptides also inhibit several secretory processes[93, 94] and, thus, the recent demonstration that loperamide, an effective agent in treating diarrhea, possesses calcium channel blocking properties is of considerable interest, especially in view of the importance of intracellular calcium in the regulation of intestinal secretory processes[95] (see Fig. 55–17). Although opiates affect intestinal electrolyte absorption and secretion, in addition to their well-known ability to prolong intestinal transit time, luminal perfusion studies suggest that the primary antidiarrheal action of codeine and loperamide is on slowing of transit time, not on electrolyte transport.[96, 97]

Somatostatin. Somatostatin, a tetradecapeptide found in both the central nervous system and the intestine, has several significant effects on intestinal functions. These include prolongation of intestinal transit time, stimulation of active sodium-chloride absorption in the ileum and colon, and inhibition of secretagogue-mediated changes in ion transport in the colon.[98–100] It is of clinical interest that the initial observation that intravenous administration of somatostatin markedly reduced diarrhea in two patients with carcinoid syndrome[101] led to the development of somatostatin analogues with longer duration of action and more gut-specific activity. One such analogue, SMS-201-995, has been used effectively in several patients with refractory watery diarrhea syndrome.[102] In such patients, SMS-201-995 has dramatically reduced diarrhea in association with an inhibition of hormone release, as well as manifesting effects on both intestinal transport and transit[103] (see pp. 1569 and 1894–1896).

Adrenergic-Cholinergic Agonists. Fluid and electrolyte movement is in part regulated by both the sympathetic and parasympathetic nervous systems. Epinephrine and alpha$_2$-adrenergic agonists specifically stimulate electroneutral sodium-chloride absorption in both the small and large intestine.[104–106] This action of epinephrine represents alpha$_2$-adrenergic activity, as beta-adrenergic agonists have little effect on intestinal ion transport. Recent studies indicate that alpha$_2$-adrenergic receptors are present on enterocytes and alpha$_2$-adrenergic agonists block calcium uptake by enterocytes.[107, 108] It is likely that this action of adrenergic agonists is related to a lowering of intracellular calcium activity. The importance of adrenergic agonists in the control of basal intestinal transport is suggested by the recent observation that, following chemical symphathectomy by 6-hydroxydopamine, there is a significant decrease in colonic and ileal water absorption.[109] Because similar changes in fluid movement were noted in rats with streptozocin-induced diabetes mellitus, as were reduced stores of tissue norepinephrine, an attractive speculation is that there is diminished noradrenergic tone in chronic diabetes mellitus. It should be noted that clonidine, an alpha$_2$-adrenergic agonist, has been shown to be effective in the treatment of watery diarrhea syndrome and in both experimental and clinical diabetic diarrhea.[110, 111] Finally, a newly developed antidiarrheal agent, lidamidine, is a potent alpha$_2$-adrenergic agonist (see pp. 21–52, 311–312, and 496–497).

Although information regarding cholinergic regulation of intestinal ion transport is less extensive than that for adrenergic agonists, there is excellent evidence that cholinergic muscarinic agonists either inhibit sodium and chloride absorption or stimulate sodium and chloride secretion by interacting with muscarinic agonists on enterocytes and by functioning as a calcium ionophore.[112, 113] As already noted, basal chloride secretion may be regulated by cholinergic agonists, and a portion of the chloride secretion induced by intrinsic nerve stimulation is cholinergic-mediated.[68] Thus, these classic neutrotransmitters modulate both absorptive and secretory processes by influencing intracellular calcium.

Vasoactive Intestinal Peptide (VIP). VIP is both a circulating peptide hormone and a neurotransmitter found in both brain and gut. Although a clear-cut physiologic function for VIP has not been identified, intravenous infusion of VIP results in net fluid secretion, and VIP is the primary circulating secretagogue responsible for the diarrhea in the so-called watery diarrhea syndrome (frequently secondary to an islet cell adenoma)[114, 115] (see pp. 303 and 1890–1891). Receptors for VIP are on the basolateral membrane of enterocytes and VIP stimulates adenylate cyclase activity; in addition, the effects of VIP on intestinal transport are mediated by cAMP[116, 117] (see pp. 80–92).

Arachidonic Acid Metabolites. Arachidonic acid is metabolized via two separate and distinct pathways, those of cyclo-oxygenase and lipoxygenase. Considerable information exists that metabolites of both pathways have important effects on small and large intestinal transport. Initial observations indicating an effect of prostaglandins (PG) (which are cyclo-oxygenase metabolites) on intestinal electrolyte movement included the frequent occurrence of diarrhea in persons receiving prostaglandins, the stimulation of active chloride secretion by the addition of certain prostaglandins, (e.g., PGE$_1$) to isolated intestinal mucosa, and the induction of net fluid secretion following the intravenous infusion of prostaglandins. These effects of PGs on electrolyte transport are a result of stimulation of adenylate cyclase with an increase in mucosal cAMP.

More recent observations provide evidence of additional importance of arachidonic acid metabolites in the regulation of intestinal transport. First, certain lipoxygenase metabolites (e.g., 5-hydroperoxyeicosatetraenoic acid, or 5-HPETE) stimulate active chloride secretion in the colon by an unidentified mechanism, as roles for cAMP, cGMP, and extracellular calcium have been excluded.[118] Second, the demonstration of increased PG and leukotriene synthesis in the rectal mucosa of patients with ulcerative colitis has suggested that mucosal PGs are responsible for the abnormal fluid and electrolyte movement in these patients.[119, 120] (It should be noted that sulfasalazine, a drug that is effective in the treatment of ulcerative colitis, inhibits PG synthesis.) Third, several studies have suggested that PGs are involved in the mechanism by which certain laxatives (e.g., bisacodyl, phenolphthalein, and ricinoleic acid) alter colonic fluid and electrolyte movement.[121] Finally, bradykinin stimulates active Cl secretion in the rabbit colon by activating membrane phospholipases with subsequent release and metabolism of arachidonic acid and the production of PGs.[122] Taken together, these several observations indicate that arachidonic acid metabolites (primarily PGs) are secretagogues and alter intestinal ion transport primarily by increasing mucosal cAMP; it is likely that arachadonic acid metabolites also affect epithelial cell transport by other mechanisms and perhaps act as an intracellular mediator of ion secretion.

DIARRHEA: ALTERED ELECTROLYTE TRANSPORT

Diarrhea is best defined as an increase in fecal water excretion. During the past two decades attempts to explain this increase in stool water excretion have been directed primarily toward identifying changes of intestinal fluid and electrolyte movement.[123, 124] Considerable attention has focused on intestinal fluid and electrolyte secretion, but even modest decreases in fluid and electrolyte absorption (without actual net fluid secretion) can cause increases in stool fluid output. Although it is likely that changes in intestinal motor activity are present in some diarrheal disorders, adequate understanding of their pathogenic importance is not available at present (see p. 1039).

The colon absorbs more than 90 per cent of the fluid that passes across the ileocecal valve, as shown in Figure 55–14. A decrease in colonic fluid absorption to the extent that stool water excretion increased to 800 ml/day would mean that the rate of efficiency of water absorption in the colon was still approximately 50 per cent. Furthermore, if it were assumed that normal small intestinal function was present, zero net colonic fluid movement would result in fecal water excretion of approximately 1.5 L/day! Conversely, if it were assumed that the disease processes responsible for the alteration in fluid and electrolyte movement were restricted to the small intestine and that colonic function were normal, water excretion would not increase until the absorptive capacity of the colon (approximately 5 L/day) was exceeded. The efficiency of small intestinal fluid absorption normally is about 80 per cent (absorption of 6.5 of 8 L entering the small intestine), but a decline to less than 40 per cent (3 of 8 L) would result in an ileocecal flow rate that was greater than the colonic absorptive capacity. Therefore, in the presence of small intestinal disease, maximal colonic absorptive capacity is the major determinant in preventing diarrhea. The ecology of the colon also affects the colon's ability to compensate for changes in small intestinal fluid and electrolyte absorp-

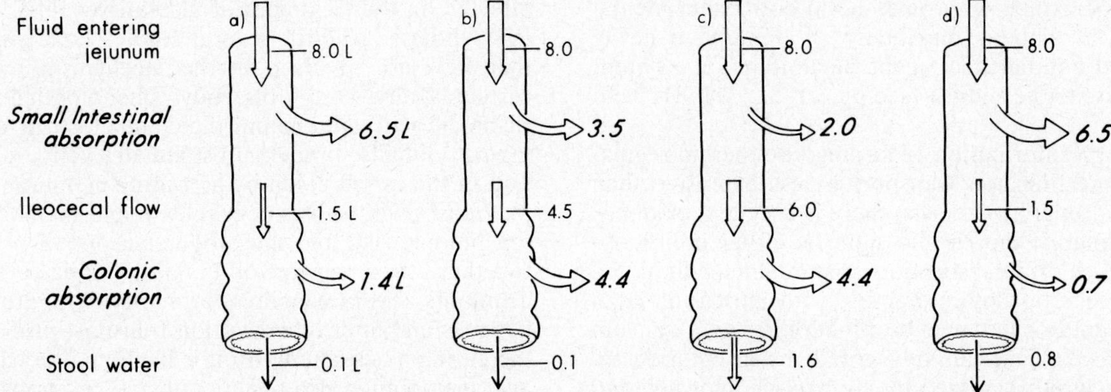

Figure 55–14. Importance of colonic absorption and colonic absorptive capacity in determining increase in stool water (i.e., diarrhea). Normal fluid balance in humans (identical to Fig. 55–1) is shown *(a)*. Significant changes in small intestinal fluid absorption will not produce diarrhea *(b)* as long as colonic fluid absorptive capacity, which is approximately 5 L per day, is not exceeded. Diarrhea occurs when ileocecal flow exceeds colonic absorptive capacity *(c)*. A decrease in colonic absorption (with normal small intestinal function) *(d)* will also result in an increase in stool water excretion.

tion and partially determines the occurrence of diarrhea.[125] Diarrhea could be considered "a failure of colonic salvage," as the colon is unable to handle the load.[126]

Although these figures indicate that net fluid and electrolyte secretion in the small intestine are not necessary for diarrhea, net fluid and electrolyte secretion* has been observed in almost every diarrheal disorder in which fluid and electrolyte movement has been measured directly by luminal perfusion Table 55–2 lists those diarrheal diseases in which net fluid and electrolyte secretion has been observed and emphasizes the heterogeneity of the disorders with documented net fluid and electrolyte secretion.[44, 115, 127–141] Net fluid and electrolyte secretion has also been observed in several experimental situations, many of which are experimental models of diarrhea.[142–147]

Net fluid and electrolyte absorption represents the difference between lumen-to-plasma movement and plasma-to-lumen movement. Either a decrease in lumen-to-plasma movement or an increase in plasma-to-lumen movement can produce changes in net fluid and electrolyte absorption. Relatively small quantitative differences in either of these oppositely directed transport processes will produce either an apparent decrease in net absorption or an actual net secretion (Fig. 55–15). The mechanisms responsible for such changes

*Confusion occurs at times because *secretion* is used to describe two different events. In one sense, secretion is often employed to describe the phenomenon in which there is an addition of fluid to a segment of intestine. In this context, secretion is the opposite of absorption and does not describe the mechanism(s) for the observed movement of fluid and electrolytes. In this chapter, the term *net fluid and electrolyte secretion* is used to refer to this phenomenon, which most frequently is best observed *in vivo*. Secretion is also used to describe the active transport process that is, for example, stimulated by cholera enterotoxin. This latter event is referred to as *active ion secretion* or *active secretory process* and often is best demonstrated in *in vitro* experiments.

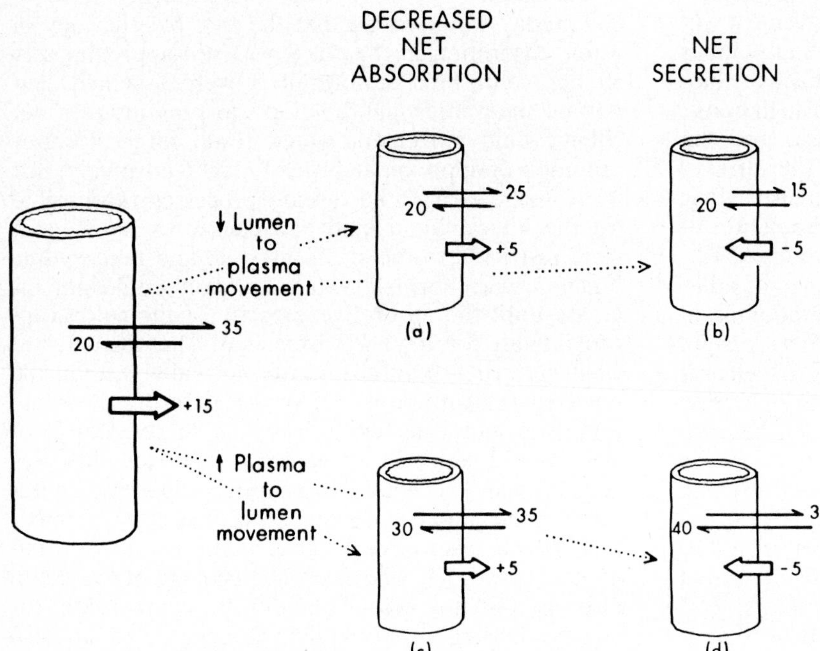

Figure 55–15. Both decreased net absorption (*a* and *c*) and net secretion (*b* and *d*) can be caused by either a decrease in lumen-to-plasma movement (*a* and *b*) or an increase in plasma-to-lumen movement (*c* and *d*). A decrease in lumen-to-plasma movement could be produced by diminished active absorption, whereas an increase in plasma-to-lumen movement could be caused by active ion secretion, increased luminal osmolality, or increased hydrostatic pressure.

Table 55–2. DIARRHEAL DISORDERS WITH DOCUMENTED NET FLUID AND ELECTROLYTE SECRETION

Lactase deficiency[127]
Celiac sprue[128]
Tropical sprue[129]
Crohn's disease[130]
Ulcerative colitis[131]
Intestinal obstruction[132]
Carcinoid syndrome[133]
Watery diarrhea syndrome (pancreatic cholera)[115]
Cholera[134]
Acute undifferentiated diarrhea (tropical)[135]
Medullary carcinoma of thyroid[136]
Ileal tuberculosis[137]
Congenital chloridorrhea[44]
Systemic sclerosis, mixed collagen disease[138, 139]
Alcoholism (when associated with folate deficiency)[140]
Collagenous colitis[141]

include *active anion secretion, decreased solute absorption, increased luminal osmolality,* and *increased hydrostatic pressure.* The importance of altered motility, increased mucosal permeability, and mucosal damage in the production of changes in fluid and electrolyte movement is unknown but also will be considered (see pp. 1039–1040).

Active Anion Secretion

Intracellular Mediators

Investigation of the pathogenesis of cholera established active anion secretion as both a physiologic and a pathophysiologic process. Cholera enterotoxin activates adenylate cyclase activity, resulting in an increasing mucosal cAMP and stimulating active electrogenic chloride secretion as well as inhibiting electroneutral sodium-chloride absorption.[148] The combined inhibition of electroneutral sodium-chloride absorption and stimulation of active chloride secretion (Fig. 55–16) results in net fluid and electrolyte secretion. However, cAMP does not inhibit glucose-stimulated sodium absorption.

The ability of glucose to increase sodium and water absorption both in cholera enterotoxin–exposed mucosa and experimentally in the presence of cAMP is the physiologic basis for the therapeutic effectiveness of oral glucose therapy with oral rehydration solution in cholera and many turista illnesses.

As already noted, absorptive processes are located in villus cells and secretory processes in crypt cells (Fig. 55–16) (see p. 1028 and Fig. 55–9 for a discussion of cellular changes associated with cAMP-stimulated active chloride secretion).[15] Similar effects on sodium and chloride transport in both small intestine and colon are produced by other enterotoxins and hormones (heat labile *E. coli* enterotoxin, VIP, PGE_1) that increase adenylate cyclase activity and increase mucosal cAMP.[117, 149] Although cholera enterotoxin (and cAMP) stimulates active chloride secretion *in vitro,* it induces active bicarbonate secretion *in vivo.* This difference has not been explained.

In addition to *cAMP,* two other intracellular mediators stimulate intestinal anion secretion and inhibit electroneutral sodium-chloride absorption: cytosolic concentration of *calcium* and *cGMP.*[32, 150] The role of calcium in the induction of secretion was initially suggested by the observation that the calcium ionophore A23187 stimulated active chloride secretion only in the presence of extracellular calcium.[151] Subsequent studies demonstrated that serotonin and be-

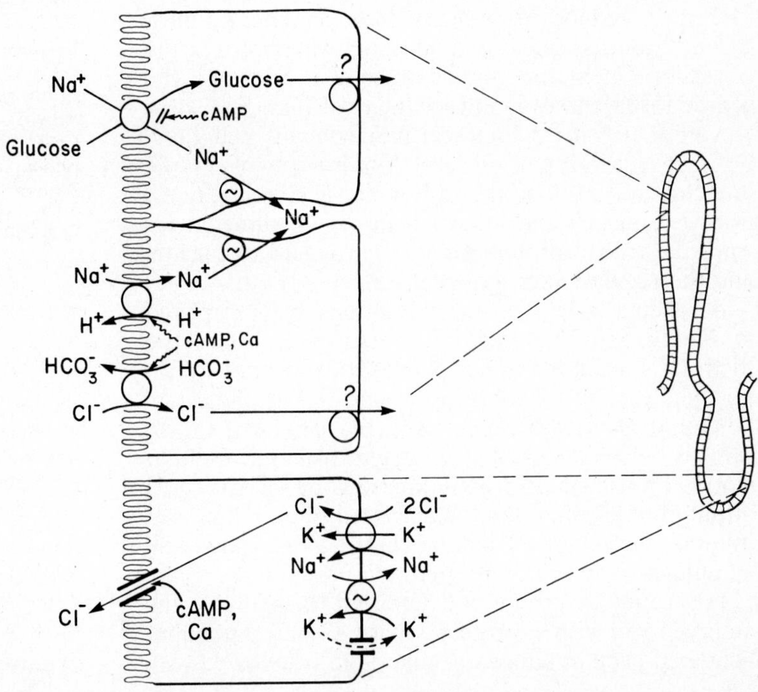

Figure 55–16. Summary of the effect of cAMP (or calcium) on sodium and chloride movement, based on the model that absorptive processes are located in villus epithelial cells and secretory ones in crypt epithelial cells. Details of glucose-stimulated sodium absorption, electroneutral sodium-chloride absorption, and electrogenic chloride secretion are provided in Figures 55–7, 55–8, and 55–9, respectively. Cyclic AMP and calcium inhibit electroneutral sodium-chloride absorption, but not glucose-stimulated sodium absorption, and stimulate electrogenic chloride secretion.

thanechol also stimulate active chloride secretion and inhibit electroneutral sodium-chloride absorption; however, these effects are also calcium-dependent and not associated with an increase in mucosal cAMP or cGMP levels.[113, 152] Other studies indicate that increases and decreases in electroneutral sodium-chloride absorption are inversely proportional to the concentration of intracellular calcium.[32] Agents such as clonidine, an alpha$_2$-adrenergic agonist, by inhibiting calcium entry into the epithelial cell, increase electroneutral Na-Cl absorption. Conversely, agents such as serotonin and acetylcholine, which increase intracellular calcium, inhibit electroneutral Na-Cl absorption.[32, 108, 152]

Increased mucosal cGMP influences intestinal transport in ways similar to cAMP and calcium ionophores. Two enterotoxins, a heat-labile (LT) (which is similar to cholera enterotoxin) and a heat-stable (ST), are produced by *E. coli*; the ST toxin binds to a brush border receptor, activates guanylate cyclase, and increases mucosal cGMP.[150] The ST toxin, similar to VIP and carbachol, also activates an apical membrane chloride channel and a basolateral membrane potassium channel[153] (see Fig. 55–9).

The cellular mechanisms by which cAMP, cGMP, and calcium alter ion transport are not known but presumably involve activation of one or more protein kinases with subsequent phosphorylation of specific apical membrane proteins, resulting in either an activation or an insertion of chloride channels in the apical membrane[154–156] (Fig. 55–17*a*). The inhibition of electoneutral sodium-chloride absorption undoubtedly also involves activation of one or more other protein kinases.[157] An attractive, although unproved, hypothesis is that cAMP alters ion transport by mobilizing calcium from intracellular calcium stores. Alternatively, ion transport might be altered by a cAMP activated protein kinase. Little information is available regarding the cellular regulation of ion transport by cGMP.

Certain agonists (e.g., serotonin, cholinergic muscarinic agonists) function as calcium ionophores at the basolateral membrane, and extracellular calcium is the source for increases in intracellular calcium.[113, 152] How elevation of intracellular calcium controls cell functions, particularly water and ion movement in the intestine and in nonintestinal tissue, is a crucial question.[156] Considerable attention has been directed toward the role of protein kinase C in regard to calcium and the regulation of ion transport.

A schema to explain these relationships is depicted in Figure 55–17*b*. Certain secretagogues induce the hydrolysis of membrane phosphatidylinositol-4,5-diphosphate (PIP$_2$) hydrolysis to inositol triphosphate (IP$_3$) and diacylglycerol (DG)[156] (Fig. 55–17*b*). IP$_3$, in turn, is believed to mobilize calcium from intracellular stores. DG activates protein kinase C by increasing its affinity for calcium, and the activated protein kinase C inhibits electroneutral sodium-chloride absorption and stimulates active chloride secretion.[154, 157–159]

Intracellular calcium modulates ion transport via the activation of either protein kinase C or calmodulin-activated protein kinases. Calmodulin is involved with

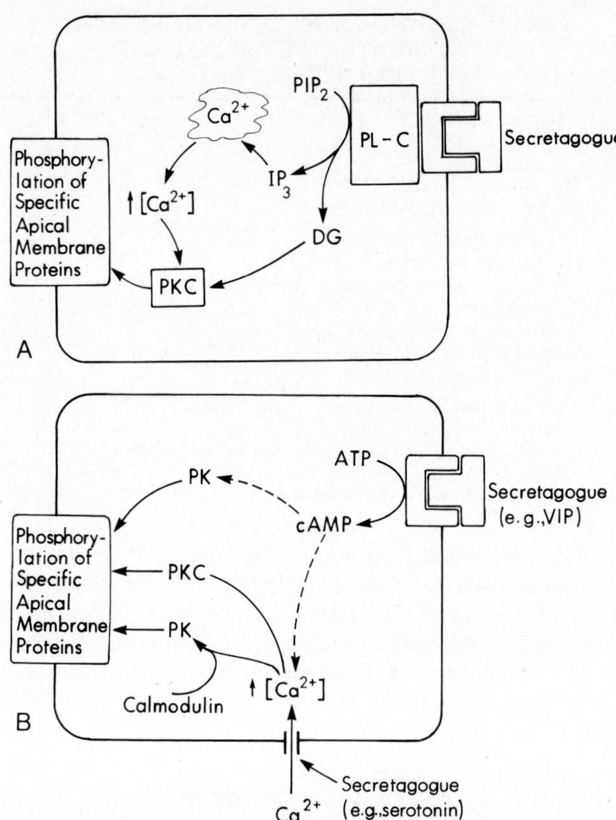

Figure 55–17. Secretagogue regulation of intestinal ion transport via multiple intracellular mediators. *A*, This diagram illustrates the present model by which both cAMP and elevation of intracellular calcium modify electrolyte transport (inhibition of electroneutral sodium-chloride absorption in villous epithelial cells and stimulation of electrogenic chloride secretion in crypt epithelial cells [see Fig. 55–16]), probably by activation of one or more protein kinases that phosphorylate specific apical membrane proteins. It is likely that different protein kinases regulate the basal and the two ion transport processes. Certain secretagogues (e.g., VIP) activate adenylate cyclase and result in an increase in mucosal cAMP. Cyclic AMP either activates a protein kinase directly or increases calcium via mobilizing intracellular calcium stores. Other secretagogues (e.g., serotonin) act as calcium ionophores and increase intracellular calcium, which may activate either a Ca-calmodulin protein kinase or protein kinase C. Heat-stable enterotoxin of *Escherichia coli* (not shown) activates guanylate cyclase and increases mucosal cyclic GMP. Little is known about the details of cyclic guanosine monophosphate (cGMP) activated protein kinases. *B*, This diagram describes the proposed role of protein kinase C (PKC) in stimulus-secretion coupling of electrolyte transport. Agonist-activated membrane phospholipase C (PL-C) hydrolyzes plasma membrane phosphatidylinositol-4,5-bisphosphate (PIP$_2$) to two second messengers: inositol-1,3,5-triphosphate (IP$_3$) and diacylglycerol (DG). IP$_3$ increases intracellular calcium by mobilizing intracellular calcium stores. Both calcium and DG activate PKC, which can stimulate active chloride secretion and inhibit electroneutral sodium-chloride absorption[157, 159] via posphorylation of specific apical membrane proteins. Athough this process is depicted in a single cell, it is generally believed that absorptive processes are located in the villous epithelial cell, whereas secretory processes are located in crypt epithelial cells (see Fig. 55–16).

basal sodium and chloride transport in the rabbit ileum, whereas protein kinase C helps regulate both sodium-chloride absorption and active chloride secretion.[154, 155, 157–159] No matter what the eventual true sequence of events, intracellular calcium is central to the control of

Table 55–3. BACTERIAL EXOTOXINS THAT PRODUCE NET FLUID SECRETION OR MUCOSAL DAMAGE, OR BOTH

Bacterium	Toxin	Intracellular Mediator
Vibrio cholerae[148]	Cholera toxin	cAMP
Escherichia coli[160, 161]	Heat-labile toxin	cAMP
	Heat-stable toxin (STa)	cGMP
Aeromonas hydrophila[162, 163]	Heat-stable toxin	Not established
	Heat-labile toxin	? cAMP
Bacillus cereus[164]	Enterotoxin	? cAMP
Campylobacter spp.[165]	Heat-labile enterotoxin	Probably cAMP
Clostridium difficile[166, 167]	Toxin A (enterotoxin)	Calcium
	Toxin B (cytotoxin)	? cGMP
Clostridium perfringens	Enterotoxin	Not established
Enterobacter cloacae[168]	Heat-stable toxin	Not established
Klebsiella pneumoniae[169]	Enterotoxin	Not established
Salmonellae typhimurium[170]	Cholera-like toxin	cAMP
Shigellae dysenteriae 1[171]	Shiga toxin	? cAMP
Staphylococcus aureus[172]	Enterotoxin a-f	? cAMP
Yersenia enterocolitica[173]	Heat-stable toxin	cGMP

cAMP, Cyclic adenosine monophosphate; cGMP, cyclic guanosine monophosphate.

basal electrolyte transport both in health and in diarrhea.

Secretagogues

Those agents that can induce net fluid and electrolyte secretion (secretagogues) by stimulating active ion secretion can be classified into three general categories: *bacterial enterotoxins, hormones,* and *detergents.*

Bacterial Enterotoxins. To date, at least 13 bacteria have been identified that elaborate an exotoxin that produces net intestinal fluid and electrolyte secretion (that is, an enterotoxin) (Table 55–3).[148, 160–173] Cholera enterotoxin, the prototype, initially binds to a brush border receptor Gm_1 ganglioside, stimulates adenylate cyclase and increases mucosal cAMP, but it does not impair absorptive function or alter mucosal histology.[148] The heat-labile toxins (LT) of *E. coli* have structures similar to those of cholera toxin and also activate adenylate cyclase. The mechanism by which cholera enterotoxin and the LT toxins of *E. coli* activate adenylate cyclase involves adenosine diphosphate (ADP) ribosylation of the enzyme.[174] Not all bacterial toxins, however, increase mucosal cAMP, and both cGMP and calcium can explain the action of certain enterotoxins on intestinal function. Cyclic GMP has been implicated as the intracellular mediator of the changes of ion transport produced by the heat-stable (ST) toxin of *Escherichia coli* and *Yersinia enterocolitica,*[161, 173] whereas calcium appears to be required for the alteration in ion transport produced by the enterotoxin of *Clostridium difficile.*[166]

Diarrhea secondary to infectious agents is not caused solely by enterotoxins. Net fluid secretion is present in experimental salmonellosis, shigellosis, and so-called transmissible gastroenteritis (produced by both coronaviruses and rotaviruses).[142, 175–177] Although the exact mechanism of net fluid secretion is not known in these experimental models, significant changes in ion transport and morphologic damage have been identified. Whether endogenously produced prostaglandins are important in the production of ion secretion associated with bacteria-induced mucosal damage requires clarification.[178] The recent demonstration that amebae release serotonin raises the additional possibility that the diarrhea in amebic colitis may in part be mediated by serotonin.[179] Thus, microorganisms can either release or result in the production of many substances (exotoxins, neurohumoral substances, arachidonic acid metabolites) that can alter ion transport (see pp. 1192–1198).

Hormones. Several hormones, when injected intravenously into humans or experimental animals or when studied *in vitro,* produce net fluid and electrolyte secretion or stimulate active ion secretion, respectively (see footnote on p. 1034) (Table 55–4).[113, 117, 122, 152, 181–189] VIP and PGE_1 stimulate adenylate cyclase, increase mucosal cAMP, and produce changes of ion transport in rabbit ileum and rat colon qualitatively similar to those observed with cAMP and cholera

Table 55–4. HORMONES AND NEUROTRANSMITTERS THAT STIMULATE ACTIVE ELECTROYTE SECRETION

Agonist	Intracellular Mediator
Vasoactive intestinal peptide	cAMP[117]
Secretin	cAMP[180, 185]
Prostaglandin E_1	cAMP[181]
Bradykinin	cAMP*[122]
Adenosine	cAMP[182]
Cholinergic muscarinic agonists	Calcium[113]
Serotonin	Calcium[152]
Substance P	Calcium[183]
Neurotensin	Calcium[183]
Peptide histidine isoleucine (PHI)	Not established[188]
Cholecystokinin	Not established[186]
Gastric inhibitory peptide	Not established[184]
Calcitonin	Not established[189]
Glucagon	Not established[187]

*Via release and metabolism of arachidonic acid.
cAMP, Cyclic adenosine monophosphate.

Table 55–5. LAXATIVES THAT PRODUCE NET FLUID AND ELECTROLYTE SECRETION

Laxative	Intracellular Mediator
Ricinoleic acid[191]	? cAMP
Dihydroxy bile acids[192]	? cAMP
Senokot[193]	Calcium
Phenolphthalein[194]	Not established
Bisacodyl[195]	Not established
Oxyphenisatin[196]	Not established
Dioctyl sodium sulfosuccinate[197]	Not established
Magnesium salts[198]	Not established
Anthraquinones[199]	Not established

cAMP, Cyclic adenosine monophosphate.

enterotoxin.[117, 181] Recent studies establish that bradykinin stimulates active chloride secretion via activation of membrane phospholipases that initiate arachidonic acid catabolism with the production of prostaglandins, which in turn activate adenylate cyclase.[122] Serotonin, calcitonin, and substance P alter active ion transport but do not increase mucosal cAMP or cGMP. The intracellular mediator of serotonin, substance P, and cholinergic-induced changes of ion transport is an increase in the cytosolic concentration of calcium.[113, 152, 183] The mechanism by which several other hormones (for example, calcitonin, glucagon) produce secretion is not related to cAMP, cGMP, or calcium and is at present unknown (see pp. 78–107).

Detergents. Detergents that alter intestinal fluid and electrolyte movement include bile acids, fatty acids, hydroxy fatty acids, and several commercial laxatives.[190] All commercial laxatives studied to date produce changes in small or large intestinal fluid and electrolyte transport (that is, they either decrease net absorption or cause net secretion) to account for their laxative action (Table 55–5).[191–199] The diarrhea associated with ileal dysfunction and steatorrhea is most likely mediated by changes in colonic fluid movement produced by dihydroxy bile acids and fatty acids, respectively.

In addition to the ability of bile acids (which have been studied more than the other detergents) either to decrease net fluid and electrolyte absorption or to produce net fluid and electrolyte secretion, detergents produce several other changes in intestinal function: They stimulate active anion secretion, increase mucosal permeability, alter colonic motility, and alter mucosal morphology.[200] There are two controversies regarding detergent-induced changes of net fluid absorption (Fig. 55–18); these relate to the mechanism by which detergents induce active anion secretion and the role of increased permeability in fluid secretion. At present there are experimental data to support several possible hypotheses for bile acid–induced active anion secretion: (1) direct stimulation of mucosal cAMP; (2) indirect stimulation via release of PGs; (3) bile acids functioning as calcium ionophores; and (4) involvement in part by enteric neurons.[201–204]

In addition to stimulating active ion secretion, bile acids increase mucosal permeability. Although controversial, it is most likely that the changes in mucosal permeability are not solely responsible for the alteration in fluid and electrolyte movement, but that net fluid secretion is the result of *both* active anion secretion and increased mucosal permeability. Regardless of any role that altered permeability may have in the genesis of fluid secretion, the increase in mucosal permeability in the colon produced by bile acids and fatty acids is responsible, however, for the increase in colonic oxalate absorption that underlies the increase in urinary oxalate excretion of patients with ileal disease (enteric hyperoxaluria).[205]

Miscellaneous. Animals sensitized to egg albumin will secrete water and electrolytes when challenged with antigen. This reaction is associated with mast cell degranulation and reduced histamine levels; doxantrazole, a mast cell–stabilizing agent, prevents this reaction.[206, 207] Previous studies have revealed that histamine (acting as an H_1 agonist) stimulates active chloride secretion *in vitro*.[208] These observations provide an experimental model to explore IgE-mediated mucosal reactions to food protein and to determine how immune reactions in the lamina propria can modify epithelial cell function. Extension of these observations should have significant impact on the clinical problems of "food allergy" (see pp. 1113–1134).

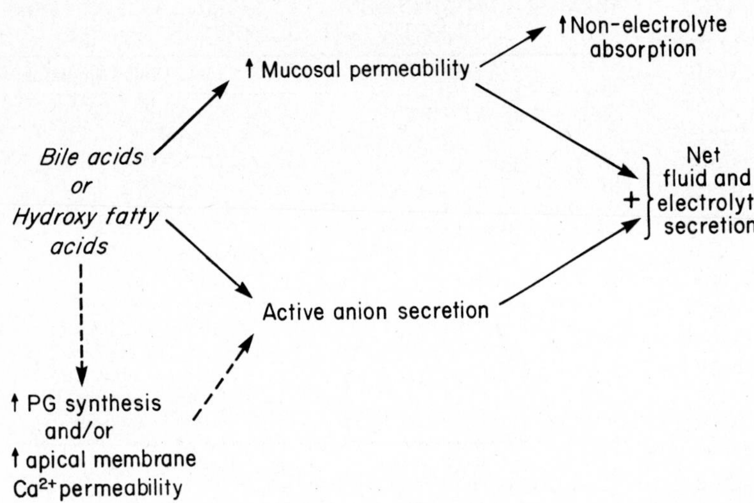

Figure 55–18. Model to explain bile acid or fatty acid induced fluid secretion. It is likely that net fluid secretion is the result of *both* active anion secretion *and* increased mucosal permeability. At least three different explanations have been advanced to explain active anion secretion. See text for additional detais. (Modified from Binder, H. J., and Sandle, G. I. *In* Johnson, L. R. [ed.]. Physiology of the Gastrointestinal Tract. 2nd ed. New York, Raven Press, 1987, p. 1389. Used by permission.)

Diminished Active Solute Absorption

Diminished solute absorption is attributable either to the effects of altered mucosal morphology or to deletion of discrete transport mechanisms. Excellent examples of net fluid secretion by damaged mucosa include *celiac sprue* and the experimental model of *viral enteritis* (TGE).[176] In celiac sprue, a "flat" mucosa is present, with absent villi, abnormal surface epithelial cells, and an increased number of crypt cells. Net fluid secretion seen in these patients is the result of diminished absorption (as a result of the decreased number of surface epithelial cells) and increased secretion (as a result of the increased number of crypt epithelial cells). In TGE a transient decrease in villus surface epithelial cells occurs that is associated with decreased glucose absorption and net sodium secretion. Within four to five days, both villus surface cells and transport processes return to normal. In this model, net fluid secretion is primarily a result of a diminished number of surface epithelial cells without any increase in crypt epithelial cells.

Congenital deletion of a transport process occurs in *congenital chloridorrhea* and in monosaccharide malabsorption.[43, 44, 209] In the former, the chloride-bicarbonate exchange in the ileum and colon is absent, resulting in an increased concentration of chloride in stool. In monosaccharide malabsorption, there is a defect in the absorption of actively transported hexoses (i.e., glucose, galactose). Recently an absence of the sodium-hydrogen exchange process in the jejunum was described in an infant with "secretory" diarrhea.[29]

Increased Luminal Osmolality

Perfusion of a segment of intestine with a hyperosmolar solution (usually over 340 mOm/kg water) results in net fluid secretion. The diarrheal disorder that represents the best clinical analogy of this experimental phenomenon is *lactase deficiency*. Catabolism of nonabsorbed disaccharides by enteric bacteria in the distal ileum and colon results in an increase in fluid osmolality and an alteration of normal fluid and electrolyte absorption in the colon.[127] The increase in luminal fluid in lactase deficiency in the jejunum is secondary to increased effective osmotic pressure as well as to diminished luminal sodium concentration and the absence of luminal glucose.

Increased Hydrostatic Pressure

Experimental elevation of mesenteric venous pressure or of volume expansion in animals clearly establishes that increased hydrostatic pressure produces net fluid and electrolyte secretion.[143, 144, 210] An increase in mucosal permeability in these models also contributes to net fluid secretion. One possible clinical analogy to experimentally induced net fluid secretion due to increased hydrostatic pressure may be seen in patients with increased intraluminal pressure and luminal distention.[211] It is possible, however, that net fluid secretion in this model is in part induced by cholinergic mechanisms elicited by distention of the intestinal wall.[212] The failure to observe changes in net fluid movement in patients with chronic portal hypertension[213] suggests that acute and chronic increases in hydrostatic pressure affect intestinal electrolyte movement differently.

Other Mechanisms That May Result in Altered Fluid and Electrolyte Movement

Considerable experimental data are available to confirm the role of the four mechanisms just discussed in producing alterations of net fluid and electrolyte movement and the genesis of diarrhea: *active ion secretion, diminished solute absorption, increased luminal osmolarity,* and *increased hydrostatic pressure.* Several other mechanisms, outlined in the next section, may be important but their roles are not clearly established.

Altered Intestinal Motility. Considerable controversy persists as to the precise importance of altered intestinal motility in the genesis of diarrhea. Diminished motor function with increased transit time can undoubtedly produce stasis and bacterial overgrowth. *Scleroderma* is an excellent example (see pp. 1289–1297), and the diarrhea in this condition is secondary to the steatorrhea produced by bacterial overgrowth.[214] In addition, it should be noted that opiates also prolong transit time. The increased contact time very likely explains the increased fluid and electrolyte absorption that is the basis for their antidiarrheal effect (see p. 1032).

It is more difficult to establish that diminished transit time produces changes in fluid and electrolyte movement. Although more rapid flow should never induce net fluid and electrolyte secretion, it could diminish fluid absorption. However, experimental data confirming such a phenomenon do not exist. Increasing perfusion speed is one way to study the effect of transit time on absorption, but it also increases fluid load. Indeed, this experimental approach increases rather than decreases fluid and sodium absorption.[215]

Changes in myoelectric activity (i.e., induction of migrating action potential complexes or repetitive bursts of action potentials, or both) have been described in several models of diarrhea produced by cholera enterotoxin, *Shigella, E. coli,* and ricinoleic acid.[216–220] It is possible that observed changes in motor function represent events that are secondary to abnormal fluid and electrolyte transport. It is evident that the relationship of (1) muscle function to intraluminal pressure, (2) intraluminal pressure to transit time, and (3) flow rate (i.e., transit time) to fluid and electrolyte absorption require additional study, probably using new methodologic approaches. Neurohumoral regulation of transit and transport are probably interrelated, and such factors must be considered in the future. The recent demonstration of an "ileal brake," which is an inhibition of motor activity with a prolongation of transit time following perfusion of the ileum with lipid, emphasizes the need to study this problem in the whole organism with particular attention to neurohumoral relationships.[221] Such studies likely will require simultaneous measurement of motor activity and fluid and electrolyte movement to define the role of altered intestinal motility in the development of diarrhea.

Increased Mucosal Permeability. Increased permeability occurs in several situations in which there is net fluid and electrolyte secretion (e.g., perfusion with bile acids and hydroxy fatty acids, volume expansion, and increased luminal distention).[143, 191, 211] Changes in mucosal permeability should not result in changes in *net* electrolyte movement *in vitro*. Increased mucosal permeability together with resting hydrostatic pressure may contribute to the observed changes of fluid and electrolyte movement that are produced in *in vivo* experimental diarrheal models.

Mucosal Damage. Although many diarrheal disorders are associated with mucosal damage and inflammation (e.g., *celiac sprue, salmonellosis,* and so on), it is unlikely that these mucosal abnormalities represent the primary *mechanism* responsible for the observed changes in fluid and electrolyte movement. Rather, the mucosal damage may result in (1) decreased solute absorption secondary to a defect in surface mucosal cells, or (2) increased ion secretion, either secondary to an increase in crypt cells (e.g., celiac sprue) or possibly mediated by increased prostaglandin synthesis (e.g., ulcerative colitis).[119]

This discussion of the several specific mechanisms that can alter fluid and electrolyte movement should not be interpreted to mean that changes in fluid movement in all diarrheal disorders are always the result of a *single* mechanism. In reality, it is most likely that the diarrhea in various gastrointestinal diseases is the result of more than one cause and that multiple mechanisms may be present simultaneously. For example, at least three separate mechanisms are responsible for the diarrhea present in *celiac sprue:* one, active ion secretion occurs in the jejunum, probably as a result of the increased number of crypt epithelial cells together with the decreased number of villous epithelial cells; two, increased luminal osmolarity occurs subsequently to secondary lactase deficiency, which is the result of mucosal damage; and three, fatty acid–induced fluid secretion in the colon is secondary to steatorrhea.

There are additional examples in which more than one mechanism can be identified as responsible for the alterations in fluid movement that results in diarrhea. Thus, in *ulcerative colitis* the mucosal inflammatory reaction is responsible for both decreased absorption as a consequence of alteration of colonic surface epithelial cells and a stimulation of active electrolyte secretion secondary to enhanced prostaglandin synthesis. In *gastrinoma,* albeit a rare condition, diarrhea is present not infrequently either with or without ulcer disease. There are at least three separate mechanisms for this diarrhea. One factor is fluid volume overload of the small intestinal absorptive capacity by the substantial increase in gastric fluid secretion. Another is the steatorrhea that is present in some patients with gastrinoma as a result of a low duodenal pH with inactivation of pancreatic lipase and precipitation of bile acids. The resulting nonabsorbed fatty acids induce fluid secretion in the colon. The third mechanism is related to enhanced plasma gastrin levels that can reduce small intestinal fluid and electrolyte absorption.[222] In all of these conditions there is undoubtedly a role for an additional contributing factor: intestinal motor function.

References

1. Phillips, S. F., and Giller, J. The contribution of the colon to electrolyte and water conservation in man. J. Lab. Clin. Med. *81*:733, 1973.
2. Kennedy, H. J., Al-Dujaili, E. A. S., Edward, C. R. W., and Truelove, S. C. Water and electrolyte balance in subjects with a permanent ileostomy. Gut *24*:702, 1983.
3. Ladas, S. D., Isaacs, P. E. T., Murphy, G. M., and Sladen, G. E. Fasting and postprandial ileal function in adapted ileostomates and normal subjects. Gut *27*:906, 1986.
4. Billich, C. O., and Levitan, R. Effects of sodium concentration and osmolality on water and electrolyte absorption from the intact human colon. J. Clin. Invest. *48*:1336, 1969.
5. Debongnie, J. C., and Phillips, S. F. Capacity of the human colon to absorb fluid. Gastroenterology *74*:698, 1978.
6. Curran, P. F., and MacIntosh, J. R. A model system for biological water transport. Nature (Lond.) *193*:347, 1962.
7. Diamond, J. M. Osmotic water flow in leaky epithelia. J. Membr. Biol. *51*:195, 1979.
8. Fordtran, J. S., Rector, F. C., Jr., and Carter, W. The mechanisms of sodium absorption in the human small intestine. J. Clin. Invest. *47*:884, 1968.
9. Persson, B. E., and Spring, K. R. Gall bladder epithelial cell hydraulic water permeability and volume regulation. J. Gen. Physiol. *79*:481, 1982.
10. Fordtran, J. S., Rector, F. C., Locklear, T. W., and Ewton, M. F. Water and solute movement in the small intestine of patients with sprue. J. Clin. Invest. *46*:287, 1967.
11. Schultz, S. G., and Zalusky, R. Ion transport in isolated rabbit ileum. I. Short-circuit current and Na Fluxes. J. Gen Physiol. *47*:567, 1964.
12. Binder, H. J., and Rawlins, C. L. Electrolyte transport across isolated large intestinal mucosa. Am. J. Physiol. *225*:1232, 1973.
13. Murer, H., and Kinne, R. The use of isolated vesicles to study epithelial transport processes. J. Membr. Biol. *55*:81, 1980.
14. Jodal, M., Lundrgen, O. Countercurrent mechanisms in the mammalian gastrointestinal tract. Gastroenterology *91*:225, 1986.
15. Welsh, M., Smith, P., Fromm, M., and Frizzell, R. F.: Crypts are the site of intestinal fluid and electrolyte secretion. Science *218*:1219, 1982.
16. Schafer, J. A., and Andreoli, T. E. Principles of water and electrolyte transport across membranes. *In* Andreoli, T. E., Hoffman, J. F., Fanestil, D. D., and Schultz, S. G. (eds.). Physiology of Membrane Disorders. 2nd edition. New York, Plenum Medical Book Company, 1986, p. 177.
17. Schultz, S. G. Cellular models of epithelial ion transport. *In* Andreoli, T. E., Hoffman, J. F., Fanestil, D. D., and Schultz, S. G. (eds.). Physiology of Membrane Disorders. 2nd edition. New York, Plenum Medical Book Company, 1986, p. 519.
18. Fordtran, J. S., Rector, F. C., Ewton, M. F., Soter, N., and Kinney, J. Permeability characteristics of the human small intestine. J. Clin. Invest. *44*:1935, 1965.
19. Schultz, S. G. A cellular model for active sodium absorption by mammalian colon. Ann. Rev. Physiol. *46*:435, 1984.
20. Schultz, S. G., and Curran, P. F. Coupled transport of sodium and organic solutes. Physiol. Rev. *50*:637, 1970.

21. Aronson, P. S. Identifying secondary active solute transport in epithelia. Am. J. Physiol. *240*:F1, 1981.
22. Frizzell, R. A., Koch, M. J., and Schultz, S. G. Ion transport by rabbit colon. I. Active and passive components. J. Membr. Biol. *27*:297, 1976.
23. Goldner, A. M., Schultz, S. G., and Curran, P. F. Sodium and sugar fluxes across the mucosal border of rabbit ileum. J. Gen. Physiol. *53*:362, 1969.
24. Hopfer, U., Sigrist-Nelson, K., Ammann, E., and Murer, H. Differences in neutral amino acid and glucose transport between brush border and basolateral membrane of intestinal epithelial cells. J. Cell. Physiol. *89*:805, 1976.
25. Turnberg, L. A., Fordtran, J. S., Carter, N. W., and Rector, F. C. Mechanism of bicarbonate absorption and its relationship to sodium transport in the human jejunum. J. Clin. Invest. *49*:548, 1970.
26. Murer, H., Hopfer, U., and Kinne, R. Sodium/proton antiport in brush-border-membrane vesicles isolated from rat small intestine and kidney. Biochem. J. *154*:597, 1976.
27. Knickelbein, R., Aronson, P. S., Atherton, W., and Dobbins, J. W. Na and Cl transport across rabbit ileal brush border. I. Evidence for Na/H exchange. Am. J. Physiol. *245*:G504, 1983.
28. Binder, H. J., Strange, G., Murer, H., Steiger, B., and Hauri, H. P. Sodium-proton exchange in colon brush-border membranes. Am. J. Physiol. *251*:G382, 1986.
29. Booth, I. W., Stange, G., Murer, H., Fenton, T. R., and Milla, P. J. Defective jejunal brush border Na^+/H^+ exchange. A cause of secretory diarrhea. Lancet *2*:1066, 1985.
30. Seiffer, J. L., and Aronson, P. S. Properties and physiologic roles of the plasma membrane sodium-hydrogen exchanger. J. Clin. Invest. *78*:859, 1986.
31. Frizzell, R. A., Field, M., and Schultz, S. G. Sodium-coupled chloride transport by epithelial tissue. Am. J. Physiol. *236*:F1, 1979.
32. Donowitz, M. Ca^{2+} in the control of active intestinal Na and Cl transport: Involvement in neurohumoral action. Am. J. Physiol. *245*:G165, 1983.
33. Ahn, J., Chang, E. B., and Field, M.: Phorbol ester inhibition of Na-H exchange in rabbit proximal colon. Am. J. Physiol. *249*:C527, 1985.
34. Turnberg, L. A., Bieberdorf, F. A., Morawski, S. G., and Fordtran, J. S. Interrelationships of chloride, bicarbonate, sodium and hydrogen transport in the human ileum. J. Clin. Invest. *49*:557, 1970.
35. Knickelbein, R. G., Aronson, P. S., Schron, C. M., Seifter, J., and Dobbins, J. W. Na and Cl transport across rabbit ileal brush border. II. Evidence for Cl:HCO_3 exchange and mechanism of coupling. Am. J. Physiol. *249*:G236, 1985.
36. Dharmsathaphorn, K., Mandel, K. G., Masui, H., and McRoberts, J. A. Vasoactive intestinal polypeptide-induced secretion by a colonic epithelial cell line. J. Clin. Invest. *75*:462, 1985.
37. Schultz, S. G., and Zalusky, R. Ion transport in isolated rabbit ileum. II. The interaction between active sodium and active sugar transport. J. Gen. Physiol. *47*:1043, 1964.
38. Binder, H. J. Sodium transport across isolated human jejunum. Gastroenterology *67*:231, 1974.
39. Fordtran, J. S. Stimulation of active and passive sodium absorption by sugars in the human jejunum. J. Clin. Invest. *55*:728, 1975.
40. Powell, D. W., Binder, H. J., and Curran, P. F. Electrolyte secretion by the guinea pig ileum *in vitro*. Am. J. Physiol. *223*:531, 1972.
41. Devroede, G. J., and Phillips, S. F. Conservation of sodium, chloride and water by the human colon. Gastroenterology *56*:421, 1969.
42. Duffey, M. Intracellular pH and bicarbonate activities in rabbit colon. Am. J. Physiol. *246*:C558, 1984.
43. Holmberg, C., Perheentupa, J., and Launiala, K. Colonic electrolyte transport in health and congenital chloride diarrhea. J. Clin. Invest. *56*:302, 1975.
44. Bieberdorf, F. A., Gordon, P., and Fordtran, J. S. Pathogenesis of congenital alkalosis with diarrhea. J. Clin. Invest. *51*:1958, 1972.
45. Donowitz, M., and Welsh, M. J. Regulation of mammalian small intestinal electrolyte secretion. *In* Johnson, L. R. (ed.). Physiology of the Gastrointestinal Tract. 2nd edition. New York, Raven Press, 1987, p. 1351.
46. Binder, H. J., and Sandle, G. I. Electrolyte absorption and secretion in the mammalian colon. *In* Johnson, L. R. (ed.). Physiology of the Gastrointestinal Tract. 2nd edition. New York, Raven Press, 1987, p. 1389.
47. Davis, G. R., Santa Ana, C. A., Morawski, S., and Fordtran, J. S. Active chloride secretion in the normal human jejunum. J. Clin. Invest. *66*:1326, 1980.
48. Heintze, K., Stewart, C., and Frizzell, R.: Sodium-dependent chloride secretion across rabbit descending colon. Am. J. Physiol. *244*:G357, 1983.
49. Cartwright, C. A., McRoberts, J. A., Mandel, K. G., and Dharmsathaphorn, K. Synergistic action of cyclic adenosine monophosphate- and calcium-chloride secretion in a colonic epithelial cell line. J. Clin. Invest. *76*:1837, 1985.
50. Dharmsathaphorn, K., Pandol, S. J. Mechanism of chloride secretion induced by carbachol in a colonic epithelial cell line. J. Clin. Invest. *77*:348, 1986.
51. Horvath, P. J., Ferriola, P. C., Weiser, M. M., and Duffey, M. E. Localization of chloride secretion in rabbit colon: inhibition by anthracene-9-carboxylic acid. Am. J. Physiol. *250*:G185, 1986.
52. Turnberg, L. A. Potassium transport in human small bowel. Gut *12*:811, 1971.
53. Foster, E. S., Hayslett, J. P., and Binder, H. J. Mechanism of active potassium absorption and secretion in the rat colon. Am. J. Physiol. *246*:G611, 1984.
54. Smith, P. L., and McCabe, R. D. Mechanism and regulation of transcellular potassium transport by the colon. Am. J. Physiol. *247*:G445, 1984.
55. Foster, E. S., Zimmerman, T. W., Hayslett, J. P., and Binder, H. J. Corticosteroid alteration of action electrolyte transport in rat distal colon. Am. J. Physiol. *245*:G668, 1983.
56. Foster, E. S., Sandle, G. I., Hayslett, J. P., and Binder, H. J. Dietary potassium modulates active potassium absorption and secretion in rat distal colon. Am. J. Physiol. *251*:G619, 1986.
57. Gustin, M. C., and Goodman, D. B. P. Isolation of brush border membrane from the rabbit descending colon epithelium: partial characterization of a unique potassium-activated ATPase. J. Biol. Chem. *256*:10651, 1981.
58. Foster, E. S., Sandle, G. I., Hayslett, J. P., and Binder, H. J. Cyclic adenosine monophosphate stimulates active potassium secretion in the rat colon. Gastroenterology *84*:324, 1983.
59. Ruppin, H., Bar-Meir, S., Soergel, K. H., Wood, C. M., and Schmitt, M. G., Jr. Absorption of short-chain fatty acids by the colon. Gastroenterology *78*:1500, 1980.
60. Bond, J. H., Currier, B. E., Buchwald, H., and Levitt, M. D. Colonic conservation of malabsorbed carbohydrate. Gastroenterology *78*:444, 1980.
61. Sellin, J. H., and DeSoignie, R. Rabbit proximal colon: a distinct transport epithelium. Am. J. Physiol. *246*:G603, 1984.
62. Sandle, G. I., Wills, N. K., Alles, W., and Binder, H. J. Electrophysiology of the human colon: evidence of segmental heterogeneity. Gut *27*:999, 1986.
63. Foster, E. S., Budinger, M. E., Hayslett, J. P., and Binder, H. J. Ion transport in proximal colon of the rat: sodium depletion stimulates neutral sodium chloride absorption. J. Clin. Invest. *77*:228, 1986.
64. Clauss, W., Schafer, H., Horch, I., and Hornicke, H. Segmental differences in electrical properties and Na-transport of rabbit caecum, proximal and distal colon *in vitro*. Pfluegers Arch. *403*:278, 1985.
65. Devroede, G. J., and Phillips, S. F. Failure of the human rectum to absorb electrolyte and water. Gut *11*:438, 1970.
66. Binder, H. J., Foster, E. S., Budinger, M. E., and Hayslett, J. P. Mechanism of electroneutral sodium-chloride absorption in distal colon of the rat. Gastroenterology *93*:449, 1987.
67. Hubel, K. A. The effects of electrical field stimulation and tetrodotoxin on ion transport by the isolated rabbit ileum. J. Clin. Invest. *62*:1039, 1978.
68. Cooke, H. J. Influence of enteric cholinergic neurons on

mucosal transport in guinea pig ileum. Am. J. Physiol. *246*:G263, 1984.

69. Cooke, H. J., Shonnard, K., Highison, G., and Wood, J. D. Effects of neurotransmitter release on mucosal transport in guinea pig ileum. Am. J. Physiol. *245*:G745, 1983.
70. Hubel, K. A., Renquist, K., and Shiragi, S. Ion transport in human cecum, transverse colon and sigmoid colon *in vitro*. Base line and response to electrical stimulation of intrinsic nerves. Gastroenterology *92*:501, 1987.
71. Cassuto, J., Jodal, M., and Lundgren, O. The effect of nicotinic and muscarinic receptor blockade on cholera toxin-induced intestinal secretion. Acta Physiol. Scand. *114*:573, 1982.
72. Cassuto, J., Jodal, M., Tuttle, R., and Lundgren, O. On the role of intramural nerves in the pathogenesis of cholera toxin-induced intestinal secretion. Scand. J. Gastroenterol. *16*:377, 1981.
73. Lenz, H. J., Mortrud, M. T., Rivier, J. E., and Brown, M. R. Central nervous system actions of calcitonin gene-related peptide on gastric acid secretion in the rat. Gastroenterology *88*:539, 1985.
74. Bueno, L., Fargeas, M. J., Fioramonti, J., and Primi, M. P. Central control of intestinal motility by prostaglandins: a mediator of the actions of several peptides in rats and dogs. Gastroenterology *88*:1888, 1985.
75. Fogel, R., Kaplan, R. B., and Arbit, E. Central action of the α aminobutyric acid ligands to alter basal water and electrolyte absorption in the rat ileum. Gastroenterology *88*:523, 1985.
76. Primi, M. P., and Bueno, L. Central nervous system influence of prostaglandin E2 on jejunal water and electrolyte transport in conscious dogs. Gastroenterology *91*:1427, 1986.
77. Primi, M. P., Bueno, L., and Fioramonti, J. Central regulation of intestinal basal stimulated water and ion transport by endogenous opiates in dogs. Dig. Dis. Sci. *311*:172, 1986.
78. Yamada, T. Local regulatory actions of gastrointestinal peptides. *In* Johnson, L. R. (ed.). Physiology of the Gastrointestinal Tract. 2nd edition. New York, Raven Press, 1987, p. 131.
79. Dockray, G. J. Physiology of enteric neuropeptides. *In* Johnson, L. R. (ed.). Physiology of the Gastrointestinal Tract. 2nd edition. New York, Raven Press, 1987, p. 41.
80. Levitan, R., and Ingelfinger, F. J. Effect of D-aldosterone on salt and water absorption from the intact human colon. J. Clin. Invest. *44*:801, 1965.
81. Sandle, G. I., and Binder, H. J. Corticosteroids and intestinal electrolyte transport. Gastroenterology *93*:188, 1987.
82. Levens, N. R. Control of intestinal absorption by the renin-angiotensin system. Am. J. Physiol. *249*:G3, 1985.
83. Charney, A. N., and Donowitz, M. Prevention and reversal of cholera enterotoxin-induced intestinal secretion by methyl prednisolone induction of Na^+-K^+-ATPase. J. Clin. Invest. *57*:1590, 1976.
84. Binder, H. J. Effect of dexamethasone on electrolyte transport in the large intestine of the rat. Gasterenterology *75*:212, 1978.
85. Bastl, C., Barnett, C., Schmidt, T., and Litwack, G. Glucocorticoid stimulation of sodium absorption in colon epithelia is mediated by corticosteroid IB receptor. J. Biol. Chem. *259*:1186, 1984.
86. Binder, H. J., White, A., Whiting, D., and Hayslett, J. P. Demonstration of specific high-affinity receptors for aldosterone in cytosol of rat colon. Endocrinology *118*:628, 1986.
87. Sandle, G. I., Hayslett, J. P., Binder, H. J. The effect of glucocorticosteroids on rectal transport in normal subjects and patients with ulcerative colitis. Gut *27*:309, 1986.
88. Dobbins, J., Racusen, L., and Binder, H. J. Effect of D-alanine$_2$ methionine enkephalin amide on ion transport in the rabbit ileum. J. Clin. Invest. *66*:19, 1980.
89. McKay, J. S., Linaker, B. D., and Turnberg, L. A. Influence of opiates on ion transport across rabbit ileal mucosa. Gastroenterology *80*:279, 1981.
90. Binder, H. J., Laurenson, J. P., and Dobbins, J. W. Role of opiate receptors in the regulation of enkephalin stimulation of active sodium and chloride absorption. Am. J. Physiol. *247*:G432, 1984.
91. Fogel, R., and Kaplan, R. B. Role of enkephalins in regulation of basal intestinal water and ion absorption in the rat. Am. J. Physiol. *246*:G386, 1984.
92. Brown, D. R., and Miller, R. J. Adrenergic mediation of the intestinal antisecretory action of opiates administered into the central nervous system. J. Pharmacol. Exp. Ther. *231*:114, 1984.
93. Coupar, I. M. Inhibition by morphine of prostaglandin-stimulated fluid secretion in rat jejunum. Br. J. Pharmacol. *63*:57, 1978.
94. Hughes, S., Higgs, N. B., and Turnbert, L. A. Loperamide has antisecretory activity in the human jejunum *in vivo*. Gut *25*:931, 1984.
95. Chang, E. B., Brown, D. R., Wang, N. S., and Field, M. Secretogogue-induced changes in membrane calcium permeability in chicken and chinchilla ileal mucosa. J. Clin. Invest. *78*:281, 1986.
96. Schiller, L. R., Davis, G. R., Santa Ana, C. A., and Morawski, S. G. Studies of the mechanism of the antidiarrheal effect of codeine. J. Clin. Invest. *70*:999, 1982.
97. Schiller, L. R., Santa Ana, C. A., Morawski, S. G., and Fordtran, J. S. Mechanism of the antidiarrheal effect of loperamide. Gastroenterology *86*:1475, 1984.
98. Dharmsathaphorn, K., Rascusen, L., and Dobbins, J. W. Effect of somatostatin on ion transport in rat colon. J. Clin. Invest. *66*:813, 1980.
99. Dharmsathaphorn, K., Binder, H. J., and Dobbins, J. W. Somatostatin stimulates sodium and chloride absorption in the rabbit ileum. Gastroenterology *78*:1559, 1980.
100. Davis, G. R., Camp, R. C., Raskin, P., and Krejs, G. J. Effect of somatostatin infusion in jejunal water and electrolyte transport in a patient with secretory diarrhea due to malignant carcinoid syndrome. Gastroenterology *78*:346, 1980.
101. Dharmsathaphorn, K., Sherwin, R., Cataland, S., Jaffe, B., and Dobbins, J. W. Somatostatin inhibits diarrhea in the carcinoid syndrome. Ann. Intern. Med. *92*:68, 1980.
102. Bonfils, S. New somatostatin molecule for management of endocrine tumors. Gut *26*:433, 1985.
103. Kraenzlin, M. E., Ch'ng, J. L. C., Wood, S. M., Carr, D. A., Bloom, S. R. Long-term treatment of a VIPoma with somatostatin analogue resulting in remission of symptoms and possible shrinkage of metastases. Gastroenterology *88*:185, 1985.
104. Field, M., and McColl, I. Ion transport in rabbit ileal mucosa. III. Effects of catecholamines. Am. J. Physiol. *225*:852, 1973.
105. Racusen, L. C., and Binder, H. J. Adrenergic interaction with ion transport across colonic mucosa: role of both α and β adrenergic agonists. *In* Binder, H. J. (ed.). Mechanisms of Intestinal Secretion. New York, Alan R. Liss, 1979, p. 201.
106. Chang, E. B., Field, M., and Miller, R. J. Alpha$_2$-adrenergic receptor regulation of ion transport in rabbit ileum. Am. J. Physiol. *242*:G237, 1982.
107. Chang, E. B., Field, M., and Miller, R. J. Enterocyte α_2-adrenergic receptors: yohimbine and p-aminoclonidine binding relative to ion transport. Am. J. Physiol. *244*:G76, 1983.
108. Donowitz, M., Cusalito, S., Battisti, L., Fogel, R., and Sharp, G. W. G. Dopamine stimulation of active Na and Cl absorption in rabbit ileum: interaction with alpha$_2$-adrenergic and specific dopamine receptors. J. Clin. Invest. *69*:1008, 1982.
109. Chang, E., Bergenstal, R. M., and Field, M. Diarrhea in streptozocin-treated rats. Loss of adrenergic regulation of intestinal fluid and electrolyte transport. J. Clin. Invest. *75*:1666, 1985.
110. McArthur, K., Anderson, D., Durbin, T., Orloff, M., and Dharmsathaphorn, K. Clonidine and lidamidine inhibit watery diarrhea in a patient with lung cancer. Ann. Intern. Med. *96*:323, 1982.
111. Chang, E. B., Fedorak, R. N., and Field, M. Experimental diabetic diarrhea in rats. Intestinal mucosal denervation hypersensitivity and treatment with clonidine. Gastroenterology *91*:564, 1986.
112. Tapper, E. J., Powell, D. W., and Morris, S. M. Cholinergic-adrenergic interactions on intestinal ion transport. Am. J. Physiol. *4*:E402, 1978.
113. Zimmerman, T. W., Dobbins, J. W., and Binder, H. J.

Demonstration of cholinergic regulation of electrolyte transport in rat colon *in vitro*. Am. J. Physiol. *242*:G209, 1982.

114. Krejs, G. J., and Fordtran, J. Effect of VIP infusion on water and ion transport in the human jejunum. Gastroenterology *78*:722, 1980.
115. Krejs, G. J., Walsh, J. H., Morawski, S. G., and Fordtran, J. S. Intractable diarrhea: intestinal perfusion studies and plasma VIP concentrations in patients with pancreatic cholera syndrome and surreptitious ingestion of laxatives and diuretics. Am. J. Dig. Dis. *22*:280, 1977.
116. Dharmsathaphorn, K., Harms, V., Yalashiro, D. J., Hughes, R. J., Binder, H. J., and Wright, E. M. Preferential binding of vasoactive intestinal polypeptide to basolateral membrane of rat and rabbit enterocytes. J. Clin. Invest. *71*:27, 1983.
117. Schwartz, C. J., Kimberg, K. V., Sheerin, H. E., Field, M., and Said, S. I. Vasoactive intestinal peptide stimulation of adenylate cyclase and active electrolyte secretion in intestinal mucosa. J. Clin. Invest. *54*:536, 1974.
118. Musch, M. W., Miller, R. J., Field, M., and Siegel, M. I. Metabolites of colonic secretion by lipoxygenase metabolites of arachidonic acid. Science *217*:1255, 1982.
119. Sharon, P., Ligumsky, M., Rachmilewitz, D., and Zor, U. Role of prostaglandins in ulcerative colitis: enhanced production during active disease and inhibition by sulfasalazine. Gastroenterology *75*:638, 1978.
120. Sharon, P., and Stenson, W. Enhanced synthesis of leukotriene B_4 by colonic mucosa in inflammatory bowel disease. Gastroenterology *86*:453, 1984.
121. Beubler, E., and Juan, H. Effect of ricinoleic acid and other laxatives on net water flux and prostaglandin E release by the rat colon. J. Pharm. Pharmacol. *31*:681, 1979.
122. Musch, M. W., Viachur, J. F., Miller, R. J., Field, M., and Stoff, J. F. Bradykinin-stimulated electrolyte secretion in rabbit and guinea pig intestine: involvement of arachidonic acid metabolites. J. Clin. Invest. *71*:1073, 1983.
123. Binder, H. J. (ed). Mechanisms of Intestinal Secretion. New York, Alan R. Liss, 1979.
124. Field, M., Fordtran, J. S., and Schultz, S. G. (eds.). Secretory Diarrhea. Washington, D.C., American Physiological Society, 1980.
125. Argenzio, R. A., Moon, H. W., Kemony, L. J., and Whipp, S. C. Colonic compensation in transmissible gastroenteritis in swine. Gastroenterology *86*:1501, 1984.
126. Read, N. W. Diarrhea: the failure of colonic salvage. Lancet *2*:481, 1982.
127. Christopher, N. L., and Bayless, T. M. Role of the small bowel and colon in lactose-induced diarrhea. Gastroenterology *60*:845, 1971.
128. Fordtran, J. S., Rector, F. C., Locklear, T. W., and Ewton, M. F. Water and solute movement in the small intestine of patients with sprue. J. Clin. Invest. *46*:287, 1967.
129. Banwell, J. G., Gorbach, S. L., Mitra, R., Casells, J. S., Guhu Mazumder, D. N., Thomas, J., and Yardley, J. H. Tropical sprue and malnutrition in West Bengal. II. Fluid and electrolyte transport in the small intestine. Am. J. Clin. Nutr. *23*:1559, 1970.
130. Atwell, J. D., and Duthie, H. L. The absorption of water, sodium and potassium from the ileum of humans showing the effects of regional enteritis. Gastroenterology *46*:16, 1964.
131. Harris, J., and Shields, R. Absorption and secretion of water and electrolytes by the intact human colon in diffuse untreated proctocolitis. Gut *11*:27, 1970.
132. Wright, H. K., O'Brien, J. J., and Tilson, M. D. Water absorption in experimental closed segment obstruction of the ileum in man. Am. J. Surg. *121*:96, 1971.
133. Donowitz, M., and Binder, H. J. Jejunal fluid and electrolyte secretion in carcinoid syndrome. Am. J. Dig. Dis. *20*:1115, 1975.
134. Banwell, J. G., Pierce, N. F., Mitra, R. C., Brigham, K. L., Caranasos, G. J., Keimowitz, R. I., Fedson, D. S., Thomas, J., Gorbach, S. L., Sack, B., and Mondal, A. Intestinal fluid and electrolyte transport in human cholera. J. Clin. Invest. *49*:183, 1970.
135. Banwell, J. G., Gorbach, S. L., Pierce, N. F., Mitra, R., and Mondal, A. Acute undifferentiated human diarrhea in the tropics. II. Alterations in intestinal fluid and electrolyte movements. J. Clin. Invest. *50*:890, 1971.
136. Isaacs, P., Whittaker, S. M., and Turnberg, L. A. Diarrhea associated with medullary carcinoma of the thyroid. Studies of intestinal function in a patient. Gastroenterology *67*:521, 1974.
137. Davis, G. R., Corbett, D. B., and Krejs, G. J. Ileal chloride secretion as a cause of secretory diarrhea in a patient with primary intestinal tuberculosis. Gastroenterology *76*:829, 1979.
138. Phillips, S. F., and Schmid, W. C. Jejunal transport of electrolytes and water in intestinal disease. Gut *10*:990, 1969.
139. Theile, D. L., and Krejs, G. J. Secretory diarrhea in mixed connective tissue disease. Am. J. Gastroenterol. *80*:107, 1985.
140. Halsted, C. H., Robles, E. A., and Mexey, E. Intestinal malabsorption in folate-deficient alcoholics. Gastroenterology *64*:526, 1973.
141. Rask-Madsen, J., Grove, O., Hansen, M. G. J., Bukhave, K., and Henrik-Nielsen, R. Colonic transport of water and electrolytes in a patient with secretory diarrhea due to collagenous colitis. Dig. Dis. Sci. *28*:1141, 1983.
142. Giannella, R. A., Gots, R. E., Charney, A. N., Greenough, W. B., and Formal, S. B. Pathogenesis of salmonella-mediated intestinal fluid secretion. Gastroenterology *69*:1238, 1975.
143. Humphreys, M. H., and Earley, L. E. The mechanism of decreased intestinal sodium and water absorption after acute volume expansion in the rat. J. Clin. Invest. *50*:2355, 1971.
144. Yablonski, M. E., and Lifson, N. Mechanism of production of intestinal secretion by elevated venous pressure. J. Clin. Invest. *57*:904, 1976.
145. Caren, J. F., Meyer, J. H., and Grossman, M. I. Canine intestinal secretion during and after distention of the small bowel. Am. J. Physiol. *227*:183, 1974.
146. Curran, P. F., Webster, E. W., and Hovsepian, J. A. The effect of x-irradiation on sodium and water transport in rat ileum. Radiat. Res. *13*:369, 1960.
147. Nelson, R. A., Code, C. F., and Brown, A. L. Sorption of water and electrolytes and mucosal structure in niacin deficiency. Gastroenterology *42*:26, 1962.
148. Field, M., Fromm, D., Al-awqati, Q., and Greenough, W. B. Effect of cholera enterotoxin on ion transport across isolated ileal mucosa. J. Clin. Invest. *51*:796, 1972.
149. Racusen, L. C., and Binder, H. J. Effect of prostaglandin on ion transport across isolated colonic mucosa. Dig. Dis. Sci. *25*:900, 1980.
150. Rao, M. C., Orellana, S. A., Field, M., Robertson, D. C., Giannella, R. A. Comparison of the biological actions of three purified heat-stable enterotoxins: effects on ion transport and guanylate cyclase activity in rabbit ileum *in vitro*. Infect. Immun. *33*:165, 1981.
151. Bolton, J. E., and Field, M. Ca ionophore-stimulated ion secretion in rabbit ileal mucosa: Relation to actions of cyclic 3′,5′-AMP and carbamylcholine. J. Membr. Biol. *35*:159, 1977.
152. Donowitz, M., Asarkof, N., and Pike, G. Calcium dependence of serotonin-induced changes in rabbit ileal electrolyte transport. J. Clin. Invest. *66*:341, 1980.
153. Huott, P. A., Liu, W., McRoberts, J. A., Giannella, R. A., and Dharmsathaphorn, K. The mechanism of action of *E. coli* heat stable enterotoxin in a human colonic cell line. (Submitted for publication.)
154. Donowitz, M., Wicks, J., Madora, J. L., and Sharp, G. W. G. Studies on role of calmodulin in Ca^{2+} regulation of rabbit ileal Na and Cl transport. Am. J. Physiol. *248*:G726, 1985.
155. Fondacaro, J. D., Henderson, L. S. Evidence of protein kinase C as a regulator of intestinal electrolyte transport. Am. J. Physiol. *249*:G422, 1985.
156. Rassmussen, H. The calcium messenger system. N. Engl. J. Med. *314*:1094, 1164, 1986.
157. Donowitz, M., Cheng, H. Y., and Sharp, G. W. G. Effects of phorbol esters on sodium and chloride transport in rat colon. Am. J. Physiol. *251*:G509, 1986.
158. Ahn, J., Chang, E., and Field, M. Phorbol ester inhibition of Na-H exchange in rabbit proximal colon. Am. J. Physiol. *249*:C527, 1985.
159. Chang, E. B., Wang, N. S., and Rao, M. C. Phorbol ester stimulation of active anion secretion in intestine. Am. J. Physiol. *249*:C356, 1985.

160. Gill, D. M., and Richardson, S. H. Adenosine diphosphate-ribosylation of adenylate cyclase catalyzed by heat-labile enterotoxins of *E. coli:* comparison with cholera toxin. J. Infect. Dis. *141*:64, 1980.
161. Giannella, R. A., Drake, K. W.: Effect of purified *E. coli* heat-stable enterotoxin on intestinal cyclic nucleotide metabolism and fluid secretion. Infect. Immun. *24*:19, 1979.
162. Chakraborty, T., Montenegro, M. A., Sanyal, S. C., Helmuth, R., Bulling, E., and Timmis, K. N.: Cloning of enterotoxin gene from *Aeromonas hydrophila* provides conclusive evidence of production of cytotonic enterotoxin. Infect. Immun. *46*:435, 1984.
163. Honda, T., Sato, M., Nishimura, T., Higashitsutsumi, M., Fukai, K., and Miwatani, T.: Demonstration of cholera toxin-related factor in cultures of aeromonas species by ELISA. Infect. Immun. *50*:322, 1985.
164. Turnbull, P. C. B.: Studies on the production of enterotoxins by *Bacillus cereus*. J. Clin. Pathol. *29*:941, 1976.
165. Walker, R. I., Caldwell, M. B., Lee, E. C., Guerry, P., Trust, T. J., and Ruiz-Palacios, G. M.: Pathophysiology of *Campylobacter* enteritis. Microbiol. Rev. *50*:81, 1986.
166. Hughes, S., Warhurst, G., Turnberg, L. A., Higgs, N. B., Giugliano, L. G., and Drasar, B. S.: *C. difficile* toxin-induced intestinal secretion in rabbit ileum *in vitro*. Gut *224*:94, 1983.
167. Vesely, D. L., Straub, K. D., Nolan, C. M., Rolfe, R. D., Finegold, S. M., and Monson, T. P.: Purified *C. difficile* cytotoxin stimulates guanylate cyclase activity and inhibits adenylate cyclase activity. Infect. Immun. *33*:285, 1981.
168. Klipstein, F. A., and Engert, R. F.: Partial purification and properties of *Enterobacter cloacae* heat-stable enterotoxin. Infect. Immun. *13*:1307, 1976.
169. Klipstein, F. A., Horowitz, I. R., Engert, R. F., and Schenk, E. A.: Effect of *Klebsiella pneumoniae* enterotoxin on intestinal transport in the rat. J. Clin. Invest. *56*:799, 1975.
170. Giannella, R. A., Grots, R. E., Charney, A. N., Greenough, W. B., III, and Formal, S. B.: Pathogenesis of salmonella-mediated intestinal fluid secretion: activation of adenylate cyclase and inhibition by indomethacin. Gastroenterology *69*:1238, 1975.
171. Keusch, G. T., Donohue-Rolfe, A., and Jacewicz, M.: Shigella toxin and the pathogenesis of shigellosis. *In* Evered, D., and Whelan, J. (eds.). Microbial Toxins and Diarrheal Disease. Ciba Foundation Symposium 112. London, Pitman Press, 1985, p. 193.
172. O'Brien, A. D., and Kapral, F. A.: Increased cAMP content in guinea pig ileum after exposure to *S. aureus* delta-toxin. Infect. Immun. *13*:152, 1976.
173. Rao, M. D., Guandalini, S., Laird, W. J., and Field, M.: Effects of heat-stable enterotoxin of *Yersinia enterocolitica* on ion transport and cyclic guanosine 3[1],5[1]-monophosphate metabolism in rabbit ileum. Infect. Immun. *26*:875, 1979.
174. Gill, D. M., and Richardson, S. H.: Adenosine diphosphate-ribosylation of adenylate cyclase catalyzed by heat-labile enterotoxins of *E. coli:* comparison with cholera toxin. J. Infect. Dis. *141*:64, 1980.
175. Rout, W. R., Formal, S. B., Giannella, R. A., and Dammin, G. J. Pathophysiology of shigella diarrhea in the rhesus monkey: intestinal transport, morphological and bacteriological studies. Gastroenterology *68*:270, 1975.
176. Butler, D. G., Gall, D. G., Kelly, M. H., and Hamilton, J. R. Transmissible gastroenteritis: mechanisms responsible for diarrhea in an acute viral enteritis in piglets. J. Clin. Invest. *53*:1335, 1974.
177. Graham, D. Y., Sackman, J. W., and Estes, M. K. Pathogenesis of rotavirus-induced diarrhea preliminary studies in miniature swine piglet. Dig. Dis. Sci. *29*:1028, 1984.
178. Giannella, R. A., Rout, W. R., and Formal, S. B. Effect of indomethacin on intestinal water transport in salmonella-infected rhesus monkeys. Infect. Immunol. *17*:136, 1977.
179. McGowan, K., Kane, A., Asarkof, N., Wicks, J., Kellum, J., Gintzler, A. R., and Donowitz, M. Isolation of serotonin from *Entamoeba histolytica*: role in diarrhea? Science *221*:762, 1983.
180. Binder, H. J., Lemp, G. F., and Gardner, J. D. Receptors for vasoactive intestinal peptide and secretin on small intestinal epithelial cells. Am. J. Physiol. *238*:G190, 1980.
181. Kimberg, D. V., Field, M., Johnson, J., Henderson, A., and Gershon, E. Stimulation of intestinal mucosal adenyl cyclase by cholera enterotoxin and prostaglandins. J. Clin. Invest. *50*:1218, 1971.
182. Dobbins, J. W., Laurenson, J. P., and Forrest, J. N. Adenosine and adenosine analogues stimulate adenosine cyclic 3',5'-monophosphate-dependent chloride secretion in the mammalial ileum. J. Clin. Invest. *74*:929, 1984.
183. Donowitz, M., Fogel, S., Battisti, L., and Asarkof, N. The neurohumoral secretogogues carbachol, substance P and neurotensin increase Ca^{2+} influx and calcium in rabbit ileum: mechanisms of action? Life Sci. *31*:1919, 1982.
184. Helman, C. A., and Barbezat, G. O. The effect of gastric inhibitory polypeptide on human jejunal water and electrolyte transport. Gastroenterology *72*:376, 1977.
185. Moritz, M., Finkelstein, G., Meshkinpour, H., Fingerut, J., and Lorber, S. Effect of secretin and cholecystokinin of the transport of electrolyte and water in human jejunum. Gastroenterology *64*:76, 1973.
186. Matuchansky, C., Huet, P. M., Mary, J. Y., Rambaud, J. C., and Bernier, J. J. Effects of cholecystokinin and metoclopramide on jejunal movements of water and electrolytes and on transit time of luminal fluid in man. Eur. J. Clin. Invest. *2*:169, 1975.
187. Hicks, T., and Turnberg, L. A. The effect of glucagon and secretin on salt and water transport in the human jejunum. Gut *13*:854, 1972.
188. Moriarty, K. J., Hegarty, J. E., Tatemoto, K., Mutt, V., Christofides, N. D., Bloom, S. R., and Wood, J. R. Effect of peptide histidine isoleucine on water and electrolyte transport in the human jejunum. Gut *25*:624, 1984.
189. Gray, T. K., Bieberdorf, F. A., and Fordtran, J. S. Thyrocalcitonin and the jejunal absorption of calcium, water, and electrolytes in normal subjects. J. Clin. Invest. *52*:3084, 1973.
190. Binder, H. J. Pharmacology of laxatives. Annu. Rev. Pharmacol. Toxicol. *17*:355, 1977.
191. Bright-Asare, P., and Binder, H. J. Stimulation of colonic secretion of water and electrolytes by hydroxy fatty acids. Gastroenterology *64*:81, 1973.
192. Mekhjian, H. S., Phillips, S. F., and Hoffmann, H. F. Colonic secretion of water and electrolytes induced by bile acids: perfusion studies in man. J. Clin. Invest. *50*:1569, 1971.
193. Donowitz, M., Wicks, J., Battisti, L., Pike, G., and DeLellis, R. Effect of Senokot on rat intestinal electrolyte transport evidence of Ca^{2+} dependence. Gastroenterology *87*:503, 1984.
194. Powell, D. W., Lawrence, B. A., Morris, S. M., and Etheridge, D. R. Effect of phenolphthalein on *in vitro* rabbit ileal electrolyte transport. Gastroenterology *78*:454, 1980.
195. Ewe, K. Effect of laxatives on intestinal water and electrolyte transport. Eur. J. Clin. Invest. *2*:282, 1972.
196. Nell, G., Overhoff, H., Forth, W., Kulenkampff, H., Specht, W., and Rummel, W. Influx and efflux of sodium in jejunal and colonic segments of rats under the influence of oxyphenisatin. Naunyn Schmiedebergs Arch. Pharmacol. *277*:53, 1973.
197. Donowitz, M., and Binder, H. J. Effect of dioctyl sodium sulfosuccinate on colonic fluid and electrolyte movement. Gastroenterology *69*:941, 1975.
198. Reichelderfer, M., Pero, B., Lorenzsonn, V., and Olsen, W. A. Magnesium sulfate-induced water secretion in hamster small intestine. Proc. Soc. Exp. Biol. Med. *176*:8, 1984.
199. Ewe, K. Effect of rhein on the transport of electrolytes, water, and carbohydrates in the human jejunum and colon. Pharmacology *20*(Suppl. 1):27, 1980.
200. Binder, H. J. Pathophysiology of bile acid- and fatty acid–induced diarrhea. *In* Field, M., Fordtran, J. S., and Schultz, S. G. (eds.). Secretory Diarrhea. Washington, D.C., American Physiological Society, 1980, p. 159.
201. Racusen, L. C., and Binder, H. J. Ricinoleic acid stimulation of active anion secretion in colonic mucosa of the rat. J. Clin. Invest. *63*:743, 1979.
202. Buebler, E., and Juan, H. Effect of ricinoleic acid and other

laxatives on net water flux and prostaglandin E release by the rat colon. J. Pharm. Pharmacol. *31*:681, 1979.

203. Maenz, D. D., and Forsyth, G. W. Ricinoleate and deoxycholate are calcium ionophores in jejunal brush border vesicles. J. Membr. Biol. *70*:125, 1982.
204. Karlstrom, L., Cassuto, J., Jodal, M., and Lundgren, O. The importance of the enteric nervous system for the bile-salt induced secretion in the small intestine of the rat. Scand. J. Gastroenterology *18*:117, 1983.
205. Dobbins, J. W., and Binder, H. J. Effect of bile salts and fatty acids on the colonic absorption of oxalate. Gastroenterology *70*:1096, 1976.
206. Perdue, M. H., Chung, M., and Gall, D. G. Effect of intestinal anaphylaxis in gut function in the rat. Gastroenterology *86*:391, 1984.
207. Perdue, M. H., and Gall, D. G. Intestinal anaphylaxis in the rat: jejunal response to *in vitro* antigen exposure. Am. J. Physiol. *250*:G427, 1986.
208. Cooke, H. J., Nemeth, P. R., and Wood, J. D. Histamine action on guinea pig ileal mucosa. Am. J. Physiol. *246*:G372, 1984.
209. Schneider, A. J., Kinter, W. B., and Stirling, C. E. Glucose-galactose malabsorption. Report of a case with audioradiographic studies of mucosal biopsy. N. Engl. J. Med. *274*:305, 1966.
210. Lifson, N. Fluid secretion and hydrostatic pressure relationships in the small intestine. *In* Binder, H. J. (ed.). Mechanisms of Intestinal Secretion. New York, Alan R. Liss, 1979, p. 249.
211. Swabb, E. A., Hynes, Z. A., and Donowitz, M. Elevated intraluminal pressure alters rabbit small intestinal transport *in vivo*. Am. J. Physiol. *242*:G58, 1982.
212. Caren, J. F., Meyer, J. H., and Grossman, M. I. Canine intestinal secretion during and after rapid distention of the small bowel. Am. J. Physiol. *227*:183, 1974.
213. Norman, D. A., Atkins, J. M., Seelig, L. L., Jr., Gomez-Sanchez, C., and Krejs, G. J. Water and electrolyte movement and mucosal morphology in the jejunum of patients with portal hypertension. Gastroenterology *79*:707, 1980.
214. Kahn, I. J., Jeffries, G. H., and Sleisenger, M. H. Malabsorption in intestinal scleroderma. N. Engl. J. Med. *274*:1339, 1966.
215. Harris, M. S., Dobbins, J. W., and Binder, H. J. Augmentation of neutral sodium chloride absorption by increased flow rate in rat ileum *in vivo*. J. Clin. Invest. *78*:431, 1986.
216. Mathias, J. R., Carlson, G. M., DiMarino, A. J., Bertiger, G., Morton, H. E., and Cohen, S. Intestinal myoelectric activity in response to live *Vibrio cholerae* and cholera enterotoxin. J. Clin. Invest. *58*:91, 1976.
217. Mathias, J. R., Martin, J. L., Burns, T. W., Carlson, G. M., and Shields, R. P. Ricinoleic acid effect on the electrical activity of the small intestine in rabbits. J. Clin. Invest. *61*:640, 1978.
218. Burns, T. W., Mathias, J. R., Matrin, J. L., Carlson, G. M., Martin, J. L., and Shields, R. P. Effect of toxigenic *Escherichia coli* on myoelectric activity of small intestine. Am. J. Physiol. *235*:E311, 1978.
219. Burns, T. W., Mathias, J. R., Martin, J. L., Carlson, G. M., and Shields, R. P. Alteration of myoelectric activity of small intestine by invasive *Escherichia coli.* Am. J. Physiol. *238*:G57, 1980.
220. Mathias, J. R., Carlson, G. M., Martin, J. L., Shields, R. P., and Formal, S. *Shigella dysenteriae* I enterotoxin: Proposed role in pathogenesis of shigellosis. Am. J. Physiol. *239*:G382, 1980.
221. Spiller, R. C., Trotman, I. F., Higgins, B. E., Ghatei, M. A., Grimble, G. K., Lee, Y. C., Bloom, S., Misiewicz, J. J., and Silk, D. B. A. The ileal brake–inhibition of jejunal motolity after ileal fat perfusion in man. Gut *25*:365, 1984.
222. Gingell, J. C., Davies, M. W., and Shields, R. Effect of synthetic gastrin-like pentapeptide upon the intestinal transport of sodium, potassium, and water. Gut *9*:111, 1968.

56

Absorption of Vitamins and Divalent Minerals

DAVID H. ALPERS

Although all required nutrients must be absorbed by the small intestine, some of these are of greater concern for the gastroenterologist. *Anemia* commonly results from malabsorption of any of three nutrients: folic acid, cobalamin, or iron. *Osteopenia* also often accompanies intestinal disease. This results from diminished mineralization of bone related to the decreased absorption of the required minerals, particularly calcium and magnesium, as well as vitamin D. Abnormalities of small bowel mucosa and decreased biliary secretion both depress mineral absorption. By decreasing bile acid reabsorption, mucosal disease also depletes the luminal concentration of bile acids below the level needed for fat-soluble vitamin absorption. Diarrhea is a common cause of zinc malabsorption, because the stool is the route of most zinc excretion under normal circumstances. Disorders of absorption of these major vitamins and minerals are commonly encountered in gastrointestinal disease. In the pages that follow, absorption of these nutrients is discussed. Diagnosis and treatment of deficiency states are discussed on pages 263 to 282 and 1983 to 2027.

ABSORPTION AND METABOLISM OF SOLUBLE VITAMINS

Folic Acid (Pteroylglutamic Acid, PteGlu$_1$)

Food Sources

Dietary *folates*, or *folacins*, occur mostly as polyglutamates, which are not absorbed intact. Folacin is a generic term of compounds having structures and functions similar to those of folic acid. All polypteroylglutamates are hydrolyzed to pteroylglutamic acid during absorption. Neither reduction nor addition of carbon fragments is needed for absorption. Folates are synthesized only by bacteria and plants. The basic pteroyl structures can be modified by reduction of the pyrazine ring, by addition of a one-carbon group to the N_5 and N_{10} positions, or by elongation of the peptide chain by the addition of glutamyl residues. Because reduction can result in the dihydro or tetrahydro form, and at least six glutamates and six possible one-carbon groups can be added, the number of possible folates is large. Only the polyglutamate forms are important in altering the rate of absorption.

Pteroylglutamic acid (PteGlu$_1$) is absorbed at a faster rate than larger polymers (PteGlu$_n$).[1] However, when the heptaglutamate form is ingested and transit time to the colon is normal, over 90 per cent of the ingested folic acid is absorbed. Therefore, hydrolysis of polyglutamate folates becomes a possible clinical problem only when the small intestine is shortened or transit is rapid. The best evidence in mammals suggests that the glutamyl residues are removed from polyglutamates one at a time.[2] Such a sequential hydrolysis of polyglutamates obviously permits folic acid to be available from polyglutamates in foods that contain from one to seven residues.

The assessment of amounts of polyglutamates in food is difficult because of rapid breakdown to pteroylglutamic acid in mammalian tissues. Because folates must be deconjugated prior to absorption, it is also difficult to estimate the availability of folacins in foods. The pentaglutamate predominates in most foods; forms with four and six residues also are common. Estimates of the percentage of folacin available as the monoglutamate form vary from 30 per cent in orange juice to 60 per cent in cow's milk.[3]

Only 25 to 50 per cent of dietary folate is thought to be available nutritionally, although these estimates may be low. Boiling destroys much of folate in milk and leads to loss of most folacin activity of vegetables. On the basis of these considerations as well as on the proportion that is in monoglutamate form (PteGlu$_1$), some foods are judged to contain folacin of high availability (for example, bananas, lima beans, liver, and yeast), whereas other foods have low folacin availability (orange juice, lettuce, egg yolk, soy beans, and wheat germ). Average diets in the United States and Canada contain from 30 to 1890 μg of folacin per day, with an average of 242 (Canada) to 689 (United States).[4] The daily requirement for folate is about 100 μg, although the recommended dietary allowance is 400 μg.

Hydrolysis of Polyglutamate Folates

Food polyglutamate forms of folate are hydrolyzed during intestinal perfusion, with a decreasing number of glutamate residues down to the monoglutamate form appearing in the gut lumen. Intestinal fluid obtained from humans contains little hydrolytic activity, and as the hydrolytic products appear rapidly in the lumen, it has been postulated that the brush border hydrolyzes polyglutamates. Most measurements of enzyme activity in intestinal cells have localized the "conjugase" activity to the lysosomal fraction, with an additional activity at a pH optimum of 7.5 in human jejunal brush borders.[5,6] Although both activities seem clearly present, it is not certain which activity represents the primary site of cleavage.

Some patients with *tropical sprue* have responded to pteroylglutamic acid while ingesting a normal diet.[7] This observation suggests that some patients with tropical sprue can absorb monoglutamates but cannot metabolize food polyglutamates. This result could be due to a decreased activity of brush border conjugase, or to the presence of natural inhibitors of conjugase activity, or to folate-binding proteins in the diet. In *celiac sprue* and *tropical sprue*, either adequate or increased levels of folate conjugase activity have been found in biopsy specimens.[2,8] These results may reflect lysosomal enzyme levels. If lysosomal activity were rate limiting for polyglutamate hydrolysis, a mechanism for transporting polyglutamate folate would be required, a system that has not yet been described. These clinical data suggest that the brush border folate conjugase may be the rate-controlling step in folate polyglutamate hydrolysis.

Absorption of Folic Acid (PteGlu$_1$)

Demonstration of a specific absorption mechanism for folic acid has been made in the rat.[9] In humans, evidence for a saturable mechanism and for transport against a concentration gradient has been obtained during luminal perfusion studies.[10] The best resolution of the data in the literature suggests that two mechanisms are present: (1) a *carrier-mediated, saturable* system that can transport against a concentration gradient at low luminal concentration and (2) *passive transport* at higher concentrations. Absorption of folates is reduced at alkaline pH,[5] a fact that may explain in part the folic acid deficiency seen after subtotal gastrectomy. The best evidence for a specific folate transport system is those rare patients with congenital folate malabsorption in the absence of other intestinal dysfunction.[11,12] Such patients have impaired absorption of all forms of folate and require high doses of oral folic acid to prevent anemia. In normal subjects, reduced folic acid is absorbed better than the oxidized form, although it is unlikely that this difference is nutritionally important. Factors that affect absorption

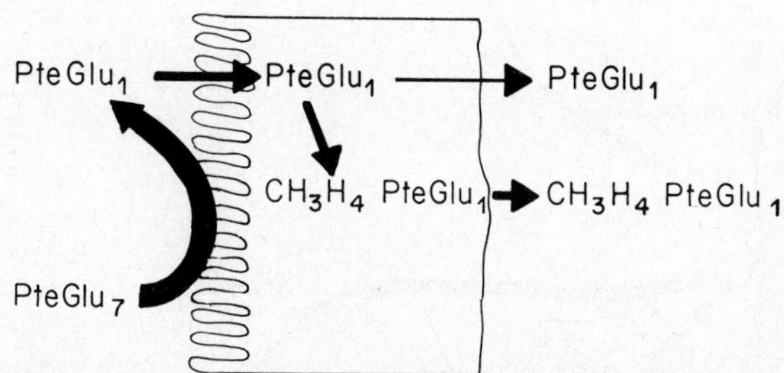

Figure 56–1. Proposed scheme of the digestion and absorption of dietary pteroylpolyglutamates. Hydrolysis of pteroylpolyglutamates (shown here as $PteGlu_7$) probably occurs outside the intestinal cell. The overall rate of absorption into the mesenteric circulation is governed by the rate of transport of the monoglutamyl product ($PteGlu_1$). At physiologic doses, a substantial amount of $PteGlu_1$ is reduced and then methylated to CH_3-$H_4PteGlu_1$ in the intestinal cell before release to the circulation. (From Rosenberg, I. H. Reprinted by permission of the New England Journal of Medicine *293*:1303, 1975.)

of folic acid include not only dietary folacins but also the tetrahydrofolic acid excreted in high concentration in the bile.[13] Within the mucosa, folic acid is usually methylated and reduced to the tetrahydro form (CH_3-$H_4PteGlu_1$). Steps in the hydrolysis and absorption of folic acid are summarized in Figure 56–1.

Inhibition of Folic Acid Absorption by Drugs

The administration of various drugs has been associated with the development of folic acid deficiency. Anticonvulsant phenytoin (Dilantin) therapy causes deficiency, but the mechanism is unclear. Alterations in absorption of both food polyglutamate and folic acid have been documented.[14, 15] Other studies have not confirmed a defect in absorption of synthetic polyglutamates.[16] Sulfasalazine has been shown to decrease folic acid absorption in humans[17] and does so presumably by competitive inhibition of the specific folate transport system.[18] Clinical folate deficiency, however, is uncommon, as inhibition is not nearly complete. Oral contraceptive drugs have not been shown to affect folic acid absorption.[19] Folic acid deficiency itself can impair folic acid absorption by producing "megaloblastic" changes in columnar epithelial cells of the gut. Alcohol ingestion is often associated with a low serum folate concentration, most likely attributable to increased renal excretion.[20] It has been suggested that an alteration in the enterohepatic circulation of folate may be related to this change, but this hypothesis has been challenged.[20] Low serum folate is also due in part to markedly diminished intake of folate in chronic alcoholism, to a direct effect of alcohol on intestinal mucosa, and to increased urinary losses of folate[21] (see also p. 1987).

Relationship of Folic Acid Absorption to Overall Folate Metabolism

An average Western diet contains 200 to 400 μg of nutritionally available folacins, to which another 100 μg of folic acid is added from the enterohepatic circulation (Fig. 56–2). In rats, after intravenous or enteric administration, 10 to 20 per cent of substituted CH_3- or CHO-) folate monoglutamates are taken up by the liver by a carrier-mediated mechanism during the first pass, and the rest are cleared by peripheral tissues.[22] Methyltetrahydrofolic acid (CH_3-$H_4PteGlu_1$) is the major form in which the vitamin seems to be excreted in the bile. Thus, malabsorption leads to folic acid deficiency more rapidly than does dietary deficiency alone. Because tissue stores are only about 5 mg, malabsorption can rapidly deplete them. However, as the liver does not secrete folate during deficiency states at an increased rate, the rate of folate depletion will fall as deficiency becomes more severe.[20] The storage form of folate is a polyglutamate form of methyltetrahydrofolic acid (CH_3-$H_4PteGlu_n$), produced in the liver and red cells, which are the major storage tissues. The major circulating form of folate, however, is the monoglutamate form of CH_3-$H_4PteGlu_1$. During mobilization from tissue stores, the glutamate residues are removed. Figure 56–2 demonstrates the major features of normal folate homeostasis. During short periods of dietary deprivation, there is decreased tissue uptake and storage of folates. The liver is the most important organ in this regulation, by virtue of its large mass, rapid folate turnover, large flux through the enterohepatic cycle, and salvage of folates from aging cells. A wide variety of extracellular folate-binding proteins have been described in serum, milk, and tissues.[23] These preferentially bind oxidized folates rather than the natural reduced forms. Soluble and membrane-bound forms also exist, the latter almost certainly related to transport findings. The absorption defect for all forms of folate seen in patients with congenital folate deficiency suggests the presence of specific folate receptors involved in folate transport. The best-studied receptor is on the choroid plexus, but a large brush border enterocyte protein has also been reported.[23]

Folate Deficiency

Severe folate deficiency is found clinically most often in chronic *alcoholism* (p. 1987), *celiac sprue* (pp. 1134–1152) or *tropical sprue* (pp. 1281–1297), or *blind loop syndrome* (pp. 1289–1297).[3] In *Crohn's disease* (pp. 1327–1358) and following partial gastrectomy (pp. 962–987), mild deficiency is found. As folate absorption is largely complete in the upper small intestine, its malabsorption is expected in disorders that affect the upper gut (nontropical sprue, duodenal bypass). However, any intestinal disorder, when accompanied by decreased dietary intake or rapid transport, may result in deficiency. Table 56–1 summarizes the major steps in folic acid absorption (and that of the other nutrients

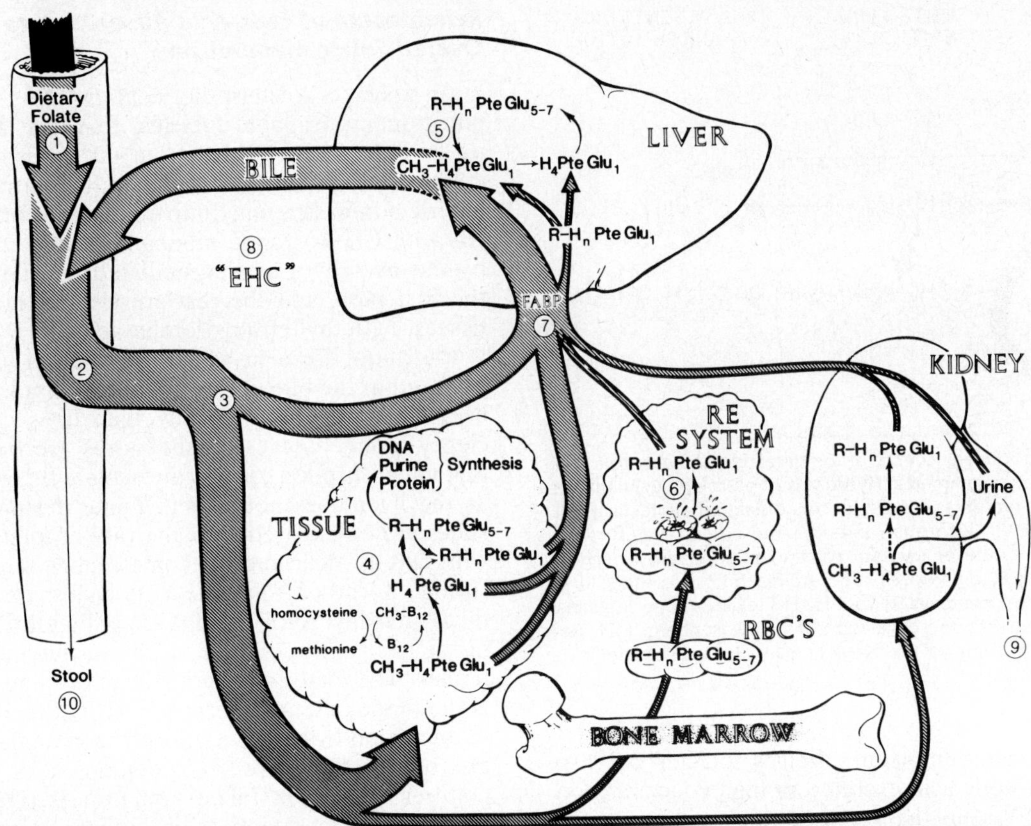

Figure 56–2. Elements of normal folate homeostasis. 1, Dietary supply. 2, Conversion of dietary polyglutamates to monoglutamates and absorption. 3, Transport to liver and other tissues, possibly involving folic acid binding proteins (FABP). 4, Intracellular conversion to polyglutamates for biochemical functions and storage. 5, Hydrolysis of polyglutamates to monoglutamates, which may be redistributed. 6, Salvage of folates from senescent cells for reutilization. 7, Return of monoglutamates (CH_3-H_4PteGlu$_1$ and partially oxidized and nonsubstituted forms, e.g., H_2PteGlu$_1$ and H_4PteGlu$_1$) to liver—possibly involving folic acid binding protein. 8, Transport of CH_3-H_4PteGlu$_1$ into enterohepatic cycle for distribution to tissues. 9, Urinary excretion of products of folate catabolism and of small amounts of folate. 10, Minimal losses of folate in stool. (From Steinberg, S. E. Am. J. Physiol. *246*:G319, 1984. Used by permission.)

discussed in this chapter) and lists the major causes of deficiency that result from disturbances in these processes.

Cobalamin (Vitamin B_{12})

Food Sources

Cobalamin (cbl) refers to the cobalt-containing compounds with a corrin ring that have biologic activity for humans. Vitamin B_{12} is the generic term for all these compounds with activity in any species. Cobalamin is now the preferred term to distinguish these compounds active in humans from the many analogues produced in bacteria. The average Western diet contains 5 to 15 μg/day. Cobalamin is produced by bacteria and enters animal tissues through ingestion of contaminated foods or by production in the rumen. Microorganisms in the human colon synthesize cobalamin, but it is not absorbed. Thus, strict vegetarians who do not eat cobalamin-containing meats will develop cobalamin deficiency.[24]

Cobalamin is bound to enzymes in food sources and must first be liberated by gastric proteases. The relative importance of food preparation, gastric acid, and pepsin in the liberation of cobalamin is unclear. Cobalamin malabsorption can be detected in patients treated with H_2 blocking drugs.[25] These patients absorb crystalline cobalamin, but not protein-bound cobalamin. However, it is not clear if any long-term effects result from chronic therapy with these agents. It is unlikely that clinical cobalamin deficiency develops solely as a result of inability to liberate food cobalamin. In nearly all cases, some defect in intrinsic factor secretion is present.[26]

Role of the Stomach and Pancreas (Fig. 56–3)

Once cobalamin is liberated from food, it is bound at acid pH to the first of three binding proteins, the R proteins, so called because of their rapid movement during electrophoresis (Table 56–2).[27] The R proteins bind cobalamin analogues better than cobalamin itself, but there is usually a large excess of cobalamin compared with analogues in food. The amount of R protein (and intrinsic factor) produced is very large compared with the cobalamin ingested so that virtually all of the vitamin becomes protein-bound. The R proteins cannot

Table 56–1. PATHOPHYSIOLOGY OF VITAMIN AND MINERAL DEFICIENCY COMMONLY ENCOUNTERED IN GASTROINTESTINAL DISEASE

Nutrient	Important Steps in Absorption	Major Causes of Deficiency
Folic acid	Hydrolysis of polyglutamate forms, carrier-mediated transport, enterohepatic circulation	Inadequate intake, alcoholism, malabsorption
Cobalamin	Receptor-mediated endocytosis (ileum), enterohepatic circulation	Ileal disease, vegetarian diets
Vitamin A	Hydrolysis of dietary esters, enterohepatic circulation of retinoic acid, solubilization of hydrophobic vitamin by bile salts and binding proteins	Malabsorption (especially bile salt loss), alcoholism
Vitamin D	Production in skin by sunlight, solubilization in mixed micelles	Malabsorption (especially bile salt loss), lack of sunlight
Vitamin E	Hydrolysis of dietary esters, passive absorption, transport in lipoproteins	Biliary obstruction, malabsorption (especially cystic fibrosis), prematurity
Vitamin K	Production by colonic flora, ileal and colonic passive transport	Malabsorption, broad-spectrum antibiotics
Iron	Active transport in duodenum	Blood loss, prematurity, pregnancy, proximal intestinal disease or bypass
Calcium	Active transport in duodenum enhanced by vitamin D and PTH, inefficient jejunal and ileal transport decreased by multiple luminal and systemic factors, obligatory fecal excretion	Malabsorption (of calcium or vitamin D), decreased intake
Magnesium	Passive, inefficient transport, decreased by multiple luminal factors	Malabsorption, alcoholism
Zinc	Inefficient absorption; intestinal secretion is major route of excretion	Malabsorption, diarrhea

PTH, Parathyroid hormone.

mediate the absorption of cobalamin, and their physiologic function is unknown. They may be present to bind in the lumen, or to remove from the blood, any noncobalamin vitamins produced by bacterial action. However, rare cases of complete R protein deficiency have occurred with no obvious hematologic effect on the patient.[28]

The cobalamin–R protein complex leaves the stomach along with free intrinsic factor.[29] In the upper small intestine, pancreatic proteases hydrolyze the R protein, thereby liberating free cobalamin. The cobalamin now binds to intrinsic factor, as R protein is no longer present to compete for binding.[30] The intrinsic factor–cobalamin complex is resistant to proteolytic digestion, allowing the complex to traverse the small bowel and reach the ileum, its site of active transport. These processes in the stomach and upper small intestine are outlined in Figure 56–3.

Although the cobalamin malabsorption in some patients with pancreatic insufficiency can be reversed by trypsin,[31] it is unlikely that pancreatic proteases are always required for cobalamin absorption, as some patients with total pancreatectomy have normal cyanocobalamin absorption.[32] Moreover, cobalamin deficiency is very unusual in patients with pancreatic insufficiency. Even in the absence of significant pancreatic proteolytic activity, enough dietary cobalamin is transferred to intrinsic factor to prevent clinical evidence of deficiency, as it binds to some extent to luminal intrinsic factor in patients with pancreatic insufficiency.[29] The explanation for this may lie in the fact that at pH 8 some cobalamin binds to intrinsic factor, even in the presence of intact R proteins.[30] Atrophic gastritis often accompanies pancreatic insufficiency in chronic alcoholic individuals. Since these patients have hypochlorhydria or achlorhydria, a pH of about 8 may be found in the upper small intestine, allowing some binding of cobalamin to intrinsic factor.

Role of the Ileum

The cobalamin–intrinsic factor complex is bound to a specific receptor in the ileum. This step is a requirement for active transport of the vitamin. The binding

Table 56–2. VITAMIN B_{12} BINDING PROTEINS

Protein	Origin	Fluid	Molecular Weight	Nature	Function
Intrinsic factor	Parietal cell	Gastric juice	44,000 (human) 50,000 (hog)	Glycoprotein	Required for ileal transport
R proteins (includes transcobalamin I and III)	Many cells	Serum, bile, milk, saliva, gastric juice, amniotic fluid	58,000-66,000	Glycoprotein	Unknown
Transcobalamin II	Liver	Serum	38,000	Polypeptide	Transports cobalamin from gut and delivers it to cells

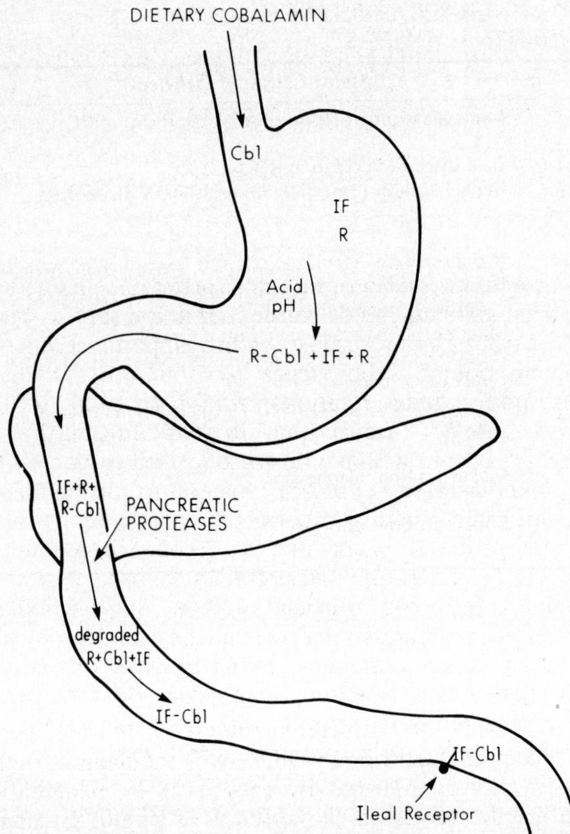

Figure 56–3. Absorption of cobalamin (Cbl) requires proteolysis and intrinsic factor (IF). The mass of intrinsic factor secreted is far in excess of that needed for binding the available cobalamin. R protein (see Table 56–1) derived from saliva is also present in great abundance. More R protein and cobalamin are added from biliary secretions into the duodenum. Note that Cbl binds initially to R protein in the stomach at acid pH. Only after R protein is degraded by proteases does Cbl bind to IF. After Cbl is absorbed in the ileum, it is bound to transcobalamin II (TC II) and perhaps to TC I and III (see Table 56–1).

occurs at neutral pH and requires calcium, but not energy. R proteins do not bind to this receptor. The receptor is located on the brush border and has been purified from dog,[33] pig, and human ileum.[33a] It has a molecular weight of about 200,000, most of which extends beyond the lipid bilayer,[34] similar to small bowel disaccharidases. Free cobalamin does not bind to the ileal receptor. The locus of the human receptor extends from at least the mid–small intestine to the ileocecal valve.[35] Although resection of the terminal 100 cm of ileum alone is not sufficient to remove entirely this active transport system, cobalamin deficiency often results.

Cobalamin does not appear in blood for three to four hours after it attaches to the ileum. The intrinsic factor–cobalamin complex is taken up by the enterocyte by receptor-mediated endocytosis,[36] and the cobalamin is released from the complex at acid pH, possibly in acid endosomes.[33, 37] After passage through the enterocytes, cobalamin is transported in blood bound to transcobalamins. The bulk of cobalamin is found on transcobalamin I and III, which deliver it to the liver (see Table 56–2). Transcobalamin II binds only a minority of total serum cobalamin, but is the protein that delivers the vitamin to the tissue where it is needed.

Role of the Liver

Cobalamins bound to R proteins are present in high concentration in the bile and participate in an enterohepatic circulation.[38] The extent of this enterohepatic circulation is unknown, but it has been estimated at 5 to 10 μg/day—that is, five or ten times the human daily requirement of cobalamin. The cobalamin enters the luminal pool, in which it is liberated and then bound to intrinsic factor, as are dietary cobalamins. Dietary lack of cobalamin alone leads to human clinical deficiency slowly, as daily requirements (1 μg) are only about 0.02 per cent of hepatic stores (about 5000 μg). Deficiency develops more rapidly in patients with malabsorption as a result of losses from the enterohepatic circulation.

Non–Intrinsic Factor–Mediated Absorption

A passive mechanism exists for absorption of cobalamin when the amount of ingested vitamin is very large, in excess of the content of a normal diet. Absorption is by diffusion, probably at all levels of the intestine. When doses over 100 μg are given, a maximum of 1.5 μg can be absorbed.[24] The non–intrinsic factor–mediated absorption does not require calcium and is independent of pH. The practical importance of this information is that oral cobalamin theoretically could suffice for the requirements in *pernicious anemia*, but not in *malabsorption*, in which losses exceed 1 μg daily. Oral therapy is not usually used for pernicious anemia because daily treatment would be required.

Alterations of Cobalamin Absorption in Disease

On the basis of available knowledge of cobalamin absorption, the clinical illnesses associated with cobalamin malabsorption and deficiency can be categorized as in Table 56–3.

Table 56–3. ABNORMALITIES IN COBALAMIN ABSORPTION PRODUCING DEFICIENCY

Physiologic Step	Disorder
1. Impaired food digestion	Gastrectomy, achlorhydria[39]
2. Decreased IF secretion	Pernicious anemia,[24] congenital absence of IF[40] Gastrectomy[26]
3. Impaired transfer to IF	Pancreatic insufficiency[41, 42] Zollinger-Ellison syndrome[43]
4. Abnormal IF	Decreased ileal binding,[40] susceptible to acid proteolysis[41]
5. Competition for uptake	Bacterial overgrowth[38]
6. Impaired attachment to ileal receptor	Ileal disease or resection[38]
7. Impaired uptake or passage through the ileal cell	Familial cobalamin malabsorption[44]
8. Impaired uptake into blood	Transcobalamin II deficiency[45]

IF, Intrinsic factor.

Malabsorption is detected by the Schilling test (>8 per cent urinary excretion).[46] The dual labeled test (^{57}Co-Cbl and ^{58}Co-Cbl-IF) for detection of IF deficiency had been thought to be more sensitive; however, an unexpected, rapid exchange of ^{58}Co-Cbl for IF-bound ^{57}Co-Cbl results in uninterpretable data in some patients, and a one-stage test involving two isotopes is not recommended.[47] Body stores are best estimated by serum cobalamin (normal is usually 120 pg/ml, but values may vary widely).[47]

Other B Vitamins and Vitamin C[5, 48]

Vitamins B_1, B_2, B_6 (thiamine, riboflavin, and pyridoxine), and C are widely distributed in foods, ranging from fruits and vegetables for vitamin C to grains and meats for riboflavin. Absorption is rapid and occurs in the upper small intestine. The mechanism of transport ranges from passive absorption (e.g., vitamins B_6 and C) to a saturable active transport system (e.g., riboflavin). Some of these vitamins exhibit both mechanisms (e.g., thiamine). The major causes of deficiency include decreased intake and alcoholism, which combines decreased intake with small intestinal damage (see also pp. 1983–1994).

FAT-SOLUBLE VITAMINS

Vitamin A[49]

Food Sources

Vitamin A as retinyl esters is found only in foods of animal origin. Beta-carotene, a vitamin A precursor, is found in vegetables. In the United States, dairy products and margarines are supplemented with retinyl esters, and these provide the major dietary source.

Absorption

Vitamin A (retinol) is ingested as the ester or as the dimer (beta-carotene) and is hydrolyzed by esterases prior to absorption. The dominant structural feature of vitamin A is a conjugated double bond system on its side chain. This structure is extremely hydrophobic and represents a major problem in absorption and transport of this vitamin through aqueous media. A complex system has evolved to handle this problem, including absorption in mixed micelles from the intestinal lumen and a series of binding proteins (Fig. 56–4). Human milk contains a milk lipase that is activated by bile salts and hydrolyzes retinyl esters. In adults, pancreatic and intestinal brush border esterases liberate free retinol, which is converted back to a retinyl ester and incorporated into chylomicrons. On the villus of an enterocyte a small protein, CRBP-II, carries all-trans-retinol and presumably delivers it to the appropriate esterifying enzyme.[50]

Carotene either is hydrolyzed in the enterocyte to two retinal molecules or is absorbed intact (about 10 per cent). These products are also carried in chylomicrons, which are taken up by the liver (Fig. 56–4). The liver is the major clearing house for vitamin A, and it consigns the esters either to storage via hydrolysis to retinol and then re-esterification, to release of retinol to the blood, or to conversion of retinol to retinoic acid (about 10 per cent). Retinoic acid is conjugated

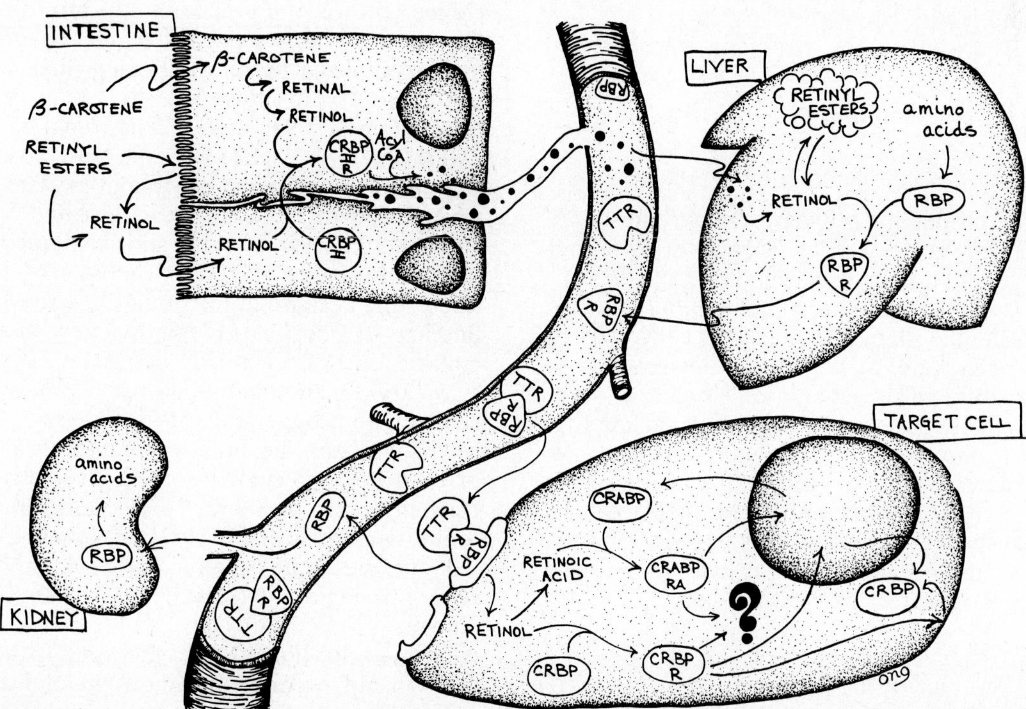

Figure 56–4. Movement of vitamin A within an animal. Abbreviations used are: CRABP, cellular retinoic acid-binding protein; CRBP, cellular retinol-binding protein; CRBP (II), cellular retinol-binding protein, type II; R, retinol; RA, retinoic acid; RBP, retinol-binding protein; TTR, transthyretin. (From Ong, D. E. Nutrition Rev. *43*:225, 1985. Used by permission.)

with glucuronide and excreted in the liver, to be reabsorbed by the intestine via the portal vein. The concentration of vitamin A metabolites in bile is proportional to hepatic stores.[51] The significance of this enterohepatic circulation in malabsorptive states is unknown, as in vitamin A deficiency little of the incoming vitamin is deposited in the liver but is delivered to depleted tissues.[52]

Retinol leaves the liver bound to retinol-binding protein (RBP), which complexes with another plasma protein, transthyretin (previously called prealbumin). This ternary complex is responsible for delivering the vitamin to body tissues. The complex prevents filtration and loss by the kidney. After delivery of retinol the apo-RBP is catabolized by the kidney. Liver disease lowers RBP and transthyretin levels, whereas renal disease raises them. In these situations serum levels of vitamin A do not correlate with those of body tissues.[53]

Inside the cell to which retinol has been delivered, there are additional binding proteins (Fig. 56–4). Some tissues (e.g., retina, testis), have cellular retinol-binding proteins specific to those tissues. These proteins are thought to permit efficient delivery to specific sites within the cell, but their precise function is not yet clear.

Deficiency

Disorders that produce *fat malabsorption*, in particular if caused by decreased intraluminal bile salt concentration, lead to vitamin A deficiency. Decreased intake is the other major cause of deficiency and can occur in patients with *anorexia nervosa* and *alcoholism*.[48] Vitamin A deficiency is uncommon in pancreatic insufficiency, a condition presenting with normal bile salt secretion.

Vitamin D

Sources

Endogenous production is the most important source of vitamin D. For this reason, deficiency owing to diet alone is less common than is suspected. 7-Dehydrocholesterol is first converted to previtamin D_3, a substance that remains in the skin and is slowly converted to vitamin D_3. This rate of conversion increases with rising temperature. The amount of vitamin D_3 produced endogenously is variable, depending on latitude, season, and exposure to sunlight, but it averages 2.5 to 10 μg/day (100 to 400 IU), values that nearly satisfy the minimum daily requirement.[54] The major natural sources are fish liver and oils, egg yolk, beef liver, fortified milk, and bread. The latter two now provide the major dietary sources in Western diets.

Absorption

The absorption of nonpolar vitamin D_3 and D_2 from animal and plant sources is by means of mixed bile acid and fatty acid micelles. Because of their initial insolubility in aqueous solution, these sterols require bile acid concentrations above their critical micellar levels for absorption. Addition of fatty acids to the micelle increases its capacity to solubilize vitamin D.

Vitamin D from skin is bound to a transport protein (vitamin D–binding protein), and this limits its uptake by the liver. It has been suggested that this binding protein carries only the vitamin, not the previtamin from the skin, further limiting the ability to produce endogenous vitamin D intoxication. However, hepatic uptake of chylomicrons from the intestine is not limited, and toxic levels of vitamin D can be absorbed following excessive ingestion. The liver adds a 25-hydroxyl group, and the kidney adds hydroxyl groups on the 1 and 24 positions (Fig. 56–5). Adipose tissue is the major storage site for these metabolites. All vitamin D metabolites can be taken up by the liver to some extent, and some of them are excreted in the bile. The contribution of an interrupted enterohepatic circulation to vitamin D deficiency in malabsorption is probably small.[55] Less than one third of highly polar metabolites, and virtually no 25-hydroxy vitamin D_3, are excreted in bile. It has been suggested that the loss of bile salts in malabsorption alters hepatic metabolism of vitamin D, producing the rapid half-life found in that condition.

Production of Active Hormone

Vitamin D is a prehormone. The active compounds, the 25-hydroxy and 1,25-dihydroxy derivatives, are produced in the body for delivery to other target organs (Fig. 56–5).

The liver hydroxylates vitamin D_3 to 25-hydroxycholecalciferol, the predominant form of vitamin D in the plasma.[56] Any feedback regulation of hepatic 25-hydroxycholecalciferol production that may exist is overcome as the intake or production of vitamin D_3 is substantially increased. The renal conversion of $25(OH)D_3$ to $1,25(OH)_2D_3$ is the most closely regulated step in the metabolism of vitamin D. The 1-α-hydroxylase found in renal cortex is inhibited by phosphate and by $1,25(OH)_2D_3$ itself and is stimulated by parathyroid hormone (PTH).[57] The role of phosphate is interesting because of the similarities between the bone findings in phosphate depletion and those of osteomalacia due to vitamin D deficiency. Both PTH and $1,25(OH)_2D_3$ stimulate bone resorption and release of calcium from bone (Fig. 56–5). These actions tend to regulate serum calcium at normal levels at the expense of total body calcium stores. Conversely, high serum calcium levels decrease PTH release and, via calcitonin, decrease $1,25(OH)_2D_3$ production.

Hormones other than parathyroid hormone affect renal production of $1,25(OH)_2D_3$.[58] Estrogens increase conversion of $25(OH)D_3$, and this result has been confirmed in humans by the finding of a positive relationship between the duration of pregnancy and $1,25(OH)_2D_3$ levels. Prolactin and growth hormone also stimulate conversion to the dihydroxy form.

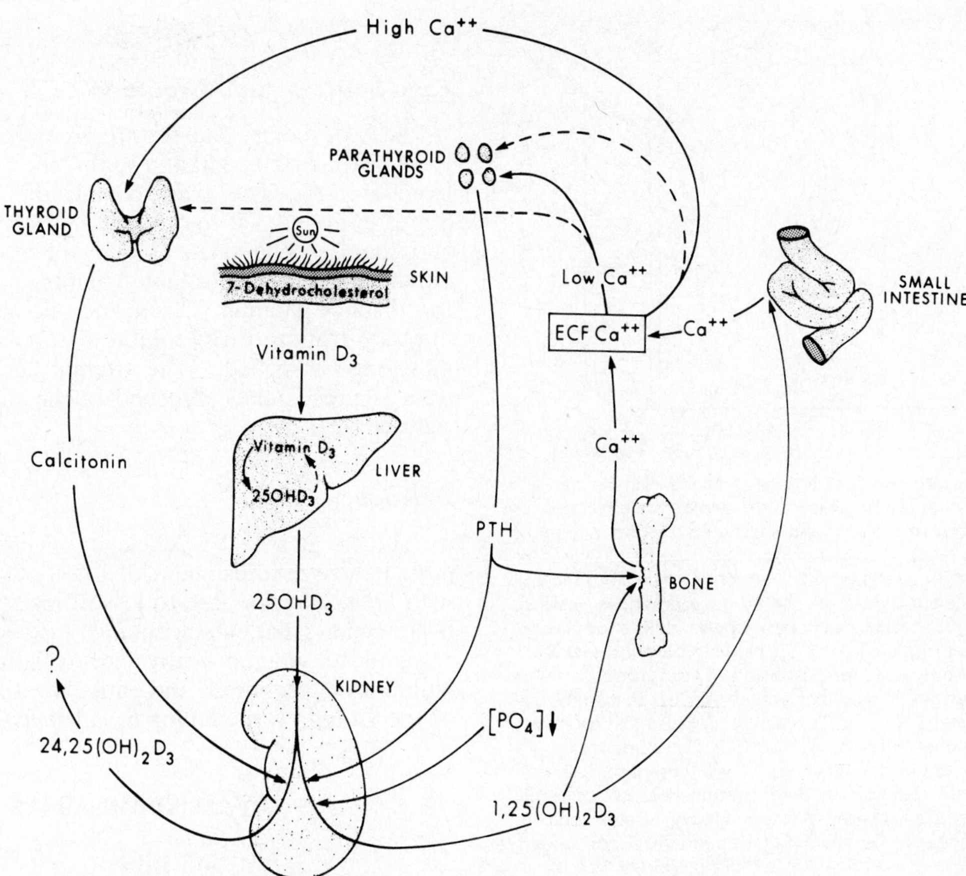

Figure 56–5. Vitamin D metabolism. A detailed description of the pathways appears in the text.

Although most studies have concentrated on generation of active forms of vitamin D, much is known about degradation of the vitamin. Side-chain cleavage and oxidation of $1,25(OH)_2D_3$ occur to form $24,25(OH)_2D_3$ or $25(OH)D_3$. This reaction is stimulated by calcitonin. It is still uncertain whether $24,25(OH)_2D_3$ represents solely a degradation product or is a physiologically important form of the hormone.[58, 59] Substantial quantities of vitamin D metabolites may appear in urine, suggesting a role for the kidney in the excretion of vitamin D metabolites.

Action on the Intestine

The best-studied effect of vitamin D is its stimulation of the intestinal transport of calcium.[60] Although vitamin D stimulates the intestinal production of macromolecules that are involved in calcium metabolism (calcium-binding proteins, Ca-Mg-ATPase, and a brush border calcium-binding complex), the likely major effect of vitamin D is to alter the permeability of the brush border membrane to Ca^{2+}. At the other end of the cell, vitamin D–stimulated mechanisms for calcium extrusion have been identified and may involve an ATP pump, or Na^+-Ca^{2+} exchange, or both (Fig. 56–6).

Alteration in Absorption During Disease

Because of its nonpolar structure and dependence upon bile acid micelles for solubilization, *vitamin D malabsorption* is found most often in disorders in which bile acid absorption is markedly decreased. Even the production of endogenous vitamin D (100 to 400 IU/day) is not sufficient in these circumstances, as some of the vitamin may be lost during its enterohepatic circulation, and the half-life of the active 1,25-dihydroxy vitamin D is shortened.[55] *Pancreatic insufficiency*, while producing steatorrhea, is not commonly associated with vitamin D deficiency, although some malabsorption may result from partitioning vitamin D in the luminal oil phase.

Vitamin E

Food Source

Vitamin E is found in lipids of green leafy plants and in oils of seeds. The richest sources for humans are salad oils, shortenings, margarines, eggs, and meat. A 1000- to 3000-kcal diet in the United States contains 8 to 11 mg equivalent of α-tocopherol, sufficient for the average adult. The ratio of vitamin E to polyun-

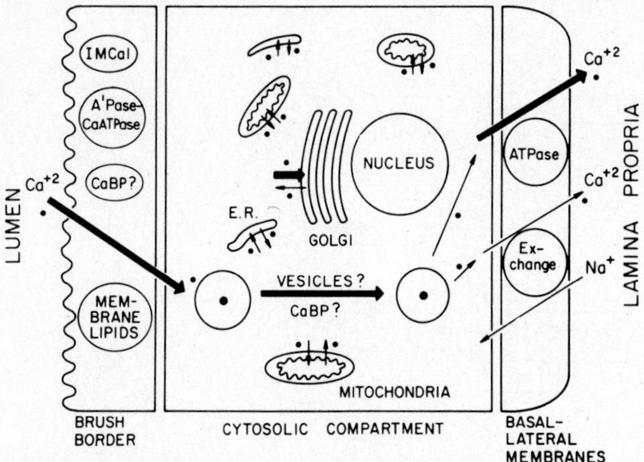

Figure 56–6. Diagram of possible events in the transfer of Ca^{2+} across the intestinal epithelial cell. Transfer across the brush border is downhill thermodynamically and facilitated by the action of vitamin D. Several factors located in this region, some of which are vitamin D–dependent, could be involved. Transfer through the cell might be in association with CaBP or by encasement in vesicles. Sequestration of intracellular Ca^{2+} by mitochondria, endoplasmic reticulum, or other organelles or by binding proteins maintains cytosolic Ca^{2+} at nontoxic levels. Extrusion of Ca^{2+} from the cell is against a thermodynamic gradient and is via a high affinity Ca-activated ATPase or by Na^{+}-Ca^{2+} exchange. IMCal, intestinal membrane calcium binding protein; ATPase-CaATPase, adenosine triphosphatase–low affinity Ca-activated ATPase complex; CaBP, vitamin D-dependent calcium binding protein; ER, endoplasmic reticulum; ATPase, Ca-activated ATPase. Heavy arrows indicate processes that appear to be vitamin D–dependent. (Reproduced, with permission, from the Annual Review of Physiology, Vol. 45. © 1983 by Annual Reviews Inc.)

saturated fatty acids in the diet determines in part its adequacy in the diet, because it functions as an antioxidant, affecting oxidation of unsaturated fatty acid.[48]

Absorption

Absorption requires biliary and pancreatic secretions, producing bile salts and esterases respectively. The natural form ingested is d-α-tocopherol acetate, which must be hydrolyzed. Only 40 per cent of dietary vitamin is absorbed passively as free tocopherol, all of which is found in intestinal lymph. In serum there is no specific protein carrier for vitamin E, which is carried in lipoproteins.[61] Thus, its serum level is proportional to total lipid concentration.[62]

Deficiency

In *malabsorption syndromes*, especially with biliary obstruction, tocopherol levels decline. In *short bowel syndrome* and abetalipoproteinemia, unsteady gait, tremor, weakness, ophthalmoplegia, cerebellar dysfunction, and proprioceptive impairment have been noted.[63] End-organ damage is probably more common than once thought, but its detection may require sophisticated techniques, such as electroretinograms or sensory evoked potentials in the extremities (see pp. 1106–1112).

Vitamin K

Food Sources and Absorption

The best dietary sources are green leafy vegetables. Roughly half of the vitamin K absorbed daily is derived from bacteria. The average daily diet in the United States contains 300 to 500 mg. Absorption is passive and requires bile salts, as with all of the fat-soluble vitamins.[64] Other fat-soluble vitamins in large amounts can displace vitamin K from the bile acid micelle and limit absorption or can inhibit metabolism of the vitamin, once absorbed.[65] The vitamin derived from bacteria is presumably absorbed in the distal ileum and right colon.

Deficiency

Subjects at risk for deficiency include *newborn infants* before establishment of intestinal flora, patients with *malabsorption* due to loss of intestine or bile salt insufficiency, patients with *liver disease* who cannot respond to vitamin K by carboxylation of selected glutamic acid residues, and patients with no oral intake of the vitamin while *taking broad-spectrum antibiotics.*

DIVALENT MINERALS

Iron

Food Sources

Food iron is available in a variety of nuts and seeds as well as in red meat and egg yolks. Many sources of iron, especially inorganic salts and vegetable iron, are not well absorbed without ascorbic acid to reduce ferric to ferrous iron. Hemoglobin iron is absorbed better than a comparable amount of vegetable iron.[66] The iron content of foods is fairly constant, about 6 mg/1000 kcal. Baked goods account for about 20 per cent of iron intake in the United States, usually added in the form of ferric orthophosphate or sodium acid sulfate salts.

Absorption

Human iron metabolism is unique, because there is no normal mechanism for the excretion of excess iron. Therefore, iron absorption and the factors that control it assume a large role in normal iron metabolism.

Iron is absorbed as heme and nonheme iron. Heme iron, largely in meat, is better absorbed (10 to 20 per cent) than is nonheme iron, found primarily in vegetables, which is absorbed at an efficiency of only 1 to 6 per cent. The average Western diet provides more nonheme iron (15 to 20 mg/day) than heme iron (1.5 to 3.0 mg/day). The factors that affect iron absorption of these two forms also differ. Heme iron absorption is unaffected by intraluminal factors or by dietary composition.[67] On the other hand, nonheme iron absorption is largely controlled by luminal events.

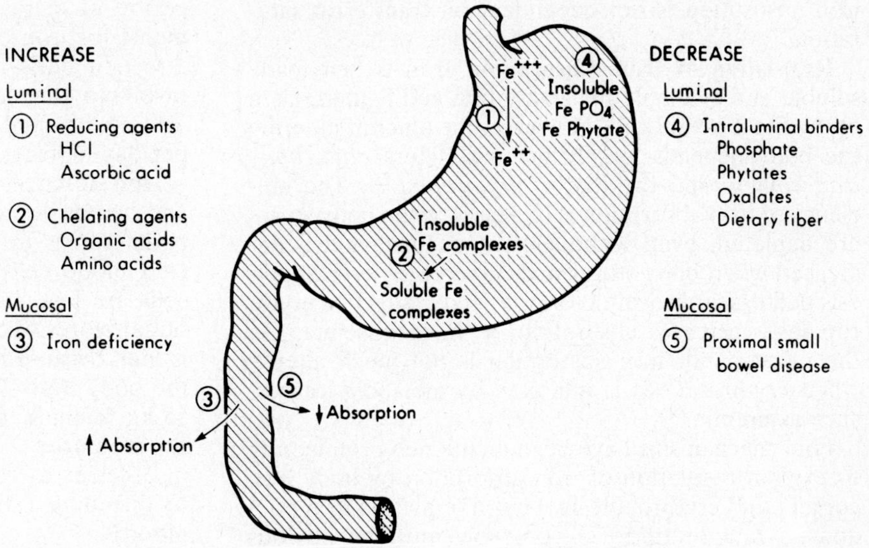

Figure 56–7. Factors that affect iron absorption. Nonheme iron absorption is affected both by intraluminal factors (1, 2, and 4) and by the total iron body content (3) as well as by small bowel disease (5). Heme iron absorption is altered only by those factors that affect the mucosa itself (3 and 5). The mechanism by which iron deficiency alters mucosal iron absorption is discussed in the text.

Luminal Factors (Fig. 56–7). Hydrochloric acid contributes to the absorption of nonheme iron from food and medications.[68] The presence of acid is not required for absorption, but it tends to prevent the formation of insoluble iron complexes. Dietary components may render nonheme iron more soluble and include reducing agents, such as ascorbic acid, and amino acids, (especially histidine and lysine), liberated during digestion of dietary protein these amino acids stabilize iron in the soluble state by forming low molecular weight complexes with it. Dietary factors that inhibit nonheme iron absorption include organic anions (phosphate, phytate) and phosphoproteins. These compounds bind ionic iron and render it insoluble. Certain components of dietary fiber (pectin, lignin, hemicelluloses) have been shown to decrease iron absorption in dogs.[69] The importance of dietary fiber in human iron absorption is unclear. Lactoferrin is the major iron-binding protein in exocrine secretion (milk, bile, pancreatic juice). It has been suggested that this protein can both inhibit and enhance[70] iron uptake by duodenal cells. However, lactoferrin itself does not seem to enter the mucosal cell. Its role in iron uptake remains uncertain.

Certain medications can interfere with iron absorption. These include antacids, zinc sulfate in multivitamin or mineral tablets, and H_2 blocking agents used in ulcer therapy.

Cellular Mechanisms. Both heme and non-heme iron are absorbed fastest in the duodenum.[67] Uptake into the cell, transport across the cell, and release from the cell into the plasma seem to be separate steps and are regulated independently. The initial step in uptake of iron by human mucosa is an active metabolic process, exhibiting the properties of an active transport process (i.e., dependent on metabolic energy and exhibiting saturation kinetics).[71] It is not known whether this uptake is a rate-controlling step in the process of iron absorption.

Two major mechanisms have been implicated in the initiation of iron absorption. One mechanism involves the secretion of apotransferrin into the gut lumen; transferrin complexes with iron, facilitating its uptake as Fe-transferrin.[72] The complexes are also thought to prevent degradation of the transferrin, which is then re-excreted into the lumen. It is not clear whether or not this process is mediated by a transferrin receptor at the brush border.[73] A second mechanism involves Fe-micromolecular (low molecular weight) complexes with citrate, ascorbate, or amino acids. This process of absorption of iron in low molecular weight complexes seems to be carrier mediated, and is followed by binding of the iron within the membrane, thus providing irreversibility of the absorption process.[74]

Normally, much of the iron taken up is either deposited as ferritin within the cell or transferred to the plasma bound to transferrin. When iron absorption is increased, less iron is deposited as mucosal ferritin. When the enterocyte defoliates, iron is lost into the intestinal lumen. However, it is likely that this mechanism is overwhelmed when large amounts of iron are ingested.

The mechanism for iron uptake is thought to be carrier mediated and exhibits specificity for other metals. When iron deficiency is present, the absorption of metals closely related to iron (cobalt, nickel, manganese, zinc, and cadmium) is enhanced.[75] Lead absorption is also increased in iron-deficient patients.[76] However, the rate of absorption of calcium, magnesium, copper, and mercury is not altered.

The events involved in the release of iron from the mucosal cell are not well understood. Most absorbed iron enters the portal blood, primarily in a low molecular weight form.[77] The amount of transferrin in the extravascular compartment of the mucosa seems insufficient to suggest a role for this protein in the removal of iron from the enterocyte. Furthermore, the rate of iron absorption is not dependent on transferrin saturation.[78]

Regulation of Iron Absorption. Iron is first made soluble and available for absorption and is then taken up by the mucosal cell. However, the amount entering the body depends largely on two factors: *total body iron content* and the *rate of erythropoiesis*. The efficiency of iron absorption is increased when body stores are depleted, even without overt anemia, and is decreased when body stores rise.[79] Increased erythropoiesis decreases absorption of iron, and ineffective erythropoiesis increases absorption, as in thalassemia. On the other hand, iron absorption is not much altered when erythropoiesis is inhibited by metabolic causes, such as uremia.[80]

Four mechanisms have been mentioned prominently to explain regulation of iron absorption by body iron content and erythropoiesis. First, the plasma iron pool and its rate of turnover somehow must be obvious factors in the consideration of control of iron absorption; however, studies indicate that neither pool size nor rate of turnover seems to affect iron absorption directly. Second, increasing degrees of plasma transferrin saturation might inhibit iron absorption; however, in *thalassemia* and *hemochromatosis*—diseases characterized by saturation of plasma transferrin—iron absorption is increased.[81] Third, as the concentration of ferritin in human duodenum is proportional to the serum ferritin concentration,[82] it might be thought that mucosal or serum ferritin content, or both, plays a role(s) in regulating iron absorption. However, duodenal ferritin concentration can increase even when body iron content and serum ferritin levels are low.[83] Thus, it seems unlikely that mucosal or serum ferritin is a major regulatory factor. Fourth, the iron content of the mucosal cells has been suggested as the regulatory factor. However, nonheme iron concentration in the human duodenum does not correlate with iron absorption.[84] In iron deficiency, the mucosal flux across the whole epithelium is increased, but mucosal iron content remains low.[85] Therefore, it is possible that the initial influx across the brush border, not any intracellular process, is the rate-limiting step. The carrier-mediated mechanism at the brush border is increased in iron deficiency and is maximal in the duodenum, consistent with such a regulatory role.[86] It has been suggested that both newly absorbed iron that is not needed and excess body iron are excreted via macrophage in the lamina propria through the goblet cells.[79]

Causes for Iron Deficiency

Increased Requirements. During the first years of life, iron requirements are affected by growth. The infant is born with excess red cells, which are temporarily converted into iron stores. As growth proceeds, these store are exhausted by the third or fourth month of life.[87] Thereafter, diet must provide the iron, explaining the clinical observation that iron deficiency due to inadequate diet in infancy is usually is seen only after three months of age. Adolescence is another period of increased requirements. The daily requirements for iron of infants and for pregnant women on a weight basis are six times that of an adult man,[81] owing to the demands of growth and development. The adult female excretes an average of 2 mg of iron per day in excess of losses in males.

Iron stores reside in those tissues that contain ferritin and hemosiderin (liver, spleen); however, most of the body iron is in tissues that require iron for function (red blood cells, marrow, muscle). When red blood cells are lost, iron is mobilized first from these functional stores. The potential for iron loss via bleeding is high because red blood cells contain the majority of the body iron—2750 mg for 70-kg males, 2180 mg for 55-kg females. Only about 5 mg of iron per day can be mobilized from cell storage tissues, an amount insufficient to compensate for acute iron loss caused by bleeding (about 250 mg of iron per 500 ml of blood).

Decreased Absorption. With disease (e.g., *celiac sprue, Whipple's disease, Crohn's disease, amyloidosis, eosinophilic gastroenteritis*, etc.) or bypass of the upper small intestine, especially the duodenum, both heme and nonheme iron absorption are diminished. The conditions that most commonly produce iron malabsorption are *celiac sprue, Billroth II anastomosis* following antrectomy, and *gastric bypass procedures* for obesity. Decreased gastric acid production (as in *pernicious anemia* or following *subtotal gastrectomy*) and intraluminal binders (e.g., phytates or phosphates, such as occurs with ingestion of large amounts of unprocessed cereal grains) affect only nonheme iron absorption. As dietary iron is limited, a meat-deficient diet will lead to decreased iron absorption, especially because heme iron is more efficiently absorbed. Occult blood loss can add to negative iron balance when persisting peptic disease complicates ulcer surgery.

Functions of Iron

Iron is required for hemoglobin synthesis and is important as a cofactor in many intracellular reactions, including those involving myoglobin, cytochromes, iron-sulfur containing dehydrogenases, the synthesis and degradation of biogenic amines, bacterial killing by neutrophils, and activation of T lymphocytes.[87] As iron deficiency progresses, depletion of oxidative enzymes and myoglobin in skeletal muscle proceeds more gradually than anemia, but it can eventually cause severe weakness. Intestinal sugar absorption can be decreased in iron deficiency, although this usually occurs in those cases in children in association with ingestion of cow's milk. There is no clear clinical counterpart to the observed alterations in biogenic amine synthesis. Likewise, despite the obvious effects of iron deficiency on the immune response, the extent and clinical significance of the impairment remain uncertain.[87] Therefore, iron deficiency is characterized not only by symptoms related to anemia but also by *angular stomatitis, atrophic lingual papillae*, and *koilonychia*. Iron deficiency in children causes *anorexia, decreased resistance to infection, decreased growth*, and *reversible protein-losing enteropathy*.

Calcium[88]

Food Sources

Because calcium salts, like those of other divalent ions, are poorly soluble in water, their form and stability in the sources of dietary calcium directly affect absorption of this important mineral. About 60 to 75 per cent of daily calcium intake in adults is derived from milk and other dairy products. At the pH of cow's milk (6.1), about 25 per cent of calcium is in the form of the citrate salt. The remaining calcium (about 70 mg/dl) is probably present as colloidal calcium phosphate, held in suspension in micelles with casein.[89] At acid pH the calcium salts become ionized and are thus readily available for absorption. It is not clear whether any of the calcium is complexed to casein, and an important role for gastric proteases in calcium absorption has never been established. In other animal products, calcium is present largely bound to protein, from which it is liberated and then absorbed. On the other hand, calcium in vegetables and grains is complexed with organic anions such as phytates, oxalates, and polysaccharides, which impair absorption of intraluminal calcium; hence calcium is less available from vegetables and grains than from animal tissues.[89]

Absorption

The absorption of calcium is very complex and the importance of the various factors is not well understood.[89] There are three major influences on calcium absorption—*intraluminal factors, cellular events*, and *systemic modulators* of cell function.

Intraluminal Factors. Following a meal, *gastric pH* rises no higher than 5 to 6. Thus, calcium carbonate, the most commonly used supplement, is probably ionized in the stomach. Although the importance of an optimum amount of acid in gastric secretion to facilitate the absorption of calcium salts has been questioned,[90] it is clear that absorption of $CaCO_3$ is decreased in fasted elderly patients who presumably have diminished acid secretion, suggesting also that $CaCO_3$ may not be ideal as a supplement for the elderly.[90, 91] Calcium is absorbed in the ionized form; hence, ideally it should be associated intraluminally with an anion that forms a soluble salt and not with one with that it will precipitate. Further, salts of divalent cations tend to precipitate in alkaline solution, especially when phosphate is the anion. As both luminal pH and phosphate concentration rise progressively along the course of the small intestine, precipitation increases and absorption is more difficult, explaining why high calcium intake in humans increases soluble concentration in the proximal bowel, but not in the ileum.[92] Because of the important roles of pH and anions in its absorption, the jejunum probably absorbs more calcium than the ileum after a meal, even though both are capable of absorbing comparable amounts of calcium.[93]

Table 56–4. EFFECT OF ORALLY INGESTED SUBSTANCES ON CALCIUM ABSORPTION

Decreased	No Effect	Increased
Phytates	Phosphates	Lactose
Cellulose	Protein	Lysine
Long-chain fatty acids	Ascorbic acid	Arginine
Alginates	Citric acid	Medium chain triglycerides
Oxalates		Penicillin, chloramphenicol
Alcohol		
Antacids		
Inorganic magnesium		
Cholestyramine		
Cortisol		
Tetracycline		

Based on data from Allen[95] and Avioli.[96]

Many compounds decrease calcium absorption when they are present in the lumen, owing to the formation of insoluble complexes (Table 56–4). These include *long-chain fatty acids* (steatorrhea), *cholestyramine, oxalic acid*, and *organic polyphosphates*. As much as 500 mg of calcium can be found in fatty acid soaps during steatorrhea. Because inorganic phosphorus is absorbed more efficiently than calcium, alterations in phosphorus intake do not have much effect on intraluminal phosphorus concentrations or calcium absorption. Intraluminal magnesium decreases calcium absorption by an unknown mechanism.

Other luminal compounds can enhance calcium absorption, presumably by forming more soluble complexes and preventing formation of less soluble calcium phosphate. These compounds include *bile acids,* certain *amino acids* (lysine, arginine), certain *antibiotics* (penicillin, chloramphenicol), and *monosaccharides* or *disaccharides*, especially lactose.[94] This may explain why milk calcium is better absorbed than equal amounts of calcium from other foods.[95]

Cellular Events. In some animal species, the duodenum is the site of a high affinity, very responsive vitamin D system for transporting calcium, whereas the ileum contains a lower affinity, less vitamin D–responsive system for transporting calcium.[97] It is not clear whether this major distinction is present in humans.[93] Uptake of calcium across the brush border is rate limiting, and this step is dependent upon vitamin D (see p. 1052). The energy-requiring pump for calcium is located in the basolateral membranes and is also vitamin D and sodium dependent (Fig. 56–6).[98] Transfer through the cell might be associated with calcium-binding protein or occur in microvesicles. Either binding by calcium-binding protein or secretion of intracellular calcium by organelles (e.g., mitochondria, endoplasmic reticulum), or both, maintains cytosolic calcium at nontoxic concentrations. Extrusion from the cell seems to occur via Ca^{2+} ATPase, by Na^+-Ca^{2+} exchange, or by both mechanisms.

The transport system for calcium can be modified by alterations in calcium intake and by age. Overall, adaptation to a low-calcium diet probably involves both increased calcium absorption and decreased release from bone, with subsequent decreased urinary excretion (Fig. 56–5). In humans, the intestinal component is more important. Older subjects absorb calcium less well than do younger subjects.[99] In addition, older subjects adapt less well to a low calcium diet because they have impaired conversion of vitamin D to $1,25(OH)_2D_3$. The exact mechanism of this defect is unknown.

Systemic Modulators of Cell Function (Fig. 56–5). $1,25(OH)_2D_3$ is the most potent modifier of calcium absorption. In vitamin D deficiency, active calcium transport is absent.[89] 25(OH)D also stimulates calcium absorption, but is only about 1 per cent as potent as the dihydroxy vitamin D. Growth hormone (GH) and parathyroid hormone (PTH) also can stimulate calcium absorption, whereas glucocorticoids, estrogens, thyroxine, phenytoin, and thiazides may decrease absorption. Systemic acidosis decreases calcium absorption; alkalosis enhances it. Calcium absorption is decreased in uremia,[57] although the exact cause is unclear.

Regulation of Body Calcium Content

The ability of the body to regulate absorption of calcium is limited because of the many factors involved. Of primary importance is the maintenance of serum calcium, which is exquisitely regulated by parathyroid hormone and vitamin D metabolites at the expense of overall body stores.

About 300 to 400 mg of calcium are absorbed each day in the adult from a total luminal content of 1200 to 1300 mg. This total luminal calcium assumes an average intake of 1000 mg, plus 200 to 300 mg entering the intestinal tract via pancreatic, biliary, and intestinal secretions. Thus, overall efficiency of absorption is only about 33 per cent.[100] The newly absorbed calcium mixes with an exchangeable calcium pool of about 1 gram in tissues and plasma. This pool is filtered through the kidneys so that about 10 gm of calcium pass through the kidneys each day. Of the filtered load, 99 per cent is reabsorbed and about 100 mg are excreted in the urine. Two hundred to 300 mg of calcium resorbed from bone each day pass through the exchangeable calcium pool. Overall calcium balance is maintained (100 mg net absorbed and excreted) but the potential exists for great losses during malabsorption because of uncompensated endogenous secretion. In healthy humans at calcium intakes of less than 3 mg/kg of body weight/day, net calcium absorption is negative.[88] This obligatory fecal calcium loss becomes significant when no dairy products are ingested.

When intestinal (or urinary) losses of calcium are excessive, the rate of bone resorption is insufficient to maintain serum calcium. Hypocalcemia develops when extracellular fluid calcium concentration falls, and the following series of events ensues[54] (Fig. 56–5): PTH is released to act on bone, kidney, and intestine. By increasing $1,25(OH)_2D$ formation in the kidney, it helps to increase calcium absorption and to mobilize calcium from bone; it increases urinary phosphate and decreases calcium excretion by reducing calcium clearance. Finally, PTH acts permissively on the intestine to increase calcium absorption in the presence of vitamin D. The $1,25(OH)_2D$ formed acts on bone to increase resorption and on intestine to increase absorption. All of these factors tend to restore extracellular calcium concentration at the expense of body stores.

Causes of Decreased Calcium Absorption

Calcium deficiency attributable to limited absorption is relatively common for the following reasons: (1) The sources in the diet are limited; (2) absorption is inefficient; and (3) the amount excreted in stool per day (1000 mg) is very high relative to the circulating pool size (about 1000 mg). Thus, malabsorption often leads to hypocalcemia, which, as discussed, leads to eventual losses of body stores of calcium.

The major causes of decreased calcium absorption include *dietary deficiency, diffuse small intestinal disease, malabsorption or decreased intake of vitamin D, steatorrhea* of any cause (with excessive binding of calcium by fatty acids), *renal failure*, and *severe magnesium depletion* (see following). Achlorhydria from any cause theoretically might lead to inefficient absorption of calcium because of decreased conversion of insoluble to soluble calcium salts. So many factors are important in calcium absorption that it is not surprising that calcium malabsorption commonly accompanies diseases of the gastrointestinal tract.

Magnesium

Food Sources

In contrast to calcium, magnesium is highly concentrated in cells and thus is widely distributed in foods, largely bound by protein and phosphate. In vegetables and green plants, magnesium is complexed with porphyrins in chlorophyll. Like calcium, it must be solubilized before it is absorbed. The milieu for achieving this is the same as for calcium: adequate protease activity, acid pH, and the presence of anions capable of forming soluble magnesium salts. The average daily intake of magnesium in a Western diet is 300 mg.

Absorption

Absorption of magnesium is relatively inefficient in a normal intake (about 30 per cent). Most magnesium in humans is absorbed in the ileum, probably owing to a long retention time in that organ. Unfortunately, most of the information regarding magnesium absorption has been obtained in experimental animals (e.g., rats, sheep), in whom there is colonic absorption and in whom net absorption is about 60 per cent.[101] Thus, the relevance of some of the data in humans is unclear. In animals, the anion associated with magnesium can alter the efficiency of absorption, but not strikingly. In fact, MgO is well absorbed by animals, although it is a cathartic in humans. Although magnesium can be absorbed at an equal rate in jejunum and ileum in humans, alterations in diet can change magnesium absorption, with a high intake (greater than 800 mg/day) decreasing net absorption by 20 to 30 per cent. Absorption is passive[102] but can be affected by vitamin D and calcium intake.[103]

Unlike calcium, net magnesium absorbed seems to be linearly related to intake, even at zero magnesium intake. In other words, no obligatory fecal magnesium loss seems to exist, although the data for intakes less than 2 mg/kg of body weight/day have not been obtained.[88]

Most magnesium salts are fairly insoluble, and it is not clear that the solubility of the ingested salt is crucial to eventual absorption. Moreover, highly insoluble salts (e.g., MgO) as well as relatively soluble ones (magnesium citrate) are both good laxatives and presumably are poorly absorbed. Gastric and small bowel pH may play important roles as they may do for calcium; low pH is more desirable in producing soluble salts, but absorption occurs only in the small intestine. Phosphate and other luminal binders can delay absorption. Transit time is probably the single most important factor in determining the efficiency of magnesium absorption, as it is a passive process.

Regulation of Magnesium Metabolism

Unlike calcium, the contribution of digestive juice to luminal magnesium is relatively small (35 mg).[88] This fact may account for the absence of a significant obligatory magnesium loss. Once absorbed, magnesium enters a large exchangeable pool, because magnesium is the major intracellular cation. The kidney is the major excretory organ of absorbed magnesium. Over one third of the ingested magnesium, or over two thirds of absorbed magnesium, is excreted in the urine each day. The kidneys can conserve magnesium avidly and can reduce excretion to less than 1 mEq/day.[104] Moreover, maximal excretion in response to magnesium loading can exceed 160 mEq/day (1920 mg). Excretion is increased by *volume expansion, hypercalcemia, diuretics, alcohol*, and *phosphate depletion* and is decreased by the action of PTH. Because of the marked urinary conservation and lack of obligatory fecal loss, magnesium deficiency is not usual in the absence of abnormal losses from the body.

Serum and extracellular magnesium content (about 250 mg) are probably regulated in part by PTH and *calcitonin*. Magnesium flux from bone is a source to replenish the exchangeable pool, but the rate of this flux per day has not been accurately assessed.

The regulatory response to a low magnesium level depends on the severity of the deficit.[105] When hypomagnesemia is not severe, PTH is stimulated to increase calcium release from bone. Moreover, low luminal magnesium may increase calcium absorption, as the absorption of these ions seems to be inversely related. Both of these effects raise the serum calcium level. On the other hand, hypomagnesemia decreases calcium mobilization from bone, so that net change in serum calcium level is small. When magnesium deficiency is severe and serum magnesium concentration is very low, PTH secretion is impaired.[105] Both the low PTH and low magnesium act together to decrease calcium mobilization from bone, and hypocalcemia results. When PTH secretion is low, calcium absorption may also decrease, even in the presence of hypomagnesemia. In this situation, hypocalcemia may be less a manifestation of depleted calcium stores than of low exchangeable magnesium. This explains the need for magnesium therapy to treat the hypocalcemia of severe malabsorption.

Causes of Decreased Magnesium Absorption

Because dietary sources are abundant and the usual daily loss (100 mg) is small relative to exchangeable pool size (about 5 gm), dietary deficiency is uncommon. However, all causes of *malabsorption* may lead to deficiency, because an obligatory fecal loss is created. Increased urinary excretion caused by reduced tubular reabsorption is seen with *diuretics* and in *diabetic ketoacidosis, primary renal disease*, and *hypercalcemia* of any cause. Urinary excretion is increased in severe *alcoholism*. In addition, three other factors contribute to hypomagnesemia in alcoholic patients: a deficient diet, vomiting and diarrhea, and ketosis that further increases urinary excretion.[106]

Zinc

Food Sources

Like the sources for calcium, but unlike those for magnesium, the zinc content of Western diets is relatively limited. The average zinc content is 10 to 15 mg/day, just adequate to provide the recommended daily allowance. In general, zinc intake is proportionate to protein intake, as most meats and seafood have the highest content and vegetable sources contain zinc-binding anions.

Absorption

About 5 to 10 per cent of ingested zinc is absorbed, largely in the proximal bowel. The mechanism of zinc absorption is not known. It is thought that brush border transport may require ATP, after which the zinc equilibrates with a "zinc pool" and is transferred to intracellular zinc-binding proteins (among which is metallothionein) or is transferred to the plasma.[107] About 0.5 per cent of body stores (1.5 to 2 mg/70 kg man) is secreted daily into the upper intestine of man.[108] This represents an amount equivalent to that absorbed from dietary intake. Overall absorption of endogenous zinc is 20 to 50 per cent, so that some of the secreted zinc is retained, but the margin of safety is small. Absorption is decreased by anions in the lumen, and by high calcium intake.[109] Inorganic iron also can decrease zinc absorption.[110] If either zinc or iron is present as the organic dietary form, such competitive inhibition does not occur.

Metabolism

The major route of excretion is in the feces (2 to 3 mg/day). Diarrheal fluid may contain over 11 mg of zinc/L. Thus, the severity of diarrhea is a good indication of the risk of zinc depletion in patients with gastrointestinal problems.[111] Urinary losses average 0.5 mg/day but are unregulated. Increased urinary losses occur in nephrosis, sickle cell disease, and cirrhosis, and after therapy with penicillamine.

Disorders Causing Zinc Deficiency[112]

Acrodermatitis enteropathica (see pp. 500–501) is a hereditary disorder of zinc absorption. Severe and chronic diarrheal disorders, however, are the most common cause of zinc deficiency, of which *Crohn's disease* is an important example. In *cirrhosis, sickle cell anemia*, and *nephrosis*, urinary losses, probably combined with decreased intake, produce deficiency. Zinc can also be lost during *hemodialysis*. The problem with identification of deficiency syndromes has been the nonspecificity of many of the manifestations of zinc deficiency (*dysgeusia, fatigue, decreased libido, anorexia, impaired glucose tolerance* (see pp. 500–501).

References

1. Halsted, C. H. Intestinal absorption and malabsorption of folates. Ann. Rev. Med. *31*:79, 1980.
2. Hoffbrand, A. V. Synthesis and breakdown of natural folates (folate polyglutamates). Hematology 9:85, 1975.
3. Davis, R. E. Clinical chemistry of folic acid. Adv. Clin. Chem. *25*:233, 1986.
4. Thenan, S. W. Food folate values. Am. J. Clin. Nutr. *28*:1341, 1975.
5. Rose, R. C. Intestinal absorption of water soluble vitamins. *In* Johnson, L. R. (ed.). Physiology of the Gastrointestinal Tract. New York, Raven Press, 1987, p. 1581.
6. Reisenhauer, A. M., Krumdieck, C. L., and Halsted, C. H. Folate conjugase: two separate activities in human jejunum. Science *198*:196, 1977.
7. Lindenbaum, J. Aspects of vitamin B_{12} and folate metabolism in malabsorption syndromes. Am. J. Med. *67*:1036, 1979.
8. Hoffbrand, A. V., Douglas, A. P., Fry, L., and Steward, J. S. Malabsorption of dietary folates (pteroyl polyglutamates) in adult coeliac disease and dermatitis herpetiformis. Br. Med. J. *4*:85, 1970.
9. Selhub, J., and Rosenberg, I. H. Demonstration of high affinity folate binding activity associated with the brush border membranes of rat kidney. Proc. Natl. Acad. Sci. USA *75*:3090, 1978.
10. Rosenberg, I. H. Absorption and malabsorption of folates. Clin. Hematol. *5*:589, 1976.
11. Chanarin, I. Disorders of vitamin absorption. Clin. Gastroenterol. *11*:73, 1982.
12. Santiago-Borrero, P. J., Santini, R., Jr., Perez-Santiago, E., and Maldonado, N. Congenital isolated defect of folic acid absorption. J. Pediatr. *82*:450, 1973.
13. Pratt, R. F., and Cooper, B. A. Folates in plasma and bile of man after feeding folic acid-^{3}H and 5-formyltetrahydrofolate (folinic acid). J. Clin. Invest. *50*:455, 1971.
14. Reizenstein, P., and Lund, L. Effect of anticonvulsive drugs on folate absorption and the cerebrospinal pump. Scand. J. Haematol. *11*:158, 1973.
15. Gerson, C. D., Hepner, G. W., Brown, N., Cohen, N., Herbert, V., and Janowitz, H. D. Inhibition by diphenylhydantoin of folic acid absorption in man. Gastroenterology *63*:426, 1972.
16. Fehling, C., Jagerstad, M., Lundstrand, K., and Westesson, A. K. The effect of anticonvulsant therapy upon the absorption of folates. Clin. Sci. *44*:595, 1973.
17. Franklin, J. L., and Rosenberg, I. H. Impaired folic acid absorption in inflammatory bowel disease: effects of salicylazosulfapyridine. Gastroenterology *64*:577, 1973.
18. Selhub, J., Dhar, G. J., and Rosenberg, I. H. Inhibition of folate enzymes by sulfasalazine. J. Clin. Invest. *61*:221, 1978.
19. Lindenbaum, J., Whitehead, N., and Reyner, F. Oral contraceptive hormones, folate metabolism and the cervical epithelium. Am. J. Clin. Nutr. *28*:246, 1975.
20. Weir, D. G., McGing, P. G., and Scott, J. M. Folate metabolism, the enterohepatic circulation and alcohol. Biochem. Pharmacol. *34*:1, 1985.
21. Green, P. H. R. Alcohol, nutrition, and malabsorption. Clin. Gastroenterol. *12*:563, 1983.
22. Steinberg, S. E. Mechanisms of folate homeostasis. Am. J. Physiol. *246*:G319, 1984.
23. Wagner, C. Folate binding proteins. Nutr. Rev. *43*:293, 1985.
24. Chanarin, I. The Megaloblastic Anemias. Oxford, Blackwell, 1979.
25. Steinbert, W. M., King, C. E., and Toskes, P. P. Malabsorption of protein bound cobalamin but not unbound cobalamin during cimetidine administration. Dig. Dis. Sci. *25*:188, 1980.
26. Hines, J. D., Hoffbrand, A. V., and Mollin, D. L. The hematologic complications following partial gastrectomy. Am. J. Med. *43*:555, 1967.
27. Marcoullis, G., and Rothenberg, S. P. Macromolecules in the assimilation and transport of cobalamin. *In* Lindenbaum, J. (ed.). Nutrition in Hematology. New York, Churchill Livingstone, 1983, p. 89.
28. Carmel, R., and Herbert, V. Deficiency of vitamin B_{12} binding alpha globulin in two brothers. Blood *33*:1, 1969.
29. Marcoullis, G., Parmentier, Y., Nicholas, J. P., Jimenez, M., and Gerard, P. Cobalamin malabsorption due to non-degradation of R proteins in the human intestine. Inhibited cobalamin absorption in exocrine pancreatic dysfunction. J. Clin. Invest. *66*:430, 1980.
30. Allen, R. H., Seetharam, B., Podell, E., and Alpers, D. H. Effect of proteolytic enzymes on the binding of cobalamin to R protein and intrinsic factor. J. Clin. Invest. *61*:45, 1978.
31. Toskes, P. P., Deren, J. J., and Conrad, M. E. Trypsin-like nature of the pancreatic factor that corrects vitamin B_{12} malabsorption associated with pancreatic dysfunction J. Clin. Invest. *52*:1660, 1973.
32. Kano, Y., Sakamoto, S., Miura, Y., and Takaku, F. Disorders of cobalamin metabolism. CRC Crit Rev Oncol. Hematol. *3*:1, 1985.
33. Seetharam, B., Alpers., D. H., and Allen, R. H. Isolation and characterization of the ileal receptor for intrinsic factor. J. Biol. Chem. *256*:3785, 1981.

33a. Seetharam, B., and Alpers, D. H. Gastric intrinsic factor and cobalamin absorption. *In* Field, M., and Frizell, R. (eds.). Section on Intestinal Absorption and Secretion. Handbook of Physiology. Washington, D.C., American Physiological Society, 1988, in press.

34. Seetharam, B., Bagur, S., and Alpers, D. H. Interaction of receptor for intrinsic factor cobalamin with synthetic and brush border lipids. J. Biol. Chem. *257*:183, 1982.
35. Hagedorn, C. H., and Alpers, D. H. Distribution of intrinsic factor-vitamin B_{12} receptors in human intestine. Gastroenterology *73*:1019, 1977.
36. Kapadia, C. R., Serfilippi, D., Voloshin, K., and Donaldson, R. M., Jr. Intrinsic factor–mediated absorption of cobalamin by guinea pig ileal cells. J. Clin. Invest. *71*:440, 1983.
37. Seetharam, B., Presti, M., Frank, B., Tiruppathi, C., and Alpers, D. H. Intestinal uptake and release of cobalamin complexed with rat intrinsic factor. Am. J. Physiol. *248*:326, 1985.

38. Kapadia, C. R., and Donaldson, R. M. Disorders of cobalamin absorption and transport. Ann. Rev. Med. *36*:98, 1985.
39. Doscherholmen, A., McMahon, J., and Ripley, D. Vitamin B_{12} assimilation from chicken meat. Am. J. Clin. Nutr. *31*:825, 1979.
40. Yang, Y.-M., Ducos, R., Rosenberg, A. J., Catrou, P. G., Levine, J. S., Podell, E. R., and Allen, R. H. Cobalamin malabsorption in three siblings due to an abnormal intrinsic factor that is markedly susceptible to acid and proteolysis. J. Clin. Invest. *76*:2057, 1985.
41. Toskes, P. P., Hansell, J., Gerda, J., and Deren, J. J. Vitamin B_{12} malabsorption in chronic pancreatic insufficiency. N. Engl. J. Med. *284*:627, 1971.
42. Allen, R. H., Seetharam, B., Allen, N. C., Podell, E. R., and Alpers, D. H. Correction of cobalamin malabsorption in pancreatic insufficiency with a cobalamin analogue that binds with high affinity to R protein but not to intrinsic factor. J. Clin. Invest. *61*:1628, 1978.
43. Schimode, S., Saunders, D. R., and Rubin, C. E. The Zollinger-Ellison syndrome with steatorrhea. II. The mechanisms of fat and vitamin B_{12} malabsorption. Gastroenterology *55*:705, 1968.
44. Burman, J. F., Jenkins, W. J., Walker-Smith, J. A., Phillips, A. D., Sourial, N. A., Williams, C. B., and Mollin, D. L. Absent ileal uptake of IF-bound vitamin B_{12} in-vivo in the Imerslund-Grasbeck syndrome (familial vitamin B_{12} malabsorption with proteinuria). Gut *26*:311, 1985.
45. Burman, J. F., Mollin, D. L., Sladden, R. A., Sourial, N., and Greany, M. Inherited deficiency of transcobalamin II causing megaloblastic anemia. Br. J. Haematol. *35*:676, 1977.
46. Fairbanks, V. F., Wahner, H. W., and Phyliky, R. L. Tests for anemia: the "Schilling Test." Mayo. Clin. Proc. *58*:541, 1983.
47. Lee, D. S. C., and Griffith, B. W. Human serum vitamin B_{12} assay methods—a review. Clin. Biochem. *18*:261, 1985.
48. Alpers, D. H., Clouse, R. E., and Stenson, W. F. Manual of Nutritional Therapeutics. 2nd edition. Boston, Little Brown, 1987.
49. Sporn, M. B., Roberts, A. B., and Goodman, D. S. (eds.) The Retinoids. Vol. 2. Orlando, Florida, Academic Press, 1984.
50. Ong, D. E. Vitamin A-binding proteins. Nutr. Rev. *8*:225, 1985.
51. Hicks, V. A., Gunning, D. B., and Olson, J. A. Metabolism, plasma transport and biliary excretion of radioactive vitamin A and its metabolites as a function of liver reserves of vitamin A in the rat. J. Nutr. *114*:1326, 1984.
52. Vitamin A in vitamin-A deficient and sufficient rats. Nutr. Rev. *42*:87, 1982.
53. Goodman, D. S. Dietary A and retinoids in health and disease. N. Engl. J. Med. *310*:1023, 1984.
54. Audran, M., and Kumar, R. The physiology and pathophysiology of vitamin D. Mayo. Clin. Proc. *60*:851, 1985.
55. The enterohepatic circulation of vitamin D is negligible. Nutr. Rev. *43*:76, 1985.
56. DeLuca, H. F. The metabolism, physiology, and function of vitamin D. *In* R. Kumar (ed.). Vitamin D: Basic and Clinical Aspects. The Hague, Martinus Nijhoff, 1984, p. 1.
57. Portale, A. A., Halloran, B. P., Murphy, M. M., and Morris, R. C., Jr. Oral intake of phosphorus can determine the serum concentration of 1,25-dihydroxy-vitamin D by determining its production rate in humans. J. Clin. Invest. *77*:7, 1986.
58. Henry, H. L., and Norman, A. W. Vitamin D: metabolism and biological functions. Ann. Rev. Nutr. *4*:493, 1985.
59. DeLuca, H. F. Recent advances in the metabolism of vitamin D. Ann. Rev. Physiol. *43*:199, 1981.
60. Wasserman, R. H., Fullmer, G. S., and Shimura, F. Calcium absorption and the molecular effects of vitamin D_3. *In* Kumar, R. (ed.). Vitamin D: Basic and Clinical Aspects. The Hague, Martinus Nijhoff, 1984, p. 233.
61. Bieri, J. G., Hoeg, J. M., Schaefer, E. J., Zech, L. A., and Brewer, H. B., Jr. Vitamin A and vitamin E replacement in abetalipoproteinemia. Ann. Intern. Med. *100*:238, 1984.
62. Sokol, R. J., Heubi, J. E., Iannaccone, S. T., Bove, K. E., and Balistreri, W. F. Vitamin E deficiency with normal serum vitamin E concentration in children with chronic cholestasis. N. Engl. J. Med. *310*:1209, 1984.
63. Vitamin E deficiency. Lancet *1*:423, 1986.
64. Olsen, R. E. The function and metabolism of vitamin K. Ann. Rev. Med. *4*:287, 1984.
65. Weber, F. Absorption mechanisms for fat soluble vitamins and the effect of other food constituents. Prog. Clin. Biol. Res. *77*:119, 1981.
66. Layrisse, M., Martinez-Torres, C., and Roche, M. Effect of interaction of various foods on iron absorption. Am. J. Clin. Nutr. *21*:1175, 1968.
67. Prasad, A. S. Iron. *In* Trace Elements and Iron Metabolism. New York, Plenum, 1978, p. 91.
68. Schade, S. G., Cohen, R. J., and Conrad, M. E. Effect of hydrochloric acid on iron absorption. N. Engl. J. Med. *279*:672, 1968.
69. Phillips, S. F., and Fernandez, R. Components of dietary fibre reduce iron absorption. Gut *21*:A904, 1980.
70. Lonnerdal, B. Biochemistry and physiological function of human milk proteins. Am. J. Clin. Nutr. *42*:1299, 1985.
71. Cox, T. M., and Peters, T. The kinetics of iron uptake in vitro by human duodenal mucosa: studies in normal subjects. J. Physiol. *289*:469, 1979.
72. Huebers, H. A., Huebers, E., Csiba, E., Rummel, W., and Finch, C. A. The significance of transferrin for intestinal iron absorption. Blood *61*:283, 1983.
73. Bomford, A. B., and Munro, H. N. Transferrin and its receptor: their roles in cell function. Hepatology *5*:870, 1985.
74. Muir, W. A., Hopfer, U., and King, M. Iron transport across brush border membrane from normal and iron-deficient mouse upper small intestine. J. Biol. Chem. *259*:4896, 1984.
75. Powell, L. W., and Halliday, J. W. Iron absorption and iron overload. Clin. Gastroenterol. *10*:707, 1981.
76. Barton, J. C., Conrad, M. E., Nuby, S., and Harrison, L. Effects of iron on the absorption and retention of lead. J. Lab. Clin. Med. *92*:1536, 1978.
77. Morgan, E. H. The role of plasma transferrin in iron absorption in the rat. Q. J. Exp. Physiol. *65*:239, 1980.
78. Wheby, M. S., and Jones, L. G. Role of transferrin in iron absorption. J. Clin. Invest. *42*:1007, 1963.
79. Refsum, S. B., and Schreiner, B. B.-I. Regulation of iron balance by absorption and excretion: a critical review and a new hypothesis. Scand. J. Gastroenterol. *19*:867, 1984.
80. Finch, C. A., and Huebers, W. Perspectives in iron metabolism. N. Engl. J. Med. *306*:1520, 1982.
81. Bothwell, T. H., Charlton, R. W., Cook, J. D., and Finch, C. A. Iron Metabolism in Man. Oxford, Blackwell Scientific Publications, 1979.
82. Halliday, J. W., Mack, U., and Powell, L. W. Duodenal ferritin content and structure: relationship with body iron stores in man. Arch. Intern. Med. *138*:1113, 1978.
83. Britten, G. M., and Raval, D. Duodenal ferritin synthesis in iron deficient rats: Response to small doses of iron. J. Lab. Clin. Med. *77*:54, 1971.
84. Allgood, L. W., and Brown, E. B. The relationship between duodenal mucosal iron concentration and iron absorption in human subjects. Scand. J. Haematol. *4*:217, 1967.
85. Cox, T. M., and Peters, T. J. Cellular mechanisms in the regulation of iron absorption by human intestine: studies in patients with iron deficiency before and after treatment. Br. J. Hematol. *44*:75, 1980.
86. Muir, A., and Hopfer, U. Regional specificity of iron uptake by small intestine brush border membrane from normal and iron-deficient mice. Am. J. Physiol. *248*:G376, 1985.
87. Dallman, P. R. Biochemical basis for the manifestation of iron deficiency. Ann. Rev. Nutr. *6*:13, 1986.
88. Nordin, B. E. C. (ed). Calcium, Phosphate and Magnesium Metabolism. Edinburgh, Churchill Livingstone, 1976.
89. Kenny, A. D. Intestinal Calcium Absorption and Its Regulation. Boca Raton, Florida, CRC Press, 1981.
90. Bo-Linn, G. W., Vendrell, D. D., Lee, E., and Fordtran, J. S. An evaluation of the importance of gastric acid secretion in the absorption of dietary calcium. J. Clin. Invest. *73*:640, 1984.
91. Recker, R. R. Calcium absorption and achlorhydria. N. Engl. J. Med. *313*:70, 1985.

92. Fordtran, J. S., and Locklear, W. Ionic constituents and osmolality of gastric and small intestinal fluids after eating. Am. J. Dig. Dis. *11*:503, 1966.
93. Vergne-Marini, P., Parker, T. R., Pak, C. Y. C., Hull, A. R., DeLuca, H. F., and Fordtran, J. S. Jejunal and ileal calcium absorption in patients with chronic renal disease. Effect of 1-hydroxycholecalciferol. J. Clin. Invest. *57*:861, 1976.
94. Wasserman, R. H., and Taylor, A. N. Gastrointestinal absorption of calcium and phosphorus. *In* Auerbach, G. D. (ed.). Handbook of Physiology, Section 7, Endocrinology. Vol VII. American Physiological Society, 1976, p. 137.
95. Allen, L. H. Calcium bioavailability and absorption: a review. Am. J. Clin. Nutr. *35*:783, 1982.
96. Avioli, L. V. Calcium and osteoporosis. Ann. Rev. Nutr. *4*:471, 1984.
97. Favus, M. J. Factors that influence absorption and secretion of calcium in the small intestine and colon. Am. J. Physiol. *28*:G147, 1985.
98. Wasserman, R. H., and Fullmer, C. S. Calcium transport proteins, calcium absorption and vitamin D. Am. Rev. Physiol. *45*:375, 1983.
99. Ireland, P., and Fordtran, J. S. Effect of dietary calcium and age in jejunal calcium absorption in humans studied by intestinal perfusion. J. Clin. Invest. *53*:2672, 1973.
100. Solomons, N. W. Calcium intake and availability from the human diet. Clin. Nutr. *5*:167, 1986.
101. Cook, D. A. Availability of magnesium: balance studies in rats with various inorganic magnesium salts. J. Nutr. *103*:1365, 1973.
102. Norman, D. A., Fordtran, J. S., Brinkley, L. J., Zerwekh, J. E., Nicar, M. J., Strowig, S. M., and Pak, C. Y. Jejunal and ileal adaptation to alteration in dietary calcium. Changes in calcium and magnesium absorption. J. Clin. Invest. *65*:1599, 1981.
103. Levin, B. S., and Coburn, J. W. Magnesium, the mimic antagonist of calcium. N. Engl. J. Med. *310*:1253, 1984.
104. Wester, P. O. Magnesium. Am. J. Clin. Nutr. *45*:1305, 1987.
105. Slatopolsky, E., Rosenbaum, R., Mennes, P., and Klahr, S. The hypocalcemia of magnesium depletion. *In* Massey, S. G., et al (eds.). Homeostasis of Phosphate and Other Minerals, New York, Plenum, 1978, p. 263.
106. Wacker, W. E. C. Magnesium and Man. Cambridge, Harvard University Press, 1980.
107. Cousins, R. J. Regulation of zinc absorption. Am. J. Clin. Nutr. *32*:339, 1979.
108. Matseshe, J. W., Phillips, S. F., Malagelada, J. R., and McCall, J. T. Recovery of dietary iron and zinc from the proximal intestine of healthy man: studies of different meals and supplements. Am. J. Clin. Nutr. *33*:1946, 1980.
109. Cousins, R. J. Absorption, transport and hepatic metabolism of copper and zinc: special reference to metallothionein and ceruloplasmin. Physiol. Rev. *65*:23, 1985.
110. Solomons, N. W., and Jacob, R. A. Studies on the bioavailability of zinc in humans: effects of heme and nonheme iron on the absorption of zinc. Am. J. Clin. Nutr. *34*:475, 1981.
111. Wolman, S. L., Anderson, G. A., Marliss, E. B., and Jeejeebhoy, K. N. Zinc in total parenteral nutrition: requirements and metabolic effects. Gastroenterology *76*:458, 1979.
112. Prasad, A. S. Clinical manifestation of zinc deficiency. Ann. Rev. Nutr. *5*:341, 1985.

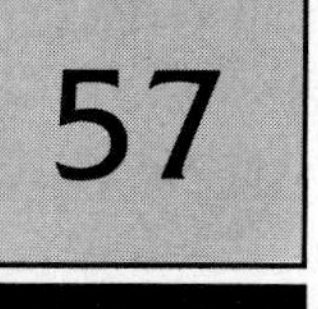

Mechanisms of Digestion and Absorption of Food

REBECCA W. VAN DYKE

A major function of the tubular gastrointestinal tract is the digestion and absorption of a wide variety of nutrients. The complex sequential array of mechanisms that have evolved to perform this function may be affected, to a greater or lesser extent, by many different diseases, resulting in malabsorption of some or all ingested materials. Because of the diversity and complexity of normal digestion and absorption of food, an orderly and systematic approach to the diagnosis and therapy of malabsorption requires an understanding of normal processes of digestion. This chapter reviews normal physiologic mechanisms of digestion and absorption of each of the major nutrients (carbohydrates, fats, and proteins) and briefly discusses inherited defects in these processes, as well as absorption of fiber and bile salts and the effects of motility, aging, and developmental changes on digestion and absorption. Fluid and electrolyte transport is covered on pages 1022 to 1045, vitamin and mineral absorption is discussed on pages 1045 to 1062, and maldigestion and malabsorption are reviewed on pages 263 to 282.

GENERAL ASPECTS OF DIGESTION

Digestion and absorption of all foodstuffs follow a series of sequential steps that occur both with time and with progression through the gastointestinal tract from mouth to colon. This overall series of events comprises (1) reduction of particle size, leading to an increase in the surface area of solid materials, (2) conversion of foods to an isotonic aqueous suspension, (3) solubilization (emulsification) of hydrophobic lipids, (4) enzymatic digestion of large macromolecules to small fragments, and (5) absorption of the small molecular weight products of digestion across the intestinal epithelial cells. The first three steps occur principally in the stomach and proximal portion of the duodenum. The stomach is primarily responsible for grinding and mixing ingested foods (see pp. 675–712). This process is efficient, solid food being consistently reduced to particles less than 1 mm in size, which are passed from stomach to duodenum at a well-regulated, constant rate (zero order kinetics) while large particles are retained for further grinding. High speed propulsion of liquid material from the stomach through the pylorus also contributes to fat emulsification by forcibly dispersing large fat globules into small droplets.[1] Finally, food particles, lipids, products of digestion, and ingested liquids are diluted to isotonicity in the duodenum and jejunum by intestinal epithelial cell-mediated secretion of ions, principally Na^+ and Cl^-, and water (see pp. 1022–1045).

The principal site of the last two stages, enzymatic digestion and absorption, is in the small intestine, with digestion conventionally divided into two phases: (1) luminal digestion in the bulk fluid phase, followed by (2) mucosal (brush border) digestion at the surface of intestinal epithelial cells (enterocytes). The final products of digestion are subsequently absorbed across the intestinal epithelial cell into the lamina propria, a process involving movement of small molecules across both the apical and basolateral cell membranes as well as the cytoplasm of the enterocyte (see Figure 54–8). Specific mechanisms for digestion and absorption of carbohydrates, lipids, and proteins are discussed in the next three sections of this chapter.

CARBOHYDRATE DIGESTION AND ABSORPTION

Carbohydrates provide the majority of the calories for most humans, principally in the form of starch (~60 per cent), sucrose (~30 per cent), and lactose (~10 per cent). Carbohydrate intake approximates 400 gm/day or more in a typical Western diet.

Starch is a polysaccharide with a molecular weight of 100,000 to 1,000,000. It is a polymer of glucose molecules that occurs in two forms: alpha-amylose, which consists of long, unbranched chains of glucose units, and amylopectin, which is a highly branched chain of glucose units (Fig. 57–1). The glucose molecules of amylose are linked in straight chains by alpha-1,4 bonds between carbon atom 1 (C1) of one glucose molecule and C4 of the next one in the chain. In amylopectin, branch points along these straight glucose chains are located at every 12 to 25 glucose residues, when C6 of one glucose molecule binds to C1 of the first glucose molecule of the branch (alpha-1,6 bonds). (In contrast, cellulose, which cannot be digested by mammalian enzymes, is an unbranched polymer of glucose molecules linked by beta-1,4 bonds.)

Sucrose and lactose, the other major dietary carbohydrates, are disaccharides (i.e., they consist of two linked monosaccharides). Sucrose, extremely abundant in plants, is a dimer of one glucose and one fructose molecule. Lactose, which is found only in milk, is a dimer of one glucose and one galactose molecule.

Luminal Digestion of Starch

Digestion of starch proceeds with both luminal and mucosal stages. Luminal digestion begins in the mouth with the action of salivary amylase, an alpha-amylase secreted by acinar cells of salivary glands, which attacks alpha-1,4 glucose linkages in the interior of the starch molecule, releasing products containing two (maltose) or three (maltotriose) glucose molecules (Fig. 57–1). The action of salivary amylase is terminated rapidly by gastric acid, and the bulk of luminal starch is digested rapidly in the duodenum, mediated by pancreatic alpha-amylase.[2] Pancreatic alpha-amylase, secreted in vast excess of that needed for normal starch digestion, is, like salivary alpha-amylase, an endoenzyme that cleaves internal alpha-1,4 bonds, but it does not split the alpha-1,6 bonds of amylopectin (Fig. 57–1). The products of alpha-amylase digestion are, therefore, maltose, maltotriose, and a series of highly branched compounds called "alpha-limit dextrins." These latter oligosaccharides average about eight glucose units each and contain one or more alpha-1,6 linkages (Fig. 57–1). Secretion of salivary and pancreatic amylase is lower in infants than in adults, although an amylase found in human milk may provide an additional mechanism for carbohydrate digestion in infants.[3]

None of the products of amylase activity can be absorbed readily by small intestinal enterocytes; all these products undergo further digestion to their component monosaccharides at the enterocyte membrane prior to absorption.

Enterocyte Digestion of Oligosaccharides

The highly specialized apical membrane (brush border) of small intestinal enterocytes contains an array of integral membrane proteins that mediate the final stages of carbohydrate digestion and absorption. Three well-characterized oligosaccharidases or disaccharidases have been identified in humans and other animal species: glucoamylase, sucrase-alpha-dextrinase (sucrase-isomaltase), and lactase (lactase-glycosylceramidase) (Table 57–1).[4–14] A fourth minor disaccharidase, trehalase, is also present in humans. All three major oligosaccharidases are large, glycosylated dimeric ectoenzymes (membrane-bound enzymes whose active site is on the outside of the cell) with two active sites. Each enzyme is synthesized initially as a single-chain proform in the rough endoplasmic reticulum, is inserted into the membrane of the endoplasmic reticulum, and is then transported to the Golgi apparatus, where it is glycosylated (Fig. 57–2). These enzymes thus follow the classic pattern for synthesis and processing of integral membrane proteins. Recent exami-

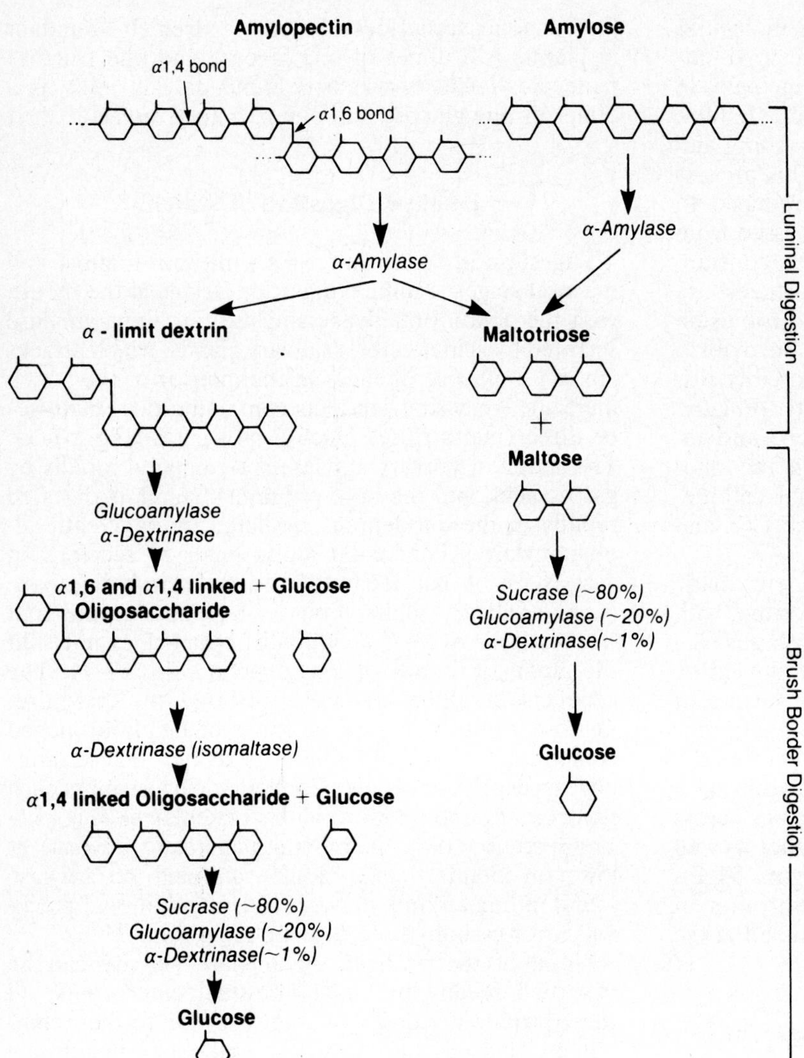

Figure 57–1. Starch digestion in the small intestine. In this schematic representation, the two major forms of dietary starch are shown: amylopectin (branched chains) and amylose (unbranched chains). Substrates are indicated in boldface type, enzymes in italic type. Luminal digestion is depicted at the top of the figure and brush border (mucosal) digestion at the bottom. Two or more enzymes are listed for those steps in digestion in which activity is attributed to several enzymes. The relative contribution of each enzyme is shown, where it is known, in parentheses.

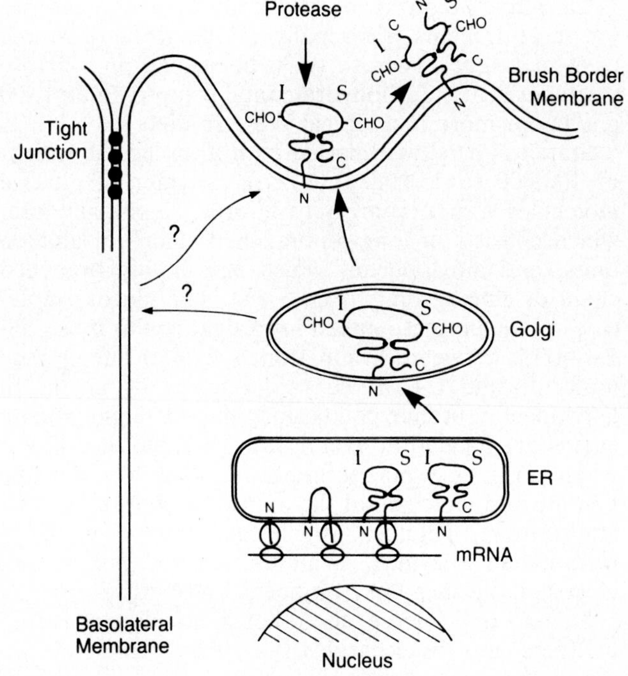

Figure 57–2. Synthesis of sucrase-isomaltase. This schema depicts the synthesis and processing of a representative enterocyte brush border oligosaccharidase: sucrase-isomaltase (alpha-dextrinase). A single proenzyme polypeptide chain is synthesized in the rough endoplasmic reticulum (ER) with the N terminus (N) on the cytoplasmic side, the C- terminus (C) on the luminal side of the ER, and noncovalent bonds (••) between the isomaltase (I) and sucrase (S) portions of the protein. The protein is transferred to the Golgi apparatus, glycosylated, and transported, by exocytosis, to the brush border membrane. (The arrows labeled with question marks indicate possible transport via the basolateral plasma membrane.) Following insertion into the brush border membrane, the protein is cleaved into its two separate subunits by pancreatic enzymes (protease), particularly elastase. (Modified from Hauri, H. P. *In* Brush Border Membranes. London, Pitman, 1983, p. 132.)

Table 57–1. SMALL INTESTINAL BRUSH BORDER GLYCOSIDASES (OLIGOSACCHARIDASES)*

Complex	Glycosidase	Activity	Products	Molecular Weight	K_m (mM)
Sucrase-alpha-dextrinase (sucrase-isomaltase)	Sucrase	Hydrolyzes sucrose	Glucose, fructose	~120,000; peripheral protein linked to isomaltase via noncovalent bonds	20 (sucrose) 3.6 (maltotriose) 2.6 (maltose)
		Sequentially splits alpha-1,4 bonds of starch, maltotriose, maltose	Glucose		
	Alpha-dextrinase (isomaltase)	Cleaves alpha-1,6 bond of alpha-limit dextrins, isomaltose†	Maltotriose, glucose, straight-chain oligosaccharides	~140,000; anchored to membrane by N-terminal region of protein	1–5 (alpha-1,6 bonds) 11 (maltotriose) 3.1 (maltose)
		Sequentially cleaves alpha-1,4 bonds of starch, maltotriose, maltose	Glucose		
Glucoamylase	Two similar glucoamylases	Sequentially cleaves alpha-1,4 bonds of oligosaccharides, maltotriose, maltose	Glucose, residual oligosaccharides with alpha-1,6 bond	Two subunits of 135,000 and 125,000; one subunit is anchored to the membrane by its N-terminal region, the other subunit is linked to it by noncovalent bonds; two active sites distinguished by heat sensitivity	1.1 (oligosaccharides) 3.8 (maltose)
Lactase (beta-glycosidase)	Lactase	Hydrolyzes lactose	Glucose Galactose	160,000 (anchored to membrane)	18 (lactose)
		Slowly hydrolyzes cellobiose, cellotriose	Glucose		
	Aryl-beta-glycosidase	Hydrolyzes glycosylceramides	Glucose Ceramide	160,000 (anchored to membrane)	—
Trehalase	Trehalase	Hydrolyzes trehalose	Glucose	—	—

*Based on data from references 4 to 14.
†Isomaltose is a disaccharide of two glucose molecules linked by an alpha-1,6 bond.

nation of the DNA coding for these proteins indicates a great deal of sequence similarity between the two active subunits of each enzyme (i.e., between sucrase and alpha-dextrinase), suggesting that each dimeric enzyme arose by gene duplication.[14]

From the Golgi apparatus, these enzymes are transported to the apical plasma membrane, presumably in Golgi secretory vesicles, and inserted into the membrane by exocytic fusion. The mechanisms responsible for sorting and transporting these enzymes to the brush border remain unclear. Interestingly, although activity of the enzymes is confined to the enterocyte brush border, immunofluorescence and pulse-chase studies indicate that sucrase-alpha-dextrinase (and perhaps other brush border proteins) is inserted, at least briefly, into the basolateral plasma membrane before ultimately arriving at the brush border.[5] The physiologic function (if any) of sucrase-alpha-dextrinase on the basolateral membrane, and the mechanism(s) responsible for movement of the enzyme from basolateral to brush border membrane, are not understood (Fig. 57–2).

Prior to insertion into the apical plasma membrane, the single-chain proform of lactase is cleaved into its two active subunits, lactase and glycosylceramidase, by intracellular protease(s), perhaps in the Golgi apparatus. In contrast, both glucoamylase and sucrase-alpha-dextrinase are first transported to the brush border membrane and are cleaved subsequently into their respective subunits by pancreatic proteases (principally elastase) (Fig. 57–3). Cleavage is not, however, essential for enzyme activity.[7]

These three oligosaccharidases, with a total of six active sites, exhibit complementary but overlapping specificities for oligosaccharide derivatives of starch and dietary disaccharides, as shown in Table 57–1 and Figure 57–4.[5–14] Trehalase, a minor and poorly understood enzyme, cleaves trehalose, a disaccharide composed of two glucose molecules, which is found in insects and mushrooms.

The brush border oligosaccharidases are distributed throughout the small intestine but are found in highest concentration in the midportion of the villus and, longitudinally, in the jejunum [15, 16] These enzymes, as well as pancreatic amylase, generally are present in amounts sufficiently large to preclude hydrolysis as the rate-limiting step for overall carbohydrate assimilation.[17] Lactase is, however, an important exception. Even in lactase-sufficient individuals, hydrolysis of lactose is the rate-limiting step for assimilation of this sugar[17, 18] (see pp. 269 and 1068).

Degradation and synthesis of brush border hydrolases can be altered by a number of factors, with implications for overall carbohydrate digestion. For

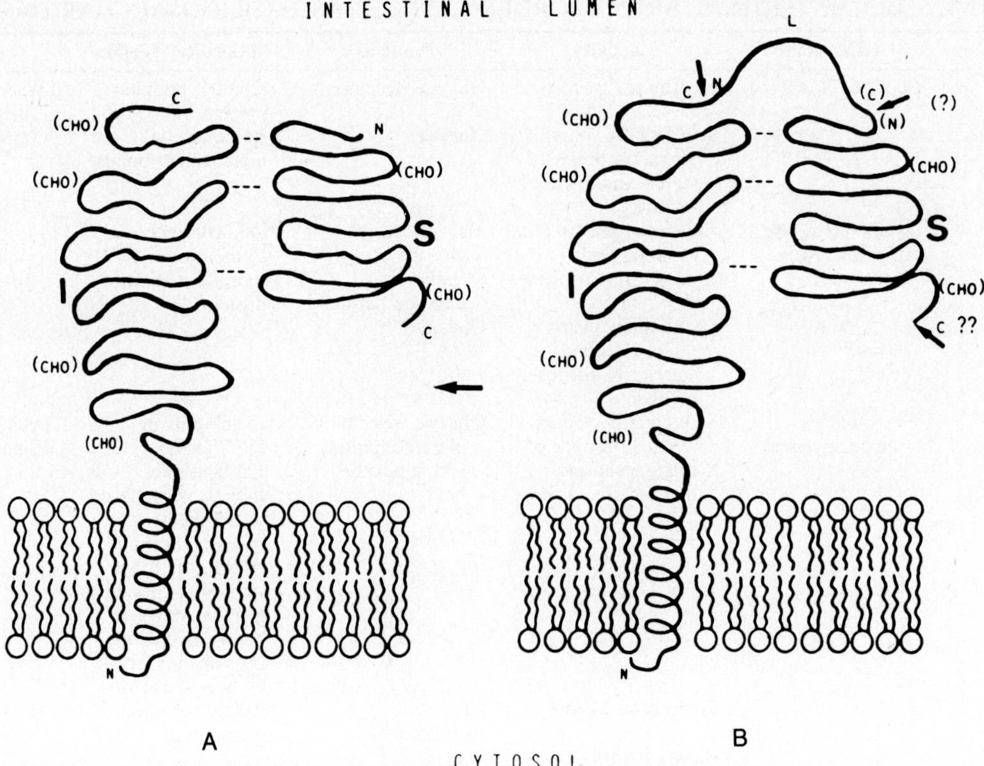

Figure 57–3. Positioning of the sucrase-isomaltase complex *(a)* and the "Pro-sucrase-isomaltase" complex *(b)* in the small intestinal brush border membrane. I, Isomaltase subunit; S, sucrase subunit; L, loop accessible to attack by pancreatic proteases at the point(s) indicated by the arrows; N,C, the N and C-termini of the complexes, respectively; (CHO), carbohydrate chains; - - -, noncovalent bonds linking the two subunits. (From Dahlqvist, A., and Semenza, G. Disaccharidases of small-intestinal mucosa. J. Pediatr. Gastroenterol. Nutr. 4:857, 1985. Used by permission.

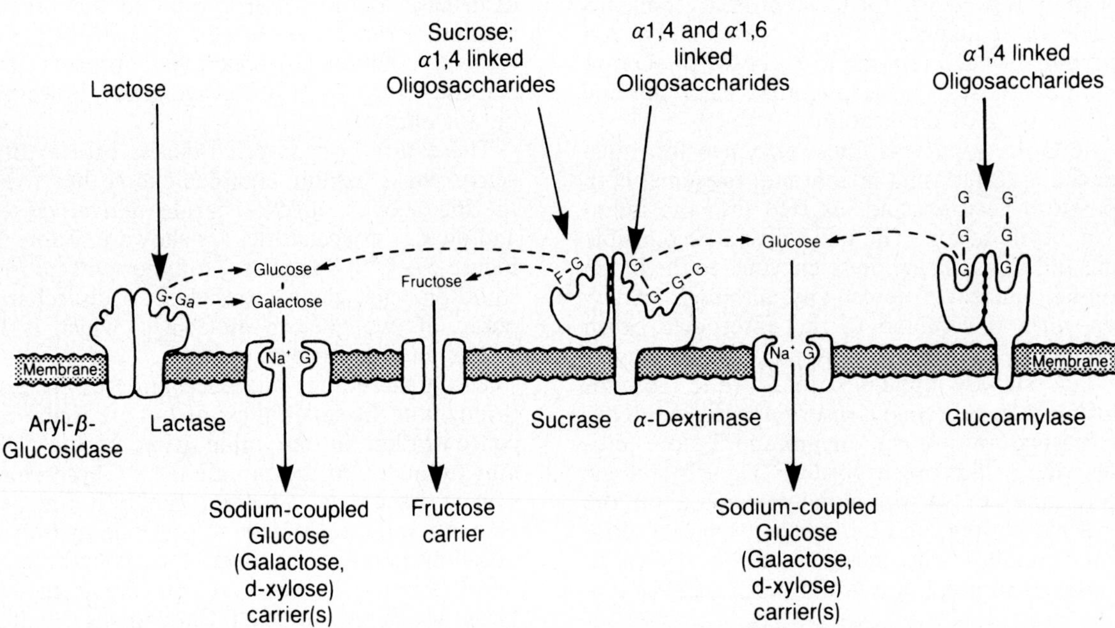

Figure 57–4. Small intestinal brush border hydrolysis of dietary carbohydrate. In this diagrammatic representation, oligosaccharides, produced by the luminal action of pancreatic amylase, and dietary disaccharides are hydrolyzed by specific integral membrane enzymes positioned in the enterocyte brush border membrane so that their active hydrolytic sites (depicted as clefts) are exposed to the luminal contents. The released monosaccharides then bind to specific carrier sites for translocation to the enterocyte cytoplasm. For clarity, simple diffusion of monosaccharides across the brush border membrane is not shown. G, Glucose; F, fructose; Ga, galactose. (Modified from Gray, G. M. N. Engl. J. Med. *292*:1225, 1975.)

example, the half-life of these enzymes is short (≤ 11 hours), in part because of degradation by luminal pancreatic proteases and bacterial proteases.[19–21] Indeed, the carbohydrate malabsorption seen in many patients with small intestinal bacterial overgrowth may be due, in part, to accelerated destruction of brush border oligosaccharidases.[21, 22] In contrast, absence of pancreatic proteases in patients with pancreatic exocrine insufficiency might lead to increased oligosaccharidase activity, rapid glucose absorption, and postprandial hyperglycemia. Finally, synthesis of sucrase-alpha-dextrinase varies with a circadian rhythm and also increases promptly after sucrose feeding, a positive feedback response that may optimize carbohydrate digestion.[23, 24] In contrast, lactose intake fails to stimulate lactase synthesis.

Enterocyte Transport of Monosaccharides

Monosaccharides produced by the action of brush border oligosaccharidases are small hydrophilic molecules that do not penetrate cell membranes rapidly. *Simple diffusion* of these compounds across membranes is slow, but it is important for glucose uptake at high luminal concentrations. *Specific active transport systems* that mediate efficient transport of these compounds from gut to blood are located on the apical (Fig. 57–4) and basolateral plasma membranes of enterocytes.[25, 26] The brush border membrane contains at least two distinct transporters that couple uptake of glucose, galactose, or xylose, but not fructose, to uptake of sodium. These *sodium-coupled transporters*, presumably integral membrane proteins, use the energy of the electrochemical sodium gradient, generated by the sodium pump Na^+,K^+-ATPase, to transport glucose and to concentrate it inside enterocytes. Two sodium-coupled glucose carriers have been tentatively identified in small intestine and are thought to bind one molecule of glucose and one or three sodium ions, respectively.[25] Similar sodium-coupled transport mechanisms exist in many different cell types, where they mediate transport of a wide variety of substances, including amino acids, organic and inorganic anions, and protons as well as monosaccharides. Indeed, the sodium-coupled glucose transporter, which is found in both kidney and intestine, was the first one of these to be recognized and characterized, and it has served as the model for this large class of important transport mechanisms.

Glucose, galactose, xylose, and fructose also enter enterocytes by means of other membrane carriers that are not coupled to any energy source, a process termed *facilitated diffusion* (Fig. 57–4).

Subsequently, all of these monosaccharides move out of enterocytes into the lamina propria through other poorly characterized facilitated diffusion pathways located in the basolateral cell membrane. The exact specificity of the various sodium-independent facilitated diffusion transporters is not known.

The sodium-coupled glucose or galactose carrier is important for intestinal glucose uptake, especially when luminal glucose concentrations are low, and, like sucrase, it increases its activity with carbohydrate feeding or diabetes by an increase in the number of functional transporters.[25–28] Because of the high affinity for glucose (Km ~ 0.03 to 0.3 mM)[25] and the active nature of this transporter, it also efficiently scavenges glucose in the distal portion of the intestine, where luminal glucose concentrations are equal to or less than plasma concentrations. With the exception of lactose, the assimilation of which is limited by lactase activity, the capacity of the hexose carriers constitutes the rate-limiting step(s) for overall carbohydrate absorption. Indeed, xylose is an excellent test substrate for detecting absorption defects because it is not digested prior to transport, and, owing to its relatively low affinity for the sodium-coupled glucose carrier, small decreases in intestinal function cause relatively large reductions in xylose uptake. On the other hand, a limited capacity for uptake of fructose and sugar alcohols, such as sorbitol, has led to symptoms of carbohydrate malabsorption in some individuals as these substances have been used increasingly as commercial sweeteners[29, 30] (see also Table 20–2, p. 296, and p. 1068).

Interactions Between Oligosaccharidases and Monosaccharide Absorption

The brush border hydrolases and monosaccharide carriers are separate, unrelated membrane proteins, yet they mediate sequential and closely related steps in carbohydrate assimilation.[31] The functions of these two classes of proteins appear to be related owing to their geographic proximity in the brush border membrane and the unstirred water layer located in and around the brush border. Thus, monosaccharides normally are released from oligosaccharides in close proximity to their membrane carriers (Fig. 57–4). This arrangement prevents development of hypertonic luminal contents during rapid carbohydrate digestion and facilitates hexose transport by markedly increasing hexose concentration in the poorly stirred milieu of the enterocyte brush border.[17–32, 33, 34] As an example of this effect, the Km for glucose transport is > 10 mM in intact tissue and is ≤ 0.1 mM in membrane vesicles for which there is no unstirred water layer.[25, 35] Finally, because the activity of brush border oligosaccharidases is inhibited by free glucose, carbohydrate hydrolysis is regulated by the hexose transporters; free glucose awaiting transport reduces the rate of glucose production from oligosaccharides, thus minimizing escape of glucose into the bulk luminal contents.[32]

Efficiency of Carbohydrate Absorption

Although carbohydrate digestion and absorption are highly efficient processes, not all dietary carbohydrate is absorbed during passage through the small intestine. Intestinal perfusion studies and H_2 breath tests indicate that, whereas in normal humans 96 to 98 per cent of sucrose is absorbed in the small intestine, 2 to 20 per cent of ingested starch is not absorbed and reaches the colon.[36–40] The source of the starch is an important factor in absorption: rice starch is virtually completely absorbed,[38, 41, 42] whereas 8, 6, 13, 10 to 20, and 18 to 20 per cent, respectively, of starch derived from oats, corn, potatoes, wheat, and dried beans is not absorbed.[38, 40, 41] Indeed, it is estimated that up to 70 gm of dietary carbohydrate, including fiber, reaches the colon each day. Carbohydrate in the colon, as in the bovine rumen, is fermented by colonic bacteria to short-chain fatty acids, H_2, and methane[36, 43–45] (see pp. 259–260). H_2 and methane contribute to flatus production, whereas short-chain fatty acids are rapidly absorbed by colonic epithelial cells and, indeed, constitute a major energy source for the epithelium.[45–49] Thus, the colon plays an important role in scavenging dietary carbohydrate. Unabsorbed sugars and fatty acids contribute to the osmotic activity of colonic contents and, under normal conditions, determine the degree of stool hydration. When malabsorption of carbohydrate is pronounced because of excessive intake or impaired small intestinal absorption (see pp. 263–282), symptoms that include excessive flatus, abdominal cramps, and watery osmotic diarrhea ensue.[50, 51] Individuals with lactase deficiency, for example (see next section), malabsorb about 50 per cent of ingested lactose and develop symptoms (flatus and diarrhea) after ingesting ≥ 20 gm of lactose (see p. 269).

Inherited Disorders of Carbohydrate Digestion

Lactase Deficiency. *Lactase deficiency* is the most common disorder of carbohydrate digestion in humans, occurring in most adults with the exception of those from Northern Europe. Indeed, deficiency of lactase, an enzyme that is nutritionally necessary only for infants prior to weaning, could be considered a normal aspect of maturation and aging. Lactase-deficient adults retain 10 to 30 per cent of intestinal lactase activity and develop symptoms (syndrome of lactose intolerance) only when they ingest sufficient lactose to overwhelm colonic conservation mechanisms. Most people would have to drink 1 to 2 glasses of milk (containing approximately 11 gm of lactose per 8-ounce serving) or more per day to exhibit symptoms. Yoghurt may be well tolerated by lactase-deficient persons, as it has considerable bacterial lactase activity.[51]

Lactase deficiency also occurs as a result of small intestinal diseases such as *viral gastroenteritis, celiac sprue,* or *tropical sprue* (see pp. 1134–1152, 1212–1215, and 1281–1289). Lactase levels appear to be depressed by small bowel diseases more readily and for a more prolonged period than other oligosaccharidases.[52]

Congenital Lactase Deficiency. This is a rare disorder in which lactase activity is low or absent at birth.[53] Infants develop symptoms (abdominal pain, watery diarrhea, and failure to thrive) as soon as milk is fed. These symptoms are seen in siblings, but not in parents, suggesting that the condition is transmitted as an autosomal recessive disorder. Therapy simply involves elimination of dietary milk.

Sucrase-Isomaltase (Sucrase-alpha-dextrinase) Deficiency. Deficiency of this enzyme complex is inherited as an autosomal recessive disorder that is rare in most populations (0.2 per cent prevalence in North Americans), but common in others, such as Eskimos, in whom 10 per cent or more of the population may be affected.[53, 54] Symptoms follow ingestion of sucrose; dietary starch, however, is well tolerated, probably because of residual isomaltase (alpha-dextrinase) activity of glucoamylase and the low osmotic activity of alpha-dextrins. In at least one case, impaired enzyme function was due to impaired transport of immunologically identifiable sucrase-isomaltase from the Golgi apparatus to the apical membrane of enterocytes.[55]

Trehalase Deficiency. Three patients have been reported who developed symptoms of carbohydrate malabsorption after ingestion of mushrooms[53] and in whom impaired trehalose absorption was documented by a trehalose tolerance test. Because mushrooms are generally ingested in small amounts (i.e., below the threshold for producing symptoms) trehalase deficiency actually may be more common than is presently believed.

Glucose-galactose Malabsorption. This rare autosomal recessive disorder of sodium-coupled monosaccharide transport causes symptoms of intractable acidic, osmotic diarrhea and glucosuria when lactose or sucrose is ingested.[53, 56, 57] Fructose is absorbed normally, whereas absorption of glucose and galactose is reduced to less than 25 per cent of normal values in both intestine and kidney tubules owing to abnormal function of the sodium-coupled glucose carrier.

Fructose Malabsorption. Symptomatic fructose malabsorption has been reported in four persons, although the underlying mechanism has not been elucidated.[53] Normal subjects, however, exhibit a limited capacity for fructose absorption,[29] and therefore fructose intolerance may appear more frequently with the increasing use of fructose to sweeten foods.

Inhibitors of Amylase and Disaccharidases

An alpha-glucosidase inhibitor has been purified from bacteria that inhibits alpha-amylase, sucrase, and maltase,[37, 58] and, in addition, an amylase inhibitor has been purified from white beans.[59] These compounds slow digestion of starch and disaccharides and may be useful in retarding glucose absorption in diabetic persons.[60] Other potential roles for these agents, such as therapy for *obesity* and the *dumping syndrome*, conceivably might be limited by symptoms of carbohydrate malabsorption (see pp. 173–185 and 964–968).

FAT DIGESTION AND ABSORPTION

Ingestion of fat, which constitutes up to 160 gm/day and up to 50 per cent of the caloric content of the Western diet, presents the intestine with a series of unique digestive challenges. Dietary fat, composed primarily of triglycerides, is, by definition, hydrophobic, yet it is a vital source of fuel as well as of the essential fatty acids linoleic acid and linolenic acid, vitamins A, D, E, and K, and cholesterol. A sequence of complex mechanisms has evolved to facilitate digestion and absorption of fat within the aqueous environment of the intestinal lumen. The overall process of fat digestion and absorption can be divided into seven phases. These are (1) *emulsification* of fat and dispersion into small particles; (2) *enzymatic hydrolysis* of fatty acid esters; (3) *dispersion* of digestion products into a form suitable for absorption; (4) *diffusion* across the unstirred water layer; (5) *absorption* across the enterocyte brush border membrane; (6) *intracellular metabolism* and packaging of lipid into lipoproteins; and (7) *transport* from epithelial cells to the lamina propria. More detailed reviews of this subject can be found in the literature on the subject.[61, 62]

Composition of Dietary Fat

Dietary fat consists mainly of triglycerides, tri-fatty acid esters of glycerol (Fig. 57–5) that are abundant in plants and animals. Most dietary triglycerides (>90 per cent) are composed of long-chain fatty acids (C16–C18). Triglycerides are essentially insoluble in water and usually form a separate oil phase or, after mixing, an unstable oil-water emulsion. Triglyceride droplets in milk, in cells, and in processed foods are stabilized by a surface coating of phospholipids or a combination of gums, phospholipids, and other agents. Although digestion and absorption of the triglycerides have been studied most extensively and these are the focus of this discussion, there are other important dietary fats. Phospholipids (Fig. 57–5), especially lecithin (phosphatidylcholine) are derived primarily from plant and animal cell membranes (4 to 8 gm/day) and from cells shed in the gastrointestinal tract as well as from bile (up to 12 gm/day). Small amounts of a variety of complex lipids, often derived from plants, are also ingested, including waxes, sterols, wax esters, and complex lipids from industrial sources. Finally, the diet also contains small amounts of cholesterol, sterol vitamins (A, D, E, and K), fatty acids, prostaglandins, and steroid hormones. Many of these are solubilized in phospholipid bilayers or micelles, whereas small amounts are found in the lipid cores of triglyceride oil droplets. Digestion and absorption of many of these

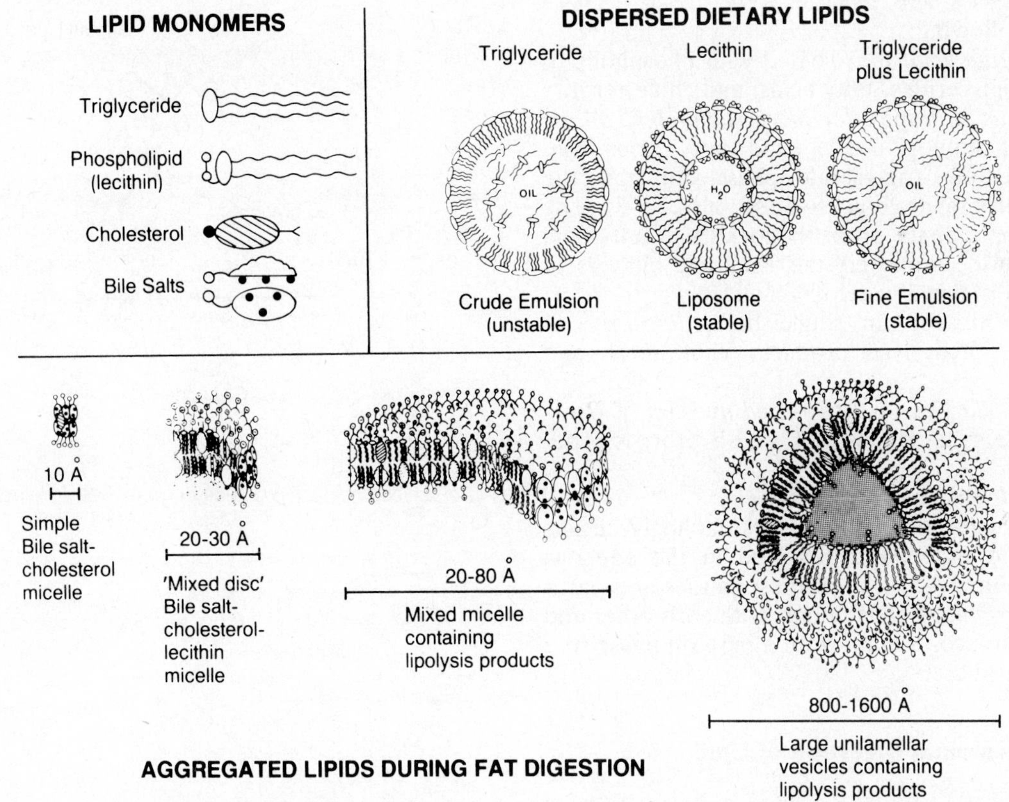

Figure 57–5. Schematic representation of the chemical structures and physical states of dietary lipids and lipolysis products in the small intestine. Lipid monomers, which are present in small amounts in aqueous solution, are depicted at the top left of the figure. In the stomach and proximal duodenum, emulsions of triglyceride and triglyceride plus phospholipid (lecithin) (shown at the top right of the figure), are thought to appear. Addition of gallbladder bile (containing bile salt micelles and small mixed micelles) to dietary lipids in the duodenum results in formtion of mixed micelles and large unilamellar liposomal vesicles. The viscous isotropic phase of lipolysis products found near triglyceride emulsions is not shown here (see Fig. 57–6). (Modified from Carey, M. C., et al. Ann. Rev. Physiol. *45*:651, 1983; Carey, M. C., *in* Arias, I., et al. [eds.]. The Liver: Biology and Pathophysiology. New York, Raven Press, Inc., 1982; and Mazer, N. A., and Carey, M. C. Biochemistry *22*:426, 1983.)

additional lipids remain poorly understood (Absorption of fat-soluble vitamins A, D, E, and K is discussed on pp. 1051–1054).

Emulsification and Solubilization of Lipid

With the exception of some short- and medium-chain fatty acids, lipids form an oil phase separate from the aqueous environment of the intestinal lumen. As digestion proceeds almost entirely at the oil-water interface, emulsification of fat to small particles, providing a large surface area for digestion, is an essential first step to efficient fat digestion. Indeed, most human lipases function only on substrates at an oil-water interface (interfacial activation) and hydrolyze dissolved lipids poorly, if at all. As triglycerides are released from food in the stomach and small intestine, they are emulsified to particles less than 0.5 μ in diameter through the mixing actions of these organs and the shear forces developed at the pylorus. Triglyceride emulsions are stabilized during the course of digestion by a coat of phospholipids (derived from ingested food and from bile), bile salts, and products of triglyceride hydrolysis (mono- and diglycerides and partially ionized fatty acids) (Fig. 57–5).

In the intestinal lumen, lipid is dispersed into a variety of phases and particles (Fig. 57–5).[1] These include the following:

1. *Triglyceride emulsions* coated with phospholipid, mono- and diglycerides, fatty acids, and cholesterol.
2. A *viscous isotropic (liquid crystalline) oil phase* composed of monoglycerides and fatty acids that "flows" from the triglyceride phase out into the aqueous environment (Fig. 57–5; see also 57–7). The viscous isotropic phase probably consists of fatty acid or monoglyceride liquid crystals (multiple bilayers of lipid with internalized water channels).
3. Large (80 to 160 nm) single-shelled *liposomes* of phospholipids, hydrolysis products, cholesterol, and bile salts.
4. Disc-shaped (2 to 8 nm) *mixed micelles* of phospholipids, bile salts, cholesterol, and hydrolysis products.
5. Small *bile salt micelles* (rare).
6. Low concentrations of bile salts, monoglycerides, and fatty acid *monomers* dissolved in the aqueous phase[1, 61–64] (Fig. 57–5). All of these phases and particles rapidly exchange constituents with each other and probably form a continuum from a pure oil phase to a pure aqueous phase.

Luminal Digestion of Lipid

Lipid digestion comprises mainly the hydrolysis of ester bonds in triglycerides and phospholipids and also in a wide range of sterols and xenobiotic lipids. Five or six human lipases mediate these reactions (Table 57–2). Lipid digestion begins in the stomach, where *lingual lipase* (and perhaps a separate *gastric lipase*), which is active at low pH, initiates hydrolysis of triglycerides[65–67] (Fig. 57–6). Because lipids remain in the stomach for up to several hours, lingual lipase may hydrolyze from 10 to 40 per cent of lipid ingested. Its primary products, fatty acids and diglycerides, become distributed on the surface of triglyceride emulsions, where they promote emulsion stability and facilitate the action of pancreatic lipase. Because of the broad pH optimum of lingual lipase (2 to 7.5), this enzyme is also active in the small intestine and plays an important role in lipid digestion in infants and in patients with cystic fibrosis or other types of pancreatic insufficiency.[68]

Intestinal lipolysis is mediated by at least four enzymes (Table 57–2). *Human milk lipase*, found only in the milk of humans and gorillas, is of great importance for infants because lipids account for up to 50 per cent of the calories in milk and pancreatic lipase production is low in young children.[69] Human milk lipase is resistant to gastric acid, is activated in the duodenum by bile salts, and hydrolyzes triglycerides and a wide variety of sterol esters.

In adults, intestinal triglyceride hydrolysis is mediated largely by *pancreatic lipase* acting in conjunction with its essential cofactor, pancreatic *(pro)colipase*.[70, 71] After secretion, procolipase is converted to its active

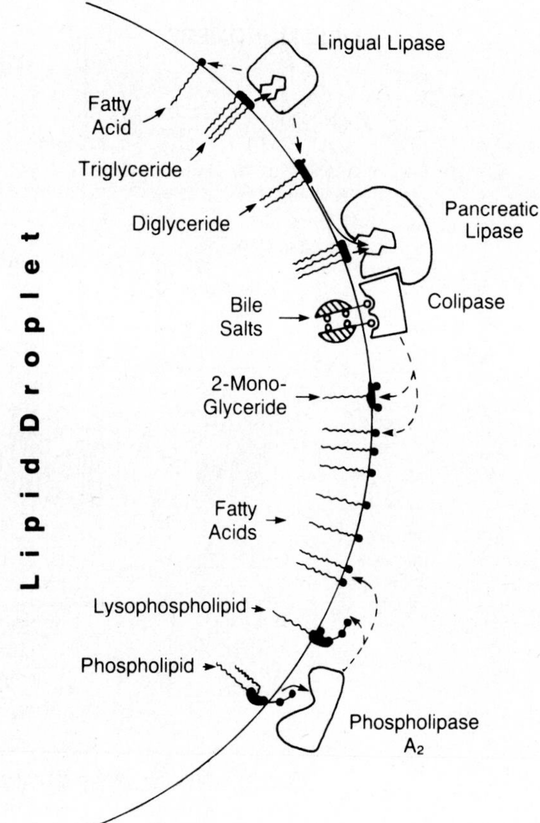

Figure 57–6. Luminal fat digestion. In this schematic representation, reactions occur on the surface of a lipid (triglyceride) droplet with both substrates and products solubilized in the surface membrane. Both gastric (lingual lipase) and small intestinal (pancreatic lipase-colipase and phospholipase A_2) lipid digestion are shown here, although these processes are sequential rather than simultaneous. →, substrate-enzyme interaction; - - -→, removal of product.

Table 57–2. LIPASE IN HUMANS*

Enzyme	Source	Characteristics	Site of Action	Physiologic Role
Human milk lipase	Milk (mammary gland)	Stable at acid pH Requires bile salts for activity Hydrolyzes long-chain triglycerides at all three bonds and sterol esters Molecular weight, 125,000 pH optimum, 8.0–9.5	Small intestine	Produces fatty acids, glycerol, monoglycerides, and free sterols Mediates triglyceride hydrolysis in infants as pancreatic lipase secretion is limited
Lingual lipase	Serous (von Ebner) glands under circumvallate papillae	Cleaves fatty acids from positions 3 (preferred) and 1 of long- and short-chain triglycerides Works only on aggregated substrate (oil droplet) ("interfacial activation") Optimal at acid pH (4–5) Does not require bile salts, phospholipid, or colipase Molecular weight, 50,000	Stomach (small intestine in patients with pancreatic insufficiency)	Produces diglycerides and fatty acids, thus further solubilizing bulk triglycerides for digestion by pancreatic lipase May contribute 10–40 per cent of lipolysis (more in infants and in patients with pancreatic insufficiency)
Gastric esterase ("lipase")	Gastric glands	Hydrolyzes short-chain triglycerides and some long-chain triglycerides	Stomach	Probably similar to lingual lipase
Pancreatic lipase-colipase	Pancreas	Colipase secreted as procolipase Cleaves fatty acids from positions 1 and 3 of long- and short-chain triglycerides Requires colipase and bile salts for binding to emulsion surface and activity Works only on aggregated substrate (oil droplet, liposome) Molecular weight, 50,000 (lipase), 10,000 (colipase)	Small intestine	Products are 2-monoglyceride and fatty acids Major intestinal lipase
Phospholipase A_2	Pancreas	Secreted as a proenzyme Hydrolyzes fatty acid from position 2 of phospholipids Works on aggregated substrate (membranes, liposomes, emulsions) Requires Ca^{2+} Requires bile salts (to form micelles) Molecular weight 14,000	Small intestine	Products are fatty acids and lysophospholipids Major intestinal phospholipase Required for optimal function of pancreatic lipase, perhaps by clearing phospholipids from emulsion surface
Pancreatic nonspecific lipase or cholesterol esterase	Pancrease ? Enterocytes	Requires bile salts to form active enzyme dimer Hydrolyzes a variety of esters: lysophospholipids, cholesterol esters, sterol vitamin (A,D,E) esters, especially when substrates are solubilized in micelles Molecular weight ~100,000	Small intestine	Hydrolyzes a wide range of sterol, vitamin, and xenobiotic esters

*Based on references 61, 62, and 65 to 72.

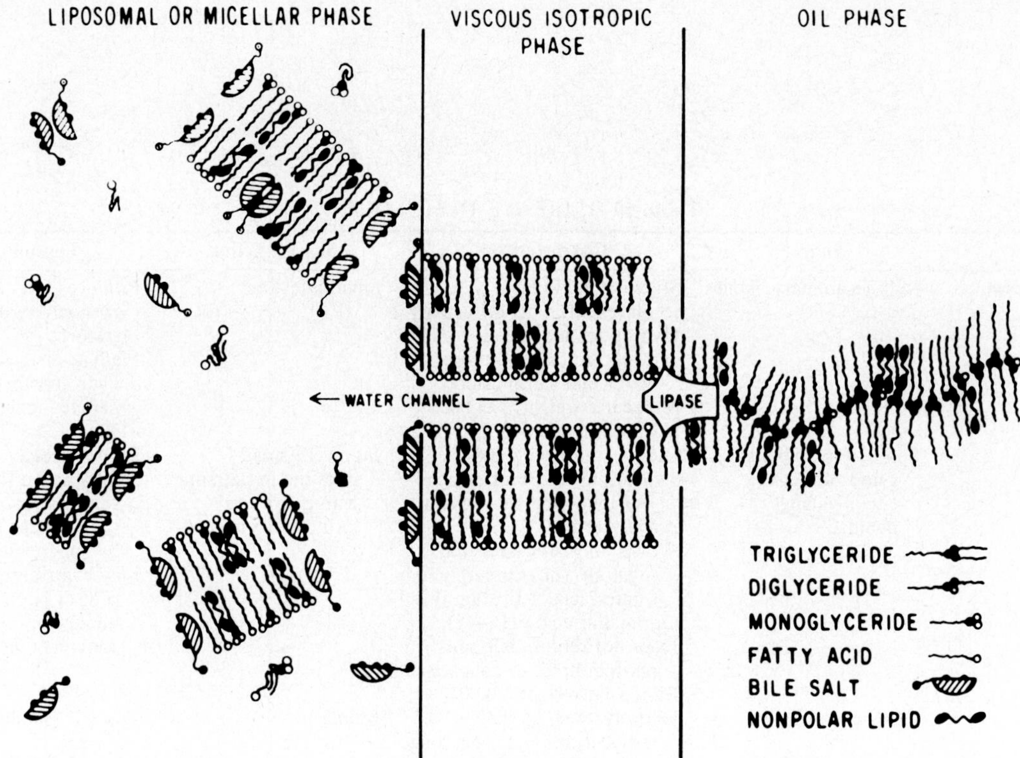

Figure 57–7. Small intestinal luminal triglyceride digestion. This schematic model depicts formation of a viscous isotropic phase composed mainly of lipolysis products. Materials in the viscous isotropic phase are subsequently solubilized as large mixed micelles and unilamellar vesicles (see Fig. 57–5) by bile salts. (From Patton, J. S. Gastrointestinal lipid digestion. *In* Johnson, L. R. [ed.]. Physiology of the Gastrointestinal Tract. New York, Raven Press, 1981, p. 1123.)

form, *colipase,* by trypsin.[72] When bile salts and phospholipids are present, colipase is required for binding of lipase to triglyceride emulsions and, therefore, for efficient lipid hydrolysis (Table 57–2 and Figs. 57–6 and 57–7).[70, 71] Pancreatic lipase activity is also, to a certain extent, dependent on phospholipase A_2 activity because high concentrations of intact phospholipids can inhibit pancreatic lipase. Pancreatic lipase hydrolyzes the ester bonds at the C1 and C3 positions of triglycerides, producing fatty acids and 2-monoglyceride, products suitable for transport by enterocytes.

Phospholipase A_2 is a Ca^{2+}-dependent, bile salt–activated lipase that is secreted by the pancreas in a proenzyme form and is activated in the intestine by trypsin. It is the major intestinal phospholipase and cleaves dietary and biliary phospholipids at the C2 position, producing fatty acids and lysophospholipids (Fig. 57–6).

The other lipase secreted by the pancreas is called *nonspecific lipase* or *cholesterol esterase.* This enzyme has a wide substrate range, but its main function is probably the hydrolysis of ester bonds in cholesterol esters and sterol vitamin (A, D, and E) esters when these compounds are solubilized in bile salt micelles. The enzyme may also be present inside enterocytes, where it could function in the re-esterification of cholesterol.[1, 61]

Overall Scheme for Lipid Digestion

Ingested lipids are released from food in the mouth and stomach, where triglyceride hydrolysis is initiated by lingual lipase. Emulsification of lipids is promoted by gastric and pyloric motility, by accumulation of hydrolysis products, and by addition of bile in the proximal duodenum. Although bile salts and biliary phospholipids are important for solubilization of dietary fats and for promoting lipase activity, bile salts are not required for triglyceride digestion and absorption.[73] Indeed, in the absence of bile salts, up to 75 per cent of triglcyeride is absorbed. In contrast, absorption of cholesterol and sterol vitamins is severely compromised by bile salt deficiency.[73, 74] Lipolysis of emulsified fats proceeds efficiently in the small intestine, mediated by pancreated lipase-colipase, phospholipase A_2, and nonspecific lipase (Figs. 57–6 and 57–7). These enzymes work together to hydrolyze surface and internal components, leading to shrinkage of the triglyceride oil phase (droplet), release of fatty acids and monoglycerides into a complex oil-water viscous isotropic phase, and subsequent "budding off" of mixed micelles and complex liposomes (Fig. 57–7).[1] Lipid exchange between all these phases is rapid, transferring hydrolysis products throughout the intestinal lumen in preparation for absorption.

Lipid Absorption

The products of lipid digestion, including fatty acids, monoglycerides, cholesterol, sterol vitamins, and other exotic lipids, pass from the intestinal lumen into the enterocyte cytoplasm. Lipolysis products move through the intestinal aqueous milieu and across the peripheral unstirred water layer and mucous gel by (1) diffusion of large liposomes and mixed micelles, (2) an extension of a viscous hydrocarbon phase, and (3) diffusion of lipid monomers in free solution. All of these processes occur, although the first two are quantitatively more important than the third in view of the substantial thickness of the intestinal unstirred water layer and the low aqueous solubility of most lipolysis products.[34] Movement of lipid across the unstirred water layer constitutes the rate-limiting step in lipid absorption and is facilitated by aggregation of lipids into micelles and liposomes, because diffusion in water of these large particles, relative to the number of contained lipid molecules, is greater than that of individual lipid monomers.[74]

Lipolysis products are all relatively soluble in cell membranes and rapidly diffuse passively into enterocytes once they reach the cell surface, either as free monomer dissociated from micelles or by contact between lipid particles and membrane surface (Fig. 57–8). Rates of transfer of fatty acids across the enterocyte membrane are related to chain length (faster rate with longer chains) and degree of ionization (protonated, uncharged molecules cross faster). In addition, a specific sodium-dependent transport mechanism for fatty acids has been demonstrated in the brush border, although its role in intestinal fatty acid absorption is not clear.[75, 76]

Uptake of cholesterol, plant and animal sterols, and sterol vitamins requires bile salts (probably for solubilization in micelles and liposomes, as these compounds are insoluble in water) and probably occurs by direct transfer from micelles after these have collided with the cell membrane. (Specific transport mechanisms for vitamins are discussed on pp. 1046–1054). Absorption is relatively inefficient, with only about 40 to 50 per cent of ingested cholesterol taken up by enterocytes.[74, 77]

Phospholipids are absorbed passively, primarily as the lipolysis product lysophospholipids (Fig. 57–8). No specific enterocyte membrane carriers for these compounds have been described.

After entering the enterocyte membrane, lipolysis products move to sites of lipid metabolism within the cell. Mechanisms for removal of these hydrophobic compounds from the plasma membrane and for transfer through the aqueous cytosol are not well understood. Fatty acid–binding protein (molecular weight, ~15,000), an abundant cytoplasmic protein found in enterocytes, hepatocytes, and other fat-metabolizing tissues, is known to facilitate intracellular transport and use of fatty acids[78, 79] and might function to transport fatty acids as well as to protect the enterocyte from the detergent effects of large concentrations of fatty acids.

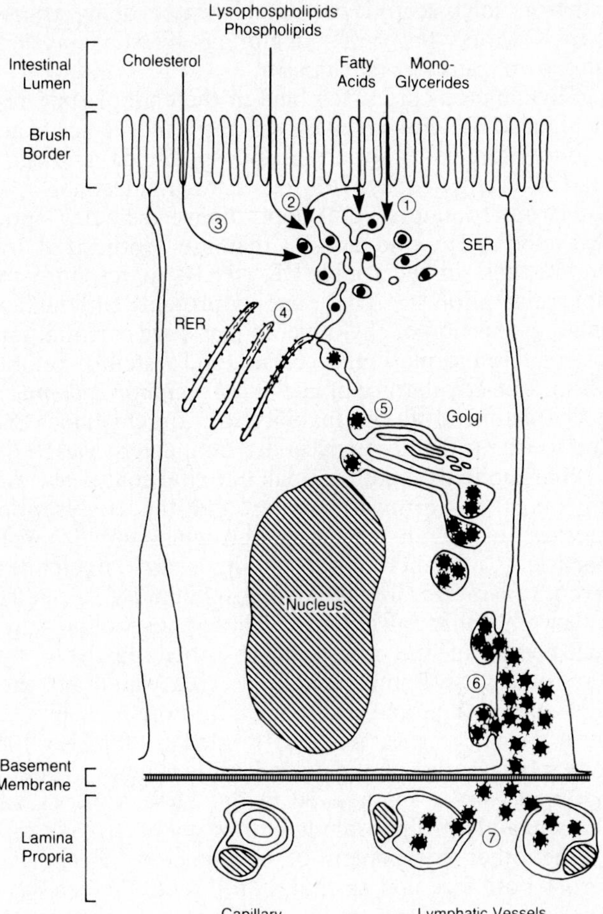

Figure 57–8. Uptake of lipolysis products; resynthesis and secretion of chylomicrons. Lipolysis products first are taken up by small intestinal enterocytes across the brush border membrane. Subsequently, (1) triglycerides are resynthesized from fatty acids and monoglycerides, via the monoacylglycerol pathway, in the smooth endoplasmic reticulum (SER) and accumulate as a dense oil droplet within the SER lumen (●); (2) phospholipids are resynthesized in the SER from lysophospholipids, glycerol, and fatty acids via acyltransferase or by the alpha-glycerophosphate pathway; (3) cholesterol is re-esterified in the SER by acyl CoA:cholesterol acyltransferase (ACAT); (4) apolipoproteins are synthesized in the rough endoplasmic reticulum (RER) (~~, protein); (5) chylomicrons (✱) are assembled within the tubular system of ER and Golgi apparatus, undergo final processing in the Golgi; (6) they are released by exocytosis of Golgi secretory vesicles across the basolateral membrane of the enterocyte, and cross the epithelial basement membrane; (7) chylomicrons enter lymphatic vessels in the lamina propria.

Chylomicron Formation and Transport

Triglycerides are resynthesized inside enterocytes from long-chain fatty acids and monoglycerides and are packaged into *chylomicrons* for export (Fig. 57–8).[80, 81] Triglyceride synthesis takes place in the apical portion of the enterocyte mediated by a complex of three enzymes (fatty acyl CoA ligase, monoacylglycerol acyltransferase, and diacylglycerol acyltransferase) located in a complex on the cytoplasmic face of the smooth endoplasmic reticulum (SER).[82–86] Triglyceride subsequently accumulates in the lumen of the smooth endoplasmic reticulum in droplets that are visible by electron microscopy, presumably after being transported across the SER membrane by some as yet unknown transport mechanism.

Chylomicrons are assembled in the endoplasmic reticulum (ER)-Golgi region of the enterocyte from apolipoproteins, triglycerides, phospholipids, and cholesterol esters (Table 57–3).[81, 87] Human intestinal chylomicrons contain several lipoproteins, including apo-A-I, apo-A-IV, and apo-B, that are synthesized by enterocytes, in the rough ER (RER) in response to lipid absorption.[88–91] These apolipoproteins, although a small proportion of chylomicron mass, are essential for chylomicron formation, secretion, and systemic metabolism. Indeed, absence of apo-B (*abetalipoproteinemia*) is characterized by the inability to form chylomicrons and to export dietary triglycerides from enterocytes.[88, 89]

Phospholipids, another small but vital component of chylomicrons, form a coat around the triglyceride particle and, with the apolipoproteins, stabilize the particle. Chylomicron phospholipids are largely derived from dietary and biliary phospholipids (especially biliary phosphatidylcholine).[92] These phospholipids are hydrolyzed in the intestine, absorbed passively by enterocytes as lysophospholipids, reacylated on the SER membrane, and transported into the SER lumen by a specific carrier protein (termed a "flippase").[93] When biliary phospholipid availability is limited, phospholipid can be synthesized in the SER de novo via the alpha-glycerolphosphate pathway.

The other component of chylomicrons is cholesterol—both free and as cholesterol ester. Free cholesterol, after transfer from intestinal lumen to enterocyte cytoplasm, is esterified by acyl CoA cholesterol acyltransferase (ACAT) in the SER[94] prior to incorporation into chylomicrons. Esterification is essential for overall absorption of dietary cholesterol,[94] and, as it is selective for cholesterol over other plant and shellfish sterols, may thus enhance cholesterol absorption. Indeed, patients with sitosterolemia and xanthomatosis exhibit marked increases in absorption of plant and shellfish sterols,[95] possibly because of nondiscriminant esterification.

Table 57–3. CHYLOMICRONS

Component	Per Cent by Weight	Site of Synthesis
Triglycerides	86–92	Enterocyte: smooth endoplasmic reticulum
Phospholipids	6–8	Enterocyte: smooth endoplasmic reticulum
Cholesterol esters	0.8–1.4	Enterocyte: ? smooth endoplasmic reticulum
Free cholesterol	0.8–1.6	—
Lipoproteins	1–2	Enterocyte: rough endoplasmic reticulum
Apolipoprotein A-I	Activates LCAT*	
Apolipoprotein A-II	Function unknown	
Apolipoprotein A-IV	Function unknown	
Apolipoprotein B-100	Essential for chylomicron secretion	

Other apolipoproteins (C-I, C-II, C-III, D, and E) are acquired during passage through lymph and blood

*LCAT; Lecithin:cholesterol acyltransferase.

Chylomicrons appear to be assembled as 75- to 600-nm particles in the endoplasmic reticulum, where triglycerides from the SER meet apolipoproteins from the RER, although the precise mechanisms involved are not known.[81, 91, 96, 97] Nascent chylomicrons subsequently move to the Golgi apparatus[97] (Fig. 57–8) for glycosylation[96] and final processing. This is the same pattern of formation and release of secretory proteins seen in many cell types. From the Golgi apparatus, secretory vesicles, each containing several chylomicrons, bud off and move to the basolateral enterocyte plasma membrane. Chylomicrons are released into the intercellular space by exocytosis, and they subsequently enter intestinal lacteals and are transported in lymph.[97] The mechanisms responsible for correct sorting of Golgi products and for the selective directional movement of secretory vesicles to the basolateral membrane are not known, although microtubules may be involved.[98] Finally, it is not clear whether chylomicrons move from enterocytes to lymph lacteals by processes other than simple diffusion.

The entire process of lipid absorption is efficient and rapid (chylomicron secretion can be seen as early as 12 minutes after lipid is placed in the intestinal lumen)[87] and is virtually identical to the mechanisms of synthesis and secretion of very low density lipoproteins (VLDL) in the liver. Enterocytes also synthesize and secrete VLDL; however, the role of these lipoproteins in dietary lipid absorption is unclear.

After transfer to lymph and blood, chylomicrons acquire additional apolipoproteins (especially apo-C and apo-E) from other lipoproteins. Apo-C activates lipoprotein lipase and stimulates hydrolysis of chylomicron triglyceride in other tissues. After depletion of chylomicron triglyceride, apo-E mediates uptake of the chylomicron remnants by liver cells.

Medium-Chain Triglycerides (MCT)

Lipids containing only short- and medium-chain fatty acids (C6–C12) are absorbed in a somewhat different manner from long-chain triglycerides.[99, 100] Approximately 30 per cent of MCT can be absorbed intact by enterocytes, presumably by passive diffusion.

MCTs are also rapidly and completely hydrolyzed by pancreatic lipase to fatty acids and glycerol, both of which are rapidly taken up by enterocytes. Medium-chain fatty acids are not re-esterified inside enterocytes, but rather exit the cell directly and enter the portal venous blood. Patients with a variety of small intestinal diseases absorb MCTs more efficiently than long-chain triglycerides, probably related to their less complex absorptive mechanism.[99]

Inherited Defects of Lipid Digestion and Absorption

Abetalipoproteinemia. Abetalipoproteinemia is an autosomal recessive disorder resulting from the absence of apo-B synthesis, in which there is no chylomicron formation, severe triglyceride malabsorption, acanthocytosis of erythrocytes, fat-soluble vitamin deficiency, and progressive neurologic disease. The enterocytes of patients with this disease contain no identifiable apo-B and, although triglyceride droplets are seen throughout the SER, the Golgi apparatus contains neither chylomicrons nor VLDLs[89, 101] (see pp. 270–271).

Sitosterolemia. Sitosterolemia is an autosomal recessive disorder in which patients hyperabsorb a variety of plant and shellfish sterols, resulting in xanthomatosis and premature cardiovascular disease. It has been proposed that the disease results from an inability of the gut and other tissues to discriminate between cholesterol, which normally is efficiently esterified and absorbed, and other ingested sterols, which are normally esterified and absorbed only in small amounts.[95]

Pancreatic Lipase or Colipase Deficiency. These deficiencies have been reported in a few patients. Congenital lipase deficiency is a rare form of inherited exocrine pancreatic insufficiency that presents in childhood with steatorrhea and that responds symptomatically to decreased fat intake and pancreatic enzyme supplementation.[102] Combined deficiency of pancreatic lipase and colipase has been reported in a child with steatorrhea[103] who absorbed 50 per cent of ingested fat despite the absence of both enzymes. Finally, two brothers who presented in childhood with steatorrhea and 50 per cent fat absorption were reported to have isolated colipase deficiency.[104] Symptoms and fat absorption in these brothers improved with pancreatic enzyme supplementation (see p. 1804).

Cystic Fibrosis. Cystic fibrosis, a common autosomal recessive disorder, is frequently associated with generalized exocrine pancreatic insufficiency and malabsorption. Steatorrhea is a major symptom in patients with this disease (see pp. 1789–1801).

Efficiency of Lipid Absorption

Lipid absorption is highly efficient; 90 to 95 per cent of ingested fat is absorbed within the first 100 cm of the small intestine. Overall, the average healthy person can absorb up to 98 per cent of dietary lipid (100 to 160 gm/day) and endogenous lipid (15 to 40 gm derived from biliary secretions and sloughed cells).[1] Lipid absorption is, however, affected by the physical form of ingested food; only 5 per cent of ingested peanut oil is excreted in the stool, but 7 per cent of fat in peanut butter and 18 per cent of the fat in whole peanuts is not absorbed.[105]

Small amounts of dietary and endogenous lipid as well as nonabsorbed complex lipids, such as calcium soaps and waxes, enter the colon.[1, 61] Volatile short-chain fatty acids are well absorbed by the colonic mucosa. Other lipids may undergo bacterial metabolism, but virtually nothing is known about this process. Fecal lipids, approximately 4 to 6 gm/day, comprise a mixture of fatty acids, calcium and magnesium fatty acid soaps, sterols, and some waxes and bacterial lipids.

PROTEIN DIGESTION AND ABSORPTION

Protein intake, which averages 70 to 100 gm/day in a standard Western diet, provides 10 to 15 per cent of the total caloric intake and, more important, supplies the essential amino acids required for protein synthesis. Indeed, to maintain positive nitrogen balance, a 70-kg man must ingest approximately 45 gm of protein per day. The gastrointestinal tract not only digests and absorbs the daily load of exogenous (dietary) protein but also digests and recycles 20 to 30 gm or more of endogenous protein derived from gastrointestinal secretions, sloughed mucosal cells, gastrointestinal mucus, and leakage of plasma proteins.[106] Protein digestion is conceptually more simple than fat digestion, as it involves repetitive hydrolysis of peptide bonds in relatively hydrophilic substrates. Absorption is, however, a complex process owing to the diversity of digestive products (20 amino acids and 400 possible dipeptides).

Overall, protein digestion and absorption can be considered in five stages: (1) *luminal digestion;* (2) *enterocyte brush border digestion;* (3) *brush border membrane transport;* (4) *cytoplasmic digestion;* and (5) *basolateral enterocyte membrane transport.* Each of these stages is discussed briefly. Excellent detailed reviews are also available.[25, 107–109]

Luminal Digestion

Protein digestion begins in the stomach, where protein is released through grinding and mixing of food particles and is denatured by acid to forms susceptible to proteolysis. Limited proteolysis in the stomach is mediated by at least two enzymes, *pepsin I* and *pepsin II* (Table 57–4). These, and perhaps additional minor proteolytic enzymes also secreted by gastric mucosal cells in precursor form, are activated by a combination of exposure to acid and autocatalysis and require an acid environment for continued activity.[110, 111] These enzymes are endopeptidases, cleaving internal peptide bonds of large proteins, particularly if these bonds are adjacent to hydrophobic amino acids. Proteolysis in the stomach is limited in extent (products are large, nonabsorbable peptides) and in duration (pepsins are inactivated in the duodenum, where the pH rises above 4), and it is probably not critical because protein digestion and absorption are essentially normal in patients with achlorhydria and in those who have undergone complete gastrectomy.

Luminal digestion occurs primarily in the small intestine, mediated by a group of five potent proteolytic enzymes, all secreted by the pancreas, that exhibit complementary specificities (Table 57–4). The pancreatic *proteases* (or *peptidases*) are essential for adequate protein digestion, and their combined action efficiently converts proteins and large polypeptides to a mixture of 30 per cent free amino acids and 70 per cent oligopeptides (average size two to six amino acid residues).[107, 115, 116]

Table 57–4. GASTRIC, PANCREATIC, AND SMALL INTESTINAL PEPTIDASES*

Enzyme	Precursor	Source	Activation	Activity	Products
Pepsin I (A) (~ 35,000)	Pepsinogen I	Gastric chief cells	Low pH causes conformational change followed by autocatalytic cleavage of 44-amino acid "activation peptide" from the inactive pepsinogen producing active pepsin	Aspartic proteinase Requires acid pH Endopeptidase cleaves internal peptide bonds at hydrophobic amino acids (phenylalanine, methionine, leucine, tryptophan, etc.)	Peptides
Pepsin II (C) (Gastricsin) (~ 35,000)	Pepsinogen II	Gastric chief cells Pyloric glands of antral mucosa	Same as pepsin I	Same as pepsin I	Peptides
Enteropeptidase (enterokinase) (~ 296,000)	None	Brush border of duodenum and proximal jejunum	None	Cleaves N-terminal octapeptide from trypsinogen, generating active trypsin	Trypsin
Trypsin (~ 25,000)	Trypsinogen	Pancreatic acinar cell	Activated by enteropeptidase primarily; minor autoactivation	Neutral serine protease Endopeptidase Cleaves internal peptide bond at lysine or arginine residues Activates other pancreatic proenzymes	Peptides
Chymotrypsin (~ 27,000)	Chymotrypsinogen	Pancreatic acinar cell	Activated by trypsin via cleavage of two peptide bonds	Neutral serine protease Endopeptidase Cleaves peptide bond at aromatic (phenylalanine, tyrosine, tryptophan) or neutral amino acids	Peptides
Elastase (~ 30,000)	Proelastase	Pancreatic acinar cell	Activated by trypsin	Neutral serine protease Endopeptidase Cleaves peptide bond at aliphatic amino acids (leucine, methionine)	Peptides
Carboxypeptidase A (~ 34,000)	Procarboxy-peptidase A	Pancreatic acinar cell	Activated by trypsin	Metalloenzyme (zinc) Cleaves carboxyterminal aromatic amino acids from proteins and peptides	Aromatic amino acids Peptides
Carboxypeptidase B (~ 34,000)	Procarboxy-peptidase B	Pancreatic acinar cell	Activated by trypsin	Metalloenzyme (Zinc) Cleaves carboxyterminal arginine and lysine from proteins and peptides	Arginine, lysine Peptides

*From references 107, 108, and 110 to 114.

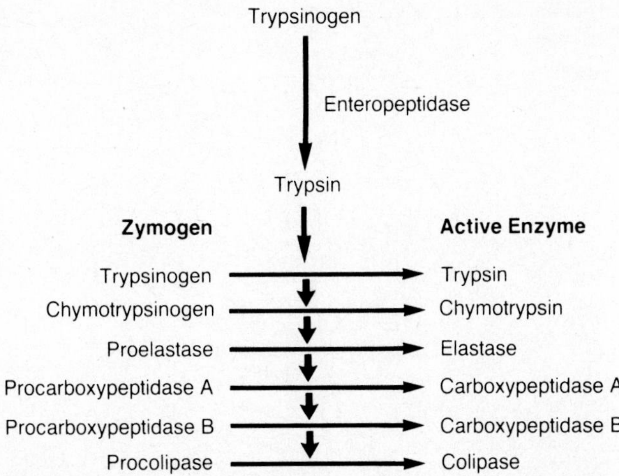

Figure 57–9. Activation cascade of pancreatic zymogens. (From Rinderknecht, H. Pancreatic secretory enzymes. *In* Go, V. L. W., Brooks, F. P., DiMagno, E. P., et al. [eds.]. The Exocrine Pancreas: Biology, Pathobiology, and Diseases. New York, Raven Press, 1986, p. 163.)

The pancreatic proteases are all synthesized by the pancreatic acinar cell as inactive proenzymes (or zymogens) and are packaged by the Golgi apparatus into dense secretory (zymogen) granules. The proenzymes are then released, after stimulation by hormonal or neuronal effectors, by exocytosis through the apical membrane of the acinar cell into the pancreatic duct (see pp. 1777–1784). These proenzymes are activated in the duodenum by a cascade of events mediated by *enteropeptidase* and *trypsin* (Fig. 57–9).[107] *Enteropeptidase* is a large membrane-bound glycoprotein produced by enterocytes in the duodenum, whose only function is activation of trypsinogen to trypsin. After being activated in the neutral or alkaline milieu of the duodenum, *trypsin* catalyzes the activation of additional trypsinogen as well as activation of chymotrypsinogen to *chymotrypsin,* proelastase to *elastase,* and procarboxypeptidase A and procarboxypeptidase B to *carboxypeptidases A* and *B* (Fig. 57–9).

Trypsin, chymotrypsin, and elastase are neutral (acid inactivated) proteases that cleave interior peptide bonds in proteins or large polypeptides (Table 57–4). Carboxypeptidases A and B, in contrast, are zinc metalloenzymes that cleave specific amino acids from the C-terminal end of proteins and peptides. The complementary actions of the five enzymes are illustrated in Figure 57–10.

The products of luminal protein digestion (amino acids and oligopeptides) are suitable substrates for digestion by enterocyte brush border peptidases or absorption by enterocytes.

Enterocyte Peptide Digestion

The brush border of small intestinal enterocytes contains a group of as many as eight peptidases that participate in peptide digestion (Table 57–5). Although not studied as extensively as the brush border oligosaccharidases, many of the brush border peptidases are probably similar dimeric integral membrane glycoproteins, attached to the enterocyte plasma membrane by a short segment, with their active site(s) located on the external (luminal) side of the plasma membrane.[6, 117–121] The peptidases are all synthesized, like the oligosaccharidases, in the RER and are transported, presumably in vesicles, through the Golgi apparatus to the brush border membrane.[5, 6, 9, 117–121] At least one oligopeptidase, amino-oligopeptidase, is known to be cleaved, like the oligosaccharidases, by pancreatic proteases. In general, these aminopeptidases are synthesized faster than the oligosaccharidases.[9]

The major brush border peptidase appears to be *amino-oligopeptidase,* an enzyme that preferentially uses medium-sized oligopeptides (containing three to eight amino acid residues) and sequentially cleaves off the N-terminal amino acids, producing a variety of free amino acids and a dipeptide (Table 57–5).[109, 122, 125–127] Another important peptidase is *dipeptidyl aminopeptidase IV,* an enzyme that cleaves the N-terminal dipeptide from larger oligopeptides and is particularly important for digestion of proline-containing proteins because few other peptidases cleave proline-associated peptide bonds.[109, 123, 127, 128] Several other *oligopeptidases* have been described, including an endopeptidase and two carboxypeptidases, but these have not been studied extensively.[117, 120, 129, 130]

The enterocyte brush border also contains several *dipeptidases,* enzymes that cleave dipeptides to free amino acids, of which the best characterized is aminopeptidase A or aspartate aminopeptidase (Table 57–5).[118–120, 122]

Collectively, the brush border peptidases reduce the oligopeptide products of luminal digestion to a series of free amino acids, dipeptides, and a few tripeptides (Figs. 57–11 and 57–12), which are suitable substrates for transport into enterocytes.

Absorption of Peptides

Specific transport mechanisms exist in the enterocyte brush border for transport of amino acids and dipeptides (Fig. 57–11). Kinetic studies indicate the presence of at least one dipeptide transport mechanism that is saturable, that is independent of sodium, and that transports a few tripeptides but no peptides of greater size.[109, 131–137] The peptide transporter is quantitatively important for nutrition because many amino acids are absorbed faster as dipeptides than as free amino acids.[135–138] Indeed, patients with amino acid transport defects such as Hartnup disease (see p. 1081) can absorb the affected amino acid(s) adequately in dipeptides.[135, 139] Peptide transport is active and transfers a positive charge to the cell interior, although the energy source for this transport process remains unclear. Recent studies suggest that peptides are cotransported with protons (H^+) and that the protons are subsequently recycled out of the enterocyte by Na^+-H^+ exchange.[140]

Inside enterocytes, peptides are rapidly cleaved to their component amino acids by a battery of poorly characterized but potent *cytoplasmic peptidases.*[108, 109,

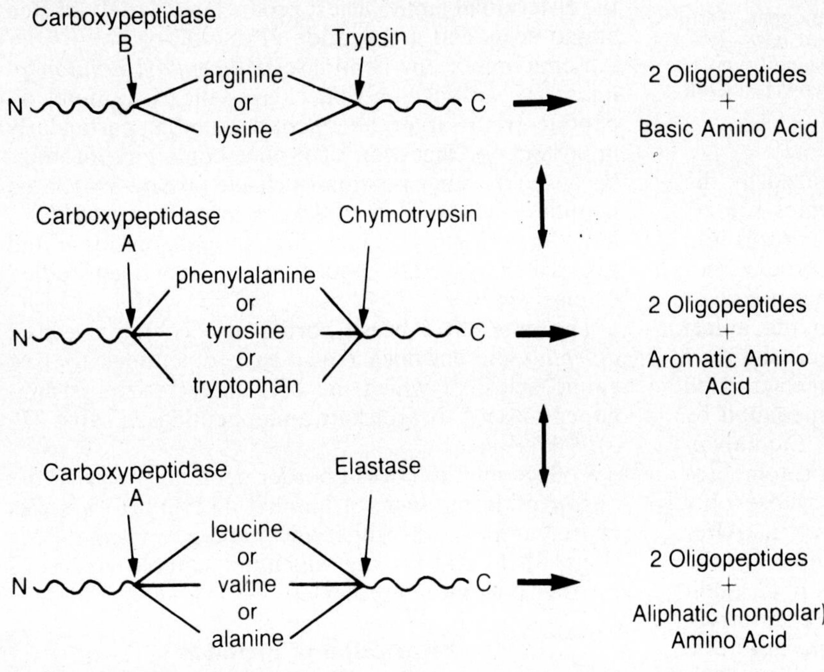

Figure 57–10. Luminal pancreatic digestion of protein. This schematic representation of luminal protein digestion illustrates the complementary and sequential action of pancreatic proteases. N, N-terminus of protein; C, C-terminus of protein; ~, protein.

Table 57–5. INTESTINAL BRUSH BORDER PEPTIDASES*

Peptidase	Molecular Weight	Structure	Activity	Products
Oligopeptidases				
Amino-oligopeptidase (aminopeptidase N)	~ 130,000 (human)	Dimeric integral membrane enzyme(s) with two active sites	Most abundant peptidase Cleaves N-terminal amino acid from 3- to 8-residue oligopeptides, particularly phenylalanine, leucine, etc. No activity for proline or D-amino acids Metalloenzyme (zinc) Hydrophobic amino acid products inhibit activity	Amino acids and dipeptides
Dipeptidyl aminopeptidase IV	~ 230,000 (human)	Dimeric glycoprotein Integral membrane protein	Cleaves N-terminal dipeptide from oligopeptide when penultimate amino acid is proline or alanine Probable serine protease	X-Proline or X-alanine and dipeptide
Endopeptidase(s)	100,000–300,000	Probably several endopeptidases At least one is a dimeric integral membrane glycoprotein	Metalloenzyme(s) (zinc) Cleaves internal peptide bonds of proteins or large peptides	Oligopeptides that are substrates for amino-oligopeptidase
Dipeptidyl carboxypeptidase	—	—	Cleaves C-terminal dipeptide, especially when proline is C-terminal residue	Dipeptide and oligopeptide
Carboxypeptidase	—	—	Cleaves C-terminal residue of peptides containing proline	Proline, other amino acids, peptides
Dipeptidases				
Aminopeptidase A (aspartate aminopeptidase)	~ 120,000 (human)	—	Cleaves dipeptides that possess an N-terminal acidic amino acid	Aspartic acid or glutamic acid and other amino acids
Gly-Leu peptidase (dipeptidase)	~ 91,000	—	Metalloenzyme (zinc) Cleaves N-terminal glycine and other neutral amino acids from dipeptides	Amino acids
Zinc-stable Asp-Lys peptidase (dipeptidase)	~ 190,000	—	Dipeptidase, especially when N-terminal amino acid is aspartic acid or methionine	Amino acids

*From references 5, 9, 108, 109, and 122 to 130.

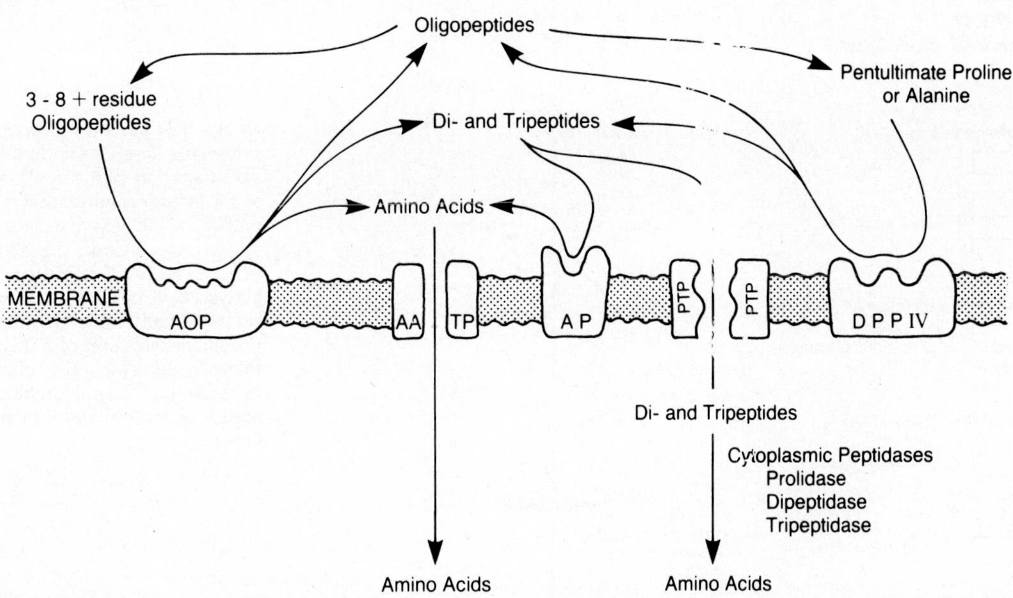

Figure 57–11. Enterocyte brush border peptide digestion and absorption. Oligopeptides, the products of luminal digestion by pancreatic proteases, are further digested to amino acids, dipeptides, and a few tripeptides (see Fig. 57–12) by brush border peptidases, integral membrane proteins oriented with their active sites located in the intestinal luman. Amino acids are taken up by several different transport systems (see Fig. 57–13). Dipeptides and some tripeptides are taken up by the peptide transport system and subsequently cleaved to their component amino acids by cytoplasmic peptidases. AOP, Amino-oligopeptidase; AP, aminopeptidase(s); DPP IV, dipeptidylpeptidase IV; AATP, amino acid transport process; PTP, peptide transport process.

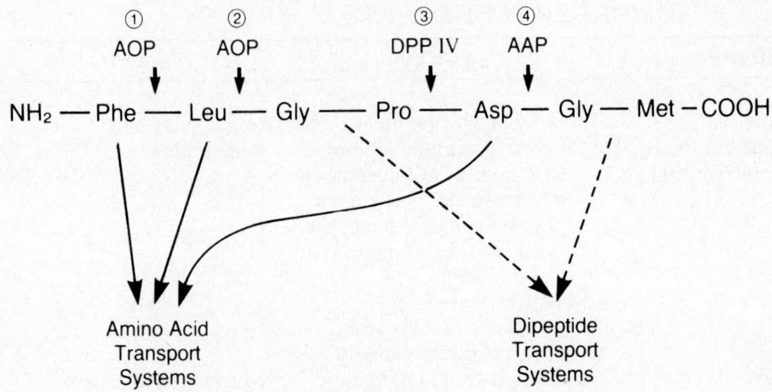

Figure 57–12. Digestion of a hypothetical oligopeptide by brush border peptidases. Initially the N-terminal amino acids phenylalanine and leucine are sequentially cleaved by amino-oligopeptidase (AOP) (1, 2), subsequently the Gly-Pro dipeptide is cleaved by dipeptidylpeptidase IV (DDP IV) (3), and finally aspartate is cleaved from the N-terminus by aspartate aminopeptidase (AAP)(4), leaving the dipeptide Gly-Met. Amino acid and peptide absorption occurs via transporters depicted in Figure 57–11 and 57–13.

[141–144] At least three such peptidases have been described: *prolidase* (one of the few peptidases that cleave peptide bonds involving proline), a *general dipeptidase,* and a *tripeptidase*.[108, 109, 143, 145] In contrast to the brush border peptidases, these enzymes cleave dipeptides preferentially. The brush border and cytoplasmic peptidases work in a complementary fashion: small peptides that are poor substrates for brush border enzymes are excellent substrates for the dipeptide carrier and for cytoplasmic peptidases. A few peptides, however, escape hydrolysis by cytoplasmic enzymes and appear intact in the blood.[146] The mechanisms responsible for transport of peptides out of enterocytes into the blood, and the physiologic importance of this pathway, are unclear.

Absorption of Amino Acids

During absorption, amino acids are transported from the intestinal lumen into the blood across two cell membranes—namely, the brush border membrane and the basolateral enterocyte plasma membrane. A complex array of transport mechanisms have been identified, including carrier-mediated active and facilitative diffusion pathways as well as simple diffusion.[25, 147–151] (Fig. 57–13). Presumably the array of different transporters reflects the wide structural diversity of amino acids as well as the importance of supplying essential amino acids for enterocyte protein synthesis during feeding and fasting.

At least four sodium-coupled amino acid transport-

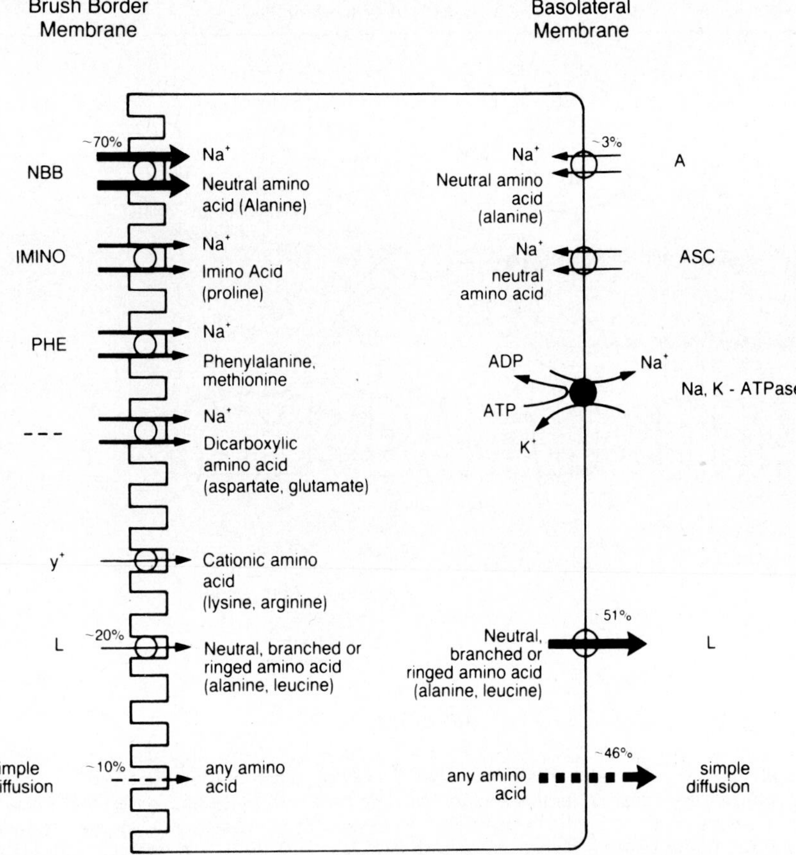

Figure 57–13. Amino acid transport. This schematic representation depicts amino acid transport pathways in a representative small intestinal enterocyte. Names of the pathways are listed beside each transport system and include the NBB, IMINO, PHE, y⁺, L, A, and ASC pathways. The Na^+-dicarboxylic acid pathway has not yet been assigned a name. The arrows depict the predominant direction of transport, with arrow thickness indicating the relative prominence of each pathway. Numbers indicate estimates of relative rates of transport of alanine.[25]

ers (NBB, IMINO, PHE, and one unnamed pathway) have been identified in the enterocyte brush border (Fig. 57–13). Analogous to the sodium-coupled glucose uptake, these transporters represent *active transport,* coupling uptake of sodium to amino acid uptake, probably in a 1:1 ratio, resulting in active, concentrative movement of amino acids and in net transfer of positive charge.[25] Two other transport systems (y^+ and L) (Fig. 57–13) mediate uptake of certain amino acids independently of sodium and constitute *facilitated diffusion* pathways.[25] Finally, *simple diffusion* also occurs and, for neutral amino acids such as alanine, may be a significant pathway for uptake, especially when luminal amino acid concentrations are high. The relative importance of these pathways with respect to alanine uptake is indicated in Figure 57–13.

The enterocyte basolateral membrane also contains an array of amino acid transporters (Fig. 57–13). Two sodium-coupled transporters, called A and ASC, closely resemble the amino acid transporters in liver and kidney and are distinct from the brush border NBB, IMINO, and PHE systems. It is thought that the A and ASC systems supply enterocytes with amino acids from the blood during periods of fasting.[25] The major pathways for efflux of absorbed amino acids out of enterocytes into the blood are the facilitated diffusion L system and simple diffusion. Although the L transporter exists on both sides of the enterocyte, its transport capacity appears to be greater on the basolateral side than on the brush border, perhaps reflecting a difference in the number of transporter molecules. As shown in Figure 57–13, it is estimated that alanine, for example, is transferred from lumen to cell primarily by the active NBB transporter, whereas transfer from cell to the blood is largely via the L transporter and by diffusion.

Efficiency of Protein Digestion and Absorption

Protein digestion takes place throughout the entire small intestine, but mainly in the jejunum and ileum.[152, 153] Indeed, the brush border peptidases are found in high concentrations in the ileum.[154] In contrast, carbohydrate digestion and oligosaccharidases are found predominantly in the proximal small intestine, suggesting that protein digestion is relatively more difficult. The overall rate-limiting step in protein digestion and absorption appears to be amino acid transport. Protein assimilation normally is efficient, with absorption of 60 per cent of an ingested test protein in the jejunum and loss of only 1 per cent to the colon.[153] Although hydrolysis and absorption of most naturally occurring proteins is efficient, digestion and absorption of artificial peptides, such as the sweetener aspartame, may be poor.[155]

Approximately 6 to 12 gm of protein (representing less than 5 per cent of dietary intake) is passed in the stool each day,[106] presumably representing undigested dietary protein and bacterial protein. Little is known about colonic digestion and absorption of protein.

Implications for Enteral Feedings

Because dipeptides are transported efficiently by intestinal enterocytes and are less active osmotically than an equivalent amino acid mixture, they may be a better tolerated and absorbed source of protein in enteral feedings.[109, 135, 136, 156] Few studies have been performed to test this hypothesis, and to date no clinically significant advantages have been demonstrated.[157]

Development and Regulation

Protein digestion and absorption appear to be functional at the time of birth.[158, 159] Peptidase activity and amino acid transport increase to adult levels after birth and can be stimulated further in adults by increased protein intake[109, 158, 160] and by corticosteroids;[161] they are reduced by starvation.[109, 162]

Uptake of Intact Proteins

Intact proteins can be taken up by a variety of cells through specific receptor-mediated endocytosis or nonspecific pinocytosis. Infant mammals take up immunoglobulin efficiently from maternal milk via endocytosis and transport immunoglobulins through small intestinal enterocytes to the blood.[163, 164] This process is limited to a short period in infancy, and the enterocytes of adults exhibit little endocytosis of luminal materials. Tiny amounts of intact protein may, however, be taken up by some individuals and may contribute to the development of certain food allergies.

Certain specialized cells of the small intestine, the M cells overlying Peyer's patches, are able to sample and transport luminal proteins and microorganisms, probably as part of the intestinal immune system[165] (see pp. 118–120).

Hereditary Defects of Protein Digestion and Absorption

A variety of inherited defects of protein assimilation have been identified (Table 57–6).[106, 139, 143, 145, 166–171] These defects can be divided into three categories: (1) deficiences of luminal digestive enzymes, enteropeptidase and trypsinogen deficiencies being the most common; therapy with pancreatic enzyme supplements is often successful in these disorders; (2) deficiency of cytoplasmic peptidase(s)—prolidase deficiency is the only identified syndrome; and (3) amino acid transport deficiencies. This is the largest recognized category of such defects, perhaps because renal aminoaciduria is a common and readily detectable feature. In *Hartnup disease* and *cystinuria,* impaired transport of amino acids across the brush border of renal and intestinal cells has been clearly shown, although protein nutrition is normal as the affected amino acids are efficiently transported in dipeptides. In contrast, patients with

Table 57–6. INHERITED DISORDERS OF PROTEIN DIGESTION AND ABSORPTION*

Disorder	Underlying Defect	Clinical Features
Enzyme Deficiencies		
Enterokinase deficiency	Absence of enzyme (< 10% of normal activity)	Failure to thrive, malabsorption; active pancreatic enzymes absent from duodenal juice
Isolated trypsin deficiency (congenital trypsinogen deficiency)	Absence of enzyme	Failure to thrive, malabsorption; active pancreatic enzymes absent from duodenal juice
Prolidase deficiency (iminopeptiduria)	Impaired cytoplasmic prolidase activity Reduced hydrolysis of di- and tripeptides containing proline	Iminopeptiduria, proline malabsorption, skin rash, bone demineralization, defective collagen metabolism
Johanson-Blizzard syndrome	Absence of most or all pancreatic digestive enzymes	Dysmorphic features, malabsorption and pancreatic insufficiency, hypothyroidism
Transport Deficiencies		
Hartnup disease	Impaired absorption of neutral amino acids (alanine, serine, threonine, asparagine, glutamine, valine, leucine, isoleucine, phenylalanine, tyrosine, tryptophan, histidine, citrulline) by small intestine and kidney	Massive aminoaciduria, pellagra-like features due to tryptophan deficiency, central nervous system toxicity from bacterial degradation products of malabsorbed amino acids, potential for essential amino acid deficiencies
Blue diaper disease (tryptophan malabsorption)	Tryptophan malabsorption	Growth retardation, blue discoloration of diapers, hypercalcemia
Oasthouse urine disease (methionine malabsorption)	Methionine malabsorption	Seizures, mental retardation, diarrhea
Cystinuria	Impaired uptake of cystine, lysine, arginine, and ornithine across the apical membrane of intestinal and renal epithelium cells	Renal calculi
Hyperdibasic aminoaciduria (lysinuric protein intolerance)	Impaired efflux of dibasic amino acids (lysine, arginine, ornithine) across basolateral membrane of intestinal and renal epithelial cells leading to impaired absorption	Urinary excretion of lysine, ornithine, arginine, citrulline (dibasic aminoaciduria); malabsorption of dibasic amino acids; clinical protein intolerance, poor growth, mental retardation; hyperammonemia after protein meals
Familial iminoglycinuria	Impaired uptake of proline, hydroxyproline, and glycine by intestinal and renal epithelial cells	Iminoglycinuria, no clinical symptoms

*Based on references 25, 106, 139, 143, 145, and 166 to 171.

hyperdibasic aminoaciduria do exhibit amino acid malnutrition because the amino acid transport defect is located on the basolateral cell membrane and other transport mechanisms cannot compensate.[170, 171]

Finally, a few children with severe, generalized malabsorption have been found to have congenital microvillus atrophy.[172–174] The enterocyte brush border in these patients is poorly formed or missing and presumably these subjects lack virtually all brush border oligosaccharidases and peptidases as well as sugar, amino acid, and peptide transport systems.

INTESTINAL TRANSPORT OF BILE SALTS

Bile salts are synthesized in the liver and are conjugated, through the carboxylic side chain, to glycine or taurine, amino acids that form peptide bonds resistant to pancreatic carboxypeptidases.[175] They are secreted in the bile, taken up by small intestinal enterocytes, and recycled, via the portal system, back to the liver where they are extracted and resecreted[176, 177] (see pp. 144–161 and 1656–1668). By recycling through this enterohepatic circulation 4 to 12 times per day, a total pool of approximately 3 gm of bile salts contributes 12 to 36 gm of bile salts to the intestinal lumen for participation in lipid digestion and absorption[176] (see pp. 150–152). Intestinal reabsorption of bile salts is efficient with only 0.2 to 0.6 gm of bile salts lost to the colon per day (2 per cent of the total amount). This daily loss is balanced by hepatic synthesis of bile salts from cholesterol.

Bile salt transport in the small intestine occurs by at least two mechanisms: (1) *passive diffusion* and (2) *active transport.* Bile salts in free solution are taken up by diffusion throughout the small intestine as lipid absorption proceeds.[178, 179] This transport process, which presumably involves passive movement across enterocytes into the blood, is particularly important for relatively hydrophobic dihydroxy bile salts and for those bile salts that have been deconjugated by bacterial action.

Enterocytes in the terminal ileum also possess an active, sodium-coupled bile salt transporter located in the brush border membrane that is functionally similar to the active bile salt transporters located in the sinusoidal membrane of hepatocytes and in renal tubule cells[177–180] (see pp. 144–152 and 1658). The ileal bile salt transporter couples uptake of bile salt and sodium, efficiently extracting bile salts from ileal fluid, and thus it serves as a salvage pathway to limit fecal loss of bile salts. The ileal bile salt transporter preferentially transports relatively hydrophilic trihydroxy bile salts and conjugated bile salts, compounds that are poorly transported by diffusion. After uptake by enterocytes, bile salts may diffuse through the basolateral membrane of these cells and enter the portal circulation. A carrier-mediated facilitated diffusion pathway has been identified in the canalicular membrane of hepatocytes[177] (see pp. 1656–1662), and an analogous transporter could exist in the basolateral membrane of enterocytes to facilitate cell-to-blood transfer of bile salts. Because of the efficient ileal bile salt transport, tests of bile salt absorption are being developed that can be used to assess overall function of the terminal ileum.[181]

Bile salts are essential for normal lipid digestion, yet they are potentially toxic detergent molecules. Normally confined within the enterohepatic circulation, they spill over into the colon in increased quantities in patients with dysfunction or loss of the terminal ileum.[182, 183] In the colon, bile salts are not absorbed actively, but they stimulate colonic motility[184, 185] and secretion of NaCl and water[184] and increase permeability of the colonic mucosa to ions and water.[186, 187] These effects lead to watery diarrhea (choleretic diarrhea)[183, 188] (pp. 153–154 and 303).

Analogous severe watery diarrhea is seen in children with congenital absence of the ileal bile salt transporter.[189] In contrast, bile salt deficiency is reported to be associated with severe constipation,[190] suggesting that a certain amount of bile salt in the colonic lumen is essential for normal colonic function.

EFFECTS OF CHANGES IN INTESTINAL MOTILITY ON NUTRIENT ABSORPTION

Intuitively it would seem that changes in intestinal motility and transit time might alter nutrient absorption by increasing or decreasing the time during which ingested food is exposed to digestive enzymes and the small intestinal absorptive surface. This issue has not been examined thoroughly, although some studies support the hypothesis.[191] For example, retrograde electrical pacing of canine intestine slows intestinal transit and increases absorption of water, sodium, and glucose, particularly in animals with the *short bowel syndrome.*[192] In humans, small intestinal transit time can be decreased by oral administration of lactulose or magnesium sulfate, with associated increases in ileal output of water, sodium, fat, carbohydrate, and protein.[191, 193] Similarly, metoclopramide decreases intestine transit time and reduces cholesterol absorption.[77] Some patients with *hyperthyroidism* also exhibit increased intestinal motility, decreased transit time, and mild steatorrhea[194, 195] (see pp. 488–489). Opiates, in contrast, increase the intestinal transit time (slowing intestinal motility), an important factor in the antidiarrheal activity of these agents.[196] Fat, when present in the ileum, also decreases motility[197, 198] and increases carbohydrate absorption[198] in the proximal small intestine—a response termed the "ileal brake." Collectively, these effects on nutrient absorption, although measurable, may not be of clinical significance in adults ingesting an adequate diet. Indeed, massive intestinal purging with laxatives or gastric saline infusion results in fecal loss of only 100 to 200 kcal/day, an amount ≤15 per cent of daily intake[199] (see p. 306).

EFFECT OF DIETARY FIBER ON NUTRIENT ABSORPTION

A high intake of dietary fiber or of bulk agents like guar gum increases fecal weight and water content. These agents also slow the small intestinal absorption of carbohydrates by decreasing the rate of gastric emptying and increasing the small intestinal unstirred water layer.[200–202] Dietary fiber, therefore, blunts the glycemic response to an oral carbohydrate load in normal volunteers and in patients with diabetes mellitus.[200, 202] This finding suggests that increased dietary fiber may help to control hyperglycemia in patients with non–insulin-dependent diabetes.[200]

EFFECTS OF AGING ON NUTRIENT ABSORPTION

The gastrointestinal tract appears to function quite well even after many years of service.[203, 204] Subtle decreases in carbohydrate, fat, and protein absorption have been documented in elderly individuals, especially when large oral test loads have been administered.[203–205] However, clinically significant malabsorption has not been found in asymptomatic elderly humans and, in one study, absorption of an essential fatty acid, linoleic acid, was actually increased in aging rats due to a decrease in the unstirred water layer.[206] For a more complete discussion of aging and the gut, the reader is referred to pages 162 to 169.

References

1. Carey, M. C., Small, D. M., and Bliss, C. M. Lipid digestion and absorption. Ann. Rev. Physiol. *45*:651, 1983.
2. Fogel, M. R., and Gray, G. M. Starch hydrolysis in man: an intraluminal process not requiring membrane digestion. J. Appl. Physiol. *35*:263, 1973.
3. Heitlinger, L. A., Lee, P. C., Dillon, W. P., and Lebenthal, E. Mammary amylase: a possible alternate pathway of carbohydrate digestion in infancy. Pediatr. Res. *17*:15, 1983.
4. Miller, D., and Crane, R. K. The digestive function of the epithelium of the small intestine. Biochem. Biophys. Acta *52*:293, 1961.
5. Kenny, A. J., and Maroux, S. Topology of microvillar membrane hydrolases of kidney and intestine. Physiol. Rev. *62*:91, 1982.
6. Danielsen, M., Cowell, G. M., Noren, O., and Sjöström, H. Biosynthesis of microvillar proteins. Biochem. J. *221*:1, 1984.
7. Dahlqvist, A., and Semenza, G. Disaccharidases of small-intestinal mucosa. J. Pediatr. Gastroenterol. Nutr. *4*:857, 1985.
8. Hauri, H.-P. Biosynthesis and transport of plasma membrane glycoproteins in the rat intestinal epithelial cell: studies with sucrase-isomaltase. *In* Brush Border Membranes. London, Pitman Books, 1983 (Ciba Foundation Symposium 95), p. 132.
9. Hauri, H.-P., Sterchi, E. E., Bienz, D., Fransen, J. A. M., and Marxer, A. Expression and intracellular transport of microvillus membrane hydrolases in human intestinal epithelial cells. J. Cell Biol. *101*:838, 1985.
10. Skovbjerg, H., Danielsen, E. M., Noren, O., and Sjöström, H. Evidence for biosynthesis of lactase-phlorizin hydrolase as a single-chain high-molecular weight precursor. Biochim. Biophys. Acta *798*:247, 1984.

11. Gray, G. M., Lally, B. C., and Conklin, K. A. Action of intestinal sucrase-isomaltase and its free monomers on an α-limit dextrin. J. Biol. Chem. *254*:6038, 1979.
12. Semenza, G., Brunner, J., and Wacker, H. Biosynthesis and assembly of the largest and major intrinsic polypeptide of the small intestinal brush borders. *In* Brush Border Membranes. London, Pitman Books, 1983 (Ciba Foundation Symposium 95), p. 92.
13. Norén, O., Sjöström, H., Cowell, G. M., Tranum-Jensen, J., Hansen, O. C., and Welinder, K. G. Pig intestinal microvillar maltase-glucoamylase. J. Biol. Chem. *261*:12306, 1986.
14. Hunziker, W., Spiess, M., Semenza, G., and Lodish, H. F. The sucrase-isomaltase complex: primary structure, membrane-orientation, and evolution of a stalked, intrinsic brush border protein. Cell *46*:227, 1986.
15. Newcomer, A. D., and McGill, D. B. Distribution of disaccharidase activity in the small bowel of normal and lactase-deficient subjects. Gastroenterology *51*:481, 1966.
16. Smith, M. W. Expression of digestive and absorptive function in differentiating enterocytes. Ann. Rev. Physiol. *47*:247, 1985.
17. Gray, G. M., and Santiago, N. A. Disaccharide absorption in normal and diseased human intestine. Gastroenterology *51*:489, 1966.
18. Dawson, D. J., Lobley, R. W., Burrows, P. C., Miller, V., and Holmes, R. Lactose digestion by human jejunal biopsies: the relationship between hydrolysis and absorption. Gut *27*:521, 1986.
19. Alpers, D. H., and Tedesco, F. J. The possible role of pancreatic proteases in the turnover of intestinal brush border proteins. Biochim. Biophys. Acta *40*:28, 1975.
20. Riepe, S. P., Goldstein, J., and Alpers, D. H. Effect of secreted *Bacteroides* proteases on human intestinal brush border hydrolases. J. Clin. Invest. *66*:314, 1980.
21. Jonas, A., Krishnan, C., and Forstner, G. Pathogenesis of mucosal injury in the blind loop syndrome. Gastroenterology *75*:791, 1978.
22. Sherman, P., Wesley, A., and Forstner, G. Sequential disaccharidase loss in rat intestinal blind loops: impact of malnutrition. Am. J. Physiol. *248*:G626, 1985.
23. Henning, S. J. Ontogeny of enzymes in the small intestine. Ann. Rev. Physiol. *47*:231, 1985.
24. Cezard, J. P., Broyart, J. P., Cuisinier-Gleizes, P., and Mathieu, H. Sucrase-isomaltase regulation by dietary sucrose in the rat. Gastroenterology *84*:18, 1983.
25. Stevens, B. R., Kaunitz, J. D., and Wright, E. M. Intestinal transport of amino acids and sugars: advances using membrane vesicles. Ann. Rev. Physiol. *46*:417, 1984.
26. Semenza, G., Kessler, M., Hosang, M., Weber, J., and Schmidt, U. Biochemistry of the Na^+, D-glucose cotransporter of the small-intestinal brush-border membrane. Biochim. Biophys. Acta *779*:343, 1984.
27. Karasov, W. H., and Diamond, J. M. Adaptive regulation of sugar and amino acid transport by vertebrate intestine. Am. J. Physiol. *245*:G443, 1983.
28. Morant, A., Turner, R. J., and Handler, J. S. Regulation of sodium-coupled glucose transport by glucose in a cultured epithelium. J. Biol. Chem. *258*:15087, 1983.
29. Ravich, W. J., Bayless, T. M., and Thomas, M. Fructose: incomplete intestinal absorption in humans. Gastroenterology *84*:26, 1983.
30. Hyams, J. S. Sorbitol intolerance: an unappreciated cause of functional gastrointestinal complaints. Gastroenterology *84*:30, 1983.
31. Sandle, G. I., Lobley, R. W., Warwick, R., and Holmes, R. Monosaccharide absorption and water secretion during disaccharide perfusion of the human jejunum. Digestion *26*:53, 1983.
32. Gray, G. M. Carbohydrate digestion and absorption. N. Engl. J. Med. *292*:1225, 1975.
33. Barry, P. H., and Diamond, J. M. Effects of unstirred layers on membrane phenomena. Physiol. Rev. *64*:763, 1984.
34. Wilson, F. A., Dietschy, J. M. The intestinal unstirred layer: its surface area and effect on active transport kinetics. Biochim. Biophys. Acta *363*:112, 1974.
35. Westergaard, H., Holtermüller, K. H., and Dietschy, J. M. Measurement of resistance of barriers to solute transport in vivo in rat jejunum. Am. J. Physiol. *250*:G735, 1986.
36. Bond, J. H., Currier, B. E., Buchwald, H., and Levitt, M. D. Colonic conservation of malabsorbed carbohydrate. Gastroenterology *78*:444, 1980.
37. Higuchi, S., Fukushi, G., Baba, T., Sasaki, D., and Yoshida, Y. New method of testing for carbohydrate absorption in man. Dig. Dis. Sci. *31*:369, 1986.
38. Anderson, I. H., Levine, A. S., and Levitt, M. D. Incomplete absorption of the carbohydrate in all-purpose wheat flour. N. Engl. J. Med. *304*:891, 1981.
39. Stephen, A. M., Haddad, A. C., and Phillips, S. F. Passage of carbohydrate into the colon. Gastroenterology *85*:589, 1983.
40. Wolever, T. M. S., Cohen, Z., Thompson, L. U., Thorne, M. J., Jenkins, M. J. A., Prokipchuk, E. J., and Jenkins, D. J. A. Ileal loss of available carbohydrate in man: comparison of a breath hydrogen method with direct measurement using a human ileostomy model. Am. J. Gastroenterol. *81*:115, 1986.
41. Levine, A. S., and Levitt, M. D. Malabsorption of starch moiety of oats, corn and potatoes (Abstract). Gastroenterology *80*:1209, 1981.
42. Kerlin, P., Wong, L., Harris, B., and Capra, S. Rice flour, breath hydrogen, and malabsorption. Gastroenterology *87*:578, 1984.
43. Bond, J. H., Jr., and Levitt, M. D. Fate of soluble carbohydrate in the colon of rats and man. J. Clin. Invest. *57*:1158, 1976.
44. Flourie, B., Florent, C., Jouany, J.-P., Thivend, P., Etanchaud, F., and Rambaud, J.-C. Colonic metabolism of wheat starch in healthy humans. Gastroenterology *90*:111, 1986.
45. Cummings, J. H. Fermentation in the human large intestine: evidence and implications for health. Lancet *2*:1206, 1983.
46. Ruppin, H., Bar-Meir, S., Soergel, K. H., Wood, C. M., and Schmitt, M. G., Jr. Absorption of short-chain fatty acids by the colon. Gastroenterology *78*:1500, 1980.
47. Cummings, J. H. Short chain fatty acids in the human colon. Gut *22*:763, 1981.
48. Cummings, J. H. Colonic absorption: the importance of short chain fatty acids in man. Scand. J. Gastroenterol. *93*(Suppl.):89, 1984.
49. Wiggins, H. S. Nutritional value of sugars and related compounds undigested in the small gut. Proc. Nutr. Soc. *43*:69, 1984.
50. Levitt, M. D., and Bond, J. H. Volume, composition, and source of intestinal gas. Gastroenterology *59*:921, 1970.
51. Levitt, M. D., Kolars, J. C., and Savaiano, D. A. Carbohydrate malabsorption and intestinal gas production. Neth. J. Med. *27*:258, 1984.
52. Gray, G. M., Walter, W. M., Jr., and Colver, E. H. Persistent deficiency of intestinal lactase in apparently cured tropical sprue. Gastroenterology *54*:552, 1968.
53. Ravich, W. J., and Bayless, T. M. Carbohydrate absorption and malabsorption. Clin. Gastroenterol. *12*:335, 1983.
54. Gudmand-Høyer, E. Sucrose malabsorption in children: a report of thirty-one Greenlanders. J. Pediatr. Gastroenterol. Nutr. *4*:873, 1985.
55. Hauri, H.-P., Roth, J., Sterchi, E. E., and Lentze, M. J. Transport to cell surface of intestinal sucrase-isomaltase is blocked in the Golgi apparatus in a patient with congenital sucrase-isomaltase deficiency. Proc. Natl. Acad. Sci. USA *82*:4423, 1985.
56. Evans, L., Grasset, E., Heyman, M., Dumontier, A. M., Beau, J.-P., and Desjeux, J.-F. Congenital selective malabsorption of glucose and galactose. J. Pediatr. Gastroenterol. Nutr. *4*:878, 1985.
57. Beyreiss, K., Hoepffner, W., Scheerschmidt, G., and Müller, F. Digestion and absorption rates of lactose, glucose, galactose, and fructose in three infants with congenital glucose-galactose malabsorption: perfusion studies. J. Pediatr. Gastroenterol. Nutr. *4*:887, 1985.
58. Radziuk, J., Kemmer, F., Morishima, T., Berchtold, P., and Vranic, M. The effects of an alpha-glucoside hydrolase inhibitor on glycemia and the absorption of sucrose in man determined using a tracer method. Diabetes *33*:207, 1984.

59. Layer, P., Carlson, G. L., and DiMagno, E. P. Partially purified white bean amylase inhibitor reduces starch digestion in vitro and inactivates intraduodenal amylase in humans. Gastroenterology *88*:1895, 1985.
60. Layer, P., Rizza, R. A., Zinsmeister, A. R., Carlson, G. L., and DiMagno, E. P. Effect of a purified amylase inhibitor on carbohydrate tolerance in normal subjects and patients with diabetes mellitus. Mayo Clin. Proc. *61*:442, 1986.
61. Patton, J. S. Gastrointestinal lipid digestion. *In* Johnson, L. R. (ed.). Physiology of the Gastrointestinal Tract. New York, Raven Press, 1981, p. 1123.
62. Borgström, B. Luminal digestion of fats. *In* Go, V. L. W., Brooks, F. P., DiMagno, E. P., Gardner, J. D., Lebenthal, E., and Scheele, G. A. (eds.). The Exocrine Pancreas. New York, Raven Press, 1986, p. 361.
63. Patton, J. S., and Carey, M. C. Watching fat digestion. Science *204*:145, 1979.
64. Borgström, B. The micellar hypothesis of fat absorption: Must it be revisited? Scand. J. Gastroenterol. *20*:389, 1985.
65. Gargouri, Y., Pieroni, G., Riviere, C., Sauniere, J.-F., Lowe, P. A., Sarda, L., and Verger, R. Kinetic assay of human gastric lipase on short- and long-chain triacylglycerol emulsions. Gastroenterology *91*:919, 1986.
66. Roberts, I. M., Montgomery, R. K., and Carey, M. C. Rat lingual lipase: partial purification, hydrolytic properties, and comparison with pancreatic lipase. Am. J. Physiol. *247*:G385, 1984.
67. Hamosh, M. Lingual lipase. Gastroenterology *90*:1290, 1986.
68. Abrams, C. K., Hamosh, M., Hubbard, V. S., Dutta, S. K., and Hamosh, P. Lingual lipase in cystic fibrosis. J. Clin. Invest. *73*:374, 1984.
69. Jensen, R. G., Clark, R. M., deJong, F. A., Hamosh, M., Liao, T. H., and Mehta, N. R. The lipolytic triad: human lingual, breast milk, and pancreatic lipases: physiological implications of their characteristics in digestion of dietary fats. J. Pediatr. Gastroenterol. Nutr. *1*:243, 1982.
70. Borgström, B. On the interactions between pancreatic lipase and colipase and the substrate, and the importance of bile salts. J. Lipid Res. *16*:411, 1975.
71. Patton, J. S., and Carey, M. C. Inhibition of human pancreatic lipase-colipase activity by mixed bile salt-phospholipid micelles. Am. J. Physiol. *241*:G328, 1981.
72. Borgström, B., Wieloch, T., and Erlanson-Albertsson, C. Evidence for a pancreatic pro-colipase and its activation by trypsin. FEBS Lett. *108*:407, 1979.
73. Porter, H. P., Saunders, D. R., Tytgat, G., Brunser, O., and Rubin, C. E. Fat absorption in bile fistula man. Gastroenterology *60*:1008, 1971.
74. Westergaard, H., and Dietschy, J. M. The uptake of lipids into intestinal mucosa. *In* Andreoli, T. E., Hoffman, J. F., Fanestil, D. D., and Schultz, S. G. (eds.). Physiology of Membrane Disorders. 2nd edition. New York, Plenum Medical, 1986, p. 597.
75. Stremmel, W., Lotz, G., Strohmeyer, G., and Berk, P. D. Identification, isolation, and partial characterization of a fatty acid binding protein from rat jejunal microvillous membranes. J. Clin. Invest. *75*:1068, 1985.
76. Stremmel, W., Strohmeyer, G., and Berk, P. D. Hepatocellular uptake of oleate is energy dependent, sodium linked, and inhibited by an antibody to a hepatocyte plasma membrane fatty acid binding protein. Proc. Natl. Acad. Sci. USA *83*:3584, 1986.
77. Ponz de Leon, M., Iori, R., Barbolini, G., Pompei, G., Zaniol, P., and Carulli, N. Influence of small-bowel transit time on dietary cholesterol absorption in human beings. N. Engl. J. Med. *307*:102, 1982.
78. Bass, N. M. Function and regulation of hepatic and intestinal fatty acid binding proteins. Chem. Phys. Lipids *38*:95, 1985.
79. Bass, N. M. The cellular fatty acid binding proteins: aspects of structure, regulation and function. Int. Rev. Cytol. *111*:141, 1988.
80. Tso, P. Gastrointestinal digestion and absorption of lipid. Adv Lipid Res *21*:143, 1985.
81. Tso, P., and Balint, J. A. Formation and transport of chylomicrons by enterocytes to the lymphatics. Am. J. Physiol. *250*:G715, 1986.
82. Mattson, F. H., and Volpenhein, R. A. The digestion and absorption of triglycerides. J. Biol. Chem. *239*:2772, 1964.
83. Kayden, H. J., Senior, J. R., and Mattson, F. H. The monoglyceride pathway of fat absorption in man. J. Clin. Invest. *46*:1695, 1967.
84. Higgins, J. A., and Barrnett, R. J. Fine structural localization of acyltransferases. J. Cell Biol. *50*:102, 1971.
85. Grigor, M. R., and Bell, R. M. Separate monoacylglycerol and diacylglycerol acyltransferases function in intestinal triacylglycerol synthesis. Biochim. Biophys. Acta *712*:464, 1982.
86. Coleman, R. A., and Bell, R. M. Topography of membrane-bound enzymes that metabolize complex lipids. *In* Boyer, P. D. (ed.). The Enzymes. Vol. 16. New York, Academic Press, 1983, p. 605.
87. Green, P. R. H., and Glickman, R. M. Intestinal lipoprotein metabolism. J. Lipid Res. *22*:1153, 1981.
88. Bisgaier, C. L., and Glickman, R. M. Intestinal synthesis, secretion, and transport of lipoproteins. Ann. Rev. Physiol. *45*:625, 1983.
89. Green, P. R. H., Lefkowitch, J. H., Glickman, R. M., Riley, J. W., Quinet, E., and Blum, C. B. Apolipoprotein localization and quantitation in the human intestine. Gastroenterology *83*:1223, 1982.
90. Christensen, N. J., Rubin, C. E., Cheung, M. C., and Albers, J. J. Ultrastructural immunolocalization of apolipoprotein B within human jejunal absorptive cells. J. Lipid Res. *24*:1229, 1983.
91. Alexander, C. A., Hamilton, R. L., and Havel, R. J. Subcellular localization of B apoprotein of plasma lipoproteins in rat liver. J. Cell Biol. *69*:241, 1976.
92. Patton, G. M., Clark, S. B., Fasulo, J. M., and Robins, S. J. Utilization of individual lecithins in intestinal lipoprotein formation in the rat. J. Clin. Invest. *73*:231, 1984.
93. Bishop, W. R., and Bell, R. M. Assembly of the endoplasmic reticulum phospholipid bilayer: the phosphatidylcholine transporter. Cell *42*:51, 1985.
94. Clark, S. B., and Tercyak, A. M. Reduced cholesterol transmucosal transport in rats with inhibited mucosal acyl CoA:cholesterol acyltransferase and normal pancreatic function. J. Lipid Res. *25*:148, 1984.
95. Gregg, R. E., Connor, W. E., Lin, D. S., and Brewer, H. B., Jr. Abnormal metabolism of shellfish sterols in a patient with sitosterolemia and xanthomatosis. J. Clin. Invest. *77*:1864, 1986.
96. Kessler, J. I., Narcessian, P., and Mauldin, D. P. Biosynthesis of lipoproteins by intestinal epithelium. Site of synthesis and sequence of association of lipid, sugar and protein moieties (Abstract). Gastroenterology *68*:1058, 1975.
97. Sabesin, S. M., and Frase, S. Electron microscopic studies of the assembly, intracellular transport, and secretion of chylomicrons by rat intestine. J. Lipid Res. *18*:496, 1977.
98. Pavelka, M., and Gangl, A. Effects of colchicine on the intestinal transport of endogenous lipid. Gastroenterology *84*:544, 1983.
99. Greenberger, N. J., and Skillman, T. G. Medium-chain triglycerides. N. Engl. J. Med. *280*:1045, 1969.
100. Ruppin, D. C., and Middleton, W. R. J. Clinical use of medium chain triglycerides. Drugs *20*:216, 1980.
101. Glickman, R. M., Green, P. H. R., Lees, R. S., Lux, S. E., and Kilgore, A. Immunofluorescence studies of apolipoprotein B in intestinal mucosa. Gastroenterology *76*:288, 1979.
102. Figarella, C., De Caro, A., Leupold, D., and Poley, J. R. Congenital pancreatic lipase deficiency. J. Pediatr. *96*:412, 1980.
103. Ghishan, F. K., Moran, J. R., Durie, P. R., and Greene, H. L. Isolated congenital lipase-colipase deficiency. Gastroenterology *86*:1580, 1984.
104. Hildebrand, H., Borgström, B., Békássy, A., Erlanson-Albertsson, C., and Helin, I. Isolated co-lipase deficiency in two brothers. Gut *23*:243, 1982.
105. Levine, A. S., and Silvis, S. E. Absorption of whole peanuts, peanut oil, and peanut butter. N. Engl. J. Med. *303*:917, 1980.
106. Freeman, H. J., Sleisenger, M. H., and Kim, Y. S. Human protein digestion and absorption: Normal mechanisms and protein-energy malnutrition. Clin. Gastroenterol. *12*:357, 1983.

107. Rinderknecht, H. Pancreatic secretory enzymes. *In* Go, V. L. W., Brooks, F. P., DiMagno, E. P., Gardner, J. D., Lebenthal, E., and Scheele, G. A. (eds.). The Exocrine Pancreas: Biology, Pathobiology, and Diseases. New York, Raven Press, 1986, p. 163.
108. Gray, G. M. Intraluminal and surface membrane digestion of dietary carbohydrate and protein. *In* Go, V. L. W., Brooks, F. P., DiMagno, E. P., Gardner, J. D., Lebenthal, E., and Scheele, G. A. (eds.). The Exocrine Pancreas: Biology, Pathobiology, and Diseases. New York, Raven Press, 1986, p. 375.
109. Adibi, S. A., and Kim, Y. S. Peptide absorption and hydrolysis. *In* Johnson, L. R. (ed.). Physiology of the Gastrointestinal Tract. New York, Raven Press, 1981, p. 1073.
110. Foltmann, B. Gastric proteinases—structure, function, evolution and mechanism of action. *In* Campbell, P. N., and Marshal, R. D. (eds.). Essays in Biochemistry. New York, Academic Press, 1981, p. 52.
111. Samloff, I. M. Pepsins, peptic activity, and peptic inhibitors. J. Clin. Gastroenterol. *3*:91, 1981.
112. Gray, G. M., and Cooper, H. L. Protein digestion and absorption. Gastroenterology *61*:535, 1971.
113. Grant, D. A. W., and Hermon-Taylor, J. The purification of human enterokinase by affinity chromatography and immunoadsorption. Biochem. J. *155*:243, 1976.
114. Hermon-Taylor, J., Perrin, J., Grant, D. A. W., Appleyard, A., Bubel, M., and Magee, A. I. Immunofluorescent localisation of enterokinase in human small intestine. Gut *18*:259, 1977.
115. Silk, D. B. A., Grimble, G. K., and Rees, R. G. Protein digestion and amino acid and peptide absorption. Proc. Nutr. Soc. *44*:63, 1985.
116. Rinderknecht, H. Activation of pancreatic zymogens. Dig. Dis. Sci. *31*:314, 1986.
117. Kenny, A. J., and Fulcher, I. S. Microvillar endopeptidase, an enzyme with special topological features and a wide distribution. *In* Brush Border Membranes. London, Pitman Books, 1983 (Ciba Foundation Symposium 95), p. 12.
118. Danielsen, E. M., and Cowell, G. M. L. Biosynthesis of intestinal microvillar proteins. Eur. J. Biochem. *152*:493, 1985.
119. Danielsen, E. M., Cowell, G. M., Sjöström, H., and Nóren, O. Translational control of an intestinal microvillar enzyme. Biochem. J. *235*:447, 1986.
120. Kenny, A. J., Fulcher, I. S., McGill, K. A., and Kershaw, D. Proteins of the kidney microvillar membrane. Biochem. J. *211*:755, 1983.
121. Quaroni, A., Kirsch, K., and Weiser, M. M. Synthesis of membrane glycoproteins in rat small-intestinal villus cells. Biochem. J. *182*:203, 1979.
122. Tobey, N., Heizer, W., Yeh, R., Huang, T.-I., and Hoffner, C. Human intestinal brush border peptidases. Gastroenterology *88*:913, 1985.
123. Erickson, R. H., Bella, A. M., Jr., Brophy, E. J., Kobata, A., and Kim, Y. S. Purification and molecular characterization of rat intestinal brush border membrane dipeptidyl aminopeptidase IV. Biochim. Biophys. Acta *756*:258, 1983.
124. Kim, Y. S., Brophy, E. J., and Nicholson, J. A. Rat intestinal brush border membrane peptidases. J. Biol. Chem. *251*:3206, 1976.
125. Gray, G. M., and Santiago, N. A. Intestinal surface amino-oligopeptidases. I. Isolation of two weight isomers and their subunits from rat brush border. J. Biol. Chem. *252*:4922, 1977.
126. Kania, R. K., Santiago, N. A., and Gray, G. M. Intestinal surface amino-oligopeptidases. II. Substrate kinetics and topography of the active site. J. Biol. Chem. *252*:4929, 1977.
127. Bella, A. M., Jr., Erickson, R. H., and Kim, Y. S. Rat intestinal brush border membrane dipeptidyl-aminopeptidase. IV. Kinetic properties and substrate specificities of the purified enzyme. Arch. Biochem. Biophys. *218*:156, 1982.
128. Kim, Y. S., and Brophy, E. J. Effect of amino acids on purified rat intestinal brush-border membrane aminooligopeptidase. Gastroenterology *76*:82, 1979.
129. Auricchio, S., Greco, L., de Vizia, B., and Buonocore, V. Dipeptidylaminopeptidase and carboxypeptidase activities of the brush border of rabbit small intestine. Gastroenterology *75*:1073, 1978.
130. Song, I.-S., Yoshioka, M., Erickson, R. H., Miura, S., Guan, D., and Kim, Y. S. Identification and characterization of brush-border membrane-bound neutral metalloendopeptidases from rat small intestine. Gastroenterology *91*:1234, 1986.
131. Sleisenger, M. H., Burston, D., Dalrymple, J. A., Wilkinson, S., and Matthews, D. M. Evidence for a single common carrier for uptake of a dipeptide and a tripeptide by hamster jejunum in vitro. Gastroenterology *71*:76, 1976.
132. Smithson, K. W., and Gray, G. M. Intestinal assimilation of a tetrapeptide in the rat. J. Clin. Invest. *60*:665, 1977.
133. Rosen-Levin, E. M., Smithson, K. W., Gray, G. M. Complementary role of surface hydrolysis and intact transport in the intestinal assimilation of di- and tripeptides. Biochim. Biophys. Acta *629*:126, 1980.
134. Rajendran, V. M., Ansari, S. A., Harig, J. A., Adams, M. B., Khan, A. H., and Ramaswamy, K. Transport of glycyl-L-proline by human intestinal brush border membrane vesicles. Gastroenterology *89*:1298, 1985.
135. Silk, D. B. A. Peptide transport. Clin. Sci. *60*:607, 1981.
136. Silk, D. B. A., Hegarty, J. E., Fairclough, P. D., and Clark, M. L. Characterization and nutritional significance of peptide transport in man. Ann. Nutr. Metab. *26*:337, 1982.
137. Steinhardt, H. J., and Adibi, S. A. Kinetics and characteristics of absorption from an equimolar mixture of 12 glycyl-dipeptides in human jejunum. Gastroenterology *90*:577, 1986.
138. Silk, D. B. A., Perrett, D., and Clark, M. L. Intestinal transport of two dipeptides containing the same two neutral amino acids in man. Clin. Sci. Molec. Med. *45*:291, 1973.
139. Asatoor, A. M., Cheng, B., Edwards, K. D. G., Lant, A. F., Matthews, D. M., Milne, M. D., Navab, F., and Richards, A. J. Intestinal absorption of two dipeptides in Hartnup Disease. Gut *11*:380, 1970.
140. Ganapathy, V., and Leibach, F. H. Is intestinal peptide transport energized by a proton gradient? Am. J. Physiol. *249*:G153, 1985.
141. Kim, Y. S., Kim, Y. W., and Sleisenger, M. H. Studies on the properties of peptide hydrolases in the brush-border and soluble fractions of small intestinal mucosa of rat man. Biochim. Biophys. Acta *370*:283, 1974.
142. Heizer, W. D., Kerley, R. L., and Isselbacher, K. J. Intestinal peptide hydrolases: differences between brush border and cytoplasmic enzymes. Biochim. Biophys. Acta *264*:450, 1972.
143. Powell, G. F., Rasco, M. A., and Maniscalco, R. M. A prolidase deficiency in man with iminopeptiduria. Metabolism *23*:505, 1974.
144. Rapley, S., Lewis, W. H. P., and Harris, H. Tissue distributions, substrate specificities and molecular sizes of human peptidases determined by separate gene loci. Ann. Hum. Genet. *34*:307, 1971.
145. Myara, I., Charpentier, C., and Lemonnier, A. Optimal conditions for prolidase assay by proline colorimetric determination: application to iminodipeptiduria. Clin. Chim. Acta *125*:193, 1982.
146. Gardner, M. L. G. Intestinal assimilation of intact peptides and proteins from the diet—a neglected field? Biol. Rev. *59*:289, 1984.
147. Stevens, B. R., Ross, H. J., and Wright, E. M. Multiple transport pathways for neutral amino acids in rabbit jejunal brush border vesicles. J. Membr. Biol. *66*:213, 1982.
148. Wright, E. M., Stevens, B. R., and Peerce, B. E. Neutral amino acid transport in rabbit intestinal brush-border membranes. Fed. Proc. *45*:2450, 1986.
149. Munck, B. G. Intestinal absorption of amino acids. *In* Johnson, L. R. (ed.). Physiology of the Gastrointestinal Tract. New York, Raven Press, 1981, p. 1097.
150. Corcelli, A., Prezioso, G., Palmieri, F., and Storelli, C. Electroneutral Na^+/dicarboxylic amino acid cotransport in rat intestinal brush border membrane vesicles. Biochim. Biophys. Acta *689*:97, 1982.
151. Schafer, J. A., and Barfuss, D. W. Membrane mechanisms for transepithelial amino acid absorption and secretion. Am. J. Physiol. *238*:F335, 1980.
152. Curtis, K. J., Kim, Y. S., Perdomo, J. M., Silk, D. B. A., and Whitehead, J. S. Protein digestion and absorption in the rat. J. Physiol. *274*:409, 1978.

153. Chung, Y. C., Kim, Y. S., Shadchehr, A., Garrido, A., MacGregor, I. L., and Sleisenger, M. H. Protein digestion and absorption in human small intestine. Gastroenterology *76*:1415, 1979.
154. Triadou, N., Bataille, J., and Schmitz, J. Longitudinal study of the human intestinal brush border membrane proteins. Gastroenterology *85*:1326, 1983.
155. Tobey, N. A., and Heizer, W. D. Intestinal hydrolysis of aspartylphenylalanine—the metabolic product of aspartame. Gastroenterology *91*:931, 1986.
156. Fairclough, P. D., Hegarty, J. E., Silk, D. B. A., and Clark, M. L. Comparison of the absorption of two protein hydrolysates and their effects on water and electrolyte movements in the human jejunum. Gut *21*:829, 1980.
157. Hegarty, J. E., Fairclough, P. D., Moriarty, K. J., Clark, M. L., Kelly, M. J., and Dawson, A. M. Comparison of plasma and intraluminal amino acid profiles in man after meals containing a protein hydrolysate and equivalent amino acid mixture. Gut *23*:670, 1982.
158. Austic, R. E. Development and adaptation of protein digestion. J. Nutr. *115*:686, 1985.
159. Thomson, A. B. R., and Keelan, M. The development of the small intestine. Can. J. Physiol. Pharmacol. *64*:13, 1986.
160. Levine, G. M. Nonspecific adaptation of jejunal amino acid uptake in the rat. Gastroenterology *91*:49, 1986.
161. Miura, S., Morita, A., Erickson, R. H., and Kim, Y. S. Content and turnover of rat intestinal microvillus membrane aminopeptidase. Effect of methylprednisolone. Gastroenterology *85*:1340, 1983.
162. Vazquez, J. A., Morse, E. L., and Adibi, S. A. Effect of starvation on amino acid and peptide transport and peptide hydrolysis in humans. Am. J. Physiol. *249*:G563, 1985.
163. Rodewald, R., and Kraehenbuhl, J. P. Receptor-mediated transport of IgG. J. Cell Biol. *99*:159s, 1984.
164. Udall, J. N., and Walker, W. A. The physiologic and pathologic basis for the transport of macromolecules across the intestinal tract. J. Pediatr. Gastroenterol. Nutr. *1*:295, 1982.
165. Owen, R. L. And now pathophysiology of M cells—good news and bad news from Peyer's patches (Editorial). Gastroenterology *85*:468, 1983.
166. Lerner, A., Heitlinger, L. A., and Lebenthal, E. Hereditary abnormalities of pancreatic function. *In* Go, V. L. W., Brooks, F. P., DiMagno, E. P., Gardner, J. D., Lebenthal, E., and Scheele, G. A. (eds.). The Exocrine Pancreas: Biology, Pathobiology, and Diseases. New York, Raven Press, 1986, p. 819.
167. Townes, P. L., and White, M. R. Identity of two syndromes. Proteolytic, lipolytic and amylolytic deficiency of the exocrine pancreas with congenital anomalies. Am. J. Dis. Child. *135*:248, 1981.
168. Stanbury, J. B., Wyngaarden, J. B., Fredrickson, D. S., Goldstein, J. L., and Brown, M. S. (eds.). The Metabolic Basis of Inherited Disease. 5th edition. (Chapters: The hyperlysinemias; Cystinuria; Familial iminoglycinuria; Hartnup disease.) New York, McGraw-Hill, 1983, pp. 439, 1774, 1792, 1804.
169. Jepson, J. B. Hartnup disease. *In* Stanbury, J. B., Wyngaarden, J. B., and Fredrickson, D. S. (eds.). The metabolic Basis of Interited Disease. 4th edition. New York: McGraw-Hill, 1978, p. 1563.
170. Desjeux, J.-F., Rajantie, J., Simell, R. O., Dumontier, A.-M., Perheentupa, J. Lysine fluxes across the jejunal epithelium in lysinuric protein intolerance. J. Clin. Invest. *65*:1382, 1980.
171. Rajantie, J., Simell, O., and Perheentupa, J. Intestinal absorption in lysinuric protein intolerance: impaired for diamino acids, normal for citrulline. Gut *21*:519, 1980.
172. Phillips, A. D., Jenkins, P., Raafat, F., and Walker-Smith, J. A. Congenital microvillous atrophy: specific diagnostic features. Arch. Dis. Child. *60*:135, 1985.
173. Davidson, G. P., Cutz, E., Hamilton, J. R., and Gall, D. G. Familial enteropathy: a syndrome of protracted diarrhea from birth, failure to thrive, and hypoplastic villus atrophy. Gastroenterology *75*:783, 1978.
174. Carruthers, L., Phillips, A. D., Dourmashkin, R., and Walker-Smith, J. A. Biochemical abnormality in brush border membrane protein of a patient with congenital microvillus atrophy. J. Pediatr. Gastroenterol. Nutr. *4*:902, 1985.
175. Huijghebaert, S. M., and Hofmann, A. F. Pancreatic carboxypeptidase hydrolysis of bile acid-amino acid conjugates: selective resistance of glycine and taurine amidates. Gastroenterology *90*:306, 1986.
176. Carey, M. C. The enterohepatic circulation. *In* Arias, I., Popper, H., Schachter, D., and Shafritz, D. A. (eds.). The Liver: Biology and Pathobiology. New York, Raven Press, 1982, p. 429.
177. Scharschmidt, B. F. Bile formation and cholestasis, metabolism and enterohepatic circulation of bile acids, and gallstone formation. *In* Zakim, D., and Boyer, T. D. (eds.). Hepatology: A Textbook of Liver Disease. 2nd edition. Philadelphia, W. B. Saunders, 1988, in press.
178. Wilson, F. A. Intestinal transport of bile acids. Am. J. Physiol. *241*:G83, 1981.
179. McClintock, C., Shiau, Y.-F. Jejunum is more important than terminal ileum for taurocholate absorption in rats. Am. J. Physiol. *244*:G507, 1983.
180. Lack, L. Properties and biological significance of ileal bile salt transport system. Environ. Health Perspec. *33*:79, 1979.
181. Ferraris, R., Jazrawi, R., Bridges, C., and Northfield, T. C. Use of a γ-labeled bile acid (^{75}SeHCAT) as a test of ileal function. Gastroenterology *90*:1129, 1986.
182. Mekhjian, H. S., Phillips, S. F., and Hofmann, A. F. Colonic secretion of water and electrolytes induced by bile acids: perfusion studies in man. J. Clin. Invest. *50*:1569, 1971.
183. Hofmann, A. F., and Poley, J. R. Role of bile acid malabsorption in pathogenesis of diarrhea and steatorrhea in patients with ileal resection. Gastroenterology *62*:918, 1972.
184. Binder, H. J. Pathophysiology of bile acid- and fatty acid-induced diarrhea. *In* Field, M., Fordtran, J. S., and Schultz, S. G. (eds.). Secretory Diarrhea. Bethesda, Maryland, American Physiological Society, 1980, p. 159.
185. Wienbeck, M., Erckenbrecht, J., and Karaus, M. Motor and secretory effects of laxatives in the colon. *In* Skadhauge, E., and Heintze, K. (eds.). Intestinal Absorption and Secretion. Falk Symposium 36. Lancaster, England, MTP Press, 1984, p. 171.
186. Freel, R. W., Hatch, M., Earnest, D. L., and Goldner, A. M. Role of tight-junctional pathways in bile salt-induced increases in colonic permeability. Am. J. Physiol. *245*:G816, 1983.
187. Loeschke, K., and Farack, U. M. Loperamide reduces deoxycholic acid-induced intestinal secretion by decreasing epithelial permeability and by stimulating fluid absorption. *In* Skadhauge, E., and Heintze, K. (eds.). Intestinal Absorption and Secretion. Falk Symposium 36. Lancaster, England, MTP Press, 1984, p. 483.
188. Dutta, S. K., Anand, K., and Gadacz, T. R. Bile salt malabsorption in pancreatic insufficiency secondary to alcoholic pancreatitis. Gastroenterology *91*:1243, 1986.
189. Heubi, J. E., Balistreri, W. F., Fondacaro, J. D., Partin, J. C., and Schubert, W. K. Primary bile acid malabsorption: defective in vitro ileal active bile acid transport. Gastroenterology *83*:804, 1982.
190. Iser, J. H., Dowling, R. H., Murphy, G. M., Ponz de Leon, M., Mitropoulos, K. A. Congenital bile salt deficiency associated with 28 years of intractable constipation. *In* Paumgartner, G., and Stiehl, A., (eds.). Bile Acid Metabolism in Health and Disease. Falk Symposium 24. Lancaster, England, MTP Press, 1977, p. 231.
191. Holgate, A. M., and Read, N. W. Is absorption of nutrients from the small intestine limited by transit time? *In* Skadhauge, E., and Heintze, K. (eds.). Intestinal Absorption and Secretion. Falk Symposium 36. Lancaster, England, MTP Press, 1984, p. 179.
192. Phillips, S. F. Motor function and nutrient absorption. *In* Skadhauge, E., and Heintze, K. (eds.). Intestinal Absorption and Secretion. Falk Symposium 36. Lancaster, England, MTP Press, 1984, p. 129.
193. Holgate, A. M., and Read, N. W. Relationship between small bowel transit time and absorption of a solid meal. Dig. Dis. Sci. *28*:812, 1983.
194. Thomas, F. B., Caldwell, J. H., and Greenberger, N. J. Steatorrhea in thyrotoxicosis. Ann. Intern. Med. *78*:669, 1973.
195. Hellesen, C., Larsen, T. F. E., and Pock-Steen, O. C. H.

Small intestinal histology, radiology and absorption in hyperthyroidism. Scand. J. Gastroenterol. *4*:169, 1969.
196. Schiller, L. R., Santa Ana, C. A., Morawski, S. G., and Fordtran, J. S. Mechanism of the antidiarrheal effect of loperamide. Gastroenterology *86*:1475, 1984.
197. Spiller, R. C., Trotman, I. F., Higgins, B. E., Ghatei, M. A., Grimble, G. K., Lee, Y. C., Bloom, S. R., Misiewicz, J. J., and Silk, D. B. A. The ileal brake—inhibition of jejunal motility after ileal fat perfusion in man. Gut *25*:365, 1984.
198. Holgate, A. M., and Read, N. W. Effect of ileal infusion of intralipid on gastrointestinal transit, ileal flow rate, and carbohydrate absorption in humans after ingestion of a liquid meal. Gastroenterology *88*:1005, 1985.
199. Bo-Linn, G. W., Santa Ana, C. A., Morawski, S. G., and Fordtran, J. S. Purging and calorie absorption in bulimic patients and normal women. Ann. Intern. Med. *99*:14, 1983.
200. Mendeloff, A. I. Dietary fiber and nutrient delivery. *In* Green, M., and Greene, H. L. (eds.). The Role of the Gastrointestinal Tract in Nutrient Delivery. Orlando, Florida, Academic Press, 1984, p. 209.
201. Vahouny, G. V., and Cassidy, M. M. Dietary fibers and absorption of nutrients. Proc. Soc. Exp. Biol. Med. *180*:432, 1985.
202. Jenkins, D. J. A., and Jenkins, A. L. Dietary fiber and the glycemic response. Proc. Soc. Exp. Biol. Med. *180*:422, 1985.
203. Rosenberg, I. H., and Bowman, B. B. Gastrointestinal function and aging. *In* Green, M., and Greene, H. L. (eds.). The Role of the Gastrointestinal Tract in Nutrient Delivery. Orlando, Florida, Academic Press, 1984, p. 259.
204. Holt, P. R. The small intestine. Clin. Gastroenterol. *14*:689, 1985.
205. Feibusch, J. M., and Holt, P. R. Impaired absorptive capacity for carbohydrate in the aging human. Dig. Dis. Sci. *27*:1095, 1982.
206. Hollander, D., Dadufalza, V. D., and Sletten, E. G. Does essential fatty acid absorption change with aging? J. Lipid Res. *25*:129, 1984.

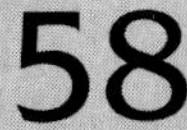

58 Movement of the Small and Large Intestine

SIDNEY COHEN
WILLIAM J. SNAPE, JR.

GENERAL CONTROL MECHANISMS

Movement of contents through the small and large intestine is controlled by the intrinsic activity of the smooth muscle together with the modulating actions of the autonomic nervous system and the gastrointestinal hormones.[1, 2]

The intestinal smooth muscle contractions are regulated by cyclic depolarizations in the muscle membrane, which are called slow waves (basic electrical rhythm, electrical control activity) (Fig. 58–1). Each portion of the gastrointestinal tract has its own intrinsic slow wave frequency that is affected by the adjacent intestinal slow wave activity. The effect of the contiguous slow wave activity of neighboring smooth muscle is called coupling (phase lock). The degree of coupling between adjacent portions of the intestine depends directly on the resistance between neighboring smooth muscle cells (Fig. 58–2). When intercellular resistance is maximal and coupling is minimal, each section of the intestine has its own slow wave frequency.

Spike potentials are rapid changes in smooth muscle membrane potential that initiate the rapid influx of calcium into the muscle cell or release calcium from intracellular binding sites. These changes in intracellular calcium then initiate contractile activity. The spike potentials always occur at one portion of the slow wave cycle. Thus, the frequency of the slow waves determines the shortest interval between spike potentials and in this manner determines the frequency of intestinal contractions. Contractions may be irregular as not every slow wave contains spike potentials. The intensity of the spike potentials determines the strength of the contraction.

Owing to these interrelations between slow waves and spike potentials, the rate and rhythm of the intestinal contractions depend on the characteristics of the smooth muscle membrane in that portion of the intestine. The pattern of these contractions then controls the movement of luminal contents in the intestinal tract.

SMALL INTESTINE

Types of Small Intestinal Movements

The movement of material within the lumen of the small intestine is a complex phenomenon that depends

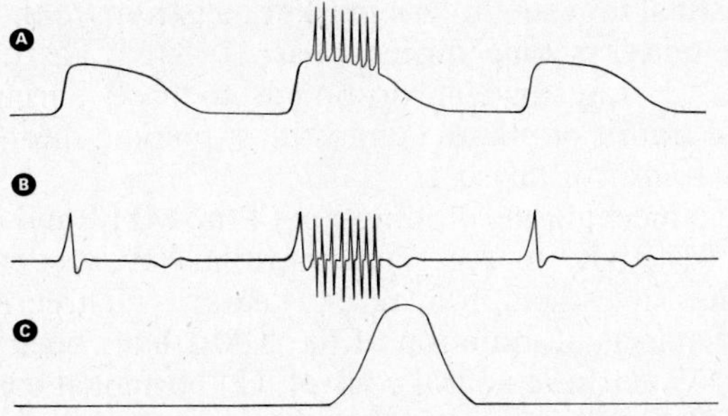

Figure 58–1. Diagram of time relations between slow waves, spike bursts, and contractions. *A* represents the electromyogram of a single smooth muscle cell, recorded with an intracellular microelectrode. *B* represents the electromyogram recorded from several such cells by a large extracellular volume-recording electrode. *C* shows tension in the muscle mass. All three traces are drawn to a common time-base. In *A*, three slow waves appear as a monophasic depolarization from a stable maximal value, the resting membrane potential. Observe that the rate of depolarization is faster than the rate of repolarization. In *B*, the slow waves appear with two components, an initial biphasic spike, which represents depolarization, and a secondary slower biphasic signal, representing repolarization. The trace shown in *B* approximates the second derivative of the trace shown in *A*. The second of the three slow waves bears a burst of spikes, appearing on the plateau of the slow wave. The tension record, in *C*, shows a contraction beginning during the spike burst, and apparently initiated by it. (From Christensen, J. Reprinted by permission of The New England Journal of Medicine, *285*:85, 1971.)

on the interaction of multiple myogenic and neurohumoral factors.[3] The slow waves in the small intestine are generated in adjacent cells of the longitudinal muscle layer and are propagated by electrotonic spread to the circular muscle layer. Slow waves occur at regular intervals and are present continuously.

The aborad movement of intestinal contents is controlled by (1) a frequency gradient of slow wave activity that is present in the small intestine, and (2) propagation of the slow wave activity through contiguous sites. Slow wave frequencies are faster in the duodenum (12 cycles/minute) compared with the ileum (8 cycles/minute). The faster contractile rate in the upper intestine pushes the intestinal contents forward. Tight coupling of neighboring sites is prominent in the duodenum and proximal jejunum, giving a constant frequency in this segment. In this segment of the small bowel, the propagation of the slow waves in an aborad direction controls the orderly movement of luminal contents. Beyond the proximal jejunum, the slow wave frequency occurs because the coupling between slow waves becomes weaker. Thus, slow wave gradient determines intestinal flow throughout the entire small bowel but is especially important distally where the gradient is greatest. Proximally, the prominent coupling of slow waves plays an important role in propulsion.

Physiologic Control of the Small Intestine

Neural Control of the Small Intestine

The small intestine receives extrinsic innervation from the parasympathetic and sympathetic systems.[4] The parasympathetic nerves increase contractions of the small bowel, whereas the sympathetic nerves decrease contractions. The extrinsic nerves act on the smooth muscle cells and on the intrinsic neural system. Intestinal smooth muscle cells possess both alpha- and beta-adrenergic receptors. Activation of either type of receptor inhibits small intestinal smooth muscle. The intrinsic nerves also contain adrenergic receptors. In some species, norepinephrine inhibits contractions by decreasing the release of acetylcholine from the intrinsic neural system.

Other neurotransmitters have been postulated in the small bowel. Serotonergic nerves have been identified in the myenteric plexus. Serotonin stimulates small intestinal contractions. Enkephalins also are present in

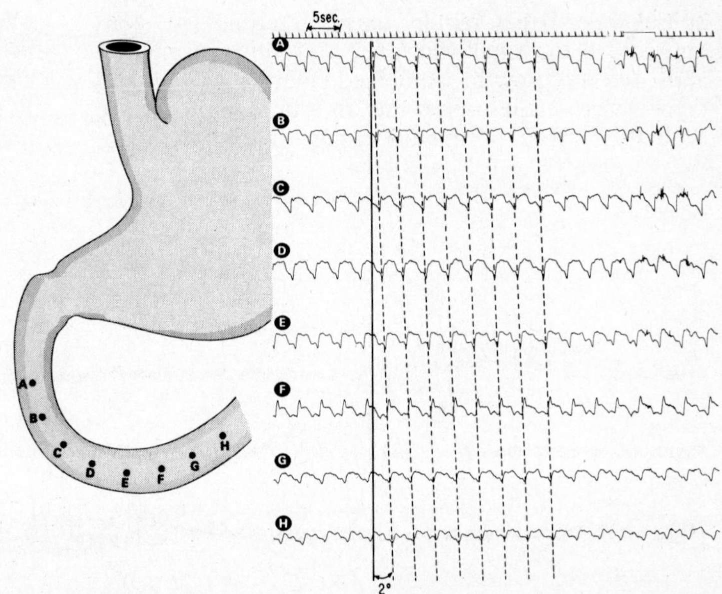

Figure 58–2. Slow waves recorded simultaneously from closely spaced electrodes in the unanesthetized cat. Eight monopolar AC-amplified records are shown as recorded from eight chronically implanted needle electrodes spaced uniformly 1 cm apart along the duodenum. Slow wave configuration is between that of the actual signal and its second derivative. The last few slow waves, at the right, carry spike bursts. Dashed lines are drawn through corresponding slow-wave cycles from each record. The angle, 2 degrees, between these lines and the solid line, the common time-base, is a function of the apparent velocity of spread of slow waves and of the paper speed of the recording polygraph. (From Christensen, J. Reprinted by permission of The New England Journal of Medicine, *285*:85, 1971.)

the myenteric plexus. The enkephalin acts on both the intestinal smooth muscle and the myenteric plexus. The "nonadrenergic inhibitory" transmitter that controls motility has been suggested to be either a purine nucleotide, such as ATP, or the peptide hormone VIP.[5]

Several intestinal reflexes are present in the small intestine.[6] The bowel responds to feeding, light touch, or distention. Reflex inhibition in response to marked distention, handling, or peritoneal irritation is carried in the splanchnic nerves with a central connection in the spinal cord. The intestinal mucosa may be excited orad and inhibited aborad through mucosal neuroreceptors. Longitudinal and circular muscle contraction can be initiated by distention of an isolated segment of intestine. These reflexes are cholinergic in type (see pp. 21–52).

The Interdigestive Motility Pattern

During the interdigestive period, the small intestine shows long periods of quiescence alternating with periods of intense activity.[7,8] This well-defined pattern of small intestinal electrical and motor activity is divided into several phases. Phase 1 is the period of quiescence in which no spike or motor activity is seen. Phase 2 is a period of random spike and motor activity. Phase 3 is characterized by intense spike activity that begins in the stomach, duodenum, or upper jejunum and migrates down the bowel (Fig. 58–3). As one complex reaches the terminal ileum, another complex is initiated in the proximal bowel. Phase 4 is a short period during which the activity returns to the phase 1 type.

The phase 3 activity has been termed the interdigestive migrating motor complex (MMC) and has now been well characterized in many species, including humans.[9] The human MMC occurs every 84 to 112 minutes and migrates down the upper small intestine about 6 to 8 cm/minute. In human beings, as compared with dogs, the site of initiation of the MMC is not constant and may begin at sites other than the proximal bowel. The MMC has been called an "intestinal housekeeper" that rapidly moves interdigestive contents down the small intestine, preventing stagnation and bacterial growth. Combined cineradiography and myoelectric studies show that intestinal contents are propelled ahead of the advancing phase 3 activity. Intestinal movement of a marker or barium took up to four times as long during phase 1 activity as during phase 3. Intestinal absorption is reduced during the rapid transit of phase 3 and is most marked during the slow transit of phase 1.

The mechanisms of initiation of the MMC and cyclic motor activity in the small intestine have undergone intense investigation in recent years.[10,11] Three major mechanisms of initiation of the MMC have been studied: (1) extrinsic neural control, (2) hormonal control, and (3) intrinsic neural control.

The initial studies focused on extrinsic neural mechanisms, with the hypothesis being that cyclic activity was programmed in the central nervous system and the signal was propagated through extrinsic nerves. The MMC continues uninterrupted after truncal vagotomy, splanchnicectomy, celiac and superior mesenteric ganglionectomy, or a combination of these procedures. MMC activity continues in isolated denervated segments of small bowel, in experimental Thiry-Vella loops, and in segments of jejunum used for esophageal replacement in humans.[12]

The central nervous does not initiate MMC activity but does modulate this activity. The central nervous system can trigger a premature MMC and delay or inhibit MMC activity.[10]

The initiation of MMC activity closely correlates with peak blood levels of the gastrointestinal peptide hormone motilin. Motilin when given exogenously can trigger a premature MMC. Immunohistochemical studies show endogenous motilin in the small intestine of the enterochromaffin cells in the duodenum and proximal jejunum. These findings suggested that MMC activity was initiated by motilin. Recent studies indicate that motilin release is associated with, but does not cause, MMC activity. Motilin antiserum in animals inhibits the action of motilin without altering MMC activity. MMC activity initiated by cholinergic or opiate agents subsequently increases motilin levels as a secondary event. Other hormones, pancreatic polypeptide and somatostatin, also cycle in conjunction with the MMC. Both peptides can initiate MMC activity. At present, MMC activity can be initiated by a variety of agents, including morphine, somatostatin, substance P, pancreatic polypeptide, histamine, metoclopramide, and erythromycin. MMC activity is interrupted by

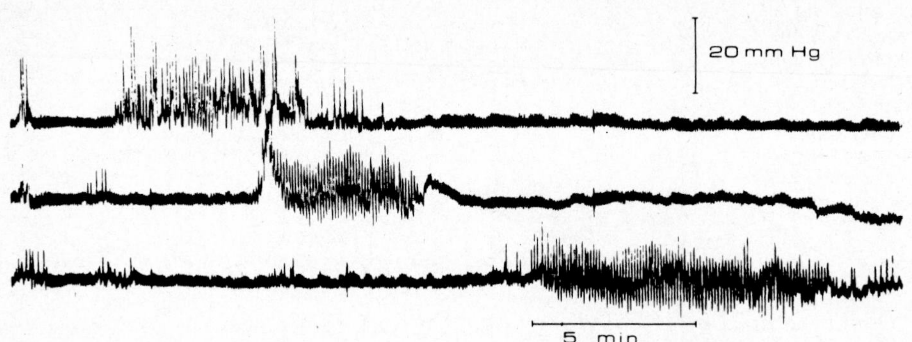

Figure 58–3. The activity front of the interdigestive motor complex is characterized on manometric tracings by a burst of rhythmic contraction waves that progress down the intestine. (From VanTrappen, G., Janssen, S. J., Hellmans, J., and Ghoos, Y. Reproduced from The Journal of Clinical Investigation, 1977, *59*:1158, by copyright permission of the American Society for Clinical Investigation.)

feeding but also by gastrin, cholecystokinin, or insulin (see pp. 78–107).

The MMC cycling phenomenon is now believed to be regulated by the intrinsic neural plexuses in the small bowel.[10, 11] The cycling phenomenon is attributable to spontaneous oscillators residing in the enteric nervous system. Transection and reanastomosis of the small bowel disrupts the coupling of these oscillators. Experimental disruption of the enteric nerves by close arterial injections of atropine, hexamethonium, and tetrodotoxin blocks the migration of the MMC.

The results of these studies indicate that cycling MMC activity is initiated by the intrinsic nerves of the small intestine but can be modulated by extrinsic nerves, hormonal factors, and drugs.

In humans, a mixed meal disrupts the interdigestive pattern for several hours, initiating the fed pattern of intestinal motility. However, the fed pattern is not easy to characterize because no distinct phases are present. The fed pattern is best characterized by the absence of the interdigestive pattern and by the presence of random bursts of spike and motor activity. Disruption of the interdigestive pattern by eating depends on the quantity and type of food ingested. The duration of interruptions is linearly related to the caloric content of a meal and the composition of the meal once a threshold for disruption is reached. Triglycerides are much more effective than an equicaloric amount of carbohydrate or protein in disrupting the migrating complex. The type of food is perhaps even more important in determining the duration of the disruption of the interdigestive MMC.[9]

Direct mucosal contact of food is not essential.[2] Distal small intestinal MMC activity is interrupted before ingested food reaches that site. MMC activity can be disrupted by the sight and smell of food. Total parenteral nutrition does not disrupt MMC cycling, which indicates that nutrients in the blood do not activate the mechanism that alters MMC activity. Disruption of MMC activity by a meal is not affected by vagotomy, splanchnicectomy, or celiac and superior mesenteric ganglionectomy. The MMC activity is disrupted by general anesthesia as well as laparotomy.[10, 11]

The start of phase 3 activity in the duodenum is coordinated with cyclic motor activity in the stomach, gallbladder, sphincter of Oddi, and the lower esophageal sphincter. The appearance of phase 3 activity in the upper small bowel is associated with gastric, pancreatic, and biliary tract secretions. Secretions begin to increase 10 to 30 minutes before the start of phase 3 activity and peak during the occurrence of phase 3 activity in the proximal duodenum. The coordination of the motor and secretory events may be due to the hormones motilin and pancreatic polypeptide or to intrinsic neural reflexes.

The caudad-moving band of intense contractions during phase 3 is believed to be the "housekeeper" in the fasted state.[7] The contractions clean the small intestine of residual food, secretions, and desquamated cells moving this material into the colon. It has been shown that no residual material remains in the small bowel after phase 3 activity. Disorders in cyclic patterns of the small intestine emphasize the importance of this physiologic function.[13, 14, 16]

Disorders of Small Intestinal Motility

Abnormalities in motility may lead to either diminished or increased movement of contents through the small intestine (Table 58–1).[13, 14] The clinical presentation in patients with disordered small bowel motility has been difficult to understand because of additional abnormalities in intestinal function in this group. If small intestinal motility is reduced, bacterial overgrowth of the bowel leads to malabsorption. In diarrheal disorders, altered patterns of small bowel motility may occur concomitantly with increased secretion or decreased absorption.

Small Intestinal Stasis Syndromes

In progressive systemic sclerosis and chronic idiopathic intestinal pseudo-obstruction, the small intestine becomes stagnant, thereby allowing bacterial overgrowth to occur.[15] In these disorders, it has been shown that small intestinal slow wave activity is normal, but the bowel fails to generate spike potentials and contractions in response to intestinal distention. This finding suggests an abnormality in the cholinergic reflex pathways. Late in the course of systemic sclerosis, the bowel also loses its responsiveness to direct-acting cholinergic drugs, indicating a stage of muscle atrophy and fibrosis. The poorly responsive small intestine becomes overgrown with bacteria, leading to malabsorption on this basis (see pp. 1289–1297).

In patients with various small intestine bacterial overgrowth syndromes, an abnormality in the migrating motility complex also has been reported.[13, 16] Fewer complexes of this "housekeeper" mechanism occur, further enhancing the potential for the overgrowth of bacteria. In patients with an absence or reduction in the MMC, bowel sterilization with antibiotics does not restore normal function. This observation indicates that loss of MMC activity is a primary disorder, not simply a response to small bowel overgrowth with bacteria.

In patients with stagnant small bowel, distention and constipation may be prominent early in the disease process. As bacterial overgrowth occurs, steatorrhea and diarrhea ensue.

Thyroid Disease

The thyroid hormones affect small intestinal slow wave frequency. In thyrotoxicosis, slow wave frequency is increased, whereas in myxedema the frequency is diminished.[17] Thyrotoxicosis may be associated with diarrhea; myxedema may be associated with constipation. The contribution of these altered states of small bowel slow wave frequency in these syndromes is not clear. (See also pp. 488–490.)

Table 58–1. ABNORMALITIES IN SMALL BOWEL MOTILITY

Bowel Disorder	Description	Disease or Etiologic Factor	Symptom
Abnormalities of Slow Wave Rhythm			
a. Tachyrhythmia	Increased slow wave frequency	Hyperthyroidism	Diarrhea
b. Bradyrhythmia	Decreased slow wave frequency	Myxedema	Constipation
c. Paroxysmal tachyrhythmia (Q complex)	Burst of regular high amplitude contractions (15–18 cpm)	Prostaglandin E_2, other diseases	Diarrhea
d. Ectopic pacemaker	Inversion of frequency gradient	Chronic idiopathic pseudo-obstruction	Pseudo-obstruction
e. Intermittent slow wave activity	Periods of absent slow waves	Familial idiopathic pseudo-obstruction	Pseudo-obstruction
Abnormalities of Interdigestive Patterns (Phase 3 Abnormalities)			
a. Absence of phase 3	Permanent or temporary absence of phase 3	Jejunal bacterial overgrowth	Malabsorption
b. Increased migration velocity in phase 3	Increased cycling frequency	Ricinoleic acids; carcinoid tumors with increased 5-hydroxytryptamine; thyrotoxicosis	Diarrhea
c. Decreased migration velocity in phase 3	Decreased cycling frequency	Intrinsic denervation in Chagas' disease, diabetes mellitus	Diarrhea or pseudo-obstruction
d. Retrograde propagation in phase 3	Slow retrograde propagation	Myotonic dystrophy	Intestinal stasis
e. Stationary phase 3	Failure of phase 3 to migrate aborad	Cisapride, cholecystokinin, idiopathic	Diarrhea, vomiting
f. Hypertonic phase 3	Exaggerated tonic component	Idiopathic	Nausea, vomiting, pain
g. Interrupted phase 3	Interrupted propagation	Myotonic dystrophy	Distention, pain
Disorders of Interdigestive Patterns (Phase 2 Abnormalities)			
a. Migrating action potential complexes	Prolonged propagated contractions	Ricinoleic acid, prostaglandins, secretory diarrhea, bacterial toxins	Diarrhea
b. Abnormal burst activity	Rhythmic burst of action potentials	Bacterial toxins	Diarrhea
c. Increased ultrarapid contractions	Ultrarapid contractions propagated over long distances	Secretory diarrhea	Diarrhea
d. Increase duration of phase 2	Prolonged phase 2	Duodenal ulcer	Peptic ulcer
e. Hypomotility pattern	Flat baseline with low amplitude contractions	Idiopathic	Nausea, vomiting
f. Hypermotility pattern	Constant phasic contractions	Idiopathic	Dyspepsia
Abnormalities of Digestive Patterns			
a. Fasting pattern	Persistent fasting pattern after meals	Diabetes mellitus, mechanical obstruction, pseudo-obstruction	Distention, stasis, dyspepsia
b. Prolonged fed pattern	Long duration of fed pattern	Duodenal ulcer	Pain
Emesis Pattern	Oral migration of contractions	Emesis of many causes	Vomiting, retching
Abnormal Intestinal Reflex Patterns	Diminished cholinergic response to distention	Diabetes mellitus, scleroderma, pseudo-obstruction	Constipation, distention, stasis syndromes

Diarrheal Disorders

In animal models, marked abnormalities in small bowel motility have been described in animals infected with diarrhea-producing bacteria or their toxins.[18] The abnormal pattern of intestinal motility has been seen with *Vibrio cholerae, Salmonella, Shigella, Escherichia coli,* and *Trichinella spiralis.* The disordered motility is not caused by mucosal destruction or by intestinal secretion per se. The motility disorder consists of powerful aborad bursts of action potentials and contractions. Similar abnormalities have not been documented in human beings. However, the presence of abnormal motility patterns in these known diarrheal diseases suggests that motility may be an important factor in the pathogenesis of the infectious diarrheas. Diarrhea is discussed more completely on pages 290–316.

Pregnancy

During pregnancy, progression of intestinal contents through the small bowel is delayed, as measured by intestinal transit studies using breath analysis. This effect may be mediated through an overall depressive effect of progesterone on smooth muscle contraction and slow wave coupling. (See also page 500.)

Ileocecal Sphincter

The ileocecal sphincter is a prominent human anatomic region. However, its physiologic role is not entirely clear. It has been shown that bacterial colony counts in the ileum immediately adjacent to the ileocecal sphincter are markedly reduced in comparison with those in the cecum. In humans, surgical resection of the ileocecal sphincter leads to increased stool volume and frequency.

Limited studies in humans indicate that the ileocecal sphincter has true sphincteric properties. It is a zone of tonically elevated pressure that relaxes with ileal distention and contracts with colonic distention. Studies in animals also demonstrate a high pressure zone with similar responses to distention.[19] The sphincter maintains an independent slow wave rhythm similar to that of the ileum. It shows spontaneous spike burst activity with phasic contractions as well as its tonic pressure elevation. The ileocecal sphincter in the cat contracts in response to vagal or splanchnic nerve stimulation. The vagal response is mediated through cholinergic nerves. The splanchnic response is mediated through an excitatory alpha-adrenergic receptor.

Ileal contractile activity and especially the intense migratory contractions seen with cholera toxin or other toxigenic bacteria migrate through the ileocecal sphincter into the colon. During these periods, baseline tonic ileocecal sphincter pressure is reduced. In contrast to the patterns seen with diarrhea-producing bacteria, the ileocecal sphincter shows an opposite response to the antidiarrheal effects of the opiates. Opiates cause an increase in baseline sphincter pressure and retrograde contractions progressing from the sphincter into the ileum. These studies in animals suggest that the ileocecal sphincter may play an important integrative role in coordinating propulsion of ileal contents into the colon and also may be important as an antidiarrheal mechanism.

COLONIC MOTILITY

The rate of movement of luminal contents through the colon provides the control for the absorption and secretion of water and electrolytes and the excretion of dietary waste products. The movement of colonic contents depends upon the slow waves and spike potentials generated by the smooth muscle cell membranes.

Myoelectric Properties of the Colon

Slow waves are generated in the cells within the innermost layer of circular muscle bordering on the submucosa in the dog.[20] In the cat, the frequency of the slow waves (5 cycles/minute) is similar throughout the entire length of the colon. A slow wave pacemaker in the transverse colon maintains regular and coordinated slow wave activity throughout the colon.[21] The slow waves in the proximal colon in the cat propagate most often from the transverse colon toward the cecum[22] (Fig. 58–4).

Two types of spike potentials occur.[22, 23] One consists of spike potentials superimposed on the slow waves, as seen in other parts of the gastrointestinal tract. Slow wave–associated spike activity appears to come from the circular muscle in most species studied. The second type consists of oscillatory potentials that appear to initiate a migrating spike burst within the transverse colon that migrates distally.[23] The oscillatory potential and the migrating spike burst originate in the longitudinal muscle of most species and are associated with a powerful contraction of the circular smooth muscle that is unrelated to the slow wave activity.[24] The migrating spike burst may move the colonic luminal contents from the transverse colon to the sigmoid colon.

In humans, a slow wave frequency plateau exists from the ascending to the descending colon at 11 cycles per minute.[25] The frequency of slow waves in the ascending colon appears more variable than in the transverse, descending, or sigmoid colon.[26] The frequency of the slow waves decreases to 6 cycles/minute in the sigmoid and rectosigmoid to the colon.[25, 27] A slower frequency of 3 cycles/minute occurs intermittently. *In vitro* studies do not demonstrate a frequency gradient for slow wave activity in the human colon.[28] However, the frequency of contractions (6 cycles/minute) in the ascending and proximal transverse colon is increased compared to the remainder of the colon (3 cycles/minute).[28] The propagation of slow waves in humans has not been studied extensively. In

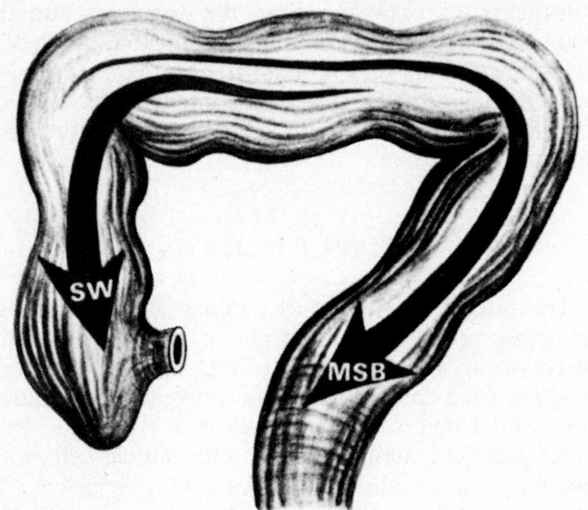

Figure 58–4. A proposed scheme relating flow in the colon to the electrical slow waves (SW) and the migrating spike bursts (MSB). Electrical slow waves are oriented in such a way that they appear to spread toward the cecum, away from the pacemaker, whose position is highly variable about midway along the colon. Since slow waves appear to pace rhythmic contractions, such contractions should tend to produce flow with a polarity in the same direction (*arrow*, SW). This polarity of slow-wave spread is probably not fixed. The migrating spike bursts begin at a variable position in the middle or proximal colon and migrate toward the rectum. Since contractions accompany migrating spike bursts, such contractions should tend to produce flow with a polarity in the same direction (*arrow*, MSB). The migrating spike burst also has the capacity for reversal of direction. (From Christensen, J., Anuras, S., and Hauser, R. L. Migrating spike bursts and electrical slow waves in the cat colon: effect of sectioning. Gastroenterology *66*:240–247. Copyright 1974 by The Williams & Wilkins Co., Baltimore.)

the ascending colon, slow waves are not phase locked in either the longitudinal or the circumferential direction, possibly because of poor intercellular electrical coupling.[21, 26]

In the human colon, spike potentials may be superimposed on the slow waves or may exist as bursts unrelated to slow wave activity.[27–32] An increase in spike activity correlates with an increase in colonic intraluminal pressure.[27, 30] Spike bursts greater than 10 seconds in duration increase after eating, and may increase transit of luminal contents through the colon in the dog.[32, 33] The long-duration spike bursts are also decreased in patients with diarrhea.[30]

In vitro myoelectric recordings from human colonic tissue suggest that spontaneous colonic myoelectric activity differs between the circular and longitudinal layers.[34, 35] The frequency range of spontaneous activity recorded *in vitro* (2 to 60 cycles/minute)[28, 34–37] is larger than *in vivo* (2.5 to 12 cycles/minute).[26, 37] Spike activity increases when the muscle is stretched[35] so that distention of the colon by intraluminal contents may control the motor activity of the intact organ. Myoelectric events more rapid than 12 cycles/minute are associated with tetanic contractions.[34, 35] Although the major control for the transit of luminal contents is exerted by the smooth muscle itself, the gastrointestinal peptides and the autonomic nervous system are important in modulating the control of the colon.

Colonic Motility and Transit of Luminal Contents

Contractions that originate in the transverse and ascending colon move toward the cecum more often than distally,[38, 39] which suggests that the proximal portion of the colon acts as a brake on the forward flow of luminal contents. The retrograde propagation of the slow waves in the proximal segment[22] allows longer mucosal exposure for the intraluminal contents, resulting in more complete absorption of salt and water.[40] In cats with diarrhea,[41, 42] the slow wave pattern in the ascending colon is irregular, with decreased coupling between neighboring segments within the ascending colon. Thus, the disruption of myoelectrical control of the ascending colon impairs the braking action on the flow of luminal contents and is associated with diarrhea.

The flow of luminal contents through the colon is not steadily progressive.[43] There is significant mixing of ileal effluent with dietary residue already present in the colon. Frequently markers that are given on different days are present in the same stool. The mechanism through which such mixture of luminal contents takes place is uncertain; however, modulation of the intrinsic myogenic activity by the enteric nervous system is necessary for the orderly progression of luminal contents through the colon.[44]

Nonpropulsive segmental movements in the colon move the luminal contents equally in a retrograde and antegrade direction.[45] Segmental activity of the colon prevents the rapid forward flow of colonic contents by producing a back-and-forth movement of the feces. Solid colonic contents are transported between 30 and 100 times more slowly than liquid or gas.[35, 46]

The use of radionuclides has enhanced understanding of gastrointestinal transit. In healthy subjects food reaches the colon approximately three hours after eating and the colon fills linearly with small intestinal contents.[47] The transverse colon may serve as the storage area for colonic contents, because luminal contents empty rapidly from the cecum and ascending colon and are retained for a long time in the transverse colon.[48] Long-chain fatty acids stimulate motility in the ascending colon, which increases the emptying rate of the ascending colon.[49]

Storage of luminal contents within the distal colon may affect the entry of intestinal contents into the colon, as rectal distention slows colonic filling.[50] This may explain why patients with constipation have slower small intestinal transit than patients with diarrhea.[47]

Increased colonic contractility is more likely to produce constipation than diarrhea.[51] Increased segmenting activity of the colon produces a functional partial obstruction of the colon, resulting in fewer movements and increased absorption of water from the fecal residua.[40] Decreased colonic contractility also can be associated with constipation. The increase in the incidence of gastrointestinal motility disturbances in women may be secondary to the slowing of colonic transit by estrogen or progesterone.[52]

Mass propulsion is a wave of contraction that moves intraluminal contents of the colon from the transverse colon to the sigmoid colon. Mass propulsion is seen in 6 per cent of subjects during fasting.

Physiologic Control of Colonic Motility

Extrinsic Neural Control of the Colon

The human proximal colon receives cholinergic fibers from the vagus, whereas the distal colon receives cholinergic input from the sacral pelvic nerves.[53, 54] These cholinergic nerves stimulate the colon, but the vagal nerve trunk also carries inhibitory fibers.

The proximal colon receives adrenergic innervation from the splanchnic nerve, of which the nerve bodies are in the superior mesenteric ganglion. The distal colon receives innervation from the inferior mesenteric ganglia via the lumbar colonic nerves. The sympathetic nervous system inhibits colonic motility by blocking cholinergic synaptic transmission to the myenteric plexus and by hyperpolarizing smooth muscle cells.[55] The beta-adrenergic system may contribute to the inhibitory control of colonic motility in humans, as beta-adrenoceptor blockers increase resting tone in the rectosigmoid region.[56] The beta-adrenergic effect on the colon may be mediated either through a direct effect on the smooth muscle (beta$_2$-receptor) or through the myenteric neurons (beta$_1$-receptor).[57]

The sympathetic inhibition of colonic motility is controlled by the prevertebral ganglia.[58, 59] Distention of the proximal portion of the colon inhibits contraction in the more distal segment of the colon through intermesenteric neurons passing between the prevertebral ganglia and paravertebral ganglia (celiac plexus, superior mesenteric ganglion, or inferior mesenteric ganglion)[60] (Fig. 58–5). Inhibition is then mediated through either the splanchnic nerves or the lumbar colonic nerves.[61] Impulses from the peripheral mechanoreceptors in the wall of the colon rarely are strong enough to depolarize ganglionic cells in the inferior mesenteric ganglia.[58] Neural impulses from the central nervous system (possibly originating from the pons)[62] and the upper gastrointestinal tract reach the colon through the spinal cord.[63, 64] Input from the central nervous system via the paravertebral ganglia or from other peripheral locations within the gastrointestinal tract augments the activity from the colonic mechanoreceptors and stimulates efferent sympathetic discharge, inhibiting colonic activity.[58] Thus, the prevertebral ganglia act as modulators of neural activity, not just as relay stations.

Patients with lumbar spinal cord lesions have increased colonic motility.[65] These data suggest that the spinal cord provides chronic neural inhibition to the colon. The supraspinal centers also appear to have a stimulatory influence on the colon, as patients with a high cord transection and an intact cord below the lesion have reduced colonic motility.

Intrinsic Neural Control of the Colon

Chronic neural inhibitory activity of the colonic smooth muscle is mediated by the myenteric plexus.[66] Anatomic differences in the myenteric plexus from different species and different locations within the colon are probably responsible for the different patterns of motility observed.[67, 68] Characterization of the neurotransmitter that is responsible for mediating the orderly contraction and relaxation of the colon is incomplete. However, substance P, vasaoactive intestinal polypeptide, met-enkephalin, and somatostatin may be important mediators of motility by (1) directly affecting the smooth muscle, (2) affecting the myenteric neural release of one of the classic neurotrans-

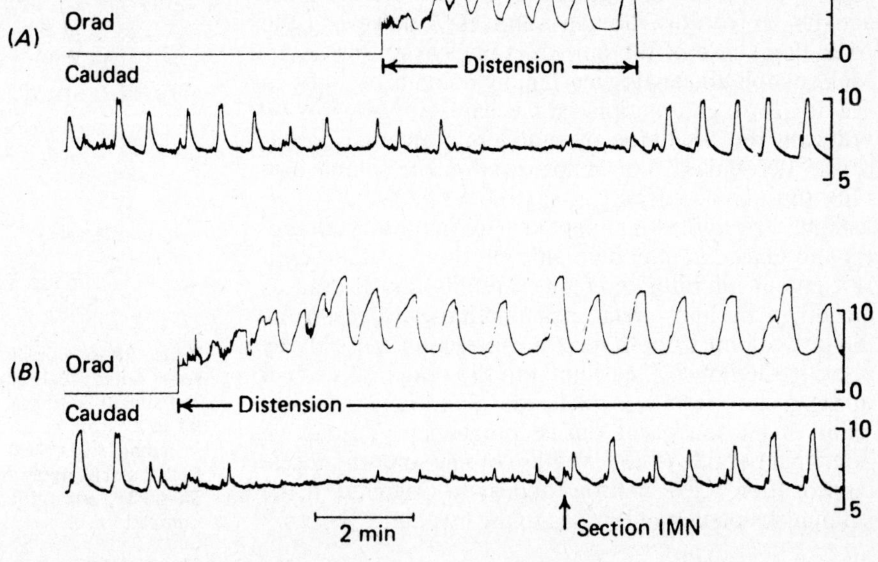

Figure 58–5. Effect of distention of orad segment of colon on contractions in caudad segment and the effect of sectioning intermesenteric nerve (IMN). The intraluminal pressure was zero before and after distention. The trace in *B* begins two minutes after the end of panel *A*. (From Kruelen, D. L., and Szurszewski, J. H. J. Physiol. *295*:21, 1979.)

mitters, or (3) serving as an interneuron[69] (see pp. 21–52).

Gastrointestinal Peptide Hormones

The gastrointestinal peptides (see also pp. 78–107) control colonic motility by acting either as hormonal agents released into the systemic circulation or as local neurotransmitters. Immunohistologic studies have shown that many of the peptides are present within the myenteric plexus of the colon.[70] Gastrin and cholecystokinin (CCK-OP) stimulate a dose-dependent increase in colonic spike activity.[71] In *in vitro* studies, CCK-OP interferes with the intrinsic rhythm of colonic muscle and stimulates an increase in spike activity that is dependent on the presence of extracellular calcium.[72] The serum level of exogenously administered gastrin that stimulates colonic motility is similar to postprandial levels. However, the increase in postprandial colonic motility occurs prior to the time when serum gastrin levels reach their peak level after a meal.[71] Thus, the physiologic role of gastrin in the control of colonic motility is unknown. The postprandial rise in CCK occurs within 45 minutes of eating,[73] which suggests that it may be involved the regulation of postprandial colonic motility.

Neurotensin is present within the mucosa and myenteric plexus of the colon.[74] Ingestion of fat increases plasma neurotensin levels and stimulates an increase in colonic motility, which is greater in the ascending colon.[75–77]

Substance P stimulates contraction of the circular smooth muscle of the colon, possibly by depolarizing the smooth muscle cell membrane by decreasing the outward potassium conductance.[78, 79] Neurons containing substance P arise within the myenteric plexus and send axons into the longitudinal and circular smooth muscle. In patients with constipation associated with a decrease in colonic enteric ganglion cells, substance P levels are decreased.[80]

Enkephalin is present within the wall of the colon and may also be a neurotransmitter controlling colonic motility.[70] Morphine stimulates an increase in spike activity in healthy human subjects;[81] however, the physiologic role of the opioids is unclear at this point. Met-enkephalin analogues inhibit colonic motility in the dog through a peripheral mechanism,[82] possibly by reducing the discharge of cholinergic myenteric neurons.[83] Leu-enkephalin analogues stimulate colonic motility through a centrally mediated mechanism.[81]

Some gastrointestinal peptides are inhibitory. Secretin and glucagon inhibit colonic motility.[84, 85] Glucagon is a potent inhibitor of colonic motility and is used as an aid in barium enema examinations. Progesterone inhibits colonic smooth muscle contraction, possibly by altering the influx of calcium into the cell.[86] This effect of progesterone may explain the alterations in bowel habit that often occur during pregnancy. Vasoactive intestinal peptide (VIP) inhibits colonic smooth muscle contractility.[87] VIP neurons appear to originate in the submucous plexus and spread to the myenteric plexus.[87] These findings suggest that VIP is an interneuron that is part of the inhibitory limb of autoregulation. Interaction between the various gastrointestinal peptides probably has a significant role in the physiologic control of colonic motility.

Effect of Eating on Colonic Motility

After eating, there is a rapid increase in colonic spike and contractile activity[88] (Fig. 58–6). The spike activity is superimposed on the slow wave. This increase in spike activity is associated with a concomitant increase in phasic intraluminal pressure, characteristic of segmenting contractions. A postprandial increase in propagating spike bursts was associated with an increase in colonic propulsive activity.[89, 90] The magnitude of the colonic response to eating increases as the total number of calories increases and the fat content of the meal increases.[88] The volume or pH of the meal does not affect colonic motility. Fat ingestion stimulates a rapid increase in colonic motility within 10 minutes. A later response also occurs 70 to 90 minutes after eating. Both intravenous and intraluminal amino acids inhibit the early and late increases in spike activity following a 1000-calorie mixed meal or fat.[91] The response to fat suggests that amino acids inhibit the late colonic response following the 1000-calorie mixed meal. The gastrocolonic response is initiated by a sensory receptor in the gastroduodenal mucosa, as intragastric procaine inhibits the gastrocolonic response.[81] Intragastric but not intravenous administration of fat stimulates colonic motility.[91] There is no cephalic phase of the gastrocolonic response because sham feeding does not stimulate

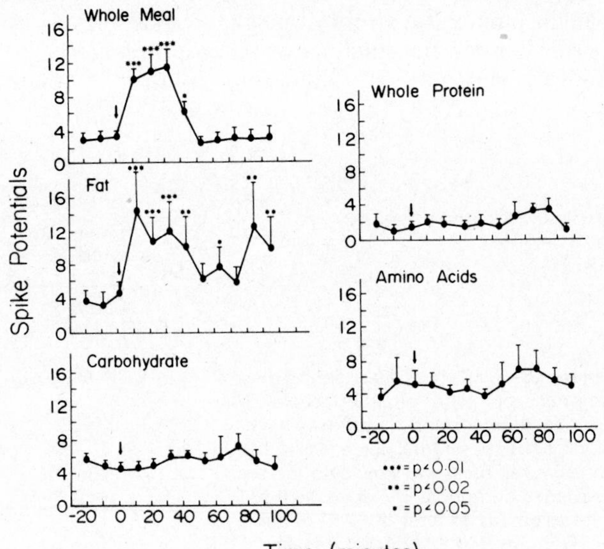

Figure 58–6. Colonic spike response following eating. Number of spike potentials is shown for ten-minute periods before and after ingesting a 1000 kcal whole meal or individual dietary components, fat (600 kcal), carbohydrate (320 kcal), whole protein (200 kcal), or amino acids (200 kcal). Arrow (↑) signifies ingestion of meal. Each point is mean ± SE for 7 normal subjects. (From Wright, S., Snape, W., and Cohen, S. Am J. Physiol. *238*:G228, 1980. Used by permission.)

an increase in colonic motility. The increase in postprandial colonic spike activity appears to be mediated by both the opioid and the cholinergic nervous system, as anticholinergics and naloxone inhibit the response to the 1000-calorie meal and also the early response to fat.[81] The response is mediated through the M_2 receptor as pirenzepine did not block the gastrocolonic response.[92] The neural reflex for the gastrocolonic response passes through the spinal cord because transection abolishes the gastrocolonic response.[64]

Dietary Fiber

Dietary fiber consists of nonabsorbable carbohydrate (lignan, cellulose, and hemicellulose) from plant material. Dietary fiber increases the speed of transit through the gastrointestinal tract. The major increase in transit occurs in the colon. Wheat bran appears to have the greatest effect on transit. Cabbage, apples, and carrots increase fecal weight and transit, but not to the same degree as wheat bran.[93]

Colonic intraluminal pressure decreases after eating wheat bran or methylcellulose.[94] The physical characteristics of the bran are important for its effects on gastrointestinal motility. A decrease in colonic motility occurred after ingesting coarse bran, whereas ingestion of fine bran increased intracolonic pressure.[95]

Bile Salts

Bile salts generally are completely reabsorbed within the ileum. When bile salt absorption is disturbed by ileal disease or administration of excessive amounts of dihydroxy bile salts, diarrhea is produced. Bile salts stimulate colonic motility in rabbits and in humans.[96, 97]

Table 58–2. ABNORMALITIES IN COLONIC MOTILITY

Disease	Mechanism	Symptom
Irritable colon syndrome	Decreased slow wave frequency	Abdominal pain
	Increased segmenting contractions	Altered bowel habit
	Delayed gastrocolonic response	
Diverticular disease	Increased slow wave frequency	Abdominal pain
	Segmental increase in colonic intraluminal pressure	Altered bowel habit
Diabetes mellitus	Absent gastrocolonic response	Constipation
Progressive systemic sclerosis	Absent gastrocolonic response	Constipation
	Early—normal response to neostigmine	
	Late—no response to neostigmine	
Idiopathic pseudo-obstruction	Absent gastrocolonic response	Diarrhea or constipation
Ulcerative colitis	Absent postprandial, increased colonic intraluminal pressure	Toxic megacolon Diarrhea

In the rabbit, deoxycholic acid stimulates a migrating propulsive wave in the colon. This increase in migrating complexes is inhibited by the intravenous administration of atropine or an alpha-adrenergic antagonist.[97] Secretion induced by deoxycholic acid is inhibited by the beta-adrenergic antagonists, suggesting different mechanisms for each effect of the bile acids[98] (see pp. 144–161 and 310).

Deoxycholic acid may increase colonic contractility in patients with the irritable bowel syndrome, reproducing their symptoms.[99]

Emotional Stress

Emotional stress caused by physical or mental discomfort alters colonic motility (Fig. 58–7).[100] Healthy subjects and patients with the irritable colon syndrome have increased spike activity and intraluminal pressure in the distal sigmoid colon during physical discomfort or emotional stress.[101] The increase in the colonic motility is associated with an increase in heart and respiratory rate. The connection of the central nervous system with the colon through the autonomic nervous system suggests a pathway through which emotional stress may alter colonic motility. Stimulation of the hypothalamus or cerebral hemispheres increases or inhibits colonic motility, depending on the area stimulated.[49]

Abnormalities of Motility

Irritable Bowel Syndrome

Previous studies[41, 42] showed that an abnormality in the slow wave rhythm is capable of altering the bowel habit (Table 58–2). Although irritable bowel patients have abdominal pain, an alteration in their bowel habit, and abnormal colonic myoelectric activity, they have no anatomic abnormality.[102]

Healthy subjects have predominantly 6 cycles/minute slow wave activity, with only 10 per cent of the total slow wave activity occurring at other frequencies. In patients with the irritable bowel syndrome, 40 per cent of the slow wave activity occurs at a frequency of 3 cycles/minute. A similar increase in slow waves with the slower rhythm occurs in patients with chronic constipation in the absence of abdominal pain.[103] As the slow wave determines the frequency of contractions, these patients also have an increase in the 3 cycles/minute contractions. A delayed increase in spike activity occurs 70 to 100 minutes after a meal.[30, 104] Associated with this delayed spike response is a delayed contractile response that consists of phasic 3 cycle/minute contractions. The patients with predominantly constipation have an increase in spike bursts lasting shorter than 3.5 seconds.[30] These short bursts were not associated with increase in the transport of luminal contents.[90] These types of motor events in the distal portion of the colon may inhibit the forward flow of the fecal stream, alter the patient's bowel habits, and produce abdominal pain[105] (see pp. 1402–1418).

Diverticular Disease of the Colon

Diverticular disease of the colon is associated with or caused by abnormalities of colonic motility. Colonic intraluminal pressure is elevated in diverticulosis.[106] This increased intraluminal pressure may force the mucosa through the weaknesses in the colonic wall at the sites of perforating vessels. Patients with the irritable colon syndrome may have a higher incidence of diverticular disease of the colon.[106] Slow wave frequency in diverticular disease may be similar to that of healthy individuals or increased.[37, 107] The postprandial increase in colonic spike activity occurs within the first 30 minutes after eating, similar to that in healthy subjects.[37] It appears that the myoelectric pattern of diverticular disease and the irritable bowel syndrome are dissimilar (see pp. 1402–1434).

Diabetes Mellitus

Constipation is common in patients with diabetes mellitus. Abnormalities in colonic motility may cause constipation,[108] whereas the less frequently occurring diarrheal syndrome probably may be secondary to an abnormality in small intestinal motility.

The response to eating is disturbed in diabetic patients with severe constipation, but not in those with normal bowel function. Patients with severe constipation have no increase in colonic spike activity after eating a 1000-calorie meal. A defect in neural control of the colonic smooth muscle appears to be present, since colonic spike activity and colonic contractions can be stimulated by parenteral administration of either neostigmine or metoclopramide[108] (see p. 1099).

Progressive Systemic Sclerosis

The movement of colonic contents is abnormal in patients with progressive systemic sclerosis. These patients develop wide-mouth colonic diverticula and may have severe fecal impactions.[109] Abnormalities in colonic motility are present in 90 per cent of patients with progressive systemic sclerosis.[110] The severity of the colonic motor disturbance is related to the length and severity of the illness. The patients show no increase in spike activity or contractile activity after eating. Patients with mild progressive systemic sclerosis respond with increased spike activity and contractions after parenteral administration of neostigmine or metoclopramide. Patients with advanced progressive systemic sclerosis generally have constipation and do not respond to exogenous drug stimulation. These studies suggest that, early in the illness, the predominant pathophysiologic abnormality involves neural transmission to the colon, similar to results of previous studies on other parts of the gastrointestinal tract. However, later in the disease, atrophy of the smooth muscle leads to a generalized lack of response (see pp. 505–506).

Intestinal Pseudo-obstruction

Idiopathic intestinal pseudo-obstruction may be caused by involvement of either the smooth muscle or the intramural nerves.[111] When the pseudo-obstruction occurs predominantly in the colon, the condition is called *Ogilvie's syndrome.* Classically, Ogilvie's syndrome consists of colonic distention secondary to malignant invasion into the prevertebral ganglia controlling colonic function.[112] However, this cause of colonic pseudo-obstruction is rare (see pp. 377–379).

Careful histologic examination may be necessary to diagnose the presence of a lesion in the myenteric plexus.[111] Physiologic studies have been performed on patients with predominantly neural involvement.[113] These patients have normal slow wave activity but have no increase in spike activity or in contractile activity of the colon after eating. They do have increased colonic spike activity and contractile activity after administration of either neostigmine or metoclo-

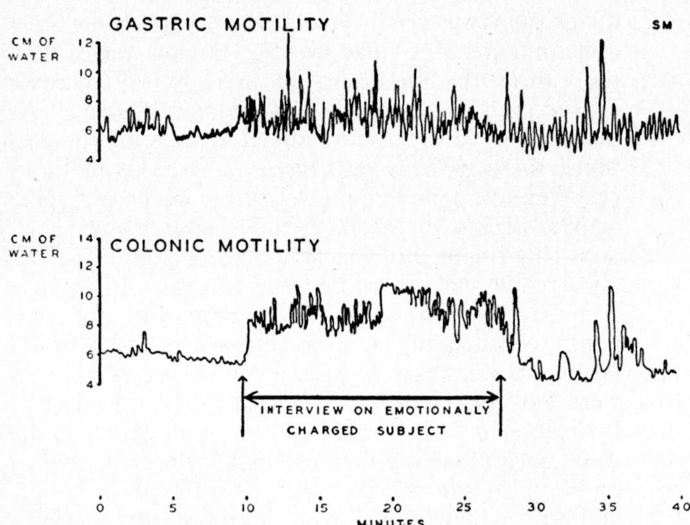

Figure 58–7. Alteration in colonic motility during discussion of a stress-producing life situation. The gastric motility tracing provides a control on the effects of respiratory changes and altered intra-abdominal pressure. (From Almy, T. P., et al. Alterations in colonic function in man under stress. Gastroenterology *12*:425–436. Copyright 1949 by The Williams & Wilkins Co., Baltimore.)

pramide. A similar decrease in the postprandial gastrocolonic response occurs in patients with multiple sclerosis.[114] An abnormality in the smooth muscle also may cause colonic pseudo-obstruction. Muscular dystrophy may involve visceral smooth muscle, resulting in colonic pseudo-obstruction.[115] The motility pattern of patients with myogenic pseudo-obstruction is well described at present.

Ulcerative Colitis

Decreased colonic contractility may be present in patients with ulcerative colitis. The decrease in contractility may contribute to the diarrhea. Myoelectric studies showed that the slow wave frequency is normal but the gastrocolonic response is abnormal. Patients with ulcerative colitis have an increase in spike activity after eating a 1000-kcal meal, but there is no concomitant increase in contractility.[116] In an experimental model of mucosal inflammation, the underlying smooth muscle also is abnormal. The muscle membrane potential is more positive than in healthy muscle and the contactile response to stimulation is decreased.[117] The electromechanical coupling of the smooth muscle appears to be abnormal in inflammatory bowel disease (see pp. 1435–1477).

Pharmacologic Effects on Colonic Motility

In recent years several drugs have been shown to have efficacy in the treatment of colonic diseases (see Table 58–3).

Table 58–3. EFFECTS OF DRUGS ON SMALL AND LARGE INTESTINAL CONTRACTILITY

Drug	Effect on Small Intestine	Effect on Colon	Mechanism of Action
Acetylcholine and analogues	Excitatory	Excitatory	Agonist muscarinic receptors on muscle cells
Neostigmine	Excitatory	Excitatory	Acetylcholine esterase inhibitor
Metoclopramide	Excitatory	Excitatory	Dopamine antagonist central, peripheral
Domperidone	Excitatory	No effect	Dopamine antagonist, peripheral
Cisapride	Excitatory	Excitatory	Unknown
Atropine	Inhibitory	Inhibitory	Antagonist muscarinic receptor
Secoverine	Inhibitory	Inhibitory	Antagonist M_2 muscarinic receptor on muscle cells
Papaverine	?	Inhibitory	Unknown
Calcium channel blockers			Blockade of voltage-operated calcium channels
Nifedipine	Inhibitory	Inhibitory	
Verapamil	Inhibitory	Inhibitory	
Nitro compounds	Inhibitory	Inhibitory	a. Blockade of receptor-operated calcium channel b. Increase of intracellular cGMP
Peppermint oil	Inhibitory	Inhibitory	Unknown

cGMP, cyclic guanosine monophosphate.

Excitatory Effects

Parasympathomimetic Agents. Acetylcholine analogues, such as bethanechol, stimulate colonic contractility through direct binding to the muscarinic receptor. Acetylcholine esterase inhibitors, such as neostigmine, stimulate colonic contractility by increasing the amounts of endogenous acetylcholine present at the myoneural junction through inhibiting the enzymatic degradation of acetylcholine. These agents are potent stimulants of colonic spike and contractile activity.[27] Parasympathomimetic stimuli or agents may be useful in treating patients with colonic inertia caused by an abnormal excitatory neural input, such as patients with diabetes mellitus, scleroderma, and pseudo-obstruction. The use of acetylcholine esterase inhibitors theoretically may be preferable to direct parasympathetic stimulation, as the distribution of acetylcholine could be predetermined by the autonomic nervous system.

Dopamine Antagonists. Metoclopramide, a centrally and peripherally acting dopamine antagonist, stimulates colonic motility in intact human subjects.[108] Increases in spike and contractile activity occur in patients with diabetes mellitus, scleroderma, and pseudo-obstruction.[108, 110, 113] Metoclopramide has not helped alleviate symptoms in patients with scleroderma or pseudo-obstruction, but patients with diabetes mellitus have noticed an increase in the frequency of bowel movements. Domperidone, a peripherally acting dopamine antagonist, does not stimulate colonic motility.[118] Therefore, this drug may have no effect in patients with colonic inertia.

Cisapride

Cisapride is a non–dopamine-blocking prokinetic agent that is presently undergoing evaluation of clinical efficacy. Cisapride stimulates contractions of colonic muscle, which are not inhibited by atropine and only marginally inhibited by tetrodotoxin.[119] The prokinetic effect of cisapride does not seem to involve the release of acetylcholine.[120] Cisapride stimulates a dose-dependent increase in colonic spike activity in healthy human subjects.[121]

Inhibitory Effects

Anticholinergic Agents. Anticholinergic agents inhibit muscarinic receptor stimulation. They should be useful in the treatment of diseases of increased colonic contractility. However, few studies have thoroughly examined the effect of anticholinergic agents on the symptoms of patients with the irritable bowel syndrome and decreased abdominal pain in patients with this syndrome.[104]

Dietary Fiber. Ingestion of increased dietary fiber is thought to be useful in patients with diverticular disease. These patients have an increase in smooth muscle contractility that causes both their abdominal pain and also the formation of the diverticula.[122] Ingestion of dietary fiber decreases intraluminal colonic pressure and decreases the abdominal pain of these patients.[123] Dietary fiber decreases abdominal pain in patients who have the irritable bowel syndrome, although not all studies agree.[124, 125]

Papaverine. Papaverine is a potent smooth muscle relaxant. It also decreases cholinergic and cholecystokinin stimulation of colonic smooth muscle.[126] These studies suggest that papaverine may well be an important agent in the treatment of patients with increased colonic motility.

Calcium Channel Blockers. Calcium is a requirement for contraction of colonic smooth muscle.[127] Several classes of calcium channel blockers, including verapamil and the dihydropyridines, are available. Most investigation has focused on nifedipine (a dihydropyridine). The dihydropyridines decrease human gastrointestinal smooth muscle contraction by inhibiting calcium influx through voltage-dependent channels.[128]

Nitrate. Nitrate compounds are potent inhibitors of smooth muscle contraction. The nitrate compounds may inhibit smooth muscle contraction by increasing the intracellular concentration of cyclic guanosine monophosphate (cGMP).[129] The nitrate compounds also may decrease calcium influx into the smooth muscle cell.[130]

Peppermint Oil. Peppermint oil is a potent relaxant of smooth muscle, which improves symptoms in some patients with the irritable bowel syndrome.[131]

Rectal Continence and Defecation

The maintenance of continence by the internal and external anal sphincters is important and complicated. Small amounts of material in the rectum will not cause reflex relaxation of the tonically contracted internal sphincter. The anal canal also remains closed when intra-abdominal pressure is increased, except during a conscious attempt to defecate. Once the internal anal sphincter relaxes, usually in response to rectal distention, material will pass into the anal canal. The anal mucosa has receptors that warn the person of pending passage of material. Voluntary contractions of the external sphincter may prevent defecation. As rectal pressure rises, the rectum adapts to its new volume of material that has moved cephalad, and the anal stimulus for defecation is relieved[132] (see pp. 321–322).

Anorectal Sphincters

The sphincters are divided into the internal anal sphincter and the external anal sphincter. The internal anal sphincter is composed of circular smooth muscle. These muscle bundles form a wall that is three to four times thicker than the circular muscle of the colon itself. The external sphincter is made up of striated muscle located at various layers; the deeper one surrounds the internal sphincter, whereas the more superficial one lies caudad and surrounds the end of the anal canal. Both sphincters contribute to the proximal border of the anorectal ring, which is composed posterolaterally by the puborectalis sling.

The striated musculature involved in the defecation mechanism consists of an anorectal ring, which is made up principally of the levatores ani, attached to the pubis anteriorly and to the ischial spine posteriorly. Several muscle groups form slings within this ring, the most important one swinging from the posterior surface of the rectum and attaching to the pubis. Its action moves the rectum forward and upward toward the pubis, providing a strong, sphincter-like mechanism at the anorectal junction. The other muscle group inserts into the fibrous thickening of the rectal sheath and binds the anal canal to the pelvic diaphragm. On contraction, it pulls the rectum upward and forward. Other muscle groups—the ileococcygeal portion of the levators—elevate the pelvic floor and provide some support for the abdominal viscera (see pp. 317–322).

Innervation of the Anorectum

The anorectal area has rich innervation (Fig. 58–8). The anus derives its normal cutaneous sensation from the branches of the pudendal nerve (S2, S3, S4). The rectum, on the other hand, derives its sensory innervation from parasympathetic fibers passing through the same nerve trunks (S2, S3, S4) via the pelvic nerves. The fibers do not mediate ordinary painful stimuli but are extremely sensitive to pressure.

Motor innervation of the external anal sphincter is by way of the perineal and inferior hemorrhoidal branches of the pudendal nerve (S2, S3, S4) as well as from branches of the coccygeal plexus (S4, S5). The levator ani is supplied by branches of both the pudendal nerve and the fourth sacral nerve.

Autonomic motor innervation of the internal anal sphincter is important because it plays such a major role in defecation. Sympathetic supply is via the hypogastric nerves from the fifth lumbar segments, and the parasympathetic supply is via the pelvic nerves, from S1, S2, and S3. The sympathetic nerve induces contraction of the sphincters, whereas the parasympathetic nerve provides an inhibitory action. On the other hand, the external sphincter receives only somatic pudendal innervation. Its relaxation is attributable to reduction in frequency of the existing motor impulses in the pudendal nerve.

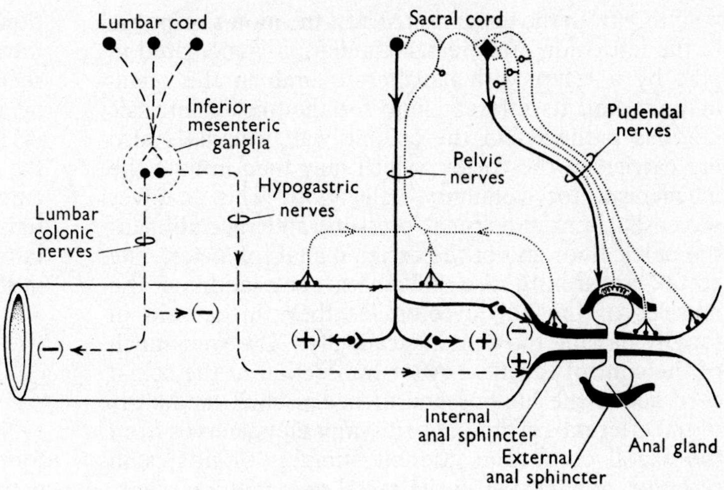

Figure 58–8. Schematic representation of the innervation of the distal colon and anal canal. The lumbar sympathetic outflow inhibits the colon and stimulates the internal anal sphincter. The sacral parasympathetic outflow in the pelvic nerves stimulates the colon and inhibits the internal anal sphincter. Afferent ingoing fibers from the tissues surrounding the anal canal and from the wall of the colon run in the pelvic nerves. The pudendal nerves innervate the external anal sphincter. Afferent fibers from the circumanal skin, from tissues surrounding the anal canal, and from the external anal sphincter run in the pudendal nerves. (From Bishop, B., et al. J. Physiol. (Lond.) *134*:229, 1956. Used by permission.)

The rectum has an efferent sympathetic supply from the hypogastric plexus (L2, L3, L4) distally and from the inferior mesenteric plexus proximally. Parasympathetic innervation is by the pelvic nerves (S2, S3, S4). The parasympathetic nerves are stimulatory for the rectum but are inhibitory for the internal anal sphincter. The sympathetic system is inhibitory for the rectum.

Motility Studies of Anorectum

A zone of elevated pressure representing the internal sphincter is found 3 to 7 cm proximal to the external anal margin. The anal canal is 2 to 5.5 cm in length and has a lower pressure anteriorly in the orad segment and posteriorly in the caudad segment.[133] Although pressure varies from person to person, the range in this segment is 25 to 85 cm H_2O. The anal sphincters are in tonus; the internal sphincter has a higher resting pressure and this pressure remains present in persons with transection of the spinal cord, indicating its autonomic control.[132] The external sphincter, although functioning at a lower baseline pressure, is also in a tonic state of contraction. Although its principal nerve supply is somatic and extrinsic, when separated from this nerve supply its muscular structure does not degenerate, as do other voluntary muscles in such a situation. The external anal sphincter responds to various changes of posture and activity. Any increase in intra-abdominal pressure is associated with an increased external anal sphincter tone. When increased intra-abdominal pressure is associated with defecation, the sphincter activity is markedly diminished. After defecation there is a rebound of increased sphincter activity, the so-called closing reflex. Micturition is also associated with inhibition of external anal sphincter activity. Dilation of the anus, especially if sudden or forceful, will elicit a marked increase in sphincter tone. The external sphincter will also close in response to stimulation of the perianal skin.

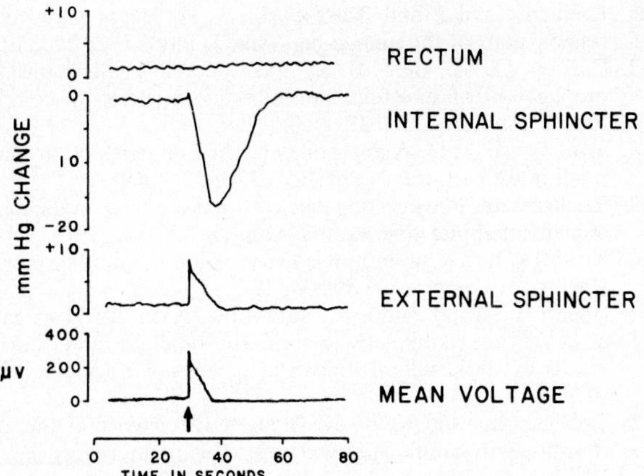

Figure 58–9. Distention of the rectum (arrow) initiates relaxation of the internal anal sphincter and contraction of the external anal sphincter. A burst of electrical activity is recorded from the external sphincter simultaneous with the increase in pressure. (From Tobon, F., Reid, N. C., Talbert, J. L., and Schuster, M. M. Reprinted by permission of The New England Journal of Medicine *278*:188, 1968.)

The anal sphincters are extremely responsive to sudden changes in intrarectal pressure. Rectal distention produces relaxation of the internal sphincter and contraction of the external sphincter[134] (Fig. 58–9). Rapid intermittent distention of the rectum produces the same effect on the internal and external sphincters, only more pronounced. Continuous and progressive distention, however, is associated with a gradual return of pressure in both sphincters to prestimulus baseline levels. Thus, the internal sphincter responds mainly to rectal distention, whereas the external sphincter responds to a number of stimuli—voluntary effort, increased intra-abdominal pressure, anal dilatation, perianal stretch, and rectal distention.

Control of Defecation

Afferent and efferent pathways between the descending colon and rectum react to local stimulus resulting from the distention. Thus, the motor response in the left colon after rectal stimulation is mediated in part by a reflex with its afferent limb in the rectal ampulla and its efferent limb terminating in intrinsic nervous pathways in the colonic wall. Impulses also are carried to the cortex, which may then initiate the mechanism for voluntary defecation. This involves increased intra-abdominal pressure and relaxation of the pelvic floor and of the external anal sphincter. The cortex apparently also influences contraction of the muscles of the pelvic colon, as they further aid in rapidly moving the contents caudally. However, much of the control is reflex. After transection of the spinal cord above the lumbosacral area, the chief mediators of the efferent arc are the parasympathetic nerves from the sacral cord. The afferent stimulus originates in receptors for tension in the rectal musculature. Thus, incontinence is controlled. However, defecation is inefficient in this situation, because contraction of the rectum and rectosigmoid is not normal, presumably because of the interruption of the pathways from the cortex that synapse with pelvic parasympathetic nerves. Appropriate stimulus of the rectum, however, such as with enemas, will usually be sufficient to result in evacuation.

ABNORMALITIES OF ANAL MOTILITY

Diabetes Mellitus

Fecal incontinence can be a major problem in some patients with diabetes mellitus, especially if they have diarrhea. The internal anal sphincter pressure is decreased in patients with incontinence associated with diabetes mellitus. The patients have impaired continence for both solids and liquids.[135] The sensation of rectal contents is decreased in incontinent diabetic patients.[136] The improvement in sensory threshold after biofeedback is associated with improvement in incontinence (see pp. 494–500).

Idiopathic (Neurogenic) Incontinence

Fecal incontinence in women with no other metabolic or anatomic cause may be secondary to pudendal nerve damage associated with childbirth or descent of the perineum with age or straining at stool. Increases in the spinal motor latency from the level of L1 to the puborectalis and the external anal sphincter in these patients suggests that the innervation to both muscles is disturbed.[137] In certain patients, perineal descent is associated with difficulty in moving bowels.[138] In these patients the anal sphincter pressure is normal; however, the rectal angle is disturbed.

Hirschsprung's Disease

Hirschsprung's disease usually presents as an acute intestinal obstruction in children or as chronic constipation in older children or young adults. The obstruction is due to a contracted distal bowel in which intramural ganglion cells are missing.[134] The disease seen in older individuals is caused by a very short aganglionic segment. The rectoanal reflex is disturbed in Hirschsprung's disease. The normal relaxation of the internal anal sphincter is absent. In the normal colon, both excitatory and inhibitory junction potentials were recorded after field stimulation. Only excitatory junction potentials occur during field stimulation in the aganglionic muscle[139] (see pp. 1390–1395).

Physiologic Aspects of Colonic Pain

The relationship between stimulus intensity (in the form of an acute distending force) and its duration with onset of visceral pain is similar to the relationship of stimulus and intensity for cutaneous pain. The duration of the threshold of pain in normal subjects when the intensity of stimulus is 100 cm H_2O averages 6.6 seconds. The relationship of rate of distention to onset of pain is uncertain; however, it is likely that a more intense stimulus (i.e., an increased rate of distention) lowers the pain threshold. On the other hand, increased intramural tension in the sigmoid associated with a decreased rate of distention might also result in an earlier onset of pain with correspondingly lowered threshold.[140]

References

1. Christensen, J. The controls of gastrointestinal movements: some old and new views. N. Engl. J. Med. *285*:85, 1971.
2. Weisbrodt, N. W. Motility of the small intestine. *In* Johnson, L. (ed.). Physiology of the Gastrointestinal Tract, Vol. 1. New York, Raven Press, 1981, p. 411.
3. Scott, L. D., and Summers, R. W. Correlation of contractions and transit in rat small intestine. Am. J. Physiol. *230*:132, 1976.
4. Kewenter, J. The vagal control of the jejunum and ileal motility and blood flow. Acta Physiol. Scand. (Suppl.) *251*:3, 1965.
5. Burnstock, G. Purinergic nerves. Pharmacol. Rev. *54*:418, 1972.
6. Kreulen, D. L., and Szurszewski, J. H. Nerve pathways in celiac plexus of the guinea pig. Am. J. Physiol. *237*:90, 1979.
7. Carlson, G. M., Bedi, B. S., and Code, C. F. Mechanisms of propagation of intestinal interdigestive myoelectric complex. Am. J. Physiol. *222*:1027, 1972.
8. Szurszewski, J. H. A migrating electrical complex of the canine small intestine. Am. J. Physiol. *217*:1757, 1969.
9. Fleckenstein, P. Migrating electrical spike activity in the fasting human small intestine. Am. J. Dig. Dis. *23*:769, 1978.
10. Sarna, S. K. Cyclic motor activity; migrating motor complex: 1985. Gastroenterology *89*:894, 1985.
11. Bueno, L., Proddaude, F., and Ruckebusch, Y. Propagation of electrical spiking activity along the small intestine: intrinsic versus extrinsic neural influence. J. Physiol. (Lond.) *292*:15, 1979.
12. Sarr, M. G., and Kelly, K. Myoelective activity of the autotransplanted canine jejunoileum. Gastroenterology *81*:303, 1981.
13. Vantrappen, G., Janssens, J., Coremans, G., and Jian, R. Gastrointestinal motility disorders. Dig. Dis. Sci. *31*(Suppl.):5, 1986.
14. Coremans, G., Janssens, J., Vantrappen, G., Cucciara, S., and Ceccatelli, P. The slow wave frequency of the human small intestine. Dig. Dis. Sci. *30*:765, 1985.

15. DiMarino, A. J., Carlson, G., Myers, A., Schumacher, H. R., and Cohen, S. Duodenal myoelectric activity in scleroderma: abnormal responses to mechanical and hormonal stimuli. N. Engl. J. Med. *289*:1220, 1973.
16. Vantrappen, G., Janssens, J., Hellemans, J., and Ghoos, Y. The interdigestive motor complex of normal subjects and patients with bacterial overgrowth of the small intestine. J. Clin. Invest. *59*:1158, 1977.
17. Christensen, J., Schedle, H. P., and Clifton, J. The basic electrical rhythm of the human duodenum in normal subjects and in patients with thyroid disease. J. Clin. Invest. *43*:1659, 1964.
18. Mathias, J. R., Carlson, G. M., DiMarino, A. J., Bertiger, G., Norton, H. E., and Cohen, S. Intestinal myoelectric activity in response to live *Vibrio cholerae* and cholera enterotoxin. J. Clin. Invest. *58*:91, 1976.
19. Ouyang, A., Snape, W. J., Jr., and Cohen, S. Myoelectric properties of the cat ileocecal sphincter. Am. J. Physiol. *240*:450, 1981.
20. Durdle, N. G., Kingma, Y. J., Bowes, K. L., and Chambers, M. M. Origin of slow waves in the canine colon. Gastroenterology *84*:375, 1983.
21. Christensen, J., and Hauser, R. L. Longitudinal axial coupling of slow waves in proximal cat colon. Am. J. Physiol. *221*:246, 1971.
22. Christensen, J., Anuras, S., and Hauser, R. L. Migrating spike bursts and electrical slow waves in the cat colon: effect of sectioning. Gastroenterology *66*:240, 1974.
23. Christensen, J. Myoelectric control of the cat colon. Gastroenterology *68*:601, 1975.
24. Huizinga, J. D., Diamant, N. E., and El-Sharkawy, T. Y. Electrical basis of contractions in the muscle layers of the pig colon. Am. J. Physiol. *246*:G482–G491, 1983.
25. Taylor, I., Duthie, I., Smallwood, R., and Linkens, D. Large bowel myoelectrical activity in man. Gut *16*:808, 1975.
26. Sarna, S. K., Bardakjian, B. L., Waterfall, W. E., and Lind, J. F. Human colonic electrical control activity (ECA). Gastroenterology *78*:1526, 1980.
27. Snape, W. J., Jr., Carlson, G. M., and Cohen, S. Human colonic myoelectrical activity in response to prostigmine and the gastrointestinal hormones. Am. J. Dig. Dis. *22*:881, 1977.
28. Gill, R. C., Cote, K. R., Bowes, K. L., and Kingma, Y. J. Human colonic smooth muscle: spontaneous contractile activity and response to stretch. Gut *27*:1006, 1986.
29. Sarna, S. K., Waterfall, W. R., Bardakjian, B. L., and Lind, J. F. Type of human colonic electrical activities recorded postoperatively. Gastroenterology *81*:61, 1981.
30. Bueno, L., Fioramonti, J., Ruckebusch, Y., Frexinos, J., and Coulom, P. Evaluation of colonic myoelectrical activity in health and functional disorders. Gut *21*:480, 1980.
31. Sarna, S., Latimer, P., Campbell, D., and Waterfall, W. E. Electrical and contractile activities of the human rectosigmoid. Gut *23*:698, 1982.
32. Frexinos, J., Bueno, L., and Fioramonti, J. Diurnal changes in myoelectrical spiking activity of the human colon. Gastroenterology *88*:1104, 1985.
33. Fioramonti, J., Garcia-Villar, R., Bueno, L., and Ruckebusch, Y. Colonic myoelectric activity and propulsion in the dog. Dig. Dis. Sci. *25*:641, 1980.
34. Duthie, H. L., and Kirk, S. Electrical activity of human colonic smooth muscle in vitro. J. Physiol. *283*:319, 1978.
35. Huizinga, J. D., Stern, H. S., Chow, E., Diamant, N. E., and El-Sharkawy, T. Y. Electrophysiologic control of motility in the human colon. Gastroenterology *88*:500, 1985.
36. Chambers, M. M., Bowes, K. L., Kingma, Y. J., Bannister, C., and Cote, K. R. In vitro electrical activity in human colon. Gastroenterology *81*:502, 1981.
37. Suchowiecky, M., Clarke, D. D., Bhsker, M., Perry, R. J., and Snape, W. J., Jr. Effect of secoverine on colonic myoelectric activity in diverticular disease of the colon. Dig. Dis. Sci. (in press).
38. Cannon, W. B. The movements of the intestines studied by means of the roentgen rays. Am. J. Physiol. *6*:251, 1902.
39. Elliott, T. R., and Barclay-Smith, E. Antiperistalsis and other muscular activities of the colon. J. Physiol. (Lond.) *31*:272, 1904.
40. Devroede, G., and Soffie, M. Colonic absorption in idiopathic constipation. Gastroenterology *641*:552, 1973.
41. Christensen, J., Weisbrodt, N. W., and Hauser, R. L. Electrical slow wave of the proximal colon of the cat in diarrhea. Gastroenterology *62*:1167, 1972.
42. Christensen, J., and Freeman, B. W. Circular muscle electromyogram in the cat colon: local effect of sodium ricinoleate. Gastroenterology *63*:1011, 1972.
43. Wiggins, H. S., and Cummings, J. H. Evidence for the mixing of residue in the human gut. Gut *17*:1007, 1976.
44. Weems, W. A., and Weisbrodt, N. W. Ileal and colonic propulsive behavior: contribution of enteric neural circuits. Am. J. Physiol. *250*:G653, 1986.
45. Ritchie, J. A. Colonic motor activity and bowel function. Part I. Normal movement of contents. Gut *9*:442, 1968.
46. Ritchie, J. A., Ardran, G. M., and Trulove, S. C. Motor activity of the sigmoid colon of humans: a combined study by intraluminal pressure recording and cineradiography. Gastroenterology *43*:642, 1962.
47. Read, N. W., Al-Janabi, M. N., Holgate, A. M., Barber, D. C., and Edwards, C. A. Simultaneous measurement of gastric emptying, small bowel residence and colonic filling of a solid meal by the use of the gamma camera. Gut *27*:300, 1986.
48. Krevsky, B., Malmud, L. S., D'ercole, F., Maurer, A. H., and Fisher, R. S. Colonic transit scintigraphy. Gastroenterology *91*:1102, 1986.
49. Spiller, R. C., Brown, M. L., and Phillips, S. F. Decreased fluid tolerance, accelerated transit, and abnormal motility of the human colon induced by oleic acid. Gastroenterology *91*:100, 1986.
50. Youle, M. S., and Read, N. W. Effect of painless rectal distension on gastrointestinal transit of solid meal. Dig. Dis. Sci. *29*:902, 1984.
51. Connell, A. The motility of the pelvic colon. Part II. Paradoxical motility in diarrhea and constipation. Gut *3*:342, 1962.
52. Ryan, J. P., and Bhojwani, A. Colonic transit in rats: effects of ovariectomy, sex steroid hormones, and pregnancy. Am. J. Physiol. *251*:G46, 1986.
53. Hulten, L. Extrinsic nervous control of colonic motility and blood flow: an experimental study in the cat. Acta Physiol. Scand., Suppl.335:1, 1969.
54. Rostad, H. Central and peripheral nervous control of colonic motility in the cat. Acta Physiol. Scand. *89*:79, 1973.
55. Cardette, B., and Gonella, J. Etude electromyographique in vivo de la commande nerveuse orthosympathique du colon chez le chat. J. Physiol. (Paris) *68*:671, 1974.
56. Lyrenas, E., Abrahamsson, H., and Dotevall, G. Effects of β-adrenoceptor stimulation on rectosigmoid motility in man. Dig. Dis. Sci. *30*:536, 1985.
57. Ek, B. A., Bjellin, L. A. C., and Lundgren, B. T. β-adrenergic control of motility in the rat colon. I. evidence for functional separation of the β_1-and β_2-adrenoreceptor-mediated inhibition of colon activity. Gastroenterology *90*:400, 1986.
58. Weems, W. A., and Szurszewski, J. H. Modulation of colonic motility by peripheral neural inputs to neurons of the inferior mesenteric ganglion. Gastroenterology *73*:273, 1977.
59. Kreulen, D. L., and Szurszewski, J. H. Nerve pathways in celiac plexus of the guinea pig. Am. J. Physiol. *237*:E90, 1979.
60. Kreulen, D. L., and Szurszewski, J. H. Reflex pathways in the abdominal prevertebral ganglia: evidence for a colocolonic inhibitory reflex. J. Physiol. *295*:21, 1979.
61. DeGroat, W. C., and Krier, J. The central control of the lumbar sympathetic pathway of the large intestine of the cat. J. Physiol. *289*:449, 1979.
62. Weber, J., Denis, P., Mihout, B., Muller, J. M., Blanquart, F., Galmiche, J. P., Simon, P., and Pasquis, P. Effect of brainstem lesion on colonic and anorectal motility. Dig. Dis. Sci. *30*:419, 1985.
63. Aaronson, M. J., Freed, M. M., and Burakoff, R. Colonic myoelectric activity in persons with spinal cord injury. Dig. Dis. Sci. *30*:295, 1985.
64. Glick, M. E., Meshkinpour, H., Haldeman, S., Hoehler, F., Downey, N., and Bradley, W. E. Colonic dysfunction in patients with thoracic spinal cord injury. Gastroenterology *86*:287, 1984.
65. Connell, A. M., Frankel, H., and Suttmann, L. The motility

of the pelvic colon following the complete lesions of the spinal cord. Paraplegia *1*:98, 1963.
66. Christensen, J., Anuras, S., and Arthur, C. Influence of intrinsic nerves on electromyogram of cat colon in vitro. Am. J. Physiol. *234*:E641, 1978.
67. Christensen, J., Stiles, G., Rick, G. A., and Sutherland, J. Comparative anatomy of the myenteric plexus of the distal colon in eight mammals. Gastroenterology *86*:706, 1984.
68. Christensen, J., Rick, G. A., Robison, B. A., Stiles, M. J., and Wix, M. A. Arrangement of the myenteric plexus throughout the gastrointestinal tract of the oppossum. Gastroenterology *85*:890, 1983.
69. Probert, L., De Mey, J., and Polak, J. M. Ultrastructural localization of four different neuropeptides within separate populations of p-type nerves in the guinea pig colon. Gastroenterology *85*:1094, 1983.
70. Jessen, K. R., Saffrey, J., Van Noorden, S., Bloom, S. R., Polak, J. M., and Burnstock, G. Immunohistochemical studies of the enteric nervous system in tissue culture and in situ: localization of vasoactive intestinal polypeptide (VIP), substance p and enkephalin immunoreactive nerves in the guinea-pig gut. Neuroscience *5*:171, 1980.
71. Snape, W. J., Jr., Matarazzo, S. A., and Cohen, S. Effect of eating and gastrointestinal hormones on human colonic myoelectrical and motor activity. Gastroenterology *75*:373–378, 1978.
72. Snape, W. J., Jr. Effect of calcium on neurohumoral stimulation of feline colonic smooth muscle. Am. J. Physiol. *243*:G134, 1982.
73. Walsh, J. H., Lamers, C. B., and Valenzuela, J. E. Cholecystokinin-octapeptide immunoreactivity in human plasma. Gastroenterology *82*:438, 1982.
74. Holzer, P., Bucsics, A., Saria, A., and Lembeck, F. A study of the concentration of substance P and neurotensin in the gastrointestinal tract of various mammals. Neuroscience *7*:2919, 1982.
75. Rosell, S., and Rokaeus, A. The effect of ingestion of amino acids, glucose and fat on circulating neurotensin-like immunoreactivity (NTLI) in man. Acta Physiol. Scand. *107*:263, 1979.
76. Thor, K., and Rosell, S. Neurotensin increases colonic motility. Gastroenterology *90*:P27, 1986.
77. Bardon, T. H., and Ruckebusch, Y. Neurotensin-induced colonic motor response in dogs: a mediation by prostaglandins. Regul. Peptides *10*:107, 1985.
78. Jessen, K. R., Polak, J. M., Van Noorden, S., Bloom, S. R., and Burnstock, G. Peptide-containing neurones connect the two ganglionated plexuses of the enteric nervous system. Nature *283*:391, 1980.
79. Sims, S. M., Walsh, J. V., and Singer, J. J. Substance P and acetylcholine both suppress the same K^+ current in dissociated smooth muscle cells. Am. J. Physiol. *251*:C580, 1986.
80. Polak, J. M., Bishop, A. E., Lake, B., Bryant, M. G., and Bloom, S. R. Abnormalities of the peptidergic nervous system in Hirschsprung's disease. Lab. Invest. *42*:143, 1980.
81. Sun, E. A., Snape, W. J., Jr., Cohen, S., and Renny, A. The role of opiate receptors and cholinergic neurons in the gastrocolonic response. Gastroenterology *82*:689, 1982.
82. Bueno, L., Fioramonti, J., Honde, C., Fargeas, M. J., and Primi, M. P. Antral and peripheral control of gastrointestinal and colonic motility by endogenous opiates in conscious dogs. Gastroenterology *88*:549, 1985.
83. Vizi, S. E., Ono, K., Adam-Zivi, V., Duncalf, D., and Foldes, F. F. Presynaptic inhibitory effect of met-enkephalin on [^{14}C] acetylcholine release from the myenteric plexus and its interaction with muscarinic negative feedback inhibition. J. Pharmacol. Exp. Ther. *230*:493, 1984.
84. Dinoso, V. P., Meshkinpour, H., Lorber, S. H., Gutierrez, J. G., and Chey, W. Y. Motor responses of the sigmoid colon and rectum to exogenous cholecystokinin and secretin. Gastroenterology *65*:435, 1973.
85. Taylor, I., Duthie, H. L., Cumberland, D. C., and Smallwood, R. Glucagon and the colon. Gut *16*:973, 1975.
86. Gill, R. C., Bowes, K. L., Kingma, Y. J. Effect of progesterone on canine colonic smooth muscle. Gastroenterology *88*:1941, 1985.
87. Strunz, U., Mitnegg, P., Domschke, S., Domschke, W., Wunsch, E., and Demling, L. VIP antagonizes motilin-induced antral contractions in vitro. *In* Duthie, H. L. (ed.). Gastrointestinal Motility in Health and Disease. Lancaster, England, MTP Press, 1978, p. 125.
88. Wright, S. H., Snape, W. J., Jr., Battle, W. M., Cohen, S., and London, R. L. Effect of dietary components on the gastrocolonic response. Am. J. Physiol. *238*:G228, 1980.
89. Schang, J. C., and Devroede, G. Fasting and postprandial myoelectric spiking activity in the human sigmoid colon. Gastroenterology *85*:1048, 1983.
90. Schang, J. C., Hemond, M., Hebert, M., and Pilote, M. Myoelectrical activity and intraluminal flow in human sigmoid colon. Dig. Dis. Sci. *31*:1331, 1986.
91. Levinson, S., Bhasker, M., Gibson, T. R., Morin, R., and Snape, W. J., Jr. Comparison of intraluminal and intravenous mediators of colonic response to eating. Dig. Dis. Sci. *30*:33, 1985.
92. Narducci, F., Bassotti, G., Daniotti, S., Del Soldato, P., Pelli, M. A., and Morelli, A. Identification of muscarinic receptor subtype mediating colonic response to eating. Dig. Dis. Sci. *30*:124, 1985.
93. Cummings, J. H., Branch, W., Jenkins, D. J. A., Southgate, D. A. T., Houston, H., and James, W. P. T. Colonic response to dietary fibre from carrot, cabbage, apple, bran and guar gum. Lancet *1*:5, 1978.
94. Findlay, J. M., Mitchell, W. D., Smith, A. N., Anderson, A. J. B., and Eastwood, M. A. Effects of unprocessed bran on colon function in normal subjects and diverticular disease. Lancet *1*:146, 1974.
95. Kirwan, W. O., Smith, A. N., Mitchell, W. D., Falconer, J. D., and Eastwood, M. A. Action of different bran preparations on colonic function. Br. Med. J. *4*:187, 1974.
96. Kirwan, W. O., Smith, A. N., Mitchell, W. D., Falconer, J. D., and Eastwood, M. A. Bile acids and colonic motility in the rabbit and the human. Part 1. The rabbit. Gut *16*:894, 1975.
97. Shiff, S. J., Soloway, R. D., and Snape, W. J., Jr. The mechanism deoxycholic acid stimulation of the rabbit colon. J. Clin. Invest. *69*:985, 1982.
98. Coyne, M. J., Bonorris, G. G., Chung, A., Conley, D., and Schoenfield, L. J. Propranolol inhibits bile acid and fatty acid stimulation of cyclic AMP in human colon. Gastroenterology *73*:971, 1977.
99. Flynn, M. M., Hammond, P., Darby, C., Hyland, J., and Taylor, I. Foecal bile acids and the irritable colon syndrome. Digestion *22*:144, 1981.
100. Almy, T. P., and Tulin, M. Alterations in colonic function in man under stress: experimental production of changes simulating the "irritable colon." Gastroenterology *8*:616, 1947.
101. Narducci, F., Snape, W. J., Jr., Battle, W. M., London, R. L., and Cohen, S. Increased colonic motility during exposure to a stressful situation. Dig. Dis. Sci. *30*:40, 1985.
102. Snape, W. J., Jr., Carlson, G. M., Matarazzo, S. A., and Cohen, S. Evidence that abnormal myoelectric activity produces colonic motor dysfunction in the irritable bowel syndrome. Gastroenterology *72*:382, 1977.
103. Giuseppe, F., Parisi, F., Corazziari, E., and Caprilli, R. Colonic electromyography in chronic constipation. Gastroenterology *84*:737, 1983.
104. Sullivan, M. A., Cohen, S., and Snape, W. J., Jr. Colonic myoelectrical activity in the irritable bowel syndrome: effect of eating and anticholinergics. N. Engl. J. Med. *298*:878, 1978.
105. Connell, A., Jones, F., and Rowland, E. Motility of the pelvic colon. Part IV. Abdominal pain associated with colonic hypermotility after meals. Gut *6*:105, 1965.
106. Arfwidsson, S. Pathogenesis of multiple diverticula of the sigmoid colon in diverticular disease. Acta Chir. Scand. (Suppl.) 342:1, 1964.
107. Taylor, I., and Duthie, H. L. Bran tablets and diverticular disease. Br. Med. J. *1*:988, 1976.
108. Battle, W. M., Snape, W. J., Jr., Alavi, A., Cohen, S., and Braunstein, S. Colonic dysfunction in diabetes mellitus. Gastroenterology *79*:1217, 1980.
109. Thompson, M. A., Jr., and Summers, R. Barium impaction as

a complication of gastrointestinal scleroderma. JAMA *235*:1715, 1976.

110. Battle, W. M., Snape, W. J., Jr., Wright, S., Sullivan, M. A., Cohen, S., Myers, A., and Tuthill, R. Abnormal colonic motility in progressive systemic sclerosis. Ann. Intern. Med. *97*:749, 1981.
111. Schuffler, M. D., Lowe, M. C., and Bill, A. H. Studies of idiopathic intestinal pseudo-obstruction. 1. Hereditary hollow visceral myopathy in clinical pathological studies. Gastroenterology *73*:327, 1977.
112. Ogilvie, H. Large-intestine colic due to sympathetic deprivation: a new clinical syndrome. Br. Med. J. *2*:671, 1948.
113. Sullivan, M. A., Snape, W. J., Jr., Matarazzo, S. A., Petrokubi, R. J., Jefferies, G., and Cohen, S. Gastrointestinal myoelectrical activity in idiopathic intestinal pseudo-obstruction. N. Engl. J. Med. *297*:233, 1977.
114. Glick, M. E., Meshkinpour, H., Haldeman, S., Bhatia, N. N., and Bradley, W. E. Colonic dysfunction in multiple sclerosis. Gastroenterology *83*:1002, 1982.
115. Nowak, T. V., Ionasescu, V., and Anuras, S. Gastrointestinal manifestations of the muscular dystrophies. Gastroenterology *82*:800, 1982.
116. Snape, W. J., Jr., Matarazzo, S. A., and Cohen, S. Abnormal gastrocolonic response in patients with ulcerative colitis. Gut *21*:392, 1980.
117. Cohen, J. D., Kao, H. W., Tan, S. T., Lechago, J., and Snape, W. J., Jr. Effect of acute experimental colitis on rabbit colonic smooth muscle. Am. J. Physiol. *251*:G538, 1986.
118. Lanfranchi, G. A., Bazzocchi, G., Fois, F., Brignola, C., Campieri, M., and Menni, B. Effect of domperidone and dopamine on colonic motor activity in patients with the irritable bowel syndrome. Eur. J. Clin. Pharmacol. *29*:307, 1985.
119. Schuurkes, J. A. J., Van Nueten, J. M., Van Daele, P. G. H., Reyntjens, A. J., and Janssen, P. A. J. Motor-stimulating properties of cisapride on isolated gastrointestinal preparations of the guinea-pig. J. Pharmacol. Exp. Ther. *234*:775, 1985.
120. Burleigh, D. E., and Trout, S. J. Evidence against an acetylcholine releasing action of cisapride in the human colon. Br. J. Clin. Pharmacol. *20*:475, 1985.
121. Snape, W. J., Jr., Clarke, D. D., and Gautsch, E. Effect of cisapride on colonic smooth muscle in vivo and in vitro. Gastroenterology *88*:1592, 1985.
122. Painter, N. S., Almeida, A. Z., and Colebourne, K. W. Unprocessed bran in treatment of diverticular disease of the colon. Br. Med. J. *2*:137, 1972.
123. Eastwood, M. A., Smith, A. N., Brydon, W. G., and Pritchard, J. Comparison of bran, ispaghula, and lactulose on colon function in diverticular disease. Gut *19*:1144, 1978.
124. Manning, A. P., Heaton, K. W., and Harvey, R. F. Wheat fibre and irritable bowel syndrome. Lancet *2*:417, 1977.
125. Soltoft, J., Gudmand-Hoyer, E., Krag, B., Kristensen, E., and Wulff, H. R. A double blind trial of the effect of wheat bran on symptoms of irritable bowel syndrome. Lancet *1*:270, 1976.
126. Snape, W. J., Jr. Influence of papaverine on bethanechol or OP-CCK stimulation on feline colonic muscle. Gastroenterology *80*:498, 1981.
127. Snape, W. J., Jr., and Tan, S. T. Role of sodium or calcium in electrical depolarization of feline colonic smooth muscle. Am. J. Physiol. *249*:G66, 1985.
128. Bortolotti, M., and Labo, G. Clinical and manometric effects of nifedipine in patients with esophageal achalasia. Gastroenterology *80*:39, 1981.
129. Lincoln, T. M., and Fisher-Simpson, V. A comparison of the effects of forskalin and nitroprusside on cyclic nucleotide and relaxation in the rat aorta. Eur. J. Pharmacol. *101*:17, 1983.
130. Karaki, H., Nakagawa, H., and Urakawa, N. Comparative effects of verapamil and sodium nitroprusside on contraction and ^{45}Ca uptake in the smooth muscle of rabbit aorta, rat aorta, and guinea-pig taenia coli. Br. J. Pharmacol. *81*:393, 1984.
131. Rees, W. D. W., Evans, B. K., and Rhodes, J. Treating irritable bowel syndrome with peppermint oil. Br. Med. J. *3*:635, 1979.
132. Schuster, M. M., and Mendeloff, A. I. Motor action of rectum and anal sphincters in continence and defecation. *In* Code, C. F., and Heidel, W. (eds.). Handbook of Physiology. Sect. 6, Vol. IV. Washington, D.C., American Physiological Society, 1968, p. 2121.
133. Taylor, B. M., Beart, R. W., and Phillips, S. F. Longitudinal and radial variation of pressure in the human anal sphincter. Gastroenterology *86*:693, 1984.
134. Schuster, M. M. The riddle of the sphincter. Gastroenterology *69*:249, 1975.
135. Schiller, L. R., Santa Ana, C. A., Schmulen, C. A., Hendler, R. S., Harford, W. V., and Fordtran, J. S. Pathogenesis of fecal incontinence in diabetes mellitus. N. Engl. J. Med. *307*:1666, 1982.
136. Wald, A., and Tunuguntla, A. K. Anorectal sensorimotor dysfunction in fecal incontinence and diabetes mellitus. Modification with biofeedback therapy. N. Engl. J. Med. *310*:1282, 1984.
137. Snooks, S. J., Henry, M. M., and Swash, M. Anorectal incontinence and rectal prolapse: differential assessment of the innervation to puborectalis and external anal sphincter muscles. Gut *26*:470, 1985.
138. Bartolo, D. C. C., Read, N. W., Jarratt, J. A., Read, M. G., Donnelly, T. C., and Johnson, A. G. Differences in anal sphincter function and clinical presentation in patients with pelvic floor descent. Gastroenterology *85*:68, 1983.
139. Kubota, M., Ito, Y., and Ikeda, K. Membrane properties and innervation of smooth muscle cells in Hirschsprung's disease. Am. J. Physiol. *244*:G406, 1983.
140. Lipkin, M., and Sleisenger, M. H. Studies of visceral pain. Measurements of stimulus intensity and duration associated with the onset of pain in esophagus, ileum and colon. J. Clin. Invest. *37*:28, 1958.

59

The Short Bowel Syndrome

JERRY S. TRIER
MARVIN LIPSKY

BACKGROUND

The absorptive and digestive surface provided by the small intestinal mucosa in healthy adults is more than is needed to maintain adequate nutrition. Therefore, resection of small amounts of small intestine usually causes no clinical symptoms. The severity of symptoms after resection of large segments of the small bowel is related to (1) the extent of the resection (i.e., the amount of functional absorptive and digestive surface remaining); and (2) the specific level of the resected small intestine. The latter is important because absorption of certain physiologically needed substances is most efficient in either the proximal portion (iron, folate, calcium) or the distal portion (bile salts, vitamin B_{12}) of the small intestine (see pp. 1062–1105). Thus, resection of up to 40 to 50 per cent of the total length of the small intestine is usually well tolerated, provided the duodenum, the proximal portion of the jejunum, the distal half of the ileum, and the ileocecal sphincter are spared. In contrast, resection of the distal two thirds of the ileum and ileocecal sphincter alone may induce severe diarrhea and significant malabsorption even though only 25 per cent of the total small intestine has been resected. Resection of 50 per cent or more of the small intestine usually results in significant malabsorption, and resection of 70 per cent or more of the small intestine often produces such catastrophic malabsorption that survival of the patient is threatened.

ETIOLOGY

The most common clinical conditions that require resection of massive portions of the small intestine to preserve the life of the patient are those compromising its blood supply. These include *thrombosis* or *embolus* of the *superior mesenteric artery, low flow ischemia* of the superior mesenteric arterial bed, *thrombosis* of the *superior mesenteric vein* and its branches, *volvulus* of the *small intestine,* and *strangulated internal* or *external hernias.* Less common causes for massive bowel resection include *Crohn's disease, neoplasm,* and *trauma.* Very rarely, surgical error, such as inadvertent *gastroileal anastomosis* in the course of surgery for peptic ulcer, may result in bypass of a major portion of the small intestine and produce a clinical picture indistinguishable from that seen after massive intestinal resection. Past efforts to treat intractable obesity and hypercholesterolemia by jejunocolic or jejunoileal anastomosis with bypass of part or all of the ileum and part of the jejunum have also produced, in some patients, catastrophic malabsorption of the type seen following massive resection; as a result, these operations are no longer recommended.[1]

PATHOPHYSIOLOGY AND CLINICAL FEATURES

The minimum amount of small intestinal absorptive surface required to sustain life seems to vary from patient to patient. Prolonged survival with oral alimentation has been recorded in a number of patients with an intact duodenum and as little as 15 to 45 cm (6 to 18 inches) of residual jejunum.[2] However, without long-term total parenteral nutrition, prolonged patient survival is the exception rather than the rule if, in addition to the entire duodenum, less than 60 cm (2 feet) of jejunum or ileum remains. Preservation of the ileocecal sphincter is important as it reduces contamination of the residual small intestine by the colonic flora, and its presence seems to increase the transit time of the small intestinal intraluminal contents. Preservation of part or all of the colon also significantly reduces fluid and electrolyte losses.

Reduction of absorption of virtually all nutrients, including water, electrolytes, fat, protein, carbohydrate, vitamins, and trace elements, after massive resection of the small intestine, creates an urgent clinical situation. Fluid loss is usually greatest during the first few days after resection, and fecal effluent frequently is in excess of 5 L/day, especially if part or all of the colon with its capacity for water and ion absorption has been lost. If vigorous fluid and electrolyte replacement is not instituted promptly, life-threatening dehydration and electrolyte imbalance may develop. As time progresses, the consequences of impaired absorption of other nutrients rapidly become evident and may affect virtually all body systems. The resulting symptoms and physical findings may closely resemble those encountered in other intestinal diseases with severe panmalabsorption, such as *celiac sprue* or *Whipple's disease,* whose manifestations have been described in detail on pages 263 to 282, 1134 to 1152, 1297 to 1306. Briefly, severe weight loss, fatigue, lassitude, and weakness may result from caloric deprivation caused by impaired fat, protein, and carbohydrate absorption. Impaired absorption of divalent cations (Ca^{2+}, Mg^{2+}) may aggravate the weakness, and frank tetany may develop. As the duration of calcium and protein malabsorption lengthens, osteopenia with bone pain and even spontaneous fractures may develop. Purpura and generalized bleeding may reflect impaired coagulation caused by malabsorption of vitamin K. In time, peripheral neuropathy may develop. Plasma proteins are usually not lost excessively into the gut; hence, severe hypoalbuminemia with ascites and peripheral edema is less common than in diffuse mucosal diseases of the small intestine, such as *celiac sprue* or *Whipple's disease,* but mild or moderate hypoalbuminemia is common.

Gastric hypersecretion may follow massive resection of the small intestine, causing serious complicating *peptic ulcer disease*[2, 3] and compromising intestinal absorption by inducing mucosal damage and impaired intraluminal lipid digestion and dispersion (see pp. 728–729 and 824–828). However, human postresection gastric hypersecretion usually is a transient phenomenon in that gastric acid secretion decreases to normal levels in most patients who survive the acute effects of massive resection.[2, 3] Both fasting and meal-stimulated gastrin levels may be elevated in patients months and even years after extensive intestinal resection.[4] The cause of this hypergastrinemia is not known, but possibilities include loss of an intestinal inhibitory factor or impaired intestinal gastrin catabolism. These elevated gastrin levels do not appear to correlate with an increase in acid secretion. Indeed, normal gastric acid secretion has been documented in concert with hypergastrinemia after massive resection.[5]

In striking contrast to massive resections, resections of small portions of the midintestine are usually well tolerated, because the residual bowel has sufficient reserve absorptive and digestive capacity. Indeed, clinical evidence of malabsorption may be absent in patients in whom up to 182 cm (6 feet) of midsmall bowel is resected. However, even when much smaller segments of either the proximal or the distal portions of the small intestine are removed, significant clinical signs and symptoms usually develop.

If the entire duodenum is resected or bypassed surgically, *anemia* caused by malabsorption of dietary iron or folate or both may develop, much as in patients who have undergone gastrojejunal anastomosis for treatment of peptic ulcer disease. Such patients may be especially at risk to develop *osteopenia,* because calcium is absorbed most efficiently by the proximal segment of the small intestine (see pp. 974–975). Resection of the distal portion of the ileum induces predictable vitamin B_{12} malabsorption, because the specific transport mechanism for intrinsic factor–mediated vitamin B_{12} absorption is localized to the ileal absorptive cells. Thus, patients with total ileal resection will, in due course, develop vitamin B_{12} deficiency and macrocytic anemia unless this vitamin is replaced parenterally. Intraluminal overgrowth of bacteria may develop in the remaining small intestine and aggravate the already severe malabsorption of fat and vitamin B_{12}, especially in patients whose ileocecal sphincter has been resected (see pp. 1289–1297).

Diarrhea After Ileal Resection

Resection of the distal small intestine may cause serious *diarrhea* and *steatorrhea.* Conjugated bile salts, essential for normal fat absorption, are absorbed most effectively by an active transport mechanism present only in the ileum. Reduction or complete removal of these active absorptive sites in patients who have undergone ileal resection disrupts the enterohepatic circulation of bile salts (see pp. 144–161).

If less than 100 cm of the distal part of the ileum has been resected, watery diarrhea termed *cholerrheic* diarrhea with little or no steatorrhea usually results. Although increased amounts of bile salts reach the colon, hepatic synthesis compensates sufficiently to maintain adequate concentrations of bile salts in the lumen of the proximal portion of the intestine for normal digestion and absorption of dietary fats to proceed. However, the excessive dihydroxy bile salts (chenodeoxycholate and deoxycholate) that enter the colon not only impair water and ion absorption but actually stimulate their secretion by the colonic mucosa when they are present in concentrations greater than 3 mM[6, 7] (see pp. 144–161 and 1037–1038). The mechanisms responsible for cholerrheic diarrhea are not fully understood, but increased mucosal cyclic adenosine monophosphate (cAMP) levels and direct damage by bile salts to the epithelium have been implicated.[6–8]

If more than 100 cm of ileum has been resected, bile salt loss in the stool is so large that even maximum hepatic synthesis is unable to maintain a sufficient bile salt pool for normal intraluminal micellar solubilization of dietary fat. As a result, fat is malabsorbed in the remaining small intestine. The fatty acids that enter the colon, like bile acids, impair colonic water and ion absorption and stimulate colonic fluid secretion, especially when they are hydroxylated by the colonic bacterial flora.[9] Here the stool contains not only water, ions, and bile acids but also excess fat, hence this has been termed *steatorrheic* diarrhea. The direct effect of bile acids on the colon is unimportant in this steatorrheic diarrhea. Dilution caused by the large intraluminal volume entering the colon and the low stool pH that accompanies steatorrhea reduces the concentration of bile salts in the aqueous phase of colonic contents to levels so low that they have little effect on colonic mucosal function.[10]

Differentiation of cholerrheic from steatorrheic diarrhea has important therapeutic implications as bile salt–binding agents alleviate cholerrheic diarrhea but aggravate steatorrheic diarrhea by depleting further the available bile salt pool.[11] Stool fat content, vitamin B_{12} absorptive capacity, and, if available, determination of aqueous fecal bile salt concentrations help distinguish these entities, but a therapeutic trial of a bile salt binder may be useful if the extent of ileal resection is not known.

It has been well documented that ileal disease and ileal resection result in lithogenic bile,[12] presumably caused by depletion of the bile salt pool. Indeed, it has been reported that the frequency of gallstones in patients with partial or total ileal resection is 25 to 32 per cent, approximately three times that of control populations[13, 14] (see pp. 1668–1676).

Physical Findings

Physical examination, as in other situations with panmalabsorption, varies with the severity and duration of the malabsorption. Initially, physical findings may be limited to poor skin turgor caused by dehydration or signs of hypocalcemia and hypomagnesemia, including a positive Chvostek's or Trousseau's sign or even frank tetany. Later, profound cachexia with purpura, increased skin pigmentation, evidence of multiple vitamin and trace element deficiencies, anemia, osteopenia, and peripheral neuropathy may be present (see pp. 263–282).

Laboratory Findings

The laboratory findings in patients with massive intestinal resection are predictable but not specific. Marked fluid and electrolyte derangements caused by massive initial fecal fluid loss are reflected in plasma volume determinations and serum electrolyte levels. Hypokalemia is common, as are sodium and water depletion. As mentioned earlier, serum gastrin levels may be elevated and excessive gastric secretion may occur and may aggravate the already immense fluid and electrolyte losses during the first few weeks after resection. Fecal calcium and magnesium losses may result in low serum levels of these divalent cations. If the patient survives the initial few weeks after massive resection, the laboratory abnormalities found in other clinical entities associated with severe panmalabsorption may develop. Xylose absorption may be diminished, and low serum prothrombin, carotene, and cholesterol levels are common. Zinc and essential fatty acid deficiency may be evident. As the patient is fed, marked steatorrhea develops. Hypoalbuminemia appears if prolonged negative nitrogen balance persists. Eventually, anemia caused by vitamin B_{12}, iron, or folate deficiency develops if these substances are not adequately replaced. Quantitation of vitamin B_{12} absorption with added intrinsic factor is particularly helpful in assessing the extent of ileal resection, although impaired vitamin B_{12} absorption both with and without added intrinsic factor may also reflect bacterial overgrowth within the lumen of the small intestine. Careful culture of intestinal fluid on selective media or a ^{14}C-xylose absorption test[15] helps to establish or exclude intraluminal bacterial overgrowth in patients with ileal resections. If these special tests are not available, a diagnostic trial of broad-spectrum antibiotics (ampicillin or tetracycline) as for blind loop syndrome may be appropriate (see pp. 1295–1296). Barium contrast studies of the small bowel may show some adaptive dilation of the bowel (Fig. 59–1) and are also helpful prognostically by providing a means of assessing the length and health of the remaining bowel.

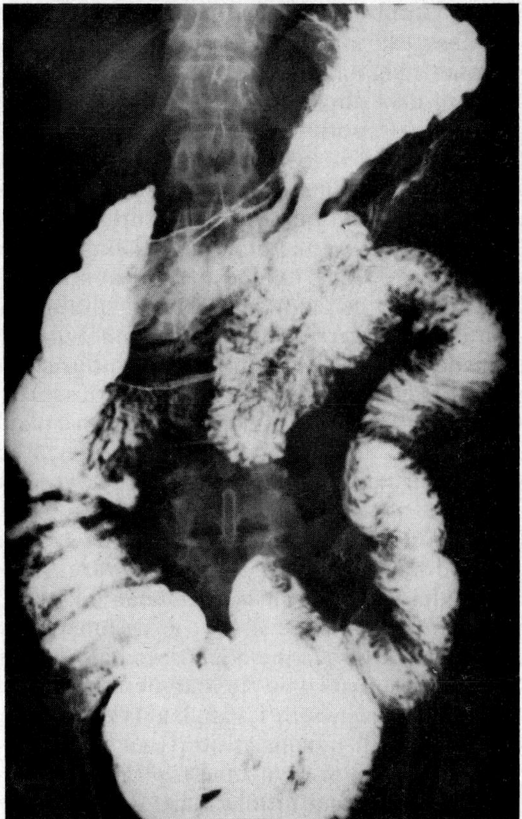

Figure 59–1. Barium contrast study of the small intestine from a patient who had undergone resection of the ileum and over half of the jejunum six months earlier. There is an increase in the caliber of the remaining small intestine, but the mucosal pattern appears normal.

Adaptation

If the patient survives the first few weeks after massive resection, the remaining small intestine adapts, facilitating efficient absorption and digestion.[16, 17] This adaptation to resection has been studied extensively in experimental animals but only to a limited degree in humans.

In experimental animals, partial intestinal resection promptly induces an increase in the mass of the remaining bowel, resulting in a substantial increase in absorptive surface. There is enlargement of the remaining villi, and the lengthened villi are lined by increased numbers of epithelial cells; however, individual epithelial cells do not increase in size. This epithelial hyperplasia is associated with accelerated epithelial cell renewal and migration.[16, 17] However, the total life span of individual absorptive cells changes little because villi are longer, and the distance that must be traversed by cells from the time of their formation in the crypts until they are extruded from the villous tips is increased. Although absorption of nutrients per unit length of remaining small intestine is generally increased substantially after resection, such improvement reflects the increase in the number of absorptive cells per unit length of the gut and is not due to increased absorptive or digestive capacity of the individual cells. Whereas total activity of enzymes involved in digestion, such as disaccharidases and enterokinase, increases per length of gut, activity of most of these enzymes in relation to protein or DNA content (that is, specific activity) remains constant or even decreases.[17, 18]

The mechanisms implicated in regulating this adaptive response include (1) the exposure of the remaining small intestine to dietary nutrients; (2) the exposure of the remaining small intestine to bile and pancreatic secretions; and (3) the effect on the remaining small intestine of trophic gut peptides. The importance of feeding is shown in several studies. Thus, starvation promptly induces mucosal atrophy in experimental animals,[19] even when nutrition is maintained by parenteral alimentation.[20] Furthermore, the adaptive response to partial intestinal resection requires the presence of nutrients in the lumen of the residual small intestine as the response was absent in rats who underwent similar resection but who were nourished by conventional parenteral alimentation.[21]

Recent efforts have been directed toward determining specific dietary elements that are instrumental in stimulating mucosal adaptation. Intraluminal administration of hydrolyzable disaccharides (sucrose, maltose, lactose) or free fatty acids has a greater stimulatory effect in rats than does administration of monosaccharides (glucose, fructose, galactose) or long-chain triglycerides, respectively.[22, 23] Intraluminal administration of amino acids of varying charge increase small intestinal growth in parenterally nourished rats.[24]

Diversion of biliary and pancreatic secretions from the jejunum to the ileum results in ileal hyperplasia and jejunal atrophy, suggesting a role for pancreatobiliary secretions in the adaptive process.[25] However, the effects both of intraluminal nutrients and endogenous secretions may be mediated, at least in part, by their stimulation of the release of gut peptides on direct contact with mucosal cells.[26, 27]

There is increasing evidence that selected peptide hormones influence small intestinal growth. Whereas mucosal structure is maintained in isolated transplanted segments of small intestine in orally alimented animals, such segments develop atrophy in parenterally alimented animals, suggesting an important role for humoral factors.[28] Although many hormones have been implicated, circulating enteroglucagon correlates best with enterocyte growth.[29] It was first suggested as a trophic factor in a patient with an enteroglucagon-producing tumor who had concomitant mucosal enlargement that regressed on removal of the tumor[30] (see pp. 1892–1894). Plasma levels of enteroglucagon have been reported to be elevated in untreated celiac sprue, infective diarrhea, and tropical sprue and after intestinal resection or jejunoileal bypass.[29] However, until it is demonstrated that mucosal growth is induced in normal subjects when pure enteroglucagon is administered in doses that produce the plasma levels found in adaptive states, evidence supporting its role in adaptive intestinal growth must be considered circumstantial.

Epidermal growth factor, a polypeptide produced by the salivary glands, increases mucosal DNA content, crypt cell labeling index, and mucosal ornithine decarboxylase activity when infused intraluminally.[31] Ornithine decarboxylase is a key enzyme controlling the synthesis of polyamines, which are required during the early phase of adaptive cell growth.[32] Administration of cholecystokinin octopeptide and secretin induces partial adaptation in parenterally fed rats,[33] but whether this effect is mediated by these peptides or by pancreatic and biliary secretions stimulated by them is not clear.

In humans, an increase in the caliber of the remaining segment of small intestine usually is seen in barium contrast X-ray films over several weeks to months after massive resection (Fig. 59–1). This dilatation of the bowel may reflect an increase in the total absorptive surface of the remaining small intestine. Whereas an increase in the length of villi following massive resection was observed in one study in humans[34] but not in another,[35] hyperplasia of the intestinal epithelial cells seems to be a consistent response.[34, 35] There is clinical evidence that absorptive function improves with time after massive resection in humans. For example, stool water and electrolyte losses appear to decrease during the first several weeks after massive resection. Intraluminal perfusion studies demonstrate a modest increase in glucose absorption in patients who have survived a massive resection.[36]

TREATMENT

Treatment is adjusted to the particular period after resection, and, in view of the foregoing discussion of adaptation, requirements for support gradually become less urgent. Vigorous parenteral replacement therapy is essential and lifesaving during the first few weeks after massive intestinal resection. Fluid and electrolyte replacement should be guided by careful quantitation of all fluid losses in the nasogastric aspirate, fecal effluent, and urine. Serial determinations of serum electrolyte, calcium, magnesium, phosphorus, and zinc levels and body weight serve as further guides to the massive replacement therapy necessary in these patients.

Medical Approach

Early initiation of total parenteral alimentation has been advocated in the treatment of patients with massive intestinal resection to prevent development of cachexia and severe nutritional deficiencies. Such alimentation should ensure balanced nutrition and should include glucose, amino acids, electrolytes, vitamins, trace minerals, and lipid, the last-named as a source of calories and to prevent essential fatty acid deficiency. The principles, techniques, and potential hazards of total parenteral alimentation are described in detail on pages 2018 to 2023. The feasibility of long-term parenteral alimentation with prolonged survival is now well documented and has proved life-saving in patients with massive intestinal resections.[37, 38] The length of time total parenteral nutrition is needed generally is inversely proportional to the length of remaining small intestine,[39] although residual disease and the presence or absence of ileum and colon are influential.

Antidiarrheal agents such as diphenoxylate (Lomotil), 5.0 mg; loperamide (Imodium), 2 mg; tincture of opium, 10 drops; codeine, 30 to 60 mg; and anticholinergics (e.g., probanthine, 15 to 30 mg) given three to four times daily may facilitate absorption by increasing intestinal transit time, thereby prolonging the duration of contact between luminal contents and mucosa and are worth trying. Reduced doses of these agents may be required permanently in some patients after stabilization.

If gastric hypersecretion has been documented, especially in the immediate postresection period, therapy with H_2-receptor antagonists should be implemented. Improved absorption after reduction of hypersecretion with the H_2-receptor antagonist cimetidine has been noted,[40] but as acid hypersecretion usually is transient and long-term therapy is rarely required, the need for continued treatment should be monitored by periodically re-examining acid secretion.

Under no circumstances should prophylactic ulcer surgery, such as vagotomy and antrectomy, be carried out at the time of initial resection. As has been indicated, many patients never develop gastric hypersecretion, and in most who do, the phenomenon is transient. Ulcer surgery may have disastrous consequences, because it may further impair the already compromised absorptive capacity in the resected patient.

Oral feedings should be initiated as soon as possible. This is especially important because, as noted earlier, intraluminal nutrients may stimulate adaptive mucosal hyperplasia of the remaining intestine directly and also stimulate release of potentially trophic gastrointestinal peptides, bile, and pancreatic juice. Initial feedings should be small but frequent and consist of foodstuffs that require no or only minimal digestion for effective absorption. Thus, initial feedings should consist primarily of simple sugars, amino acid preparations, and readily absorbable lipids such as medium-chain triglycerides. Commercial preparations of elemental diets such as Vivonex and Flexical are useful. However, such formulations are hypertonic and should be diluted initially to avoid aggravation of the patient's diarrhea owing to administration of an excessive osmolar load. If the patient is able to tolerate these simple foodstuffs, additional, more complex foods, including polymeric supplements such as Ensure and Isocal, should be added gradually until optimal nutrition is achieved. Polymeric foods, whether taken in formula form or as a native food, present a smaller osmotic load than do elemental diets, but if they are to be absorbed, they require sufficient intestinal length to permit both intraluminal digestion and mucosal absorption. Milk must be added cautiously to the diet, because the total amount of lactase-bearing epithelium is markedly reduced after massive resection, and large amounts of milk may aggravate diarrhea.

A dietary regimen in which 50 to 75 per cent of long-chain fat has been replaced by medium-chain triglyceride has been beneficial in some patients in whom a reduction in fecal water and electrolyte loss and improved overall nutrition have been noted.[41] Recently, more liberal inclusion of dietary fats has been recommended as they are an excellent source of calories, are more palatable, and often are well tolerated.[42] Optimal fat intake may vary not only with extent of resection but also from patient to patient. Thus, dietary therapy must be individualized and may require trials of a number of different nutritional regimens in problem patients. Because some steatorrhea will always persist in patients with massive resections, total caloric intake will ultimately have to exceed that of normal individuals if the resected patient is to maintain a reasonable weight. Ideally these patients will eat at least five or six meals per day rather than the customary three. Intraluminal infusion of formula diets during the night has been helpful in some patients.

The administration of vitamin supplements, especially fat-soluble vitamins, is essential. Calcium supplements, and in many patients magnesium and zinc supplements as well, may be needed, as in other patients with severe malabsorption (see Table 18–7, p. 279). The reader is also referred to pages 1971–2027 for detailed information relating to nutritional deficiencies and their management.

Orally administered drugs may be absorbed poorly and, when indicated, plasma levels should be monitored closely (i.e., antibiotics, digoxin). If there is clinical and laboratory evidence of intraluminal bacterial overgrowth in the small intestinal remnant, intermittent courses of appropriate broad-spectrum antibiotics such as tetracycline or ampicillin should be administered (see pp. 1289–1297 for details of diagnosis and treatment of bacterial overgrowth).

In patients with limited resection of the small intestine, therapy is less complex. Patients with duodenal bypass or resection may require iron, folate, and calcium supplements (see Table 18–7, p. 279).

In patients who have undergone ileal resections of less than 100 cm, cholestyramine in doses of 8 to 12 gm/day or aluminum hydroxide, 15 to 30 ml four times daily, is often effective in controlling diarrhea caused by bile salt malabsorption.[11, 43] Both agents bind conjugates of dihydroxy bile salts effectively *in vitro*.[44] In patients with more extensive ileal resections, cholestyramine and aluminum hydroxide are usually ineffective; in fact, they may aggravate already severe steatorrhea by further depleting the patient's bile acid pool. A therapeutic trial may be needed in those patients in whom the extent of ileal resection and the contribution to diarrhea of direct interaction of bile salts with colonic mucosa are unclear. Patients who have undergone sufficiently extensive ileal resection to have impaired vitamin B_{12} absorption should receive monthly injections of vitamin B_{12}. In questionable cases, a stage II Schilling test should be performed to document malabsorption of cobalamine (Table 18–5, p. 275).

Surgical Approach

Some physicians have advocated surgical intervention in patients who fail to maintain adequate nutrition and who have persistent, life-threatening malabsorption and continued weight loss several months after initiation of oral feeding as outlined earlier. Reversal of a short segment of bowel at the distal margin of the remaining small intestine has been tried. Optimally, this procedure induces partial intestinal obstruction and facilitates absorption by increasing the transit time. Alternatively, construction of a recirculating loop with some of the remaining small intestine has been attempted in the hope that such loops would permit nutrients to pass several times along the same segment of bowel, thus facilitating absorption. In isolated instances, such surgical intervention has appeared helpful, but more often it has been of no benefit or deleterious.[45] Such operations predispose to stasis and may induce severe bacterial overgrowth in the remaining segment of small intestine, compromising absorption even further. Attempts to increase the duration of contact between nutrients and sucrose by intestinal tapering and lengthening procedures have been helpful in only a few instances.[45] Moreover, there is always the risk that manipulation of the remaining intestinal segment may impair its blood supply, necessitate additional resection, and further reduce the available absorptive surface.

Small bowel transplantation may ultimately offer an alternative in these patients, but not for some time. Better methods for donor organ preservation and controlling graft versus host disease and graft rejection are needed.[46] At present, surgical treatment of massive intestinal resection must be considered experimental and should be attempted only in desperate situations.[45]

PROGNOSIS AND COMPLICATIONS

The prognosis in patients with massive resection varies directly with the length and location of the remaining intestine and its freedom from disease. Patients who still have 25 per cent or more of morphologically and functionally normal small intestine after resection have a good prognosis, especially if the remaining intestine includes duodenum, proximal jejunum, and distal ileum. Patients with less than 25 per cent of their small intestine have a much poorer prognosis. Patients in the later group often are nutritionally crippled unless adequate nutrition can be maintained with supplemental parenteral alimentation or supplemental peroral formula diets or both. In addition to the diverse complications they may develop related to their nutritional deficiencies (see earlier discussion), chronic infections such as *tuberculosis* may complicate their already stormy course.[2]

Hyperoxaluria frequently occurs in patients with severe steatorrhea, especially if associated with ileal resection or ileal disease, and may result in calcium oxalate urinary tract stones. These form only in patients whose colon remains in continuity with the small intestine, not in patients with ileostomies or jejunostomies, and excessive colonic absorption of oxalate appears to be responsible.[47] Two mechanisms have been implicated: (1) exposure of the colonic mucosa to excessive concentrations of bile salts and perhaps fatty acids increases its permeability to oxalate, and (2) excessive quantities of fatty acids in the gut form soaps with calcium, reducing its availability for formation of insoluble calcium oxalate and leading to persistence of soluble and absorbable oxalate in the colon. A low oxalate diet, oral calcium supplements, and maintenance of a high urinary volume are helpful in the control of this complication.

Patients with short gut or jejunoileal bypass may develop lactic acidosis. The elevated blood lactate is D-lactate, generated by anaerobic colonic bacteria, predominantly *Lactobacillus, Eubacterium,* and *Bifidobacterium.* Presumably these organisms are exposed to high concentrations of unabsorbed carbohydrate. Clinically, these patients present with central nervous system symptoms—particularly altered personality, confusion, and stupor. Diagnosis is made by finding a profound metabolic acidosis and elevated D-lactate levels in the serum. Treatment consists of reducing dietary carbohydrate and administering a broad-spectrum antimicrobial agent for 10 days to 2 weeks.[48]

References

1. Hocking, M. P., Duerson, M. C., O'Leary, J. P., and Woodward, E. R. Jejunoileal bypass for morbid obesity. N. Engl. J. Med. *308*:995, 1982.
2. Winawer, S. J., and Zamcheck, N. Pathophysiology of small intestinal resection in man. *In* Glass, G. B. J. (ed.). Progress in Gastroenterology. Vol. 1. New York, Grune & Stratton, 1968, p. 339.
3. Windsor, C. W. O., Fejfar, J., and Woodward, D. A. K. Gastric secretion after massive small bowel resection. Gut *10*:779, 1969.
4. Strauss, E., Gerson, C. D., and Yalow, R. S. Hypersecretion of gastrin associated with short bowel syndrome. Gastroenterology *66*:175, 1974.
5. Williams, N. S., Evans, P., and King, R. F. G. J. Gastric acid secretion and gastrin production in the short bowel syndrome. Gut *26*:914, 1985.
6. Chadwick, V. S., Gaginella, T. S., Carlson, G. L., Debongnie, J. C., Phillips, S. F., and Hofmann, A. F. Effect of molecular structure on bile acid–induced alterations in absorptive function, permeability and morphology in the perfused rabbit colon. J. Lab. Clin. Med. *94*:661, 1979.

7. Binder, H. J., Filburn, C., and Volpe, B. T. Bile salt alteration of colonic electrolytes induced by the bile acids: perfusion studies in man. J. Clin. Invest. *50*:1569, 1971.
8. Saunders, D. R., Hedges, J. R., Sillery, J., Matsumura, E. K., and Rubin, C. E. Morphological and functional effects of bile salts on rat colon. Gastroenterology *68*:1236, 1975.
9. Bright-Asare, P., and Binder, H. J. Stimulation of colonic secretion of water and electrolytes by hydroxy fatty acids. Gastroenterology *64*:81, 1973.
10. McJunkin, B., Fromm, H., Sarva, R. P., and Amin, P. Factors in the mechanism of diarrhea in bile acid malabsorption: fecal pH—a key determinant. Gastroenterology *80*:1454, 1981.
11. Hoffman, A. F., and Poley, J. R. Cholestyramine treatment of diarrhea associated with ileal resection. N. Engl. J. Med. *281*:397, 1969.
12. Dowling, R. H., Bell, G. D., and White, J. Lithogenic bile in patients with ileal dysfunction. Gut *13*:415, 1972.
13. Heaton, K. W., and Read, A. E. Gallstones in patients with disorders of the terminal ileum and disturbed bile salt metabolism. Br. Med. J. *3*:394, 1969.
14. Hill, G. L., Masir, W. S. J., and Goligher, J. C. Gallstones after ileostomy and ileal resection. Gut *16*:932, 1975.
15. King, C. E., and Toskes, P. P. Comparison of the 1-gram ^{14}C-xylose, 10-gram lactulose-H^2, and 80-gram glucose-H^2 breath tests in patients with small intestine bacterial overgrowth. Gastroenterology *91*:1447, 1986.
16. Weser, E. Nutritional aspects of malabsorption. Short gut adaptation. Am. J. Med. *67*:1014, 1979.
17. Williamson, R. C. N. Intestinal adaptation. Structural, functional and cytokinetic changes. N. Engl. J. Med. *298*:1393, 1978.
18. McCarthy, D. M., and Kim, Y. S. Changes in sucrase, enterokinase and peptide hydrolase after intestinal resection. J. Clin. Invest. *52*:942, 1973.
19. Altmann, G. G. Influence of starvation and refeeding on mucosal size and epithelial renewal in rat small intestine. Am. J. Anat. *133*:391, 1972.
20. Eastwood, G. L. Small bowel morphology and epithelial proliferation in intravenously alimented rabbits. Surgery *82*:613, 1977.
21. Levine, G. M., Deren, J. J., and Yezdimer, E. Small bowel resection: oral intake is the stimulus for hyperplasia. Am. J. Dig. Dis. *21*:441, 1976.
22. Weser, E., Babbitt, J., Hoban, M., and Vandeventer, A. Intestinal adaptation. Different growth responses to disaccharides compared with monosaccharides in rat small bowel. Gastroenterology *91*:1521, 1986.
23. Grey, V. L., Garofalo, C., Greenberg, G. R., and Morin, C. L. The adaptation of the small intestine after resection in response to free fatty acids. Am. J. Clin. Nutr. *40*:1235, 1984.
24. Levine, G. M. Nonspecific adaptation of jejunal amino acid uptake in the rat. Gastroenterology *91*:49, 1986.
25. Altmann, G. G. Influence of bile and pancreatic secretions on the size of the intestinal villi in the rat. Am. J. Anat. *132*:167, 1971.
26. Miazza, B. M., Al-Mukhtar, M. Y. T., Salmeron, M., Ghate, M. A., Felce-Dachez, M., Filali, A., Villet, R., Wright, N. A., Bloom, S. R., and Rambaud, J. C. Hyperenteroglucagonaemia and small intestinal mucosal growth after colonic perfusion in glucose in rats. Gut *26*:518, 1985.
27. Al-Mukhtar, M. Y. T., Sasgor, G. R., Ghatei, M. A., Bloom, S. R., and Wright, N. A. The role of pancreatico-biliary secretions in intestinal adaptation after resection, and its relationship to plasma enteroglucagon. Br. J. Surg. *70*:398, 1983.
28. Dworkin, L. D., Levine, G. M., Farber, N. J., and Spector, M. H. Small intestinal mass of the rat is partially determined by indirect effects of intraluminal nutrition. Gastroenterology *71*:626, 1976.
29. Bloom, S. R. Gut hormones in adaptation. Gut *28*(Suppl. 1):31, 1987.
30. Bloom, S. R. An enteroglucagon tumor. Gut *13*:520, 1972.
31. Ulshen, M. H., Lyn-Cook, L. E., and Raasch, R. H. Effects of intraluminal epidermal growth factor on mucosal proliferation in the small intestine of adult rats. Gastroenterology *91*:1134, 1986.
32. Luk, G. D., and Baylin, S. B. Inhibition of intestinal epithelial DNA synthesis and adaptive hyperplasia after jejunectomy in the rat by suppression of polyamine biosynthesis. J. Clin. Invest. *74*:698, 1984.
33. Weser, E., Bell, D., and Tawil, T. Effects of octapeptide-cholecystokinin, secretin, and glucagon on intestinal mucosal growth in parenterally nourished rats. Dig. Dis. Sci. *26*:409, 1981.
34. Dowling, R. H., and Gleason, M. H. Cell turnover following small bowel resection and bypass. Digestion *8*:190, 1973.
35. Porus, R. L. Epithelial hyperplasia following massive small bowel resection in man. Gastroenterology *48*:753, 1965.
36. Dowling, R. H., and Booth, C. C. Functional compensation after small bowel resection in man. Lancet *2*:146, 1966.
37. Jeejeebhoy, K. N., Langer, B., Tsallas, G., Chu, R. C., Kuksius, A., and Anderson, G. H. Total parenteral nutrition at home: studies in patients surviving four months to five years. Gastroenterology *71*:943, 1976.
38. Heizer, W. D., and Orringer, E. P. Parenteral nutrition at home for five years via arteriovenous fistulae. Supplemental intravenous feedings for a patient with severe short bowel syndrome. Gastroenterology *72*:527, 1977.
39. Gouttebel, M. C., Saint-Aubert, B., Astre, C., and Joyeux, H. Total parenteral nutrition needs in different types of short bowel syndrome. Dig. Dis. Sci. *31*:718, 1986.
40. Cortot, A., Fleming, C. R., and Malagelada, J. R. Improved nutrient absorption after cimetidine in short-bowel syndrome with gastric hypersecretion. N. Engl. J. Med. *300*:79, 1979.
41. Bochenek, W., Rodgers, J. B., and Balint, J. A. Effects of changes in dietary lipids on intestinal fluid loss in the short bowel syndrome. Ann. Intern. Med. *72*:205, 1970.
42. Woolf, G. M., Miller, C., Kurian, R., and Jeejeebhoy, K. N. Diet for patients with a short bowel: high fat or high carbohydrate? Gastroenterology *84*:823, 1983.
43. Sali, A., Murray, W. R., and MacKay, C. Aluminum hydroxide in bile-salt diarrhea. Lancet *2*:1051, 1977.
44. Clain, J. E., Malagelada, J. R., Chadwick, V. S., and Hofmann, A. F. Binding properties in vitro of antacids for conjugated bile acids. Gastroenterology *73*:556, 1977.
45. Thomson, J. S. Surgical therapy for the short bowel syndrome. J. Surg. Res. *39*:81, 1985.
46. Pritchard, T. J., and Kirkman, R. L. Small bowel transplantation. World J. Surg. *9*:860, 1985.
47. Dobbins, J. W., and Binder, H. J. Importance of the colon in enteric hyperoxaluria. N. Engl. J. Med. *296*:298, 1977.
48. Stolberg, L., Rolfe, R., Gitlin, N., Merritt, J., Mann, L., Jr., Linder, J., and Finegold, S. D-Lactic acidosis due to abnormal gut flora. N. Engl. J. Med. *306*:1344, 1982.

60 Food Sensitivity and Eosinophilic Gastroenteropathies

MELVIN B. HEYMAN

Adverse reactions to ingested substances have been noted throughout recorded time. Indeed, over 2000 years ago, Lucretius wrote, "What is food to one is to others bitter poison."[1] People carefully choose the foods they eat by personal preference, often with regard to previous positive or negative reactions. Investigation of the variety and pathophysiologic mechanisms of such reactions has been initiated only recently. This chapter discusses current information regarding the pathophysiology of and approach to gastrointestinal sensitivity to food.

Terminology

Terminology in the literature concerning adverse reactions to foods is confused. For the sake of uniformity, in this chapter the term food *sensitivity* reflects any adverse *immunologic* response (reaginic or nonreaginic) to ingested food. Food *allergy* will be used synonymously with food sensitivity. Food *anaphylaxis* is an acute food sensitivity reaction involving IgE antibody and chemical mediator activity. Food *intolerance* encompasses any adverse reaction to food, and here the implied mechanism is nonimmunologic.[2, 3] Food *toxicity* (poisoning) results from direct nonimmunologic action of an ingested food or food additive, which may be contained within the food or released by organisms contaminating the food. An *anaphylactoid reaction* to a food or food additive results from nonimmune release of chemical mediators and mimics food anaphylaxis. Some food substances contain natural or added chemicals that produce adverse *pharmacologic reactions,* whereas other foods or food additives result in *metabolic reactions* owing to aberrant metabolism by the host recipient.[4] The term "*pseudoallergy*" occasionally is applied to nonimmunologically mediated reactions to food.

Types of Reactions to Food

Clinical reactions to specific foods have been well described, although the mechanisms involved are poorly understood. The clinical presentation may be an expression of local gastrointestinal reactions (for example, diarrhea or gastrointestinal bleeding) or of systemic allergic reactions (such as urticaria or anaphylaxis). The severity and nature of the allergic response is dependent on the sensitivity of the patient and the amount of allergen ingested.

Two general types of food sensitivity reactions are encountered. *Immediate (anaphylaxic) reactions* to ingestants are usually dramatic, easily recognized, and often very serious; these include urticaria and laryngeal edema, occasionally leading to asphyxia. Because they can be life-threatening, early recognition and therapy are absolutely essential. IgE-mediated, nonanaphylactic *intermediate reactions* occurring within two hours of antigen exposure are less dangerous and are manifested by gastrointestinal symptoms, urticaria, asthma, and rhinitis. By comparison, the more prevalent *delayed responses* (non–IgE-mediated), appearing at least two hours after antigen exposure, can be difficult to diagnose and may produce nonspecific and diverse symptoms, such as failure to thrive, chronic (in some subjects, migraine) headaches, recurrent abdominal pain, fatigue, nocturnal enuresis, pain and swelling of joints, aphthous ulcers, seizures, and chronic respiratory symptoms often misdiagnosed as infections.[5]

GUT DEFENSE MECHANISMS

A complex arrangement of specialized immunologic tissue protects the human body from the environment within the gastrointestinal lumen (see pp. 114–144). Peyer's patches are lymphoid aggregates that contain B and T lymphocytes; most of the T lymphocytes are of the suppressor-cytotoxic subset. Many lymphocytes are distributed throughout the epithelium and lamina propria. Microfold membrane (M) cells are located in the epithelium overlying the Peyer's patches. Immunoglobulins are derived primarily from plasma cells located around the crypts, with some contribution from the circulating pool. IgA is the predominant immunoglobulin, found in over 80 per cent of intestinal plasma cells. IgM and IgE are found fairly commonly, and IgG rarely in gut plasma cells. IgE does not predominate in the mucosa of normal subjects, but it increases in patients with type 1 hypersensitivity reactions.[6]

The Mucosal Barrier

The intestinal mucosa functions as a barrier to foreign substances. The integrity of this barrier is vital to protect the host against intrusion of foreign substances into intestinal cells and, ultimately, into the remainder of the body. The mucosal barrier consists of both nonimmunologic and immunologic components (Table 60–1).[7] Nonimmune mechanisms inhibit absorption of

Table 60–1. COMPONENTS OF THE GUT MUCOSAL BARRIER

Immunologic:
Local immunoglobulins
Secretory IgA
Local cell-mediated immune mechanisms
Gut-associated lymphoid tissue (GALT)
Mast cell activation
Nonimmunologic:
Normal intestinal flora
Gastric barrier (acid, pepsin)
Intestinal secretions (glycoproteins, glycolipids, bile salts, lysozymes)
Epithelial cell renewal
Gastrointestinal peristalsis
Hepatic reticuloendothelial system ("filter")

Adapated from Stern, M., and Walker, W. A. Pediatr. Clin. North Am. *32*:471, 1985.

ingested antigens generally by hindering exposure of these substances to the mucosa or, if antigens cross the mucosa, to immunologically active sensitizing cells. Primarily involved are the hydrolytic gastric barrier; native intestinal flora that inhibits overgrowth of pathogens; intestinal secretions, which cover and protect the mucosa; gastrointestinal peristalsis, which minimizes the time antigens are exposed to the mucosa; and the reticuloendothelial system, particularly in the liver, which filters absorbed substances from portal venous blood.[7] Glycoproteins overlying the mucosa may be especially important by inhibiting attachment of microorganisms to epithelial cells and by interacting with allergens and enterotoxins to minimize epithelial cell penetration.

Of the immune mechanisms, secretory IgA is the primary immunoglobulin preventing absorption of incompletely digested food antigens. Circulating immune complexes and milk precipitins have been found in the majority of subjects with IgA deficiency,[8] supporting the important role for secretory IgA in the protective mechanism. Furthermore, intraepithelial and mucosal lymphocytes inhibit local and systemic immune reactions to absorbed food particles. High levels of IgE found in mesenteric lymph nodes may also act as a secondary line of defense.

Antigen Uptake and Sensitization. Deficiencies in the gastrointestinal protective barrier system may result from immaturity of the gastrointestinal tract (in premature infants), inherited abnormalities, particularly those relating to the gut immune system and mucosal abnormalities, and injury to the mucosa from chemotherapy and irradiation therapy, ischemic bowel damage, and infection (bacterial, viral, parasitic, and other types) (Table 60–2).

Mucosal Leakage. Immaturity of the gastrointestinal mucosa in infants, especially premature newborns, enhances the risk of sensitization owing to increased permeability of the intestinal mucosa and a poorly developed secretory IgA system.[9, 10] Food sensitivity appears to resolve by 1 to 3 years of age, when the gastrointestinal tract has more mature barrier function, at which time children tolerate previously offending agents.

The mechanism of absorption of macromolecules across the intestinal mucosa underlying sensitivity reactions in infants and young children is unclear. Macromolecules appear to be absorbed across intestinal epithelium by *pinocytosis,* by *transport* directly through and between cells (persorption), and by active *M cell uptake.* The general mechanism involves endocytosis of macromolecules, a process that is energy dependent. Membrane-bound vesicles (phagosomes) containing the macromolecules combine with lysosomes to form large vacuoles (phagolysosomes), the site of normal intracellular digestion of macromolecules. Some of the ingested macromolecules may escape digestion and migrate to the basolateral surface of the cell. Exocytosis (reverse endocytosis) subsequently results in deposition of these macromolecules into the intercellular space[11, 12] (Fig. 60–1).

Increased antigen absorption has been demonstrated after acute gastroenteritis clinically in animals as well as in infants and in organ culture, as detected by horseradish peroxidase.[13–15] Radiation and chemotherapy cause intestinal mucosal damage, which may predispose to increased antigen uptake.[16] Similarly, a high osmotic load owing to an elemental diet or alcohol may damage the intestinal surface sufficiently to enhance antigen uptake.[17, 18] Increased macromolecular uptake is also found in helminthic infestations of the gastrointestinal tract.[6] Anaphylaxis has also been shown to predispose to increased antigen uptake in animals.[19] Except in celiac sprue, small intestinal damage from food ingestion has not been documented in adults (see pp. 1134–1152) (Table 60–2).

Once macromolecules cross the gastrointestinal barrier, sensitivity reactions may be caused by excess antigen entry, resulting in overstimulation of the immune system.[20] Alternatively, minimally increased antigen entry may result in antigen exposure sufficient to stimulate a reaginic response, which normally is suppressed.

Reactions to Absorbed Antigens. Absorbed antigens induce mucosal and systemic immune reactions, which may be protective or harmful. The mucosal immunity involves sensitization and production of specific secretory IgA to retard further absorption of macromole-

Table 60–2. FACTORS LEADING TO ENHANCED UPTAKE OF MACROMOLECULES ACROSS THE INTESTINAL MUCOSA

Local antibody deficiency
Secretory IgA deficiency
Altered mucosal barrier
Changes in surface membrane charge
Inflammation
Ulceration
Lysosomal dysfunction
?Storage diseases
?Corticosteroids
Intraluminal factors
Decreased gastric acidity
Pancreatic insufficiency

Modified from Walker, W. A. *In* Johnson, L. R. (ed.), Physiology of the Gastrointestinal Tract. New York, Raven Press, 1981, p. 1282.

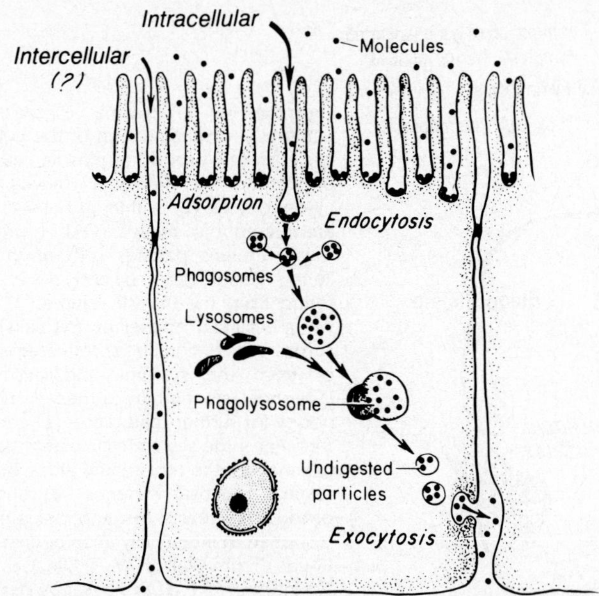

Figure 60–1. General mechanisms for the uptake and transport of macromolecules by the intestine. In *intracellular* uptake, after adsorption and endocytosis by the microvillus membrane, macromolecules are transported in small vesicles and larger phagosomes. Intracellular digestion occurs when lysosomes combine to form phagolysosomes. Intact molecules that remain after digestion are deposited in the intercellular space by reverse endocytosis (exocytosis). Alternatively, in *intercellular* uptake, macromolecules may cross the "tight junction" barrier between cells and diffuse into the intercellular space. (From Walker, W. A., and Isselbacher, K. J. Uptake and transport of macromolecules by the intestine. Gastroenterology *67*:531–550. Copyright by Williams & Wilkins, 1974.)

cules by binding to food antigens. Thus, IgA deficiency predisposes to enhanced antigen uptake (Fig. 60–2). Systemically, antibodies to food antigens can often be found in the plasma of nonallergic persons. Food antibodies therefore do not always indicate food allergies but may also have protective functions that currently are unclear.[6]

In most persons, food substances normally cross the mucosa. Systemic T suppressor cells may induce systemic tolerance to antigens and possibly suppress harmful cell-mediated immune reactions in the gastrointestinal tract; however, T cell suppression and tolerance to food antigens (which usually develop in normal subjects) may fail to develop in food-sensitive persons.[7] Thus, absorbed antigens result in signs and symptoms caused by an immune system that is insufficiently modulated.

SENSITIVITY (ALLERGIC) REACTIONS TO FOODS

Definition of Types of Reactions

Food sensitivity reactions are characterized by local gastrointestinal or systemic symptoms and signs subsequent to food ingestion, caused by an immunologically mediated reaction originating within the gastrointestinal tract.[21] The gastrointestinal symptoms may be local effects or may be responses to neurologic or endocrinologic stimuli resulting from the effect of foods on another target organ (e.g., vomiting in migraine induced by food sensitivity).[21] Alternatively, food sensitivity responses resulting from entrance of food substances into the circulation via the gastrointestinal tract may be devoid of gastrointestinal symptoms. Thus, symptoms of skin and respiratory tract involvement frequently accompany gastrointestinal signs and symptoms.

Because they are not based on an immunologic response, neither *toxic reactions* to mushrooms, shellfish, or bacterial toxins (among other substances) nor *idiosyncratic reactions* to galactose in patients with galactosemia and to beans in patients with favism are "food allergies." Furthermore, the symptoms and signs of reactions to chemicals found naturally in foods (e.g., tyramine in cheddar cheese, chocolate, caffeine, and histamine in tuna, sauerkraut, and cooked pork meats) or food additives (e.g., monosodium glutamate and nitrite compounds) are also unrelated to the immune system (see p. 1119). Specific food intolerances of certain malabsorption syndromes (e.g., to lactose in lactase deficiency and to gluten in celiac sprue) are not discussed in this chapter (see pp. 269 and 1138–1140).

Epidemiology

Precise prevalence data of responses to ingested foods are not available, as many reactions are unreported or are subclinical. Immediate and delayed hypersensitivity reactions to food conceivably are present in as high as 10 to 20 per cent of the population in the United States, or between 25,000,000 and 50,000,000 persons.[5]

Patients with food allergy often have a positive family history for allergic disorders. Twin studies show inconclusive evidence for a genetic predisposition for food sensitivity, but the environmental setting and feeding practices early in life appear to influence the development of food sensitivity significantly.

Tests can frequently identify patients with type 1 (IgE-mediated) reactions. However, probably fewer than 10 to 30 per cent of food reactions are of type 1. Delayed reactions to food account for the remaining 70 to 90 per cent and are much more difficult to document.

Prevalence data must be viewed with the realization that many nonimmune reactions to food are often interpreted as allergic reactions. Examples of such nonimmune reactions to ingested substances include lactose intolerance from milk and milk products, malabsorption, reactions to caffeine, food poisoning, psychologic influences, and idiosyncratic reactions.[5]

The prototype for hypersensitivity reactions to ingested foods is cow's milk protein sensitivity. The frequency of cow's milk protein intolerance is estimated to range from 0.3 to 7.5 per cent[4] and may be as high as 25 per cent in atopic children with eczema

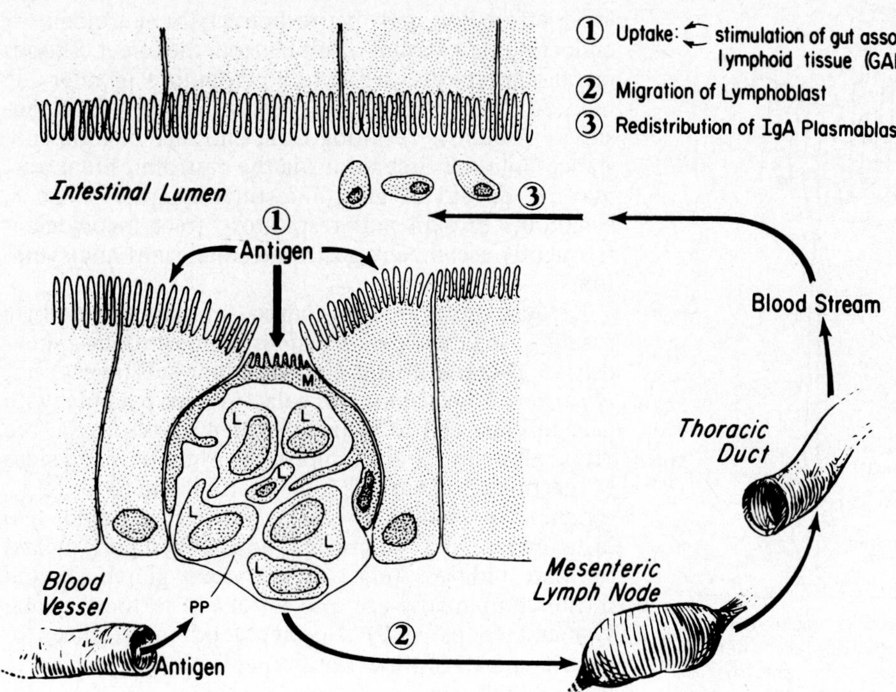

Figure 60–2. IgA plasma cell cycle. Schematic representation of the cell cycle for IgA-producing plasma cells populating the intestinal mucosa. Lymphocytes (L) within gut-associated lymphoid tissues (GALT), primarily Peyer's patches (PP) of the ileum, are stimulated by antigens entering from the intestinal lumen (1) via specialized epithelium (M cells), across conventional absorptive cells, or from the systemic circulation. Lymphoblasts migrate to mesenteric nodes for further maturation (2) and then enter the systemic circulation as plasmablasts to redistribute along intestinal mucosal surfaces (3) and produce secretory IgA antibodies in response to intestinally absorbed antigens. (From Walker, W. A. Clin. Gastroenterol. *15*:1, 1986. Used by permission.)

or asthma.[22] It is manifested most commonly in the first 6 months of life, with over 50 per cent of cases presenting in the first month. Cow's milk protein sensitivity rarely occurs in older children or adults and should not be confused with the much more common entity, lactose intolerance (see p. 269). Gluten-sensitive enteropathy (celiac sprue) is discussed on pages 1134 to 1152.

Etiology and Pathogenesis of Food Sensitivity Reactions

Food allergies are caused by over 6000 antigens, 400 of which are nutrient foodstuff, and may involve any organ system in the body.[5] This contrasts dramatically with inhalant allergies, in which respiratory symptoms are the response to approximately 150 dust, pollen, and epidermal allergens.

Food antigens cause gastrointestinal or systemic allergic and toxic reactions after traversing the mucosal barrier. Macromolecular uptake of antigens is enhanced by several conditions, listed in Table 60–2. These factors were discussed in more detail earlier.

Food Allergens. Allergic responses in the gastrointestinal tract depend on a reaction of the immune system to an ingested substance. The most common food allergens are listed in Table 60–3. Nonprotein substances have not been demonstrated to cause allergic phenomena, although any ingested substance may incite a nonallergic response. Food allergens tend to be glycoproteins (molecular weight, 18,000 to 36,000), which induce immediate hypersensitivity responses when small amounts are injected subcutaneously. Many food allergens are resistant to heat and proteolytic enzymes. Heat treatment will denature and reduce the antigenicity of some proteins, but conversely it may increase antigenicity of other proteins.

Food allergens known to induce *IgE-mediated reactions* include substances found in cow's milk, soybeans, egg white, codfish, cottonseed, crab, shrimp, peanuts, and tomatoes. Casein, alpha-lactalbumin, beta-lactoglobulin, bovine gamma globulin, and bovine serum albumin, the five most common proteins in cow's milk, are highly allergenic.[23] Milk proteins often retain allergenicity after enzymatic digestion,[24] and the process of enzymatic digestion of milk proteins with pepsin and trypsin has even been shown to uncover some new antigens.[25, 26] Psyllium, commonly ingested as a laxative preparation, has also been documented to cause IgE-mediated anaphylaxis.[27]

Any food should be suspected as an etiologic agent in the individual patient. Once a food has been impli-

Table 60–3. COMMON FOOD ALLERGENS

Allergen	Percentage*
Milk	65
Chocolate, cola	45
Corn	30
Legumes	26
Egg	26
Citrus	25
Tomato	16
Wheat, rice	11
Pork	10
Cinnamon	8

*Percentage of patients with known food allergy who react to the offending allergen tested.

Other foods include: fish, potato, onion, apple, beef, crustaceans (especially shrimp), black pepper, and banana.

Adapted from Speer, F. Food Allergy. Littleton, MA, PSG Publishing Company, 1978, pp. 111–113.

Table 60–4. CLASSIFICATION OF IMMUNE RESPONSES UNDERLYING HYPERSENSITIVITY REACTIONS

Immediate Hypersensitivity Reactions:		
Type 1 Anaphylactic		
	Mediators:	IgE, eosinophil, mast cell
		Histamine, heparin
		Slow-reacting substance A
		Bradykinins
		5-Hydroxytryptamine
	Reactions:	Systemic anaphylaxis
		Respiratory symptoms (asthma, rhinitis)
		Dermatologic symptoms (urticaria)
		Gastrointestinal symptoms
Type 2. Cytolytic or Cytotoxic		
	Mediators:	Cytotoxic or cytolytic
		Antibodies versus cell-associated antigen; complement activation
	Reactions:	Foreign substance (drug, food) which attaches to erythrocyte, leukocyte, or platelet membrane
		Transfusion reactions
		Autoimmune hemolytic anemia
Type 3. Toxic Complex		
	Mediators:	Antigen-antibody complexes
		Chemotactic factors
		Vasoactive amines
	Reactions:	Serum sickness (systemic)
		Arthus reaction (local)
		Gastrointestinal symptoms
Delayed Hypersensitivity Reactions		
Type 4. Cell-mediated hypersensitivity		
	Mediators:	Sensitized T cells
		Chemotactic factors
		Lymphokines
		Lymphocyte migration inhibition factor (LIF)
	Reactions:	Mixed cellular reactions
		Dermatologic symptoms
		Gastrointestinal symptoms

cated to cause the clinical problems in a patient, botanically similar foods that may have cross-reacting antigens should be considered as well. (Lists of related and cross-reacting foods can be found elsewhere.[4, 28])

Immune Mechanisms of Hypersensitivity (Table 60–4). Food sensitivities could be mediated by any of the four classic hypersensitivity reactions, although type 2 hypersensitivity reactions have not been linked definitively to food-related allergic reactions.

Type 1 Hypersensitivity Reactions. The *IgE-mediated mast cell-dependent immediate hypersensitivity* (type 1) *reaction* accounts for most of the clinical manifestations of food allergy.

IgE antibodies to specific foods, especially cow's milk protein, wheat, soy, nuts, eggs, and seafood, can be detected in many patients by the radioallergosorbent test (RAST). Specific IgE antibodies determined by RAST correlate well with clinical signs and symptoms of immediate-onset hypersensitivity reactions to food antigens in some subjects.[2, 29] However, IgE antibody to suspected allergens is not detectable in many patients with immediate hypersensitivity reactions. Additionally, IgE antibodies occasionally are found in patients with delayed hypersensitivity reactions. Thus, precise determination of the type of immunologic reaction to a food antigen in an individual patient may be difficult.

IgE appears to interact with gastrointestinal mucosal and circulating mast cells to cause a local and systemic immune response by inducing mast cell degranulation. Degranulation of mast cells releases chemical mediators of inflammation, particularly histamine and heparin, which account for many of the signs and symptoms occurring after exposure to offending ingestants. The proposed pathogenesis of the mast cell–IgE-mediated immune reaction is discussed further on pages 1123 to 1124.

Type 2 Hypersensitivity Reactions. *Cytotoxic and cytolytic reactions* (type 2) to food antigens have not been well demonstrated in patients with allergic reactions to ingestants. Type 2 reactions are initiated by attachment of a foreign substance (antigen) to a cell wall. Antibody to the antigen coats the sensitized cell, and subsequent destruction of the cell is caused by complement activation or phagocytosis by the reticuloendothelial system. The Mexican fava bean, for example, causes this type of reaction with red blood cells in patients with glucose-6-phosphate dehydrogenase (G-6-PD) deficiency, and some medications and endotoxins (e.g., from *Salmonella* organisms) may cause a hemolytic anemia by this mechanism.

Type 3 Hypersensitivity Reactions. *Immune complex–complement mediated hypersensitivity reactions* (type 3) probably cause intermediate and delayed responses seen several hours to days after exposure to food allergens.[30] IgE and IgG complexes are detectable in food-allergic patients. These complexes accumulate in the gastrointestinal mucosa and in other organs, leading to a local inflammatory response, complement activation, and anaphylotoxin generation. Extraintestinal reactions may be due to absorbed antigens or antigen-antibody complexes carried in the circulation to organs such as the skin or respiratory tract.[31] Precipitating serum antibodies are found more commonly in patients with malabsorption or pulmonary involvement (hemosiderosis) than in atopic forms of protein sensitivity.[31] IgA complexes are found in normal subjects and are cleared rapidly.

Type 4 Hypersensitivity Reactions. Sensitized circulating lymphocytes mediate *delayed (cell-mediated) hypersensitivity reactions* (type 4). Exposure of sensitized lymphocytes to food antigens causes release of lymphokines responsible for the cell-mediated immune response. Lymphokines are relatively low molecular weight effector molecules, such as macrophage migration inhibition factor (MIF), lymphotoxin (which inhibits cell division), skin-reactive factor, and blastogenic factor. Some of these factors are detected by recently developed *in vitro* tests for delayed food-hypersensitivity reactions (see p. 1121).

Eosinophilic Infiltration. Eosinophils migrate into affected tissues by several processes.[32] Inflammatory mediators, including the vasoactive amines, alter vascular permeability and allow migration of eosinophils through the vessel walls by diapedesis. Chemotactic factors derived from complement activation, immune complexes, and mast cell degranulation as well as lymphocyte secretory factors (lymphokines) promote accumulation of eosinophils in tissues. The pathologic role of eosinophils in the gastrointestinal tract is discussed on pages 1123 to 1131.

Clinical Manifestations of Food Sensitivity

Clinical manifestations of food sensitivity range from acute anaphylactic reactions, which may lead to death as a result of airway obstruction, to minor symptoms (Table 60–5). The extreme variability may make diagnosis difficult. The characteristics of the clinical presentation depend on the type and amount of food ingested, the age of the subject, and often the organ site of initial exposure to the offending agent (usually gastrointestinal tract, skin, or lungs). In infancy, many of the gastrointestinal syndromes associated with ingested foods are transient. Food allergies, particularly those involving other systems, tend to be more persistent and permanent in older children and adults.

Table 60–5. CLINICAL MANIFESTATIONS OF FOOD SENSITIVITY

- Gastrointestinal
  - Vomiting
  - Diarrhea
  - Protein-losing enteropathy
  - Malabsorption
  - Abdominal pain
  - Rectal bleeding; proctocolitis
  - Edema of lips, palate, or oral mucosa
  - Constipation
  - Pruritis ani
- Respiratory
  - Nasal stuffiness and sneezing
  - Allergic rhinitis
  - Serous otitis media
  - Chronic cough; bronchitis
  - Asthma; wheezing
  - Airway obstruction
- Skin
  - Atopic eczema
  - Angioedema
  - Urticaria
  - Localized swellings
- Urinary tract?
  - Enuresis
  - Nephrotic syndrome; albuminuria
- Neuropsychiatric syndromes?
  - Headache (migraine)
  - Hyperkinesis
  - Learning disorders
  - Tension-fatigue syndrome
  - Altered spatial perception
- Arthritis or Arthralgias?
- Secondary effects
  - Iron deficiency anemia
  - Failure to thrive
  - Malnutrition
  - Hypoproteinemia
  - Thrombocytopenia
  - Eosinophilia

Data from references 21, 125, and 126.

Acute Reactions to Foods. Anaphylaxis with urticaria and potentially fatal laryngeal edema is the most severe acute reaction and is seen after exposure to specific proteins. Cow's and soy milk, shellfish, wheat, egg, nuts, and chocolate are the antigens most commonly implicated (Table 60–3). Other immediate reactions involving the gastrointestinal tract include vomiting, sometimes with eczema, urticaria, or swollen lips and tongue associated with cow's milk sensitivity; vomiting with diarrhea, abdominal pain, and nausea with egg sensitivity; acute abdominal pain with fish sensitivity; and abdominal pain and oral mucosal lesions with peanut ingestion. Some persons react with vomiting, urticaria, and wheezing to several different food substances. These subjects often have a family history of atopy, peripheral eosinophilia, elevated total serum IgE, and positive RAST and skin tests to specific foods.

Delayed Reactions to Foods. Patients with delayed-onset hypersensitivity are reported to manifest joint or muscle pain, fatigue, tension, serous otitis, or altered spatial perception in addition to signs and symptoms similar to those seen in acute reactions (Table 60–5). Proving that the delayed hypersensitivity reactions are attributable to specific foods is often difficult.

Acute gastroenteritis occasionally precedes the development of delayed gastrointestinal reactions to foods, although the relationship of these two intestinal disorders is unclear. Acquired food allergy may prolong symptoms of a gastroenteritis. Altered gut immune function, such as transient IgA deficiency or increased antigen entry across damaged enterocytes,[33] may result in food sensitivity. Some foods cause acute reactions, which progress to chronic, delayed allergic responses.

Sensitivity Reactions to Specific Proteins in Infants. In infancy, food-sensitive enteropathies have been shown to be induced by cow's milk, wheat (gluten), and soy protein. By injuring mucosal epithelial cells, acute severe gastroenteritis increases the ability of these proteins to enter the circulation, predisposing young children to sensitivity to these antigens. Fortunately, sensitivity reactions to fish, rice, egg,[34] and chicken meat[35] tend to be transient.

Cow's Milk Protein Sensitivity. Cow's milk protein sensitivity usually appears within the first 6 months of life and may present acutely or with gradual onset of vomiting, diarrhea, and other gastrointestinal symptoms after introduction of cow's milk protein into the diet. A family history of atopy or cow's milk protein sensitivity is uncommon. When infants present with acute symptoms, protein sensitivity must be distinguished from acute gastroenteritis and from postenteritis lactose malabsorption. As discussed earlier, infectious gastroenteritis may particularly predispose young infants to uptake of an offending protein and subsequent sensitivity reactions.[11] Occasionally infants present with an acute or chronic mild to severe *ulcerative proctocolitis,* having blood-tinged stools or bloody diarrhea.[36]

A high index of suspicion is necessary to diagnose insidious onset of protein sensitivity in infants. Children may manifest *chronic diarrhea* with failure to thrive and malabsorption, suggestive of celiac disease or cystic fibrosis.

Patients with milk protein sensitivity have been documented to have type 1 or type 3 hypersensitivity reactions (Table 60–4); however, the pathogenesis in many patients with milk or soy protein intolerance is unknown.

Soy Protein Sensitivity. Soy protein sensitivity is similar to cow's milk protein sensitivity and may exist alone or as a sequel to cow's milk protein sensitivity.[37] Twenty to 50 per cent of infants with reactions to cow's milk protein also have adverse responses to soy protein.

Transient Gluten Sensitivity. Some infants with *chronic diarrhea* respond to a gluten-free diet as if they had celiac sprue. However, in contrast to patients with celiac sprue, these children tolerate a normal diet without clinical or pathologic abnormalities by about age two years.[21]

Colic. *Infantile colic* is a syndrome of paroxysms of prolonged crying and irritability in the first three to four months of life. Abdominal discomfort is often thought to cause these symptoms and has been surmised to result from sensitivity to ingested proteins, mainly cow's milk. However, studies are not conclusive.[21, 38] Although some infants with cow's milk protein sensitivity have colic, not all infants with colic have cow's milk protein sensitivity.

There is little evidence to support reports that *irritable bowel syndrome*[39] (see pp. 1435–1477) and *chronic constipation*[40] (see pp. 331–368) are related to food hypersensitivity reactions.

Extraintestinal Reactions to Ingested Antigens. Manifestations of extraintestinal involvement are prevalent in food sensitivity reactions. In individual patients, the *respiratory tract* may be involved to a greater extent than the gastrointestinal tract. This is particularly true in children, in whom rhinitis, chronic serous otitis media, and cough are common. Other respiratory symptoms secondary to food sensitivity include asthma, bronchitis, chronic or recurrent pulmonary disease, and upper airway obstruction by pharyngeal lymphoid hyperplasia.[41] Heiner and coworkers reported a nonreaginic syndrome of chronic respiratory disease, characterized by pulmonary infiltrates and hemosiderosis, wheezing, tachypnea, chronic rhinitis, otitis media, failure to thrive, and anemia due to gastrointestinal blood loss. Patients responded to withdrawal of cow's milk or, occasionally, peanuts and pork.[42]

Immediate *dermatologic reactions* to ingested antigens are frequent and include urticaria, angioedema, and lip swelling. Food antigens also cause chronic urticaria, but an association of a specific ingestant to the reaction is usually difficult to establish.[43] The relationship of *atopic dermatitis* to food sensitivity is controversial; double-blind studies have demonstrated that elimination of milk, eggs, peanuts, wheat, and other foods from the diets of possibly as many as 70 to 75 per cent of children with atopic dermatitis may provide relief of symptoms.[44–46]

Sketchy evidence suggests a possible link between food sensitivity and *psychologic alterations.* Soy and rice were related to gastrointestinal and neurologic disturbances in an infant,[47] and gluten withdrawal resulted in a dramatic response in some schizophrenic patients.[48] Similarly, the association of migraine, behavioral disorders such as hyperactivity,[49] sudden infant death syndrome, and urinary and cardiovascular disease with food allergies is tenuous at best. Controlled studies are necessary before conclusions can be made regarding the role of food allergy with these clinical problems.

Nonimmunologic Reactions. A brief comment should be made concerning nonfood substances which, when ingested, can induce reactions often confused with food allergy. Food contaminants, such as mold (on fruits, cheeses, yoghurts, and wines), bacteria, bacterial toxins, and drugs are included in this group of substances. Scombroid poisoning follows ingestion of spoiled tuna or related fish containing high levels of histamine and saurine.[50, 51] Food additives, such as dyes (tartrazine), preservatives (sodium benzoate, sulfites), antimicrobials, and flavors (monosodium glutamate), cause phenomena often indistinguishable from food sensitivity reactions. Finally, foods containing pharmacologically active agents may precipitate episodes that also resemble allergic reactions. Such substances include vasoactive amines (e.g., pineapples, wine, banana [peel], and avocados), methylxanthines, chocolate, and alcohol[52] (see pp. 1986–1987).

Diagnosis of Food Sensitivity (Fig. 60–3)

Criteria. Three criteria must be satisfied to diagnose an allergic response to food:

1. Identification of an offending antigen and amelioration of symptoms on withdrawal of the antigen.
2. Reappearance of symptoms on re-exposure to the antigen.
3. Documentation of an immunologic mechanism.

Diagnosis depends on recognition of clinical features that may be produced by ingested substances. A thorough history and physical examination is often the most important and informative step in the process of evaluating patients for potential food sensitivities and in excluding other disorders in the differential diagnosis (Table 60–6). All intake, including foods with additives and potential contaminants, the source and method of preparation, and the timing of signs and symptoms with consumption should be considered in detail. A dietary diary, attempting to correlate reactions with ingested substances, is especially helpful in this assessment and may provide useful clues for selection of appropriate *in vitro* antigen testing.

Objective Tests of Food Sensitivity. Dependence on history alone to make a diagnosis of food sensitivity is often unreliable. Therefore, objective tests of food sensitivity reactions are desirable. However, none of the tests described in this section has proved to be 100 per cent free of false negative or false positive results.

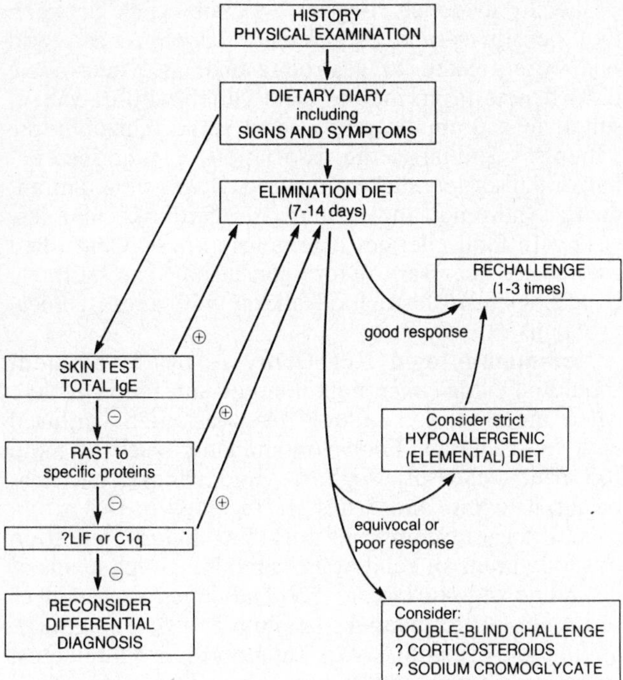

Figure 60–3. Suggested protocol for evaluation of suspected food sensitivity. (Modified from McCarty, E. P., and Frick, O. L. J. Pediatr. *102*:645, 1983. Used by permission.)

Food Challenge. Double-blind, placebo-controlled food challenge is the most definitive method and has the lowest false-positive rate for diagnosing food sensitivity.[46] It is extremely useful for excluding the presence of reactions to specific food antigens. However, differentiation of immunologic from nonimmunologic reactions to foods or food additives is not possible by this method. The patient must be monitored carefully after the challenge, as patients may experience severe reactions to the ingested substance. Other tests that are not as time-consuming or risky are preferable.

Skin Tests. *Direct skin testing* is the most sensitive method for detecting specific IgE antibodies in the skin. This test is performed by inoculating small amounts of food antigen extracts and control solutions into the skin (by prick, scratch, or intradermal injection). A positive response is indicated by induration and erythema (wheal and flare) within 20 minutes. Correlation of direct skin testing with double-blind food challenges varies depending on the study conditions. One study in patients with atopic dermatitis demonstrated that skin testing is a reliable means of eliminating immediate food hypersensitivity but, because of a high false positive rate, is a poor indicator of sensitizing antigens.[53]

Immediate-reacting skin tests to proteins are most often positive in patients sensitive to milk, eggs, peanuts, soy, fish, and shellfish. Direct skin tests will demonstrate the presence of reaginic (IgE) antibody in the skin but do not always indicate specific sensitivity to antigens in the gastrointestinal tract. Skin tests may remain positive even though subjects are able to tolerate sensitizing foods without symptoms. A negative skin test usually excludes an IgE-mediated hypersensitivity reaction to a particular food but does not eliminate a delayed hypersensitivity reaction. For instance, only approximately 10 per cent of milk sensitive individuals demonstrate positive skin tests.[54]

Indirect skin testing (Prausnitz-Kustner or P-K transfer test) is performed by introducing serum from a sensitized subject into the skin of a nonallergic volunteer. Subsequent oral challenge or a local direct skin test with antigen at the injection site will produce a wheal and flare response if the serum contains specific reaginic antibodies to the antigen. This test is rarely used owing to its inherent risk of transferring hepatitis antigen or other contaminants.[4]

Tests for Antibodies. The radioallergosorbent test (RAST) detects serum IgE antibodies to specific antigens. It is especially useful in patients with severe skin disease, such as extensive eczema, in whom skin testing would be contraindicated. RAST is less sensitive and does not correlate well with skin tests except for eggs, nuts, and fish. Patients with cow's milk protein sensi-

Table 60–6. DIFFERENTIAL DIAGNOSIS OF FOOD SENSITIVITY REACTIONS

Gastrointestinal
Feeding problems
Disaccharidase deficiency, primary or secondary
Gastroesophageal reflux
Cystic fibrosis
Celiac disease
Ulcerative colitis
Crohn's disease
Eosinophilic gastroenteropathy
Parasitic infestation
Galactosemia
Shwachman syndrome
Lead poisoning
Psychologic factors
Pulmonary
Foreign body
Congenital anomalies (e.g., vascular ring, tracheomalacia)
Cystic fibrosis
Alpha-1-antitrypsin deficiency
Hypersensitivity
Aspiration pneumonia
Bronchopulmonary aspergillosis
Asthma unrelated to food
Skin
Irritation rashes
Seborrhea
Ichthyosis
Acrodermatitis enteropathica
Leiner disease
Nonallergic urticarial syndromes
Nasal
Eosinophilic nonallergic rhinitis
Vasomotor rhinitis
Immunologic
Immunoglobulin deficiencies
Combined immunodeficiency
Complement deficiency
Hereditary angioedema
Food additives and toxins
Other allergens, penicillin, dyes
Natural vasoactive amines
Monosodium glutamate
Food contaminants, preservatives

Modified from McCarty, E. P., and Frick, O. L. J. Pediatr. *102*:624, 1983.

tivity (milk-sensitive enteropathy) often have normal total serum IgE levels and negative RAST for antigen-specific IgE.[55] In contrast, IgG anti-milk antibodies are commonly detectable.[55] IgG_4 RAST has been proposed to diagnose food allergy in some subjects, but its clinical usefulness requires confirmation. The enzyme-linked immunosorbent assay (ELISA) test can also be used to detect food-specific serum IgE antibodies.

Cytotoxic IgG antibodies, resulting in type 2 hypersensitivity reactions, can be detected with a double-antibody assay using a solid-phase carrier (an APT-activated disk) containing various food antigens.[56] This test is seldom used in clinical situations.

Eosinophils and mast cells in the nasal smear may be helpful to characterize an IgE-mediated cause for atopic disease, but this test has low sensitivity.[57]

Tests of Cell Mediated Immune Reactions. Leukocyte inhibition factor (LIF), which causes white blood cell migration, and solid-phase C1q binding to test for levels of C1q, the protein initiating the complement cascade, have been proposed and may be useful as *in vitro* tests of delayed hypersensitivity when skin test results are negative or challenge test results are equivocal.[2] More data are needed, however, to assess the reliability, especially the false negative and false positive rates, of these tests.

Relating Foods to Sensitivity Reactions

Elimination and Challenge Tests. Suspected antigens should be eliminated from the diet for 7 to 14 days to document relief of symptoms. When multiple or unknown foods are implicated, a strict hypoallergenic diet may become necessary (Table 60–7). Unequivocal diagnosis of a specific agent causing food allergy is made by rechallenge with the food substance leading to demonstrable relapse, often with associated laboratory abnormalities. Patients, especially infants, should be observed closely during a challenge test, as reactions can be extreme. Most severe reactions appear within the first hour after administration of an allergen, although severe delayed reactions may develop up to several days later. Challenge tests should be avoided when anticipated reactions are unusually severe (e.g., anaphylaxis). Double-blind challenge tests, in which suspected foods are administered in capsules, are rarely necessary, but may be helpful when results of the initial evaluation are in doubt. An elemental diet can be useful as a diagnostic tool to determine whether patients truly have a sensitivity to ingested food substances. Furthermore, if a clinical remission can be attained, the elemental diet can be used as a complete nutrient source while food challenges are initiated.[58]

Table 60–7. SAMPLE ELIMINATION DIET

Foods Allowed*	Foods to Be Avoided
Lamb	Milk
	Tea
Rice	Coffee
	Cola
Pears	Soft drinks
Blueberries	
Peaches	
Apricots	Candy
	Chewing gum
Lettuce	
Artichokes	All medications (except as prescribed by physician)
Beets	
Spinach	
Celery	
Parsnips	All other foods not listed in column 1
Salt	
Sugar (cane or beet)	
Water	
Any vegetable oil except oleomargarine	

*Note: All fruits and vegetables, except lettuce, must be cooked.

Adapted from American Academy of Allergy and Immunology Committee on Adverse Reactions to Foods. *In* Anderson, J. A., and Sogn, D. D. (eds.). Adverse Reactions to Foods. NIH Publication No. 84–2442. Washington, National Institute of Allergy and Infectious Diseases, U.S. Department of Health and Human Services, Public Health Service, National Institutes of Health, 1984.

A standardized procedure to challenge children with suspected cow's milk or soy protein sensitivity has been proposed by Powell.[59] Prior to challenge, carbohydrate (lactose or sucrose) malabsorption is excluded, usually by hydrogen breath test, and baseline blood and stool samples are obtained. Patients should not have received the suspected allergen for at least two weeks prior to testing and should be asymptomatic. A standard dose (e.g., 100 ml) of milk (cow's or soy) is administered while the child is monitored carefully for acute reactions. Subsequent stool specimens are analyzed for blood, leukocytes, and reducing sugars, and a repeat cell blood count with differential count is obtained six to eight hours later. The challenge is considered positive (i.e., indicative of protein sensitivity) when diarrhea appears within 24 hours of challenge, fecal samples contain leukocytes or blood not present prior to challenge, or the six- to eight-hour post-challenge total polymorphonuclear leukocyte count in the blood is increased by over 4000 cells/cu mm above baseline.[59] Patients should be followed carefully for several days after challenge, as life-threatening reactions may not appear acutely.

Delayed reactions to food substances can be difficult to diagnose, as the relationship of symptoms to administration of the allergen is not as clear. Challenge with food allergens for several days may be required before a reaction becomes evident.

Evaluation of Gastrointestinal Function. Intestinal function can be adversely affected by mucosal injury. Iron deficiency anemia due to gastrointestinal blood loss is common among milk-sensitive infants.[60, 61] Measuring serum iron concentration and testing stool samples for occult blood loss may be useful to determine whether a patient has adverse gastrointestinal reactions (mucosal damage) to specific antigens. Protein-losing enteropathy has been documented using ^{51}Cr-labeled human serum albumin in the stool after intravenous injection of the isotopically labeled protein.[62] Fecal alpha-1-antitrypsin may also be a useful marker for gastrointestinal protein loss[63, 64] (see pp. 283–290). D-xylose absorption may be abnormal, but it appears to be an insensitive indicator of intestinal damage of protein-induced enteritis.[65]

Gastrointestinal endoscopy, particularly in type 1 (IgE-mediated) hypersensitivity reactions, may reveal hyperemia, nodularity, edema, thickened folds, and excess mucus production.[6] Small intestinal biopsies are seldom useful in patients with food sensitivity except to exclude other gastrointestinal disorders. Serial biopsies of the small intestine in conjunction with elimination and challenge infrequently provide objective evidence of food-sensitive disorders involving the small intestinal mucosa. Celiac sprue is the most common exception (see pp. 1134–1152). Cow's milk protein sensitivity can result in a variable and patchy pattern of small intestinal mucosal damage and a thin mucosal surface.[66] Eosinophilic infiltrates in the mucosa and submucosa are substantial, and patchy villus damage is common.[55] The number of intraepithelial lymphocytes in subjects with cow's milk protein sensitivity is increased with milk exposure and falls below that of normal controls (non–milk-sensitive individuals) with a milk-free diet.[67] Altered microvilli are correlated with diminished disaccharidase activity. Minimal morphologic changes, principally decreased villus-crypt ratio, have also been described in patients with eczema attributable to food sensitivity.[68]

Protein-Induced Proctocolitis. Proctocolitis associated with food sensitivity, primarily to cow's milk, soy, and, in one case, beef[69] protein, appears primarily in infants. This entity must be differentiated from colitis due to infection, inflammatory bowel disease, and, particularly in infants and young children, hemolytic uremic syndrome and Henoch-Schönlein purpura. Colonoscopy typically reveals loss of vascular pattern, friability, and minimal mucosal ulcerations. Biopsy results show acute and chronic inflammatory changes that may suggest ulcerative colitis, although eosinophils, plasma cells, and IgE-containing monocytes (if counted) tend to predominate (Fig. 60–4). Except in severe cases, crypt architecture is usually maintained, and crypt abscesses and goblet cell mucus depletion are uncommon.[69] Eosinophilic infiltrates, although not pathognomonic, are usually moderate.[36, 69, 71] Cow's milk sensitivity enteropathy and cow's milk–induced colitis seldom coexist in the same patient.[20]

Treatment and Prognosis

Elimination Diets. Treatment is based on recognition of the offending agent(s) and the elimination of all implicated allergens from the diet. Elimination of related foods may limit the diet unnecessarily, however. Care should be taken to ensure that a nutritionally appropriate, palatable, and complete diet is instituted. Infants, in particular, are frequently placed on restrictive diets that are dangerously inadequate.

Protein Sensitivity in Infancy. Cow's milk–sensitive infants are often placed on soy protein formulas. However, as 20 to 50 per cent of patients with cow's milk sensitivity also react to soy protein, a cow's milk– and soy-free "hypoallergenic" formula (e.g., Pregestimil or Nutramigen) should probably be initiated until the problems resolve. Goat's milk is not suitable for patients with sensitivity to casein because of a high degree of cross reactivity between bovine and goat's milk proteins (Casein constitutes 80 per cent of the milk protein in both animals). However, some patients with sensitivity to the whey protein fraction of cow's milk will tolerate goat's milk. Because lactose intolerance often accompanies cow's milk protein sensitivity, lactose-free formulas may have to be provided. Rechallenge at 6- to 12-month intervals may eventually demonstrate disappearance of the cow's milk protein sensitivity in many young children, usually by one to three years of age. When prior antigen exposure led

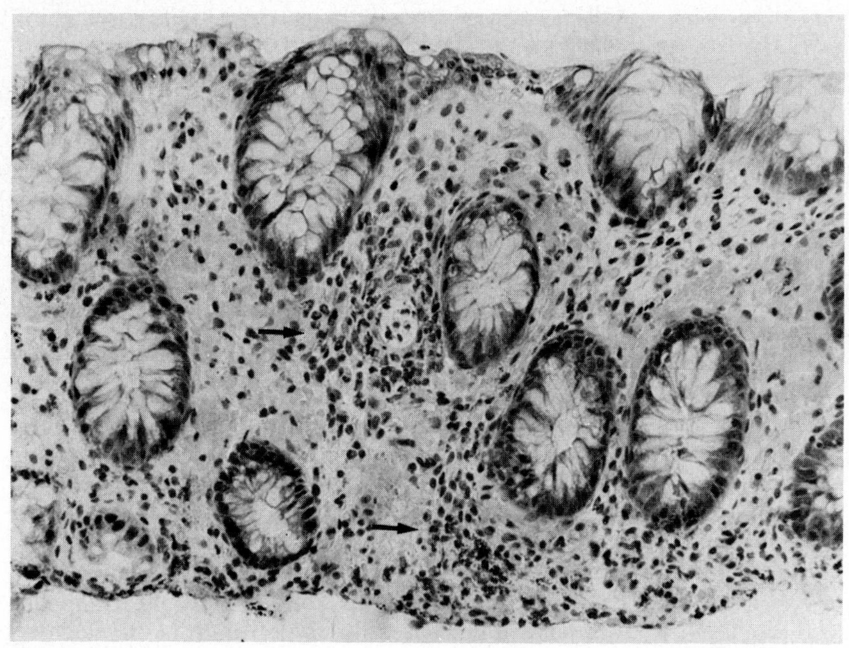

Figure 60–4. Rectal biopsy from a three-week-old infant with milk-induced colitis. In addition to a diffusely increased eosinophilic infiltrate, there is a dense perivascular collection of eosinophils *(arrow)* extending also to the base of the mucosa *(arrow)*. × 280. (Courtesy of Alan M. Leichtner, M.D., and Richard J. Grand, M.D., Children's Hospital Medical Center, Boston.)

to a severe reaction, such as anaphylaxis or urticaria, reintroduction of the potential allergen should be performed under close medical supervision, and with treatment immediately available.

Although clinical tolerance to ingested allergens may develop in the majority of young children, histologic and immunologic abnormalities in the intestinal mucosa and skin reactivity may persist.[54, 72] The significance of this subclinical sensitivity reaction is unknown. Many of the children who have reactions to foods early in life appear to have a predilection for developing reactions to a variety of allergens as they grow older.

Food Sensitivity in Children and Adults. Older children and adults presenting with food sensitivities after infancy are much less likely to outgrow them.[54] Dietary avoidance of offending antigens is the primary goal of therapy in any patient with food sensitivity. Avoidance of hidden antigens in prepared foods (e.g., "nonfat milk solids," "hydrolyzed vegetable protein," flavorings, and other additives) is frequently difficult.

In situations in which stringent elimination diets have been successful, single foods are reintroduced into the diet every three to seven days, depending on the patient's condition. Foods causing reactions can be deleted from the diet systematically. When milk is eliminated from the diet of infants and young children, a good source for calcium and possibly vitamin D must be provided.[73] Older children and adults with milk protein sensitivity may require supplemental calcium.

Elemental formulas as a sole source of nutrients are effective in some patients with severe reactions to foods,[74] including atopic dermatitis[75] or asthma,[76] which are uncontrollable with other therapies.

Pharmacologic agents do not usually prevent gastrointestinal symptoms in patients with food sensitivity reactions. Antihistamines administered prior to meals may decrease rhinitis or urticaria, and theophylline may be of benefit for chronic respiratory symptoms in selected patients.[31] Sodium cromoglycate, which may act in part by inhibiting mast cell degranulation, has effectively prevented food sensitivity reactions in some patients. High doses (200 to 400 mg or up to 800 mg 30 to 60 minutes before food ingestion) may be required to achieve a beneficial effect.[77–79] Epinephrine is useful in acute reactions, such as anaphylaxis, bronchospasm, or laryngeal edema. Corticosteroids are rarely indicated and should be reserved only for severe cases when avoidance therapy is ineffective or not feasible. Ketotifen, an anti-allergic, anti-anaphylactic agent that inhibits eosinophil degranulation,[80] may prove to be beneficial in selected patients.

Hyposensitization therapy has no proved efficacy for food sensitivity.

Prevention of Food Sensitivity in Susceptible Infants

Prevention of food allergic disease is directed toward the four stages in the development of reactions.[81] Its tenets are as follows: 1. Avoid exposure to antigens toward which a host has previously been sensitized; 2. prevent uptake of the antigen from the gastrointestinal tract; 3. Induce hyposensitization or modification of the allergic reaction; and 4. avoid damaging sensitization.

Dietary restriction is required for the first (avoidance of antigenic exposure) and is discussed earlier, whereas hyposensitization has no proved role in the prevention of food sensitivity reactions. Prevention of antigen uptake and avoidance of sensitization can best be instituted in the first months of life.

Breast Feeding and Food Sensitivity. Strong arguments can be made for early identification of infants at risk for development of atopic disease and food sensitivity. Exposure to cow's milk protein early in life increases the risk for developing sensitivity to it. In contrast, breast feeding during the first few months of life appears to prevent the development of some allergic reactions.[82] Exclusive breast feeding should therefore be recommended for four months or more, especially in infants with a strong family history for atopy. At-risk infants who are unable to breast feed may benefit from a casein-hydrolysate, hypoallergenic formula until six months old.[83] The same formulas should also be considered for use in infants recovering from acute gastroenteritis, as milk protein may further injure or sensitize an already damaged mucosa.[84] The long-term outcome of these recommendations remains to be determined.

Milk and other foreign proteins (e.g., egg, citrus fruits, wheat, and chocolate[85]) may be carried into breast milk, resulting in allergic phenomena in breast-fed infants, including protein sensitivity–induced colitis.[86, 87] Therefore, lactating mothers must also consider altering their own dietary intake if symptoms and signs suggestive of protein sensitivity appear in their breast-feeding infant.

EOSINOPHILIC GASTROENTEROPATHY

Definition

Patients with eosinophilic gastroenteropathy have gastrointestinal symptoms associated in some types of the disease with peripheral blood eosinophilia and in all with variable eosinophilic infiltration of the gastrointestinal tract, particularly of the stomach and small intestine.

Epidemiology

Over 150 cases have been reported in the literature. The peak age of presentation is in the third decade. Approximately 15 to 20 per cent of the reported cases are in children, and several cases have been documented in early infancy.

Etiology and Pathogenesis

IgE-Mediated Hypersensitivity. The cause of eosinophilic gastroenteropathy is unknown, although the

Table 60–8. EVIDENCE FOR IMMUNOLOGIC MEDIATION IN EOSINOPHILIC GASTROENTEROPATHY

Peripheral eosinophilia
Lymphocyte involvement in eosinophilopoiesis
Gastrointestinal tract eosinophilic infiltrates
Lymphocyte-derived factors and complement fragments that are chemotactic for eosinophils
Increased incidence of allergic disorders (asthma, rhinitis, eczema, urticaria)
Correlation of food sensitivity with direct skin tests and indirect tests for skin sensitizing (reaginic; IgE) antibody
Symptomatic response to food (especially milk) elimination and challenge
Response to corticosteroid therapy

association with systemic allergic symptoms, elevated serum IgE concentrations, and response to corticosteroid therapy in some patients suggests a relationship with type 1 hypersensitivity reactions (Table 60–8). Food sensitivity, especially to milk, appears to play a role in at least some of these patients, whose gastrointestinal symptoms are exacerbated with a food challenge.[55, 63, 88, 89] RAST for IgG anti-milk antibodies and IgE tests for whole milk, lactalbumin, and beta-lactoglobulin often give positive results.[55] Some patients have strongly positive results of direct skin tests, RAST, and IgE to specific food substances and respond symptomatically to elimination of these foods. Results of challenge tests with food antigens to which patients believe they are intolerant are often positive, although there are few reports of good double-blind studies of challenge tests in patients with this disease.[90–92] Moreover, the observation that elimination diets do not resolve the intestinal disorder in most patients attests to a poorly understood and complex pathophysiologic mechanism.

Immunologic Dysfunction. Besides a sensitized immune system mediating this disorder, altered immune function has also been proposed as an underlying mechanism for eosinophilic gastroenteropathy. However, no consistent abnormalities of the immune system have been shown, and serum immunoglobulins and complement components, total lymphocyte counts, and responses to phytohemagglutinin, pokeweed mitogen, and concanavalin A are usually normal.[93]

Eosinophilic Infiltration of the Gastrointestinal Tract. Three mechanisms, involving hypersensitivity reactions described earlier (Table 60–4), have been postulated to explain the development of eosinophilic infiltration in the intestinal tract of patients with severe gastrointestinal symptoms and specific food allergies:[94] (1) Arthus-type immediate hypersensitivity (type 3) reactions in the walls of small blood vessels activate the standard complement pathway, which may attract eosinophils to the site of antigen-antibody complexes; (2) T cells specifically sensitized to antigens release lymphokines, including eosinophilic chemotactic factor of anaphylaxis (ECF-A), eosinophil-stimulating promoter (ESP), and ECF-G (extracted from eosinophilic hepatic granulomas caused by schistosomiasis in mice), all of which attract peripheral eosinophils from the circulating blood;[32] and (3) food antigens may react in the gut wall with IgE antibodies to specific food substances bound to tissue mast cells at Fc receptor sites. Resulting mast cell degranulation generates histamine and ECF-A, which attract eosinophils to the site of tissue injury. The mast cells, rather than the eosinophils, may be responsible for the local tissue injury by releasing these plus other toxic substances, such as bradykinin and leukotrienes (slow-reacting substance of anaphylaxis or SRS-A) (Fig. 60–5).

Other studies suggest a more important pathogenetic role for eosinophils in eosinophilic gastroenteropathy. Cytotoxicity appears when eosinophils degranulate.[32] In one report of two affected siblings, activated degranulating eosinophils in the gastrointestinal mucosa correlated with the degree of histologic change.[95] Tox-

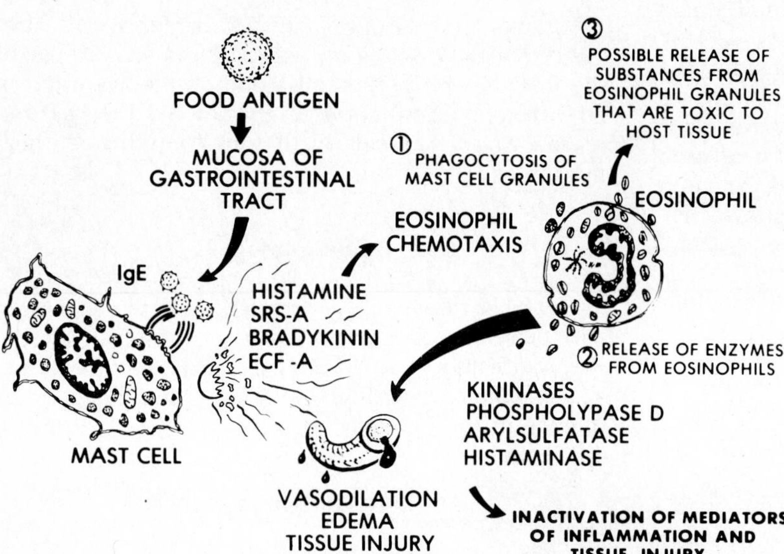

Figure 60–5. Hypothetical scheme of the pathophysiology of eosinophilic gastroenteropathy. Antigen passes through the mucosa of a sensitized patient and binds to two molecules of mast cell–bound IgE. Degranulating mast cell attracts eosinophils through release of SRS-A. Eosinophils play a largely homeostatic role, neutralizing the tissue-damaging effects of the mast cell degranulation. (From Cello, J. P. Am J Med *67*:1097, 1979. Used by permission.)

icity induced by eosinophils is postulated to be due to tissue-toxic substances such as eosinophil cationic protein and major basic protein released by the eosinophils. However, the major role of eosinophils is believed to be one of homeostasis and modulation of inflammation rather than tissue damage. Enzymes such as histaminase and arylsulfatase (which inactivate SRS-A), major basic protein (which inactivates heparin), and others such as kininase, phospholipase D, and lysophospholipase may neutralize or inactivate the effects of the inflammatory substances released by mast cells.[32]

In sum, the pathogenesis of eosinophilic gastroenteropathy remains to be clarified. As the symptoms, signs, and laboratory presentation of many patients with eosinophilic gastroenteropathy are often analogous to findings in patients with sensitivity ("allergy") to ingested antigens described in the previous section, there is a high probability that these disorders share a similar pathophysiology. The spectrum of disease defined by the nonspecific findings of signs and symptoms of gastrointestinal dysfunction associated with eosinophilic involvement of the gastrointestinal tract may eventually be sorted into several disorders.

Pathology

Three pathologic groups of patients have been described (Table 60–9). The most common group has primarily mucosal involvement, leading to malabsorption and gastrointestinal protein loss. Less frequently, patients have eosinophilic infiltration of the muscle layers, causing marked thickening and rigidity of the intestine, which may lead to pyloric or intestinal obstruction. The rarest group has predominant involvement of the serosal surface, presenting with eosinophilic ascites and peritonitis.[90]

Eosinophilic infiltration in all three groups of patients usually involves the stomach and small intestine. The esophagus and colon may be affected alone or in combination with the stomach and small intestine. Infrequently, the gallbladder, pancreas,[96] liver, spleen,[97] urinary bladder,[98] and prostate may also be involved. Eosinophilic cystitis, characterized by recurrent episodes of sterile cystitis, may also accompany eosinophilic gastroenteropathy.[98] A diffuse mucosal and submucosal inflammatory process is suggested by an irregular bladder wall by excretory urography, and marked eosinophilic infiltrates are seen in cystoscopic biopsies. Mesenteric eosinophilic lymphadenopathy[99] and eosinophilic infiltration of the appendix[100] have also been reported.

Clinical and Laboratory Manifestations

General Presentation. Because the gastrointestinal mucosa from esophagus to colon may be involved, signs and symptoms depend on the depth of bowel wall involvement and the presence of esophagitis, gastritis, enteritis, or colitis. Manifestations therefore may consist of nausea, vomiting, recurrent and crampy abdominal pain, weight loss from diarrhea, protein-losing enteropathy, steatorrhea, and generalized malabsorption, pallor due to anemia from gastrointestinal blood loss, and melena or hematochezia. Most commonly, patients present with symptoms of gastritis and enteritis. Accompanying signs and symptoms include allergic phenomena, especially eczema, rhinitis, and asthma, hepatomegaly, splenomegaly, or evidence of gallbladder, urinary bladder, or prostate involvement. Young children may present with anasarca and severe anemia owing to the gastrointestinal protein and blood loss.

Three clinical patterns predominate, corresponding to the three pathologic types of involvement (Table 60–9).

Eosinophilic Gastroenteropathy with Predominant Mucosal Disease. Symptoms include intermittent nausea, emesis, diarrhea, weight loss, and abdominal and back pain, which may be exacerbated by ingestion of specific food antigens. A history of atopy (asthma, rhinitis) is present in as many as 50 per cent of patients. Atopic eczema, urticaria, and pedal edema may be noted on physical examination. Laboratory studies usually demonstrate a moderate to marked eosinophilia, usually greater than 20 per cent, low erythrocyte sedimentation rate, iron deficiency anemia, Charcot-Leyden crystals on otherwise negative stool examinations for ova and parasites, and low serum albumin levels. Severe protein loss via the gut, documented by fecal ^{51}Cr-labeled albumin, $^{51}CrCl_3$, or alpha-1-antitrypsin clearance,[63, 64] may occasionally lead to low immunoglobulin levels. Steatorrhea and abnormal D-xylose absorption may also be found in the presence of damaged intestinal mucosa.

Radiographs may be normal or demonstrate nonspecific mucosal edema, owing in part to hypoproteinemia, and coarse, irregular, nodular folds ("cobblestoning"), most frequently involving the gastric antrum and jejunum and resulting from infiltration of the mucosa with eosinophils and other inflammatory cells. The valvulae conniventes are usually diffusely thickened.[101] The polypoid filling defects and luminal narrowing of the antrum often suggest polypoid gastritis or even lymphosarcoma[101, 102] (Fig. 60–6). Spasm, irritability, and increased secretion may also be evident.[102] Intestinal loops may be separated, and the intestine may appear rigid during fluoroscopy. Esophageal involvement may be manifested as strictures or polypoid lesions[103] or can be difficult to distinguish radiologically and manometrically from achalasia.[104] Abdominal sonogram or computed tomographic scan may reveal thickened intestinal walls and intraperitoneal fluid if the serosa is involved.

Endoscopically, the mucosa may vary in appearance from normal to ulcerated, hemorrhagic and nodular. Gastric[71, 105] and jejunal biopsies demonstrate mild to severe villus injury and eosinophilic infiltration of the mucosa, particularly the lamina propria.

Eosinophilic Gastroenteropathy with Predominant Muscle Layer Disease. Patients with this pattern pres-

Table 60–9. CLINICAL PATTERNS OF EOSINOPHILIC GASTROENTEROPATHY

I. Predominant Mucosal Disease
- A. History
  - Nausea, emesis, abdominal pain
  - History of atopy (asthma, allergic rhinitis) in approximately 50%
  - Occasional diarrhea, weight loss, growth failure, delayed puberty, amenorrhea
- B. Physical Examination
  - Atopic dermatitis, urticaria, pedal edema
  - Evidence of nutritional deficiencies
- C. Laboratory Studies
  - Peripheral eosinophilia
  - Iron deficiency anemia
  - Stool specimens positive for occult blood
  - Stool specimens positive for Charcot-Leyden crystals
  - Steatorrhea (usually mild)
  - Abnormal D-xylose absorption
  - Hypoproteinemia; hypoalbuminemia
  - Normal or decreased levels of serum immunoglobulins IgG, IgM, IgA
  - Increased fecal loss of ^{51}Cr-labeled albumin and increased fecal alpha-1-antitrypsin clearance
  - Positive skin tests to specific food antigens
  - Elevated IgE levels in serum and duodenal fluid
  - Normal erythrocyte sedimentation rate
- D. Radiography
  - Normal to irregular, thickened, nodular folds
  - Edematous bowel walls
  - Abnormal (diminished) peristalsis
- E. Endoscopy
  - Normal to nodular, ulcerated, or hemorrhagic mucosa
- F. Histology
  - Eosinophilic infiltration of the mucosa and lamina propria, especially in gastric antrum and jejunum; mild to severe villus injury
- G. Diagnosis
  - Peripheral eosinophilia
  - Eosinophilic infiltrate on gastrointestinal, especially gastric antral, biopsy specimens
  - Exclude disorders in differential diagnosis
- H. Therapy
  - Trial of elimination diet
  - Corticosteroids as indicated (usually effective)

II. Predominant Muscle Layer Involvement*
- A. History
  - Especially nausea, emesis, crampy abdominal pain
  - Pyloric outlet or small intestinal obstruction
  - Allergic history in approximately 40%
- B. Physical Examination
  - Evidence of obstruction
- C. Laboratory Studies
  - As described for mucosal disease

II. Predominant Muscle Layer Involvement *Continued*
- D. Radiography
  - 1. Localized ("monoenteric") form:
    - Focal irregular narrowing of antral (70%) or small intestinal (30%) mucosa
  - 2. Diffuse ("polyenteric") form:
    - Thickened, indurated stomach and small intestine; may also involve colon; terminal ileum usually distensible
- E. Endoscopy
  - Nodular, indurated, poorly compliant mucosa
- F. Histology
  - Eosinophilic infiltrates extending through the muscle layers often to the serosa
- G. Diagnosis
  - Peripheral eosinophilia
  - Full-thickness biopsy often necessary to demonstrate eosinophilic infiltrates
- H. Therapy
  - Corticosteroids usually effective
  - Rarely: surgical resection

III. Predominant Subserosal Infiltration* (<10% of eosinophilic gastroenteropathy)
- A. History
  - Abdominal distention, with pain
- B. Physical Examination
  - Ascites
- C. Laboratory Studies
  - Normal results on liver enzyme and function studies
  - Paracentesis: exudative ascites with eosinophilia, sometimes bloody, usually sterile unless complicated by peritonitis
- D. Radiography
  - Radiography may or may not show mucosal involvement;
  - CT scan and ultrasonography confirm intraperitoneal fluid and may reveal enlarged mesenteric nodes
- E. Endoscopy
  - As for mucosal and muscle layer involvement; variable involvement
- F. Histology
  - Eosinophilic infiltrates in the subserosa, serosa, and mesenteric lymph nodes
- G. Diagnosis
  - Peripheral and ascitic eosinophilia
  - Laparotomy may be required to exclude other disorders
- H. Therapy
  - Corticosteroids, usually intermittent although sometimes low-dose maintenance required
  - Diuretics may be useful for ascites

IV. Extraintestinal involvement associated with eosinophilic gastroenteropathy:

Liver	Prostate
Spleen	Urinary bladder (cystitis)
Pancreas	Pleural effusions
Gallbladder	Lymphatic system (cervical, mesenteric)

*These patterns may have identical presentations to those of predominant mucosal disease. In addition, deeper infiltration by eosinophils can alter the clinical pattern.

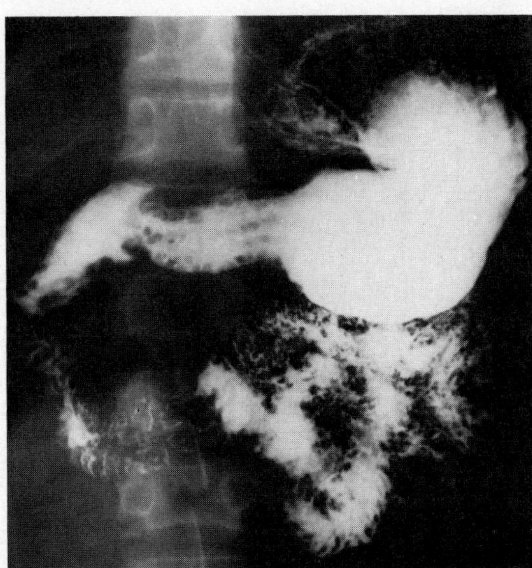

Figure 60–6. The distal portion of the stomach is noted to be cobblestoned with multiple polypoid filling defects. Similar defects are noted in the upper duodenum with coarsening of folds in the upper small intestine. (Courtesy of M. H. Sleisenger, M.D.)

ent between the second and fifth decades and typically manifest signs and symptoms of intermittent pyloric outlet or incomplete small intestinal obstruction owing to thickening and rigidity of the wall of the stomach and small intestine. The nausea, emesis, and crampy abdominal pain are not relieved by antacids or anticholinergic drugs. Some patients give a history of specific food intolerances, and an allergic history is positive in approximately 40 per cent.

Involvement may be localized ("monoenteric") or diffuse ("polyenteric").[106] Localized muscle layer disease is more common and is usually limited to the gastric antrum and pylorus (Fig. 60–7). Radiologically,

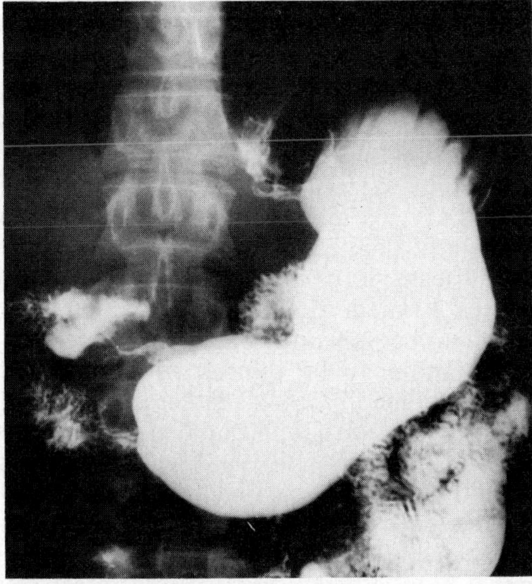

Figure 60–7. Narrowing of distal antrum in eosinophilic gastroenteropathy caused by hypertrophy of the muscle layer and eosinophilic infiltration. (Courtesy of M. H. Sleisenger, M.D.)

this form of the disease may be difficult to distinguish from pyloric stenosis or scirrhous carcinoma.[102] The diffuse form, found in approximately one third of these patients, is characterized by extensive thickening and induration of the stomach and small intestine. Some areas appear firm and cartilaginous. Differentiation from Crohn's disease may be difficult, especially if mesenteric nodes are hyperplastic. Enteric protein loss and iron-deficiency anemia are seen in patients with gastric involvement alone as well as in those with intestinal involvement.

Eosinophilic Gastroenteropathy with Predominant Subserosal Disease. Patients with eosinophilic gastroenteropathy may develop an exudative ascites containing 12 to 95 per cent eosinophils.[107] This form of eosinophilic gastroenteropathy is relatively uncommon (less than 10 per cent of the reported cases). It may appear alone or in combination with either of the other clinicopathologic patterns.

Table 60–9 summarizes the recognized clinical patterns of eosinophilic gastroenteropathy. The classification is based on clinical and pathologic findings depending on the tissue layer involved in the primary disease process. However, patients often have manifestations of mixed forms of disease—for example, ascites (serosal involvement) and obstruction (muscular involvement).

Diagnosis

Eosinophilic Gastroenteropathy with Predominant Mucosal Disease. Diagnosis of mucosal disease is best made by biopsy of the involved area of gastrointestinal mucosa (Fig. 60–8). Most frequently, antral biopsies performed perorally or endoscopically will demonstrate eosinophilic infiltrates.[71, 105] Although infiltration of the mucosal layer is predominant, significant eosinophilic infiltration may also be found in the submucosal and muscle layers. As the pathologic findings may be patchy, specimens from at least eight different sites within the small intestine should be examined histologically to exclude this diagnosis.[94, 108] Some children have been noted to have severe eosinophilic infiltrates localized only within the esophagus (Fig. 60–9), with normal gastric and duodenal biopsy findings.

Differential diagnosis includes malabsorptive disorders such as celiac sprue; other causes of protein-losing enteropathy such as parasitic infestations, intestinal lymphangiectasia, ischemic enteritis, radiation enteritis, and Crohn's disease; neoplastic diseases such as lymphosarcoma; toxic reactions (e.g., to gold[109]); and connective tissue disorders such as polyarteritis nodosa. Crohn's disease, visceral lymphoma, and polyarteritis nodosa in particular can mimic eosinophilic gastroenteropathy. Isolated eosinophilic esophagitis should be differentiated from eosinophilic infiltrates found associated with gastroesophageal reflux.[110, 111]

The hypereosinophilic syndrome should also be excluded. In this condition, multiple organs are involved, especially the cardiovascular, pulmonary, hemato-

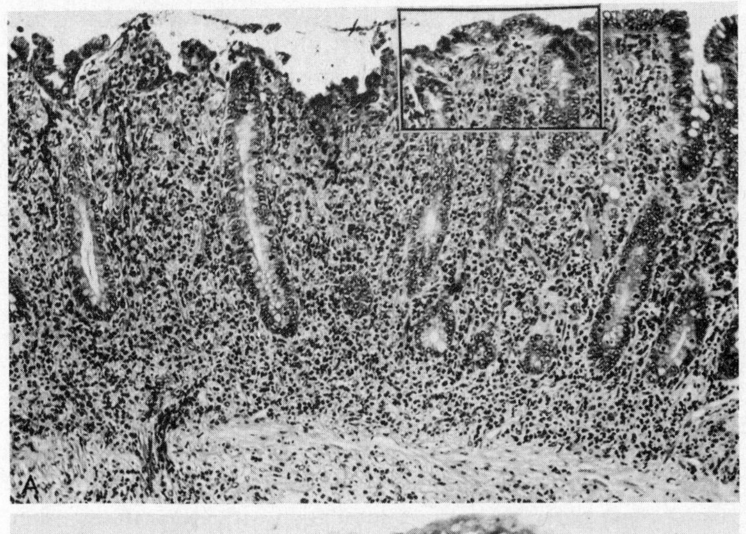

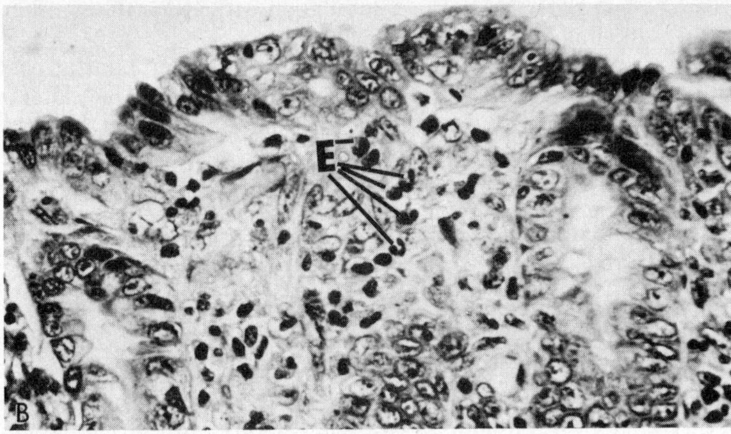

Figure 60–8. *A*, Small bowel suction biopsy specimen, revealing absence of villi and massive infiltration of the lamina propria with eosinophilic leukocytes. Hematoxylin and eosin stain, × 100. *B*, Enlargement of boxed area in *A*. Note the surface epithelial abnormalities and the eosinophils (E). (From Leinbach, G. E., and Rubin, C. E. Eosinophilic gastroenteritis: a simple reaction to food allergens? Gastroenterology *59*:874–889. Copyright by Williams & Wilkins, 1970.)

poietic, and central and peripheral nervous systems, and to lesser degrees the liver, gastrointestinal tract, skin, and kidneys.[112] Damage is presumably attributable to eosinophilic infiltrates. Only 40 per cent of patients with this disorder survive more than three years,[112] and aggressive therapy is indicated.[113] In patients with atopy, the hyper-IgE (Job's) syndrome should be excluded. Considerable overlap appears to exist between eosinophilic gastroenteropathy and the Churg-Strauss syndrome, characterized by allergic rhinitis and asthma, systemic vasculitis, multisystem involvement, and eosinophilia.[114] Differentiation is based on clinical, histologic, and angiographic assessment.

Distinguishing eosinophilic gastroenteropathy from cow's milk protein sensitivity can sometimes be difficult.[55] Although patients with either disorder may present with peripheral eosinophilia, iron deficiency anemia, malabsorption, protein-losing enteropathy, and eosinophilic infiltration of the gastrointestinal tract, children with cow's milk protein sensitivity are younger (usually under one year old), do not have elevated serum and duodenal fluid IgE levels, and respond immediately to withdrawal of milk. By three years of age, these patients generally will tolerate milk. In contrast, patients with eosinophilic gastroenteropathy present later in childhood, have elevated IgE levels, and do not uniformly respond to dietary manipulation.[55]

Proctitis is rarely associated with eosinophilic gastroenteropathy and histologically consists only of minimal eosinophilic infiltrates, in contrast to milk protein-induced proctocolitis (discussed earlier).[71]

Eosinophilic Gastroenteropathy with Predominant Muscle Layer Disease. Patients with predominantly muscularis layer involvement often have radiographic evidence of focal irregular narrowing of the antral or small intestinal mucosa. These features may resemble an infiltrating gastric carcinoma, antral gastritis secondary to acid peptic disease, Menetrier's disease, or Crohn's disease involving the stomach (Fig. 60–7). Colonic involvement resulting in obstruction may occur alone or in conjunction with small intestinal disease,[99, 115] and may be difficult to distinguish from colonic carcinoma or Crohn's disease.

Biopsy diagnosis of infiltrated muscularis is often more difficult than in mucosal disease, as the eosinophilic infiltrates may be beyond the depth of the biopsy instruments used. Diagnosis is usually established by full-thickness biopsies of stomach or intestine, or both. Operative biopsies may be necessary in selected patients to exclude gastric carcinoma and lymphoma. Histologic examination of deep endoscopic or surgical

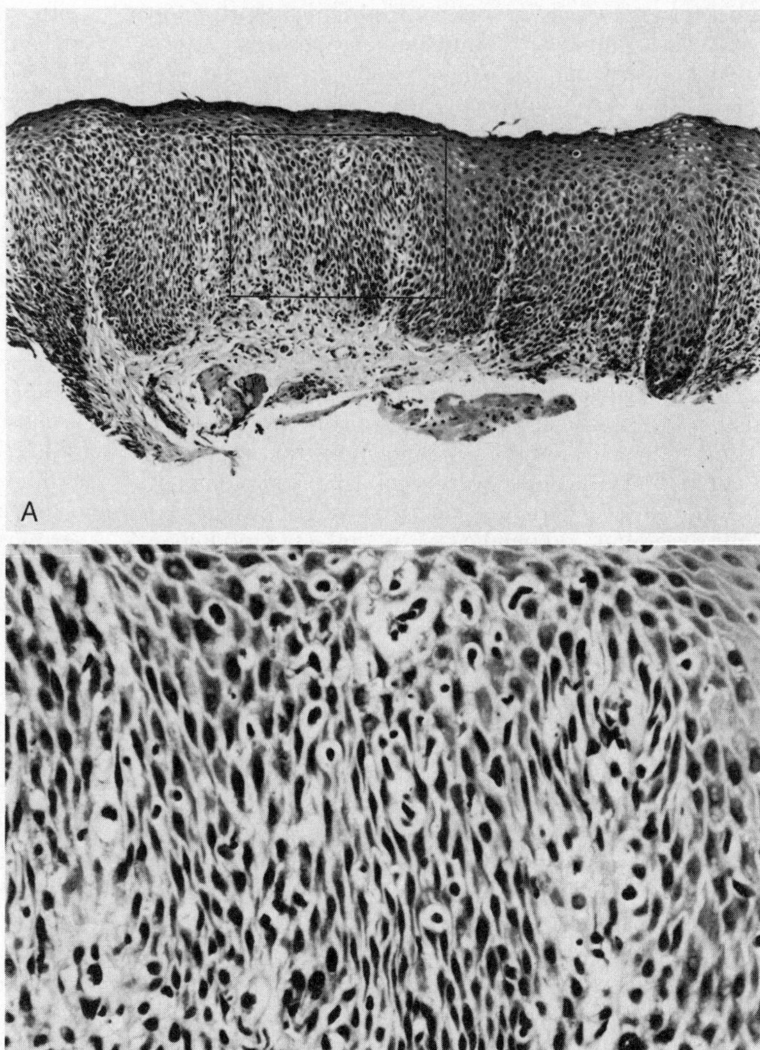

Figure 60–9. *A,* Endoscopic esophageal biopsy specimen in a 2-year-old with eosinophilic gastroenteropathy, demonstrating diffuse eosinophilic mucosal infiltrates. Antral and duodenal biopsy results were normal, and gastroesophageal reflux was excluded. Hematoxylin and eosin stain, × 100. *B,* Enlargement (× 350) of boxed area in *A.* Many eosinophils (E) can be identified throughout the mucosa.

biopsy specimens reveals diffuse eosinophilic infiltration of the submucosa, often extending through the muscle layers to the serosa. Differential diagnosis of these histologic findings includes gastric polyps, particularly inflammatory fibrous polyps, amyloidosis, variable combined immunodeficiency, Waldenström's macroglobulinemia, alpha-chain disease, polyarteritis nodosa, lymphosarcoma, parasitic infections (including giardiasis, schistosomiasis, strongyloidiasis, gnathostomiasis, and anisakiasis), and Crohn's disease. Differentiation of eosinophilic gastroenteropathy with muscle layer involvement from Crohn's disease may be quite difficult,[99] as patients may present with iron deficiency anemia, stools positive for occult blood, leukocytosis, and radiographic abnormalities of the terminal ileum and cecum, and they may respond favorably to corticosteroids. In contrast to Crohn's disease, patients with eosinophilic gastroenteropathy typically reveal an open ileocecal valve and distensible terminal ileum on barium enema, and multiple areas with predominant eosinophilic infiltrates on colonoscopic biopsies.

Eosinophilic involvement of esophageal muscle layers has also been reported to produce signs, symptoms, and manometric findings similar to those of achalasia[116] and esophageal spasm.[117] Patients with disorders of esophageal motility should have biopsies performed to exclude eosinophilic gastroenteropathy as an etiologic factor. Conversely, patients with eosinophilic infiltration of the gastrointestinal tract may develop subsequent motility dysfunction and its sequellae.

Collagen Vascular Disease and Eosinophilic Gastroenteropathy. A small number of patients have eosinophilic muscle layer disease in conjunction with connective tissue disorders, in particular scleroderma, dermatomyositis, or polymyositis.[118] Biopsies from such patients reveal increased mast cell infiltration and degranulation adjacent to degenerating muscle cells in the muscularis mucosae, supporting the hypothesis that cytotoxic effects of the eosinophils and mast cells have a pathogenetic role in the gastrointestinal manifestations of collagen vascular disorders. One patient treated with sodium cromoglycate for eosinophilic gastroenteropathy was reported to subsequently develop polyarteritis nodosa.[119] Thus, the relationship of eosinophilic gastroenteropathy with collagen vascular diseases is provocative but unclear.

Gastrointestinal Eosinophilic Granulomas. Gastrointestinal eosinophilic granulomas are localized, sessile, or pedunculated polypoid lesions that are most frequently located near the pylorus, although they may be found throughout the gastrointestinal tract as well as in the urinary bladder. They are not associated with food sensitivities or peripheral eosinophilia[120] and are most likely attributable to local inflammatory processes. Histologically, the eosinophilic granuloma is sharply localized and intermingled with connective tissue stroma. Such lesions occasionally are found in association with the parasitic infections noted earlier. Patients may present with signs and symptoms of pyloric outlet obstruction owing to gastric lesions, or intussusception, appendicitis, or an acute abdomen from intestinal involvement. Recurrence has not been reported after surgical excision of these granulomas.

Eosinophilic Gastroenteropathy with Predominant Subserosal Disease. Serosal infiltration with eosinophils resulting in ascites may exist concomitant with mucosal and muscularis involvement, although commonly it occurs alone. Barium studies may not reveal any mucosal abnormalities. Abdominal paracentesis yields sterile, sometimes bloody fluid high in eosinophils and protein. At laparotomy, a thickened serosa with subserosal eosinophilic infiltration (Fig. 60–10) and enlarged mesenteric lymph nodes containing eosinophils are found. Eosinophilic pleural effusions have also been reported to be associated with this form of the disease. Differential diagnosis includes abdominal lymphoma, collagen vascular disorders such as polyarteritis nodosa, ruptured hydatid cyst, or peritoneal dialysis.

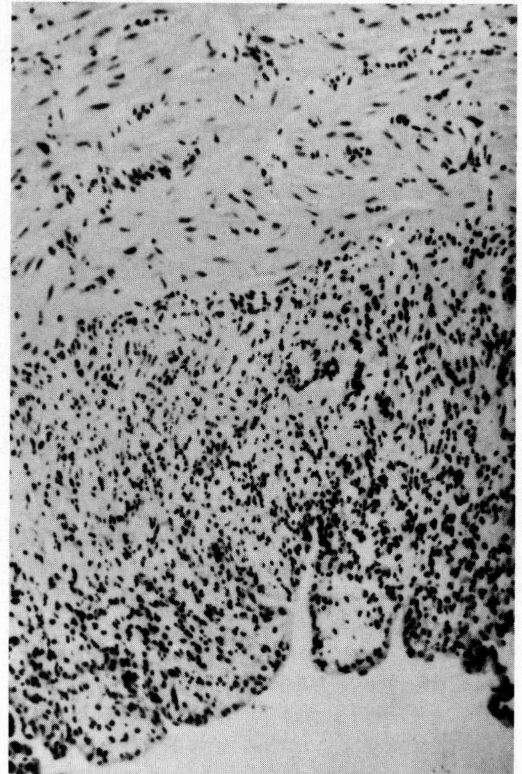

Figure 60–10. Histologic section of the upper small intestine showing infiltration with eosinophils in a thickened serosa and also in the muscle layer. Hematoxylin and eosin stain, × 200. (Courtesy of M. H. Sleisenger, M.D.)

Food Sensitivity in Eosinophilic Gastroenteropathy. All patients manifesting clinical and laboratory findings consistent with eosinophilic gastroenteropathy should be evaluated for food sensitivities. Many patients with eosinophilic gastroenteropathy have findings suggestive of allergic disorders.[105] Markedly elevated serum IgE levels (greater than 1000 IU/ml), positive results of skin tests and RAST to multiple foods and inhalants, and normal findings on immunologic function tests are characteristic.[55] Immunoglobulin levels may be low secondary to mucosal protein loss.

Treatment

Diet Therapy. Dietary manipulation alone is usually unsuccessful in alleviating signs and symptoms. However, if skin tests or RAST suggest specific food sensitivities, elimination of the specific antigens should be instituted. If there are no known or suspected food sensitivities, a trial of sequential elimination of milk (especially in children), eggs, pork, beef, and gluten-flour products should be attempted. Sufficient time (two to four weeks) should be allowed between challenges to be certain no delayed reactions to the ingested material appear. Elimination of specific food antigens often produces only temporary relief of symptoms. Elimination diets occasionally result in prolonged remission of symptoms,[91] although sustained responses generally are uncommon.[90, 92] Three factors may account for the lack of effectiveness of diet therapy alone: (1) the precipitating factors of flare-ups are unknown and may include environmental factors and ingestion of nonfood substances; (2) elimination diets, in addition to being impractical and difficult to comply with, frequently are effective only temporarily; and (3) corticosteroids are often added to a regimen to maintain a remission. However, elimination diets, being the simplest potentially effective treatment, should be attempted in patients with this entity.

Pharmacologic Management. Oral prednisone is usually required to induce a remission. No controlled trials have documented its efficacy, although treatment with corticosteroids ameliorates or resolves symptoms and signs in most patients.[71, 88, 90–92, 94] Treatment is initiated at a dose of 20 to 40 mg (1 to 2 mg/kg in children) of prednisone daily in single or divided doses. Many patients respond rapidly and require only a short-term, 7- to 10-day course, particularly for treatment of an acute exacerbation. Some require maintenance prednisone therapy on low-dose daily (5 to 10 mg every day) or alternate day (10 to 20 mg every other day) regimens, whereas others can be placed on prednisone therapy periodically for symptomatic flares.

Ketotifen is a recently introduced agent that inhibits eosinophil degranulation.[80] Its effectiveness in patients with eosinophilic gastroenteropathy requires further investigation.

Associated atopic symptoms such as rhinitis or asthma typically continue until specific medications are provided. Antihistamine and antispasmodic agents generally are not beneficial for the gastrointestinal symptoms. Sodium cromoglycate has not been successful in treating the gastroenteropathy, although it may rarely be effective in children with allergic gastroenteropathy.[77] In patients with serosal involvement, diuretics in addition to corticosteroids may help resolve ascites.

Elimination of all foods can provide relief of signs and symptoms. Enteral alimentation using elemental (hypoallergenic) formulas has been effective in some patients, whereas other patients may require total parenteral nutrition to achieve a remission. Parenteral nutrition may be necessary in patients with severe symptoms induced by any oral intake or with significant steroid dependence and toxicity.

Prognosis

The prognosis for remission generally is favorable, although the condition is lifelong and chronic. Symptoms may wax and wane, unrelated to diet and therapy. The longest duration of eosinophilic gastroenteritis reported is 32 years.[121] Mortality is rare and results from complications of the disease. Acute complications include obstruction and, rarely, perforation. Significant but not life-threatening hemorrhage has been reported. Chronic malnutrition leading to severe cachexia, reported for example in one patient with small intestinal bacterial overgrowth secondary to gastrointestinal dysmotility,[122] should not lead to death in this era of aggressive nutrition support. Children treated for eosinophilic gastroenteropathy often have persistent growth failure,[55] although the efficacy of aggressive nutritional support and judicious use of steroids remains to be determined. Many of the deaths reported in patients with alleged eosinophilic gastroenteropathy may actually be due to polyarteritis nodosa, visceral lymphoma, gastric cancer, or the hypereosinophilic syndrome.[94] Patients with eosinophilic gastroenteropathy appear to have no increased risk of gastrointestinal malignancies. The significance of hepatic eosinophilic granulomas, reported in one patient with eosinophilic gastroenteropathy,[123] is unclear.

Acknowledgments

Information for portions of this chapter has been extracted from the chapter written by Dr. Norton Greenberger for the third edition of this textbook. The author appreciates the helpful suggestions of Drs. Oscar L. Frick and Elizabeth Gleghorn.

References

1. Lucretius (95–55 B.C.) De Rerum Natura. IV, 637. *In* Bartlett, J. Familiar Quotations. 15th ed. Boston, Little, Brown and Company, 1980, p.101.
2. McCarthy, E. P., and Frick, O. L. Food sensitivity: keys to diagnosis. J. Pediatr. *102*:645, 1983.
3. Bock, S. A. More on food sensitivity or intolerance. (letter). J. Pediatr. *103*:1011, 1983.
4. American Academy of Allergy and Immunology Committee on Adverse Reactions to Foods. *In* Anderson, J. A., and Sogn, D. D. (eds.). Adverse Reactions to Foods. NIH Publication No. 84-2442. Washington, D.C.: National Institute of Allergy and Infectious Diseases, U.S. Department of Health and Human Services, Public Health Service, National Institutes of Health, 1984.
5. Breneman, J. C. Immunology of food allergy. *In* Breneman, J. C. (ed.). Handbook of Food Allergies. New York, Marcel Dekker, 1987, p. 1.
6. Jain, V. K., and Chandra, R. K. Food allergy in adults. *In* Breneman, J. C. (ed.). Handbook of Food Allergies. New York, Marcel Dekker, 1987, p. 71.
7. Stern, M., and Walker, W. A. Food allergy and intolerance. Pediatr. Clin. North Am. *32*:471, 1985.
8. Eastham, E. J., and Walker, W. A. Adverse effects of milk formula ingestion on the gastrointestinal tract. Gastroenterology *76*:365, 1979.
9. Roberton, D. M., Paganelli, R., Dinwiddie, R., and Levinsky, R. J. Milk antigen absorption in the preterm and term neonate. Arch. Dis. Child. *57*:369, 1982.
10. Rieger, C. H. L., and Rothberg, R. M. Development of the capacity to produce specific antibody to an ingested food antigen in the premature infant. J. Pediatr. *87*:515, 1975.
11. Walker, W. A. Antigen handling by the small intestine. Clin. Gastroenterol. *15*:1, 1986.
12. Walker, W. A., and Isselbacher, K. J. Uptake and transport of macromolecules by the intestine. Possible role in clinical disorders. Gastroenterology *67*:531, 1974.
13. Keljo, D. J., Butler, D. G., and Hamilton, J. R. Altered jejunal permeability to macromolecules during viral enteritis in the piglet. Gastroenterology *88*:998, 1985.
14. Gruskay, F. L., and Cooke, F. E. The gastrointestinal absorption of unaltered protein in normal infants and in infants recovering from diarrhoea. Pediatrics *16*:763, 1955.
15. Jackson, D., Walker-Smith, J. A., and Phillips, A. D. Macromolecular absorption by histologically normal and abnormal small intestinal mucosa in childhood: an in vitro study using organ culture. J. Pediatr. Gastroenterol. Nutr. *2*:235, 1983.
16. Hampton, J. C., and Rosario, B. The distribution of exogenous peroxidase in irradiated mouse intestine. Radiat. Res. *34*:209, 1968.
17. Cooper, M., Teichberg, S., and Lifshitz, F. Alterations in rat jejunal permeability to a macromolecular tracer during a hyperosmotic load. Lab. Invest. *38*:447, 1978.
18. Worthington, B. S., and Syrotuck, J. Intestinal permeability to large particles in normal and protein-deficient rats. J. Nutr. *106*:21, 1976.
19. Walker, W. A., Wu, M., Isselbacher, K. J., and Bloch, K. J. Intestinal uptake of macromolecules. IV. The effect of pancreatic duct ligation on the breakdown of antigen and antigen-antibody complexes on the intestinal surface. Gastroenterology *69*:1123, 1975.
20. Walker-Smith, J. A. Food sensitive enteropathies. Clin. Gastroenterol. *15*:55, 1986.
21. Walker-Smith, J. A., Ford, R. P. K., and Phillips, A. D. The spectrum of gastrointestinal allergies to food. Ann. Allergy *53*:629, 1984.
22. Heiner, D. C. Allergy to cow's milk. N. Engl. Soc. Allergy Proc. *2*:192, 1981.
23. Bachman, K. D., and Dees, S. C. Milk allergy. I. Observations on incidence and symptoms in "well" babies. Pediatrics *20*:393, 1957.

24. Schwartz, H. R., Nerurkar, L. S., Spies, J. R., Scanlon, R. T., and Bellanti, J. A. Milk hypersensitivity: RAST studies using new antigens generated by pepsin hydrolysis of beta-lactoglobulin. Ann. Allergy *45*:242, 1980.
25. Haddad, Z. H., Kalra, V., and Verma, S. IgE antibodies to peptic and peptic-tryptic digests of betalactoglobulin: significance in food hypersensitivity. Ann. Allergy *42*:368, 1979.
26. Spies, J. R., Stevan, M. A., Stein, W. J., and Coulson, E. J. The chemistry of allergens. XX. New antigens generated by pepsin hydrolysis of bovine milk proteins. J. Allergy *45*:208, 1970.
27. Zaloga, G. P., Hierlwimmer, U. R., and Engler, R. J. Anaphylaxis following psyllium ingestion. J. Allergy Clin. Immunol. *74*:79, 1984.
28. Speer, F. Food Allergy. Littleton, MA, PSG Publishing Company, 1978, p. 111–113.
29. Bock, S. A. Food sensitivity: a critical review and practical approach. Am. J. Dis. Child. *134*:973, 1980.
30. Matthews, T. S., and Soothill, J. F. Complement activation after milk feeding in children with cow's milk allergy. Lancet *2*:893, 1970.
31. Goldman, A. S., and Heiner, D. C. Clinical aspects of food sensitivity. Pediatr. Clin. North Am. *24*:133, 1977.
32. Ottesen, E. A., and Cohen, S. G. The eosinophil, eosinophilia, and eosinophil-related disorders. *In* Middleton, E., Jr., et al. (eds.). Allergy—Principles and Practice. St. Louis, C. V. Mosby, 1983, p. 701.
33. Jackson, D., Walker-Smith, J. A., and Phillips, A. D. Macromolecular absorption by histologically normal and abnormal small intestinal mucosa in childhood: an *in vitro* study using organ culture. J. Pediatr. Gastroenterol. Nutr. *2*:235, 1983.
34. Iyngkaran, N., Abidin, Z., Meng, L. L., and Yadav, M. Egg-protein-induced villous atrophy. J. Pediatr. Gastroenterol. Nutr. *1*:29, 1982.
35. Vitoria, J. C., Camarero, C., Sojo, A., Ruiz, A., and Rodriguez-Soriano, J. Enteropathy related to fish, rice, and chicken. Arch. Dis. Child. *57*:44, 1982.
36. Gryboski, J. D. Gastrointestinal milk allergy in infants. Pediatrics *40*:354, 1967.
37. Ament, M. E., and Rubin, C. E. Soy protein—another cause of the flat intestinal lesion. Gastroenterology *62*:227, 1972.
38. Jacobsson, I., and Lindberg, T. Cow's milk as a cause of infantile colic in breast-fed infants. Lancet *2*:437, 1978.
39. Jones, V. A., McLaughlin, P., Shorthouse, M., Workman, E., and Hunter, J. O. Food intolerance: a major factor in the pathogenesis of irritable bowel syndrome. Lancet *2*:1115, 1982.
40. Chin, K. C., Tarlow, M. J., and Allfree, A. J. Allergy to cow's milk presenting as chronic constipation. Br. Med. J. *287*:1593, 1983.
41. Bahna, S. L., and Heiner, D. C. Allergies to Milk. New York, Grune & Stratton, 1980.
42. Heiner, D. C., Sears, J. W., and Kniker, W. T. Multiple precipitins to cow's milk in chronic respiratory disease. A syndrome including poor growth, gastrointestinal symptoms, evidence of allergy, iron deficiency anemia, and pulmonary siderosis. Am. J. Dis. Child. *103*:634, 1962.
43. Hannuksela, M. Food allergy and skin diseases. Ann. Allergy *51*:269, 1983.
44. Atherton, D. J., Sewell, M., Soothill, J. F., Wells, R. S., and Chilvers, C. E. D. A double-blind controlled crossover trial of an antigen-avoidance diet in atopic eczema. Lancet *1*:401, 1978.
45. Bock, S. A., Lee, W. Y., Remigio, L., Holst, A., and May, C. D. Appraisal of skin tests with food extracts for diagnosis of food hypersensitivity. Clin. Allergy *8*:559, 1978.
46. Sampson, H. A. Role of immediate food hypersensitivity in the pathogenesis of atopic dermatitis. J. Allergy Clin. Immunol. *71*:473, 1983.
47. Strunk, R. C., Pinnas, J. L., John, T. J., Hansen, R. C., and Blazovich, J. L. Rice hypersensitivity associated with serum complement depression. Clin. Allergy *8*:51, 1978.
48. Ross-Smith, P., and Jenner, F. A. Diet (gluten) and schizophrenia. J. Hum. Nutr. *34*:107, 1980.
49. Stare, F. J., Whelan, E. M., and Sheridan, M. Diet and hyperactivity: is there a relationship? Pediatrics *66*:521, 1980.
50. Gilbert, R. J., Hobbs, G., Murray, C. K., Cruickshank, J. G., and Young, S. E. Scombrotoxic fish poisoning: features of the first 50 incidents to be reported in Britain (1976–9). Br. Med. J. *281*:71, 1980.
51. Merson, M. H., Baine, W. B., Gangarosa, E. J., and Swanson, R. C. Scombroid fish poisoning. Outbreak traced to commercially canned tuna fish. JAMA *228*:1268, 1974.
52. Atkins, F. M., and Metcalfe, D. D. The diagnosis and treatment of food allergy. Ann. Rev. Nutr. *4*:233, 1984.
53. Sampson, H. A., and Albergo, R. Comparison of results of skin tests, RAST, and double-blind, placebo-controlled food challenges in children with atopic dermatitis. J. Allergy Clin. Immunol. *72*:26, 1984.
54. Bock, S. A. The natural history of food sensitivity. J. Allergy Clin. Immunol. *69*:173, 1982.
55. Katz, A. J., Twarog, F. J., Zeiger, R. S., and Falchuk, Z. M. Milk-sensitive and eosinophilic gastroenteropathy: similar clinical features with contrasting mechanisms and clinical course. J. Allergy Clin. Immunol. *74*:72, 1984.
56. Dockern, R. J. Laboratory tests for food hypersensitivity. *In* Breneman, J. C. (ed.). Handbook of Food Allergies. New York, Marcel Dekker, 1987, p. 163.
57. Kajosaari, M., and Saarinen, U. M. Evaluation of laboratory tests in childhood allergy. Total serum IgE, blood eosinophilia and eosinophil and mast cells in nasal mucosa of 178 children aged 3 years. Allergy *36*:329, 1981.
58. Hughes, E. C. Use of a chemically defined diet in the diagnosis of food sensitivities and the determination of offending foods. Ann. Allergy *40*:393, 1978.
59. Powell, G. K. Milk- and soy-induced enterocolitis of infancy. J. Pediatr. *93*:553, 1978.
60. Wilson, J. F., Heiner, D. C., and Lahey, M. E. Milk-induced gastrointestinal bleeding in infants with hypochromic microcytic anemia. JAMA *189*:568, 1964.
61. Wilson, J. F., Lahey, M. E., and Heiner, D. C. Studies on iron metabolism. V. Further observations on cow's milk-induced gastrointestinal bleeding in infants with iron-deficiency anemia. J. Pediatr. *84*:335, 1974.
62. Waldmann, T. A., Wochner, R. D., Laster, L., and Gordon, R. S., Jr. Allergic gastroenteropathy. A cause of excessive gastrointestinal protein loss. N. Engl. J. Med. *276*:762, 1967.
63. Florent, C., L'Hirondel, C., Desmazures, C., Aymes, C., and Bernie, J. J. Intestinal clearance of a_1-antitrypsin. A sensitive method for the detection of protein-losing enteropathy. Gastroenterology *81*:777, 1981.
64. Perrault, J., and Markowitz, H. Protein-losing gastroenteropathy and the intestinal clearance of serum alpha-1-antitrypsin. Mayo Clin. Proc. *59*:278, 1984.
65. McDonald, P. J., Powell, G. K., and Goldblum, R. M. Serum D-xylose absorption tests: reproducibility and diagnostic usefulness in food-induced enterocolitis. J. Pediatr. Gastroenterol. Nutr. *1*:533, 1982.
66. Maluenda, C., Phillips, A. D., Briddon, A., and Walker-Smith, J. A. Quantitative analysis of small intestinal mucosa in cow's milk sensitive enteropathy. J. Pediatr. Gastroenterol. Nutr. *4*:349, 1984.
67. Phillips, A. D., Rice, S. J., France, N. E., and Walker-Smith, J. A. Small intestinal intraepithelial lymphocyte levels in cow's milk protein intolerance. Gut *20*:509, 1979.
68. McCalla, R., Savilahti, E., Perkkio, M., Kuitunen, P., and Backman, A. Morphology of the jejunum in children with eczema due to food allergy. Allergy *35*:563, 1980.
69. Jenkins, H. R., Pincott, J. R., Soothill, J. F., Milla, P. J., and Harries, J. T. Food allergy: the major cause of infantile colitis. Arch. Dis. Child. *59*:326, 1984.
70. No entry.
71. Goldman, H., and Proujansky, R. Allergic proctitis and gastroenteritis in children. Clinical and mucosal biopsy features in 53 cases. Am. J. Surg. Pathol. *10*:75, 1986.
72. Shiner, M., Brook, C. G. D., Ballard, J., and Herman, S.

Intestinal biopsy in the diagnosis of cow's milk protein intolerance without acute symptoms. Lancet *1*:1060, 1975.
73. David, T. J., Waddington, E., and Stanton, R. H. J. Nutritional hazards of elimination diets in children with atopic eczema. Arch. Dis. Child. *59*:323, 1984.
74. Dockhorn, R. J., and Smith, T. C. Use of a chemically defined hypoallergenic diet (Vivonex) in the management of patients with suspected food allergy/intolerance. Ann. Allergy *47*:264, 1981.
75. Villaveces, J. W., and Heiner, D. C. Experience with an elemental diet. Ann. Allergy *55*:783, 1985.
76. Hoj, L., Osterballe, O., Bundgaard, A., Weeke, B., and Weiss, M. A double-blind controlled trial of elemental diet in severe, perennial asthma. Allergy *36*:257, 1981.
77. Kocoshis, S., and Gryboski, J. D. Use of cromolyn in combined gastrointestinal allergy. JAMA *242*:1169, 1979.
78. Canonica, G. W., Ciprandi, G., Bagnasco, M., and Scordamaglia, A. Oral cromolyn in food allergy: in vivo and in vitro effects. Clin. Immunol. Immunopathol. *41*:154, 1986.
79. Bahna, S. L. Management of food allergies. Ann. Allergy *53*:678, 1984.
80. Podleski, W. K., Panaszek, B. A., Schmidt, J. L., and Burns, R. B. Inhibition of eosinophils degranulation by Ketotifen in a patient with milk allergy, manifested as bronchial asthma—an electron microscopic study. Agents Actions *15*:177, 1984.
81. Soothill, J. F. Prevention of food allergic disease. Ann. Allergy *53*:689, 1984.
82. Kajosaari, M., and Saarinen, U. M. Prophylaxis of atopic disease by six months' total solid food elimination. Evaluation of 135 exclusively breast-fed infants of atopic families. Acta Paediatr. Scand. *72*:411, 1983.
83. Eastham, E. J., Lichauco, T., Grady, M. I., and Walker, W. A. Antigenicity of infant formulas: role of immature intestine on protein permeability. J. Pediatr. *93*:561, 1978.
84. Iyngkaran, N., Robinson, M. J., Sumithran, E., Lam, S. K., Puthucheary, S. D., and Yadav, M. Cow's milk protein-sensitive enteropathy. An important factor in prolonging diarrhoea of acute infective enteritis in early infancy. Arch. Dis. Child. *53*:150, 1978.
85. Gerrard, J. W., and Shenassa, M. Food allergy: two common types as seen in breast and formula fed babies. Ann. Allergy *50*:375, 1983.
86. Warner, J. O. Food allergy in fully breast-fed infants. Clin. Allergy *10*:133, 1980.
87. Lake, A. M., Whitington, P. F., and Hamilton, S. R. Dietary protein-induced colitis in breast-fed infants. J. Pediatr. *101*:906, 1982.
88. Caldwell, J. H., Tennenbaum, J. I., and Bronstein, H. A. Serum IgE in eosinophilic gastroenteritis. Response to intestinal challenge in two cases. N. Engl. J. Med. *292*:1388, 1975.
89. Scudamore, H. H., Phillips, S. F., Swedlund, H. A., and Gleich, G. J. Food allergy manifested by eosinophilia, elevated immunoglobulin E level, and protein-losing enteropathy: the syndrome of allergic gastroenteropathy. J. Allergy Clin. Immunol. *70*:129, 1982.
90. Klein, M. C., Hargrove, R. L., Sleisenger, M. H., and Jeffries, G. H. Eosinophilic gastroenteritis. Medicine *49*:299, 1970.
91. Greenberger, N. J., Tennenbaum, J. I., and Ruppert, R. D. Protein-losing enteropathy associated with gastrointestinal allergy. Am. J. Med. *43*:777, 1967.
92. Leinbach, G. E., and Rubin, C. E. Eosinophilic gastroenteritis: a simple reaction to food allergens. Gastroenterology *59*:874, 1970.
93. Thomas, E., Lev, R., McCahan, J. F., and Pitchumoni, C. S. Eosinophilic gastroenteritis with malabsorption, extensive villous atrophy, recurrent hemorrhage and chronic pulmonary fibrosis. Am. J. Med. Sci. *269*:259, 1975.
94. Cello, J. P. Eosinophilic gastroenteritis—a complex disease entity. Am. J. Med. *67*:1097, 1979.
95. Keshavarzian, A., Saverymuttu, S. H., Tai, P. -C., Thompson, M., Barter, S., Spry, C. J. F., and Chadwick, V. S. Activated eosinophils in familial eosinophilic gastroenteritis. Gastroenterology *88*:1041, 1985.
96. Vazquez-Rodriguez, J. J., Saez, E. S., Vega, J. S., and Serrano, M. C. L. Pancreatitis and eosinophilic gastroenteritis. Int. Surg. *58*:415, 1973.
97. Robert, F., Omura, E., and Durant, J. Mucosal eosinophilic gastroenteritis with systemic involvement. Am. J. Med. *62*:139, 1977.
98. Gregg, J. A., and Utz, D. C. Eosinophil cystitis associated with eosinophilic gastroenteritis. Mayo Clin. Proc. *49*:185, 1974.
99. Haberkern, C. M., Christie, D. L., and Haas, J. E. Eosinophilic gastroenteritis presenting as ileocolitis. Gastroenterology *74*:896, 1978.
100. Jona, J. Z., Belin, R. P., and Burke, J. A. Eosinophilic infiltration of the gastrointestinal tract in children. Am. J. Dis. Child. *130*:1136, 1976.
101. Goldberg, H. I., O'Kieffe, D., Jenis, E. H., and Boyce, H. W. Diffuse eosinophilic gastroenteritis. AJR *119*:342, 1973.
102. Marshak, R. H., Lindner, A., Maklansky, D., and Gelb, A. Eosinophilic gastroenteritis. JAMA *245*:1677, 1981.
103. Feczko, P. J., Halpert, R. D., and Zonca, M. Radiologic abnormalities in eosinophilic esophagitis. Gastrointest. Radiol. *10*:321, 1985.
104. Matzinger, M. A., and Daneman, A. Esophageal involvement in eosinophilic gastroenteritis. Pediatr. Radiol. *13*:35, 1983.
105. Katz, A. J., Goldman, H., and Grand, R. J. Gastric mucosal biopsy in eosinophilic (allergic) gastroenteritis. Gastroenterology *73*:705, 1977.
106. Ureles, A. L., Alschibaja, T., Lodico, D., and Stabins, S. J. Idiopathic eosinophilic infiltration of the gastrointestinal tract, diffuse and circumscribed. Am. J. Med. *30*:899, 1961.
107. McNabb, P. C., Fleming, C. R., Higgins, J. A., and Davis, G. L. Transmural eosinophilic gastroenteritis with ascites. Mayo Clin. Proc. *54*:119, 1979.
108. Leinbach, G. E., and Rubin, C. E. Eosinophilic gastroenteritis: a simple reaction to food allergens? Gastroenterology *59*:874, 1970.
109. Martin, D. M., Goldman, J. A., Gilliam, J., and Nasrallah, S. M. Gold-induced eosinophilic enterocolitis: response to oral cromolyn sodium. Gastroenterology *80*:1567, 1981.
110. Winter, H. S., Madara, J. L., Stafford, R. J., Grand, R. J., Quinlan, J., and Goldman, H. Intraepithelial eosinophils: a new diagnostic criterion for reflux esophagitis. Gastroenterology *83*:818, 1982.
111. Lee, R. G. Marked eosinophilia in esophageal mucosal biopsies. Am. J. Surg. Pathol. *9*:475, 1985.
112. Chusid, M. J., Dale, D. C., West, B. C., and Wolff, S. M. The hypereosinophilic syndrome: analysis of fourteen cases with review of the literature. Medicine *54*:1, 1975.
113. Parrillo, J. E., Fauce, A. S., and Wolff, S. M. Therapy of the hypereosinophilic syndrome. Ann. Intern. Med. *89*:167, 1978.
114. Lanham, J. G., Elkon, K. B., Pusey, C. D., and Hughes, G. R. Systemic vasculitis with asthma and eosinophilia: a clinical approach to the Churg-Strauss syndrome. Medicine *63*:65, 1984.
115. Naylor, A. R., and Pollet, J. E. Eosinophilic colitis. Dis. Colon Rectum *28*:615, 1985.
116. Landres, R. T., Kuster, G. G. R., and Strum, W. B. Eosinophilic esophagitis in a patient with vigorous achalasia. Gastroenterology *74*:1298, 1978.
117. Dobbins, J. W., Sheahan, D. G., and Behar, J. Eosinophilic gastroenteritis with esophageal involvement. Gastroenterology *72*:1312, 1977.
118. DeSchryver-Kecskemeti, K., and Clouse, R. A previously unrecognized subgroup of "eosinophilic gastroenteritis." Association with connective tissue diseases. Am. J. Surg. Pathol. *8*:171, 1984.
119. Heatley, R. V., Harris, A., and Atkinson, M. Treatment of a patient with clinical features of both eosinophilic gastroenteritis and polyarteritis nodosa with oral sodium cromoglycate. Dig. Dis. Sci. *25*:470, 1980.
120. Salmon, P. R., and Paulley, J. W. Eosinophilic granuloma of the gastrointestinal tract. Gut *8*:8, 1967.
121. Weisberg, S. C., and Crosson, J. T. Eosinophilic gastroenter-

itis—report of a case of thirty-two years' duration. Am. J. Dig. Dis. *18*:1005, 1973.
122. Tytgat, G. N., Grijm, R., Dekker, W., and Den Hartog, N. A. Fatal eosinophilic enteritis. Gastroenterology *71*:479, 1976.
123. Everett, G. D., and Mitros, F. A. Eosinophilic gastroenteritis with hepatic eosinophilic granulomas. Am. J. Gastroenterol. *74*:519, 1980.
124. Walker, W. A. Intestinal transport of macromolecules. *In* Johnson, L. R. (ed.). Physiology of the Gastrointestinal Tract. New York, Raven Press, 1981, p. 1282.
125. Katz, A. J. Gastroenterology of food hypersensitivity. *In* Breneman, J. C., (ed.). Handbook of Food Allergies. New York, Marcel Dekker, 1987, p. 37.
126. Bahna, S. L., and Gandhi, M. D. Pediatric food allergy. *In* Breneman, J. C., (ed.). Handbook of Food Allergies. New York, Marcel Dekker, 1987, p. 55.

Celiac Sprue

JERRY S. TRIER

DEFINITION

A precise definition of *celiac sprue* is essential; without one, classification of intestinal malabsorptive disease becomes hopelessly confused. The many other names used to identify patients with this disease (celiac disease, adult celiac disease, idiopathic steatorrhea, nontropical sprue, gluten-induced enteropathy, and so on) provide testimony to the confusion of the past. Because this disease has the same clinical features, etiology, pathology, and response to treatment in children and in adults, the term celiac sprue[1] seems the most suitable and will be used in this chapter, although the term gluten-sensitive enteropathy is an acceptable alternative.

Celiac sprue is a disease in which there is (1) malabsorption of nutrients by that portion of the small intestine which is damaged, (2) a characteristic though not specific lesion of the small intestinal mucosa, and (3) prompt clinical improvement following withdrawal of certain gluten-containing cereal grains from the diet. The prevalence of the disease, which in most of Europe has been estimated to be approximately 0.05 to 0.2 per cent of the general population,[2] is not really known, because the typical intestinal celiac sprue lesion and the potential for eventually developing overt disease is present in apparently asymptomatic individuals.[3] However, the prevalence and incidence appear to vary considerably in different parts of the world; the highest prevalence (1 in 300) has been reported in West Ireland.[4] The disease must now be considered worldwide in its distribution, because there have been convincing descriptions of celiac sprue occurring in natives of tropical countries.[5]

HISTORY

Although the literature pertaining to celiac sprue is quite voluminous, a few reports have provided particularly important conceptual contributions to our understanding of this disease. Gee,[6] in 1888, and Thaysen,[7] in 1932, provided clinical descriptions of the disease in children and adults, respectively, although they were totally unaware of the intestinal pathologic features. In 1950, Dicke suggested, in a landmark study, that certain dietary cereal grains were harmful to children with celiac sprue.[8] He astutely noted that the incidence of celiac sprue in children in Holland during World War II was markedly reduced and that previously diagnosed celiac patients improved during the war years. During that time, grain products such as wheat and rye flour were in short supply in Holland, and dietary carbohydrate was obtained from vegetable sources. In other European countries where, during the same period, cereal grains were more available, the incidence of celiac sprue did not appear reduced. Moreover, when cereal grains became plentiful in Holland after the war, the prevalence of celiac sprue returned rapidly to prewar levels. Subsequently, van de Kamer, Weijers, and Dicke[9] showed that the water-insoluble protein or gluten moiety of wheat was the substance that damaged the small intestine of patients with celiac sprue.

In 1954, Paulley, studying surgical biopsy material, provided the first accurate description of the characteristic intestinal lesion in patients with celiac sprue.[10] With the development of effective peroral suction biopsy instruments in the late 1950s, Rubin and coworkers[11] demonstrated convincingly that celiac disease in children and idiopathic or nontropical sprue in adults were identical diseases with the same clinical and pathologic features.

PATHOLOGY

Celiac sprue affects primarily the mucosa of the small intestine; the submucosa, muscularis, and serosa are usually not involved. The mucosal lesion of the small intestine in patients with celiac sprue may vary considerably in both severity and extent.[11] This spectrum of pathologic involvement helps explain the striking variability of the clinical manifestations of this disease.

Examination of the mucosal surface of biopsy specimens from untreated celiac sprue patients with severe lesions with a hand lens or a dissecting microscope reveals a flat mucosal surface with complete absence of normal intestinal villi.

Histologic examination of tissue sections confirms this loss of normal villous structure (Fig. 61–1*A*). The intestinal crypts are markedly elongated and open onto a flat absorptive surface. The total thickness of the mucosa is only slightly reduced in most cases, because hyperplasia of the crypts compensates for the absence or shortening of the villi. As shown by Rubin and coworkers,[11] these architectural changes decrease the amount of epithelial surface available for digestion and absorption in the involved bowel. Striking cytologic abnormalities characterize the relatively few absorptive cells that line the luminal surface. These cells, which appear columnar in normal biopsy specimens, are cuboidal or, at times, squamoid in celiac sprue biopsy specimens. Their cytoplasm is more basophilic, the basal polarity of the nuclei is lost, and the brush or striated border is markedly attenuated (Fig. 61–1*B*). When viewed with the electron microscope, the microvilli of the absorptive cells appear significantly shortened and often fused (Fig. 61–2). The number of free ribosomes is increased, reflecting impaired differentiation and resulting in the increase in cytoplasmic basophilia evident in histologic preparations. Moreover, degenerative changes, including cytoplasmic and mitochondrial vacuolization and the presence of many large lysosomes, are obvious in many of the absorptive cells (Fig. 61–2).[12] Structural abnormalities of tight junctions between damaged absorptive cells suggest that the barricade that normally separates luminal contents from the paracellular space and the underlying mucosal vasculature is focally disrupted and more permeable in celiac sprue.[13]

Many mucosal enzymes that may contribute to digestive-absorptive processes are altered in these damaged

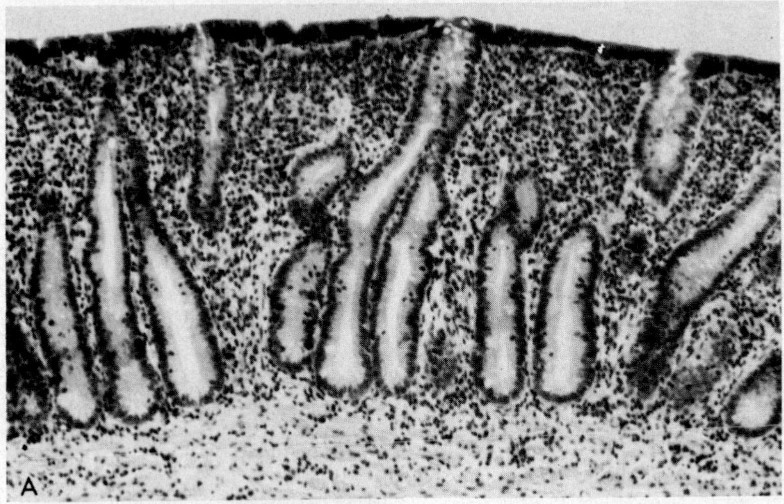

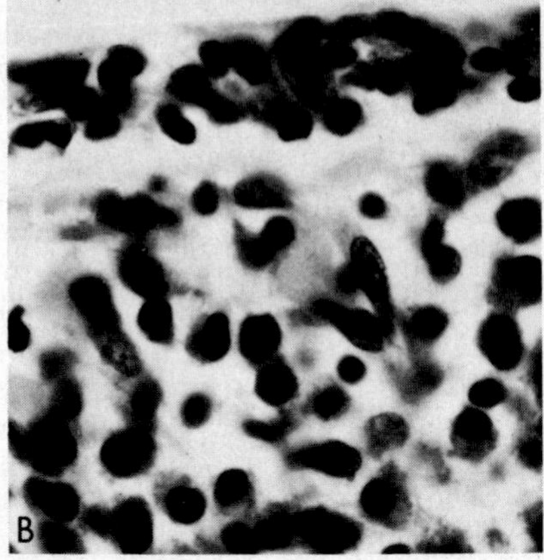

Figure 61–1. Mucosal pathology in celiac sprue. *A,* Mucosa from the duodenojejunal junction of a man with untreated celiac sprue. The mucosal surface is flat, villi are absent, and the crypts are markedly hyperplastic. There is increased cellularity of the lamina propria. (× 80.) *B,* Higher magnification of surface absorptive cells shown in *A.* The cells are cuboidal, without a well-defined apical striated border. There is marked loss of nuclear polarity. (× 650.)

Illustration continued on following page

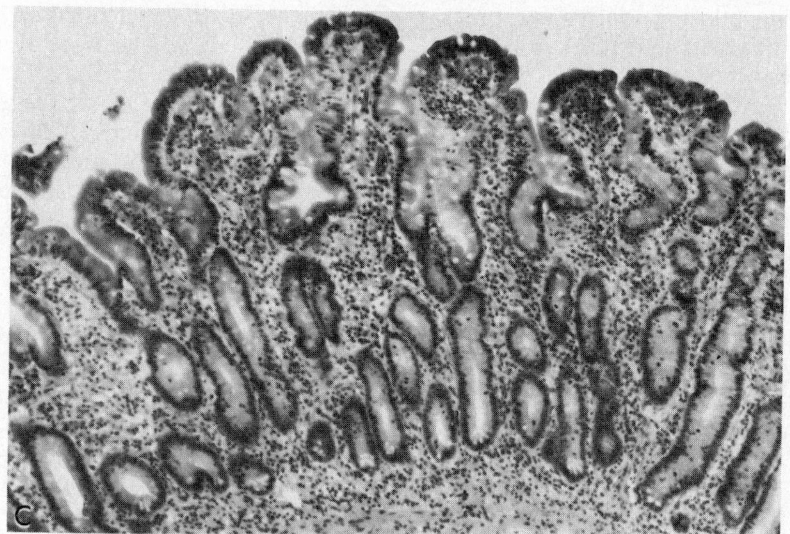

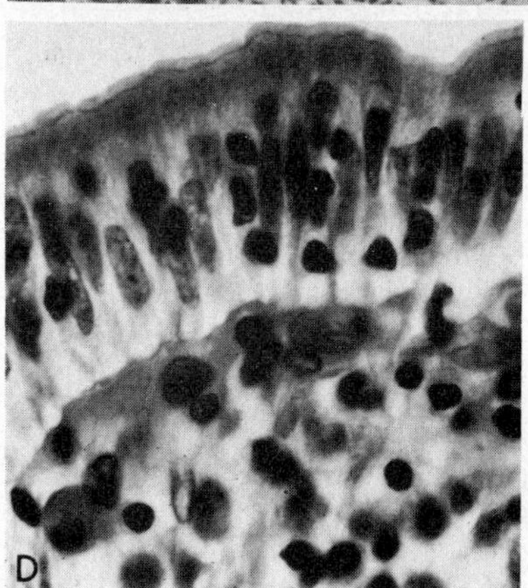

Figure 61–1. *Continued. C,* Mucosa from the duodenojejunal junction from the same patient shown in *A* after four weeks of gluten withdrawal. The mucosal architecture is definitely improved. Villi can be recognized, but mucosal architecture is still abnormal because villi are short and crypt hyperplasia and increased cellularity of the lamina propria persist. (× 80.) *D,* Higher magnification of the surface absorptive cells from the biopsy specimen shown in *C.* The absorptive cells are columnar, with basally located nuclei and a well-defined striated border after four weeks of gluten withdrawal. (× 650.)

absorptive cells. Disaccharidases, peptidases, alkaline phosphatase, adenosine triphosphatase, and esterases are decreased.[14, 15] Activities of acid hydrolases (lysosomal enzymes) are increased.[15] Thus, not only are mature absorptive cells reduced in number in celiac sprue patients, but also those that remain are functionally compromised.

Unlike the absorptive cells, the undifferentiated crypt cells are markedly increased in number in severe untreated celiac sprue, and this accounts for the marked lengthening of crypts. Moreover, the number of mitoses in crypts is strikingly increased.[14, 16] The cytologic features and histochemistry of the crypt cells are normal by both light and electron microscopy.[12] Thus, there are usually normal numbers of normal-appearing Paneth and goblet cells, whereas endocrine cells appear abundant in the crypts of patients with severe lesions.[17] Whether this represents true endocrine cell hyperplasia or impaired release of endocrine cell secretory products is not established.

The cellularity of the lamina propria is regularly increased in the involved small intestine. The cellular infiltrate consists largely of immunoglobulin-producing plasma cells and lymphocytes. Generally, the number of IgA-, IgM-, and IgG-producing cells is increased, but as in normal mucosa, IgA-producing cells predominate.[18] Polymorphonuclear leukocytes, eosinophils, and mast cells may contribute substantially to the increased cellularity of the lamina propria.[19] The number of intraepithelial lymphocytes per unit length of absorptive epithelium is increased in untreated celiac sprue;[20] however, the total number of intraepithelial lymphocytes is not increased, for the absorptive surface is markedly reduced.[21]

The length of small intestine with the celiac sprue lesion in untreated patients varies from patient to patient and correlates with the severity of clinical symptoms.[22] Thus, the patient with a severe lesion that involves the full length of the small intestine will be much sicker and have far greater malabsorption than the patient with a severe duodenal lesion, a milder jejunal lesion, and a histologically normal ileum. When the intestinal lesion does not involve the entire length of the small gut, the proximal intestine is the most severely involved and the lesion decreases in severity toward the distal small intestine. Sparing of the proximal intestine with involvement of the distal small intestine does not occur in celiac sprue.

In some untreated patients with relatively mild or clinically latent celiac sprue, not even the proximal

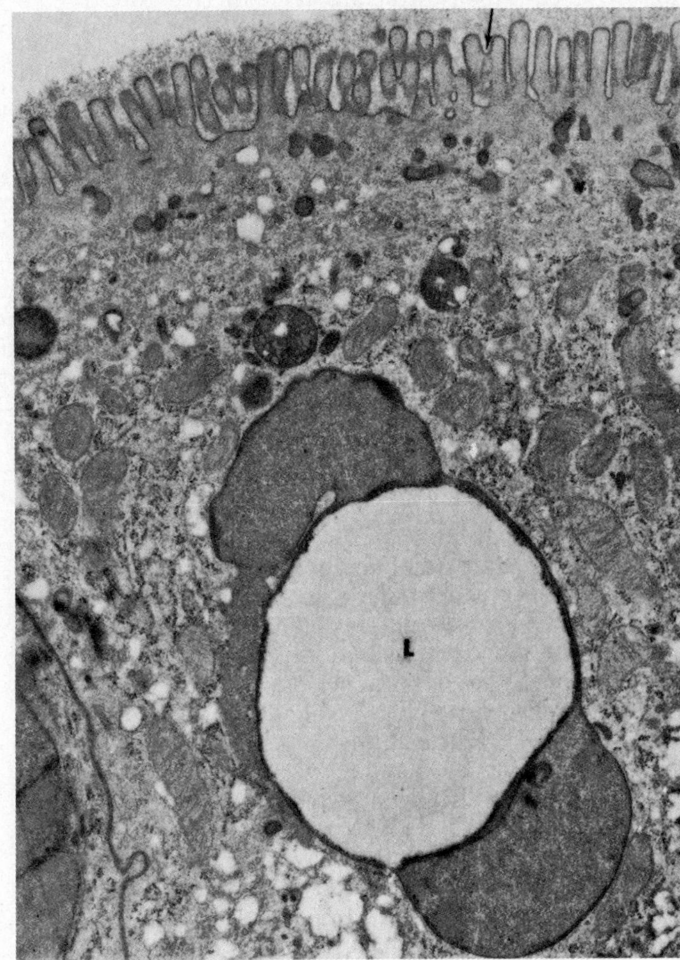

Figure 61–2. Electron micrograph of apical cytoplasm of a surface absorptive cell from a man with untreated celiac sprue. The microvilli are markedly shortened and some are fused *(arrow)*, although the surface coat is well developed. A huge lysosome-like body (L) is prominent in the cytoplasm. There are more free ribosomes and fewer elements of membraneous endoplasmic reticulum than in normal absorptive cells. (× 10,000.)

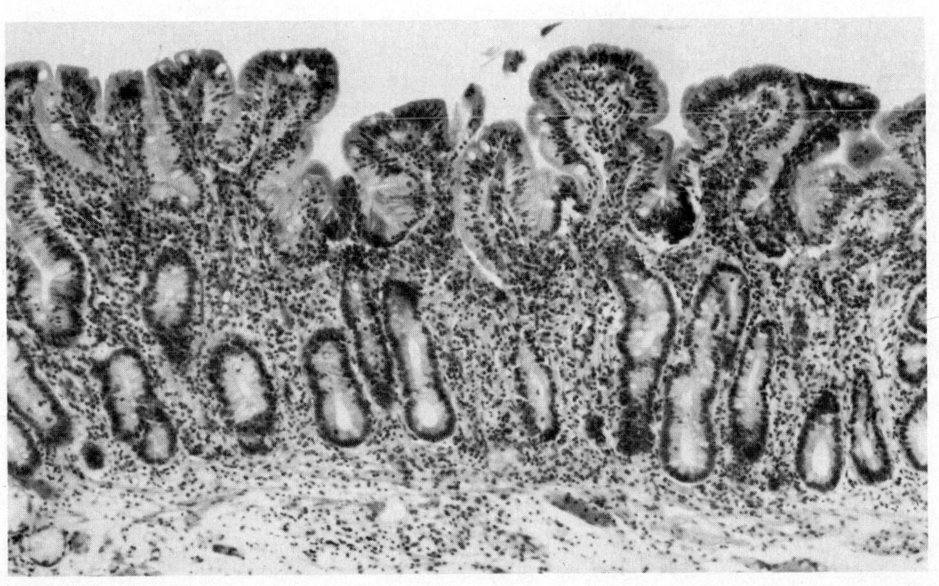

Figure 61–3. Mucosal biopsy section from a patient with a moderate sprue lesion and dermatitis herpetiformis. Villi are present, but they are significantly shorter than normal and the crypts are hyperplastic. The cellularity of the lamina is increased, and the absorptive epithelium is infiltrated by mononuclear cells. (× 80.)

intestine shows the typical severe flat lesion. Rather, some residual villous structure remains (Fig. 61–3), and the absorptive surface, although less than normal, is greater than that seen in severely diseased mucosa.[1] However, some shortening of the villi, hyperplasia of the crypts, cytologically abnormal surface cells, and increased cellularity of the lamina propria must be present in biopsy specimens from patients with untreated disease in order to establish the diagnosis.

Appropriate treatment with a gluten-free diet results in significant improvement in intestinal structure in celiac sprue patients (Fig. 61–1*C*). The cytologic appearance of the surface absorptive cells improves first, often within a few days.[16] Tall, columnar absorptive cells with basal nuclei and well-developed brush borders replace the abnormal cuboidal surface cells that were exposed to gluten, and the ratio of intraepithelial lymphocytes to absorptive cells decreases (Fig. 61–1*D*).[20] Subsequently, villous architecture reverts toward normal, with lengthening of the villi, shortening of the crypts, and a decrease in the cellularity of the lamina propria. The mucosa of the distal small intestine improves more rapidly than that of the severely involved proximal bowel.[22] Months or even years of gluten withdrawal may be required in some patients before mucosal structure reverts maximally toward normal; indeed, some residual abnormality, which may be striking or subtle and may be due in part to inadvertent gluten ingestion, persists in the proximal intestine of many patients.

There are patients who have mucosal intestinal lesions which are indistinguishable from the lesion observed in patients with celiac sprue but who fail to respond to gluten withdrawal. These patients appear to have a mucosal disease that *resembles* celiac sprue but that has a different response to treatment and often a grave prognosis. They should not be confused with typical celiac sprue patients.[23, 24] Initially responsive celiac sprue in a few patients may evolve into this refractory disease.[24] (See discussion of refractory sprue on p. 1150.)

Another extremely rare condition that may cause confusion is *collagenous sprue*. These patients may present initially with symptoms and biopsy findings consistent with celiac sprue. However, they fail to respond to dietary gluten withdrawal and, with time, develop extensive deposition of collagen in the lamina propria just beneath the absorptive epithelium (Fig. 61–4).[25] In contrast to celiac sprue, the prognosis in collagenous sprue is grim; all reported patients have died from the disease.

In addition to the typical lesion of the small intestine, mild, nonspecific histologic changes are seen in the rectal mucosa of some but not all celiac sprue patients.[26] These mimic the changes of mild proctitis and may include branching and disorganization of the rectal glands and an increase in the cellularity of the lamina propria.

In the severely depleted patient with severe untreated celiac sprue, pathologic changes may be present in many other organ systems besides the digestive tract. Detailed description and discussion of these diverse pathologic changes are not within the scope of this chapter, but some of the more commonly encountered extraintestinal manifestations are listed in Table 61–1.

ETIOLOGY AND PATHOGENESIS

The interaction of the water-insoluble protein moiety (gluten) of certain cereal grains with the mucosa of the small intestine is crucial in the pathogenesis of celiac sprue. Instillation of wheat, barley, or rye flour into a histologically normal-appearing segment of small intestine of an asymptomatic patient with treated celiac sprue produces bloating, malaise, abdominal cramps, and diarrhea within a few hours.[9, 27] The fecal fat excretion increases acutely, and the intestinal segment exposed to the gluten develops the typical mucosal lesion of celiac sprue within eight to 12 hours. In contrast, instillation of rice or corn flour into a normal-

Table 61–1. EXTRAINTESTINAL MANIFESTATIONS OF CELIAC SPRUE

Organ System	Manifestation	Probable Cause(s)
Hematopoietic	Anemia	Iron, folate, vitamin B_{12}, or pyridoxine deficiency
	Hemorrhage	Hypoprothrombinemia and, rarely, thrombocytopenia due to folate deficiency
Skeletal	Osteopenia	Malabsorption of calcium and vitamin D
	Pathologic fractures	Osteopenia
	Osteoarthropathy	Unknown
Muscular	Atrophy	Malnutrition due to panmalabsorption
	Tetany	Calcium, vitamin D, and/or magnesium malabsorption
	Weakness	Generalized muscle atrophy, hypokalemia
Nervous	Peripheral neuropathy	Vitamin deficiencies such as thiamine and vitamin B_{12}
	Demyelinating central nervous system lesions	Unknown
Endocrine	Secondary hyperparathyroidism	Calcium and vitamin D malabsorption causing hypocalcemia
	Amenorrhea, infertility, impotence	? Malnutrition due to panmalabsorption, ? hypothalamic-pituitary dysfunction
Integument	Follicular hyperkeratosis and dermatitis	Vitamin A malabsorption, ? vitamin B complex malabsorption
	Petechiae and ecchymoses	Hypoprothrombinemia and, rarely, thrombocytopenia
	Edema	Hypoproteinemia
	Dermatitis herpetiformis	Unknown

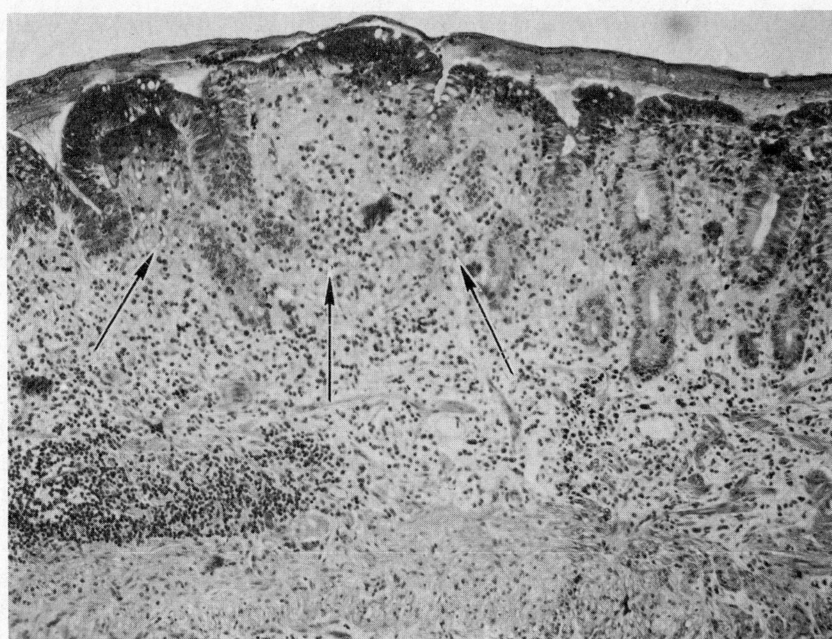

Figure 61–4. The histologic appearance of jejunal mucosa from a patient with collagenous sprue. Note the deposition of collagen in the lamina propria, particularly beneath the absorptive epithelium *(arrows)*. Crypts are decreased in number. (Masson trichrome stain, × 80.) (Courtesy of L. L. Brandborg, M.D.)

appearing segment produces neither clinical symptoms nor histologic changes. Instillation of oat flour seems toxic to some but not all celiac sprue patients, although the symptoms and histologic changes are always less pronounced than those produced by wheat, barley, or rye flour.

Gliadin, a complex mixture of glutamine- and proline-rich proteins obtained by alcohol extraction of wheat gluten,[28] will also produce symptoms and histologic lesions when instilled into the small intestine of asymptomatic celiac sprue patients. Gliadin can be separated electrophoretically into four major fractions; these have been designated α-, β-, γ-, and ω-gliadins. There is general agreement that α-gliadin is toxic to celiac sprue patients, but whether or not all fractions are toxic is controversial.[29] However, the peptide structure seems essential for toxicity, because gliadin that has been hydrolyzed to its constituent amino acids is nontoxic and produces neither symptoms nor an intestinal lesion when fed to asymptomatic celiac sprue patients (Table 61–2).[30] The amino acid sequences of α-type gliadin proteins have recently been determined.[31] Such clarification of the chemical structure of toxic gluten fractions may ultimately lead to precise definition of the molecular interaction between gluten and susceptible mucosal cells in celiac sprue.

How gluten damages the intestinal mucosa is not known. Four possible mechanisms that have been suggested are (1) that celiac sprue is caused by an immune response to dietary gluten, (2) that genetic factors facilitate the adverse effect of gluten, (3) that celiac sprue is a metabolic disease in which gluten is incompletely digested, resulting in the accumulation of toxic substances that damage the mucosa, and (4) that toxicity is mediated by a lectin-like interaction between gluten and intestinal epithelial cells.

Immune Mechanisms. Evidence implicating immune mechanisms in the pathogenesis of celiac sprue is substantial but not conclusive. As mentioned earlier, increased numbers of immunocytes are present in the lamina propria of the small intestine of untreated celiac sprue patients.[18, 32] Although the greatest relative increase is among immunocytes that produce IgM, cells that produce IgA and IgG are also increased.[18] In addition, serum IgA levels are increased, whereas serum IgM levels are diminished in the majority of untreated patients but not in treated patients with celiac sprue, although IgA is not crucial for development of the disease because patients with selective IgA deficiency and celiac sprue have been described.[33] Circulating antibodies to gliadin fractions are found in the serum of many celiac sprue patients[34, 35] and frequently persist for years in asymptomatic, treated

Table 61–2. TOXICITY OF GRAINS AND WHEAT FRACTIONS TO PATIENTS WITH CELIAC SPRUE DISEASE

Grains	Toxicity
Wheat	+
Barley	+
Rye	+
Oats	±
Rice	−
Corn	−
Wheat Fractions	
Aqueous extract of wheat	−
Alcohol extract of wheat (gliadin)	+
Deaminated gliadin	−
Amino acids obtained by complete acid hydrolysis of gliadin	−
α-gliadin	+
β-, γ-, ω-gliadins	?

patients.[35] Thus, the presence of these circulating antibodies correlates poorly with the severity of the disease. Moreover, some celiac sprue patients have circulating antibodies to nongluten dietary proteins, such as milk and egg proteins, and circulating antibodies to gluten fractions and other foodstuffs are found in diseases other than celiac sprue that involve intestinal mucosa, as well as in some normal individuals.[35]

That antigliadin antibodies are synthesized by the diseased mucosa in patients with untreated celiac sprue has been shown by exposing biopsies to gluten *in vitro*.[36, 37] The role of antigliadin antibodies in the pathogenesis of celiac sprue is, however, unclear. Because they are present in treated patients in remission, the antibodies by themselves do not seem harmful, but they may participate in an antibody-dependent cell-mediated cytotoxic reaction directed against absorptive cells or may form immune complexes following gluten ingestion.[29] Alternatively, such circulating antibodies may simply reflect nonspecific responses to the passage of incompletely digested dietary proteins across an abnormally permeable intestinal epithelium.[13] Antibodies directed against reticulin have been detected in many but not all patients with celiac sprue[38, 39] as well as in occasional patients with Crohn's disease.[40] Like antigliadin antibodies, their significance, if any, in the pathogenesis of celiac sprue is unknown.

Cell-mediated immune responses may play a role in the pathogenesis of celiac sprue. However, subset distribution among circulating T lymphocytes appears comparable in healthy individuals and patients with celiac sprue.[41] T lymphocytes are abundant in the lamina propria of the small intestine, and most intraepithelial lymphocytes, which are so abundant in untreated celiac sprue, are T lymphocytes which bear the marker of suppressor cytotoxic lymphocytes (OKT8).[41] However, there is no convincing evidence that T cell subset distribution differs in the epithelium or lamina propria of the small intestine of patients with untreated or treated celiac sprue from that observed in the mucosa of normal individuals. It has been noted that biopsies from untreated celiac sprue patients produce a substance or substances that inhibit migration of leukocytes when the biopsies are exposed to gluten fractions, whereas biopsies from treated patients produce no such substance.[42, 43] Such factors, presumably produced by sensitized T cells, have been implicated in the pathogenesis of the mucosal lesion in celiac sprue,[42, 43] but additional studies are needed to define the role of cell-mediated immune responses in this disease.

Genetic Factors. There is no doubt that genetic factors play a role in the etiology of celiac sprue. The incidence of the disease in relatives of celiac sprue patients is significantly greater than in control populations. MacDonald and coworkers[3] found as many as four biopsy-proved cases of celiac sprue in a single family and noted a total of 11 affected relatives among 96 people studied from 17 families. The symptoms were often either absent or so mild that some affected relatives were not aware of any abnormality. A prevalence of latent celiac sprue in approximately 10 per cent of first-order relatives has subsequently been reported in several other studies.[44] The detection of these "asymptomatic" celiac sprue patients casts doubt on the accuracy of available incidence and prevalence figures and suggests that "mild" or latent celiac sprue may be common. Although several relatives were affected in some kindreds, only a single case could be found in other carefully studied large families. Moreover, both concordance and discordance for celiac sprue have been documented in identical twin pairs.

That genetic factors play a role in celiac sprue is supported further by the distribution of a number of genetic markers. The class I histocompatibility antigen, HLA-B8, and the class II histocompatibility antigen, HLA-DR3, are present in 60 to 90 per cent of patients with celiac sprue, compared with 20 per cent or less of normal individuals.[45–47] In many celiac sprue patients, HLA-DR7 is present in conjunction with HLA-DR3. More recently, HLA-DQw2 was noted to be present in 80 to 100 per cent of celiac sprue patients.[48, 49] It is of interest that a polymorphic 4.0 kb DNA fragment was detected in nuclei of lymphoblastoid B cell lines in 18 of 20 HLA-DQw2 positive celiac sprue patients but in only two of the cell lines established from 10 HLA-DQw2 positive control subjects.[49] However, not all individuals with HLA-B8, HLA-DR3, HLA-DR7, and/or HLA-DQw2 develop celiac sprue, nor do all celiac sprue patients carry one or more of these antigens. In that regard, it is of interest that other genetic markers have been identified, including alloantigens on the surface of B cells[50] and Gm allotype markers on the IgG heavy chain.[51, 52] In recent studies, all treated celiac sprue patients with antigliadin antibody and all HLA-B8 and HLA-DR3 negative patients had the IgG heavy chain phenotype, G2m(n), suggesting that this marker is associated with persistence of antigliadin antibodies and may predispose to celiac sprue in HLA-B8 and HLA-DR3 negative individuals.[51, 52]

The unusual interrelationship of *dermatitis herpetiformis* and celiac sprue has relevance in any discussion of the etiology of celiac sprue. If the proximal small intestine is sampled at several sites, almost all patients with dermatitis herpetiformis have at least a mild mucosal lesion consistent with celiac sprue, even though many patients with mild intestinal lesions have no symptoms (see Fig. 61–3).[53–55] Yet, the majority of patients with celiac sprue do not develop skin lesions of dermatitis herpetiformis. Thus, dermatitis herpetiformis and celiac sprue appear to be distinct diseases, with the curious relationship that all or almost all patients with the skin disease also have at least latent celiac sprue, whereas only relatively few patients with celiac sprue have dermatitis herpetiformis. It is of interest that, as in celiac sprue without skin disease, the prevalence of the histocompatibility antigens HLA-B8, HLA-DR3, and HLA-DQw2 is much higher in patients with dermatitis herpetiformis than in normal individuals.[56]

Enzyme Deficiency. There is essentially no evidence that celiac sprue represents a metabolic disorder that results from accumulation of toxic material in the intestinal lumen or mucosa, owing to incomplete gluten digestion. It has been shown that levels of some specific peptidases, important in the digestion of gliadin, are reduced in the mucosa of untreated celiac sprue patients. However, following successful treatment, levels of these peptidases revert to normal in the histologically normal-appearing mucosa, even though reingestion of gluten promptly induces clinical symptoms and recurrence of the celiac sprue lesion.[57] If deficiency of a specific peptidase were causative, deficiency of the enzyme would be apparent in *treated* as well as untreated patients. Thus, the documented peptidase deficiencies are nonspecific and reflect only the mucosal damage. Knowledge of the amino acid sequences of toxic gliadin polypeptides[31] should facilitate definitive studies to establish or exclude a peptidase deficiency in patients with celiac sprue.

Lectin Interaction. It has been suggested that a primary abnormality in the composition of the surface glycoproteins (glycocalyx) on epithelial cell apical membranes results in exposure of distinctive sugar residues that selectively bind toxic gliadin fractions in celiac sprue patients.[58] The gliadin fraction might then damage the intestinal epithelium[58] much as cytotoxic plant lectins damage cells after binding to their surface glycoconjugates.[59] That plant lectins are capable of damaging intestinal epithelium has been clearly demonstrated.[60] However, at present there is little evidence that gliadin fractions have lectin-like activity directed against epithelial cells isolated from normal intestine or from intestinal biopsies obtained from untreated or treated celiac sprue patients.[61]

Composite Hypothesis. A provocative hypothesis of the possible pathogenesis of celiac disease which invokes immunologic, genetic, and dietary factors but also requires exposure to a suitable environmental factor has recently been developed by Kagnoff and coworkers.[29, 62] This hypothesis is based on the finding of sequence homology of a 12–amino acid segment in a human adenovirus protein and in an α-gliadin fraction as well as cross-reactivity of antibody to the viral protein and appropriate gliadin fractions.[62] It is proposed that environmental exposure to the intestinal viral infection may sensitize the genetically predisposed host to antigenic determinants in gluten that closely resemble those of the viral protein. This attractive hypothesis, if true, provides explanations for the observed discordance of the disease in monozygotic twins[29] as well as the recently reported decline in incidence of celiac sprue among children in some, but not all, geographic regions.[2]

Although the mechanism by which gluten produces its toxic effect on the mucosa is not known, certain aspects of the interaction of the mucosa with gluten merit comment, because they help clarify the histogenesis of the mucosal lesion. There seems little doubt that certain gluten fractions are toxic to the intestinal mucosa and result ultimately in damage to intestinal absorptive cells. The damaged and dying absorptive cells are sloughed from the mucosal surface into the gut lumen more rapidly than normal. To compensate for this excessive loss of mature cells, the number of proliferating cells increases and the crypts become hyperplastic. Thus, in the fully developed celiac sprue lesion, the absorptive cells are damaged and diminished in number, villi are blunted or absent, the number of proliferating undifferentiated crypt cells is markedly increased, the crypts are markedly elongated, and cell renewal and migration are more rapid than normal.[63]

CLINICAL FEATURES AND DIAGNOSIS

The clinical manifestations of celiac sprue vary tremendously from patient to patient. Moreover, because most of the symptoms result from intestinal malabsorption, they are not specific for celiac sprue, but resemble those seen in other diseases with intestinal malabsorption (see pp. 263–282).

The patient with a severe lesion involving the entire small intestine from proximal duodenum to distal ileum will present with devastating and life-threatening panmalabsorption. Such a patient may develop secondary involvement of many organ systems as a consequence of the extensive absorptive defects. In striking contrast, the patient with a limited lesion involving only the duodenum and proximal jejunum may have no overt gastrointestinal symptoms and may present only with anemia caused by iron or folate deficiency or both, or with evidence of osteopenic bone disease. Clearly, the severity of the celiac sprue lesion and its extent govern, at least in part, the severity of the clinical manifestations of the disease. However, other as yet undefined factors may be important, for the natural history of *untreated* celiac sprue is one of intermittent exacerbations and relative remissions.

The disease may first become apparent in infants when gluten ingestion, usually in the form of cereals, begins. Symptoms may persist throughout childhood if treatment is not begun, but they often diminish or disappear completely during adolescence. Symptoms generally reappear in early adult life (third and fourth decades).

In other patients, symptoms are not noted and the diagnosis is not established until middle or even old age. Whether these patients had asymptomatic or undetected celiac sprue with some degree of gluten intolerance since birth or whether they first develop gluten intolerance and the intestinal lesion as adults is not known. The finding of the typical lesion in asymptomatic relatives of celiac sprue patients[3] and the unmasking of asymptomatic disease by surgery that induces rapid gastric emptying (gastric resection, pyloroplasty)[64] suggest that adults may have clinically inapparent celiac sprue for some time.

Gastrointestinal Symptoms. The most common symptoms in patients with extensive disease include *diarrhea, flatulence, weight loss,* and *weakness*. The frequency and nature of the stools vary considerably from patient to patient. Those with extensive intestinal involvement may have in excess of ten stools per day.

Severe dehydration, electrolyte depletion, and even acidosis may develop, especially in infants and young children. The stools may be watery or semiformed, light tan or gray, or oily and frothy and have a characteristic foul, rancid odor. Not all patients have diarrhea; some even complain of constipation. But when they do have a bowel movement, they excrete large quantities of putty-like stool that may be difficult to flush down the toilet. Because of their high gas content, the stools of celiac sprue patients often float on water.

The mechanisms of diarrhea in symptomatic celiac sprue are not fully understood, but several factors probably contribute. First, the stool volume and osmotic load delivered to the colon are increased by the malabsorption of fat, carbohydrate, protein, water, electrolytes, and, indeed, all nutrients. In addition, the delivery of excessive dietary fat into the large bowel probably results in the production by bacteria of hydroxy fatty acids. These hydroxy fatty acids are potent, irritating cathartics. Water and electrolytes are actually *secreted* into, rather than absorbed from, the lumen of the upper small intestine in celiac sprue patients.[65] This secretion further increases stool volume in an intestine with already compromised absorptive capacity. There is also evidence that cholecystokinin and secretin release in response to a meal are impaired in celiac sprue, diminishing delivery of bile and pancreatic secretions into the gut lumen and possibly compromising intraluminal digestions.[66–68] Alterations in the secretion of other gut peptides have been noted and may contribute to the observed diarrhea. For example, basal and postprandial plasma enteroglucagon concentrations are higher in untreated celiac sprue patients than in treated patients or control subjects.[69] Finally, if the disease extends to and involves the ileum, impaired absorption of conjugated bile salts may further aggravate the diarrhea by the direct cathartic action of the bile salts on the colon.

The amount of weight loss in a celiac sprue patient depends upon the severity and extent of the intestinal lesion that governs the degree of malabsorption and upon the ability of the patient to compensate for the malabsorption by increasing dietary intake. Many celiac sprue patients with significant malabsorption have enormous appetites and lose little or no weight. A careful dietary history of such patients often reveals tremendous hyperphagia, with daily caloric intakes well in excess of normal. In severe disease, anorexia may develop with associated rapid and severe weight loss. In such debilitated patients, some of the weight loss may be masked by fluid retention caused by hypoproteinemia. In infants and young children with untreated celiac sprue, failure of weight gain and growth retardation may be the counterpart of weight loss in the adult.

In most celiac sprue patients, the weakness, lassitude, and fatigue commonly observed are not specific and are related to the general poor nutrition. In some patients, severe anemia may contribute to the weakness. In occasional patients, severe hypokalemia resulting from loss of potassium in the stool may cause severe muscle weakness.

Severe abdominal pain is uncommon in patients with uncomplicated celiac sprue. Rather, many patients have no abdominal pain whatever. However, abdominal distention with excessive amounts of malodorous flatus is a common complaint and occurs in over half of patients with clinically apparent disease. Nausea and vomiting are uncommon in uncomplicated celiac sprue.

Extraintestinal Symptoms. The metabolic defects that may develop because of defective absorption of nutrients from the gut may involve virtually all organ systems (see Table 61–1). Thus, although the gastrointestinal symptoms are often prominent, the symptoms most distressing to the patient may involve other organ systems. Many celiac sprue patients present initially with complaints not referable directly to the gastrointestinal tract. The alert physician may establish a diagnosis of celiac sprue in patients with such diverse findings as fatigue associated with refractory iron deficiency anemia or severe back pain owing to a collapsed lumbar vertebra (see Table 61–1).

Anemia commonly occurs in adults with severe celiac sprue. Usually it is caused by impaired iron and/or folate absorption from the proximal intestine; in severe disease with ileal involvement, vitamin B_{12} absorption is also impaired. Purpura and gastrointestinal, vaginal, nasal, or renal bleeding may occur in patients with extensive disease. Such bleeding may further aggravate pre-existing anemia and is most often caused by impaired blood coagulability resulting from prothrombin deficiency secondary to impaired intestinal absorption of fat-soluble vitamin K. In one series, thrombocytosis was noted in roughly 50 per cent of patients,[70] and hyposplenism that improves with elimination of gluten from the diet has been documented in some patients.[71]

Osteopenic bone disease may develop in patients with celiac sprue. Calcium absorption is impaired by (1) defective calcium transport by the diseased small intestine, (2) vitamin D deficiency caused by impaired absorption of this fat-soluble vitamin, and (3) binding of intraluminal calcium to unabsorbed dietary fatty acids, forming insoluble calcium soaps, which are then excreted in the feces. Bone pain, especially of the low back, rib cage, and pelvis, may develop. Pathologic fractures that occur without trauma are uncommon but have been described. Calcium depletion and magnesium depletion may cause paresthesias, muscle cramps, and even frank tetany.

Neurologic symptoms caused by lesions of the central or peripheral nervous system are not common, but occur occasionally in patients with severe disease. Muscle weakness, paresthesias with sensory loss, and ataxia are the most common symptoms encountered. Pathologic evidence of peripheral neuropathy and, very rarely, patchy demyelinization of the spinal cord, cerebellar atrophy, and capillary proliferation suggestive of Wernicke's encephalopathy have been described (see Table 61–1). The cause of these phenomena is not at all clear. In most patients with neurologic findings, serum vitamin B_{12} levels have been normal, although vitamin B_{12} absorption might be defective. Causative roles for thiamine, riboflavin, and pyridoxine deficiencies, although suggested, have not been established. Night blindness caused by vitamin A deficiency may occur.

Secondary hyperparathyroidism may develop in patients with severely impaired calcium absorption. The hyperparathyroidism results in mobilization of calcium from the bones in response to the low serum calcium level and may contribute to the osteopenia seen in such patients.

Amenorrhea, delayed menarche, and infertility in women and impotence and infertility in men with untreated celiac sprue have been described.[72, 73] Malnutrition related to malabsorption may contribute. Abnormalities in hypothalamic-pituitary regulation of gonadal function and gonadal androgen resistance that disappears upon gluten withdrawal have been incriminated in men.[73]

Physical Findings. Physical findings, like symptoms, may vary considerably among patients with celiac sprue. In the patient whose lesion is limited to the proximal small intestine, physical findings may be entirely absent or limited to pallor caused by anemia. On the other hand, the patient who has an extensive lesion involving most or all of the small intestine may have many of the findings described below.

Emaciation with evidence of recent weight loss, including loose skin folds and muscle wasting, may be prominent in patients with severe celiac sprue. Hypotension may be related to fluid and electrolyte depletion.

Careful examination of the integument of celiac sprue patients is important, because it is often the site of significant physical signs. *Clubbing* of the nails is seen in severe disease. The skin may be dry with poor turgor if there is dehydration. There may be *edema*, especially of the lower extremities, if there is hypoproteinemia caused by deficient albumin synthesis or enteric loss of serum proteins. Increased skin pigmentation may be obvious in severely ill patients. Other findings may include spontaneous *ecchymoses* related to hypoprothrombinemia, *hyperkeratosis follicularis* caused by vitamin A deficiency, and pallor caused by anemia. The coexistence of celiac sprue and dermatitis herpetiformis has been discussed (see p. 1140). All patients with dermatitis herpetiformis should be evaluated for celiac sprue.

Examination of the mouth may show *cheilosis* and *glossitis* with decreased papillation of the tongue.

The abdomen is often protuberant and tympanic, and has a characteristic doughy consistency when palpated owing to distention of intestinal loops with fluid and gas. Hepatomegaly is uncommon, but ascites occasionally may be detected in patients with significant hypoproteinemia. Abdominal tenderness is uncommon.

The extremities may reveal loss of various sensory modalities, including light touch, vibration, and position, usually caused by peripheral neuropathy and, very rarely, demyelinating spinal cord lesions. If the neuropathy is severe, deep tendon reflexes are diminished or even absent. Hyperpathia may be present, and an ataxic gait in severely ill patients is not uncommon.

A positive *Chvostek* or *Trousseau* sign may be elicited in patients with severe calcium or magnesium depletion. In such individuals, bone tenderness related to osteopenia may be present, especially if collapsed vertebrae or other fractures are present.

It must be emphasized that these physical findings are not specific for celiac sprue, because they may be elicited with malabsorption caused by other diseases.

LABORATORY FINDINGS

The laboratory findings in celiac sprue, like the symptoms and signs, vary with the extent and severity of the intestinal lesion. Moreover, like other clinical findings in this disease, similar laboratory abnormalities may often be seen in patients with other diseases producing intestinal malabsorption (see Table 18–4, p. 273).

Stool Examination. If malabsorption is sufficient to produce significant steatorrhea, the appearance and the odor of the stools may be typical. A watery or bulky, semiformed, light tan or grayish, greasy-appearing stool with a rancid odor is characteristic. Microscopic evaluation of the fat content of a stool suspension stained with Sudan III or IV after hydrolysis with acetic acid and heat is a helpful bedside screening test.

To document steatorrhea unequivocally, the amount of fat in stool may be determined quantitatively, using a reliable method such as the van de Kamer chemical method. The recently introduced ^{14}C-triolein breath test can also be used to test for steatorrhea, but it is less sensitive and specific. Steatorrhea is present in most patients with symptomatic celiac sprue, and its severity correlates reasonably well with the severity and the extent of the intestinal lesion. Steatorrhea is absent, however, in some patients with disease limited to the proximal small intestine.

Hematologic Tests. The anemia of celiac sprue may be secondary to iron, folate, or, rarely, vitamin B_{12} deficiency; hence red blood cell morphologic appearance may range from microcytic to macrocytic. A low serum iron level is very common, because the duodenal lesion often impairs iron absorption in the untreated patient. Leukopenia and thrombocytopenia are uncommon but may occur if severe folate or vitamin B_{12} deficiency is present. Under such circumstances, the serum vitamin B_{12} absorption test is valuable in determining whether or not the sprue lesion involves the distal ileum. If severe ileal disease is present, vitamin B_{12} absorption is abnormally low both with and without added intrinsic factor. Thrombocytosis may be present and may reflect hyposplenism.

The prothrombin time may be prolonged in celiac sprue owing to malabsorption of vitamin K. It is essential that the prothrombin time be evaluated prior to intestinal biopsy in patients with possible celiac sprue, because serious intestinal bleeding may occur from the biopsy site if blood coagulation is abnormal. Parenteral administration of vitamin K or one of its analogues should rapidly correct the prothrombin time if the patient has no liver disease.

Oral Tolerance Tests. Certain oral tolerance tests are helpful in the evaluation of absorptive function in patients with suspected intestinal malabsorption, but they must be interpreted cautiously, because altered gastric emptying, renal function, and metabolism of the test substance may affect the test results. Administration of the test substance through a tube placed in the duodenum eliminates the variable of gastric emptying.

The most useful tests are the xylose and lactose tolerance tests. Xylose is absorbed preferentially by the proximal small intestine; hence, xylose excretion in the urine is usually markedly depressed in patients with severe, untreated celiac sprue, because the proximal intestine is most severely affected. The xylose tolerance test is therefore the most sensitive and useful oral tolerance test for evaluating patients with suspected celiac sprue. Similarly, the absorptive cell lesion also results in secondary lactase deficiency in patients with a celiac sprue lesion; thus blood glucose may fail to rise normally after lactose ingestion. Measurement of breath hydrogen excretion after oral lactose administration is used increasingly in place of the lactose tolerance test (see p. 1295).

Blood Chemistries. Because many organ systems may be involved in celiac sprue, it is not surprising that many blood chemical determinations may be abnormal in these patients. If diarrhea is severe, marked electrolyte depletion with low serum levels of sodium, potassium, chloride, and bicarbonate can occur. In occasional patients, significant metabolic acidosis can develop in association with bicarbonate loss in the stool. Serum calcium, magnesium, and even zinc may be decreased in patients with diarrhea and steatorrhea. Serum phosphorus may be decreased and alkaline phosphatase may be increased in patients with osteopenia. Serum albumin and, to a lesser degree, serum globulins may be diminished owing to excessive leakage of serum protein into the gut lumen. In patients with sufficient intestinal involvement to produce steatorrhea, serum cholesterol and serum carotene levels are often depressed.

Miscellaneous. Abnormal tryptophan metabolism, perhaps caused by pyridoxine (vitamin B_6) deficiency, may result in elevated urinary excretion of 5-hydroxyindoleacetic acid and indican in patients with malabsorption. Detection of antigliadin antibodies in the serum has been advanced as a diagnostic test for celiac sprue.[74] However, reported sensitivity and specificity have varied considerably with different methods and in different laboratories.[75, 76] Hence, this test should not be substituted for intestinal mucosal biopsy in the diagnostic evaluation of patients with suspected celiac sprue.

Roentgenographic Studies. Barium contrast roentgenograms of the gastrointestinal tract should be obtained in any patient with malabsorption. X-ray films of the small intestine after a barium meal are particularly helpful in evaluating patients suspected of having untreated celiac sprue. Abnormal findings usually include dilatation of the small intestine, replacement of the normal delicate mucosal pattern with either marked coarsening or complete obliteration of the mucosal folds, and fragmentation and flocculation of the barium meal within the gut lumen, although the latter are less common with currently used barium suspensions (Figs. 61–5 and 61–6). The distorted mucosal fold pattern is related to the mucosal lesion, and its distribution correlates with the histologic involvement of the mucosa. In patients with mild or moderate disease, the mucosal pattern is usually distorted in the proximal small intestine, whereas the ileal mucosa appears normal. In patients with severe disease, the mucosal pattern appears abnormal throughout the small intestine, including the ileum. Excessive secretion of fluid into the proximal small intestine, coupled with defective absorption of intraluminal contents, probably causes dilution of the barium meal and results in decreased contrast of the barium in the more distal small intestine. A somewhat different X-ray picture suggesting rigidity of the bowel wall may be seen in the rare disease known as collagenous sprue (Fig. 61–7). Occasionally, patients with relatively mild celiac sprue may have normal barium contrast studies of the small bowel. Hence, radiologic study is not as sensitive as small intestinal biopsy in providing diagnostic information.

X-ray films of the bones may reveal diffuse demineralization with a generalized decrease in bone density. In addition, secondary effects of osteopenic bone disease, including compression fractures of vertebrae and pseudofractures (Milkman's lines), are seen occasionally.

Intestinal Biopsy. Since its introduction in the mid-1950s, peroral biopsy has become an invaluable diagnostic procedure in the evaluation of patients with gastrointestinal malabsorption. Indeed, this procedure is the most valuable single diagnostic maneuver in establishing whether or not celiac sprue may be the cause of malabsorption in a given patient. A variety of biopsy instruments are now available that permit relatively safe peroral biopsy of the proximal small intestine. Some now advocate endoscopic biopsy over suction biopsy for all suspected diseases that merit small intestinal mucosal biospy.[77] However, this author much prefers the multipurpose biopsy tube (also called the Rubin or the Quinton tube). It has proved safe, provided there is no tendency to bleed, and it can be positioned rapidly and visualized easily under the fluoroscope.[78] Moreover, two to four untraumatized mucosal samples are excised routinely with one passage of the tube, permitting extensive sampling. These biopsies, in the author's experience, are larger, easier to orient, and less traumatized than most endoscopic

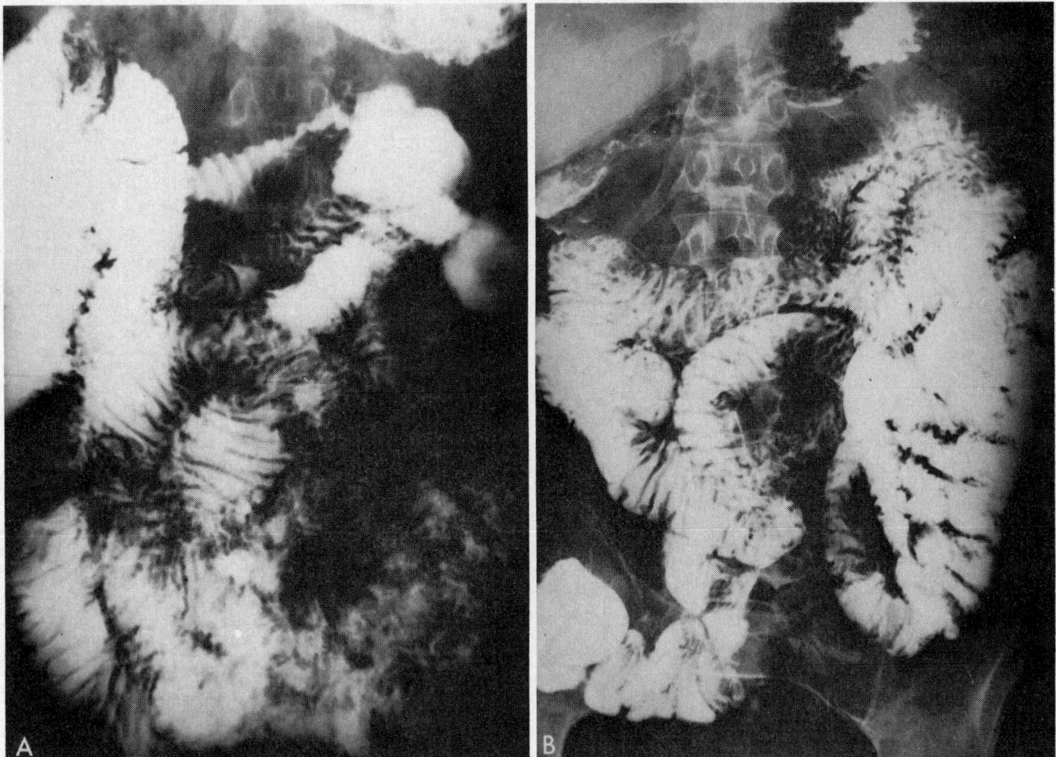

Figure 61–5. Barium contrast studies from a patient with celiac sprue. Before treatment *(A)*, there is significant dilatation of some of the loops of small bowel as well as marked distortion and coarsening of the mucosal pattern. After six weeks of maintenance on a gluten-free diet *(B)*, there is a significant reduction in the dilatation and improvement in the mucosal pattern, although it has not yet returned to normal.

biopsies. Moreover, endoscopic biopsies are often obtained from the more proximal duodenum, where Brunner's glands and lymphoid follicles are abundant and may compromise histologic interpretation.[79] Although direct visualization of the biopsy site is sometimes useful in diseases that cause focal disease in the small intestine, it is of no benefit in diffuse mucosal disease such as celiac sprue.

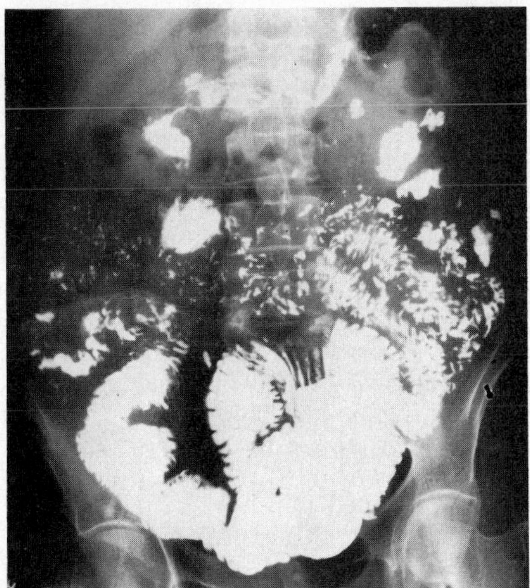

Figure 61–6. Barium contrast study from a patient with untreated celiac sprue. Note the dilated loops, coarsened mucosal folds, and "puddling" of the barium. (Courtesy of M. H. Sleisenger, M.D.)

To be definitive and, indeed, informative, peroral biopsy must be done correctly and the tissue must be processed and interpreted properly. Requirements essential for biopsies to be of maximum diagnostic value include (1) precise localization of the biopsy site, (2) proper orientation and prompt fixation of the biopsy samples, and (3) careful study not of one or two but of serial sections of the well-oriented central half or two thirds of each biopsy. As Perera and coworkers have stressed,[79] the techniques of the embryologist, not the pathologist, must be used.

Biopsy material should be obtained from the duodenal junction at the ligament of Treitz. The bowel in this area is retroperitoneal and fixed; thus biopsy specimens from the same intestinal segment can be obtained serially and compared. This is of particular value in documenting histologic improvement in a celiac sprue patient after treatment with a gluten-free diet. Moreover, this area is almost invariably involved in diffuse mucosal diseases such as celiac sprue and Whipple's disease.

The biopsy findings in celiac sprue patients are described in detail on pages 1135 to 1137 (see Figs. 61–1 and 61–3).

DIFFERENTIAL DIAGNOSIS

Although the presenting signs and symptoms are not specific and may resemble those seen with malabsorption from other causes, the diagnosis of celiac sprue can be established readily. The initial step is the

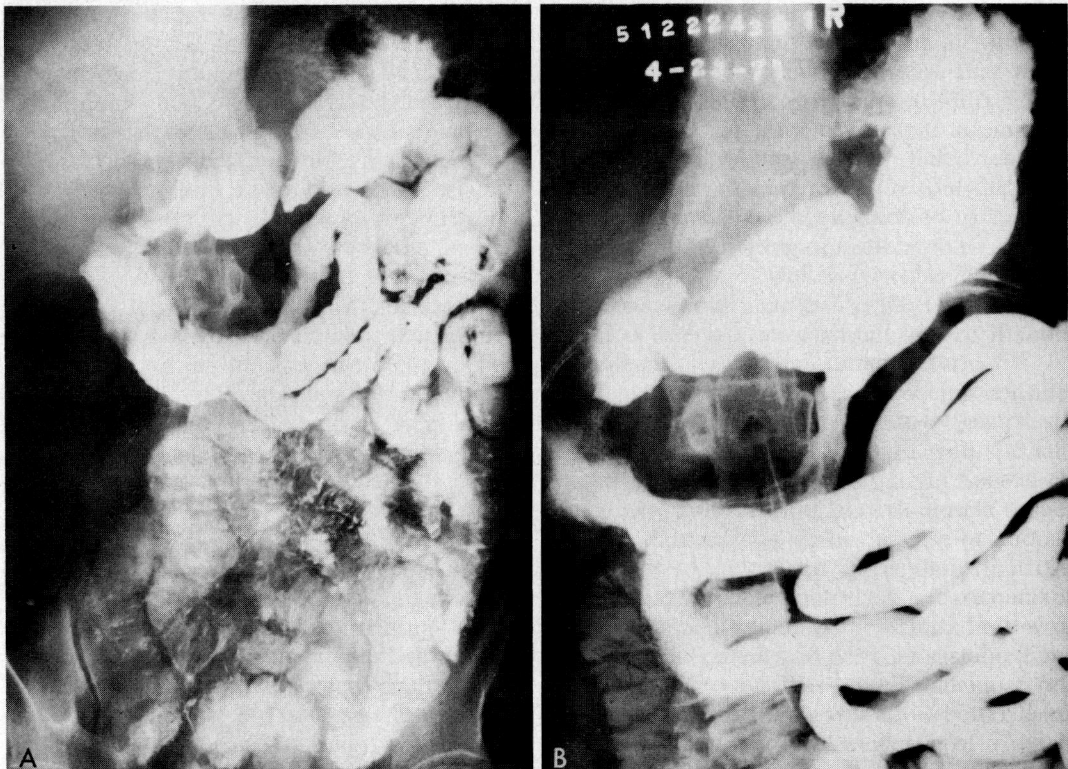

Figure 61–7. Barium contrast studies of a patient with collagenous sprue *(A)* and again seven years later *(B)*. Note the progressive rigidity of the small bowel loops. (Courtesy of L. L. Brandborg, M.D.)

suspicion of defective intestinal absorption. Malabsorption is obvious in the patient with a severe, extensive intestinal lesion and severe panmalabsorption. Its recognition in the patient with a limited lesion without steatorrhea and only subtle evidence of malabsorption, such as refractory anemia, requires a high index of suspicion and an awareness that celiac sprue can present extremely diverse clinical manifestations (see pp. 1141 to 1143).

Once malabsorption has been established, the clinician must determine the nature of the underlying absorptive defect. Steatorrhea and depressed serum cholesterol, carotene, calcium, and prothrombin levels in themselves do not differentiate primary intestinal mucosal diseases, such as celiac sprue, from other diseases that may cause malabsorption. Indeed, these findings can all be abnormal in patients with defective intraluminal digestion caused by previous gastric or ileal resection or pancreatic insufficiency.

The presence of an abnormal xylose tolerance test is helpful in the differential diagnosis of primary mucosal disease, because xylose is usually absorbed normally by patients with defective intraluminal digestion so long as mucosal structure is normal. X-ray films of the small intestine after a barium meal also help differentiate mucosal malabsorption from that of other causes; the presence of an *abnormal mucosal pattern* and *dilatation* as well as dilution of the barium meal strongly suggests mucosal disease.

A normal biopsy sample obtained from the proximal small intestine effectively excludes the diagnosis of clinically significant untreated celiac sprue, whereas a biopsy that demonstrates the typical celiac sprue lesion strongly suggests this diagnosis. Biopsies that demonstrate the characteristic histologic findings of *Whipple's disease* exclude the diagnosis of celiac sprue in patients with diffuse mucosal disease in whom the clinical picture itself is not diagnostic. Patients with *hypogammaglobulinemia* may have an architectural lesion that resembles celiac sprue, but plasma cells are absent or markedly diminished.

Because the histologic appearance of the mucosa in untreated celiac sprue patients is not absolutely specific, demonstration of the mucosal histologic appearance typical of celiac sprue cannot, in itself, be considered diagnostic of this disease. A mucosal lesion identical to or closely resembling that of celiac sprue may be seen in persons with *tropical sprue*, although this disease occurs only in patients who have resided or traveled in areas of the world endemic for tropical sprue (see p. 1282). In addition, it may be difficult or impossible to distinguish the celiac sprue lesion from that seen occasionally in patients with *diffuse lymphoma* of the small intestine, the *Zollinger-Ellison syndrome* with marked gastric hypersecretion, *eosinophilic gastroenteritis*, intraluminal *bacterial overgrowth, unclassified sprue*, and, especially in infants and young children, *viral gastroenteritis*.

Therefore, to establish unequivocally the diagnosis of celiac sprue, a clinical response by the patient to treatment with a gluten-free diet is needed in addition to a biopsy showing the typical celiac sprue lesion. If the diet used is completely free of toxic gluten, a clinical response is usually evident within a few weeks. Indeed, some improvement in mucosal histologic appearance accompanies this early clinical response, although reversion of the mucosa to normal usually requires months or even years of gluten withdrawal. A mucosal lesion suggestive of celiac sprue may be even less specific in young children, for a similar lesion may accompany gastroenteritis; thus, rechallenge with gluten following an apparent response to gluten withdrawal is desirable in infants and young children to establish the diagnosis unequivocally.

In summary, the diagnosis of celiac sprue is made by (1) demonstrating impairment of small intestinal mucosal function, (2) documenting the presence of the typical mucosal lesion, and (3) observing a prompt clinical response and, ideally, improvement in mucosal histologic appearance upon withdrawal of toxic gluten from the diet.

TREATMENT

Diet. Removal of toxic gluten from the diet is essential for the treatment of patients with celiac sprue (Table 61–3). The need for gluten withdrawal was established by Dicke, van de Kamer, and Weijers' astute studies some 30 years ago in which the toxicity of wheat protein in children with celiac sprue was documented convincingly.[8, 9] Some ten years later, Rubin and coworkers demonstrated that instillation of wheat, barley, and rye flour into histologically normal-appearing small intestine of treated celiac sprue patients rapidly induced spruelike symptoms and that these symptoms were accompanied by the development of the typical celiac sprue lesions in the exposed mucosa.[27]

Although complete dietary removal of all cereal grains known to contain toxic gluten (wheat, barley, rye, and probably oats) sounds simple enough, such a diet is in reality very difficult for most patients to achieve and maintain.[80] Obvious sources of toxic gluten, such as baked goods, wheat- or oat-containing dry cereals, noodles, or spaghetti are easily avoided. But toxic glutens, especially wheat flour, are virtually ubiquitous in the normal American diet. Wheat is often used as an extender in processed foods and is present in many brands of commercially available ice cream, in salad dressing, and in many canned foods, including vegetables and soups. Indeed, wheat flour is even contained in many brands of instant coffee, catsup, mustard, and most candy bars, to give only a few examples (Table 61–4). The rising popularity of processed foods such as frozen vegetables with wheat-containing sauces has further compounded the problem. As a result, the institution of an effective gluten-free diet requires extensive and repeated indoctrination of the patient by the physician and the dietician, as well as a motivated and basically suspicious, label-reading patient.

Table 61–3. PRINCIPLES OF INITIAL DIETARY THERAPY FOR CELIAC SPRUE PATIENTS

- Avoid all foods containing wheat, rye, and barley gluten
- Avoid oat gluten initially
- Use only rice, corn, buckwheat, potato, soybean, or tapioca flours, meals, or starches
- Wheat starch from which gluten has been removed can be tried after the diagnosis is established
- Read all labels and study ingredients of processed foods
- Beware of gluten in food additives, emulsifiers, or stabilizers
- Limit milk and milk products initially

Table 61–4. REPRESENTATIVE FOODS THAT MAY OR MAY NOT CONTAIN GLUTEN, DEPENDING UPON MANUFACTURER

Ice cream	Cheese spreads
Nondairy creamer	Chip and dip mixes
Yogurts with fruit	Luncheon meats
Hot chocolate mixes or cocoa	Weiners and other sausage products
	Processed canned meats and poultry
Chocolates and candy bars	Meat sauces (soy, Worcestershire, etc.)
Instant coffee and tea	
Boullion cubes	Mustard
Soup mixes	Catsup
Canned soups	Tomato sauce
Salad dressings	Peanut butter

Aside from containing no wheat, rye, barley, or oat gluten, the diet should be well balanced and contain normal amounts of fat, protein (initially at least 100 gm per day), and carbohydrates.

It is not clear whether oats are toxic to all patients with celiac sprue. Some patients who are very sensitive to ingestion of small amounts of wheat flour tolerate oats without ill effects; others develop symptoms within a few hours after eating oat-containing foods. Therefore, oats are best eliminated from the diet initially, but can be tried carefully once remission has been achieved.

Rice, soybean, and corn flours are clearly nontoxic, and baked goods and cereals containing these flours can be eaten safely by celiac sprue patients. Helpful recipes as well as detailed instructions regarding gluten-free diets have been published by Marion Wood in two valuable books entited *Gourmet Food on a Wheat-Free Diet*[81] and *Delicious and Easy Rice Flour Recipes*.[82]

Because treatment with a gluten-free diet represents a lifetime commitment for patients with celiac sprue and may carry with it significant social liability, especially in childen, it should not be undertaken casually as a therapeutic trial in a patient prior to biopsy. Rather, the probable diagnosis should be established first by biopsy. Thereafter, institution of a gluten-free diet serves two functions: it initiates treatment and, if followed by clinical improvement, confirms the histologic diagnosis.

Responses to Diet. If a patient fails to improve within a few weeks following institution of a gluten-free diet, the physician must review the patient's dietary intake

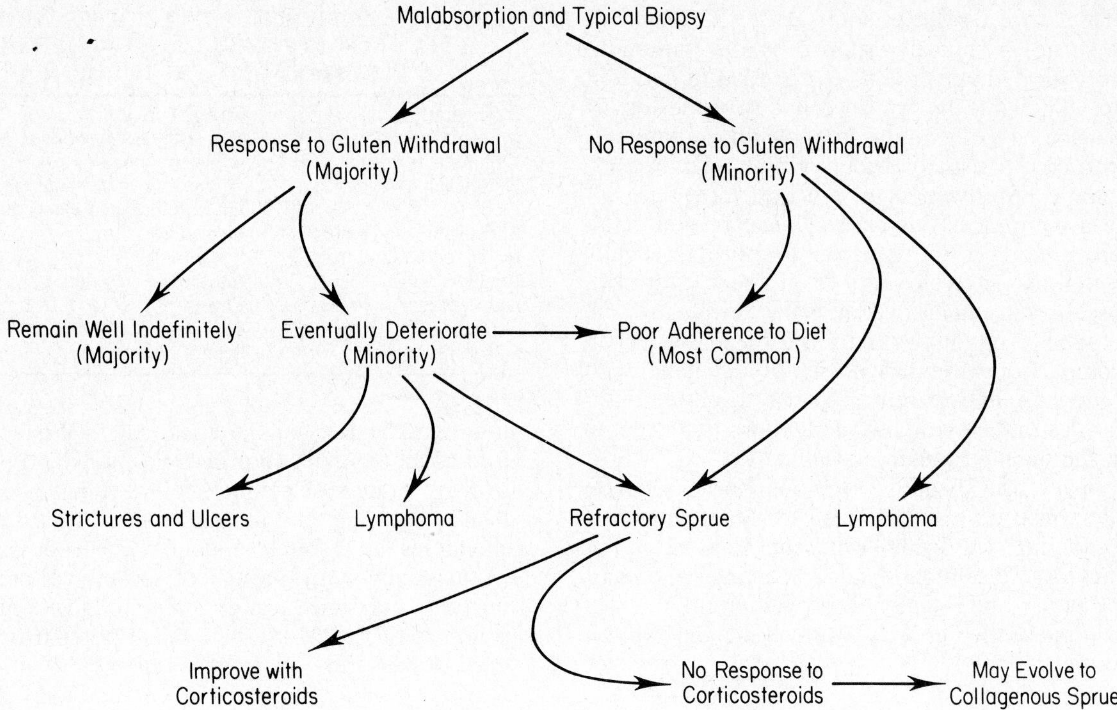

Figure 61–8. Variations in clinical course that may be observed in patients with malabsorption and a biopsy characteristic of celiac sprue, in whom other potential causes for such a biopsy (tropical sprue, viral gastroenteritis, bacterial overgrowth, and so forth) have been excluded. (Reprinted with permission from: Celiac sprue and refractory sprue, by Trier, J. S., Falchuk, A. Z., Carey, M. C., and Schreiber, D. S. Gastroenterology *75*(2):307–316. Copyright 1978 by The American Gastroenterological Association.)

meticulously. The most common cause of failure to respond to a gluten-free diet is incomplete removal of gluten from the diet (Fig. 61–8). Even patients hospitalized in sophisticated medical centers are often challenged inadvertently with gluten-containing foods while they are supposedly receiving gluten-free diets. It is sometimes necessary to hospitalize a patient who has not responded to gluten withdrawal under the supervision of a knowledgeable dietician to be certain that rigid gluten exclusion is in effect. By definition, celiac sprue patients respond to gluten withdrawal. Therefore, if a given patient fails to improve on a gluten-free diet, either the diet is inadequate or the mucosal lesion is caused by another disease in which the intestinal histologic appearance closely resembles that of celiac sprue (Fig. 61–8). If the patient has refractory sprue, an attempt to identify a causative dietary agent other than gluten may be worthwhile,[83] although none can be identified in most instances. Long-term treatment with corticosteroids is helpful to some but not all patients with refractory sprue.[24]

There is considerable variation among patients with celiac sprue in their ability to tolerate small amounts of toxic gluten. This difference is most apparent after patients have responded to gluten withdrawal and intestinal absorptive function has reverted to normal or near-normal. Under such circumstances, some patients can tolerate ingestion of small amounts of toxic gluten and still maintain their remission without developing symptoms. Such individuals may stray from their diets from time to time without ill effect. Other patients are exquisitely sensitive to ingestion of even minute amounts of toxic gluten and may develop massive watery diarrhea reminiscent of acute cholera within hours after ingesting as little gluten as is contained, for example, in a couple of pieces of bakery bread. The diarrhea in such patients may be so severe that it can induce clinical shock resulting from acute dehydration and be life-threatening; indeed, the term "gliadin shock" has been applied to this condition.[84]

MacDonald and coworkers[22] have shown that during treatment with a gluten-free diet, the less severely damaged distal intestine recovers more rapidly than the maximally damaged proximal intestine. Clinical improvement correlates better with the length of histologically improved intestine than with the severity of the lesion in the proximal intestine. This helps explain the common observation that a clinical response to gluten withdrawal may precede by many months reversion of the proximal intestinal lesion to normal. Eventually, even the proximal biopsy specimens revert to normal or almost normal in about 50 per cent of patients maintained on a gluten-free diet. Most of the remaining patients show partial reversion of proximal mucosa toward normal.[22, 85] In a few patients, the proximal intestinal lesion fails to revert toward normal despite a good clinical response to prolonged gluten withdrawal. It is usually impossible to be certain that such patients are not ingesting any gluten without subjecting them to prolonged hospitalization.

Lactase Deficiency. Some patients with untreated celiac sprue develop aggravation of their symptoms, with bloating, cramps, and diarrhea, after ingesting milk and milk products. The probable cause of this milk intolerance is secondary lactase deficiency. Lactase and other disaccharides are located in the brush border membrane of intestinal absorptive cells, and since these cells are both reduced in number and damaged in patients with celiac sprue, the occurrence of secondary lactase deficiency is not surprising. However, milk and milk products should be omitted from the diet of celiac sprue patients only if they produce unpleasant symptoms. These foods are an excellent source of protein, calories, and calcium for the nutritionally depleted patient. Many severely ill celiac sprue patients will tolerate some milk initially, and most develop increased tolerance as intestinal structure and function revert toward normal with gluten withdrawal.

Supplemental Therapy. Patients with severe disease should receive appropriate replacement therapy, in addition to a gluten-free diet, to help correct deficiencies caused by the absorptive defects.

Anemic patients should receive supplemental iron, folate, or vitamin B_{12}, depending upon the specific deficiency or deficiencies responsible for their anemia. If there is purpura or other evidence of bleeding or if there is significant prolongation of the prothrombin time, administration of vitamin K or one of its analogues is indicated.

Vigorous intravenous replacement of fluid and electrolytes may be essential in patients with dehydration and electrolyte depletion caused by severe diarrhea. Hypokalemia should be treated with parenteral potassium chloride if the deficiency is severe and with oral potassium supplements if it is mild.

Intravenous calcium gluconate should be administered promptly to the rare patient who develops tetany. If there is no response to 1 or 2 gm of intravenously administered calcium gluconate, the tetany may be due to hypomagnesemia. If so, 0.5 gm of magnesium sulfate may be given very slowly in dilute solution, although oral administration of 100 mEq of magnesium chloride daily in divided doses is much safer and usually sufficient. All patients with hypocalcemia or with clinical or radiologic evidence of osteopenic bone disease should receive oral calcium in the form of calcium gluconate or calcium lactate, 6 to 8 gm per day, as well as oral vitamin D or 25-hydroxyvitamin D. In fact, it is probably desirable to administer some supplemental calcium and vitamin D to all celiac sprue patients with significant steatorrhea to help prevent mobilization of skeletal calcium until the malabsorption has responded to gluten withdrawal. Of course, overtreatment with vitamin D and calcium may be harmful. Therefore, serum calcium must be monitored and supplementation discontinued promptly if hypercalcemia develops.

Vitamin A, thiamine, riboflavin, niacin, pyridoxine, vitamin C, and vitamin E, in the form of a therapeutic formula multivitamin preparation, should probably be administered to celiac sprue patients with malabsorption, although the need for supplementation of these vitamins is not fully established (see Table 18–7, p. 279).

Corticosteroid administration is advocated by some authorities for all severely ill celiac sprue patients, although in this author's experience it is rarely needed. Treatment with a gluten-free diet is safer and more specific and usually results in equally rapid and more lasting improvement, even in severely ill patients. Therefore, steroids are rarely needed in the treatment of celiac sprue and then only for the acute treatment of transient adrenal insufficiency which may accompany severe malnutrition and depletion in the severely ill patient.

Finally, it must be mentioned that drugs, like nutrients, may be absorbed capriciously by patients with severe celiac sprue. Medications considered essential for the patient's well-being should be administered parenterally until improved absorption is induced by treatment with a gluten-free diet.

PROGNOSIS AND COMPLICATIONS

Prognosis

If not recognized and properly treated, celiac sprue, if severe, may be fatal. Patients may develop marked malnutrition and debilitation and die of complications such as hemorrhage or intercurrent infection. On the other hand, death caused by celiac sprue among patients in whom the diagnosis has been established is exceedingly uncommon, because the response to gluten withdrawal is both specific and rapid. Therefore, the prognosis for patients with correctly diagnosed and treated celiac sprue is excellent. Intestinal absorptive defects disappear promptly in infants and young children upon institution of a gluten-free diet. Growth and development usually proceed normally with continued effective treatment. The natural history of celiac sprue is such that the disease often becomes quiescent as the children approach adolescence. At this point, patients may stray from their gluten-free diet, often without apparent ill effects. However, their inability to tolerate gluten remains, and if gluten ingestion continues into adult life, most, if not all, of these patients eventually develop recurrent clinical evidence of celiac sprue, most often in the third or fourth decade of life. The recurrent disease may manifest itself as mild refractory iron deficiency anemia, blatant panmalabsorption, or anything in between. Therefore, patients with unequivocal evidence of celiac sprue in childhood should be encouraged to remain on a gluten-free diet indefinitely if recurrent clinical disease is to be avoided during adult life.

The prognosis also seems good for patients who develop clinically apparent celiac sprue as adults. As absorptive function returns to normal on a gluten-free diet, both the primary and secondary manifestations of celiac sprue disappear. A few of the complications seen in celiac sprue, such as peripheral neuropathy and pathologic fractures caused by severe osteopenia, may not be totally reversible, but these are the exception, not the rule.

Complications

Three serious complications that have been associated with celiac sprue merit mention (Fig. 61–8). First, there have been a number of reports which suggest that the incidence of *malignant disease* is greater in adults with celiac sprue than in the general population. In two studies,[86, 87] malignancy was reported to develop in 13 per cent and 11 per cent of patients with celiac sprue, respectively. *Lymphomas* and *squamous carcinomas* of the esophagus were most common, but other gastrointestinal and extraintestinal malignancies were noted. Mean follow-up time was not clearly stated in one study, but was nine years in the Australian series. In a recent retrospective multicenter collaborative study from Great Britain of 259 malignancies in 235 celiac sprue patients, 133 were lymphomas.[88] Of the remaining neoplasms, 19 were *small intestinal adenocarcinomas*, an 80-fold increase over the expected incidence. For a number of years it was considered likely that most celiac sprue–associated lymphomas were derived from monocyte-macrophages (malignant histiocytosis),[89] but recent evidence suggests that many of these lymphomas originate from T lymphocytes.[90, 91] Mesenteric lymphadenopathy with central cavitation has been described recently in celiac sprue, both in concert with[92] and in the absence of[93] lymphoma.

However, it seems doubtful that over 10 per cent of *all* celiac sprue patients followed for nine or more years might be expected to develop malignant disease, as these reports might suggest. Other clinicians with extensive experience have not noted such a high incidence of malignancy in patients with a documented diagnosis of celiac sprue, especially children and young adults, although sporadic cases of coexisting celiac sprue and malignancy have been observed by many. Interpretation of the data regarding the incidence of lymphoma in patients with celiac sprue is particularly difficult, because patients with primary diffuse lymphoma of the small intestine may present initially with symptoms of malabsorption and with peroral biopsy findings that are difficult or impossible to differentiate from those of patients with untreated celiac sprue. Thus, some patients initially diagnosed as having celiac sprue may, in fact, have had intestinal lymphoma simulating celiac sprue. In any case, patients with documented celiac sprue merit a careful search for a gastrointestinal malignancy if, after initially improving with gluten withdrawal, they subsequently develop symptoms such as weight loss, malabsorption, abdominal pain, or intestinal bleeding despite strict adherence to a gluten-free diet. It is not known whether treatment with a gluten-free diet reduces the incidence of intestinal lymphoma or other malignancies in patients with celiac sprue (see pp. 1519–1560).

The second serious complication that may develop in a very small percentage of celiac sprue patients is evolution of their disease with time, into a syndrome arbitrarily termed *refractory* or *unclassified sprue*.[23, 24] Such patients respond early in their disease to gluten withdrawal, but after a period of remission they relapse despite continued adherence to a strict gluten-free diet. A few of these unusual patients subsequently respond at least partially to treatment with corticosteroids[24] or other immunosuppressive drugs such as azathioprine or cyclophosphamide. Others who initially respond to gluten withdrawal for as long as several years will be unaffected by all known treatments, and their course is characterized by a persistence of a flat mucosal lesion and relentless and often progressive malabsorption, usually culminating in death. Occasionally, patients with a flat mucosa histologically indistinguishable from celiac sprue will be refractory to all therapies, including gluten withdrawal, from the onset (Fig. 61–8).

The third reported serious complication associated with celiac sprue is that of *ulceration* and *stricture* of the small intestine.[94] Whether this rare complication is truly an entity has been questioned, as lymphoma is ultimately diagnosed in many of these patients by careful study or with the passage of time.[95] On the other hand, there are a few seemingly well-documented patients with celiac sprue and localized intestinal ulceration in whom no evidence of malignancy develops and who respond to surgical extirpation of the diseased bowel. The characteristic clinical findings are diarrhea, abdominal pain, intestinal bleeding, and intestinal obstruction. The ulcers occur at any level of the small intestine, and perforation with peritonitis may occur. The histologic appearance of the ulcerations is nonspecific and provides no clue to their pathogenesis unless lymphoma can be diagnosed. In the initially reported series, 75 per cent of reported patients have died as a direct result of this complication, emphasizing its seriousness (see pp. 1320–1327).[94]

References

1. Rubin, C. E. Malabsorption: Celiac sprue. Ann. Rev. Med. *12*:39, 1961.
2. Logan, R. F. A., Rifkind, E. A., Busuttil, A., Gilmour, H. M., and Ferguson, A. Prevalence and "incidence" of celiac disease in Edinburgh and the Lothian region of Scotland. Gastroenterology *90*:334, 1986.
3. MacDonald, W. C., Dobbins, W. O., and Rubin, C. E. Studies of the familial nature of celiac sprue using biopsy of the small intestine. N. Engl. J. Med. *272*:448, 1965.
4. McCarthy, C. F., Mylotte, M., Stevens, F., Egan-Mitchell, B., Fottrell, P. F., and McNicholl, B. Family studies on coeliac disease in Ireland. *In* Hekkens, W. Th. J. M., and Pena, A. S. (eds.). Coeliac Disease: Proceedings of the Second International Coeliac Symposium. Leiden, Stenfert Korese, 1974, p. 311.
5. Misra, R. C., Kasthuri, S., and Chuttani, H. K. Adult coeliac disease in tropics. Br. Med. J. *2*:1230, 1966.
6. Gee, S. On the celiac affection. St. Bartholomews Hosp. Rep. *24*:17, 1888.
7. Thaysen, T. E. H. Non-Tropical Sprue. Copenhagen, Levin and Munksgaard, 1932.
8. Dicke, W. K. Coeliac disease: Investigation of harmful effects of certain types of cereal on patients with coeliac disease. Doctoral thesis, University of Utrecht, Netherlands, 1950.
9. van de Kamer, J. H., Weijers, H. A., and Dicke, W. K. Coeliac disease. IV. An investigation into the injurious constituents of

wheat in connection with their action on patients with coeliac disease. Acta Paediatr. *42*:223, 1953.

10. Paulley, L. W. Observations on the aetiology of idiopathic steatorrhea. Br. Med. J. *2*:1318, 1954.
11. Rubin, C. E., Brandborg, L. L., Phelps, P. C., and Taylor, H. C., Jr. Studies of celiac disease. I. The apparent identical and specific nature of the duodenal and proximal jejunal lesion in celiac disease and idiopathic sprue. Gastroenterology *38*:28, 1960.
12. Rubin, W., Ross, L. L., Sleisenger, M. H., and Weser, E. An electron microscopic study of adult celiac disease. Lab. Invest. *15*:1720, 1966.
13. Madara, J. L., and Trier, J. S. Structural abnormalities of jejunal epithelial cell membranes in celiac sprue. Lab. Invest. *43*:254, 1980.
14. Padykula, H. A., Strauss, E. W., Ladman, A. J., and Gardner, F. H. A morphologic and histochemical analysis of the human jejunal epithelium in non-tropical sprue. Gastroenterology *40*:735, 1961.
15. Peters, T. J., Heath, J. R., Wansbrough-Jones, M. H., and Doe, W. F. Enzyme activities and properties of lysosomes and brush borders in jejunal biopsies from control subjects and patients with coeliac disease. Clin. Sci. Molec. Med. *48*:259, 1975.
16. Yardley, J. H., Bayless, T. M., Norton, J. H., and Hendrix, T. R. A study of the jejunal epithelium before and after a gluten-free diet. N. Engl. J. Med. *267*:1173, 1962.
17. Polak, J. M., Pearse, A. G. E., van Norden, S., Bloom, S. R., and Rossiter, M. A. Secretin cells in coeliac disease. Gut *14*:870, 1973.
18. Baklien, K., Brandtzaeg, P., and Fausa, O. Immunoglobulins in jejunal mucosa and serum from patients with adult coeliac disease. Scand. J. Gastroenterol. *12*:149, 1977.
19. Marsh, M. N., and Hinde, J. Inflammatory component of celiac sprue mucosa. I. Mast cells, basophils and eosinophils. Gastroenterology *89*:92, 1985.
20. Ferguson, A., and Murray, D. Quantitation of intraepithelial lymphocytes in human jejunum. Gut *12*:988, 1971.
21. Niazi, N. M., Leigh, R., Crowe, P., and Marsh, M. N. Morphometric analysis of small intestinal mucosa. Virchows Arch. [Pathol. Anat.] *404*:49, 1984.
22. MacDonald, W. C., Brandborg, L. L., Flick, A. L., Trier, J. S., and Rubin, C. E. Studies of celiac sprue. IV. The response of the whole length of the small bowel to a gluten-free diet. Gastroenterology *47*:573, 1964.
23. Rubin, C. E., Eidelman, S., and Weinstein, W. M. Sprue by any other name. Gastroenterology *58*:409, 1970.
24. Trier, J. S., Falchuk, Z. M., Carey, M. C., and Schreiber, D. S. Celiac sprue and refractory sprue. Gastroenterology *75*:307, 1978.
25. Weinstein, W. M., Saunders, D. R., Tytgat, G. N., and Rubin, C. E. Collagenous sprue—an unrecognized type of malabsorption. N. Engl. J. Med. *283*:1279, 1970.
26. Dobbins, W. O., and Rubin, C. E. Studies of the rectal mucosa in celiac sprue. Gastroenterology *47*:471, 1964.
27. Rubin, C. E., Brandborg, L. L., Flick, A. L., MacDonald, W. C., Parkins, R. A., Parmentier, C. M., Phelps, P., Sribhibhadh, S., and Trier, J. S. Biopsy studies on the pathogenesis of celiac sprue. *In* Wolstenholme, G. E. W., and Cameron, M. P. (eds.). Intestinal Biopsy. Boston, Little, Brown & Co., 1962, p. 67.
28. Kasarda, D. D., Bernardin, J. E., and Nimmo, C. C. Wheat proteins. *In* Pomeranz, Y. (ed.). Advances in Cereal Science and Technology. Vol. I. St. Paul, American Association of Cereal Chemists, 1976, pp. 158–236.
29. Cole, S. G., and Kagnoff, M. F. Celiac disease. Ann. Rev. Nutr. *5*:241, 1985.
30. Kowlessar, O. D., and Sleisenger, M. H. The role of gliadin in the pathogenesis of adult celiac disease. Gastroenterology *44*:357, 1963.
31. Kasarda, D. D., Okita, T. W., Bernardin, J. E., Baecker, P. A., Nimmo, C. C., Lew, E. J. L., Dietler, M. D., and Greene, F. C. Nucleic acid (cDNA) and amino acid sequences of α-type gliadins from wheat (triticum aestivum). Proc. Natl. Acad. Sci. USA *81*:4712, 1984.
32. Rubin, W., Fauci, A. S., Sleisenger, M. H., and Jeffries, G. H. Immunofluorescent studies in adult celiac disease. J. Clin. Invest. *44*:475, 1965.
33. Crabbé, P. A., and Heremans, J. F. Selective IgA deficiency with steatorrhea. Am. J. Med. *42*:319, 1967.
34. Taylor, K. B., Truelove, S. C., Thompson, D. L., and Wright, R. An immunological study of coeliac disease and idiopathic steatorrhea. Br. Med. J. *2*:1727, 1961.
35. Levenson, S. D., Austin, R. K., Dietler, M. D., Kasarda, D. D., and Kagnoff, M. F. Specificity of antigliadin antibody in celiac disease. Gastroenterology *89*:1, 1985.
36. Loeb, P. M., Strober, W., Falchuk, Z. M., and Laster, L. Incorporation of L-leucine-^{14}C into immunoglobulins by jejunal biopsies of patients with celiac sprue and other gastrointestinal diseases. J. Clin. Invest. *50*:559, 1971.
37. Falchuk, Z. M., and Strober, W. Gluten-sensitive enteropathy: Synthesis of antigliadin antibody in vitro. Gut *15*:947, 1974.
38. Eade, O. E., Lloyd, R. S., Lang, C., and Wright, R. IgA and IgG reticulin antibodies in celiac and non-celiac patients. Gut *18*:991, 1977.
39. Volta, U., Lenzi, M., Lazzari, R., Cassani, F., Collina, A., Bianchi, F. B., and Pisi, E. Antibodies to gliadin detected by immunofluorescence and a micro-ELISA method: Markers of active childhood and adult coeliac disease. Gut *26*:667, 1985.
40. Alp, M. H., and Wright, R. Autoantibodies to reticulin in patients with idiopathic steatorrhoea, coeliac disease and Crohn's disease, and their relation to immunoglobulins and dietary antibodies. Lancet *2*:682, 1971.
41. Selby, W. S., Janossy, G., Bofill, M., and Jewell, D. P. Lymphocyte subpopulations in the human small intestine. The findings in normal mucosa and in the mucosa of patients with adult coeliac disease. Clin. Exp. Immunol. *52*:219, 1983.
42. Ferguson, A., McClure, J. P., MacDonald, T. T., and Holden, R. J. Cell-mediated immunity to gliadin within the small intestinal mucosa in coeliac disease. Lancet *1*:895, 1975.
43. Howdle, P. D., Bullen, A. W., and Losowsky, M. S. Cell-mediated immunity to gluten within the small intestinal mucosa in coeliac disease. Gut *23*:115, 1982.
44. Ellis, A. Coeliac disease: Previous family studies. *In* McConnell, R. B. (ed.). The Genetics of Coeliac Disease. Lancaster, England, MTP Press, 1981, pp.197–200.
45. Falchuk, Z. M., Rogentine, G. N., and Strober, W. Predominance of histocompatibility antigen HL-A8 in patients with gluten-sensitive enteropathy. J. Clin. Invest. *51*:1603, 1972.
46. Keuning, J. J., Peña, A. S., van Hooff, J. P., van Leeuwen, A., and van Rood, J. J. HLA-DW3 associated with coeliac disease. Lancet *1*:506, 1976.
47. DeMarchi, M., Carbonara, A., Ansaldi, N., Santini, B., Barbera, C., Borelli, I., Rossino, P., and Rendine, S. HLA-DR3 and DR7 in coeliac disease: Immunogenetic and clinical aspects. Gut *24*:706, 1983.
48. Tiwari, J. L., and Terasaki, P. I. HLA and Disease Associations. New York, Springer Verlag, 1985.
49. Howell, M. D., Austin, R. K., Kelleher, D., Nepom, G. T., and Kagnoff, M. F. An HLA-D region restriction fragment length polymorphism associated with celiac disease. J. Exp. Med. *164*:333, 1986.
50. Mann, D. L., Katz, S. I., Nelson, D. L., Abelson, L. D., and Strober, W. Specific B-cell antigens associated with gluten-sensitive enteropathy and dermatitis herpetiformis. Lancet *1*:110, 1976.
51. Weiss, J. B., Austin, R. K., Schanfield, M. S., and Kagnoff, M. F. Gluten-sensitive enteropathy. J. Clin. Invest. *72*:96, 1983.
52. Kagnoff, M. F., Weiss, J. B., Brown, R. J., Lee, T., and Schanfield, M. S. Immunoglobulin allotype markers in gluten-sensitive enteropathy. Lancet *1*:952, 1983.
53. Marks, J., Shuster, S., and Watson, A. J. Small-bowel changes in dermatitis herpetiformis. Lancet *2*:1280, 1962.
54. Brow, J. R., Parker, F., Weinstein, W. M., and Rubin, C. E. The small intestinal mucosa in dermatitis herpetiformis. I. Severity and distribution of the small intestinal lesion and associated malabsorption. Gastroenterology *60*:355, 1971.
55. Weinstein, W. M., Brow, J. R., Parker, F., and Rubin, C. E. The small intestinal mucosa in dermatitis herpetiformis. II.

Relationship of the small intestinal lesion to gluten. Gastroenterology *60*:362, 1971.
56. Sachs, J. A., Awad, J., McCloskey, D., Navarrele, C., Feslenstein, H., Elliot, E., Walker-Smith, J. A., Griffiths, C. E., Leonard, J. N., and Fry, L. Different HLA associated gene combinations contribute to susceptibility for coeliac disease and dermatitis herpetiformis. Gut *27*:515, 1986.
57. Douglas, A. P., and Booth, C. C. Digestion of gluten peptides by normal human jejunal mucosa and by mucosa from patients with adult coeliac disease. Clin. Sci. *38*:11, 1970.
58. Weiser, M. M., and Douglas, A. P. An alternative mechanism for gluten toxicity in coeliac disease. Lancet *1*:367, 1976.
59. Nicholson, G. L., and Blaustein, J. The interaction of *Ricinus communis* agglutinin with normal and tumor cell surfaces. Biochim. Biophys. Acta *266*:543, 1972.
60. Lorenzsonn, V., and Olsen, W. A. *In vivo* responses of rat intestinal epithelium to intraluminal dietary lectins. Gastroenterology *82*:838, 1982.
61. Colyer, J., Farthing, M. J. G., Kumar, P. J., Clark, M. L., Ohannesian, A. D., and Waldron, N. M. Reappraisal of the "lectin hypothesis" in the aetiopathogenesis of coeliac disease. Clin. Sci. *71*:105, 1986.
62. Kagnoff, M. F., Austin, R. K., Hubert, J. J., Bernardin, J. E., and Kasarda, D. D. Possible role for a human adenovirus in the pathogenesis of celiac disease. J. Exp. Med. *160*:1544, 1984.
63. Trier, J. S., and Browning, T. H. Epithelial-cell renewal in cultured duodenal biopsies in celiac sprue. N. Engl. J. Med. *283*:1245, 1970.
64. Hegberg, C. A., Melnyk, C. S., and Johnson, C. F. Gluten enteropathy appearing after gastric surgery. Gastroenterology *50*:796, 1966.
65. Fordtran, J. S., Rector, F. C., Locklear, T. W., and Ewton, M. F. Water and solute movement in the small intestine of patients with sprue. J. Clin. Invest. *46*:287, 1967.
66. DiMagno, E. P., Go, V. L. W., and Summerskill, W. H. J. Impaired cholecystokinin-pancreozymin secretion, intraluminal dilution, and maldigestion of fat in sprue. Gastroenterology *63*:25, 1972.
67. Rhodes, R. A., Tai, H. H., and Chey, W. Y. Impairment of secretin release in celiac sprue. Am. J. Dig. Dis. *23*:833, 1978.
68. Maton, P. N., Selden, A. C., Fitzpatrick, M. L., and Chadwick, V. S. Defective gallbladder emptying and cholecystokinin release in celiac disease. Reversal by gluten-free diet. Gastroenterology *88*:391, 1985.
69. Kilander, A. F., Dotevall, G., Lindstedt, G., and Lundberg, P.-A. Plasma enteroglucagon related to malabsorption in coeliac disease. Gut *25*:629, 1984.
70. Nelson, E. W., Ertran, A., Brooks, F. P., and Cerda, J. J. Thrombocytosis in patients with celiac sprue. Gastroenterology *70*:1042, 1976.
71. O'Grady, J. G., Stevens, F. M., Harding, B. O'Gorman, T. A., McNicholl, B., and McCarthy, C. F. Hyposplenism and gluten-sensitive enteropathy. Natural history, incidence, and relationship to diet and small bowel morphology. Gastroenterology *87*:1326, 1984.
72. Ferguson, R., Holmes, G. K. T., and Cooke, W. T. Coeliac disease, fertility and pregnancy. Scand. J. Gastroenterol. *17*:65, 1982.
73. Farthing, M. J., Rees, L. J., and Dawson, A. M. Male gonadal function in coeliac disease: III. Pituitary regulation. Clin. Endocrinol. *19*:661, 1983.
74. Stenhammar, L., Kilander, A. F., Nilsson, L. A., Stromberg, L., and Tarkowski, A. Serum gliadin antibodies for detection and control of childhood coeliac disease. Acta Paediatr. Scand. *73*:657, 1984.
75. Burgin-Wolff, A., Bertele, R. M., Berger, R., Gaze, H., Harms, H. K., Just, M., Khanna, S., Schurmann, K., Signer, E., and Tomovic, D. A reliable screening test for childhood celiac disease: Fluorescent immunosorbent test for gliadin antibodies. J. Pediatr. *102*:655, 1983.
76. O'Farrelly, C., Kelly, J., Hekkens, W., Bradley, B., Thompson, A., Feighery, C., and Weir, D. G. Alpha gliadin antibody levels: A serological test for coeliac disease. Br. Med. J. *286*:2007, 1983.
77. Achkar, E., Carey, W. D., Petras, R., Sivak, M. V., and Revta, R. Comparison of suction capsule and endoscopic biopsy of small bowel mucosa. Gastrointest. Endosc. *32*:278, 1986.
78. Brandborg, L. L., Rubin, C. E., and Quinton, W. E. A multipurpose instrument for suction biopsy of the esophagus, stomach, small bowel and colon. Gastroenterology *37*:1, 1959.
79. Perera, D. R., Weinstein, W. M., and Rubin, C. E. Small intestinal biopsy. Hum. Pathol. *6*:157, 1975.
80. Bye, W. A., and Trier, J. S. Treatment of celiac sprue and related diseases. *In* Bayless, T. M. (ed.). Current Therapy in Gastroenterology and Liver Disease, 1984–1985. Philadelphia, B. C. Decker, 1984, pp. 147–152.
81. Wood, M. N. Gourmet Food on a Wheat-Free Diet. Springfield, Charles C Thomas, 1967.
82. Wood, M. N. Delicious and Easy Rice Flour Recipes. Springfield, Charles C Thomas, 1972.
83. Baker, A. L, and Rosenberg, I. H. Refractory sprue: Recovery after removal of nongluten dietary products. Ann. Intern. Med. *89*:505, 1978.
84. von Krainick, H. G., Debatin, F., Gautier, E., Tobler, R., Velasco, J. A., and von Schwenk, M. Weitere Untersuchung über der schadlichen Voizenmehlaffekt bei der Coeliakie. I. Die akute Gliadinreaktion (gliadin shock). Helv. Pediatr. Acta *13*:432, 1958.
85. Benson, G. D., Kowlessar, O. D., and Sleisenger, M. H. Adult celiac disease with emphasis upon response to the gluten-free diet. Medicine *43*:1, 1964.
86. Holmes, G. K. T., Stokes, P. L., Sorahan, T. M., Prior, P., Waterhouse, J. A. H., and Cooke, W. T. Coeliac disease, gluten-free diet, and malignancy. Gut *17*:612, 1976.
87. Selby, W. S., and Gallagher, N. D. Malignancy in a 19 year experience of adult celiac disease. Dig. Dis. Sci. *24*:684, 1979.
88. Swinson, C. M., Slavin, G., Coles, E. C., and Booth, C. C. Coeliac disease and malignancy. Lancet *1*:111, 1983.
89. Isaacson, P. Primary gastrointestinal lymphoma. Virchows Arch. *391*:1, 1981.
90. Isaacson, P. G., O'Connor, N. T., Spencer, J., Bevan, D. H., Connolly, C. E., Kirkham, N., Pollock, D. J., Wainscoat, J. S., Stein, H., and Mason, D. Y. Malignant histiocytosis of the intestine: A T-cell lymphoma. Lancet *2*:688, 1985.
91. Loughran, T. P., Jr., Radin, M. E., and Joachim Deeg, H. T-cell intestinal lymphoma associated with celiac sprue. Ann. Intern. Med. *104*:44, 1986.
92. Freeman, H. J., and Chiu, B. K. Small bowel malignant lymphoma complicating celiac sprue and the mesenteric lymph node cavitation syndrome. Gastroenterology *90*:2008, 1986.
93. Matuchansky, C., Colin, R., Hemet, J., Touchard, G., Babin, P., Eugene, C., Bergue, A., Zeitoun, P., and Barboteau, M. A. Cavitation of mesenteric lymph nodes, splenic atrophy and a flat small intestinal mucosa. Gastroenterology *87*:606, 1984.
94. Bayless, T. M., Kapelowitz, R. F., Shelly, W. M., Ballinger, W. F., II, and Hendrix, T. R. Intestinal ulceration—A complication of celiac disease. N. Engl. J. Med. *276*:996, 1967.
95. Baer, A. N., Bayless, T. M., and Yardley, J. H. Intestinal ulceration and malabsorption syndromes. Gastroenterology *79*:754, 1980.

62

Parasitic Diseases

ROBERT L. OWEN

Intestinal parasitic infections in humans are important health problems.[1] Frequently they are not considered in the differential diagnosis of intestinal diseases, because it is commonly held that they are largely confined to the tropics, underdeveloped areas, and areas of inadequate sanitation. The prevalence of these infections in temperate zones is growing because of increasing international travel and migration from Southeast Asia and other areas with a high incidence of intestinal parasites. Changes in life-style, including sexual habits (see pp. 1233–1280) and crowding in institutions, have increased transmission of parasites in urban areas.

The parasites infecting the intestine may be divided into three broad groups. These include the *protozoa*, the *roundworms*, and the *flatworms*. The flatworms may be further divided into *cestodes* or *tapeworms* and *trematodes* or *flukes*.

PROTOZOA

Giardia lamblia

Giardia lamblia was the first protozoan parasite to be described. Van Leeuwenhoek of Delft, who had intermittent chronic diarrhea, observed *Giardia* in his own stool and described it in a letter to the Royal Society of Medicine in 1681.[2] He also made the important clinical observation that when he had liquid stools he could identify the "animalcules," but they were not identifiable in normal formed stool. *Giardia lamblia* is a cosmopolitan parasite with worldwide distribution. It is the most frequently reported gut parasite in the United Kingdom. Incidences vary between 2 and 25 to 30 per cent.[3] In many surveys the incidences are underestimates, because they depended upon examination of a single stool specimen.

Most patients harboring this parasite are asymptomatic, but there is general agreement that it is a pathogen and not simply a commensal. Malabsorption that is clinically identical to celiac sprue and cured by eradication of the parasite[4, 5] may occur in children. Steatorrhea is a less common finding in otherwise healthy adults.[6, 7] *Giardia lamblia* has been incriminated and is considered to be one of the most important intestinal parasites responsible for travelers' diarrhea. Travelers have contracted it in virtually every part of the world.[8] There are particularly high attack rates in travelers to the Soviet Union, especially Leningrad. Several community-wide epidemics have occurred in the United States. In these epidemics the parasite has been demonstrated in water systems that fail to filter out cysts that resist chlorination.[9] There is a particularly high incidence of giardiasis acquired by campers and backpackers in the mountainous West in the United States. The parasite appears to be especially prevalent in the Rocky Mountains and in the Northern Cascades.[9] The infection apparently is acquired through drinking water from the pristine mountain streams contaminated by feces from humans, dogs, and other species that are susceptible to *Giardia lamblia*. Infected beavers may be particularly important in amplifying infection because of defecation directly into water supplies.[10] Infection may be prevented by disinfecting water, using 13 ml of a saturated solution of iodine added to 1 liter of clear water or 26 ml added to 1 liter of cloudy water. In 15 minutes, virtually all pathogens will be killed at 20° C, but at 3° C, this and other common disinfectant methods may not be totally effective.[11] Bringing water to boiling kills all cysts.

Giardia is frequently spread by sexual or other close person-to-person contacts in which fecal contamination may occur, especially in day care centers and institutions for the retarded. Rarely, *Giardia* infection has been spread by contaminated food.[12]

Pathogenesis

Giardia lamblia exists in two forms, the encysted form and the trophozoite (Fig. 62–1). No intermediate hosts are required. Several animal species harbor organisms of the *Giardia* genus. There appears to be some degree of host specificity for the three major recognized species of *Giardia*, but cross-transmission of *Giardia duodenalis*, the species infecting man, has also been demonstrated with dogs, cats, rats, gerbils, guinea pigs, beavers, raccoons, bighorn sheep, and pronghorn sheep.[10] Infection is acquired by ingestion of cysts that excyst and multiply in the duodenum and proximal small intestine.

The pathogenesis of diarrhea and steatorrhea in giardiasis is unknown. Possible factors include mechanical occlusion of the mucosa by massive numbers of the organism preventing passage of nutrients, competition of the parasite and host for nutrients,[6] epithelial damage, altered motility, and excess mucus secretion.[13] Mucosal invasion has been proved,[14] and the organism has been found within epithelial cells, by electron microscopy.[7] The degree of invasion appears to reflect

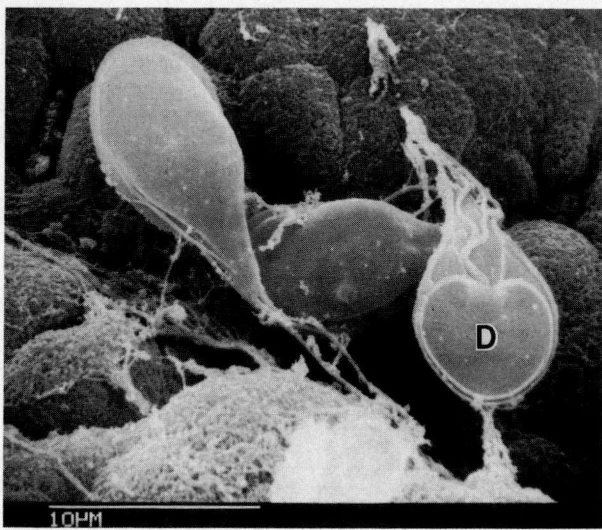

Figure 62–1. Three *Giardia lamblia* trophozoites on the surface of a jejunal biopsy from a patient with giardiasis. *Giardia* absorb nutrients through their rounded dorsal surfaces seen on the left and in the center. The ventral adhesive disc (D) seen on the right allows *Giardia* to attach and remain in the nutrient-rich upper small intestine, unlike most other microorganisms, which are swept caudally by peristalsis. (From Carlson, J. R., Heyworth, M. F., and Owen, R. L. Surv. Dig. Dis. *2*:201, 1984. Used by permission of S. Karger AG, Basel, Switzerland.)

numbers of trophozoites in the lumen and is enhanced by processes, such as coexisting gastroenteritis or malnutrition, which reduce the integrity of the intestinal barrier. The major significance of invasion may be exposure of *Giardia* to intestinal immune surveillance.[15] Although activation of immune processes may contribute to pathogenesis, it appears also to eliminate intestinal *Giardia* infection (see pp. 1153–1155).[16] Other phenomena that have been observed include reversible vitamin B_{12} and folate malabsorption, bile salt deconjugation in patients with an otherwise sterile proximal small intestine, and reduced pancreatic proteolytic enzyme activity following stimulation with a standard meal or cholecystokinin.

A striking association occurs between giardiasis and the dysgammaglobulinemias (gastrointestinal immunodeficiency syndromes). In most patients with these entities there are deficiencies of both IgA and IgM with variable levels of IgG. These immunoglobulin abnormalities occur with or without nodular lymphoid hyperplasia of the intestine.[17] Symptomatic patients with isolated IgA deficiency may also have giardiasis. A reversible disaccharidase deficiency occurs in some patients with the immunodeficiency syndromes[18] as well as in patients who have normal immunoglobulin levels.[6] This reversible brush border enzyme deficiency suggests injury to brush border by the parasite. In the immunodeficiency syndromes, bacterial overgrowth has not seemed to be important, because therapy with broad-spectrum antibiotics produces no apparent benefit until the parasite is eradicated.[18]

Diagnosis

History. Patients with symptomatic giardiasis often complain of diarrhea, which may be acute or chronic, continuous or intermittent, and may alternate with constipation. The stools are loose or watery and contain mucus but rarely blood. In a few patients, the stool may have the characteristic appearance of steatorrhea. Other symptoms include abdominal colic, nausea and vomiting, anorexia, flatulence, fatigue, weight loss, and nonspecific "nervous" symptoms. Children may have growth retardation. Otherwise healthy patients with domestically acquired giardiasis from sexual or other close personal contact commonly present with gas and cramps but no frank diarrhea.

Physical Examination. Physical examination does not contribute to the diagnosis of giardiasis. There may be some evidence of weight loss. Sigmoidoscopy may demonstrate a nonfriable, somewhat hyperemic mucosa with a mucoid secretion in the bowel.

Laboratory Findings. The routine laboratory tests, e.g., blood counts and electrolytes, are normal in most patients. Eosinophilia is not found. Steatorrhea may be present on chemical examination for fecal fat. Serum carotene in the presence of steatorrhea may be depressed. Serum folate is low in some patients, as is vitamin B_{12} urinary excretion; these are reversible in most instances after eradication of the giardia (these patients are not anemic). Protein-losing enteropathy is a rare finding and is reversible after therapy. Disaccharidase deficiency is diagnosed by a lactose tolerance test after feeding 100 gm of lactose or assay of biopsy for enzyme activity. If the true blood glucose rises more than 20 mg per 100 ml, the test is considered to be normal. Serum electrophoresis in patients with immunoglobulin deficiency diseases will reveal very low to absent gamma globulin. Immunoelectrophoresis will demonstrate the marked reduction or absence of IgA, IgM, and, in some instances, IgG. Antibody to *G. lamblia* surface-exposed antigens can be detected in serum of some patients with giardiasis, but no serologic test is generally available for diagnostic use.[19]

Radiology. A nonspecific radiographic abnormality of the small intestine is seen in some patients with giardiasis. The changes consist of thickening and distortion of the mucosal folds of the duodenum and jejunum, hypersecretion, and hypermotility. These changes are reversible after therapy. On the other hand, randomized, coded films of 16 patients with invasive giardiasis compared with 16 normal control subjects revealed no abnormalities (personal observations).

Mucosal Biopsy. ***Duodenal Aspiration.*** Patients with *Giardia* infection and without immunodeficiency diseases most often have a structurally normal small bowel mucosa.[14] A focal acute inflammatory reaction may be present, particularly in the crypts and remote from the organisms.[20] However, these changes are seen in only a few subjects. Patients with isolated IgA deficiency may have a normal villous structure, or the mucosa may have varying degrees of abnormality and occasionally may even be flat. By light microscopy some of these individuals have absent to markedly reduced plasma cells. If normal numbers of plasma cells are present, they are producing IgM by anti-IgM fluorescent antibody staining. Patients with giardiasis and the immunodeficiency diseases have a patchy intestinal lesion of variable severity, ranging from a normal villous structure to a severely abnormal flat mucosa similar to that seen in patients with celiac sprue.[18] The major difference from celiac sprue is the absence of plasma cells in the lamina propria.

With conventional formalin fixation and hematoxylin and eosin staining, giardia may be very difficult to recognize, even in the luminal aspects of the biopsy.[14] They tend to stain very similar or identical to the host's tissue and, on occasion, resemble droplets of mucus between the villi and overlying the surface. Occasionally, their identity can be resolved by examination of the specimens under the oil immersion lens.

By utilizing small bowel mucosal biopsies that are fixed in Bouin's solution, serially sectioned in their entirety, and stained with a modification of Masson's trichrome stain, giardia are easily recognizable in the luminal aspects of the biopsy.[14] By *careful* searching, small numbers of invasive giardia may be seen in all levels of the specimen from the epithelium to below the muscularis mucosae.[14] In lightly infected individuals, identification of the parasite may require exhaustive search through multiple serial sections.

Diagnosis is more easily accomplished by examining the duodenal contents[18] and by gently wiping the luminal aspect of the biopsy on glass slides, which are then air-dried for one hour, fixed in methanol for 30 minutes, washed in tap water, and stained with Giemsa stain. The giardia found in this preparation are a violet-purple in color and are easily recognized. Microscopic examination of unstained jejunal aspirate beneath a cover slip may reveal tear-shaped motile trophozoites, confirming the diagnosis of giardiasis. When small bowel biopsy equipment is unavailable or jejunal intubation is not feasible, jejunal fluid may be retrieved by aspiration during endoscopy or from a string carried into the intestine within a capsule (Enterotest, Hedeco, Mountain View, California 94043).[21]

Stool Examination. If *Giardia lamblia* cysts or trophozoites are present on examination of feces, the diagnosis of giardiasis is established. However, as many as 50 per cent of stool specimens in patients proved to have giardiasis by duodenal intubation do not contain the parasite.[18] In some patients the organism is never found in the stool. In addition to direct fecal smears in physiologic saline, a stool concentration technique and permanent slides, such as trichrome stains of Schaudinn-fixed material, should be used.

Although enzyme-linked immunosorbent assay (ELISA) examination of stool for disrupted fragments of *Giardia* has been shown to be feasible, such a definitive diagnostic test is not yet generally available. Consequently, the true prevalence of giardiasis is not known, owing to the insensitivity of the diagnostic tests that are available.

Treatment

Although the majority of patients harboring giardiasis are asymptomatic, treatment is indicated, particularly if conditions are unhygienic or if there is close contact through which other individuals might become infected. The treatment of choice in both asymptomatic and symptomatic patients is quinacrine (Atabrine), 100 mg given by mouth three times daily for seven days, or 6 mg per kg per day for children divided into three doses (maximum 300 mg per day).[22] An initial course will cure between 90 and 95 per cent of the infections. An excellent alternative drug is metronidazole (Flagyl), administered in dosages of 250 mg three times daily for a week or 15 mg per kg per day, divided in three doses, for children.

Therapy with metronidazole at this dosage for six to eight weeks in patients with giardiasis and gastrointestinal immunodeficiency syndrome results in reversal of the mucosal abnormality to or toward normal (Figs. 62–2 and 62–3).[18] Some immunodeficient patients may require treatment for as long as six months before giardia are cleared from the stool. Patients with hypogammaglobulinemic sprue without *Giardia lamblia* infection have no improvement of the mucosal abnormality on this same regimen.

Giardia do not generally become resistant *in vitro* to these antibiotics, but occasional patients without identifiable immune deficiency or sources of reinfection have failed to clear their infections with standard drug dosages. A combination regimen of quinacrine, 100 mg three times daily, and metronidazole, 750 mg three times daily, for two weeks has been effective in such cases.[23]

AMEBIASIS

Amebiasis is an acute and chronic disease caused by the organism *Entamoeba histolytica*. Although multiple organs may be involved, the colon is the usual site of initial disease. The manifestations of illness may vary from the asymptomatic carrier state to a severe fulminating illness with mucosal inflammation and ulceration, occasionally with a fatal outcome. The disease is worldwide in distribution but is most prevalent in the tropics and in areas where sanitation and living conditions are suboptimal.

Etiology

There are numerous species of amebae that inhabit the human intestinal tract, including *Entamoeba coli, E. polecki, Iodamoeba buetschlii,* and *Endolimax nana*; however, with rare exceptions, *E. histolytica* seems to be the only variety pathogenic for man. *Dientamoeba fragilis,* which resembles an ameba and occasionally causes mild intestinal symptoms, has been shown by electron microscopy to be related to flagellates and not to amebae.[24] Within the *E. histolytica* group there are morphologic differences in the size of the organism,

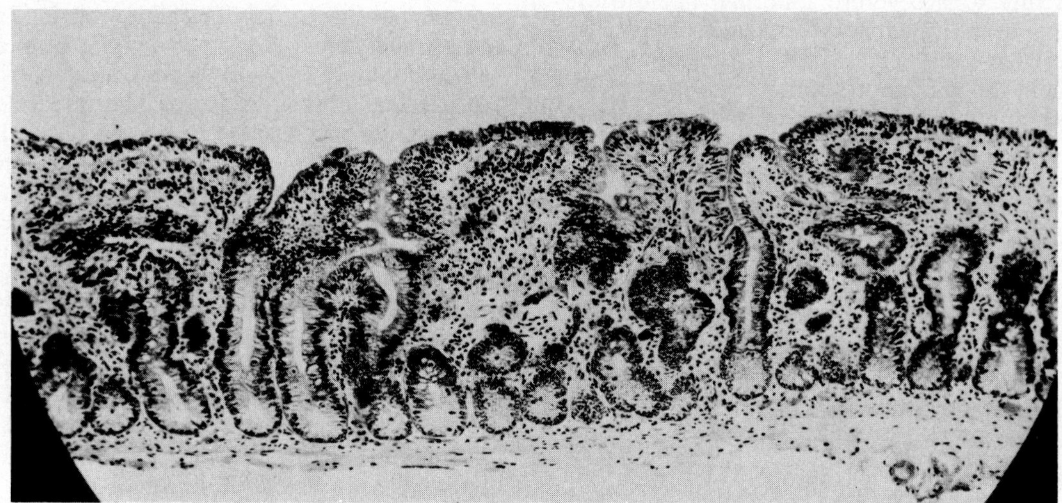

Figure 62–2. Severely abnormal intestinal lesion from a patient with a gastrointestinal immunodeficiency syndrome and giardiasis. (× 120.) (From Ament, M. E., and Rubin, C. E. Relation of giardiasis to abnormal intestinal structure and function in gastrointestinal immunodeficiency syndromes. Gastroenterology *62*:216–226. © by Williams & Wilkins, 1972.)

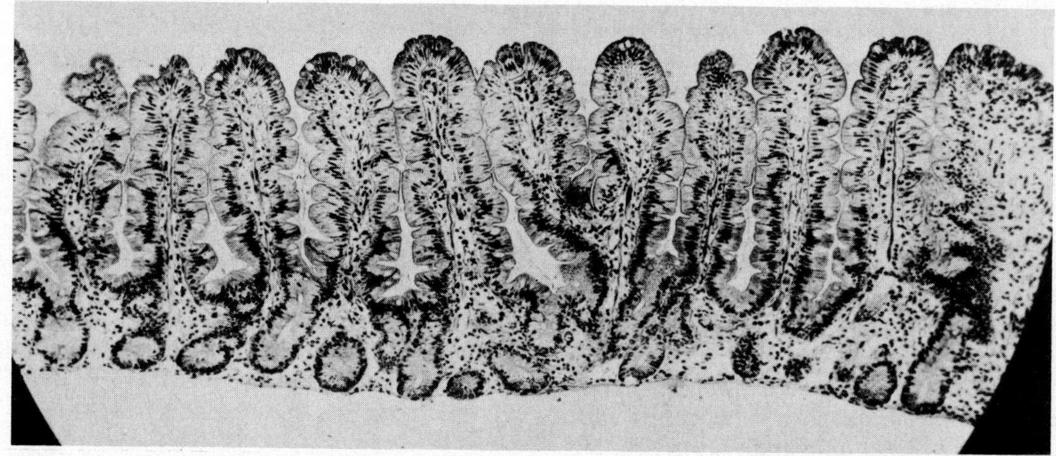

Figure 62–3. Reversal to a normal villous architecture in the same patient as in Figure 62–2 after eradication of *Giardia.* (× 120.) (From Ament, M. E., and Rubin, C. E. Relation of giardiasis to abnormal intestinal structure and function in gastrointestinal immunodeficiency syndromes. Gastroenterology *62*:216–226. © by Williams & Wilkins, 1972.)

and there has been a subdivision of this group. The strain characterized by small size and lack of virulence is *E. hartmanni*. True *E. histolytica*, previously known as the large race, is generally recognized as the ameba pathogenic for man.

Epidemiology

The worldwide average incidence of amebiasis has been estimated at 10 per cent. However, there is a wide variation of incidence figures, depending upon the population studied. In the tropics, where the disease is prevalent, 50 to 80 per cent of the population have been reported to harbor the organism.[25] Unsanitary conditions, close living, and poor personal hygiene all contribute to the spread of the disease. In the United States, amebiasis is often thought of as a tropical disease to be looked for only in other areas of the world or in travelers returning from abroad. It is estimated, however, that at least 5 per cent of the untraveled population of the United States are infected with *E. histolytica*.[26] In urban areas in the United States and elsewhere, transmission of ameba infection occurs by direct fecal-oral contamination during sexual contact and with fecal soilage in day care centers caring for children in diapers and in institutions for the retarded[27] (see pp. 1258–1260).

Asymptomatic patients with no evidence of tissue invasion harbor only cysts in their stools. The cyst form of the organism can resist the outside environment, whereas the trophozoite, passed by patients with acute or chronic invasive disease, cannot survive outside the host. The disease can therefore be transmitted by individuals who are unaware of their infective potential. On the other hand, there are patients with gastrointestinal complaints of nonamebic origin who harbor cysts in their stools but who are living in a peaceful symbiotic relationship with the organism. These patients are often erroneously diagnosed as having symptomatic amebiasis.

Analysis of the isoenzyme patterns of amebae isolated from humans has allowed them to be classified into 18 or more groups or zymodemes, of which only types II and XI are associated with intestinal ulceration or hepatic abscess formation.[28] As many as 20 to 30 per cent of homosexual males surveyed in venereal disease clinics may be infected with *E. histolytica*, but dysentery and extraintestinal infection are exceedingly rare, even in AIDS patients. *E. histolytica* isolates from homosexual men are rarely of invasive zymodemes, and prevalence of serum antibodies to *E. histolytica* is low[29] (pp. 1258–1260).

Life Cycle

Entamoeba histolytica exists in the human colon in two forms, the motile trophozoite and the nonmotile cyst. The cyst is the infective form that is ingested, resulting in colonization of the host. Cyst forms predominate in the stools of individuals who are asymptomatic carriers or who have a mild form of the illness. They vary greatly in size, containing refractile masses of chromatin or chromatoid bodies. Early cyst forms contain one nucleus, which divides by binary fission to form the mature quadrinucleate cyst; thus cysts found in the stools will contain one to four nuclei. Cysts may survive outside the body for as long as ten days if kept cool and moist. Otherwise they die quickly. The cyst is important because it is the infective stage of the life cycle, and through it infection is conveyed from one host to another. This occurs when food or water that has been contaminated with fecal material containing *E. histolytica* cysts is ingested. Upon entering the bowel, there is a division resulting in eight trophozoites from one cyst. On excystation the parasites transform to motile trophozoites, the active, potentially pathogenic stage that causes amebic colitis. They are recognized by their occurrence in clumps or masses and their uneven distribution throughout stool specimens. The trophozoite appears as a clear transparent organism with an eccentric nucleus about three to five times the diameter of a red corpuscle. The presence of trophozoites with intracytoplasmic red blood cells is pathognomonic for infection by *E. histolytica* and serves to distinguish it from the nonpathogenic amebae, e.g., *E. coli*. Movement is accomplished by pseudopods and is brisk, unidirectional, and seemingly purposeful in warm, fresh specimens. Binary fission then produces the precystic forms, which develop into fully mature cysts in the period of a few hours in the lumen of the bowel. These are passed out into the stools and are ingested by a new host, and the cycle continues.

Pathogenesis of Colitis

In germ-free animals the virulence of *E. histolytica* is dependent upon the introduction of bacteria, and this fact is the basis for the rationale of using antibiotic therapy in the early stages of treatment.[1, 30] The majority of individuals who harbor amebae remain asymptomatic passers of cysts, which, however, may yield invasive trophozoites at any time. The contributing factors leading to emergence of virulence of the organism are not yet fully defined.[1] Some postulate that nonvirulence is due to failure to form trophozoites. Others feel that perhaps an unrecognized virulence factor may be brought into play as a result of the phagocytosis of certain bacteria. Still others suggest that some change in the host allows a trophozoite to assume invasive potential, especially with immunosuppression from steroids, in pregnancy, or from other causes. Invasion and tissue destruction correlate with the zymodeme (pattern of isoenzymes) from *E. histolytica* isolates. Change from a nonpathogenic to a pathogenic zymodeme has been observed *in vitro*, and it is not yet clear whether zymodemes represent stable inherent properties of amebic strains *in vivo*.[31] The mechanism of invasion is also not clearly understood.

It has been postulated that toxic products are liberated from amebae either through the release of lysosomal vesicles from the surface membrane or from rupture of the whole organism. The released toxic products provoke a generalized inflammatory response that progresses to mucosal destruction.[32] With continued damage, the classic ulcer with undermined edges is formed. As amebae move into the bowel wall, they are picked up in the portal circulation and become disseminated systemically. The organ distant from the bowel most frequently involved is the liver, which is often the site of abscess formation. With widespread disease, however, especially in individuals treated with corticosteroids, amebae can be found in virtually every organ of the body, including the brain, lung, and eyes. Surprisingly, neither giardiasis nor amebiasis has been reported to cause major problems in AIDS patients despite their heightened susceptibility to the protozoan *Pneumocystis carinii* in the lungs (see pp. 1237–1238).

Pathology

The frequently described pathologic lesions of amebiasis are ulcers, which first appear covered with small yellow hemispheric elevations of exudate. These are scattered throughout the large intestine, most frequently involving the cecum and ascending colon, with the descending colon, sigmoid, rectum, and hepatic flexure following in that order. Rarely, the disease may involve the terminal ileum. As the disease progresses, the size of the ulcers may grow to an inch or more in diameter. With increasing size, the edges become more undermined and the base extends from the submucosa into the muscular coat. The craters may be filled by necrotic tissue. On rare occasions, involvement of the blood vessels at the base of the ulcer may produce brisk bleeding. More rarely, the patient may perforate and die of peritonitis. In contrast to bacillary dysentery and ulcerative colitis, the intervening mucosa between ulcers may appear relatively normal. However, diffuse inflammation has also been described, making firm diagnosis on gross appearance difficult.[33]

Histologically, there is a diffuse inflammatory lesion that is indistinguishable from the nonspecific inflammation seen in other types of colitis. The lamina propria contains an infiltrate of plasma cells, lymphocytes, neutrophils, histiocytes, and eosinophils. There is edema and focal hemorrhage from distended capillaries. The infiltrate also involves the surface epithelium, and frequently there is an overlying exudate within which amebae may be residing. Focal ulcerations, varying from mild to severe, are present, and amebae may be found at the surface or in the adjacent exudate. Changes seen on electron microscopic examination include extensive damage to the microvillous border, which may account in part for the diarrhea of amebic colitis. As the disease advances, the classically described flask-shaped ulcers with undermined edges are formed.

On histologic section, the amebae can be seen at the leading edge of the ulceration (Fig. 62–4). Occasionally, an ulcer may penetrate deep enough to involve the circular and longitudinal muscle layers of the bowel. For unknown reasons, a dense, fibrous, and granulomatous reaction may be induced in some cases, leading to the formation of a mass lesion called an ameboma, important clinically because of its resemblance to carcinoma.

Clinical Picture

Patients harboring amebae may vary clinically from being completely asymptomatic to being acutely ill with an ulcerative colitis-type picture. The asymptomatic carrier lives in good relationship with the organism; however, cysts are passed in the stool, and the patient is at some risk of infecting others as well as becoming acutely ill. Among patients found to have *E. histolytica* by incidental culture in a sigmoidoscopy clinic, there was no correlation with symptoms or

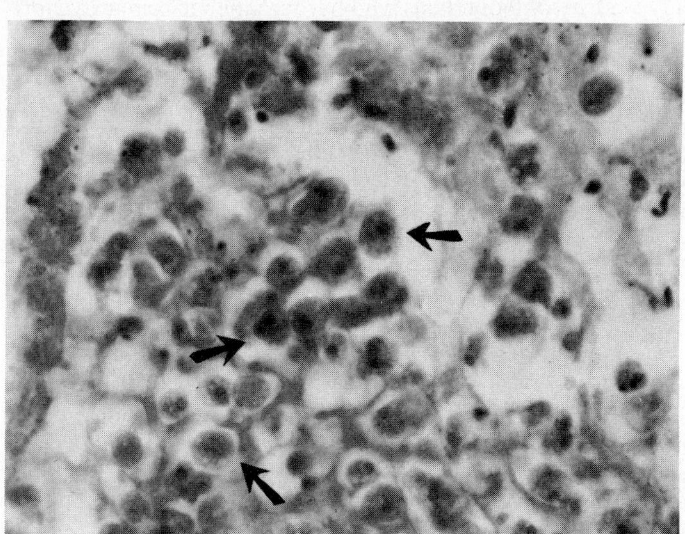

Figure 62–4. *E. histolytica* trophozoites in an ameboma *(arrows)*. The appearance is the same at the edge of amebic ulcers. Note lack of inflammatory response in their immediate vicinity. (Hematoxylin and eosin stain, × 400.) (Courtesy of Frank R. Dutra, M.D.)

histologic or serologic features. During follow-up without treatment of 15 culture-positive patients, none developed symptoms of invasive amebiasis, and all spontaneously eradicated the parasite within 18 months.[34] The type and severity of complaints in the symptomatic patients vary with the location and extent of bowel disease. Often there is abdominal pain, intermittent diarrhea, anorexia, and malaise. In the chronic form these symptoms may wax and wane for months or weeks and may alternate with constipation. The acute, fulminant picture is similar to, and must be differentiated from, other acute inflammatory bowel diseases such as ulcerative colitis and bacillary dysentery. Diarrhea is common, containing blood and mucus; the stools number around seven to ten per 24 hours. They are usually associated with cramping abdominal pain; tenesmus is associated with rectal involvement.

On physical examination, tenderness may be localized anywhere in the lower abdomen but is usually over the cecum, transverse colon, or sigmoid. The liver may be slightly enlarged and tender. If untreated, the patient may go on to develop extreme dilatation of the bowel similar to the toxic megacolon of ulcerative colitis, accompanied by high fever, rapid dehydration, vomiting, and circulatory collapse. One of the most common and grave complications of this state is perforation, leading to peritonitis, overwhelming sepsis, shock, and death. In some areas of the world the mortality rate of amebic colitis is as high as 3 per cent, and perforation probably accounts for about 30 per cent of these deaths. Other bowel complications include massive hemorrhage, which is rare; ameboma formation in any part of the colon, which may lead to obstruction or intussusception; stricture formation during the healing stage; and postdysenteric colitis, which usually resolves over a period of weeks or months without specific therapy. The systemic dissemination of infection may involve other organs, such as brain, lung, pericardium, and liver. The most common extraintestinal infection by amebae is liver abscess.

Diagnosis

The diagnosis of amebiasis is important, not only because it is readily made in most acute cases but also because therapy is highly effective. It is also necessary to distinguish amebiasis from inflammatory bowel disease such as ulcerative colitis or Crohn's colitis, because steroids are often prescribed in the latter and these drugs may be lethal in patients with acute invasive amebiasis.

Microscopic examination of repeated (three to six) fresh stool specimens, if done correctly, will reveal trophozoites and establish the diagnosis in 90 per cent of patients with symptomatic amebiasis. In acute infection with *E. histolytica*, trophozoites will be seen to contain ingested red blood cells when invasion of the bowel wall has occurred, making the diagnosis virtually certain. Confusion with macrophages containing red blood cells may be avoided by observing for the motility characteristic of amebae, which display direct, seemingly purposeful movement. This is true only in fresh warm stools, and examination of nuclear characteristics in stained preparations by trained observers is necessary to confirm the presence of ameba trophozoites.[26] Other amebae, such as *E. hartmanni, E. coli, E. nana*, and *I. buetschlii*, can be found in the human gastrointestinal tract and rarely are pathogenic.[35] Some experience is necessary to distinguish them from the pathogenic *E. histolytica.*

The traditional method of examining stools is a saline wet-mount preparation, which is satisfactory in most cases. Experienced laboratories use concentration techniques and make permanent mounts using stains such as trichrome stain for improved identification of cysts. Stool examination should be completed before barium studies are performed, because the yield is markedly decreased for days to weeks after introduction of barium into the colon. Prior treatment with mineral oil or broad-spectrum antimicrobial agents will also hinder the search for the parasite.

Sigmoidoscopy will be helpful in some, but not all, patients with acute amebiasis, because rectal involvement is less frequent than cecal involvement. The examination should be performed initially, without bowel preparation, prior to therapy. The ulcers are small, discrete, flat, and shallow-based with undermined edges and are often covered with an elevated yellow-white collection of exudate. The intervening mucosa is strikingly normal in contrast to that in patients with ulcerative colitis and bacillary dysentery. However, in those with acute fulminant amebiasis, the rectum can become markedly involved and amebiasis may be easily mistaken for either of the latter two entities. Trophozoites may be obtained from the base of the ulcers by scraping or aspiration of the material into a pipette. A warm saline wet-mount is then made with the specimen and examined microscopically for the parasite. Charcot-Leyden crystals may also be seen in the colonic exudate of patients with amebic colitis. It is thought that they are formed from disintegrating eosinophils. Although they are not entirely specific for amebiasis, their presence should increase the index of suspicion for the disease. Biopsy may be helpful if trophozoites are seen; however, they may not be apparent in 50 per cent or more of cases, even with multiple sectioning. The histologic picture may otherwise resemble other types of colitis. As an adjunct to diagnosis, the indirect hemagglutination test has been found to be of significant value in detecting patients with invasive disease.[25, 26] Asymptomatic cyst passers frequently have low or negative titers. The test is most useful in differentiating amebic colitis from other types of inflammatory bowel disease or in the evaluation of a hepatic mass.

The roentgen features of enteric amebiasis are many, varied, and nonspecific.[36, 37] Identification of amebae in the stool may be precluded after barium is administered. With severe involvement, abdominal films may show toxic dilatation of the colon. Mucosal changes on

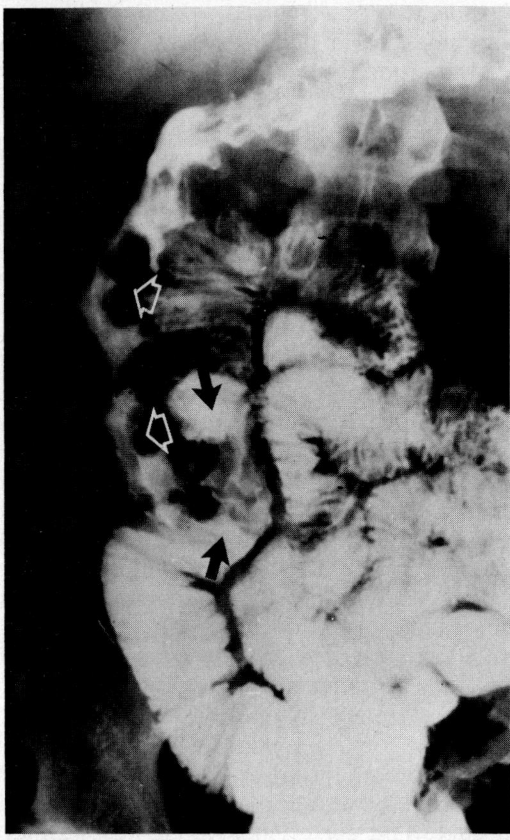

Figure 62–5. Narrowing, ulceration, and nodular contour defects of the cecum and ascending and transverse colon in a patient with amebic colitis. The large filling defects *(open arrows)* were due to extensive submucosal infiltration and hemorrhage. Note the *relative* sparing of the terminal ileum *(closed arrows),* although terminal ileal ulceration is present. (Courtesy of H. I. Goldberg, M.D.)

barium enema can vary from fine granularity and irregularity of the bowel margins to "collar-button" ulcers, deep spike-like penetrating ulcers, pseudopolyps, cobblestoning, and thumbprinting. Haustral changes include spasm and irritability, reduction or loss of haustral pattern, and stricture formation (Figs. 62–5 and 62–6). The cecum is involved in 90 per cent of cases of chronic amebiasis and can become concentrically narrowed—i.e., the "coned cecum." Any portion of the colon, including the appendix, may be involved, and multiple skip lesions are found in 50 per cent of cases. Other findings include perforation, sinuses, fistulas, and pericolic abscesses. An ameboma appears as a mass lesion that is often impossible to distinguish from a neoplasm (Fig. 62–7). The terminal ileum is only rarely involved, and the association of a "coned cecum," a grossly patent ileocecal valve, and terminal ileal distention is an important sign in amebiasis.

The most important differential diagnosis lies in distinguishing acute amebiasis from ulcerative colitis or Crohn's disease of the colon (see pp. 1327–1358 and 1435–1477). Acute, severe parasitic infection may closely resemble these diseases; on occasion, patients with ulcerative colitis harbor amebae. Another condition to consider in the differential diagnosis is bacillary

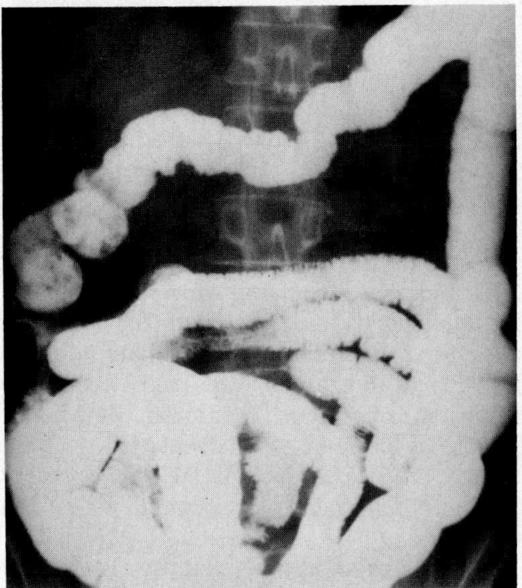

Figure 62–6. Acute amebic colitis of eight days' duration, characterized radiographically by loss of the normal haustral pattern and mucosal ulceration of the right and transverse colon. (Courtesy of H. I. Goldberg, M.D.)

dysentery, clinically confirmed by an appropriate stool culture. Ischemic colitis and acute diverticulitis usually occur in the older age group and have rather characteristic findings, as does diverticulosis with bleeding (see pp. 1327–1358 and 1903–1932). Acute appendicitis (see pp. 1382–1389), carcinoma (see pp. 1519–1560), and tuberculosis (see pp. 1221–1224) must also be included in the differential diagnosis.

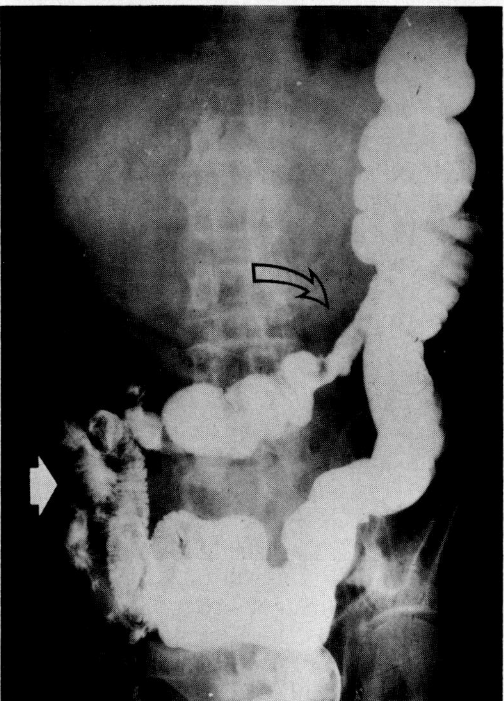

Figure 62–7. Colonic stricture due to ameboma. The midtransverse colon is narrowed secondary to fibrous tissue proliferation induced by chronic amebic infection *(open arrow).* These lesions can be virtually indistinguishable from carcinoma of the colon. The cecum is also diseased with narrowing and contraction *(closed arrow).*

Treatment

The recommended treatment of amebiasis has varied considerably over the years, chiefly because numerous drugs have been employed and none has been found to be entirely satisfactory, either because of toxicity or an unacceptably low cure rate. The emergence of metronidazole (Flagyl) as an antiamebic drug was initially met with great enthusiasm, because it appeared to be highly effective and was less toxic than drugs that have long been given for this disease. However, reports have described some treatment failures with metronidazole, stressing the need for careful follow-up. In addition, there is evidence to suggest that it is carcinogenic in rodents and mutagenic in bacteria in larger than therapeutic doses, and it should not be used in pregnant women. Currently, metronidazole is considered by many to be the drug of choice for invasive amebiasis; however, it is ineffective against organisms within the bowel lumen. Iodoquinol (diiodohydroxyquin) is therefore advised as an accompanying agent in most regimens.[22]

The conventional therapeutic agents available for treatment of amebiasis act as selected sites: intraluminally, intramurally, or systemically. Iodoquinol is an effective agent that acts against amebae that are located intraluminally, but it has been reported to cause optic atrophy in rare instances. Diloxanide furoate (Furamide) is effective only against cysts but appears safe for use in asymptomatic cyst passers. Paromomycin (Humatin) is an aminoglycoside antibiotic that has been used for many years for acute and chronic intestinal amebiasis. It is amebicidal both *in vivo* and *in vitro,* acting directly on amebae, and is antibacterial as well. In patients with mild to moderate nondysenteric amebiasis, paromomycin is effective as a single drug with low toxicity.[38] Tetracycline has also been of value and presumably acts by altering the gastrointestinal flora. Since bacteria may facilitate colonization of the gut by *E. histolytica* as well as heighten its invasive potential, an antibiotic may act to depress the overall virulence of the organism. It may also be useful in controlling postulated secondary bacterial invasion of the damaged gut wall. Chloroquine diphosphate (Aralen) is of value primarily in treating amebae in the liver. Emetine hydrochloride is a toxic but effective amebicidal agent, which is used in severe colitis, amebic-hepatic abscess, or apparent systemic dissemination. The physician and the patient should be aware that all these drugs have a multiplicity of side effects. Emetine, in particular, must be used with caution, because it may be cardiotoxic; fatal myocarditis has been reported with this agent. Although T-wave changes are noted in two thirds of patients receiving emetine, arrhythmias are the prime indication for withdrawing the drug. Dehydroemetine, an analogue of emetine, has been shown to be effective and is less toxic than emetine. It can be used instead of emetine in equivalent doses. Recommended dosage schedules for treatment of intestinal amebiasis are as follows:[22, 39]

Asymptomatic Intestinal Infection. Iodoquinol (diiodohydroxyquin), 650 mg three times daily for 20 days, *or* diloxanide furoate (Furamide),* 500 mg three times a day for 10 days, or paromomycin 25 to 30 mg per kg three times a day for seven days.

Mild to Moderate Intestinal Disease. Metronidazole (Flagyl), 750 mg three times a day for 10 days, plus iodoquinol (diiodohydroxyquin), 650 mg three times daily for 20 days. An alternative is paromomycin (Humatin), 25 to 30 mg per kg per day in three doses for seven days.

Severe Intestinal Disease. Metronidazole (Flagyl), 750 mg three times daily for 10 days; *or* paromomycin (Humatin), 25 to 35 mg per kg per day in three doses for seven days, *plus* iodoquinol, 650 mg three times daily for 20 days.

Alternative drugs that can be used in severe intestinal disease are dehydroemetine,* 1 to 1.5 mg per kg per day (maximum, 90 mg per day) for up to five days, *or* emetine, 1 mg per kg per day (maximum 60 mg per day) for up to five days. These should be accompanied by iodoquinol in the dosage listed above.

Intestinal Complications

A rare patient with severe diffuse inflammation of the colon may progress to a fulminant condition before antiamebic therapy can take effect. The clinical picture then is virtually indistinguishable from fulminant ulcerative colitis. The bowel is dilated, particularly in its transverse portion, to a diameter greater than 9 cm. The patient is extremely febrile and toxic, and shows signs of hypovolemia and electrolyte imbalance. It is remarkable that despite the severity of the illness, amebae may not be readily recovered from the stools in these individuals. If examination and flat films of the abdomen reveal no change in the degree of distention over a period of several days and if evidence of increasing peritoneal inflammation appears, surgery should be considered. The risk of surgery is high, as in ulcerative colitis; however, in good hands a subtotal colectomy may be carried out as antiamebic therapy is continued.

Another classic indication for surgical intervention in this disease is colonic perforation while the patient is receiving antiamebic therapy. This catastrophe, requiring immediate laparotomy, is very similar to its counterpart in fulminant ulcerative colitis. The patient will suddenly have an increase in abdominal pain, usually generalized, evidence of free air in the peritoneal cavity on flat film of the abdomen, and a rapidly progressing picture of septic peritonitis. In some instances, the perforation may not be quite so dramatic and the abdominal signs are more localized. In either

*Available from Parasitic Disease Drug Service, Center for Disease Control, Atlanta, Georgia. Telephone 404-639-3670 (days) or 404-639-2888 (emergency calls outside of regular business hours). Metronidazole can be used as an alternative drug in all three groups with careful follow-up.

event, if it is clinically apparent or justifiably suspicious that the colon has perforated, the abdomen should be explored. Closure of the rent in the colon, drainage of the peritoneal cavity, and exteriorization of the perforated bowel are indicated. With continued antiamebic therapy, these patients will usually recover and the colostomy can be subsequently closed. Alternatively, if the involved segment is irreversibly damaged, exteriorization and colostomy may be followed by a resection and anastomosis.

Another amebic lesion that may be mistaken for a surgically correctable lesion is colonic narrowing produced by an ameboma (Fig. 62–7). Every effort should be made to achieve accurate diagnosis before surgery in any patient with a mass lesion of the colon in whom there is historical or other reason to suspect previous or current amebic infection, because ameboma must be treated medically. Surgery for this lesion is usually followed by complications such as perforation, fistula, peritonitis, and death. Although the parasite is usually absent in stools, the indirect hemagglutination test is usually positive in those with amebomas and should be done when the diagnosis is suspected. If ameboma is likely to be present, the patient should be treated with the drugs outlined earlier, which will resolve the majority of cases. If the lesion does not disappear after a course of such treatment, surgery should then be undertaken under cover of continuing antiamebic therapy.

Prophylaxis of Amebiasis

The best prophylaxis is correction of unsanitary conditions. Houseflies should be eradicated, unboiled water should not be drunk, and raw vegetables or other foods that might have been contaminated by human feces should be avoided. Enteric studies of food handlers and treatment, if indicated, should be carried out when disease investigation suggests possible transmission by food. If water that is suspected of being contaminated is going to be used on a large scale, measures aside from boiling may be employed, including the addition of aluminum sulfate, 400 to 600 mg per gallon, filtration, and, finally, chlorination. Prophylaxis for travelers to endemic areas is not recommended. Iodochlorohydroxyquin (Entero-Vioform) is ineffective and can cause severe neurologic disease, including paralysis and blindness. Although withdrawn from the United States, it is widely available elsewhere and should be advised against. Neither metronidazole nor iodoquinol should be used prophylactically because of the risk of carcinogenesis with prolonged use of the former or of optic atrophy with prolonged use of the latter drug. For those who insist on prophylactic medication, bismuth subsalicylate (Pepto-Bismol), which ameliorates common travelers' diarrhea associated with *Escherichia coli*, can be recommended.[25]

Amebiasis is best prevented by sanitary measures and avoidance of potentially contaminated ingestibles. Stool examination for ova and parasites should be performed upon those who return from endemic areas.

AMEBIC ABSCESS OF THE LIVER

Although the major manifestations of amebiasis are enteric in location, the pathogenicity of the organism is not limited to the intestinal tract and other anatomic sites may be affected. The liver is the most commonly involved extraintestinal organ, and hepatic abscess is a major complication, which, if untreated, often proceeds to a fatal outcome. Amebic abscess of the liver is a well-known entity that is frequently observed in many countries of the world. It may present in a variety of ways as well as manifest a number of unusual complications. The prognosis for eradication of the organism with today's drugs is excellent; if amebic abscess of liver is diagnosed while confined, present modes of treatment are curative.

Epidemiology

The incidence of *hepatic amebic abscess* varies widely according to population and geographic location. It is highest in tropical countries and in areas where sanitary conditions are poor, because these conditions favor a high incidence of intestinal infection. Less than 1 per cent of patients with intestinal amebiasis develop amebic abscess of the liver,[30] yet some institutions are reporting an increasing incidence of amebic abscess of the liver, possibly because of a combination of advanced techniques for scanning the liver in a selected population with high risk of endemic exposure to amebiasis. Thus, hospitals that employ up-to-date techniques and that care for migrant workers or military returnees from the tropics may be expected to encounter increasing numbers of patients with amebiasis and liver abscess. There are differing opinions regarding racial susceptibility to amebiasis and liver abscess; however, no convincing evidence is available on the subject. In general, for unknown reasons males seem to be more frequently afflicted than females, and the peak incidence of the disease is in the third, fourth, and fifth decades of life. Hepatic abscess, although uncommon, has been reported in homosexual males with sexually acquired amebic colitis[41] (see pp. 1258–1260).

Pathogenesis and Pathology

Although it is not always possible to consistently document liver involvement in relationship to intestinal infection, presumably it occurs from migration of the organism from the bowel to the liver by way of the portal circulation. The predisposing factors leading to this type of invasion and spread are unknown, as are the pathogenetic mechanisms for abscess formation. The right lobe of the liver is most often involved. Usually the abscess is solitary, but the formation of multiple abscesses in both lobes is not rare. Whether or not abscess formation is preceded by an active phase of amebic hepatitis is debatable. Most observers believe that right upper quadrant pain and slight enlargement of the liver may be seen during the course of acute intestinal amebiasis; however, this clinical event may represent a nonspecific reaction rather than diffuse dissemination of organisms throughout the liver. In one extensive pathologic study of 145 patients with acute or recent amebiasis, no examples of amebic hepatitis were found.[42]

Gross pathologic changes include an enlarged liver with an abscess cavity that may be quite large, occupying at times almost an entire lobe. The material from the abscess cavity is typically thick and brown and is often described as anchovy sauce–like. It is usually sterile, and *E. histolytica* organisms are absent. Rarely, the abscess may become secondarily infected with bacteria, its content becomes more purulent, and the invading bacterial organism may be cultured. Microscopically, the amebae may be seen limited to the outer wall of the abscess as they invade the normal surrounding parenchyma.

Clinical Features

Amebic abscess of the liver may present in a variety of ways. It may accompany an acute attack of intestinal amebiasis or may appear weeks to years later. Often there is no clear-cut history of amebiasis or diarrhea, and fewer than 50 per cent of patients will have *E. histolytica* in their stools at the time the abscess is diagnosed. The onset of symptoms may be slow and insidious or may be quite rapid. Fever, right upper quadrant pain, and malaise are among the most prominent symptoms. The temperature may vary from low-grade elevation to spiking fevers accompanied by chills and diaphoresis. The right upper quadrant pain may be dull and constant but can also be sharp and stabbing, accentuated by coughing or breathing. Radiation to the right shoulder, aggravated by inspiration, signifies diaphragmatic involvement. Anorexia, weight loss, nausea, vomiting, and fatigue may all be present. Jaundice is rare; it is usually present only in advanced cases.

The most common finding on physical examination is an enlarged tender liver. Splenomegaly is rare; if it is present, other diagnoses must be seriously considered. If the abscess is in the left lobe, tenderness and a palpable liver edge will be felt in the epigastric area. Occasionally, a bulge in the abdominal or chest wall will indicate the site of an abscess that is "pointing." The right diaphragm may appear elevated to percussion, and its excursion is poor. A friction rub may also be heard over the pleura and, occasionally, over the liver as well. Some patients may present with complications of hepatic amebic abscess, most of which are manifestations of rupture of the abscess into adjacent structures. Rupture through the diaphragm into the pleural cavity is a common complication and results in empyema. When the process extends into the lung parenchyma, bronchopleural as well as bronchohepatic fistulas may result, the latter manifested by periodic expectoration of thick, dark, anchovy sauce–like material. Rupture into the peritoneal cavity results in peritonitis; it is a most serious complication with a mortality rate of 75 per cent. Abscess of the left hepatic lobe may perforate into the pericardial sac, precipitating sudden tamponade, vascular collapse, and, in most cases, death. Rupture through the abdominal wall may be further complicated by draining fistulous tracts. Other sites of perforation include the stomach, intestine, vena cava, and biliary tree. All these situations require intensive therapy, including rapid evacuation of the abscess.

Diagnosis and Differential Diagnosis

The key to diagnosis of amebic abscess of the liver is a high degree of suspicion of the condition, particularly in individuals who have resided in an endemic area and present with fever and an enlarged, tender liver. It should be emphasized that often the patient does not have a prior history of amebic dysentery (or even of diarrhea), and the physician must never dismiss the diagnosis on the basis of absence of diarrhea and *E. histolytica* in the stools.

Laboratory features include a moderate anemia and polymorphonuclear leukocytosis. Eosinophilia, in contrast to some other parasitic diseases, is not a feature of this disease. Liver function tests in general are nonspecific. The alkaline phosphatase is elevated in 50 per cent of patients, and the serum aspartate transaminase (AST) may also be abnormal.[43] Hyperbilirubinemia is rare. Serum albumin may be depressed and the globulin elevated. If readily available, the indirect hemagglutination determination (IHAA) is helpful, because it is positive in over 95 per cent of cases. Serologic testing is particularly useful in the United States because of the low prevalence of positive antibody levels.[44] Most state health department laboratories and an increasing number of other centers have available the IHAA or other serologic tests for amebiasis. Treatment must not be withheld pending results in the face of an abundance of clinical evidence that indicates that an abscess is present. Eighty per cent of patients have roentgenographic abnormalities, most commonly elevation and poor mobility of the right diaphragm with obliteration of the right cardiophrenic angle.

Photoscanning techniques have been of major importance in dealing with amebic abscess of the liver (Fig. 62–8). In addition, ultrasound (sonography) and computerized axial tomography (CAT or CT scanning) are of great value. The identification of one or more filling defects with fever and a tender liver is highly suggestive of hepatic abscess. Not only are these studies used in diagnosing and localizing the site of disease, but they are also valuable in assessing the results of therapy.

Needle aspiration of the abscess has been used as a maneuver to establish the diagnosis of an abscess. The type of material contained within it is noted, and the aspirate should be carefully examined microscopically for *E. histolytica*. The latter is often unrewarding unless the specimen is from the edge of the abscess, where

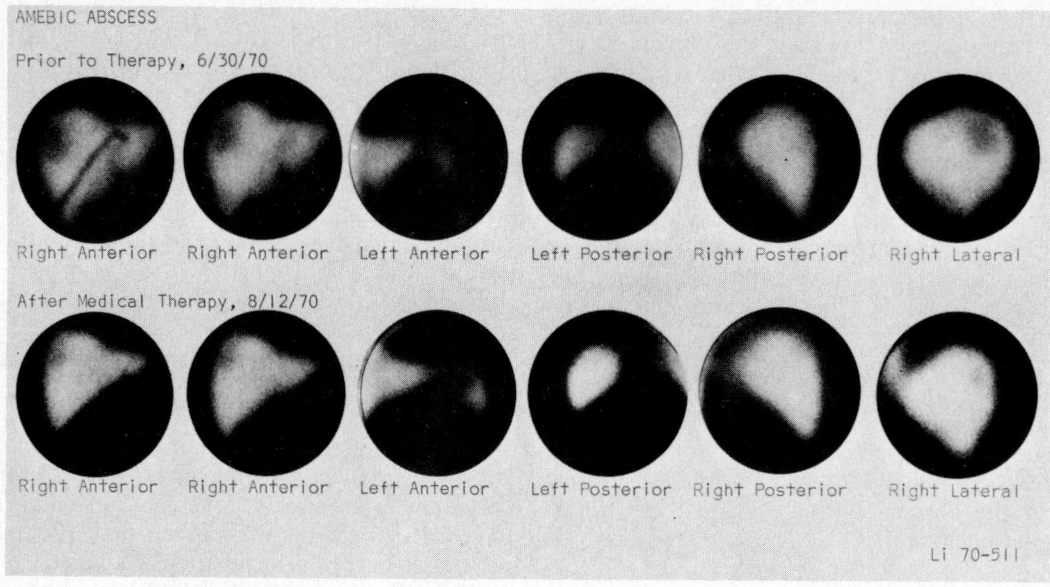

Figure 62–8. Scintigrams of amebic abscess in the liver. (Courtesy of M. Powell, M.D.)

most of the organisms are concentrated. Biopsy of the edge of the abscess with a Vim-Silverman needle to obtain material with the organism has become progressively less important because of the availability of serologic testing and liver scanning and the effectiveness of a trial of drug therapy. The advantage of aspiration is the detection of superimposed bacterial infection and possibly the prevention of rupture of a large abscess.

Amebic abscess of the liver must be distinguished from pyogenic abscess of the liver, tumors in the liver, biliary tract infection, and subphrenic abscess. Non-amebic hepatic abscesses will usually feature a history of antecedent intra-abdominal septic disease (e.g., ruptured appendix, ulcer, diverticulum) or of biliary tract disease, usually with jaundice (acute cholecystitis and cholangitis), that will point the clinician toward the correct diagnosis.

An interesting condition that enters into the differential diagnosis is carcinoma of the liver, which may present with fever, hepatomegaly, weight loss, and a filling defect on liver scan (Fig. 62–9); usually, however, the patient does not have leukocytosis. Further evaluation by means of arteriography is indicated in such cases (Fig. 62–10). In the past several years, sonography has been successful in diagnosis (Fig. 62–11); the CT scan has also been helpful. Liver biopsy may be helpful but is hazardous. The rapid response to medical therapy for amebic abscess is of great diagnostic value, distinguishing it from tumors. Patients who do not respond to amebicidal drugs should be explored for a diagnosis.

Treatment

Amebic abscess of the liver can be treated successfully with drugs alone in the vast majority of patients, provided that it has not ruptured.[39]

Preferred treatment is metronidazole (Flagyl), 750

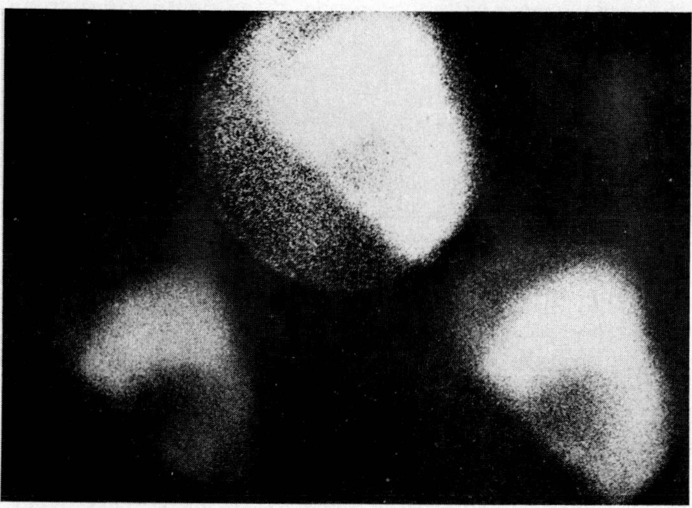

Figure 62–9. Scintigram of the liver, right lateral view. This patient, who presented with fever and hepatomegaly, was first thought to have an hepatic amebic abscess. The final diagnosis was hepatoma.

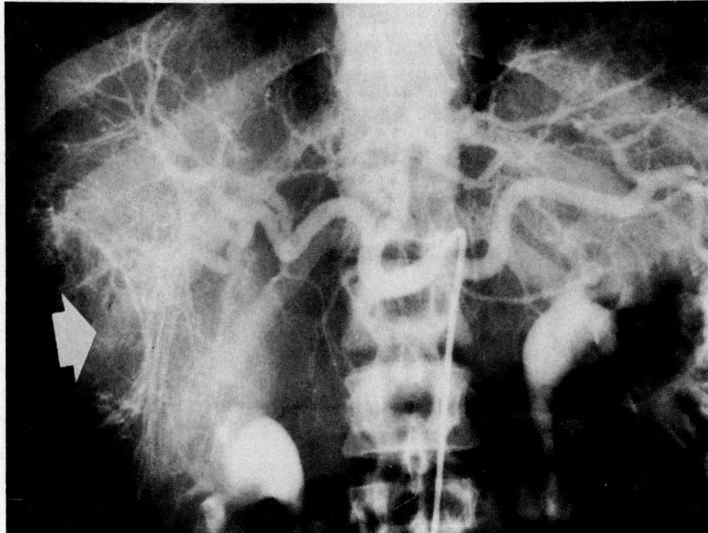

Figure 62–10. Celiac arteriogram in the same patient shown in Figure 62–9. There is a mass displacing and separating the hepatic vasculature in the lateral aspect of the right lobe of the liver *(arrow).*

mg three times a day for ten days, plus iodoquinol, 650 mg three times a day for 20 days.

Alternative regimens include:

1. Dehydroemetine, 1 to 1.5 mg per kg per day intramuscularly (maximal dose, 90 mg per day) for up to five days, *or* the more toxic but more commonly available emetine hydrochloride, 1 mg per kg (maximal dose, 60 mg) intramuscularly for up to five days, *followed by*

2. Chloroquine phosphate, 500 mg twice daily for two days and then 250 mg twice daily for two to three weeks, *plus*

3. Iodoquinol, 650 mg three times daily for 20 days, *or* diloxanide furoate (Furamide), 500 mg three times a day for ten days.

Dehydroemetine and diloxanide are available in the United States from the Parasitic Disease Drug Service, Center for Disease Control, Atlanta, Georgia; telephone 404-639-3670.

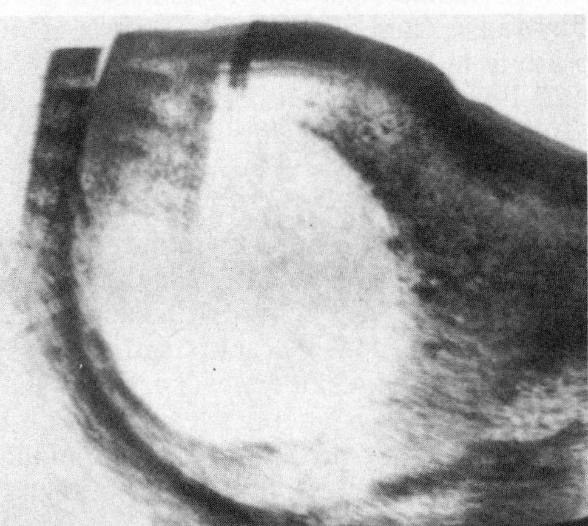

Figure 62–11. Sonogram of large amebic abscess of the liver (echo-free circular area). (Courtesy of George R. Leopold, M.D., University of California, San Diego.)

Nearly all patients with amebic abscess of the liver will respond to medical therapy with a fall in temperature within 72 hours. Failure of such response demands further diagnostic evaluation to rule out other septic or malignant disease in the liver, particularly hepatoma. Early drug therapy is strongly recommended in suspected patients who are moderately to severely ill, because the danger of rupture and death is real. The trial of therapy is quite safe and, if amebic abscess is present, effective, constituting an attractive mode for simultaneous diagnosis and treatment.

Surgical drainage is no longer indicated in the treatment of uncomplicated hepatic amebic abscess, as it may lead to secondary bacterial infection and prolonged drainage. Routine needle aspiration of the abscess has its proponents, but many feel it is an unnecessary procedure. It may be beneficial, however, in large abscesses with impending rupture or in cases of treatment failure, when it may be both diagnostic and therapeutic.

COCCIDIOSIS

Coccidia are protozoa from the suborder Eimeriorina in the phylum Apicomplexa. Within this suborder members of three families are currently known to cause disease in humans. These are *Isospora belli* and *Isospora natalensis* in the family Eimeriidae, *Cryptosporidium* species in the family Cryptosporidiidae, and *Sarcocystis* and *Toxoplasma* in the family Sarcocystidae.[45] Only *Isospora* and *Cryptosporidium* will be considered here.

This order of parasites is an important cause of morbidity and mortality in domestic and wild animals. Their distribution is limited only by the availability of hosts. Virtually every animal examined has been found to harbor its own species-specific coccidium. Some animals may be infected by several different species of coccidia. Infection is acquired by ingestion of viable oocysts. No vectors are required, and the oocysts may persist for long periods of time in soil.

Coccidiosis is infrequently recognized as the cause of disease in man in the United States. However, endemic areas exist in South America, Africa, and the Middle East; Chile, Rotterdam, and the Western Pacific appear to have particularly high incidences.[46] Failure to diagnose coccidiosis elsewhere may be due not so much to its rarity as to the failure to recognize these parasites as a cause of human disease.

Pathogenesis

Sporulated oocysts excyst in the proximal small intestine, where the sporozoites that are released invade the epithelium. They become round trophozoites that enter the asexual stage of development, schizogony. The merozoites (Fig. 62–12) depart the mature schizont and invade adjacent epithelial cells. On invasion, they may either undergo further schizogony or become sexual gametocytes. On fertilization, the macrogametocyte (female) becomes a nonsporulated oocyst that is extruded into the intestinal lumen and eliminated in the feces. Sporulated oocysts have also been observed in intestinal aspirates, raising the possibility of direct person-to-person transmission, as well as infection by ingestion of fecally contaminated material containing oocysts which have sporulated outside the host.[47]

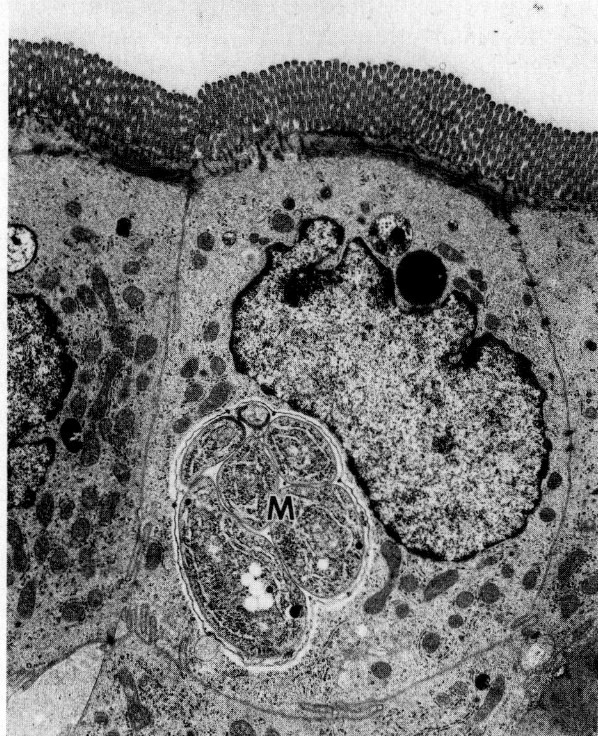

Figure 62–12. *Isospora belli* merozoites (M) clustered together in the vacuole where they were formed by division of a trophozoite. These fusiform motile forms invade adjacent enterocytes in the asexual proliferative phase of this infection. Transmission electron micrograph of a jejunal biopsy. (× 5700.)

In animals, the symptoms may be explained by the amount of intestinal epithelial destruction. Most coccidia are strictly intestinal parasites. Chickens and lambs infected with their own species-specific coccidia have been shown to develop "villus atrophy" when compared with suitable control animals. Some species develop a necrotizing enteritis.

Human intestinal pathologic changes in coccidiosis represent a spectrum of damage. Included are necrotizing enterocolitis,[48] a flat mucosa similar to celiac sprue, tall clubbed villi with a marked excess of collagen and dilated vessels in the lamina propria, "stubby" residual villi with elongated crypts, eosinophilic infiltration similar to eosinophilic enteritis, and mild nonspecific changes in lightly infected patients.[49] Organisms are not found in postmortem specimens, possibly because of autolysis. One patient is recorded to have had a reversal of the severe intestinal pathologic changes caused by chronic coccidiosis of many years' duration, following successful therapy.[50] This is strong circumstantial evidence that the spectrum of pathology is caused by the parasite (see below).

Diagnosis

History. Coccidiosis usually has an acute onset, with fever, headache, and asthenia. Diarrhea occurs in 98 per cent of patients, weight loss in 86 per cent, and colicky abdominal pain in 61 per cent. Tetany, muscle cramps, paresthesias, and night blindness may occur.[49] The stools frequently contain undigested food and often appear grossly steatorrheal. Steatorrhea has been proved in a small number of patients.[49, 50] The illness is usually of limited duration, rarely more than six months.

Physical Examination. Physical examination does not contribute to the diagnosis of coccidiosis. If the disease has been chronic, there may be evidence of weight loss, which at times is profound. Characteristically, there is no tenderness on palpation of the abdomen.

Laboratory Findings. Depending upon the severity of the diarrhea and steatorrhea, electrolyte abnormalities may range from none to very severe. The blood counts are usually within normal limits, except for the differential white blood cell count, in which there are both a relative and an absolute eosinophilia in 54 per cent of patients. (This is extremely unusual in other protozoan infections.)

The diagnosis may be made by finding oocysts in the stool. This may prove to be extremely difficult, because they are frequently very scanty or absent even in the presence of severe diarrhea and steatorrhea. In contrast to usual techniques, the fecal specimen should be incubated for two days at room temperature to allow maturation of oocysts. Concentration techniques such as sucrose or zinc sulfate flotation should be used. Oocysts fluoresce bright yellow with auramine-rhodamine stain and appear pink with red-purple sporocysts with a modified acid-fast stain.[51]

The mature oocyst of *I. belli* is a thick-walled ovoid structure that is elongated at one end and somewhat constricted at the other. The dimensions range between 11 to 16 μm and 22 to 33 μm. The mature forms contain two sporocysts that measure 7 to 9 μm by 12 to 14 μm, each containing four sporozoites and a large residual mass.

Mucosal Biopsy. Peroral small bowel mucosal biopsy is probably the most sensitive way of making the diagnosis of coccidiosis.[49] The pathologic changes are variable, ranging from a flat mucosa to mild nonspecific abnormalities. The mucosal morphologic appearance is not diagnostic. However, various forms of the parasites may be seen within epithelial cells.[49] All the various stages of the life cycle of the organism are present, but the most easily recognizable forms are the various stages of schizogony, which are also the most numerous (Figs. 62–13 to 62–15).

Great care must be taken in handling, preparation, and examination of the biopsy specimen. Because coccidia in the epithelium in humans are not nearly so numerous as in many animal species, the specimen should be processed in the following manner. Bouin's fixed specimens (two hours following which they are transferred to 70 per cent alcohol and run up in the usual techniques to paraffin embedding) are used. Each biopsy should be, serially and entirely, sectioned perpendicular to the luminal surface at 4 μm. Giemsa stain or colophonium Giemsa offers the best differential stain for recognizing the various forms of schizogony. *Multiple* sections must be scanned before coccidiosis is discarded as a diagnosis.

Duodenal Drainage. Examination of the intestinal secretions may provide the diagnosis. Immature schizonts and unsporulated and sporulated oocysts are present in the intestinal secretions in some patients.

Radiology. Few data are available on the radiographic appearance of the small intestine in patients with coccidiosis. In some patients, the small bowel series is normal. In some there is obstruction of the duodenum. There may be thickened folds in the duodenum and proximal jejunum with an infiltrated, rigid appearance, excessive secretions within the small bowel, and a rapid transit time.

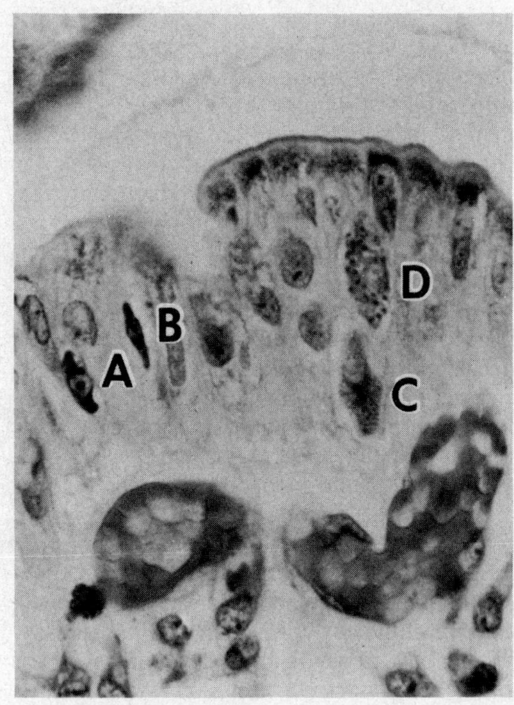

Figure 62–13. Merozoites that are developing into either schizonts or gametocytes (A and B), immature schizont (C), and macrogametocyte (D). (Colophonium Giemsa stain, × 1000.) (From Brandborg, L. L., Goldberg, S. G., and Breidenbach, W. C. N. Engl. J. Med. *283*:1306, 1970. Reprinted by permission of the New England Journal of Medicine.)

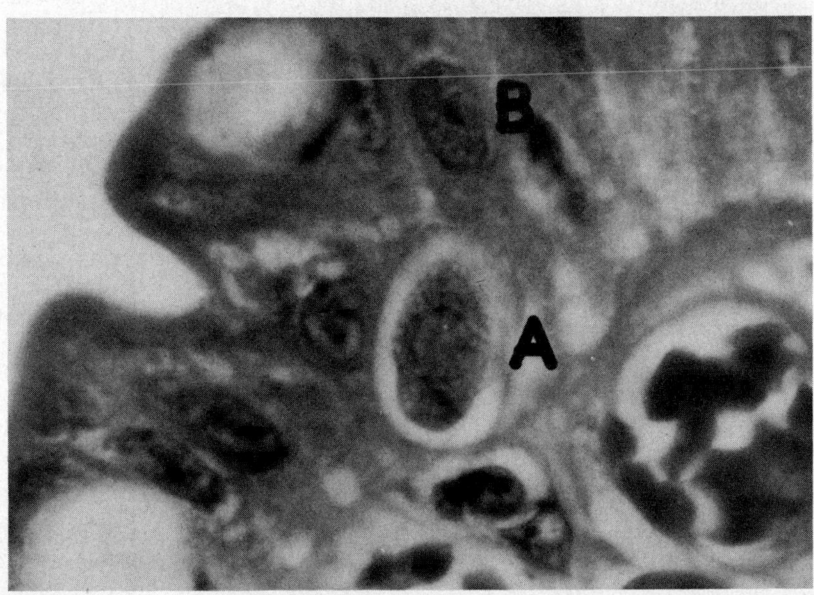

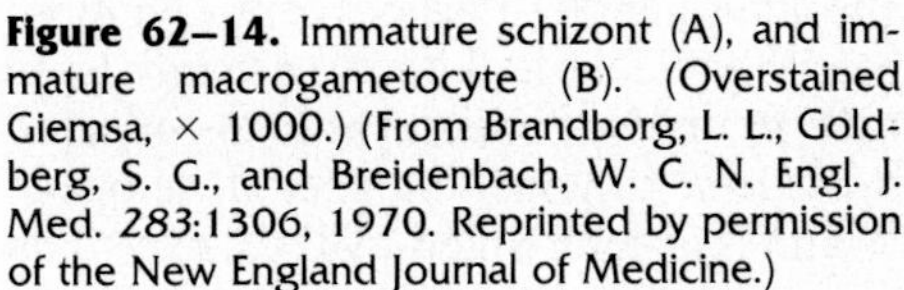

Figure 62–14. Immature schizont (A), and immature macrogametocyte (B). (Overstained Giemsa, × 1000.) (From Brandborg, L. L., Goldberg, S. G., and Breidenbach, W. C. N. Engl. J. Med. *283*:1306, 1970. Reprinted by permission of the New England Journal of Medicine.)

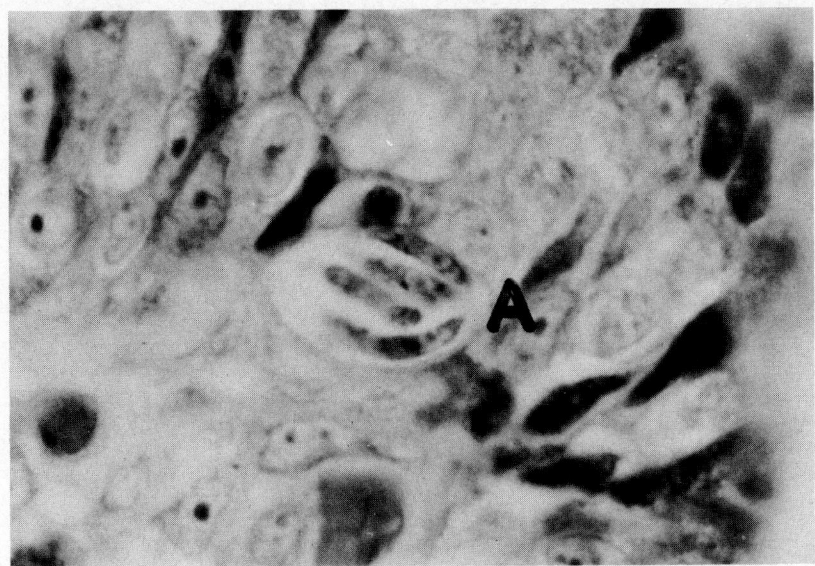

Figure 62–15. Mature schizont containing merozoites (A). (Colophonium Giemsa stain, × 1000.) (From Brandborg, L. L., Goldberg, S. G., and Breidenbach, W. C. N. Engl. J. Med. *283*:1306, 1970. Reprinted by permission of the New England Journal of Medicine.)

Treatment

Most patients with coccidiosis have a benign and self-limited illness of a few days' to six months' duration. Trimethoprim, 160 mg, and sulfamethoxazole, 800 mg, four times a day for ten days, then twice daily for three weeks, is recommended.[22] In patients with AIDS, this regimen eliminated abdominal pain and diarrhea after two days. In 47 per cent of patients symptoms recurred, but again responded to repeat treatment.[52] In those who are allergic to trimethoprim-sulfamethoxazole, furazolidone, 100 mg four times a day for ten days, can be tried. One patient is described whose chronic coccidiosis, associated with severe malabsorption of many years' duration, was cured with antimalarial drugs. The regimen administered was pyrimethamine, 75 mg, plus sulfadiazine, 4 gm daily for 21 days, followed by pyrimethamine and sulfadiazine at a dosage of 37.5 mg and 2 gm per day for 28 days.[47]

No data are available, but in patients with the benign and less chronic diseases whose diarrhea is troublesome, diphenoxylate with atropine (Lomotil) in doses of 2.5 to 5 mg every six hours may be of some benefit.

Cryptosporidia

Cryptosporidia are protozoa classified with the coccidia. They have been recognized as a common cause of diarrhea in calves and in many other mammals, reptiles, and birds. Some species specificity may exist, but infection is transmissible among humans, calves, pigs, and mice.[53] Cryptosporidia infection has been recognized as a cause of diarrheal disease in humans only in the past ten years. Most reported cases have occurred in patients with congenital immunoglobulin deficiency or immunologic incompetence produced by medications, concurrent viral infection, acquired immunodeficiency syndrome (AIDS) (see pp. 1243–1250), or idiopathic causes. As serologic and stool methods of detection develop, milder self-limited cases of cryptosporidiosis are being diagnosed in patients with normal immune competence, especially after contact with farm animals or in day care centers.[53] As with Legionnaires' disease and *Campylobacter* infection, cryptosporidiosis can be expected to be recognized more often as diagnostic capability increases.[54]

Pathogenesis

Cryptosporidia are spherical parasites 2 to 5 μm in diameter, which are excreted in the stool as oocysts. These oocysts are immediately infective without further maturation outside the host and remain infective for weeks to months. After oocysts are ingested, cryptosporidia trophozoites attach to intestinal epithelial cells through the small and large intestine, destroying microvilli and attaching firmly to epithelial cells. In light microscopy they appear as multiple round basophilic bodies, lying in the brush border over villi in the small intestine (Fig. 62–16) and over the surface and crypts of colon. Cryptosporidia lie just beneath the luminal enterocyte membrane but, unlike *Isospora*, remain extracytoplasmic (Fig. 62–17). Villi are reduced in height and crypts lengthened. Plasma cells, lymphocytes, and polymorphonuclear leukocytes are increased in the lamina propria. In experimental animals infected with cryptosporidia from humans, diarrhea develops in three to five days and is accompanied by fecal excretion of oocysts.[53]

Diagnosis

Nausea, low-grade fever, abdominal cramps, and profuse watery diarrhea accompany cryptosporidial infection. Vomiting and mild rectal bleeding subsequent to five to ten watery bowel movements a day

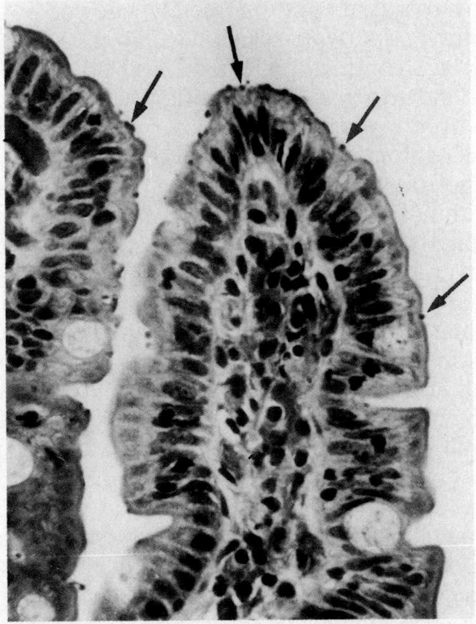

Figure 62–16. Darkly stained, rounded cryptosporidia embedded in the microvilli on the surface of jejunal villi of an immunodeficient patient with malabsorption. × 264. (From Heyworth, M. F., and Owen, R. L. Surv. Dig. Dis. *3*:197, 1985. Used by permission of S. Karger AG, Basel, Switzerland.)

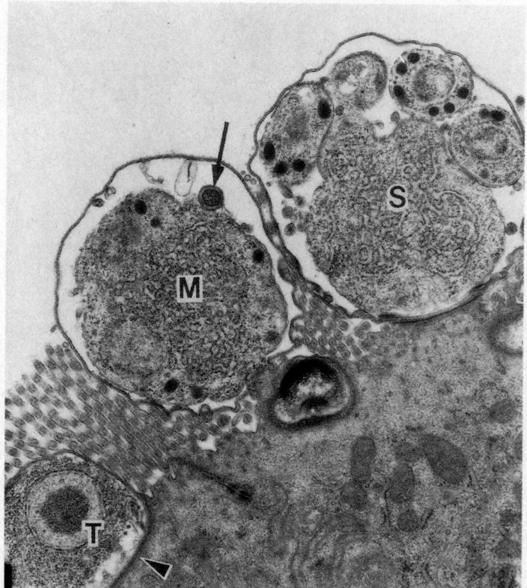

Figure 62–17. Three *Cryptosporidium* stages embedded in the microvillus border of an enterocyte. On the left is an immature trophozoite (T) with a dense attachment zone *(arrowhead)* through which it feeds from the host cell. In the center is a microgamont (M) with multiple nuclei in the periphery of its cytoplasm and a microgamete (male sexual reproductive form) at its surface *(arrow)* within the parasitophorous vacuole surrounded by host cell membranes. On the right is an asexual reproductive form or schizont (S) with four merozoites, which depart the parasitophorous vacuole and invade adjacent enterocytes, perpetuating the infection. Transmission electron micrograph. (× 9300.)

may occur. Patients frequently demonstrate physical signs of dehydration, hyperactive bowel sounds, diffuse abdominal tenderness, and lethargy. Sigmoidoscopy has demonstrated a reddened nonfriable mucosa without ulcers. Urinary excretion of a test dose of D-xylose is decreased, and stool fat is increased. Barium X-ray studies are nonspecific. With experience, cryptosporidial oocysts can be detected in modified acid-fast–stained smears of feces, especially after oocyst concentration by sugar flotation.[53, 54] Oocysts are approximately 4 μm in diameter with eccentrically located red granules. In unstained concentrates, oocysts float to the cover slip; they are 5 to 6 μm in diameter with granular cytoplasm and a black dot near the center. In most hospitals, the diagnosis is best made by mucosal biopsy and examination of the microvillous border for embedded basophilic bodies. The diagnosis can be confirmed by the distinctive appearance of the cryptosporidia in electron micrographs.

Treatment

Treatment consists of correction of fluid and electrolyte abnormalities. In patients with normal immunologic status, infection is self-limited and clears in approximately 14 days. When immunosuppression is present, clearance of infection can be anticipated only if the immunologic status can be corrected. Pharmacologic agents may eliminate coexisting intestinal infections, but none has been identified that prevents or eliminates cryptosporidiosis. Patients with cryptosporidia in the current epidemic of acquired immunodeficiency syndrome (AIDS) have been treated with a wide variety of chemotherapeutic agents but have continued to have profuse watery diarrhea. Cryptosporidiosis has not been identified as the direct cause of death but has contributed to death through severe malnutrition (see pp. 1243–1250).

Microsporidia

Microsporidia are obligatory intracellular protozoa, which occur widely in fish and in insects. They are also found in humans and other mammals.[55] A large number of genera and species of microsporidia have been identified which vary in host specificity, tissue predilection, and pathogenetic potential. Human infections have been described in normal and immunodeficient patients. In the intestine spores within host enterocytes (Fig. 62–18) pass into the lumen when enterocytes are desquamated.[54] Spores in feces contaminate food and other material ingested by new hosts. Spores within muscle, brain, or other tissues may be released by digestion when infected animals are ingested by carnivores. Intestinal microsporidial infections in humans have been recognized only rarely, possibly because spores are very small (1 to 2 μm) and are not detected by stool parasite examination. Intestinal infections are being recognized with increasing frequency in AIDS patients. In Sweden a screening study found positive serologic evidence of microsporidia in one third of homosexual men in an AIDS clinic[56] (see p. 1246). Twelve per cent of an unselected group of Swedish

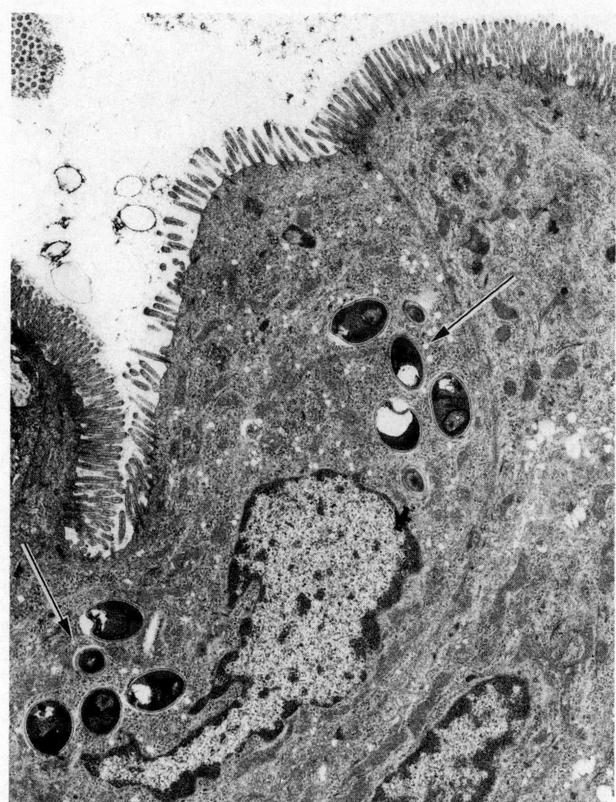

Figure 62–18. Oval microsporidia spores *(arrows)* in the jejunum of a man with AIDS, intractable diarrhea, and malabsorption. When infected enterocytes desquamate into the lumen, spores are released to infect other enterocytes endogenously or to pass into the feces where they may be ingested by another host. (× 6050.) (From Current, W. L., and Owen, R. L.: Cryptosporidiosis and microsporidiosis. *In* Farthing, M. J. G., and Keusch, G. T. [eds.]. Enteric Infection: Mechanisms, Manifestations, and Management. London, Chapman and Hall, 1988.)

adults returning from travel to tropical areas also had antibody to microsporidia, but no Swedes without a history of travel outside of Europe were positive.[57] Among tropical disease clinic patients, 42.7 per cent of Nigerians with tuberculosis, 35.9 per cent of Ghanians with malaria, and 18.6 per cent of Malaysians with filariasis also had antibody to microsporidia.[58] These studies of selected patient populations suggest that microsporidia infection may be much more common than usually suspected.

Pathogenesis

Microsporidia spores contain a coiled polar tubule which everts in response to environmental stimuli, penetrating adjacent cells, usually in the gastrointestinal tract. The nucleus and cytoplasm of the spore are then injected through the polar tubule, initiating infection. Proliferation of microsporidia in host cells leads to direct extension to nearby cells or to vascular dissemination to other tissues including liver, muscle, brain, and kidneys. Although most infections begin in the gastrointestinal tract, the life cycles of different genera and species of microsporidia vary widely and in many cases are not completely known. Spores of the genus *Pleistophora* which develop in skeletal muscle displace contractile elements and provoke inflammation and scarring.[59] In an infant with thymic hypoplasia, severe diarrhea, and later ileus, postmortem sections of stomach, small intestine, and colon showed microsporidia of the genus *Nosema* in the interstitium and within smooth muscle cells in all layers of the muscularis.[60] Organisms were also seen in mesenteric ganglia and nerve fibers and within media of small muscular arteries. Infection in the mucosa could not be evaluated because of autolysis. Numerous parasites in intestinal musculature and nerves may have impeded strength and coordination of muscle contractility, contributing to altered intestinal motility in this patient. Intestinal biopsy in an AIDS patient with weight loss and severe diarrhea showed microsporidia within 10 per cent of enterocytes,[61] but there was little evidence of epithelial cell injury or alteration of villus architecture. This genus of microsporidia, which seems to be restricted to enterocytes, has been tentatively designated *Enterocytozoon*.[62]

Diagnosis

In patients with AIDS or other immunodeficiencies with severe diarrhea, weight loss, epigastric pain, and watery nonbloody bowel movements, microsporidiosis should be considered when no other pathogens are identified. In one such patient D-xylose and vitamin B_{12} were malabsorbed and stool fat was three times greater than the upper limit of normal.[63] No lesions were evident at endoscopy, but biopsies showed partial villus atrophy and mild inflammatory infiltrate. By light microscopy identification of microsporidia is difficult because of their small size and the variable staining characteristics of various genera. Microsporidia in muscle stain with Gomori's methenamine-silver stain, tissue Gram stain, PAS, and acid-fast stains,[60] but microsporidia in intestinal mucosa are very difficult to discern in paraffin-embedded sections with any light microscopic stain.[54, 61] In electron micrographs sections of the coiled polar tubule resemble stacked erythrocytes (Fig. 62–19). At present, electron microscopy is the only available diagnostic tool for detecting microsporidia in intestinal biopsies. Although an indirect immunofluorescence test for microsporidia using rabbit *Encephalitozoon cuniculi* as an antigen has been applied to epidemiologic screening,[56–58] no serologic test is available for use in diagnosis. Until sensitive and specific tests become available, it is not possible to know whether or how often microsporidia cause acute self-limited gastrointestinal infection in patients with normal immune systems.

Treatment

Symptoms in the AIDS patient with myositis were stabilized after the patient was given trimethoprim, 20 mg/kg, and sulfisoxazole, 100 mg/kg per day.[59] We found that trimethoprim-sulfamethoxazole was tem-

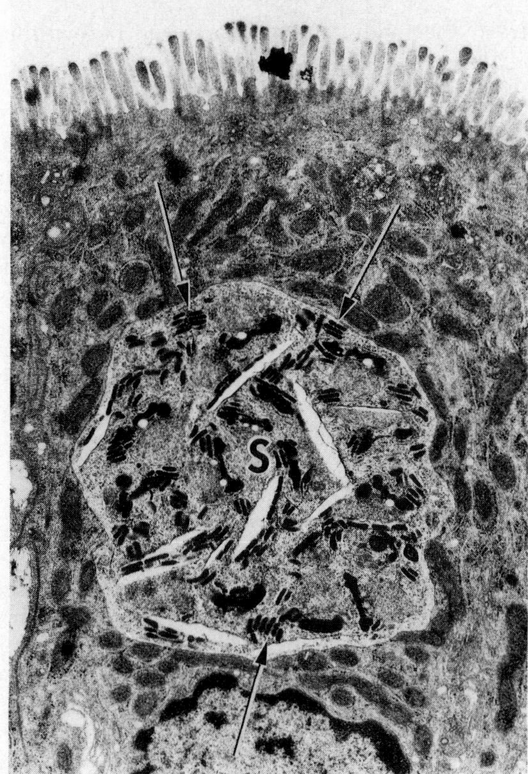

Figure 62–19. In a jejunal enterocyte a microsporidia sporont (S) dividing within a vesicle contains at least 11 nuclei, each associated with an elongated vacuole and a coiled polar tubule which in section resembles stacked erythrocytes *(arrows)*. After division is complete, each nucleus with its organelles will form a spore. (× 9740.)

porarily effective in controlling diarrhea in an AIDS patient with microsporidia; however, as in many AIDS patients, skin rash and fever developed, limiting use of this combination.[54] Neither tetracycline nor spiramycin was helpful. Symptoms were partially controlled by loperamide and other antimotility drugs (see also pp. 1245–1248).

BALANTIDIASIS

Although human infection with the organism *Balantidium (B. coli)* is rare, it is important to recognize, because it is a curable disease that may produce severe intestinal symptoms and even death.

Etiology

Balantidium coli is a protozoan and the only member of the class Ciliata known to infect humans.[25] The trophozoite is quite large and may occasionally be seen with the naked eye. It averages 50 to 100 μm in length. The organism is oval in shape, and the anterior end contains a funnel-shaped cytosome leading to the cytopharynx. The organism is covered with cilia, which act to propel it as well as to direct food into its digestive passage. A large, variably shaped macronucleus, an adjacent small micronucleus, and numerous vacuoles that may contain red blood cells, starch granules, and other inert substances may be seen in the cytoplasm. The cyst, which is the infective form, develops when the organism is passed in the feces and is exposed to the outside environment. It is a round, thick-walled, ovoid structure 40 to 65 μm in diameter, within which the organism can be seen.

Epidemiology

The majority of reported cases of balantidiasis have been found in the tropics; however, the organism is encountered in the United States and has been identified as far north as Sweden and Norway.[64] There are several antigenically distinguishable species of *Balantidium*, and these may reside in numerous animals, particularly monkeys and hogs. The evidence linking infection in humans with exposure to pigs in an unsanitary environment is suggestive but not conclusive.[65] The *Balantidium* found in hogs is morphologically indistinguishable from the organism in humans, but there are antigenic differences; further, the exact mode of transmission remains unclear. Epidemiologically significant outbreaks of *Balantidium* infection have occurred in mental institutions where poor sanitation and neglected personal hygiene are prevalent.

Pathogenesis and Pathology

Infection presumably begins when the *Balantidium* cyst is ingested. The parasite excysts in the small intestine, and the new trophozoite passes into the colon, where it penetrates the mucosal epithelium. The organism produces an enzyme, hyaluronidase, which apparently aids in invasion of the tissue. The gross pathologic appearance is similar to that in amebiasis.[66] Usually only the colon is involved, although rarely the terminal ileum may also be infected. The gross pathologic changes consist of multiple superficial ulcers with necrotic bases and undermined edges; the intervening mucosa ranges from normal to hemorrhagic. In some infections, the ulcers are deep and may perforate.

The balantidia may be seen microscopically clustered at the bases of the crypts, where they penetrate through the intact mucosal epithelium. They progress through the muscularis mucosae to the submucosa, where they may become lodged in capillaries and dilated lymph channels. The protozoan may also be seen in the bases and edges of the ulcer. Round cells dominate the inflammatory response, and eosinophils may be numerous. Rarely, the organism may be seen in the regional lymph nodes.

Clinical Picture

Generally, balantidiasis presents one of three differing clinical states. (1) The patient may be a completely asymptomatic carrier, capable of spreading the infection, particularly in an institutional environment. (2) The patient may have chronic diarrhea with loose, frequent bowel movements alternating with periods of constipation. Mucus may be present, but blood or pus rarely appears. The organism is not easily recovered in this stage, and multiple fresh stool specimens must be examined to make the diagnosis. It may cause appendicitis. (3) The patient may be acutely ill with the sudden onset of frequent stools containing mucus and blood; the patient complains of epigastric pain, tenesmus, nausea, and abdominal tenderness. Weight loss and dehydration are common. In its extreme form the illness is severe and fulminant with rectal hemorrhage, which, along with rapid dehydration and fever, leads to shock and death within a few days.[67] Extraintestinal involvement in this form may be noted: peritonitis, urinary tract infection, vaginitis, liver abscess, pleuritis, and even pneumonia have been described.

Diagnosis

The sigmoidoscopic picture of *B. coli* infection may be difficult to distinguish from that of acute amebiasis or bacillary dysentery. At colonoscopy ulcers may be shallow and "aphthoid" or deep and coalescent with normal intervening mucosa.[68] The diagnosis is best made by examination of scrapings of the bases of the ulcers for the trophozoites. Rectal biopsy may reveal the organism that has penetrated the epithelial surface (Fig. 62–20). Stool examination will also provide the diagnosis; however, it must be emphasized that multiple fresh specimens must be analyzed before the disease can be excluded.

Treatment

The drug of choice for treatment of *Balantidium* infection is tetracycline, 500 mg four times a day for 10 days. An alternative is iodoquinol (diiodohydroxyquin), 650 mg three times daily for 20 days, or metronidazole, 750 mg three times a day for seven days.[39] Treatment should be directed toward asymptomatic carriers as well as the acutely or chronically ill in order to eradicate the organism and prevent its spread.

BLASTOCYSTIS HOMINIS

B. hominis was previously considered an intestinal yeast and of interest only because it might be confused with *E. histolytica*. Ultrastructural and physiologic studies now support reclassification of this organism as a protozoan.[69] It has been associated with gastrointestinal signs and symptoms, although debate continues whether it is the cause of symptoms or is only an indicator of exposure to fecal contamination and infection with *E. histolytica* or other "true" pathogens. Both positions may be correct, depending on extent of infection. Watery diarrhea associated with frequent penetration of the intestinal epithelium by *B. hominis* has been demonstrated in germ-free guinea pigs inoculated with *B. hominis* (Fig. 62–21).[70]

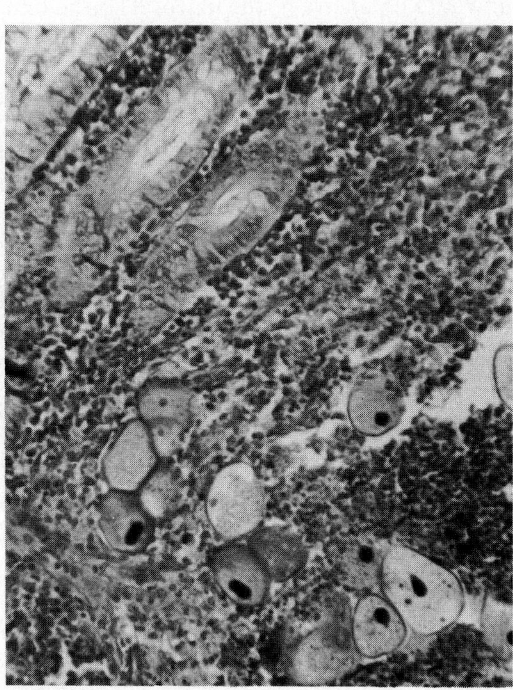

Figure 62–20. *B. coli* parasites in intestinal ulcer. (Photomicrograph by Zane Price. From Markell, E. K., Voge, M., and John, D. T. Medical Parasitology. Ed. 6. Philadelphia, W. B. Saunders Company, 1986.)

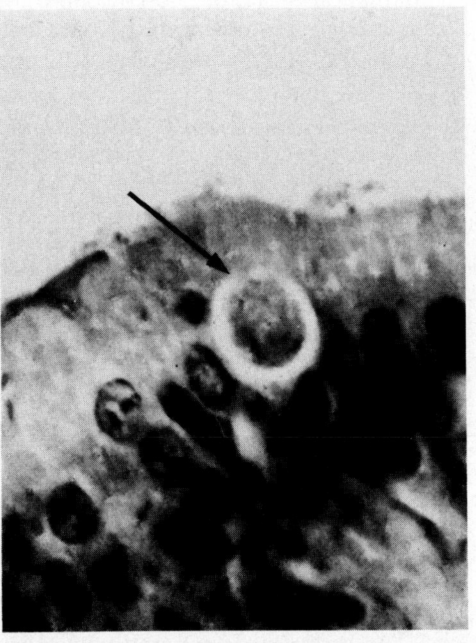

Figure 62–21. Ameba-like form of *Blastocystis hominis (arrow)* surrounded by a halo in the colonic epithelium of an experimentally infected germ-free guinea pig. (× 328.) (From Phillips, B. P., and Zierdt, C. H. Exp. Parasitol. *39*:358, 1976.)

Clinical Presentation

B. hominis has been reported in epidemics of gastrointestinal disease in subtropical areas, sporadic diarrhea throughout the world, and chronic diarrhea in higher primates. Among 2360 patients who submitted stools for parasitologic examination at UCLA over a 20-month period, 289 (12 per cent) had *B. hominis*.[71] An analysis of 36 of these men and women who were negative for bacterial pathogens and parasites other than *B. hominis* revealed that 56 per cent had underlying disease associated with some degree of immunosuppression or deficiency. Two thirds had symptoms, including diarrhea, pain, cramps, nausea, fever, vomiting, headache, gas, chills, and malaise. Symptoms usually lasted three to ten days but ranged from a few hours to three years. At least one death has been associated with *B. hominis* infection in a man with severe prolonged diarrhea.[72]

Diagnosis

Purged or spontaneous stools are examined in unstained wet mounts or permanent stained smears. Over a five-month period, 62 of 389 consecutive patients referred to a New York parasitology laboratory had *B. hominis*. Among the 43 with five or more *B. hominis* organisms per high-power field in their stools, 20 also had other intestinal parasites, but 23 had only *B. hominis*. Clinical symptoms were rare in patients with less than five *B. hominis* cells per high-power (×40) field, but were common with five or more *B. hominis* organisms.[73] It appears reasonable to treat symptomatic patients in whom no other stool pathogens have been identified and in whom moderate to heavy *B. hominis* infection is found.

Treatment

When physicians choose to treat *B. hominis*, metronidazole is prescribed most commonly, in doses from 250 mg to 750 mg three to four times a day by mouth for one week. In adults and children this approach has been reported to eliminate both symptoms and *B. hominis*.[74, 75] Furazolidone, trimethoprim-sulfamethoxazole, and emetine have also been found to be inhibitory in *in vitro* evaluation of ten antiprotozoal drugs against four axenic strains of *B. hominis*.[76] Iodoquinol, 650 mg three times daily by mouth for 10 to 20 days, eliminated diarrhea and other symptoms but not *B. hominis* in 32 patients with *B. hominis*, of whom 27 had at least one other known pathogen (*E. histolytica, G. lamblia*, or *D. fragilis*).[77] If symptoms are relieved, most patients will, however, be grateful whether the mechanism is elimination of *B. hominis,* elimination of an undetected coexisting pathogen, or a change in bowel flora affecting the pathogenicity of *B. hominis*.

INTESTINAL ROUNDWORMS* (NEMATODES)

Ascariasis

Ascaris lumbricoides is a large (over 20 cm long) roundworm with a worldwide distribution. The highest prevalence is in the hot and humid tropics. Infection is through the ingestion of embryonated eggs contaminating food or drink. The larvae emerge from the ovum in the duodenum, from which they migrate through the epithelium of the small bowel into the portal venous system and pass through the liver into the lungs. The incubation period is not precisely known, but within 4 to 16 days after infection a pneumonitis develops, with fever, cough, sputum production, and pulmonary infiltrates. At this time, the larvae may be found in the sputum.

After several days in the lung, the larvae break through the pulmonary capillaries into the alveoli and migrate up the bronchioles and bronchi to the pharynx, whence they are ultimately swallowed. On arrival in the small intestine, they develop into the adult males and females.

Pathogenesis

The pulmonary lesions are produced as the larvae rupture into the alveoli and include small hemorrhages at each site. An inflammatory reaction or a hypersensitivity reaction to various components of the larvae may also occur, which is more severe on reinfection.

The adult worms in the small intestine may produce either traumatic or toxic damage.[3, 25] Large masses of worms may produce intestinal obstruction, usually in the region of the ileocecal valve. There may be perforation of the bowel wall with peritonitis or penetration into other ectopic areas. *Ascaris* organisms in the appendix may lead to appendicitis and in the common bile duct to obstructive jaundice or pancreatitis. The lungs, heart, and genitourinary systems have been invaded.[3] Sensitization and allergic symptoms may be caused by absorption of products of the living or dead worm. Massive numbers of worms, particularly in children, may lead to malnutrition caused by competition of the organism with the host.[3]

Diagnosis

Clinical Features. The most common symptoms caused by *Ascaris* infestation are vague abdominal discomfort and abdominal colic, which is usually epigastric.[3] Occasionally, diarrhea is present. Children characteristically have fever. The symptoms may suggest abdominal tumor or peptic ulcer disease.

---

*For illustrations of eggs and larvae of roundworms, flatworms, and flukes, the reader is referred to Figure 62–22.

When worms migrate, perforation, appendicitis, and peritonitis may occur.[78] On migration into the biliary or pancreatic ducts, jaundice, right upper quadrant pain, and colic and epigastric pain boring through to the back may occur. During general anesthesia, worms may migrate to the larynx, interfering with respiration.

Allergic reaction such as asthma, hay fever, urticaria, or conjunctivitis may also be the result of absorption of toxins derived from the worm.

Individuals harboring only a small number of worms may have few or no symptoms.

Physical Examination. Unless there are complications caused by the *Ascaris* infestation, there are no helpful physical findings. With bowel obstruction, the abdomen is distended with hyperactive, obstructive, high-pitched bowel sounds. Tenderness may or may not be present. If worms have perforated the intestine into the peritoneal cavity, tenderness to light percussion and rebound tenderness are found. The findings of acute appendicitis caused by *Ascaris* cannot be differentiated from other appendicitis. If the worm has migrated into the common bile duct or pancreatic ducts, the patient may be jaundiced. However, no specific physical findings will differentiate obstructive jaundice or pancreatitis caused by *Ascaris* from that of other causes.

Laboratory Findings. Routine laboratory data are of little value in diagnosing ascariasis. There may be a mild eosinophilia ranging between 5 and 10 per cent of the differential white blood cell count.[3, 25] The diagnosis is based mainly on finding eggs, adult worms, or larvae. Since each female worm excretes 200,000 eggs per day, two or three direct fecal smears are ordinarily sufficient to make the diagnosis. The eggs vary in appearance; fertilized eggs are ovoid, have a thick, double transparent mammilated wall, and are 50 to 75 μm in diameter. When first passed, the fertilized egg contains a mass of granular amorphous protoplasm. Unfertilized eggs are longer and narrower, contain a thin inner shell, and measure 40 to 90 μm. If the outer shell of the egg is lost, it can be confused with the ova of hookworm (Fig. 62–22). If only male worms are present, no ova will be recovered and diagnosis depends upon demonstration of the adult worm, its detection by radiographic methods, or a therapeutic trial. Occasionally, adult worms have been vomited, been aspirated into the lungs, and caused asphyxiation, the diagnosis being made on postmortem examination. Adult worms may also be recovered from sputum and from vomitus.

Radiographic Features. Small bowel and colon barium studies may reveal the presence of the worm as a long, translucent filling defect. If large numbers of worms are present, they may be seen as parallel filling defects in either the small bowel or the colon. After the bowel is emptied of barium, the diagnosis of ascariasis may be made upon finding the intestinal tract of the worm filled with barium.

Treatment. The first choice for treatment is pyrantel pamoate, 11 mg per kg, to a maximum of 1 gm in a single dose.[22] Alternative treatment is piperazine citrate, 75 mg per kg, with a maximum of 3.5 gm daily for two days. If hookworm is present, mebendazole, a broad-spectrum anthelmintic, at a dose of 100 mg, is given twice daily for three days. It is also effective in trichuriasis, hookworm, and pinworm infections.[79]

Bowel obstruction may be treated by a long intestinal tube through which piperazine citrate is injected. If the drug does not cause the bolus of worms to be passed spontaneously and the obstruction is unrelieved, laparotomy is indicated. With perforation and peritonitis, hemorrhagic pancreatitis, or obstructive jaundice caused by *Ascaris*, laparotomy is indicated.

Strongyloidiasis

Strongyloides stercoralis exists in two forms, the free-living and parasitic forms.[3, 25] It exists in warm, moist climates in areas where there is frequent fecal contamination of the soil. In the free-living cycle, the male and female rhabditoid larvae develop into free-living adults and repeat the cycle. The rhabditoid larvae may develop into the infective form, the filariform larvae, which are capable of penetrating the skin or buccal mucosa.

Pathogenesis

On penetration of the skin, the filariform larvae are carried in the circulation to the lungs. They rupture into the alveoli and develop into adolescent worms. Occasionally, females may invade the bronchial or tracheal mucosa and deposit eggs. Usually they are swallowed and invade the small bowel mucosa, where they reside. The parasitic males are rhabditoid forms, are not tissue parasites, and soon disappear in the feces. Parasitic females invade the mucosa. Infection usually occurs in the proximal small intestine but may extend from the stomach to the anus. The female deposits thin-walled, ovoid eggs, which are 50 to 60 μm long, within tissue. The eggs usually develop into rhabditoid larvae (Fig. 62–22), which escape into the gut and are passed in the stool. The transformation to filariform larvae usually occurs in soil. If transformation to this stage occurs within the intestine, autoinfection or hyperinfection results. Mucosal destruction or migration of the worm to other sites is responsible for the clinical features of strongyloidiasis.

Clinical Features

History. After cutaneous invasion by the filariform larvae, *petechial hemorrhages, pruritus, papular rashes, edema*, and *urticaria* occur.[3, 25] The pulmonary symptoms result from the pneumonitis and, depending upon the severity of the infection, include fever, cough, dyspnea, hemoptysis, chest pain, and pleural effusions. Symptoms, however, are usually less severe than in ascariasis. There may also be malaise and anorexia; in severe infections, pulmonary edema and bronchial asthma may occur. The cutaneous and pulmonary symptoms are usually of one to two weeks' duration.

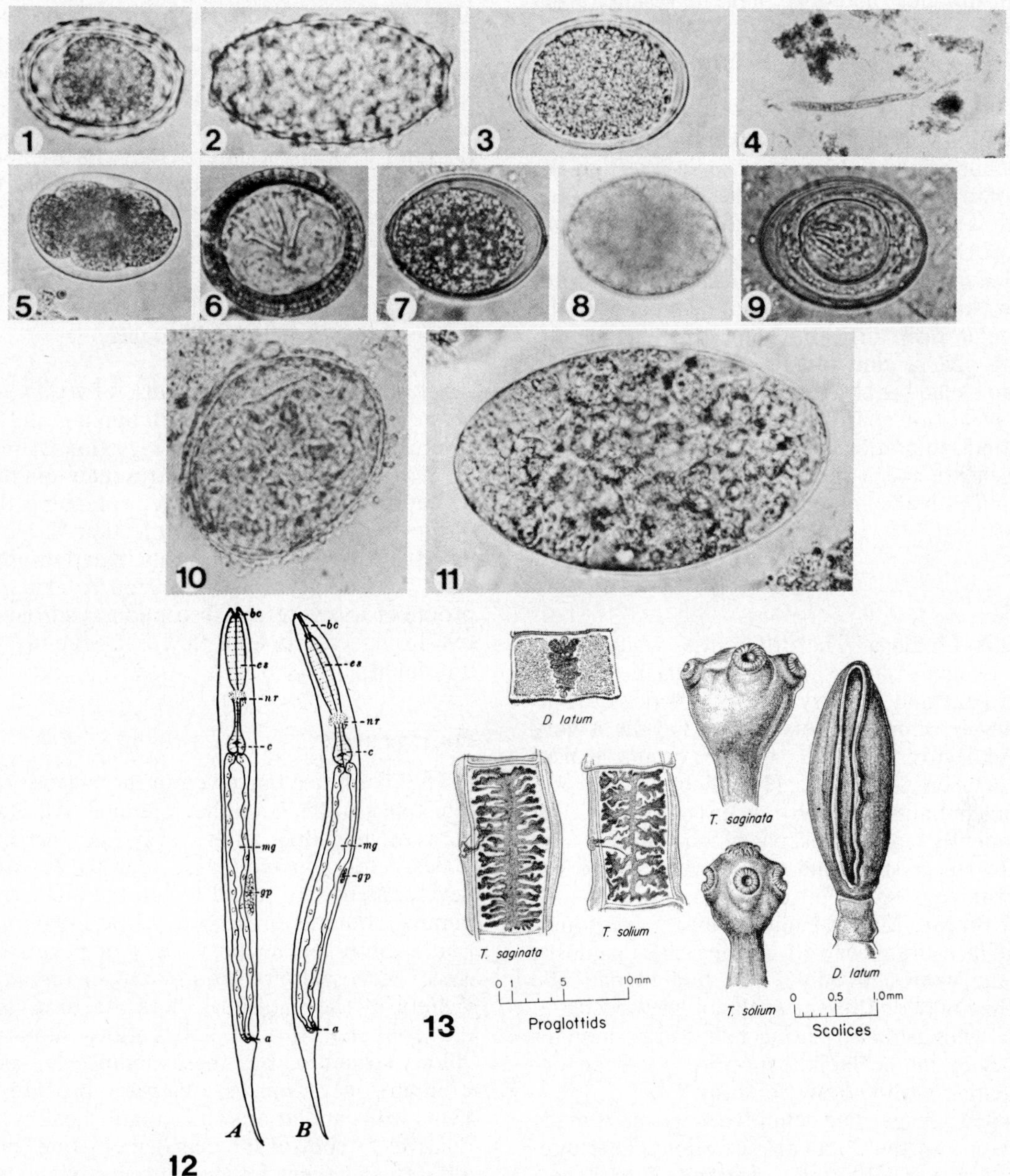

Figure 62–22. *1, Ascaris lumbricoides,* fertilized egg. (× 500.) *2,* Ascaris, unfertilized egg. (× 500). *3,* Ascaris, decorticated egg. (× 500.) *4,* Rhabditiform larva of *Strongyloides stercoralis.* (× 75.) *5,* Hookworm egg. (× 500.) *6,* Taenia sp. ovum. (× 750.) *7, Diphyllobothrium latum* ovum. (× 500.) *8, D. latum* ovum. (× 500.) *9, Hymenolepis nana* ovum. (× 7.50.) *10, Schistosoma japonicum* ovum. (× 500.) *11, Fasciolopsis buski* ovum. (× 500.) *12,* Diagram of rhabditoid larvae of *(A) S. stercoralis* and *(B)* hookworm: a, anus; bc, buccal chamber; c, cardiac bulb of esophagus; es, esophagus; gp, germinal primordia; mg, midgut. (× 400.) *13,* Scolices and gravid proglottids of some tapeworms of man. (Adapted from Hunter, G. W., III, Swartzwelder, J. C., and Clyde, D. F. Tropical Medicine. Ed. 4. Philadelphia, W. B. Saunders Company, 1966.)

Light infections of the intestine may cause no symptoms. More severe involvement results in malaise, fever, nausea, weight loss, vomiting, and abdominal pain, which is usually epigastric. Strongyloidiasis may resemble acute tropical sprue with severe diarrhea and steatorrhea. Hepatomegaly, jaundice, bloody diarrhea, intestinal obstruction, and death have all resulted from strongyloidiasis.

Because of the autoinfection, symptoms may be present for up to 40 or more years.[80] Since infective filariform larvae may be present in stool, venereal transmission may occur in regions where *Strongyloides* is not endemic (see p. 1261). In chronic infection the most common complaints are nausea and abdominal pain, which is usually epigastric and may be similar to peptic ulcer. Diarrhea may or may not be present.

Physical Examination. Physical examination is not specific for strongyloidiasis. In acute infections, the maculopapular rash, urticaria, and petechial hemorrhages may give a clue to the diagnosis. Once the worm is established in the small intestine, the physical findings may include epigastric tenderness to palpation. Rapid dermal migration produces cutaneous larval tracts, which are much more common (84 per cent) than gastrointestinal symptoms (5 per cent) in chronic carriers.[80]

Diagnosis

Laboratory Findings. The differential white blood cell count typically shows an eosinophilia between 8 and 10 per cent and, in very severe infections, up to 50 per cent. In some patients, there may be a very marked leukocytosis. Anemia, when it occurs, is usually iron deficiency in type. Hypoalbuminemia and hypergammaglobulinemia have been observed. The stools frequently contain occult blood, mucus, and Charcot-Leyden crystals, and may contain larvae but rarely contain eggs except in severe diarrhea.

Mucosal Biopsy. Mucosal suction biopsy is an inefficient and inaccurate way of making the diagnosis, detecting the worms in only 2 per cent of patients, although they may be present in the biopsy specimen. Duodenitis, with as many plasma cells and eosinophils as lymphocytes in the lamina propria, has been observed in patients with strongyloidiasis.[81]

Duodenal Drainage. The definitive diagnosis is made by examination of the duodenal secretions. One duodenal drainage is equal to ten concentrated stool specimens as a means of diagnosing strongyloidiasis. Another means of recovering larvae is using a weighted gelatin capsule containing a nylon string (Enterotest).[21] After recovery of the string, the intestinal secretions are expressed from it by the fingers and placed on a slide for examination. (This technique is also useful in detecting *Giardia lamblia.*)

Radiology. The radiographic features of strongyloidiasis are nonspecific and include irritability and thickening of the mucosal folds of the duodenum and proximal jejunum. In very heavy infections, the entire intestine may be involved.

Treatment

The therapy of choice is thiabendazole, 25 mg per kg twice daily (maximum 3 gm per day) for two days. Therapy should be continued five days or longer in disseminated strongyloidiasis.[22] Mebendazole, 100 mg twice daily for three days, has been suggested as an alternative in patients with renal failure who cannot tolerate thiabendazole, but cure rates with this dosage and duration have been only 50 per cent or less.[79] Strongyloidiasis should always be treated, even in asymptomatic patients when detected, because of the possibility of hyperinfectivity. Corticosteroid drugs should *never* be administered to patients with strongyloidiasis, because such therapy results in a fatal dissemination of the organism to all areas of the body.[82]

Capillariasis

Intestinal capillariasis is caused by *Capillaria philippinensis* and is found in the Philippines and Thailand.[83] Infection appears to follow ingestion of infected raw freshwater fish. Fish-eating birds maintain the infection in nature in a fish-bird cycle, spreading the parasite during migration. Human infection has been recognized in Japan and can be anticipated in other parts of Asia where raw fish are eaten.[83] This roundworm produces a severe malabsorption syndrome with protein-losing enteropathy that is frequently fatal when untreated.

Pathogenesis

The worm lies burrowed in the mucosa of the small intestine, particularly the jejunum. All stages of the parasite, including adult worms, larviparous adult females, embryonated eggs, and all stages of larval development, are found within the mucosa and in the luminal contents of the gut. Little inflammatory reaction is observed in the vicinity of penetrating organisms. Mucosal destruction may be apparent in the vicinity of the parasite. There are disorganization of the epithelial surface and various abnormalities of villous structure, but these findings are not specific. Comparison of mucosal biopsies procured from patients with capillariasis and suitable healthy, uninfected relatives as control subjects demonstrates no histologic differences except for the presence of the worm.[84]

Clinical Features

History. The symptoms of capillariasis are borborygmi, diarrhea of up to eight to ten voluminous, watery stools daily, recurrent vague abdominal pain, weight loss, malaise, anorexia, and vomiting. Diarrhea usually begins two to six weeks after the onset of abdominal pain and borborygmi.

Physical Examination. Most patients have evidence of muscle wasting and weakness. The weakness is so profound that half the patients are unable to stand up.

They are hypotensive with distant heart sounds, gallop rhythms, and pulsus alternans. Borborygmi are prominent, as is abdominal distention. About half the patients have abdominal tenderness. Edema and hyporeflexia are usual. Hepatosplenomegaly does not occur.

Diagnosis

Laboratory Findings. Anemia, when it occurs, is iron deficiency in type. Macrocytic anemia has not been described. The major electrolyte abnormalities are hypocalcemia and hypokalemia, which may be severe and associated with nephropathy, neuropathy, and cardiomyopathy. The total plasma protein levels are reduced. Fecal fat is increased to a mean of 25 gm per day. (Stool weight averages 1200 gm per day.) The D-xylose excretion is reduced in most patients and approximates 2.5 gm in a five-hour urine specimen after a 25-gm oral dose. ^{51}Chromium-labeled albumin studies document the protein-losing enteropathy, with stool radioactivity ranging from 6 to 43 per cent of the injected dose in five days.

The eggs of *C. philippinensis* are somewhat similar to those of *T. trichiura.* However, they are somewhat smaller, 45 by 21 μm in size. They are shaped like a peanut and are not operculated; the shell is pitted rather than smooth.

Small bowel mucosal biopsies have demonstrated the worms in approximately 50 per cent of specimens. Thus, biopsy is not a sensitive technique for making the diagnosis. Examination of the duodenal contents will reveal ova, larvae, and adult capillaria and will aid in the diagnosis.

Treatment

Mebendazole, 200 mg twice daily for 20 days for the initial infection and for 30 days for patients who have relapsed, is now the treatment of choice for intestinal capillariasis.[22] Following the onset of therapy, stool egg counts decrease dramatically, the quantity of stool decreases, and the clinical condition improves. In contrast to therapy of most roundworms, therapy should be continued for 30 days. Drugs appear to act on adult but not on larval forms so that prolonged treatment is necessary to eliminate larval forms as they mature.[85] Relapses are heralded by the reappearance of ova in the stools prior to the recurrence of clinical symptoms. If relapses persist, mebendazole dosage should be increased and duration of treatment extended.

Hookworm Disease

Intestinal hookworm disease in humans is caused by *Ancylostoma duodenale* and *Necator americanus.*[3, 25] The life cycles of these species are similar. Eggs in feces, when deposited in soil, hatch in one to two days to rhabditoid larvae, which develop into filariform larvae within a week. On penetration of the skin, the larvae reach venules and are carried to the lung. When they break out of the alveolar capillaries, they pass up the respiratory tree and are swallowed. On arrival in the small intestine, they attach themselves to the mucosa and mature in approximately six weeks. Occasionally, female worms have been found to be depositing eggs in the submucosa. As with other worm infections, hookworm is common where warm, moist soil is present, fecal contamination is common, and shoes are not worn.

Pathogenesis

The worm, on attachment to the small intestinal mucosa, may remove as much as 0.67 ml of blood per worm per day.[3] This may be reduced with worms that have been in the intestine for months or years. Mechanical blood loss from the site of attachment also contributes to the anemia. Disruption of the mucosa and heavy hookworm infestation may also contribute to the hypoproteinemia. Increased fecal loss of albumin and decreased synthesis, presumably caused by malnutrition, occurs in some patients. Whether the worms produce intestinal pathologic changes other than at the site of attachment is unknown. The intestinal pathologic changes and malabsorption in malnourished patients are reversible with a nutritious diet even though the hookworm disease is not treated.[86] In the vicinity of the worm, there is an increase in plasma cells, lymphocytes, and eosinophils. There are associated erosions, ulcerations, and, occasionally, secondary bacterial infection.[3]

Whether or not hookworm disease results in malabsorption is controversial. Malabsorption associated with hookworm disease occurs in regions of endemic tropical sprue and malnutrition. In patients with steatorrhea caused by pancreatic exocrine insufficiency, hookworm infestation does not contribute to the malabsorption.[87] The consensus is that hookworm disease does not cause malabsorption.[88]

Patient resistance is important in the production of hookworm disease. Most patients suffering from severe hookworm disease are malnourished, which appears to enhance their susceptibility to infection.

Clinical Features

History. On penetration of the skin, hookworm larvae produce local tissue reactions with pruritus, which may be aggravated by secondary bacterial infections. Pneumonitis and pulmonary symptoms are not so common as those seen in strongyloidiasis and ascariasis.[3, 25] Small worm loads do not produce symptoms. Moderate or severe infestation may result in anorexia or a voracious appetite, abdominal discomfort, flatulence, and epigastric pain, which is peculiarly relieved by eating bulky food or ingesting clay (geophagia). In the heavier infections, there may be abdominal distention, weight loss, nausea and vomiting, and intermittent constipation and diarrhea. With very heavy infections, edema of the face and extremities and emaciation are present.

Physical Examination. Lightly infected patients have no significant physical findings. In the presence of moderate to severe hookworm disease, the skin is dry and has a yellow pallor that is striking in light-skinned patients. Perspiration is decreased. There is edema, particularly of the face and extremities. The abdomen may be distended with prominent borborygmi. There may be tenderness to palpation, which in some patients will be limited to the upper abdomen. Rebound tenderness is unusual. In very severe, untreated cases, there may be marked congestive heart failure and anasarca.

Diagnosis

Laboratory Findings. Anemia occurring in hookworm disease is a classic iron deficiency anemia. Folic acid–deficient megaloblastic anemia may be masked by the severe iron deficiency. The differential white blood cell count generally demonstrates an eosinophilia of 7 to 15 per cent, and it may exceed 50 per cent in severe cases. There is hypoalbuminemia, hypercholesterolemia, and occasionally proteinuria.

The eggs of all the species of hookworm are very similar. They are ovoid with a thin hyaline shell and rounded ends; they measure 35 to 40 μm by 55 to 75 μm (Fig. 62–22). Within the egg, varying stages of development may be observed. There may be a morula, or they may contain differentiated larvae. In light infections, concentration techniques are required to identify the ova. In heavy infections, direct fecal smears will contain sufficient eggs to permit diagnosis. Stool specimens that are allowed to stand for several hours may contain rhabditoid larvae that have hatched from the eggs. These may be differentiated from the rhabditoid larvae of other roundworms.

Adult worms, when recovered, may be identified by the anatomy of the buccal capsule. *A. duodenale* has a buccal capsule containing ventral teeth, and *N. americanus* has semilunar plates.

Mucosal Biopsy—Duodenal Drainage. Pathologic findings vary in the small bowel mucosa biopsy, ranging from a normal mucosa to a severely abnormal flat mucosa. Occasionally a specimen may be obtained to which an adult worm is attached. The pathologic appearance is not diagnostic of hookworm disease and probably represents the severe malnutrition from which most of these patients are suffering. Occasionally, adult worms may be recovered in the duodenal contents.

Radiographic Findings. Nonspecific radiographic findings are seen in hookworm disease. These include thickening and coarsening of the mucosal folds, flocculation and segmentation of barium, and hypermotility.

Treatment

The therapy of choice for *A. duodenale* is mebendazole, 100-mg tablets that should be chewed before swallowing twice a day for three days. Pyrantel pamoate, 11 mg per kg of body weight (maximum of 1 gm) in a single dose, however, is effective for *Ancylostoma duodenale*. For *Necator americanus*, however, the dose must be repeated for three days, especially in heavy infections (over 2000 ova per gm of feces).[22, 79] In the United States, pyrantel pamoate is an investigational drug for treatment of hookworm. After treatment, stools should be rechecked in two weeks and patients retreated if necessary.

WHIPWORM

Life Cycle: Epidemiology

Trichuris trichiura has a worldwide distribution but is most commonly found in the tropics and in areas with poor sanitary conditions. It has been estimated that there are 2.2 million individuals in the United States with trichuriasis. Prevalence is highest in the rural Southeast.[89] *Trichuris trichiura* belongs to the group Nematoda or roundworms. Although it is found in other animals, man is the principal host. Commonly referred to as whipworm, the parasite is aptly named. Its whip-like appearance consists of a long, thin anterior segment containing the esophagus and a thick posterior portion harboring the digestive and reproductive organs (Fig. 62–23). Adult worms range from 3 to 5 cm in length. The egg is barrel- or lemon-shaped with a plug at either end and contains an unsegmented embryo. Infection occurs through the ingestion of stale fecal material, the embryo requiring a period of three to five weeks outside the body to reach the infective stage. Once the egg is ingested, the digestive juices dissolve the shell, releasing larvae in the small intestine. The larvae reside in the small intestinal mucosa for three to ten days and then emerge to relocate in the cecal area. Here they attach themselves to the mucosa with the attenuated anterior end and mature in 30 to 90 days. The adult egg-laying worm may survive in this location for several years. In heavy infestations, the entire colon extending down to the rectum may be involved.

Clinical Picture

Trichuris infections are quite common in the tropics; the majority of patients are asymptomatic, although an eosinophilia may occur. Heavy infestations may result in right lower quadrant abdominal pain, abdominal distention, blood-streaked stools, diarrhea, weakness, emaciation, and anemia. Appendicitis and rectal prolapse have been described as direct consequences of whipworm infection.

Diagnosis and Treatment

Diagnosis is best made by finding the characteristic barrel-shaped ova in the feces. In severe infections, the clinging, writhing worms may be seen on the rectal mucosa during sigmoidoscopy.

Mebendazole (Vermox) is highly effective against not only *Trichuris* but also other worms, including

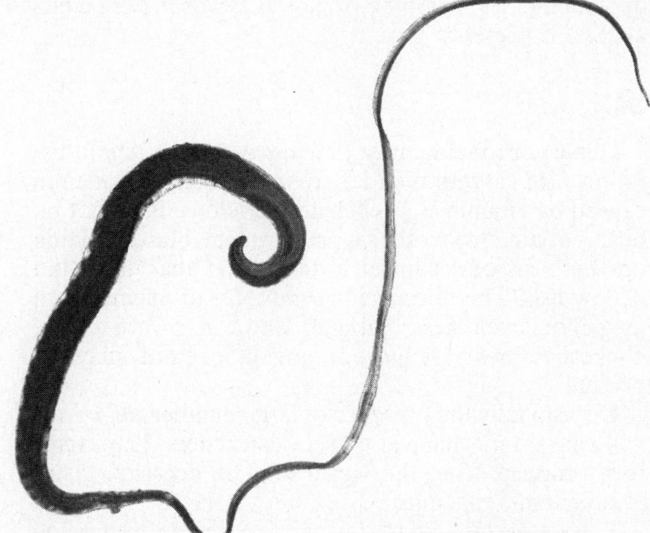

Figure 62–23. *T. trichiura*, adult male. (Photomicrograph by Zane Price. From Markell, E. K., and Voge, M. Medical Parasitology. Ed. 3. Philadelphia, W. B. Saunders Company, 1971.)

pinworm *(Enterobius vermicularis)*, hookworm *(Necator americanus)*, and *Ascaris lumbricoides.*[79] Cure rates for trichuriasis range from 60 to 80 per cent, and reduction of egg output occurs in 90 to 99 per cent of cases. Retreatment is often necessary for cure. Mebendazole is poorly absorbed from the human gastrointestinal tract, and side effects appear to be minimal. It is contraindicated in pregnancy because of teratogenicity. It is not recommended for children less than two years old because of limited experience with the drug in this age group. Mebendazole is given in a dosage of 100 mg twice a day for three days.[22, 79] Asymptomatic individuals with light infection do not require therapy.

Enterobius vermicularis

Enterobius vermicularis infection is discussed on page 1260.

TAPEWORMS OR CESTODES OF MAN

A number of adult tapeworms parasitize the intestinal tract of man.[3, 25] Some depend primarily or exclusively on man as the definitive host. The more important intestinal tapeworms of man are *Diphyllobothrium latum, Taenia saginata, Taenia solium,* and *Hymenolepis nana. Echinococcus* disease caused by *Echinococcus granulosus* and *Echinococcus multilocularis* will not be considered, because the manifestations of these diseases are not intestinal.

Infection is acquired through the ingestion of infected flesh of the intermediate host that is raw or inadequately cooked. Infection with *H. nana* occurs through contact with human feces; it is the most common tapeworm found in the southern United States.

Adult tapeworms consist of a scolex, or head, that anchors the worm to the intestinal mucosa of the host. The egg-producing units, which are known as proglottides, develop from the distal end of the scolex. The proglottides include immature, mature, and gravid forms. The worm does not contain an intestinal system and absorbs its nutrients through the integument from the host's intestinal mucosa. The entire tapeworm is called a strobila.

Diphyllobothrium latum

D. latum, the fish tapeworm, is 3 to 10 m long and may contain as many as 3000 or more proglottides. The scolex is a small spatulate structure with a pair of deep sulci that provide the attachment to the intestine. As with the other tapeworms, *D. latum* is hermaphroditic. Each proglottid contains both the male and the female genitalia.

Pathogenesis

Infection in humans results from ingestion of infected raw fish. The patient may harbor single or multiple worms. The presence of more than one worm probably represents repeated consumption of the infected source.

The host may harbor large numbers of *D. latum* for decades without symptoms or ill effects. A small proportion of patients, most of whom are reported from Finland, develop tapeworm pernicious anemia. The worm most frequently attaches to the wall of the ileum, occasionally to the jejunum, and seldom to the colon. It has been found in the gallbladder.

The worm produces vitamin B_{12} deficiency in the host by competing with the host for available vitamin B_{12}. Both the host and the worm are capable of taking up vitamin B_{12} whether or not tapeworm pernicious anemia is present.

Diagnosis

History. Probably most patients with *D. latum* infestation are asymptomatic. If megaloblastic anemia caused by vitamin B_{12} deficiency develops, it cannot be differentiated from other types of megaloblastic anemia on the basis of a clinical history other than ingestion of raw fish. The nonspecific symptoms of anemia such as pallor, weakness, fatigue, and, in severe cases, congestive heart failure or angina pectoris may be present.

Occasionally the presence of large numbers of worms will cause a mechanical bowel obstruction. The excretory products from the worm may on occasion result in a systemic toxemia.

Laboratory Findings. Diagnosis is made by finding the ova or proglottides of *D. latum* in the feces. The ovum measures 40 to 50 μm by 58 to 76 μm. It has a small operculum at one end of the egg and a tiny knob at the other (Fig. 62–22). The proglottides may crawl around and deposit eggs in the perianal area. They may be found by swabbing or using cellophane tape to sample this particular region of the body. The proglottides of *D. latum* are somewhat wider than they are long. The mature proglottides are packed with genital organs. There are myriads of testes and a symmetric bilobed ovary. A convoluted uterus is present, which terminates in the uterine pore. A single worm may discharge as many as 1,000,000 ova per day.

Routine laboratory data are of little use in making a specific diagnosis of *D. latum* infection. There may be a mild eosinophilia, between 5 and 10 per cent, in the differential white blood cell count. When it is present, anemia is macrocytic and the bone marrow is megaloblastic.

Radiographic Features. The worm may cause some mild irritation of the intestinal mucosa at the point of attachment. This may be manifest by some minor thickening of the mucosal folds and perhaps some motor abnormalities. In small bowel barium studies and barium enemas, the worm may be apparent as a long, thin, translucent filling defect extending over a long length of intestine.

Treatment

The drug of choice is niclosamide, four 500-mg tablets chewed thoroughly in a single dose after a light meal.*[22] Praziquantel, 10 mg per kg in a single dose, also cures 97 to 100 per cent of cases.[79] Another drug of equal efficacy is paromomycin given in four doses of 1 gm 15 minutes apart, followed by a purgative in one hour.

On passage of the worm, cure should not be assumed unless the scolex can be found and identified. If more than 10 m of worm is recovered, it is likely that more than one worm is parasitizing the host. With niclosamide, the scolex may be digested and unrecognizable. Cure cannot be presumed for three to five months when no further segments have appeared in stool.

Taenia solium (Pork Tapeworm)

Pathogenesis

Humans acquire pork tapeworm infection through ingestion of raw or inadequately cooked pork. The larvae are digested from the pork flesh; the heads evaginate from the cysticerci and attach to the wall of the small intestine, developing into adult worms in 5 to 12 weeks. Patients usually harbor only one adult worm, although more than one may be present. They may live up to 25 years or more and be resistant to multiple attempts to evacuate them. Hyperinfection in untreated patients is common and leads to cysticercosis.

Cysticercosis occurs when humans or other mammals ingest the egg of *T. solium.* On contact with gastric juices and subsequently with intestinal contents, the emergent oncospheres penetrate through the intestinal wall into the mesenteric vasculature and are distributed throughout the body. They are typically filtered out between muscles, where in 60 to 70 days they become cysticerci. This larval stage of the worm has been found in every organ and tissue of the body. The symptoms produced depend upon the location and the number present. Most frequently they are found in subcutaneous tissues, followed in frequency by eye, brain, musculature, heart, liver, lungs, and abdominal cavity.[3] The larvae provoke a typical cellular reaction, including infiltration of neutrophils, eosinophils, lymphocytes, plasma cells, and, occasionally, giant cells. Fibrosis follows necrosis of the capsule, with caseation and calcification of the larvae as the final events.

Clinical Features

History. Human infection with the pork tapeworm is frequently encountered in the southwestern United States and in immigrants from Mexico and Central and South America residing in other parts of the United States.[90] The adult worm does not result in serious illness, and its presence may provoke no symptoms. Occasionally, vague abdominal discomfort, hunger pains, "chronic indigestion," and diarrhea or alternating diarrhea and constipation may occur.[3] It may be responsible for anorexia, hyperesthesia, and nervous disorders caused by absorption of toxic substances from the worm. Rarely, the scolex perforates the intestinal wall and peritonitis results.

Cysticercosis from ingestion of eggs shed by chronic carriers may be more common at present in the United States than tapeworm from infected meat.[90] The symp-

*This drug is available in the United States from the Parasitic Diseases Division, Center for Disease Control, Atlanta, Georgia 30333; telephone 404-639-3670 (days) or 404-639-2888 (night emergencies only).

toms of cysticercosis depend upon the location of the parasite. The precysticercus larvae in the brain may produce little functional or symptomatic abnormality. When the larvae die, tissue reactions result in a great variety of cerebral symptoms and may eventuate in a rapidly fatal course. Convulsive disorders are the most common manifestation of cerebral cysticerci, but they may also produce behavioral disorders, paresis, obstructive hydrocephalus, dysequilibrium, meningoencephalitis, and failing vision.[3] Ocular cysticercosis results in uveitis, iritis, retinitis, choroidal atrophy, palpebral conjunctivitis, or cyst formation.

Physical Examination. Physical examination does not contribute to the diagnosis of *T. solium* infection. Occasionally the presence of proglottides may be found on the finger following a rectal examination, or they may be seen through the sigmoidoscope.

The physical manifestations of cysticercosis do not permit differentiation from other space-occupying lesions, whether cerebral or visceral. Ocular involvement of cysticercosis may be detected by retinoscopy.

Diagnosis

Laboratory Findings. Other than a moderate eosinophilia, up to 13 per cent, the routine laboratory studies are usually within normal limits. The ova of *T. solium* are spherical or slightly ovoid in configuration and measure 31 to 43 μm in diameter. The ova have a thick-walled shell consisting of many truncated prisms and originally are provided with a thin, hyaline mother embryonic membrane. The fully developed oncosphere within the ova usually has three pairs of hooklets. The ova of *T. solium* cannot be distinguished from those of *T. saginata* (Fig. 62–22). Definitive diagnosis depends upon the recovery of typical gravid proglottides. They are longer than they are wide, and the main lateral side arms of the uterus number from 7 to 13 on each side. Identification of the scolex on evacuation differentiates it from that of *T. saginata.* It is about 1 mm in diameter, and has four large, deeply cupped suckers and a conspicuous rounded rostellum with a double row of large and small hooklets.

The definitive diagnosis of cysticercus disease depends on excision and microscopic examination. The invaginated scolex of the larvae has four suckers and anterior hooklets that are an exact miniature of the scolex of the adult.[3]

Radiographic Features. The worm may be detected in the intestine on barium studies. Radiographs are useful in making a diagnosis of cysticercosis after the parasite has calcified. They may be found in the musculature and in the central nervous system by high-penetration X-ray films. Although calcification usually occurs in the scolex, the cyst wall may resemble an enveloping eggshell.

Treatment

The treatment for *T. solium* in the intestine is the same as for *D. latum* (see above). For cysticercus disease excision is indicated whenever possible. Praziquantel is reported to decrease seizures associated with cerebral cysticercosis. Although optimal dosage remains to be determined, 50 mg per kg in three divided doses for 14 days is currently recommended.[22, 90] Ocular cysticercosis may be treated by removal of the cyst rather than enucleation of the eye. Optimal therapy is removal of the cysticercus while it is still living.[3]

Taenia saginata (Beef Tapeworm)

Pathogenesis

Infection with *Taenia saginata* is through the ingestion of inadequately cooked or raw beef containing viable cysticercus larvae. Because of the popularity of rare steak and other uncooked or inadequately cooked beef dishes, human infection with *T. saginata* continues to be frequent in the United States.[25] The mature eggs are ingested by cattle; on hatching in the duodenum they penetrate the intestinal mucosa and are carried in the circulation to the striated muscle. They develop into *Cysticerus bovis* in 60 to 75 days. On digestion of the infected flesh in the intestine, the cysticercus is released and the scolex evaginates and attaches to the intestinal wall. The adult lives with its scolex embedded in the mucosa of the small bowel.

T. saginata is considerably longer than *T. solium* and may attain lengths of 25 m or more. Ordinarily, the worms measure between 12 and 15 feet and have between 1000 and 2000 proglottides at any given time. Their effects on the host are due to their large size, which may result in mechanical bowel obstruction, undernutrition, and release of toxic metabolites that are absorbed.

Clinical Picture

History. The worm produces substantial disturbance in normal intestinal function. It derives its nutrition by diverting digested material from the host. Diarrhea and hunger pains frequently develop, and loss of weight may occur. Its presence may result in hyperphagia or in anorexia. Occasionally it may produce acute intestinal obstruction. Proglottides lodged in the appendix have caused acute appendicitis. Absorption of toxic products of the worm may result in allergic symptoms in the form of edema of the face, abdomen, and lower limbs. The most common symptoms are the discomfort and embarrassment of proglottides crawling from the anus.

Cysticercosis caused by the larvae of *T. saginata* is not nearly so common as that occurring in the presence of *T. solium.* Beef cysticercosis, however, has the same manifestations, depending upon the site and number of cysticerci present.

Physical Examination. There may be edema of the face and extremities in patients having allergic reactions to absorbed toxins. Physical evidence of weight loss may occasionally be present. Proglottides may be observed around the anus, may be recovered on the examining finger following rectal examination, or may be seen occasionally at sigmoidoscopy.

Diagnosis

Laboratory Findings. Except for a moderate eosinophilia of the differential white blood cell count, the laboratory findings are usually normal. The presence of ova in feces establishes infection with a species of *Taenia*, but differentiation from *T. solium* is not possible. No eggs may be present in the stool, but all patients pass gravid proglottides. The definitive diagnosis is established by examining the proglottid, which is pressed between two slides, and counting the main lateral arms of the uterus. There are usually 15 to 20 main lateral branches on each side of the main uterine stem in *T. saginata* (Fig. 62–22). Overripe proglottides lose the distinctive appearance. Administration of a purgative will cause discharge of more proximal proglottides and aid in establishing the diagnosis. Identification of the scolex after therapy also aids diagnosis and ensures that the entire worm has been evacuated. The head is quadrate with a diameter of 1 to 2 mm and has four hemispherical suckers. The apex is somewhat concave and may be pigmented. There are no hooklets. Diagnosis of cysticercosis depends upon excision and microscopic examination.

Radiographic Features. The radiographic appearance of *T. saginata* is the same as that of *T. solium.*

Treatment

The treatment of *T. saginata* is the same as that of *D. latum*, given above.

Hymenolepis nana (Dwarf Tapeworm)

Pathogenesis

H. nana is the only human tapeworm that has no intermediate host. Infection is direct from patient to patient upon ingestion of embryonated eggs. It occurs more often in children than in adults and has a higher incidence in family and institutional groups. The worms hatch in the stomach or small intestine, and the free oncospheres penetrate the villi and metamorphose into cercocysts. When the larvae migrate into the lumen of the intestine, they become attached by their scolices to the mucosa and mature into adult worms in two weeks. Continued heavy infection in humans is probably due to internal autoinfection.[25]

Clinical Picture

History. Large numbers of *H. nana* within the intestine produce considerable irritation. The more common symptoms are due to absorption of metabolic waste products of the parasite.[3] The major symptoms are headache, dizziness, anorexia, inanition, pruritus of the nose and anus, intermittent diarrhea, and abdominal distress. Most patients are restless and irritable, and a few have convulsive disorders.

Physical Examination. There are no specific physical findings to indicate *H. nana* infection. Evidence of weight loss may be seen.

Diagnosis

Laboratory Findings. The laboratory findings are nonspecific. An eosinophilia of 5 to 15 per cent of the differential white blood cell count may be observed.

The diagnosis is based upon finding characteristic eggs of *H. nana*. They are spherical, having a hyaline membrane, and measure 30 to 40 μm in diameter (Fig. 62–22). The egg contains an oncosphere enclosed in an inner envelope with two polar thickenings each having four to eight polar filaments.[3] Within the oncosphere are three pairs of lancet-shaped hooklets. The adult worm is 25 to 30 mm in length by 1 mm in diameter. The tiny scolex is 0.2 mm in diameter, is rhomboidal, and has four hemispherical suckers. There is a short rostellum containing 20 to 30 spines in one ring.

Radiographic Features. Few data are available of the small intestinal appearance in *H. nana* infection. There may be nonspecific changes, including thickening and coarsening of the mucosal folds, excess secretions within the intestine, and rapid transit of barium.

Treatment

The drug of choice is praziquantel, 25 mg per kg, given once. An alternative is niclosamide, four tablets (2 gm) in a single dose daily for seven days, or paromomycin, 45 mg per kg once daily for seven days.[22, 79] Prolonged treatment with the latter two drugs is necessary because they do not kill ova, and autoinfection can occur from viable ova that continue to pass into stool.[25]

SCHISTOSOMIASIS

Schistosomiasis is a disease produced by trematodes belonging to the family Schistosomatidae. The three principal species affecting humans are *Schistosoma mansoni, S. japonicum,* and *S. haematobium.* It has been estimated that more than 200 million of the world's population are affected with schistosomiasis. Conditions that contribute to the prevalence of the disease include poor sanitation, contaminated water, and a specific snail host required to complete the life cycle. These requirements are best met in the tropical and subtropical climates. *S. mansoni* is prevalent in Africa, the Arabian peninsula, Brazil, and Puerto Rico. *S. japonicum* is found primarily in the Far Eastern countries: Japan, China (including Taiwan), and the Philippines. *S. haematobium* is centered in the Nile Valley but also causes disease throughout Africa.

Life Cycle

Humans acquire the infection by exposure to water contaminated by the cercaria form of the organism, which emerges in large numbers from the snail host. If they locate a human host within 48 hours, they penetrate the skin and find their way to the peripheral venules. The metacercariae, as they are now termed, are carried to the right side of the heart and lungs, where they enter the systemic circulation by an as yet undetermined pathway. They eventually reach the intrahepatic portal bed, where, in four to six weeks, they mature into the adult forms. As fertilization takes place between the male and female, the worms migrate upstream together into the terminal mesenteric vein and venules. Once situated, the female deposits the fertilized eggs. Each worm pair may produce 300 to 3000 eggs per day over a period of several years. The egg secretes a lytic substance and migrates into the surrounding tissue partly by destroying it. Approximately 50 per cent of the eggs erode through the gut wall into the lumen and are excreted in the feces; those remaining reside trapped in the tissues. If the eliminated eggs reach fresh water, they hatch and release miracidia, which seek out and then penetrate a specific snail host. Each miracidium develops into a sporocyst, which in turn produces several daughter sporocysts. Within weeks, the sporocysts begin to release thousands of cercariae, which escape into the surrounding water to actively seek out a human host and repeat the cycle.

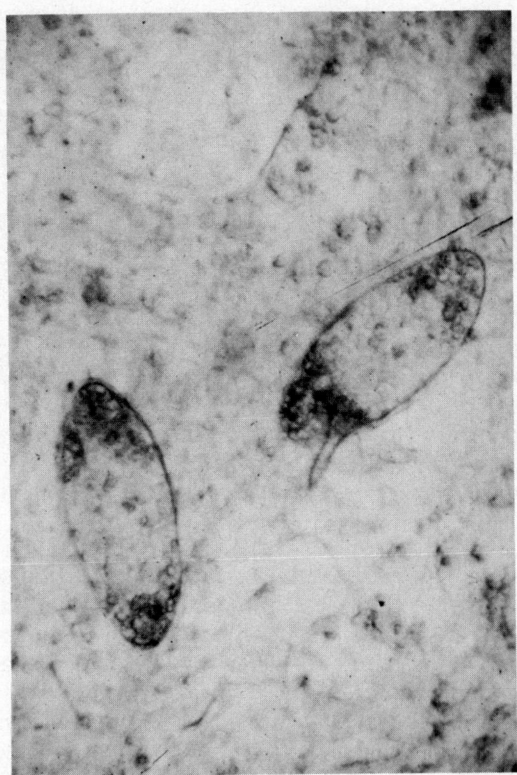

Figure 62–24. *S. mansoni* ovum as it appears microscopically in the bowel wall. (× 200.) (Courtesy of C. M. Knauer, M.D.)

Pathology

The severity of the disease varies considerably from country to country. This may reflect virulence of the organism or such factors as exposure, worm burden, nutrition, or host defense. Currently, there is great interest in the immunologic aspects of schistosomiasis with regard to both pathogenesis and therapy. Enzymes and other antigens secreted by eggs in tissue provoke granulomatous cellular immune responses and fibrosis. Continued antigen release suppresses the immunologic response modulating the pathogenic effect. This suppressor effect offers hope of immunologic intervention to reduce tissue damage subsequent to infection.[91]

As the adult worms traverse the portal system, *S. japonicum* preferentially finds its way into the superior mesenteric veins, *S. mansoni* to the inferior mesenteric veins, and *S. haematobium* to the vesical plexus. Because of this interesting anatomic migration, *S. japonicum* tends to involve the small intestine but also the descending colon and rectum, *S. mansoni* the descending colon, and *S. haematobium* the bladder, pelvic organs, and rectum.

Pathologic changes result from the deposition of large numbers of eggs in the intestinal submucosa (Figs. 62–22 and 62–24). As the eggs enzymatically digest their way through the intestinal mucosa, they provoke an inflammatory response. Grossly, the mucosal surface appears hyperemic, granular, and friable. Punctate hemorrhages as well as small, shallow ulcerations may be present. In cases of *S. mansoni, S. japonicum,* and, to a lesser degree, *S. haematobium* infection, patchy areas of the rectal mucosal surface may have a sandpaper appearance.[92] In later stages of the disease, papillomas and polyps may develop. These are frequently multiple and most often are found in the rectum and sigmoid, although they may also be present in the proximal colon. Polyps may be associated with chronic blood loss and protein-losing enteropathy. Fistulas have also been described in the advanced disease state. Rarely, acute schistosomal dysentery may be fatal. In these cases the bowel and lumen contain blood and mucus; the mucosal surface is intensely congested, and multiple punctate hemorrhages and small ulcerations are present. Microscopically, the picture varies with the severity of the disease. In many cases of schistosomiasis, there may be ova or their remnants present in the mucosa and submucosa, accompanied by little or no inflammatory or fibroblastic response. In more advanced disease there may be focal areas of mucosal necrosis. Ova in the mucosa and submucosa form the nucleus for a pseudotuberculoid reaction and are surrounded with foreign-body giant cells, epithelial cells, eosinophils, plasma cells, and lymphocytes. The "sandy patch" lesions of schistosomal involvement of the rectum appear to be large collections of calcified ova lying in the submucosa. Histologic examination of the polyps reveals large numbers of ova in various stages of degeneration, evoking a hyperplastic, ade-

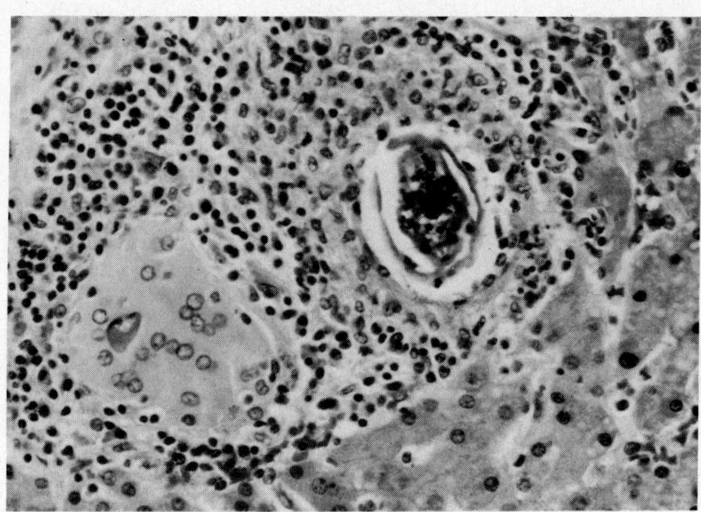

Figure 62–25. Granulomatous pseudotubercle of the liver in a patient with schistosomiasis. Note the ovum on the right and foreign body giant cell on the left. (× 150.) (Courtesy of S. H. Choy, M.D.)

nomatous response with an inflammatory infiltrate made up of lymphocytes, eosinophils, and plasma cells.

Intestinal obstruction is a possible outcome in *S. japonicum* infection. Although few data are available, there appears to be interference with digestion and absorption with extensive parasitization of the intestine. *S. japonicum* infection should be considered in any patient with liver or bowel disease who has resided in an endemic area in Asia. Living *S. japonicum* ova have been demonstrated in such a patient in whom there was no possibility of reinfection for 47 years.[93]

In addition to involving the intestine, the *Schistosoma* ova are carried by the portal circulation to the liver, where they become entrapped in the portal areas. Granulomatous pseudotubercles then develop around the ova (Fig. 62–25). With continued deposition of the ova in the portal areas, progressive portal and periportal fibrosis ensues, with relative sparing of hepatic parenchyma. The late stages of the disease were first described in 1904 by Symmers, who described the cut surface of the liver as appearing as though a number of white clay pipestems had been pushed through the organ at various angles. The severe involvement of the portal areas results in so-called presinusoidal portal hypertension (Fig. 62–26).

Clinical Picture

The initial clinical picture is associated with penetration of the skin of the host by the cercariae. Most of the cercariae die at this stage, and repeated exposures provoke a hypersensitivity response characterized by pruritus and a papular rash. Approximately four to six weeks after the initial infection, the flukes mature, migrate from the portal area to the bowel, and deposit eggs in the intestinal submucosa. In heavy infestations, the large numbers of eggs will damage the bowel wall, resulting in lower abdominal cramping pain and diarrhea with the passage of bloody mucus. Allergic-type responses such as urticaria, swelling of the face and lips, cough, and fever with a daily spike of temperature of 101 to 102°F may develop. Some patients suffer tenderness and enlargement of the liver as well as of

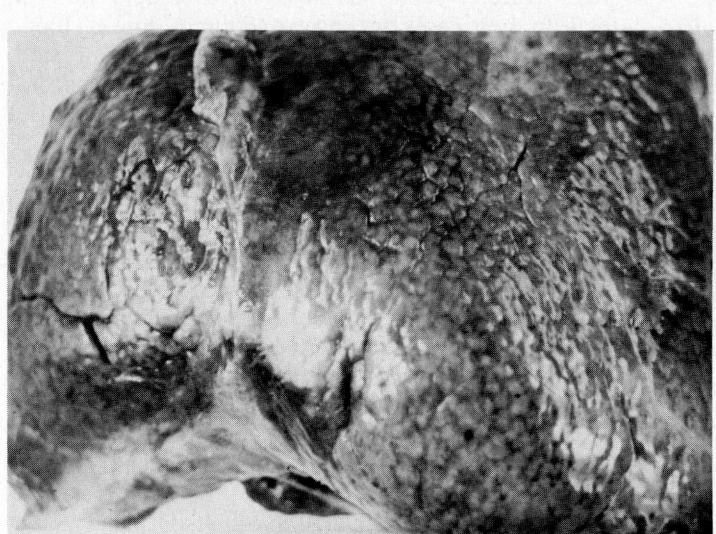

Figure 62–26. Cirrhosis of the liver in a patient with schistosomiasis. Note the coarse nodules. (Courtesy of S. H. Choy, M.D.)

the spleen and lymph nodes. Peripheral blood eosinophilia is invariably present. In Japan, where *S. japonicum* is prevalent, a severe form of this reaction is known as Katayama fever. It appears somewhat earlier after cercarial invasion than is noted in *S. mansoni* infection and may be fatal, particularly in children with heavy infestations. Many feel that the clinical features of this phase of the illness are consistent with a serum sickness–like response. If the initial exposure is heavy and the disease is left untreated, or if there are repeated infections, both acute and chronic intestinal disease may follow. Children in particular may succumb to the acute dysentery. In the chronic form of the illness, the mucous membrane of the colon thickens, being sufficiently pronounced and discrete on occasion to give the appearance of a papilloma on sigmoidoscopic examination. Ulcers may also be noted and may be due to the sloughing of these pedunculated papillomas. Polyps in the cecum may lead to intussusception. Occasionally, eggs infiltrate the appendix, causing a syndrome akin to acute appendicitis. If the infection is virulent and widespread in the bowel, the parasite may penetrate the serosa with the formation of multiple nodules resembling tuberculomas, and regional lymph nodes may be infiltrated with *Schistosoma* eggs. Rectal prolapse and colonic obstruction are also late complications of advanced disease.

Eggs that are laid in the mesenteric venous system can travel through the portal systems to the liver. They lodge in the portal areas, forming granuloma-like lesions, which with accompanying fibrosis produce presinusoidal obstruction.[94] Thus, wedged hepatic vein pressure is normal, as in obstruction or cavernous transformation of the portal vein. The course is slow and progressive, and patients are often asymptomatic. It is characterized by hepatosplenomegaly and, in advanced stages, by portal hypertension with ascites and variceal bleeding. Liver function, despite widespread involvement of the liver, appears to be much better than in most types of cirrhosis. With altered hemodynamics secondary to liver disease, eggs may bypass the liver to lodge in the pulmonary bed, giving rise to pulmonary hypertension. Central nervous system symptoms may also occur with secondary involvement of the brain and spinal cord.

Diagnosis

During the acute stage of the disease, the diagnosis may be readily made by finding ova in freshly passed stools; concentration techniques improve the yield significantly. *S. mansoni* may be easily recognized by its oval shape and prominent lateral spine. By comparison, *S. japonicum* is somewhat diminished in size and the spine is small and difficult to see. *S. haematobium* has a conspicuous terminal spine. Because the eggs of all three types are present in the mucosa in a high percentage of patients, a rectal biopsy is often successful in making the diagnosis. This is performed by taking a small mucosal snip from the surface of one of the valves of Houston. This specimen is compressed with a small amount of warm saline between a glass slide and coverslip and examined by light microscopy for ova (Fig. 62–24). Needle biopsy of the liver may be diagnostic in patients with liver involvement. The biopsy may be examined by routine histologic techniques; the pathologic picture, as previously described, is very characteristic. Part of the specimen should also be crushed between a slide and coverslip and examined for eggs as carried out with the rectal tissue. Characteristically, the wedged hepatic vein pressure is normal in those patients with portal hypertension and cirrhosis, affording indirect evidence for the diagnosis of schistosomiasis of the liver. A skin test and numerous serologic tests are currently available for the diagnosis of schistosomiasis.[25, 95] Probably the best of these is the complement fixation test, although some experienced laboratories find the indirect hemagglutination test useful as well. However, reliance upon serologic testing alone to make the diagnosis is hazardous, because false positive tests may result from cross-reactions with other antibodies generated by other parasitic infections. Also, false negative reactions may be obtained. The radiologic picture of colonic schistosomiasis varies from an edematous mucosal pattern with tiny ulcerations and spasm to loss of haustration and the presence of multiple polyps (Fig. 62–27).

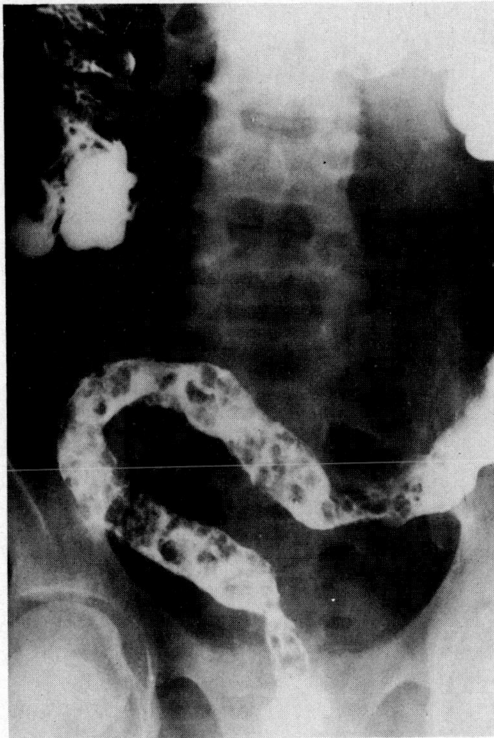

Figure 62–27. *S. mansoni* infestation of the colon in a 20-year-old Egyptian man with bloody diarrhea and tenesmus. Note the multiple polypoid lesions throughout the rectosigmoid colon, which is displaced out of the pelvis by a large pericolic bilharzial abscess. There is a generalized narrowing of the left colon with scattered areas of stricture formation. Note also the spasm, mural spiculation, and loss of haustration in the less involved descending colon, whereas the proximal colon appears relatively normal. (From Reeder, M. M., and Hamilton, L. C. Radiol. Clin. North Am. 7:55, 1969.)

Treatment

Praziquantel is the first drug which has proved both safe and effective for all types of schistosome infection. The dosage is 20 mg per kg three times a day for one day. Tablets are taken after a meal and should not be chewed but should be swallowed quickly with fluid, because the tablets are bitter and can induce vomiting. Mild and transient side effects occur in 50 per cent of adults after this regimen. These side effects include drowsiness, dizziness, malaise, headache, and anorexia. Consequently, driving and other tasks requiring alertness should be avoided on the day of treatment.[79]

The alternative drug for *S. mansoni* is oxamniquine (Vansil). The dose is 15 mg per kg of body weight as a single oral dose, which may be given after the evening meal. This dose has been effective in the Western Hemisphere, but cases originating in Africa have required the same dose twice a day for two days for satisfactory rates of cure. This drug can be used without severe side effects even in the presence of liver disease.[79]

An alternative drug for *S. haematobium* is metrifonate (Bilarcil) in a dosage of 7.5 mg per kg of body weight (maximum 600 mg) every other week for three doses.[79] In the United States, this drug is available only from the Center for Disease Control, Atlanta, Georgia (telephone 404-639-3670).

An alternative drug for *S. japonicum* is niridazole (Ambilhar). Numerous side effects are common, and, in the United States, where this drug is available only from the CDC Parasitic Disease Drug Service, hospitalization is required for its use. In particular, its use is contraindicated in the presence of hepatocellular disease. Dosage is 25 mg per kg per day (maximum of 1.5 gm) divided in two or three fractions and given with meals. Treatment is continued for five days with *S. japonicum* because of the severity of side effects, even though cure rates may be limited.[79]

Surgery may be considered for advanced cases with portal hypertension and recurrent bleeding varices. In general, patients with schistosomiasis tolerate bleeding better than patients with portal hypertension secondary to cirrhosis. Portal decompression should be reserved for the recurrent bleeder who is difficult to manage conservatively. Although some reports indicate that patients with schistosomiasis may tolerate bypass very well, the preponderant evidence indicates that they often have diminished liver function with encephalopathy after the procedure. Accordingly, great caution should be exercised in selection of cases and type of procedure.

Fasciolopsis buski (Giant Intestinal Fluke)

F. buski is a common parasite in the Orient. Indigenous cases have not been described elsewhere. It is a common parasite of humans and swine.[3]

Pathogenesis

Humans are infected when they ingest the raw pods, roots, stems, and bulbs of certain water plants that grow in endemic foci containing the appropriate molluscan hosts.[3] Water in the shallow ponds or lakes containing the plant vectors is contaminated by human or swine feces that contain immature viable eggs. The eggs mature, hatch, and infect suitable snails. The cercariae escape the snails and encyst on the plants. The larvae of *F. buski* excyst in the duodenum and attach to the duodenal and jejunal mucosa. In about 90 days they develop into large, elongated, ovidal worms measuring 20 to 75 mm in length, 8 to 20 mm in breadth, and 0.5 to 3 mm in thickness. They damage the mucosa and cause deep ulcerations at the site of attachment; large numbers may produce intestinal obstruction. Systemic symptoms have been attributed to absorption of toxic products from the worms but are probably caused by protein-losing enteropathy due to mucosal damage.[25] In very heavy infections, the organisms may be found adherent to the pyloric mucosa and even in the large bowel. Erosions lead to hemorrhage, abscesses may develop, and large numbers of parasites result in acute ileus.[3]

Clinical Picture

History. Initial symptoms of diarrhea with hunger pains occur toward the end of the incubation period. In light infections these may be the only symptoms. In heavy infections, pain may mimic peptic ulcer and the patient may become asthenic. Edema of the face, abdominal wall, and lower extremities is common. Ascites commonly develops, accompanied by generalized abdominal pain. There may be intermittent constipation. The stool is typically greenish yellow and foul-smelling and contains undigested food. There may be hyperphagia or anorexia with nausea and vomiting. Ultimately, there is extreme prostration, which may be followed by death in untreated patients.[3]

Physical Examination. Edema of the face and extremities may be prominent. Ascites is present frequently. There may be severe weakness or even coma.

Diagnosis

Laboratory Findings. Leukocytosis is often found with an absolute eosinophilia and a neutrophilic leukopenia. Occasionally there is lymphocytosis. Other laboratory abnormalities depend upon the duration and magnitude of the diarrhea.

The diagnosis rests specifically on recovery of the eggs. They are large, shaped like hens' eggs, measuring 130 to 140 μm by 80 to 85 μm (Fig. 62–22), and are operculated and unembryonated when passed. Each worm is capable of discharging 25,000 eggs per day. The miracidium does not develop within the egg until it is deposited in water.

Treatment

Praziquantel in the standard dosage of 25 mg per kg three times a day for one day is effective against *Fasciolopsis buski* as well as against *Clonorchis sinensis* (Chinese liver fluke).[22, 79]

MISCELLANEOUS PARASITIC INFECTIONS

A number of other parasites whose major manifestations are primarily nonintestinal may produce small bowel symptoms. Some of these organisms gain access to the body through the intestinal tract.

Trichinella spiralis

Pathogenesis

Humans acquire trichinosis through the ingestion of raw or rare flesh infected with cysts of *Trichinella spiralis*.[3, 25] These cysts are digested from the meat in the stomach, and on passage into the small intestine they excyst and the larvae invade the intestinal mucosa. The larvae mature into adults in five to seven days, at which time the adult worms mate and the female begins discharging larvae in the tissues. The larvae have a predilection for striated muscle and myocardium, where they ultimately encyst. Although both adults and encysted larvae of *T. spiralis* may develop in the same host, two hosts are required to complete the life cycle. The infection is propagated in nature by the black rat and the brown rat, which are cannibalistic. Although pork is the main source of infection in man, trichinosis has resulted from the ingestion of flesh from wild boars, bears, and other mammals.

Diagnosis

History. The intestinal symptoms of trichinosis may begin within 24 hours of ingestion of the infective organism. During the five- to seven-day incubation period, irritation and inflammation of the intestine occur at the site of larval invasion. The symptoms of nausea, vomiting, diarrhea or dysentery, colic, and profuse diaphoresis may mimic acute food poisoning or bacterial infection. Bright scarlet macules or maculopapular rashes may occur on the trunk and limbs.

During the period of larval migration to the muscles, there are muscular pains, dyspnea, difficulty with mastication, pharyngeal and laryngeal dysfunction, and, at times, spastic paralysis. There is frequently a tender lymphadenopathy, at times salivary gland enlargement mimicking mumps, and a remittent fever of 40 to 41° C. There may be periorbital edema. Central nervous system symptoms include those of encephalitis and meningitis, ophthalmoplegia, or deafness; the infection may also resemble amyotrophic lateral sclerosis.

During the period of encystation, there may be cachexia, edema, and extreme dehydration. There may be protean neurologic signs resulting from cerebral damage. In severe cases, the patient may die from toxemia, myocarditis, pneumonitis, peritonitis, pleurisy, nephritis, or central nervous system involvement.

The great majority of patients with trichinosis do not have any symptoms, the clinical disease occurring in only approximately 5 per cent of individuals infected.[3]

Physical Examination. During the incubation or diarrheal phase, there may be few or no physical findings to suggest trichinosis. During the phase of larval migration, the cardinal physical finding is muscle tenderness. There may be spasticity of the limbs. Periorbital edema may be prominent. There is frequently a tender lymphadenitis. Cardiac arrhythmias may occur, and congestive heart failure may be present.

Laboratory Findings. The white blood cell count typically reveals a leukocytosis with a marked hypereosinophilia ranging between 20 and 75 per cent or more. Rarely, adult worms may be recovered in the feces during the diarrheal stage of the disease. Larvae may rarely be found in the blood or spinal fluid or in the mother's milk during migration. The definitive diagnosis is made by muscle biopsy after the larvae have lodged in muscle. If they cannot be identified in small compressed samples of deltoid, biceps, pectoralis, or gastrocnemius muscle, digestion with artificial gastric juice will provide a concentrate, increasing diagnostic accuracy. Several serologic tests are available.[95]

Treatment

Trichinosis is frequently not considered during the incubation period. However, it should be included in the differential diagnosis in any patient presenting with the aforementioned symptoms and findings. It is particularly important to procure a history of ingestion of raw meat, particularly pork. Thiabendazole has been shown to be of effect in experimental animals when given 24 hours after inoculation. Corticosteroids should be used for severe symptoms during the period of migration and encystation. Prednisone in dosages of 20 to 40 mg daily and tapered after three to five days is customarily used. Thiabendazole in dosages of 25 mg per kg (maximum 1.5 gm single dose) chewed well twice daily for five successive days is currently recommended.[22, 79] There will be prompt defervescence and general relief of muscle pain, tenderness, and edema. This occurs within 24 to 48 hours after the thiabendazole treatment. Mebendazole prevents tissue infection and appears to be effective against the established tissue phase of the disease in a dose of 1 gm in three divided doses for 14 days.[79, 96]

American Trypanosomiasis (Chagas' Disease)

Although symptomatic Chagas' disease has been confined to the South American continent and Central

America, two indigenous cases and nine seropositive asymptomatic patients have been diagnosed in south Texas.[97, 98] In patients surviving acute infection with *Trypanosoma cruzi* and developing the chronic form of illness, myocardial disease is the most common manifestation. Megaesophagus and megacolon are the most common intestinal manifestations of American trypanosomiasis. However, small intestinal dilatation and aperistalsis are also seen. At postmortem examination, even in patients with asymptomatic *T. cruzi* involvement of the intestine, the small intestine has a significant reduction in submucosal and myenteric autonomic plexuses.[98, 99]

American trypanosomiasis could prove to be a significant health problem in the United States. There is a large reservoir of *T. cruzi* infection in animals in the southern United States. Infection has been detected in Arizona, California, New Mexico, Texas, Louisiana, Georgia, Florida, and Maryland.[97] The epidemiologically important insects, the reduviid bugs of the Triatominae group, also have the same wide geographic distribution. Infection is transmitted when the reduviid bug infected with *T. cruzi* bites the victim. On biting, the arthropod discharges feces. The parasite is introduced through the skin by the patient scratching the bite. The apparent difference between the South American reduviid bugs and those found in the United States is that the species in the United States do not defecate upon biting. It is possible that effective vectors may be introduced in the United States.

Pathogenesis

Metacyclic trypanosomes are deposited from the feces of the bug during the time it is taking a blood meal.[3] Characteristically, deposition occurs on or near mucous membranes, particularly on the outer canthus of the eye or around the nose or lips. The invading organisms are phagocytosed by histiocytes in the corium and invade adipose and subcutaneous muscle cells. They multiply in this location in the amastigote forms previously called *Leishmania* forms. When the histiocytes and other parasitized cells rupture on the fourth or fifth day, the amastigote forms are taken up by regional lymph nodes, from where, at variable intervals, they are discharged through the blood and lymphatic circulation and spread to diverse areas of the body.

The signs and symptoms of Chagas' disease are due to the intracellular amastigote forms. When the host cell ruptures, large numbers escape and temporarily enter the circulation as trypanosome forms. In the intestine, escaping amastigotes apparently result in release of a toxin that destroys the submucosal and the myenteric plexuses. The end result is enteromegaly, which at times may be massive.[99]

Diagnosis

History. Acute Chagas' disease occurs most often in children. It is characterized by high fever and marked edema, particularly with a periorbital distribution and often involving the entire body. The acute stage lasts approximately 20 to 30 days.

Chronic Chagas' disease depends upon the major involvement within the body. Most commonly the symptoms are cardiac, primarily manifested as arrhythmias and congestive heart failure. With megaesophagus, the history is indistinguishable from that of achalasia. With megacolon, infrequent bowel movements and chronic constipation are the cardinal symptoms. With dilatation of the small intestine, diarrhea or constipation may be part of the picture. Data are not available, but in the presence of stasis one could speculate that bacterial overgrowth may play an important part in the pathogenesis.

Physical Examination. In patients with acute Chagas' disease, the periorbital edema of one or both eyes is spectacular. The victim may appear to be suffering from myxedema. There is usually enlargement of the thyroid, lymph nodes, and salivary glands, and hepatosplenomegaly is present. In chronic Chagas' disease involving the intestine, there may be evidence of weight loss and abdominal distention caused by the markedly dilated bowel.

Laboratory Findings. Routine laboratory data provide no clue to the diagnosis of Chagas' disease. Diagnosis depends upon demonstration of the trypanosome forms in blood during periods when the amastigotes rupture cells.[3] During febrile periods, if the blood films are negative, guinea pig inoculation will frequently recover the organism. Amastigote forms may be detected in bone marrow, spleen, or enlarged lymph nodes. The most usual immunologic method for diagnosis of American trypanosomiasis is a complement fixation technique. Other immunologic tests are under investigation but not widely applied. Xenodiagnosis has been used but is relatively insensitive, diagnosing fewer than 50 per cent of patients infected with chronic Chagas' disease. In this technique, trypanosome-free laboratory reduviid bugs are allowed to bite suspected victims. The trypanosomes multiply rapidly in the intestinal tract of the insect, and examination of the intestine will reveal flagellated trypanosomes in 10 to 30 days.

Treatment

Nifurtimox, available from the Center for Disease Control Parasitic Disease Drug Service, Atlanta, Georgia, may be given in a dose of 8 to 10 mg per kg orally in four divided doses.[22] Treatment is continued for 120 days.[25] Patients with achalasia caused by Chagas' disease may be treated with either brusque pneumatic dilation of the esophagus or esophagomyotomy. Occasionally, aperistaltic segments of intestine that are responsible for symptoms may be resected.

Other Pathogenic Intestinal Parasites

An astonishingly large number of other parasites have been identified and incriminated in human intestinal disease.[3] Many are primary parasites of animals, or even plants, and human infection has been accidental. In others, the intestinal involvement has been coincidental with a wider systemic parasitism.

A fatal leishmanial enteritis occurs during epidemic kala-azar.[100] Sections and scrapings of the intestinal mucosa contain myriads of Donovan bodies. It is likely that many patients with visceral leishmaniasis terminating with a fatal enteritis have parasitism of the small intestine. In the past this has been dismissed as typhoid fever.

Nonpathogenic Parasites

A number of parasites are frequently recovered in stool for which no evidence of pathogenicity exists.[3, 25] Even though they are most frequently found in diarrheal stools, it is probable that they are not responsible for the patient's symptoms. These are most commonly protozoa and include *Retortamonas intestinalis, Enteromonas hominis, Chylomastix mesnili, Trichomonas hominis,* and a large number of nonpathogenic amebae. If these sorts of organisms are detected and are the only ones present in feces, no treatment is indicated.

References

1. Knight, R., and Wright, S. G. Intestinal protozoa. Gut *19:*940, 1978.
2. Dobell, C. Discovery of intestinal protozoa in man. Proc. R. Soc. Med. *13:*1, 1920.
3. Strickland, G. T. Hunter's Tropical Medicine. Ed. 6. Philadelphia, W. B. Saunders Co., 1984.
4. Veghelyi, P. Celiac disease imitated by giardiasis. Am. J. Dis. Child. *57:*894, 1939.
5. Cortner, J. A. Giardiasis, a cause of celiac syndrome. J. Dis. Child. *98:*311, 1959.
6. Hoskins, L. C., Winawer, S. J., Broitman, S. A., Gottlieb, L. S., and Zamcheck, N. Clinical giardiasis and intestinal malabsorption. Gastroenterology *53:*265, 1967.
7. Morecki, R., and Parker, J. G. Ultrastructural studies of the human *Giardia lamblia* and subadjacent mucosa in a subject with steatorrhea. Gastroenterology *52:*151, 1967.
8. Wolfe, M. S. Giardiasis. JAMA *233:*1362, 1975.
9. Barbour, A. G., Nichols, C. R., and Fukushima, T. An outbreak of giardiasis in a group of campers. Am. J. Trop. Med. Hyg. *25:*384, 1976.
10. Davies, R. B., and Hibler, C. P. Animal reservoirs and cross-species transmission of *Giardia. In* Proceedings of National Symposium on Waterborne Transmission of Giardiasis. Cincinnati, Ohio, U.S. Environmental Protection Agency, 1978, pp. 104–126.
11. Jarroll, E. L., Bingham, A. K., and Meyer, E. A. Giardia cyst destruction: Effectiveness of six small-quantity water disinfection methods. Am. J. Trop. Med. Hyg. *29:*8, 1980.
12. Osterholm, M. T., Forfang, J. C., Ristinen, T. L., Dean, A. G., Washburn, J. W., Godes, J. R., Rude, R. A., and McCullough, J. G. An outbreak of foodborne giardiasis. N. Engl. J. Med. *304:*24, 1981.
13. Meyer, E. A., and Radulescu, S. Giardia and giardiasis. Adv. Parasitol. *17:*1, 1979.
14. Brandborg, L. L., Tankersley, C. B., Gottlieb, S., Barancik, M., and Sartor, V. E. Histological demonstration of mucosal invasion by *Giardia lamblia* in man. Gastroenterology *52:*143, 1967.
15. Owen, R. L., Allen, C. L., and Stevens, D. P. Phagocytosis of *Giardia muris* by macrophages in Peyer's patch epithelium in mice. Infect. Immun. *33:*591, 1981.
16. Carlson, J. R., Heyworth, M. F., and Owen, R. L. Giardiasis: Immunology, diagnosis and treatment. Surv. Dig. Dis. *2:*201, 1984.
17. Hermans, P. G., Huizenga, K. A., Hoffman, H. N., Brown, A. L., Jr., and Markowitz, H. Dysgammaglobulinemia associated with nodular lymphoid hyperplasia of the small intestine. Am. J. Med. *40:*78, 1966.
18. Ament, M. E., and Rubin, C. E. Relation of giardiasis to abnormal intestinal structure and function in gastrointestinal immunodeficiency syndromes. Gastroenterology *62:*216, 1972.
19. Taylor, G. D., and Wenman, W. M. Human immune response to *Giardia lamblia* infection. J. Infect. Dis. *155:*137, 1987.
20. Yardley, J. H., Takano, J., and Hendrix, T. R. Epithelial and other mucosal lesions of the jejunum in giardiasis. Jejunal biopsy studies. Bull. Johns Hopkins Hosp. *116:*413, 1964.
21. Bezjak, B. Evaluation of a new technique for sampling duodenal contents in parasitologic diagnosis. Am. J. Dig. Dis. *17:*848, 1972.
22. Drugs for parasitic diseases. Med. Lett. *28:*9, 1986.
23. Smith, P. D., Gillin, F. D., Spira, W. M., and Nash, T. E. Chronic giardiasis: Studies on drug sensitivity, toxin production and host immune response. Gastroenterology *83:*797, 1982.
24. Yang, J., and Scholten, T. *Dientamoeba fragilis:* A review with notes on its epidemiology, pathogenicity, mode of transmission, and diagnosis. Am. J. Trop. Med. Hyg. *26:*16, 1977.
25. Markell, E. K., Voge, M., and John, D. T. Medical Parasitology. Ed. 6. Philadelphia, W. B. Saunders Co., 1986.
26. Krogstad, D. J., Spencer, H. C., Healy, G. R., Gleason, N. N., Sexton, D. J., and Herron, C. A. Amebiasis: Epidemiologic studies in the United States, 1971–1974. Ann. Intern. Med. *88:*89, 1978.
27. Thacker, S. B., Simpson, S., Gordon, T. J., Wolfe, M., and Kimball, A. M. Parasitic disease control in a residential facility for the mentally retarded. Am. J. Pub. Health *69:*1279, 1979.
28. Sargeaunt, P. G., and Jackson, T. F. H. G. Biochemical homogeneity of *Entamoeba histolytica* isolates, especially those from liver abscess. Lancet *1:*1386, 1982.
29. Allason-Jones, E., Mindel, A., Sargeaunt, P., and Williams, P. *Entamoeba histolytica* as a commensal intestinal parasite in homosexual men. N. Engl. J. Med. *315:*352, 1986.
30. Dupont, H. L., and Pickering, L. K. Infections of the Gastrointestinal Tract. New York, Plenum Medical Book Company, 1980, pp. 21–46.
31. Mirelman, D., Bracha, R., Chayen, A., Aust-Kettis, A., and Diamond, L. S. *Entamoeba histolytica:* Effect of growth conditions and bacterial associates on isoenzyme patterns and virulence. Exp. Parasitol. *62:*142, 1986.
32. Pittman, F. E., El-Hashimi, W. K., and Pittman, J. C. Studies of human amebiasis. II. Light and electron-microscopic observations of colonic mucosa and exudate in acute amebic colitis. Gastroenterology *65:*588, 1973.
33. Pittman, F. E., El-Hashimi, W. K., and Pittman, J. C. Studies of human amebiasis. I. Clinical and laboratory findings in eight cases of amebic colitis. Gastroenterology *65:*581, 1973.
34. Nanda, R., Baveja, U., and Anand, B. S. *Entamoeba histolytica* cyst passers: Clinical features and outcome in untreated subjects. Lancet *2:*301, 1984.
35. Stauffer, J. Q., and Levine, W. L. Chronic diarrhea related to *Endolimax nana:* Response to treatment with metronidazole. Am. J. Dig. Dis. *19:*59, 1974.
36. Balikian, J. P., Uthman, S. U., and Khouri, N. F. Intestinal amebiasis. A roentgen analysis of 19 cases including 2 case reports. Am. J. Roentgenol. Radium Ther. Nucl. Med. *122:*245, 1974.
37. Kolawole, M. B., and Lewis, E. A. Radiologic observation of intestinal amebiasis. Am. J. Roentgenol. Radium Ther. Nucl. Med. *122:*257, 1974.
38. Sullam, P. M., Slutkin, G., Gottlieb, A. B., and Mills, J. Paromomycin therapy of endemic amebiasis in homosexual men. Sex. Transmiss. Dis. *13:*151, 1986.
39. Katzung, B. G., and Goldsmith, R. S. Antiprotozoal drugs. *In* Katzung, B. G. (ed.). Basic and Clinical Pharmacology, Ed. 3. Norwalk, Connecticut, and Los Altos, California, Appleton and Lange, 1987, pp. 618–640.

40. Levine, S. M., Stover, J. F., Warren, J. G., Chapelka, A. R., and Burke, E. L. Ameboma, the forgotten granuloma. JAMA *215:*1461, 1971.
41. Ylvisaker, J. T., and McDonald, G. B. Sexually acquired amebic colitis and liver abscess. West. J. Med. *132:*153, 1980.
42. Kean, B. H., Gilmore, H. R., Jr., and Van Stone, W. W. Fatal amebiasis: Report of 148 fatal cases from the Armed Forces Institute of Pathology. Ann. Intern. Med. *44:*831, 1956.
43. Viranuvatti, V., Harinasuta, T., Plengvanit, U., Choungchareon, P., and Viranuvatt, V. Liver function tests in hepatic amebiasis based on 274 clinical cases. Am. J. Gastroenterol. *39:*345, 1963.
44. Healy, G. R. Immunologic tools in the diagnosis of amebiasis: Epidemiology in the United States. Rev. Infect. Dis. *8:*239, 1986.
45. Long, P. L. (ed.). The Biology of the Coccidia. Baltimore, University Park Press, 1982.
46. Smitskamp, H., and Oey-Muller, E. Geographical distribution and clinical significance of human coccidiosis. Trop. Geogr. Med. *18:*133, 1966.
47. Trier, J. S., Moxey, P. C., Schimmel, E. H., and Robles, E. R. Chronic intestinal coccidiosis in man: Intestinal morphology and response to treatment. Gastroenterology *66:*923, 1974.
48. Webster, B. H. Human isosporiasis: A report of three cases with necropsy findings in one case. Am. J. Trop. Med. Hyg. *6:*86, 1957.
49. Brandborg, L. L., Goldberg, S. G., and Breidenbach, W. C. Human coccidiosis—A possible cause of malabsorption. The life cycle in small bowel, mucosal biopsies as a diagnostic feature. N. Engl. J. Med. *283:*1306, 1970.
50. Westerman, E. L., and Christensen, R. P. Chronic *Isospora belli* infection teated with cotrimoxazole. Ann. Intern. Med. *91:*413, 1979.
51. Garcia, L. S., Owen, R. L., and Current, W. L. *Isospora belli. In* Balows, A., Hausler, W. J., Jr., and Lennette, E. H. (eds.). The Laboratory Diagnosis of Infectious Disease: Principles and Practice. New York, Springer Verlag, 1988.
52. DeHovitz, J. A., Pape, J. W., Boncy, M., and Johnson, W. D. Clinical manifestations and therapy of *Isospora belli* infection in patients with the acquired immunodeficiency syndrome. N. Engl. J. Med. *315:*87, 1986.
53. Reese, N. C., Current, W. L., Ernst, J. V., and Bailey, W. S. Cryptosporidiosis of man and calf: A case report and results of experimental infections in mice and rats. Am. J. Trop. Med. Hyg. *31:*226, 1982.
54. Current, W. L., and Owen, R. L. Cryptosporidiosis and microsporidiosis. *In* Farthing, M. J. G., and Keusch, G. T. (eds.). Enteric Infection: Mechanisms, Manifestations and Management. London, Chapman and Hall, 1988.
55. Canning, E. U., and Lom, J. The Microsporidia of Vertebrates. London, Academic Press, 1986.
56. Bergquist, R., Morfeldt-Månsson, L., Pehrson, P. O., Petrini, B., and Wasserman, J. Antibody against *Encephalitozoon cuniculi* in Swedish homosexual men. Scand. J. Infect. Dis. *16:*389, 1984.
57. WHO Parasitic diseases surveillance. Antibody to *Encephalitozoon cuniculi* in man. WHO Weekly Epidem. Rec. *58:*30, 1983.
58. Singh, M., Kane, G. J., Mackinlay, L., Quaki, I., Hian, Y. E., Chuan, H. B., Chuen, H. L., and Chew, L. K. Detection of antibodies to *Nosema cuniculi* (protozoa: Microsporidia) in human and animal sera by the indirect fluorescent antibody technique. Southeast Asia J. Trop. Med. Publ. Health *13:*110, 1982.
59. Ledford, D. K., Overman, M. D., Gonzalvo, A., Cali, A., Mester, S. W., and Lockey, R. F. Microsporidiosis myositis in a patient with acquired immunodeficiency syndrome. Ann. Intern. Med. *102:*628, 1985.
60. Margileth, A. M., Strano, A. J., Chandra, R., Neafie, R., Blum, M., and McCully, R. M. Disseminated nosematosis in an immunologically compromised infant. Arch. Pathol. *95:*145, 1973.
61. Dobbins, W. O., III, and Weinstein, W. M. Electron microscopy of the intestine and rectum in acquired immunodeficiency syndrome. Gastroenterology *88:*738, 1985.
62. Desportes, I., Le Charpentier, Y., Galian, A., Bernard, F., Cochand-Priollet, B., Lavergne, A., Ravisse, P., and Modigliani, R. Occurrence of a new microsporidian: *Enterocytozoon bieneusi* n. g., n. sp., in the enterocytes of human patient with AIDS. J. Protozool. *32:*250, 1985.
63. Modigliani, R., Bories, C., Le Charpentier, Y., Salmeron, M., Messing, B., Galian, A., Rambaud, J. C., Lavergne, A., Cochand-Priollet, B., and Desportes, I. Diarrhea and malabsorption in acquired immune deficiency syndrome: A study of four cases with special emphasis on opportunistic protozoan infestations. Gut *26:*179–187, 1985.
64. Arean, V. M., and Koppish, E. Balantidiasis, a review and report of cases. Am. J. Pathol. *32:*1089, 1956.
65. Walzer, P. D., Judson, F. N., Murphy, K. B., Healy, G. R., English, D. K., and Schultz, M. G. Balantidiasis outbreak in Truk. Am. J. Trop. Med. Hyg. *22:*33, 1973.
66. Baskerville, L. Balantidium colitis. Report of a case. Am. J. Dig. Dis. *15:*727, 1970.
67. Dorfman, S., Rangel, O., and Bravo, L. G. Balantidiasis: Report of a fatal case with appendicular and pulmonary involvement. Trans. R. Soc. Trop. Med. Hyg. *78:*833, 1984.
68. Castro, J., Vazquez-Iglesias, J. L., and Arnal-Monreal, F. Dysentery caused by *Balantidium coli*—report of two cases. Endoscopy *15:*272, 1983.
69. Zierdt, C. H. *Blastocystis hominis,* a protozoan parasite and intestinal pathogen of human beings. Clin. Microbiol. Newsletter *5:*57, 1983.
70. Phillips, B. P., and Zierdt, C. H. *Blastocystis hominis:* Pathogenic potential in human patients and in gnotobiotes. Exp. Pathol. *39:*358, 1976.
71. Garcia, L. S., Bruckner, D. A., and Clancy, M. N. Clinical relevance of *Blastocystis hominis*. Lancet *1:*1233, 1984.
72. Zierdt, C. H., and Tan, H. K. Ultrastructure and light microscope appearance of *Blastocystis hominis* in a patient with enteric disease. Z. Parasitenkd. *50:*277, 1976.
73. Sheehan, D. J., Raucher, B. G., and McKitrick, J. C. Association of *Blastocystis hominis* with signs and symptoms of human disease. J. Clin. Microbiol. *24:*548, 1986.
74. Vannatta, J. B., Adamson, D., and Mullican, K. *Blastocystis hominis* infection presenting as recurrent diarrhea. Ann. Intern. Med. *102:*495, 1985.
75. Gallagher, P. G., and Venglarcik, J. S., III. *Blastocystis hominis* enteritis. Pediatr. Infect. Dis. *4:*556, 1985.
76. Zierdt, C. H., Swan, J. C., and Hosseini, J. In vitro response of *Blastocystis hominis* to antiprotozoal drugs. J. Protozool. *30:*332, 1983.
77. Markell, E. K., and Udkow, M. P. *Blastocystis hominis:* Pathogen or fellow traveler? Am. J. Trop. Med. Hyg. *35:*1023, 1986.
78. Bustamante-Sarabia, J., Martuscelli, A., and Tay, J. Ectopic ascariasis: Report of a case with adult worms in the kidney. Am. J. Trop. Med. Hyg. *26:*568, 1977.
79. Goldsmith, R. S. Clinical pharmacology of the antihelminthic drugs. *In* Katzung, B. G. (ed.). Basic and Clinical Pharmacology, Ed. 3. Norwalk, Connecticut, and Los Altos, California. Appleton and Lange, 1987, pp. 641–664.
80. Gill, G. V., and Bell, D. R. *Strongyloides stercoralis* infection in former Far East prisoners of war. Br. Med. J. *2:*572, 1979.
81. Corachan, M., Oomen, H. A. P. C., and Sutorius, F. J. M. Parasitic duodenitis. Trans. R. Soc. Trop. Med. Hyg. *75:*385, 1981.
82. Civantos, F., and Robinson, M. J. Fatal strongyloidiasis following corticosteroid therapy. Am. J. Dig. Dis. *14:*643, 1969.
83. Cross, J. H., and Bhaibulaya, M. Intestinal capillariasis in the Philippines and Thailand. *In* Croll, N., and Cross, J. H. (eds.). Human Ecology and Infectious Diseases. New York, Academic Press, 1983, pp. 103–136.
84. Watten, R. H., Beckner, W. M., Cross, J. H., Gunning, J.-J., and Jarimillo, J. Clinical studies of capillariasis philippinensis. Trans. R. Soc. Trop. Med. Hyg. *66:*828, 1972.
85. Alcantara, A. K., Uylangco, C. V., and Cross, J. An obstinate

case of intestinal capillariasis. Southeast Asian J. Trop. Med. Publ. Health *16:*410, 1985.

86. Mayoral, L. G., Tripathy, K., Garcia, F. T., and Ghitis, J. Intestinal malabsorption and parasitic disease. The role of protein malnutrition. Gastroenterology *50:*856, 1966.
87. Banwell, J. G., Marsden, P. D., Blackman, V., Leonard, P. G., and Hutt, M. S. R. Hookworm infection and intestinal absorption among Africans in Uganda. Am. J. Trop. Med. Hyg. *16:*304, 1967.
88. Tandon, B. N., Kohli, R. K., Saroya, A. K., Ramachandran, K., and Prakash, P. M. Role of parasites in the pathogenesis of intestinal malabsorption in hookworm disease. Gut *10:*293, 1969.
89. Warren, K. S., and Mahmoud, A. A. F. Algorithms in the diagnosis and management of exotic diseases. IX. Trichuriasis. J. Infect. Dis. *133:*240, 1976.
90. Brown, W. J., and Voge, M. Cysticercosis—a modern day plague. Pediatr. Clin. North Am. *32:*953, 1985.
91. Mahmoud, A. A. F. Schistosomiasis. *In* Warren, K. S., and Mahmoud, A. A. F. (eds.). Tropical and Geographical Medicine. New York, McGraw-Hill Book Co., 1984, pp. 443–457.
92. Bhagwandeen, S. B. The Clinico-pathological Manifestations of Schistosomiasis in the African and the Indian in Durban. Pietermaritzburg, University of Natal Press, 1968.
93. Hall, S. C., and Kehoe, E. L. Prolonged survival of *Schistosoma japonicum.* Calif. Med. *113:*75, 1970.
94. Hidayst, M. A., and Wanid, H. A. A study of the vascular changes in bilharzic hepatic fibrosis and their significance. Surg. Gynecol. Obstet. *132:*997, 1971.
95. Higashi, G. I. Immunodiagnostic tests for protozoan and helminthic infections. Diagn. Immunol. *2:*2, 1984.
96. McCracken, R. P., and Taylor, D. D. Mebendazole therapy of parenteral trichinellosis. Science *207:*1220, 1980.
97. Woody, N. C., and Woody, H. B. American trypanosomiasis. I. Clinical and epidemiologic background of Chagas' disease in the United States. J. Pediatr. *58:*568, 1961.
98. Winslow, D. J., and Chaffee, E. F. Preliminary investigations on Chagas' disease. Milit. Med. *130:*826, 1965.
99. Köberle, F. Enteromegaly and cardiomegaly in Chagas' disease. Gut *4:*399, 1963.
100. Sati, M. H. Leishmanial enteritis as a cause of intractable diarrhoea and death. Sudan Med. J. *1:*(NS) 216, 1962.

63

Infectious Diarrhea

SHERWOOD L. GORBACH

Our knowledge of infectious diarrheal diseases has expanded exponentially in the past ten years.[1] Advances have come from a number of disciplines, with an integration of epidemiologic, clinical, and laboratory studies to produce new understanding of this ancient group of diseases.

Changes in Normal Flora Caused by Diarrhea

The proximal small bowel, including the stomach, duodenum, jejunum, and upper ileum, has a sparse microflora. The concentrations of bacteria are generally less than 10^4 organisms per milliliter.[2] Most of the organisms are derived from the oropharynx, coming down with each meal and passing through the upper bowel in a wave-like fashion. Colonization of the upper intestine by coliform organisms is an abnormal event, one characteristic of diseases caused by pathogens such as *Vibrio cholerae* and toxigenic *Escherichia coli*[3,4] (see also p. 1162).

The large bowel contains a luxuriant microflora, with total concentrations of 10^{11} bacteria per gram. Anaerobes, such as *Bacteroides, anaerobic Streptococcus,* and *Clostridium,* outnumber aerobic bacteria, such as coliforms, 1000-fold. During an episode of acute diarrhea, regardless of the etiology, the colonic flora changes, becoming less anaerobic because of the rapid transit. As a result, strict anaerobic bacteria are decreased in number, with an increase in coliforms—often aberrant types like *Klebsiella, Enterobacter,* and *Proteus.* The pathogen itself rises to ascendancy in the flora, so that the major isolate from the feces might be *V. cholerae* or *Shigella.*

Not only is there a longitudinal distribution of bacteria in the gastrointestinal tract, there is also a cross-sectional arrangement with regard to the mucosal surface. The microflora is found within the lumen and overlying the epithelial cells, adhering to the mucus layer. Penetration of bacteria through the mucosal surface is an abnormal event that can be caused by invasive agents such as *Shigella, Salmonella, Campylobacter,* and *Yersinia.*[5]

Control Mechanism

The same mechanisms that control the normal flora also serve to protect the bowel from invasion by pathogens. At the portal of entry, gastric acid suppresses most organisms that are swallowed. Individuals with reduced or absent gastric acid show a high incidence of bacterial colonization in their upper small bowel and are more susceptible to bacterial diarrheal diseases. Bile has antibacterial properties, and this may be another factor in controlling the flora. A key element in maintaining the sparse flora of the upper bowel is forward propulsive motility. Finally, the microflora, by producing its own antibacterial substances, maintains stability of the normal populations and prevents implantation of pathogens (see pp. 107–114).

Classifications of Bacterial Diarrhea

Acute bacterial diarrhea can be classified into *toxigenic* types, in which an enterotoxin is the major if not exclusive pathogenic mechanism, and *invasive* types, in which the organism penetrates the mucosal surface as the primary event, but enterotoxin may be produced as well. Many organisms elaborate enterotoxins that cause fluid and electrolyte secretion in the gut. That an organism produces an enterotoxin is established in the laboratory by *in vivo* tests, such as the rabbit ileal loop model and the suckling mouse model,[6–8] or by *in vitro* tests involving a tissue culture line such as Y-1 adrenal cells or Chinese hamster ovary cells.[9, 10]

The recognized diarrheal toxins can be grouped broadly into two categories:[11] *cytotonic*—producing fluid secretion by activtion of intracellular enzymes such as adenylate cyclase, without any damage to the epithelial surface; and *cytotoxic*—causing injury to the mucosal cell, as well as inducing fluid secretion, but not primarily by activation of cyclic nucleotides (Table 63–1). Several organisms produce both cytotonic and cytotoxic toxins, e.g., *Aeromonas, Campylobacter,* and *V. parahaemolyticus.*

TOXIGENIC DIARRHEAS

The prototype organisms in this group are *Vibrio cholerae* and enterotoxigenic *Escherichia coli* (ETEC). These pathogens elaborate enterotoxins of the cytotonic type that cause dehydrating diarrhea.

Diarrheal disease caused by *Vibrio cholerae* and ETEC has the following characteristics: (1) The entire disease consists of intestinal fluid loss which is related to the action of the enterotoxin on the small bowel epithelial cell. (2) The organism itself does not invade the mucosal surface; rather, it colonizes the upper small bowel, "sticking" to the epithelial cells, and elaborates an enterotoxin. The mucosal architecture remains intact, with no evidence of cellular destruction. Bacteremia is not a complication. (3) The fecal effluent is watery and often voluminous, producing clinical features of dehydration. The origin of the fluid is the upper small bowel, where the enterotoxin has its greatest activity.

Table 63–1. CLASSIFICATION OF BACTERIAL TOXINS ASSOCIATED WITH DIARRHEA

Cytotonic	Cytotoxic
Vibrio cholerae	*Shigella*
Escherichia coli (LT and ST)	*Clostridium perfringens* types (A and C)
Bacillus cereus	*Clostridium difficile*
Other *Vibrio* species	*Staphylococcus aureus*
Aeromonas	*Campylobacter*
? Coliforms	? *Yersinia*
? *Yersinia*	

Cholera

Cholera is a severe diarrheal disorder that can cause dehydration and death within three to four hours of onset. Stool output can exceed 1 L per hour, with daily fecal outputs of 15 to 20 L, if parenteral fluid replacement is kept up. The acutely ill patient has marked signs of dehydration, poor skin turgor, "washerwoman's hands," absent pulses, reduced renal function, and hypovolemic shock. It has been said that cholera is a disease that begins where other diseases end—with death.

Cholera is the prototypic toxigenic diarrhea. Its importance derives not necessarily from its incidence, for cholera is confined to certain areas of the world and tends to be epidemic, but from its role as a model of secretory diarrhea. More has been learned about pathophysiology—and normal intestinal function—from cholera than from any other intestinal disease. Treatment programs have been devised, including an oral rehydration regimen; the enterotoxin has been purified; the immunology and epidemiology have been clarified; and vaccines have been developed. Experimental and therapeutic successes and failures mirrored in the study of cholera have been realized with other forms of diarrhea as well.

Microbiology. *Vibrio cholerae* is a gram-negative, short, curved rod that is shaped like a comma.[12] It is actively motile by means of a single polar flagellum. These organisms are strongly aerobic, preferring alkaline and high salt environments.

There are two major biotypes—*classic* and *El Tor.* The El Tor strain is responsible for the current pandemic. It is differentiated from classic strains by its ability to hemolyze sheep and goat red blood cells, its reactivity to certain phages, and its resistance to polymyxin. El Tor vibrios are somewhat hardier in nature. The clinical disease is similar with both biotypes, although as a rule, El Tor infections are somewhat milder. Antigenic serotypes are identified by the somatic antigen. The major serotypes associated with clinical disease are Inaba and Ogawa; there also exists a third, rare, type, Hikojima.

Cholera Toxin. All wild strains of *Vibrio cholerae* elaborate the same enterotoxin, a protein molecule with a molecular weight of 84,000 daltons.[13] Like the diphtheria toxin, it is composed of two types of subunits. Each toxin molecule contains five B subunits that encircle a single A subunit.[14] The B subunit is responsible for binding to the receptor on the mucosa.[15]

The A subunit is responsible for binding and activation of adenylate cyclase located on the inner cellular membrane.[16]

Pathogenesis. The entire clinical syndrome of cholera is caused by the action of the toxin on the intestinal epithelial cell.[17] Fluid loss in cholera originates in the small intestine. The most sensitive areas are the upper bowel, particularly the duodenum and upper jejunum; the ileum is less affected, and the colon is usually in a state of absorption because it is relatively insensitive to the toxin. This is a form of "overflow" diarrhea, with a large volume of fluid produced in the upper intestine that overwhelms the capacity of the lower bowel to absorb. Cholera toxin increases adenylate cyclase activity, resulting in elevated levels of cyclic AMP in the intestinal mucosa.[18] There appears to be differential action on the mucosal cells, in that there is a direct secretory effect on the crypt cells and an antiabsorptive effect on the villous cells.

The visual appearance of cholera stools resembles "rice water"; that is, the stool has lost all pigment and becomes a clear fluid with small flecks of mucus. The electrolyte composition is isotonic with plasma, and the effluent has a low protein concentration (Table 63–2). On microscopic examination, there are no inflammatory cells; all that can be seen are small numbers of shed mucosal cells.

Cholera vibrios do not invade the mucosal surface, and bacteremia is virtually unknown in this disease. There are no histologic abnormalities in the intestinal epithelium. A biopsy specimen of the mucosa during acute cholera shows only evidence of dehydration, with maintenance of normal architecture. This is in sharp contrast to the invasive and ulcerating lesions associated with *Salmonella* and *Shigella*.

Clinical Features. Like many other infectious diseases, there is a spectrum of clinical manifestations—from an asymptomatic carrier state to a desperately ill patient with severe dehydration. The initial stage is characterized by vomiting and abdominal distention. This is followed rapidly by diarrhea, which accelerates over the next few hours to frequent purging with large volumes of rice-water stools. All the clinical signs and symptoms can be ascribed to the fluid and electrolyte losses. Patients present profound dehydration and hypovolemic shock, usually leading to renal failure. The stool is isotonic with plasma, although there is an inordinate loss of potassium and bicarbonate, producing hypokalemic acidosis.[17] Mild fever may be present, but there are no signs of sepsis.

Table 63–2. FLUID COMPOSITIONS IN INFECTIOUS DIARRHEA

	Electrolyte Concentrations (mm/L)			
	Sodium	*Potassium*	*Chloride*	*Bicarbonate*
Stool				
Cholera, adult	124	16	90	48
Cholera, child	101	27	92	32
Nonspecific, child	56	25	55	14
Intravenous therapy				
Ringer's lactate	130	4	109	28*
5:4:1 solution	129	11	97	44
2:1 solution	141	—	94	47
Oral rehydration therapy				
WHO formula†	90	20	80	30

*Equivalent from lactate conversion.
†Add glucose, 110 mm/L.

Immunologic Responses. Following acute cholera, serum antibody can be demonstrated against two components: a vibriocidal antibody directed against somatic antigen and antitoxin antibody against the enterotoxin. Vibriocidal titers rise and fall rapidly, and by six months only 1 per cent of individuals have high levels. In areas of high endemicity, such as the Indian subcontinent, the level of vibriocidal titer rises with age; by the tenth year of life, 50 per cent of individuals have measurable titers. Infectivity is related to the presence and actual level of vibriocidal antibody. High titers of this antibody are associated with significant protection. From these observations, it follows that acute cholera in endemic areas is a disease largely of young children, primarily those who lack vibriocidal antibody. Antitoxin titers rise somewhat slowly after acute infection and remain elevated for many months.[19]

Exposure to vibrios, either by actual infection or by asymptomatic carriage, causes an elevation of vibriocidal antibody. In field situations, the clinical case rate is approximately 0.26 per cent; that is, for every clinical case of cholera there are approximately 400 asymptomatic individuals who have contact with the organism, as demonstrated by a rise in vibriocidal antibody titer.

Epidemiology. For many centuries, the Bay of Bengal has been considered the "cradle of cholera." The disease has raged in the Indian subcontinent and Asia since recorded history. Western countries were relatively free of cholera epidemics until the nineteenth century. Since then, six pandemics have been reported, and we are currently in the seventh. This outbreak started in 1961, initially in the Celebes Island in Indonesia, then made its way to the Philippines, Hong Kong, Japan, Korea, Thailand, India, Pakistan, and the Middle East, and finally passed across the African continent to engulf the entire region.

The present pandemic has introduced a new dimension to the spread of cholera, namely intercontinental passage by air travel. This route is the only explanation for the introduction of cholera to Guinea in the summer of 1970. Since that time, the disease has spread throughout the African continent, and finally into southern Europe, with epidemics in Spain, Portugal, and Italy. The organism associated with the current pandemic is an El Tor biotype. This disease, is, in general, milder than that seen with "classic" strains, and there is a higher incidence of inapparent infection. Cholera occurs sporadically along the Gulf Coast of the United States, primarily in Texas and Louisiana.[20] Among 5 million American travelers to endemic areas only 10 cases of cholera were reported in the period 1961–1982.

The major vehicle for spreading cholera is contaminated water and food. Infection by person-to-person contact is uncommon, and it is rare for physicians, nurses, ward attendants, and laboratory workers who come in contact with the microorganism to acquire the clinical disease. The inoculum required to cause acute cholera is very large, approximately 10^9 organisms. Even this number cannot cause disease in a healthy individual without bicarbonate or some substance to buffer the acidity of the stomach. In nature, people with low gastric acid, such as that associated with malnutrition, are more easily infected than those with normal acidity.

Human beings are the only host for cholera vibrios. Asymptomatic carriers are responsible for overwintering of the organism. The carrier rate is approximately 5 per cent following acute exposure, although long-term carriers are much less common. The site of harboring the cholera vibrios is the gallbladder.

Therapy. Fluid and electrolyte replacement is the mainstay of therapy for cholera. Fluid repletion was first advocated in 1830 by two workers at the Institute for Artificial Mineral Waters in Moscow. Dr. William O'Shaughnessy, working in Scotland in 1831, measured stool electrolyte losses in cholera and echoed the suggestion that fluids and electrolytes should be effective treatment for cholera. In the next 120 years, however, irrational therapy prevailed. Misdirected suggestions for "abstraction of blood" or exchange transfusions set back the application of rational, effective management.

Treatment of acute cholera is based upon physiologic principles of restoring fluid and electrolyte balance and maintaining intravascular volume. This can be accomplished with intravenous solutions or oral fluids that contain electrolytes in isotonic concentrations[17] (Table 63–2; see pp. 290–316).

Particular attention is paid to administration of bicarbonate and potassium, which are lost excessively in the stool. An oral rehydration regimen has been developed for treating mild to moderate cases and is especially useful in underdeveloped regions.[21, 22]

Antimicrobial agents are useful as ancillary measures in the treatment of cholera.[23, 24] The dose of tetracycline is 40 mg per kilogram of body weight per day orally, up to a maximum of 4 gm per day, in four divided doses for two days. Intravenous therapy is indicated for patients unable to take medication by mouth. There is no proven value in lengthening the duration of treatment to four days.[25]

In a recent cholera epidemic in Tanzania, patients were reported to have excreted *V. cholerae* after a full course of tetracycline, while others developed cholera during or soon after tetracycline chemoprophylaxis.[26] A survey of 110 isolates of El Tor *V. cholerae* from this outbreak documented a 75 per cent incidence of tetracycline-resistant strains after five months of extensive therapeutic and prophylactic use of this drug in Tanzania.

The simple therapeutic principles of fluid replacement and antibiotics can save many lives. This knowledge has been available only in the past 30 years, before which time the cholera mortality rate was 50 to 75 per cent. Application of these physiologic principles reduces the mortality rate in adults to below 1 per cent. Children still suffer a mortality rate of approximately 3 to 5 per cent from cholera because of the lack of fluid reserve in the young child.

Vaccines. A commercial vaccine has been prepared to the somatic antigen of the two major serotypes of *V. cholerae.* Studies in Bangladesh have shown that the vaccine is approximately 70 per cent effective for three to five months.[27] Following vaccination, an elevation in antibody titer can be seen within eight days in individuals who had demonstrable antibody titer; this indicates an anamnestic response. Young children, presumably having had no prior contact with the vibrio, show a more delayed response and often do not develop significant titers until a second injection is administered, approximately three to four weeks later. Thus, the vaccine has limited effectiveness in epidemic situations, because by the time the initial cases are seen there is already widespread infection in the community. Application of vaccine at this stage requires days to weeks before immunity can be produced in children. There had been a field trial of a toxoid vaccine made from cholera toxin that was inactivated with glutaraldehyde. Initial field trials with this toxoid preparation have proved disappointing in Bangladesh.[28]

Other Vibrios

Beside the cholera vibrios, other vibrios have important pathogenic significance (Table 63–3).[20, 29] Of the ten species in nature, at least seven have been related to human infection. These organisms are all isolated from surface water. They tend to be halophilic (prefer high salt concentration) and are associated primarily with mollusks such as oysters, crabs, and mussels. Strains within the same species may produce different toxins, including enterotoxins, cytotoxins, and hemolysins. The diversity of toxin production is matched by the diversity of clinical symptoms, which range from watery, dehydrating diarrhea to frank dysentery. Some strains penetrate the intestinal mucosa, producing bacteremia. Others have been incriminated in wound infections acquired while swimming in ocean water.

These organisms are gram-negative, straight or curved rods that are pleomorphic, oxidase-positive, and highly motile. They are members of the Vibrionaceae, which also includes the cholera vibrios.

Table 63–3. OTHER VIBRIOS ASSOCIATED WITH DIARRHEA

V. cholerae non-O:1*†
*V. parahaemolyticus**†
V. fluvialis
*V. vulnificus**†
*V. mimicus**
V. hollisae†
V. furnissii

*Also causes wound and ear infections.
†Also causes septicemia.

Vibrio Parahaemolyticus

This organism is associated with seafood, causing acute diarrheal disease after consumption of raw fish or shellfish. Recognized as an important pathogen in the Far East, it has been isolated in the United States, although the exact incidence is unknown.[30]

Strains of *V. parahaemolyticus* produce a number of distinct hemolysins, the most significant of which appears to be responsible for the "Kanagawa phenomenon" that causes hemolysis of human red blood cells in bacteriologic medium.[31] Kanagawa-positive isolates are pathogenic for humans, whereas Kanagawa-negative strains are nonpathogenic, being isolated from marine sources as part of the flora.

Pathogenic strains produce a number of other toxins. A lethal toxin, which is also hemolytic, has been described.[31] In other studies, these organisms produce an enterotoxin that causes fluid accumulation in the rabbit ileal loop model.[32] A cytotoxic toxin that causes damage to HeLa cells also has been discovered. Finally, some strains invade the mucosa and cause bacteremia in experimental animals.[33] It is clear that more studies are required to clarify the multitude of toxins and hemolysins as well as the invasive properties of this organism.

Clinical Features. The diversity in toxins and virulence is reflected in the variation in signs and symptoms observed in laboratory-confirmed outbreaks in the United States.[34–36] Explosive, watery diarrhea is the cardinal manifestation in over 90 per cent of the cases. Abdominal cramps, nausea, vomiting, and headaches are common. Fever and chills occur in approximately 25 per cent of cases. Clinically, this illness resembles that produced by nontyphoidal *Salmonella.* However, in come cases a bloody dysenteric syndrome is observed, with fecal leukocytes and superficial mucosal ulcerations on sigmoidoscopic examination.

The duration of illness generally has been short, with a median of three days (range, two hours to ten days). There have been no deaths in the 1000 cases reported in the United States. This has generally been the experience in Japan, although in the first outbreak reported in Japan, 20 of 272 clinically ill patients died.[37] The diarrhea is usually not profuse, as with *V. cholerae.* Yet hypotension and shock have been noted in some patients.[38]

Subclinical cases have been demonstrated in fewer than 1 per cent of healthy individuals. In addition, this infection is rare in the winter, suggesting that the carrier state is probably transient. Individuals do not continue to harbor the organism in their stools once symptoms have disappeared.

Epidemiology. Most outbreaks of *V. parahaemolyticus* gastroenteritis have been reported in Japan; indeed, during the warm months, when the incidence is higher, this organism is responsible for most episodes of bacterial food poisoning in that country. Other countries in Asia, as well as Australia and Great Britain, have documented this infection. In the United States, there is a striking geographic association, with most cases seemingly confined to coastal states such as Maryland, Massachusetts, Louisiana, New Jersey, and Washington.[30] The organism itself is ubiquitous in marine waters and can be found along the coastline of most countries in which cases have been reported.

The attack rate in a specific epidemic has varied between 24 and 86 per cent of exposed individuals. The mean incubation period for most outbreaks has been 13 to 23 hours, but the range is quite variable, from four to 48 hours.

Most infections have been associated with seafish or seawater. Occasionally, boiled sardines, salted vegetables (contaminated from salt water), or crabs, shrimp, and oysters (both cooked and uncooked) have been incriminated. The common factor in most outbreaks appears to be food kept for several hours without proper refrigeration, at an inadequate holding temperature.

Therapy. Although explosive in onset, this disease is generally rather shortlived, and no deaths have been reported in the United States. Patients generally are treated symptomatically. The organism is sensitive to several antibiotics, including tetracycline, but there is no evidence that antimicrobial therapy has any role in the management of this infection.

***Vibrio cholerae* Non-O:1.** These strains represent a diverse group of organisms which are identical morphologically and biochemically to *V. cholerae,* but they do not agglutinate with the O-group antiserum of the three cholera serotypes.[29, 39] The non-O:1 cholera vibrios produce several toxins *in vitro,*[40] and they cause a wider range of infection than cholera vibrios, including watery diarrhea, dysentery, wound and ear infections, and septicemia.[20, 29]

The non-O:1 cholera vibrios can be isolated from salty coastal waters of the United States, most commonly in the summer and fall when the temperature rises.[41] Mollusks, particularly oysters, which have a reported contamination rate of 10 to 15 per cent, are the major source; clams, mussels, and crabs have also been implicated.

In the Far East non-O:1 cholera vibrios have been associated mainly with severe, dehydrating diarrhea. Reported cases in the United States, however, include wound and ear infections, septicemia, and infections of the lung and biliary tract.[29] The most common antecedent history is consumption of raw oysters within the previous 72 hours. In outbreaks, there is a high attack rate, with incubation periods ranging from very rapid onset (six to 12 hours) to as long as three days. A one-week course of diarrheal illness is common. Because the gastrointestinal disease is self-limited and relatively benign in the United States, antibiotics are not recommended.[41] However, septicemia, wound infections, and deep organ infections should be treated with appropriate antibiotics.

V. fluvialis, previously designated as enteric group EF-6, has been isolated mostly in the Orient from patients with severe, watery diarrhea.[20, 29] The isolates produced a range of toxins, including an enterotoxin similar to classic cholera toxin. It is only rarely found in other parts of the world, including the United States. *V. vulnificus* has been seen in two clinical settings, wound infections in people swimming in salt waters, and septicemia in patients with liver disease who had consumed raw shellfish, usually oysters. The disease can be highly lethal in the patients with underlying liver disease. *V. mimicus* acquires its name from its similarity to cholera vibrios, even to producing an enterotoxin which resembles cholera toxin.[42] The organism has been isolated from patients in the United States suffering from diarrhea or ear infection. *V. hollisae,* also known as enteric EF-13, is a rare isolate from stool and occasionally blood cultures. *V. furnissii* is found in the Orient. Its most celebrated outbreak was during an airflight from Tokyo to Seattle, in which 23 passengers developed severe diarrhea, resulting in one death and two hospitalizations.

Aeromonas

Aeromonas species are ubiquitous environmental organisms found principally in fresh and brackish water, especially in the summer months. These organisms are often mistaken for coliforms in the laboratory, leading to a falsely low reported incidence. *A. salmonicida* is a fish pathogen, whereas *A. hydrophila* causes disease in human beings; the latter group is divided by some authors into three species: *A. hydrophila, A. caviae,* and *A. sobria.* This taxonomy is not completely agreed upon, but it appears that the last three species are all potential human pathogens.[43, 44] *Aeromonas* strains produce an array of toxins, including heat-labile enterotoxin, hemolysin, and cytotoxin.[45]

Epidemiology. A recent study emphasized that *Aeromonas* infections were most likely associated with drinking untreated water such as well water or spring water just before onset of symptoms.[46] Several studies have reported a high incidence of stool isolation in children with diarrhea; for example, the incidence of *Aeromonas* in Western Australia was 10.2 per cent in over 1000 cases of childhood diarrhea, compared to 0.06 per cent in control subjects.[43] Other studies have found a high carrier rate in healthy individuals, ranging from 0.7 per cent to 3.2 per cent and up to 27 per cent in Thailand. This finding has raised some question about the pathogenicity of these organisms.[44]

Clinical Features. *Aeromonas* has long been recognized as a cause of wound infection following swimming in fresh or brackish water and of bacteremic or deep organ infections in immunocompromised hosts.[47] Most isolates in recent years, however, come from intestinal infections. There is a range of illness, from mild diarrhea, seen mostly in children, to severe illness, requiring hospitalization. In the study from Western Australia, 22 per cent of patients had blood and mucus in their stool, and one third required hospitalization for severe illness.[43] Most cases resolved within one week, but 37 per cent of these children had symptoms for two or more weeks. In adults, chronic diarrhea is even more common, lasting an average of 42 days in a nationwide U.S. study.[46]

Treatment. These organisms are consistently resistant to beta-lactam antibiotics, such as penicillin, ampicillin, and cephalosporins. In fact, some cases of *Aeromonas* diarrhea have been activated apparently by prior treatment with ampicillin.[46] The organisms tend to be sensitive to trimethroprim-sulfamethoxazole, tetracyclines, and chloramphenicol. There is no convincing evidence that mild cases are improved by antibiotic treatment, but it may be possible to shorten a chronic infection by appropriate use of these drugs.

Plesiomonas shigelloides is also a member of the family Vibrionaceae, but is isolated less frequently in the United States than *Aeromonas.*[44] Most cases have been associated with consumption of raw oysters or recent travel to Mexico or the Orient.[48] The antibiotic sensitivity pattern is similar to that of *Aeromonas,* but little information is available on efficacy of treatment.

Escherichia Coli

These organisms are major components of the normal intestinal microflora in human beings and animals. Although most strains are relatively harmless in the bowel, others possess virulence factors that are linked to diarrheal disease. At least five types of *E. coli* intestinal pathogens have been recognized (Table 63–4). Their virulence factors include toxin production, adherence to epithelial cells, invasiveness, and specific

Table 63–4. TYPES OF *E. COLI* INTESTINAL PATHOGENS

Strains	Mechanisms	Types of Patients	Clinical Features
Enteropathogenic (EPEC)	Shiga-like toxin Adherence O serogroups	Children Newborn nursery outbreaks	Watery diarrhea
Enterotoxigenic (ETEC)	Heat-labile toxin (LT) and/or Heat-stable toxin (ST) Adherence (fimbriae) O serogroups	Children (developing countries) Travelers Food and water outbreaks	Watery diarrhea
Enteroinvasive (EIEC)	Shiga-like toxin Epithelial cell invasion O serogroups (eight types, many related to *Shigella*)	Children and adults Food and water outbreaks	Dysentery (WBCs and RBCs in feces)
Enterohemorrhagic (EHEC)	Shiga-like toxin (large quantities) O serogroups (usually 0157:H7)	Children and adults Food (hamburger) outbreaks	Bloody diarrhea Hemolytic-uremic syndrome
Enteroadherent (EAEC)	Adherence to HEp-2 cells O serogroups (0119, 0125ac; in children with chronic diarrhea)	Children (protracted illness) Travelers	Chronic diarrhea or Watery diarrhea (acute)

genetic elements (plasmids or chromosomal) that determine pathogenicity.

Enteropathogenic *E. coli* (EPEC). Severe epidemics of diarrhea raged in neonatal nurseries for decades, starting in the 1920s and continuing to the present time. Although uncommon in recent years, such outbreaks had a high mortality rate in infants. The development of a serotyping system for *E. coli* facilitated understanding of the epidemiology of the outbreaks. The serotyping system designed by Kauffmann and White is based on O, H, and K antigens. Over 150 somatic O antigens have been recognized. There is considerable crossover with other enterobacteria, including *Salmonella* and *Shigella.* More than 40 flagellar H antigens have been described. The K antigen is a surface or capsular material that interferes with O antigen agglutination.

Certain O serotypes have been associated epidemiologically with outbreaks of neonatal diarrhea. Approximately 14 serotypes were identified, including the well-known types 055, 0111, and 0119.[49, 50] Although EPEC are undoubtedly causative agents in nursery outbreaks of diarrhea and some community-wide epidemics, their role in sporadic diarrhea is uncertain. A high carrier rate in asymptomatic individuals, at least in some communities, has confused the picture. Nevertheless, an anlaysis of published case-controlled studies showed that EPEC was recovered more frequently from sick individuals than healthy control subjects in almost every report.[49]

Recent studies on pathogenic mechanisms have shown that adherence to intestinal epithelial cells and toxin production are critical virulence factors.[50] Most EPEC adhere to an epithelial cell line known as HEp-2. In germ-free piglets these organisms attach to the epithelial cells of the intestine. Some EPEC elaborate a Shiga-like toxin, similar to the toxin associated with *Shigella.* Although the search for virulence factors has been somewhat elusive with EPEC, their pathogenicity has been established conclusively in human volunteer studies in which diarrhea is produced in a high proportion of cases.[51]

Although diagnosis can be established by serotyping the isolates of *E. coli* in the feces, routine testing for EPEC is not warranted in sporadic cases of diarrhea owing to the high carrier rate and the uncertain role of these organisms. In the past, neonates with severe EPEC diarrhea have been treated orally with nonabsorbable antibiotics such as neomycin and gentamicin, and this remains a therapeutic indication; however, there is no need for treatment of sporadic diarrhea in older children or adults because the disease appears to be self-limited.

Toxigenic *E. coli* (ETEC). Inspired by the discoveries in cholera, investigators directed their attention to *Escherichia coli* as a cause of acute toxigenic diarrheal disease. Originally in India, and thereafter in many parts of the world, strains of *E. coli* were found to elaborate an enterotoxin somewhat similar to the toxin of *Vibrio cholerae.*[52–54] ETEC is a group of *E. coli* not belonging to serotypes previously recognized as EPEC. ETEC infections occur mostly as sporadic cases but may cause a large outbreak.

Pathologic Mechanism of Infection. The first requirement for ETEC diarrhea is colonization of the upper small intestine by the pathogen. These organisms are acquired through contaminated food and liquids and must pass the acid barrier of the stomach. They colonize the surface of the small bowel epithelium without penetrating below the epithelial layer. As in cholera, there is no mucosal damage and no bacteremia.

The process of colonization is related to specific protein antigens on the surface of the bacterial cell, known as pili or fimbriae. These fimbriae are capable of hemagglutination in the presence of mannose. They are variously known as adherence antigens or colonization factor antigens (CFA).[55]

The antigenic structure of the adherence pili determines the host specificity of the ETEC strains. For example, those bearing a K88 antigen are pathogenic for piglets, while others bearing a K99 antigen cause disease in calves and lambs. The ETEC pathogenic strains for humans have another group of antigens.[50, 55, 56] The enterotoxins, on the other hand, are similar in the human and animal strains.

Enterotoxins: Pathophysiology of ETEC. Two types of enterotoxins are produced by ETEC.[57] The *heat-labile* toxin (LT) is a protein that is destroyed by heat and acid and has a molecular weight of approximately 80,000 daltons. It acts pathophysiologically like cholera toxin by activating adenylate cyclase, causing secretion of fluid and electrolytes into the intestinal lumen. LT also shares antigenic components with cholera toxin.[58] The second toxin is *heat stable* (ST), being able to withstand heating to 100°C. It has a low molecular weight of approximately 4500 daltons, fails to activate adenylate cyclase, and has no biochemical similarity to cholera toxin. It appears that guanylate cyclase is activated by ST, producing fluid secretion in the small intestine.[59, 60] ETEC can elaborate LT only, ST only, or both toxins. Not only do these toxins cause diarrhea in humans, but similar types of toxigenic *E. coli* cause dehydrating diarrhea in domestic animals such as pigs, cows, and sheep.[61]

Clinical Features. There is nothing distinctive about the clinical presentation of ETEC diarrhea. The incubation period is 24 to 48 hours, and the disease often begins with upper intestinal distress, followed soon thereafter by watery diarrhea. The infection can be extremely mild, with only a few loose movements, or it can be quite severe, mimicking a case of cholera with severe dehydration and even rice-water stools. Indeed, the initial demonstration of toxigenic diarrhea came from studies in Calcutta of a serious form of diarrheal disease called "acute undifferentiated diarrhea."[52] Such patients were admitted to the cholera ward until it was determined that vibrios were not present. ST-only strains cause a milder attack of diarrhea, but these patients suffer from more vomiting and constitutional complaints.[62]

Immunologic Responses. Antibodies against the enterotoxins and colonization factors have been demonstrated in individuals infected with ETEC. It also appears that people residing in areas at high risk for ETEC infection acquire some protection over time. Thus, students at a college in Mexico tended to develop ETEC diarrhea, depending upon their country of origin; those from South America had a relatively low risk of ETEC diarrhea; and those from North America had a high risk.[63]

Epidemiology. ETEC are of human origin, because the animal strains are rather host-specific. The major vehicles of infection appear to be contaminated food and beverages. ETEC infection affects primarily children, particularly in the tropics. There have been varying reports of infection in the United States, with high incidences in Chicago and Dallas, but low incidences in other American cities and in Canada. Even in developing countries, the incidence of ETEC infection has varied between 15 and 50 per cent.

Much of the confusion over epidemiologic studies of *E. coli* diarrhea relates to the difficulty with toxin assays and the high frequency of infection with multiple pathogens, especially in developing countries. ETEC infections are particularly important in travelers from North America and Northern Europe to areas of the world where diarrheal disease is prevalent. Indeed, it is generally accepted that ETEC are responsible for 50 to 70 per cent of travelers' diarrhea.

Treatment. Most patients with ETEC diarrhea have only mild dehydration, although in children and older people even small amounts of intestinal purging can produce serious consequences. The stool electrolyte losses in ETEC diarrhea are similar to those in cholera, and fluid replacement should follow the same principles. These organisms tend to be sensitive to many antimicrobial drugs, especially ampicillin and tetracycline. However, evidence that antibiotics shorten the disease is only marginal.[62]

Enteroinvasive *E. coli* (EIEC). Originally described in Asia, EIEC is recognized as a rare cause of the dysentery syndrome. During 1971 there was an outbreak caused by EIEC related to contaminated imported cheese.[64] The presenting symptoms of EIEC infection are diarrhea, tenesmus, fever, and intestinal cramps. The fecal effluent shows multiple polymorphonuclear leukocytes. EIECs have been recognized in at least eight *E. coli* serogroups, most of which are related biochemically and antigenically to *Shigella.* Virulence factors include the ability to invade epithelial cells and production of a Shiga-like toxin. Diagnosis in a routine bacteriologic laboratory is rather difficult and generally impractical. Surveys for EIEC in the United States have shown low isolation rates, except in a few celebrated outbreaks.

Enterohemorrhagic *E. coli* (EHEC). Acute hemorrhagic colitis has been associated with a specific serotype of *E. coli* 0157:H7. Two outbreaks were described in 1982,[65] caused by contaminated hamburgers in a restaurant chain. The patients presented with grossly bloody stool and crampy, abdominal pain, generally without fever. Subsequently, sporadic cases, without gross blood in the stool, have been described.[66] Most patients have a benign course, although hospitalization, because of the bloody stools, has often been recommended. Examination of the colon by endoscopy demonstrates a friable, inflamed mucosa. X-rays show mucosal involvement with submucosal edema and "thumbprinting" in the ascending and transverse colon. A potent cytotoxin, resembling the toxin produced by *Shigella,* has been demonstrated in the EIHC strains using tissue culture lines, such as Vero cells and HeLa cells.

The hemolytic-uremic syndrome (HUS) seen in young children has been associated with EHEC. An episode of diarrhea may precede HUS, or there may be no antecedent history of bowel disorders. In either situation the incriminated *E. coli* serotype (0157:H7) can be isolated from the feces, and the organism is positive in the Vero cell test for toxin production.[67] Other *E. coli* serotypes occasionally can cause hemorrhagic colitis and HUS.

Detection of EIHC in fecal specimens is rather difficult. A useful marker is the inability of this organism to ferment sorbitol. Serotyping and testing for Vero cell toxin should be performed in a reference laboratory.

Enteroadherent *E. coli* (EAEC). Adherence to the intestinal epithelium was described as a virulence factor in *E. coli* producing a diarrheal disease in rabbits (RDEC).[68] A similar phenomenon has been observed in children with chronic, mild diarrhea, resulting in failure to thrive.[69, 70] Small bowel biopsies reveal normal mucosal morphologic appearance by light microscopy. Electron microscopy shows a layer of *E. coli* bacterial cells attached to the mucosal surface; the microvilli are grossly distorted—some missing, others shortened, and others elongated. Treatment with antibiotics has not necessarily proved effective, although these children do improve slowly over time.

EAEC has also been associated with some cases of travelers' diarrhea in Mexico, according to one report.[71] The incriminated *E. coli* strains showed adherence to HEp-2 tissue culture cells in approximately 30 per cent of travelers in whom other pathogens could not be found. Although adherence seems to be an important virulence factor, other pathogenic mechanisms have not been described in the EAEC strains.

INVASIVE PATHOGENS

These organisms make their main impact on the host by invading the intestinal epithelium. Although the toxigenic organisms characteristically involve the upper intestine, the invasive pathogens target the lower bowel, particularly the distal ileum and colon. The main histologic finding is mucosal ulceration, with an acute inflammatory reaction in the lamina propria. Principal pathogens in this group are *Salmonella, Shigella,* enteroinvasive *E. coli, Campylobacter,* and *Yersinia.* Although there are important differences among these organisms, they all share the property of mucosal invasion as the initiating event.

The precise mechanism of fluid production in invasive diarrhea is not known, but three theories have been invoked:

1. An enterotoxin may be responsible for fluid production, at least in the initial phase of the illness. Most *Shigella* strains elaborate an enterotoxin that differs significantly from cholera toxin, but also causes fluid and electrolyte secretion by the intestine.[72] A similar toxin has been proposed for *Salmonella,* and there is evidence that *Campylobacter* and *Yersinia* elaborate enterotoxins.

2. Invasive organisms increase local synthesis of prostaglandins at the site of the intense inflammatory reaction. In experimental animals, fluid secretion can be blocked by prostaglandin inhibitors, such as indomethacin.[73] This theory suggests that prostaglandins are responsible for fluid secretion and subsequent diarrhea.

3. Damage to the epithelial surface may prevent reabsorption of fluids from the lumen. It does not appear that transudation of fluid from the colon is a significant factor; however, a decrease in colonic absorption of fluid, with the same level of secretion, would produce a net accumulation of fluid, resulting in diarrhea.

Shigella

Shigella organisms cause bacillary dysentery, a disease that has been described since early recorded history. The inhabitants of Athens in the second year of the Peloponnesian War were revaged by dysentery: "the disease descended to the bowels, producing violent ulceration and uncontrollable diarrhea." In the American Civil War, over 1,700,000 soldiers suffered from dysentery, with 44,500 deaths. World War I also produced a very high incidence of dysentery: 3.7 per 1000 total casualties in France and up to 486 per 1000 casualties in East Africa. Although dysentery is a disease that becomes more prevalent in wartime, there is a constant endemic incidence in tropical countries as well as in temperate zones.

Microbiology. Shigellae compose a group of gram-negative enteric organisms that are included in the Enterobacteriaceae and most closely resemble *Escherichia coli.* They are differentiated from *E. coli* by being nonmotile, not producing gas in glucose, and generally being lactose-negative. There are four major subgroups:

Group A: Serotypes of *S. dysenteriae* (10 types)
Group B: Serotypes of *S. flexneri* (six types)
Group C: Serotypes of *S. boydii* (15 types)
Group D: Serotypes of *S. sonnei* (one type)

Group A (*S. dysenteriae I*), also known as the Shiga bacillus, produces the severest form of dysentery. An outbreak in Central America in 1971 and 1972 caused over 10,000 deaths, mostly in young children.[74] *S. sonnei* produces the mildest disease.

There have been recent shifts in the incidence of dysentery as well as in the prevalence of specific serotypes. In the tropics, dysentery is mostly a disease of late summer. The better developed countries, such as the United States and those in Europe, have noted a steady increase in the incidence of dysentery, and the seasonal prevalence has shifted to winter. *S. flexneri* is the most frequent organism in tropical countries; however, in the United States and Europe, *S. flexneri* has decreased in prevalence so that *S. sonnei* is now the most common serotype causing 60 to 80 per cent of *Shigella* dysentery in the United States.

Pathogenicity. All strains of *Shigella* cause dysentery, a term that refers to a diarrheal stool that contains inflammatory exudate composed of polymorphonuclear leukocytes and blood. The dysentery of *Shigella* is also called shigellosis. The exudative character of the stool is a point to be emphasized: this is not mere watery diarrhea, but rather loose bowel movements that contain pus. The inflammatory exudate is related to the main pathologic event—namely, invasion of the colonic epithelium.[75]

Human beings are the only natural host for the dysentery organism, although monkeys and chimpanzees can become infected in captivity. Experimental infections can be produced in monkeys and guinea pigs. Mucosal invasion is demonstrated in the conjunctival sac of guinea pigs (Sereny test), and direct invasion of HeLa cells is observed in tissue culture. In experimental animal infections, the disease is made worse by starving the animals, feeding them antibiotics, or administering opium to reduce forward propulsive motility of the bowel.[76]

The major site of attack of *Shigella* is the colon. Scattered ulcerations can be seen in the terminal ileum as well. Although stomach and small bowel involvement has been noted in animal experiments and occasionally in fatal human infections, these areas are usually spared in clinical cases.

Shigellae cause intestinal disease by two mechanisms: adherence to the mucosal surface and invasion of the epithelial lining. Lacking either of these characteristics, the organisms would be rapidly cleared from the gut.[77]

Having penetrated the mucosal surface, the organisms multiply within the epithelial cells and extend the infected area by "cell-to-cell transfer" of bacilli. Time-lapse phase-contrast cinemicroscopy of HeLa cells infected with *Shigella* has shown bacilli vigorously moving throughout the cytoplasm and migrating to adjacent cells by filopodium-like protrusions.[78] Shigellae rarely penetrate beyond the intestinal mucosa and generally do not invade the blood stream. (Bacteremia does occur, however, in malnourished children and immunocompromised patients.) Presumably, both attached and intracellular organisms are elaborating toxic products. Although the initial lesions are confined to the epithelial layer, the local inflammatory response is severe, involving polymorphonuclear leukocytes and macrophages. There is edema, microabscess formation, loss of goblet cells, degeneration of normal cellular architecture, and mucosal ulceration. These events give rise to the characteristic clinical picture of bloody, mucopurulent diarrhea. As the disease progresses, the lamina propria is involved extensively with inflammatory response. Crypt abscess is a prominent feature (Fig. 63–1).

Enterotoxins. Until recently, only *S. dysenteriae* I was known to elaborate an enterotoxin. This toxin, first identified by Shiga, has since been shown to display a variety of biologic effects depending upon the experimental model employed. In brief, these include cytotoxicity (but not adenyl cyclase activation, as with cholera toxin), neurotoxicity in mice, and enterotoxicity (secretion of fluid and electrolytes). The toxin inhibits protein synthesis by irreversible inactivation of the 60S ribosomal subunit.[79]

A toxin with similar antigenic and physiologic effects has been found in strains of *S. flexneri* and *S. sonnei.*[80] It has been suggested that this toxin is more than an innocent bystander; the watery diarrhea preceding the dysenteric stage, the presence of large numbers of organisms in the terminal ileum, and the development of toxin-specific neutralizing antibody all provide evidence of a primary role for the toxin in bacillary dysentery.[81, 82]

Shigellosis is a major diarrheal disease throughout the world. The incidence of 10 to 20 per cent among all cases of diarrhea is remarkably similar from country to country. Dysentery is a disease mostly of children between the ages of six months and five years. It is rare in infants less than six months of age. In the six months to five years age group, the disease tends to be less severe than in adults. There is a synergistic relationship with malnutrition so that children with nutritional deficiencies can have severe and even fatal infections.[83]

Epidemiology. Shigellae are present in large numbers in feces, and the route of infection is oral. The organisms survive best in alkaline conditions, being very sensitive to heat and drying. Fecal specimens are the best source of positive culture; blood and urine are only rarely positive in acute cases.

Most of the transmission is person to person and is related to close human contact. There also have been dramatic epidemics related to milk, ice cream, other food, and occasionally water. The Shiga epidemic in Central America in recent years was probably related to water contamination, although such outbreaks are uncommon.[74] The incidence of infection among laboratory workers who come in contact with this organism is high.

Measurements of inoculum size in volunteers reveal that 10^5 organisms produce a 75 per cent attack rate. Inoculums above this number do not, however, increase it. There is not a good dose-response curve with *Shigella* (as contrasted with *Salmonella*); indeed, dysentery can be produced with as few as 200 bacteria.[84] Person-to-person transmission, facilitated by the low infective dose, accounts for rapid spread of *Shigella* among people living in conditions of poor hygiene. These factors also explain the high frequency of dysentery among male homosexuals[85] (see p. 1261).

Clinical Features. The classic presentation of bacillary dysentery is crampy abdominal pain, rectal burning, fever, and multiple, small volume, bloody mucoid stools.[82] However, this constellation is seen in only a minority of patients. The most constant findings are lower abdominal pain and diarrhea. Fever is present in about 40 per cent of patients, and the typical dysentery stool, consisting of blood and mucus, is seen in only one third. Many patients demostrate a biphasic illness. The initial symptoms are fever, abdominal pain, and watery diarrhea without gross blood; this stage may be related to the action of the enterotoxin. The second phase, starting three to five days after onset, is featured by tenesmus (pain upon defecation) and small volume, bloody stools. This period corresponds to invasion of the colonic epithelium and acute colitis. Although some patients have a toxic, highly febrile illness, this is usually associated with a more severe form of colitis; bacteremia, even in this setting, is distinctly uncommon. Malnutrition, especially in young children, and infection with the Shiga bacillus are

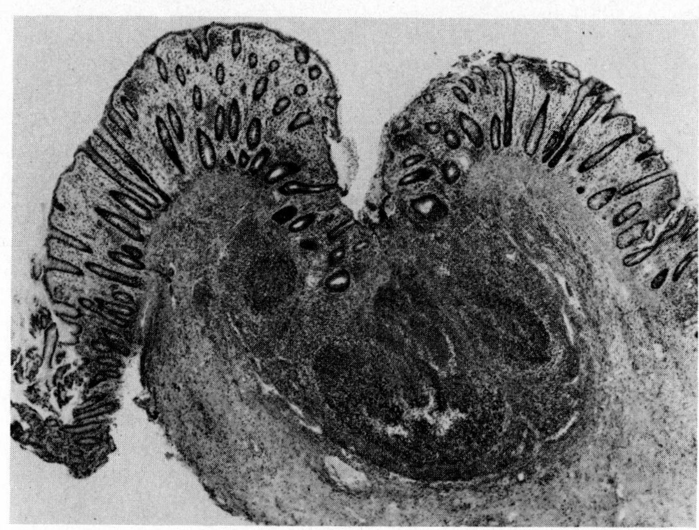

Figure 63–1. Shigellosis. This low-power magnification of the mucosa and submucosa of the colon from a patient with shigellosis shows an ulcer with central necrosis and a polymorphonuclear leukocyte infiltrate.

factors associated with a more severe course. Among the intestinal complications are intestinal perforation, toxic megacolon, and severe protein loss (see pp. 283–290).

An extensive list of extraintestinal complications is associated with bacillary dysentery.[86] Many patients complain of respiratory symptoms, such as cough and coryza, although pneumonia is rather rare. In children, several neurologic findings can dominate the clinical picture, even before the diarrheal symptoms. Stiff neck, referred to as meningismus because the cerebrospinal fluid is normal, and seizures have been noted with shigellosis, although there is not direct involvement of the central nervous system.[87] These findings have been related to the high fever, but there seems to be something unusual about their occurrence in dysentery, even when the fever is not extraordinarily high. During the acute phase, there may be a hemolytic-uremic syndrome.[88] Thrombocytopenia and a severe leukemoid reaction also have been reported.[89] Several types of rash have been noted during the acute phase of shigellosis.

Following an acute attack of dysentery, usually two to three weeks after the onset, arthritis can appear. The presentation of pain or actual effusion is usually asymmetric, with involvement of large joints. The joint complaints usually are present by themselves, without the other signs of Reiter's syndrome. Recent studies have shown that the joint complaints and other findings of Reiter's syndrome are associated more often with histocompatibility type HLA-B27.[90]

The course of shigellosis is extremely variable. Children tend to have mild infections, lasting no more than one to three days. The average length of symptoms in adults is about seven days. More severe cases have persistent symptoms for three to four weeks, often associated with relapses. Untreated bacillary dysentery, particularly with a more prolonged course, can be confused with ulcerative colitis.

Chronic carriers of *Shigella* have been identified, and they pass their organism for as long as a year or more. Such carriers are distinctly uncommon, and they usually lose the organism spontaneously. It is important to note that carriers of *Shigella* are prone to intermittent attacks of the disease. This is in contrast to *Salmonella* carriers, who rarely become infected with their own strain.

The diagnosis of shigellosis is suspected in the first instance by the constellation of lower abdomial pain, rectal burning, and diarrhea. Microscopic examination of the fecal effluent is extremely useful because it reveals multiple polymorphonuclear leukocytes and red blood cells. This information is sufficient to make diagnosis of bacillary dysentery, although the identification of the specific bacterial pathogen must await culture, because other microorganisms can cause the dysentery syndrome (*Campylobacter, Vibrio parahaemolyticus, Salmonella, Entamoeba histolytica, Balantidium coli*) (see pp. 300–302). Antibiotic sensitivity of the infecting organism should also be done to help direct therapy.

Sigmoidoscopy can confirm the diagnosis of colitis, but this procedure is not necessary in most cases of shigellosis. It is also extremely uncomfortable to have this instrument introduced into a flaming hot rectum that has been assaulted by the dysentery bacillus. If there is an urgent need to distinguish between dysentery and the acute presentation of idiopathic ulcerative colitis, a colonic biopsy may be useful when taken within four days from onset of symptoms.[91] Serologic tests are not useful in diagnosing acute cases of dysentery, although they are available for epidemiologic investigations.

A subacute presentation of dysentery can masquerade as ulcerative colitis. The patient may have endured bloody diarrhea, cramps, and rectal pain for two to four weeks. At this stage, sigmoidoscopy, barium enema, and even mucosal biopsy specimens are indistinguishable from those of patients with idiopathic ulcerative colitis (Fig. 63–2). The two major differences are a positive culture for *Shigella* and dramatic improvement in symptoms following treatment with appropriate antimicrobial agents (see pp. 1445–1446).

Deaths are rare in healthy persons, particularly adults, with bacillary dysentery; death is usually seen in very young, often malnourished children or in debilitated patients, particularly the elderly or those with immunodeficiency diseases.

Therapy. There are certain general principles in the therapeutic approach to bacillary dysentery: (1) Rehydration must be appropriately managed in any diarrheal disease, regardless of etiology; this maxim holds for dysentery. (2) The general supportive measures require attention; in the case of dysentery, children may have seizures related to fever or aseptic meningitis. (3) Narcotic-related drugs should be avoided, including tincture of opium, paregoric, diphenoxylate

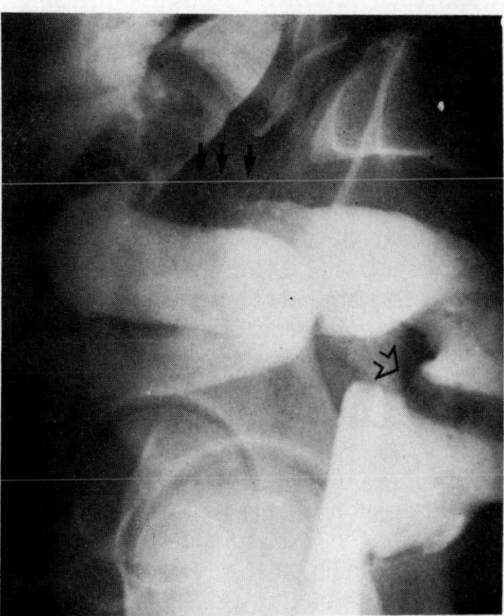

Figure 63–2. Shigellosis. The lateral view of the rectum shows narrowing and mucosal ulceration similar to that seen in ulcerative colitis. (Courtesy of H. I. Goldberg, M.D.)

(Lomotil), and loperamide (Imodium). (4) Antibiotic treatment is indicated for most individuals with shigellosis.

Fluid and Electrolyte Therapy. Most patients with dysentery can be managed with oral rehydration. It is generally suggested that glucose-containing products be administered, such as decarbonated beverages, Karo syrup plus water, the commercially available oral solutions (Lytren or Pedialyte), or the beverage Gatorade. If available, the packaged carbohydrate-electrolyte powder, mixed with drinking water, is the preferred solution (see Table 63–2). The indications for IV fluid replacement are high-volume diarrhea, with dehydration, or severe vomiting that prevents oral administration. The composition of intravenous fluids is described in Table 63–2. Fluid losses can be repaired within a few hours by intravenous solutions, and oral replacement should be encouraged as soon as possible.

High fever in children should be treated with tepid water sponges or baths. Phenobarbital is recommended (short-term) for children with seizures or aseptic meningitis. Antidiarrheal remedies are generally worthless and may even aggravate a case of bacillary dysentery. Kaolin and pectate and other "water-binding" agents do not diminish stool volume or frequency. Narcotic-containing drugs are interdicted because they can prolong the diarrhea and even provoke toxic megacolon, a dire complication of dysentery.

Antimicrobial Agents. The major determinant in the decision to employ antibiotics is the severity of the disease. In practice, moderate and severe cases of dysentery should receive antibiotic therapy.[92, 93] Mild cases often pass as self-limited events, without coming to a physician's attention. If such cases are seen in the clinic or in the doctor's office, antibiotic therapy may not be required in view of the relatively benign course. A reappraisal in such cases is made when the culture report has been returned as positive for *Shigella.* In many cases, diarrhea has already ceased. Patients with persistent diarrhea should receive antibiotics.

Ampicillin, 500 mg orally, four times daily, or 1 gm intravenously every six hours, is preferred for drug-sensitive strains when a decision has been made to begin therapy. Children should receive 50 to 100 mg per kilogram of body weight per day. Duration of therapy is five days.

R factor–mediated resistance of *Shigella* strains, particularly *S. sonnei* and *S. flexneri,* to ampicillin is widespread in some geographic areas. Resistance to ampicillin is found in 95 per cent of strains from the Washington, D.C. area; over one half of the isolates were multiply resistant to sulfonamides, tetracycline, carbenicillin, cephaloridine, and streptomycin.[94] Other centers in the United States have reported resistance to ampicillin in 30 to 70 per cent of *Shigella* strains.

When isolates in a community are known to be resistant to ampicillin, the drug of choice is trimethoprim-sulfamethoxazole, at a dose of 10 mg trimethoprim per kilogram of body weight per day and 50 mg sulfamethoxazole per kilogram of body weight per day for five days. This combination should be used also for patients with penicillin allergy. An evaluation of patients with ampicillin-sensitive strains showed no differences in clinical or bacteriologic response between trimethoprim-sulfamethoxazole and ampicillin.[95, 96] However, patients with ampicillin-resistant strains continued to have diarrhea and positive stool cultures when treated with ampicillin, but such patients responded to treatment with trimethoprim-sulfamethoxazole. Although resistance to sulfamethoxazole is common in *Shigella* strains (greater than 60 per cent), these organisms remain consistently sensitive to trimethoprim. Encouraging preliminary results in treating shigellosis have been reported with the new quinolone antibiotics, such as norfloxacin and ciprofloxacin.[97]

A single oral dose of 2.4 gm of tetracycline is effective treatment for shigellosis in adults.[98] In a reported study, eight patients with strains sensitive to tetracycline treated in this fashion had good clinical and bacteriologic responses. Sixteen of 18 symptomatic patients infected with tetracycline-resistant strains and 15 of 16 asymptomatic patients with positive stool cultures also responded to a single-dose therapy. No trial comparing this treatment regimen with standard therapy is yet available.

Antibiotics for shigellosis must be absorbed from the bowel in order to reach the population of organisms within the intestinal wall and the lamina propria, and the only effective delivery system is the blood stream.[99] Nonabsorbable drugs, such as neomycin, kanamycin, paromomycin, colistin, and polymyxin, are clinically ineffective, despite *in vitro* sensitivity. Intravenous cefamandole also has proved disappointing. Curiously, amoxicillin, which is very well absorbed and achieves higher serum levels than ampicillin, is not effective therapy for shigellosis.[100]

Chronic carriers of *Shigella* are unusual. Postinfection carriage is generally less than three to four weeks and rarely exceeds three to four months. In circumstances in which eradication of the carrier state is deemed necessary, trimethoprim-sulfamethoxazole is very effective, having eliminated the carrier state in about 90 per cent of patients.[101] The dose of trimethoprim was 5 mg per kilogram of body weight per day and for sulfamethoxazole it was 25 mg per kilogram of body weight per day for 28 days.

Mild, grinding diarrhea and cramps may continue for many days after treatment of bacillary dysentery, even when the organism is no longer present and the acute episode seems to have passed. These symptoms are not necessarily a cause for alarm, as the bowel may have sustained severe mucosal injury that requires a certain period of time for repair.

Instances of *chronic ulcerative colitis* have been traced to a proven attack of dysentery, but such cases are rare. It should be recalled that certain antibiotics, especially ampicillin, have a high incidence of intestinal side effects, including *Clostridium difficile*–associated diarrhea, and a persistent diarrhea must be evaluated in terms of a possible untoward drug reaction (see pp. 1307–1320 and 1435–1477). Finally, shigellosis is a highly contagious disease. Spread within a family is common. Secondary cases can occur in hospitals, both among other hapless patients and among nurses and physicians. Careful hand washing should avoid dissemination of this disease.

Nontyphoidal Salmonellosis

Nontyphoidal salmonellosis refers to disease caused by any serotype of the genus *Salmonella,* with the exception of *S. typhi.* Approximately 1700 serotypes and variants are potentially pathogenic for animals and human beings. Recently, the salmonellae have been classified into three primary species: *Salmonella typhi, S. cholerae-suis,* and *S. enteritidis.* The first two species have only one serotype each, leaving the other 1700 serotypes in the species *S. enteritidis.* Using this formal taxonomic classifiction, one would designate serotypes as follows: *S. enteritidis* sertoype *typhimurium* or *S. enteritidis* serotype *agona.* For convenience, most workers bypass this awkward formality in favor of the more familiar convention of designating an organism by the genus and serotype, such as *S. typhimurium* or *S. agona.*

Microbiology. *Salmonella* is a large group of gram-negative bacilli that compose one of the six divisions in the family of Enterobacteriaceae. Most strains are motile and produce acid and gas from glucose, mannitol, and sorbitol (except *S. typhi* and rare others that produce only acid); they are active elaborators of hydrogen sulfide, and they are closely related to each other by somatic and flagellar antigens. These organisms are primarily intestinal parasites, although some can be found in the blood stream and internal organs or invertebrates; they are frequently isolated in sewage, river water, seawater, and certain foods. Most salmonellae have a wide range of hosts.

These bacteria grow on several types of artificial media. However, they can be separated on differential media by the inclusion of certain chemicals that favor their growth and suppress other coliforms; i.e., brilliant green, selenite, tetrathionate, lithium, and bile salts. Most strains die at 55°C in one hour, or at 60°C in 15 to 20 minutes.

The initial separation of *Salmonella* from other bacteria is based on biochemical characteristics. The biochemically positive organisms have antigenic similarity to other *Salmonella* strains, and it is the antigenic structure that confers the species designation. It must be emphasized that the possession of *Salmonella* antigens does not automatically qualify an organism for inclusion in this group. To qualify as a *Salmonella* requires the proper antigens and the biochemical characteristics.

Antigens. There are now nearly 1700 serotypes and variants of *Salmonella.* The typing scheme is based on the antigenic structure, but in recent years the name of the strain has been derived from the city in which it was first isolated; i.e., Montivideo, Heidelberg, Dublin, Newport, and so on. Most salmonellae are flagellated; utilizing the proper growth conditions, the H (flagellar) and O (somatic) antigens can be tested separately.

In addition to H and O antigens, some strains, notably typhoid bacilli, have an additional somatic antigen associated with virulence (V_1). The V_1 antigen prevents agglutination with O antigen. A positive correlation exists between virulence in mice and the amount of V_1 antigen in a specific strain. However, this correlation does not necessarily carry over to human beings because even typhoid bacilli without measurable V_1 antigen can be pathogenic for humans. A bacteriophage typing system against the V_1 antigen is used for epidemiologic investigation of typhoid outbreaks. Over 70 anti-V_1 phage types have been identified.

For convenience in the laboratory, a series of Kauffmann-White groups containing several serotypes has been developed, and these are based on shared antigens among the most common *Salmonella* types. There are now some 40 recognized groups. Human cases generally fall into groups A to E; 90 per cent of *Salmonella* pathogenic for human beings are in groups B, C, and D.

Pathogenic Mechanisms. Many serotypes are restricted to animals and have narrow host preferences. Some strains, however, are less fastidious and can cause serious human infection. Their main portal of entry is via the mouth and gastrointestinal tract. These organisms are unique in attacking the ileum and to a lesser extent, the colon. They cause mild mucosal ulcerations and rapidly make their way through the epithelial surface to the lamina propria, and thence to the lymphatics and blood stream. Histologic sections show edematous, shortened crypts; invasion of the lamina propria by polymorphonuclear leukocytes; and rapid spread of infection to other organs by hematogenous dissemination.[102, 103]

Two virulence factors in *Salmonella* strains affect the bowel: one involves mucosal invasion and the other causes net fluid and electrolyte secretion into the bowel lumen. The invasive factor produces mucosal wall infection and bacteremia, and the other causes diarrhea.[104]

The exact mechanisms responsible for diarrhea are not clear, although penetration and inflammation appear to be important components. Studies in a rabbit ligated loop model have demonstrated that nonpenetrating strains of *Salmonella* fail to produce diarrhea.[104] Certain strains are capable of invading the mucosa, but they are unable to cause fluid accumulation if they lack the "secretory" factor. Studies have shown that cyclic AMP can be stimulated by some strains that produce fluid accumulation. Indomethacin, which blocks prostaglandin synthesis, inhibits intestinal secretion in experimental *Salmonella* infections.[73, 105] Thus, *Salmonella* may produce prostaglandin-stimulating factors that in turn act on the adenylate cyclase system.

The infectivity of a specific strain is related to its serotype and the inoculum size. For example, 10^5 *S. newport* organisms produce illness in some volunteers, whereas 10^9 *S. pullorum* organisms are unable to do so.[106, 107] The latter strain is poorly adapted to humans, as suggested by its rarity in clinical infections, but it is well adapted to chickens, from which it is frequently isolated. A dose-response curve has been determined for certain strains of *Salmonella.* An approximately 50 per cent infection rate is seen with 10^7 organisms, whereas the infectivity raises to 90 per cent at 10^9 organisms.

In experimental animals, the number of bacteria required to produce infections can be reduced by pretreating the animals with antibiotics. In addition, reduced or absent gastric acid is known to increase the susceptibility to infection because acid in the stomach kills off many of the challenge organisms.

Clinical Features. Five clinical syndromes are seen with *Salmonella* (Table 63–5): (1) gastroenteritis, noted in 75 per cent of *Salmonella* infections; (2) bacteremia, with or without gastrointestinal involvement, seen in approximately 10 per cent of the cases; (3) typhoidal or "enteric fever," seen with all typhoid strains and in approximately 8 per cent of other *Salmonella* infections; (4) localized infections, i.e., in bones, joints, and meninges, seen in approximately 5 per cent; and (5) a carrier state in asymptomatic individuals (the organism is usually harbored in the gallbladder).[108]

The most common syndrome is *gastroenteritis.* The usual incubation period is six to 48 hours, although latency could last as long as seven to 12 days. The initial symptoms are nausea and vomiting, followed by abdominal cramps and diarrhea. The diarrhea usually lasts three or four days and is accompanied by fever in about 50 per cent of individuals. In general, the pain of *Salmonella* gastroenteritis is located in the periumbilical area or the right lower quadrant. The diarrhea can vary from a few loose stools to dysentery with grossly bloody and purulent feces, to a cholera-like syndrome.[109, 110] The latter condition, with massive purging, has been described in patients with achlorhydria.[111] Persistent fever or specific findings on physical examination suggest bacteremia or focal infection. *Salmonella* bacteremia is similar to sepsis from any other gram-negative bacteria, although there is an impression that it is less severe. A persistent form of *Salmonella* bacteremia is seen in patients with AIDS[112] (see pp. 1245–1248).

Table 63–5. CLINICAL SYNDROMES OF *SALMONELLA* INFECTION

Syndrome	Incidence (%)
Gastroenteritis	75
Mild	
Dehydrating	
Colitis ("dysenteric")	
Bacteremia	5–10
With or without gastroenteritis	
Endocarditis	
Arteritis	
AIDS	
Typhoidal ("enteric fever")	5–10
With or without gastroenteritis	
Localized	5
Meninges	
Bones, joints	
Wounds	
Abscesses	
Gallbladder	
Carrier state (> one year)	<1

Table 63–6. PREDISPOSING CONDITIONS IN *SALMONELLA* INFECTION

Hemolytic anemia
Sickle-cell disease
Malaria
Bartonellosis
Malignancy
Lymphoma
Leukemia
Disseminated carcinoma
Immunosuppression
AIDS
Steroid therapy
Chemotherapy
Radiation
Achlorhydria
Gastroduodenal surgery
Idiopathic
Ulcerative colitis
Schistosomiasis

Once the organism invades the blood stream, almost any organ can become involved. Meningitis, arteritis, endocarditis, osteomyelitis, wound infections, septic arthritis, and focal abscesses all have been recorded.[108–110]

Patients become chronic carriers of nontyphoidal *Salmonella* as a consequence of either symptomatic or asymptomatic infections. The overall carrier rate is between 2 and 6 per 1000 infected individuals. Children, especially neonates, and patients over age 60 years tend to become carriers more frequently. Also, structural abnormalities in the biliary tract, such as cholelithiasis, or in the urinary tract, such as nephrolithiasis, predispose and perpetuate the carrier state.[113]

Predisposing Conditions. A number of associated conditions seem to increase the risk of salmonellosis (Table 63–6). The relationship between sickle cell anemia and *Salmonella* osteomyelitis has been well documented.[114] Indeed, several forms of hemolytic anemia predispose to this infection, including malaria, bartonellosis, and louse-borne relapsing fever.[109, 114]

The presumed mechanism of increased susceptibility is blockage of the reticuloendothelial system by macrophages ingesting breakdown products of red blood cells, thereby reducing their ability to phagocytize salmonellae.[115] Recent studies also have shown a decreased capacity for patients with sickle cell anemia to opsonize salmonellae because of defective activation of the alternative complement pathway.[116]

Neoplastic disease has been associated with an increased risk of salmonellosis. *Leukemia, lymphomas,* and *disseminated malignancy* appear to predispose patients to blood stream invasion by this organism.[117, 118] Use of corticosteroids, chemotherapy, and radiotherapy also is associated with *Salmonella* sepsis. In AIDS patients persistent *Salmonella* bacteremia, only temporarily yielding to antibiotic therapy, is related to the profound suppression of cell-mediated immunity[112] (see pp. 1245–1248).

Gastric surgery appears to be an important predisposing condition in the development of *Salmonella* infection.[119] The obvious implication is that destruction of the gastric acid barrier enhances the host's susceptibility to infection.

All three forms of schistosomiasis have been associated with invasive salmonellosis.[120] Salmonellae, as well as other gram-negative bacteria, are capable of penetrating and multiplying within the parasites, which then serve as a source for recurrent bacteremia or bacilluria.

Ulcerative colitis may predispose to *Salmonella* infection and an increased carrier state, although this implication is based upon only a few retrospective studies. One such analysis found that 5 per cent of patients with idiopathic ulcerative colitis harbored *Salmonella* in their stool.[121]

***Salmonella* Colitis.** Involvement of the colon in the course of *Salmonella* gastroenteritis probably is rather common, at least on the basis of animal studies and proctoscopy examinations in selected patients.[122] Although the great majority of patients with *Salmonella* present with mild diarrhea and watery bowel movements, in a small but important group colonic involvement dominates the clinical picture. Patients with *Salmonella* colitis typically have 10 to 15 days of diarrhea before the diagnosis is established. In contrast, patients with the usual form of gastroenteritis are symptomatic for five days or less. In the colonic form, the diarrhea is more persistent, even though the organism may have disappeared from the feces. Bowel movements are grossly bloody in approximately half the patients. Proctoscopic findings include hyperemia, granularity, friability, and ulcerations. Rectal biopsy specimens reveal mucosal ulcerations, hemorrhage, and crypt abscesses. Barium enema films confirm these findings, usually showing a patchy, global colitis. In the acute period, there is no reliable method to distinguish idiopathic ulcerative colitis from *Salmonella* colitis, except by positive stool culture. However, a patient with an acute onset of colitis, without a past history, who has symptoms of three weeks' or less duration should be considered to have an infectious form of colitis, and *Salmonella,* as well as *Shigella* and *Campylobacter,* must be important considerations.

The course of *Salmonella* colitis is variable. It can last for as short a time as one week or go on for two to three months. The average duration of illness is three weeks. Complications include toxic megacolon, bleeding, and overwhelming sepsis.

Although no prospective trial evaluating antibiotic therapy in *Salmonella* colitis has been performed, it seems reasonable to administer antibiotics, at least to eradicate the organisms from the stool. It is also important to recognize this disease so that inappropriate therapy is not administered. Corticosteroids can exacerbate *Salmonella* colitis, producing silent perforation and septicemia.[123] Finally, patients can be reassured of the self-limited course of *Salmonella* colitis, as opposed to the chronic, relapsing course of idiopathic ulcerative colitis.

Immunology (see pp. 1233–1248). Mucosal immunity plays a key role in protection against *Salmonella* infection. Macrophages in Peyer's patches and the lamina propria, activated by T-lymphocytes through the release of lymphokines, phagocytose and destroy the organism.[124] Certain virulent strains, such as *S. typhi* and *S. cholerae-suis,* are able to survive in macrophages and make their way to the blood stream. During the hematogenous stage of dissemination, circulating organisms are removed from the blood stream and are sequestered in the reticuloendothelial cells of the liver and spleen. If the host is successful in containing the infection, the organisms are killed in these cells. If the organism is particularly virulent, it may divide and multiply within the reticuloendothelial cells and then break out for another phase of bacteremia. Antibiotics have difficulty in penetrating reticuloendothelial cells, and the organisms are somewhat protected from drugs in this location. Deficiencies in cell-mediated immunity and sequestration in reticuloendothelial cells are the explanations for continued infection with relapses and remissions often seen in *Salmonella* infections.

Antibody is formed against both somatic and flagella antigens. The anti-O antibody is the first to rise, reaching its peak in the third week of infection and falling off during the subsequent weeks. The H antibody rises more slowly after several weeks of infection, but it maintains a high level for many months following infection. These humoral antibodies, while impressively high in some people, are not correlated well with protection against *Salmonella* infection. The laboratory examination for H and O antibody is called the Widal test.

Epidemiology. *Salmonella* is one of the great foodborne infections.[125] The major route of passage is by five Fs: flies, food, fingers, feces, and fomites. The disease can cause large outbreaks, often associated with common-source routes of spread. A frequent setting is an institution supper or a barbecue. Community outbreaks may persist for several months. For example, Riverside, California, experienced an epidemic involving 16,000 persons that raged for many months and was related to a contaminated municipal water supply.[126]

In the United States, there are approximately 500 isolates of *Salmonella* per week from humans and approximately 400 from nonhuman sources. The incidence in England is 28 times higher, presumably related to the superior English reporting system rather than to inferior hygiene. The most common serotype in the United States is *S. typhimurium,* followed by *S. enteritidis, S. newport, S. heidelberg,* and *S. infantis.*

The marked similarity in the frequency of serotypes isolated from human and animal sources suggests that nonhuman reservoirs play a crucial role in the transmission of the disease (Table 63–7). When one examines recognized common-source outbreaks, the importance of animal reservoirs is easily discerned. In 500 outbreaks investigated over a ten-year period, almost 50 per cent were related to animals or animal products.

Table 63–7. THE 20 MOST FREQUENTLY REPORTED *SALMONELLA* SEROTYPES FROM HUMAN AND NONHUMAN SOURCES,* 1978

Human					Nonhuman			
Rank	*Serotype*	*Number*	*Per Cent*	*Rank Last Year*	*Rank*	*Serotype*	*Number*	*Per Cent*
1	*typhimurium*†	10,015	34.8	1	1	*typhimurium*	222	10.8
2	*heidelberg*	2,078	7.2	3	2	*derby*	180	8.8
3	*enteritidis*	1,934	6.7	4	3	*agona*	158	7.7
4	*newport*	1,879	6.5	2	4	*manhattan*	127	6.2
5	*agona*	1,229	4.3	6	5	*panama*	119	5.8
6	*infantis*	1,225	4.3	5	6	*heidelberg*	103	5.0
7	*montevideo*	703	2.4	9	7	*tennessee*	103	5.0
8	*typhi*	604	2.1	8	8	*london*	79	3.9
9	*saint-paul*	602	2.1	7	9	*meleagridis*	73	3.6
10	*javiana*	528	1.8	11	10	*infantis*	68	3.3
	Subtotal	20,797	72.3			Subtotal	1,232	60.1
11	*blockley*	494	1.7	14	11	*habana*	66	3.2
12	*oranienburg*	487	1.7	10	12	*montevideo*	62	3.0
13	*derby*	346	1.2	12	13	*worthington*	59	2.9
14	*muenchen*	293	1.0	13	14	*anatum*	56	2.7
15	*anatum*	262	0.9	16	15	*enteritidis*	42	2.0
16	*java*	257	0.9	20	16	*newport*	33	1.6
17	*thompson*	245	0.9	18	17	*kentucky*	29	1.4
18	*panama*	220	0.8	15	18	*weltevreden*	25	1.2
19	*bredeney*	218	0.8	22	19	*oranienburg*	23	1.1
20	*braenderup*	204	0.7	21	20	*choleraesuis*‡	23	1.1
	Subtotal	23,823	82.9			Subtotal	1,650	80.3
All other serotypes		4,925			All other serotypes		398	
	Total	28,748				Total	2,048	

*Reported to the Center for Disease Control.
†Includes var. copenhagen.
‡Includes var. kunzendorf.
From the Center for Disease Control: *Salmonella* Surveillance, Annual Summary 1978. U.S. Department of Health and Human Services, Public Health Service, Jan., 1981.

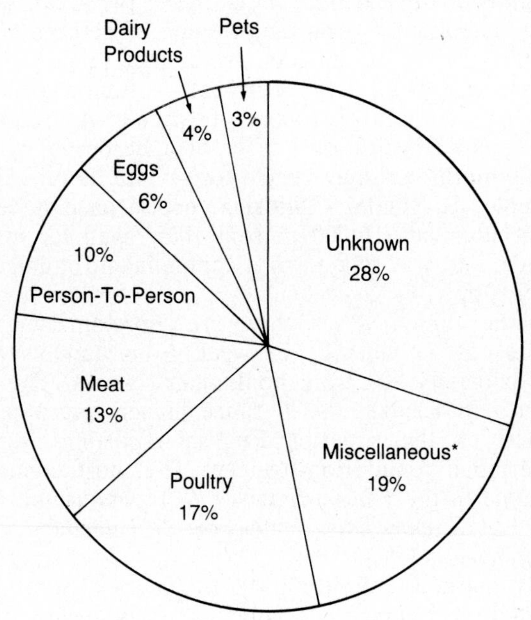

Figure 63–3. Mode of transmission in 500 human salmonellosis outbreaks between 1966 and 1975. (Redrawn from the Center for Disease Control, Salmonella Surveillance, Annual Summary, 1976. Washington, D.C., U.S. Department of Health, Education and Welfare, Public Health Service, 1977.)

Poultry, meats, eggs, and dairy products are most frequently involved (Fig. 63–3).

Salmonellae have a tendency to colonize domestic animals. Poultry has the highest incidence of *Salmonella* carriage, particularly chickens and ducks. Pigs and cattle also are heavily contaminated. Many of these animals can cohabit peacefully with their salmonellae and are usually asymptomatic. Among the other animals that have been known to harbor *Salmonella* are buffalo, sheep, dog, cat, rat, mouse, guinea pig, hamster, seal, donkey, turkey, dove, pigeon, parrot, sparrow, lizard, whale, tortoise, house fly, tick, louse, flea, and cockroach, to name but a few.

Commercially prepared food may be contaminated with salmonellae: 40 per cent of turkeys examined in California, 50 per cent of chickens in Massachusetts, and 20 per cent of commercial egg whites have been shown in surveys to harbor these organisms. Large national and international outbreaks have been traced to commercially prepared chocolate balls, precooked roast beef, smoked whitefish, frozen eggs, and powdered milk. Other commercial products not directly related to foods, such as carmine dye or brewer's yeast, can be contaminated and may be transmitted to humans. Contaminated pets, especially turtles, have been implicated in the transmission of salmonellosis. These microorganisms have been isolated from many types of animals, and all pets should be considered potential carriers whether or not they show signs of illness.

Salmonellae are so ubiquitous in our environment that it is extraordinary that so few human infections are encountered.

Attack rates of *Salmonella* show a strong relationship to age. Children younger than one year of age have the highest attack rate, especially in the subset of three to five-month-old infants. The susceptibility of infants may be related to immunologic immaturity. There is also a high attack rate and increased mortality rate in individuals over age 70 years (Fig. 63–4).

Treatment. Although a large number of antibiotics have been used to treat nontyphoidal *Salmonella* gastroenteritis, all have failed to alter the rate of clinical recovery. In fact, antibiotic therapy increases the incidence and duration of intestinal carriage of these organisms. In one report,[127] 185 patients with *S. typhimurium* gastroenteritis were treated with either chloramphenicol or ampicillin; stools from 65.4 per cent were still positive for the organism 12 days after exposure, and 27 per cent were positive at 31 days. In contrast, of 87 who were not treated, only 42.5 per cent and 11.5 per cent of stool cultures were positive at 12 and 31 days, respectively. *Salmonella* strains resistant to one or more antibiotics were isolated from 9.7 per cent of patients treated with antibiotics, whereas no resistant strains were obtained from untreated patients. On the basis of this study, as well as others,[128, 129] it is apparent that antimicrobial therapy should not be employed in most cases of *Salmonella* gastroenteritis.

Despite this general rule, some clinical situations dictate that antibiotics should be used when a disorder is complicated by *Salmonella* gastroenteritis (Table 63–8); lymphoproliferative disorders; malignancies; immunosuppressed hosts (AIDS and congenital forms); transplant patients; known or suspected abnormalities of the cardiovascular system, such as prosthetic heart valves, vascular grafts, aneurysms, and rheumatic or congenital valvular heart disease; individuals with foreign bodies implanted in the skeletal system; patients with hemolytic anemias; and patients at the extreme ages of life. In addition, treatment should be used in patients with *Salmonella* gastroenteritis when they exhibit findings of severe sepsis, that is, high fever, rigors, hypotension, decreased renal function, and systemic toxicity.

If a decision is made to initiate therapy in these selected patients, ampicillin or trimethoprim-sulfamethoxazole is an appropriate drug. The dose of ampicillin is 50 to 100 mg per kilogram of body weight per day in divided doses, orally or parenterally, for 10 to 14 days. Trimethoprim-sulfamethoxazole is administered at a dose of 10 mg per kilogram of body weight per day for trimethoprim and 50 mg per kilogram of body weight per day for sulfamethoxazole, to a maximum of four tablets (320 mg and 1600 mg) per day for two weeks.

Resistance to more than one drug among nontyphoidal species of *Salmonella* appears to be increasing. The results of a nationwide study published in 1968

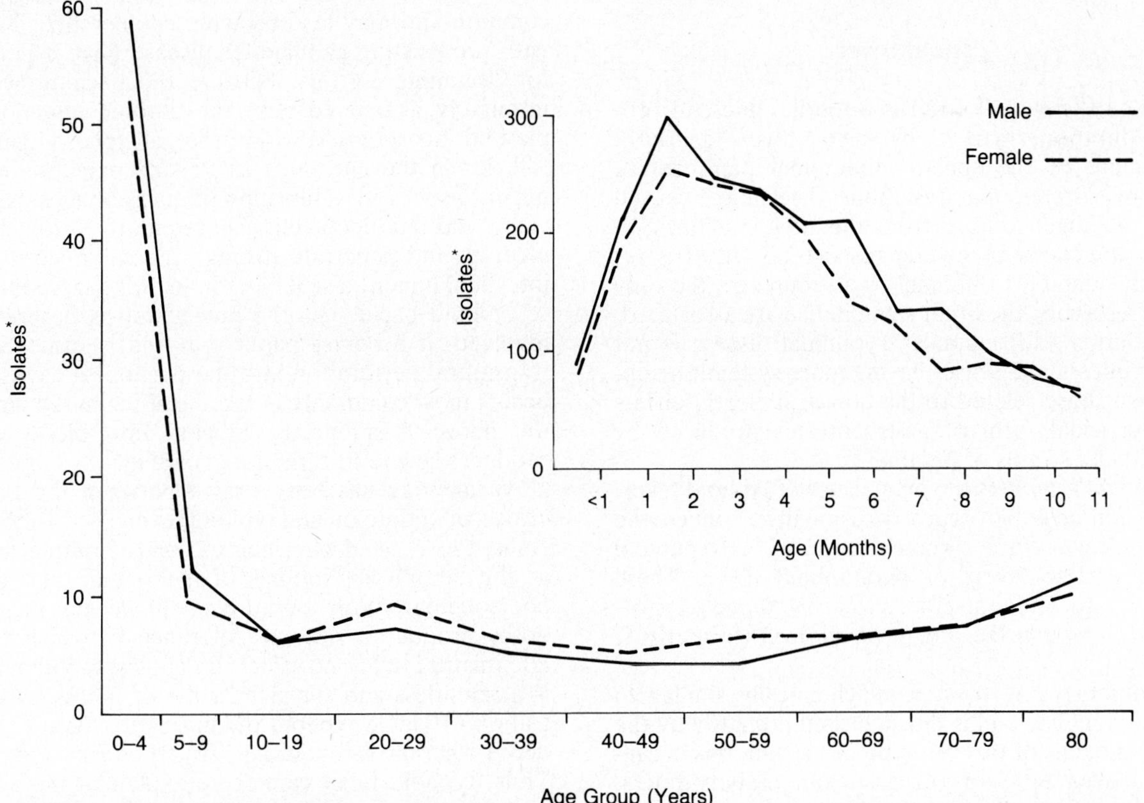

Figure 63–4. Salmonella attack rates, by age, in the United States during 1978. (Redrawn from the Center for Disease Control, Salmonella Surveillance, Annual Summary, 1978. Washington, D.C., U.S. Department of Health and Human Services, Public Health Service, 1981.)

Table 63–8. INDICATIONS FOR THERAPY IN *SALMONELLA* GASTROENTERITIS

Lymphoproliferative disorders
Leukemia
Lymphoma
Malignancies
Immunosuppression
AIDS
Congenital and other acquired forms
Corticosteroids
Transplant patients
Abnormal cardiovascular system
Prosthetic heart valves
Vascular grafts
Aneurysms
Valvular heart disease
Prosthetic orthopedic devices
Hemolytic anemia
Extreme ages of life
Severe sepsis, toxicity

demonstrated that 22 per cent of nontyphoidal strains of *Salmonella* were resistant to one or more antibiotics. Resistance to streptomycin, tetracycline, sulfathiazole, and ampicillin were most common, occurring in 8 to 14 per cent of strains. A study from New York in 1975 documented resistance to four or more drugs in 50 per cent of isolates of *S. typhimurium* and *S. newport.*[130] However, the incidence of chloramphenicol resistance in nontyphoidal strains of *Salmonella* in the United States is still very low, and this drug should be used in the event of multiple drug resistance.

Typhoid Fever

Typhoid ("cloudy") fever is a febrile illness of prolonged duration, marked by hectic fever, delirium, enlargement of the spleen, abdominal pain, and a variety of systemic manifestations. The illness caused by this pathogen differs from the nontyphoidal *Salmonella* infections in several respects. *S. typhi* is remarkably adapted to humans, who represent the only natural reservoir; the other salmonellae are associated, by and large, with animals. Typhoidal disease is not truly an intestinal disease, having more systemic symptoms than those related to the bowel; it clearly differs from the usual form of gastroenteritis produced by nontyphoidal strains of *Salmonella*.

Although *S. typhi* is the main cause of typhoid fever, other *Salmonella* serotypes occasionally produce the same clinical features, known variously as typhoidal disease, enteric fever, or paratyphoid fever. These serotypes are *S. paratyphi* A, *S. schottmuelleri* (formerly *S. paratyphi* B), and *S. hirschfeldii* (formerly *S. paratyphi* C).

Microbiology. *S. typhi* is biochemically similar to other salmonellae and is distinguished primarily by the specific antigens of this serotype. As a rule, this organism produces little or no gas from carbohydrates, elaborates only small amounts of hydrogen sulfide, and bears the V_1 antigen on its surface. These biochemical characters should alert the laboratory to the possibility of this pathogen; confirmation of *S. typhi* is accomplished by serologic testing.

Pathogenic Mechanisms. The pathologic events of typhoid fever are initiated in the intestinal tract following oral ingestion of typhoid bacilli.[131] The organism penetrates the small bowel mucosa, sparing the stomach, and makes its way rapidly to the lymphatics, the mesenteric nodes, and within minutes, to the blood stream. There is a paucity of local inflammatory findings, which explains the lack of intestinal symptoms at this stage. This sequence of events is in marked contrast to that of other forms of salmonellosis and to shigellosis, in which the intestinal findings are prominent at the onset.

Following the initial bacteremia, the organism is sequestered in macrophages and monocytic cells of the reticuloendothelial system. It undergoes multiplication, and re-emerges several days later in recurrent waves of bacteremia, an event that initiates the symptomatic phase of infection. Now in great numbers, the organism is spread throughout the host, infecting many organ sites. The intestinal tract may be seeded by direct bacteremic spread, as, for example, to Peyer's patches in the terminal ileum. Alternatively, the gallbladder contains a large number of bacilli, and contaminated bile is another method of infecting the gut.[132]

Hyperplasia of the reticuloendothelial system, including lymph nodes, liver, and spleen, is characteristic of typhoid fever. The liver contains discrete, micronodular areas of necrosis, surrounded by macrophages and lymphocytes. Inflammation of the gallbladder is common and may lead to acute cholecystitis. Patients with pre-existing gallbladder disease have a penchant for becoming carriers, because the bacillus becomes intimately associated with the chronic infection and may be incorporated within the gallstones. Lymphoid follicles in the gut, such as Peyer's patches, become hyperplastic, with infiltration of macrophages, lymphocytes, and red blood cells. Subsequently, a follicle may ulcerate and penetrate through the submucosa to the intestinal lumen, discharging in its wake large numbers of typhoid bacilli. As the bowel wall is progressively involved, it becomes paper thin and is susceptible to transmural perforation into the peritoneal cavity. This occurs most commonly in the distal ileum, 24 cm from the ileocecal sphincter. Erosion into blood vessels produces severe intestinal hemorrhage.

An analogy has been drawn between the biologic effects of endotoxin and typhoid fever.[131, 133] Both cause chills, fever, headache, nausea, and vomiting, as well as the laboratory findings of leukopenia and thrombocytopenia. With endotoxin, however, increasing doses produce a state of tolerance in which further administration has no effect. By contrast, typhoid fever is a relentless and sustained state of illness. Administration of viable typhoid organisms to volunteers rendered tolerant to endotoxin still produces symptoms. Thus, typhoid fever cannot be explained merely as a reaction to endotoxin, although this material may play some role in the disease state.

Clinical Features. In its classical form without treatment, typhoid fever lasts about four weeks, evolving in a manner consistent with the pathologic events. The illness is described traditionally as a series of one-week stages, although this pattern may be altered in mild cases and by antibiotic treatment.[134–136] The incubation period is generally seven to 14 days, with wide variations at either extreme. During the first week, high fever, headache, and abdominal pain are commonly encountered. The pulse is often slower than would be expected for the degree of temperature elevation. The abdominal pain is localized to the right lower quadrant in most instances, although it can be diffuse. In approximately 50 per cent of patients, there is no change in bowel habits; in fact, constipation is more common than diarrhea in children with typhoid fever. Near the end of the first week, enlargement of the spleen is noticeable, and an evanescent, classic rash, "rose spots," becomes manifest at this time.

During the second week, the fever becomes more continuous, and the patient looks sick and withdrawn. During the third week the patient's illness evolves into the "typhoidal state," with disordered mentation and, in some cases, extreme toxemia. In this period there is often intestinal involvement, manifested clinically by greenish, "pea-soup" diarrhea and the dire complications of intestinal perforation and hemorrhage. The fourth week brings slackening of the fever and improvement in the clinical status.

Typhoid fever is a less severe illness in previously healthy adults who seek medical attention for the earliest symptoms of fever, lassitude, and headache. Prompt diagnosis and appropriate therapy interrupt the classic four-week scenario, producing an aborted illness consisting of little more than a few days of fever and malaise.

Because the typhoid bacillus is widely disseminated through recurrent waves of bacteremia, many organ sites are involved. Thus, patients with typhoid fever can have pneumonia, headache, delirium, pyelonephritis, and metastases to bone, large joints, and the brain. The gallbladder and liver are involved with inflammatory changes. Acute cholecystitis can occur during the initial two to three weeks, and jaundice, because of diffuse hepatic inflammation, has been observed in some patients.

The pre-eminent complications are intestinal hemorrhage and perforation.[137] These events are most apt to occur in the third week during convalescence and are not closely related to the severity of the disease. However, they tend to occur in the same patient, with the bleeding serving as a harbinger of a possible perforation. Bleeding may be either sudden and severe, or may be a slow ooze. Prior to chemotherapy, the incidence of hemorrhage was 7 to 20 per cent in various series; it is somewhat less frequent since specific treatment has been available. The ileum is the main site of bowel perforation. The onset may be sudden, with signs of an acute abdomen, or there may be a leak of intraluminal contents to form an abscess in the lower quadrant or pelvis, producing a more chronic, insidious course. Approximately 3 per cent of patients with typhoid fever experience intestinal perforation.

After defervescence has occurred and the patient has apparently "ridden through the storm," a potential for recurrence remains. The relapse generally occurs eight to ten days after cessation of drug therapy and consists of a re-enactment of the major manifestations. The organism is the same as the one causing the original infection, maintaining the identical antimicrobial susceptibility pattern.

Carriers. After six weeks, approximately 50 per cent of typhoid victims are still shedding the organism in their feces. This figure progressively declines so that after three months only 5 to 10 per cent are excretors, and by one year the incidence is 1 to 3 per cent.[136, 138] The chronic carrier is identified by positive stool cultures for *S. typhi* at least one year following the episode or, in some cases, positive stool cultures without a documented history of disease. The probability of spontaneously aborting the carrier state is very unlikely after this time. Chronic carriers are more common in older age groups, in women (a 3:1 ratio of women to men), and in people with gallbladder disease. The organism is usually harbored in the gallbladder, often forming part of the gallstones. Occasionally, the organism is carried in the large intestine, without involvement of the biliary tract.

Diagnosis. The diagnosis of typhoid fever is established by isolating the organism. The blood culture is the primary diagnostic test; it is positive in 90 per cent of the patients during the first week and remains positive for several weeks thereafter if the patient is untreated. Bone marrow culture also has a high yield, even in the treated patient.[139] Stool cultures become positive in the second and third weeks. By the third week, urine cultures reveal the organism in approximately one third of the patients. The titer of agglutinins (Widal test) against somatic (O) antigen rises during the third week of illness. An O titer of 1:80 or more in nonimmunized individuals is suggestive of typhoid fever. Higher initial titers or a fourfold rise provides stronger evidence. The H antigen is more nonspecific and is likely to be elevated from prior immunization or by infection with other enteric bacteria. There are many false positive and occasional false negative Widal reactions, so that a diagnosis based on titer rise alone is tenuous.

Epidemiology. Improvements in environmental sanitation have reduced the incidence of typhoid fever in the industrialized nations. Approximately 500 cases occur each year in the United States, chiefly in young people. Most cases are sporadic but they are invariably related to a human carrier. Large-scale epidemics of typhoid occur on a regular basis; they are usually traced to contaminated food that may be imported from an endemic area or to contaminated water supplies.

Because *S. typhi* cohabits exclusively with human beings, the appearance of a single case means the presence of a carrier. An investigation by public health authorities should be instituted to determine the source and the presence of other cases. As they are discovered, chronic carriers are registered with the health authorities, and the microorganism is phage-typed so that it can be traced in the event of an outbreak. However, the registered carriers represent only a minority of the potential reservoir and do not take account of the "imported" cases of typhoid, which include nearly half the acute infections in the United States.

Treatment. Drug resistance, mediated by plasmids, can occur among typhoid bacilli. Most strains are susceptible to chloramphenicol and ampicillin, although notable epidemics with strains resistant to either of these drugs have been reported in recent years. Hence, a great effort should be made in each case to isolate the organism and to perform drug susceptibility tests. Chloramphenicol remains the standard therapy because of its proved efficacy and its high activity against most clinical isolates of typhoid bacilli. The response to therapy is remarkably constant, as defervescence regularly occurs three to five days after initiating treatment.[137] The clinical condition improves within one to two days, with decreased toxemia and slowly declining fever. In adults, chloramphenicol should be given in a total daily dose of 2 to 4 gm, administered in four equally divided doses. Occasionally, in very sick patients, it may be necessary to give the drug by the intravenous route, and the same total daily dose of 2 to 4 gm should be used. Oral medication can then be given after improvement in the clinical status. Chloramphenicol is well absorbed from the intestinal tract, but is rather poorly absorbed from intramuscular sites. Thus, the intramuscular route is to be avoided. The duration of treatment is two weeks; prolongation of this treatment does not reduce the incidence of complications or carriers. Intestinal perforation and hemorrhage can occur during what is apparently successful treatment. Relapse may follow an otherwise uneventful course and should be treated with the same drug.

Ampicillin has been recommended as an alternative therapy, but it has been somewhat disappointing in comparison with chloramphenicol.[134, 140, 141] The dose is 6 gm per day, intravenously, in four to six divided doses. Amoxicillin, a closely related drug, provides better absorption and increased efficacy. Several studies have shown that amoxicillin, in doses of 4 gm per day in four divided doses, has good activity.[142, 143] Trimethoprim-sulfamethoxazole also has been used in the therapy of typhoid fever, and the results are promising.[144, 145]

Corticosteroids are administered for severe toxemia and fever and may produce a dramatic response in the patient with profound sepsis.[146] The treatment should be given in high doses, 60 mg per day of prednisone divided in four doses, and rapidly tapered over the next three days. The wide experience with steroid treatment has failed to show any adverse effects, although the potential for masking intestinal perforation is still present. Thus, steroids are best reserved for patients with severe toxicity.

Intestinal perforation is managed by standard surgical practices. All patients should be treated with nasogastric suction. Indications for operation are progressive peritoneal signs or localization of an abscess. Simple closure of the perforation is the treatment of choice. However, the ileum may be riddled with multiple perforations, and resection or exteriorization of the intestinal loop may be required. Recent studies have emphasized the importance of aggressive surgical intervention in typhoid fever.[147, 148]

Good nursing care plays a major role in the recovery from typhoid fever. The pyrexia can be managed with tepid baths and sponging. Salicylates and antipyretics should be avoided, as they cause severe sweating and may lower the blood pressure.

A chronic carrier who has been discharging *S. typhi* for longer than one year can be treated with antimicrobial agents in an attempt to eliminate the infection. One regimen that works in approximately two thirds of patients is 6 gm of ampicillin per day in four divided doses for six weeks.[138] Reappearance of the carrier state following such treatment is generally associated with gallbladder disease. In persons with gallstones or chronic cholecystitis, cholecystectomy eliminates the carrier state in 85 per cent. This procedure, however, is recommended only for those whose profession is not compatible with the typhoid carrier state—food handlers and health care providers.

Vaccines. Typhoid vaccine affords 70 per cent protection. This relative immunity can be overcome by a large inoculum of bacilli. The most active vaccine is the acetone-dried product, which is administered in two doses of 0.5 ml, subcutaneously, at four-week intervals. The phenol-inactivated product has somewhat reduced immunogenicity, but it produces less local discomfort, a problem which is prominent with the acetone-dried vaccine. There is no relationship between serum antibody levels measured against O, H, or V_1 antigens and resistance to disease, relapse, or reinfection. The major forces of immunity act at the intestinal mucosal surface. Owing to its limitations, the standard typhoid vaccine is recommended only for travelers to endemic regions who plan a prolonged visit; revaccination should be done every three years with a single 0.5-ml dose. An oral live typhoid vaccine currently is undergoing field testing, with initial rather favorable results.[149]

Campylobacter

The most important *Campylobacter* species found in human infections are *C. jejuni,* a major cause of diarrhea; *C. fetus* ssp. fetus, generally found in immunocompromised patients; *C. coli,* a rare cause of gastroenteritis; *C. pylori,* associated with gastritis and peptic ulcerations; and *Campylobacter*-like organisms (CLOs), found in homosexual males with diarrhea.

Epidemiology. The incidence and importance of human *Campylobacter* gastroenteritis only recently are recognized. It is estimated that 5 to 11 per cent of all diarrhea cases are caused by *C. jejuni.* A study from Denver has shown that *Campylobacter jejuni* infection is the most frequent cause of bacterial diarrhea; this organism was isolated from 5 per cent of patients with diarrhea, exceeding the numbers of both *Salmonella* and *Shigella*.[150] Studies in Canadian children confirm the importance of *Campylobacter* gastroenteritis, where it was second only to nontyphoidal *Salmonella* in isolation rate.[151] Furthermore, data from one district in Great Britain show an incidence of 0.3 per 100,000, with 50 per cent of all bacterial diarrhea due to this pathogen.[152]

The organism has been only rarely isolated from fecal samples of asymptomatic individuals in these surveys. In the tropics, however, where the incidence of *Campylobacter* infections is even higher, there is also a substantial incidence of asymptomatic carriers of the organism.

The most common route of transmission appears to be from infected animals to human beings. Several epidemics have been related to farm animals and their food products, such as raw milk and eggs. The reservoir for *Campylobacter* is enormous because many animals in nature can be infected: cattle, sheep, swine, fowl, and dogs. Furthermore, the organism has been isolated from fresh and salt water.[153] The hypothesis is that most of the human infections are from consumption of improperly cooked or contaminated foodstuffs. Chickens seem to be the major source, accounting for 50 per cent of infections in some surveys. In this regard, *Campylobacter jejuni* is very similar to *Salmonella*.

Clinical Features. The incubation period is 24 to 72 hours after ingestion of organisms, but this can be quite variable and may extend up to ten days. There is a wide spectrum of clinical illness, from frank dysentery to watery diarrhea to asymptomatic excretion.[150, 154, 155] Diarrhea and fever are almost invariable (90 per cent). Abdominal pain is usually present (70 per cent), and the patient may note bloody stools (50 per cent). Frequently other constitutional symptoms are present, such as headache, myalgias, backache, malaise, anorexia, and vomiting. Stool examination confirms a colitis by the presence of fecal leukocytes on methylene blue staining and the presence of occult blood.[156]

Although certain clinical features suggest the diagnosis of *Campylobacter* rather than other pathogens, it must be appreciated that in many cases the clinical picture mimics other forms of diarrhea and the diagnosis can be established only by culture. The suggestive features, however, are (1) a prodrome consisting of constitutional symptoms, with coryza, headache, and generalized malaise; (2) a prolonged diarrheal illness, often with a biphasic character, with initial diarrhea, slight improvement, and then increasing severity; and (3) many white and red blood cells upon microscopic examination of the stool, indicating an invasive disease of the large bowel. The duration of illness usually is less than one week, although symptoms can persist for several days, and relapses occur in as many as 25 per cent of patients. It is not unusual for symptoms to last two weeks or longer.

The most reliable way to diagnose *Campylobacter* gastroenteritis is by stool culture. A selective isolation medium containing antibiotics must be used, and the plates are grown at 42°C under CO_2 and reduced oxygen conditions. Dark field or phase-contrast microscopy of fresh diarrhea stool shows the organism as a curved, highly motile rod, with darting, corkscrew movements.

Therapy. Although *C. jejuni* is sensitive to erythromycin *in vitro*, three controlled therapeutic trials with this drug showed no effect on the clinical course when compared to placebo.[93] One study, however, showed some clinical benefit when the antibiotic was started within three days of onset of symptoms. A delay of therapy beyond four days produces no clinical improvement. Fecal excretion of the organism, however, is reduced by erythromycin therapy, in a dose of 250 to 500 mg four times per day for seven days. The new quinolone antibiotics are also active against these organisms, and clinical trials are currently in progress.[97] The penicillins, cephalosporins, sulfamonides, and other drugs conventionally used to treat diarrhea have little effect on *Campylobacter*.

Yersinia

Yersinia enterocolitica is an important intestinal pathogen that causes a spectrum of clinical illnesses from simple gastroenteritis to invasive ileitis and colitis.[157] It is a nonlactose-fermenting, urease-positive, gram-negative rod. Thirty-four serotypes and five biotypes have been identified.[158, 159]

The pathogenic mechanisms include the ability to invade epithelial cells and the production of a heat-stable enterotoxin, which is elaborated at 25°C but not at 37°C.[160] Not all strains have these pathogenic properties.

Epidemiology. *Yersinia* gastroenteritis has been reported more frequently in Scandinavian and other European countries than in the United States. Several epidemics were related to the consumption of contaminated milk and ice cream.[161] The organism can be found in stream and lake water, and it has been isolated from many animals, including puppies, cats, cows, chickens, and horses. It is generally believed that animals, either as pets or food sources, are involved in the transmission of this disease.

The serotypes most frequently involved in Scandinavia and Europe are O3 and O9. Canada also has many serotype O3 isolates, but most of those isolated in the United States are serotype O8. A recent study from Canada reported that several serotypes of *Yersinia* are involved in human infections.[162]

Clinical Features. Several clinical syndromes have been described with *Yersinia,* and they tend to vary with the age of the patient and the underlying disease state.[159, 163, 164] Enterocolitis is the most common clinical condition, accounting for two thirds of all reported cases. This illness occurs most frequently in children less than five years of age.[155] Its presentation is nonspecific, with fever, abdominal cramps, and diarrhea, usually lasting one to three weeks. Microscopic exam-

Table 63–9. GASTROINTESTINAL INVESTIGATIONS IN PATIENTS WITH CULTURE-POSITIVE *YERSINIA ENTEROCOLITICA* INFECTION

Investigation	Total No.	Per Cent	Acute Symptoms[a]	Per Cent
Flexible sigmoidoscopy	62	50.4	20	35.1
Normal	46		10	
Inflammatory changes	13		7	
Pseudomembranous colitis	3		3	
Rectal biopsy	46	37.4	13	22.8
Normal	26		4	
Inflammatory changes	20		9	
Barium imaging of ileum	20	16.3	4	7.0
Normal	18		4	
Abnormal[b]	2		0	
Gastroduodenoscopy	27	22.0	2	3.5
Normal	17		0	
Inflammatory changes	8		1	
Frank ulceration	2		1	
Gastric and duodenal biopsy	25	20.3	2	3.5
Normal	6		0	
Inflammatory changes	16		2	
Other[c]	3		0	

[a]Arbitarily defined as < two weeks in duration.
[b]Narrowing and mucosal ulceration.
[c]Celiac sprue, gastric polyp, and dysplasia.
Reprinted with permission from: Gastrointestinal features of culture-positive *Yersinia enterocolitica* infection, by Simmonds, S. D., Noble, M. A., and Freeman, H. J. Gastroenterology *92*:112. Copyright 1987 by The American Gastroenterological Association.

ination of the fecal effluent reveals leukocytes and red blood cells in most instances. Profuse watery diarrhea, possibly related to the enterotoxin, also can occur. The diarrheal condition can persist for several weeks, raising the possibility of inflammatory bowel disease. Radiographic findings, particularly in prolonged cases, are most intense in the terminal ileum, and may resemble Crohn's disease[165] (see pp. 1327–1358). The majority of patients, however, have normal findings on endoscopy, intestinal biopsy, and barium X-ray studies (Table 63–9).[162]

In children over five years of age, mesenteric adenitis and associated ileitis have been described. Accompanying symptoms include nausea, vomiting, and aphthous ulcers in the mouth. These children often undergo a laparotomy, at which time enlarged mesenteric nodes and an ulcerated ileitis are observed. *Yersinia* is less likely to cause disease in adults; the illness is acute diarrhea, which may be followed two to three weeks later by joint symptoms and rash (erythema nodosum or erythema multiforme).[166] The joint symptoms are reminiscent of Reiter's syndrome, and this symptom complex is associated with the HLA-B27 histocompatibility antigen.

Yersinia bacteremia, a relatively uncommon condition, is seen in patients with underlying diseases such as malignancies, diabetes, anemia, and liver disease. Metastatic foci can occur in bones, joints, and lungs.[167]

The diagnosis is established by culture of stool or body fluids. Because the organism is easily missed on the culture plate, the laboratory should be advised of the suspicion of this infection. Serologic tests have proved useful in Europe and Canada, but do not provide much help for the cases reported in the United States.[168]

Therapy. *Yersinia enterocolitica* strains are susceptible to several antimicrobial agents, including chloramphenicol, gentamicin, tetracycline, and trimethoprim-sulfamethoxazole, but they are resistant to penicillins and cephalosporins. There is no substantial evidence that antibiotics alter the course of the gastrointestinal infection; indeed, the diagnosis often is established rather late in the course, when the patient is improving spontaneously. For the chronic, relapsing form of diarrhea, antibiotic therapy has not proved useful. The septicemic patients suffer a high mortality rate, with no apparent benefit from antibiotics.

VIRAL DIARRHEA

The decade of the 1970s witnessed the exciting discovery of specific viral agents associated with diarrheal disease.[169] Although suspected in the past, the proof of these agents and their pathogenicity has been a recent event. Even now, workers in this field are hampered by the inability to grow most of these agents in simple tissue cultures and by the lack of animal models.

Two groups of viruses have attracted most attention: the rotavirus that causes endemic diarrhea in children generally less than two years of age and the Norwalk virus that appears in epidemics, attacking all age groups; enteric adenovirus has emerged recently as an important group as well (Table 63–10). These viruses have been identified in the fecal effluent of infected patients. The rotaviruses and enteric adenoviruses, being somewhat larger, can be seen directly by electron microscopy (EM), but the smaller Norwalk viruses require an immune electron microscopy (IEM) technique in which antiserum from a recently infected patient is mixed with the fecal specimen to produce aggregation of the viral particles.

Rotaviruses

This group of viruses was discovered in 1973 in studies from Australia, in which the viral agents were visualized by EM in duodenal biopsy specimens from children with acute diarrhea. This infection is now recognized to be cosmopolitan in distribution, occurring in virtually every part of the world where it has been studied.

Microbiology. These viruses measure 70 nm in diameter and contain a double-walled outer capsid without an envelope.[170] They are related structurally to reoviruses and orbiviruses; however, the structure of the agents causing disease in humans is somewhat different, resembling the spokes of a wheel—hence the name "rota." These are RNA-containing viruses that are stable to heat, ether, and mild acids. They can be maintained in prolonged storage; indeed, an agent isolated by Hodes in 1943 from an infection in infants

Table 63–10. CLINICAL AND LABORATORY CHARACTERISTICS OF HUMAN GASTROENTERITIS VIRUSES OF MEDICAL IMPORTANCE*

Feature	Norwalk Virus	Rotavirus	Enteric Adenovirus
Biologic characteristics			
Diameter, shape	27 nm, round	70 nm, with double-shelled capsid	70 nm
Nucleic acid	Not known	Double-stranded, segmented RNA	DNA
Number of serotypes	At least three	At least four	Two (40 and 41)
Replication in cell culture	No	Yes	Yes
Clinical characteristics			
Epidemiology	Family and community epidemics	Sporadic cases, usually in winter, occasionally epidemic	Sporadic cases
Age primarily affected	Older children, adults	Infants, young children	Infants, young children
Method of transmission	Fecal-oral, contaminated water, and shellfish	Fecal-oral	Unknown
Incubated period	1–2 days	1–3 days	Unknown
Duration of illness	Usually 1–2 days	Usually 5–8 days	Usually 5–10 days
High fever (>39° C)	50% (usually low-grade)	30%	5%
Vomiting	Common	80%	80%
Upper respiratory signs	Absent	20–40%	20%
Pathogenic characteristics			
Attack rate in adult volunteers	About 50%	Low	Unknown
Site of human infection	Small bowel	Small bowel	Unknown
Mechanism of immunity	? Nonimmune genetic factors; not local or systemic antibody	Local intestinal IgA antibody, not systemic antibody	Unknown
Disease production in animals	No	Yes, particularly young animals	No
Major diagnostic tests	Immune electron microscopy, radioimmunoassay	Electron microscopy, radioimmunoassay, enzyme-linked immunosorbent assay, counter immunoelectrophoresis; cell-culture antigen production; serologic adaptation of some of the above tests	Electron microscopy; solid phase immunoassays of stool; direct cell culture; serum antibody by hemagglutination inhibition

*Data from Blacklow, N. R., and Cukor, G. N. Engl. J. Med. *304*:397, 1981; Cukor, G., and Blacklow, N. R. Microbiol. Rev. *48*:157, 1984.

was maintained in a freezer until 1977 when it was examined by EM and shown to contain rotavirus particles.[171]

Rotaviruses can be visualized in a fecal specimen by EM, but they do not grow in conventional tissue cultures or organ cultures (Fig. 63–5). Recently, special techniques involving roller cultures have been used. There are four serotypes, based on outer glycoproteins and two, possibly three, subgroups, based on inner proteins.

Pathology and Pathogenesis. Duodenal biopsy specimens of young children with rotavirus infection have demonstrated a patchy abnormality, confined mostly to the epithelial cells of the upper intestine.[172, 173] In its severe form, the infection can produce denuded villi and flattening of the epithelial surface. These changes persist for three to eight weeks. The morphologic changes are accompanied by physiologic abnormalities, such as decreased xylose absorption and reduced levels of disaccharidase enzymes.

Clinical Features. A range of clinical illness, from asymptomatic carriers to severe dehydration and even fatalities, has been seen with rotavirus infections.[174, 175] The disease occurs principally in children aged six to 24 months. Vomiting often heralds the disease process, followed soon by watery diarrhea. The average duration is three to five days, although some instances of chronic diarrhea have been noted. Loss of fluids and electrolytes appears to be the main pathologic event.

Diagnosis. Rapid diagnosis, by detection of rotavirus antigen in the feces, is achieved with solid-phase immunoassay, such as an ELISA test kit known as Rotazyme. This method gives comparable results to electron microscopic techniques, although Rotazyme produces some false positive results in neonates and false negative results in infected adults.

Epidemiology. It has been recognized for many years that viral diarrhea is a major cause of disease and death in young children. Since discovery of the rotaviruses, a great number of studies have established that many cases of infantile diarrhea are caused by this group of agents. Incidence studies have shown that 30 to 70 per cent of hospitalized children under two years of age with acute diarrhea are infected with rotavirus.[176] The virus appears to be spread by a fecal-oral route. In the temperate zones, the disease is more common in the wintertime, but in the tropics it is endemic year-round. Within a family grouping, the young child is often afflicted with the clinical illness, although older siblings and adults can excrete the virus, albeit asymptomatically.[177] However, adults occasionally can become ill with this infection.[178]

Immunity. Serum antibodies to rotavirus are found in older children and adults, apparently having been formed during the period of peak infection, six to 24 months of age.[176] Type-specific antibody also has been demonstrated in intestinal secretions, and it appears that this antibody is responsible for protection. The different serogroups do not induce cross-reacting antibodies, although infection with one strain seems to reduce the severity of infection with other strains.[179] Evidence that secretory antibody of the IgA type

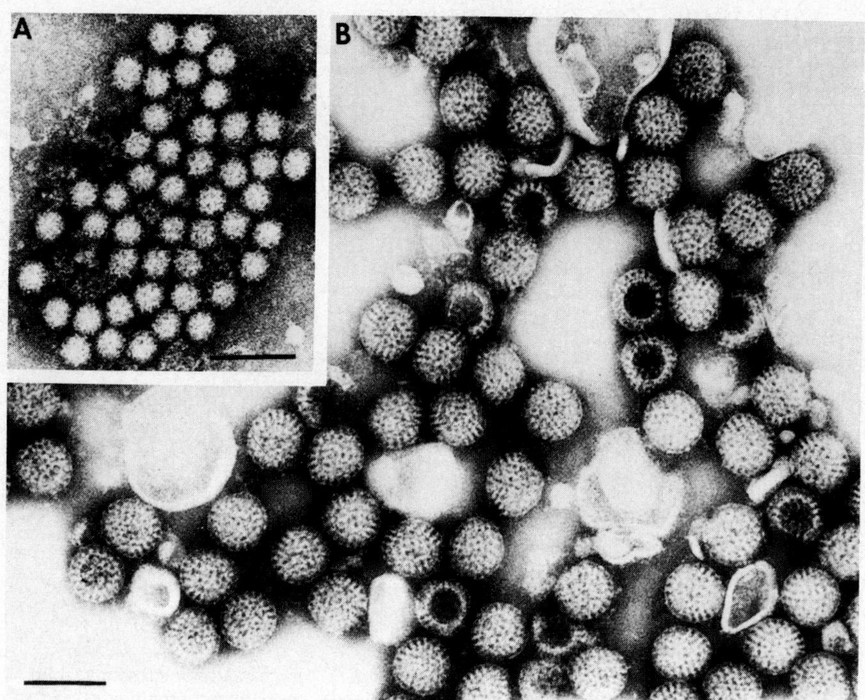

Figure 63–5. *A*, The Norwalk virus particle and aggregate, observed after incubation of 0.8 ml of Norwalk stool filtrate (prepared from a stool of a volunteer administered the Norwalk agent) with 0.2 ml of a 1:5 dilution of a volunteer's prechallenge serum and further preparation for electron microscopy. The quantity of antibody on these particles was rated as 1+. Bar equals 100 nm. *B*, Human rotavirus particles observed in the stool filtrate (prepared from the stool of an infant with gastroenteritis) after incubation with PBS and further preparation for electron microscopy. The particles appear to have a double-shelled capsid. Occasional "empty" particles are seen. Bar equals 100 nm. (Courtesy of A. Kapikian, M.D. Previously published in Lennete, E. H., and Schmidt, N. J. Diagnostic Procedures for Viral, Rickettsial, and Chlamydial Infections. Ed. 5. New York, American Public Health Association, 1979, p. 933.)

provides protection is suggested by the relative immunity of breastfeeding infants to rotavirus infection.[180] A promising vaccine from an attenuated bovine rotavirus strain, RIT 4237, is undergoing clinical trials.[181]

Therapy. Rehydration is the mainstay of therapy for this infection. Field studies have established that the oral rehydration fluid consisting of glucose and electrolytes is effective in restoring fluid balance.[182]

Norwalk Virus

Named for a 1968 outbreak of "winter vomiting disease" in Norwalk, Ohio, this group of viruses is recognized as the pathogen in approximately 40 per cent of nonbacterial epidemics in the United States. It has also been encountered in Hawaii, England, Australia, and Japan.[169]

Microbiology. Because these viruses have defied growth in cell cultures, our current knowledge is based on direct observations by EM in fecal material from infected patients or volunteers[183, 184] (Fig. 63–5). This is a small agent, measuring 27 nm in diameter, which is highly resistant to ether, acid, and heat. Most evidence suggests that it is a DNA-containing virus, similar to parvoviruses, although this point remains controversial. Unlike the rotaviruses, which have many counterparts as diarrheal agents in animals, the Norwalk agent is not related, so far as we know, to any other group of pathogens. It appears that at least three serotypes, and possibly more, are included in this group.

Pathology and Pathogenesis. Intestinal biopsies have been performed in volunteers receiving a challenge of the infective agent. The upper small intestine is the focus of attack, with sparing of the stomach and large bowel.[185] Patchy mucosal lesions are noted in the proximal small bowel in all symptomatic volunteers, in addition to some of the asymptomatic subjects. Being so small, the virus particles cannot be observed in EM sections, as can be done with the rotavirus. Among the physiologic abnormalities observed during this illness are malabsorption of fat and xylose, diminished activity of disaccharidase enzymes, and delayed gastric emptying. Both the morphologic and physiologic abnormalities are reversed within one to two weeks.

Clinical Features. In one outbreak, diarrhea was noted in 92 per cent of proven cases, nausea in 88 per cent, abdominal cramps in 67 per cent, vomiting in 66 per cent, and muscle aches in 56 per cent.[186] The spectrum of other signs and symptoms, all rather mild, includes low-grade fever, myalgias, anorexia, and malaise. Generally, the clinical illness lasts no longer than 24 to 48 hours.

There are no simple diagnostic tests to identify this agent. The virus can be seen in fecal effluent by using the immune electron microscopy technique, with the aid of serum from a convalescent subject. There is also a radioimmunoassay for identifying the virus in the feces and antibody in the serum.[169, 187]

Epidemiology. The Norwalk virus causes explosive epidemics of diarrhea that sweep through a community with a high attack rate.[188] It shows no respect for age, as it preys on virtually all age groups except infants. Transmission occurs by person-to-person contact, with the fecal-oral route being the primary method. Raw shellfish is a major source of infection; for example, during an eight-month period in 1982, 103 outbreaks of Norwalk virus infection in New York State were related to ingestion of raw clams or oysters.[189]

Immunity. Radioimmunoassay has established that serum antibody is not generally present in children but appears in adolescents and peaks in adults, with approximately two thirds of the older age groups possessing antibodies.

Volunteer studies have revealed an unusual form of immunity that apparently is not related to antibody formation.[190] Volunteers who became sick during initial challenge were the same ones who became ill when rechallenged 24 to 42 months later. Those who resisted the initial challenge, on the other hand, also resisted the subsequent challenge. Measurement of antibody in serum and intestinal juice showed higher levels of antibody in the volunteers who became ill, both on the initial and subsequent challenge. This antibody has some protective value, albeit short-lived, because early rechallenge at six to 14 weeks after the initial dose produced protection in the subjects with antibody. Yet this protection did not persist, for the same group with antibody became ill when rechallenged several months later. Thus, it is postulated that nonimmune mechanisms in the intestine resist infection by this virus. This also implies that people can have repeated infections by this virus.

Therapy. No specific treatment is available. The disease is usually mild, but it can produce dehydration in elderly patients, which occasionally requires hospitalization. Bismuth subsalicylate was unimpressive in a controlled trial for treatment of disease induced in volunteers; there was some decrease in abdominal cramps, but vomiting episodes, the rate of purging, and other symptoms were unaffected.[191]

Miscellaneous Viral Agents

The medical literature is replete with reports of viruses that are associated with gastroenteritis in humans.[169] Unfortunately, it is not clear whether these viruses are truly the infective agents or merely bystanders, either as normal flora or as a carrier state. Surely, new viral agents will be described in the future, because two thirds of what are presumably viral epidemics are undiagnosed by the available techniques. In sporadic diarrhea, in 30 to 50 per cent of the cases the cause cannot be identified even when our best methods for bacteriologic and virologic techniques are employed.

Adenovirus, both respiratory types and newly recognized enteric Adenovirus or fastidious types (serotypes 40 and 41), have been identified in 5 to 15 per cent of cases of infantile diarrhea.[192] As with rotavirus, enteric Adenovirus infection is most common in children under two years of age.

The classic enteroviruses, such as echovirus and coxsackievirus, are rare causes of gastroenteritis; they tend to cause diarrhea in association with other organ systems, such as respiratory, central nervous, and myocardial involvement. Cytomegaloviruses (CMV) have been recognized as the cause of diarrhea in some patients. Intestinal X-ray films have shown punctate ulcerations in the stomach and small intestine, especially the ileum.

Calicivirus infections in community and hospital settings have been reported in several countries, primarily in young children. Astrovirus and coronavirus have been associated sporadically with diarrhea, although the incidence is yet unknown. A diverse group of viruses, identified in stools of patients with diarrhea as small, round viral particles, similar in size to Norwalk virus, are known variously as Hawaii, W-Ditchling, Snow Mountain, Marin County, and Otofluke agents.[169] A paucity of information on their overall significance currently exists.

TRAVELERS' DIARRHEA

Diarrheal illness has plagued travelers for centuries. It has given rise to numerous theories of causation and achieved worldwide fame by its various euphemisms. Within the glossary of descriptive epithets that have been applied to the intestinal agonies of travelers are GI trots, gyppy tummy, Casablanca crud, Aden gut, Barsa belly, Turkey trot, Hong-Kong dog, Delhi belly, Aztec two-step, Montezuma's revenge, and turista. Most recently, a disease associated with *Giardia* infection acquired by travelers to the Soviet Union has been called "the Trotskys."

Annually, more than one quarter of a billion people travel from one country to another, of which at least 16 million persons from industrialized countries travel to developing countries. United States travelers to Mexico alone number 3 million annually. With an attack rate of 25 to 50 per cent, diarrheal illness may affect upward of 4 million visitors yearly, close to 30 per cent of whom are ill enough to require confinement to bed and another 40 per cent of whom must alter their scheduled activities.[193]

Clinical Features. Typically, the traveler is well for the first two to three days, with the onset of illness beginning four to six days after arrival.[194] The disease begins abruptly, with abdominal cramps followed by watery diarrhea, numbering most often between three and eight stools per day, but rarely more than 15 per day. By the second or third day, diarrhea usually has lessened and normal activity gradually resumes. Duration of illness is variable, averaging two days in some studies (one to three days in 90 per cent of patients),[195, 196] whereas others report a median duration of five days.[197] Certain beleaguered travelers experience two to three such episodes of diarrhea, even during a relatively short stay. In some instances, diarrhea persists and may last for weeks. Besides loose bowel movements, a series of associated symptoms is involved with travelers' diarrhea (Table 63–11).

Microbiology. Elucidation of the microorganisms responsible for travelers' diarrhea has come only recently, as laboratory techology has advanced in this field. Studies from several parts of the world—Mexico, Morocco, Salvador, Kenya, Bangladesh—have shown the same litany of pathogens associated with this condition (Table 63–12).

The leading pathogen in virtually all studies conducted in recent years has been toxigenic *Escherichia*

Table 63–11. ASSOCIATED SYMPTOMS IN TRAVELERS' DIARRHEA

Symptoms	%	Symptoms	%
Gas	79	Headache	39
Fatigue	74	Chills	38
Cramps	68	Backache	35
Nausea	61	Dizziness	34
Fever	56	Vomiting	29
Abdominal pain	55	Malaise	24
Anorexia	53	Arthralgia	23

coli, including those organisms that elaborate the heat-labile toxin (LT), the heat-stable toxin (ST), or both.[198] As noted in Table 63–12, many cases still lack an etiologic diagnosis. In other individuals, more than one potential pathogen is isolated from the diarrheal stool, and it is difficult to assign a causal role to a specific organism.[193, 199] There also is a high incidence of asymptomatic infections; for example, approximately 15 per cent of healthy travelers acquire toxigenic *E. coli,* and a similar number may acquire *Shigella.* Despite these reservations, the studies of antibiotic prophylaxis (discussed later) demonstrate protection in 90 per cent of the treated travelers, suggesting that approximately 90 per cent of such infections are caused by bacteria sensitive to these drugs. Even though our laboratory technology still is imperfect, it can be assumed that most cases of travelers' diarrhea are caused by an infectious microorganism, probably a coliform bacterium.

Special epidemiologic circumstances may produce a different range of pathogens. On cruise ships there have been epidemics of *Shigella, Salmonella,* and *V. parahaemolyticus* that have caused large numbers of cases. American and Scandinavian travelers to the Soviet Union have experienced a high infection rate with *Giardia,* representing in some series 20 to 40 per cent of all visitors to that country.[200]

Amebic dysentery is an uncommon form of diarrhea, despite the tendency to associate every type of diarrhea in travelers with this pathogen.[201] This gave rise to the incisive remark by Elsdon-Dew that "amebiasis is the refuge of the diagnostically destitute." In unfortunate travelers who acquire an amebic infection, the major symptom is intermittent diarrhea associated with blood and mucus in the stool. There may be alternating periods of constipation and diarrhea, as well as symptom-free periods (see pp. 1155–1162).

Table 63–12. PATHOGENS IN TRAVELERS' DIARRHEA

Microorganisms	Frequency in Travelers' Diarrhea (%)
Toxigenic *E. coli*	40–70
Invasive *E. coli*	0–4
Shigella	5–15
Salmonella	0–15
Campylobacter jejuni	Variable
Vibrio parahaemolyticus	0–2
Aeromonas	Variable
Giardia lamblia	0–2
Entamoeba histolytica	0–2
Cryptosporidium	Rare
Rotavirus	Rare
Norwalk virus	Rare
Enterovirus	Rare
Undiagnosed	10–35

Epidemiology. The most important determinant in the acquisition of travelers' diarrhea is the destination of the trip.[196, 202] Certain countries have a low risk, such as those in northern Europe, and other areas have a higher risk, especially the tropical or developing countries. The incidence of diarrhea among North American travelers in Mexico has varied between 25 and 50 per cent.[196, 198, 203] Such high incidences have been reported for other Latin American (Salvador, Peru), African (Morocco, Kenya), Mediterranean (Spain, Greece), Middle Eastern (Iran, Egypt), and Far Eastern (Pakistan, India, Bangladesh, Thailand) countries. In contrast, low-risk areas are the British Isles, Scandinavia, northern and western Europe, the United States, and Canada. In one investigation, simultaneous interviews were carried out at the San Francisco airport of North American travelers returning from Hawaii or Mexico; the travelers from Hawaii had an attack rate of diarrhea of 7 per cent, whereas travelers from Mexico reported an incidence of 33 per cent.[203] A warm climate *per se* is not the important factor; besides the low incidence in Hawaii, another study from Miami showed an incidence of 2 per cent of travelers' diarrhea at an international conference in that city.[204]

The origin of the traveler is another important factor in liability to develop diarrhea. In international meetings held in Teheran and Mexico City, an incidence of 40 to 50 per cent of diarrhea was reported by North Americans, South Africans, and western Europeans, compared with 1 to 8 per cent among visitors from Asia, South America, and southern Europe.[202]

The purpose of travel and style of eating play significant roles. The highest incidence of diarrhea occurs in people traveling for study purposes or tourism, whereas the lowest incidence is seen in those visiting relatives. Intermediate risk is associated with business travel. More diarrhea occurs in people eating in restaurants and school cafeterias, with a particularly high risk, as might be imagined, in those who succumb to the wares of street vendors.[205] The safest place to eat is in a private home.

Travelers' diarrhea is acquired through ingestion of fecally contaminated food or beverages. Both cooked and uncooked foods may be implicated if improperly handled. Especially risky foods include raw vegetables and uncooked meat and seafood. Tap water, ice, unpasteurized milk, dairy products, and unpeeled fruits are associated with increased risk. Safe products include bottled carbonated beverages (especially flavored beverages), beer, wine, hot coffee or tea, and water boiled or appropriately treated with iodine or chlorine.

Advancing age is associated with a lower incidence of travelers' diarrhea. It is not known whether this protection is due to immunity gained after frequent attacks or from differences in eating habits.

Therapy. Rehydration is the major therapeutic consideration. Travelers experience voluminous purging, but the period of severe fluid loss usually is brief. In addition, travelers tend to be rather healthy, and they are able to sustain these losses, so long as there is some replenishment.[206]

Bismuth subsalicylate, an over-the-counter product, has been used successfully to treat travelers' diarrhea in Mexico.[207] The recommended dose for mild to moderate travelers' diarrhea (<3 bowel movements in an eight-hour period) is 30 to 60 ml doses (1 or 2 tablets) every eight hours for eight doses; this regimen reduced the fecal evacuation by 50 per cent, compared with the placebo control.

Antimotility agents (narcotic analogs), all related to opiates, are useful in providing symptomatic relief for acute travelers' diarrhea.[208] Several caveats should be inserted regarding the use of the narcotic analogs for travelers' diarrhea. These drugs should be avoided in patients with acute bacillary dysentery. There is considerable evidence that they potentiate any form of ulcerating process involving the colon, such as caused by shigellae, salmonellae, and amebae, and they may provoke the serious complication of toxic megacolon. Fortunately, bacillary dysentery is a uncommon form of travelers' diarrhea. In one study of American travelers to Mexico, loperamide was beneficial in treating diarrhea, without any significant untoward reactions.[209]

Antimicrobial drugs are recommended for treatment of moderate to severe travelers' diarrhea; for example, three or more loose stools in an eight-hour period, especially if associated with nausea, vomiting, abdominal cramps, fever, or bleeding.[210] A typical three- to five-day illness can be reduced to approximately one day by using trimethoprim-sulfamethoxazole (TMP-SMZ) in a dose 160 mg of TMP and 800 mg of SMZ, or TMP alone, 200 mg, each taken twice daily for three to five days.[211] Some evidence suggests that doxycycline (100 mg twice daily) and ciprofloxacin (500 mg twice daily) are effective as well.[212, 213]

Prevention. Four approaches to preventing travelers' diarrhea can be conceived: instruction regarding food and beverage comsumption, immunization, use of anti-infective drugs, and use of nonanti-infective medications.

Although it is obviously beneficial to prevent an attack of diarrhea during an overseas journey, such prevention is not easy to accomplish. The only certain way is to travel with sterile, hermetically sealed containers of food and drink. More practically, certain precautions regarding eating habits will not only help to prevent diarrhea, but also other food- and water-borne diseases. Thus, in high-risk areas it is advisable to avoid tap water, ice cubes, salads, unpeeled fruits and vegetables, custards and cream desserts, unpasteurized milk and dairy products, items offered by street vendors, and buffet foods. Thirsty travelers should rely on bottled carbonated beverages, wines, beer, tea, and coffee. Although these precautions reduce the risk of diarrhea, even the most fastidious travelers will be plagued occasionally by a bout of intestinal upset. Others are unable to maintain perfect vigilance during a pleasure trip and suffer a definite risk for acquiring travelers' diarrhea.

In experimental studies, bismuth subsalicylate (BSS) has been shown to reduce active secretion caused by toxigenic *E. coli* and *Vibrio cholerae*.[214, 215] The subsalicylate component may exert its effect by antiprostaglandin activity, a mechanism that has proved to be important in other forms of experimental diarrhea. Bismuth subsalicylate was efficacious in a field trial among U.S. citizens newly arrived from Mexico; they took it as a prophylactic agent in a dose of 2 oz (60 ml) four times a day. Untreated students had a 61 per cent incidence of diarrhea, compared with 23 per cent in the treated individuals, a difference that is statistically significant.[216] The limitation on such prophylactic use is the requirement to pack one bottle per day, or 14 eight-oz bottles for a two-week voyage. An extra suitcase perhaps would suffice, and this would permit additional room on the return trip for souvenirs.

Even if these bottles could be accommodated in a 44-lb weight allotment, many tourists would be reluctant to face this drug four times a day during what should be a vacation. However, the minimal dose has not been determined, and it may be possible to use less of this drug.[209] When considering a lower dose, it should not be overlooked that in the study mentioned earlier, 23 per cent of students developed diarrhea even on the higher dose schedule.[216]

In 1963 a classic study in Mexico showed that either neomycin or a nonabsorbable sulfa drug, when used as a prophylactic agent, reduced the frequency of diarrhea by 70 per cent among North American travelers.[217] Two other antimicrobial drugs, doxycycline and TMP-SMZ, when taken prophylactically proved to be consistently effective in reducing the frequency of travelers' diarrhea by 50 per cent to 90 per cent.[218, 219] In one study, TMP alone also was effective. It is necessary, however, to weigh the benefits of widespread prophylactic use of antimicrobial drugs in millions of travelers against the potential drawbacks. The known risks of doxycycline and TMP-SMZ include allergic reactions, including skin rashes, photosensitivity of the skin, various adverse hematologic responses, Stevens-Johnson syndrome, staining of the teeth in children, and susceptibility to other infections, such as antibiotic-associated colitis, candidal vaginitis, and possibly *Salmonella* enteritis. In addition, excessive use of these agents would stimulate bacterial resistance to antimicrobial drugs in general. Thus, antimicrobial agents are not recommended for universal use by travelers.

Available data support only the instruction of travelers with regard to sensible dietary practices as a prophylactic measure.[193] Antimicrobial agents are not recommended for universal use by travelers. This is justified by the excellent results of early and aggressive treatment of travelers' diarrhea as outlined above. By avoiding prophylactic antimicrobial agents, only those people traveling to high-risk areas who actually develop moderate to severe travelers' diarrhea (less than 30%

of travelers at risk) will be exposed to the side effects of antimicrobial agents, and the exposure will be restricted to a treatment period of three days or less in those individuals. Some may wish to consult with their physicians and may elect to use prophylactic antimicrobial agents for travel under special circumstances, once the risks and benefits are clearly understood.

A legendary mystique, passed on by word of mouth to successive generations of international travelers, has surrounded the drug iodochlorhydroxyquin (Enterovioform). In a well-designed study of prophylactic use among North American students in Mexico, no benefits from iodochlorhydroxyquin could be demonstrated over a placebo.[220] Other studies, poorly designed under the drug company's auspices, did show a protective effect among British rugby players engaged in matches on five continents. Besides the considerable controversy over efficacy, a more important issue of toxicity has been raised, because iodochlorhydroxyquin has been implicated in subacute myelo-optic neuropathy (SMON), a condition associated with neurologic dysfunction and blindness. Currently, iodochlorhydroxyquin is not recommended for therapeutic or prophylactic use, and it is not licensed for use in the United States at present.

DIAGNOSIS OF DIARRHEAL DISEASE

A pathophysiologic approach can be used to make a presumptive etiologic diagnosis in patients with infectious diarrhea (Table 63–13). Perhaps the most convenient approach is to separate pathogens that involve the upper small intestine from those that attack the large bowel. Toxigenic bacteria (*E. coli, V. cholerae*), viruses, and the parasite *Giardia* are examples of small bowel pathogens. These organisms produce watery diarrhea, which may lead to dehydration. Abdominal pain, although often diffuse and poorly defined, is generally periumbilical. Microscopic examination of the stool fails to reveal formed cellular elements, such as erythrocytes and leukocytes.

Table 63–13. CLINICAL FEATURES OF DIARRHEAL DISEASES

	Location of Infection	
	Small Bowel	***Large Bowel***
Pathogens	*V. cholerae*	*Shigella*
	E. coli (ETEC, EPEC)	*E. coli* (EIEC, EHEC)
	Rotavirus	*Campylobacter*
	Norwalk virus	*Entamoeba histolytica*
	Giardia	
Location of pain	Midabdomen	Lower abdomen, rectum
Volume of stool	Large	Small
Type of stool	Watery	Mucoid
Blood in stool	Rare	Common
Leukocytes in stool	Rare	Common (except in amebiasis)
Proctoscopy	Normal	Mucosal ulcers; hemorrhage; friable mucosa

A large bowel pathogen, the major one being *Shigella,* is an invasive organism that causes the clinical syndrome of dysentery. Characteristic rectal pain, known as tenesmus, strongly implicates colonic involvement. Although initially the fecal effluent may be watery, by the second or third day of illness it becomes a relatively small-volume stool, often bloody and mucoid. Microscopic examination almost invariably reveals abundant erythrocytes and leukocytes. Proctoscopy shows a diffusely ulcerated, hemorrhagic, and friable colonic mucosa. Other organisms fitting into this category are *Campylobacter*, *E. coli* (EIEC, EHEC).

Certain pathogens involve principally the lower small bowel but may invade the colon as well. *Salmonella* and *Yersinia* make up this group. Although watery diarrhea is the usual presentation, depending on the focus of infection, the spectrum extends from dehydrating diarrhea to a frank colitis. Vibrios produce different clinical presentations, apparently related to the virulence factors in each infecting strain. *Entamoeba histolytica* attacks the large bowel, producing an invasive disease. Curiously, there is a paucity of polymorphonuclear leukocytes, although occasional macrophages are present in the stool (see pp. 290–316 and 1155–1162).

Laboratory Diagnosis. Infectious diarrhea is a major cause of illness throughout the world, leading to a high morbidity rate with loss of time from school and work in Western countries, and a high mortality rate in developing countries. Surveys of diarrhea incidence in the United States indicate that each person suffers one to two episodes per year, and even higher frequencies are reported in young children.[221] In developing countries the figures are greater, up to four episodes of diarrhea per year in children. A specific laboratory diagnosis is useful epidemiologically, diagnostically, and therapeutically.

A specific diagnosis of infectious diarrhea is obtained mainly through study of fecal specimens, e.g., bacteriologic culture, viral culture (or direct electron microscopic examination), and identification of microbial antigens (viruses, bacteria, parasites, or toxins). Although some diseases can be diagnosed by rising serum antibody titers, it is usually retrospective and often inaccurate.

Standard stool cultures for pathogens cost $25 to $50, depending on the laboratory and the need for antibiotic sensitivities or special tests. Fecal exams for ova and parasites cost an additional $20 to $40. If a physician were to order the full range of diagnostic tests for a stool specimen, it could easily cost $150. Conventional methods of hospital laboratories yield very few specific diagnoses of diarrhea. At the Massachusetts General Hospital the isolation rate of bacterial pathogens from 2000 fecal cultures in 1980 was 2.4 per cent, producing a cost per positive test of $952.[222]

Most patients with infectious diarrhea, even with a recognized pathogen, have a mild, self-limited course. It follows that neither a stool culture nor specific treatment is required for most such patients. An al-

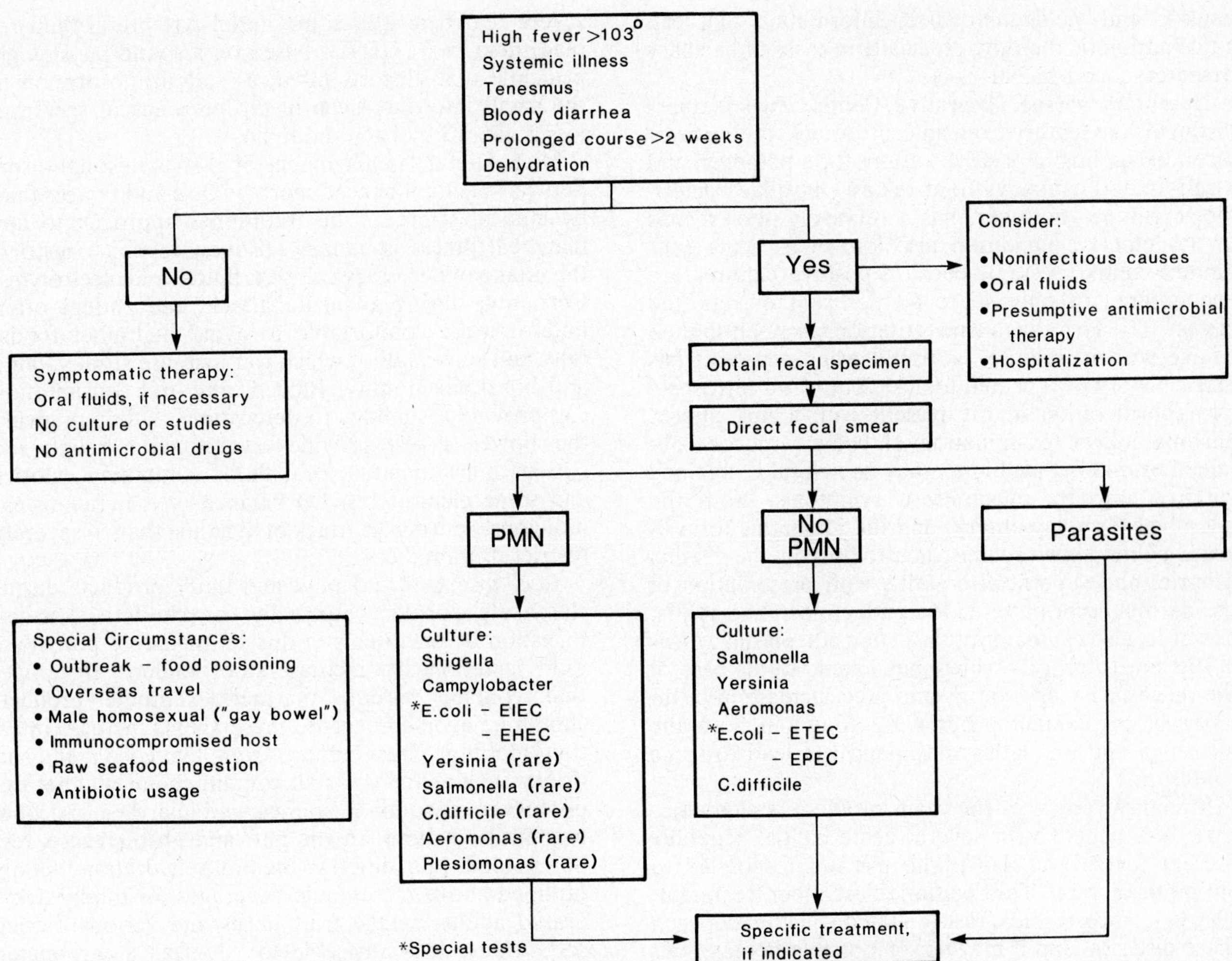

Figure 63–6. Algorithm for the diagnosis and treatment of infectious diarrhea.

gorithm for diagnosis is presented to help decide which patients should be treated symptomatically and which require further diagnostic studies and treatment (Fig. 63–6). Approximately 90 per cent of acute diarrhea falls into the "no studies–no treatment" category.

Fecal Leukocytes. A particularly useful technique to establish a presumptive diagnosis in infectious diarrhea is microscopic examination of the stool[223, 224] (Table 63–14). Using two drops of Loeffler's methylene blue mixed with a small amount of stool on a slide, one searches for leukocytes and erythrocytes. (An experienced observer can do the examination without the stain, thereby looking for protozoa and other parasites on the same slide.) Invasive pathogens, such as *Shigella* and *Campylobacter,* produce a "sea of polys," easily visible in every field, as well as red blood cells. The toxigenic organisms, viruses, and food poisoning bacteria cause a watery stool that harbors very few formed elements.

Several organisms produce variable findings on microscopic stool examination, depending on the invasive properties of the strain and the degree of colonic involvement. This category includes *Salmonella, Yersinia,* and *V. parahaemolyticus.* Pseudomembranous colitis and antibiotic-associated diarrhea, caused by *Clostridium difficile,* have unpredictable findings with regard to cellular elements in the stool. Most cases show a profusion of sloughed epithelial and red blood cells, but only rare polymorphonuclear leukocytes.

An acute exacerbation of ulcerative colitis can produce a great discharge of leukocytes and erythrocytes into the stool, resulting in an exudative microscopic appearance that resembles bacillary dysentery.

Although the fecal microscopic examination is neither infallible nor even helpful in all cases, it is inex-

Table 63–14. FECAL LEUKOCYTES IN INTESTINAL INFECTIONS

Present	Variable	Absent
Shigella	*Salmonella*	*V. cholerae*
Campylobacter	*Yersinia*	Toxigenic *E. coli* (ETEC)
Invasive *E. coli*	*V. parahaemolyticus*	Enteropathogenic *E. coli* (EPEC)
	Clostridium difficile (antibiotic-associated colitis)	Rotavirus
		Norwalk virus
		Giardia lamblia
		Entamoeba histolytica
		Food poisoning
		Staphylococcus aureus
		Clostridium perfringens
		Bacillus cereus

pensive and yields immediate information that can guide antibiotic therapy, especially in cases of bacillary dysentery (see pp. 290–316).

Dysentery versus Ulcerative Colitis. Two features distinguish dysentery from an acute attack of idiopathic ulcerative colitis: a positive culture for a pathogen and a self-limited course without relapse. Positive bacteriologic culture, however, has a relatively poor record in dysentery, a condition also known as acute self-limited colitis (ASLC), because positive cultures are encountered in only 40 to 60 per cent of reported cases.[91, 225] The diagnostic criterion of "self-limited course without relapse" is useful when a patient has had a history of repeated attacks, but it is a retrospective consideration in the patient with a first attack. Histopathologic examination of colonic mucosa obtained by endoscopic biopsy may be helpful if obtained within four days of onset of symptoms. Both the microbial form (dysentery) and the idiopathic form of acute colitis show edema, neutrophils in the lamina propria, and superficial cryptitis with preservation of the normal crypt pattern. Idiopathic ulcerative colitis, however, also causes crypt distortion and plasmacytosis in the lamina propria which may extend to the base of the mucosa. Focal cryptitis and mild increase in cellularity of the lamina propria are found in both the microbial and idiopathic forms and can lead to some confusion.[91]

In clinical practice, the main problem is characterized by a patient with severe, acute colitis, generally present for several days, who has not responded to antibiotic therapy. The decision to use other treatment, such as corticosteroids, rests on the distinction between these diseases, and it may not be possible to make this distinction based on culture or histopathologic findings. Herein lies the conundrum, which is yet unresolved.

TREATMENT OF INFECTIOUS DIARRHEA

Fluid Therapy. The most devastating consequences of acute infectious diarrhea result from fluid losses.[17] Toxigenic organisms, such as *V. cholerae* and certain strains of *E. coli,* can be associated with extreme forms of dehydration due to production of large amounts of isotonic fluid in the small bowel which overwhelms the ability of the lower intestine to reabsorb (see Table 63–2). Children with toxigenic diarrhea lose somewhat less sodium and bicarbonate than adults, but they excrete significantly more potassium. Nonspecific diarrhea, usually caused by viruses, causes less fluid loss and a lower electrolyte concentration in the fecal effluent.

The major aim of treatment is replacement of fluid and electrolytes. The traditional route of administration has been intravenous, but in recent years oral rehydration therapy (ORT) has been proved equally effective physiologically[17] and more practical logistically in developing countries.[21, 22] Indeed, ORT is the treatment of choice for mild to moderate diarrhea in both children and adults, and it can be used even in severe diarrhea after some initial parenteral fluid replacement.[226, 227] ORT is based on a sound physiologic principle that glucose enhances sodium absorption in the small intestine, even in the presence of secretory losses caused by bacterial toxins.

Diet. Dietary management of gastrointestinal disorders has been influenced more by fads and fancies than by clinical science. The traditional approach to any diarrheal illness is dietary abstinence, which restricts the intake of necessary calories, fluids, and electrolytes. Certainly, during an acute attack, the patient often finds it more comfortable to avoid high-fiber foods, fats, and spices, all of which can increase stool volume and intestinal motility. Indeed, any oral consumption can provide a stimulus to defecation. Although giving the bowel a rest provides symptomatic relief, the patient must maintain oral fluids containing calories and some electrolytes. On balance, it is better to eat judiciously during an attack of diarrhea than to severely restrict oral intake.

It is wise to avoid milk and dairy products during the acute episode, especially for children, because ingestion of such items in this setting could potentiate fluid secretion and increase stool volume. Beverages that contain caffeine or methylxanthine products should be avoided because these agents increase intestinal motility. Thus, coffee, strong tea, cocoa, and soft drinks such as the colas all contain chemicals that can potentiate abdominal cramps and diarrhea. Alcohol has similar actions on the gut, and abstinence is recommended. In addition to the oral rehydration therapy outlined above, acceptable beverages for mildly dehydrated adults include fruit juices and various bottled soft drinks. It is advisable to "de-fizz" a carbonated drink by letting it stand in a glass before consuming it. Soft, easily digestible foods are most acceptable to the patient with acute diarrhea.

Antimicrobial Drugs. Less than 5 per cent of cases of acute diarrhea can be treated successfully with antimicrobial drugs (Table 63–15). In the United States it is reckoned that 90 per cent of acute diarrhea is caused by viral agents, unresponsive to any current specific therapy. Shigellosis should be treated with

Table 63–15. ANTIMICROBIAL THERAPY OF BACTERIAL DIARRHEA

Recommended in symptomatic cases
Shigella
Clostridium difficile
Travelers' diarrhea
E. coli (EPEC and EAEC in infants)
Typhoid fever
Cholera
Not generally recommended due to inconclusive findings or no studies
Campylobacter
Yersinia
Aeromonas
Vibrios, noncholera species
E. coli (EPEC in adults, EHEC, EIEC)
Not recommended (except in unusual cases)
Nontyphoidal *Salmonella*
E. coli (ETEC)

antibiotics. There are conflicting studies concerning the efficacy of antimicrobial drugs in several important infections, such as those caused by *Campylobacter,* and insufficient data for infections caused by *Yersinia, Aeormonas, Vibrio,* and several forms of *E. coli.*[93]

The choice of antimicrobial drugs is based on *in vitro* sensitivity patterns, which are related to geographic prevalence. One new group of antimicrobial drugs that appears to possess broad-spectrum activity against virtually all important diarrheal pathogens (except *C. difficile*) is the quinolones, including norfloxacin and ciprofloxacin.[97] In general, the burden of proof is on the physician who decides to treat a simple case of diarrhea. More complicated cases, however, may trip the balance in favor of treatment (see algorithm, Fig. 63–6).

Nonspecific Therapy. The first line of therapeutic defense against acute diarrhea is nonspecific therapy[208, 209, 228] (Table 63–16). Antimotility drugs are particularly useful in controlling moderate to severe diarrhea. These agents decrease jejunal motor activity, thereby disrupting forward propulsive motility. Opiates decrease fluid secretion, enhance mucosal absorption and increase rectal sphincter tone. The overall effect is to normalize fluid transport, slow transit time, reduce fluid losses, and ameliorate abdominal cramping. Loperamide is arguably the best agent because it does not cross the blood-brain barrier, thereby reducing the risk for habituation and for depressing the respiratory center.

The antimotility drugs have proved safe for use in infectious diarrhea, even when inadvertently given for *Shigella;* as noted above, these drugs should not be used when this condition is strongly suspected or established.[209, 228] The treatment regimen for loperamide which proved successful in travelers' diarrhea was an initial dose of two 2-mg capsules, followed by a single capsule after each bowel movement for 48 hours, not to exceed eight capsules in 24 hours.

Bismuth subsalicylate (BSS) is a useful over-the-counter preparation for treating mild to moderate diarrhea. The effect is dose-dependent, with a larger dose (60 ml or 2 tablets, every half hour, for eight doses) more effective than a smaller dose (half this amount).[207, 209] The salicylate moiety is felt to be the active agent, but the bismuth has antibacterial activity which also may play a beneficial role. Bismuth subsalicylate is safe, inexpensive, and easily available, making it nearly ideal for treating mild diarrhea. In moderate to severe acute diarrhea loparamide is more effective than BSS.[209]

Literally hundreds of antidiarrheal nostrums can be found in pharmacies, apothecary shops, herbal stands, homeopathy stores, soothsayers' booths, witchcraft dispensaries, and assorted medical establishments throughout the world. Each country has its own brand names and labeling requirements. Many products contain a combination of drugs, most of them therapeutically worthless, others potentially dangerous. Various starches, talcs, and chalks have been prescribed for diarrheal illnesses for as long as recorded history. Kaolin and pectin, alone or in combination, are popular remedies. Theoretically, they absorb water, converting a loose bowel movement into a mushy movement with lumps. Although this may have some aesthetic appeal and perhaps produce a more formed stool, there is no evidence that these preparations diminish the number of evacuations or reduce intestinal fluid losses.[208, 228] Most of these traditional remedies have proved ineffective in treating acute infectious diarrhea.

Table 63–16. NONSPECIFIC THERAPY OF INFECTIOUS DIARRHEA

Effective
Fluid
Intravenous
Oral rehydration therapy
Food
Continue nutrition intake
Avoid lactose, caffeine, and methylxanthines
Antimotility drugs
Codeine, paragoric, tincture of opium
Loperamide
Diphenoxylate
Bismuth subsalicylate
Not effective
Lactobacilli
Kaolin, pectin, charcoal
Anticholinergics
Cholestyramine
Hydroxyquinolones (enterovioform, diiodolydroxyquin)
Warning: Hydroxyquinolones may be harmful

TUBERCULOSIS OF THE GASTROINTESTINAL TRACT

Any region of the gastrointestinal tract can be involved with tuberculosis. This complication is still prevalent in the developing countries where tuberculosis is a common health problem. In most countries, however, gastrointestinal tuberculosis has become relatively uncommon, and many of the classical findings no longer apply. In addition, the older literature does not separate Crohn's disease from tuberculosis, so there is some confusion about incidence and clinical course of early studies.[229]

Pathogenesis. The major pathogen is *Mycobacterium tuberculosis.* Some parts of the world still report cases caused by *M. bovis,* an organism found in dairy products, but it is an uncommon human pathogen in Western countries. The major route of infection is by swallowed organisms directly penetrating through the intestinal mucosa. In the past, intestinal tuberculosis was associated with active pulmonary infection and especially with active laryngeal involvement. Autopsies of patients with pulmonary tuberculosis, before the era of effective treatment, demonstrated intestinal involvement in 55 to 90 per cent of fatal cases.[230] The frequency of intestinal disease was related to the severity of pulmonary involvement: 1 per cent of patients with minimal pulmonary tuberculosis had gastrointestinal infection, compared to 4.5 per cent with moderately advanced pulmonary disease, and 25 per cent with far advanced disease.[231] There was also a higher risk of intestinal involvement with pulmonary cavitation and positive sputum smears, again reflecting the risk of a high inoculum with swallowed organisms. In modern series, however, pulmonary involvement is seen in less than 50 per cent of patients with intestinal tuberculosis.[232–234] Indeed, the chest X-ray is completely unremarkable in the majority of patients now being seen with intestinal tuberculosis.

Classification and Distribution of Disease. The most frequent site of intestinal involvement is the cecum, with 85 to 90 per cent of patients having disease at this site. Multiple areas of the bowel can be involved, but the ileocecal region is clearly the most frequent. The other locations, in order of incidence, are ascending colon, jejunum, appendix, duodenum, stomach, sigmoid colon, and rectum. Because of frequent involvement of both sides of the ileocecal valve, this structure is apt to become incompetent, a point that sometimes distinguishes tuberculosis from Crohn's disease.

Pathology. The gross appearance of intestinal tuberculosis has been divided into three categories: (1) Ulcerative, seen in 60 per cent of patients. There are multiple superficial lesions confined largely to the epithelial surface. It is considered a virulent process which in the past was associated with a high mortality rate. (2) Hypertrophic, occurring in 10 per cent of patients. This condition consists of scarring, fibrosis, and heaped-up mass lesions that mimic a carcinoma. (3) Ulcerohypertrophic, seen in 30 per cent. This type has mucosal ulcerations combined with healing and scar formation.[229]

At surgery tuberculous lesions often can be recognized by an experienced observer. The bowel wall appears thickened, and there is an inflammatory mass surrounding the ileocecal region (Fig. 63–7). Active inflammation is apparent, as well as strictures and even fistula formation (Fig. 63–8). The serosal surface is covered with multiple tubercules (Fig. 63–9). The mesenteric lymph nodes are frequently enlarged and thickened; upon sectioning, caseous necrosis is seen. The mucosa itself is hyperemic, cobblestoned, edematous, and in some cases, ulcerated. In contrast to Crohn's disease, the superficial ulcers tend to be circumferential, with the long axis perpendicular to the lumen. When these ulcers heal, the associated fibrosis causes stricture and stenosis of the lumen.

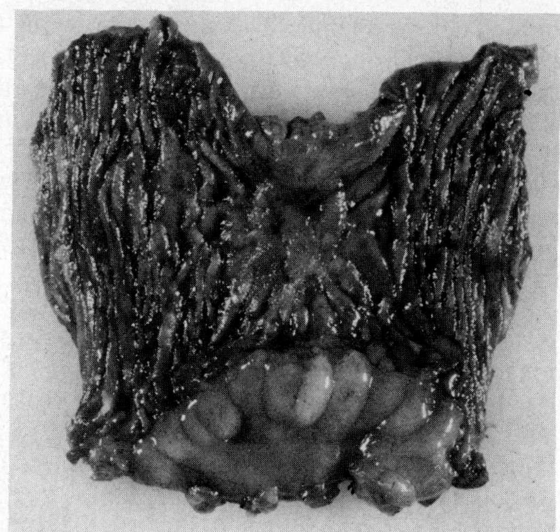

Figure 63–8. Tuberculosis of the terminal ileum. Segmental involvement, mucosal ulceration, and thickening of the bowel wall with stricture formation are apparent.

Histologically, the distinguishing lesion is a granuloma (Fig. 63–10). Caseation is not always seen, especially in the mucosa, although caseating granulomas are found with regularity in regional lymph nodes. The muscularis usually is spared (Fig. 63–11). Sections of the involved region sometimes show acid-fast bacilli, using the Ziehl-Neelsen stain, a finding which is noted in about one third of patients. The organism also can be recovered in a culture of the involved tissues.

Clinical Features. Only a minority of patients with intestinal tuberculosis have specific symptoms. The most common complaint is chronic abdominal pain, which is nonspecific in character and is reported in about 80 to 90 per cent of individuals. An abdominal mass, usually in the right lower quadrant of the abdomen, deep and rather posterior, can be appreciated in two thirds of patients, and approximately the same number report constipation.

Laboratory findings show a mild anemia with a normal white blood cell count. The tubercle bacillus can be isolated from the stool in about one third of patients, but this finding is not helpful in patients with coexisting pulmonary tuberculosis because it may represent only swallowed organisms.

Complications include hemorrhage, perforation, obstruction, fistula formation, and malabsorption syn-

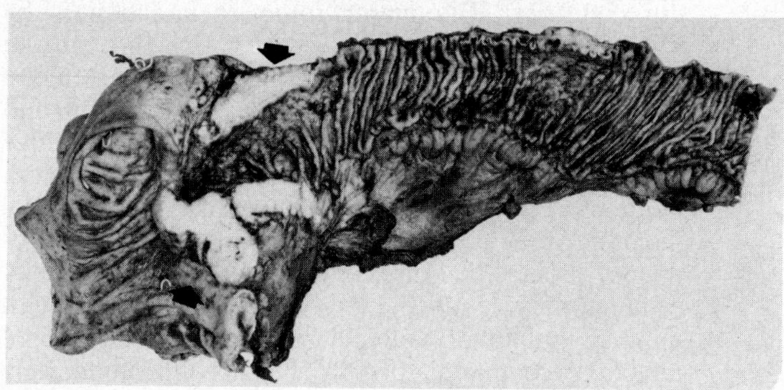

Figure 63–7. Tuberculosis of the ileocecal region and terminal ileum. Note the mucosal destruction and thickening of the bowel wall by multiple discrete and coalescent granulomas *(arrows)*. This ultimately led to stenosis and obstruction in this patient.

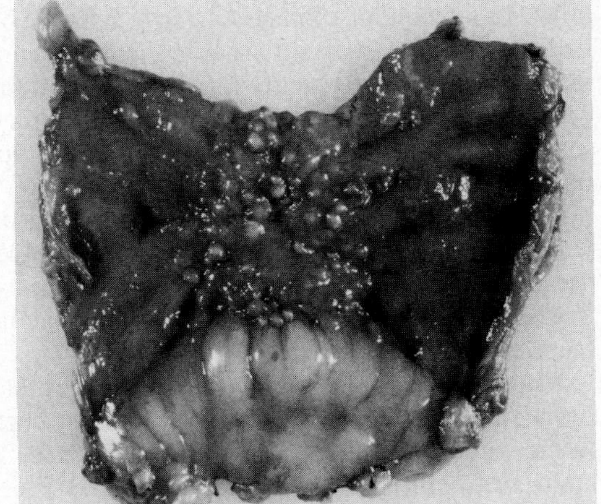

Figure 63–9. Serosal surface of tuberculous small bowel with tubercle formation.

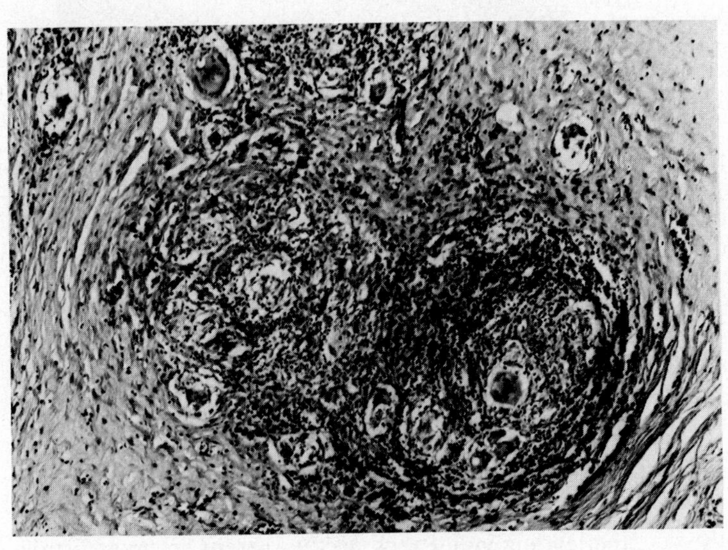

Figure 63–10. High-power view of small early miliary-sized granuloma with Langhans type giant cells in tuberculosis of the bowel. (Hematoxylin and eosin stain, × 100.)

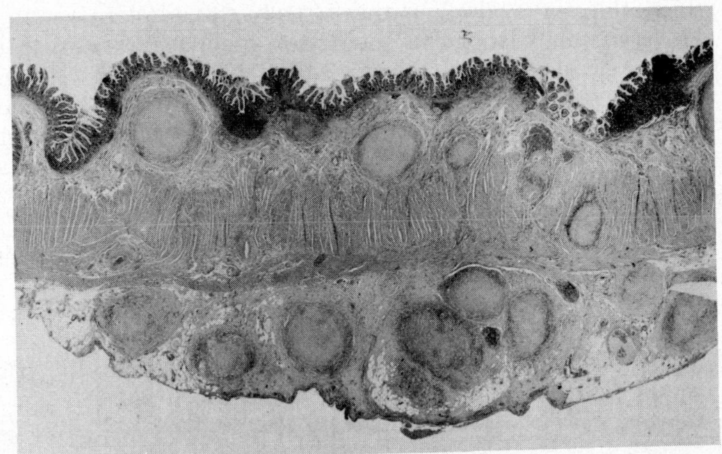

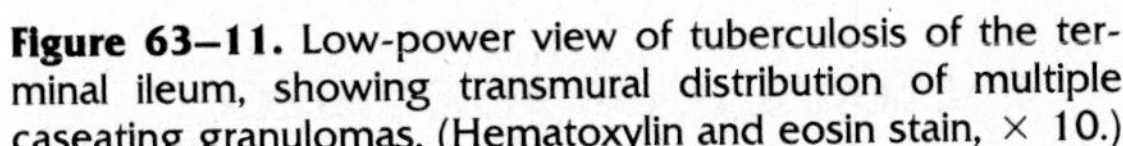

Figure 63–11. Low-power view of tuberculosis of the terminal ileum, showing transmural distribution of multiple caseating granulomas. (Hematoxylin and eosin stain, × 10.)

drome.[235] Free perforation is rather uncommon, certainly less frequent than in Crohn's disease, but it can happen in intestinal tuberculosis even during treatment. Intestinal obstruction is a more common finding, occurring in a segmental, stenotic form. It may require surgical intervention for relief, even with appropriate drug therapy. Malabsorption can be caused by obstruction that leads to proximal bacterial overgrowth, a variant of the stagnant loop syndrome. Involvement of the mesenteric lymphatic system, known as "tabes mesenterica," is also associated with malabsorption (see pp. 263–282).

Diagnosis. The definitive diagnosis of intestinal tuberculosis is made by identification of the organism in tissue, either by direct visualization with an acid-fast stain, or by culture of the excised tissue. A presumptive diagnosis can be established in a patient with active pulmonary tuberculosis who has radiographic and clinical findings suggestive of intestinal involvement. At laparotomy, an experienced surgeon can raise the high suspicion of tuberculosis, although it should be emphasized that this disease can simulate several others. The tuberculin skin test is less helpful because a positive test does not necessarily mean active disease. In addition, many patients, especially older individuals with weight loss and inanition, have a negative skin test in the face of active intestinal tuberculosis.

Roentgenographic examination of the bowel reveals a thickened mucosa, with distortion of the mucosal folds, ulcerations, various degrees of thickening and stenosis of the bowel, and pseudopolyp formation[236, 237] (Fig. 63–12). The cecum is contracted with disease on both sides of the valve, and the valve itself is often distorted and incompetent. Tuberculosis tends to involve small segments of the intestine with stenosis and fistula formation. In the hypertrophic form a mass can be seen that resembles a cecal carcinoma. Calcified mesenteric lymph nodes and an abnormal chest X-ray are other signs that aid in the diagnosis of intestinal tuberculosis.

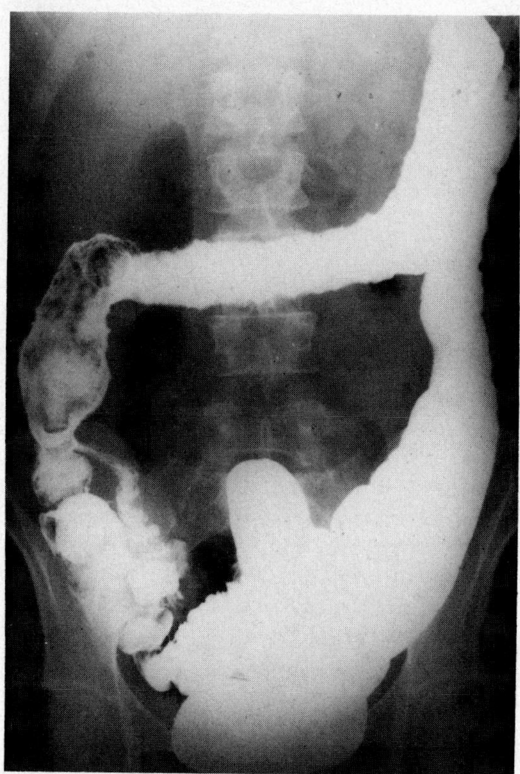

Figure 63–12. A barium enema of tuberculous colon shows extensive involvement of the cecum and ascending and transverse colon. The ulcerated, narrowed, ahaustral appearance is typical of granulomatous infiltration of the bowel. (Courtesy of H. I. Goldberg, M.D.)

Several diseases can resemble intestinal tuberculosis.[238] Crohn's disease gives virtually all the changes of intestinal tuberculosis, except for the presence of the organism which makes the definitive diagnosis of *Mycobacterium* infection. *Yersinia enterocolitica* can produce mesenteric adenopathy, as well as ulcerations and thickening of the bowel mucosa. Usually, this infection has a shorter history and cures itself spontaneously. Involvement of the cecum with carcinoma or amebiasis can be confused with the tuberculosis. Syphilis and lymphogranuloma venereum should be considered, but intestinal involvement with these infections is now rather uncommon.

Treatment. Standard antituberculosis treatment gives a high cure rate for intestinal tuberculosis. There are no controlled studies to determine the optimum type of therapy or duration, but extrapolation from other forms of extrapulmonary tuberculosis suggests that a three-drug regimen for a period of 18 months would be adequate treatment. The drugs are isoniazid (300 mg per day), ethambutol (15 mg/kg per day), and rifampin (600 mg per day). More recently the treatment of pulmonary tuberculosis includes pyrazinamide to replace ethambutol and a shorter treatment course (12 months). This regimen has not been studied in intestinal tuberculosis.

Surgical intervention often was required for intestinal tuberculosis in the past, especially in cases involving the ileum.[233] Obstruction and fistula formation were the leading indications. In the current era most fistulas respond to medical management, as do the ulcerative complications. However, mass lesions associated with the hypertrophic form still may necessitate an operative approach, for they can lead to compromise of the lumen, strictures, and eventually complete obstruction. Because of the similarity to carcinoma of the cecum, patients with undiagnosed disease may undergo exploratory laparotomy and right hemicolectomy, although only minimal resection is suggested for tuberculous disease because the condition often improves dramatically with appropriate drug therapy.

BACTERIAL FOOD POISONING*

Bacterial food poisoning is defined as an illness caused by the consumption of food contaminated with bacteria or bacterial toxins. Food poisoning also can

*David R. Snydman joined me in writing this section.

be related to parasites (i.e., trichinosis), viruses (i.e., hepatitis), and chemicals (i.e., mushrooms), but these considerations are not within the scope of this chapter. Food poisoning caused by bacteria constitutes approximately two thirds of the outbreaks in the United States for which an etiology can be determined.[239] However, it must be noted that only 44 per cent of such outbreaks fulfill the microbiologic standards for confirmed etiology.

A food-borne disease outbreak generally is defined by two criteria: similar illness, usually gastrointestinal, in two or more individuals; and epidemiologic or laboratory investigation that implicates food as the source. The major recognized causes of bacterial food poisoning are limited to 11 bacteria: *Clostridium perfringens, Staphylococcus aureus, Vibrio* (including *V. cholerae* and *V. parahaemolyticus*), *Bacillus cereus, Salmonella, Clostridium botulinum, Shigella,* toxigenic *Escherichia coli,* and certain species of *Campylobacter, Yersinia,* and *Aeromonas.* Other bacteria such as *Streptococcus, Arizona,* and *Listeria* have been implicated in some outbreaks.

In the 1980–1981 reporting period in the United States, 1180 food-borne outbreaks affected 28,000 people.[240] Surveillance suggests that the true scope of infection related to food is probably 10 to 100 times more frequent. *Salmonella* outbreaks predominate and constitute almost 33 per cent of reported cases of food-borne illness. This may be due in part to the ease of recognition and to the awareness of general physicians and the public. *Staphylococcus aureus* is the next most frequent cause of food-borne outbreaks, associated with 25 per cent of reported cases. Although there have been almost as many outbreaks due to *Staphylococcus* as to *Salmonella,* fewer individuals have been affected in each outbreak of *Staphylococcus* poisoning. *Clostridium perfringens* is the next most common, constituting 17 per cent. Several pathogens are rarely reported, namely *B. cereus* and *V. parahaemolyticus,* which have been well studied in other parts of the world. Their contribution to food-borne diarrheal illness in the United States has been recognized only recently, and their recovery from stool or food requires special laboratory procedures.[241]

This section deals with *Clostridium perfringens, Staphylococcus aureus, and Bacillus cereus;* the other bacterial agents are discussed in previous sections.

Clostridium perfringens

Clostridium perfringens is a major food-borne pathogen that causes vomiting and diarrhea in a high percentage of exposed individuals. The disease is related to an enterotoxin elaborated by strains of *C. perfringens* type A. A more severe and often lethal food-borne illness, known variously as enteritis necroticans (Darmbrand) and pigbel, is caused by *C. perfringens* type C. (This group of diseases is discussed on p. 1226.)

Microbiology. Clostridia are gram-positive, spore-forming, obligate anaerobes that can be found in the intestinal flora of humans and animals and in the soil. Although all species grow better under anaerobic conditions, *C. perfringens* is remarkably aerotolerant and may survive exposure to oxygen for as long as 72 hours. It was originally thought that food poisoning strains were heat-resistant and hemolytic, but more recent studies have shown that heat-sensitive and nonhemolytic strains can cause this illness as well.[242]

C. perfringens is known to produce 12 toxins, mostly active in tissues, as well as several enterotoxins. The gastrointestinal disease is caused by a heat-labile, protein enterotoxin with a molecular weight of approximately 34,000. The enterotoxin is a structural component of the spore coat, formed during sporulation;[243] it causes fluid accumulation in the rabbit ileal loop model.[244] Although both cholera vibrios and *C. perfringens* produce enterotoxins, they differ in the following respects: clostridial enterotoxin has its maximum activity in the ileum and has minimal activity in the duodenum, just opposite to that of cholera toxin. Clostridial enterotoxin inhibits glucose transport, damages the intestinal epithelium, and causes protein loss into the intestinal lumen, all of which are not observed with cholera toxin.[245]

Pathogenic Mechanisms. Almost every outbreak of clostridial food poisoning is associated with roasted, boiled, stewed, or steamed meats or poultry as the vehicle of infection.[246] Usually the meat is cooked in bulk so that heat gain and internal pressure are not sufficient to kill the spores. The implicated food invariably undergoes a period of inadequate cooling, at which time the oxidation-reduction of the food is in a reduced state that allows the spores to germinate. This usually happens below 50°C. Unless the food is reheated to a very high temperature, it will contain many viable organisms.

Once the organisms endure the initial heating, they must be ingested in large quantities in order to cause disease. It also appears that older cultures are more readily able to withstand the acid pH of the stomach than younger cultures. Therefore, food that has been allowed to cool for some period of time may be a better medium to produce disease.

Clinical Features. *C. perfringens* food poisoning is characterized by watery diarrhea and severe, crampy abdominal pain, usually without vomiting, beginning eight to 24 hours after the incriminating meal. Fever, chills, headache, or other signs of infection usually are not present. The illness is of short duration—14 hours or less. Rare fatalities have been recorded in debilitated or hospitalized patients.[247]

Epidemiology. Epidemics are characterized by high attack rates, with a large number of affected individuals, usually 40 to 50 per outbreak.[248] The incubation period in most outbreaks varies between eight and 14 hours but can be as long as 22 hours. Such outbreaks are most frequently reported from institutions or after large gatherings. The pathogenesis of infection requires a meat or fish dish to be precooked and then reheated to be served. Beef, turkey, and chicken are the most frequent vehicles of infection.

Therapy. No specific treatment is required for this illness. The symptoms last no longer than 24 hrs to 36 hours.

Enteritis Necroticans. This disease was described originally in post–World War II Germany, in an outbreak affecting over 400 people who consumed rancid meat.[249] Similar outbreaks, associated with consuming poorly cooked pork, have been described in New Guinea and are labeled pigbel.[250] The disease is caused by strains of *C. perfringens* type C, which elaborate an enterotoxin similar, and possibly identical, to the one described for type A strains.[251]

Outbreaks of pigbel have been related to origiastic consumption of pig in large native feasts. The pig is improperly cooked, and large quantities are consumed over three or four days. Other cases, most often in children under ten years of age, occur in villages.

Compared with the usual form of clostridial food poisoning seen in the United States and Europe, pigbel is a much more severe, necrotizing disease of the small intestine with a high mortality rate. After a 24-hour incubation period, the illness ensues, with intense abdominal pain, bloody diarrhea, vomiting, and shock. The mortality rate in this disease is about 40 per cent, usually due to intestinal perforation.

Staphylococcus aureus

Food poisoning caused by coagulase-positive strains of *Staphylococcus aureus* is the second most common type in the United States, and prior to 1973 it was the leading cause.

Microbiology. Five immunologically distinct enterotoxins have been associated with food-poisoning strains of *S. aureus.* These enterotoxins, termed A, B, C, D, and E, are heat-resistant, single polypeptide chains that range in molecular weight from 28,000 to 34,000. When tested in a rat intestinal loop model, net secretion of water and electrolytes is observed.[252] Vomiting is induced in monkeys and in human volunteers using the enterotoxins or culture filtrates of the organism.

Pathogenic Mechanisms. Three requisites are necessary for staphylococcal food poisoning to occur: (1) contamination of a food with enterotoxin-producing staphylococci; (2) suitable growth requirements of the food for the organism; and (3) an allotment of time and temperature in which the organism can multiply.

The emetic dose of enterotoxin A or B for human beings has been estimated to be between 1 and 25 μg (assuming 100 gm of food is consumed). Clearly, individuals have different sensitivities to the enterotoxins, because studies in volunteers show a varying dose response among individuals. However, in outbreaks in which the implicated food has a large concentration of toxin, the attack rate is very high, approaching 100 per cent.

Clinical Features. The symptoms of staphylococcal food poisoning are primarily profuse vomiting, nausea, and abdominal cramps, often followed by diarrhea. Vomiting is the dominant initial symptom, and it can lead to a severe metabolic alkalosis. Rarely, hypotension and marked prostration occur. Fever is not a common accompaniment, but a low-grade fever may be present in more severe cases. Fatalities are unusual, and recovery is complete within 24 to 48 hours.[253, 254]

Epidemiology. Staphylococcal food poisoning has a short incubation period, approximately three hours (range, one to six hours). The disease usually is clustered within a family or group, with a high attack rate observed. Many different foods have been implicated in this form of food poisoning. However, foods with a high salt concentration, such as ham or canned meat, or with a high sugar content, such as custard and cream, selectively favor the growth of staphylococci. The major mode of transmission is from a food handler to the food product. Involved foods usually have been cut, sliced, grated, mixed, or ground by workers who are carriers of toxin-producing strains of *S. aureus.*

Therapy. Most people with staphylococcal food poisoning suffer in silence, without reporting their symptoms to a physician. More severe cases may require supportive care, particularly rehydration and correction of alkalosis. No specific therapy is available.

Bacillus cereus

This organism is an aerobic, spore-forming, gram-positive rod that has been associated with two clinical types of food poisoning—a *diarrhea* syndrome and a *vomiting* syndrome.[255] Although the organisms appear similar by biochemical tests, those responsible for the two syndromes produce distinct toxins and have different epidemiologies.

Diarrhea Syndrome. The original report of *B. cereus* causing diarrheal disease was associated with consumption of contaminated meatballs in a sanatorium. Subsequent studies have demonstrated production of an enterotoxin by this organism that causes fluid accumulation in the rabbit ileal loop.[256] The mechanism appears to be activation of adenlyate cyclase in intestinal epithelial cells, similar to the action of cholera toxin.[257] Cultures of the strains elaborating this enterotoxin cause diarrhea when fed to rhesus monkeys.

The median incubation period appears to be nine hours, with a range of six to 14 hours. The clinical illness is characterized by diarrhea (96 per cent), generalized cramps (75 per cent), and vomiting (23 per cent).[255] Fevers are uncommon. The duration of illness ranges from 20 to 36 hours, with a median of 24 hours. The strains of *B. cereus* associated with diarrhea are found in about 25 per cent of many foodstuffs sampled, including cream, pudding, meat, spices, dried potatoes, dried milk, vanilla sauces, and spaghetti sauces, all of which are contaminated prior to cooking.[258] If the food is prepared so that the temperature is maintained at

30 to 50°C, vegetative growth is permitted. Spores can survive extreme temperatures, and when allowed to cool relatively slowly, they germinate, multiply, and elaborate toxin. There is no evidence that human carriage of the organism or other means of contamination plays a role in transmission.

Whether the diarrheogenic, heat-labile enterotoxin is actually ingested or produced *in vivo* is not known; however, several pieces of evidence suggest the latter mechanism. The incubation of diarrheal illness is too long for performed toxin, and a large inoculum (10^6) is required to cause illness, suggesting a requirement for intestinal colonization.

Vomiting Syndrome. Although the organism associated with the vomiting disease appears the same, a different type of toxin has been implicated.[259] Cell-free culture filtrates from these strains do not produce fluid accumulation in the rabbit ileal loop, nor do they stimulate adenylate cyclase; however, they produce vomiting when fed to rhesus monkeys. This vomiting toxin is stable to heat.

The vomiting syndrome has a short incubation period, approximately two hours. Virtually all affected individuals have vomiting and abdominal cramps. Diarrhea is present in only one third of these persons. The length of illness ranges from eight to ten hours with a median of nine hours. This illness usually is a mild, self-limited, condition. Nearly all reported cases involving the vomiting toxin have implicated fried rice as the vehicle.[255]

In England, almost 90 per cent of uncooked rice was found to be colonized by *B. cereus,* although the number of organisms was relatively low.[260] The disease has been ascribed to the common practice in Chinese restaurants of allowing large portions of boiled rice to drain unrefrigerated in order to avoid clumping. Flash-frying during the final preparation of the fried rice does not produce enough heat to destroy what seems to be preformed heat-stable toxin. It appears that the emetic illness is caused by preformed toxin, for the incubation period is very short, and there is an extremely high attack rate in outbreaks, approaching 100 per cent.

References

1. Gorbach, S. L. (ed.). Infectious Diarrhea. Boston, Blackwell Scientific Publications, 1986.
2. Simon, G. L., and Gorbach, S. L. Intestinal flora in health and disease: A review. Gastroenterology *86*:174, 1984.
3. Gorbach, S. L., Banwell, J. G., Jacobs, B., Chatterjee, B. D., Mitra, R., Brigham, K. L., and Noegy, K. N. Intestinal microflora in asiatic cholera. II: The small bowel. J. Infect. Dis. *121*:38, 1970.
4. William-Smith, H., and Jones, J. E. T. Observations on the alimentary tract and its bacterial flora in healthy and diseased pigs. J. Pathol. Bacteriol. *86*:387, 1963.
5. Formal, S. B., Gemski, P., Giannella, R. A., and Takechui, A. Studies on the pathogenesis of enteric infections caused by invasive bacteria. *In* Acute Diarrhea in Childhood. New York, Elsevier Press, 1976, pp. 27–43.
6. De, S. N., Battacharya, K., and Sarkar, J. K. A study of the pathogenicity of strains of *Bacterium coli* from acute and chronic enteritis. J. Pathol. Bacteriol. *71*:201, 1956.
7. Dean, A. G., Ching, Y. C., Williams, R. G., and Hardin, L. B. Test for *Escherichia coli* enterotoxin using infant mice: Application in a study of diarrhea in children in Honolulu. J. Infect. Dis. *125*:407, 1972.
8. Giannella, R. A. Suckling mouse model for detection of heat-stable *Escherichia coli* enterotoxin. Characteristics of the model. Infect. Immun. *14*:95, 1976.
9. Donta, S. T., and Smith, S. M. Stimulation of steroidogenesis in tissue cultures by enterotoxigenic *Escherichia coli* and its neutralization by specific antiserum. Infect. Immun. *9*:500, 1974.
10. Guerrant, R. L., Brunton, L. L., Schnaitman, T. C., Rebhun, L. I., and Gilman, A. G. Cyclic adenosine monophosphate and alteration of Chinese hamster ovary cell morphology: A rapid, sensitive in vitro assay for the enterotoxin of *Vibrio cholerae* and *Escherichia coli.* Infect. Immun. *10*:320, 1974.
11. Keusch, G. T., and Donta, S. T. Classification of enterotoxins on the basis of activity in cell culture. J. Infect. Dis. *131*:58, 1975.
12. Finkelstein, R. A. Cholera. CRC Crit. Rev. Microbiol. *2*:553, 1973.
13. Levine, M. M., Kaper, J. B., Black, R. E., and Clements, M. L. New knowledge of pathogenesis of bacterial enteric infections as applied to vaccine development. Microbiol. Rev. *47*:510, 1983.
14. Gill, D. M. The mechanisms of action of cholera toxin. Adv. Cyclic Nucleotide Res. *8*:85, 1977.
15. Holmgren, J., Lonnroth, I. and Svennerholm, L. Tissue receptor for cholera exotoxin. Postulated structure from studies with GM, ganglioside and related glycolipids. Infec. Immun. *8*:208, 1973.
16. Fishman, D. H. Mechanism of action of cholera toxin: Events on the cell surface. *In* Field, M., Fordtran, J. S., and Schultz, S. G. (eds.): Secretory Diarrhea. Bethesda, American Physiological Society, 1980, pp. 85–106.
17. Carpenter, C. C. J. Clinical and pathophysiologic features of diarrhea caused by *Vibrio cholerae* and *Escherichia coli. In* Field, M., Fordtran, J. S., and Schultz, S. G. (eds.): Secretory Diarrhea. Bethesda, American Physiological Society, 1980, pp. 66–73.
18. Field, M. Secretion of electrolytes and water by mammalian small intestine. *In* Johnson, L. R. (ed.): Physiology of the Gastrointestinal Tract. Vol. 2. New York, Raven Press, 1981, pp. 963–982.
19. Mosley, W. H. The role of immunity in cholera. A review of epidemiological and serological studies. Texas Rep. Biol. Med. *27*(suppl. 1):227, 1969.
20. Morris, J. G., and Black, R. E. Cholera and other vibrios in the United States. N. Engl. J. Med. *312*:343, 1985.
21. Pierce, N. F., and Hirschhorn, N. Oral fluid—a simple weapon against dehydration in cholera. WHO Chron. *31*:87, 1977.
22. World Health Organization. A Manual for the Treatment of Acute Diarrhea. Geneva, World Health Organization, 1984.
23. Carpenter, C. C. J., Sack, R. B., Mondal, A., and Mitra, P. P. Tetracycline therapy in cholera. J. Indian Med. Assoc. *43*:309, 1964.
24. Greenough, W. B., Gordon, R. S., Rosenberg, I. S., Davies, B. I., and Beneson, A. S. Tetracycline in the treatment of cholera. Lancet *1*:355, 1964.
25. Wallace, C. K., Anderson, P. N., Brown, T. C., Khanra, S. R., Lewis, G. W., Pierce, N. F., Sanyal, S. N., Segré, G. V., and Waldman, R. H. Optimal antibiotic therapy in cholera. Bull. WHO *39*:239, 1968.
26. Mhalu, F. S., Mmari, P. W., and Ijumba, J. Rapid emergence of El Tor *Vibrio cholerae* resistant to antimicrobial agents during first months of fourth cholera epidemic in Tanzania. Lancet *1*:345, 1979.
27. Joo, I. Cholera vaccines. *In* Barua, D., and Burrows, W. (eds.): Cholera. Philadelphia, W. B. Saunders Company, 1975, pp. 335–355.
28. Curlin, G. Cholera toxoid field trial. *In* Fukumi, H., and Zinnaka, Y. (eds.): Twelfth Joint Conference on Cholera. The United States–Japan Cooperative Medical Science Program Symposium on Cholera, Sapporo, Japan, 1976, pp. 276–285.

29. Blake, P. A., Weaver, R. E., and Hollis, D. G. Diseases of humans (other than cholera) caused by Vibrios. Ann. Rev. Microbiol. *34*:341, 1980.
30. Barker, W. H. Vibrios parahaemolyticus outbreaks in the United States. Lancet *1*:551, 1974.
31. Kato, T., Obara, H., Ichinose, H., Yamai, S., Nagashimak, H., and Sakazahi, R. Hemolytic activity and toxicity of *Vibrio parahaemolyticus*. Jpn. J. Bacteriol. *21*:442, 1966.
32. Twedt, R. M., and Brown, D. F. Toxicity of *Vibrio parahaemolyticus. In* Schlessenger, D. (ed.): Microbiology 1974. Washington, D.C., American Society for Microbiology, 1975, pp. 241–245.
33. Calia, F. F., and Johnson, D. E. Bacteremia in suckling rabbits after oral challenge with *Vibrio parahaemolyticus*. Infect. Immun. *11*:1222, 1975.
34. Bolen, J. L., Zamiska, S. A., and Greenough, W. B., III. Clinical features in enteritis due to *Vibrio parahaemolyticus*. Am. J. Med. *57*:638, 1974.
35. Lawrence, D. N., Blake, P. A., Yashuk, J. C., Wells, J. G., Creech, W. B., and Hughes, J. H. *Vibrio parahaemolyticus* gastroenteritis outbreaks aboard two cruise ships. Am. J. Epidemiol. *109*:71, 1979.
36. Joseph, S. W., Colwell, R. R., and Kaper, J. B. *Vibrio parahaemolyticus* and related halophic vibrios. CRC Crit. Rev. Microbiol. *10*:77, 1983.
37. Fujino, T., Okuno, Y., Nahada, D., Aoyama, A., Fukai, K., Mukai, T., and Ueno, T. On the bacteriological examination of Shirasu food poisoning. Med. J. Osaka Univ. *4*:299, 1953.
38. Peffers, A. S. R., Baily, J., Barrow, G. I., and Hobbs, B. C. *Vibrio parahaemolyticus* gastroenteritis and international air travel. Lancet *1*:143, 1973.
39. Hughes, J. M., Hollis, D. G., Gangarosa, E. J., and Weiner, R. E. Non-cholera vibrio infections in the United States. Ann. Intern. Med. *88*:602, 1978.
40. Craig, J. P., Yamamoto, K., Takeda, Y., and Miwatani, T. Production of cholera-like enterotoxin by *Vibrios cholerae* non-O strain isolated from the environment. Infect. Immun. *34*:90, 1981.
41. Morris, J. G., Wilson, R., Davis, B. R., et al. Non-O group 1 *Vibrio cholerae* gastroenteritis in the United States. Ann. Intern. Med. *94*:656, 1981.
42. Shandera, W. X., Johnston, J. M., Davis, B. R., and Blake, P. A. Disease from infection with *Vibrios mimicus,* a newly recognized vibrios species. Ann. Intern. Med. *99*:169, 1983.
43. Gracey, M., Burke, V., and Robinson, J. *Aeromonas*-associated gastroenteritis. Lancet *2*:1304, 1982.
44. Holmberg, S. D., and Farmer, J. J., III. *Aeromonas hydrophila* and *Plesiomonas shigelloides* as causes of intestinal infections. Rev. Infect. Dis. *6*:633, 1984.
45. Ljungh, A., and Wadström, T. Aeromonas toxins. Pharmacol. Ther. *15*:339, 1981.
46. Holmberg, S. D., Schell, W. L., Fanning, G. R., Wachsmuth, K., Kickman-Brenner, F. W., Blake, P. A., Brenner, D. J., and Farmer, J. J., III. Aeromonas infections in the United States. Ann. Intern. Med. *105*:683, 1986.
47. Daris, W. A., II, Kane, J. G., and Garagusi, V. F. Human aeromonas infections: A review of the literature and a case report of endocarditis. Medicine (Baltimore) *57*:267, 1978.
48. Holmberg, S. D., Wachsmuth, K., Hickman-Brenner, F. W., Blake, P. A., and Farmer, J. J., III. Plesiomonas enteric infections in the United States. Ann. Intern. Med. *105*:690, 1986.
49. Levine, M. M., and Edelman, R. Enteropathogenic *Escherichia coli* of classic serotypes associated with infant diarrhea: Epidemiology and pathogenesis. Epidemiol. Rev. *6*:31, 1984.
50. Robins-Browne, R. M. Traditional enteropathogenic *Escherichia coli* of infantile diarrhea. Rev,. Infect. Dis. *9*:28, 1987.
51. Levine, M. M., Nalin, D. R., Hornick, R. B., Berquist, E. J., Waterman, D. H., Young, C. R., Sotman, S., and Rowe, B. *Escherichia coli* strains that cause diarrhoea but do not produce heat-labile or heat-stable enterotoxins and are noninvasive. Lancet *1*:1119, 1978.
52. Gorbach, S. L., Banwell, J. F., Chatterjee, B. D., Jacobs, B., and Sack, R. B. Acute undifferentiated human diarrhea in the tropics. I. Alterations in intestinal microflora. J. Clin. Invest. *50*:881, 1971.
53. Sack, R. B. Human diarrheal disease caused by enterotoxigenic *Escherichia coli*. Ann. Rev. Microbiol. *29*:333, 1975.
54. Clements, J. D., and Finkelstein, R. A. Immunological cross-reactivity between a heat-labile enterotoxin(s) of *Escherichia coli* and subunits of *Vibrio cholerae* enterotoxin. Infect. Immun. *21*:1036, 1978.
55. Evans, D. G., Silver, R. P., Evans, D. J., Jr., Chase, D. G., and Gorbach, S. L. Plasmid-controlled colonization factor associated with virulence in *Exchерichia coli* enterotoxigenic for humans. Infect. Immun. *12*:656, 1975.
56. Deneke, C. F., Thorne, G. M., and Gorbach, S. L. Serotypes of attachment pili of enterotoxigenic *Escherichia coli* isolated from humans. Infect. Immun. *19*:1254, 1981.
57. Sack, R. B. Enterotoxigenic *Escherichia coli:* Identification and characterization. J. Infect. Dis. *142*:279, 1980.
58. Aldrete, J. F., and Robertson, D. C. Purification and chemical characterization of the heat-stable enterotoxin produced by porcine strains of enterotoxigenic *Escherichia coli*. Infect. Immun. *19*:1021, 1978.
59. Hughes, J. M., Murad, F., Chang, B., and Guerrant, R. L. Role of cyclic GMP in the action of heat-stable enterotoxin of *Escherichia coli*. Nature *271*:755, 1978.
60. Field, M., Graf, L. H., Jr., Laird, W. J., and Smith P. L. Heat-stable enterotoxin of *Escherichia coli:* In vitro effects on guanylate cyclase activity, cyclic GMP concentration, and ion transport in small intestine. Proc. Nat. Acad. Sci. USA *75*:2800, 1978.
61. Smith, H. W., and Linggood, M. A. Further observations on *Escherichia coli* enterotoxins with particular regard to those produced by atypical piglet strains and by calf and lamb strains. J. Med. Microbiol. *5*:243, 1972.
62. Merson, M. H., Sack, R. B., Islam, S., Saklayen, G., Huda, N., Huq, I., Zulich, A. W., Yolken, R. H., and Kapikian, A. Z. Disease due to enterotoxigenic *Escherichia coli* in Bangladeshi adults: Clinical aspects and a controlled trial of tetracycline. J. Infect. Dis. *141*:702, 1980.
63. Evans, D. J., Jr., Ruiz-Palacios, G., Evans, D. G., DuPont, H. L., Pickering, L. H., and Olarte, J. Humoral immune response to the heat-labile enterotoxin of *Escherichia coli* in naturally acquired diarrhea and antitoxin determination by passive immune hemolysis. Infect. Immun. *16*:781, 1977.
64. Tulloch, E. F., Ryan, K. J., and Formal, S. B. Invasive enterohepatic *Escherichia coli* dysentery: An outbreak in 28 adults. Ann. Intern. Med. *79*:13, 1973.
65. Riley, L. W., Remis, R. S., Helgerson, S. D., McGee, H. B., Wells, J. G., Davis, B. R., Hebert, R. J., Olcott, E. S., Johnson, L. M., Hargrett, N. T., Blake, P. A., and Cohen, M. L. Hemorrhagic colitis associated with a rare *Escherichia coli* serotype. N. Engl. J. Med. *308*:681, 1983.
66. Remis, R. S., MacDonald, K. L., Riley, L. W., Puhr, N. D., Wells, J. G., Davis, B. R., Blake, P. A., and Cohen, M. L. Sporadic cases of hemorrhagic colitis associated with *Escherichia coli* 0157:H7. Ann. Intern. Med. *101*:624, 1984.
67. Grandsen, W. R., Damm, M. A. S., Anderson, J. D., Carter, J. E., and Lior, H. Further evidence associating hemolytic uremic syndrome with infection by Verotoxin-producing *Escherichia coli* 0157:H7. J. Infect. Dis. *154*:522, 1986.
68. Canty, J. R., and Blake, R. K. Diarrhea due to *Escherichia coli* in the rabbit: A novel mechanism. J. Infect. Dis. *35*:454, 1977.
69. Ulshen, M. H., and Rollo, J. L. Pathogenesis of *Escherichia coli* gastroenteritis in man—another mechanism. N. Engl. J. Med. *302*:99, 1981.
70. Rothbaum, R., McAdams, A. J., Giannella, R., and Partin, J. C. A clinicopathologic study of enterocyte-adherent *Escherichia coli:* A cause of protracted diarrhea in infants. Gastroenterology *83*:441, 1982.
71. Mathewson, J. J., Johnson, D. C., DuPont, H. L., Morgan, D. R., Thornton, S. A., Wood, L. V., and Ericsson, C. D. A newly recognized cause of travelers' diarrhea: Enteroadherent *Escherichia coli*. J. Infect. Dis. *151*:471, 1985.
72. Keusch, G. T., Grady, G. F., Mata, L. J., and McIver, J. Pathogenesis of shigella diarrhea. I. Enterotoxin production by *Shigella dysenteriae* I. J. Clin. Invest. *51*:1212, 1972.
73. Gots, R. E., Formal, S. B., and Giannella, R. A. Indomethacin inhibition of *Salmonella typhimurium, Shigella flexneri,* and

cholera-mediated rabbit ileal secretion. J. Infect. Dis. *130*:280, 1974.

74. Mata, J., Gangarosa, E. J., Caceres, A., Perera, D. R., and Mejicanos, M. L. Epidemic Shiga bacillus dysentery in Central America. 1. Etiologic investigations in Guatemala. J. Infect. Dis. *122*:170, 1970.
75. LaBrec, E. H., Schneider, H., and Magnani, T. J., Jr. Epithelial cell penetration as an essential step in the pathogenesis of bacillary dysentery. J. Bacteriol. *88*:1503, 1964.
76. Takeuchi, A., Sprinz, H., LaBrec, E. H., and Formal, S. B. Experimental bacillary dysentery: An electron microscopic study of the response of the intestinal mucosa to bacterial invasion. Am. J. Pathol. *47*:1011, 1965.
77. Gorbach, S. L., and Thorne, G. M. Shigella vaccines, Shigella pathogens—Dr. Jekyll and Mr. Hyde. J. Infect. Dis. *136*:601, 1977.
78. Ogawa, H., Nakamura, A., and Nakaya, R. Cinemicroscopic study of tissue cultures infected with *Shigella flexneri*. Jpn. J. Med. Sci. Biol. *21*:259, 1968.
79. Keusch, G. T., Donohue-Rolfe, A., and Jacewicz, M. Shigella toxin and the pathogenesis of shigellosis. *In* Evered, D., and Whelan, K. (ed.): Microbial Toxins and Diarrheal Disease. London, Ciba Foundation Symposium No. 112, 1985.
80. Keusch, G. T., and Jacewicz, M. The pathogenesis of shigella diarrhea. VI. Toxin and antitoxin in *Shigella flexneri* and *Shigella sonnei* infections in humans. J. Infect. Dis. *135*:552, 1977.
81. Rout, W. R., Formal, S. B., Giannella, R. A., and Damin, G. J. Pathophysiology of Shigella diarrhea in the rhesus monkey. Intestinal transport; morphological and bacteriological studies. Gastroenterology. *68*:270, 1975.
82. DuPont, H. L., Hornick, R. B., Dawkins, A. T., Snyder, M. J., and Formal, S. B. The response of man to virulent *Shigella flexneri* 2a. J. Infect. Dis. *119*:296, 1969.
83. Shiga, K. The trend of prevention, therapy, and epidemiology of dysentery since the discovery of its causative organism. N. Engl. J. Med. *215*:1205, 1936.
84. DuPont, H. L., Hornick, R. B., Snyder, M. J., Libonati, J. P., Formal, S. B., and Gangarosa, E. J. Protection induced by oral live vaccine or primary infection. J. Infect. Dis. *125*:12, 1972.
85. Quinn, T. C., Stamm, W. E., Goodell, S. E., et al. The polymicrobial origin of intestinal infections in homosexual men. N. Engl. J. Med. *309*:576, 1983.
86. Barrett-Connor, E., and Conner, J. D. Extra-intestinal manifestations of shigellosis. Am. J. Gastroenterol. *52*:234, 1970.
87. Ashkenazi, S., Dinari, G., Weitz, R., and Nitzan, R. Convulsions in shigellosis. Evaluation of possible risk factors. Am. J. Dis. Child. *137*:985, 1983.
88. Koster, F. T., Boonpuncknavig, V., Sujaho, S., and Gilman, R. H. Renal histopathology in the hemolytic-uremic syndrome following shigellosis. Clin. Nephrol. *21*:126, 1984.
89. Butler, T., Islam, M., and Bardhan, P. K. The leukemoid reaction in shigellosis. Am. J. Dis. Child. *138*:162, 1984.
90. Calin, A., and Fries, J. F. An "experimental" epidemic of Reiter's syndrome revisited: Follow-up evidence on genetic and environmental factors. Ann. Intern. Med. *84*:564, 1976.
91. Nostrant, T. T., Kumar, N. B., and Appleman, H. D. Histopathology differentiates acute self-limited colitis from ulcerative colitis. Gastroenterology *92*:318, 1987.
92. Weissman, J. B., Gangarosa, E. J., DuPont, H. L., Nelson, J. D., and Haltalin, K. C. Shigellosis: To treat or not to treat? JAMA *229*:1215, 1974.
93. Levine, M. M. Antimicrobial therapy for infectious diarrhea. Rev. Infect. Dis. *8*:S207, 1986.
94. Ross, S., Controni, G., and Khan, W. Resistance of shigellae to ampicillin and other antibiotics. JAMA *221*:1239, 1976.
95. Nelson, J. D., Kusmiesz, H., Jackson, L. H., and Woodman, E. Trimethoprim-sulfamethoxazole therapy for shigellosis. JAMA *235*:1239, 1976.
96. Chang, M. J., Dunkle, L. M., Van Reken, D., Anderson, D., Wong, M. L., and Feigin, R. D. Trimethoprim-sulfamethoxazole compared to ampicillin in the treatment of shigellosis. Pediatrics *59*:726, 1977.
97. Ruiz-Palacios, G. M. Norfloxacin in the treatment of bacterial enteric infections. Scand. J. Infect. Dis. *48*(suppl.):55, 1986.
98. Pickering, L. K., DuPont, H. L., and Olarte, J. Single dose tetracycline therapy for shigellosis in adults. JAMA *239*:853, 1978.
99. Haltalin, K. C., Nelson, J. D., Hinton, L. V., Kusmiesz, H. T., and Sladoje, M. Comparison of orally absorbable and nonabsorbable antibiotics in shigellosis. J. Pediatr. *72*:708, 1968.
100. Nelson, J. D., and Haltalin, K. C. Amoxicillin less effective than ampicillin against Shigella in vitro and in vivo: Relationship of efficacy to activity in serum. J. Infect. Dis. *129*:S222, 1974.
101. Robertson, R. P., Wahab, M. F. A., and Raasch, F. 0. Evaluation of chloramphenicol and ampicillin in salmonella enteric fever. N. Engl. J. Med. *278*:171, 1968.
102. Takeuchi, A. Electron microscope studies of experimental salmonella infection. I. Penetration into the intestinal epithelium by *S. typhimurium*. Am. J. Pathol. *50*:109, 1966.
103. Takeuchi, A., and Sprinz, H. Electron microscope studies of experimental salmonella infection in the preconditioned guinea pig. II. Response of the intestinal mucosa to the invasion by *S. typhimurium*. Am. J. Pathol. *51*:137, 1967.
104. Giannella, R. A., Formal, S. B., Dammin, G. J., and Collins, H. Pathogenesis of salmonellosis. J. Clin. Invest. *52*:441, 1973.
105. Giannella, R. A., Gots, R. E., Charney, A. N., Geenough, W. B., III, and Formal, S. B. Pathogenesis of salmonella-mediated intestinal fluid secretion: Activation of adenylate cyclase and inhibition by indomethacin. Gastroenterology *69*:1238, 1975.
106. McCullough, N. B., and Eisele, C. W. Experimental human salmonellosis. III. Pathogenicity of strains of *Salmonella newport, Salmonella derby,* and *Salmonella bareilly* obtained from spray-dried whole egg. J. Infect. Dis. *89*:209, 1951.
107. McCullough, N. B., and Eisele, C. W. Experimental human salmonellosis. IV. Pathogenitity of strains of *Salmonella pullorum* obtained from spray-dried whole egg. J. Infect. Dis. *89*:259, 1951.
108. Rubin, H. R., and Weinstein, L. Salmonellosis: Microbiologic, Pathologic, and Clinical Features. New York, Stratton Intercontinental Medical Book Corporation, 1977.
109. Black, P. H., Kunz, L. J., and Swartz, M. N. Salmonellosis—a review of some unusual aspects. N. Engl. J. Med. *262*:811, 1960.
110. Saphra, I., and Winter, J. W. Clinical manifestations of salmonellosis in man. N. Engl. J. Med. *256*:1128, 1957.
111. Gray, J. I., and Trueman, A. M. Severe salmonella gastroenteritis associated with hypochlorhydria. Scot. Med. J. *16*:255, 1971.
112. Glaser, J. B., Morton-Kute, L., and Berger, S. R. Recurrent Salmonella typhimurium bacteremia associated with the acquired immune deficiency syndrome. Ann. Intern. Med. *102*:189, 1985.
113. Musher, D. N., and Rubenstein, A. D. Permanent carriers of nontyphosa salmonellae. Arch. Intern. Med. *132*:869, 1973.
114. Hook, E. W. Salmonellosis: Certain factors influencing the interaction of salmonella and the human host. Bull. N.Y. Acad. Med. *37*:499, 1961.
115. Kaye, D., Gill, F. A., and Hook, E. W. Factors influencing host resistance to salmonella infections: The effects of hemolysis and erythrophagocytosis. Am. J. Med. Sci. *254*:205, 1967.
116. Hand, W. L., and King, N. L. Serum oponization of salmonella in sickle cell anemia. Am. J. Med. *64*:388, 1977.
117. Han, T., Sokal, J. E., and Neter, E. Salmonellosis in disseminated malignant diseases. N. Engl. J. Med. *276*:1045, 1967.
118. Wolfe, M. S., Armstrong, D., Louria, D. B., and Blevins, A. Salmonellosis in patients with neoplastic disease. Arch. Intern. Med. *128*:546, 1971.
119. Waddell, W. R., and Kunz, L. J. Association of salmonella enteritis with operations on the stomach. N. Engl. J. Med. *255*:555, 1956.
120. Rocha, H., Brazil, S., Kirk, J. W., and Hearey, C. D. Prolonged salmonella bacteremia in patients with *Schistosoma mansoni* infection. Arch. Intern. Med. *128*:254, 1971.

Acute HIV Infection

Approximately one to six weeks after exposure to HIV, some (but not necessarily all) infected patients may manifest an acute, nonspecific, and self-limiting illness.[23, 24] Fevers, sweats, myalgias, arthralgias, headaches, anorexia, nausea, vomiting, lymphadenopathy, rash, and diarrhea are quite typical. Symptoms and signs last for 3 to 14 days. Routine laboratory parameters are nonspecific. It is difficult to distinguish this syndrome from many similar self-limiting illnesses caused by other common microbes, particularly viruses. Immunologic profiles done for research purposes during the acute illness show elevated suppressor/cytotoxic T lymphocyte counts, and HIV can be cultured from blood and cerebrospinal fluid. Anti-HIV antibodies detectable by enzyme-linked immunosorbent assay (ELISA) techniques become positive 3 to 12 weeks after exposure.

Asymptomatic HIV Infection

Following the acute, self-limiting retroviral infection, patients are asymptomatic for months or years. As noted above, it is not clear what factors determine how long patients remain asymptomatic. Over years, an increasing number of patients will develop AIDS-related manifestations (about 20 per cent over five years) or AIDS (an additional 13 per cent over six years).[11, 12] It is unclear at present what percentage of seropositive individuals will develop AIDS over an extended period of time.[11, 12] During the asymptomatic period there may be no laboratory manifestation other than a positive HIV serology and positive HIV blood culture. In some infected patients serologic studies may be negative but evidence of infection can be found by newer diagnostic techniques such as polymerase chain reaction. Some asymptomatic patients develop varying degrees of immunosuppression.

The principal epidemiologic importance of HIV-infected asymptomatic individuals is that they represent a reservoir for potential HIV transmission.

AIDS-Related Syndromes

HIV can produce a wide range of clinical manifestations that do not meet the surveillance definition of AIDS. These manifestations range in severity from modest increase in the size of lymph nodes in otherwise healthy individuals to severe, life-threatening fevers associated with extraordinary inanition and organ dysfunction. Many of these syndromes are designated as AIDS-related complex (ARC), but this designation covers such a broad range of disorders that it is not helpful clinically or prognostically. There are many times more patients with these AIDS-related syndromes than there are AIDS patients.

Generalized lymphadenopathy, often called progressive generalized lymphadenopathy (PGL) or lymphadenopathy syndrome (LAS), is seen in many otherwise asymptomatic HIV-positive individuals.[25–29] More than two extrainguinal sites are usually involved, especially anterior cervical, posterior cervical, and axillary chains. Lymph nodes are characteristically firm but not tender and may vary in size from month to month. Biopsy of lymph nodes usually demonstrates a relatively nonspecific hyperplasia, although some reports suggest that these nodes can be histologically distinguished from nodes taken from HIV-negative individuals. Occasionally, biopsy of these nodes will show Kaposi's sarcoma despite the absence of skin lesions. It is relatively uncommon to find infectious agents such as mycobacteria or fungi in these nodes in patients who are truly asymptomatic. Thus, the trend in clinical practice is to avoid biopsy of firm, nontender nodes that do not progressively enlarge in an HIV-positive individual who is asymptomatic with normal blood count and chemistry profile. In assessment of patients who are symptomatic, especially with fever and weight loss, patients with very asymmetric nodes, or patients whose nodes are suspicious because of tenderness or physical characteristics, a biopsy is appropriate.

Leukopenia, thrombocytopenia, and anemia are often recognized in asymptomatic HIV-positive individuals or in patients with more advanced HIV-related disorders.[30] Leukopenia and thrombocytopenia can be substantial with total peripheral leukocyte and platelet counts of 1500 to 2500/mm^3 and 10,000 to 100,000/mm^3, respectively, being quite common. Even when patients have only 500 to 1000 neutrophils/mm^3 and fewer than 50,000 platelets/mm^3, infection due to common bacterial pathogens and clinical bleeding have not often been major problems. Bone marrow examination usually reveals a normal or mildly hypocellular marrow in these asymptomatic individuals, with adequate precursors and maturation. There is some evidence linking these cytopenias to immune complex–mediated mechanisms.[30]

Weight loss, malaise, fatigue, fever, and night sweats are often recognized in HIV-seropositive individuals. Some of these individuals also have generalized lymphadenopathy or cytopenias. These constitutional symptoms, fevers, and weight declines can be mild or can be so severe as to disable the patient completely. Anorexia and diarrhea can be impressive aspects of the syndrome. In Africa this wasting syndrome is especially frequent and has been called "slim disease."[31] Extensive evaluations of these individuals for infections and tumors may reveal AIDS-defining criteria. In many of these patients, however, only HIV infection is found. They are often (but not invariably) seropositive and culture-positive for cytomegalovirus and Epstein-Barr virus. It is not yet clear whether eradication of one or both of these herpes viruses with chemotherapeutic agents could improve the performance status of any of these individuals. Specific enteric pathogens may be found in association with the diarrhea, but eradication or suppression of these pathogens often has no impact on the volume or frequency of stools. Total parenteral nutrition has been attempted in individuals with the most severe wasting and inanition, but anecdotal reports suggest that such nutritional support rarely appears to have a major impact on patient performance status or longevity. Individuals who are the most severely disabled with fever, weight loss, and malaise may be more immunologically impaired than some patients who meet the definition of AIDS. It is not uncommon for these severely disabled individuals to have helper/inducer T lymphocyte counts below 100/mm^3, and to have a very short survival. Some will die without ever developing an AIDS-defining opportunistic process.

Dementia, aseptic meningitis, and peripheral neuropathy are recognized both in AIDS patients and in HIV-seropositive individuals who do not yet have an AIDS-defining process.[32–34] The dementia can be mild or severe. Computerized tomography (CT) scans of the head characteristically show cortical atrophy and ventricular enlargement. Spinal fluid may show a mild pleocytosis with an elevated protein and a normal glucose, and HIV can be cultured intermittently from the fluid.[35] A few of these demented patients may ultimately turn out to have focal cerebral lesions due to lymphoma or toxoplasmosis, and occasionally a chronic fungal or mycobacterial meningitis will be recognized. The peripheral neuropathy associated with HIV may be manifested as mild tingling and numbness of the lower extremities or may produce such severe dysesthesias that patients have difficulty walking. The cause of the dementia and neuropathy is unclear, although there is evidence pointing toward direct involvement of brain and peripheral nerves by HIV.

Candida stomatitis, hairy leukoplakia, dermatomal herpes zoster, and *Mycobacterium tuberculosis* infection all occur with increased frequency in HIV-infected patients.[15, 36–38] Each can be recognized as an initial clinical manifestation of HIV infection in otherwise asymptomatic individuals or as persistent or recurrent problems in patients who clearly meet the definition of AIDS. *Candida* stomatitis is a very uncommon entity in individuals who are not immunosuppressed, receiving antibiotics or corticosteroids, or diabetic. The presence of *Candida* stomatitis in an individual who is not in one of these categories should raise an immediate concern for HIV infection. Over 50 per cent of HIV-seropositive patients who present with *Candida* stomatitis will develop an AIDS-defining disease within 6 months.[36] The stomatitis may be associated with *Candida* esophagitis. *Candida* proctitis and vaginitis are also recognized. Hairy leukoplakia consists of asymptomatic white lesions that characteristically occur on the lateral aspects of the tongue and is associated with Epstein-Barr virus. A high percentage of individuals with hairy leukoplakia will also develop an AIDS-defining disease within 6 to 12 months of presentation.[37] Dermatomal herpes zoster and pulmonary or extrapulmonary tuberculosis are also predictive of AIDS, although there may be a longer interval until the development of AIDS-defining diseases than is the case for *Candida* stomatitis and hairy leukoplakia.

The distinction between AIDS-related syndromes and AIDS is not clear-cut from a biologic perspective. Some patients with AIDS-related syndromes are clinically sicker and immunologically more suppressed than patients who meet the surveillance definition of AIDS. Thus, decisions about the use of prophylactic drugs and advice about how readily to seek medical care for new symptoms and how long survival will likely be must be made on the basis of the clinical situation, immunologic data, and the results of prospective studies (as they become available) rather than on rigid and somewhat arbitrary classification schemes.

AIDS

The most common diseases that present as the initial AIDS-defining illness are *Pneumocystis* pneumonia (64 per cent) and Kaposi's sarcoma (14 per cent). A variety of other opportunistic infections (Table 64–1) and lymphomas are the initial manifestations in the remaining 22 per cent of cases.[39] The opportunistic infections and tumors that occur in AIDS may behave differently in their clinical presentation and their response to therapy than do the identical pathogens in other immunosuppressed populations.[40]

Pneumocystis pneumonia usually presents in AIDS patients as a very subtle cough or sensation of shortness of breath.[41] Because the progression of dyspnea, shortness of breath, and cough is not as fulminant as that seen in non-AIDS patients who are receiving immunosuppressive drugs, patients often wait for relatively long periods of time (several weeks or months) before they seek medical attention. Because AIDS-related *Pneumocystis* pneumonia is so characteristically indolent, the chest roentgenogram and arterial blood gases are often normal or close to normal at the time of presentation. It is often difficult to decide whether an invasive diagnostic procedure is indicated or whether the patient has a self-limiting viral process. Pulmonary function tests and gallium citrate scanning are often not helpful in this regard in that they are relatively insensitive and nonspecific. It seems likely that prognosis for survival of *Pneumocystis* pneumonia is improved by early institution of therapy. Thus, aggressive attempts to induce sputum or to perform bronchoalveolar lavage with transbronchial biopsy should be instituted for any patients with suggestive symptoms.[41–43] Sputum induction should permit identification of organisms in 50 to 90 per cent of cases. Bronchoalveolar lavage with transbronchial biopsy when properly performed should provide a diagnosis in almost 100 per cent of cases of *Pneumocystis* pneumonia. Treatment of *Pneumocystis* pneumonia (Table 64–2) should

Table 64–1. OPPORTUNISTIC INFECTIONS IN 16,500 AIDS CASES

Opportunistic Infections	Frequency (%)
Pneumocystis pneumonia	63
Candida esophagitis	14
Cytomegalovirus disease	7
Cryptococcosis	7
Mucocutaneous herpes simplex	4
Cryptosporidiosis	4
Toxoplasmosis	3
Others	3

Percentages show frequency of infections at time of initial report to Centers for Disease Control, June 1981 to January 1986.

Table 64–2. THERAPY FOR FREQUENT INFECTIOUS DISEASES IN AIDS PATIENTS

Pathogen and Clinical Manifestation	Drug	Usual Daily Adult Dose	Interval between Divided Doses	Route	Minimum Duration*
Protozoa					
Pneumocystis pneumonia	Trimethoprim-sulfamethoxazole	20 mg/kg trimethoprim with 100 mg/kg sulfamethoxazole	q 8 h	IV, PO	21 days
	Pentamidine isethionate	4 mg/kg	qd	IV	21 days
Toxoplasmosis	Pyrimethamine and	75 mg once, then 25 mg	qd	PO	28 days
	sulfadiazine or trisulfapyrimidines	4 gm	q 6 h	PO	28 days
Cryptosporidiosis	?Spiramycin*	4 gm	q 6 h	PO	14 days
Fungi					
Oral thrush *(Candida)*	Nystatin or	3×10^6 units	q 4 h	PO	7–10 days
	ketoconazole	200–400 mg	q 12 h	PO	7–10 days
Candida esophagitis	Amphotericin B or	0.6 mg/kg	qd	IV	7–10 days
	ketoconazole	400 mg	q 12 h	PO	7–10 days
Disseminated candidiasis	Amphotericin B	0.6 mg/kg	qd	IV	42 days
Cryptococcosis	Amphotericin B and	0.3–1 mg/kg	qd	IV	42 days
	flucytosine	150 mg/kg	q 6 h	PO	42 days
Viral					
Mucocutaneous herpes simplex	Acyclovir	15 mg/kg	q 8 h	IV or PO	7 days
Disseminated herpes zoster	Acyclovir	30 mg/kg	q 8 h	IV	7 days
Cytomegalovirus	Gancyclovir	10 mg/kg	q 12 h	IV	14–21 days
Bacteria					
Mycobacterium avium-intracellulare	No drug combinations are known to be effective				
	?Ansamycin* and	150–? mg	q 24 h	PO	?
	?Clofazimine* and	100–600 mg	q 24 h	PO	?
	?Amikacin	15 mg/kg	q 24 h	IV	?
Mycobacterium tuberculosis	INH and	300 mg	q 24 h	PO, IM	18 months
	rifampin and	600 mg	q 24 h	PO, (IV)	18 months
	ethambutol	15 mg/kg	q 24 h	PO	18 months

*Investigational drugs.

be trimethoprim-sulfamethoxazole (oral or intravenous) or pentamidine isethionate (intravenous).[44] These two drugs appear to be equally effective. The former has traditionally been preferred because it is better tolerated in many patients. However, AIDS patients have an unusually high and as yet unexplained intolerance of trimethoprim-sulfamethoxazole; 60 per cent of patients develop rash, leukopenia, hepatitis, nausea, or fever.[45] On the other hand, pentamidine, which is approved only as a parenteral agent, is associated with nephrotoxicity and neutropenia. Trimethoprim-sulfamethoxazole, administered for 14 to 21 days, is thus the preferred therapy, although several new agents currently being tested, such as aerosolized pentamidine and intravenous trimetrexate, are highly promising.

Cytomegalovirus infection occurs in virtually all AIDS patients who are homosexual, bisexual, or intravenous drug abusers, and in many of the remaining patients as well. Most of these patients ultimately have cytomegalovirus that can be isolated from oral secretions, urine, blood, and probably semen. Cytomegalovirus can cause retinitis, pneumonitis, colitis, esophagitis, and adrenal insufficiency, and may be associated with central and peripheral neurologic disorders. Blindness and copious diarrhea can be very disabling and disheartening complications for patients who already have substantial medical problems. The diagnosis of cytomegalovirus retinitis must be based on clinical grounds since the retina is obviously inaccessible for biopsy, and aspirations of the aqueous or vitreous can be hazardous. Cytomegalovirus esophagitis, pneumonitis, or colitis must be diagnosed by demonstration of typical cytomegalovirus inclusion bodies in the appropriate tissue. Cytomegalovirus cultures are not helpful in the diagnosis of organ involvement since so many patients are viremic without cytomegalovirus-induced organ dysfunction, and a positive culture may not be related to the cause of the colitis, pneumonitis, or esophagitis. Therapy of cytomegalovirus disease with 9-(1,3-dihydroxy 2-propoxymethyl)guanine (DHPG or Gancyclovir) and with phosphoformate (Foscarnet) appears to be effective in containing the disease process. However, lifelong suppressive therapy may be necessary to avoid prompt recurrences or relapses.[46, 47]

Mycobacterium avium-intracellulare occurs with unprecedented frequency among AIDS patients.[40] At least 40 per cent of patients have evidence of this mycobacterium at autopsy, in contrast to non-AIDS patients, among whom disseminated *Mycobacterium avium-intracellulare* is a distinct rarity. *Mycobacterium avium-intracellulare* can be found in large quantities in the blood, the bowel wall, the bone marrow, and less often in other organs. The extent to which this mycobacterium contributes to fever, weight loss, or specific organ dysfunction is difficult to determine since some heavily infected patients are asymptomatic and since there is no effective therapy to determine if suppression of the microorganisms will be associated with disappearance of such signs and symptoms. Other atypical mycobacteria have also been recognized in AIDS patients, including *M. kansasii, M. fortuitum, M. hemophilum*, and *M. chelonei. M. tuberculosis* is particularly common among Haitian and African patients. *M. tuberculosis* presents as either pulmonary or extrapulmonary disease and has quite typical antibiotic sensitivity patterns.[38]

Cerebral toxoplasmosis is the most common cause of central nervous system mass lesions in AIDS patients.[48] Lymphoma, *Cryptococcus* and mycobacterial infections, and bacterial abscesses are much less common causes. Toxoplasmosis outside of the central nervous system occurs but is uncommon. Patients usually present with focal neurologic deficits and have one or multiple contrast-enhancing lesions on CT scan. There is no definitive diagnostic test other than biopsy. Most clinicians will attempt an empiric trial of sulfadiazine and pyrimethamine for two to three weeks before performing a diagnostic biopsy. For patients unable to tolerate sulfa there is no approved therapy that is effective. Therapy must be continued for the patient's lifetime.

Cryptococcus neoformans is the most common cause of meningitis in AIDS patients, occurring in at least 5 to 10 per cent of patients.[49, 50] Patients often present with unimpressive headaches which are not invariably associated with fever. Cryptococcal infection less often presents as pneumonia, abdominal pain, skin lesions, or focal brain abscess. Most (but not all) patients with cryptococcal disease are fungemic and have a positive serum cryptococcal antigen test. Diagnosis is usually established by lumbar puncture, blood culture, bronchoalveolar lavage, or a screening serum cryptococcal antigen test. Therapy consists of amphotericin B for a total dose of at least 1.0 gm. It is unclear if flucytosine enhances efficacy. Because flucytosine is toxic to the bone marrow and excreted renally, it is often difficult to administer to AIDS patients because of bone marrow suppression. Relapses of cryptococcal disease are quite common after amphotericin B therapy is discontinued, and thus some type of chronic suppressive therapy (amphotericin B or perhaps fluconazole) is needed for most patients.

Herpes simplex causes perirectal lesions with or without proctitis in at least 5 to 10 per cent of AIDS patients. The extensive perirectal and sacral lesions are often mistaken for decubitus ulcers. Oral lesions (especially lip ulcers) and herpetic whitlow also occur. Herpes simplex lesions usually respond readily to oral acyclovir, but they have a high likelihood of recurrence when therapy is stopped.

Candida species cause stomatitis, esophagitis, and proctitis in AIDS patients. Most patients ultimately develop *Candida* stomatitis, which can be uncomfortable and interfere with nutrition. Esophagitis occurs in 5 to 10 per cent of patients and should be diagnosed by endoscopic biopsy since cytomegalovirus, herpes simplex, lymphoma, and Kaposi's sarcoma can cause similar syndromes (see pp. 640–642). Stomatitis usually responds to topical therapy with nystatin or clotrimazole. For esophagitis or proctitis, ketoconazole or amphotericin B is appropriate. Relapses are common when therapy is stopped.

Kaposi's sarcoma is the most common neoplastic manifestation of AIDS.[51–53] It occurs almost exclusively in homosexual males; lesions in females or heterosexual males are distinctly unusual. Kaposi's sarcoma, when it occurs, most often presents as the initial manifestation of AIDS. Less often lesions occur after opportunistic infections have been manifested. The clinical behavior of this tumor in AIDS patients is quite distinct from that of the disease recognized in HIV-seronegative Africans or elderly North American males of Mediterranean extraction. Most patients present with skin lesions that appear as purple nodules that are not always easy to distinguish from various nevi. Kaposi's sarcoma lesions probably occur as often on mucosal surfaces as on cutaneous surfaces. They can frequently be noted during examination of the oropharynx or during endoscopic procedures of the upper or lower gastrointestinal tract. These cutaneous and mucosal lesions rarely cause symptoms unless they occur at anatomic sites where they produce pain (e.g., soles of the feet), obstruction (larynx, colon), or social-cosmetic problems (face, hands). In some patients with advanced disease, Kaposi's sarcoma lesions can be so extensive and bulky that they appear to contribute to the patient's inanition. Occasionally visceral organs will be extensively involved, resulting in dysfunction such as pneumonia or diarrhea or bowel obstruction that can be life-threatening (see p. 1244). Any therapy should be regarded as palliative, not curative, for this multifocal tumor. Radiation therapy is effective for individual lesions such as those on the face, over joints, or on the feet. Alpha interferon can produce partial or complete remission in 40 per cent of patients for up to one year, especially those with good immunologic function.[54] Single- or multiple-agent chemotherapy can be palliative and improve the quality of life in many patients.

Lymphoma can present in HIV-infected individuals as primary central nervous system lesions, as adenopathy, as bone marrow tumors, or as disseminated lesions.[55–57] A variety of non-Hodgkin's lymphoma histologies have been described. Radiation therapy appears to have a palliative role for central nervous system lesions. Combination chemotherapy has been used for therapy of lymphoma, but its role in extending survival is not clear.

DIAGNOSIS

The surveillance definition of AIDS is more suited for epidemiologic purposes than for diagnosis of individual patients. In individual patients, it is more useful to document whether or not HIV infection is present, and then to determine whether the symptoms, signs, or laboratory abnormalities observed are due to HIV infection alone. The presence of HIV infection is strongly suspected when a screening test of high sensitivity such as an ELISA test is positive on two or more determinations, using the same sample or serial samples. The ELISA test is readily available and highly sensitive, but is not completely specific. The presence of HIV infection is usually confirmed by the highly specific (but less sensitive) Western blot test, which confirms the specificity of the immunologic reactions between the antibodies and the virally encoded proteins. A substantial fraction of ELISA-positive and ELISA-negative patients will, however, have Western blot tests that are indeterminate. These patients must have serial follow-up tests. Radioimmunoprecipitation assay can also confirm a positive ELISA test. The precise sensitivity and specificity of each technique and each commercial test is impossible to determine precisely since there is no absolute standard. Some research techniques such as polymerase chain reaction suggest that evidence of HIV infection can be detected months before ELISA or Western blot tests become positive in some high-risk individuals. Culture of HIV is available only at research laboratories, and in the best of hands will not yield virus in all patients who unequivocally have AIDS as determined by clinical criteria. The vast majority of patients who are seropositive can be shown to have virus in their blood if cultures are done carefully on more than one occasion. Certain virus antigens such as p24 can be detected in blood by commercially available tests.

The presence of antibody to HIV specifically indicates that an individual has been exposed to HIV or is infected with it. The presence of lymphopenia with a selective deficiency in the helper/inducer (OKT4/Leu-3) T lymphocyte subset is the characteristic immune defect in patients with HIV infection. This generally results in a reversal of the T4 to T8 lymphocyte ratio. It is important to point out that reversal of the T4 to T8 lymphocyte ratio can also be seen in other infections such as cytomegalovirus and Epstein-Barr virus. However, in the latter cases the reversal is almost invariably due to an increase in number of T8 lymphocytes and not to a selective depletion of T4 cells.

When a patient presents with an opportunistic infection or Kaposi's sarcoma and no apparent cause of immunosuppression, the most direct technique for determining whether or not the patient has AIDS is to perform a serologic test for HIV antibody. On rare occasions Kaposi's sarcoma will present in an otherwise healthy North American male under the age of 60 years who does not have HIV infection and who thus does not have AIDS. Other than in association with AIDS, *Pneumocystis* pneumonia almost never presents in adults who do not have an obvious cause of immunosuppression such as cancer, corticosteroid therapy, or an organ transplant. *Pneumocystis* pneumonia can, however, be the initial manifestation of congenital immunodeficiencies in infants. Similarly, cerebral toxoplasmosis, disseminated *Mycobacterium avium-intracellulare*, perirectal herpes simplex, and cytomegalovirus retinitis or colitis occur only in the setting of a recognized immunosuppressive disease. These particular infectious processes are especially characteristic of AIDS as opposed to other immunodeficiency disorders. In contrast, disseminated cryptococcosis, histoplasmosis, or tuberculosis occur often in patients who are immunologically normal and who have no underlying disease.

TREATMENT AND PROGNOSIS

There is no clear answer concerning the fraction of HIV-infected individuals who will ultimately develop AIDS or AIDS-related disorders. The best current estimate is that during the initial 6 to 8 years of follow-up about 40 to 60 per cent will develop AIDS or related disorders.[11, 12] Once AIDS develops, prognosis is discouraging. The median cumulative probability of survival for patients presenting with Kaposi's sarcoma is 107 weeks; for those presenting with *Pneumocystis* pneumonia, 45 weeks; for those presenting with other opportunistic infections, 30 weeks.[58] Advances in diagnosis and therapy of AIDS-related infections and tumors may be extending these survival figures modestly. It is very unusual for patients to survive more than 24 months after an episode of *Pneumocystis* pneumonia. Of note is the fact that approximately 20 per cent of patients with Kaposi's sarcoma seem to survive for several years. Their ultimate outcome is unknown. There are, however, no reports of spontaneous reversal of the immunologic defect associated with AIDS.

Several agents have been identified which have activity against HIV *in vitro*, including 3′-azido-3′deoxythymidine (AZT), didoxycytidine, alpha interferon, ribavirin, and phosphonoformate.[59–62] Initial trials suggest that at least one of these agents, 3′-azido-3′deoxythymidine, during a six-month placebo-controlled trial does reduce the number of deaths in patients with AIDS who have had *Pneumocystis carinii* pneumonia. The long-term benefits of 3′-azido-3′deoxythymidine or the precise mechanism by which it exerts its beneficial effect are unknown. Other antiretroviral agents are currently being tested.[63] Immunomodulation using natural or recombinant interferons and interleukins has also been attempted in HIV-infected patients without dramatic impact on *in vivo* immune function or on patient survival.[19, 61] Bone marrow transplantation to reconstitute immune response has been attempted in identical twins.[19] However, the long-term benefits of this approach have yet to be determined. Thus, at this time, AIDS must be regarded as an incurable, inevitably fatal disease for which new therapeutic approaches are just beginning to offer some hope.[63]

PREVENTION

It is clear that HIV is transmitted by sexual intercourse, by contaminated blood associated with intravenous drug abuse, by infected blood or biologic products, and by mother to infant perinatally.[11] Education of the general public has the potential, therefore, for decreasing spread by changing behavior.[63] It is likely that the use of condoms will decrease sexual transmission of HIV. To encourage sexually active individuals to consider the drug and sexual histories of their sexual partners will permit these individuals to at least be aware of the consequences of their sexual activity. Unfortunately, drug abusers are notoriously difficult to reach with education campaigns. Even if public education were completely successful in eradicating the spread of HIV, it is important to keep in mind that several hundred thousand North Americans already infected with HIV will still progress to AIDS over the next five to ten years unless an effective therapy is discovered.

References

1. Centers for Disease Control. Revision of the case definition of acquired immunodeficiency syndrome for national reporting—United States. MMWR *34*:373, 1985.
2. Centers for Disease Control. Classification system for human T-lymphotropic virus type III/lymphadenopathy-associated virus infections. MMWR *35*:334, 1986.
3. Centers for Disease Control. Revision of the CDC surveillance case definition for acquired immunodeficiency syndrome. MMWR *36*(15):1, 1987.
4. Barre-Sinnousi, F., Chermann, C., Rey, F., et al. Isolation of a T-lymphocyte retrovirus from a patient at risk for acquired immune deficiency syndrome (AIDS). Science *220*:868, 1983.
5. Popovic, M., Sarngadharan, M. G., Reed, E., and Gallo, R. C. Detection, isolation, and continuous production of cytopathic retrovirus (HTLV-III) from patients with AIDS and pre-AIDS. Science *224*:497, 1984.
6. Levy, J. A., Hoffman, A. D., Kramer, S. M., et al. Isolation of lymphocytopathic retroviruses from San Francisco patients with AIDS. Science *225*:840, 1984.
7. Lowy, D. R. Transformation and oncogenesis: retroviruses. *In* Fields, B. N. (ed.). Virology. New York, Raven Press, 1985, pp. 235–263.
8. Poiesz, B. J., Ruscetti, F. W., Gazdor, A. F., et al. Detection and isolation of type C retrovirus particles from fresn and cultured lympnocytes of a patient with cutaneous T cell lymphoma. Proc. Natl. Acad. Sci. USA *77*:7415, 1980.
9. Wayne-Hobson, S., and Montagnier, L. Genetic structure of the lymphadenopathy-AIDS virus. Cancer Rev. *1*:18, 1986.
10. Wong-Staal, F., and Gallo, R. C. Human T lymphotropic retroviruses. Nature *317*:395, 1985.
11. Curran, J. W., Morgan, W. M., and Hardy, A. M. The epidemiology of AIDS: current status and future prospects. Science *229*:1352, 1985.
12. Jaffe, H. W., Darrow, W. W., Echenberg, D. R., et al. The acquired immunodeficiency syndrome in a cohort of homosexual men. Ann. Intern. Med. *103*:210, 1985.
13. Centers for Disease Control. Human T lymphotropic virus type III/lymphadenopathy associated virus antibody prevalence in U.S. military recruit applicants. MMWR *35*:421, 1986.
14. Public Health Service. Coolfont report: a PHS plan for prevention and control of AIDS and the AIDS virus. Public Health Rep. *101*:341, 1986.
15. Polk, B. F., Fox, R., Brookmeyer, R., et al. Predictors of the acquired immunodeficiency syndrome developing in a cohort of seropositive homosexual men. N. Engl. J. Med. *310*:61, 1987.
16. Ward, J. W., Deppe, D. A., Samson, S., et al. Risk of human immunodeficiency virus infection from blood donors who later developed the acquired immunodeficiency syndrome. Ann. Intern. Med. *106*:61, 1987.
17. Henderson, D. K., Saah, A. J., Zak, B. J., et al. Risk of nosocomial infections with human T lymphotropic virus III in a large cohort of intensively exposed health care workers. Ann. Intern. Med. *104*:644, 1986.
18. Gallin, J. I., and Fauci, A. S. (eds.). Advances in Host Defense Mechanisms, Vol. 5. Acquired Immunodeficiency Syndrome (AIDS). New York, Raven Press, 1985.
19. Fauci, A. S. (moderator). The acquired immunodeficiency syndrome: an update. Ann. Intern. Med. *102*:800, 1985.
20. Lane, H. C., Masur, H., Gelman, E. P., et al. Correlation between immunologic function and clinical subpopulations of patients with the acquired immune deficiency syndrome. Am. J. Med. *78*:417, 1985.
21. Lane, H. C., Masur, H., Edgar, L. C., et al. Abnormalities of B-cell activation and immunoregulation in patients with the acquired immunodeficiency syndrome. N. Engl. J. Med. *309*:453, 1983.
22. Goedert, J. J., Biggar, R. J., Melbye, M., et al. Effect of T4 count and cofactors on the incidence of AIDS in homosexual men infected with human immunodeficiency virus. JAMA *257*:331, 1987.
23. Cooper, D. A., MacLean, P., Finlayson, R., et al. Acute AIDS retrovirus infection, definition of a clinical illness associated with seroconversion. Lancet *1*:537, 1985.
24. Tindall, B., Barker, S., Donovan, B., et al. Characterization of the acute clinical illness associated with human immunodeficiency virus infection. Arch. Intern. Med. *148*:945, 1988.
25. Centers for Disease Control. Persistent, generalized lymphadenopathy among homosexual males. MMWR *31*:249, 1982.
26. Abrams, D. I. AIDS-related lymphadenopathy. The role of biopsy. J. Clin. Oncol. *4*:126, 1986.
27. Metroka, C. E., Cunningham-Rundles, S., Pollack, M. S., et al. Generalized lymphadenopathy in homosexual men. Ann. Intern. Med. *99*:585, 1983.
28. Mathur-Wagh, U., Spigiel, I., Sachs, H. S., et al. Longitudinal study of persistent generalized lymphadenopathy in homosexual men: relation to acquired immunodeficiency syndrome. Lancet *1*:1033, 1984.
29. Fishbein, D. B., Kaplan, J. E., Spira, T. J., et al. Unexplained lymphadenopathy in homosexual men. A longitudinal study. JAMA *245*:930, 1985.
30. Abrams, D. I., Kiprov, D. D., Goldest, J. J., et al. Antibodies to human T lymphotropic virus type III and development of the acquired immunodeficiency syndrome in homosexual men presenting with immune thrombocytopenia. Ann. Intern. Med. *104*:47, 1986.
31. Serwadda, D., Mugerwa, R. D., and Sewankambo, N. K. Slim disease: a new disease in Uganda and its association with HTLV-III infection. Lancet *2*:849, 1985.
32. Navia, B. A., Jordan, B. D., and Price, R. W. The AIDS dementia complex: I. Clinical features. Ann. Neurol. *19*:517, 1986.
33. Snider, W. D., Simpson, D. M., Nielsen, S., et al. Neurologic complications of acquired immune deficiency syndrome, analysis of 50 patients. Ann. Neurol. *14*:403, 1983.
34. Goldstick, L., Mandybur, T. I., and Bode, R. Spinal cord degeneration in AIDS. Neurology *35*:103, 1985.
35. Ho, D., Rota, T. R., Schooley, R. T., et al. Isolation of HTLV-III from cerebrospinal fluid and neural tissues of patients with neurologic syndromes related to the acquired immunodeficiency syndrome. N. Engl. J. Med. *313*:1493, 1985.
36. Klein, R. S., Harris, C. A., Small, C. B., et al. Oral candidiasis in high risk patients as the initial manifestation of the acquired immune deficiency syndrome. N. Engl. J. Med. *311*:358, 1984.
37. Greenspan, J. S., Greenspan, D., Lennette, E. T., et al. Replication of Epstein-Barr virus within the epithelial cells of oral "hairy" leukoplakia, an AIDS-associated lesion. N. Engl. J. Med. *313*:1564, 1985.
38. Sunderam, G., McDonald, R. J., Maniatis, T., et al. Tuberculosis as a manifestation of the acquired immunodeficiency syndrome. JAMA *256*:362, 1986.
39. Centers for Disease Control. Update: acquired immunodeficiency syndrome—United States. MMWR *35*:17, 1986.
40. Kovacs, J. A., and Masur, H. Opportunistic infections. *In* Gallin, J. I., and Fauci, A. S. (eds.). Advances in Host Defense Mechanisms, Vol. 5. Acquired Immunodeficiency Syndrome. New York, Raven Press, 1985, pp. 35–58.
41. Kovacs, J. A., Hiemenz, J. W., Macher, A. M., et al. *Pneumocystis carinii* pneumonia: a comparison between patients with the acquired immunodeficiency syndrome and patients with other immunodeficiencies. Ann. Intern. Med. *100*:663, 1984.
42. Kovacs, J. A., Ng, V., Masur, H., et al. Diagnosis of Pneumocystis pneumonia: improved detection in sputum using monoclonal antibodies. N. Engl. J. Med. *318*:589, 1988.

43. Ognibene, F. P., Shelhamer, J., Macher, A. M., et al. The diagnosis of *Pneumocystis carinii* pneumonia in patients with the acquired immunodeficiency syndrome using subsegmental bronchoalveolar lavage. Am. Rev. Respir. Dis. *129*:929, 1984.
44. Small, C. B., Harris, C. A., Greedland, G. H., et al. The treatment of *Pneumocystis carinii* pneumonia. Arch. Intern. Med. *145*:837, 1985.
45. Gordin, F. M., Simon, G. L., Wofsy, C. B., et al. Adverse reactions to trimethoprim-sulfamethoxazole in patients with the acquired immunodeficiency syndrome. Ann. Intern. Med. *100*:495, 1984.
46. Masur, H., Lane, H. C., Palestine, A., et al. Effect of 9-(1,3-dihydroxy-2-propoximethyl) guanine on serious cytomegalovirus disease in eight immunosuppressed homosexual men. Ann. Intern. Med. *104*:41, 1986.
47. Collaborative DHPG Treatment Study Group. Treatment of serious cytomegalovirus infections with 9-(1,3-dihydroxy-2-propoxymethyl) guanine in patients with AIDS and other immunodeficiencies. N. Engl. J. Med. *314*:801, 1986.
48. Navia, B. A., Petito, C. K., Gold, J. W., et al. Cerebral toxoplasmosis complicating the acquired immune deficiency syndrome: clinical and neuropathological findings in 27 patients. Ann. Neurol. *19*:224, 1986.
49. Kovacs, J. A., Kovacs, A. A., Polis, M., et al. Cryptococcosis in the acquired immunodeficiency syndrome. Ann. Intern. Med. *103*:533, 1985.
50. Zyer, A., Louie, E., Holzman, R. S., et al. Cryptococcal disease in patients with the acquired immunodeficiency syndrome, diagnostic features and outcome of treatment. Ann. Intern. Med. *104*:234, 1986.
51. Volberding, P. A. Kaposi's sarcoma and the acquired immunodeficiency syndrome. Med. Clin. North Am. *70*:665, 1986.
52. Muggia, F. M., and Lonberg, M. Kaposi's sarcoma and AIDS. Med. Clin. North Am. *70*:139, 1986.
53. Freidman-Kien, A. E., Laubenstein, L. J., Rubinstein, P., et al. Disseminated Kaposi's sarcoma in homosexual men. Ann. Intern. Med. *96*:693, 1982.
54. Krown, S. E., Rial, F. X., Cunningham-Rundles, S., et al. Preliminary observations on the effect of recombinant leukocyte A interferon in homosexual men with Kaposi's sarcoma. N. Engl. J. Med. *308*:1071, 1983.
55. Levine, A. M., Meyre, P. R., Byandy, M. K., et al. Development of B-cell lymphoma in homosexual men. Ann. Intern. Med. *100*:7, 1984.
56. Ziegler, J. L., Beckstead, J. A., Volberding, P. A., et al. Non-Hodgkin's lymphoma in 90 homosexual men, relation to generalized lymphadenopathy and the acquired immunodeficiency syndrome. N. Engl. J. Med. *311*:565, 1984.
57. So, Y. T., Beckstead, J. A., and Davis, R. L. Primary central nervous system lymphoma in acquired immune deficiency syndrome: a clinical and pathological study. Ann. Neurol. *20*:566, 1986.
58. Rothenberg, R., Woelfel, M. Stoneburner, R., et al. Survival with the acquired immunodeficiency syndrome: experience with 5833 cases in New York City. N. Engl. J. Med. *317*:1297, 1987.
59. Fischl, M. A., Richman, D. D., Grieco, M. H., et al. The efficacy of azidothymidine in the treatment of patients with AIDS and AIDS related complex. N. Engl. J. Med. *317*:1, 1987.
60. McCormick, J. B., Getchell, J. P., Mitchell, S. W., and Hicks, D. R. Ribavirin suppresses replication of lymphadenopathy-associated virus in cultures of human adult T-lymphocyte. Lancet *2*:1367, 1984.
61. DeVita, V. (moderator). Drug development for acquired immunodeficiency syndrome. Ann. Intern. Med. *106*:568, 1987.
62. Yarchoan, R., and Broder, S. Development of antiretroviral therapy for the acquired immunodeficiency syndrome and related disorders. N. Engl. J. Med. *316*:557, 1987.
63. Francis, D. P., and Chin, J. The prevention of acquired immunodeficiency syndrome in the United States—an objective strategy for medicine, public health, business, and the community. JAMA *257*:1357, 1987.

Gastrointestinal Manifestations of AIDS and Other Sexually Transmissible Diseases

SCOTT L. FRIEDMAN
ROBERT L. OWEN

GASTROINTESTINAL MANIFESTATIONS OF AIDS*

FREQUENCY OF GASTROINTESTINAL SYMPTOMS

See also pages 1233 to 1242.

Gastrointestinal and hepatobiliary symptoms are among the most frequent complaints in AIDS, and a methodical effort is required to identify those symptoms which are treatable. Best estimates suggest that 50 to 93 per cent of all AIDS patients will have marked gastrointestinal symptoms during the course of their illness.[1, 2] The most frequent symptom in AIDS is

*Recognizing the rapidly changing state of knowledge in the field of AIDS, a portion of the material in this chapter, used with permission of BRS Colleague, Inc, is also available on-line in the San Francisco General Hospital AIDS Knowledgebase. On-line updates will be made quarterly.

diarrhea, which is usually chronic and associated with weight loss and malnutrition. Odynophagia and dysphagia, abdominal pain, and jaundice are less frequently seen, but present equally difficult diagnostic and management challenges to the clinician caring for the AIDS patient. Gastrointestinal bleeding is rare, and is as likely to be due to non–AIDS-related pathology as to specific opportunistic infections or neoplasms.

EVALUATION OF GASTROINTESTINAL SYMPTOMS

Three general points must be considered when evaluating gastrointestinal symptoms in AIDS:

1. The clinical signs and symptoms alone rarely suggest a specific etiology, so that all notable gastrointestinal complaints must be investigated in hopes of identifying specific infections or neoplasms associated with AIDS.
2. The overriding goal of evaluation is promptly to identify infectious agents amenable to specific therapy. These include *Salmonella, Shigella, Campylobacter,* herpes virus, and cytomegalovirus. Homosexual men with AIDS are more likely than other AIDS patients to have gastrointestinal complications of protozoal and bacterial infections associated with sexual promiscuity, including amebiasis, giardiasis, and chlamydial and treponemal infections.[3] Changing sexual habits in response to the AIDS epidemic have, however, resulted in decreasing rates of sexually transmitted disease within this population, and with it a decrease in "gay bowel" infections[4] (see pp. 1258–1260).
3. Multiple gastrointestinal infections are the rule, so it is important to distinguish between true pathogens and secondary colonization. Evidence of tissue invasion by an infectious agent is the principal hallmark of pathogenicity.

It can be difficult to decide how extensively one should investigate gastrointestinal symptoms in the patient with AIDS. The clinician must weigh the discomfort and invasiveness of additional procedures against the severity of the patient's complaints and the likelihood that the procedure will identify a treatable condition. Noninvasive methods of diagnosis such as stool collection should always be employed first.

PRECAUTIONS FOR GASTROINTESTINAL PROCEDURES

Epidemiologic studies underscore the lack of transmissibility of the human immunodeficiency virus (HIV) by casual contact.[5] Furthermore, no cases have been reported in which AIDS has been transmitted to health care personnel or patients via contaminated endoscopic instruments. Nonetheless, high standards of instrument care and protection must be maintained to ensure the safety of patients and health professionals. In accordance with established guidelines, personnel performing or observing any gastrointestinal procedures in a patient with AIDS or AIDS-related complex (ARC) should wear gowns, gloves, masks, and protective eyewear to avoid splatter with body fluids.[6] Needles must be disposed of carefully. Lensed instruments must be thoroughly washed and disassembled to remove secretions and debris and then disinfected or sterilized after each use. A variety of disinfectants are suitable for this purpose, including 1 per cent glutaraldehyde, 6 per cent hydrogen peroxide, or 25 per cent ethanol for 10 to 30 minutes. Both glutaraldehyde and 25 per cent ethanol have been shown to inactivate reverse transcriptase activity of HIV.[7] Iodophors should be avoided because of their inability to kill mycobacteria.[8] Alternatively, instruments may be sterilized using ethylene oxide or glutaraldehyde for 10 hours, or 6 per cent hydrogen peroxide for 6 hours.

ENTERIC AND HEPATOBILIARY MANIFESTATIONS OF AIDS

Infections

Enteric infections are a major cause of morbidity in AIDS and ARC (see pp. 1238–1239). Decreased numbers of small intestinal T lymphocytes and a reversal in the normal mucosal "helper/suppressor" T cell ratio have now been recognized in homosexual men with AIDS or ARC; these changes may facilitate infection by a wide array of opportunistic enteric pathogens.[9]

Protozoa are among the most frequent gastrointestinal pathogens identified in AIDS. *Cryptosporidium* is a major cause of morbidity due to intractable diarrhea, resulting in profound weight loss and malnutrition. In one series, *Cryptosporidium* was identified in one third of all patients with diarrhea in association with AIDS.[10] Overall, 3 to 4 per cent of AIDS patients will harbor this organism.[11] *Isospora belli* is a protozoan related to *Cryptosporidium* that is occasionally identified in AIDS patients with diarrhea (see p. 1168). Microsporidia are small (1 to 5 μ) organisms that have been seen in the intestinal mucosa of AIDS patients (see p. 1169).

Viral infections of the gastrointestinal tract also occur frequently in AIDS. Cytomegalovirus (CMV) is, overall, the most common pathogen identified in autopsy series.[12] All patients with CMV will have gastrointestinal involvement,[13] predominantly in the colon.[14, 15] Gastrointestinal herpes simplex infections in AIDS involve the oropharynx, anus, or esophagus. Distal herpetic proctitis associated with proctalgia and bladder or bowel dysfunction is seen in AIDS patients, but *per se* is not an opportunistic infection, since herpetic proctitis is commonly seen among otherwise healthy gay men.[16] However, severe mucocutaneous herpes infection persisting for one month without healing is considered an opportunistic infection, thereby establishing an AIDS diagnosis.[17]

Infection of the esophagus by *Candida albicans* is the most frequent manifestation of fungal disease in the gastrointestinal tract. *Histoplasma* and *Cryptococcus* commonly infect the liver, always in the setting of disseminated infection.[18]

Bacterial infections by *Mycobacterium avium-intracellulare* and *Salmonella* can cause severe diarrhea. *Mycobacterium avium-intracellulare* is also the most frequent hepatic finding in AIDS.[19]

Neoplasms

Kaposi's Sarcoma

Incidence. Gastrointestinal involvement by Kaposi's sarcoma (KS) is frequent in AIDS. In autopsy series, gastrointestinal KS was seen in 56 to 70 per cent of all patients who had KS.[12, 20] Most clinical series probably underestimate the overall incidence of luminal gastrointestinal involvement with KS, since intestinal lesions rarely cause symptoms. In a prospective endoscopic evaluation of 50 homosexual men with AIDS and skin or lymph node KS, 20 patients (40 per cent) had evidence of gastrointestinal KS within the range of the flexible sigmoidoscope or upper endoscope.[21] The clinical pattern of gastrointestinal KS in AIDS resembles the disease in African patients with AIDS.[22] In contrast, the indolent variant of KS previously recognized in elderly men of European origin only rarely is associated with gastrointestinal involvement.[23]

The location of nonvisceral sites of KS (skin versus lymph nodes) does not predict the likelihood of gastrointestinal KS, although in general, patients with extensive cutaneous lesions are more likely to have gastrointestinal involvement.[21, 24] The absence of skin or lymph node KS, however, does not exclude the possibility of gastrointestinal involvement.[25] Gastrointestinal KS is not more common in patients with concurrent oral KS lesions than in those without oral lesions.[21]

Clinical Features. Gastrointestinal KS, although often widely disseminated, rarely leads to symptoms. KS lesions are usually small and multiple, but occasionally bulky masses may be seen.[21] Several autopsy series have failed to demonstrate a single instance of death primarily due to a gastrointestinal KS lesion.[20, 26] Similarly, in a prospective study of 20 patients with endoscopic evidence of KS, none had proven clinical sequelae of gastrointestinal lesions.[21]

Rarely, luminal KS lesions have clinical consequences. Many of these complications are likely to be seen more frequently as the AIDS epidemic spreads. Gastrointestinal bleeding from ulcerated KS lesions has been reported in one AIDS patient,[27] as well as the variants of KS in patients with renal allografts[28] and in African[29] and European[30] patients with KS. Bowel involvement in non-AIDS patients has on rare occasion led to obstruction,[31] perforation with peritonitis,[32] or mesenteric cyst formation.[33] Intestinal KS has also been described in association with celiac disease,[34] protein-losing enteropathy,[35, 36] and malabsorption.[37] Hepatobiliary and pancreatic KS have also been reported. In fact, KS has been found in every solid organ except kidneys, heart, and brain.[38]

Evaluation. Most gastrointestinal KS lesions are discovered incidentally during endoscopic procedures.

Table 65–1. SURVIVAL OF PATIENTS WITH AND WITHOUT GASTROINTESTINAL KAPOSI'S SARCOMA AT SIX-MONTH INTERVALS

Months after Diagnosis	Number of Patients Alive		
	With GI KS	*Without GI KS*	*p Value*
6	15/16 (94%)	21/21 (100%)	<0.01
12	11/16 (69%)	20/21 (95%)	<0.005
18	4/13 (31%)	15/16 (94%)	<0.001
24	1/9 (11%)	7/8 (88%)	<0.005

p values using one sided Fisher's exact test.
Reprinted with permission from: Gastrointestinal Kaposi's sarcoma in patients with acquired immune deficiency syndrome: endoscopic and autopsy findings by Friedman, S. L., Wright, T. L., and Altman, D. F. Gastroenterology *89*:102–108. Copyright 1985 by The American Gastroenterological Association.

Three distinct luminal KS lesions have been reported: *maculopapular* (often hemorrhagic) lesions, *polypoid* lesions, and *umbilicated nodular* lesions (Color Figs. 65–1 and 65–2, p. xl).[39] Each has a characteristic appearance, although cytomegalovirus infection, especially in the colon, may resemble the appearance of hemorrhagic KS lesions.[14]

Endoscopic biopsy of KS lesions is safe; no complications, including perforation or bleeding, have been reported since KS was recognized as a manifestation of AIDS. The yield of endoscopic biopsy of a characteristic lesion is only 23 per cent,[21] probably because most enteric lesions are submucosal. Sigmoidoscopic biopsies are positive for KS in 36 per cent of patients with visible lesions, whereas the smaller endoscopic biopsies are positive in only 13 per cent.[21] Radiologic contrast studies may demonstrate KS lesions;[40] however, the low specificity and sensitivity of this technique compared with endoscopy make it a less desirable means of evaluating gastrointestinal KS.

Prognosis. Even though visceral KS lesions rarely cause symptoms, AIDS patients with gastrointestinal involvement by KS have a poorer prognosis than those patients who have KS without gastrointestinal involvement. The 24-month survival in those without gastrointestinal KS was significantly greater than in those with gastrointestinal KS at the time of initial evaluation (Table 65–1).[21]

The reason for the poorer prognosis in patients with gastrointestinal KS is unclear. It is possible that the extent of visceral involvement by KS parallels the severity of immunosuppression and thus also parallels the susceptibility to life-threatening infections.

There is little reason to treat most gastrointestinal KS lesions because so few are symptomatic. In those patients who develop biliary or luminal obstruction or perforation due to KS lesions, surgery may be indicated (see p. 1252).

Lymphoma

A striking increase in the incidence of lymphoma in AIDS has been recognized, often with enteric or hepatobiliary involvement. In two separate series, gastrointestinal involvement by non-Hodgkin's lymphoma occurred in 17 and 28 per cent, respectively, of patients with AIDS and extranodal lymphoma.[41, 42] The tumors are of B lymphocyte origin in practically all cases.[43] The tumors involve all sites of the gastrointestinal tract, including the esophagus[44] and rectum.[45, 46]

Anorectal Carcinoma

Anorectal carcinomas are more common in homosexual men; however, expression of these tumors may not necessarily require immune deficiency. Epidemiologic studies also demonstrate an increased incidence of anal carcinomas in young unmarried males compared with married males,[47, 48] and several recent reports have described this tumor specifically in homosexual men,[49–53] some of whom had AIDS. Furthermore, anorectal dysplasia in homosexual men is associated with presence of serum antibodies to HIV, and a depressed T4/T8 lymphocyte ratio.[54] It is not certain, however, whether the dysplasia results from immune supression or if both these findings reflect a high frequency of anal-receptive intercourse. These neoplasms appear to result from chronic *perianal herpes* or *papillomavirus* infections acquired through sexual contact. Morphologic studies have documented histologic progression, often in the same lesion, from benign condyloma acuminatum to marked dysplasia or *squamous carcinoma.*[55, 56] Immune deficiency might enhance this progression; immunocompromised renal transplant patients display a 100-fold increase in the incidence of carcinoma of the vulva and anus compared with the general population.[57] No increased incidence of anorectal carcinoma has been recognized in other AIDS subgroups apart from homosexual men (i.e., in hemophiliacs or intravenous drug users).

CLINICAL ASPECTS OF GASTROINTESTINAL AND HEPATOBILIARY INVOLVEMENT IN AIDS

Diarrhea

Diarrhea is the most common gastrointestinal symptom in AIDS, reported in 50 per cent[58] to 90 per cent[2] of all AIDS patients.

Differential Diagnosis

A wide variety of protozoal, viral, and bacterial organisms have been implicated as diarrheal pathogens in AIDS (Table 65–2). Some, like *Mycobacterium avium-intracellulare,* are unique to AIDS; others, like *Cryptosporidium,* cause self-limited diarrheal illness in healthy hosts but chronic diarrhea in immunosuppressed patients. Other organisms, like *Shigella,* produce clinical illnesses indistinguishable from those occurring in healthy hosts (see pp. 1199–1203).

The majority of AIDS patients with diarrhea have one or more identifiable pathogens. In a recent study, gastrointestinal infection was identified in 15 of 21 AIDS patients with diarrhea.[1] Simultaneous infections with more than one organism in this study were common, emphasizing the need to exclude all pathogens thoroughly when evaluating diarrhea in these patients. Some AIDS patients with diarrhea will have no clear explanation for their symptoms, despite extensive evaluation. This subset of patients has been described as having "idiopathic AIDS enteropathy" (see p. 1248).

Table 65–2. DIARRHEA IN AIDS: DIFFERENTIAL DIAGNOSIS

Infections
Protozoan
*Cryptosporidium**
Isospora belli
Microsporidium
Giardia
Entamoeba histolytica
Bacterial
*Mycobacterium avium-intracellulare**
*Salmonella**
Shigella
Campylobacter
Clostridum difficile
Bacterial small bowel overgrowth
Viral
*Cytomegalovirus**
?Rotavirus
?Norwalk agent
Fungal
Candida
Neoplasms
Lymphoma
Kaposi's sarcoma
Idiopathic
"AIDS enteropathy"*

*More frequent.

Protozoa are the most frequent diarrheal pathogens identified in AIDS (see p. 1237). Diarrhea due to *Cryptosporidium,* for example, may result in profound weight loss and malnutrition. The small bowel is the most common site of luminal involvement,[59] but cryptosporidial organisms have also been identified in the appendix,[60] the rectal mucosa, and the stomach, as well as the biliary tree[59] and respiratory tract.[61] The site of involvement within the gastrointestinal tract does not appear to affect the clinical presentation, except when cryptosporidial cholecystitis is present.[62]

Although patients with cryptosporidiosis are almost always symptomatic, a rare asymptomatic carriage of the organism has been identified.[63] Prominent clinical features include diarrhea (up to 17 liters per day) associated with frank malabsorption[10] and evidence of intestinal secretion.[64] Abdominal pain is seen in one half to two thirds of all patients, and is usually dull, crampy, and predominantly epigastric or upper abdominal.[10, 59] The mechanism of diarrhea in cryptosporidiosis is unknown; it has been suggested that the organisms impair cell function by releasing cellular toxins, but none have been identified. A culture system facilitating complete growth of cryptosporidia *in vitro* has been developed that should enable investigators to clarify the pathogenetic features of this infection[65] (see pp. 1165–1169).

Isospora belli is a protozoan related to *Cryptosporidium* that is occasionally identified in AIDS patients with diarrhea. In general, the organism causes weight loss and watery diarrhea similar to that occurring in disease due to *Cryptosporidium*.[66] The pathogenetic mechanisms and significance of these infections are unclear[10] (see pp. 1165–1168).

Microsporidia are small (1 to 5 μ) protozoa that have been seen in the intestinal mucosa of AIDS patients and are associated with nonbloody diarrhea. They can best be recognized by their characteristic ultrastructure[67, 68] (see pp. 1169–1171).

Mycobacterium avium-intracellulare is a highly prevalent AIDS-associated pathogen with protean manifestations. The hallmark of intestinal *M. avium* infection, as in other tissues, is the relative paucity of tissue response. Intestinal involvement with *M. avium* is common but often asymptomatic. Of patients with *M. avium* identified at autopsy, up to 60 per cent have gastrointestinal involvement, yet few clinical series recognize *M. avium* as an intestinal pathogen antemortem. The small bowel is the most common site of infection (Fig. 65–3*A* and *B*); however, organisms have been identified in the colon as well.[69, 70] A small subset of patients with intestinal *M. avium* will develop a clinical syndrome strikingly similar to *Whipple's disease*.[71] As in Whipple's disease, patients with pseudo-Whipple's disease due to *M. avium* develop severe malabsorption and small bowel is infiltrated with submucosal and lamina propria macrophages laden with organisms, but in *M. avium* these organisms are acid-fast bacilli instead of the Whipple's bacillus.[72] Pseudo-Whipple's disease due to *M. avium* can also be distinguished by the absence of both arthralgias and biopsy evidence of dilated small bowel villous lacteals, two common features of Whipple's disease.[72]

Recurrent *Salmonella* infection, with or without clinical enteritis, has a twentyfold higher incidence in patients with AIDS than in a healthy population[73] and may be the presenting finding of AIDS.[74] There is an increased likelihood of bacteremia associated with non-*typhi* infections in AIDS, whereas healthy hosts rarely develop bacteremia. *Salmonella* serogroup B, *Salmonella choleraesuis,* and *Salmonella* serogroup D have been isolated thus far, and most have been sensitive to chloramphenicol, tetracycline, and ampicillin.[74, 75] AIDS patients with salmonellosis have watery, nonbloody diarrhea and positive stool cultures for *Salmonella.* No clear explanation has been established for the increased incidence of this bacterial infection in AIDS (see p. 1262). *Candida* and other fungal organisms have not been clearly established as diarrheal pathogens in AIDS. Yeasts are often present in areas of intestinal pathology, most likely representing secondary colonization rather than fungus-induced disease.

Infection of the gastrointestinal tract by cytomegalovirus (CMV) most commonly affects the colon, where it causes a patchy or diffuse colitis associated with ulceration, in association with watery diarrhea[14] (Color Figs. 65–4 and 65–5, p. xl). Diarrhea results from mucosal vasculitis via invasion of vascular endothelium; the sequence may ultimately lead to perforation or infarction.

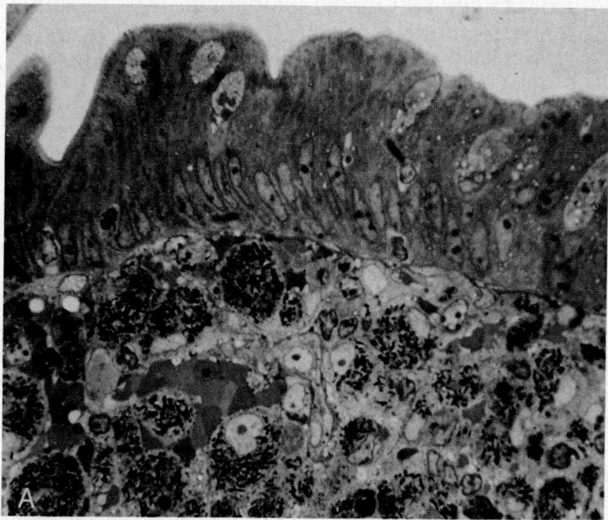

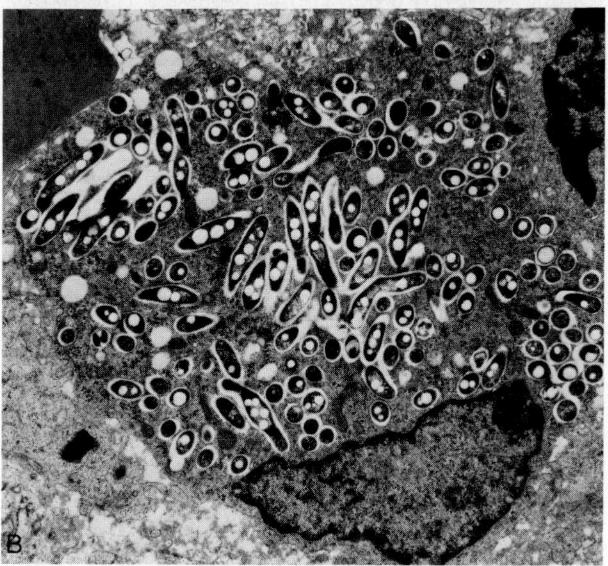

Figure 65–3. Endoscopic duodenal biopsy from an AIDS patient with malabsorption and diarrhea. *A,* Macrophages distended with acid-fast *Mycobacterium avium-intracellulare* beneath the villus epithelium produce an appearance similar to Whipple's disease. ×56. *B,* Rodlike longitudinal profiles and round cross-sectional profiles of *M. avium-intracellulare* fill the cytoplasm of a lamina propria macrophage in this AIDS patient. Transmission electron micrograph, ×332.

Herpes simplex virus does not cause diarrhea via enteric infection; however, AIDS patients may develop chronic perianal ulcerations with a mucopurulent discharge that may be interpreted as diarrhea.[76] Herpes virus is often cultured from enteric ulcerations in association with other pathogens in AIDS patients. Such findings, however, do not exclude herpes as a secondary infection.[77]

Neoplasms rarely cause diarrhea in AIDS. Intestinal lymphoma may lead to lymphatic obstruction and enteropathy with protein loss (see pp. 263–290, and 1519–1560). Kaposi's sarcoma has never been clearly identified as a cause of diarrhea in this population.

Evaluation

History and Physical Examination. The clinical history is not highly useful for establishing a specific diagnosis in AIDS patients with diarrhea, since co-infection by more than one enteric pathogen at the time of evaluation is the rule.[58] A careful history can, however, aid in localizing the segment of luminal gastrointestinal tract most severely involved. For example, symptoms of cramps, bloating, and nausea suggest gastric or small bowel involvement or both, raising the possibility of infection with *Cryptosporidium, Isospora belli,* or *Giardia.* Hematochezia usually implies large bowel inflammation; most commonly this results from colonic infection by cytomegalovirus, *Shigella,* or *Campylobacter.* Tenesmus can occur as a result of herpes, *Shigella,* or *Campylobacter* infections. The character, frequency, color, and odor of the stool are nonspecific in AIDS, and are therefore of little value in identifying specific infections.

A history of sexual promiscuity, especially when it includes multiple anonymous homosexual contacts, broadens the differential diagnosis of diarrhea to include the spectrum of infections commonly seen in many healthy homosexual men[3, 78, 79] (see pp. 1258–1262).

The physical exam also provides few diagnostic clues in the evaluation of diarrhea in AIDS. Peripheral lymphadenopathy, hepatosplenomegaly, and abdominal tenderness are commonly seen yet they have little diagnostic value.

Laboratory Evaluation. The overriding goal in the evaluation of diarrhea is to identify treatable infections while minimizing diagnostic invasiveness. The following outline is useful in evaluating diarrhea in a patient with AIDS:

1. All patients with diarrhea should have stool specimens cultured for *Salmonella, Shigella,* and *Campylobacter.* If no treatable infection is found or if diarrhea persists after treatment, stool specimens are stained for the acid-fast organisms *Cryptosporidium* and *Isospora belli.* A specimen is also cultured for *Mycobacterium avium-intracellulare.*

2. If diarrhea and weight loss persist in an otherwise functioning patient, upper endoscopy is performed with aspiration of secretions for ova and parasites and for bacterial culture and colony count. A small bowel mucosal biopsy is also done to identify *Cryptosporidium, Mycobacterium avium intracellulare,* or neoplasm.

3. If the patient has rectal bleeding, tenesmus, or both, flexible sigmoidoscopy is carried out with biopsy of the mucosa for pathology, particularly involving cytomegalovirus and herpes virus. Cultures are sent for bacteria, acid-fast bacilli, viruses, and *Clostridium difficile* toxin assay.

All patients with symptomatic diarrhea (defined here in functional terms as a significant increase in the frequency and decrease in the consistency of the patient's stools) should have multiple stool specimens cultured for bacterial pathogens and examined for ova and parasites. Specific pathogens should be treated, and if no improvement follows, stool should be re-examined with Ziehl-Neelsen stain in order to identify cryptosporidia[80] or *Isospora belli,*[81] cultured for mycobacteria, and evaluated for *Clostridium difficile* toxin. In practical terms, there is no urgency in finding cryptosporidia or *M. avium,* since no effective treatment is presently available. In contrast, *Isospora belli* infection will respond initially to trimethoprim-sulfamethoxazole, but is associated with a high rate of recurrence.[66] Even if noninvasive studies do not identify a pathogen, it is reasonable to offer a two- to three-week empiric trial of antibiotics prior to undertaking invasive workup, provided that diarrhea is not debilitating and is not associated with gastrointestinal blood loss. We have seen responses in this setting to trimethoprim-sulfamethoxazole, tetracycline, and norfloxacin. Responses may be due to eradication of small bowel bacterial overgrowth, occuring in the setting of gastric achlorhydria.[312, 313] Milk products should be avoided, since lactose intolerance is not unusual in this population.

If stool exams are negative or identify untreatable infections, the decision to undertake more extensive evaluation should be based on the degree to which diarrhea alone contributes to the patient's overall debility. For example, it would be reasonable further to evaluate the AIDS patient who has severe diarrhea and weight loss, but who otherwise feels well and remains active. Upper endoscopy or small bowel capsule biopsy could be performed to obtain mucosal samples for pathologic exam, and intestinal fluid for cytology, ova and parasite exam, and culture. Tests used to identify fat malabsorption, such as fecal fat quantitation and the D-xylose test, are not specific, since they are abnormal in almost all AIDS patients with diarrhea, regardless of etiology.[58, 82] Similarly, hypokalemia and true intestinal fluid secretion have been observed commonly but are not associated with any single infection.[82]

A second circumstance that may justify an invasive work-up exists when symptoms suggest colitis or proctitis, or both. Flexible sigmoidoscopy with mucosal biopsy may reveal pathologic hallmarks of cytomegalovirus or herpesvirus infection. Tissue should be cultured for bacterial enteric pathogens, *Chlamydia,* and viruses. Infections or noninfectious colitis not unique to AIDS (see p. 1267) may also be identified. Barium contrast studies of the gastrointestinal tract are not helpful in the evaluation of diarrhea, since nonspecific multifocal abnormalities are almost always present.[83]

Treatment. When the evaluation of diarrhea identifies an enteric pathogen, specific therapy, if available, should be administered. Prolonged antibiotic therapy (weeks to months) for *Salmonella, Shigella,* or *Campylobacter* infections may be necessary to prevent recurrence.[314] There are no effective antimicrobial therapies for cryptosporidial infections in AIDS, despite early enthusiasm for using spiramycin for cryptosporidial enteritis.[84] *Isospora belli* infections are sensitive to trimethoprim/sulfamethoxazole, but are associated with high relapse rates.[66] Acyclovir and a related drug, DHPG, show promise in treating herpes and cytomegalovirus infections, respectively, but early relapses are also common.[85, 86] A patient whose work-up fails to identify a treatable infection should be treated symptomatically with an antidiarrheal drug such as Lomotil or Imodium. If clinical signs of dehydration are present, intravenous fluid repletion is indicated. Nutritional support may be important for these patients, and should be given to those patients with reversible infections (see pp. 1994–2027), to those who feel well despite diarrhea and weight loss, and to children with AIDS who are failing to thrive (see pp. 1249–1250).

Idiopathic AIDS Enteropathy

Definition and Clinical Findings

A substantial number of AIDS patients have diarrhea and wasting without evidence of enteric infections; such patients are described as having idiopathic AIDS enteropathy. No standard definition of this entity exists, and patients with idiopathic diarrhea are clinically indistinguishable from those in whom an enteric pathogen is identified. It remains uncertain whether patients with idiopathic diarrhea have a noninfectious cause for their diarrhea, or simply an infectious diarrhea caused by one or more as yet unidentified pathogens. Often the idiopathic diarrhea is associated with AIDS-related complex before an AIDS diagnosis is established. This is a troubling and often ominous sign in the patient at risk for AIDS, and invasive evaluation at this stage is usually fruitless.

Few studies have systematically evaluated AIDS patients with unexplained diarrhea. The largest reported series compares findings in 12 gay men with AIDS and unexplained diarrhea with those in 13 "healthy" homosexual controls.[87] Patients with diarrhea have moderate to marked increases in stool weight associated with weight loss and occasional fevers. Diarrhea tends to be worse at night. Evidence of malnutrition in association with impaired D-xylose absorption is invariably present in all patients with diarrhea as well as histopathologic abnormalities of the small intestines. Partial villous atrophy associated with crypt hyperplasia is the finding most commonly seen in the small bowel. Rectal abnormalities include decreased plasma cells and the presence of focal viral inclusions. Increased numbers of intraepithelial lymphocytes are seen in both small bowel and rectal biopsies, suggesting that the syndrome might be due to immunologically mediated intestinal injury. It is likely, however, that enteric viral infections and *Cryptosporidium* are not definitively excluded in many of these patients. Moreover, subsequent studies have suggested that many of the morphologic findings described could have been a direct result of malnutrition itself.[88]

Investigators have used electron microscopy to demonstrate "tubuloreticular particles" in the intestinal mucosa of AIDS patients.[68] The particles are thought to be condensations of endoplasmic reticulum and are often associated with immunologically mediated tissue injury. However, it would be surprising if the severely impaired cellular immune responses associated with AIDS were capable of inducing autoimmune intestinal injury. Furthermore, many viral and possibly protozoal pathogens exist that are not detectable by the diagnostic methods currently employed. For example, no studies of AIDS patients have excluded infection by rotavirus or Norwalk agent, two diarrheal pathogens that have been well characterized in healthy hosts.[89] Indeed, evidence of virus-like particles in the ileal and rectal mucosa has been found in a few patients with AIDS.[90] As the sensitivity of our diagnostic methods improves and the full spectrum of infections seen in AIDS is appreciated, it is likely that fewer patients will be considered to have "idiopathic" diarrhea.

Management

AIDS patients with idiopathic diarrhea should be treated symptomatically. Antidiarrheals such as Imodium or Lomotil are often required. Bulk-forming agents, including Metamucil or bran, may be helpful in some cases. Narcotics such as codeine should be avoided if possible, since they are more likely to induce drowsiness or altered mental status in the debilitated patient. Nutritional repletion will increase the patient's sense of well-being, although it has not been demonstrated to prolong survival. In severe cases, short-term or long-term intravenous fluid repletion may be indicated.

Weight Loss

Weight loss is the most common, and at times most disturbing, general symptom associated with AIDS. Its presence is almost universal, reported in 95 to 100 per cent of all patients.[58, 91] Striking weight loss often precedes the actual diagnosis of AIDS.[92] The mean weight loss varies in clinical series from 25 to 35 pounds, but may be more severe if associated with watery diarrhea.[58, 84, 92] *Anorexia* associated with weight loss is the rule, although weight loss may be profound even in the presence of adequate caloric intake.[93]

Differential Diagnosis

Weight loss in AIDS is so common, and the variety of illnesses so great, that it is impossible to ascribe this symptom to a single opportunistic infection or neoplasm. The few clinical studies specifically investigating weight loss have noted that it tends to be greater if diarrhea is present, although patients still lose weight in the absence of diarrhea.[87, 94] Thus, the differential diagnosis of weight loss in the AIDS patient is similar to that of diarrhea. In addition, profound weight loss should direct attention to the possibility of steatorrhea due to fat malabsorption, which is most often associated with infiltrative or infectious small bowel disease due to *Mycobacterium avium-intracellulare, Cryptosporidium,* or cytomegalovirus (CMV). A more treatable, although less common cause of fat malabsorption is pancreatic insufficiency, resulting either from chronic pancreatitis unrelated to AIDS, from opportunistic infection of the pancreas by cytomegalovirus, or from drug-induced pancreatitis, especially following use of pentamidine.

Adrenal insufficiency is a rare but treatable cause of wasting in the AIDS patient, which, in most cases, is due to CMV infection of the adrenals;[95] this may precede the diagnosis of AIDS.[96] All patients have weight loss, fever, hypotension, hyperkalemia, and hyponatremia. Hypoglycemia, eosinophilia, and hyperpigmentation are not always present.[97] The ACTH stimulation test is always abnormal in this setting, and affected patients respond to steroid replacement.

It must be remembered that weight loss and generalized wasting are common consequences of any overwhelming illness, including AIDS, and that such weight loss will often progress without evidence of malabsorption or anorexia.

Evaluation

Specific investigation of weight loss without diarrhea is rarely indicated in AIDS patients, since an extensive evaluation is unlikely to identify a single cause. There are three notable exceptions: (1) patients whose laboratory and clinical features suggest adrenal insufficiency (see Differential Diagnosis above); (2) patients with clinical and laboratory evidence of pancreatitis (increased amylase, abdominal pain, history of chronic alcohol abuse, pancreatic calcifications), in whom fat malabsorption may indicate pancreatic insufficiency; and (3) patients who otherwise feel relatively well and are ambulatory, but have profound weight loss and diarrhea out of proportion to their general state of health.

An ACTH stimulation test is indicated if the clinical data suggest adrenal insufficiency. Empiric therapy with pancreatic enzyme replacement should be considered as a diagnostic and therapeutic maneuver when pancreatic insufficiency is suspected. Noninvasive imaging of the pancreas (CT scan or ultrasonography) is also appropriate.

A reasonable work-up for the relatively well AIDS patient who has disproportionate weight loss is the same as for the AIDS patient who has diarrhea. Emphasis should be placed on identifying treatable infections, using noninvasive means where possible, emphasizing careful stool exams and culture. Tests of small bowel absorptive function such as D-xylose absorption, fecal fat quantitation, and serum vitamin B_{12} are not specific, since results are abnormal in over half of all AIDS patients with diarrhea and weight loss regardless of which pathogens are present.[58, 94, 98]

Nutritional Abnormalities Associated with Weight Loss in AIDS

See also pages 1045 to 1062 and 1994 to 2006.

Malnutrition is common in AIDS patients and tends to be worse when diarrhea is present. AIDS patients with weight loss all have depressed serum albumin, with significantly lower values in those with diarrhea.[87] Hypoalbuminemia has also been observed in Haitians[93] and children with AIDS.[99] Few other parameters of nutritional status have been studied. In 11 Haitians with AIDS, 6 weighed less than 80 per cent of ideal body weight and 9 had triceps skin fold thicknesses below the 30th percentile.[93] No assessment of nitrogen balance in AIDS patients has been reported. Animal studies have shown that low zinc levels result in depressed T cell function and reduced IgM production.[100, 101] In humans, a statistical correlation has been noted between zinc levels and lymphocyte proliferation,[102] and zinc repletion in patients with considerable gastrointestinal fluid losses results in improved nitrogen retention.[103] Although it has been reported that zinc deficiency in AIDS patients may contribute to impaired immune function, little direct evidence supports the hypothesis. Clinical surveys of AIDS patients do not consistently report depressed zinc levels.[93, 103]

Protein malabsorption *per se* may cause intestinal mucosal atrophy, which further exacerbates malnutrition. This phenomenon has been clearly demonstrated in children with marasmus[104] as well as in patients with AIDS.[105] In each instance, nutritional repletion resulted in reversal of small bowel mucosal abnormalities.

Treatment

The primary therapeutic goal in the AIDS patient with weight loss is to identify all treatable infections contributing to diarrhea or general debility. When possible, specific antimicrobial therapy should be instituted for enteric protozoal or bacterial pathogens.

Few studies address the role of intravenous nutritional supplementation; however, its indications are best limited either to AIDS patients who appear relatively well, but whose weight loss and diarrhea are disproportionately severe, or to young children with AIDS who fail to thrive. Regardless, no clear evidence supports the notion that hyperalimentation will prolong survival, although it may increase the patient's sense of well-being. Enteral supplementation should be attempted initially, since intravenous hyperalimentation imposes the additional risk of catheter infections, bleeding, or thrombosis. No published studies are available that compare different enteral formulas; at least 30 per cent of the total calories should be provided as fat, usually as medium-chain triglycerides. Formulas should be lactose-free and contain trace metals, including zinc and selenium. A reasonable end point for enteral supplementation is either meaningful improvement or the appearance of a contraindication to further nutritional support (e.g., intractable diarrhea not responsive to antidiarrheal medications).

At present, intravenous hyperalimentation for AIDS patients is rarely indicated. Two groups, children or adult patients with severe diarrhea, may require short-term alimentation if enteral formulas are not tolerated. Perioperative intravenous hyperalimentation may be appropriate to enhance wound healing and speed recovery in the AIDS patient who requires surgery. The most effective hyperalimentation formulas for these patients have not been established; however, as previously stated, any formula employed should contain adequate trace metals (see pp. 1994–2027).

Ultimately the decision to offer parenteral nutritional supplementation is highly subjective. The needs or desires of the debilitated patient must be weighed against the additional morbidity of nasogastric or intravenous catheter placement. The patient should be made cognizant of the lack of evidence that such supplementation will substantially alter the overall course of the disease.

Odynophagia and Dysphagia

Differential Diagnosis

Dysphagia and *odynophagia* due to esophagitis are very common in AIDS, both having been recognized as prominent symptoms in early reports of the disease.[106] Their exact frequencies have not been established, since not all patients with esophagitis are symptomatic[12] (see pp. 640–656).

The majority of patients with dysphagia/odynophagia have *Candida* esophagitis alone or in association with other infectious pathogens (Table 65–3). Cytomegalovirus and herpes virus are the only other pathogens that cause esophagitis. *M. avium* has rarely been cultured in patients with esophageal disease, but is not clearly pathogenic. AIDS patients may also have esophageal symptoms due to diseases not unique to AIDS, including esophagitis due to reflux or medications (see pp. 594–619).

The incidence of *Candida* esophagitis varies with the AIDS risk group being studied. Many studies fail to distinguish between colonization and true infection by *Candida,* making it difficult to compare data from different studies. Ninety-three per cent of Haitians with AIDS have oral thrush or *Candida* esophagitis,[2] whereas in one series of homosexual men, the incidence of *Candida* esophagitis was only 40 per cent.[92] The association of oral thrush with *Candida* esophagitis approaches 100 per cent. Some observers believe that all patients with oral lesions consistent with thrush will have endoscopic evidence of candidal involvement of the esophagus.[107] While oral thrush often predicts concurrent esophagitis, it is clearly established that the absence of thrush does not exclude the possibility of esophageal candidiasis.[108] Oral *Candida* probably is overdiagnosed, since it is difficult for the inexperienced clinician to distinguish between thrush and hairy leukoplakia, a tongue lesion associated with herpes and papilloma viruses, whose appearance is similar to that of *Candida* infection[109] (see pp. 533–534).

Table 65–3. DIFFERENTIAL DIAGNOSIS OF DYSPHAGIA/ODYNOPHAGIA IN AIDS

*Candida**
Cytomegalovirus (CMV)
Herpes simplex*
Mycobacterium avium-intracellulare
Neoplasm: Kaposi's sarcoma, lymphoma
Non-AIDS esophageal disease (e.g., reflux esophagitis)

*More common.

Although cytomegalovirus is the most commonly identified pathogen in AIDS, its association with esophageal disease is relatively uncommon. When recognized, CMV infection may appear either as a diffuse distal esophagitis or occasionally as a large mucosal ulcer.[110]

Herpesvirus is an occasional cause of esophagitis in AIDS and has also been reported as a rare cause of esophagitis in immunocompetent patients.[111] In healthy patients, esophagitis is usually due to herpes simplex, type I;[111] however, AIDS patients may have esophagitis due to either type I or type II herpes. The disease is similar to herpetic infections of other mucous membranes in that the pathogenetic features follow a predictable sequence: discrete vesicles form, then shallow ulcers, which finally coalesce into regions of diffuse inflammation indistinguishable from those resulting from other causes of esophagitis. It is during this late stage of diffuse esophagitis that most patients with herpes are usually evaluated. The esophagitis of herpes infection, in comparison with that of *Candida,* is more commonly associated with severe odynophagia (see pp. 640–643).

Esophageal lymphoma can cause odynophagia or dysphagia.[44] Tumors may be ulcerated or polypoid, causing bleeding or obstruction. Histologic diagnosis based on endoscopic biopsy may be difficult if significant necrosis is present.

A self-limited syndrome in homosexual men has been described of acute esophageal ulceration in association with a maculopapular skin rash and oral ulcers.[112] The syndrome in most cases occurs coincident with both HIV seroconversion and inversion of the T lymphocyte helper/suppressor ratio, and may represent a direct pathogenic effect of HIV. Electron microscopy of affected tissue reveals retrovirus-like particles at the ulcer site, without characteristic features of cytomegalovirus or herpes infections. The significance of this syndrome with respect to AIDS is uncertain, since these patients do not have clinical criteria consistent with AIDS.

Evaluation

There is no way to identify the specific cause of odynophagia in the AIDS patient based on symptoms or physical examination alone. As with other gastrointestinal symptoms, the presence of multiple coinfecting organisms makes it impossible to ascribe a symptom or sign to a single pathogen.

As seen in Table 65–4, endoscopy, with biopsy and specific culture, is the only method of establishing a specific etiology for the cause of dysphagia/odynophagia.

Evidence of tissue invasion is required to establish definitely the pathogenicity of an infectious agent.

Candida appears grossly as a thick, cheesy, white exudate, often in association with marked mucosal friability and hemorrhage[113] (see Color Fig. 65–6, p. xl). Brushings display evidence of pseudomycelia, and biopsies are diagnostic, showing mucosal invasion by fungi.[113] *Candida* serology is not useful in the AIDS

Table 65–4. EVALUATION OF DYSPHAGIA/ODYNOPHAGIA IN AIDS

1. Barium swallow
   Suggestive, but not diagnostic
2. Endoscopy
   Gross: *Candida*: white plaques, friability
   CMV: single ulcer or diffuse esophagitis
   HSV: vesicles or shallow ulcers
   Micro: Look for tissue invasion by specific organism
   Candida: yeast forms
   CMV: inclusions in endothelial cells
   HSV: inclusions in epithelial cells
   Brush: May reveal specific organism
   Culture: Supportive evidence, but doesn't exclude superinfection
3. Serology
   Not diagnostic

patient, even though it may have utility in the immunocompetent host.[114]

Cytomegalovirus usually produces single deep ulcerations or very large superficial ulcerations of the esophagus. Microscopically, CMV esophagitis displays evidence of vascular endothelial cell invasion, often in association with a vasculitis.[14]

Early herpes esophagitis appears as characteristic discrete vesicles that gradually resolve, leaving shallow ulcers. Biopsies and brushings for cytology from the margin of the ulcers (the sites of active viral replication) are most likely to show epithelial cell invasion and nuclear changes typical of herpes infections.[111]

In general, cultures of esophageal biopies for fungi and viruses are less useful than is histologic study of the tissue, since cultures alone do not distinguish between true pathogens and secondary colonizers.

Conventional barium swallow radiography in the patient with odynophagia may reveal typical features of *Candida,*[83] cytomegalovirus,[115] or herpes,[116] but the technique has a lower sensitivity than endoscopy. Studies of non-AIDS patients with *Candida* esophagitis suggest a false negative rate of between 20 and 80 per cent.[117, 118] Enhanced sensitivity has been reported with use of a multiphasic double-contrast technique[119, 120] (see pp. 640–642).

Treatment

An empiric approach to the management of esophageal symptoms is most reasonable in the AIDS patient. Given the preponderance of *Candida* infection, patients with odynophagia who have oral thrush should be treated empirically with ketoconazole, 200 mg/day. (Nystatin lozenges alone are rarely efficacious in this setting.) If symptoms persist, endoscopy with biopsy and brushings should be performed to exclude CMV or herpes. Esophageal symptoms due to *Candida* will sometimes improve with treatment even though endoscopic evidence of infection persists.[121] However, eradication of invasive candidiasis does not necessarily prolong survival. Furthermore, symptomatic improvement of esophageal symptoms is probably the most important goal, since it leads to greater comfort, increased oral intake, and better nutritional status.

Patients with *Candida* esophagitis not responsive to ketoconazole have been reported,[121] and persistent symptoms in these patients should be treated with miconazole or amphotericin B. Herpes esophagitis will respond to acyclovir, although resolution is often followed by relapse. Effectiveness of DHPG, an experimental antiviral drug related to acyclovir,[86] in treating CMV esophagitis is unknown.

Endoscopy often establishes a definitive cause for esophagitis. The main difficulty arises in identifying the culprit when two or more infections coexist. Evidence of tissue invasion by *Candida,* CMV, or herpes should be sought. If two pathogens appear invasive, initial treatment for the one that is histologically more aggressive should be chosen. If symptoms persist, a trial of therapy for the remaining organism should be undertaken.

Abdominal Pain

The exact frequency of abdominal pain in patients with AIDS is unknown; however, when acute, it may portend a catastrophic complication.

Differential Diagnosis

In the differential diagnosis, the physician evaluating the AIDS patient with abdominal pain must consider

Table 65–5. ABDOMINAL PAIN: DIFFERENTIAL DIAGNOSIS

Organ	Causes	References
Stomach		
Gastritis	CMV*, *Cryptosporidium*	59, 124, 125
Focal ulcer	CMV*, *Candida*, MTB	126, 127
Outlet obstruction	*Cryptosporidium**, CMV, lymphoma	41, 59, 115, 128
Small bowel		
Enteritis	*Cryptosporidium**, CMV, MAI	38, 59
Obstruction	Lymphoma*, KS	31, 129
Perforation	CMV*, lymphoma	15, 129, 130
Colon		
Colitis	CMV*, HSV	15, 16
	Salmonella	1, 73
Obstruction	Lymphoma*, KS, intussusception	42, 129, 131
Perforation	CMV*, lymphoma, HSV	132
Appendicitis	KS*, *Cryptosporidium*	105, 133
Anorectum		
Proctitis	Herpes*, *Candida**	16, 134
Tumor	KS, lymphoma, condyloma	45, 46, 53
Liver, spleen		
Infiltration	Lymphoma*, CMV, MAI	41, 122
Biliary tract		
Cholecystitis	CMV*, *Cryptosporidium**	59, 126
Papillary stenosis	CMV*, *Cryptosporidium**, KS, Lymphoma	59, 126, 135, 136
Cholangitis	CMV*	135, 136
Pancreas		
Inflammation	CMV*, KS, Pentamidine	26
Mesentery		
Infiltration	MAI*, *Cryptococcus*, KS, lymphoma	12, 122

*More frequent.

CMV, cytomegalovirus; MTB, *Mycobacterium tuberculosis;* MAI, *Mycobacterium avium-intracellulare*; KS, Kaposi's sarcoma.

not only the manifestations of opportunistic infections and neoplasms, but also the more common causes of abdominal pain in the general population (see pp. 238–257).

The differential diagnosis for abdominal pain in AIDS, presented in Table 65–5, is organized by the site of origin of the pain. For each organ system, a list of potential complications with their likely causes is offered. This information is based primarily on case reports, which are noted in the third column. In some instances causes are listed because of their known ability to produce symptoms by involving a particular organ. The table does not include non–AIDS-specific diagnoses, which overall are equally common causes of abdominal pain in AIDS.

Two studies have been published specifically addressing the evaluation of abdominal pain in AIDS; both underscore the broad spectrum of potential causes of abdominal pain in this population.[122, 123]

Evaluation

The history is important in localizing the origin of abdominal pain. Associated symptoms and signs should suggest the particular organ involved, and the same work-up as for a patient without AIDS should be undertaken. Abdominal sonography and computerized tomography (CT) scanning are useful early in the assessment of abdominal pain, and may highlight regions of disease not suspected clinically (Figs. 65–7 and 65–8).[137, 138] These unsuspected findings often include thickening of the gallbladder wall, focal hepatic lesions, biliary ductal dilatation, adenopathy, or peritoneal thickening.

Table 65–6 defines abdominal pain in terms of the five most common pain syndromes, their most likely causes, and the diagnostic methods indicated. The duration and severity of symptoms will dictate the urgency of evaluation. For example, patients with dull, insidious abdominal pain can be evaluated with less urgency than the patient who develops acute, severe abdominal pain with evidence of peritonitis (see pp. 238–250).

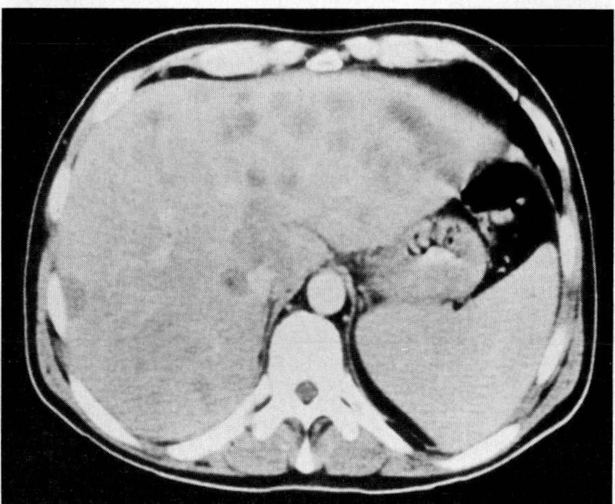

Figure 65–7. CT scan of the abdomen in a patient with AIDS and non-Hodgkin's lymphoma, showing multiple hepatic lymphomatous lesions. (From Nyberg, D. A., Jeffrey R. B., Federle, M. P., et al. AIDS-related lymphomas: evaluation by abdominal CT. Radiology *159*:59–63, 1986. Used with permission.)

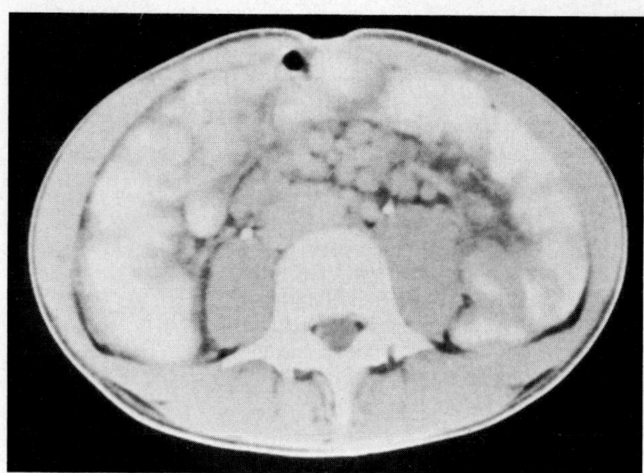

Figure 65–8. CT scan of the abdomen in a patient with AIDS, demonstrating mesenteric adenopathy and colonic wall thickening, with luminal narrowing. (From Jeffrey, R. B., Nyberg, D. A., Bottles, K., et al. Abdominal CT in acquired immunodeficiency syndrome. American Journal of Roentgenology *146*(1):7–13. © by American Roentgen Ray Society, 1986.)

Treatment

See also pages 238 to 250.

Management of abdominal pain falls broadly into surgical versus nonsurgical options. Indications for surgical intervention in AIDS patients are the same as for patients without AIDS. Specifically, intestinal perforation or obstruction must be managed surgically, despite the increased perioperative and postoperative risk for AIDS patients (Fig. 65–9). All tissue specimens must be submitted for viral and fungal culture and for pathologic examination, and biopsy of mesenteric nodes should be performed.[123] The main goal of surgery should be the palliation of symptoms; prolonged anesthesia time and extensive tissue resection should be avoided if possible.

The nonsurgical management of abdominal pain will be determined by the clinical evaluation. Treatable

Table 65–6. EVALUATION OF ABDOMINAL PAIN: "PAIN SYNDROMES"

Symptoms	Suspect	Diagnostic Method
Dull pain, diarrhea, mild nausea, vomiting	Infectious enteritis	Stool cultures, ova and parasites, sigmoidoscopy
Acute, severe pain, peritonitis	Perforation	Abdominal plain films, surgical consultation
Right upper quadrant pain, abnormal liver function tests	Cholecystitis, cholangitis, hepatic infiltrates	Liver function tests, CT/ultrasound, ERCP, liver biopsy
Subacute pain, severe nausea/vomiting	Obstruction	Contrast study
Anorectal pain	Proctitis, tumor	Anoscopy, sigmoidoscopy with biopsy and culture

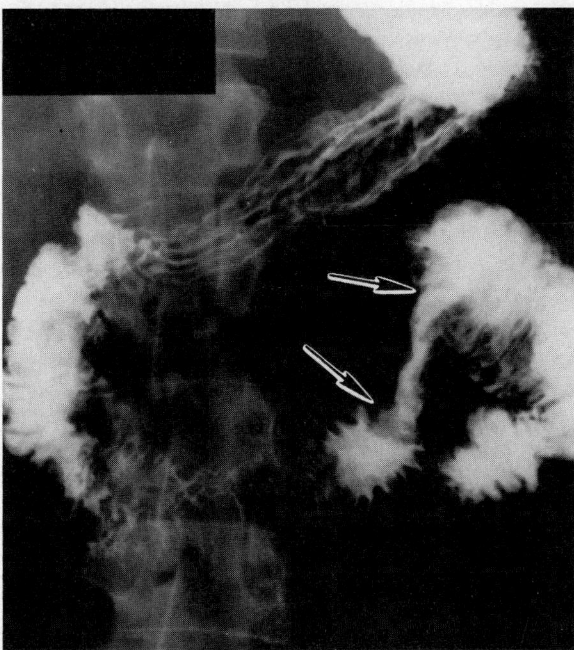

Figure 65–9. Upper gastrointestinal X-ray in an AIDS patient with clinical evidence of proximal bowel obstruction, demonstrating severe narrowing of the distal duodenum (*arrows*). Exploratory laparotomy revealed an obstructing primary duodenal lymphoma; asymptomatic Kaposi's sarcoma lesions were also present in the duodenum.

infections contributing to the symptoms should be managed with appropriate antimicrobial agents. Symptoms due to lymphoma or Kaposi's sarcoma may respond to chemotherapy or radiation therapy. Symptomatic treatment with analgesics may be indicated in addition to specific antimicrobial or antineoplastic drug regimens.

Jaundice and Hepatomegaly

See also pages 454 to 467.

Hepatomegaly, with or without jaundice, is a frequent finding in AIDS. Hepatomegaly may be present clinically in over 50 per cent of patients.[18] The clinical examination always underestimates its true incidence, which has been found to be up to 84 per cent of patients at post mortem. Hepatomegaly is usually associated with one or more liver function test abnormalities, although significant jaundice due to parenchymal disease is uncommon.

Differential Diagnosis

AIDS-related pathology accounts for the majority of cases of hepatomegaly (Table 65–7). Although it can be caused by multiple diseases, a specific diagnosis can usually be established if tissue is obtained. No features are common to all patients with hepatic disease in AIDS.[139]

Mycobacterium avium-intracellulare is consistently the most frequent specific hepatic finding in AIDS, affecting 19 to 70 per cent of patients.[140, 141] The pathologic hallmark of the infection is the presence of poorly formed granulomas containing acid-fast bacilli.[142] Organisms are rarely seen outside of granulomas.

Table 65–7. DIFFERENTIAL DIAGNOSIS OF JAUNDICE/HEPATOMEGALY IN AIDS

Hepatic Parenchymal Disease
M. avium intracellulare
Cryptococcus
Kaposi's sarcoma
Cytomegalovirus
Histoplasmosis
Lymphoma
Drug-induced, esp. sulfa
Hepatitis B
Microsporidia
Chronic active hepatitis (in children)
Biliary Disease
Cholangitis due to:
Cytomegalovirus
Cryptosporidium
Lymphoma
Kaposi's sarcoma

In each group, causes list in order from most to least common.

Cytomegalovirus is the most frequent infectious pathogen in AIDS, and the liver is involved in 5 to 25 per cent of liver biopsies.[12, 18] Typical viral inclusions are usually identified in Kupffer cells but can sometimes be seen in hepatocytes or sinusoidal endothelial cells.[18, 26]

Histoplasma has recently been recognized as an opportunistic pathogen in AIDS and the liver is occasionally affected in patients with disseminated fungal disease.[143] Biopsies may also show caseating granulomas containing fungal organisms, also subsequently confirmed by culture.

Cryptococcus commonly infects the liver and always occurs in the setting of disseminated infection.[18] Typically the organism is found in the sinusoids and is associated with a poor inflammatory response.

Kaposi's sarcoma (KS) has a predilection for periportal regions of the liver and is seen in 10 to 15 per cent of liver biopsies.[12, 18] Tumor nodules appear grossly as violaceous or hemorrhagic masses within hepatic parenchyma. Microscopically, the characteristic spindle cells and vascular slits of KS usually directly abut normal-appearing liver tissue.[24]

Primary hepatic involvement by non-Hodgkin's lymphoma can be found in about 10 per cent of homosexual men with extranodal lymphoma and AIDS.[41] The lesions are usually focal and may be large.[137, 144] In addition, Hodgkin's disease in the AIDS patient tends to be more aggressive histologically and clinically, spreading rapidly to extranodal sites, making liver involvement more likely.[145]

Drug-induced liver dysfunction in AIDS is most commonly due to sulfonamides used to treat *Pneumocystis* infections.[139] The increased frequency of adverse reactions to these medications is now well recognized in AIDS,[146] and liver biopsy typically yields evidence of granulomas containing eosinophils.[139]

A single case of hepatitis due to *Microsporidium* has been reported.[315] Laboratory data were consistent with parenchymal infiltration, and election microscopy of liver tissue demonstrated direct contact between the organism and host cell cytoplasm.

Acute or chronic liver disease attributable to hepatitis B infection is surprisingly rare, given the high prevalence of serologic markers for this infection in the homosexual community[147] (see p. 1255).

Children with AIDS or ARC may have an unusual form of chronic active hepatitis not yet seen in adults with AIDS. Four children were reported with piecemeal necrosis (the hallmark of chronic active hepatitis) in the absence of serologic markers for past hepatitis B infection.[148] Inflammation is prominent and consists primarily of T suppressor lymphocytes. The pathologic features are distinctly different from non-A, non-B hepatitis, and it is unclear whether these findings reflect an infection not previously associated with AIDS, a noninfectious consequence of AIDS, or a direct result of HIV infection itself.

Biliary tract involvement in AIDS may result in marked jaundice and right upper quadrant symptoms. A syndrome resembling sclerosing cholangitis with papillary stenosis has been described in homosexual men with AIDS.[135, 136, 149] Patients develop significant upper abdominal pain in association with marked elevation of alkaline phosphatase, moderate elevations of bilirubin, aspartate aminotransferase (AST), and alanine aminotransferase (ALT), and evidence of ductal abnormalities on abdominal ultrasound exam. ERCP reveals characteristic intra- and extrahepatic ductal dilatation with focal strictures and pruning of the intrahepatic ducts. The etiology of this syndrome is uncertain, but it may result from biliary CMV or cryptosporidial infection. Although patients appear to respond well to endoscopic sphincterotomy, symptoms may recur. Neoplastic biliary obstruction due to lymphomatous nodes or KS must also be considered in the patient with AIDS and suspected biliary disease.

An appreciable number of nonspecific findings are often present in liver biopsies of AIDS patients, in the absence of obvious infection or neoplasm. Their significance is uncertain. Sinusoidal dilatation in association with hepatic plate atrophy in a pattern similar to that of peliosis hepatitis is commonly found at autopsy.[12, 149] Granulomas are occasionally present in the absence of fungal or bacterial organisms.[19, 140] Kupffer cell hyperplasia may be present.[150] Inflammatory activity is surprisingly minimal even when large numbers of granulomas or microorganisms are present. Microvesicular and macrovesicular steatosis may be due to malnutrition, since the findings are similar to those seen in patients with kwashiorkor.[19, 139]

Evaluation

In evaluating the AIDS patient with jaundice, hepatomegaly, or both, the initial determination to be made is whether the findings are due to intrahepatic or extrahepatic disease. Simultaneous disease in both sites must also be considered. A history of mild jaundice, often in association with fever and constitutional symptoms, is more consistent with intrahepatic disease, whereas symptoms of deep jaundice associated with pain of relatively acute onset suggest extrahepatic disease.

Because the clinical history and the finding of symptomatic hepatomegaly are nonspecific, further evaluation is always necessary. Elevations of ALT, AST, or both are seen in 35 to 40 per cent of patients, but neither the pattern nor the extent of elevation of these tests correlates with specific findings in the liver.[19, 139] In contrast, marked elevation of alkaline phosphatase correlates statistically with the presence of *M. avium* infection in the liver in AIDS when extrahepatic obstruction is absent.[19] Nonetheless, an imaging procedure of the liver and biliary ducts is almost always indicated. Abdominal CT and sonography should be employed early because they are especially useful in identifying ductal dilatation, gallbladder pathology, and focal hepatic lesions.[137] Liver and spleen scintigraphy may be helpful in assessing liver and spleen size or parenchymal abnormalities[151] but is less useful than CT (see pp. 460–462).

The indications for liver biopsy in the patient in whom intrahepatic disease is suspected are not well defined. Biopsy is appropriate when symptomatic, treatable disease of the liver is suspected or when a specific diagnosis of hepatic disease is needed. Liver biopsies are abnormal in 90 to 100 per cent of patients with AIDS,[19, 139, 152] yet in a careful retrospective review, liver biopsy identified a previously undiagnosed infection or neoplasm in only 2 of 26 patients, suggesting that the liver is rarely the site of disease not manifest elsewhere.[19] Specific infections or neoplasms are usually evident on tissue sections of appropriately stained biopsy material. *M. avium* is almost always present within hepatic granulomas, although it may occasionally be detectable only after culture of biopsy material for acid-fast bacilli.[19, 142] *Cryptococcus* and *Histoplasma* are also associated with granulomas.[18, 143]

Cytomegalovirus nuclear inclusions can be localized within Kupffer cells or hepatocytes.[18] Kaposi's sarcoma and lymphomas are easily identified by their homogeneous neoplastic appearance.[18, 144] When lymphoma is suspected, material should be fixed in paraformaldehyde to allow for thin plastic sections, in order to define the histologic type. Drug-induced hepatitis may be recognized on occasion by the presence of eosinophils within granulomas.[139]

An extrahepatic cause for jaundice is suggested on CT by the presence of dilated ducts or other biliary abnormalities. The possibility of papillary stenosis associated with CMV infection or cryptosporidiosis must promptly be considered once extrahepatic obstruction is recognized. Further evaluation, when indicated, may include ERCP if CT or ultrasound demonstrates dilatation of extrahepatic ducts extending to the duodenum. Ampullary and biopsy specimens collected during ERCP should be examined for the presence of viruses, protozoa, or neoplastic cells, and cultured for viruses, particularly CMV.

Management

Biliary obstruction may respond to endoscopic papillotomy if papillary stenosis or tumor is present at the ampulla of Vater. On rare occasion, neoplastic extrahepatic obstruction not amenable to papillotomy can be treated by transhepatic percutaneous drainage or endoscopic stent placement. However, the high risk of bacterial infection created by an indwelling catheter makes this a highly morbid procedure in the AIDS patient. Surgery is indicated in patients with clinical evidence of cholecystitis and occasionally in those with severe cholangitis.

Hepatitis B Virus and AIDS

Prevalence

The prevalence of positive serology indicating past or present infection with hepatitis B is high in AIDS patients, but is no different from that in patients without AIDS who are homosexuals or intravenous drug users. Among 46 homosexual men with Kaposi's sarcoma or *Pneumocystis carinii* pneumonia, 94 per cent were positive for HB_sAg, HB_sAb, and/or HB_cAb, compared with 88 per cent of 114 homosexual controls.[153] The majority of patients have had past hepatitis B infection, as indicated by HB_sAb positivity in the absence of hepatitis B surface antigen.

The likelihood of past or present hepatitis B infection was well recognized in the male homosexual population before the AIDS epidemic. It has been related to the duration of homosexual activity, the number of nonsteady sexual partners, and the frequency of anal, genital, or oral-anal contact.[147] Subsequent clinical and autopsy studies in AIDS patients have confirmed a prevalence of positive hepatitis B serology approaching 90 per cent.[18, 154] An early study has suggested an unusually high prevalence of positive HB_cAb in serum, suggesting that ongoing hepatitis B virus replication may be more common with AIDS (see below).[155]

Clinical Features of Type B Viral Hepatitis in AIDS

Symptomatic liver disease related to hepatitis B virus infection is rare in AIDS, despite the high prevalence of serum markers reflecting past or present hepatitis B infection. Homosexual men who are HBV carriers and seropositive for HIV appear to be less immunologically responsive to hepatitis B virus and have higher rates of viral replication. Thus, histologic injury is less severe, while DNA polymerase levels are significantly elevated compared with carriers who are HIV negative.[156, 157] Of 30 patients with AIDS, 27 were seropositive for hepatitis B virus, yet only 3 patients had chronic surface antigenemia, and no patients had antibodies to the delta agent.[154] One of the 3 patients in this study who was HB_sAg positive subsequently died, and postmortem exam showed no evidence of chronic hepatitis even though core antigen was identified within hepatocytes. Similarly, in a large combined clinical and autopsy series, only 5 of 85 patients with positive hepatitis B virus serology had pathologic evidence of chronic active hepatitis or cirrhosis, a prevalence rate no different from that reported in immunocompetent groups infected with hepatitis B virus.[19] Based on the surprisingly low incidence of chronic liver disease in AIDS patients with type B viral hepatitis, it has been suggested that the lack of an adequate immune response in AIDS may result in decreased T lymphocyte–mediated liver injury.[154] This intriguing notion demands further study, as it may have implications for understanding the pathogenesis of type B viral hepatitis.

Hepatitis B Virus: A Cofactor in the Etiology of AIDS?

Before the identification of the human immunodeficiency virus (HIV) in 1984, several authors had suggested that hepatitis B virus might be etiologic in AIDS.[155, 158, 159] This suggestion was based on the parallel epidemiology of AIDS and hepatitis B and the identification of hepatitis B viral DNA in Kaposi's sarcoma tissue of two patients with AIDS.[160] The importance attributed to hepatitis B virus in AIDS receded with the identification of HIV; however, it has now become clear that many factors aside from HIV seroconversion alone may determine which patients will develop AIDS. The risk of the development of AIDS after HIV seroconversion varies among different cohorts: seropositive homosexuals in Manhattan had a 34 per cent risk of AIDS, compared with a risk of 8 per cent in Danish homosexuals.[161] Although a longer duration of seropositivity in Manhattan patients may have accounted for some increased risk, it remains possible that other factors, including hepatitis B infection, may act as cofactors in the development of AIDS.

Two recent studies have provided more direct evidence for the importance of hepatitis B virus in AIDS by demonstrating that hepatitis B virus DNA is present in circulating lymphoid cells from patients with AIDS or ARC.[162, 163] There is controversy over whether hepatitis B virus DNA exists primarily as an integrated form within the genome, or extrachromosomally. Hepatitis B virus DNA was seen even in lymphocytes of patients who had no serologic markers of hepatitis B, suggesting that hepatitis B virus may be present in more patients than is suggested based on serologic studies alone.

Many questions remain unanswered with regard to the role of hepatitis B in AIDS. Future studies will undoubtedly address the molecular mechanisms responsible for hepatitis virus infection of lymphoid cells, and the pathogenetic significance of this phenomenon.

Hepatitis B Vaccine and AIDS

No evidence exists of any risk of AIDS after use of the hepatitis B vaccine, Heptavax-B. This concern was raised initially because the hepatitis vaccine was produced largely from the serum of homosexual men, a known risk group for AIDS.[164, 165] This lack of association between AIDS and the hepatitis B vaccine was clearly established when investigators in New York demonstrated that of 642 patients in New York who received the vaccine, only 2 developed AIDS, or an incidence of 2.4 cases per 1000, compared with an incidence of 4.4 cases per 1000 in an unvaccinated homosexual control population.[166] If the theories implicating hepatitis B as a cofactor in AIDS are correct, then using the vaccine in seronegative high-risk patients might reduce the risk of AIDS. Furthermore, the growing availability of recombinant hepatitis B virus vaccines should eliminate any concern, however unfounded, over the safety of hepatitis B virus vaccination.

At present, the indications for hepatitis B vaccination remain unchanged. All individuals should be vaccinated who are or will be at increased risk for hepatitis B, including health care personnel, hemodialysis and hemophilia patients, and intimate contacts of hepatitis B carriers, as well as populations with a high incidence of the disease such as drug users, homosexuals, and prostitutes.

Table 65–8. DIFFERENTIAL DIAGNOSIS OF GASTROINTESTINAL BLEEDING IN AIDS (EXCLUDING NON–AIDS-SPECIFIC DIAGNOSES)

Upper Gastrointestinal Tract
Esophagitis
Candida*
Cytomegalovirus*
Herpes
Gastritis
Cryptosporidiosis
Cytomegalovirus
Enteritis
Cytomegalovirus
Bacterial infections:
Salmonella
Shigella
Neoplasms
Kaposi's sarcoma
Lymphoma
Lower Gastrointestinal Tract
Colitis
Cytomegalovirus
E. histolytica
Neoplasms
Kaposi's sarcoma
Lymphoma

*More frequent.

Gastrointestinal Bleeding

See also pages 397–427.

Gastrointestinal bleeding complicates AIDS in less than 1 per cent of patients. Several clinical and autopsy series fail to cite a single case of serious gastrointestinal hemorrhage in a combined total of 118 patients.[2, 12, 38, 91]

Differential Diagnosis

Gastrointestinal bleeding in AIDS is as likely to arise from sources not unique to AIDS as from opportunistic infections or neoplasms. These lesions, including peptic or stress ulcerations, variceal hemorrhage, inflammatory bowel disease, diverticular disease, and colonic polyps, are not more common in AIDS. Infections and neoplasms seen exclusively with AIDS can rarely cause gastrointestinal bleeding, and are listed in Table 65–8.

Cytomegalovirus involvement of the gastrointestinal tract causes bleeding by inducing a vasculitis in affected tissue. This complication results in ischemia, infarction, or both, most commonly in the colon or distal small bowel.[14, 15, 167] A similar mechanism probably accounts for the bleeding associated with cytomegalovirus infection of the esophagus and stomach.[115] Hemorrhage from colonic or esophageal infection may be due to either focal or diffuse inflammation.[14, 115] Occasionally, patients can develop a pancolitis that is clinically similar to the colitis seen in patients with inflammatory bowel disease or mesenteric ischemia.[116]

Candida albicans infection may sometimes induce esophageal hemorrhage via direct fungal invasion, causing a severe erosive esophagitis.[117] About 3 per cent of patients dying from cancer with established *Candida* esophagitis will have esophageal bleeding.[117] To date, no such bleeding has been reported in AIDS patients with this infection.

Herpes esophagitis has also rarely been associated with esophageal hemorrhage in non-AIDS patients.[167] The later stages of herpes infection of the esophagus are associated with mucosal ulcerations that may coalesce into a diffuse hemorrhagic esophagitis.

Cryptosporidiosis may rarely cause enteritis associated with hematochezia,[168] although the majority of patients with cryptosporidiosis have severe diarrhea with little or no bleeding.[10]

Salmonella enteritis is associated with watery diarrhea that may be grossly or microscopically bloody.[169]

Several enteric pathogens, including *Campylobacter, Shigella, Entamoeba histolytica*, and *Chlamydia*, often cause rectal bleeding. These infections are common, of course, in sexually active homosexual men whether or not they have AIDS.[78]

Enteric Kaposi's sarcoma lesions may ulcerate and bleed spontaneously.[122, 123] In general, however, Kaposi's sarcoma lesions are asymptomatic. No episodes of gastrointestinal bleeding were noted either spontaneously or after endoscopic biopsy in a series of 20 patients with AIDS and intestinal KS at this institution.[21] More recently, we have seen intestinal hemorrhage from enteric Kaposi's sarcoma on rare occasions. Bleeding from intestinal lymphoma in AIDS has not yet been reported.

Evaluation

The evaluation of gastrointestinal bleeding in a patient with AIDS parallels the approach taken in otherwise healthy patients (see pp. 397–427). The rate of blood loss and its approximate source must be assessed promptly. Orthostatic vital signs and placement of nasogastric tube are appropriate initial diagnostic maneuvers. Upper endoscopy is usually necessary to define a bleeding site if the upper tract hemorrhage is severe. Colonoscopy is less practical for evaluating acute lower tract hemorrhage; flexible sigmoidoscopy is preferred. If no source is evident and bleeding is severe, a nuclear red blood cell scan may help to identify the region of blood loss. Endoscopic mucosal biopsy of briskly bleeding lesions is not appropriate because of the risk of precipitating more severe hemorrhage. Once a lesion is initially identified, the patient should be managed on the basis of the gross findings, and the examination, including mucosal biopsy, should be repeated after bleeding subsides. It is often difficult to make a specific diagnosis during active hemorrhage, but endoscopy or sigmoidoscopy is useful to establish whether the bleeding arises from a focal lesion or diffuse inflammation.

Less invasive diagnostic methods, including stool examination and culture, are indicated if blood loss is not severe enough to require endoscopy or sigmoidoscopy. However, mucosal biopsy demonstrating tissue invasion by infection or neoplasm is a more specific means of identifying potential causes of gastrointestinal bleeding. The utility of barium contrast studies in evaluating acute gastrointestinal bleeding is limited.

Treatment

Appropriate management of severe gastrointestinal bleeding due to AIDS-related diseases does not require a specific diagnosis. Treatment consists of blood product support, and, if necessary, surgery (see pp. 397–427).

The patients with chronic gastrointestinal blood loss in whom no treatable infection or neoplasm is found must be managed symptomatically. Intermittent blood product replacement may be required to prevent symptomatic anemia. Surgery should be avoided, if possible.

INTESTINAL DISEASES SEXUALLY TRANSMISSIBLE IN IMMUNOCOMPETENT PATIENTS

EPIDEMIOLOGY OF SEXUALLY RELATED INTESTINAL DISEASES

Since the 1960s sexual behavior has been a major factor in urban transmission of bacterial, protozoal, and viral enteric diseases among immunocompetent adults.[170–172] Protozoal diseases that had been largely eliminated by improvements in sanitation and water treatment have been diagnosed frequently in major metropolitan areas. This shift in pattern of intestinal parasitic diseases from rural, lower economic groups to urban, middle, and upper economic populations reflects direct person-to-person transmission of infectious agents, especially during oral-anal sexual contact but also by manual contact with the partner's anus and carriage of infective organisms to the mouth by fingers.[173] Migration of large numbers of single adults to metropolitan areas and relaxation of social and sexual inhibitions converged to produce hyperendemic levels of often asymptomatic intestinal infection, especially among young adult homosexual males.

Sexually transmitted diseases now include protozoal, helminthic, bacterial, viral, and in some cases malignant diseases not previously recognized as transmissible during close sexual contact. In a venereal disease clinic in New York, 26 per cent of 89 homosexual men carried *Giardia lamblia* or *Entamoeba histolytica*.[174] A history of anilingus was found in 100 per cent of those with stool pathogens, but 12 patients who never engaged in anilingus had no protozoa in their stools. Self-selected patients in venereal disease clinics are not necessarily representative of the general population of those who engage in anal sexual activity. Sexually transmitted enteric diseases do not invariably follow anal erotic behavior, which may be more prevalent than generally recognized. Anal sexual activity, including anilingus, was reported by 25 per cent of 526 consecutive gynecologic patients, none of whom had enteric symptoms or signs of anal disease.[175]

The preponderance of sexually transmitted enteric disease in homosexual men appears to reflect not only a greater prevalence of oral-anal sexual activity but also a higher endemic rate of carriage of intestinal infectious agents. Reasons suggested for this higher endemic rate of intestinal parasites in homosexual men are greater numbers of sexual contacts,[176, 177] greater discretional income for foreign travel, and opportunity for anonymous sexual contacts.[178] When infections are asymptomatic or only mildly symptomatic, these factors may have a cumulative effect in maintaining a hyperendemic level of enteric infections.

With inception of the AIDS epidemic, it rapidly became apparent that multiple sexual contacts, economic resources for international travel, and anal erotic activity (especially anal intercourse) placed homosexual males in a very-high-risk category for AIDS. Following a major national and international educational campaign regarding the relationship between specific sexual behaviors and AIDS risk, there have been major modifications in sexual activity among male homosexuals that have drastically altered epidemiologic patterns of sexually transmitted enteric infection. Rates of rectal gonorrhea and syphilis have fallen precipitously.[179–181] These reduced rates correlate with adherence to "safe sex" guidelines and marked changes in self-reported behavior among homosexual and bisexual men.[182] Although published surveys of parasitic infection among homosexual men continue to show high prevalence of potential intestinal pathogens,[183–188] the incidence of new parasitic infections in homosexual men is falling. In Los Angeles, where amebiasis occurs principally among homosexual men and in recent immigrants from developing countries, amebiasis among white males aged 15 to 54 dropped 75 per cent from 1983 to 1986, and the ratio of cases in males to cases in females fell from 9:1 to 2:1.[189] A reduction in prevalence rates can be expected to lag behind the drop in incidence of new infections, owing to delayed publication of surveys carried out prior to safe sex guidelines, persistence of infections acquired prior to changes in sexual behavior, recrudescence of intestinal infection among patients with developing immunodeficiency syndrome, and self-selection of patients presenting to diagnostic centers because of concern that intestinal parasites might contribute to susceptibility to AIDS.[190]

AIDS, as the most devastating sexually transmissible intestinal infection, has decreased both the relative significance of other sexually related intestinal diseases and the absolute incidence of new intestinal infections. In patients presenting with intestinal complaints and a history of high-risk sexual activity, intestinal manifestations of AIDS discussed above in the first part of this chapter must be differentiated from other sexually acquired intestinal infections. Consequently the differential diagnosis of proctitis in homosexual men, the recognition of classical sexually transmitted diseases, and the identification of new presentations of sexually transmissible infection in patients with AIDS-related complex or AIDS remain important problems. An additional challenge is the education and treatment of homosexual adolescents who may not be aware of risks of specific sexual behaviors.[191]

SEXUALLY TRANSMITTED DISEASE SYNDROME

Homosexual men report more gastrointestinal symptoms, including diarrhea, cramps, mucus in stools, and gas, than heterosexual males, but these symptoms show no correlation with infection by specific protozoal pathogens.[173] Even though gastrointestinal symptoms do not correlate with the presence or absence of protozoal cysts, they may reflect infection with bacterial or viral agents acquired by the same behavioral patterns that have established hyperendemic levels of protozoal infection. Homosexual patients frequently are not distinguishable by appearance, behavior, occupation, or even marital status. Physicians should consider the sexually transmitted disease syndrome when protozoal stool infections are observed in patients without a recent travel history, or when multiple enteric infections occur simultaneously or sequentially in male patients between ages 20 and 40 years. It is important to recognize the sexually transmitted disease syndrome so that proper diagnostic tests can be carried out, probable mechanisms of disease transmission explained to patients, and reinfection differentiated from treatment failures, which might result in unnecessarily toxic drug regimens. Any infectious agent that does not require a period of maturation outside the primary host may be transmitted during sexual contact (Table 65–9). The likelihood of specific infection depends upon the required infective dose and prevalence of the infective agent; the likelihood of diagnosis depends upon the nature and severity of symptoms produced and the availability of appropriate diagnostic techniques for identification.

PROTOZOAL AND HELMINTHIC INFECTIONS

Amebiasis

In a prospective study of 89 gay men who volunteered stool specimens in New York, 20 per cent had *E. histolytica*. Gastrointestinal symptoms were relatively nonspecific, including diarrhea, cramping, and flatulence.[174] It is difficult to correlate gastrointestinal symptoms with *E. histolytica* because of the increased prevalence of nonspecific gastrointestinal complaints in homosexual patients. Increased likelihood of blood or mucus in stools, however, is noted with *E. histolytica*. Compared with the more severe presentation among the rural poor or in infants, the relatively mild clinical presentation of venereally transmitted amebic infection appears to reflect the noninvasive zymodemes of *E. histolytica* strains carried by homosexual men.[192] Those symptoms that are seen may reflect coinfection with additional undetected enteric organisms acquired by these same transmission mechanisms.

Systemic complications of sexually transmitted amebiasis are uncommon, but liver abscesses have been reported in sexually acquired amebic colitis.[193] Nonpathogenic amebas detected in stool specimens are indicators of fecal-oral transmission, and *E. histolytica* often can be found following examination of purged specimens.[172, 174] Intestinal symptoms, including diarrhea and mucus in stools, have been reported in *Endolimax nana* infection, with resolution of symptoms after treatment of patients with negative serology for *E. histolytica*. Noninvasive amebas may infect the rectal wall when it has been traumatized during sexual activity or because of coexisting enteric infection with damage to the mucosal barrier.

The mechanism of transmission in sexually acquired amebiasis is the ingestion of amebic cysts during direct oral-anal sexual contact or carriage of infective cysts from the anal and perianal area to the mouth on fingers after touching the partner's anal area. In public baths and other locations where multiple sexual partners are available, cysts may be ingested during oral contact with an inadequately washed penis following anal intercourse. Not only cysts but also trophozoites are found within the rectal ampulla and may be carried directly from one anus to the next on fingers, penises, dildos, or other objects inserted into a second anus without adequate cleansing. This facilitates direct rectal transplantation of trophozoites, as in amebic colitis transmitted by colonic irrigation equipment.[172–174, 194]

Explicit details of sexual activity usually will not be

Table 65–9. SEXUALLY TRANSMISSIBLE ENTERIC INFECTIONS

	Presumed Portal of Entry			**Gastrointestinal Site of Infection**			
	Oral	***Rectal***	***Other***	***Oropharynx***	***Intestine***	***Anorectum***	***Liver***
Protozoal							
Amebiasis	+	?			+	+	+
Giardiasis	+				+		
Cryptosporidiosis	+				+	+	+ (biliary tree)
Helminthic							
Pinworms	+				+	+	
Strongyloidiasis	+		?			+	
Cysticercosis (eggs of *T. solium* and *T. saginata*)	+				+ (migrates to brain and muscle)		
Hymenolepis nana	+				+	+	
Bacterial							
Shigellosis	+				+	+	
Salmonellosis	+				+	+ (gallbladder)	
Campylobacteriosis	+				+	+	
Streptococcal infection	+	+		+	+	+	
Mycoplasma	+	+		+		+	
Gonorrhea	+	+	+	+		+	+
Meningococci	+	+		+		+	
Chlamydial infection	+	+		+		+	
Syphilis	+	+	+	+	+	+	+
Viral							
Herpes simplex virus	+	+	+	+	+	+	+
Condyloma acuminatum	+	+		+		+	
Cytomegalovirus	+	?					+
Hepatitis A	+				+		+
Hepatitis B	?	+	+				+
Non-A, non-B hepatitis	?	?	+				+
Human immunodeficiency virus	?	+	+	?	?	?	?

volunteered because of apprehension of the physician's disapproval of patients' behavior, because patients do not recall their behavior while intoxicated, because they do not associate sexual activity during previous weeks or months with present intestinal complaints, or because the physician also cares for parents, wives, or other family members who are unaware of the patient's sexual activities. A careful sexual history is appropriate to investigate nonspecific gastrointestinal complaints that may reflect sexual anxieties as well as sexually transmitted infection. A sexual history *must* be taken and *amebiasis* looked for in all cases of *proctitis* or *inflammatory bowel disease* (see below).

It has been postulated that chronic intestinal parasitism in homosexual men, especially with amebiasis, may contribute to immunosuppression and susceptibility to AIDS.[190] This concept has received wide publicity, and consequently many persons at risk for AIDS have urged their physicians to search for intestinal parasites. Although 82 per cent of homosexual men with AIDS-related conditions had some parasite,[190] such high prevalence may be merely a marker of prior high-risk sexual behavior, which is known to be critical in development of AIDS or AIDS-related complex. Occurrence of AIDS in transfusion recipients, children of drug addicts, hemophiliacs, and others without high parasite prevalence indicates that parasites are indeed not a necessary cofactor in AIDS.

An argument can be made that any parasite, whether of known pathogenicity or not, should be treated in persons at risk for AIDS because of possible problems parasites might cause as opportunistic agents should AIDS develop. Surprisingly, even *E. histolytica* has caused remarkably few problems in AIDS patients, possibly because *E. histolytica* isolates found in homosexual men are usually commensal noninvasive strains.[192] A cost-effective strategy for screening asymptomatic homosexual men for intestinal parasites has been proposed based on the association between *E. histolytica* and nonpathogenic protozoa.[185] If *E. histolytica* is found in the first sample for ova and parasite exam or if the sample is negative for any ova or parasites, no more samples are taken. If a nonpathogen is found, one more sample is collected. This strategy was 85 per cent as effective as the traditional three-stool exam, but was only 60 per cent as expensive. In another approach small portions of stool from three successive days are pooled in a single collection bottle.[184] Although the yield of parasites was high (48.5 per cent), this method was not compared with other strategies.

When sexually acquired pathogenic and nonpathogenic amebas in patients with mild to moderate nondysenteric symptoms are treated, a luminal drug with minimal toxicity should be used, such as paromomycin. This drug, given 25 to 35 mg/kg daily in three divided doses for seven days, has been found effective in eliminating both symptoms and parasites.[195] There is little information available on treatment of nonpathogenic amebas. In patients with mixed parasitic infection, metronidazole 750 mg three times a day for 10 days and iodoquin 650 mg three times a day for 20 days cleared both pathogens and nonpathogens in 57 per cent but failed to clear the nonpathogens in 19 per cent.[184] (For further diagnostic and therapeutic approaches to amebiasis, see pages 1155–1165.)

Giardiasis

Giardia lamblia is a particular problem in sexually associated gastrointestinal illness because of large numbers of asymptomatic carriers and the low infective dose. Giardiasis is an upper small intestinal infection, in which diagnosis may frequently be difficult or impossible from stool specimens. As with amebiasis, sexually transmitted giardiasis has been most widely recognized in homosexual patients. From 4 per cent[172] to 13 per cent[173, 174] of stool specimens volunteered by homosexual men have shown *Giardia* cysts despite the known intermittent excretion of such cysts among chronic carriers and the insensitivity of a single stool specimen for detecting infection.

The infective dose of *Giardia* cysts required to establish infection may be as few as 10 to 100.[196] Unlike bacteria, which are inactivated by the gastric acid barrier, excystation and jejunal colonization with *Giardia* is facilitated by gastric acid.[197] The high prevalence of *Giardia* in stools of children in day-care centers[198] suggests that many adults may have had prior *Giardia* infection during childhood. If acquired immunity exists, it must be limited, because all adults were infected when at least 1000 cysts were given during a prospective study of prison volunteers.[196] Symptoms usually do not appear for at least one week and may be minimal or nonspecific, so that the infected persons are unaware that they are subjecting sexual partners to possible risk of infection.[196]

Direct transmission of giardiasis among adults sharing living space reflects oral-anal sexual contact and not shared food preparation or fomites.[199] *Giardia* cysts in stools of prospectively surveyed adults in a venereal disease clinic showed no correlation with frequency of restaurant meals. There is no evidence that homosexual food service workers following the usual hygienic practices pose any danger of infection to patrons.[172, 173, 199] Attribution of infection to consumption of meals in restaurants may be a convenient explanation for parasitic infection among adults who are unaware of, or choose to deny, sexual exposure to infection. *Giardia* colonizes the upper small intestinal mucosa rather than the colon and is thus unlikely to be transplanted directly during anal manipulation or rectal intercourse. Trophozoites may be carried to the colon during the rapid transit of diarrhea but do not colonize the rectal mucosa. Proctitis has been attributed to *Giardia* infection,[200] but there is no evidence to substantiate an etiologic role of *Giardia* in proctitis.

Because *Giardia* is often found in combination with other enteric pathogens, symptoms may be variable, nonspecific, and difficult to assign to this particular organism. The patient may have diarrhea, but more commonly has gas and cramps.

Because of nonspecific and intermittent symptoms with *Giardia*, diagnosis may be difficult. Unfortunately, purging is of little assistance in increasing efficiency of stool examination. Elimination of symptoms following a clinical therapeutic trial does not confirm specific diagnosis because of the broad antiprotozoal and antibacterial spectrum of available antiprotozoal agents (pp. 1153–1155).

Homosexual men at risk for AIDS are often concerned that intestinal symptoms might indicate parasite infestation because of the unconfirmed hypothesis that parasites increase likelihood of immune decompensation.[190] Following treatment of sexually acquired giardiasis and amebiasis many such patients continue to complain of symptoms, especially excessive gas production, despite negative stool examination for ova and parasites. It is unclear what causes these persistent intestinal symptoms. Exhaustive and expensive bacteriologic and parasitologic investigations often fail to reveal additional intestinal pathogens. In some patients persisting symptoms may be related to changes in the intestinal microecology subsequent to elimination of normal intestinal flora by metronidazole and other antiparasitic drugs. These effects are perpetuated by repeated empiric trials of antibiotics in patients with persisting symptoms when no parasites are found in stools. In an effort to improve their health, some patients attempt dietary manipulations, including change to a high-fiber, high-bulk diet, which can increase flatulence, regardless of its other beneficial effects. In attempts to be as "healthy" as possible, other patients take megadoses of vitamin C. Patients taking more than 1 gm of vitamin C may develop diarrhea, which stops when vitamin C intake is reduced. Capsules containing vitamins and dietary supplements from health food stores often contain lactose as a filler. Large numbers of such capsules can provide enough lactose to induce symptoms of lactose intolerance, which can be mistaken for persistent giardiasis. When no parasites are found on follow-up stool exam but symptoms persist, patients should be encouraged to avoid antibiotics, gas-forming foods, and over-the-counter medications until intestinal equilibrium returns. These patients should be followed for development of lymphadenopathy, fever, weight loss or other evidence that persistent intestinal symptoms may represent AIDS-related complex (see pp. 1245–1250).

Helminthic Infections

Only those helminths that do not require a period of maturation outside the host are susceptible to direct person-to-person transmission. *Enterobius* and *Strongyloides* have been associated with sexual transmission.

Enterobius. *Enterobius vermicularis*, known as pinworm in the United States or thread-worm in the United Kingdom, resides in the colon. Fully embryonated eggs are deposited by female worms on the skin around the anus. Although infection may cause intense pruritus in those who are hypersensitive to the worm, the majority of adults with infection are asymptomatic. In patients with inflammatory bowel disease or other intestinal diseases with reduced integrity of the intestinal wall, *E. vermicularis* can penetrate the colon and appear in ectopic locations. This is very rare. This parasite may be acquired during sexual contact by contamination of the fingers or by oral-anal contact with carriers.[201, 202] Reported prevalence of *Enterobius* in stool surveys of homosexual men has been low,[174] but the actual prevalence is probably much higher since eggs are usually present only on the perianal skin and not in stool.[203] Diagnosis is made by microscopic examination of cellophane tape that has been pressed against the unwashed external anus. This infection is treated with pyrantel pamoate in a single dose of 11 mg/kg (maximum 1 gm) or with mebendazole 100 mg. Regular sexual partners and household members should be treated at the same time. Eggs can remain viable in the environment up to two weeks. Consequently, with either regimen treatment should be repeated in two weeks, in case reinfection has occurred.

Strongyloides. *Strongyloides stercoralis* infects the human host by penetration of the skin as filariform larvae, which travel through capillaries to enter the lumen of the lungs. They are coughed up, are swallowed, and reach the small intestine, where they release eggs that may develop into infective filariform larvae. These larvae penetrate the intestinal wall, producing cycles of autoinfection and chronic carriage in urban residents, 30 years or more after leaving endemic areas. These carriers may be asymptomatic except for linear dermal lesions produced by migrating larvae. During rectal intercourse, filariform larvae within the rectal lumen may penetrate the skin of the penis directly, producing minor lesions that may not be noted.[203] Penetration of the oral mucosa by infective larvae may also occur. *Strongyloides* infection has been associated with oral-anal sexual exposure in both homosexual and heterosexual patients[172] and has been observed in patients in the Los Angeles area who have never traveled to tropical endemic areas but have had sexual exposure to chronic carriers from such areas.[204] (See also pp. 1174–1176.)

Taenia Solium and T. Saginata (Cysticercosis). *Tapeworms* that produce embryonated eggs within the human intestine do not require subsequent development in an intermediate host. These eggs will be infective when ingested during oral-anal sexual contact. The pork tapeworm *Taenia solium* is uncommon in the United States but is prevalent in parts of Mexico and may persist in immigrants and visitors. The beef tapeworm *Taenia saginata* is acquired by eating inadequately cooked beef containing living larvae, which mature into adult worms in the human intestine. When eggs from either of these two species of tapeworms are ingested during sexual contact, the larvae penetrate the intestinal wall, forming cysts in muscle or brain.[203, 205] This condition, known as *cysticercosis*, may be asymptomatic and is an end-stage human infection, since encysted larvae cannot develop into adult worms in people infected by eggs. Cysticercosis should be considered in any new onset of seizures in patients with a history of oral-anal sexual exposure. Diagnosis of cysticercosis must be made by biopsy or serology examinations; stool surveys are not helpful for determining the prevalence of such infection in patients with oral-anal sexual exposure. Fortunately, cysticercosis from the beef tapeworm, which is the more prevalent in the United States, is uncommon. Serologic tests are available, but no serum surveys of populations at risk have been carried out to determine the extent of asymptomatic infection.

Hymenolepis nana. The dwarf tapeworm, *Hymenolepis nana*, is prevalent in human beings in Latin America and Central Europe. After ingestion of eggs of this species, larvae penetrate the walls of villi but do not migrate further to muscle or brain. After development, they break through the wall back into the intestinal lumen and grow into adult worms, producing eggs that can complete the cycle of human infection if fecally contaminated material is ingested as in oral-anal sexual contact. Infection with this tapeworm can be determined from stool examination.[203] (For further information regarding diagnosis and treatment of helminth infections, see pages 1173–1182.)

BACTERIAL INFECTIONS

Shigella

Sexual transmission of *Shigella* was recognized in an outbreak of cases in young homosexual men in San Francisco without a common food source and the predominant serotype changed to *Shigella flexneri*.[170] In contrast to sexually transmitted amebiasis, cases of shigellosis were frequently quite severe and resistant to multiple antibiotics. This shift in distribution of cases from parents of infected children and foreign travelers to young, sexually active men and of serotype from *S. sonnei* to *S. flexneri* was demonstrated in Seattle with 44 per cent of cases in adult males, compared with 16 per cent in previous years.[206] Either fellatio or oral-anal contact was reported by 90 per cent of infected homosexual males. Only 10 to 100 organisms are required to establish infection because of the resistance of *Shigella* to inactivation by gastric acid. Consequently, the likelihood of ingestion of a sufficient infective dose of *Shigella*, as with *E. histolytica* and *G. lamblia*, is great. Sexually transmitted shigellosis can present with abrupt onset of fever, nausea, and crampy diarrhea, which may be watery or contain blood, mucus, and pus. Sigmoidoscopic examination shows nonspecific mucosal inflammation. Diagnosis is by culture. Long-term carriage of both *S. sonnei* and *S. flexneri* 2a may follow colonization of the colon.[207] Treatment with antibiotics does not appear to prolong secretion of *Shigella* and is indicated from a public health standpoint in persons who may be a source of sexual transmission even when symptoms of fever or bloody diarrhea are absent. (Treatment regimens are discussed on pages 1201–1203.)

Salmonella

Possibly because of a higher required infective dose of 10^4 to 10^6 organisms, salmonellosis has not been a problem in populations in which other enteric organisms have been transmitted by sexual contact. Acute *typhoid fever*, however, has been traced to sexual partners who were asymptomatic carriers with whom the symptomatic patients shared neither food nor housing.[208]

Despite the low prevalence of *Salmonella* in homosexual men,[3] bacteremia with *Salmonella* species has been frequently reported in AIDS patients.[73, 209, 210] Bacteremia thus appears to reflect the importance of cellular immunity in containing *Salmonella* infection rather than an association with sexual transmission, since *Salmonella* infection has been reported in AIDS patients who are Haitians and intravenous drug users[210] as well as in homosexuals[209] (see p. 1246).

Streptococcus

Streptococcal pharyngitis may occur following sexual exposure to anal carriers of group A, beta-hemolytic streptococci. Streptococcal pyoderma also follows orogenital sexual contact.[211] The pharynx may be infected with both streptococci and gonococci in patients with a history of fellatio. Selective cultures for both organisms are thus necessary for diagnosis. In young adults, arthritis may be associated with either streptococcal or gonococcal pharyngitis[212] but quite different therapeutic approaches are required (see Pharyngeal Gonorrhea, below).

Campylobacter

Campylobacter has been increasingly recognized as a cause of acute gastroenteritis (see p. 1210). *Campylobacter* has been identified in homosexual males with mild inflammatory proctitis, consisting of congestion of the rectal mucosa, but also in one patient with bloody diarrhea, fecal leukocytes, erythematous mucosa with decreased vascular pattern, and mucopurulent material.[213] Infection by sexual contact was not proved, but presentation with proctitis rather than systemic symptoms or abdominal pain was associated with acknowledged receptive anal intercourse. No outbreaks in homosexual men are known, but *Campylobacter*-like species have been isolated more frequently from symptomatic than from asymptomatic homosexual men.[214, 215]

Mycoplasma

Mycoplasma hominis, but not T strain mycoplasmas, has been identified in women with clinical proctitis, diagnosed by the presence of ten or more polymorphonuclear leukocytes per high power field.[216] The presence of mycoplasma in the rectum may be a risk factor for urethritis in sexual contacts, but efforts to correlate the presence of mycoplasma with clinical proctitis in homosexual men have been unsuccessful.[217]

INTESTINAL MANIFESTATIONS OF VENEREAL DISEASE

Gonorrhea

Pharyngeal Gonorrhea

Clinical Presentations. Most infections of the pharynx by *Neisseria gonorrhoeae* are asymptomatic.[218, 219] Stratified squamous epithelium is usually resistant to penetration by gonococci, which, within the pharynx, are most common over the tonsillar surfaces. Following dental manipulation and disruption of the mucosal barrier, gonococcal gingivitis has been reported.[220] Symptoms of sore throat are commonly found in women and men who acknowledge fellatio, but such symptoms alone do not indicate the presence or absence of gonococci and may reflect trauma to the pharynx by the penis or infection with other sexually transmitted organisms. Gonococcal infection can produce exudative tonsillitis with cervical lymphadenopathy,[221] stomatitis, and ulceration of the tongue and buccal mucosa.[222] Among 30 men and women with pharyngeal gonorrhea, 25 were asymptomatic, 3 had slight sore throats, and 2 had severe sore throats, one of which was associated with lymphadenitis and systemic arthritic symptoms.[223] Even when asymptomatic, pharyngeal gonorrhea may be the source for disseminated gonococcal infection.[220]

Epidemiology. The prevalence of oropharyngeal gonorrhea varies greatly among the populations surveyed. As expected, rates are highest among venereal disease clinic patients who are self-selected by symptoms or history of possible pharyngeal exposure to infection.[220] Transmission of the gonococcus to the pharynx was observed in 20 per cent of women and men who acknowledged fellatio but in only 3.1 per cent who did not. Other mechanisms of transmission include kissing[224] and carriage of the organism to the mouth on contaminated fingers. Pharyngeal infection during pregnancy may reflect changes in sexual behavior and substitution of fellatio for vaginal intercourse.[219] In a general medical setting, only 1 per cent of patients with sore throats and none of patients with upper respiratory infections had gonococci, indicating that screening of such populations with elective culture for *Neisseria* is not cost effective in the absence of a history of orogenital sexual contact.[225] Cunnilingus appears to be a less frequent source of pharyngeal infection than is fellatio and is an even less frequent source of symptomatic infection, possibly because of the absence of pharyngeal trauma.

Nongonococcal Neisseria. Gram stains of pharyngeal exudate that reveal gram-negative intracellular diplococci frequently represent species of *Neisseria* other than *N. gonorrhoeae*, including *N. meningitidis* and *N. lactamicus*. Thus, interpretation of positive Gram stains is uncertain, although clearly an indication for specific culture and possibly for treatment when symptoms are present and are associated with a clinical history of pharyngeal exposure to gonorrheal infection.

Patients with *N. gonorrhoeae* cultured at other sites

are also more than twice as likely to have *Neisseria meningitidis* in their pharynx.[226] Whether this indicates an individual susceptibility to *Neisseria* or whether those with frequent close personal contacts have a greater likelihood of exposure to both types of *Neisseria* is uncertain. In male homosexual patients with frequent sexual contacts, there is a very high rate of oropharyngeal carriage of *N. meningitidis* (42.5 per cent). Of 46 patients with gonococci in the oropharynx, only 23.9 per cent had meningococci present at the same time, suggesting competition among the *Neisseria* for colonization of the pharynx.[227] Neither form of *Neisseria* infection is commonly associated with pharyngeal symptoms. Discrimination of *N. gonorrhoeae* from *N. meningitidis* in the pharynx is necessary because of possible gonorrheal dissemination and because more rigorous antibiotic treatment is necessary for its elimination in this site.

Diagnosis. Since neither physical signs nor clinical symptoms are characteristic of gonococcal infection, diagnosis depends upon specific culture of tonsillar surfaces or patches of exudate. Ideally, swabs should be streaked directly onto culture plates for immediate incubation in a candle jar or other increased carbon dioxide atmosphere. Specimens delayed up to four hours before plating also may give positive cultures, but observable growth and diagnosis can be delayed by 24 to 48 hours.

Although less effective than immediate plating, transport systems for gonococci are available. If gonococci can be definitively cultured in 1 to 2 hours, they may be briefly transported on swabs or in holding medium. Methods are under development for gonococcus identification that do not require live organisms or culture. These methods depend on detection of gonococcal enzymes, antigens, DNA, or polysaccharides, but none has yet proved effective for detection of rectal, pharyngeal, or cervical infection.[228] There are no immediate prospects for serologic diagnostic tests for acute gonococcal infection.

Treatment. Gonococcal infection in the pharynx is often resistant to drug regimens that are effective in other sites. Most pharyngeal infections respond to a single dose of 4.8 million units of procaine penicillin G, together with 1.0 gm of probenecid orally. Response is not satisfactory to a single 4-gm intramuscular dose of spectinomycin, which is effective in other sites.[220] Alternative regimens are doxycycline, 100 mg by mouth twice a day for seven days,[229] or two oral doses of ampicillin, 3.5 gm, with 1.0 gm of probenecid 8 to 16 hours apart.[230] In regions where tetracycline and penicillin-resistant strains are present, ceftriaxone, 250 mg intramuscularly, is recommended. Pharyngeal gonorrhea may resolve without treatment, but in prospective experimental infections has been shown to persist for at least eight weeks.[231] Infection should be treated to prevent arthritis and other disseminated infection,[232] as well as possible transmission of infection to the genitals.[233] After three weeks of asymptomatic pharyngeal carriage, gonococci remain infective for the cervix.[231] Pharyngitis also has been reported with *N. lactamicus*, and physicians may wish to treat *Neisseria* species other than *N. gonorrhoeae* when symptomatic pharyngitis is present.[234]

Rectal Gonorrhea

Rectal gonorrhea has been known since 1884, when the gonococcus was first demonstrated in smears taken from the rectum and stained by the process described in that year.[235] Asymptomatic rectal carriers, both women and homosexual men, provide a reservoir for perpetuation and spread of gonorrheal urethritis. Carriers not only are a risk to others, but also are at risk of developing gonococcal sepsis, endocarditis, myocarditis, meningitis, or arthritis.[236]

Autoinfection of the rectum occurs in women with genitourinary gonorrhea by the use of contaminated thermometers and enema nozzles or by direct spread from the vagina. Almost all rectal infections in men and many in women result from rectal sexual exposure. In women, rectal coitus has long been known as a method of contraception. Physicians, however, did not usually recognize rectal coitus in men as a significant possibility prior to Kinsey's report in 1948 of the widespread incidence of male homosexuality. There has been a dramatic reduction in reported new cases of rectal gonorrhea in homosexual men, following identification of the human immunodeficiency virus (HIV) as the cause of AIDS and of unprotected anal intercourse as a major risk factor in HIV transmission. This reduction has followed emphasis on "safe sex guidelines," which include reduction in numbers of sexual partners, avoidance of sexual contacts in which semen or other body fluids are exchanged, and use of condoms during rectal or vaginal intercourse.[181]

Clinical Presentation. Unfortunately, there is no characteristic clinical picture. Some patients will have rectal burning, itching, a bloody or mucoid discharge, or diarrhea, but most people infected with rectal gonorrhea will have no symptoms.[218, 237] In homosexual men seen in a general medical practice, rectal symptoms were as frequent in those who were not infected as in those who were, suggesting that symptoms reflect anxiety, sexual trauma, or other infection.

In a venereal disease clinic, where patients were self-referred because of anorectal symptoms or possible exposure to gonorrhea, mucus in the stools was the only symptom significantly associated with a positive rectal culture for gonorrhea. In patients with rectal symptoms and a history of receptive anal intercourse, other infectious agents to consider include herpes simplex, syphilis, *Giardia, E. histolytica, Chlamydia, Campylobacter*, and nontreponemal spirochetes.[238]

Neisseria meningitidis has been found in the rectums of 2 per cent of homosexual men, but in only 0.2 per cent of rectums of women cultured in venereal disease clinics.[227, 239] Of these infections 20 to 25 per cent are associated with symptoms that include mild to moderate pain or burning. As with *N. gonorrhoeae*, the relationship of symptoms to infection with *N. meningitidis* is variable. Rectal colonization by *N. meningi-*

than by *E. histolytica*, which is usually a noninvasive zymodeme in the setting of sexual transmission. Fecal leukocytes may suggest an infectious etiology, but diagnosis is made by stool culture for enteric pathogens or by stool examination for ova and parasites.

Proctitis is defined as anorectal symptoms associated with sigmoidoscopic findings limited to the distal 15 cm of the rectum. Typically infectious proctitis follows direct implantation of infectious agents by the penis during anal intercourse. When the anal mucosa is involved, such infections can be quite painful, especially with herpes simplex. Fever, constipation, urinary symptoms, sacral neuralgias, and rectal ulceration suggest primary herpes infection. When acute rectal pain, fever, and anal discharge are accompanied by bloody diarrhea, *Lymphogranuloma venereum* should be considered. This diagnosis should be ruled out before a diagnosis of Crohn's disease is made, especially in homosexual men. Histologic changes consistent with idiopathic inflammatory bowel disease may be produced by *Treponema pallidum* or *Chlamydia trachomatis.*[79] Syphilis may cause painful ulcers in the anal mucosa. Syphilitic ulcers higher in the rectum are painless and may be associated with a rash and nonspecific intestinal symptoms. Diagnosis is made by serology, darkfield exam of exudate, or silver stain of biopsy material. Rectal infection with *N. gonorrhoeae* or non-LGV serotypes of *C. trachomatis* produces nonspecific symptoms but can be detected by sigmoidoscopy and histology. Gram stain of exudate may be diagnostic for gonorrhea if Gram negative intracellular diplococci are found, but diagnosis is usually made by culture.

When sigmoidoscopic findings extend above 15 cm, proctocolitis is present, which is produced by ingested infectious agents, including *E. histolytica, Shigella, Campylobacter*, and *Salmonella* (in AIDS patients). When patients have been recently treated with antibiotics, pseudomembranous enterocolitis should be considered.

References

1. Budhraja, M., Levendoglu, H., and Sherer, R. Spectrum of sigmoidoscopic findings in AIDS patients with diarrhea. Am. J. Gastroenterol. *80*:828, 1985.
2. Malenbranche, R., Guerin, J. M., Laroche, A. C., et al. Acquired immunodeficiency syndrome with severe gastrointestinal manifestations in Haiti. Lancet *2*:873, 1983.
3. Quinn, T. C., Stamm, W. E., Goodell, S. E., et al. The polymicrobial origin of intestinal infections in homosexual men. N. Engl. J. Med. *309*:576, 1983.
4. Carne, C. A., Johnson, A. M., Pearce, F., et al. Prevalence of antibodies to human immunodeficiency virus, gonorrhoea rates, and changed sexual behaviour in homosexual men in London. Lancet *1*:656, 1987.
5. Friedland, G. H., Saltzman, B. R., Rogers, M. F., et al. Lack of transmission of HTLV-III/LAV infection to household contacts of patients with AIDS or AIDS-related complex with oral candidiasis. N. Engl. J. Med. *314*:344, 1986.
6. Gerberding, J. L. Recommended policies for patients with human immunodeficiency virus infection. An update. N. Engl. J. Med. *315*:1562, 1986.
7. Spire, B., Barre-Sinoussi, F., Montagnier, L., and Chermann, J. C. Inactivation of lymphadenopathy associated virus by chemical disinfectants. Lancet *2*:899, 1984.
8. Nelson, K. E., Larson, P. A., Schraufnagel, D. E., and Jackson, J. Transmission of tuberculosis by flexible fiberbronchoscopes. Am. Rev. Respir. Dis. *127*:97, 1983.
9. Rodgers, V. D., Fassett, R., and Kagnoff, M. F. Abnormalities in intestinal mucosal T cells in homosexual populations including those with the lymphadenopathy syndrome and acquired immunodeficiency syndrome. Gastroenterology *90*:552, 1986.
10. Whiteside, M. E., Barkin, J. S., May, R. G., et al. Enteric coccidiosis among patients with the acquired immunodeficiency syndrome. Am. J. Trop. Med. Hyg. *33*:1065, 1984.
11. Navin, T. R., and Hardy, A. M. Cryptosporidiosis in patients with AIDS. J. Infect. Dis. *155*:150, 1987.
12. Welch, K., Finkbeiner, W., Alpers, C. E., et al. Autopsy findings in the acquired immunodeficiency syndrome. JAMA *252*:1152, 1984.
13. Reichert, C. M., O'Leary, T. J., Levens, D. L., et al. Autopsy pathology in the acquired immunodeficiency syndrome. Am. J. Pathol. *112*:357, 1983.
14. Meiselman, M. S., Cello, J. P., and Margaretten, W. Cytomegalovirus colitis. Report of the clinical, endoscopic and pathologic findings in two patients with acquired immune deficiency syndrome. Gastroenterology *88*:171, 1985.
15. Foucar, E., Mukai, K., Foucar, K., et al. Colon ulceration in lethal cytomegalovirus infection. Am. J. Clin. Pathol. *76*:788, 1981.
16. Goodell, S. E., Quinn, T. C., Mkrtichian, E., et al. Herpes simplex proctitis in homosexual men. Clinical, sigmoidoscopic and histopathological features. N. Engl. J. Med. *308*:868, 1983.
17. Centers for Disease Control. Update on acquired immunodeficiency syndrome (AIDS) in the United States. MMWR *24*:507, 1982.
18. Glasgow, B. J., Anders, K., Layfield, L. J., et al. Clinical and pathologic findings of the liver in the acquired immune deficiency syndrome (AIDS). Am. J. Clin. Pathol. *83*:582, 1985.
19. Schneiderman, D. J., Arenson, D. M., Cello, J. P., Margaretten, W., and Weber, T. E. Hepatic disease in patients with the acquired immune deficiency syndrome (AIDS). Hepatology, *7*:925, 1987.
20. Guarda, L. A., Luna, M. A., Smith, J. L., et al. Acquired immune deficiency syndrome: postmortem findings. Am. J. Clin. Pathol. *181*:549, 1984.
21. Friedman, S., Wright, T., and Altman, D. Gastrointestinal Kaposi's sarcoma in acquired immunodeficiency syndrome: endoscopic and autopsy findings. Gastroenterology *89*:102, 1985.
22. Lothe, F., and Murray, J. F. Kaposi's sarcoma: autopsy findings in the African. Acta Un. Int. Cancrum *18*:429, 1962.
23. Rothman, S. Some clinical aspects of Kaposi's sarcoma in the European and North American population. Acta Un. Int. Cancrum *18*:364, 1962.
24. Saltz, R. K., Kurtz, R. C., Lightdale, C. J., et al. Kaposi's sarcoma: gastrointestinal involvement and correlation with skin findings and immunologic function. Dig. Dis. Sci. *29*:817, 1984.
25. Gottlieb, M. S., Groopman, J. E., Weinstein, W. E., et al. The acquired immunodeficiency syndrome. Ann. Intern. Med. *99*:208, 1983.
26. Mobley, K., Rotterdam, H. Z., Lerner, C. W., and Tapper, M. L. Autopsy findings in the acquired immune deficiency syndrome. Pathology *20*:45, 1985.
27. Potter, D. A., Danforth, D. N., Macher, A. M., et al. Evaluation of abdominal pain in the AIDS patient. Ann. Surg. *199*:332, 1984.
28. Stribling, J., Weitzner, S., and Smith, G. V. Kaposi's sarcoma in renal allograft recipients. Cancer *42*:442, 1978.
29. Templeton, A. C. Studies in Kaposi's sarcoma, post mortem findings and disease patterns in women. Cancer *30*:854, 1972.
30. Nesbitt, S., Mark, P. F., and Zimmerman, H. M. Disseminated visceral idiopathic hemorrhagic sarcoma (Kaposi's disease): report of a case with necropsy findings. Ann. Intern. Med. *22*:601, 1945.
31. White, J. A. M., and King, M. H. Kaposi's sarcoma presenting with abdominal symptoms. Radiology *46*:197, 1964.
32. Mitchell, N., and Feder, I. Kaposi's sarcoma with secondary involvement of the jejunum, with perforation and peritonitis. Ann. Intern. Med. *31*:324, 1949.

33. Sherwin, B., and Gordimer, H. Kaposi's sarcoma. Case report with unique visceral manifestations. Ann. Surg. *135*:118, 1952.
34. Sunter, J. P. Visceral Kaposi's sarcoma. Occurrence in a patient suffering from celiac disease. Arch. Pathol. Lab. Med. *102*:543, 1978.
35. Laine, L., Politoske, E. J., and Gill, P. Protein losing enteropathy in acquired immunodeficiency syndrome due to intestinal Kaposi's sarcoma. Arch. Intern. Med. *14*:1174, 1987.
36. Perrone, V., Pergola, M., Abate, G., et al. Protein-losing enteropathy in a patient with generalized Kaposi's sarcoma. Cancer *47*:588, 1981.
37. Bryk, D., Farman, J., Dalleman, S., et al. Kaposi's sarcoma of the intestinal tract: roentgen manifestations. Gastrointest. Radiol. *3*:425, 1978.
38. Urmacher, C., and Nielsen, S. The histopathology of the acquired immune deficiency syndrome. Pathology *20*:197, 1985.
39. Ahmed, N., Nelson, R. S., Goldstein, H. M., and Sinkovics, J. G. Kaposi's sarcoma of the stomach and duodenum: endoscopic and roentgenologic correlations. Gastrointest. Endosc. *21*:149, 1975.
40. Rose, H. S., Balthazar, E. J., Megibow, A. J., et al. Alimentary tract involvement in Kaposi's sarcoma: radiographic and endoscopic findings in 25 homosexual men. Am. J. Roentgenol. *139*:661, 1982.
41. Ziegler, J. L., Beckstead, J. A., Volberding, P. A., et al. Non Hodgkin's lymphoma in 90 homosexual men: relation to generalized lymphadenopathy and the acquired immunodeficiency syndrome. N. Engl. J. Med. *311*:565, 1984.
42. Ioachim, H. L., Cooper, M. C., and Hellman, G. C. Lymphomas in men at high risk for acquired immune deficiency syndrome (AIDS). Cancer *56*:2831, 1985.
43. Levine, A. M., Meyer, P. R., Begandy, M. K., Parker, J. W., Taylor, C. R., Irwin, L., and Lukes, R. J. Development of B cell lymphoma in homosexual men. Clinical and immunologic findings. Ann. Intern. Med. *100*:7, 1984.
44. Bernal, A., and del Junco, G. W. Endoscopic and pathologic features of esophageal lymphoma: a report of four cases in patients with acquired immune deficiency syndrome. Gastrointest. Endosc. *329*:96, 1986.
45. Burkes, R. L., Meyer, P. R., Gill, P. S., Parker, J. W., Rasheed, S., and Levine, A. M. Rectal lymphoma in homosexual men. Arch. Intern. Med. *146*:913, 1986.
46. Lee, M. H., Waxman, M., and Gillooley, J. F. Primary malignant lymphoma of the anorectum in homosexual men. Dis. Colon Rectum *29*:413, 1986.
47. Daling, J. R., Weiss, N. S., Hislop, G. Sexual practices, sexually transmitted diseases, and the incidence of anal cancer. N. Engl. J. Med. *317*:973, 1987.
48. Peters, R. K., and Mack, T. M. Patterns of anal carcinoma by gender and marital status in Los Angeles County. Br. J. Cancer *48*:629, 1983.
49. Li, F. P., Osborn, D., and Cronin, C. M. Anorectal squamous carcinoma in two homosexual men. Lancet *2*:391, 1982.
50. Croxson, T., Chabon, A. B., Rovat, E., and Barash, I. Intraepithelial carcinoma of the anus in homosexual men. Dis. Colon Rectum *27*:325, 1984.
51. Longo, W. E., Ballantyne, G. H., Gerald, W. L., and Modlin, I. M. Squamous cell carcinoma in situ in condyloma acuminatum. Dis. Colon Rectum *29*:503, 1986.
52. Conant, M. A., Volberding, P., Fletcher, V., Lozada, F. I., and Silverman, S. Squamous cell carcinoma in sexual partner of Kaposi sarcoma patient. Lancet *1*:286, 1982.
53. Read, E. J., Orenstein, J. M., Chorba, T. L., Schwartz, A. M., Simon, G. L., Lewis, J. H., and Schulef, R. S. *Listeria monocytogenes* sepsis and small cell carcinoma of the rectum: an unusual presentation of the acquired immunodeficiency syndrome. Am. J. Clin. Pathol. *83*:383, 1985.
54. Frazer, I. H., Medley, G., Crapper, R. M., Brown, T. C., and Mackay, I. R. Association between anorectal dysplasia, human papilloma virus, and human immunodeficiency virus in homosexual men. Lancet *2*:657, 1986.
55. Kovi, J., Tillman, R. L., and Lee, S. M. Malignant transformation of condyloma acuminatum. A light microscopic and ultrastructural study. Am. J. Clin. Pathol. *61*:702, 1974.
56. Bogomoletz, W. V., Potet, F., and Molas, G. Condylomata acuminata, giant condyloma acuminatum (Buschke-Lowenstein tumour) and verrucous squamous carcinoma of the perianal and anorectal region: a continuous precancerous spectrum? Histopathology *9*:1155, 1985.
57. Penn, I. Cancers of the anogenital region in renal transplant patients. Analysis of 65 cases. Cancer *58*:611, 1986.
58. Dworkin, B., Wormser, G. P., Rosenthal, W. S., et al. Gastrointestinal manifestations of the acquired immunodeficiency syndrome: a review of 22 cases. Am. J. Gastroenterol. *80*:774, 1985.
59. Pitlik, S. D., Fainstein, V., Garza, D., et al. Human cryptosporidiosis: spectrum of disease. Arch. Intern. Med. *143*:2269, 1983.
60. Guarda, L. A., Stein, S. A., Cleary, K. A., and Ordonez, N. G. Human cryptosporidiosis in AIDS. Arch. Pathol. Lab. Med. *107*:562, 1983.
61. Forgacs, P., Tarshis, A., Ma, P., et al. Intestinal and bronchial cryptosporidiosis in an immunodeficient homosexual man. Ann. Intern. Med. *99*:793, 1983.
62. Pitlik, S. D., Fainstein, V., Rios, A., et al. Cryptosporidial cholecystitis. N. Engl. J. Med. *308*:967, 1983.
63. Current, W. L., Reese, N. C., Ernst, J. V., et al. Human cryptosporidiosis in immunocompetent and immunodeficient persons: studies of an outbreak and experimental transmission. N. Engl. J. Med. *308*:1252, 1983.
64. Andreani, T., LeCharpentier, Y., Brovet, J.-C., et al. Acquired immunodeficiency with intestinal cryptosporidiosis: possible transmission by Haitian whole blood. Lancet *1*:1187, 1983.
65. Current, W. L., and Haynes, T. B. Complete development of *Cryptosporidium* in cell culture. Science *224*:603, 1984.
66. DeHovitz, J. A., Pape, J. W., Boucy, M., and Johnson, W. D. Clinical manifestations and therapy of *Isospora belli* infection in patients with the acquired immunodeficiency syndrome. N. Engl. J. Med. *315*:87, 1986.
67. Desportes, I., LeCharpentier, Y., Galian, A., Bernard, F., Cochand-Priollet, B., Lavergne, A., Ravisse, P., and Modigliani, R. Occurrence of a new microsporidium: *Enterocytozoon bieneusi*; n.g., n. sp., in the enterocytes of a human patient with AIDS. J. Protozool. *32*:250, 1985.
68. Dobbins, W. O., and Weinstein, W. M. Electron microscopy of the intestine and rectum in acquired immunodeficiency syndrome. Gastroenterology *88*:738, 1985.
69. Sohn, C. S., Schroff, R. W., Kliewer, K. E., et al. Disseminated *Mycobacterium avium-intracellulare* infection in homosexual men with acquired cell-mediated immunodeficiency: a histologic and immunologic study of two cases. Am. J. Clin. Pathol. *79*:247, 1983.
70. Wolke, A., Meyers, S., Adelsberg, B. R., et al. *Mycobacterium avium intracellulare* associated colitis in a patient with acquired immunodeficiency syndrome. J. Clin. Gastroenterol. *6*:225, 1984.
71. Gillin, J. S., Urmacher, C., West, R., and Shike, M. Disseminated *Mycobacterium avium-intracellulare* infection in acquired immunodeficiency syndrome mimicking Whipple's disease. Gastroenterology *85*:1187, 1983.
72. Roth, R. I., Owen, R. L., Keren, D. F., and Volberding, P. A. Intestinal infection with *Mycobacterium avium* in acquired immune deficiency syndrome (AIDS). Dig. Dis. Sci. *30*:497, 1985.
73. Smith, P. D., Macher, A. M., Bookman, M. A., et al. *Salmonella typhimurium* enteritis and bacteremia in the acquired immunodeficiency syndrome. Ann. Intern. Med. *102*:207, 1985.
74. Fischl, M. A., Dickinson, G. M., Sinave, C., Pitchenik, A. E., and Chlearly, T. J. *Salmonella* bacteremia as manifestation of acquired immunodeficiency syndrome. Arch. Intern. Med. *146*:113, 1986.
75. Bottone, E. J., Wormser, G. P., and Duncanson, F. P. Nontyphoidal *Salmonella* bacteremia as an early infection in acquired immunodeficiency syndrome. Diagn. Microbiol. Infect. Dis. *2*:247, 1984.
76. Siegel, F. P., Lopez, C., Hammer, G. S., et al. Severe acquired immunodeficiency in male homosexuals manifested by chronic

perianal ulcerative herpes simplex lesions. N. Engl. J. Med. *305*:1439, 1981.
77. Gertler, S. L., Pressman, J., Price, P., et al. Gastrointestinal cytomegalovirus infection in a homosexual man with severe acquired immunodeficiency syndrome. Gastroenterology *85*:1403, 1983.
78. Baker, R. W., and Peppercorn, M. A. Gastrointestinal ailments of homosexual men. Medicine *61*:390, 1982.
79. Surawicz, C. M., Goodell, S. E., Quinn, T. C., et al. Spectrum of rectal biopsy abnormalities in homosexual men with intestinal symptoms. Gastroenterology *91*:651, 1986.
80. Garcia, L. S., Bruckner, D. A., Brewer, T. C., and Shimizu, R. Y. Techniques for the recovery and identification of *Cryptosporidium* oocysts from stool specimens. J. Clin. Microbiol. *18*:85, 1983.
81. Ng, E., Markell, E. K., Fleming, R. L., and Fried, M. Demonstration of *Isospora belli* by acid-fast stain in a patient with acquired immune deficiency syndrome. J. Clin. Microbiol. *20*:384, 1984.
82. Modigliani, R., Bories, C., LeCharpentier, Y., et al. Diarrhea and malabsorption in acquired immune deficiency syndrome: a study of four cases with special emphasis on opportunistic protozoan infestations. Gut *26*:179, 1985.
83. Wall, S. D., Ominsky, S., Altman, D. F., et al. Multifocal abnormalities of the gastrointestinal tract in AIDS. AJR *146*:1, 1986.
84. Portnoy, D., Whiteside, M. E., Buckley, E., and MacLeod, C. L. Treatment of intestinal cryptosporidiosis with spiramycin. Ann. Intern. Med. *101*:202, 1984.
85. Shepp, D. H., Newton, B. A., Dandliker, P. S., Flournoy, N., and Meyers, J. D. Oral acyclovir therapy for mucocutaneous herpes simplex virus infections in immunocompromised marrow transplant recipients. Ann. Intern. Med. *102*:783, 1985.
86. Masur, H., Lane, H. C., Palestine, A., et al. Effect of 9-(1,3-dihydroxy-2-propoxymethyl) guanine on serious cytomegalovirus disease in eight immunosuppressed homosexual men. Ann. Intern. Med. *104*:41, 1986.
87. Kotler, D. P., Gaetz, H. P., Lange, M., et al. Enteropathy associated with the acquired immunodeficiency syndrome. Ann. Intern. Med. *101*:421, 1984.
88. Brinson, R. R. Hypoalbuminemia, diarrhea, and the acquired immunodeficiency syndrome. Ann. Intern. Med. *102*:413, 1985.
89. Blacklow, N. R., and Cukor, G. Viral gastroenteritis. N. Engl. J. Med. *304*:397, 1981.
90. Chandler, F. W., White, E. H., Callaway, C. S., Spira, T. J., and Ewing, E. P. Unidentified virus like particles in the intestine of patients with the acquired immunodeficiency syndrome. Ann. Intern. Med. *100*:851, 1984.
91. Rene, E., Marche, C., Regnier, B., et al. Manifestations digestives du syndrome d'immunodeficience acquise (SIDA); etude chez 26 patients. Gastroenterol. Clin. Biol. *9*:327, 1985.
92. Gottlieb, M. S., Groopman, J. E., Weinstein, W. E., et al. The acquired immunodeficiency syndrome. Ann. Intern. Med. *99*:208, 1983.
93. Pitchenik, A. E., Fischl, M. A., Dickinson, G. M., et al. Opportunistic infection and Kaposi's sarcoma among Haitians: evidence of a new acquired immunodeficiency state. Ann. Intern. Med. *98*:277, 1983.
94. Gillin, J. S., Shike, M., Alcode, N., et al. Malabsorption and mucosal abnormalities of the small intestine in the acquired immunodeficiency syndrome. Ann. Intern. Med. *102*:619, 1985.
95. Tapper, M. L., Rotterdam, H. Z., Lerner, C. W., et al. Adrenal necrosis in the acquired immunodeficiency syndrome. Ann. Intern. Med. *100*:239, 1984.
96. Guenthner, E. E., Rabinowe, S. L., Van Niel, A., et al. Primary Addison's disease in a patient with the acquired immunodeficiency syndrome. Ann. Intern. Med. *100*:847, 1984.
97. Green, L. W., Cole, W., Greene, J. B., et al. Adrenal insufficiency as a complication of the acquired immunodeficiency syndrome. Ann. Intern. Med. *101*:497, 1984.
98. Smith, P. D., Lane, H. C., Gill, V. J., Fauci, A. S., and Masur, H. Evaluation and therapy of intestinal infections in the acquired immunodeficiency syndrome (AIDS). Clin. Res. *35*:414A, 1987.
99. Scott, G. B., Buck, B. E., Leterman, J. G., et al. Acquired immunodeficiency syndrome in infants. N. Engl. J. Med. *310*:76, 1984.
100. Fernandez, G., Nair, M., Onoe, K., et al. Impairment of cell-mediated immunity functions by dietary zinc deficiency in mice. Proc. Natl. Acad. Sci. USA *76*:457, 1979.
101. Beach, R. S., Gershwin, M. E., and Hurley, L. S. Gestational zinc deprivation in mice: persistence of immunodeficiency for three generations. Science *218*:469, 1982.
102. Cunningham-Rundles, C., Cunningham-Rundles, S., Iwata, T., et al. Zinc deficiency, depressed thymic hormones, and T lymphocytes dysfunction in patients with hypogammaglobulinemia. Clin. Immunol. Immunopathol. *21*:387, 1981.
103. Wolman, S. L., Anderson, G. H., Marliss, E. B., and Jeejeebhoy, K. N. Zinc in total parenteral nutrition: requirements and metabolic effects. Gastroenterology *76*:458, 1979.
104. Brunser, O., Castillo, C., and Araya, M. Fine structure of the small intestine mucosa in infantile marasmic malnutrition. Gastroenterology *70*:495, 1976.
105. Benkov, K. J., Stawski, C., Sirlin, S. M., et al. Atypical presentation of childhood acquired immune deficiency syndrome mimicking Crohn's disease: nutritional considerations and management. Am. J. Gastroenterol. *80*:260, 1985.
106. Masur, H., Michelis, M., Greene, J. B., et al. An outbreak of community acquired *Pneumocystis carinii* pneumonia. Initial manifestations of a cellular immune dysfunction. N. Engl. J. Med. *305*:1431, 1981.
107. Tavitian, A., Rauffman, J., and Rosenthal, L. E. Oral candidiasis as a marker for esophageal candidiasis in the acquired immunodeficiency syndrome. Ann. Intern. Med. *104*:54, 1986.
108. Scherl, E., Siegel, F., Geller, S., and Waye, J. Gastrointestinal manifestations of acquired immunodeficiency syndrome. Gastroenterology *86*:1235, 1984.
109. Greenspan, D., Conant, M., Silverman, S., et al. Oral "hairy leucoplakia" in male homosexuals: evidence of association with both papillomavirus and a herpes group virus. Lancet *2*:831, 1984.
110. St. Onge, G., and Bezahler, G. H. Giant esophageal ulcer associated with cytomegalovirus. Gastroenterology *83*:127, 1982.
111. Solammedevi, S. V., and Patwardhan, R. Herpes esophagitis. Am. J. Gastroenterol. *77*:48, 1982.
112. Rabeneck, L., Boyko, W. J., McLean, D. M., McLeod, W. A., and Wong, K. K. Unusual esophageal ulcers containing enveloped virus-like particles in homosexual men. Gastroenterology *90*:1882, 1986.
113. Trier, J. S., and Bjorkman, D. J. Esophageal, gastric and intestinal candidiases. Am. J. Med. *77*:39, 1984,
114. Kodsi, B. E., Wickremesinghe, P. C., Kozinn, P. J., et al. *Candida* esophagitis, a prospective study of 27 cases. Gastroenterology *71*:715, 1976.
115. Balthazar, E. J., Megibow, A. J., and Hulnick, D. H. Cytomegalovirus esophagitis and gastritis in AIDS. AJR *144*:1201, 1985.
116. Lerner, C. W., and Tapper, M. L. Opportunistic infection complicating acquired immune deficiency syndrome. Medicine *63*:155, 1984.
117. Eras, P., Goldstein, M. J., and Sherlock, P. J. *Candida* infection of the gastrointestinal tract. Medicine *51*:367, 1972.
118. Holt, H. *Candida* infection of the esophagus. Gut *9*:227, 1968.
119. Levine, M. A., Macones, A. J., and Laufer, I. *Candida* esophagitis: accuracy of radiographic diagnosis. Radiology *154*:581, 1985.
120. Vahey, T. N., Maglinte, D. D. T., and Chernish, S. State-of-the-art barium examination in opportunistic esophagitis. Dig. Dis. Sci. *31*:1192, 1986.
121. Tavitian, A., Kaufman, J., Rosenthal, L. E., et al. Ketoconazole resistant *Candida* esophagitis in patients with acquired immunodeficiency syndrome. Gastroenterology *90*:443, 1986.
122. Potter, D. A., Danforth, D. N., Macher, A. M., et al. Evaluation of abdominal pain in the AIDS patient. Ann. Surg. *199*:332, 1984.
123. Barone, J. E., Gingold, B. S., Nealon, T. F., and Arvanitis, M. L. Abdominal pain in patients with acquired immune deficiency syndrome. Ann. Surg. *204*:619, 1986.
124. Caya, J. G., Cohen, E. B., Allendorph, M. M., et al. Atypical

mycobacterial and cytomegalovirus infection of the duodenum in a patient with acquired immunodeficiency syndrome: endoscopic and histopathologic appearance. Wis. Med. J. *83*:33, 1984.

125. Elta, G., Turnage, R., Eckhauser, F. E., Agha, F., and Ross, S. A submucosal central mass caused by cytomegalovirus infection in a patient with acquired immunodeficiency syndrome. Am. J. Gastroenterol. *81*:714, 1986.
126. Kavin, H., Jonas, R. B., Chowdury, L., and Kabins, S. Acalculous cholecystitis and cytomegalovirus infection in the acquired immunodeficiency syndrome. Ann. Intern. Med. *104*:53, 1986.
127. Scott, B. B., and Jenkins, D. Gastro-oesophageal candidiasis. Gut *23*:137, 1982.
128. Victoria, M. S., Nangia, B. S., and Jindrak, K. Cytomegalovirus pyloric obstruction in a child with acquired immunodeficiency syndrome. Pediatr. Infect. Dis. *4*:550, 1985.
129. Steinberg, J. J., Bridges, N., Feiner, H. D., and Valensi, Q. Small intestinal lymphoma in three patients with acquired immune deficiency syndrome. Am. J. Gastroenterol. *80*:21, 1985.
130. Kram, H. B., Hino, S. T., Cohen, R. E., Desautis, S. A., and Shoemaker, W. C. Spontaneous colonic perforation secondary to cytomegalovirus in a patient with acquired immunodeficiency syndrome. Crit. Care Med. *12*:469, 1984.
131. Balthazar, E. J., Reich, C., and Pachter, H. L. The significance of small bowel intussusception in acquired immune deficiency syndrome. Am. J. Gastroenterol. *81*:1073, 1986.
132. Collier, P. E. Small bowel lymphoma associated with AIDS. J. Surg. Oncol. *32*:131, 1986.
133. Baker, M. S., Wille, M., Goldman, H., and Kim, H. K. Metastatic Kaposi's sarcoma presenting as acute appendicitis. Military Med. *151*:45, 1986.
134. Kalb, R. E., and Grossman, M. E. Chronic perianal herpes simplex in immunocompromised hosts. Am. J. Med. *80*:486, 1986.
135. Margulis, S. J., Honig, C. L., Soave, R., Govani, A. F., Mouradian, J. A., and Jacobson, I. M. Biliary tract obstruction in the acquired immunodeficiency syndrome. Ann. Intern. Med. *105*:207, 1987.
136. Schneiderman, D. J., Cello, J. P., and Laing, F. C. Papillary stenosis and sclerosing cholangitis in patients with the acquired immune deficiency syndrome (AIDS). Ann. Intern. Med. *106*:546, 1987.
137. Jeffrey, R. B., Nyberg, D. A., Bottles, K., et al. Abdominal CT in acquired immunodeficiency syndrome. AJR *146*:7, 1986.
138. Albin, J., Lewis, E., Eftekhari, F., and Shirkhoda, A. Computed tomography of rectal and perirectal disease in AIDS patients. Gastrointest. Radiol. *12*:67, 1987.
139. Lebovics, E., Thung, S. N., Schaffner, F., and Radensky, P. W. The liver in the acquired immunodeficiency syndrome: a clinical and histologic study. Hepatology *5*:293, 1985.
140. Orenstein, M. S., Tavitian, A., Yonk, B., et al. Granulomatous involvement of the liver in patients with AIDS. Gut *26*:1220, 1985.
141. Kahn, S. A., Saltzman, B. R., Klein, R. S., Mahadevia, P. S., Friedland, G. H., and Brandt, L. J. Hepatic disorders in the acquired immune deficiency syndrome: a clinical and pathological study. Am. J. Gastroenterol. *81*:1145, 1986.
142. Greene, J. B., Sidhu, G. S., Lewin, S., et al. *Mycobacterium avium intracellulare:* a cause of disseminated life-threatening infection in homosexuals and drug abusers. Ann. Intern. Med. *97*:539, 1982.
143. Wheat, L. J., Slama, T. G., and Zeckel, M. L. Histoplasmosis in the acquired immune deficiency syndrome. Am. J. Med. *78*:203, 1985.
144. Caccamo, D., Pervez, N. K., and Marchcusky, A. Primary lymphoma of the liver in the acquired immunodeficiency syndrome. Arch. Pathol. Lab. Med. *110*:553, 1986.
145. Jaffe, E. S., Clark, J., Steis, R., et al. Lymph node pathology of HTLV and HTLV-associated neoplasms. Cancer Res. *45*:4662s, 1985.
146. Gordin, F. M., Simon, G. L., Wofsy, C. B., et al. Adverse reactions to trimethoprim-sulfamethoxazole in patients with the acquired immunodeficiency syndrome. Ann. Intern. Med. *100*:494, 1984.
147. Schreeder, M. T., Thompson, S. E., Hadler, S. C., et al. Hepatitis B in homosexual men: prevalence of infection and factors related to transmission. J. Infect. Dis. *146*:7, 1982.
148. Duffy, L. F., Daum, F., Kahn, E., et al. Hepatitis in children with acquired immune deficiency syndrome. Histopathologic and immunocytologic features. Gastroenterology *90*:173, 1986.
149. Czapar, C. A., Weldon-Linne, M., Moore, D. M., and Rhone, D. P. Peliosis hepatis in the acquired immunodeficiency syndrome. Arch. Pathol. Lab. Med. *110*:611, 1986.
150. Nakanuma, Y., Liew, C. T., Petus, R. L., and Govindarajan, S. Pathologic features of the liver in acquired immune deficiency syndrome (AIDS). Liver *6*:158, 1986.
151. Smith, R. Liver-spleen scintigraphy in patients with acquired immunodeficiency syndrome. AJR *145*:1201, 1985.
152. Gordon, S. C., Reddy, K. R., Gould, E. E., McFadden, R., O'Brien, C., DeMedina, M., Jeffers, L. J., and Schiff, E. R. The spectrum of liver diseases in the acquired immunodeficiency syndrome. J. Hepatol. *2*:475, 1986.
153. Rogers, M. F., Morens, D. M., Stewart, J. A., et al. National case control study of Kaposi's sarcoma and *Pneumocystis carinii* pneumonia in homosexual men. Part 2: Laboratory results. Ann. Intern. Med. *99*:151, 1986.
154. Rustgi, V. K., Hoofnagle, J. H., Gerin, J. L., et al. Hepatitis B virus infection in the acquired immunodeficiency syndrome. Ann. Intern. Med. *101*:795, 1986.
155. Wright, T., Friedman, S., and Altman, D. Hepatitis B virus infection is implicated in the pathogenesis of Kaposi's sarcoma in homosexual men. Gastroenterology *84*:1402, 1983.
156. Perrillo, R. P., Regenstein, F. G., and Roodman, S. T. Chronic hepatitis B in asymptomatic homosexual men with antibody to the human immunodeficiency virus. Ann. Intern. Med. *105*:382, 1986.
157. Krogsgaard, K., Lindhart, B. O., Nielsen, J. O., Andersson, P., Kryger, P., Aldershville, J., Gerstof, J., and Pedersen, C. The influence of HTLV III infection on the natural history of hepatitis B virus infection in male homosexual HBsAg carriers. Hepatology *7*:37, 1987.
158. Ravenholt, R. T. Role of hepatitis B virus in acquired immunodeficiency syndrome. Lancet *2*:885, 1983.
159. McDonald, M. I., Hamilton, J. D., and Durack, D. T. Hepatitis B surface antigen could harbor the infective agent of AIDS. Lancet *2*:882, 1983.
160. Siddiqui, A. Hepatitis B virus DNA in Kaposi's sarcoma. Proc. Natl. Acad. Sci. USA *80*:4681, 1983.
161. Goedert, J. J., Biggar, R. J., Weiss, S. H., et al. Three-year incidence of AIDS in five cohorts of HTLV-III infected risk group members. Science *231*:992, 1986.
162. Laure, F., Zagury, D., Saimot, A. G., et al. Hepatitis B virus DNA sequence in lymphoid cells from patients with AIDS and AIDS-related complex. Science *229*:561, 1985.
163. Noonan, C. A., Yoffe, B., Mansell, P. W. A., Melnick, J. L., and Hollinger, F. B. Extrachromosomal sequences of hepatitis B virus DNA in peripheral blood mononuclear cells of acquired immune deficiency patients. Proc. Natl. Acad. Sci. USA *83*:5698, 1986.
164. Golden, J. A. No increased incidence of AIDS in recipients of hepatitis B vaccine. N. Engl. J. Med. *308*:1163, 1983.
165. Szmuness, W., Stevens, C. E., Harley, E. J., et al. Hepatitis B vaccine: demonstration of efficacy in a controlled clinical trial on a high-risk population in the United States. N. Engl. J. Med. *303*:833, 1980.
166. Stevens, C. E. No increased incidence of AIDS in recipients of hepatitis B vaccine. N. Engl. J. Med. *308*:1163, 1983.
167. Fishbein, P. G., Tuthill, R., Kressel, H., et al. Herpes simplex esophagitis: a cause of upper gastrointestinal bleeding. Am. J. Dig. Dis. *24*:540, 1979.
168. Babb, R. R., Differding, J. L., and Trollope, M. L. Cryptosporidia enteritis in a healthy professional athlete. Am. J. Gastroenterol. *77*:833, 1982.
169. Glaser, J. B., Morton-Kute, L., Bergeo, S. R., et al. Recurrent *Salmonella typhimurium* bacteremia associated with the acquired immunodeficiency syndrome. Ann. Intern. Med. *102*:189, 1985.
170. Dritz, S. K., Ainsworth, T. E., Back, A., Boucher, L. A., Garrard, W. F., Palmer, R. D., and River, E. Patterns of sexually transmitted enteric diseases in a city. Lancet *2*:3, 1977.

171. Owen, R. L., Dritz, S. K., and Wibbelsman, C. J. Venereal aspects of gastroenterology. Western J. Med. *130*:236, 1979.
172. Phillips, S. C., Mildvan, D., William, D. C., Gelb, A. M., and White, M. C. Sexual transmission of enteric protozoa and helminths in a venereal-disease clinic population. N. Engl. J. Med. *305*:603, 1981.
173. Keystone, J. S., Keystone, D. L., and Proctor, E. M. Intestinal parasitic infections in homosexual men: prevalence, symptoms and factors in transmission. Can. Med. Assoc. J. *123*:512, 1980.
174. William, D. C., Shookhoff, H. B., Felman, Y. M., and DeRamos, S. W. High rates of enteric protozoal infections in selected homosexual men attending a venereal disease clinic. Sex. Transm. Dis. *5*:155, 1978.
175. Bolling, D. R. Prevalence, goals and complications of heterosexual anal intercourse in a gynecologic population. J. Reprod. Med. *19*:120, 1977.
176. Drusin, L. M., Magagna, J., Yano, K., and Ley, A. B. An epidemiologic study of sexually transmitted diseases on a university campus. Am. J. Epidemiol. *100*:8, 1974.
177. Szmuness, W., Much, M. I., Prince, A. M., Hoofnagle, J. H., Cherubin, C. E., Harley, E. J., and Block, G. H. On the role of sexual behavior in the spread of hepatitis B infection. Ann. Intern. Med. *83*:489, 1975.
178. Judson, F. N. Sexually transmitted disease in gay men. Sex. Transm. Dis. *4*:76, 1977.
179. Declining rates of rectal and pharyngeal gonorrhea among males—New York City. MMWR *33*:295, 1984.
180. Rectal gonorrhea in San Francisco, October 1984–September 1986. San Francisco Epidemiologic Bulletin *2*(12):1, 1986.
181. Handsfield, H. H. Decreasing incidence of gonorrhea in homosexually active men—minimal effect on risk of AIDS. Western J. Med. *143*:469, 1985.
182. Self-reported changes in sexual behaviors among homosexual and bisexual men from the San Francisco City Clinic cohort. MMWR *36*:187, 1987.
183. Bienzle, U., Coester, C. H., Knobloch, J., and Guggenmoos-Holzmann, I. Protozoal enteric infections in homosexual men. Klin. Wochenschr. *62*:323, 1984.
184. Peters, C. S., Sable, R., Janda, W. M., Chittom, A. L., and Kocka, F. E. Prevalence of enteric parasites in homosexual patients attending an outpatient clinic. J. Clin. Microbiol. *24*:684, 1986.
185. Levinson, W., Dunn, P. M., Cooney, T. G., and Sampson, J. H. Parasitic infections in asymptomatic homosexual men: cost-effective screening. J. Gen. Intern. Med. *1*:150, 1986.
186. Jokipii, L., Pohjola, S., Valle, S.-L., and Jokipii, M. M. Frequency, multiplicity and repertoire of intestinal protozoa in healthy homosexual men and in patients with gastrointestinal symptoms. Ann. Clin. Res. *17*:57, 1985.
187. Håakansson, C., Thoren, K., Norkrans, G., and Johannisson, G. Intestinal parasitic infection and other sexually transmitted diseases in asymptomatic homosexual men. Scand. J. Infect. Dis. *16*:199, 1984.
188. Ortega, H. B., Borchardt, K. A., Hamilton, R., Ortega, P., and Mahood, J. Enteric pathogenic protozoa in homosexual men from San Francisco. Sex. Transm. Dis. *11*:59, 1984.
189. Sorvillo, F., Lieb, L., Tormey, M., Mascola, L., and Run, G. Declining rates of amebiasis among gay men in Los Angeles County—an indicator of changed sexual behavior due to AIDS? American Public Health Association Abstracts, Annual Meeting, October 1987.
190. Pearce, R. B., and Abrams, D. I. *Entamoeba histolytica* in homosexual men. N. Engl. J. Med. *316*:690, 1987.
191. Owen, W. F., Jr. Medical problems of the homosexual adolescent. J. Adolescent Health Care *6*:278, 1985.
192. Allason-Jones, E., Mindel, A., Sargeaunt, P., and Williams, P. *Entamoeba histolytica* as a commensal intestinal parasite in homosexual men. N. Engl. J. Med. *315*:353, 1986.
193. Ylvisaker, J. T., and McDonald, G. B. Sexually acquired amebic colitis and liver abscess. Western J. Med. *132*:153, 1980.
194. Istre, G. R., Kreiss, K., Hopkins, R. S., Healy, G. R., Benziger, M., Canfield, T. M., Dickinson, P., Englert, T. R., Compton, R. C., Mathews, H. M., and Simmons, R. A. An outbreak of amebiasis spread by colonic irrigation at a chiropractic clinic. N. Engl. J. Med. *301*:339, 1982.
195. Sullam, P. M., Slutkin, G., Gottlieb, A. B., and Mills, J. Paromomycin therapy of endemic amebiasis in homosexual men. Sex. Transm. Dis. *13*:151, 1986.
196. Rendtorff, R. C. The experimental transmission of human intestinal protozoan parasites. II. *Giardia lamblia* cysts given in capsules. Am. J. Hyg. *59*:209, 1954.
197. Bingham, A. K., and Meyer, E. A. *Giardia* excystation can be induced *in vitro* in acidic solutions. Nature *277*:301, 1979.
198. Black, R. E., Dykes, A. C., Sinclair, S. P., and Wells, J. G. Giardiasis in day-care centers; Evidence of person-to-person transmission. Pediatrics *60*:486, 1977.
199. Meyers, J. D., Kuharic, H. A., and Holmes, K. K. *Giardia lamblia* infection in homosexual men. Br. J. Vener. Dis. *53*:54, 1977.
200. Kacker, P. P. A case of *Giardia lamblia* proctitis presenting in a V. D. clinic. Br. J. Vener. Dis. *49*:318, 1973.
201. Waugh, M. A. Threadworm infestation in homosexuals. Tr. St. Johns Hosp. Dermatol. Soc. (London) *58*:224, 1972.
202. McMillan, A. Threadworms in homosexual males. Br. Med. J. *1*:367, 1978.
203. Markell, E. K., Voge, M., and John, D. T. Medical Parasitology. 6th ed. Philadelphia, W. B. Saunders Company, 1986.
204. Sorvillo, F., Mori, K., Sewake, W., and Fishman, L. Sexual transmission of *Strongyloides stercoralis* among homosexual men. Br. J. Vener. Dis. *59*:342, 1983.
205. Brown, W. J., and Voge, M. Cysticercosis: a modern day plague. Pediatr. Clin. North Am. *32*:953, 1985.
206. Bader, M., Pedersen, A. H. B., Williams, R., Spearman, J., and Anderson, H. Venereal transmission of shigellosis in Seattle, King County. Sex. Transm. Dis. *4*:89, 1977.
207. Levine, M. M., DuPont, H. L., Khodabandelou, M., and Hornick, R. B. Long-term *Shigella*-carrier state. N. Engl. J. Med. *288*:1169, 1973.
208. Dritz, S. K., and Braff, E. H. Sexually transmitted typhoid fever. N. Engl. J. Med. *296*:1359, 1977.
209. Jacobs, J. L., Gold, J. W. M., Murray, H. W., Roberts, R. B., and Armstrong, D. *Salmonella* infections in patients with the acquired immunodeficiency syndrome. Ann. Intern. Med. *102*:186, 1985.
210. Glaser, J. B., Morton-Kute, L., Berger, S. C., Weber, J., Siegal, F. P., Lopez, C., Robbins, W., and Landesman, S. H. Recurrent *Salmonella typhimurium* bacteremia associated with the acquired immunodeficiency syndrome. Ann. Intern. Med. *102*:189, 1985.
211. Drusin, L. M., Wilkes, B. M., and Gingrich, R. D. Streptococcal pyoderma of the penis following fellatio. Br. J. Vener. Dis. *51*:61, 1975.
212. Cherian, S., Tabatabai, M. R., and Cummings, N. A. Rheumatic fever and gonococcal pharyngitis in an adult. South. Med. J. *72*:319, 1979.
213. Quinn, T. C., Corey, L., Chaffee, R. G., Schuffler, M. D., and Holmes, K. K. *Campylobacter* proctitis in a homosexual man. Ann. Intern. Med. *93*:458, 1980.
214. Quinn, T. C., Goodell, S. E., Fennell, C., Wang, S.-P., Schuffler, M. D., Holmes, K. K., and Stamm, W. E. Infections with *Campylobacter jejuni* and *Campylobacter*-like organisms in homosexual men. Ann. Intern. Med. *101*:187, 1984.
215. Fennell, C. L., Totten, P. A., Mkrtichian, E. E., et al. Characterization of *Campylobacter*-like organisms isolated from homosexual men. J. Infect. Dis. *149* 58, 1984.
216. Dunlop, E. M. C., Hare, M. J., Jones, B. R., and Taylor-Robinson, D. Mycoplasmas and 'non-specific' genital infections. II. Clinical aspects. Br. J. Vener. Dis. *45*:274, 1969.
217. Goldmeier, D. A study on non-specific proctitis in homosexual men. M.D. Thesis, University of London, 1976.
218. Owen, R. L., and Hill, J. L. Rectal and pharyngeal gonorrhea in homosexual men. JAMA *220*:1315, 1972.
219. Corman, L. C., Levison, M. E., Knight, R., Carrington, E. R., and Kaye, D. The high frequency of pharyngeal gonococcal infection in a prenatal clinic population. JAMA *230*:568, 1974.
220. Wiesner, P. J., Tronca, E., Bonin, P., Pedersen, A. H. B., and Holmes, K. K. Clinical spectrum of pharyngeal gonococcal infection. N. Engl. J. Med. *288*:181, 1973.
221. Jamsky, R. J. Gonococcal tonsillitis: report of a case. Oral Surg. *44*:197, 1977.

222. Kohn, S. R., Shaffer, J. F., and Chomenko, A. G. Primary gonococcal stomatitis. JAMA *219*:86, 1972.
223. Stolz, E., and Schuller, J. Gonococcal oro- and nasopharyngeal infection. Br. J. Vener. Dis. *50*:104, 1974.
224. Tikjøb, G., Petersen, C. S., Ousted, M., and Øhlenschlaeger, J. Localization of gonococci in the anterior oral cavity—a possible reservoir of the gonococcal infection? Ann. Clin. Res. *17*:73, 1985.
225. Komaroff, A. L., Aronson, M. D., Pass, T. M., and Ervin, C. T. Prevalence of pharyngeal gonorrhea in general medical patients with sore throats. Sex. Transm. Dis. *7*:116, 1980.
226. Odegaard, K., and Gedde-Dahl, T. W. Frequency of simultaneous carriage of *Neisseria gonorrhoeae* and *Neisseria meningitidis*. Br. J. Vener. Dis. *55*:334, 1979.
227. Janda, W. M., Bohnhoff, M., Morello, J. A., and Lerner, S. A. Prevalence and site-pathogen studies of *Neisseria meningitidis* and *N. gonorrhoeae* in homosexual men. JAMA *244*:2060, 1980.
228. Hook, E. W., and Holmes, K. K. Gonococcal infections. Ann. Intern. Med. *102*:229, 1985.
229. Sands, M. Treatment of gonococcal pharyngeal infections in men. Western J. Med. *131*:338, 1979.
230. Hutt, D. M., and Judson, F. N. Epidemiology and treatment of oropharyngeal gonorrhea. Ann. Intern. Med. *104*:655, 1986.
231. Thurner, J., Poitschek, C., and Weninger, A. Experimenteller Beitrag zum Thema Rachengonorrhoe. Zeit. Hautkr. *53*:787, 1978.
232. Metzger, A. L. Gonococcal arthritis complicating gonorrheal pharyngitis. Ann. Intern. Med. *73*:267, 1970.
233. Evrard, J. R. Spread of gonococcal pharyngitis to the genitals. Am. J. Obstet. Gynecol. *117*:856, 1973.
234. Fisher, L. S., Edelstein, P., and Guze, L. B. *Neisseria lactamicus* pharyngitis. JAMA *233*:22, 1975.
235. Harkness, A. H. The pathology of gonorrhoea. Br. J. Vener. Dis. *24*:137, 1948.
236. Holmes, K. K., Counts, G. W., and Beaty, H. N. Disseminated gonococcal infection. Ann. Intern. Med. *74*:979, 1971.
237. Lebedeff, D. A., and Hochman, E. B. Rectal gonorrhea in men: diagnosis and treatment. Ann. Intern. Med. *92*:463, 1980.
238. Quinn, T. C., Corey, L., Chaffee, R. G., Schuffler, M. D., Brancato, F. P., and Holmes, K. K. The etiology of anorectal infections in homosexual men. Am. J. Med. *71*:395, 1981.
239. Judson, F. N., Ehret, J. M., and Eickhoff, T. C. Anogenital infection with *Neisseria meningitidis* in homosexual men. J. Infect. Dis. *137*:458, 1978.
240. Zellner, S. R., and Trudeau, W. L. Anorectal gonorrhea presenting as ulcerative proctitis. South. Med. J. *66*:706, 1973.
241. Goodman, K. J. Radiologic findings in anorectal gonorrhea. Gastrointest. Radiol. *3*:223, 1978.
242. Sands, M. Treatment of anorectal gonorrhea infections in men. JAMA *243*:1143, 1980.
243. STD Treatment Guidelines. MMWR *34*(Suppl. 4S):75S, 1985.
244. Antibiotic-resistant strains of *Neisseria gonorrhoeae.* Policy guidelines for detection, management, and control. MMWR *36*(Suppl. 5S):1S, 1987.
245. von Knorring, J., and Nieminen, J. Gonococcal perihepatitis in a surgical ward. Ann. Clin. Res. *11*:66, 1979.
246. Rutkow, I. M. Gonococcal perihepatitis (The Fitz-Hugh–Curtis syndrome): a diagnostic dilemma. Am. Surgeon *45*:369, 1979.
247. Kimball, M. W., and Knee, S. Gonococcal perihepatitis in a male. N. Engl. J. Med. *282*:1082, 1970.
248. Lassus, A., and Kousa, M. Gonococcal perihepatitis and gonococcaemia: presentation of a case with cutaneous manifestations. Br. J. Vener. Dis. *49*:48, 1973.
249. Auman, G. L., and Waldenberg, L. M. Gonococcal periappendicitis and salpingitis in a prepubertal girl. Pediatrics *58*:287, 1976.
250. Semchyshyn, S. Fitz-Hugh and Curtis syndrome. J. Reproduct. Med. *22*:45, 1979.
251. Reichert, J. A., and Valle, R. F. Fitz-Hugh–Curtis syndrome: a laparoscopic approach. JAMA *236*:266, 1976.
252. Chapel, T. A. The variability of syphilitic chancres. Sex. Transm. Dis. *5*:68, 1978.
253. Drusin, L. M., Singer, C., Valenti, A. J., and Armstrong, D. Infectious syphilis mimicking neoplastic disease. Arch. Intern. Med. *137*:156, 1977.
254. Fiumara, N. J. Oral lesions of gonorrhea and syphilis. Cutis *17*:689, 1976.
255. Chapel, T. A. Occult anatomic presentations of syphilitic chancres. Med. Aspects Hum. Sex. *13*(7):99, 1979.
256. Chapel, T. A. The signs and symptoms of secondary syphilis. Sex Transm. Dis. *7*:161, 1980.
257. Sachar, D. B., Klein, R. S., Swerdlow, F., Bottone, E., Khilnani, M. T., Waye, J. D., and Wisniewski, M. Erosive syphilitic gastritis: dark-field and immunofluorescent diagnosis from biopsy specimen. Ann. Intern. Med. *80*:512, 1974.
258. Drusin, L. M. The role of surgery in primary syphilis of the anus. Ann. Surg. *184*:65, 1976.
259. Nazemi, M. M., Musher, D. M., Schell, R. F., and Milo, S. Syphilitic proctitis in a homosexual. JAMA *231*:389, 1975.
260. Akdamar, K., Martin, R. J., and Ichinose, H. Syphilitic proctitis. Am. J. Dig. Dis. *22*:701, 1977.
261. Haburchak, D. R., and Davidson, H. Anorectal lesions and syphilitic hepatitis. Western J. Med. *128*:64, 1978.
262. Kaplan, L. R., and Takeuchi, A. Purulent rectal discharge associated with a nontreponemal spirochete. JAMA *241*:52, 1979.
263. Campisi, D., and Whitcomb, C. Liver disease in early syphilis. Arch. Intern. Med. *139*:365, 1979.
264. Tiliakos, N., Shamma'a, J. M., and Nasrallah, S. M. Syphilitic hepatitis. Am. J. Gastroenterol. *73*:60, 1980.
265. Feher, J., Somogyi, T., Timmer, M., and Jozsa, L. Early syphilitic hepatitis. Lancet *2*:896, 1975.
266. Takeuchi, A., Jervis, H. R., Nakazawa, H., and Robinson, D. M. Spiral-shaped organisms on the surface colonic epithelium of the monkey and man. Am. J. Clin. Nutr. *27*:1287, 1974.
267. Henrik-Nielsen, R., Lundbeck, F. A., Teglbjaerg, P. S., Ginnerup, P., and Hovind-Hougen, K. Intestinal spirochetosis of the vermiform appendix. Gastroenterology *88*:971, 1985.
268. Kaplan, L. R., and Takeuchi, A. Purulent rectal discharge associated with a nontreponemal spirochete. JAMA *241*:52, 1979.
269. Tompkins, D. S., Waugh, M. A., and Cooke, E. M. Isolation of intestinal spirochaetes from homosexuals. J. Clin. Pathol. *34*:1385, 1981.
270. McMillan, A., and Lee, F. D. Sigmoidoscopic and microscopic appearance of the rectal mucosa in homosexual men. Gut *22*:1035, 1981.
271. Schachter, J. Chlamydial infections. N. Engl. J. Med. *298*:428, 1978.
272. Annamunthodo, H. Rectal lymphogranuloma venereum in Jamaica. Dis. Colon Rectum. *4*:17, 1961.
273. Schachter, J., Causse, G., and Tarizzo, M. L. Chlamydiae as agents of sexually transmitted diseases. Bull. WHO *54*:245, 1976.
274. Greaves, A. B. The frequency of lymphogranuloma venereum in persons with perirectal abscesses, fistulae in ano, or both. Bull. WHO *29*:797, 1963.
275. Quinn, T. C., Goodell, S. E., Mkrtichian, E., Schuffler, M. D., Wang, S. P., Stamm, W. E., and Holmes, K. K. *Chlamydia trachomatis* proctitis. N. Engl. J. Med. *305*:195, 1981.
276. Schachter, J. Confirmatory serodiagnosis of lymphogranuloma venereum proctitis may yield false-positive results due to other chlamydial infections of the rectum. Sex. Transm. Dis. *8*:26, 1981.
277. Goldmeier, D., and Darougar, S. Isolation of *Chylamydia trachomatis* from throat and rectum of homosexual men. Br. J. Vener. Dis. *53*:184, 1977.
278. Schachter, J., and Atwood, G. Chlamydial pharyngitis? J. Am. Vener. Dis. Assoc. *2*:12, 1975.
279. Dunlop, E. M. C., Hare, M. J., Darougar, S., and Jones, B. R. Chlamydial isolates from the rectum in association with chlamydial infection of the eye or genital tract. II. Clinical aspects. *In* Nichols, R. L. (ed.). Trachoma and Related Disorders. Amsterdam, Excerpta Medica, 1971, p. 507.
280. Reeves, W. C., Corey, L., Adams, H. G., Vontver, L. A., and Holmes, K. K. Risk of recurrence after first episodes of genital herpes: Relation to HSV type and antibody response. N. Engl. J. Med. *305*:315, 1981.
281. Chang, T.-W. Herpetic angina following orogenital exposure. J. Am. Vener. Dis. Assoc. *1*:163, 1975.
282. Tustin, A. W., and Kaiser, A. B. Life-threatening pharyngitis

caused by herpes simplex virus, type 2. Sex. Transm. Dis. *6*:23, 1979.

283. Nash, G., and Ross, J. S. Herpetic esophagitis: a common cause of esophageal ulceration. Human Pathol. *5*:339, 1974.
284. Jacobs, E. Anal infections caused by herpes simplex virus. Dis. Colon Rectum *19*:151, 1976.
285. Goldmeier, D. Proctitis and herpes simplex virus in homosexual men. Br. J. Vener. Dis. *56*:111, 1980.
286. Corey, L., and Spear, P. G. Infections with herpes simplex viruses. N. Engl. J. Med. *314*:686 and *314*:749, 1986.
287. Rompalo, A. M., Mertz, G. J., Mkrtichian, E. E., Price, C. B., Stamm, W. E., and Corey, L. Oral acyclovir versus placebo for treatment of herpes simplex proctitis in homosexual men. Abstracts of the Sixth International Meeting of the International Society for STD Research, Brighton, England, July 31–August 2, 1985.
288. Keane, J. T., Malkinson, F. D., Bryant, J., and Levin, S. Herpesvirus hominis hepatitis and disseminated intravascular coagulation: occurrence in an adult with pemphigus vulgaris. Arch. Intern. Med. *136*:1312, 1976.
289. Corey, L., and Holmes, K. K. Sexual transmission of hepatitis A in homosexual men: incidence and mechanism. N. Engl. J. Med. *302*:435, 1980.
290. Villarejos, V. M., Visona, K. A., Gutierrez, D. A., and Rodriguez, A. A. Role of saliva, urine and feces in the transmission of type B hepatitis. N. Engl. J. Med. *291*:1375, 1974.
291. Wright, R. A. Hepatitis B and the HB_sAG carrier. JAMA *232*:717, 1975.
292. Alter, M. J., Ahtone, J., Weisfuse, I., Starko, K., Vacalis, T. D., and Maynard, J. E. Hepatis B virus transmission between heterosexuals. JAMA *256*:1307, 1986.
293. Ellis, W. R., Murray-Lyon, I. M., Coleman, J. C., Evans, B. A., Fluker, J. L., Bull, J., Keeling, P. W. N., Simmons, P. D., Banatvala, J. E., Willcox, J. R., and Thompson, R. P. H. Liver disease among homosexual males. Lancet *1*:903, 1979.
294. Murphy, B. L., Schreeder, M. T., Maynard, J. E., Hadler, S. C., and Sheller, M. J. Serological testing for hepatitis B in male homosexuals: special emphasis on hepatitis B e antigen and antibody by radioimmunoassay. J. Clin. Microbiol. *11*:301, 1980.
295. Shah, N., Ostrow, D., Altman, N., and Baker, A. L. Evolution of acute hepatitis B in homosexual men to chronic hepatitis B: prospective study of placebo recipients in a hepatitis B vaccine trial. Arch. Intern. Med. *145*:881, 1985.
296. Novick, D. M., Lok, A. S. F., and Thomas, H. C. Diminished responsiveness of homosexual men to antiviral therapy for HBsAg-positive chronic liver disease. J. Hepatol. *1*:29, 1984.
297. Carr, G., and William, D. C. Anal warts in a population of gay men in New York City. Sex. Transm. Dis. *4*:56, 1977.
298. Oriel, J. D. Genital warts. Sex. Transm. Dis. *4*:153, 1977.
299. Thomson, J. P. S., and Grace, R. H. The treatment of perianal and anal condylomata acuminata: a new operative technique. J. Roy. Soc. Med. *71*:180, 1978.
300. Abcarian, H., and Sharon, N. The effectiveness of immunotherapy in the treatment of anal condyloma acuminatum. J. Surg. Res. *22*:231, 1977.
301. Drew, W. L., Mintz, L., Miner, R. C., Sands, M., and Ketterer, B. Prevalence of cytomegalovirus infection in homosexual men. J. Infect. Dis. *143*:188, 1981.
302. Marino, A. W. M., and Mancini, H. W. N. Anal eroticism. Surg. Clin. North Am. *58*:513, 1978.
303. Sohn, N., Weinstein, M. A., and Gonchar, J. Social injuries of the rectum. Am. J. Surg. *134*:611, 1977.
304. Abcarian, H., and Lowe, R. Colon and rectal trauma. Surg. Clin. North Am. *58*:519, 1978.
305. Sohn, N., and Robilotti, J. G. The gay bowel syndrome, a review of colonic and rectal conditions in 200 male homosexuals. Am. J. Gastroenterol. *67*:478, 1977.
306. Barone, J. E., Sohn, N., and Nealon, T. F. Perforations and foreign bodies of the rectum: report of 28 cases. Ann. Surg. *184*:601, 1977.
307. Cooper, H. S., Patchefsky, A. S., and Marks, G. Cloacogenic carcinoma of the anorectum in homosexual men: an observation of four cases. Dis. Colon Rectum *22*:557, 1979.
308. Eftaiha, M., Hambrick, E., and Abcarian, H. Principles of management of colorectal foreign bodies. Arch. Surg. *112*:691, 1977.
309. Owen, W. F. Sexually transmitted diseases and traumatic problems in homosexual men. Ann. Intern. Med. *92*:805, 1980.
310. Fisher, A. A., and Brancaccio, R. R. Allergic contact sensitivity to propylene glycol in a lubricant jelly. Arch. Dermatol. *115*:1451, 1979.
311. Quinn, T. C., and Holmes, K. K. Proctitis, proctocolitis, and enteritis in homosexual men. *In* Holmes, K. K., Måardh, P. -A., Sparling, P. F., and Wiesner, P. J. (eds.). Sexually Transmitted Diseases. New York, McGraw-Hill, 1984.
312. Budhraja, M., Levendoglu, H., Kocka, F., Mangkornkanok, M., and Sherer, R. Duodenal mucosal T cell subpopulation and bacterial cultures in acquired immune deficiency syndrome. Am. J. Gastroenterol. *82*:427, 1987.
313. Lake-Bakaar, G., Beidas, S., El-Sakir, R., Iyer, S., and Straus, E. Impaired gastric acid secretion in AIDS. Gastroenterology *92*:1488, 1987.
314. Armstrong, D. Opportunistic infections in the acquired immune deficiency syndrome. Seminars in Oncology *14*(Suppl. 3):40, 1987.
315. Terada, S., Reddy, K. R., Jeffers, L. J., Cali, A., and Schiff, E. R. Microsporidian hepatitis in the acquired immunodeficiency syndrome. Ann. Intern. Med. *107*:61, 1987.

66

Tropical Sprue

FREDERICK A. KLIPSTEIN

Following colonization of India and Southeast Asia by the European maritime powers in the late 1700s, many European expatriates became afflicted with a hitherto unrecognized malady characterized by chronic diarrhea followed by anorexia and weight loss, and eventually glossitis, profound weakness, and emaciation.[1] Initially recognized by British military physicians, who referred to it as the white flux, diarrhea alba, or chronic diarrhea of the tropics, the disorder was subsequently described among the Dutch in Java (1837), the French in Indochina (1877), and Europeans in China (1880). By the time Manson anglicized the Dutch term *Indische sprouw* to tropical sprue (1880), it was realized that the same syndrome was afflicting expatriates in all of these locations. Only somewhat later did it become apparent that tropical sprue is not confined to Asia, when, following the Spanish-American War, it was seen among American expatriates in the Philippines (1902) and Puerto Rico (1913). Although the overall geographic distribution and characteristics of tropical sprue were thus well known early in the present century, it has only recently become generally appreciated that, rather than being a disorder that affects primarily expatriates in the tropics, sprue occurs equally often among the indigenous populations of these areas.

DEFINITION

Advancing knowledge regarding the natural history and pathophysiology of tropical sprue has resulted in modifications of its definition. It was initially defined solely on the basis of its clinical characteristics; this undoubtedly led to the inclusion of other disorders as well as rather meaningless subclassifications, such as "incomplete sprue" for cases lacking all the usual manifestations. Following recognition of the megaloblastic nature of the anemia in sprue in the early 1920s, the presence of this abnormality was regarded by many as a sine qua non for its diagnosis. However, studies conducted among large groups of European expatriates in India during the Second World War and then in Puerto Rico showed that anemia is the consequence of prolonged malabsorption and hence present only in chronic, advanced disease.[2, 3] The application of techniques developed during the next two decades, which permitted precise evaluation of small bowel structure and function, led to the proposal in 1970 that tropical sprue be considered a syndrome that is characterized by jejunal structural abnormalities accompanied by malabsorption of two distinct substances.[4] Subsequently, however, it has become apparent that this definition would encompass significant proportions both of the indigenous population and of expatriates living in rural tropical areas for more than six months who are found to have subclinical malabsorption.[5–7]

The definition of tropical sprue, therefore, must take into consideration the following features that distinguish it from the intestinal abnormalities present among many relatively asymptomatic residents of the tropics. (1) Most persons with tropical sprue have gastrointestinal symptoms; those with subclinical malabsorption usually do not. (2) The abnormalities of intestinal structure and function in tropical sprue get relentlessly worse until specific therapy is instituted, whereas those in subclinical malabsorption appear to vary spontaneously over time, either improving or worsening. (3) The intestinal malabsorption in tropical sprue consistently becomes so severe that it eventually results in the development of nutritional deficiencies, whereas the milder defects in subclinical malabsorption result in deficiencies only among those whose dietary intake is marginal or inadequate. (4) The intestinal abnormalities of subclinical malabsorption eventually spontaneously revert to normal when expatriates or native residents move to a temperate zone,[8, 9] but those of tropical sprue do so only rarely, if ever.[10–12] (5) The intestinal abnormalities in sprue nearly always improve with specific therapy with folic acid and/or tetracycline, whereas this response is unusual in persons with subclinical malabsorption.[13]

Pending clarification of its etiology, a workable definition of tropical sprue is a chronic disorder acquired in endemic tropical areas that is characterized by abnormalities of small bowel structure and function that become progressively more severe, eventually lead to the development of and manifestations of nutritional deficiencies, and are either ameliorated or cured by treatment with folic acid and/ tetracycline.

OCCURRENCE

Knowledge is limited concerning the location of those tropical areas where sprue is endemic and concerning its prevalence. Reasons for this include failure to consider the disorder and unavailability of the necessary diagnostic techniques. The presence of sprue among native populations in a number of locations, such as Haiti[14] and Rhodesia,[15] was established only when research workers undertook the studies necessary to identify it.

Tropical sprue usually involves isolated cases, but it can occur in epidemic form among large groups of expatriates or native residents as a sequela of outbreaks of acute diarrheal disease.[16, 17] It is more common among adults than children. It can develop among expatriates within a week after arrival in the tropics but more commonly occurs only after residence there for two or more years.[10, 11] Sprue has a peak seasonal incidence among both indigenous and expatriate populations that varies in different geographic areas but consistently is unrelated to the rainy season.[18] Occasionally, it does not become overtly symptomatic until months or years after expatriates or native residents have moved to a temperate climate.[11]

Tropical sprue has a scattered distribution in the West Indies (Fig. 66–1): It is endemic in Puerto Rico, Cuba, and Hispaniola (the Dominican Republic and Haiti), but it has not been seen in Jamaica; whether it occurs on any of the other islands is unknown. Elsewhere in the Western Hemisphere, the disease is endemic in the northern part of South America, but its prevalence in Central America or Mexico is uncertain. Tropical sprue is common in the Indian subcontinent[19] and elsewhere in Asia: in Sri Lanka, Burma, Malaya, Vietnam, Singapore, Hong Kong, Borneo, Indonesia, and the Philippines. It was common among European expatriates living in the southern provinces of China before the Second World War, but no information is available concerning whether it exists there now. Long thought to be either rare or nonexistent in Africa, the occurrence of the disease among native populations living in the central and southern parts of this continent (Nigeria, Zimbabwe, and South Africa) is now well established.[15] Tropical sprue is rare among the indigenous population of the Middle East; it has been described among persons who visited there.[20]

There is no evidence that tropical sprue occurs among persons who have never visited or lived in endemic areas of the tropics. It was described among native residents of the southern part of the continental United States during the early 1900s,[21] but the diagnostic techniques necessary to differentiate tropical sprue from other chronic intestinal disorders were not then available and subsequently the disorder has not been recognized there. Individuals have been seen in England who, usually after a summer visit to the continent, complained of chronic diarrhea, anorexia, and weight loss and were found to have malabsorption in the absence of detectable enteric pathogens.[22] This was considered to be postinfectious malabsorption, since spontaneous recovery occurred in most within several weeks.

Most information regarding the prevalence of tropical sprue is derived from observations among military personnel serving in the tropics. During the Second World War, it was a major cause of morbidity among British troops serving in India and Burma,[23] but rare among American forces operating in the Pacific. Thereafter, it was commonplace among British troops serving in Malaya and Hong Kong[24] and over a one-year period afflicted as many as 8 per cent of one military compound of North Americans stationed in Puerto Rico.[10] Recurrent widespread annual attacks of acute enteritis have been followed by a high prevalence of tropical

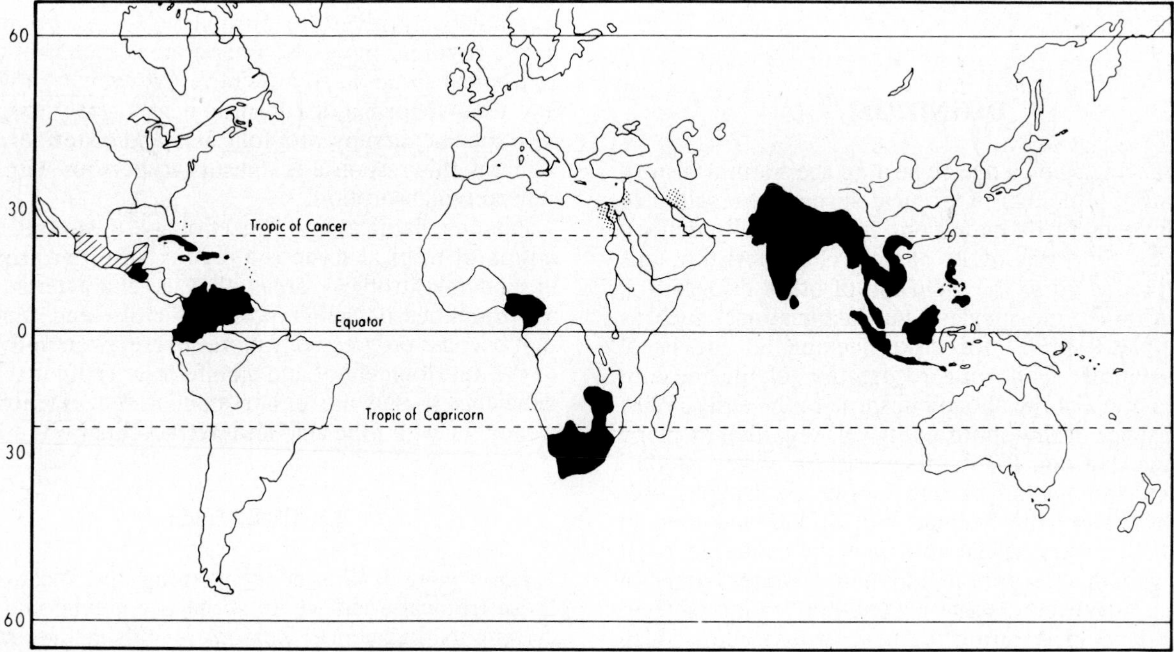

Figure 66–1. Geographic distribution of tropical sprue. *Black* indicates areas where sprue occurs; *cross hatching,* areas where a disorder resembling sprue occurs; and *stippling,* areas where mostly subclinical malabsorption is present. (From Klipstein, F. A. Tropical sprue. *In* Bockus, H. L. (ed.). Gastroenterology. Ed. 3. Philadelphia, W. B. Saunders Company, 1976. Used by permission.)

sprue among American military personnel serving at Clark Air Force Base in the Philippines.[16] Tropical sprue is also common among European expatriates traveling overland in Asia;[12] in contrast, its prevalence among American forces in Vietnam was lower than that experienced previously by military personnel serving in Asia,[25] and the disorder occurs infrequently among Peace Corps volunteers working in tropical areas. The frequent early usage of antibiotics for acute diarrheal disorders probably accounts for the low prevalence among the latter two groups.

ETIOLOGY

The factors responsible for the development of tropical sprue remain to be defined clearly. Nutritional deficiencies of folate, vitamin B_{12}, or protein, which can cause small bowel abnormalities under certain circumstances, do not appear to play a primary role in the pathogenesis of this disease, which often develops in well-nourished individuals. On the other hand, considerable evidence favors the concept that tropical sprue is an infectious disease caused by persistent, chronic intestinal contamination with one or more enteric pathogens.

In most instances, either in isolated individual cases or in epidemic outbreaks, tropical sprue occurs as the sequela to an episode of acute diarrhea for which no enteric pathogen can be identified. In epidemic outbreaks in South Indian villages, the acute diarrhea often involves multiple persons within the same household, with evidence of propagation within families; about one half of affected persons develop chronic diarrhea, which remits spontaneously within three months of onset in most but persists in about 10 per cent to develop into overtly recognizable tropical sprue.[17] In similar annual seasonal epidemics of acute diarrhea among American military personnel in the Philippines, many affected persons develop chronic diarrhea with abnormalities of intestinal structure and function; this spontaneously resolves in some but persists in others to become overt tropical sprue, requiring treatment with folic acid and/or tetracycline.[16]

Viral, fungal, or algal pathogens have not been isolated from persons with tropical sprue, but most individuals with this disorder (including native residents of the West Indies and India and expatriates traveling in Asia) have bacterial contamination of the small bowel, usually with strains of *Klebsiella pneumoniae* or, less often, of *Escherichia coli* or *Enterobacter cloacae*.[26–28] The bacterial overgrowth is clearly not just the result of constant exposure to a contaminated environment, since (1) most healthy native residents of the tropics are not found to harbor coliform bacteria within their proximal small bowel,[26, 27] although some in southern India apparently do;[29] (2) the bacterial population in individual cases of tropical sprue is not heterogeneous, including anaerobic bacteria as in the blind loop syndrome, but consists of either a single or several species, serotypes, and biotypes of coliform bacteria;[27] and (3) the jejunal contamination persists in expatriates with sprue following their return to a temperate climate[28] (see pp. 1289–1297).

The *Klebsiella* and other coliform bacteria isolated from cases of tropical sprue are not invasive, when tested either by the Sereny test or instillation into ligated intestinal loops, but they differ from the coliform contaminants in the blind loop syndrome in that they produce toxins.[30] Most strains produce a large or low molecular weight toxin, either singly or together, both of which can cause water and electrolyte secretion and impaired absorption of xylose when perfused in vivo through the ileum,[30, 31] and structural abnormalities with fluid secretion when instilled into ligated ileal loops of experimental animals.[27, 31] These toxins have not been purified, and it remains to be determined whether they are enterotoxins or cytotoxins; it is known that they are dissimilar from the heat-labile (LT) and heat-stable (ST) enterotoxins produced by enterotoxigenic strains of *Escherichia coli* (ETEC), which just cause acute diarrhea.

These observations have led to the proposal that chronic contamination of the small bowel by toxigenic strains of coliform bacteria is responsible for the small bowel abnormalities in tropical sprue. This would account for the progressive nature of the intestinal abnormalities, due to continued exposure to the toxins, and for the fact that the abnormalities are cured when the bacteria are eradicated by antimicrobial therapy. By contrast, the variable and milder intestinal abnormalities present in persons with subclinical malabsorption are thought to result from repeated self-limited episodes of small bowel infection by a variety of enteric pathogens, including bacteria and viruses. This concept does not explain the relative rarity of sprue among children or its varied geographic distribution. Further, it remains uncertain whether tropical sprue is caused in some patients (or geographic areas) by other, still unidentified pathogenic agents, such as a virus;[32] the low prevalence of coliform contamination among patients with this disorder examined in South India[29] and South Africa[33] suggests that such may be the case in these locations.

Acute infectious diarrhea due to a variety of infectious enteric pathogens can be associated with transient jejunal overgrowth by coliform bacteria;[34] it seems probable, but remains to be proved, that this is the initiating event responsible for persistent chronic small bowel contamination by coliforms in tropical sprue. The factors responsible for failure to clear these organisms from the small bowel in sprue are unknown. No defect in the immunologic protective systems responsible for ridding the gut of enteric pathogens has been found.[35] There is suggestive evidence that the coliforms involved may be unusually adherent to the intestinal mucosa but no specific mechanism for this has been identified.[36] Small bowel transit time is delayed in tropical sprue,[37] and this has been attributed by one group to excess levels of the tropic hormone enteroglucagon.[38] Certain epidemiologic aspects of tropical sprue (its geographic distribution in the West Indies, its attack rate among different groups of expatriates whose dietary intake of lipids varies qualitatively, and its seasonal incidence in Puerto Rico), together with the results of in vitro studies,[39] have led to the suggestion that excess dietary intake of long-chain unsaturated fatty acids, particularly linoleic acid, abets coliform colonization by altering the gastrointestinal ecosystem responsible for resistance to colonization by alien enteric organisms.[18]

The beneficial effect of treatment with folic acid (or with vitamin B_{12}) on the intestinal abnormalities indicates that folate deficiency plays a role in perpetuating the intestinal lesion in tropical sprue. This unique role of folate deficiency in sprue may perhaps be explained by its concurrence with the intraluminal elaboration of ethanol within the small bowel by the contaminating coliform bacteria.[27] Folate deficiency due exclusively to inadequate dietary intake does not cause mucosal abnormalities in humans, but it does when combined with excessive ethanol intake.[40] It is noteworthy that although treatment with folic acid usually improves the intestinal abnormalities, it only rarely results in complete cure among residents of the tropics;[41] eradication of the coliform bacteria by antimicrobial therapy is necessary to achieve this.[26, 28]

NATURAL HISTORY

The natural history of tropical sprue has been delineated principally by investigations conducted among expatriates who developed the disorder in isolated cases[24] or in epidemic outbreaks.[16] Most expatriates can pinpoint the onset of the disease, which usually consists of an acute episode of watery, nonbloody diarrhea that is sometimes accompanied by malaise, fever, and weakness. After about a week, these acute symptoms resolve into a milder form of chronic diarrhea often associated with abdominal cramps and borborygmi as well as excessive flatus. Somewhat later, most persons become intolerant to milk because of the development of lactase deficiency and some become intolerant to alcohol. Jejunal morphologic appearance either remains normal or is slightly deranged during the first several weeks of illness; thereafter, structural abnormalities become progressively more severe and are associated with the development of malabsorption. Within two to three months, jejunal malabsorption results in the development of mild folate deficiency; this causes *anorexia* resulting in decreased food intake which, coupled with *malabsorption*, is responsible for the onset of *weight loss*.[42] After a variable period of time, usually about six months, severe depletion of tissue folate stores coupled with the development of vitamin B_{12} deficiency results in *glossitis* and symptoms attributable to a *megaloblastic anemia;* clinical manifestations of other nutritional deficiencies, such as edema due to *hypoalbuminemia,* may also become apparent at this time. In about 10 per cent of patients, malabsorption results in deficiencies in the absence of diarrhea (see pp. 263–282).

The severity and rapidity with which nutritional deficiencies develop are related to nutritional reserves prior to the onset of illness and the duration and severity of the malabsorption. Deficiencies usually are milder and develop later in expatriates than in poorly nourished indigenous populations.

PHYSICAL EXAMINATION

Abnormal physical findings during the early stages of tropical sprue are usually confined to hyperactive bowel sounds. Subsequently, there may be evidence of recent *weight loss, pallor,* and *glossitis,* and, in some elderly persons who develop severe anemia, cardiac decompensation. Abnormal physical findings are often more prominent among native residents who were initially marginally or poorly nourished; these can include *night blindness, stomatitis, hyperpigmentation, emaciation,* and *edema.* Neurologic manifestations of vitamin B_{12} deficiency are unusual in tropical sprue and, if present, are usually confined to mild changes of proximal muscle weakness or peripheral neuropathy.

LABORATORY ABNORMALITIES

Deficiencies. The *megaloblastic anemia* of advanced tropical sprue is usually due to combined deficiencies of folate and vitamin B_{12}, although there is some variation among different populations; among Haitians, for example, folate deficiency is rare.[14] Increased requirement for folate results in more rapid and severe deficiency in women who develop sprue during pregnancy or the puerperium. Serum concentrations of carotene, vitamin A, cholesterol, calcium, and albumin are usually reduced and deficiencies of magnesium and alpha-tocopherol may develop. Tropical sprue differs from celiac disease in that serum calcium values only rarely fall to levels that produce tetany; osteomalacia is unusual; and marked elevation of the prothrombin time is uncommon (see pp. 1141–1145).

Intestinal Function. Most persons with tropical sprue have net secretion of water, sodium, and chloride into the jejunum and ileum.[43] Defective absorption of water and electrolytes also occurs in the colon;[44] this has been attributed to inhibition of ATPase activity by excessive amounts of fecal free fatty acids.[45]

Xylose, fat, and vitamin B_{12} are the most commonly used substances to test absorptive capacity. *Xylose* absorption of a 25 gm oral dose is always reduced. *Steatorrhea* is found in from 50 to 90 per cent of cases in various series; it is less common among expatriates. The basic defect is in transport through the mucosa rather than abnormal intraluminal events such as occur in the blind loop syndrome. Bile salts are not deconjugated by the contaminating coliform bacteria.[46] The re-esterification of fatty acids to triglycerides is impaired,[19] and histochemical studies show accumulation of lipid particles within or immediately subjacent to the enterocytes.[47] *Vitamin B_{12} malabsorption* is present in nearly all cases; it is not corrected by the addition of intrinsic factor. Prompt reversal to normal absorption following antibiotic therapy incriminates bacterial uptake as the causal factor in some, whereas delayed improvement in others implies impaired ileal transport as the principal abnormality.[48]

The absorption of multiple other substances is usually also impaired. (1) *Carbohydrate.* Lactase levels of the jejunal brush border and lactose tolerance tests are uniformly reduced; sucrose levels and absorption are reduced in about one third of cases. The glucose tolerance test is subnormal in about 50 per cent. (2) *Folate.* Both impaired hydrolysis of dietary polyglutamate folate by the brush border and reduced transport through the enterocyte of monoglutamate folate contribute to folate malabsorption, which is present in nearly all cases.[49] In contrast to their uptake of vitamin B_{12}, the coliform bacteria produce folate.[50] (3) *Calcium.* The absorption of calcium is usually reduced, owing principally to impaired absorption and deficiency of vitamin D. (4) *Protein.* Both excessive protein loss into the gut (protein-losing enteropathy) and impaired absorption of amino acids and dipeptides contribute to the development of protein deficiency.[51, 52] (5) *Vitamin A.* Tolerance tests show reduced absorption in most patients.

RADIOLOGIC EXAMINATION

Radiologic abnormalities of the small bowel consisting of thickening and coarsening of the mucosal folds, flocculation and segmentation of the barium meal, and dilation of the intestinal diameter are present in about three quarters of cases within two to three months after the onset of the disorder.[24] Analysis of large groups of patients has shown a general correlation between the severity of radiologic changes and morphologic and functional abnormalities, but no good correlation with any specific test of function.[53] The radiologic abnormalities are not specific for sprue and are of diagnostic value only by virtue of indicating the presence of diffuse small bowel disease and excluding the presence of other, specific chronic bowel disorders.

MORPHOLOGY

Oral. Epithelial cells of the buccal mucosa commonly have enlarged nuclei, which, unlike those in pernicious anemia, often persist along with megalocytic changes present in jejunal crypt cells after replacement therapy with folic acid or vitamin B_{12}.

Stomach. Superficial or, less often, complete atrophic gastritis is common, frequently leading to reduced gastric acidity or, less commonly, to complete achlorhydria and absent intrinsic factor secretion.

Small Bowel. Abnormalities are more prominent in the jejunum than in the ileum during the early phase of tropical sprue, but thereafter the entire small bowel is equally affected.

Gross Abnormalities. When visualized under the dissecting microscope, the villi usually appear to be thickened and coalesced to form leaves, which in some instances fuse to give the more abnormal appearance of ridges or convolutions; the flat appearance that is characteristic of celiac disease is extremely unusual. There is usually a correlation between the severity of the gross and histologic abnormalities in untreated patients.

Histology. The changes consist of lengthening of crypt area, broadening and shortening of the villi, epithelial cell changes, and infiltration by chronic inflammatory cells (plasma cells, lymphocytes, eosinophils, and histiocytes) (Fig. 66–2). Abnormalities of the surface epithelium are usually related to the severity of villus structural changes. Electron microscopy shows distortion and grouping of the microvilli, fragmentation of the terminal web, increased lysosomes, and mitochondrial changes in the enterocytes.[19, 54] Enzymatic activity, as detected by histochemical techniques, is usually reduced but not absent; the degree of decrease is usually related to the severity of abnormality of enterocyte structure.[47] In the crypts, cell nuclei show megalocytic changes; argentaffin cells are increased, but Paneth cells are normal in number. The basement membrane usually appears thickened, staining as collagen on light microscopy;[47] the basal lamella itself is normal when visualized by electron microscopy, but subjacent to it is a dense material of unknown composition.[54]

Lipid stain with oil-red-O of biopsy specimens from most fasting patients with tropical sprue shows an accumulation of lipid droplets subjacent to the surface epithelium (Color Fig. 66–3*C*, p. xli); on electron microscopy, the lipid appears as large discrete membrane-bound droplets within the thickened collagenous material beneath the basement membrane.[19, 54] This location differs from that present in normal subjects, in whom the lipid droplets are located principally in lymphatic channels within the lower half of the lamina propria (Color Fig. 66–3*A*, p. xli) and from that in patients with untreated celiac disease, where lipid accumulates principally within the enterocyte (Color Fig. 66–3*B*, p. xli). Although this abnormal pattern of lipid accumulation is characteristically present in sprue, it cannot be considered pathognomonic since it is occasionally observed in other small bowel disorders. In persons with tropical sprue, treatment with folic acid and/or tetracycline restores the lipid distribution to normal within several weeks.[55]

DIFFERENTIAL DIAGNOSIS

Tropical sprue should be considered in any person, living in or returned from an endemic tropical area, who develops chronic diarrhea and is found to have malabsorption. In evaluating such patients, disorders of the small bowel that are seen most often in temperate climates must be excluded. This can usually be done by radiologic examination of the small bowel and

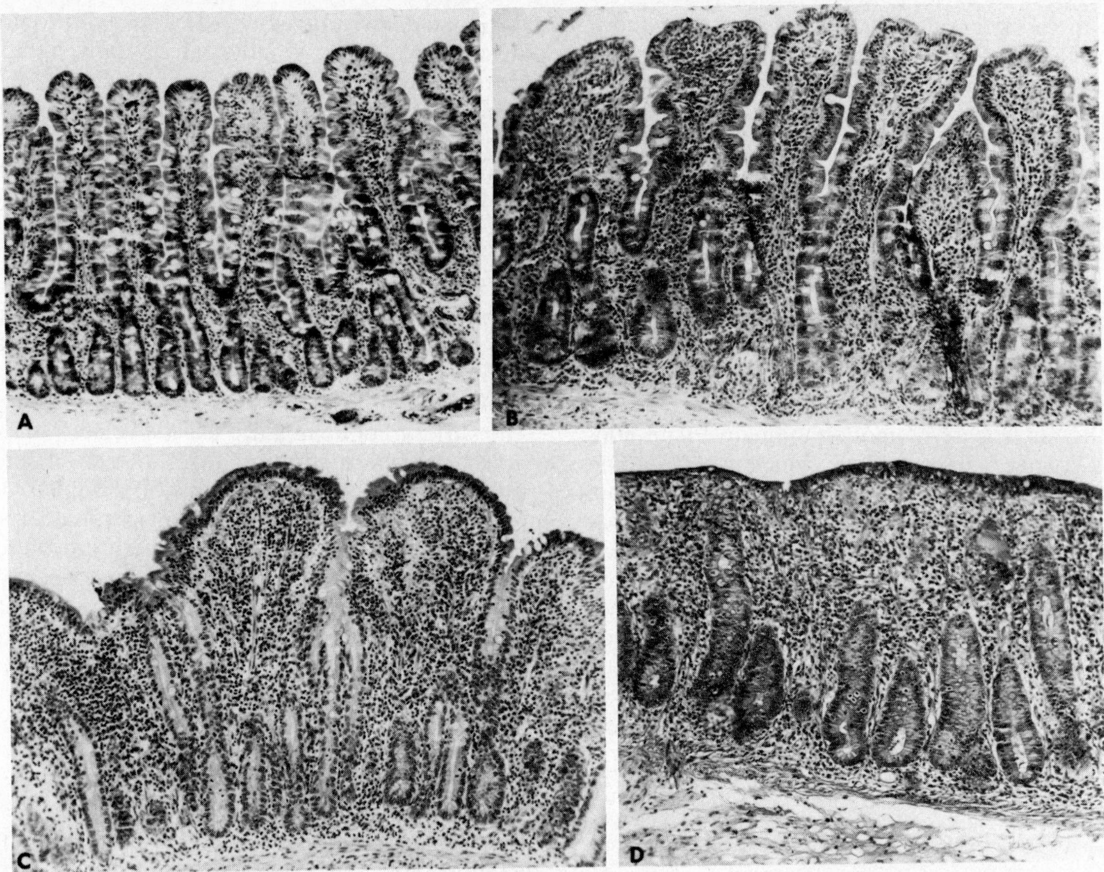

Figure 66–2. Jejunal morphology in tropical sprue. *A*, Normal control. *B*, Tropical sprue with moderate (2+) abnormalities. *C*, Tropical sprue with severe (3+) abnormalities. *D*, Tropical sprue with a flat mucosa (4+ abnormalities). (From Klipstein, F. A. Tropical sprue. *In* Bockus, H. L. (ed.). Gastroenterology. Ed. 3. Philadelphia, W. B. Saunders Company, 1976. Used by permission.)

by jejunal biopsy. In addition, infestation by those parasites that can cause chronic diarrhea and malabsorption must be excluded: *Giardia lamblia, Strongyloides stercoralis, Coccidia isospora, Capillaria philippinensis* (present only in the Philippines), and the fluke *Metagonimus yokogawai* (pp. 1153–1191). None of these parasites causes deficiency of folate or vitamin B_{12}, which is the hallmark of advanced tropical sprue.

The differential diagnosis varies with the circumstance. Most expatriates seek medical attention within several weeks to months after onset of the disease, thus presenting with chronic diarrhea, malabsorption, and sometimes weight loss but few, if any, deficiencies. Here the differential diagnosis usually rests between tropical sprue and giardiasis, which can lead to similar clinical and intestinal abnormalities.[56] Favoring the diagnosis of tropical sprue would be the presence of a subnormal serum folate concentration and accumulation of lipid subjacent to the surface epithelium in the jejunal biopsy, which do not occur in giardiasis. Culture of jejunal aspirates is not particularly helpful in differential diagnosis, since bacterial contamination of the jejunum by *Klebsiella* or other coliforms has been found in returned expatriates who have either sprue or giardiasis[28, 57] (raising the possibility that in this circumstance the mucosal abnormalities in giardiasis may be caused by both the parasite and these bacteria). *Giardia* are notoriously difficult to detect in stool samples but can be found more readily by examination of jejunal aspirates and mucosal imprints. If none of these procedures establishes a diagnosis, then the only recourse is to determine the effect of specific therapy, metronidazole (Flagyl) or quinacrine (Atabrine) (either singly or sequentially) for giardiasis, or folic acid and/or tetracycline for tropical sprue.

The diagnosis of tropical sprue does not usually pose any difficulty among well-nourished native residents who can give an articulate history. These individuals usually present with advanced sprue and thus have deficiencies, including megaloblastic anemia, as well as multiple abnormalities of intestinal structure and absorption that are usually more severe than those of the general population (Table 66–1). The diagnosis is confirmed by demonstrating improvement after treatment with folic acid and/or tetracycline. It is among those indigenous populations who are poorly nourished (often with hypoalbuminemia), who have a high prevalence of moderate to severe intestinal abnormalities, and who cannot give a clear history regarding onset of symptoms that the diagnosis of tropical sprue is often unclear. In this circumstance, such as in Haiti,[14] it is sometimes difficult to make a clear-cut distinction between those with tropical sprue and those whose deficiencies and intestinal abnormalities may be due to

Table 66–1. CLINICAL AND LABORATORY ABNORMALITIES AMONG NATIVE RESIDENTS OF PUERTO RICO

	Tropical Sprue* (%)	**General Population†** (%)
Clinical		
Diarrhea	90	9
Weight loss	96	0
Glossitis	27	0
Edema	14	0
Deficiencies		
Anemia‡	95	0
Folate	80	6
Vitamin B_{12}	86	1
Cholesterol	70	7
Albumin	50	4
Malabsorption		
Xylose	100	24
Fat	85	4
Vitamin B_{12}	96	28
Jejunal morphology		
Normal	0	18
Mild (1 +)	2	52
Moderate (2 +)	40	26
Severe (3 +)	52	4
Flat (4 +)	8	0

*Fifty-nine patients (Klipstein, F. A., and Corcino, J. J., unpublished observations).
†Ninety-six subjects.[7]
‡Megaloblastic anemia.

inadequate protein intake. Treatment with folic acid and/or tetracycline usually improves the intestinal abnormalities in those thought to have sprue and occasionally achieves this in malnourished persons as well.[13] Treatment with hospitalization and a high-protein diet has also resulted in improved intestinal structure and function in some Colombians who presented with severe protein deficiency and malabsorption.[58]

TREATMENT

The prognosis for persons with tropical sprue was bleak prior to the advent of specific therapy. The mortality rate was high among those who remained in the tropics (although spontaneous remissions sometimes occurred), and the disease often caused chronic disability among those who returned to a temperate climate.[11] The outlook was drastically altered by the introduction of liver extract (1931), folic acid (1946), and antimicrobials (1960's) for treatment. The beneficial effects of folic acid (or vitamin B_{12}) and the antimicrobials differ in persons with *chronic* sprue: Folic acid results in prompt clinical improvement by correcting the symptoms due to vitamin deficiencies but yields only marginal improvement of the intestinal lesion;[41] antimicrobials eradicate the coliform bacteria, thus producing improvement in the intestinal abnormalities and eventual correction of the vitamin deficiencies as a consequence of improved absorption.[28, 55]

Folic Acid. Treatment with pharmacologic doses of folic acid (or of vitamin B_{12}) uniformly results in a prompt hematologic remission of the megaloblastic anemia, disappearance of glossitis, and return of appetite, which results in the onset of weight gain even prior to improvement in absorption.[42] This is usually then followed by a decrease in gastrointestinal symptoms. Improvement in jejunal structural abnormalities, particularly in the crypts, is evident within three to six days in those who had marked abnormalities but may be delayed for up to several weeks in those who had mild abnormalities.[59] The absorption of xylose is often improved, but steatorrhea and malabsorption of vitamin B_{12} usually persist.[41] Mucosal activities of sucrase and maltase increase rapidly; lactase levels often remain low for months or years, but, despite this, lactose tolerance tests usually improve.

The results of treatment with folic acid appear to depend on the chronicity of the intestinal lesion. Treatment can be curative in those who have had the disease for only a few months (as is usually the case in expatriates), but, even in this circumstance, intestinal structure and function may not revert to normal until after one to two years of therapy.[10, 24] In contrast, even extended treatment of chronic disease among native residents often fails to correct completely the intestinal abnormalities and symptoms often persist.[41]

Antimicrobials. The British found that treatment with sulfaguanidine alleviated or halted the symptoms of tropical sprue among military personnel in India and Burma during the Second World War.[23] Subsequent studies in Puerto Rico showed that antimicrobial therapy, if extended for a sufficient period of time, can cure the intestinal lesion of sprue.[60, 61] Tetracycline and nonabsorbable sulfonamides are equally effective; lincomycin was reported effective in two of four patients treated; erythromycin is ineffective; and the value of other antimicrobial agents has not been evaluated. Short-term therapy for about one month results in improved jejunal morphologic appearance with eventual return of absorption to normal in most expatriates treated either in the tropics or after return to a temperate climate.[10, 11, 24] Such is usually not the case among native residents treated in the tropics; their disease is more chronic, and prolonged treatment for up to six months is often necessary.[19, 60–62]

When antibiotic therapy is used alone, water and electrolyte secretion return to normal and gastrointestinal symptoms improve within one to three weeks. During this period, villus architecture improves, enzyme activity in the brush border of the surface epithelium increases, xylose absorption improves, and fecal fat values fall.[55] Vitamin B_{12} absorption returns to normal within 10 days in some, but only after weeks or months in others. Striking clinical improvement (reversal of glossitis, return of appetite, gain of weight, and correction of megaloblastic anemia) is delayed, however, until vitamin stores are repleted as a result of improved absorption.[42, 55] The first vitamin to be repleted in Puerto Ricans treated in New York City was folate, whereas in those treated in Puerto Rico it was vitamin B_{12}.[55, 63]

Optimal Therapy. Combined therapy with folic acid and tetracycline (or a sulfonamide) has the advantage of resulting in both prompt clinical improvement and eventual healing of the intestinal lesion. The usual dose of folic acid is 5 mg by mouth per day and of tetracycline, 250 mg by mouth four times a day. In those patients in whom there is vitamin B_{12} deficiency (or when serum levels cannot be obtained), treatment should include 1000 μg of this vitamin given parenterally for several days to replete tissue stores and 1000 μg intramuscularly monthly thereafter. Other forms of treatment, such as modification of diet, are usually unnecessary. Treatment should be continued for several months or until evidence is obtained that intestinal function has returned to normal.

Prognosis. The prognosis for complete and permanent healing of the intestinal lesion is excellent among expatriates treated either in the tropics or after their return to a temperate climate. Such is also usually the case among native residents of the tropics who receive treatment after moving to a temperate climate.[11] On the other hand, the limited information available indicates that recurrences can happen among residents treated in the tropics: Significant malabsorption was detected in one half of a group of Puerto Ricans examined five years after their intestinal abnormalities had been healed by antibiotic therapy.[64]

Unlike celiac disease, diffuse lymphoma of the small bowel does not appear to occur as a consequence of tropical sprue.

References

1. O'Brien, W. Historical survey of tropical sprue affecting Europeans in South-East Asia. *In* Tropical Sprue and Megaloblastic Anaemia. London, Churchill Livingstone, 1971, pp. 13–24.
2. Stefanini, M. Clinical features and pathogenesis of tropical sprue: Observations on a series of cases among Italian prisoners of war in India. Medicine *27*:379, 1948.
3. Gardner, F. H. Tropical sprue. N. Engl. J. Med. *258*:791, 835, 1958.
4. Klipstein, F. A., and Baker, S. J. Regarding the definition of tropical sprue. Gastroenterology *58*:717, 1970.
5. Baker, S. J. Subclinical intestinal malabsorption in developing countries. Bull. WHO *54*:485, 1976.
6. Lindenbaum, J., Kent, T. H., and Sprinz, H. Malabsorption and jejunitis in American Peace Corps volunteers in Pakistan. Ann. Intern. Med. *65*:1201, 1966.
7. Klipstein, F. A., Beauchamp, I., Corcino, J. J., Maldonado, M., Tomasini, J. T., Maldonado, N., Rubio, C., and Schenk, E. A. Nutritional status and intestinal function among rural populations of the West Indies. II. Barrio Nuevo, Puerto Rico. Gastroenterology *63*:758, 1972.
8. Lindenbaum, J., Gerson, C. D., and Kent, T. H. Recovery of small-intestinal structure and function after residence in the tropics. I. Studies in Peace Corps Volunteers. Ann. Intern. Med. *74*:218, 1971.
9. Gerson, C. D., Kent, T. H., Saha, J. R., Siddiqi, N., and Lindenbaum, J. Recovery of small-intestinal structure and function after residence in the tropics. II. Studies in Indians and Pakistanis living in New York City. Ann. Intern. Med. *75*:41, 1971.
10. Sheehy, T. W., Cohen, W. C., Wallace, D. K., and Legters, L. J. Tropical sprue in North Americans. JAMA *194*:1069, 1965.
11. Klipstein, F. A., and Falaiye, J. M. Tropical sprue in expatriates from the tropics living in the continental United States. Medicine *48*:475, 1969.
12. Tomkins, A. M., James, W. P. T., Walters, J. H., and Cole, A. C. E. Malabsorption in overland travellers to India. Br. Med. J. *3*:380, 1974.
13. Klipstein, F. A., Samloff, I. M., Smarth, G., and Schenk, E. A. Treatment of overt and subclinical malabsorption in Haiti. Gut *10*:315, 1969.
14. Klipstein, F. A., Samloff, I. M., and Schenk, E. A. Tropical sprue in Haiti. Ann. Intern. Med. *64*:575, 1966.
15. Thomas, G., and Clain, D. J. Endemic tropical sprue in Rhodesia. Gut *17*:877, 1976.
16. Jones, T. C., Dean, A. G., and Parker, G. W. Seasonal gastroenteritis and malabsorption at an American military base in the Philippines. II. Malabsorption following the acute illness. Am. J. Epidemiol. *95*:128, 1972.
17. Mathan, V. I., and Baker, S. J. An epidemic of tropical sprue in southern India. I. Clinical features. Ann. Trop. Med. Parasitol. *64*:439, 1970.
18. Klipstein, F. A., and Corcino, J. J. Seasonal occurrence of overt and subclinical tropical malabsorption in Puerto Rico. Am. J. Trop. Med. Hyg. *23*:1189, 1974.
19. Baker, S. J., and Mathan, V. I. Tropical sprue in southern India. *In* Tropical Sprue and Megaloblastic Anaemia. London, Churchill Livingstone, 1971.
20. Haeney, M. R., Montgomery, R. D., and Schneider, R. Sprue in the Middle East: Five case reports. Gut *15*:377, 1974.
21. Wood, E. J. The occurrence of sprue in the United States. Am. J. Med. Sci. *150*:692, 1915.
22. Montgomery, R. D., Beale, D. J., Sammons, H. G., and Schneider, R. Postinfective malabsorption: A sprue syndrome. Br. Med. J. *2*:265, 1973.
23. Keele, K. D., and Bound, J. P. Sprue in India: Clinical survey of 600 cases. Br. Med. J. *1*:77, 1946.
24. O'Brien, W., and England, N. W. J. Tropical sprue amongst British servicemen and their families in South-East Asia. *In* Tropical Sprue and Megaloblastic Anaemia. London, Churchill Livingstone, 1971, pp. 25–60.
25. Sheehy, T. W. Digestive disease as a national problem. VI. Enteric disease among United States troops in Vietnam. Gastroenterology *55*:105, 1968.
26. Gorbach, S. L., Mitra, R., Jacobs, B., Banwell, J. G., Chatterjee, B. D., and Guha Mazunder, D. N. Bacterial contamination of the upper small bowel in tropical sprue. Lancet *1*:74, 1969.
27. Klipstein, F. A., Holdeman, L. V., Corcino, J. J., and Moore, W. E. C. Enterotoxigenic intestinal bacteria in tropical sprue. Ann. Intern. Med. *79*:632, 1973.
28. Tomkins, A. M., Drasar, B. S., and James, W. P. T. Bacterial colonisation of jejunal mucosa in acute tropical sprue. Lancet *1*:59, 1975.
29. Bhat, P., Shantakumari, S., Rajan, D., Mathan, V. I., Kapadia, C. R., Swarnara, C., and Baker, S. J. Bacterial flora of the gastrointestinal tract in southern Indian control subjects and patients with tropical sprue. Gastroenterology *62*:11, 1972.
30. Klipstein, F. A., Engert, R. F., and Short, H. B. Enterotoxigenicity of colonising coliform bacteria in tropical sprue and blind-loop syndrome. Lancet *2*:342, 1978.
31. Klipstein, F. A., Horowitz, I. R., Engert, R. F., and Schenk, E. A. Effect of *Klebsiella pneumoniae* enterotoxin on intestinal transport in the rat. J. Clin. Invest. *56*:799, 1975.
32. Baker, S. J., Mathan, M., Mathan, V. I., and Swaminathan, S. P. Chronic enterocyte infection with coronavirus. One possible cause of the syndrome of tropical sprue? Dig. Dis. Sci. *11*:1039, 1982.
33. Applebaum, P. C., Moshal, M. G., Hift, W., and Chatterton, S. A. Intestinal bacteria in patients with tropical sprue. S. Afr. Med. J. *57*:1081, 1980.
34. Klipstein, F. A. Jejunal bacterial overgrowth in acute and persistent infectious diarrhea. J. Pediatr. Gastroenterol. Nutr. *5*:683, 1986.
35. Ross, I. N., and Mathan, V. I. Immunological changes in tropical sprue. Q. J. Med. *200*:435, 1981.
36. Drasar, B. S., Agostini, C., Clarke, D., Mann, G., Mhuala, F., Montgomery, F., and Tomkins, A. M. Adhesion of enteropathogenic bacteria to cells in tissue culture. Dev. Biol. Stand. *46*:83, 1980.
37. Cook, G. C. Delayed small-intestinal transit in tropical malabsorption. Br. Med. J. *2*:238, 1978.
38. Besterman, H. S., Cook, G. C., Sarson, D. L., Christofides, N. D., Bryant, M. G., Gregor, M., and Bloom, S. R. Gut hormones in tropical malabsorption. Br. Med. J. *2*:1252, 1979.

39. Mickelson, M. J., and Klipstein, F. A. Enterotoxigenic intestinal bacteria in tropical sprue. IV. Effect of linoleic acid on growth interrelationships of *Lactobacillus acidophilus* and *Klebsiella pneumoniae*. Infect. Immun. *12*:1121, 1975.
40. Klipstein, F. A. Folate in tropical sprue. Br. J. Haematol. *23*(suppl.):119, 1972.
41. Sheehy, T. W., Baggs, B., Perez-Santiago, E., and Floch, M. H. Prognosis of tropical sprue. A study of the effect of folic acid on the intestinal aspects of acute and chronic sprue. Ann. Intern. Med. *57*:892, 1962.
42. Klipstein, F. A., and Corcino, J. J. Factors responsible for weight loss in tropical sprue. Am. J. Clin. Nutr. *30*:1703, 1977.
43. Corcino, J. J., Maldonado, M., and Klipstein, F. A. Intestinal perfusion studies in tropical sprue. I. Transport of water, electrolytes, and d-xylose. Gastroenterology *65*:192, 1983.
44. Ramakrishna, B. S., and Mathan, V. I. Water and electrolyte absorption by the colon in tropical sprue. Gut *23*:843, 1982.
45. Tiruppathi, C., Balasubramian, K. A., Hill, P. G., and Mathan, V. I. Faecal free fatty acids in tropical sprue and their possible role in the production of diarrhoea by inhibition of ATPases. Gut *24*:300, 1983.
46. Bevan, G., Engert, R., Klipstein, F. A., Maldonado, N., Rubio, C., and Turner, M. D. Bile salt metabolism in tropical sprue. Gut *15*:254, 1974.
47. Schenk, E. A., Samloff, I. M., and Klipstein, F. A. Morphologic characteristics of jejunal biopsies in celiac disease and in tropical sprue. Am. J. Pathol. *47*:765, 1965.
48. Tomkins, A. M., Smith, T., and Wright, S. G. Assessment of early and delayed responses in vitamin B_{12} absorption during antibiotic therapy in tropical malabsorption. Clin. Sci. Mol. Med. *55*:533, 1978.
49. Corcino, J. J., Reisenauer, A. M., and Halsted, C. H. Jejunal perfusion of simple and conjugated folates in tropical sprue. J. Clin. Invest. *58*:298, 1976.
50. Klipstein, F. A., and Samloff, I. M. Folate synthesis by intestinal bacteria. Am. J. Clin. Nutr. *19*:237, 1966.
51. Vaish, S. K., Ignatius, M., and Baker, S. J. Albumin metabolism in tropical sprue. Q. J. Med. *34*:15, 1965.
52. Hellier, M. D., Ganapathy, V., Gammon, A., Mathan, V. I., and Radhakrishnan, A. M. Impaired intestinal absorption of dipeptide in tropical sprue patients in India. Clin. Sci. *58*:431, 1980.
53. Caldwell, W. L., Swanson, V. L., and Bayless, T. M. The importance and reliability of the roentgenographic examination of the small bowel in patients with tropical sprue. Radiology *84*:227, 1965.
54. Brunser, O., Eidelman, S., and Klipstein, F. A. Intestinal morphology of rural Haitians. A comparison between overt tropical sprue and asymptomatic subjects. Gastroenterology *58*:655, 1970.
55. Klipstein, F. A., Schenk, E. A., and Samloff, I. M. Folate repletion associated with oral tetracycline therapy in tropical sprue. Gastroenterology *51*:317, 1966.
56. Klipstein, F. A. Tropical sprue in travelers and expatriates living abroad. Gastroenterology *80*:590, 1981.
57. Tomkins, A. M., Wright, S. G., Drasar, B. S., and James, W. P. T. Bacterial colonization of jejunal mucosa in giardiasis. Trans. R. Soc. Trop. Med. Hyg. *72*:22, 1978.
58. Mayoral, L. G., Tripathy, K., Balanos, O., Lotero, H., Duque, E., Garcia, F. T., and Ghitis, J. Intestinal, functional and morphologic abnormalities in severely protein-malnourished adults. Am. J. Clin. Nutr. *25*:1084, 1972.
59. Swanson, V. L., Whelby, M. S., and Bayless, T. M. Morphologic effects of folic acid and vitamin B_{12} on the jejunal lesion of tropical sprue. Am. J. Pathol. *49*:167, 1966.
60. Guerra, R., Whelby, M. S., and Bayless, T. M. Long-term antibiotic therapy in tropical sprue. Ann. Intern. Med. *63*:619, 1965.
61. Maldonado, N., Horta, E., Guerra, R., and Perez-Santiago, E. Poorly absorbed sulfonamides in the treatment of tropical sprue. Gastroenterology *57*:559, 1969.
62. Sheehy, T. W., and Perez-Santiago, E. Antibiotic therapy in tropical sprue. Gastroenterology *41*:208, 1961.
63. Horta, E. O., Maldonado, N., Fradera, J., Santini, R., and Velez-Garcia, E. Response of tropical sprue to poorly absorbed sulfonamides and oxytetracycline. Am. J. Clin. Nutr. *24*:1327, 1971.
64. Rickles, F. R., Klipstein, F. A., Tomasini, J., Corcini, J. J., and Maldonado, N. Long-term follow-up of antibiotic-treated tropical sprue. Ann. Intern. Med. *76*:203, 1972.

67

The Blind Loop Syndrome

PHILLIP P. TOSKES
ROBERT M. DONALDSON, JR.

The development of malabsorption in a patient with overgrowth of bacteria within the small intestine is known as the blind loop, stagnant loop, or stasis syndrome.

HISTORY

In 1890, White first suspected a relation between strictures of the small intestine and an anemia resembling pernicious anemia, but it was not until 1924 that Seyderhelm and his colleagues demonstrated clearly that removal of an intestinal stricture cured the associated anemia. It soon became apparent that this anemia and its attendant neurologic defects responded to liver therapy; that other small intestinal abnormalities such as diverticula, blind pouches, and enteroenterostomies could cause anemia; and that various small intestinal lesions were often associated not only with anemia but also with steatorrhea. By 1939, Barker and Hummel[1] were able to document in their classic review all the salient clinical features of the blind loop syndrome. Subsequently, many workers have demonstrated that malabsorption of cobalamin (vitamin B_{12}) and steatorrhea in patients with small intestine bacterial overgrowth can be corrected by administration of antibiotics or by appropriate surgical therapy. Ellis and Smith[2] have provided a detailed description of the history of the blind loop syndrome.

ETIOLOGY AND PATHOGENESIS

As described on pages 107 to 114 the small intestinal lumen normally harbors sparse numbers of gram-positive aerobes or facultative anaerobes. Any abnormality of the small intestine that results in local stasis or "recirculation" of intestinal contents is likely to be accompanied by marked proliferation of intraluminal microorganisms. In this situation there develops a complex small intestinal flora that is predominantly anaerobic and that closely resembles the colonic flora.

A large number of disorders have been associated with proliferation of enteric microorganisms in the small intestine.[3–5] It is important to recognize, however, that not every patient with these disorders necessarily develops a small intestinal flora that is clinically and metabolically significant. Many patients who have intestinal abnormalities definitely conducive to bacterial overgrowth do not in fact develop malabsorption.

Those disorders associated with bacterially induced malabsorption are listed in Table 67–1.

Anatomic (Structural) Abnormalities

Blind pouches of the small intestine formed surgically by creation of an end-to-side enteroenteric anastomosis frequently produce small intestine bacterial overgrowth (Fig. 67–1).[6] Similarly, stagnant loops of intestine resulting from *fistulas* or *surgical enterostomies* allow for continuous recirculation of small intestinal contents and consequent bacterial overgrowth (Fig. 67–2). Fol-

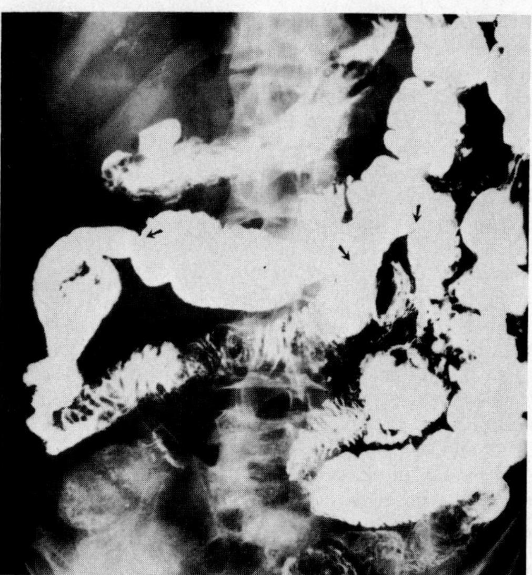

Figure 67–1. Small bowel series in a 55-year-old man with recurrent Crohn's disease obstructing a prior enterocolic anastomosis *(left arrow)* in whom a proximal enterocolic bypass was performed *(right arrows)*, creating a blind loop. (Courtesy of M. H. Sleisenger, M.D.)

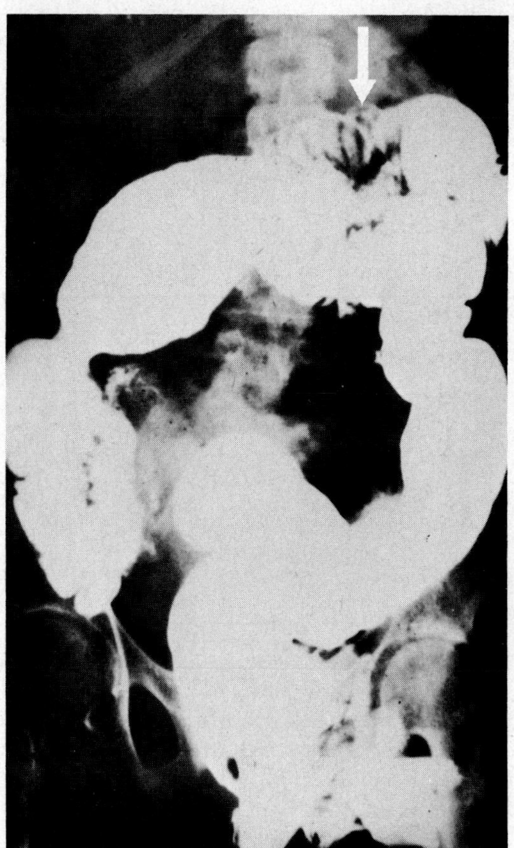

Figure 67–2. Barium enema in a 26-year-old woman with granulomatous colitis and malabsorption syndrome. Note the jejunocolic fistula and loop of jejunum *(arrow)*. (Courtesy of M. H. Sleisenger, M.D.)

Table 67–1. CLINICAL CONDITIONS ASSOCIATED WITH BACTERIAL OVERGROWTH

Gastric proliferation
Hypo- or achlorhydria, especially when combined with motor or anatomic disturbances
Small intestinal stagnation
Anatomic
Afferent loop of Billroth II partial gastrectomy
Duodenal jejunal diverticulosis
Surgical blind loop (end-to-side anastomosis)
Surgical recirculating loop (side-to-side anastomosis)
Obstruction (stricture, adhesion, inflammation, cancer)
Motor
Scleroderma
Idiopathic intestinal pseudo-obstruction
Derangements of interdigestive motor complex
Diabetic autonomic neuropathy
Abnormal communication between proximal and distal gastrointestinal tract
Gastrocolic or jejunocolic fistula
Resection of ileocecal valve
Miscellaneous
Hypogammaglobulinemia
Chronic pancreatitis

lowing partial *gastrectomy* and *Billroth II anastomoses*, dysfunction and stasis in the afferent loop may result in marked intraluminal proliferation of bacteria and consequent seeding of the remainder of the small intestine.[7] *Diverticula* of the small intestine serve as a source for bacterial overgrowth and constitute an increasingly frequent cause of the blind loop syndrome, especially in the setting of hypo- or achlorhydria (Fig. 67–3).[8] Partial chronic *small intestinal obstruction* caused by Crohn's disease, adhesions, radiation damage, lymphoma, or tuberculosis frequently leads to increased numbers of bacteria within the small intestinal lumen.[9–12] Patients with gastric ulcers, ulcerating carcinomas of the stomach or transverse colon, or stomach ulcers following subtotal gastrectomy may develop *gastrocolic* or *gastrojejunocolic fistulas* (Fig. 67–4). In this situation, food and intestinal contents are not diverted from the stomach directly into the colon, but rather colonic contents pass into the stomach and small intestine. Thus, there results a massive bacterial seeding of the small intestine, which emanates from the colon.[13] Recently, patients have been shown to have malabsorption associated with overgrowth of bacteria in and proximal to surgically constructed *Kock distal ileal pouches* (continent ileostomy).[14, 15]

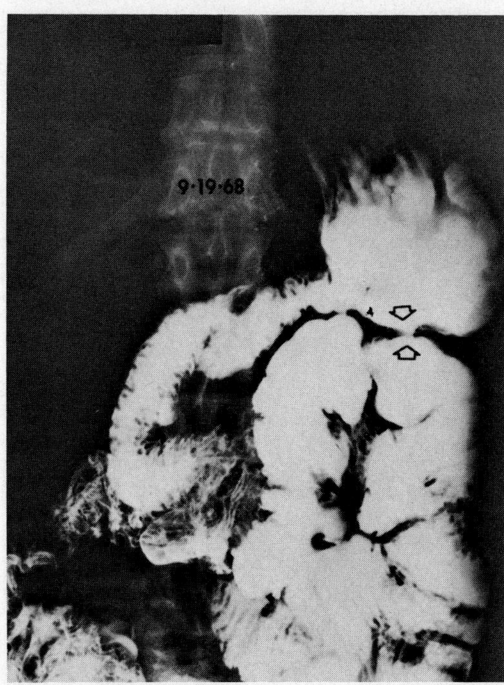

Figure 67–4. Upper gastrointestinal series in a 46-year-old man with a gastrocolic fistula *(arrows)* due to peptic ulcer disease causing malabsorption. (Courtesy of M. H. Sleisenger, M.D.)

Impaired Motor Function

In addition to structural abnormalities conducive to localized stasis, more generalized alterations in *small intestinal motor function* may favor bacterial proliferation and consequent metabolic abnormalities. Thus, malabsorption resulting from small intestine bacterial overgrowth has been documented in patients with *intestinal scleroderma* and marked hypomotility (Fig. 67–5)[16] (see pp. 505–506). Idiopathic intestinal *pseudo-obstruction* (see pp. 377–379) can also result in significant bacterial overgrowth and associated malabsorption (Fig. 67–6).[17] Some patients with *diabetic autonomic neuropathy* develop malabsorption secondary to bacterial overgrowth[18] (see pp. 494–500). Patients may develop malabsorption secondary to bacterial overgrowth with no anatomic abnormality. One example is the recent demonstration of abnormalities in the interdigestive motor complex (intestinal housekeeper of Code) in patients suspected of having bacterial overgrowth on the basis of an abnormal cholylglycine breath test.[19] Some of these patients had no recognizable anatomic lesions. Another recent example of malabsorption secondary to bacterial overgrowth in patients without anatomic lesions is the finding of positive cholylglycine breath tests or abnormal intestinal cultures in elderly patients with unexplained malnutrition and malabsorption.[20, 21] All other tests (including small intestine biopsy) for other causes of malabsorption were normal. These patients manifested a "failure to thrive" and made a striking recovery after treatment with antibiotics. Bacterial overgrowth in the elderly in all likelihood is secondary to altered motility of the small intestine and/or decreased gastric acid secretion.

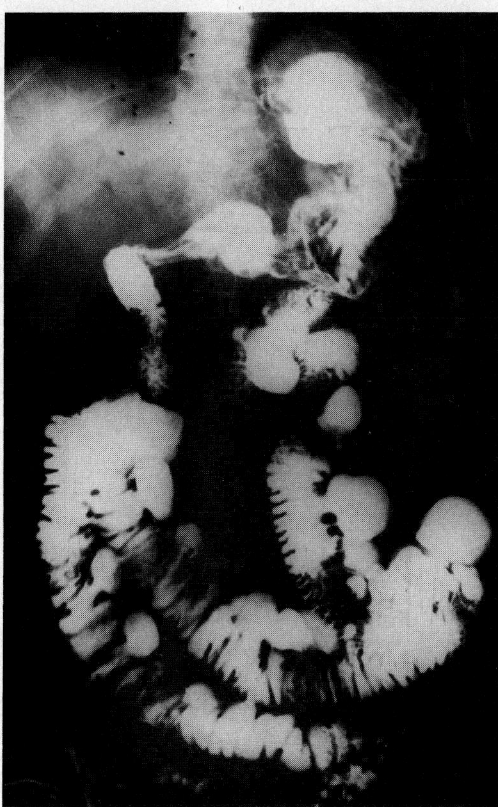

Figure 67–3. Small bowel series in an elderly male patient with blind loop syndrome due to multiple large jejunal diverticula. (Courtesy of M. H. Sleisenger. M.D.)

The pathogenesis of the bacterial overgrowth in patients with hypogammaglobulinemia and *chronic pancreatitis* is ill understood. A recent study docu-

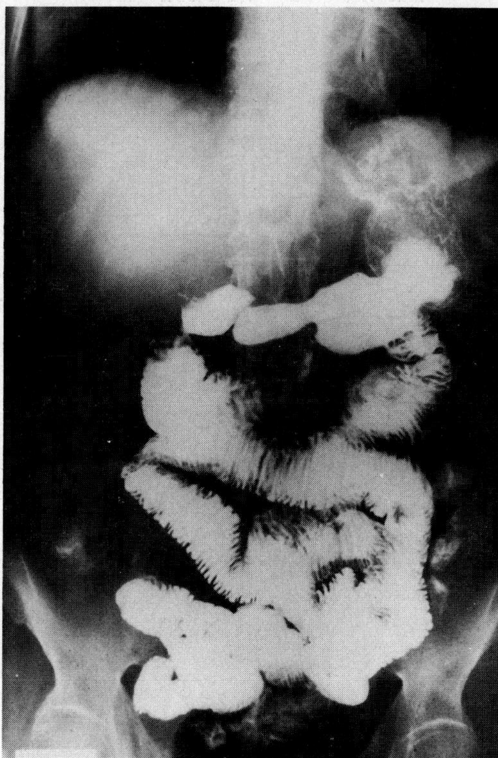

Figure 67–5. A small bowel series at one hour in a 46-year-old woman with scleroderma of the small intestine and blind loop syndrome. Note dilated loops of jejunum, delay in transit, and mucosal spiculation. (Courtesy of M. H. Sleisenger, M.D.)

mented abnormal ^{14}C-cholylglycine breath tests in 8 of 20 patients with chronic pancreatitis with and without steatorrhea.[22] Steatorrhea persisting after pancreatic extract therapy administration to patients with chronic pancreatitis may be in part due to associated bacterial overgrowth, possibly responsive to antimicrobial therapy.

The mechanisms whereby bacteria proliferating within the small intestine result in nutrient malabsorption have been studied extensively and are discussed in detail on pages 107 to 114 and 263 to 282. It is now clear that the malabsorption observed in the setting of bacteria overgrowth results not only from abnormalities within the intraluminal environment (e.g., bacterial hydrolysis of conjugated bile salts) but also from damage to the small intestine enterocyte.

CLINICAL FEATURES

Clinical manifestations vary greatly and depend, at least in part, upon the nature of the small intestine abnormality causing the bacterial overgrowth. Patients with *small intestinal diverticula* are relatively asymptomatic until small intestinal bacterial populations are sufficiently established to cause steatorrhea with increased numbers of bowel movements, weight loss, and anemia. Because most patients with steatorrhea and anemia associated with small intestine diverticula are elderly, an interval of many years has been assumed between the development of the diverticula and the appearance of metabolic abnormalities. It seems likely that hypo- or achlorhydria, which is relatively common in the elderly, permits increased bacterial overgrowth in many cases. Although most symptomatic patients have multiple diverticula, development of the complications of bacterial overgrowth has been observed in some patients with a single large diverticulum.

Patients with strictures or *surgically formed blind pouches* of the small intestine may note abdominal discomfort, bloating, and crampy periumbilical pain before diarrhea, steatorrhea, and the symptoms of anemia develop. In general, an interval of months or years may elapse between the time a blind pouch is formed and the onset of symptoms attributable to small intestinal bacterial overgrowth. When patients have *strictures* or *fistulas* caused by Crohn's disease of the small intestine or have hypomotility caused by *scleroderma* or *intestinal pseudo-obstruction*, the clinical features of the primary disease may completely overshadow any manifestations of intraluminal microbial proliferation. Furthermore, it may be difficult to determine in patients with *Crohn's disease* (pp. 1327–1358), *radiation enteritis* (pp. 1369–1382), *short bowel syndrome* (pp. 1106–1112), or *lymphoma* (pp. 1519–1560) the extent to which malabsorption is due to primary intestinal disease or insufficiency or secondary bacterial overgrowth.

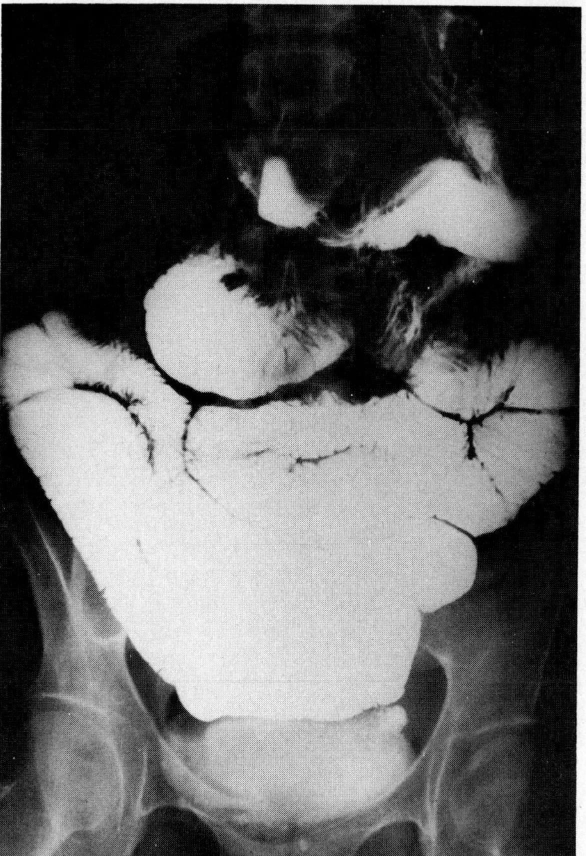

Figure 67–6. A small bowel series in a patient wtih idiopathic intestinal pseudo-obstruction and malabsorption associated with bacterial overgrowth. Note the dilated loops throughout the small bowel. (Courtesy of N. Greenberger, M.D.)

Whatever the cause of the abnormal proliferation of microorganisms within the small intestine lumen, the consequences for the patient are the same. Weight loss associated with clinically apparent steatorrhea has been observed in about one third of patients with small intestine bacterial overgrowth severe enough to cause cobalamin deficiency.[23] Osteomalacia, vitamin K deficiency, night blindness, and even hypocalcemic tetany have been known to develop as a consequence of lipid malabsorption in patients with this disorder. Appropriate therapy or surgical correction of the small intestine lesion conducive to stasis promptly reduces fecal fat excretion to normal or near normal levels (see pp. 279–280).

Ample evidence indicates that the anemia that develops in patients with the blind loop syndrome is due to cobalamin deficiency. The anemia is megaloblastic and macrocytic, and serum cobalamin levels are low. Furthermore, neurologic changes indistinguishable from those of pernicious anemia may develop, and the anemia can be corrected by physiologic doses of the vitamin.[24] In the experimental blind loop syndrome and in some patients with overgrowth, iron deficiency is secondary to blood lost through the gastrointestinal tract, perhaps secondary to ulcerated areas within stagnant loops.[25] Under these circumstances, the patient may have guaiac-positive stools together with a microcytic and hypochromic anemia or, in some instances, anemia with two populations of red blood cells: microcytic and macrocytic. On the other hand, folate deficiency is not a common occurrence in the blind loop syndrome. Unlike the situation with cobalamin, folate synthesized by microorganisms in the small intestine appears to be available for the host, and in patients with small intestine bacterial overgrowth, serum folate levels tend to be high rather than low.[26]

Hypoproteinemia is a frequent manifestation of the blind loop syndrome and is occasionally severe enough to cause edema. The etiology of the hypoproteinemia is multifactorial and may result from decreased uptake of amino acids by the damaged small intestine, intraluminal breakdown of protein and protein precursors by bacteria, and antibiotic-reversible protein-losing enteropathy.[27]

Decreased urinary xylose excretion is frequently seen in both the clinical and experimental blind loop syndrome. Although studies employing ^{14}C-xylose in the experimental blind loop syndrome have shown that the decreased urinary xylose excretion was due primarily to intraluminal catabolism of xylose to carbon dioxide, the decreased absorption of xylose in the setting of bacterial overgrowth may be secondary to both intraluminal catabolism of xylose by bacteria and diminished absorption due to small intestine mucosal dysfunction (see pp. 107–114 and 263–282).

In addition to steatorrhea, patients with the blind loop syndrome frequently complain of watery diarrhea. Just as with the other clinical manifestations of this condition, diarrhea may result from several causes. Both disturbances of the intraluminal environment (deconjugated bile acids, hydroxylated fatty acids, and organic acids) and direct changes in gut motility appear to be important (see pp. 107–114 and 290–316).

DIAGNOSIS

Overgrowth of bacteria within the small intestine should be considered in the differential diagnosis of any patient who presents with diarrhea, steatorrhea, weight loss, or macrocytic anemia, particularly if the patient is elderly or has had previous abdominal surgery. The development of diarrhea, weight loss, and macrocytic anemia months to years after gastric surgery suggests that the patient may have *afferent loop dysfunction* or a *gastrojejunocolic fistula*. A history of previous surgery for *small intestinal obstruction* should raise the question of whether the obstruction was bypassed by an end-to-side anastomosis, leaving a *blind pouch*, or a side-to-side anastomosis, resulting in recirculation of small intestine contents. On the other hand, a past history of recurrent bouts of intestinal obstruction may indicate stasis caused by a *small intestinal stricture* or adhesions. The presence of dysphagia should suggest the diagnosis of *scleroderma*, or repeated bouts of intestinal obstruction without obvious organic cause suggest *intestinal pseudo-obstruction*. In any event, a complete small intestinal series should be obtained in patients with diarrhea, steatorrhea, or macrocytic anemia to exclude the possibility of enteric stasis and consequent bacterial overgrowth.

When the history and small intestine X-ray films suggest that proliferation of microorganisms in the small intestine lumen may cause or contribute to malabsorption, further evaluation is necessary for optimal management. The presence of steatorrhea should be documented. If the patient has clinically significant bacterial overgrowth, cobalamin absorption is frequently impaired, even though the patient may not yet have become cobalamin-deficient. Intrinsic factor will not improve cobalamin absorption in these patients (see Table 18–5, p. 275). The urinary excretion of xylose may be decreased and the serum folate increased in some but not all patients with the blind loop syndrome.

A small intestine biopsy is of value in excluding primary mucosal disease as the cause of the malabsorption. Although striking histologic abnormalities of jejunal mucosa are not usually seen in patients with bacterial overgrowth, the biopsy is often abnormal[28] (Fig. 67–7). A patchy lesion of variable severity may be observed. Increased infiltration of the lamina propria with lymphocytes, plasma cells, and polymorphonuclear leukocytes, together with thickening and blunting of villi, may be seen. However, one does not find the diffuse alterations of the surface absorptive cells regularly present in celiac sprue. Although in some cases the biopsy specimen from a patient with the blind loop syndrome may show changes suggestive of tropical sprue, the history and intestinal culture should differentiate these two disorders.

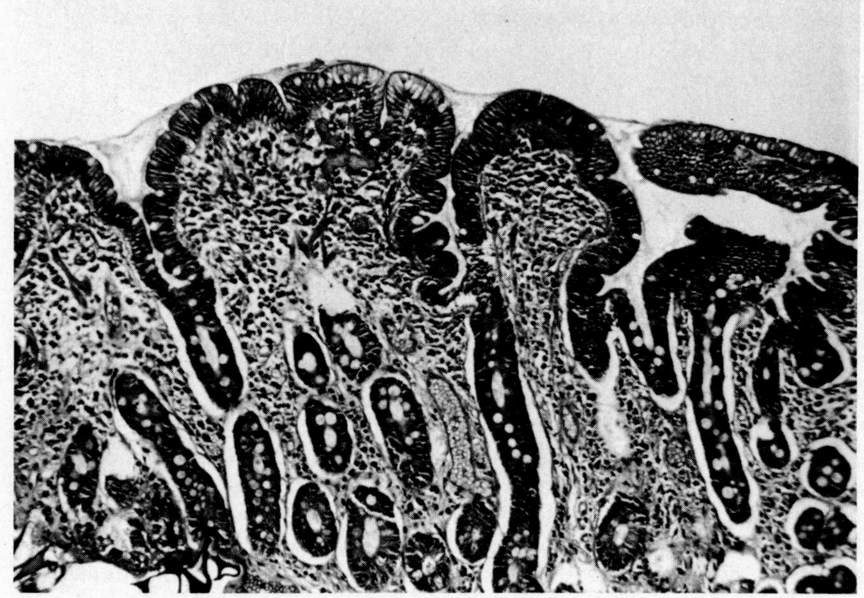

Figure 67–7. Abnormal broadened villi in a patient with severe malabsorption and bacterial overgrowth. The malabsorption was corrected with antibiotic therapy. (From King, C. E., and Toskes, P. P. *In* Bushkin, F. L., and Woodward, E. R. Postgastrectomy Syndromes. Philadelphia, W. B. Saunders Co., 1976.)

Specific Diagnosis

The sine qua non for the diagnosis of bacterial overgrowth is a properly collected and appropriately cultured aspirate from the proximal small intestine. The specimen should be obtained under anaerobic conditions, serially diluted, and cultured on several selective media. In patients with clinically significant bacterial overgrowth, a number of different species are found, and the total concentration of bacteria generally exceeds 10^5 organisms per milliliter. Bacteroides, anaerobic lactobacilli, coliforms, and enterococci are all likely to be present in varying numbers. Although in most patients the intraluminal microbial proliferation can be documented in the proximal jejunum, it is important to recognize that pockets of overgrowth may be missed by a single culture and that bacterial overgrowth may occur only in the more distal portions of the small intestine. An intestinal culture requires intubation of the small intestine and time-consuming microbiologic analyses.

A number of laboratory tests based on the metabolic actions of enteric bacteria have been proposed to assist in the diagnosis of the blind loop syndrome. Table 67–2 compares a number of these tests with the gold standard—the intestinal culture—with respect to ease of performance, sensitivity, specificity, and safety. The conclusions are based on a number of different studies from several laboratories throughout the world.

Quantitation of urinary excretion of indican, phenols, drug metabolites, and conjugated PABA does not adequately distinguish patients with bacterial overgrowth from those with other kinds of malabsorption.[3] Analyses of intestinal aspirates for deconjugated bile acids or volatile fatty acids are difficult and suffer from many of the limitations previously stated for intestinal cultures.[29, 30] Increased free serum bile acids have been noted in several patients with the blind loop syndrome.[29, 31] Although of potential use as a diagnostic aid, this test depends on the presence of bacteria that have the capability of deconjugating bile salts (e.g., *Bacteroides*).

Breath Tests

Another approach to diagnosing bacterial overgrowth is the timed analysis of breath excretion of volatile metabolites produced by intraluminal bacteria. Both measurement of expired labeled CO_2 after oral administration of ^{14}C- or ^{13}C-labeled substrates and breath hydrogen after administration of nonlabeled fermentable substrate have been employed.[32]

The bile acid or *^{14}C-cholylglycine breath test* was the first ^{14}C breath test used to diagnose bacterial overgrowth.[33, 34] Although frequently able to detect bacterial overgrowth, the bile acid breath test does not differentiate bacterial overgrowth from ileal damage or resection with excessive breath $^{14}CO_2$ production due to bacterial deconjugation within the colon of unabsorbed ^{14}C bile salt. This creates clinical difficulties, because bacterial overgrowth may be superimposed upon ileal damage in conditions such as *Crohn's disease, lymphoma*, and *radiation enteritis*. In addition,

Table 67–2. TESTS FOR BACTERIAL OVERGROWTH

Test	Simplicity	Sensitivity	Specificity	Safety
Culture	Poor	Good	Excellent	Good
Urinary indican	Good	Poor	Poor	Excellent
Jejunal fatty acids	Poor	Fair	Excellent	Good
Jejunal bile acids	Poor	Fair	Excellent	Good
^{14}C-bile acid BT	Excellent	Fair	Poor	Good
^{14}C-xylose BT	Excellent	Excellent	Excellent	Good
Lactulose-H_2 BT	Excellent	Fair-good	Fair-good	Excellent

BT, breath test.

false negative results have been described in 30 to 40 per cent of patients with culture-proved overgrowth.[35–37]

A 1 gm ^{14}*C-xylose breath test* appears to be a sensitive and specific test to diagnose the presence of bacterial overgrowth.[36, 38] Elevated $^{14}CO_2$ levels appear in the breath in 85 per cent of patients within the first 60 minutes of the test. Xylose as a substrate is attractive because (1) xylose is catabolized by gram-negative aerobes, which are always part of the overgrowth flora, (2) xylose is predominantly absorbed in the proximal small bowel as contrasted to the predominant ileal absorption of bile salts, leading to virtually no "dumping" of xylose into the colon, and (3) xylose is metabolized substantially less than other proximally absorbed substrates, such as glucose. Comparison with the bile acid breath test in a series of patients with culture-proved overgrowth demonstrated no false negative results with the xylose breath test.[36] Extensive clinical experience with this test is being accumulated, and a number of laboratories have documented its reliability in detecting small intestine bacterial overgrowth.[38–40]

Breath hydrogen analysis allows a distinct separation of metabolic activity of the intestinal flora from that by the host, for hydrogen production in mammalian tissue is unknown. Excessive breath hydrogen production has been noted in patients with bacterial overgrowth following the administration of either 50 gm or 80 gm of glucose or 10 gm of lactulose.[41–43] It should be pointed out that some patients with bacterial overgrowth may have elevated fasting levels of breath hydrogen.[44]

Still needed are systematic assessments of sensitivity and specificity, as well as investigations to determine which substrate is optimal for detecting bacterial overgrowth. In addition, it must be emphasized that the factors that affect hydrogen production by intestinal bacteria both in normal subjects and in patients with malabsorption require further attention. Thus, two recent studies demonstrated that 27 per cent of normal persons fail to show any rise in breath hydrogen following a test dose of lactulose. Further, the failure of abnormal H_2 expiration in patients with malabsorption may be due to production of organic acids or a "wash-out" effect of their diarrhea.[45, 46] The 27 per cent incidence is in sharp contrast to the 2 per cent of non-hydrogen production that is usually quoted. Such persons apparently do not have enteric flora that can produce hydrogen from carbohydrates.

A recent study compared the 1 gm ^{14}C-xylose breath test to a 10 gm lactulose-H_2 test and an 80 gm glucose-H_2 test in 20 subjects with culture-proved bacterial overgrowth and 10 control subjects.[42] The ^{14}C-xylose breath test was positive (abnormal) in 19 of 20 subjects with bacterial overgrowth and 0 of 10 control subjects. In contrast, the H_2 breath tests demonstrated: (1) uninterpretable tests (absence of H_2-generating bacteria) in 2 of 20 subjects with bacterial overgrowth and 1 of 10 control subjects, and (2) nondiagnostic increases in H_2 production in 3 of 18 80 gm glucose-H_2 tests and 7 of 18 lactulose-H_2 breath tests in subjects with bacterial overgrowth. Thus, in these patients with culture-proved bacterial overgrowth, the 1 gm ^{14}C-xylose breath test was positive in 95 per cent; the 80 gm glucose-H_2 test was positive in 75 per cent; and the 10 gm lactulose-H_2 test was positive in 55 per cent.

The nonradioactive nature, ease of performance, and inexpensiveness of H_2 breath tests make them attractive, but there appear to be significant problems with sensitivity and specificity in trying to detect the presence of small intestine bacterial overgrowth when an incompletely absorbed test probe is used.

The excellent sensitivity and specificity of the 1 gm ^{14}C-xylose breath test makes it the test of choice to detect bacterial overgrowth. Indeed, the Clinical Efficacy Committee of the American College of Physicians suggested that only two breath tests—the 1 gm ^{14}C-xylose test for bacterial overgrowth and the 50 gm lactose-H_2 test for lactose intolerance—are appropriate for routine clinical use.

TREATMENT

The aim of therapy is the reduction of the bacterial overgrowth and consists of antibiotic administration, or when feasible, correction of the small intestine abnormality leading to stasis and microbial proliferation. Unfortunately, however, surgery is often impractical (e.g., scleroderma, multiple diverticula, and so on) or unacceptable to the patient. Thus, management of many patients with bacterial overgrowth is lifelong. It is important to emphasize again that bacterial overgrowth may be a treatable component of the malabsorption seen in patients with diseases such as *Crohn's disease, intestinal lymphoma*, or *radiation enteritis*. Deterioration in such patients may not be due to their primary disease process but to associated overgrowth. It also must be stressed that bacterial overgrowth may be present without causing any disease. An abnormal breath test or a pathologic culture must be put in perspective by the clinician and appropriate decisions made.

Selection of an antimicrobial agent based on the sensitivity of the microorganisms present in the small bowel lumen is attractive in theory, but this approach is often difficult because there are usually many different bacterial species present, often with very different sensitivities. Under such circumstances, it may be extremely difficult to select what could be considered the most appropriate antibiotic on the basis of microbial sensitivity. Traditionally, treatment has been initiated with tetracycline, 250 mg four times daily by mouth. If the antibiotic is to be considered effective, diarrhea should subside and the absorption of fat and cobalamin should be distinctly improved within a week of beginning therapy. Unfortunately, up to 60 per cent of patients with clinically significant malabsorption associated with bacterial overgrowth no longer respond to tetracycline, and treatment often must include other antimicrobial agents, some of which may have serious side effects. Thus it behooves the physician to establish the diagnosis, rather than employ empirical therapy.

scribed involvement of the endocardium in Whipple's disease and concluded that the characteristic macrophages contained glycoprotein or mucopolysaccharide, not lipid, since they were periodic acid–Schiff positive.[2] Upton subsequently demonstrated the typical foamy macrophages in peripheral lymph nodes, liver, adrenal gland, and valves of the heart in a patient with Whipple's disease.[3] Sieracki and Fine then documented the presence of typical macrophages in many nonintestinal tissues in four patients, clearly establishing the systemic nature of this disorder.[4]

For 45 years after its initial description, the disease was considered to be a uniformly fatal and untreatable primary disorder of fat metabolism. However, in 1952, Paulley described a patient with histologically documented Whipple's disease in whom the disease remitted for a prolonged period following administration of the antibiotic chloramphenicol.[5] Despite his report, antibiotic therapy for this disease was not widely used over the next decade and many patients in whom the diagnosis had been established received only supportive treatments and, in some instances, ACTH or corticosteroids with only limited success.[6, 7]

In the early 1960s, rod-shaped bacilli with identical morphologic features were found within the intestinal mucosa of patients with untreated Whipple's disease in independent studies from several laboratories.[8–11] At about the same time, dramatic remission of clinical symptoms followed treatment of acutely ill Whipple's disease patients with a variety of antibiotic regimens in a number of medical centers.[11–13] Now, bacilli structurally identical to those seen in the intestine have been observed in many nonintestinal tissues in patients with Whipple's disease.[14–20] Moreover, many additional reports have clearly established that severely ill patients respond dramatically to antibiotic treatment. Thus, if properly diagnosed, this previously fatal disease can now be effectively treated in most instances.

PATHOLOGY

The pathologic appearance of Whipple's disease is distinctive; therefore, histologic examination of biopsies from involved tissues is usually diagnostic.

Small Intestine. The small intestine has been involved in the great majority of cases. Grossly, the bowel wall appears thickened and edematous. When examined with a hand lens or a dissecting microscope, the mucosa may resemble that seen in celiac sprue, in that the surface may appear flat or convoluted without apparent villi. More often, the villi are visible but markedly widened. Enlarged, whitish yellow villi have been noted endoscopically in the proximal intestine.[21]

The abnormality in mucosal structure is readily apparent in histologic sections in which extensive infiltration of the lamina propria with large macrophages markedly distorts villous architecture (Fig. 68–1). The cytoplasm of these macrophages is filled with many large glycoprotein granules that stain with the periodic acid–Schiff (PAS) technique.[22] The lamina propria may also contain accumulations of polymorphonuclear leukocytes. The cellular elements normally seen in the lamina such as plasma cells, lymphocytes, and eosinophils are usually decreased, because they have been displaced by the large number of macrophages. Sarcoid-like granulomas have been noted in the small intestine as well as in other involved tissues including lymph nodes, liver, and lungs.[23]

Mucosal and submucosal lymphatic vessels are dilated and, in sections not exposed to lipid solvents, are filled with fat. Fat droplets are also in the extracellular spaces of the lamina. This lymphatic dilatation and fat accumulation probably reflects lymphatic obstruction caused by enlarged mesenteric lymph nodes.

Although villous architecture is often markedly distorted, the absorptive epithelium shows variable and often patchy histologic abnormalities. These may include some attenuation of the brush border, some

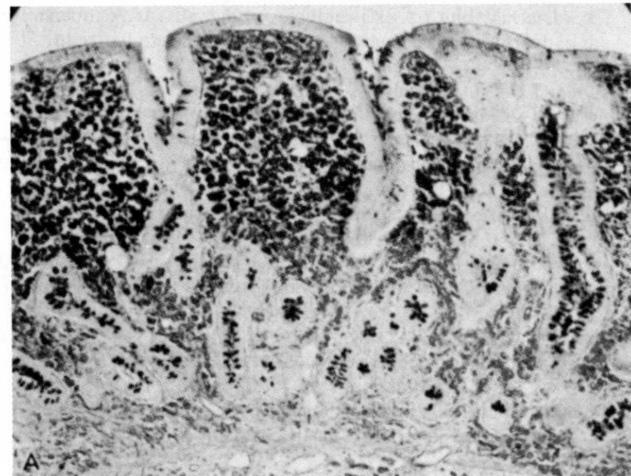

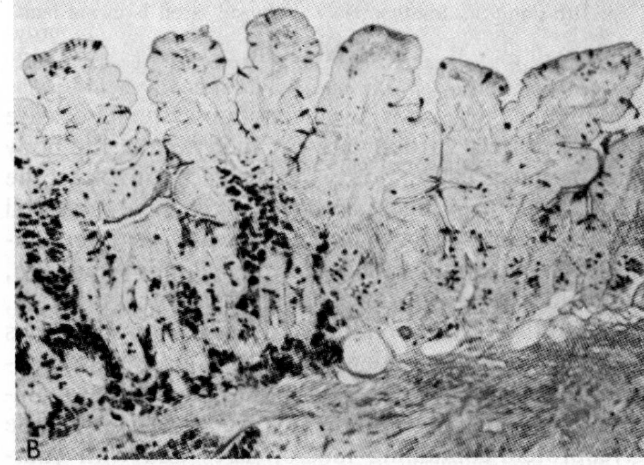

Figure 68–1. Jejunal biopsies from a patient with Whipple's disease before treatment *(A)* and 19 months after antibiotic therapy *(B)*. Before treatment, there are no normal villi and there is tremendous infiltration of the lamina propria with PAS-positive macrophages. After treatment, more normal-appearing villi are present and the lamina propria contains only focal accumulation of the PAS-positive macrophages. In fact, cores of some of the villi contain no apparent macrophages. PAS stain. Approximately × 75. (From Trier, J. S., Phelps, P. C., Eidelman, S., and Rubin, C. E. Whipple's disease: light and electron microscope correlation of jejunal mucosal histology with antibiotic treatment and clinical status. Gastroenterology *48*:684–707. © by Williams & Wilkins, 1965.)

decrease in cell height, and accumulation of a moderate amount of lipid within the cytoplasm. Diffuse, severe cytoplasmic abnormalities of absorptive cells, such as are seen in patients with celiac sprue, are not a regular feature of the intestinal lesion of Whipple's disease.

With high-resolution light microscopy (Fig. 68–2) and with the higher magnification of the electron microscope, many bacilli are seen in the lamina propria of the small intestine of patients with untreated Whipple's disease (Figs. 68–3 and 68–4). These tiny bacilli (0.25 μm wide and 1 to 2.5 μm long) may be located anywhere in the lamina but are usually most abundant just beneath the absorptive epithelium and around vascular channels in the upper half of the mucosa. Their fine structure, which is identical in different patients, conclusively establishes their bacterial nature (Fig. 68–4). They have a characteristic bacterial cell wall and a pale central nucleoid and, in favorable sections, may be seen undergoing binary fission. Moreover, these bacilli are seen within the PAS-positive macrophages by which they have been phagocytosed and in which they undergo degeneration and disintegration (Fig. 68–3). It seems likely that much of the PAS-positive glycoprotein within the macrophage granules represents remnants of the cell wall of degenerated phagocytosed bacilli. The bacilli may be seen within villous absorptive cells, usually within large lysosomes in the apical cytoplasm, and within polymorphonuclear leukocytes, plasma cells, endothelial cells, and mast cells in the lamina propria.[24] The bacilli cannot be identified with certainty with the light microscope in routinely processed paraffin-embedded tissues; instead, electron microscopic or special high-resolution light microscopic techniques must be used for positive identification.[13]

Upon treatment with effective antibiotics, the mucosa of the small intestine gradually reverts toward normal (Fig. 68–1*B*). Viable-appearing bacilli disappear from the intercellular spaces within a few days, and after four to eight weeks only degenerating organisms can be identified within the cytoplasm of the PAS macrophages. Following effective treatment, the num-

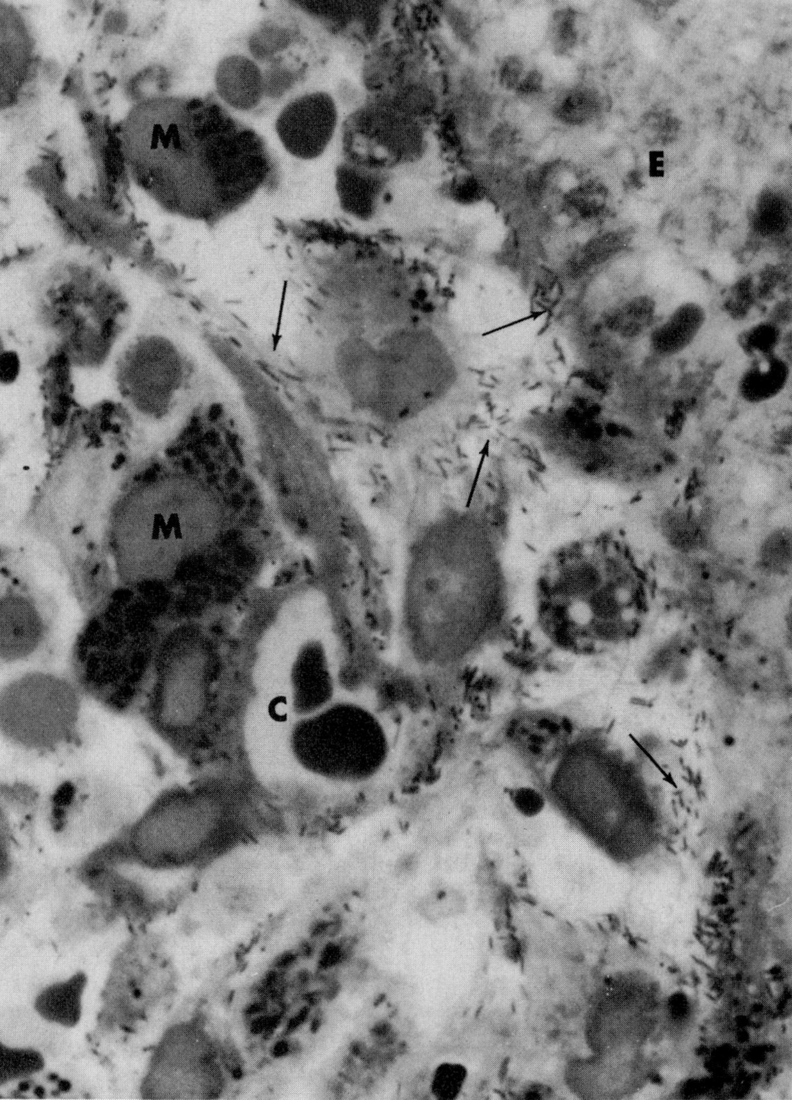

Figure 68–2. High-resolution light micrograph of the interface between epithelium and lamina propria from a patient with untreated Whipple's disease. The epithelium (E) is to the right. Numerous bacilli *(arrows)* are seen beneath the epithelium and between the cellular elements of the lamina propria. Several typical macrophages (M) can be seen. C, capillary. Osmium-fixed, epoxy embedded tissue, toluidine blue stain. Approximately × 1500. (From Trier, J. S., Phelps, P. C., Eidelman, S., and Rubin, C. E. Whipple's disease: light and electron microscope correlation of jejunal mucosal histology with antibiotic treatment and clinical status. Gastroenterology *48*:684–707. © by Williams & Wilkins, 1965.)

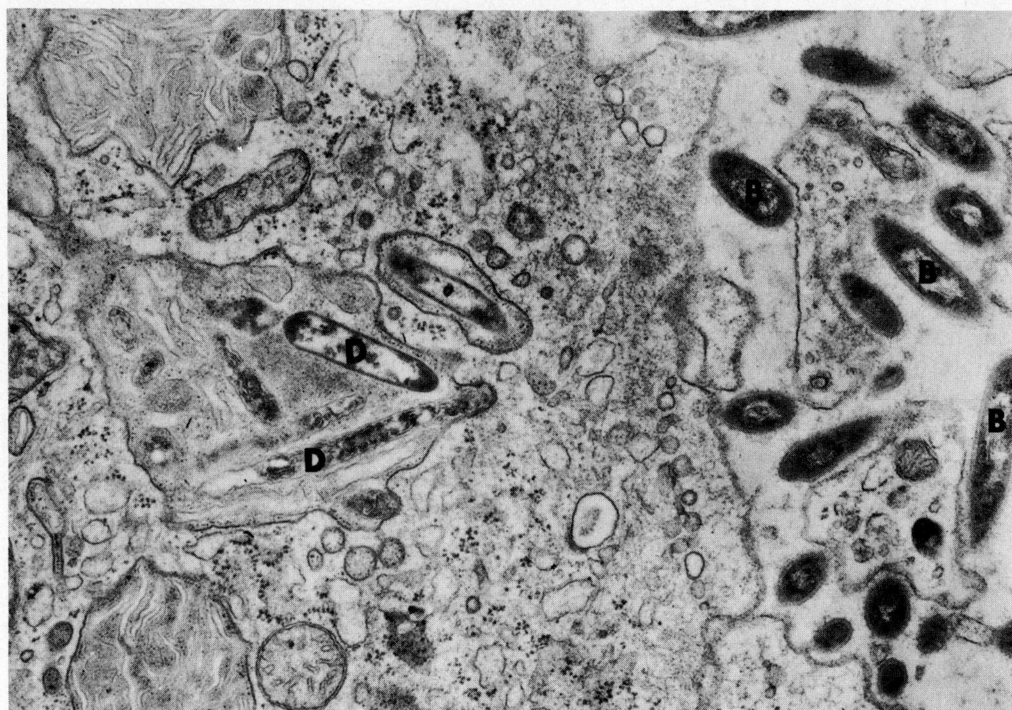

Figure 68–3. Electron micrograph of a portion of the cytoplasm of a PAS-positive macrophage and its extracellular space from a pretreatment biopsy. Many bacilli (B) are seen outside the macrophage. Within its cytoplasm, several disintegrating bacilli (D) are undergoing degeneration and contributing membranous material to a PAS-positive lysosomal granule. Portions of two other typical PAS-positive granules with their closely packed membranous material are visible above and below the granule that contains the degenerating organisms. Approximately × 23,000. (From Trier, J. S., Phelps, P. C., Eidelman, S., and Rubin, C. E. Whipple's disease: light and electron microscope correlation of jejunal mucosal histology with antibiotic treatment and clinical status. Gastroenterology *48*:684–707. © by Williams & Wilkins, 1965.)

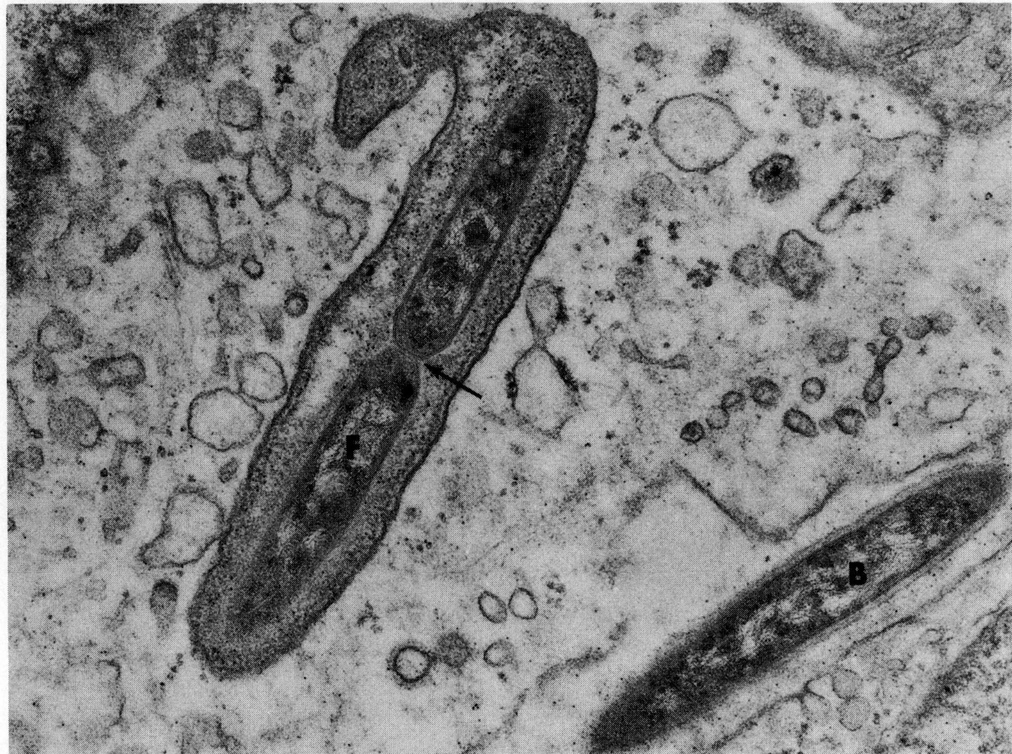

Figure 68–4. A portion of a PAS-positive macrophage from a patient with untreated Whipple's disease. A bacillus (B) is seen in the extracellular space. Within the cytoplasm of the macrophage, an organism (F) is undergoing binary fission (arrow). Approximately × 55,000. (From Trier, J. S., Phelps, P. C., Eidelman, S., and Rubin, C. E. Whipple's disease: light and electron microscope correlation of jejunal mucosal histology with antibiotic treatment and clinical status. Gastroenterology *48*:684–707. © by Williams & Wilkins, 1965.)

ber of PAS-positive macrophages in the lamina propria gradually decreases, and plasma cells, lymphocytes, and eosinophils reappear in normal numbers. Concomitantly, villous architecture and absorptive cell structure return toward normal. However, in many patients, mucosal histologic appearance may not revert completely to normal for years, if ever. Patchy accumulations of PAS-positive macrophages persist, especially around intestinal crypts, and dilated mucosal lymphatics and large lipid droplets may be found in the lamina propria of biopsies obtained from asymptomatic patients years after successful antibiotic treatment.

The colonic mucosa may or may not be involved in Whipple's disease. When involved, infiltration with PAS-positive macrophages and bacilli has been documented.[25] However, the finding of PAS-positive macrophages *without* demonstration of the bacilli in the colon is neither diagnostic nor specific; macrophages that contain cytoplasmic PAS-positive glycoprotein are occasionally seen in rectal and colonic mucosa of healthy individuals and are regularly found in patients with *colonic histiocytosis* or *melanosis coli.*

Extraintestinal Pathology. Systemic involvement in Whipple's disease is thoroughly documented. PAS-positive macrophages have been identified with the light microscope in most body tissues, including heart, lung, spleen, liver, endocrine glands, central nervous system (including cerebrum, cerebellum, thalamus, hypothalamus and spinal cord), bone, lymph nodes, and kidney.[2–4] The heart lesions are of particular interest, because endocardial infiltration of macrophages may cause grossly obvious vegetative endocarditis on the heart valves leading to functional stenosis or insufficiency. In some of these patients, secondary subacute streptococcal bacterial endocarditis has been noted at autopsy.

The typical bacilli have now been demonstrated with the electron microscope in many nonintestinal tissues, including peripheral and mesenteric lymph nodes, lung, liver, heart, artery, eye, synovial membrane, and brain of some patients with active disease.[14–20]

In Whipple's disease, as in other diseases that cause severe panmalabsorption, nonspecific pathologic changes secondary to severe malabsorption of nutrients may involve many organ systems. Thus *osteopenia*, severe *muscle wasting*, and *follicular hyperkeratosis* of the skin may be seen as secondary manifestations of the disease.

ETIOLOGY AND PATHOGENESIS

Although significant advances toward our understanding of the etiology and pathogenesis of Whipple's disease have been made in the past 25 years, many questions remain unanswered.

It is known that the mucosa of the small intestine and other involved tissues is invaded by numerous small, gram-positive bacilli in patients with active disease. The dramatic clinical improvement that parallels disappearance of these organisms during effective antibiotic therapy indicates that these bacilli play a significant role in the etiology of the disease. However, their exact role in the pathogenesis of this most unusual infection is not fully understood.

Attempts in a number of laboratories to isolate the responsible organism have yielded conflicting and, as yet, inconclusive results. Organisms that have been isolated from involved tissues and claimed to be the specific etiologic agent include aerobic corynebacteria, a *Hemophilus* species, a *Brucella*-like organism, and *l*-form streptococci.[26–30] In other laboratories, a specific organism could not be isolated consistently from multiple tissue samples known to contain many bacilli.[31] The PAS-positive material in intestinal mucosa reacts with antisera to group B and G streptococci and *B. shigella*.[29, 32, 33] The consistency of this reactivity coupled with the uniform ultrastructural features of the bacilli in involved tissues provides compelling evidence that a single distinctive bacterial species contributes to the course of Whipple's disease. However, identification of this organism awaits elucidation of its in vitro growth requirements and its consistent isolation from tissues of patients with Whipple's disease that are known to contain the bacillus.

Other factors, in addition to the difficulties in identifying the responsible organism, suggest that Whipple's disease is a most unusual infectious disease. It occurs sporadically and is so uncommon that it has been impossible to establish any epidemiologic pattern. Unlike most infectious diseases, there are no established cases of direct transmission of the illness from one patient to another, although on two occasions the disease has been reported in brothers. It seems likely that host susceptibility factors must play an important role in the pathogenesis of Whipple's disease in those few individuals who develop this disorder.

However, it has been difficult to define specific immunologic defects in this disease. Limited studies suggest a threefold increase in frequency of the class I histocompatibility antigen, HLA-B27.[33, 34] Serum immunoglobins are decreased in only a few patients during active disease and probably reflect protein leakage into the gut rather than a synthetic defect. Secretory IgA levels in intestinal secretions are also normal.[34, 35] Alterations of T cell function, including decreased responsiveness of lymphocytes to mitogens, impaired cutaneous responses to antigens, and delayed rejection of skin homografts, not explained by debilitating illness before effective treatment, have been reported by some,[34–36] but have been contested by others.[29, 30, 37] It is interesting that patients with Whipple's disease do not seem predisposed to other infections or diseases that might reflect impaired T cell function. Clearly, identification of a clear-cut T cell defect has not been simple and, if present, may be clarified only by studies in which abnormal T cell subsets are characterized in patients with Whipple's disease.

The nature and derivation of the peculiar macrophage that infiltrates affected tissues in Whipple's disease are also not clear. In a recent provocative report, impaired degradation of killed bacteria and zymosan particles by monocytes and peripheral blood monocyte-derived macrophages from a patient with treated Whipple's disease was described.[38] If confirmed, this defect would imply impaired macrophage function and help explain the long-term retention in macrophages of PAS-positive material derived from the Whipple's bacillus. In any case, the extensive infiltration of affected tissues with these large macrophages probably contributes to the clinical symptoms observed in patients. For example, infiltration of the lamina propria probably interferes with intestinal absorption, distorting villous architecture and impairing transport through the diseased lamina propria to vascular channels. Transport is further impaired by the extensively infiltrated and enlarged mesenteric lymph nodes that compromise the lymphatic drainage of the small intestine and prevent normal egress of absorbed material.

CLINICAL FEATURES AND DIAGNOSIS

The clinical presentation of patients with Whipple's disease may vary a great deal, depending upon which organ systems are involved and whether the disease is early or advanced. For example, the initial diagnosis has been established occasionally in patients with fever or joint or neurologic symptoms but without significant gastrointestinal complaints[39, 40] and, rarely, without evidence of intestinal involvement.[18, 41] In most patients, however, the diagnosis is not suspected until patients have prominent gastrointestinal symptoms. The disease may occur at any age, but is most common in the fourth and fifth decades of life. Men are affected much more often than women. Most reported cases have occurred in Caucasians, but the disease has been diagnosed in blacks and American Indians.

Symptoms. The gastrointestinal symptoms of Whipple's disease are not specific and resemble, in general, those seen in patients with other diseases in which generalized malabsorption is a feature. Diarrhea is usually but not invariably a prominent complaint, and the passage of as many as five to ten large, watery or semiformed, malodorous steatorrheal stools per day is common. Melena and hematochesia have been reported but are infrequent, whereas occult blood in the stool is common. Abdominal bloating and poorly localized, ill-defined abdominal cramps are often present. Anorexia is more common than in patients with celiac sprue and, together with malabsorption, may produce precipitous weight loss leading to profound cachexia. Fatigue, lassitude, and weakness are particularly severe in patients with severe anorexia and diarrhea. If the malabsorption continues unchecked, specific deficiencies usually develop, and these may cause extraintestinal symptoms as in other causes of malabsorption (see pp. 263–282). Thus, *paresthesias* and *hyperpathia* related to peripheral neuropathy, *tetany* caused by hypocalcemia or hypomagnesemia, and *purpura* caused by impaired coagulation may be present. Loss of substantial quantities of albumin into the intestinal lumen regularly accompanies severe diarrhea in Whipple's disease, especially when lymphatic obstruction from involved mesenteric nodes is pronounced; hence, peripheral edema and ascites may be prominent complaints (see pp. 283–290).

Extraintestinal symptoms may precede gastrointestinal complaints by many years in Whipple's disease. Of these, arthritis and fever are most common. About two thirds of patients have joint symptoms, and in one large series over 30 per cent had these symptoms for over five years before the diagnosis of Whipple's disease was established.[42] The severity of the arthropathy varies from patient to patient. An intermittent migratory arthritis that may affect both large and small joints is most common. Usually, a synovial reaction that waxes and wanes is evident with tenderness, redness, swelling, and increased heat of the affected joint. Unlike rheumatoid arthritis, permanent joint deformity is rare in Whipple's disease. Many patients have arthralgia only. Severe back pains suggest the presence of spondylitis, which has been documented in occasional patients. Significant fever is noted in over half the cases of Whipple's disease. The fever is usually low grade and intermittent, although it may be high, either spiking or sustained in advanced disease.

Chronic cough, present in Whipple's original patient,[1] is quite common. Pleuritic pain has also been noted, and both symptoms may reflect pulmonary involvement.[17, 43] Rarely, a sarcoid-like pulmonary illness may precede overt manifestations of Whipple's disease for several years.[23]

Because the endocardium, myocardium, pericardium, and even the coronary arteries may be involved in Whipple's disease,[16, 44] it is not surprising that these patients may have *congestive failure* and *symptomatic pericarditis*. Valvular lesions, especially of the mitral and aortic valves, may be sufficiently severe to cause hemodynamically significant stenosis or insufficiency. However, many patients with involvement of the heart have no cardiac symptoms.

Symptomatic involvement of the central nervous system may be present in up to 10 per cent of patients with Whipple's disease.[40, 41, 45–47] Neurologic symptoms may occur at the time of initial presentation in concert with those of other tissues (i.e., intestinal, musculoskeletal), as isolated symptoms in the absence of evident involvement of other organs,[41, 47, 48] or as the first sign of relapse following apparently effective treatment.[45, 49] A broad range of symptoms has been reported, for virtually all portions of the brain or spinal cord may be involved. Symptoms may include *dementia* with disorientation and loss of memory, *headache, lethargy* progressing to coma, *convulsions, muscle weakness, sensory deficits, incoordination, polydipsia*, and various cranial nerve symptoms such as *deafness, tinnitus, dysarthria, facial numbness, diplopia*, and *diminished visual acuity*. Visual symptoms may also reflect involvement of the eyes. The bacillus and PAS-positive macrophages have been identified in vitreous aspirates, and vitreous opacities, uveitis, and chorioretinitis have been described.[15, 50]

Physical Findings. Many of the physical findings in Whipple's disease are related to severe intestinal panmalabsorption and are identical to those discussed on pages 263 to 282. These findings may include profound emaciation with fat and muscle wasting, clubbing of the fingernails, hypotension caused by fluid and electrolyte loss, increased skin pigmentation, peripheral edema related to enteric protein loss, purpura, cheilosis and glossitis, increased muscular irritability or even frank tetany caused by hypocalcemia, and loss of sensory modalities in the extremities related to peripheral neuropathy.

Palpable, moderately enlarged peripheral lymph nodes are common; these nodes are usually firm, nontender, and freely movable. Peripheral joints may be swollen, warm, reddened, and tender if arthritis is present. Heart murmurs, when present, may be caused by valvular involvement, but functional systolic murmurs caused by anemia are more common. The presence of secondary acute or subacute bacterial endocarditis must be considered in febrile patients with Whipple's disease who have diastolic murmurs. Pleural or pericardial friction rubs signal involvement of these serosal membranes.

The abdomen is usually distended and, in about half of reported cases, is slightly to moderately tender. Periumbilical fullness or an ill-defined mass may be palpated and may be due to enlargement of the mesenteric lymph nodes. Ascites is uncommon and, when present, is usually associated with severe hypoalbuminemia. Hepatosplenomegaly is uncommon.

Neurologic signs, other than those caused by malabsorption-induced peripheral neuropathy, include confusion, dementia, nystagmus and ophthalmoplegia, other cranial nerve signs, ataxia, muscle weakness, sensory loss, and posterior column signs.[41, 45–49] Meningeal signs, though rare, may occur.[45] Patients in remission, in particular, must be carefully monitored for the appearance of neurologic symptoms or signs heralding relapse.

Laboratory Findings. Most of the laboratory abnormalities found in Whipple's disease patients are causally related to severe intestinal malabsorption (see pp. 272–279). Thus, *steatorrhea, defective xylose absorption*, and *low serum carotene* and *cholesterol* levels are common. In patients with severe diarrhea and malabsorption, hypokalemia, hypocalcemia, hypomagnesemia, and significant hypoalbuminemia are common.

Anemia is common and is usually associated with iron deficiency. Microcytic, hypochromic red blood cells and low serum iron levels accompany the anemia. In some patients there is macrocytosis caused by folate deficiency. In others serum iron, folate, and vitamin B_{12} are normal, and anemia may be of the type seen in chronic infections. Stools often contain occult blood. Mild to moderate leukocytosis may be present, especially in febrile patients. In patients with neurologic manifestations, pleocytosis, including PAS-positive mononuclear cells, has been observed in the spinal fluid of some,[41] but not all,[45] patients. Low density, contrast enhancing lesions may be evident by computed tomography, which has led to diagnostic brain biopsy in the absence of demonstrable disease in other organs.[48]

X-ray films of the small intestine following a barium meal are generally abnormal.[51] The most characteristic finding is marked thickening of the mucosal folds (plicae circulares), especially in the duodenum and proximal jejunum, suggesting infiltrative disease (Fig. 68–5*A*). In most patients there is a gradient of decreasing involvement as the distal jejunum is approached, and the ileum may appear normal. In severe disease the ileum may also appear abnormal. Dilatation of the small intestine is not usually as prominent as in other primary intestinal malabsorptive diseases such as celiac sprue. Following successful treatment with antibiotics, the thickening of the mucosal folds becomes less marked (Fig. 68–5); in fact, the radiologic appearance of the small intestine often reverts to normal.

Biopsy Studies. Although Whipple's disease may often be suspected on the basis of symptoms, physical signs, and laboratory findings, its diagnosis can be established only by histologic examination of the involved tissues.

Prior to the development of peroral intestinal biopsy methods, the diagnosis was usually established by biopsy of small intestine or involved mesenteric lymph nodes at laparotomy. Occasionally, biopsies of enlarged peripheral lymph nodes established the diagnosis. Now, the biopsy procedure of choice for establishing or excluding the diagnosis of Whipple's disease is peroral biopsy of the small intestine in the region of the duodenojejunal junction. This portion of the small bowel is involved in the great majority of symptomatic patients, even early in the disease when steatorrhea may be mild or absent.[39, 40] Moreover, the infiltration of the lamina propria of the small intestine by PAS-positive macrophages containing gram-positive, acid-fast negative bacilli accompanied by lymphatic dilatation is specific and diagnostic for Whipple's disease. As noted, enlarged whitish villi may be seen endoscopically.

In contrast, rectal biopsy may be misleading and is not a substitute for peroral small intestinal biopsy. PAS-positive macrophages resembling closely those seen in Whipple's disease may be found in the rectal lamina propria in benign conditions, such as melanosis coli, as well as in normal patients.

DIFFERENTIAL DIAGNOSIS

The lack of specificity of the gastrointestinal symptoms in Whipple's disease precludes definitive diagnosis without histologic confirmation. However, the coexistence of malabsorption, arthritis, adenopathy, fever, and the rather characteristic radiologic appearance of the small intestine should alert the clinician to the possible diagnosis and lead to biopsy of the mucosa of the small intestine.

It must be emphasized that joint symptoms often

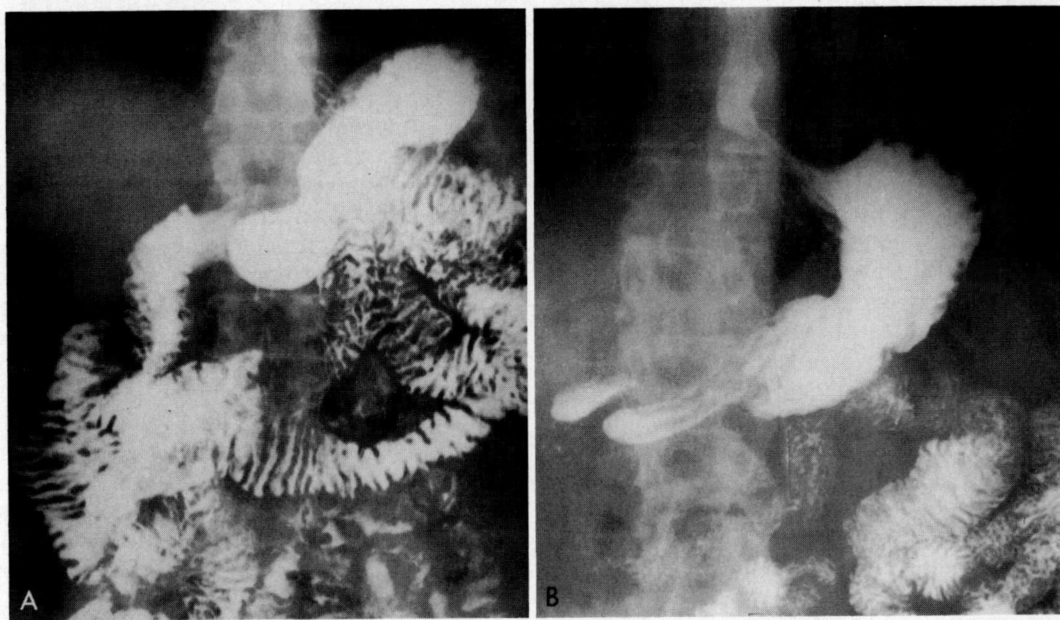

Figure 68–5. Barium contrast studies of the small intestine from a patient with Whipple's disease before *(A)* and after *(B)* treatment with antibiotics. Before treatment, there are marked thickening of the plicae circulares and a loss of the normal delicate mucosal relief pattern. There is less dilatation of the small intestine than is usually seen in films of patients with severe untreated celiac sprue. After treatment, the mucosal pattern appears much more normal, with a reduction in the thickness of the plicae circulares and partial return of the normal mucosal pattern. (Courtesy of Elihu Schimmel, M.D.)

precede by months or years the onset of intestinal symptoms in patients with Whipple's disease.[42] Such patients may initially seek medical care in arthritis clinics. Clearly, the diagnosis of Whipple's disease must be considered in any patient with arthralgia or arthritis who develops diarrhea, malabsorption, or unexplained weight loss, especially if the arthritis cannot be precisely categorized. Tests for rheumatoid factor are negative in patients with arthritis caused by Whipple's disease, and the serum uric acid level is usually normal.[42] The fever of Whipple's disease may occasionally precede gastrointestinal symptoms by months. Thus, Whipple's disease must be included among the ever-growing list of entities that may present with fever of unknown origin.

Increasingly, patients who present with CNS symptoms,[41, 47, 48] ocular involvement,[50] and pulmonary manifestations[23] in the absence of intestinal symptoms are being identified; hence, a high index of suspicion is needed if the physician is to make a timely diagnosis of Whipple's disease. If there is histologic involvement of the small intestine, the diagnosis is then established by peroral intestinal biopsy that readily permits differentiation of Whipple's disease from other diffuse mucosal diseases such as celiac sprue. Particular care must be taken to distinguish between patients with Whipple's disease and patients with acquired immunodeficiency syndrome (AIDS) who have developed intestinal infection with *Mycobacterium avium intracellulare*. The lesions in these two conditions are histologically similar; both show infiltration of the lamina propria with PAS-positive macrophages.[52, 53] Both conditions may present with malabsorption and diarrhea; however, they can be readily distinguished by an acid-fast stain of biopsy sections because the Whipple's bacillus is not acid-fast, as is *Mycobacterium avium intracellulare* (see p. 1246). In the rare instances in which the small intestine is spared, biopsy of other organs whose involvement is suggested by symptoms or physical findings may be needed to establish the diagnosis of Whipple's disease.[18, 41, 47, 48, 50]

TREATMENT AND PROGNOSIS

Treatment. The administration of effective antibiotic therapy in patients with Whipple's disease is lifesaving and results in prompt and dramatic clinical improvement. The fever and joint symptoms disappear within a few days, and the diarrhea and malabsorption disappear within two to four weeks or even sooner.

Many antibiotic regimens, administered for a few months to several years, have been used successfully. These include penicillin alone, penicillin and streptomycin in combination, erythromycin, ampicillin, tetracyclines, chloramphenicol, and trimethoprim-sulfamethoxazole.[5, 12, 13, 19, 45, 54–56] However, the optimal regimen, in regard to both agent and duration of treatment, has not been established. The initial response of patients without CNS disease to any antibiotic effective against gram-positive organisms is predictably good. However, relapses are common and may occur months or years after apparently successful treatment, even after prolonged administration of antibiotics or while therapy is still in progress.[13, 49, 55] In a recent survey of 88 patients responding to antibiotic treatment, 31 showed evidence of relapse.[55] The increasing recognition of neurologic sequelae months or years following successful treatment suggests that the central nervous system may provide a safe haven for residual Whipple's bacilli unless an antibiotic that readily penetrates the blood-brain barrier is used. That such agents can reverse significant neurologic disease has recently been well documented.[45, 56] It would seem prudent to treat newly diagnosed patients or patients in relapse with trimethoprim-sulfamethoxazole for four to six months and, if there was intestinal involvement, to obtain an intestinal biopsy before discontinuing therapy to document disappearance of the Whipple's bacillus. If trimethoprim-sulfamethoxazole cannot be tolerated, use of chloramphenicol is an option, although this potentially toxic agent may not be required by the majority of patients. Another alternative in the patient intolerant to trimethoprim-sulfamethoxazole is to initiate treatment with penicillin or ampicillin, but carefully monitor the patient indefinitely and introduce chloramphenicol immediately should CNS symptoms develop. Until controlled prospective studies are available, it is impossible to recommend dogmatically an ideal antibiotic regimen.

As in other diseases with severe intestinal malabsorption, appropriate replacement therapy designed to correct specific deficiencies is indicated in Whipple's disease. Because absorptive function improves rapidly after initiation of antibiotic treatment, such supplementation, discussed in detail on pages 279 to 280, usually need not be protracted. Fluid and electrolyte replacement should be administered when needed, anemic patients should receive iron or folate as indicated, vitamin D and calcium should be given at least until steatorrhea disappears, and parenteral calcium or magnesium or both are indicated in patients who develop tetany. Because most patients in whom the diagnosis is established are malnourished, the diet should be high in calories and protein and should be supplemented with a therapeutic formula vitamin preparation until absorptive function has returned to normal. Long-term parenteral alimentation is rarely indicated.

Prognosis. The prognosis for patients with this previously fatal disease is now excellent, and most patients are completely asymptomatic within one to three months after the start of antibiotic treatment. After antibiotics are discontinued, patients must be carefully observed for symptoms of relapse. Recurrence may be heralded by intestinal symptoms or by symptoms involving other organ systems in the absence of intestinal symptoms. Relapse with neurologic symptoms is the most ominous and may lead to permanent sequelae.[46, 49] In our experience, some residual lymphatic dilation and persistence of a few PAS-positive macrophages in the absence of bacilli are seen in jejunal biopsies obtained up to ten years after antibiotic treatment in some asymptomatic patients. Thus, the presence of macrophages alone in the absence of bacilli does not imply active disease. Relapse may be preceded by the reappearance of the typical bacilli in the mucosa of the small intestine. In fact, the bacilli have been noted to reappear several months before the recurrence of overt clinical symptoms of relapse and, when recognized, permit prediction of an impending relapse in an asymptomatic patient.[13]

References

1. Whipple, G. H. A hitherto undescribed disease characterized anatomically by deposits of fat and fatty acids in the intestinal and mesenteric lymphatic tissues. Bull. Johns Hopkins Hosp. *18*:382, 1907.
2. Hendrix, J. P., Black-Schaffer, B., Withers, R. W., and Handler, P. Whipple's intestinal lipodystrophy. Arch. Intern. Med. *85*:91, 1950.
3. Upton, A. C. Histochemical investigation of the mesenchymal lesions in Whipple's disease. Am. J. Clin. Pathol. *22*:755, 1952.
4. Sieracki, J. C., and Fine, G. Whipple's disease—observations on systemic involvement. II. Gross and histologic observations. Arch. Pathol. *67*:81, 1959.
5. Paulley, J. W. A case of Whipple's disease (intestinal lipodystrophy). Gastroenterology *22*:128, 1952.
6. Gross, J. B., Wollaeger, E. E., Sauer, W. G., Huizenga, K. A., Dahlin, D. C., and Power, M. H. Whipple's disease. Gastroenterology *36*:65, 1959.
7. Puite, R. H., and Tesluk, H. Whipple's disease. Am. J. Med. *19*:383, 1955.
8. Cohen, A. S., Schimmel, E. M., Holt, P. R., and Isselbacher, K. J. Ultrastructural abnormalities in Whipple's disease. Proc. Soc. Exp. Biol. Med. *105*:411, 1960.
9. Chears, W. C., and Ashworth, C. T. Electron microscopic study of the intestinal mucosa in Whipple's disease. Gastroenterology *41*:129, 1961.
10. Yardley, J. H., and Hendrix, T. R. Combined electron and light microscopy in Whipple's disease. Bull. Johns Hopkins Hosp. *109*:80, 1961.
11. Kurtz, S. M., Davis, T. D., Jr., and Ruffin, J. M. Light and electron microscopic studies of Whipple's disease. Lab. Invest. *11*:653, 1962.
12. Davis, T. D., Jr., McBee, J. W., Borland, J. L., Kurtz, S. M., and Ruffin, J. M. The effect of antibiotics and steroid therapy in Whipple's disease. Gastroenterology *44*:112, 1963.
13. Trier, J. S., Phelps, P. C., Eidelman, S., and Rubin, C. E. Whipple's disease: Light and electron microscope correlation of jejunal mucosal histology with antibiotic treatment and clinical status. Gastroenterology *48*:694, 1965.
14. Kojecky, Z., Malinsky, J., Kodousek, R., and Marsalek, E. Frequency of occurrence of microbes in the intestinal mucosa and in the lymph nodes during long-term observations of a patient suffering from Whipple's disease. Gastroenterologica *101*:163, 1964.
15. Selsky, E. J., Knox, D. L., Maumenee, A. E., and Green, W. R. Ocular involvement in Whipple's disease. Retina *4*:103, 1984.
16. Lie, J. T., and Davis, J. S. Pancarditis in Whipple's disease. Am. J. Clin. Pathol. *66*:22, 1976.
17. Winberg, C. D., Rose, M. E., and Rappaport, H. Whipple's disease of the lung. Am. J. Med. *65*:873, 1978.
18. Mansbach, C. M., II, Shelburne, J. D., Stevens, R. D., and Dobbins, W. O., III. Lymph-node bacilliform bodies resembling those of Whipple's disease in a patient without intestinal involvement. Ann. Intern. Med. *88*:64, 1978.
19. Viteri, A. L., Stinson, J. C., Barnes, M. C., and Dyck, W. P. Rod-shaped organism in the liver of a patient with Whipple's disease. Am. J. Dig. Dis. *24*:560, 1979.
20. Johnson, L., and Diamond, I. Cerebral Whipple's disease. Diagnosis by brain biopsy. Am. J. Clin. Pathol. *74*:486, 1980.
21. Riemann, J. F., and Rosch, W. Synopsis of endoscopic and related morphological findings in Whipple's disease. Endoscopy *10*:98, 1978.
22. Black-Schaffer, B. The tinctoral demonstration of a glycoprotein in Whipple's disease. Proc. Soc. Exp. Biol. Med. *72*:225, 1949.
23. Cho, C., Linscheer, W. G., Hirschkorn, M. A., and Ashutosh, K. Sarcoidlike granulomas as an early manifestation of Whipple's disease. Gastroenterology *87*:941, 1984.
24. Dobbins, W. O., III, and Kawanishi, H. Bacillary characteristics

in Whipple's disease: An electron microscopic study. Gastroenterology *80*:1469, 1981.
25. Gonzales-Licea, A., and Yardley, J. H. Whipple's disease in the rectum. Am. J. Pathol. *52*:1191, 1969.
26. Caroli, J., Julien, C., Eteve, J., Prévot, A. R., and Sebald, M. Trois cas de maladi de Whipple. Remarques cliniques, biologiques, histologiques et thérapeutiques. Étudie au microscope électronique de al muqueuse jéjunale. Démonstrations de l'origine bactérienne de l'affection, isolement et identification du germe en cause. Sem. Hop. (Paris) *39*:1457, 1963.
27. Kok, N., Dybkaer, R., and Rostgaard, J. Bacteria in Whipple's disease. I. Results of cultivation from repeated jejunal biopsies prior to, during and after effective antibiotic treatment. Acta Pathol. Microbiol. Scand. *60*:431, 1964.
28. Carache, P., Bayless, T. M., Shelley, W. M., and Hendrix, T. R. Atypical bacteria in Whipple's disease. Trans. Assoc. Am. Phys. *69*:399, 1966.
29. Clancy, R. L., Tomkins, W. A. F., Muckle, T. J., Richardson, H., and Rawls, W. E. Isolation and characterization of an aetiological agent in Whipple's disease. Br. Med. J. *3*:569, 1975.
30. Tytgat, G. N., Hoogendijk, J. L., Agenant, D., and Schelekens, P. T. Etiopathogenetic studies in a patient with Whipple's disease. Digestion *15*:309, 1977.
31. Sherris, J. C., Roberts, C. E., and Porus, R. L. Microbiological studies of intestinal biopsies taken during active Whipple's disease. Gastroenterology *48*:708, 1965.
32. Keren, D. F., Weisberger, W. R., Yardley, J. H., Salyer, W. R., Arthur, R. R., and Charache, P. Whipple's disease: Demonstration by immunofluorescence of similar bacterial antigens in macrophages from three cases. Johns Hopkins Med. J. *139*:51, 1976.
33. Kent, S. P., and Kirkpatrick, P. M. Whipple's disease: Immunological and histochemical studies of eight cases. Arch. Pathol. Lab. Med. *104*:544, 1980.
34. Dobbins, W. O., III. Whipple's Disease. Springfield, Illinois, C. C. Thomas, 1987, pp. 64–73.
35. Groll, A., Valberg, L. S., Simon, J. B., Eidinger, D., Wilson, B., and Forsdyke, D. R. Immunological defect in Whipple's disease. Gastroenterology *63*:943, 1972.
36. Martin, F. F., Vilsek, J., Dobbins, W. O., Buckley, C. E., and Tyor, M. P. Immunological alterations in patients with treated Whipple's disease. Gastroenterology *63*:6, 1972.
37. Keren, D. F., Weinrieb, I. J., Bertovich, M. J., and Brady, P. G. Whipple's disease: No consistent mitogenic or cytotoxic defect in lymphocyte function from three cases. Gastroenterology *77*:991, 1979.
38. Bjerknes, R., Laerum, O. D., and Odegaard, S. Impaired bacterial degradation by monocytes and macrophages from a patient with treated Whipple's disease. Gastroenterology *89*:1139, 1985.
39. Hargrove, M. D., Jr., Verner, J. V., Jr., Patrick, R. L., and Ruffin, J. M. Intestinal lipodystrophy without diarrhea. JAMA *173*:1125, 1960.
40. Moorthy, S., Nolley, G., and Hermos, J. A. Whipple's disease with minimal intestinal involvement. Gut *18*:152, 1977.
41. Feurle, G. E., Volk, B., and Waldherr, R. Cerebral Whipple's disease with negative jejunal histology. N. Engl. J. Med. *300*:907, 1979.
42. Kelly, J. J., III, and Weisiger, B. W. The arthritis of Whipple's disease. Arth. Rheum. *6*:615, 1963.
43. Symmons, D. P., Shepherd, A. N., Boardman, P. L., and Bacon, P. A. Pulmonary manifestations of Whipple's disease. Q. J. Med. *56*:497, 1985.
44. James, T. N., and Bulkley, B. H. Abnormalities of the coronary arteries in Whipple's disease. Am. Heart J. *105*:481, 1983.
45. Feldman, M., Hendler, R. S., and Morrison, E. B. Acute meningoencephalitis after withdrawal of antibiotics in Whipple's disease. Ann. Intern. Med. *93*:709, 1980.
46. Schmitt, B. P., Richardson, H., Smith, E., and Kaplan, R. Encephalopathy complicating Whipple's disease. Failure to respond to antibiotics. Ann. Intern. Med. *94*:51, 1981.
47. Romanul, F. C. A., Radvany, J., and Rosales, R. K. Whipple's disease confined to the brain: A case studied clinically and pathologically. J. Neurol. Neurosurg. Psychiatr. *40*:901, 1977.
48. Halperin, J. J., Landis, D. M., and Kleinman, G. M. Whipple disease of the nervous system. Neurology *32*:612, 1982.
49. Knox, D. L., Bayless, T. M., and Pittman, F. E. Neurologic disease in patients with treated Whipple's disease. Medicine *55*:467, 1976.
50. Avila, M. P., Jalkh, A. E., Feldman, E., Trempe, C. L., and Schepens, C. L. Manifestations of Whipple's disease in the posterior segment of the eye. Arch. Ophthalmol. *102*:384, 1984.
51. Philips, R. L., and Carlson, H. C. The roentgenographic and clinical findings in Whipple's disease. Am. J. Roentgenol. Radium Ther. Nucl. Med. *123*:269, 1975.
52. Billen, J. S., Urmacher, C., West, R., and Shike, M. Disseminated *Mycobacterium avium-intracellulare* infection in acquired immunodeficiency syndrome mimicking Whipple's disease. Gastroenterology *85*:1187, 1983.
53. Roth, R. I., Owen, R. L., Keren, D. F., and Valberding, P. A. Intestinal infection with *Mycobacterium avium* in acquired immune deficiency syndrome (AIDS). Histological and clinical comparison with Whipple's disease. Dig. Dis. Sci. *30*:497, 1985.
54. Elsborg, L., Gravgaard, E., and Jacobsen, N. O. Treatment of Whipple's disease with sulphamethoxazole-trimethoprim. Acta Med. Scand. *198*:141, 1975.
55. Keinath, R. D., Merrell, D. E., Vlietstra, R., and Dobbins, W. O., III. Antibiotic treatment and relapse in Whipple's disease. Long-term follow-up of 88 patients. Gastroenterology *88*:1867, 1985.
56. Ryser, R. J., Locksley, R. M., Eng, S. C., Dobbins, W. O., III, Schoenknecht, F. D., and Rubin, C. E. Reversal of dementia associated with Whipple's disease by trimethoprim-sulfamethoxazole, drugs that penetrate the blood-brain barrier. Gastroenterology *86*:745, 1984.

69

The Pseudomembranous Enterocolitides

JOHN G. BARTLETT

Pseudomembranous enterocolitis (PMC) was first described in the nineteenth century and has subsequently been recognized with increasing frequency as a serious, sometimes lethal, gastrointestinal disease. The common thread, regardless of clinical setting, is gross or histologic evidence of pseudomembranous exudative plaques attached to the mucosal surface of the small intestine, colon, or both. A variety of seemingly unrelated risk factors have been identified, suggesting that this represents a nonspecific response to heterogeneous insults. However, the vast majority of cases reported during the past three decades have occurred in association with antibiotic exposure. The etiology of antibiotic-associated pseudomembranous enterocolitis was commonly ascribed to *Staphylococcus aureus* in the 1950s, but more recent studies implicate a toxin or toxins produced by *Clostridium difficile* in the great majority of cases.

HISTORICAL PERSPECTIVE

Studies of pseudomembranous enterocolitis may be divided into three periods with somewhat differing observations (Table 69–1). The initial period dates from the original report by Finney in 1893 to the beginning of the antibiotic era.[1–3] There were a variety of associated risk factors in these patients, but nearly all had debilitating diseases. The most common setting at this time was intestinal surgery, which was usually for colonic carcinoma and was often complicated by hypotension.[3] A typical presentation was a patient who underwent surgery, appeared to do well postoperatively, and then suddenly deteriorated with abdominal pain, distention, diarrhea, vomiting, and hypotension. Autopsy studies showed typical pseudomembranous lesions of the small and large bowel, e.g., "enterocolitis." The incidence of the disease was relatively low as reflected in the experience at the Mayo Clinic and Mount Sinai Hospital in New York which showed an average of only four cases annually.[2, 3]

The second period of study followed shortly after the availability of antibiotics and lasted until the late 1960s. Antibiotics, primarily chloramphenicol, tetracyclines, and oral neomycin, became recognized risk factors; many of the patients had received these agents prophylactically for surgery, and *Staphylococcus aureus* became a commonly accepted pathogen.[4–10] During this period, the terms "pseudomembranous colitis," "postoperative enterocolitis," "antibiotic-associated colitis," and "staphylococcal enterocolitis" were often used interchangeably. Evidence implicating *S. aureus* was usually based on cultures, and Gram stains of stool,[4–8] studies of an enterotoxin produced by implicated strains,[11–13] and work with the chinchilla model.[14, 15] Many patients were treated with oral vancomycin with good results to provide further support for the etiologic role of *S. aureus*.[16] "Staphylococcal enteritis" was a frequent diagnosis, especially in postoperative patients receiving broad-spectrum antibiotics, in whom incidence reports ranged as high as 14 per cent in one study[6] and 27 per cent in another.[7] However, critical analysis of these reports cast doubt on the frequency of this complication, and some authorities questioned the etiologic role of *S. aureus* at that time.[17, 18]

The third period of study is from the early 1970s to the present when there was major progress in case detection, epidemiology, etiology, and therapy. The initial reports showed incidence data and anatomic descriptions made possible by the extensive use of endoscopy.[19–25] Several large series were published and there was considerable attention to the frequency with which clindamycin was implicated. A notable feature of the reports was that *S. aurues* was rarely recovered in stool cultures. It was concluded that if this organism was once an agent of antibiotic-associated colitis as

Table 69–1. STUDIES OF PSEUDOMEMBRANOUS ENTEROCOLITIS

	Preantibiotic Era	1952–1965	1970–1982
Major risk	Intestinal surgery (others, see text)	Antibiotics—especially chloramphenicol, tetracycline, and oral neomycin	Antibiotics—especially clindamycin, ampicillin, and cephalosporins
Suspected cause	Ischemia	*S. aureus*	*C. difficile*
Etiologic diagnosis	None	Stool culture and stain	*C. difficile* toxin assay
Location	Small bowel and/or colon	Small bowel and/or colon	Colon
Anatomic diagnosis	Autopsy	Usually not done	Endoscopy
Treatment	None	Vancomycin	Vancomycin, metronidazole
Prognosis	Poor	Variable	Good

previously suggested, it no longer appeared to play an important role.[25] This experience led to the use of experimental animals to detect a transferrable agent and resulted in compelling evidence that a toxin produced by *C. difficile* was responsible for most cases.[26–29]

PATHOLOGY

Pseudomembranous enterocolitis is a pathologic diagnosis which may take a variety of forms, depending on the nature of the associated condition and the time frame in which the patient is examined. The common denominator is the presence of pseudomembranes on the intestinal mucosa, which may be located in the small bowel (pseudomembranous enteritis), colon (pseudomembranous colitis, or PMC), or both (pseudomembranous enterocolitis). Most cases have been associated with antimicrobial usage in which changes are nearly always restricted to the colon, e.g., antibiotic-associated PMC. This is in contrast to pseudomembranous enterocolitis that is not associated with antibiotic usage and "staphylococcal enterocolitis" in which small bowel involvement was relatively common.[1–3, 7, 30–33] On gross inspection there are multiple elevated yellowish white plaques which vary in size from a few millimeters to 10 to 20 mm (Fig. 69–1). The intervening mucosa appears normal or shows hyperemia and edema. Early lesions are punctate, and with advanced disease, the pseudomembranes may coalesce and eventually slough to leave large denuded areas. According to recent studies, antibiotic-associated PMC is rarely a segmental disease, and pseudomembranes are usually distributed throughout the colon.

Histologic studies show the pseudomembrane typically arises from a point of superficial ulceration and is accompanied by an acute or chronic inflammatory infiltrate in the lamina propria[34, 35] (Fig. 69–2). The pseudomembrane is composed of fibrin, mucin, sloughed mucosal epithelial cells, and acute inflammatory cells. The spectrum of changes have been classified by Price and Davis into three categories, which appear to be rather uniform in any individual patient.[35] The earliest and most mild form consists of focal necrosis with a polymorphonuclear infiltrate and eosinophilic exudate in the lamina propria. Splaying out from the necrotic focus is a collection of fibrin and polymorphonuclear cells to form a characteristic "summit lesion." The second category, which appears to represent more advanced disease, shows glandular disruption and a focal polymorphonuclear cell infiltrate surmounted by typical pseudomembranes which may appear as a volcanic eruption (Fig. 69–2*B*). With both these lesions there are areas of intervening mucosa which appear normal, and the inflammatory infiltrate is generally limited to the superficial portion of the lamina propria, predominantly subepithelial in location. The third and most advanced form of the disease shows complete structural necrosis with extensive involvement of the lamina propria, which is overlaid by a thick confluent pseudomembrane. Bacterial invasion of the bowel mucosa was not found in the earlier studies ascribed to *S. aureus* or the more recent studies implicating *C. difficile*. Similarly, no typical bacterial morphotype is usually seen within the pseudomembrane.

UNDERLYING AND ASSOCIATED CONDITIONS

The initial reports of pseudomembranous enteritis antedated the antibiotic era, and a number of risk factors have been identified. The most common clinical setting in cases not associated with antimicrobial agents is surgery, primarily colonic, gastric, or pelvic.[1–3, 7, 30] Other risk factors include spinal fracture, intestinal obstruction, colonic carcinoma, leukemia, severe burns, shock, uremia, heavy metal poisoning, the hemolytic-uremic syndrome, ischemic cardiovascular dis-

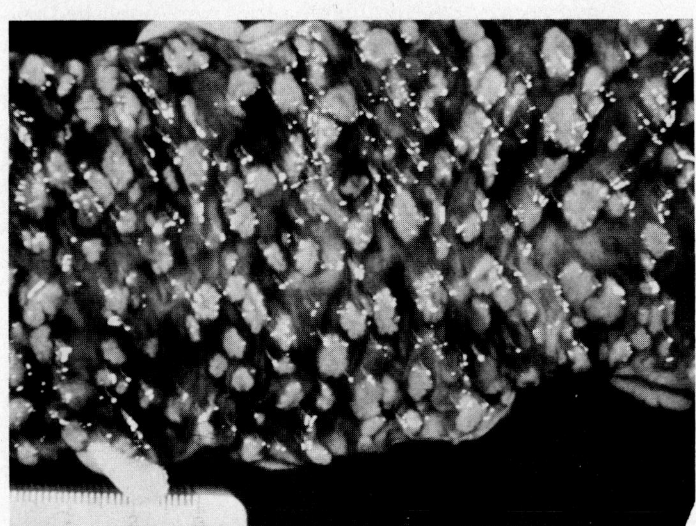

Figure 69–1. Pseudomembrane formation in colon. Note the flat, raised lesions, varying in size from a few millimeters to 8 mm. The intervening mucosa is hyperemic.

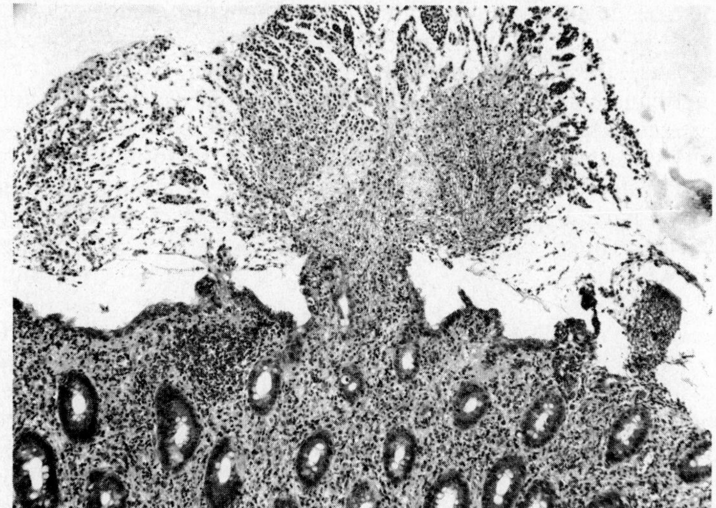

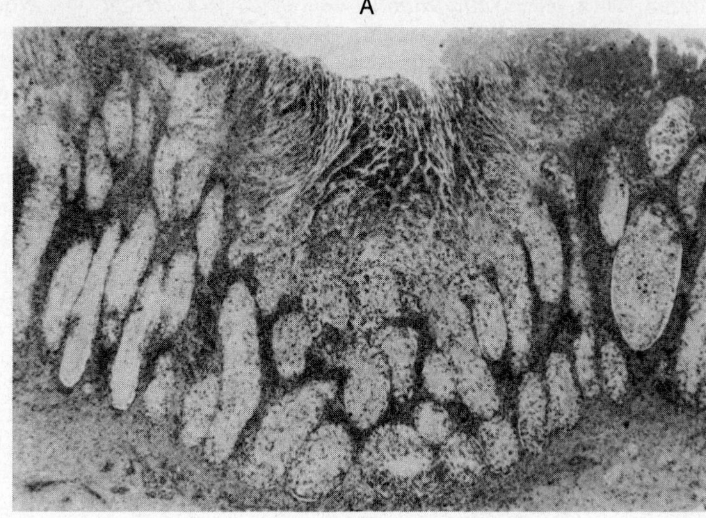

Figure 69–2. *A,* Microscopic pathologic appearance of a pseudomembrane in colon of a homosexual male who had received ampicillin and developed toxic megacolon. (Courtesy of M. Sleisenger, San Francisco.) *B,* Microscopic pathologic changes of pseudomembrane in colon associated wtih clindamycin. The pseudomembrane, composed of fibrin and inflammatory cells, arises on top of a mucosal ulceration. The surrounding mucosa is intact but filled with a mixed inflammatory infiltrate. (From Sumner, H. W., and Tedesco, F. J. Arch. Pathol. *99*:238, 1975. Copyright © 1975, American Medical Association.)

ease, Crohn's disease, shigellosis, severe infection, neonatal necrotizing enterocolitis, ischemic colitis, and Hirschsprung's disease.[36–42] Additionally, occasional cases have been encountered in previously healthy individuals in whom there was no recent antimicrobial exposure and no other identifiable risk factor.[43–45]

Despite the diversity of clinical settings noted above, the vast majority of pseudomembranous colitis cases observed during the past four decades have occurred in association with antimicrobial usage.[4–10, 19–25, 27–34] Nearly all antimicrobial agents with an antibacterial spectrum of activity have been implicated in PMC. Reports in the 1970s emphasized the role of clindamycin and its parent compound, lincomycin. The incidence of this complication with clindamycin or lincomycin varies from 0.01 per cent to as high as 10 per cent, depending on a large extent on the frequency of endoscopy and the epidemiologic patterns of *C. difficile*, which is the major pathogen.[23, 25, 46] However, it is important to recognize that many other antimicrobial agents may be associated with this disease (Table 69–2). More recent studies show that cephalosporins and ampicillin are implicated even more frequently than clindamycin, although the incidence with these agents is probably less than that with clindamycin when relative utilization rates are taken into account.[47–49] Antineoplastic compounds which have antibacterial activity have also been implicated.[42] There is a curious paucity

Table 69–2. ANTIMICROBIALS IMPLICATED IN *CLOSTRIUM DIFFICILE*–INDUCED DIARRHEA OR COLITIS*

	Number of Patients	Single Agent†
Ampicillin or amoxicillin	109	82
Clindamycin	87	56
Cephalosporins	94	55
Penicillins other than ampicillin and amoxicillin	49	19
Sulfamethoxazole-trimethoprim	16	8
Other antimicrobial agents	38	13

*Analysis of 329 patients with antibiotic-associated diarrhea or colitis and positive toxin assays including 136 with confirmed PMC. Systemically administered aminoglycosides were omitted owing to lack of evidence that these agents are implicated.

†Designated drug was the exclusive antimicrobial agent given during six weeks prior to symptoms.

From Bartlett, J. G. Johns Hopkins Med. J. *149*:6, 1981. Used by permission.

of cases involving tetracyclines, chloramphenicol, and oral neomycin in the more recent reports, curious because these drugs were the most common agents incriminated during the period in which *S. aureus* was the suspected agent.[4-6, 9, 10] We are not aware of cases of PMC which may be clearly ascribed to parenterally administered aminoglycosides, vancomycin, or agents which have a spectrum of activity restricted to mycobacteria, fungi, or parasites.

CLINICAL FINDINGS

In the preantibiotic era, pseudomembranous enterocolitis was regarded as a catastrophic complication, but the high mortality rate may reflect the fact that the diagnosis was often established only at autopsy examination. The clinical course in these patients was fulminant with *fever, abdominal pain, ileus, irreversible shock*, and *death*, usually within two to three days.[2, 3, 30-32] Diarrhea was found in only 25 to 40 per cent of these patients according to most large series. During the early antibiotic era, when *S. aureus* was commonly implicated, this was regarded as a relatively serious complication in which patients often presented with diarrhea and fever, but the course and outcome were variable. The anatomic diagnosis was not clearly established in most cases so that clinical descriptions and mortality data must be considered unreliable.

The extensive use of endoscopy in more recent years has permitted far more accurate assessment of the clinical spectrum found in patients with an established diagnosis of pseudomembranous colitis. The single symptom which is found in nearly all patients is *diarrhea*. The onset of this symptom is initially noted during the course of antibiotic treatment in two thirds of patients; the remaining third never detect a change in bowel habits until the offending drug has been discontinued. The temporal limit in time between discontinuation of an antimicrobial and its implication as a cause of diarrhea and colitis appears to be four to six weeks. We have encountered occasional patients with PMC at autopsy who had no history of diarrhea, so this diagnosis is a consideration in the patient who has fever of unknown origin (FUO) following antibiotic exposure, although this is distinctly unusual. The incidence of antibiotic-associated diarrhea according to prospective studies is 7 to 26 per cent for clindamycin,[23, 50-55] and for ampicillin it is 5 to 10 per cent.[51-56] Similar data from prospective studies using adequate surveillance methods are not available for most other antimicrobials. The diarrhea ascribed to antibiotics usually consists of loose or watery stools, sometimes containing mucus, but rarely with grossly evident blood. The severity of diarrhea varies considerably between different individuals ranging from a trivial, self-limited bout of loose stools to severe diarrhea with up to 30 stools per day for a protracted period of four weeks or longer.[23, 25] Studies of antibiotic-associated diarrhea that predated studies implicating *C. difficile* in some cases showed the average duration of diarrhea (with or without colitis) followed discontinuation of the implicated agent in 10 to 12 days.[51-53]

Most patients with antibiotic-associated diarrhea have a benign self-limited course in which symptoms generally resolve within five to ten days when the implicated agent is simply discontinued. *C. difficile* is the most commonly implicated agent of this form of nuisance diarrhea, but it only accounts for about 15 to 20 per cent of cases. Occasional cases are ascribed to enterotoxin-producing strains of *C. perfringens*,[57] *Salmonella*,[58] or other established enteric pathogens, but the majority of cases have no identifiable cause. These latter cases, which are enigmatic with respect to an identifiable pathogen, tend to develop during antibiotic administration, are dose related, are infrequently associated with signs of inflammation, and tend to resolve when the implicated antibiotic is discontinued or lowered in dose.[59] Clinical features that favor *C. difficile* are severe diarrhea, persistent diarrhea, diarrhea that begins after the implicated drug is stopped, and diarrhea accompanied by signs of colitis including fever, leukocytosis, abdominal cramps, and fecal leukocytes. There are obvious correlations between the selected antibiotics and the likelihood of *C. difficile*–induced enteric disease, but the dose, duration, and route of administration of these agents are relatively unimportant. Another diagnostic clue in some settings is that *C. difficile* may be responsible for outbreaks of diarrhea in locations where antibiotics are used extensively including hospitals, nursing homes, and day care centers.

The concern of the clinician is magnified when antibiotic-associated diarrhea is accompanied by findings suggesting colitis, especially its most characteristic form, PMC. Most patients complain of abdominal pain, and they often have tenderness in association with fever and leukocytosis.[20-25, 60] These findings may suggest intra-abdominal sepsis and occasionally lead to an unwarranted laparotomy.[61] Fever, when present, is usually low grade but may be as high as 106°F, and the peripheral leukocyte count is usually in the range of 10,000 to 20,000 per cu mm, but may be 40,000 per cu mm or greater. Serious complications include severe dehydration, electrolyte imbalance, hypotension, hypoalbuminemia with anasarca, toxic megacolon, and colonic perforation. Extraintestinal symptoms are rare with antibiotic-associated colitis, except for the complications noted previously that are ascribed to fluid, albumin, or electrolyte losses. Polyarthritis involving large joints has been reported.[62, 63] The three findings that are somewhat idiosyncratic to *C. difficile*, as opposed to other bacterial agents of diarrhea, are its penchant to cause prolonged diarrhea, its prevalence in PMC, and the apparent protein loss with hypoalbuminemia at presentation. Nevertheless, most patients with *C. difficile*–induced enteric disease do not have prolonged diarrhea, PMC, or hypoalbuminemia.

DIAGNOSIS

Pseudomembranous enterocolitis might be suspected in any of the patients with the defined risk factors noted above, but the most common clinical setting is recent exposure to an antimicrobial agent. As noted, the suspicion of PMC is magnified in antibiotic recipients in whom diarrhea is severe, prolonged, or associated with systemic signs of infection. Stool findings are nonspecific, although gross evidence of blood is unusual and patients with pancolitis will usually have fecal leukocytes. Stool Gram stains are not useful and stool leukocyte examination is neither sensitive nor specific. Radiologic findings are often nonspecific, but may be helpful in specifically suggesting PMC in up to one half of patients with advanced disease.[64–67] Plain films of the abdomen may show a markedly edematous colon, distorted haustral markings, and distention of the entire colon (Fig. 69–3). Occasionally, there are small irregularities which represent pseudomembranous plaques in profile. Contrast studies may show rounded filling defects which outline the plaques, but the findings are often nondiagnostic owing to underpenetration of barium, excessive mucus secretions, confluence of the pseudomembrane, or minimal involvement. The diagnostic accuracy is improved with air-contrast studies, which must be performed with caution because of the potential complication of colonic perforation. Computerized tomography often shows a thickened colon that often suggests idiopathic inflammatory bowel disease (Fig. 69–4).

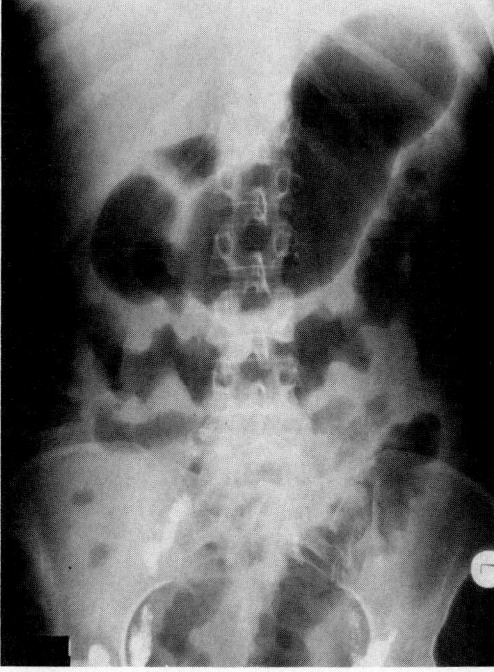

Figure 69–3. Plain abdominal film of antibiotic-associated pseudomembranous colitis. Note the involvement of the entire colon, the markedly edematous folds, and the lack of dilatation. The small bowel is normal. Severe edema and increased thickness of the colon wall is indicated by the distance between the gastric air shadow above and the colon below.

The preferred method to establish the diagnosis of PMC is with endoscopy to detect typical mucosal plaque-like lesions (Fig. 69–5). The distal colon is involved in most patients so that sigmoidoscopy is usually adequate, but up to one third of patients have lesions restricted to the right colon, necessitating colonoscopy.[68, 69] Endoscopy often requires the expertise of an experienced endoscopist. Copious amounts of mucus must be removed to recognize the plaques, and this must be done cautiously to avoid separation of loosely adherent stalks. Similar precautions are necessary for colon preparation prior to the procedure for the same reasons. There must also be care to include the entire lesion in any biopsy because the stalk attachment may be narrow, fragile, and easily dislodged. Endoscopic changes other than PMC that may be observed in patients with antibiotic-associated diarrhea include erythema, edema, a friable mucosa, colonic ulceration, or hemorrhage. In some instances, the changes noted on both gross inspection and biopsy may be highly suggestive of idiopathic ulcerative colitis.[70–72]

ETIOLOGY—*CLOSTRIDIUM DIFFICILE*

C. difficile was initially implicated as the major identifiable agent of antibiotic-associated colitis in 1978.[27] Since that time there have been extensive studies to define the role of this organism in various enteric diseases, the spectrum of pathologic changes, the clinical features, epidemiology, and diagnostic methods. A striking conclusion from this work is that *C. difficile* appears to cause disease almost exclusively in the presence of antibiotic-exposure (Fig. 69–6). The contributing factors in pathogenesis of disease are the requirements for (1) a source of the organism, presumably from the host's normal flora or from an epidemic source; (2) an altered normal flora, which is the apparent role of antibiotics; (3) toxin production that appears to reflect rapid growth of toxigenic strains at a time that the competing flora is suppressed; and (4) age-related susceptibility.

C. difficile. This organism was originally described by Hall and O'Toole in 1935 as a component of the normal fecal flora of newborn infants.[73] The difficulty the investigators experienced in recovering and maintaining these bacteria account for the original appellation, *Bacillus difficilis*. The early studies noted that the organism was responsible for a toxin that was highly lethal with subcutaneous injection to various animals,[74] and epidemiologic studies showed it was widespread in nature.[75] Nevertheless, *C. difficile* played no clearly defined role in clinical or veterinary medicine until it was recognized as an enteric pathogen.[76]

Colonization Rates. The recognition of *C. difficile* as a potentially important enteric pathogen has led to the development of improved methods for selective recovery from the complex fecal flora. A preferred method is use of antibiotic-incorporated agar media containing cycloserine and cefoxitin as originally described by George et al.[77, 78] The isolation rate of *C.*

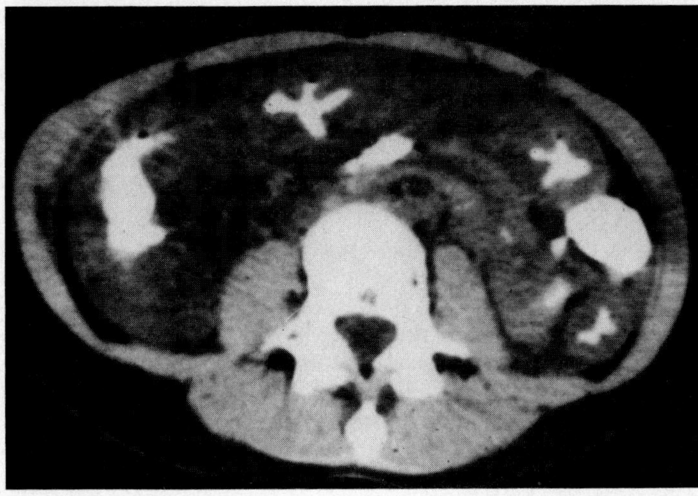

Figure 69–4. Computerized tomography of the abdomen with contrast material in the colon demonstrating thickening of the bowel wall.

difficile shows considerable variation according to the population studied (Table 69–3). Combining data from multiple investigations, the recovery rate from healthy adults is 2 to 3 per cent, from patients with antibiotic-associated diarrhea or colitis with positive toxin assays it is 90 to 100 per cent, from hospitalized patients without diarrhea it is 10 to 15 per cent, and from adults who have recently received antimicrobials without diarrhea it is 5 to 15 per cent. This organism has not been found with an increased frequency among patients with a variety of diarrheal diseases which are ascribed to conditions other than antibiotic exposure. The largest series[49] examining such individuals is from a reference laboratory in Sweden in which stool samples were routinely examined for a variety of enteric pathogens, and the overall recovery rate for *C. difficile* among 2390 samples was 3 per cent; this approximates the recovery rate noted in healthy adults. The isolation rate in infants ranges from 5 to 70 per cent, but in controlled studies the rate of carriage is similar in children with or without disease.[28,73,74,81,87–90] Relatively high carriage rates persist during the first eight months of life until the "normal flora" becomes established.[74,75,87] Isolation rates in children over one year approximates the rate noted in healthy adults, e.g., 2 to 3 per cent.

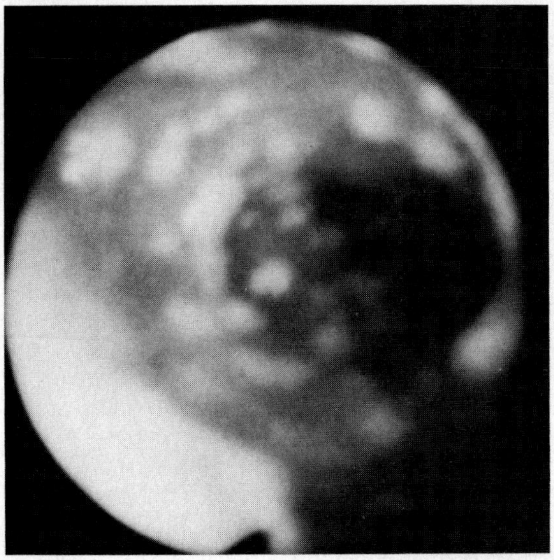

Figure 69–5. Colonoscopic appearance of pseudomembranes. Note that the lesions are only slightly raised and are single or confluent. A thick layer of mucus covers some of the folds.

In Vitro Susceptibility Tests. An assumption is commonly made that *C. difficile*–induced diarrhea or colitis occurring in association with antibiotic exposure represents a superinfection with a resistant microbe. However, experiments in hamsters have shown little correlation between in vitro activity against *C. difficile* and the propensity to cause lethal colitis.[91–93] A similar paradox appears to apply to many patients. In vitro sensitivity tests of clinical isolates indicate the most active drugs are metronidazole, vancomycin, ampicillin, and penicillin G.[94–97] Cephalosporins are considerably less active, with cefoxitin and moxalactam being especially inactive. Most strains are sensitive to tetracycline. Activity of clindamycin is variable in that approximately 50 per cent of strains are sensitive and 10 to 20 per cent are highly resistant.[96] It is especially noteworthy that ampicillin, which is one of the most common agents responsible for this complication, is active in vitro against virtually all strains, including those recovered from patients with ampicillin-associated colitis. These observations indicate that the sensitivity profiles of *C. difficile* isolates are not useful in determining which drugs are most likely to cause this complication. Nevertheless, this type of information may be potentially useful as therapy when fecal concentrations of the drug are also taken into account.

Epidemiology. *C. difficile* is a sporulating organism that survives well in nature and, like other clostridia, is found widely distributed in the environment.[75] Unlike other anaerobes including other clostridia, there is compelling evidence that *C. difficile* is a transferrable pathogen which poses a threat to hospitalized patients exposed to a nosocomial source of the organism and rendered susceptible with antibiotic administration.

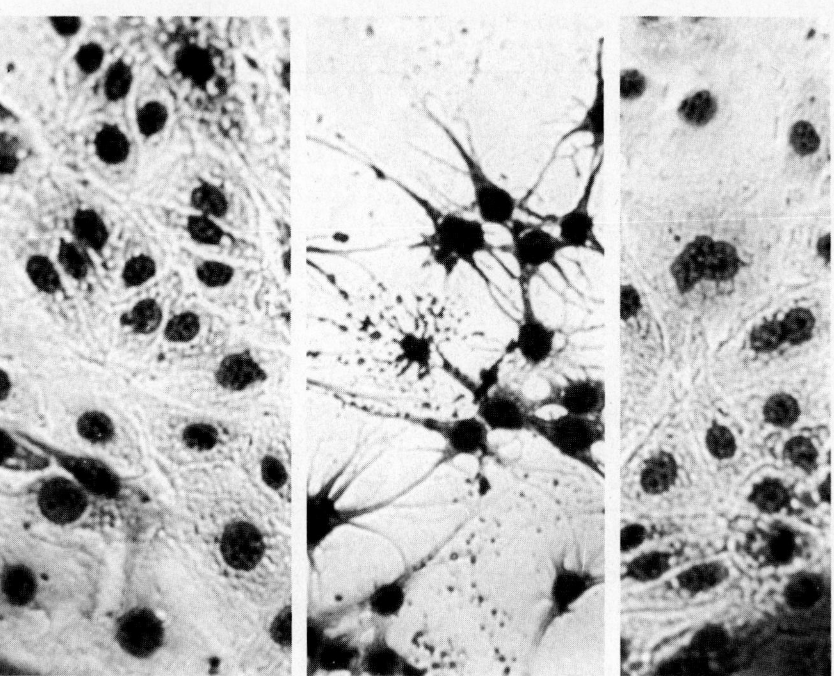

Figure 69–6. Tissue culture assay for *Clostridium difficile* toxin using primary human amnion cells. The left panel shows normal cells, the center panel shows typical actinomorphic changes after application of stool containing *C. difficile* toxin, and the right panel shows the tissue cultured cells with the same specimen after neutralization with *C. sordellii* antitoxin. Identical changes are noted with inocula of stools from experimental animals with antibiotic-induced cecitis, stools from patients with pseudomembranous colitis, cell-free supernatant fluid of *C. difficile* in broth culture, and *C. difficile* purified toxin A or toxin B. Toxin B is approximately 1000 times more active in the tissue culture assay.

This conclusion is based on several "outbreaks" of antibiotic-associated PMC which have been reported from hospitals in St. Louis,[23] Dallas,[46] Chicago,[98] Birmingham, England,[60] and London.[99] Extensive studies at the General Hospital in Birmingham, England, showed *C. difficile*–induced colitis in 67 patients located on two surgical wards during a four-year period.[60, 78, 100] Analogous problems within selected wards have been reported in a nursing home in Baltimore[101] and a Veterans Hospital in St. Paul, Minnesota.[102, 103] In each instance, extensive efforts to control epidemiologic spread proved extremely frustrating. These efforts include institution of antibiotic control programs,

Table 69–3. ISOLATION RATES OF *C. DIFFICILE* IN STOOLS

Patient Category	Reference	Isolation Rate of *C. difficile*
Antibiotic-associated diarrhea or colitis with positive assay for *C. difficile* toxin	27–29, 60, 77, 79–83, 85, 102, 106	90–100%
Antibiotic-associated diarrhea	79–81, 85, 102, 106	15%
Antibiotic exposure or hospitalization without diarrhea	48, 80, 81, 86, 102	10–20%
Gastrointestinal diseases unrelated to antibiotic exposure	28, 48, 49, 80–82, 84, 85	0–3%
Healthy adults	28, 48, 49, 77, 80, 81	2–3%
Children		
Neonates (≤1 month)	28, 73, 74, 81, 87, 89, 90	30–70%
1 to 8 months	80, 81, 87, 90	30–70%
>1 year	80, 81, 87	3%

sequestering of patients, extensive use of enteric precautions, and treatment of *C. difficile* carriers. Several investigators have found environmental sources of *C. difficile*, especially in areas of patients with *C. difficile*–induced diarrheal disease.[104–106] Mulligan et al. isolated the organism in environmental samplings from 37 of 114 (32 per cent) case-associated sites compared to 6 of 445 (1.3 per cent) control sites.[104] Similar findings were reported by Fekety et al.[105] In both investigations, the primary sources for positive cultures were toilets, bedpans, and floors. *C. difficile* was also found with hand and stool cultures from asymptomatic hospital personnel who worked in area-associated cases. Cultures of air, food, and walls were uniformly negative. As a result of these observations, the Communicable Disease Center now recommends enteric isolation precautions for patients with diarrhea accompanied by positive toxin assays or cultures for *C. difficile*, but guidelines for cleansing of potentially contaminated surfaces in rooms or methods to decontaminate endoscopes are not available.[107]

***Clostridium difficile* Toxin Assays.** The preferred method to establish the diagnosis of *C. difficile*–induced disease is toxin detection. Stool cultures are sometimes advocated, but the best clinical correlations are with the toxin. The standard toxin assay requires tissue cultures to demonstrate a cytopathic toxin, which is neutralized by *Clostridium sordellii* or *C. difficile* antitoxin (see Fig. 69–6). Detailed descriptions concerning technical aspects of performing the test and guidelines for sending specimens to reference laboratories are available elsewhere.[108, 109] The clinical experience with the tissue culture assay shows 95 to 100 per cent of patients with a confirmed diagnosis of antibiotic-associated PMC have positive tests (Table

Table 69–4. TISSUE CULTURE ASSAYS OF STOOLS FOR *C. DIFFICILE* TOXIN

Patient Category	Reference	Positive Results
Antibiotic-associated PMC	27–29, 48, 49, 60, 77, 79–83, 85, 95, 102, 108	95–100%
Antibiotic-associated diarrhea without confirmed PMC	48, 49, 79–81, 85, 95, 102, 106, 108	15–25%
Antibiotic exposure without diarrhea	49, 80, 81, 86	2–8%
Gastrointestinal disease		
Unrelated to antimicrobial exposure	49, 79–81, 83–85, 95	0
Inflammatory bowel disease in relapse	110–114	0–18% (see text)
Healthy adults	49, 80, 81, 83, 84	0
Healthy neonates	80, 81, 88–90	5–63%

69–4). The toxin titer in these individuals ranges from 10^{-1} to 10^{-7} dilutions (1:10 to 1:10,000,000) with mean titers of 10^{-3} to 10^{-4} dilutions. There is no correlation between the severity of disease and toxin titers. Positive assays with similar titers are noted in 17 to 25 per cent of patients with antibiotic-associated diarrhea without PMC, and 5 to 60 per cent of healthy neonates (Table 69–4). As noted above, the carrier rate for *C. difficile* in healthy adults is 2 to 3 per cent, but the toxin has not been detected in these individuals. Asymptomatic carriage of the toxin has been noted in 2 to 8 per cent of patients who have received antimicrobial agents without apparent gastrointestinal complications and for up to nine months or longer after recovery from *C. difficile*–induced colitis.[110] Attempts to detect *C. difficile* in enigmatic intestinal diseases other than antibiotic-associated diarrhea or colitis have been strikingly unrewarding. A possible exception is relapses of inflammatory bowel disease, but reports showing positive toxin assays in as many as 25 to 50 per cent of patients with severe relapses[111, 112] have not been supported by the studies of others.[80, 110, 113, 114] The one population in which there does appear to be a high incidence of *C. difficile* toxin is patients with PMC unassociated with antimicrobial exposure. This complication was noted long before the antibiotic era, and although such patients are infrequently encountered at the present time, the available evidence indicates that most have positive toxin assays.[43–45]

The tissue culture assay advocated poses a disadvantage for most physicians owing to the requirement for facilities which are generally not available in most clinical microbiology laboratories. This necessitates the submission of specimens to reference laboratories, often at distant locations. Studies of specimens stored in various conditions indicate the cytopathic toxin is thermolabile, and biologic activity is reduced in direct correlation with time and temperature.[108] The usual recommendation for transport is delivery within 24 hours or storage in frozen state if specimens require a more prolonged delay. Alternatives to the tissue culture assay which are being developed include the counterimmunoelectrophoresis (CIE),[115] the enzyme immunoassay (EIA),[116] and a latex particle agglutination assay.[117] The CIE and EIA methods are designed to detect *C. difficile* toxins A and B. The particle agglutination assay recognizes another protein; this test is commercially available, and the results of the initial tests are variable.[117, 118]

***Clostridium difficile* Toxins.** *Clostridium difficile* appears to produce two toxins, designated toxins A and B.[119–122] Both toxins are large molecular weight proteins that are cytopathic to tissue culture cells and lethal to experimental animals. The lethal dose for either toxin A or B to mice is about 1/100 the lethal dose noted for botulism, and this makes these among the most potent bacterial toxins. Nevertheless, there is no evidence that these toxins are absorbed into the systemic circulation, so their primary action would appear to be on the gut mucosa where they are produced in the colonic lumen. Differences between toxins A and B are based on their separation with anion exchange chromatography, antigenic differences, and variations in biologic properties.

Toxin B is a highly potent cytopathic toxin that is cytopathic to virtually all cell lines examined. With fibroblasts there are very characteristic actinomorphic changes, reflecting disruption of actin microfilaments of the cytoskeleton. As little as 0.2 pg causes typical changes, which possibly accounts for the high sensitivity of tissue culture assays for disease detection.

Toxin A is also cytopathic, but is substantially less potent. The major difference is that toxin A induces a fluid flux and causes intense mucosal inflammation in the animal loop assays used to detect enterotoxins.[119] These observations have led some to conclude that toxin B is most useful for disease detection, but that toxin A may be primarily responsible for clinical expression. This is a debated issue.[123] There is also preliminary evidence for a third toxin that alters intestinal motility.[124]

It appears that *C. difficile* strains that are toxigenic produce both toxins, and toxin production is maximal during logarithmic growth of vegetative forms. This may account for the observation that toxin production in vivo occurs when rapid growth of vegetative forms is favored by reduction of the competitive flora as with newborn infants, monoassociated germ-free mice, or antibiotic administration. Although most strains are toxigenic, there is considerable strain variation in the amount of toxins produced, which may account for vagaries in disease severity in both sporadic and epidemic forms of the disease.

Age-Related Risk. Studies cited above show that infants and young children up to one year commonly harbor *C. difficile* and its toxin with no deleterious consequences. It appears that infants are especially susceptible to colonization with this organism just as they are with *C. botulinum*, and this age corresponds to age of risk for sudden infant death syndrome and infant botulism.[125, 126] A major difference is that infants appear to be susceptible to *C. botulinum*, but they appear to be protected from *C. difficile* toxin for reasons that are obscure. Older children may develop antibiotic-associated PMC,[127] but it is clear that the incidence is less than for adults. Population-based studies in Sweden showed that the incidence of *C. difficile* toxin positive stools increase 20- to 100-fold in comparing persons aged 10 to 20 years and those over 60 years.[49] Serologic assays show that most healthy persons over 5 to 10 years have circulating antibody to toxin A and B, but this apparently fails to confer protection.[128] The suggestion is that the aging process promotes susceptibility to colonization, toxin production, or disease.

TREATMENT

The therapy of PMC includes discontinuation of any implicated antimicrobial agents, nonspecific supportive measures, and agents directed against identifiable pathogens, primarily *C. difficile* (Table 69–5). Supportive measures include intravenous fluids to correct fluid losses, electrolyte imbalance, and hypoalbuminemia. This sometimes requires hyperalimentation. Antiperistaltic agents, such as Lomotil, should be avoided because they have been noted to increase in incidence of antibiotic-associated diarrhea and worsen symptoms among those patients with established disease.[129, 130] Systemic administration of corticosteroids is sometimes advocated for critically ill patients, although treatment with methylprednisolone in the animal model of antibiotic-induced colitis failed to delay death, and the clinical experience is limited.[131, 132] Patients with *C. difficile*–induced disease who are in acute or chronic care facilities should be placed on enteric isolation precautions.[107]

Table 69–5. TREATMENT OF *C. DIFFICILE*–INDUCED DIARRHEA AND COLITIS

Nonspecific measures

1. Discontinue implicated antimicrobial agent (alternatives are to change to another agent that is infrequently associated with this complication or continue implicated agent while giving oral vancomycin
2. Supportive measures (see text)
3. Avoid antiperistaltic agents
4. Enteric isolation precautions for hospitalized patients

Specific treatment

1. Antimicrobial agents (advocated only if symptoms are severe or persist)
   a. Oral agent (preferred)
      (1) Vancomycin: 125–500 mg po qid 7–14 days*
      (2) Metronidazole: 250 mg po tid, 7–14 days*
      (3) Bacitracin: 25,000 units po qid, 7–14 days*
   b. Parenteral agents (to be used only until oral agents are tolerated): metronidazole: 500 mg IV q 6 h
2. Alternative treatments
   a. Anion exchange resins
      (1) Cholestryamine, 4 gm packet po tid, 5–10 days*
      (2) Cholestipol, 5 gm packet po tid, 5–10 days*
   b. Alter fecal flora
      (1) Lactinex (or alternative lactobacillus preparation): 1 gm packet po qid, 7–14 days
      (2) Fecal enema: fresh feces via enema once or twice separated by 3 days

Multiple relapses

1. Vancomycin or metronidazole po 7–14 days followed by:
   a. Cholestyramine (above dose), 3 weeks
   b. Lactobacillus (above dose), 3 weeks
   c. Vancomycin, 125 mg po qod, 3 weeks

*Indicates efficacy is established.

Surgery. Oral antimicrobial agents are advocated for patients with advanced disease, but some seriously ill patients who have fulminant or intractable symptoms may require colectomy or a diverting ileostomy.[133, 134] The necessity for surgical intervention is relatively infrequent, but patients with a profound ileus or toxic megacolon are generally unable to take oral medications, and the experience with parenteral drugs in this setting is limited. When surgery is deemed necessary in cases due to *C. difficile*, some authorities recommend the use of parenteral vancomycin or metronidazole in the perioperative period, as well as intraluminal instillation of vancomycin at the time of surgery.[133, 134]

Antibiotic Treatment. Specific antimicrobial agents are available for diarrhea and colitis caused by *S. aureus* and *C. difficile*. For *S. aureus*, the only drug with an established track record is vancomycin given orally; the usual dose is 500 mg four times daily for one to two weeks. This diagnosis is difficult to establish, it appears to be very rare, and the need for the high dose is not established. The majority of patients with antibiotic-associated colitis and especially those with PMC will have positive toxin assays implicating *C. difficile*. Antimicrobial options in these cases include vancomycin, metronidazole, or bacitracin (Table 69–5). Comparative clinical trials indicate these drugs are therapeutically equivalent,[79, 102, 135–137] although most authorities advocate vancomycin for patients who are seriously ill.[137] Vancomycin or metronidazole are also advocated for patients with moderately advanced clinical symptoms who have negative toxin assays for *C. difficile* based on a limited but favorable anecdotal experience. Possible explanations for the response in these cases are a low toxin titer that will be missed using dilutional techniques that are standard in some laboratories, reliance on assays that are not adequately studied, recent therapy that may include drugs that are not advocated for treatment but may reduce toxin production, undetectable levels of toxin, or implication of another vancomycin-responsive pathogen such as *S. aureus* or another clostridial species. All recommended antimicrobial treatments are potentially complicated by relapses when the therapy is discontinued, and the frequency of relapse appears comparable with the drugs suggested.[79, 102, 135–137] No treatment with these agents is recommended for patients who are mildly ill or spontaneously improving, in part to avoid the complication of relapse.

Orally administered vancomycin has been used extensively with almost uniformly good results.[102, 135–141] This includes patients in older studies who were felt to have *S. aureus* enterocolitis.[16] Most studies show a response rate of 95 to 100 per cent for those with *C. difficile*–induced colitis. In vitro tests of over 200 strains of *C. difficile* indicate all are susceptible at concentrations of 16 μg/ml or less.[94–96] The drug is poorly absorbed with oral administration so that the mean stool level with 500 mg doses is approximately 3000 μg/gm,[140] and with 125 mg doses it is 350 to 500 μg/gm.[94, 141] *C. difficile* is found only in the lumen of the intestine and does not invade the mucosa, making high fecal levels an appropriate goal. Serum levels are negligible with oral administration of vancomycin so that systemic toxicity is essentially nil.[140] Nevertheless, careful monitoring is advised in patients with renal failure and an inflamed bowel because small amounts of absorbed drug could conceivably accumulate in this setting. A review of our experience with 189 patients, most of whom received 2 gm daily, showed 183 (97 per cent) responded.[140] There was usually a prompt defervescence within 24 to 48 hours and resolution of diarrhea over 1 to 13 days with a mean of 4.5 days. The major problem in our patients was relapse characterized by a recurrence of symptoms following discontinuation of vancomycin[135, 137, 139, 140] and the high cost of treatment.

Bacitracin shares many of the advantages noted with vancomycin. Virtually all strains of *C. difficile* are sensitive, and the drug is poorly absorbed with oral administration to provide high colonic levels without the risk of systemic toxicity. Two comparative trials in patients with *C. difficile*–induced colitis showed equivalent results to those achieved with vancomycin.[135, 136] Potential advantages are reduced cost and availability in many countries where vancomycin cannot be purchased. Metronidazole is very active in vitro,[94–96] and a comparative clinical trial showed therapeutic responses comparable to that with vancomycin.[102] A theoretical disadvantage is that *C. difficile* is retained within the gut lumen, and metronidazole levels in stool with oral administration are extremely low.[142] Perhaps more disturbing is the observation that metronidazole has been implicated as a cause of *C. difficile*–induced colitis in at least 10 patients.[143, 144] Despite this concern, metronidazole has become an accepted agent for treatment, due largely to a notable cost advantage.

Anion Exchange Resins. The potential utility of cholestyramine in antibiotic-associated colitis was initially reported before the role of *C. difficile* was known.[145] Subsequent studies have shown that this drug, like other anion exchange resins, binds the toxins produced by *C. difficile*.[146] The clinical experience by different investigators has shown marked variation in results with these resins. Some have reported excellent response in virtually all patients, the only side effect being constipation.[147] By contrast, others have noted an exceptionally high rate of failures with either cholestyramine[148] or cholestipol.[140] Cholestyramine is distinctly inferior to vancomycin in the hamster model.[139] However, it is substantially less expensive, and relapses appear to be very uncommon among patients who do respond. Thus, cholestyramine along with metronidazole may be preferred for initial treatment of some patients with less serious disease. It is theoretically attractive to use both vancomycin and cholestyramine owing to the distinctive mechanisms of activity, but the resin also binds vancomcyin to produce a marked reduction in colonic levels of antibiotic.[146] Analogous drug interactions between cholestyramine and metronidazole or bacitracin have not been examined.

Relapses. Patients treated with antimicrobial agents often do well during therapy, but suffer a recurrence of symptoms when treatment is discontinued. The frequency of relapses is reported to be 5 to 50 per cent.[79, 135, 136, 138, 139, 149] In the largest reported series there were 46 relapses among 189 patients (24 per cent) treated with vancomycin; these patients responded well to a second course of vancomycin, but 22 (46 per cent) suffered a second relapse.[139] There are now many patients who have suffered five to ten relapses with sequential courses of treatment, the largest number being 19 relapses in a single year. The incidence of relapses varies in different reports, but comparative trials have shown no difference in the incidence with different agents.[79, 102, 135, 136] Thus, bacitracin, metronidazole, and vancomycin treatment have all been complicated by relapses, the frequency is about the same, and there is no reason to consider one to be an advantage for the patient who has relapsed following treatment with another.

The typical clinical pattern is a recurrence of diarrhea with or without fever, cramps, and leukocytosis at three to ten days after treatment is discontinued. Stool assays with relapses following vancomycin treatment are positive for *C. difficile* toxin, and cultures show organisms that are highly susceptible to vancomycin. It is of interest to note that either vancomycin or metronidazole alone induces lethal colitis due to *C. difficile* in experimental animals, and several clinical reports show that metronidazole may cause this disease in patients. This observation illustrates the paradox of the same agent as cause and cure of *C. difficile*–induced enteric disease. With regard to relapses, the two suggested mechanisms are that the organism is never eradicated and vegetative forms flourish when antibiotic treatment is suspended. The alternative possibility is acquisition of a new strain. Studies in monoassociated germ-free mice show that toxin production stops, but spores persist during vancomycin treatment,[150] and clinical studies show that *C. difficile* can be recovered from stool after vancomycin treatment despite stool levels several hundredfold higher than the minimum inhibitory concentration.[149] These data support microbial persistence as the mechanism of relapse.

Suggested treatment of relapses include careful observation with no specific treatment, a second course of the same antimicrobial agent, or another course of cholestyramine. In many instances it is appropriate simply to observe the patient. Studies of clindamycin-induced PMC prior to the detection of *C. difficile* showed virtually all patients eventually improved without specific therapy, although many had prolonged courses of illness.[23] Toxin assays are usually positive at the end of treatment, even among patients who do well clinically.[138] Thus, the decision to treat with an antibiotic should be based on clinical observations. When this is deemed necessary for patients with multiple relapses, the recommendation is to give an antimicrobial agent for 7 to 14 days to control the disease and then follow this with another agent for three weeks to promote disease control while the normal flora becomes re-established. This second agent may be cholestyramine (4 gm orally tid), lactobacilli (one tablet orally qid), *or* low dose "pulse" treatment with vancomycin (125 mg orally every second day).[136, 151]

References

1. Finney, J. M. T. Gastroenterology for cicatrizing ulcer of the pylorus. Bull. Johns Hopkins Hosp. *4*:53, 1893.
2. Penner, A., and Bernheim, A. Acute postoperative enterocolitis. Arch. Pathol. *27*:966, 1939.
3. Petter, J. D., Baggenstoss, A. H., Dearing, W. H., and Judd, E. S. Postoperative pseudomembranous enterocolitis. Surg. Gynecol. Obstet. *8*:546, 1954.
4. Altemeier, W. A., Hummell, R. P., and Hill, E. O. Staphylococcal enterocolitis following antibiotic-therapy. Ann. Surg. *157*:847, 1963.
5. Azar, H., and Drapanas, T. Relationship of antibiotics to wound infection and enterocolitis in colon surgery. Am. J. Surg. *115*:209, 1968.
6. Hummel, R. P., Altemeier, W. A., and Hill, E. O. Iatrogenic staphylococcal enterocolitis. Ann. Surg. *160*:551, 1964.
7. Wakefield, R. D., and Sommers, S. C. Fatal membranous staphylococcal enteritis in surgical patients. Ann. Surg. *138*:249, 1953.
8. Prohaska, J. V., Long, E. T., and Nelson, T. S. Pseudomembranous enterocolitis: Its etiology and the mechanism of the disease process. Arch. Surg. *72*:977, 1956.
9. Reiner, L., Schlesinger, M. J., and Miller, G. M. Pseudomembranous colitis following aureomycin and chloramphenicol. Arch. Pathol. *54*:39, 1952.
10. Hale, H. W., Jr., and Cosgriff, H. J., Jr. Pseudomembranous colitis. Am. J. Surg. *94*:710, 1957.
11. Surgalla, M. J., and Dach, G. M. Enterotoxin produced by micrococci from cases of enteritis after antibody therapy. JAMA *158*:149, 1955.
12. Prohaska, J. V., Jacobson, M. J., and Prohaska, J. V. Staphylococcus enterotoxin enteritis. Surg. Gynecol. Obstet. *109*:73–77, 1959.
13. Tan, T. L., Drake, C. T., Jacobson, M. J., and Prohaska, J. V. The experimental development of pseudomembranous colitis. Surg. Gynecol. Obstet. *108*:415–410, 1959.
14. Warren, S. E., Sugiyama, H., and Prohaska, J. V. Correlation of staphylococcal enterotoxins with experimentally induced enterocolitis. Surg. Gynecol. Obstet. *114*:29–33, 1963.
15. Wood, J. S., Bennett, I. L., and Yardley, J. H. Staphylococcal enterocolitis in chinchillas. Bull. Johns Hopkins Hosp. *98*:454, 1956.
16. Kahn, M. Y., and Hall, W. H. Staphylococcus enterocolitis treatment with oral vancomycin. Ann. Intern. Med. *65*:1–7, 1966.
17. Cummins, A. J. Pseudomembranous enterocolitis and the pathology of nosology. Am. J. Dig. Dis. *6*:429, 1961.
18. Dearing, W. H., Baggenstoss, A. H., and Weed, L. A. Studies on the relationship of *Staphylococcus aureus* to pseudomembranous enteritis and to post-antibiotic enteritis. Gastroenterology *38*:441–451, 1960.
19. Slagle, G. W., and Boggs, H. W. Drug induced pseudomembranous enterocolitis. Dis. Colon Rectum *19*:253, 1976.
20. Stroehlein, J. R., Sedlack, R. E., Hoffman, H. N., and Newcomer, A. D. Clindamycin-associated colitis. Mayo Clin. Proc. *49*:240, 1974.
21. Scott, A. J., Nicholson, G. I., and Kerr, A. R. Lincomycin as a cause of pseudomembranous colitis. Lancet *2*:1232, 1973.
22. Totten, M. A., Gregg, J. A., Fremont-Smith, P., and Legg, M. Clinical and pathologic spectrum of antibiotic-associated colitis. Am. J. Gastroenterol. *69*:311, 1978.
23. Tedesco, F. J., Barton, R. W., and Alpers, H. D. Clindamycin-associated colitis. Ann. Intern. Med. *81*:429, 1974.
24. LeFrock, J. L., Klainer, A. S., Chen, S., Gainer, R. B., Omar, M., and Anderson, W. The spectrum of colitis associated with lincomycin and clindamycin therapy. J. Infect. Dis. *131*:S108, 1975.
25. Keusch, G. T., and Present, D. H. Summary of workshop on clindamycin colitis. J. Infect. Dis. *133*:578, 1976.
26. Bartlett, J. G., Onderdonk, A. B., Cisneros, A. B., and Kasper, D. L. Clindamycin-associated colitis due to toxin producing species of clostridium in hamsters. J. Infect. Dis. *136*:701–705, 1977.
27. Bartlett, J. G., Chang, T. W., Gurwith, M., Gorbach, S. L., and Onderdonk, A. B. Antibiotic-associated pseudomembranous colitis due to toxin producing clostridia. N. Engl. J. Med. *298*:531, 1978.
28. Larson, H. E., Price, A. B., Hanour, P., and Borriella, S. P. *Clostridium difficile* and the aetiology of pseudomembranous colitis. Lancet *1*:1063, 1978.
29. George, R. H., Symonds, J. M., Dimock, F., Browne, J., Arabi, Y., Keighley, M. R. B., Alexander-Williams, J., and Burdon, D. W. Identification of *Clostridium difficile* as a cause of pseudomembranous colitis. Br. Med. J. *1*:695, 1978.
30. Dixon, C. F., and Weismann, R. E. Acute pseudomembranous enteritis or enterocolitis: A complication following intestinal surgery. Surg. Clin. North Am. *28*:999, 1948.
31. Kay, A. W., Richards, R. L., and Watson, A. J. Acute necrotizing (pseudomembranous) enterocolitis. Br. J. Surg. *46*:45, 1958.
32. Kleckner, M. S., Jr., Bargen, J. A., and Baggenstoss, A. H. Pseudomembranous enterocolitis: Clinicopathologic study of fourteen cases in which the disease was not preceded by an operation. Gastroenterology *21*:212, 1952.
33. Goulston, S. J. M., and McGovern, V. J. Pseudomembranous colitis. Gut *6*:207, 1965.
34. Summer, H. W., and Tedesco, F. J. Rectal biopsy in clindamycin-associated colitis. Arch. Pathol. *99*:237, 1975.
35. Price, A. B., and Davies, D. R. Pseudomembranous colitis. J. Clin. Pathol. *30*:1–12, 1977.
36. Kelber, M., and Ament, M. E. Shigella disenteriae I: A forgotten cause of pseudomembranous colitis. J. Pediatr. *89*:595, 1976.
37. Hardaway, R. M., and McKay, D. G. Pseudomembranous enterocolitis. Arch. Surg. *78*:446, 1959.
38. Prolla, J. C., and Kirsner, J. B. The gastrointestinal lesions and complications of the leukemias. Ann. Intern. Med. *67*:1084, 1964.
39. Dosik, G. M., Luna, M., Valdivieso, M., and McCredie, K. B. Necrotizing colitis in patients with cancer. Am. J. Med. *67*:646, 1979.
40. Margaretten, W., and McKay, D. G. Thrombotic ulceration of the gastrointestinal tract. Arch. Intern. Med. *127*:250, 1971.
41. Bartlett, J. G., and Gorbach, S. L. Pseudomembranous enterocolitis (antibiotic-related colitis). *In* Stollerman, G. H. (ed.): Advances in Internal Medicine. Chicago, Year Book Medical Publishers, 1977, pp. 455–446.
42. Cudmore, M. A., Silva, J., Fekety, R., Liepman, M. K., and Kim, K.-H. *Clostridium difficile* colitis associated with cancer chemotherapy. Arch. Intern. Med. *142*:333–335, 1982.
43. Moskovitz, M., and Bartlett, J. G. Recurrent pseudomembranous colitis unassociated with prior antibiotic therapy. Arch. Intern. Med. *141*:663, 1981.
44. Peikin, S. R., Galdibini, J., and Bartlett, J. G. Role of *Clostridium difficile* in a case of nonantibiotic-associated pseudomembranous colitis. Gastroenterology *79*:948, 1980.
45. Wald, A., Mendelow, H., and Bartlett, J. G. Nonantibiotic-associated pseudomembranous colitis due to toxin-producing clostridia. Ann. Intern. Med. *92*:798, 1980.
46. Ramirez-Ronda, C. H. Incidence of clindamycin-associated colitis. Ann. Intern. Med. *81*:860, 1974.
47. Bartlett, J. G. Antimicrobial agents implicated in *Clostridium difficile* toxin associated diarrhea or colitis. Johns Hopkins Med. J. *149*:6, 1981.
48. George, W. L., Rolfe, R. D., Finegold, S. M. *Clostridium difficile* and its cytotoxin in feces of patients with antimicrobial agent–associated diarrhea and miscellaneous conditions. J. Clin. Microbiol. *15*:1049, 1982.

49. Aronsson, B., Mollby, R., Nord, C. E. Antimicrobial agents and *Clostridium difficile* in acute enteric disease: epidemiological data from Sweden, 1980–1982. J. Infect. Dis. *151*:476, 1985.
50. Swartzberg, J. E., Maresca, R. M., and Remington, J. W. Gastrointestinal side effects associated with clindamycin. Arch. Intern. Med. *136*:876, 1976.
51. Neu, H. C., Prince, A., Neu, C. O., and Garvey, G. J. Incidence of diarrhea and colitis associated with clindamycin therapy. J. Infect. Dis. *135*:S120, 1977.
52. Gurwith, M., Rabin, H. R., and Love, K. Diarrhea associated with clindamycin and ampicillin therapy. J. Infect. Dis. *135*:S104, 1977.
53. Lusk, R. H., Fekety, R., Jr., Silva, J., Jr., Bodendorfer, T., Devine, B. J., Kawanishi, H., and Korff, L. Gastrointestinal side effects following clindamycin or ampicillin therapy. J. Infect. Dis. *135*:S111–S119, 1977.
54. Brause, B. D., Romankiewicz, J. A., Gotz, V., and Franklin, J. E., Jr. Comparative study of diarrhea associated with clindamycin and ampicillin therapy. Am. J. Gastroenterol. *73*:244, 1980.
55. Leigh, D. A., Simmons, K., and Williams, S. Gastrointestinal side effects following clindamycin and lincomycin treatment—a follow-up study. J. Antimicrob. Chemother. *6*:639–645, 1980.
56. Tedesco, F. J. Ampicillin-associated diarrhea—a prospective study. Dig. Dis. *20*:295, 1975.
57. Borriello, S. P., Larson, H. E., and Welch, A. R. Enterotoxigenic *Clostridium perfringens*: A possible cause of antibiotic-associated diarrhoea. Lancet *1*:305, 1984.
58. Sun, M. In search of salmonella's smoking gun. Science *226*:30, 1984.
59. Giannella, R. A., Serumaga, J., Walls, D., and Drake, K. W. Effect of clindamycin on intestinal water and glucose transport in the rat. Gastroenterology *80*:907–913, 1981.
60. Mogg, G. M., Keighley, M., Burdon, D., Alexander-Williams, J., et al. Antibiotic-associated colitis—a review of 66 cases. Br. J. Surg. *66*:738, 1979.
61. Tedesco, F. J., Anderson, C. B., and Ballinger, W. F. Drug-induced colitis mimicking an acute surgical condition of the abdomen. Arch. Surg. *110*:481, 1975.
62. Rollins, D. E., and Moeller, D. Polyarthritis associated with clindamycin-induced colitis. JAMA *231*:1228, 1975.
63. Fairweather, S. D., George, R. H., Keighley, M. R. B., Youngs, D., and Burdon, D. W. Arthritis in pseudomembranous colitis associated with an antibody to *Clostridium difficile* toxin. J. R. Soc. Med. *73*:524, 1980.
64. Stanley, R. J., Melson, G. L., and Tedesco, F. J. The spectrum of radiographic findings in antibiotic-related pseudomembranous colitis. Radiology *111*:519, 1974.
65. Tully, T. E., and Feinberg, S. B. Those other types of enterocolitis. Am. J. Roentgenol. *121*:291, 1974.
66. Stanley, R. J., Melson, G. L., Tedesco, F. J., and Saylor, J. L. Plain-film findings in severe pseudomembranous colitis. Radiology *118*:7, 1976.
67. Hakkal, H. G. Pseudomembranous colitis associated with antibiotics. Am. J. Gastroenterol. *65*:78, 1976.
68. Tedesco, F. J., Corless, J. K., and Brownstein, R. E. Rectal sparing in antibiotic-associated pseudomembranous colitis: A prospective study. Gastroenterology *83*:1259–1260, 1982.
69. Burbige, E. J., and Radigan, J. J. Antibiotic-associated colitis with normal appearing rectum. Dis. Colon Rectum *23*:198, 1981.
70. Pittman, F. E., Pittman, J. C., and Humphrey, C. D. Colitis following oral lincomycin therapy. Arch. Intern. Med. *134*:368, 1974.
71. Manashil, G. B., and Kern, J. A. Nonspecific colitis following oral lincomycin therapy. Am. J. Gastroenterol. *60*:394, 1973.
72. Koltz, A. P., Palmer, W. L., and Kirsner, J. B. Aureomycin proctitis and colitis: A report of five cases. Gastroenterology *25*:44, 1953.
73. Hall, I. C., and O'Toole, E. Intestinal flora in newborn infants with description of a new pathogenic anaerobe, *Bacillus difficilis*. Am. J. Dis. Child. *49*:390, 1935.
74. Snyder, M. L. The normal fecal flora of infants between two weeks and one year of age. I. Serial studies. J. Infect. Dis. *66*:1, 1940.
75. Hafiz, S. L. *Clostridium difficile* and its toxins. Ph.D. Thesis, University of Leeds, 1974.
76. Smith, L. D., and King, O. Occurrence of *Clostridium difficile* in infections of man. J. Bacteriol. *84*:65, 1962.
77. George, W. L., Sutter, V. L., Citron, D., and Finegold, S. M. Selective and differential medium for isolation of *Clostridium difficile*. J. Clin. Microbiol. *9*:214, 1979.
78. Willey, S. H., and Bartlett, J. G. Cultures for *Clostridium difficile* in stools containing a cytotoxin neutralized by *Clostridium sordellii* antitoxin. J. Clin. Microbiol. *10*:880, 1979.
79. Keighley, M. R. B., Burdon, D. W., Arabi, U., Alexander-Williams, J., Thomson, H., Youngs, D., Johnson, M., Bentley, S., George, R. H., and Mogg, G. A. G. Randomized controlled trial of vancomycin for pseudomembranous colitis and postoperative diarrhoea. Br. Med. J. *2*:1667, 1978.
80. Bartlett, J. G., Taylor, N. W., Chang, T. W., and Dzink, J. A. Clinical and laboratory observations in *Clostridium difficile* colitis. Am. J. Clin. Nutr. *33*:2521–2526, 1981.
81. Viscidi, R., Willey, S., and Bartlett, J. G. Isolation rates and toxigenic potential for *Clostridium difficile* isolates from various patient populations. Gastroenterology *81*:5–9, 1981.
82. Gilligan, P. H., McCarthy, L. R., and Genta, V. M. Relative frequency of *Clostridium difficile* in patients with diarrhea disease. J. Clin. Microbiol. *14*:26, 1981.
83. Lishman, A. H., Al-Jumaili, I. J., and Record, C. O. Spectrum of antibiotic-associated diarrhea. Gut *22*:34–37, 1981.
84. Falsen, E., Kaijser, B., Nehls, L., and Nygren, B. *Clostridium difficile* in relation to enteric bacterial pathogens. J. Clin. Microbiol. *12*:297, 1980.
85. Boriello, S. P. *Clostridium difficile* and its toxin in the gastrointestinal tract in health and disease. Res. Clin. Forums *1*:33–36, 1979.
86. Varki, N. M., and Aquino, T. I. Isolation of *C. difficile* from hospitalized patients without antibiotic-associated diarrhea or colitis. J. Clin. Microbiol. *16*:659, 1982.
87. Holst, E., Helin, I., and Mardh, P. -A. Recovery of *Clostridium difficile* from children. Scand. J. Infect. Dis. *13*:41, 1981.
88. Rietra, P. J., Souterus, K. W., and Zanen, H. C. Clostridial toxin in faeces of healthy infants. Lancet *2*:319, 1978.
89. Larson, H. E., Barclay, F. E., Honour, P., and Hill, I. D. Epidemiology of *Clostridium difficile* in infants. J. Infect. Dis. *146*:727, 1982.
90. Welch, D. F., and Marks, M. I. Is *Clostridium difficile* pathogenic in infants? J. Pediatr. *100*:393, 1982.
91. Bartlett, J. G., Chang, T. W., Moon, N., and Onderdonk, A. B. Antibiotic-induced lethal enterocolitis in hamsters: Studies with eleven agents and evidence to support the pathogenic role of toxin producing clostridia. Am. J. Vet. Res. *38*:1525, 1978.
92. Silva, J., Jr. Animal models of antibiotic-induced colitis. *In* Microbiology—1979. Washington, D.C., American Society of Microbiology, 1979, p. 258.
93. Ebright, J. R., Fekety, R., Silva, J., Jr., and Wilson, K. Evaluation of eight cephalosporins in hamster colitis model. Antimicrob. Agents Chemother. *19*:980, 1981.
94. Burdon, D. W., Brown, J. D., Youngs, D., Arabi, Y., and Keighley, M. Antibiotic susceptibility of *Clostridium difficile*. J. Antimicrob. Chemother. *5*:307, 1979.
95. George, W. L., Sutter, V. L., and Finegold, S. M. Toxicity and antimicrobial susceptibility of *Clostridium difficile*, a cause of antimicrobial agent-associated colitis. Curr. Microbiol. *1*:55, 1978.
96. Dzink, J. A., and Bartlett, J. G. *In vitro* susceptibility of *Clostridium difficile* isolates from patients with antibiotic-associated diarrhea or colitis. Antimicrob. Ag. Chemother. *17*:695, 1980.
97. Shuttleworth, R., Taylor, M., and Jones, D. M. Antimicrobial susceptibilities of *Clostridium difficile*. J. Clin. Pathol. *33*:1002, 1980.
98. Kabins, A., and Spira, T. J. Outbreak of clindamycin-associated colitis. Ann. Intern. Med. *83*:830–831, 1975.

99. Greenfield, C., Szawathowski, M., Noone, P., Burroughs, A., Bass, N., and Pounder, R. Is pseudomembranous colitis infectious? Lancet *1*:371, 1981.
100. Keighley, M. R. B. Antibiotic-associated pseudomembranous colitis: Pathogenesis and management. Drugs *20*:49, 1980.
101. Bender, B. S., Laughon, B. E., Gaydos, G., Forman, M. S., Bennett, R., Greenough, W. B., III, Sears, S. D., and Bartlett, J. G. Is *Clostridium difficile* endemic in chronic care facilities? Lancet *2*:11, 1986.
102. Teasley, D. G., Olson, M. M., Gebhard, R. L., Gerding, D. N., Peterson, L. R., Schwartz, M. J., and Lee, J. T. Prospective randomized trial of metronidazole versus vancomycin for *Clostridium difficile*–associated diarrhoea and colitis. Lancet *2*:1444, 1983.
103. Gerding, D. N., Olson, M. M., Peterson, L. R., Teasley, D. G., Gebhard, R. L., Schwartz, M. L., and Lee, J. T. *Clostridium difficile*–associated diarrhea and colitis in adults. Arch. Intern. Med. *146*:95, 1986.
104. Kim, K. -H., Fekety, R., Botts, D. H., and Brown, D. Isolation of *Clostridium difficile* from the environment and contacts of patients with antibiotic-associated colitis. J. Infect. Dis. *143*:42, 1981.
105. Mulligan, M. E., George, W. L., Rolfe, R. D., and Finegold, S. M. Epidemiological aspects of *Clostridium difficile*–induced diarrhea and colitis. Am. J. Clin. Nutr. *33*:2533, 1981.
106. Fekety, R., Kim, K. -H., Brown, D., Batts, D. H., Cuctmore, M., and Silva, J., Jr. Epidemiology of antibiotic-associated colitis. Am. J. Med. *70*:906–908, 1981.
107. Communicable Disease Center. Guidelines for isolation precautions in hospitals. Infect. Control *4*:267, 1983.
108. Chang, T. W., Lauermann, M., and Bartlett, J. G. Cytotoxicity assay in antibiotic-associated colitis. J. Infect. Dis. *140*:765, 1979.
109. Bartlett, J. G. Laboratory diagnosis of antibiotic-associated colitis. Lab. Med. *12*:347, 1981.
110. Bartlett, J. G. *Clostridium difficile* and inflammatory bowel disease. Gastroenterology *80*:863, 1981.
111. Trnka, Y. M., and LaMont, J. T. Association of *Clostridium difficile* toxin with symptomatic relapse of chronic inflammatory bowel disease. Gastroenterology *80*:693, 1981.
112. Bolton, R. P., Sherrief, R. J., and Read, A. E. *Clostridium difficile* associated diarrhoea: A role in inflammatory bowel disease? Lancet *1*:383, 1980.
113. Keighley, M. R. B. *Clostridium difficile* and inflammatory bowel disease. J. Antimicrob. Chemother. *11*:493–494, 1983.
114. Meyers, S., Mayer, L., Bottone, E., Desmond, E., and Janowitz, H. D. Occurrence of *Clostridium difficile* toxin during the course of inflammatory bowel disease. Gastroenterology *80*:697, 1981.
115. Wu, T. C., and Fung, J. C. Evaluation of the usefulness of counterimmunoelectrophoresis for diagnosis of *Clostridium difficile*–associated colitis in clinical specimens. J. Clin. Microbiol. *17*:610–613, 1983.
116. Laughon, B. E., Viscidi, R. P., Gdovin, S. L., Yolken, R. H., and Bartlett, J. G. Enzyme immunoassays for detection of *Clostridium difficile* toxins A and B in fecal specimens. J. Infect. Dis. *149*:781, 1984.
117. Peterson, L. R., Holter, J. J., Shanholtzer, C. J., Garrett, C. R., and Gerding, D. N. Detection of *Clostridium difficile* toxins A (enterotoxin) and B (cytotoxin) in clinical specimens. Am. J. Clin. Pathol. *86*:208, 1986.
118. Lyerly, D. M., and Wilkins, T. D. Commercial latex test for *Clostridium difficile* toxin A does not detect toxin A. J. Clin. Microbiol. *23*:622, 1986.
119. Taylor, N. S., Thorne, G., and Bartlett, J. G. Comparison of two toxins produced by *Clostridium difficile*. Infect. Immun. *34*:1036, 1981.
120. Banno, U., Kobayashi, T., Kono, H., et al. Biochemical characterization and biologic actions of two toxins (D-1 and D-2) from *Clostridium difficile*. Rev. Infect. Dis. *6*:511, 1984.
121. Sullivan, N. M., Pettett, S., and Wilkins, T. D. Purification and characterization of toxins A and B of *Clostridium difficile*. Infect. Immun. *35*:1032, 1982.
122. Pothoulakis, C., Barone, L. M., Ely, R., Faris, B., Clark, M. E., Franzblau, C., and LaMont, T. Purification and properties of *Clostridium difficile* cytotoxin B. J. Biol. Chem. *261*:1316, 1986.
123. Libby, J. M., Jortner, B. S., and Wilkins, T. D. Effects of the two toxins of *Clostridium difficile* in antibiotic-associated cecitis in hamsters. Infect. Immun. *36*:822–829, 1982.
124. Justus, P. G., Martin, J. L., Goldberg, D. A., Taylor, N. S., Bartlett, J. G., Alexander, R. W., and Mathias, J. R. Myoelectric effects of *Clostridium difficile*: Motility-altering factors distinct from its cytotoxin and enterotoxin in rabbits. Gastroenterology *83*:836, 1982.
125. Rolfe, R. D., and Iaconis, J. P. Intestinal colonization of infant hamsters with *Clostridium difficile*. Infect. Immun. *42*:480, 1983.
126. Chang, T.-W., Sullivan, N. M., and Wilkins, T. D. Insusceptibility of fetal intestinal mucosa and fetal cells to *Clostridium difficile* toxins. Acta Pharmacol. Sin. *5*:448, 1986.
127. Viscidi, R. P., and Bartlett, J. G. Antibiotic-associated pseudomembranous colitis in children. Pediatrics *67*:381, 1981.
128. Viscidi, R., Laughon, B. E., Yolken, R., Bo-Linn, P., Moench, T., Ryder, R. W., and Bartlett, J. G. Serum antibody response to toxins A and B of *Clostridium difficile*. J. Infect. Dis. *148*:93, 1983.
129. Novak, E., Lee, J. E., Seckman, C. E., Phillips, J. P., and DiSanto, A. R. Unfavorable effect of atropine-diphenoxylate (Lomotil) therapy in lincomycin-caused diarrhea. JAMA *235*:1451, 1976.
130. Pittman, E. F. Lomotil and antibiotic colitis. Ann. Intern. Med. *83*:124, 1975.
131. Bartlett, J. G., Chang, T. W., and Onderdonk, A. B. Comparison of five regimens of treatment of experimental clindamycin-associated colitis. J. Infect. Dis. *138*:81–86, 1978.
132. Viteri, A. L., Howard, P. H., and Dyck, W. P. The spectrum of colitis associated with lincomycin and clindamycin therapy. J. Infect. Dis. *131*:S1135, 1974.
133. Jackson, B. T., and Anders, C. J. Idiopathic pseudomembranous colitis successfully treated by surgical excision. Br. J. Surg. *59*:154, 1972.
134. Saylor, J. L., Anderson, C. B., and Tedesco, F. J. Pseudomembranous colitis treated with completely diverting ileostomy. Arch. Surg. *111*:596, 1976.
135. Young, G. P., Ward, P. B., and Bayley, N. Antibiotic-associated colitis due to *Clostridium difficile*: Double-blind comparison of vancomycin with bacitracin. Gastroenterology *89*:1038–1045, 1985.
136. Dudley, M. N., McLaughlin, J. C., Carrington, G., Frick, J., Nightingale, C. H., and Quintiliani, R. Oral bacitracin vs. vancomycin therapy for *Clostridium difficile*–induced diarrhea. Arch. Intern. Med. *146*:1101, 1986.
137. Bartlett, J. G. Treatment of *Clostridium difficile* colitis. Gastroenterology *89*:1192, 1985.
138. Fekety, R., Silva, J., Armstrong, J., Allo, M., Browne, R., Ebright, J., Lusk, R., Rifkin, G., and Toshniwal, R. Treatment of antibiotic-associated enterocolitis with vancomycin. Rev. Infect. Dis. *3*:S273, 1981.
139. Bartlett, J. G., Tedesco, F. J., Shull, S., Lowe, B., and Chang, T. Symptomatic relapse after oral vancomycin therapy of antibiotic-associated pseudomembranous colitis. Gastroenterology *78*:431, 1980.
140. Bartlett, J. G. Treatment of antibiotic-associated pseudomembranous colitis. Rev. Infect. Dis. *6*:S235, 1984.
141. Mogg, G. A. G., Arabi, Y., Youngs, D., Johnson, M., Bentley, S., Burdon, D. W., and Keighley, M. R. B. Therapeutic trials of antibiotic associated colitis. Scand. J. Infect. Dis. *22*(suppl.):41–45, 1980.
142. Arabi, Y., Dimock, F., Burdon, D. W., and Alexander-Williams, J. Influence of neomycin and metronidazole on colonic microflora of volunteers. J. Antimicrob. Chemother. *5*:531, 1979.
143. Thompson, G., Clark, A. H., Hare, K., and Spilg, W. G. S. Pseudomembranous colitis after treatment with metronidazole. Br. Med. J. *282*:804, 1981.

144. Saginur, R., Hawley, C. R., and Bartlett, J. G. Colitis associated with metronidazole therapy. J. Infect. Dis. *141*:772, 1980.
145. Burbige, E. J., and Milligan, F. D. Pseudomembranous colitis. JAMA *213*:1157, 1975.
146. Taylor, N. S., and Bartlett, J. G. Binding of *Clostridium difficile* cytotoxin and vancomycin by anion exchange resins. J. Infect. Dis. *141*:92, 1980.
147. Kreutzer, E. W., and Milligan, F. D. Treatment of antibiotic-associated pseudomembranous colitis with cholestyramine resin. Johns Hopkins Med. J. *143*:67, 1978.
148. Tedesco, F. J., Napier, J., Gamble, W., Chang, T.-W., and Bartlett, J. G. Therapy of antibiotic-associated pseudomembranous colitis. J. Clin. Gastroenterol. *1*:51, 1979.
149. Walters, B. A. J., Roberts, R., Stafford, R., and Seneviratne, E. Relapse of antibiotic associated colitis: Endogenous persistence of *Clostridium difficile* during vancomycin therapy. Gut *24*:206, 1983.
150. Onderdonk, A. B., Cisneros, R. L., and Bartlett, J. G. *Clostridium difficile* in gnotobiotic mice. Infect. Immun. *28*:277, 1980.
151. Tedesco, F. J. Treatment of recurrent antibiotic-associated pseudomembranous colitis. Am. J. Gastroenterol. *77*:220, 1982.

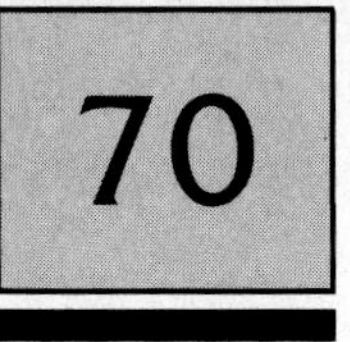

Small Intestinal Ulcers and Strictures: Isolated and Diffuse

THEODORE M. BAYLESS

Ulcers of the small intestine distal to the duodenum are not common, but they can at times be responsible for abdominal pain, intestinal obstruction, perforation, or hemorrhage. Stricturing or stenosis of the intestine may lead to obstruction and become the presenting problem. Although some ulcers and strictures are associated with known diseases, such as lymphoma, carcinoma, vasculitis, ischemia, radiation enteritis, incarcerated hernias, tuberculosis, or Crohn's disease, others are of unknown etiology and are without a distinctive or diagnostic pathologic appearance. This chapter will discuss both isolated and diffuse ulceration of the small intestines with emphasis on these idiopathic enteric ulcerations.

Some patients present with discrete or isolated, usually single, ulcerations in an otherwise normal small bowel mucosa; we will refer to those as *isolated nonspecific ulcers.*[1] These ulcers are often self-limited and usually don't recur after limited bowel resection. Other patients have a seemingly quite different syndrome with *diffuse ulceration* of the *jejunum* and *ileum,* often in association with a flattened jejunal mucosa and generalized malabsorption. Some, especially patients in their 50s and 60s, have a recognizable underlying disorder, usually *celiac sprue* (see pp. 1134–1152).[2] Others have a *chronic nongranulomatous ulcerating jejunoileitis,*[3] also known as *idiopathic chronic ulcerative enteritis.*[4] In contrast to the patients with isolated nonspecific ulcers, patients with the diffusion ulcerations often die either of complications of the ulcers or of seemingly concomitant *intestinal lymphoma.*

ISOLATED NONSPECIFIC ULCERS

Background

Primary nonspecific ulceration of the small intestine beyond the duodenum is rare. The discrete lesions may be single or multiple, are of unknown etiology, and most resemble lesions due to ischemic injury.

Small intestinal ulcers were first described in 1795, and they were considered to be infectious in nature until Crohn reported on noninfectious ulceration of the small intestine in 1932 (see p. 1327). Since then, known causes of isolated small bowel ulcers include congenital stenoses, tuberculosis, syphilis, cytomegalovirus, typhoid, *Campylobacter* infection, Crohn's disease (aphthous ulcer), Behçet's syndrome, celiac sprue, diverticulitis, ulcerated heterotopic gastric mucosa, previous irradiation, ischemia (including emboli without infarction), vasculitis, trauma, vascular abnormalities, jejunal ulcers of gastrinoma, arsenic poisoning, lymphoma, carcinoma, and enteric-coated potassium tablets, wax-matrix potassium products, and indomethacin.[5]

Ulcers that cannot be explained by such specific mechanisms are included in the category of nonspecific or idiopathic small bowel intestinal ulcers. In a 1963 review, Watson enumerated 170 cases of nonspecific or idiopathic ulcer of the small intestine in the world literature.[6] That these ulcers were not idiopathic, however, became apparent when the enteric-coated potassium chloride tablets were identified as the cause of many of these isolated ulcers in the early to mid 1960s. By 1965, a retrospective review of 484 patients with primary nonspecific ulceration revealed that over half (57 per cent) had received enteric-coated potassium chloride, a diuretic, or both.[7] The frequency of small bowel lesions was estimated to be 40 to 50 per 100,000 patient years.[7]

Since the removal of enteric-coated potassium chloride tablets from the market, the incidence has declined so much that nonspecific small bowel ulceration is again an unusual and rarely diagnosed disease. A review of 59 patients at the Mayo Clinic from 1956 to 1979 documents an overall incidence of four patients per 100,000 new patients registered at that institution; however, the yearly rate fell from 3.6 new cases per year from 1960 to 1969 to 1.2 cases per year in the decade from 1970 to 1979.[1]

Reports of intestinal ulceration, hemorrhage, and perforation in patients taking nonsteroidal anti-inflammatory drugs (NSAIDs) are appearing with increasing frequency.[8] In one study of 268 patients admitted with small or large bowel perforation or hemorrhage (excluding idiopathic inflammatory bowel disease and cancer), NSAID intake was more than twice as common in the patients as in matched control subjects.[9] Slow release formulations and coexistent inflammatory bowel disease are situations that would seem to increase the risk of NSAID-induced intestinal injury.[8]

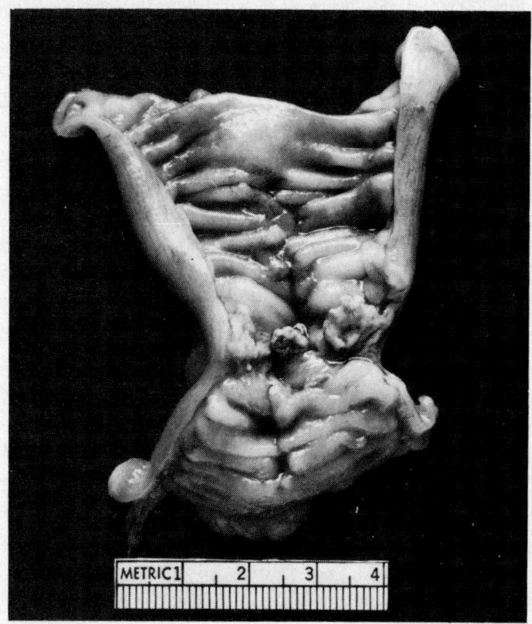

Figure 70–1. Isolated ileal ulcer. Resected specimen of ileal segment showing solitary, nonspecific, annular ulcer with necrotic, fibrinous surface. Fibrous scar formation has produced narrowing of the lumen. (From Boydston, J. S., Jr., Gaffery, T. A., and Bartholomew, L. G. Clinicopathologic study of nonspecific ulcers of the small intestine. Dig. Dis. Sci. *26*:911, 1981. Used by permission of Plenum Publishing Corp.)

Pathology of Idiopathic Small Intestinal Ulcers

The ulcers are usually single but may be multiple and clustered, and are twice as common in the ileum as in the jejunum. In the 1981 Mayo Clinic report, ileal ulcers constituted 78 per cent of the series, jejunal ulcers constituted 15 per cent, and jejunoileal ulceration made up 7 per cent.[1] These ulcers tend to be discrete and free of surrounding inflammatory response. They start as small oval lesions with sharp, punched-out edges, resembling a simple peptic ulcer. Occasionally, they extend circumferentially, becoming an annular ulcer, which then frequently becomes a fibrotic, obstructive stricture (Fig. 70–1).[10] Microscopically, the inflammatory infiltrate suggests chronicity: rarely, striking eosinophilia has been seen.[11] No disease of blood vessels is evident, and, interestingly, the bowel between ulcers is uniformly normal.

Perforation is not uncommon, especially in jejunal ulcers. In the Mayo Clinic series, 78 per cent of the jejunal ulcers had perforated, in contrast to 11 per cent of the ileal ulcers.

The differential diagnosis of nonspecific ulcer includes *Crohn's disease* (aphthous ulcers), *ischemic injury, embolization* without infarction, *incarcerated inguinal hernia, vasculitis, syphilis, typhoid fever, tuberculosis, Campylobacter* infection, *lymphoma, arsenic* poisoning, *ulceration* of *heterotopic gastric mucosa,* and *jejunal ulcers associated with gastrinomas* (Zollinger-Ellison syndrome).[12]

Etiology and Pathogenesis

With the exception of ulcerations due to potassium chloride and, more recently, indomethacin,[5] the etiology of primary nonspecific ulceration is unknown. The most prominent possibilities have included *vascular disease* (other than vasculitis, or obvious vascular abnormalities), *central nervous system disease, infection, trauma,* and *hormonal influences.*[10] Experimentally, ulcerative lesions can be produced in the small bowel of monkeys with enteric-coated potassium tablets. The lesions are due to a localized high concentration of potassium in the region of a rapidly dissolving tablet, with bowel wall injury and subsequent ulceration, hemorrhage, perforation, or obstruction. Because of this toxicity, enteric-coated potassium tablets with or without diuretics have been withdrawn from the market. However, a new series of slow-release, wax-matrix potassium chloride tablets and microencapsulated potassium chloride tablets are now being prescribed. Although the slow or controlled release of potassium chloride minimizes the possibility of a high local concentration of potassium near the bowel wall, some instances of small bowel lesions, bleeding, perforation, and obstruction with wax-matrix and microencapsulated tablets have been reported although at a rate of less than 1 per 100,000 patient years.[13] Concern is greatest in the presence of any arrest or delay in passage through the gastrointestinal tract. Because of the gastric and intestinal lesions, the use of delayed release potassium tablets is reserved for patients intolerant to liquid or effervescent products.

Indomethacin is ulcerogenic to the small intestine of rats, although the dosages have been far in excess of comparable dosages used in humans. It has been suggested that inhibition of prostaglandin synthetase causes a prostaglandin deficiency with a decreased resistance of the intestinal mucosa. This increased permeability may allow deleterious agents such as bacteria, bacterial toxins, or bile acids to penetrate the mucosa and eventually cause ulceration.[14] There are a number of reports of small intestinal ulcerations in patients taking indomethacin, phenylbutazone, and other NSAID, especially in slow release formulations. Although some had complicating problems such as previous *irradiation, tuberculosis,* concomitant *corticosteroid ingestion, Crohn's disease,* or in one patient, *celiac disease,*[5] the association of ulceration and perforation, and hemorrhage seems to be valid.[8, 9]

Postbulbar duodenal ulcerations have been reported in a patient who took salicylsalicylic acid, a nonsteroidal anti-inflammatory agent, for two days, but the patient had had a duodenal bulb ulcer four weeks earlier.[15]

Clinical Features

The clinical picture of isolated small intestinal ulcers usually consists of the symptoms of intermittent *small bowel obstruction.* Sixty-three per cent of the 59 patients at the Mayo Clinic presented in this way. *Bleeding* and an *acute abdominal crisis* associated with *perforation* were the two other major forms of presentation, representing 25 per cent and 12 per cent of the Mayo Clinic patients, respectively.[1] The 59 patients ranged from 17 to 77 years of age, with a mean age of 51 years; 31 patients were men. Many patients had no prior complaint, but some had a history of chronic periumbilical colic, nausea, or vomiting.[1] The preexistence of delayed bowel transit, concomitant corticosteroid usage, or *celiac sprue* might have been clues to drug-induced ulcerations. At times there was a lag between the use of potassium tablets and the onset of bowel obstruction. The signs on physical examination were usually minimal unless the patient had an obstructed or perforated gut. In the absence of these complications, the abdomen was not tender. There were usually no laboratory aids in the diagnosis except in the presence of bleeding, severe vomiting due to obstruction, or perforation.

Diagnosis

Preoperative diagnosis is unusual, partly because of the low index of suspicion for this problem. Plain films of the abdomen help to diagnose small bowel obstruction due to strictures. Barium contrast examinations in uncomplicated cases usually do not demonstrate the ulcerations, although carefully directed small bowel clysis studies through a tube may be helpful. Areas of obstruction or stricture may be identified either by small bowel series or by barium enema in the case of distal ileal lesions.

Increased use of small bowel endoscopy via longer instruments that permit peroral examination of the upper jejunum, or at laparotomy, has facilitated diagnosis of small bowel ulceration in some patients. Isolated ileal ulceration has been identified and biopsied via colonoscopy.

Associated Medications and Conditions

The frequent association with enteric-coated potassium tablets was an important factor in the mid-1960s. However, the Mayo Clinic series reported only 6 of 59 patients had taken such medications. Eleven had cardiovascular disease, while three had previously had peptic ulcers. Nine had other systemic diseases.[1] Indomethacin and other nonsteroidal anti-inflammatory medications may become a more important factor in the future.

Treatment

Therapy of the isolated complicated ulcer is surgical excision of the stenotic lesion. The entire intestine should be examined very carefully, because these ulcers may be multiple, although more often they are solitary. Increasingly, with growing awareness of multiple aphthous ulcerations as a manifestation of *Crohn's disease,* care must be taken not to remove extensive sections of small bowel because of small ulcers located in separate segments of the bowel. The natural history of isolated nonspecific small bowel ulcerations seems to be relatively self-limited, so that in the absence of complications a conservative approach seems warranted. Short-term reports of the effect of corticosteroid therapy of isolated ileal ulcers are difficult to evaluate because Crohn's disease has not clearly been ruled out in these patients.[16]

Discontinuation of any possible offending pharmacologic agent is indicated. The recent introduction of wax-matrix potassium chloride tablets causes concern that the incidence of small bowel ulceration will again rise. The drug companies suggest that such tablets be reserved for those patients who cannot tolerate or who refuse to take liquid or effervescent potassium preparations. As a generalization, one would feel that solutions of potassium are a safer form of potassium supplementation, especially if there is any suspicion of an alteration in gastrointestinal tract motility and transit time that prolong the contact of a potassium-containing tablet with the mucosa of jejunum. Special care should be exercised when prescribing NSAIDs, especially in the slow release forms, in patients with strictures or inflammatory bowel disease.[8]

Prognosis

Although isolated nonspecific ulcers are generally self-limited and do not recur after resection, patients with complications, especially perforation, are at great risk because of the associated *peritonitis* or *abscesses.* Five of 13 patients with perforations in the series from the Mayo Clinic died during the operative or postoperative period. Two others died with ulcer-related problems in the next one to six months. Of the 50 patients known to have survived over six months after surgery, 28 are still alive two to 25 years later, and only seven of these 28 have gastrointestinal problems. Although four (approximately 10 per cent) have proved or suspected ulcer recurrences, this type of problem is usually self-limited. Most of the deaths were due to cardiovascular disease or unrelated neoplasia. Even these patients were generally without gastrointestinal problems after ulcer resection.[1]

DIFFUSE ULCERATION OF JEJUNUM AND ILEUM

Background and Definition of Types

Multiple nonmalignant ulcers of the small intestine are an uncommon, but frequently fatal, complication of *celiac sprue* (gluten-induced enteropathy).[2, 17] Along with the development of lymphoma, this type of intestinal ulceration is the leading cause of premature death of patients in celiac disease. The patients are usually in the sixth or seventh decade at the time of diagnosis of the ulceration. The ulcers are predominantly jejunal; pathologically, they are nonspecific. The mucosa often displays subtotal villous atrophy, as in celiac sprue, but it may be normal, as it often is, in the ileum (see pp. 1135–1138).

Similar ulcerations have been described in patients with malabsorption associated with diffuse or patchy jejunal villous atrophy who did not respond to a gluten-free diet or to adrenocortical steroids. The terms "chronic ulcerative nongranulomatous jejunoileitis"[3, 18] and "idiopathic chronic ulcerative enteritis"[4, 19] have been applied to many of these latter patients. Confusion has resulted from the use of these nonspecific terms, which suggests an identifiable nosologic entity. However, since patients with primary diseases or disorders such as well-documented *celiac sprue, common variable hypogammaglobulinemia,* and *lymphoma* of the small intestine also display lesions identical with those of "chronic ulcerative nongranulomatous jejunoileitis," the use of this term should be carefully limited. Perhaps patients with diffuse ulceration and malabsorption who do not have celiac sprue or lymphoma, but who have flattening or patchy villous blunting of the jejunal mucosa with diffuse inflammation of jejunal and ileal mucosa might be considered to have *idiopathic chronic ulcerative enteritis*.[19, 20]

Ulcerations in some patients with *celiac sprue* who subsequently develop intestinal lymphomas can be deceptive, for histologically these lesions may be benign or "atypical" but not diagnostic of the underlying lymphoma. One or two years may elapse before the presence of a lymphoma is either proved or obvious.[17, 21]

The most important concept related to intestinal ulceration now being considered is that most of the intestinal lymphomas in patients with intestinal inflammation and malabsorption are T-cell lymphomas.[22] It is suggested that small intestinal ulcers in patients with *celiac sprue* and in those with *idiopathic ulcerative enteritis* are harbingers of *intestinal T-cell lymphoma*.[22, 23] It is possible that lymphokines from abnormal T-cells are responsible for some of the mucosal injury at sites distant from the obvious lymphomas.[22]

Pathology

The small intestinal ulcers are most always multiple; most are in the jejunum, some are in the ileum, and a few are in the duodenum and colon (Fig. 70–2). The ulcers vary in depth, penetrating to the muscularis propria in most cases and causing serosal scarring and contraction in some. Perforation is common, being about equal in jejunum and ileum (Fig. 70–3). The inflammatory response is limited in some instances,

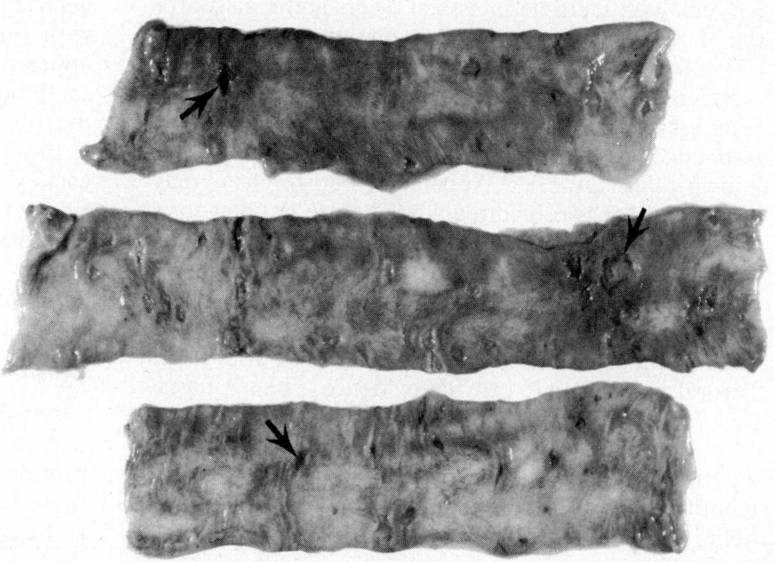

Figure 70–2. Ulceration in "unclassified sprue." Diffuse ileal ulceration in a 74-year-old patient with malabsorption, flattened jejunal mucosa, and dermatitis herpetiformis but without sustained response to a gluten-free diet or adrenal cortical steroids. The ileum at autopsy showed multiple punched-out ulcers *(arrows)*; more than 40 are seen in this figure. (Courtesy of Alan N. Baer, M.D.)

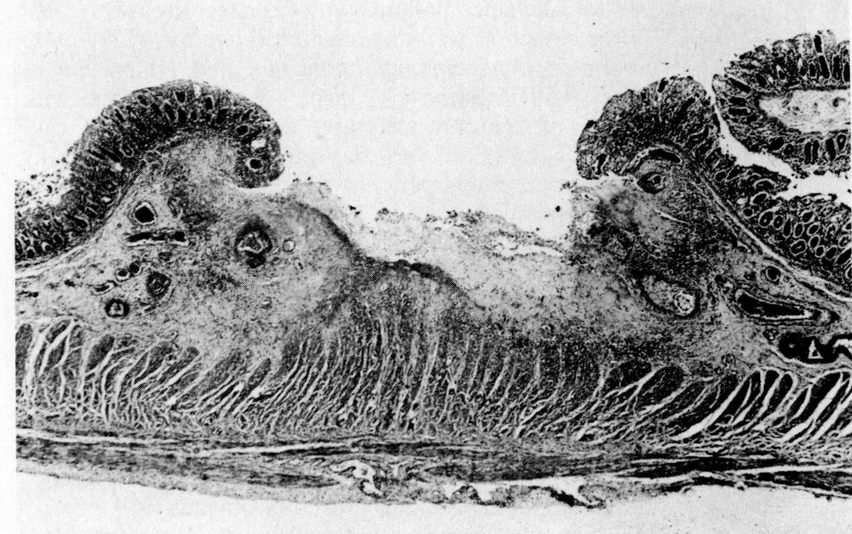

Figure 70–3. Ulceration in "unclassified sprue." Photomicrograph of autopsy specimen of ileum shown in Figure 70–2, showing undermined ulceration of the mucosa and submucosa. The adjacent mucosa shows blunted villi. (Hematoxylin and eosin stain, × 13.)

while in others there is extensive submucosal edemas and fibrosis with patchy areas of thickened bowel wall. The inflammatory infiltrate is largely confined to the bases of the ulcers and is typically a mixture of lymphocytes, plasma cells, histiocytes, and polymorphonuclear leukocytes.[3, 17, 20] Granulomas and focal inflammation suggestive of *Crohn's disease* are absent. Gastric metaplasia has been noted as a nonspecific reaction at the edge of some ulcerations. The intervening mucosa in the jejunum is usually flattened with marked villous blunting, but about one third of patients have normal-sized jejunal villi. (Some, but not all, patients who have been studied were on a gluten-free diet.) Patchy villous blunting is found in some patients with "unclassified sprue" and ulceration. Peroral jejunal biopsies usually show a flat mucosa, but a few patients with multiple intestinal ulcers and malabsorption have had normal findings on jejunal biopsies.[17] These patients could be classified as *ulcerative enteritis.*

Pathologically nonspecific benign ulcerations may progress to *T-cell* or to *histiocytic* or *mixed lymphocytic-histiocytic lymphomas,* especially in patients with known *celiac sprue.*[21–25] Apparently benign ulcers may be present for two or three years before the diagnosis of lymphoma is made.[17, 21] Indeed, areas of histiocytic cells in pleomorphic atypical ulcers are noted, in all likelihood representing areas of lymphoma. As noted above, benign ulcers may be found in one part of the bowel, and obvious lymphoma may be seen elsewhere. Peroral biopsies may provide evidence, either suggestive or diagnostic, of lymphoma, but full-thickness resection biopsies are needed to exclude lymphoma in a patient with intestinal ulceration. In the future T-cell identification or other lymphoma cell markers may help localize malignant tissue in such patients.

DIFFUSE ULCERATION IN PATIENTS WITH CELIAC SPRUE

Clinical Features

Presentations include (1) a worsening of the symptoms of malabsorption and abdominal pain in a patient with proven *celiac sprue* in his or her fifth or sixth decade; (2) an unexplained, often long-standing, malabsorption syndrome in a patient with a flat jejunal biopsy; (3) occurrence of abdominal pain, fever, intestinal obstruction, intestinal perforation, or hemorrhage in an individual with malabsorption or protein-losing enteropathy. Weight loss is prominent and often marked (see pp. 1141–1142). The diagnosis of diffuse *small intestinal ulceration* in these patients has usually been demonstrated only at exploratory laparotomy with full-thickness biopsy, at resection of abnormal-appearing small bowel, or at autopsy.[1] Endoscopy and small bowel clysis occasionally may prove to be helpful diagnostically.

Physical Examination. The findings often reflect the cachexia associated with severe malabsorption or the signs of chronic intestinal obstruction. Signs of peritonitis usually indicate free perforation. Lymphadenopathy is unusual, even in patients who have developed lymphomas.

Laboratory Diagnosis

Hypoalbuminemia, hypocalcemia, and steatorrhea due to the worsening of malabsorption and advent of protein-losing enteropathy are often the hallmarks of these patients on presentation. Anemia is common as is the presence of occult blood in the stools. The white blood cell count is variable, ranging between 3600 and 20,000 cells per cu mm, most often with a normal differential. Hyposplenism may complicate active celiac sprue.

Radiographic Features. Most patients with celiac sprue with enteric ulcerations and malabsorption have an abnormal small bowel series with dilatation, flocculation, segmentation, and edema of jejunal folds, but the ulcerations are usually not demonstrated. The exception is patients with strictures, in whom an accompanying ulcer might on occasion be recognized. In a few patients areas of dilatation and narrowing or a diffuse jejunal nodularity may be noted.[26] These findings have led to laparotomy or multiple intestinal biopsies in some of these individuals. Small bowel clysis studies have also helped demonstrate small bowel ulcers or strictures. One patient with *celiac sprue,* who subsequently developed ulcerative enteritis and gastrointestinal lymphoma, initially presented with multiple gastric ulcers refractory to medical therapy.[27]

Abdominal lymphadenopathy may be demonstrable by CT scan in patients with ulcerative enteritis without lymphoma as well as in patients with active but uncomplicated celiac sprue,[28] thus complicating the diagnosis of lymphoma.

Endoscopy. Upper intestinal fiberoptic endoscopy, performed either at laparotomy or orally via new, longer endoscopes can more readily demonstrate jejunal and ileal ulcerations. A few patients have had colonic ulcers (demonstrated by colonoscopy or flexible sigmoidoscopy), or gastric ulcers as well as jejunoileal ulcers. The recently increased awareness that aphthous ulcers are present in the esophagus, stomach, small bowel, and colon in patients with *Crohn's disease* will make differential diagnosis more difficult.

Treatment

Exclusion of gluten from the diet has not affected the ulcerations. Surgical resection of all the recognized ulcers has apparently cured four of 13 patients with celiac sprue and ulceration. Although corticosteroid therapy induced prolonged remissions in two of 13 individuals, it was associated with intestinal perforation in 10 patients receiving steroids. Thus, the decision of whether or not to use steroids is difficult. Patients who responded had relatively superficial ulcerations and were without complications.[17] Antibiotic therapy has not been helpful. Because of the difficulty in making a diagnosis of multiple ulcerations and in excluding lymphoma and because of the therapeutic usefulness of surgical resection, it seems reasonable to recommend a laparotomy with biopsy followed by resection of the involved small bowel and mesenteric lymph nodes when intestinal ulceration appears to underlie malabsorption. Repeat laparotomy with biopsy may also be needed in individuals who fail to improve, or who relapse, because lymphoma may become apparent only months or years later. Abdominal lymphadenopathy on CT scan is usually not diagnostic of lymphoma in the patient with celiac sprue.[28] The nutritional status of these patients both pre- and postoperatively can usually be improved with parenteral hyperalimentation.

IDIOPATHIC DIFFUSE ULCERATIVE NONGRANULOMATOUS ENTERITIS

These patients have been designated by Jeffries, Steinberg, and Sleisenger as having nongranulomatous ulcerative jejunoileitis[3] and by others as having *idiopathic chronic ulcerative enteritis*[20] or *unclassified sprue.*[17] The etiology and pathogenesis are not known. Gluten does not seem to play an identifiable role in the flattened jejunal mucosa, at least at the time of acute ulceration. Gluten withdrawal or steroids have not altered the course of the ulceration, which in turn makes evaluation of the absorptive status difficult. There are no other known disease associations, although one patient had hypogammaglobulinemia and a number of others developed lymphomas one or two years after diagnosis.

Review of 11 such patients[17] revealed an average age of 56 years, eight years older than 22 patients in the same institution with celiac sprue and multiple ulcerations. The majority of these patients, nine of 11, had malabsorption for over one and a half years before the onset of the ulcers. The history of preceding malabsorption, on average for 4.6 years, lends credence to the idea that at least some patients might have had underlying but unproved celiac sprue.[20] The pathologic appearance of the ulcerations is nonspecific and is similar to that described for the patients with diffuse ulcerations and celiac sprue.[17, 19] Mucosa between the ulcers as well as much of the jejunal mucosa sometimes shows severe flattening similar to celiac sprue, although these changes are patchy.[17]

Clinical Features

The clinical picture is often one of severe, unresponsive malabsorption or protein-losing enteropathy in a patient with a flattened jejunal mucosa. Although, as mentioned, most of the patients had a long history of gastrointestinal symptoms often suggestive of malabsorption, they either had not been studied prior to the onset of the ulcerations and their associated clinical complications or had not responded to gluten withdrawal. Some had also not responded to adrenocortical steroids, but these therapies were often instituted late, well after complications of the disease had become apparent. Presenting symptoms in some of these patients include melena, intestinal obstruction, or perforation in a setting of malabsorption.

The course is usually quite severe and rapidly fatal. Most of the patients described in the literature have died within one or two years of the recognition of the intestinal ulceration.[11, 13, 15] Thus far, surgical resection of the most affected segments of small bowel has been the only effective treatment in a few patients.[4, 19]

Ulcerations and Lymphoma

A number of patients with celiac sprue and small bowel ulcers or patients with chronic idiopathic ulcerative enteritis subsequently are found to have intestinal lymphoma. The sequence may begin with benign intestinal ulceration, benign ulceration with atypical inflammation, gastric ulceration or benign ulceration in one part of the small intestine, and lymphoma in another site.[29] These associations further strengthen the recommendation for laparotomy and resection in patients with suspected ulcerative enteritis or celiac sprue and ulceration. The progression from apparently benign ulceration to lymphoma may take one to three years. Other patients present initially with intestinal perforation or obstruction due to the lymphoma. In one series of 133 patients with malignant lymphoma and biopsy-proved celiac disease, the long-term survivors (over five years) all presented with a small intestinal lesion, and seven underwent an initial resection. Chemotherapy and radiotherapy were added subsequently. This suggests that in some patients the lymphoma may be confined to the intestine at presentation and that an initial resection can be curative.[24]

Prognosis

Patients with diffuse intestinal ulceration and malabsorption generally have a poor prognosis. In a 1980 review, 29 of 40 patients with benign ulceration were known to have died as a result of the ulcers, usually secondary to perforation, sepsis, hemorrhage, or inanition.[17] Other patients with seemingly benign ulcers have gone on to develop malignant lymphoma.[3, 17] Some of these latter patients have responded well to intestinal resection and chemotherapy directed at their lymphoma.[25]

Table 70–1. CAUSES OF INTESTINAL ULCERATION AND/OR STRICTURES

Isolated Intestinal Ulceration and/or Stricture	Stricture
Infections:	
Tuberculosis	Mechanical congenital stenosis
Syphilis	Intussusception
Cytomegalovirus	
Inflammatory:	
Crohn's disease	Infections: tuberculosis
Behçet's syndrome	Inflammatory:
Celiac disease	Crohn's disease
Ulcerative enteritis	Celiac disease and ulcerations
Ischemia	Ulcerative enteritis
Vasculitis	Ischemia
Radiation enteritis	Radiation enteritis
Drug-induced:	
Potassium	Drug-induced: potassium
Indomethacin	
Phenylbutazone	
Salicylsalicylate	
Neoplastic:	Neoplastic:
Lymphoma	Lymphoma
Adenocarcinoma	Adenocarcinoma
Melanoma	

Intestinal Strictures

Any of the isolated or diffuse ulcerating conditions discussed in this chapter can cause an isolated area of bowel narrowing (Table 70–1). These strictures may cause intestinal obstruction. The other causes include *adenocarcinoma* and *lymphoma,* both of which might cause a loss of folds and irregular filling defects (see pp. 1519–1560). Prolonged ischemia of the small bowel may cause a concentrically scarred and narrowed segment, varying from 5 to 15 cm in length (see pp. 1903–1932). The stenotic areas associated with *Crohn's disease* (see pp. 1327–1358) and *tuberculosis* (see pp. 1221–1224) may be associated with fistulization or mass formation, as identifiable on CT scan. *Congenital stenosis* may result in a diaphragm-like narrowing. An occasional adult with recurrent episodes of abdominal pain and vomiting is found, at surgery, to have a congenital stenotic segment of the intestine (see pp. 1011–1013).

References

1. Boydstun, J. S., Jr., Gaffey, T. A., and Bartholomew, L. G. Clinicopathologic study of nonspecific ulcers of the small intestine. Dig. Dis. Sci. *26*:911, 1981.
2. Bayless, T. M., Kapelowitz, R. F., Shelley, W. M., Ballinger, W. F., and Hendrix, T. R. Intestinal ulceration: A complication of celiac disease. N. Engl. J. Med. *276*:996–1002, 1967.
3. Jeffries, G. H., Steinberg, H., and Sleisenger, M. H. Chronic ulcerative (nongranulomatous) jejunitis. Am. J. Med. *44*:47, 1968.
4. Jewell, D. P. Ulcerative enteritis. Br. Med. J. *287*:1740, 1983.
5. Venturatos, S. G., Hines, C., Jr., and Blalock, J. B. Ulceration of the small intestine in a patient with celiac disease. Southern Med. J. *77*:520–522, 1984.
6. Watson, M. R. Primary nonspecific ulceration of the small bowel. Arch. Surg. *87*:600, 1963.
7. Lawrason, F. D., Alpert, G., Mohr, F. L., and McMahon, F. G. Obstructive-ulcerative lesions of the small intestine. JAMA *191*:641, 1965.
8. Rampton, D. S. Review. Non-steroidal anti-inflammatory drugs and the lower gastrointestinal tract. Scand. J. Gastroenterol. *22*:1–4, 1987.
9. Langman, M. J. S., Morgan, L., and Worrall, A. Use of anti-inflammatory drugs by patients admitted with small or large bowel perforations and haemorrhage. Br. Med. J. *290*:347–349, 1985.
10. Morson, B. C., and Dawson, I. M. P. Gastrointestinal Pathology. Oxford, Blackwell Scientific Publications, 1972, pp. 285–286.
11. Morgenstern, L., Freilich, M., and Panish, J. F. The circumferential small-bowel ulcer: Clinical aspects in 17 patients. JAMA *191*:637, 1965.
12. Kiser, J. L. Focal lesions of the small intestine. Am. J. Surg. *112*:48, 1966.
13. Physicians' Desk Reference, 1987. Oradell, N. J. Medical Economics Company, 1987, pp. 530–531.
14. Bjarnason, I., Williams, P., Smethurst, P., Peters, T. J., and Levi, A. J. Effect of non-steroidal anti-inflammatory drugs and prostaglandins on the permeability of the human small intestine. Gut *27*:1292–1297, 1986.
15. Souza Lima, M. A. Ulcers of the small bowel associated with stomach-bypassing salicylates. Arch. Intern. Med. *145*:1139, 1985.
16. Borsch, B., Jahnke, A., Bergbauer, M., and Nebel, W. Solitary non-specific ileal ulcer. Diagnosis by coloileoscopy in a patient with previously assumed irritable bowel syndrome. Dis. Colon Rectum *26*:734–737, 1983.

17. Baer, A. N., Bayless, T. M., and Yardley, J. H. Intestinal ulceration and malabsorption syndromes. Gastroenterology *79*:754, 1980.
18. Smitskamp, H., and Kuipers, F. C. Steatorrhoea and ulcerative jejuno-ileitis. Acta Med. Scand. *177*:1, 1965.
19. Mills, P. R., Brown, I. L., and Watkinson, G. Idiopathic chronic ulcerative enteritis: Report of five cases and review of the literature. Q. J. Med. *194*:133, 1980.
20. Robertson, D. A. F., Dixon, M. F., Scott, B. B., Simpson, F. G., and Losowsky, M. S. Small intestinal ulceration: Diagnostic difficulties in relation to coeliac disease. Gut *24*:565–574, 1983.
21. Isaacson, P., and Wright, D. H. Malignant lymphoma of mucosa-associated lymphoid tissue. A distinctive type of B-cell lymphoma. Cancer *52*:1410, 1983.
22. Isaacson, P., O'Connor, N. T., Spencer, J., et al. Malignant histiocytosis of the intestine. A T-cell lymphoma. Lancet *2*:688–691, 1985.
23. Loughran, T. P., Jr., Kadin, M. E., and Deeg, H. J. T-cell intestinal lymphoma associated with celiac sprue. Ann. Intern. Med. *104*:44–47, 1986.
24. Swinson, C. M., Slavin, G., Coles, E. C., and Booth, C. C. Coeliac disease and malignancy. Lancet *1*:111–115, 1983.
25. Morgan, D. R., Holgate, C. S., Dixon, M. F., and Bird, C. C. Primary small intestinal lymphoma: A study of 39 cases. J. Pathol. *147*:211–221, 1985.
26. Lamont, C. M., Adams, F. G., and Mills, P. R. Radiology in idiopathic chronic ulcerative enteritis. Clin. Radiol. *33*:283–287, 1982.
27. Roehrkasse, R. L., Roberts, I. M., Wald, A., Talamo, T. S., and Mendelow, H. Celiac sprue complicated by lymphoma presenting with multiple gastric ulcers. Gastroenterology *91*:740–745, 1986.
28. Jones, B., Bayless, T. M., Fishman, E. K., and Siegelman, S. S. Lymphadenopathy in celiac disease: Computed tomographic observations. Am. J. Radiol. *142*:1127–1132, June 1984.
29. Brunton, F. J., and Guyer, P. B. Malignant histiocytosis and ulcerative jejunitis of the small intestine. Clin. Radiol. *34*:291–295, 1983.

71

Crohn's Disease

ROBERT M. DONALDSON, JR.

DEFINITION

Crohn's disease is an indolent, chronic inflammatory disorder capable of involving the entire alimentary tract from mouth to anus. The etiology and pathogenesis remain unknown, and Crohn's disease might represent more than one etiologically distinct entity. The term "Crohn's disease" is preferable to "granulomatous enteritis" or "regional enteritis" because granulomas are not required for diagnosis and because other inflammatory disorders can affect "regions" of the bowel. Inflammation extends through all layers of the gut wall and involves the adjacent mesentery and lymph nodes. Distal ileum and colon are the most common sites, and the inflammatory process is characteristically discontinuous. The disease is characterized by its prolonged and variable course, by its diversity of clinical manifestations, by its perianal and systemic complications, and by its remarkable tendency to recur after surgical resection of involved gut.

HISTORY

Isolated cases closely resembling Crohn's disease were described as early as 1813, but the disease was not recognized as an entity until 1932, when Crohn, Ginzburg, and Oppenheimer first defined the clinical and pathologic features of "regional ileitis." Because their earliest patients were clinically suspected of having acute appendicitis, Crohn and his colleagues believed that the disorder was confined to the ileum. They soon recognized, however, that any region of small bowel could be affected. Subsequently, when it became apparent that the disease process could also involve duodenum, stomach, or esophagus, its name was changed from regional ileitis to regional enteritis. Considered at first to be curable by surgery, the disease soon established its reputation for recurrence, with surgery indicated only as a last resort. Although others described patients with colonic involvement as early as 1932, it was difficult to exclude ulcerative colitis in such patients. In fact, the question of whether Crohn's disease truly involved the colon remained unsettled until 1960, when Lockhart-Mummery and Morson[1] demonstrated that Crohn's disease, unequivocally distinct from ulcerative colitis, could be confined to the colon. Crohn[2] has provided a detailed history of the disease that bears his name.

PATHOLOGY

An inflammatory process that involves all layers of the bowel wall is the key pathologic feature of Crohn's disease.[3, 4] During the earliest phases of the disease, microscopic examination demonstrates (1) hyperplasia of perilymphatic histiocytes and autonomic nerves, (2) diffuse granulomatous infiltration most intense in the region of small lymphatic vessels, (3) discrete noncaseating granulomas in the submucosa and lamina propria, (4) edema and lymphatic dilatation, and (5) monocytic infiltration and histiocytic proliferation within lymph nodules and Peyer's patches on the serosal surface of the bowel. Adjacent mesentery and lymph nodes frequently demonstrate similar histopathologic changes. Axonal necrosis of autonomic nerves composes a feature recently observed by electron microscopy which may distinguish Crohn's disease from other inflammatory processes.[5]

Certain pathologic features of Crohn's disease tend to distinguish it from chronic ulcerative colitis (Table 71–1). However, no single pathologic feature is truly pathognomonic of Crohn's disease, and pathologists are unable to make a definitive diagnosis in every case. Indeed, it is impossible to distinguish ulcerative colitis from Crohn's disease on pathologic grounds in 15 to 25 per cent of cases of chronic colitis.[6]

Once the disease becomes established, the bowel is thickened and leathery, and stenosis is common. Macroscopic features are similar whether the small intestine (Fig. 71–1) or colon (Fig. 71–2) is involved. The mesentery is markedly thickened, fatty, and edematous. Finger-like projections of thick mesentery characteristically extend over the serosal surface toward the antimesenteric border of the bowel (Fig. 71–3).

Table 71–1. PATHOLOGIC FEATURES OF CROHN'S DISEASE

	Frequency of Occurrence*	
Abnormality	***Crohn's Disease***	***Ulcerative Colitis***
Macroscopic		
Thickened bowel wall	+ + +	+
Narrowing of bowel lumen	+ + +	+
Discontinuous (skip) lesions	+ +	0
Discrete mucosal ulcers	+ +	0
Confluent linear ulcers	+ +	0
Deep fissures and fistulas	+ +	0
Microscopic		
Transmural inflammation	+ + +	+
Submucosal infiltration	+ + +	+
Submucosal thickening, fibrosis	+ + +	0
Ulceration through mucosa	+ + +	+ +
Fissures	+ + +	+
Focal granulomas	+ +	0

*Frequencies represent rough estimates compiled from descriptions[3] that compare the pathology of Crohn's disease and ulcerative colitis. Abnormalities are categorized as being present rarely (0), infrequently (+), frequently (+ +), or consistently (+ + +). None of these abnormalities should be considered as always present in Crohn's disease or always absent in ulcerative colitis.

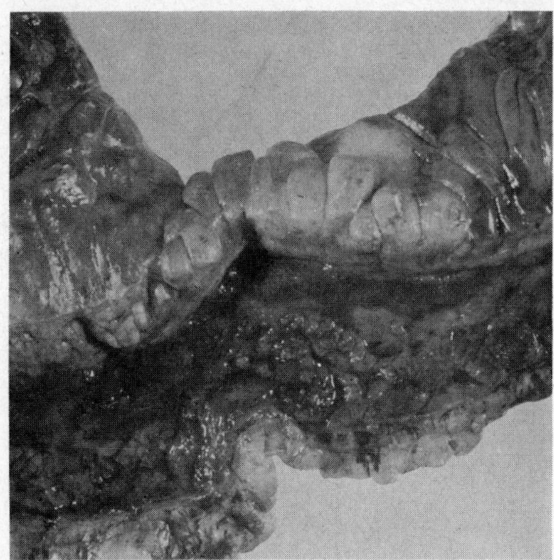

Figure 71–1. Gross specimen of ileum resected from a patient with Crohn's disease. The bowel wall is thickened as a result of involvement of all layers. Prominent mesenteric fat extends over the serosal surface. "Cobblestone" appearance of mucosa results from edema combined with ulceration.

The thick fibrotic mesentery is often contracted so as to angulate and "fix" the involved intestinal segment. Mesenteric nodes are enlarged and firm and are often matted together to form an irregular mass (Fig. 71–4). Dilated lymphatic vessels are frequently visible in the involved mesentery and serosal surface of the bowel.

When the diseased segment is opened, all layers of the bowel wall appear thickened, particularly the submucosa. The lumen is correspondingly narrowed. The mucosa may appear relatively normal to the naked eye except for hyperemia and edema. In advanced cases, however, normal mucosal architecture is completely destroyed by nodular swelling intermingled with deep ulcerations (Figs. 71–1 to 71–3). The combination of deep mucosal ulceration and nodular submucosal thickening gives a characteristic "cobblestone" appearance to the mucosal surfaces. Ulcers are frequently elongated or even linear and tend to lie in the long axis of the bowel. Ulcers usually extend at least into the submucosal layer where they often coalesce to form a single large intramural channel.

Serosal and mesenteric inflammation cause involved bowel loops to be firmly matted together by fibrotic peritoneal and mesenteric bands. Fistula formation often accompanies this adhesion. Presumably, fistulas begin as ulcerations that gradually burrow through the serosa and into adjacent loops of bowel. Fistulous tracts may penetrate small bowel, colon, abdominal wall, perineum, bladder, vagina, or indeed, any intra-abdominal organ. Most often, however, fistulas end, not in another organ, but blindly in indolent abscess cavities. These are embedded in dense inflammatory tissue and may be located within the peritoneal cavity, in the mesentery, or in retroperitoneal structures.

Segments of small or large intestine involved with Crohn's disease are often separated by "skip areas" of apparently normal bowel (Figs. 71–5 and 71–6).

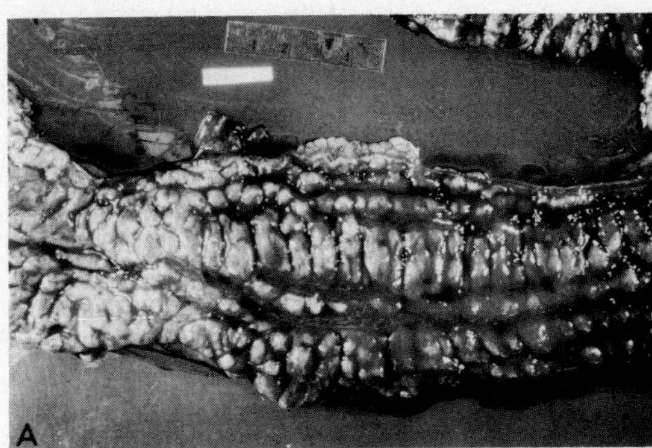

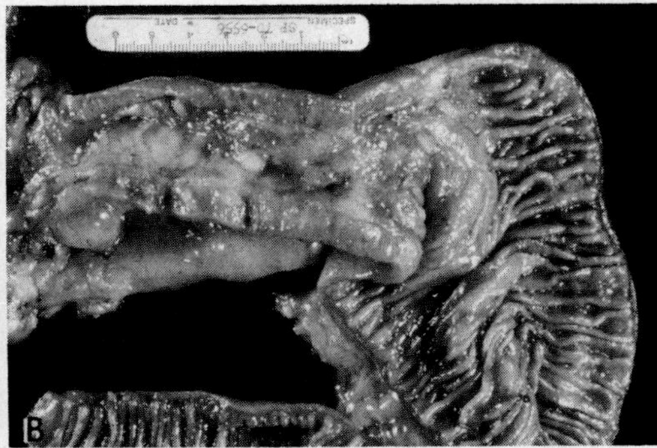

Figure 71–2. Resected specimens of colon from patients with Crohn's colitis. *A,* Note "cobblestone" mucosa formed by protuberant mucosa between confluent linear ulcers. Also note thickened colonic wall. *B,* Note segment of narrowed, thickened bowel giving "hose pipe" appearance on X-ray. Adjacent normal bowel is on the right. (Courtesy of Carolyn Montgomery, M.D.)

Whether skip areas are actually disease-free remains a key question so far as the nature of Crohn's disease is concerned.

Microscopic examination of involved intestine characteristically demonstrates a transmural inflammatory process which is most marked in the submucosa and which consists of infiltration with lymphocytes, histiocytes, and plasma cells (Fig. 71–7). Edema, endothelial and lymphatic swelling, and infiltration of the submucosa are followed by vascular hyalinization and fibrosis. Microscopic ulcerations and fissures frequently penetrate through the mucosal layer. Although seen occasionally, crypt abscesses containing polymorphonuclear leukocytes do not constitute a feature of Crohn's disease and are much more characteristic of ulcerative colitis.

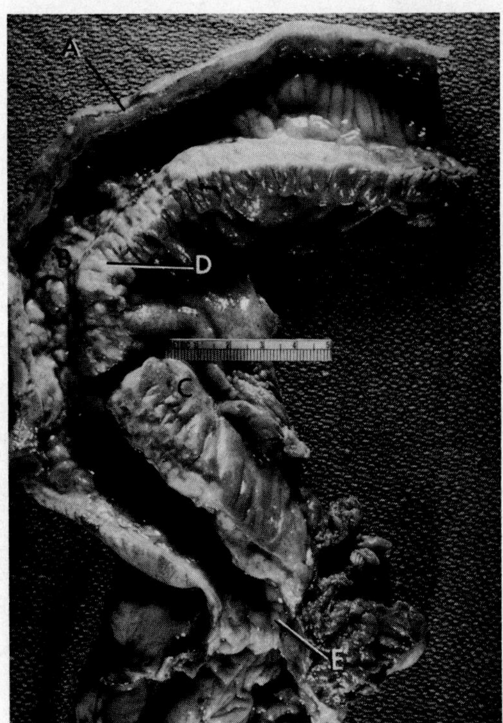

Figure 71–3. Crohn's disease. Terminal ileum is shown with thickened fibrous wall with inflammatory and proliferative changes involving all layers from the mucosa to the serosa (A). Ulcerated mucosa gives the "cobblestone" appearance (B). The mesentery is short, thick, and retracted (C), sharply angulating the loop of intestine, and adipose tissue extends onto the wall of the intestine (D). The diameter of the ileocecal valve (E) is decreased. (From Mottet K. Histopathologic Spectrum of Regional Enteritis and Ulcerative Colitis. Philadelphia, W. B. Saunders Company, 1971.)

Particularly helpful in the pathologic diagnosis of Crohn's disease is the finding of discrete granulomas (Fig. 71–7*B*). Although most numerous in the submucosa, granulomas can also be identified in mucosal biopsies.[7] Morphologically indistinguishable from sarcoid granulomas (Fig. 71–8), the discrete lesions in Crohn's disease lack the caseation necrosis and microorganisms found in tuberculosis and other infectious granulomas. Granulomas can be found in all layers of bowel wall as well as in involved lymph nodes, mesentery, peritoneum, liver, and lung. On occasion they also occur in bones, joints, and skeletal muscle.[3] These granulomas consist of epithelioid cells arranged in focal aggregates vaguely limited by an outer rim of lymphocytes. One or more multinucleated giant cells may be present in the periphery. Hyalinized connective tissue occasionally occupies the central region of the granuloma, but caseation does not occur. In about 10 per cent of cases one can identify Schaumann bodies, the birefringent crystals and basophilic particles that tend to aggregate within foreign body giant cells.

Although the presence of identifiable granulomas greatly assists in distinguishing Crohn's disease from other inflammatory bowel disorders, failure to find discrete granulomas does not by itself argue against the diagnosis of Crohn's disease. About 25 per cent of surgical specimens from patients with well-documented Crohn's disease show nonspecific transmural inflammation. A diffuse granulomatous reaction is found in another 25 per cent. In only about one half of the cases are "typical" focal granulomas identified. More important than granulomas for diagnosis is the demonstration of inflammation *in all layers* of the gut wall.[3, 4]

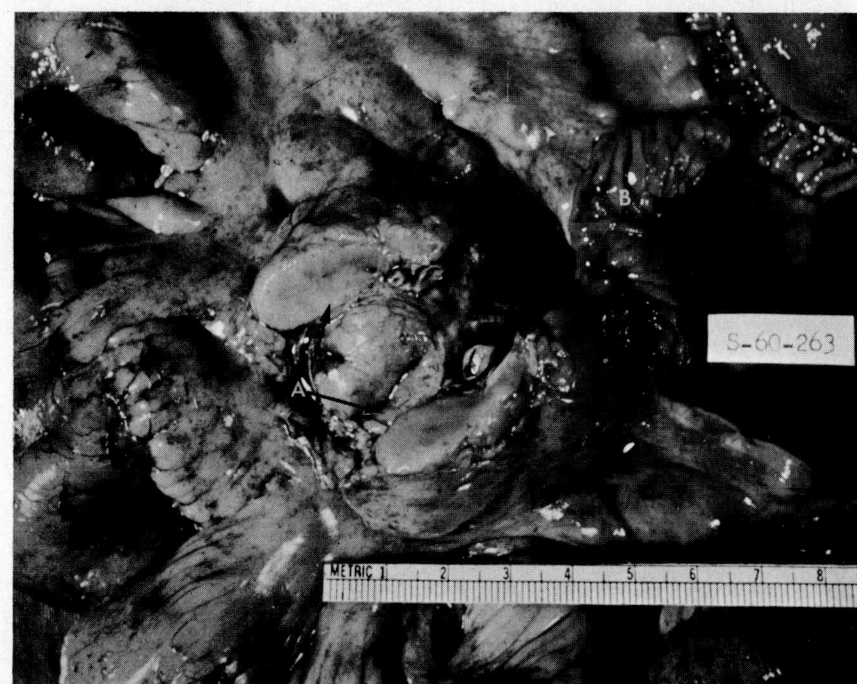

Figure 71–4. A transected enlarged mesenteric lymph node (A) and portion of mucosa (B) are shown. (From Mottet, K. Histopathologic Spectrum of Regional Enteritis and Ulcerative Colitis. Philadelphia, W. B. Saunders Company, 1971.)

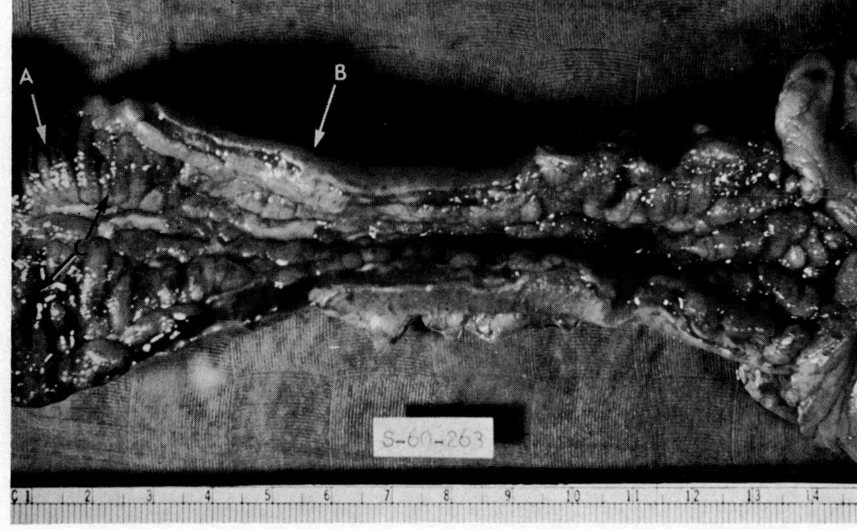

Figure 71–5. The terminal ileal lesion of relatively advanced Crohn's disease. Uninvolved bowel (A). Thick involved bowel (B). Ulcers at the bases of mucosal folds (C). (From Mottet, K. Histopathologic Spectrum of Regional Enteritis and Ulcerative Colitis. Philadelphia, W. B. Saunders Company, 1971.)

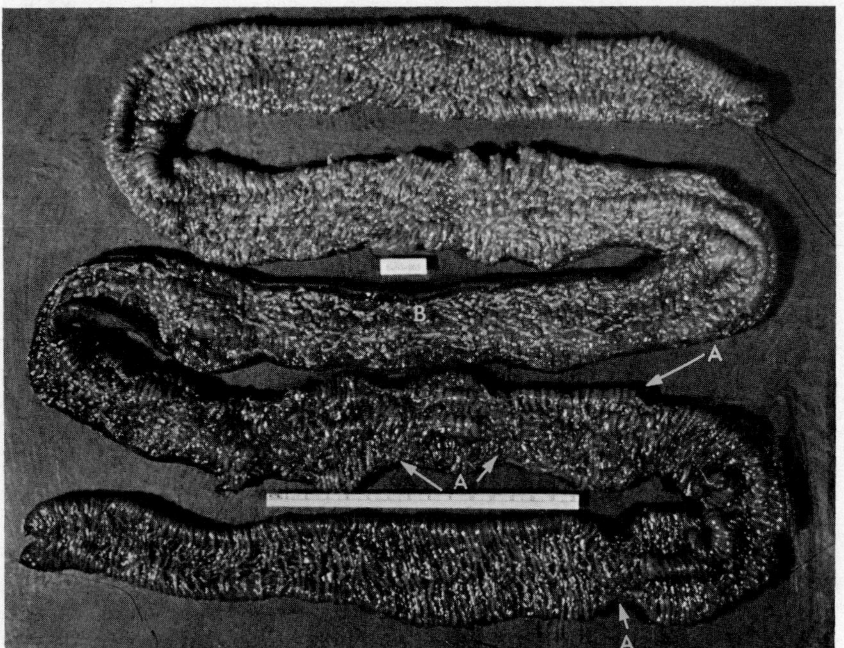

Figure 71–6. A more proximal segment of small intestine from the same patient shown in Figure 71–5, revealing the presence of multiple skip area strictures (A) and a less typical diffuse ulcerated lesion (B). (From Mottet, K. Histopathologic Spectrum of Regional Enteritis and Ulcerative Colitis. Philadelphia, W. B. Saunders Company, 1971.)

ANATOMIC DISTRIBUTION

In general, one can divide patients with Crohn's disease into those with small bowel disease alone, those with ileocolitis, those with disease involving only the colon, and a small group with disease restricted to the anorectal area (Table 71–2). The distribution and extent of disease is difficult to ascertain, however, because histologic abnormalities are often discovered in segments of bowel that appear normal by X-ray or even by endoscopy. More than two thirds of cases have grossly demonstrated disease involving the terminal ileum. In many instances, perhaps 10 to 20 per cent of cases, other areas of small bowel are also affected.

The colon is involved in two thirds of patients with Crohn's disease. The diffuse nature of the disorder is illustrated by the fact that in only 10 to 25 per cent of cases is the colon affected without concomitant small bowel disease. The distribution of disease within the colon is summarized in Table 71–3. It is apparent that any portion of the colon can be involved, that in about 25 per cent of cases the entire colon is affected, and that skip lesions are present in about 25 per cent.

Table 71–2. ANATOMIC DISTRIBUTION OF CROHN'S DISEASE IN 1699 PATIENTS*

Major Site of Involvement	Number of Cases	Per Cent
Small bowel only	501	29
Small bowel and colon	851	50
Colon only	312	19
Anorectal area only	35	2

*Data compiled from reports by Farmer et al.[38] and by Mekhjian et al.[37]

Table 71–3. DISTRIBUTION OF COLONIC LESIONS IN CROHN'S DISEASE

Site of Involvement	Diseases Limited to the Colon (% of 130 cases)	Ileocolitis (% of 89 cases)
Rectum	58	44
Sigmoid	72	35
Descending colon	59	30
Transverse colon	65	38
Ascending colon	54	26
Cecum	34	38
Entire colon	28	17
Skip areas	22	25

*Data compiled from series reported in reference 1 and in Gornes, J. S., and Stecher, M. Gut 2:189, 1961, and McGovern, V. J., and Goulston, S. J. M. Gut 9:164, 1968.

Patients afflicted with colonic disease alone tend to have more frequent involvement of the distal colon than those who have ileocolitis. Although absence of rectal disease is more characteristic of Crohn's disease than of ulcerative colitis, the rectum is grossly involved in fully half of patients with Crohn's colitis. Moreover, discrete granulomas are demonstrable in nearly 30 per cent of patients with Crohn's disease, whether or not the rectum appears grossly normal.[7]

EPIDEMIOLOGY

Problems arise whenever one tries to compare the frequency of Crohn's disease among different populations primarily because the groups being surveyed may be poorly defined and because of unrecognized differences in rates of diagnosis and reporting.[8] Neverthe-

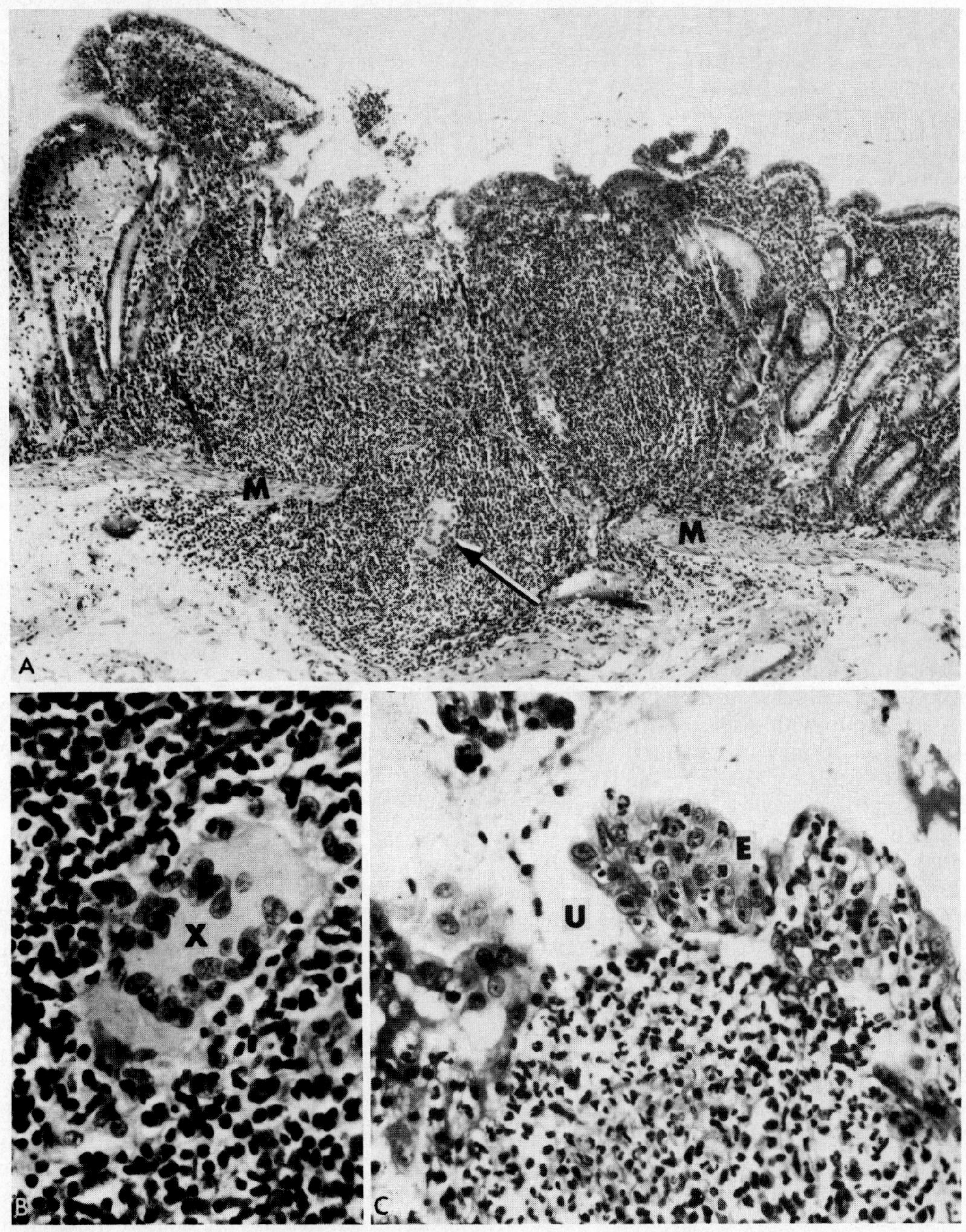

Figure 71–7. Small bowel biopsy specimen from a patient with duodenal involvement. Hematoxylin and eosin stain. *A,* The arrow indicates a multinucleated giant cell within a typical granuloma. The granuloma extends from submucosa to mucosa and disrupts the muscularis mucosae (M). The villous pattern is obliterated and the lamina propria heavily infiltrated with leukocytes in the region adjacent to the granuloma. (× 85.) *B,* Higher magnification of the giant cell (X) surrounded by mononuclear cells. (× 400.) *C,* In the region adjacent to the granuloma there is extensive infiltration of polymorphonuclear leukocytes among surface epithelial cells (E); a small ulceration (U) is present. (× 400.) (From Hermos, J. A., Cooper, H. L., Kramer, P., et al. Histological diagnosis by peroral biopsy of Crohn's disease of the proximal intestine. Gastroenterology *59*:868–873. © by Williams & Wilkins, 1970.)

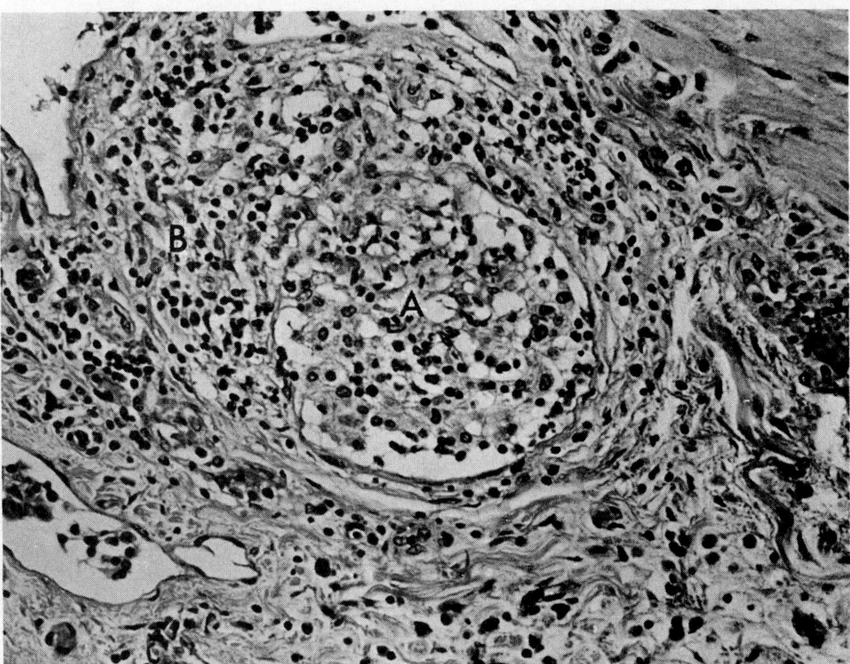

Figure 71–8. A Crohn's disease granuloma located in the submucosa. A patch of histiocytes (A) is surrounded by numerous lymphocytes (B). (× 64.) (From Mottet, K. Histopathologic Spectrum of Regional Enteritis and Ulcerative Colitis. Philadelphia, W. B. Saunders Company, 1971.)

less, some reasonably consistent trends can be discerned on the basis of demographic information from Great Britain, Europe, Israel, South Africa, and the United States (Table 71–4). Crohn's disease, with its prevalence of 10 to 70 cases per 100,000 population, occurs most frequently among peoples of European origin. In all countries surveyed, Crohn's disease is three to eight times more common among Jews than non-Jews and is consistently much more common among whites than nonwhites. On the other hand, the disease may begin at an earlier age and run a more severe course when it afflicts nonwhites.[9] In some surveys, males and females are about equally afflicted, while in others females predominate by as much as 1.6 to 1. Although the disorder can begin at any age, several surveys agree that its onset most often occurs at 15 to 30 years of age.

Many investigators have observed a familial aggregation of patients with Crohn's disease, and can elicit a positive family history in as many as 20 to 30 per cent of cases. The family history often includes relatives with ulcerative colitis as well as those with Crohn's disease. Frequency is greater among siblings than more distant relatives, suggesting a role for environmental factors, but Crohn's disease occurs more often in concordant than in discordant twins[10] and has only rarely been described in husband and wife.[11]

Table 71–4. CROHN'S DISEASE: CONSISTENTLY OBSERVED DEMOGRAPHIC FEATURES

Worldwide distribution
Prevalence: 10–70 cases/10^5 population
Incidence: 0.5–6.3 cases/10^5 population/year
Increased frequency among European stock
More common among Jews than non-Jews (3–8 times)
More common among whites than nonwhites
Most frequent age of onset: 15–30 years
Aggregation in families
Increasing incidence over past 20 years (1.4–4 times)

The incidence of Crohn's disease has increased dramatically over the past 20 years, whereas the frequency of ulcerative colitis has not changed.[8, 12, 13] The rising incidence of Crohn's disease might be more apparent than real, however, and might merely reflect increased diagnostic awareness. Indeed, interpretation of epidemiologic data concerning Crohn's disease cannot be overemphasized. For example, the frequency of this disorder is substantially lower in Israel than in several European countries and in the United States, despite its consistently increased occurrence rate among Jews in all countries surveyed. In Israel, Crohn's disease is four times more prevalent among Ashkenazi Jews than among non-Ashkenazim, with a greatly increased frequency among Israeli Jews born in Europe or the United States. Nevertheless, the prevalence even among this latter group is three- to tenfold less than among Jews living outside Israel. In contrast, the frequency of lactase deficiency among Ashkenazi Jews living in Israel, Canada, and the United States is about the same. Given the perplexities of observations such as these, one immediately recognizes how difficult it is to sort out artifactual, genetic, and environmental factors that complicate currently available epidemiologic data concerning Crohn's disease.

ETIOLOGY AND PATHOGENESIS

Crohn's disease has no known cause, despite a long and intensive search.[14] Lack of progress is understand-

Table 71–5. THE ETIOLOGY OF CROHN'S DISEASE: FACTORS EXAMINED FOR A POSSIBLE PATHOGENETIC ROLE

- Infectious agents
  - Bacteria
    - Mycobacteria
    - L-form variants
  - Viruses
    - Unidentified "transmissible" agents
    - Unidentified "cytopathic" agents
- Altered host susceptibility
  - Impaired cell-mediated immunity
    - Altered suppressor T-cell activity
  - Monocyte-macrophage dysfunction
  - Impaired neutrophil function
- Immune-mediated intestinal damage
  - Antibody-initiated reactions
    - Autoantibodies
    - Antigen-antibody immune complexes
    - Immediate hypersensitivity
  - Lymphocyte-mediated injury
    - Sensitized T cells
    - Antibody-dependent (K) cell-mediated
- Psychologic factors
- Dietary and environmental factors

able, for no single pathognomonic feature unquestionably identifies patients as having the disease. Although what we now call Crohn's disease may therefore turn out to be more than one entity, hypotheses concerning pathogenesis are at present being tested on the basis that the etiology is the same in all patients. When "pathogenetic factors" are discovered, however, they are often present in patients with ulcerative colitis as well as Crohn's disease. Moreover, when investigators describe an arrangement in patients with inflammatory bowel disease, it is usually very difficult to know whether the abnormality is important in pathogenesis or is merely a consequence of the disease. Because Crohn's disease is an inflammatory disorder, research has recently focused on the concept that the disease develops when a microbe or other antigen penetrates other intestinal epithelium and generates a cytopathic immune response in a constitutionally susceptible individual. Table 71–5 lists some of the factors that have been investigated.

Infectious Agents

The original description of Crohn's disease included a speculation that incriminated mycobacteria[15] as a possible cause, given the resemblance to intestinal tuberculosis. Efforts to culture mycobacterial agents, however, have been largely unsuccessful until recently. Table 71–6 shows that different kinds of mycobacteria have been isolated from some patients with Crohn's disease and that results vary considerably from laboratory to laboratory. Workers can undoubtedly culture mycobacteria and their spheroplasts from tissues of patients with Crohn's disease. Further investigation is necessary, however, to determine whether these microorganisms constitute a single etiologic agent capable of inducing granulomatous disease of the ileum experimentally[16, 17] or they are merely diverse kinds of bowel mycobacteria which happened to invade already diseased tissue.[18] *M. paratuberculosis* produces a granulomatous intestinal disease in goats known as Johne's disease, but the association between this bacterium and Crohn's disease still requires clarification.

Cell wall–defective variants of other enteric bacteria have also been implicated. Orr[19] reported that direct inoculation of an L-form of *Streptococcus fecalis* into the terminal ileum of rabbits produced focal granulomas, and Parent and Mitchell[20] have described a *Pseudomonas* variant cultured from eight consecutive patients with Crohn's disease but not from control tissues, including those obtained from five patients with ulcerative colitis.

Interest in an infectious etiology was particularly stimulated by reports[21] of rabbits developing a granulomatous disease when their intestines were injected with bacteria-free filtrates obtained from diseased tissues of patients with Crohn's disease. Moreover, the intestinal lesion could be serially transmitted from animal to animal via bacteria-free filtrates. The excitement initially generated by these findings has declined considerably, however, because some workers have been unable to duplicate these results while others have demonstrated that granulomatous lesions can also be induced by filtrates obtained from intestines involved with ulcerative colitis as well as from apparently

Table 71–6. MYCOBACTERIA ISOLATED FROM PATIENTS WITH CROHN'S DISEASE

	Van Patter, 1932	Burnham et al.,[16] 1978	Chiodini et al.,[17, 17a] 1984, 1985	Graham et al.,[18] 1987
Positive cultures/cases				
Crohn's disease	3/43	22/27	16/26	21/59
Ulcerative colitis		7/13	0/9	12/19
Control subjects		1/11	0/14	18/27
Tissue sources	Resected intestine mesenteric nodes (2)	Mesenteric nodes	Resected intestine	Resected intestine (47), intestinal biopsies (58)
Organism	Mycobacterium, unidentified type	Spheroplasts containing acid-fast material	Mycobacterium closely related to *M. paratuberculosis*	Mycobacteria, several different types
Comment	Organism could not be subcultured	Also cultured *M. kansasii* from 1/27 Crohn's disease cases	Spheroplasts only in 12 of 16 positive isolates	More isolates from biopsies (39/58) than from resected intestine (12/47)

normal specimens.[14] Moreover, no one has been able to characterize even partially the putative transmissible agent or agents involved. Similar difficulties have attended attempts to isolate pathogenic viruses from the tissues of patients with Crohn's disease. Identifiable human viral pathogens have occasionally been cultured from such tissues, but none has been convincingly associated with inflammatory bowel disease.[14] Cultures have also yielded unidentified cytopathic agents that are presumed to be viruses and that can apparently be serially transmitted in tissue culture lines.[23] Although provocative, these observations need wider confirmation with further characterization of the cytopathic agent or agents as well as electron microscopic documentation of the consistent presence of viral particles in tissues obtained from patients with Crohn's disease.

Altered Host Susceptibility

Crohn's disease may ultimately prove to be caused by infection, but there is very little epidemiologic evidence that it is contagious.[24, 25] An alternative possibility is that the basic defect in patients with Crohn's disease is altered susceptibility or responsiveness to a microorganism that is not ordinarily pathogenic or usually carries only an acute, self-limited infection. Thus, impaired immune or inflammatory responses to an infectious agent could conceivably play an important role in pathogenesis. Immune mechanisms in inflammatory bowel disease have been reviewed in detail[26] and are fully discussed on pages 114 to 144. In summary, four major findings suggest a primary role for immune responses in the pathogenesis of Crohn's disease. These include (1) the prominence of lymphocytes, plasma cells, and mast cells in the inflammatory process, (2) the association of Crohn's disease with other diseases with readily apparent immune disturbances, (3) the diverse extraintestinal manifestations indicating that Crohn's disease, like ulcerative colitis, is a systemic disease, and (4) the clinical improvement which attends treatment with agents known to alter or suppress immune responses. In addition, one can document in patients with Crohn's disease a variety of changes in immune function, mediated by humoral as well as by cellular mechanisms. None of these changes, however, can be considered essential to the development of Crohn's disease. Whether one talks about autoantibodies, immune complexes, or T cell responses, the immune phenomena described thus far occur only in some cases of Crohn's disease, are demonstrable in at least some patients with ulcerative colitis, and are more likely to be the result of the chronic inflammatory process than its cause.

If defective white blood cell function is a reason for increased intestinal susceptibility to injury, then the defect must be a subtle one or one that is strictly limited to the bowel. Overall production of monocyte-macrophage cells is unchanged, and monocyte functional activity is increased as assessed by indirect techniques such as serum lysozyme activity.[27] One report describes diminished phagocytic activity of leukocytes collected from patients with Crohn's disease.[28] This diminished phagocytic capacity was also observed in patients with ulcerative colitis, and its possible pathogenetic role needs further investigation. The inflammatory process results in increased production of prostaglandins, prostacyclines, and other metabolites of arachidonic acid. These mediators undoubtedly participate in the vascular and secretory responses characteristic of inflammation.[29] Still uncertain is whether these mediators account for continuing tissue damage in Crohn's disease.

Still under investigation is the possibility that susceptibility to Crohn's disease may be related to genetically determined histocompatibility (HLA) haplotypes or immunoglobulin allotypes.[26] Concordant HLA-A and HLA-B haplotypes were observed in four of five pairs of siblings with Crohn's disease in one study,[30] but another group found no such concordance.[31] Although reports continue to appear suggesting aggregation of HLA haplotypes in Crohn's disease,[32] findings are inconsistent from one study to another, and there is as yet no truly convincing evidence of genetic transmission of specific histocompatibility antigens or immunoglobulin allotypes in inflammatory bowel disease.[26]

Psychologic Factors

As in the case of ulcerative colitis, emotional factors have been implicated in the pathogenesis of Crohn's disease, but the supporting evidence is, if anything, even weaker than that for ulcerative colitis. Evidence to support this theory is derived from anecdotal, retrospective studies reporting frequent occurrence of repressed hostility and dependency among patients with Crohn's disease as well as associations between psychologic stress and clinical exacerbations of the disease. Documentation of a real association between psychologic factors, emotional or physical stress, and Crohn's disease, however, requires investigations that eliminate or reduce the possibility of bias. When such studies have, in fact, been done, no evidence has been found to indicate that emotional factors or stressful events precede Crohn's disease.[33] Also difficult to identify are behavioral or psychosocial characteristics which are specific for Crohn's disease.[34] On the other hand, a carefully conducted trial indicates that depression more frequently accompanies Crohn's disease than it does other chronic diseases.[35]

Dietary Factors

The relatively recent discovery of Crohn's disease, its apparently increasing incidence in recent years, and its relatively high incidence in industrialized countries have all stimulated investigators to consider a possible pathogenetic role for dietary changes that have occurred in modern industrialized countries.[36] Investigations have been concerned with chemical food additives such as carrageenan, reduced intake of dietary fiber, and increased consumption of refined sugars. Dietary surveys among patients with Crohn's disease have produced conflicting data,[14] however, and there is no firm epidemiologic or experimental evidence that directly links dietary or other environmental factors to intestinal damage.

From this review it is apparent that understanding of the fundamental nature of Crohn's disease has not progressed greatly over the past 50 years. Investigation of pathogenesis has been intense, but it seems likely that most of the phenomena thus far demonstrated in patients with Crohn's disease constitute results rather than specific causes. Still to be answered are fundamental questions about the nature of Crohn's disease. Is it really distinct from ulcerative colitis, or do the two disorders merely express different manifestations of the same disease process? Is Crohn's disease a specific clinical-pathologic entity with its own unique etiology, or does it have several different etiologies, each of which produces the same sort of inflammatory response? One fact is clear: We remain very much at the frontier of our understanding of the "nonspecific" or "idiopathic" inflammatory bowel diseases, including Crohn's disease.

CLINICAL FEATURES AND NATURAL HISTORY

Diarrhea and *abdominal pain* are common features of Crohn's disease and occur in more than 75 per cent of patients (Table 71–7). More than half have fever.[37] Although manifestations vary greatly from patient to patient, the "typical" patient, such as the first case encountered by Crohn,[2, 15] is a young adult whose illness begins with right lower quadrant pain, diarrhea, and low-grade fever. Tenderness, guarding, and a palpable mass are present in the right lower quadrant. If the illness is relatively acute and diarrhea is not prominent, these findings together with an elevated white blood cell count often lead to a clinical diagnosis of appendicitis, consequent laparotomy, and the discovery of Crohn's disease.

Although dramatic and thought of as typical, this clinical picture is actually relatively uncommon. More often, Crohn's disease begins insidiously. Clinical features are related to the sites and severity of involvement (Table 71–7), but patients most often have recurrent episodes of *diarrhea, abdominal pain,* and *fever* lasting from days to weeks. When the disease is confined to the ileum, diarrhea tends to be moderate in severity, with usually no more than five or six bowel movements per day. Movements may be watery but more often are soft and loose. When the disease involves the colon, urgency and incontinence are frequent and rectal bleeding occurs in about half the patients.[37, 38]

Abdominal pain usually reflects an indolent inflammatory process in the ileocecal area and thus tends to be steady and localized to the right lower quadrant. Superimposed upon this steady pain is intermittent periumbilical colic, often noted just before and during bowel movements. When the colon is involved, cramping pain may occur in one or both lower abdominal quadrants. Transient episodes of partial or complete intestinal obstruction with nausea and vomiting occur in a substantial proportion of patients with ileal or ileocolic disease. Large bowel obstruction, although less frequent, can also occur when strictures are present.

Fever occurs in more than half the cases[37] but in the absence of complications rarely exceeds 102°F. Because patients may have fever without any signs or symptoms of gastrointestinal disease, Crohn's disease must be considered in the differential diagnosis of cases of fever of unknown origin.

Weight loss that exceeds 5 per cent of body weight occurs in 25 to 40 per cent of cases. Although often incriminated, the metabolic cost of ongoing inflammation does not account for this loss of weight.[39] The clinical course of Crohn's disease varies greatly, depending largely on the site of disease. In most patients, gradual deterioration occurs over a period of years.

Table 71–7. CLINICAL FEATURES OF CROHN'S DISEASE*

	Site of Disease†		
Disease Manifestations	***Small Bowel Only***	***Small Bowel and Colon***	***Colon Only***
Diarrhea	87	92	88
Abdominal pain	78	79	74
Hematochezia	10	22	46
Intestinal obstruction	34	44	17
Fissures and fistulas			
Anal, perirectal	22	50	51
Internal, cutaneous	18	34	13
Systemic manifestations			
Arthritis, arthralgia	18	19	27
Iritis, uveitis	3	4	7
Liver disease	3	5	5
Skin lesions	3		8

*Compiled and adapted from three large series of cases.[37, 38, 58]
†Percentage of 1767 cases.

Asymptomatic intervals gradually decrease as weight loss and lassitude become more prominent. Slow but persistent blood loss combined with poor food intake leads to anemia. A patient is particularly likely to experience intermittent episodes of partial or even complete bowel obstruction. Progression to surgery occurs more rapidly among patients with ileocolitis than among those in whom only the small bowel or only the colon is involved.[38, 39]

Although progression is characteristic of Crohn's disease, 10 to 20 per cent of patients remain completely asymptomatic for as long as 20 years after the first, or even the second, episode of active Crohn's disease.[38, 40] Another 10 to 15 per cent of individuals present for the first time with perirectal disease, fever, or one of the extraintestinal manifestations described subsequently. Because some form of perianal or perirectal disease develops in at least half the patients at some time during the course of Crohn's disease, it is not surprising that the first indication of the disorder may be perianal or perirectal lesions, sometimes occurring long before there is evidence of abdominal pain or diarrhea. Occasionally, the illness begins with temperatures of 101 to 103°F resulting from intra-abdominal abscess formation or with the sudden appearance of frankly bloody or mahogany stools as the first indication of the disease.

Whatever the clinical picture, one expects the inflammatory process to be recurrent. On the other hand, it is difficult to predict when an asymptomatic patient is likely to develop symptomatic recurrence of active disease. Although increases in sedimentation rate and levels of acute phase proteins may signal a recurrence,[41] we still lack a truly reliable laboratory indication of the activity of Crohn's disease.[42]

Once the disease has advanced to a stage that is serious enough to require surgery, subsequent recurrence is common. In three large series[43–45] 70 to 90 per cent of patients operated upon needed reoperation within 15 years. The rate of reoperation was somewhat higher among patients who had bypass surgery than among those whose first surgery was a complete resection. The rate was also higher among those operated on for ileocolitis, those who had internal fistulas, and those with perianal disease. The rate is lower among those operated on for disease limited to the colon. The interval between operations appears to be shorter after the second or third operation than after the initial resection. Recurrence after surgery is much more likely to occur at the anastomotic site than anywhere else.[46]

When Crohn's disease begins in childhood or adolescence, the manifestations and course are much the same as those observed when the disease begins later in life. In one large series of children and adolescents,[47] colonic disease caused considerable disability. Toxic megacolon, for example, developed in 12 per cent of these young patients. Except for more severe growth retardation in childhood, the disease is not greatly different whether it begins in childhood or adolescence.

Because Crohn's disease afflicts young adults, it is often encountered in pregnant women.[48] Pregnancy does not have any readily predictable effect on the course of the bowel disease, although patients are somewhat less likely to do well when Crohn's disease is active at the onset of pregnancy. Similarly, the pregnancy is twice as likely to end in spontaneous abortion if active inflammation of the bowel is present at the time of conception. Under other circumstances, there does not appear to be any convincing direct relation between the pregnancy and the bowel disease. During pregnancy, patients require rigorous care, but the basic principles of managing patients with inflammatory disease remain the same and should be followed even more closely than at other times. It is just as important to carry out diagnostic procedures, including X-ray examinations, promptly when they are indicated as it is to avoid such procedures if they are not necessary. Optimal treatment, including sulfasalazine and steroids if necessary, should be promptly initiated when the disease becomes active. Treatment should not be compromised because the patient is pregnant. Indeed, outcome of both disease and pregnancy depends primarily on whether active inflammation can be adequately suppressed. Experience with agents other than steroids and sulfasalazine is very limited, however, and one should certainly avoid drugs such as azathioprine during pregnancy. Certainly there is no need to use drugs of any sort in the absence of overt inflammation.

Although Crohn's disease occurs most often in young adults, the elderly are by no means spared, and investigators are increasingly reporting cases beginning in the eighth or ninth decade. In one large series,[49] onset of symptoms occurred after age 60 in 8 per cent of cases. The disease shows no striking differences when it appears in older patients, but physicians are less likely to think of the diagnosis and the interval between onset of complaints and diagnosis is unequivocally prolonged.[49, 50]

Despite the progressive course and severe complications of Crohn's disease, only 10 to 20 per cent of patients ultimately die because of it or its complications.[51] The risk of death is particularly high during the first two or three years after diagnosis and again after the disease has been present for more than 14 years. Mortality rates do not appear to have diminished over the past half century despite major advances in treatment.

The course of Crohn's disease is best described as unpredictable. Although most patients have recurrent, symptomatic episodes with gradual progression, in perhaps 15 per cent the course of disease is rather benign. Occasionally, patients have none of the characteristic symptoms of Crohn's disease and first present with extraintestinal manifestations or one of the "late" complications. Under these circumstances, it is obvious that meaningful evaluation of any treatment for Crohn's disease requires carefully controlled observations in relatively large numbers of comparable patients.

COMPLICATIONS

Management of Crohn's disease is a constant challenge because of the diversity and frequency of its complications. *Small bowel obstruction* is the most common reason for surgery when Crohn's disease involves the small intestine.[37, 45, 52] Obstruction is usually a result of inflammation and edema in an already strictured segment of bowel and is therefore most often partial and transient. Progression to complete obstruction, when it occurs, tends to be slow. Sudden, complete obstruction may also occur, however, when the small bowel becomes kinked or pinched off in an adhesive inflammatory process that involves mesentery or peritoneum.

Fistulas form so frequently that they constitute a cardinal feature of Crohn's disease, and fistulas themselves lead to additional complications. Perianal and perirectal fistulas and fissures are particularly common. In some patients (Fig. 71–9), perianal and perirectal fistulas and infection may be so severe that they completely overshadow other clinical manifestations. Internal and enterocutaneous fistulas occur more frequently among patients with ileocolonic involvement than among those with Crohn's disease involving only the small intestine or only the colon. Fistulas between loops of small bowel contribute to nutritional problems when they cause nutrients to bypass extensive areas of small bowel absorptive surface. In addition, enteroenteric fistulas can lead to recirculation of intestinal contents, and the consequent stasis promotes bacterial overgrowth within the small bowel (see pp. 1289 to 1297). Fistulas between bowel and the urinary bladder, although infrequent, invariably cause persistent urinary tract infection and, if left unattended, will lead to irreversible renal damage. On rare occasions, pneumaturia with associated urinary symptoms can be the initial manifestation of Crohn's disease.

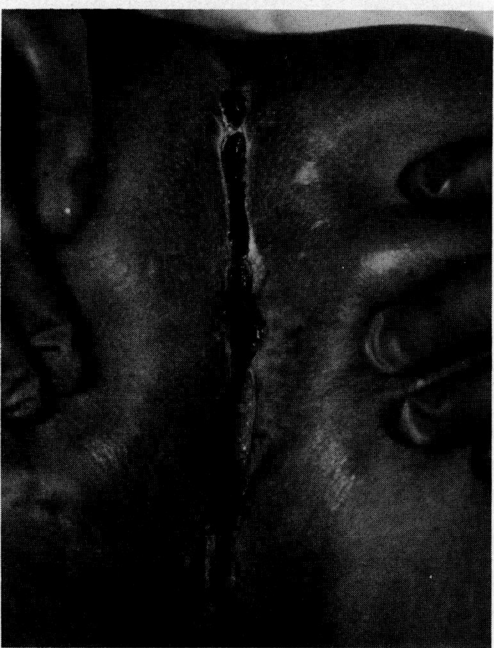

Figure 71–9. Extensive undermining of perirectal tissue in a patient with Crohn's colitis and perianal abscess.

Free perforation is unusual in Crohn's disease, in contrast to the frequent occurrence of fistulas and walled-off abscesses. Nevertheless, perforation with frank diffuse peritonitis does occur,[53] and published reports provide many examples of patients who first come to attention with all the features of a perforated viscus.

Frank *bleeding,* with the appearance of dark red or bright red blood in the stool, occurs at one time or another in 25 to 50 per cent of patients with colonic disease. Even when disease is limited to the small intestine, however, massive bleeding may occur; on occasion, this complication may be the first manifestation of Crohn's disease of the ileum. Most of the time, however, bleeding is insidious and slowly leads to iron deficiency anemia without hematochezia or melena.

Carcinoma of the bowel complicates Crohn's disease sufficiently often that the risk is distinctly increased (three- to 20-fold in various series) compared with that of the general population. Small series of cases continue to be published.[54, 55] In two surveys,[56, 57] each involving more than 500 cases of Crohn's disease, the frequency of bowel malignancy was 3.0 to 3.5 per cent. Overall frequency of colon cancer in ulcerative colitis is fourfold greater than that observed in Crohn's disease.[57]

Patients who have colonic involvement develop *extraintestinal manifestations* about as often as do patients with ulcerative colitis.[58] Those with one such manifestation are statistically at risk for developing a second. In one series of cases with extraintestinal features,[59] 25 per cent had more than one of these conditions. Systemic features also occur somewhat more often among patients with perianal disease.

The most common extraintestinal manifestation is arthritis, which may present as migratory arthritis involving large joints, sacroiliitis, or ankylosing spondylitis. Spondylitis or sacroiliitis is often present for years before bowel symptoms appear, and there is no obvious relation between its course and the course of Crohn's disease. Migratory monoarthritis involving large joints afflicts patients with ulcerative colitis or Crohn's disease, but joint and bowel symptoms more often exacerbate or remit simultaneously in cases of ulcerative colitis. Among patients with Crohn's disease, however, the arthritis tends to be less severe and seems to run a course that is relatively independent of the state of intestinal disease. As is true for other associations between bowel disease and arthritis, the frequency of haplotype HLA-BW27 is greater than expected among patients with Crohn's disease who have spondylitis or sacroiliitis.

Inflammatory disorders of the eye, skin, and mucous membranes may also develop during the course of Crohn's disease. Iritis and episcleritis are the most common ocular manifestations, while erythema nodosum and pyoderma gangrenosum constitute the major skin manifestations of inflammatory bowel disease.

Aphthous ulcerations of the buccal mucosa and tongue may be particularly troublesome.

Clinically important liver disease is relatively unusual among patients with Crohn's disease, but mild abnormalities of liver function occur commonly. When the liver is involved, biopsy samples most often show mild pericholangitis. Diffuse or focal granulomatous inflammation occurs less often, but may be helpful in establishing the diagnosis in difficult cases. Sclerosing cholangitis occurs with increased frequency in patients with Crohn's disease, and associated cholangiocarcinomas may also be seen. Fatty liver is most often seen when patients are severely ill and malnourished. The prevalence of cholelithiasis (Fig. 71–10) has not been determined in large numbers of patients with Crohn's disease, but in general the frequency appears to be about 30 per cent. The prevalence is approximately the same whether or not patients have undergone ileal resection. This apparently high incidence is intriguing, because such patients are likely to be deficient in bile salts and to produce bile that is conducive to cholesterol gallstone formation (see pp. 1668–1676).

Renal disorders have increasingly been recognized as complications of Crohn's disease. In addition to urinary tract infections resulting from enterovesical fistulas, bowel inflammation may involve the ureters with consequent urinary obstruction and hydronephrosis. Nephrolithiasis occurs in 25 to 35 per cent of patients with Crohn's disease. Oxalate stones and hyperoxaluria (Fig. 71–11) have been related to steatorrhea and hyperoxaluria. As discussed on page 270, fat malabsorption increases the availability of dietary oxalate for absorption, particularly from the colon. It is not at all certain, however, whether the resulting hyperoxaluria fully accounts for the formation of oxalate stones, because urinary oxalate excretion correlates poorly with stone formation in patients with Crohn's disease.[60] Additional factors, including calcium and fluid intake, are undoubtedly involved in determining which patients with Crohn's disease, steatorrhea, and hyperoxaluria will develop renal stones.

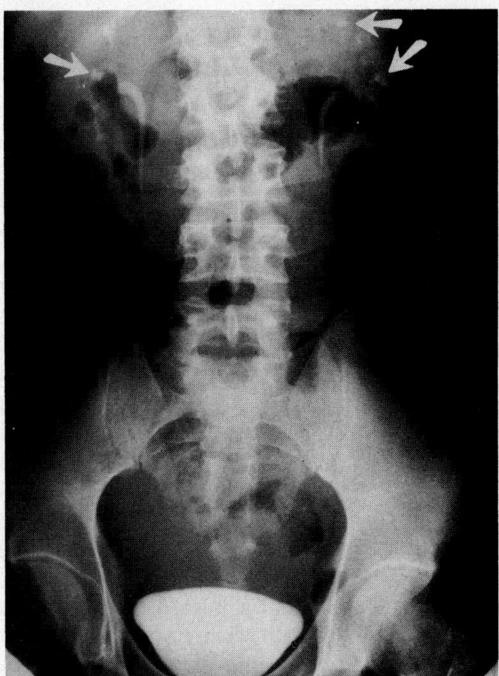

Figure 71–11. Intravenous pyelogram in a 34-year-old patient with regional enteritis and renal colic. Arrows point to oxalate kidney stones that were associated with hyperoxaluria. (Courtesy of M. H. Sleisenger, M.D.)

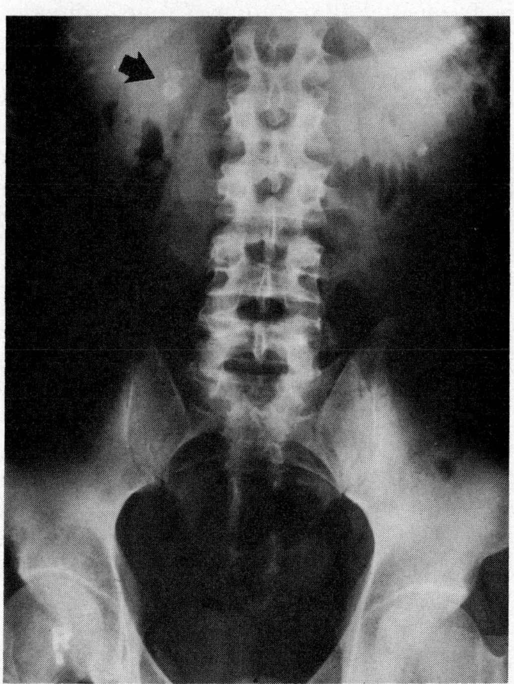

Figure 71–10. Flat film of abdomen shows gallstones in same case illustrated in Figure 71–20. (Courtesy of M. H. Sleisenger, M.D.)

Amyloidosis is a serious complication of Crohn's disease. Although the disorder is considered rare, most physicians with extensive experience in caring for patients with Crohn's disease have encountered more than one in whom "secondary" amyloidosis has developed. The appearance of the nephrotic syndrome or hepatosplenomegaly or both warrants a search for tissue evidence of this complication. The diagnosis can often be established by rectal or liver biopsy, although renal biopsy may be necessary. Because, in isolated case reports, resection of diseased intestine has resulted in apparent arrest or reversal of amyloidosis, the presence of this complication argues for surgical resection of diseased bowel, particularly when Crohn's disease is symptomatic.

Thromboembolic complications occur in about 1 per cent of cases of chronic inflammatory bowel disease,[61] and activation of clotting factors is readily demonstrable among patients with active Crohn's disease.[62] The physician should therefore constantly keep in mind the possibility of thromboembolic phenomena when managing patients with active recurrences of Crohn's disease. Of interest with respect to interactions between Crohn's disease and thrombosis is the fact that the risk of developing Crohn's disease may be increased among users of oral contraceptives.[63]

NUTRITIONAL ASPECTS

Several pathophysiologic mechanisms contribute to nutritional problems in patients with Crohn's disease (Table 71–8). Probably most important, however, are the deficiencies that result from diminished food intake because of anorexia or self-imposed dietary restrictions.[64] Inflammatory infiltration can decrease the capacity of small bowel mucosa to absorb multiple nutrients, including folate, water-soluble vitamins, carbohydrates, amino acids, lipids, and lipid-soluble vitamins. Diseased terminal ileum may occasionally be responsible for cobalamin (vitamin B_{12}) malabsorption, but the vitamin is often absorbed surprisingly well, even in patients with severe distal bowel disease. Disaccharidase deficiency, particularly lactase deficiency, frequently occurs as part of the small bowel involvement, and patients with Crohn's disease may tolerate milk poorly. Protein-losing enteropathy may be striking in extensive disease, particularly when ulcerations are present. Protein loss may be substantial even when the disease involves only the colon. Chronic blood loss from diseased mucosa also frequently leads to iron deficiency. Extensive involvement of intestinal and mesenteric lymphatics is characteristic of Crohn's disease, and lymphatic obstruction undoubtedly contributes to impaired fat absorption.

Strictures and internal fistulas, extremely common in Crohn's disease, are conducive to stasis of intestinal contents and thus frequently lead to overgrowth of enteric microorganisms within the small bowel lumen.

Table 71– 8. MECHANISMS RESPONSIBLE FOR MALABSORPTION AND MALNUTRITION IN CROHN'S DISEASE

Inadequate dietary intake
- Anorexia
- Specific dietary restrictions

Inflammatory involvement of small bowel
- Decreased absorption of diverse nutrients
- Acquired disaccharidase deficiency
- Lymphatic obstruction, decreased lipid transport
- Protein-losing enteropathy
- Iron deficiency due to chronic blood loss

Small bowel bacterial overgrowth due to strictures and fistulas
- Malabsorption of cobalamin
- Increased intraluminal catabolism of carbohydrate and protein
- Altered bile salt metabolism with fat malabsorption

Intestinal surgery
- Loss of absorptive surface area due to resection or bypass surgery
- Ileal resection causing cobalamin malabsorption, bile salt deficiency, and steatorrhea
- Enteroenterostomies or blind pouches causing bacterial overgrowth

Diarrhea
- Fluid and electrolyte losses

Catabolic effects of chronic inflammation and superimposed infection

Combination of above factors

On the basis of mechanisms described in detail on pages 1289 to 1297, this bacterial overgrowth results in impaired assimilation of cobalamin, carbohydrate, and protein as well as altered bile salt metabolism, with consequent fat malabsorption.

Nutritional problems may be further complicated by surgical therapy. Resection or bypass of diseased intestine necessarily decreases the absorptive surface area and may be sufficient to decrease substantially the absorption of multiple nutrients. Because the distal small bowel is the major site for reabsorption of conjugated bile salts, resection of the ileum leads to their loss into the colon. The total bile salt pool contracts and biliary secretion of bile salts decreases. There results an inadequate concentration of bile salts in the proximal gut lumen to form mixed bile salt micelles with the products of fat digestion. Moreover, unabsorbed bile salts entering the colon stimulate mucosal secretion and thus reduce net absorption of water and electrolytes. The overall effect is further diarrhea (see pp. 290–316). Resection of more than 2 feet of ileum also regularly produces cobalamin malabsorption, which may ultimately lead to deficiency of this vitamin. Finally, operations that result in enteroenterostomies, surgical blind loops, or loss of the protective mechanisms of the ileocecal valve create intraluminal conditions that favor bacterial overgrowth and its nutritional consequences (see pp. 1289–1297).

Caloric deficits and protein malnutrition may be further intensified by the catabolic effects of chronic inflammation and superimposed infection, although the quantitative effect of catabolism may be less than previously thought.[39] In most cases, deficiency of any one nutrient results from a combination of the aforementioned mechanisms. Folate deficiency, for example, is frequently observed in Crohn's disease and occurs both because of decreased dietary intake and because of impaired absorption by diseased bowel. Sulfasalazine, frequently used in the treatment of Crohn's disease, also diminishes absorption of folate, probably by competing for sites on intestinal folate conjugase (see pp. 1046–1048). In addition, demand for folate may be increased because of increased catabolism as well as chronic blood loss.

Whatever combination of mechanisms impairs absorption and brings about nutritional deficiencies in Crohn's disease, the clinical consequences are diverse and can consist of any combination of diarrhea, steatorrhea, microcytic or megaloblastic anemia, hypoproteinemia, edema, demineralization of bone and hypocalcemic tetany (vitamin D malabsorption), hypoprothrombinemia with a bleeding diathesis (vitamin K malabsorption), acid-base disturbances, hypokalemia and dehydration (excess water and electrolyte loss), and inanition resulting from inadequate assimilation of dietary calories (see pp. 1983–1994). The consequences of these complex absorptive and nutritional disturbances are particularly serious in children with Crohn's disease.[64–67] Retardation of growth with delayed sexual maturation occurs in 20 to 30 per cent of young patients and is often severe. Although prolonged administration of corticosteroids contributes importantly to growth retardation, aggressive nutritional therapy can reverse the process and restore growth rate in children. Precise mechanisms involved in growth retardation remain to be identified, but it is clear that somatomedin-C levels are decreased in children and adolescents with impaired growth and return to normal with nutritional repletion and increased growth rates.[68] Thus, somatomedin-C serves as a marker for growth retardation in Crohn's disease, and further studies should elucidate its role as a mediator.

DIAGNOSIS

Because Crohn's disease is a "nonspecific" inflammatory bowel disease lacking a defined etiology and curative treatment, it must be diagnosed by excluding treatable causes of bowel inflammation. When the illness begins with acute diarrhea, abdominal pain, and stools that contain blood, mucus, and pus, then treatable causes of dysentery must be excluded (e.g., amebiasis, *Salmonella* infection, shigellosis, *Campylobacter* infection). If the patient does not improve rapidly, biopsies of the colon provide the best means of distinguishing a first attack of nonspecific inflammatory bowel disease from an acute episode of self-limited colitis.[69] During acute phases of the disease, stools should also be tested for *Clostridium difficile* toxin, particularly if patients have been treated with antibiotics.[70] When the onset is more insidious and acute colitis is less prominent, then the physician also needs to examine or culture stools and rectal mucosa for chlamydiae, *Entamoeba histolytica, Yersinia enterocolitica, Giardia lamblia,* and schistosomes, all of which cause bowel disorders capable of simulating various features of Crohn's disease.

Once specific etiologic agents have been excluded, the diagnosis depends not upon any truly pathognomonic feature but upon the nature of the clinical manifestations, including the course of the patient's illness and sites of bowel involvement, together with a combination of laboratory, radiologic, endoscopic, and histologic findings.

Laboratory Tests. Although no specific laboratory test is capable of establishing the diagnosis of Crohn's disease, many tests are used to determine whether or not the inflammatory process is active. Leukocytosis, thrombocytosis, and an elevated erythrocyte sedimentation rate are the abnormalities most often used as evidence of disease activity, but other measurements also have been recommended. These include various acute phase proteins, lysozyme, and transcobalamin II levels in monocytes. These tests, alone or in combination, provide some indication as to whether disease is active, but they cannot reliably quantitate the severity or extent of the inflammatory process.[42]

Because of chronic blood loss, stools may be guaiac-positive and the patient may have a microcytic anemia with a low serum iron and ferritin concentration and decreased or absent stainable iron in the bone marrow. Macrocytic, megaloblastic anemia will suggest deficiency of folic acid or cobalamin, and serum levels of these nutrients should be measured in patients with nutritional problems. Urinalysis may indicate a urinary tract infection secondary to ureteral obstruction or an enterovesicular fistula. In patients with proteinuria, the possibility of renal amyloidosis should be pursued. The serum albumin level provides a useful indication of the patient's overall condition. It is likely to be low in patients who are not eating, as well as in those who have extensive malabsorption or whose disease is causing significant enteric loss of protein. Liver function tests may be abnormal and lead to a diagnosis of pericholangitis. The xylose tolerance test; the Schilling test; measurement of carotene, calcium, and phosphorus in the serum; and examination of the stool for fat are all useful in determining whether or not the patient has clinically significant malabsorption. Bacterial cultures of fluid aspirated from the jejunum provide an indication of whether the disease is complicated by significant small bowel bacterial overgrowth, but this procedure is time-consuming and should be reserved for cases in which clinical suspicion is high. Other "screening tests," including breath tests, may also be useful in assessing a contributory role of bacteria proliferating within the small bowel lumen. In persons with diarrhea not readily controlled by usual therapy, a lactose tolerance test or an H_2 breath test after lactose administration may be helpful in deciding whether the patient should avoid milk and milk products because of lactase deficiency (see p. 1295).

Endoscopy. In 50 to 70 per cent of patients with Crohn's disease, the mucosa of the distal colon appears unremarkable except for mild edema and erythema, which one might see in any patient with diarrhea. On the other hand, even those patients without obvious rectosigmoidal involvement may exhibit advanced anal or perianal disease with fissures, fistulas, and abscesses involving the perianal and perirectal area.

When the colon is involved with Crohn's disease, one may find a variety of endoscopic abnormalities during sigmoidoscopy or colonoscopy. Most often, mucosa is seen protruding into the colonic lumen because of submucosal inflammation and edema. In addition, one can see distinct ulcerations of the mucosa which vary in size and may appear round and punched-out, serpiginous, or linear. Characteristically, and quite different from what is seen in most patients with ulcerative colitis, relatively normal mucosa usually separates distinct ulcerations. When prominent islands of mucosa are separated by linear ulcerations, the rectosigmoid assumes a "cobblestone" appearance. Because Crohn's disease is characteristically discontinuous, the proctoscopist often finds obviously diseased areas interrupted by normal-appearing bowel. It should be emphasized, however, that up to 25 per cent of patients with clinical histologic features characteristic of Crohn's disease may demonstrate uninterrupted involvement with denudation of mucosa, which is indistinguishable from that observed in ulcerative colitis. As emphasized below, rectal biopsies obtained at the time of proctoscopy frequently provide useful diagnostic information.

When the radiologic picture is unequivocally typical of Crohn's colitis, colonoscopy does not usually add useful diagnostic information. The fact that colonoscopy may document a greater extent of disease than was seen by X-ray is not likely by itself to influence medical management, but may assist in planning for surgery. When the X-ray appearance is atypical, and particularly when it raises the question of malignancy, colonoscopy provides a means of looking directly at mucosal changes as well as obtaining washings and biopsies for cytologic diagnosis. The procedure often requires insufflation of the colon with large amounts of air and therefore should be avoided in acute phases of Crohn's colitis or when deep ulcerations or fistulas are known to be present.

Radiologic Findings. Adequate radiologic examinations play a major role in the diagnosis of patients suspected of Crohn's disease. The plain film of the abdomen may demonstrate dilated bowel loops when partial obstruction is present (Fig. 71–12). Intra-abdominal masses resulting from matted, inflamed loops of bowel or from abscesses are also frequently documented on plain film. The plain film may also detect intramural infiltration and edema, which causes "thumb printing" of the bowel wall.

Early or subtle colonic changes are best detected by double-contrast examinations, in which the thoroughly cleansed colon is visualized by a thin coating of barium followed by introduction of air.[71] As illustrated in Figure 71–13, this technique is capable of demonstrating shallow aphthous ulcers with normal intervening mucosa. In addition to detecting early subtle lesions, barium enema may be helpful by demonstrating typical patterns of disease (Figs. 71–14 and 71–15), including colonic narrowing, fistula formation, "skip areas" of involved colon, deep linear ulcerations, short sinus tracts, and a cobblestone appearance of the mucosa (Fig. 71–16). The pathologic basis for these features is described on pages 1328 to 1330. The finding of simultaneous involvement of proximal colon and ileum (Fig. 71–14) greatly increases the likelihood of a diagnosis of Crohn's disease. Particularly characteristic is the eccentric involvement of the colon (Fig. 71–17), resulting from focal ulcerations accompanied by localized swelling primarily due to submucosal infiltration.

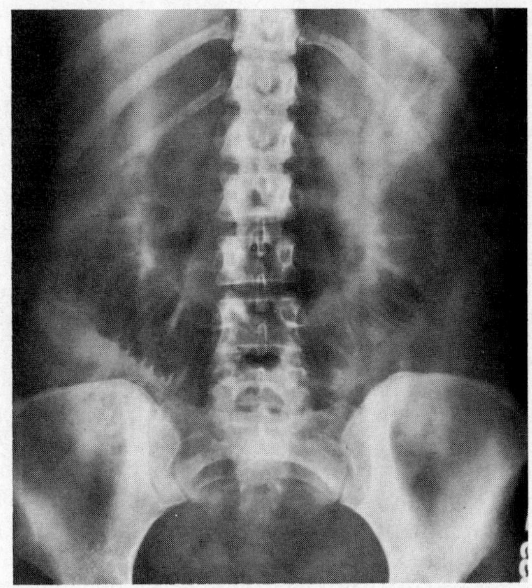

Figure 71–12. Flat film of abdomen of the same patient shown in Figure 71–20 at the time of complete small bowel obstruction. Note dilated small bowel. (Courtesy of M. H. Sleisenger, M.D.)

Although barium enema may demonstrate disease in the terminal ileum as a result of reflux of barium past the ileocecal valve, determination of the extent of small bowel involvement requires administration of the contrast medium orally or by enteroclysis in difficult

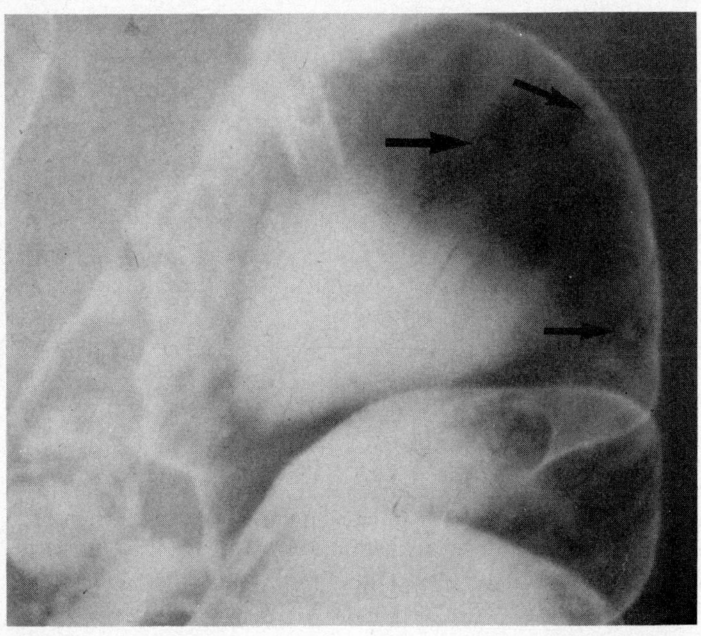

Figure 71–13. Air-contrast barium enema showing multiple discrete "aphthoid" ulcers (arrows), with ulcer craters surrounded by radiolucent areas representing adjacent edema. (Courtesy of Albert A. Moss, M.D.)

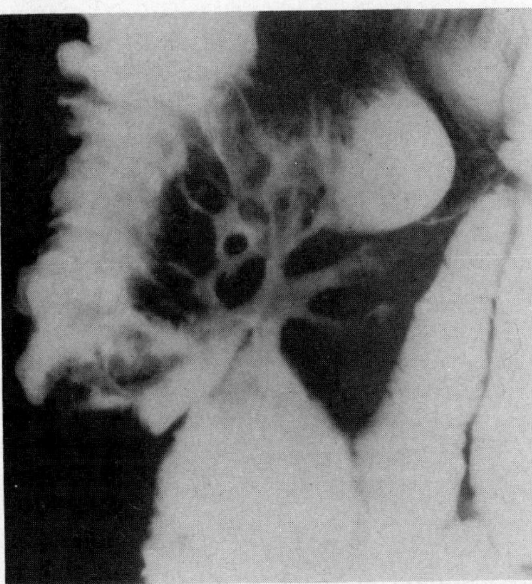

Figure 71–14. Narrowed terminal ileum and ileocecal fistula. (Courtesy of H. I. Goldberg, M.D.)

cases. Obviously, barium should not be delivered into the upper gastrointestinal tract when clinically important intestinal obstruction is suspected. Small bowel abnormalities are similar to those observed in the colon and include a characteristic cobblestone appearance (Fig. 71–18), cicatricial stenosis producing the so-called string sign (Fig. 71–19), diseased segments (skip lesions) separated by small bowel that appears to be relatively normal (Fig. 71–20), burrowing linear ulcerations (Fig. 71–21), and internal fistulas (Fig. 71–22).

Barium enema should be deferred in patients acutely ill with Crohn's colitis, because the examination is not crucial for immediate management decisions and because the risk of perforation or toxic megacolon—although not so great as in acute ulcerative colitis—is appreciable when the inflammatory process is active.

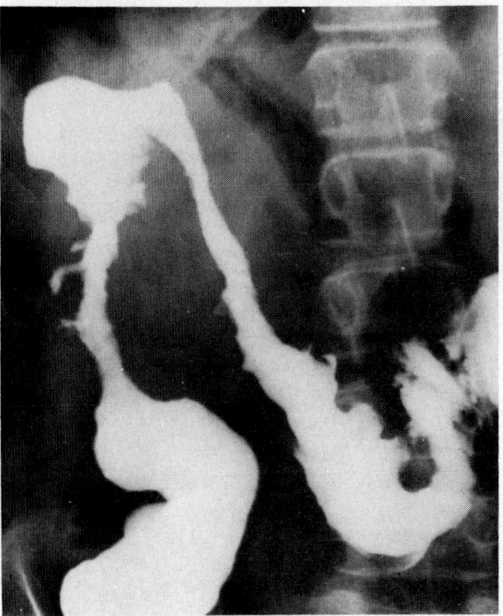

Figure 71–15. Crohn's colitis producing narrow segments of ascending and transverse colon. The hepatic flexure is not involved so that narrowed segments are "skip areas" of disease. Barium extends through the wall of the ascending colon in short sinus tracts.

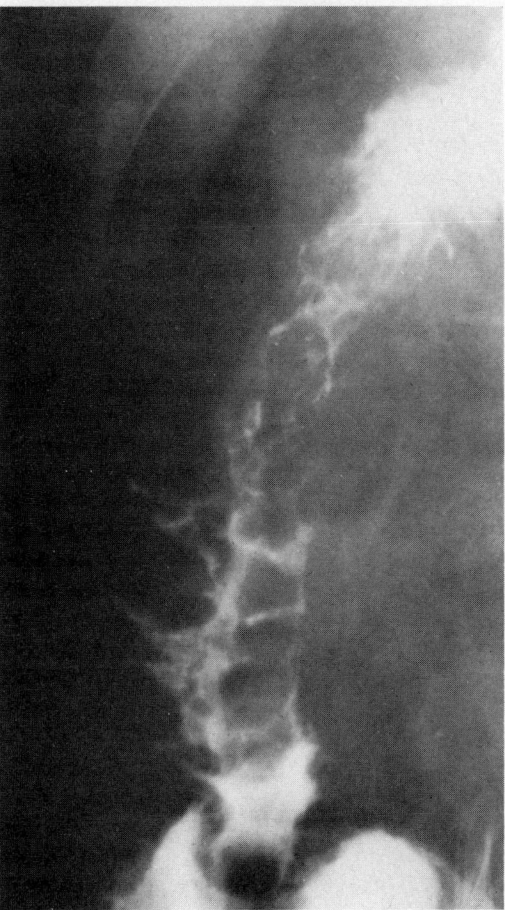

Figure 71–16. Cobblestoning of the mucosa of ascending colon. The rectangular areas result from intersections of transverse fissures and deep longitudinal ulcers. (Courtesy of H. I. Goldberg, M.D.)

X-ray abnormalities are most often detected in the terminal ileum with or without involvement of cecum and ascending colon (Fig. 71–21). Also commonly observed is radiologic evidence of disease at the site of previous surgical anastomosis (see Fig. 71–19). In one large series,[72] however, 22 per cent of cases demonstrated abnormalities of the duodenum, and in 8 per cent these were characteristic of Crohn's disease. Figures 71–22 and 71–23 exemplify extensive radiologic abnormalities involving duodenum, jejunum, and ileum.

Although contrast X-rays of the bowel provide useful diagnostic information and assist in determining the extent of Crohn's disease, it should be emphasized that changes in X-ray appearance correlate poorly, if at all, with the course of the disease.[72] There appears to be no reason for "routine" repetition of X-ray examinations when one is evaluating a patient's progress or response to therapy.

Nuclear Imaging. Investigators are also beginning to use radionuclide scanning techniques to assess the

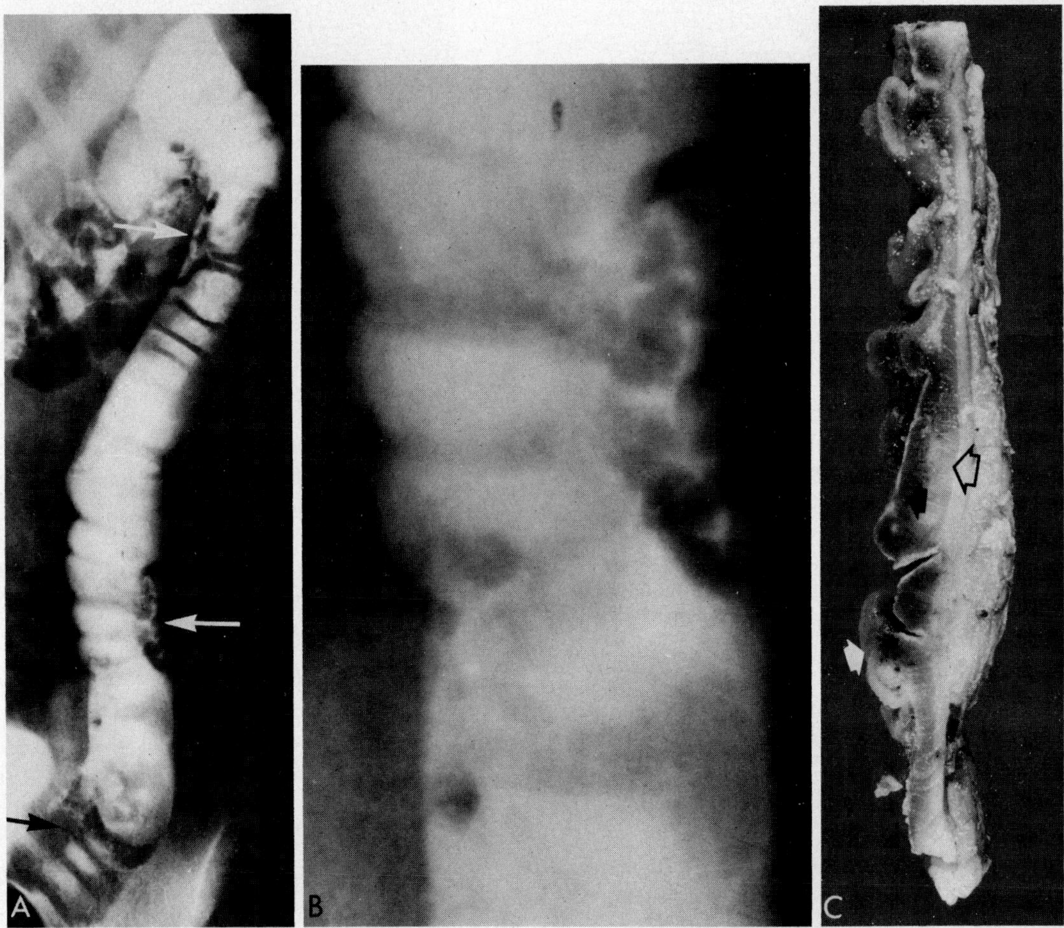

Figure 71–17. *A*, Eccentric segmental narrowing of the colonic wall *(arrows)* with plaque-like ulcerations. *B*, Close-up of middle lesion in *A*, showing a transmural mass with surface ulceration. *C*, Gross pathologic specimen of the same lesion, showing transition between normal and diseased mucosa *(solid white arrow)*, extensive submucosal infiltrate *(solid black arrow)* with denudation of overlying mucosa, and thickened muscularis *(open arrow)*. (From Goldberg, H. I. Focal ulcerations of the colon in granulomatous colitis. AJR *101*:296–300. © by the American Roentgen Ray Society, 1967.)

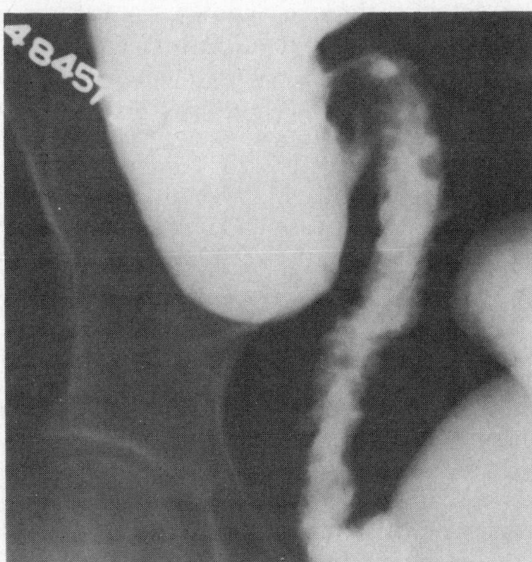

Figure 71–18. Moderate involvement of terminal ileum with typical cobblestone appearance. (Courtesy of P. Kramer, M.D.)

extent of active bowel inflammation in cases of Crohn's disease and ulcerative colitis. When indium-111–labeled granulocytes are injected, they accumulate in inflamed bowel and yield images that correlate well with the location and extent of involvement as determined by X-ray or colonoscopy.[73, 74] Variations of this approach include labeling autologous phagocytes (monocytes as well as granulocytes) with technetium-99–labeled stannous chloride[75] or feeding labeled sucralfate which adheres to injured, mucus-secreting tissue.[76] While attracting considerable attention, these approaches must be considered investigational until a much wider experience is gained.

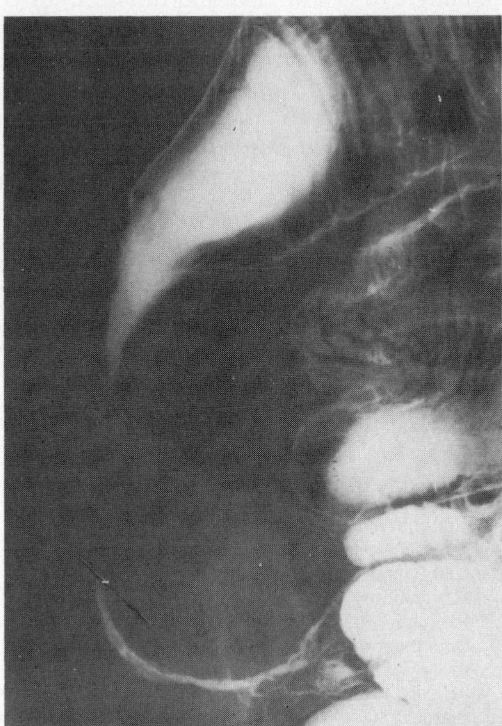

Figure 71–19. Postoperative recurrence of Crohn's disease. The small bowel at the site of anastomosis is involved and shows the typical "string" sign. (Courtesy of J. Wittenberg, M.D.)

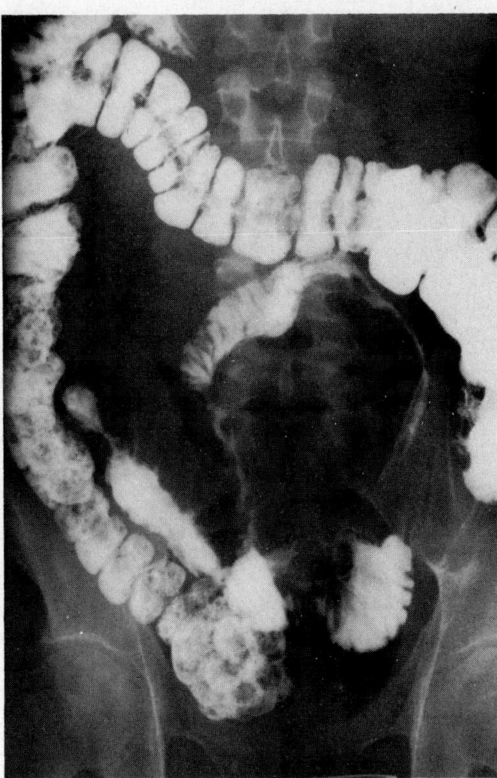

Figure 71–20. Small bowel barium study showing narrow segments of ileum by Crohn's disease. Note the cobblestones and linear ulcers. The patient had symptoms of small bowel obstruction. (Courtesy of M. H. Sleisenger, M.D.)

Mucosal Biopsy. Histologic documentation of granulomatous inflammation of bowel mucosa argues strongly for a diagnosis of Crohn's disease, particularly

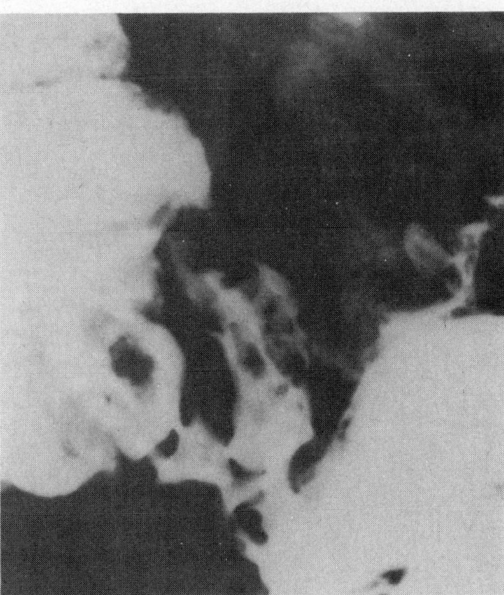

Figure 71–21. Extensive involvement of terminal ileum with burrowing ulceration, cobblestoning, and fistula formation.

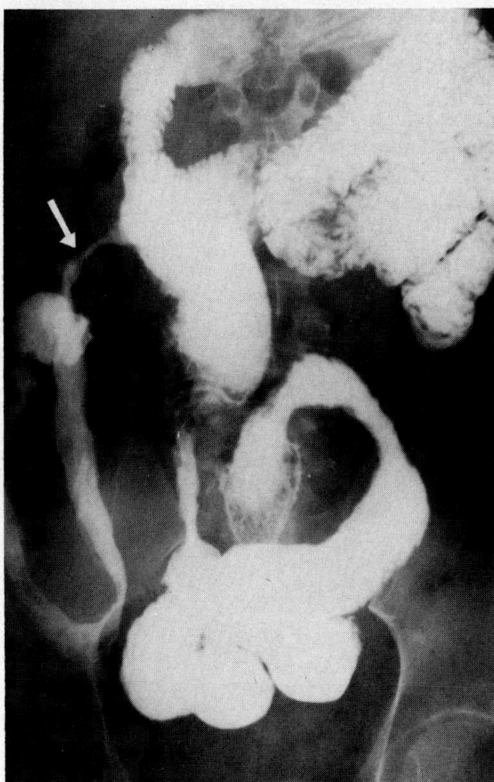

Figure 71–22. Crohn's disease of distal jejunum and proximal ileum, demonstrating narrowed, rigid loops of bowel. Arrow indicates a fistulous tract between two loops of bowel.

when discrete noncaseating granulomas are found and other causes of granulomatous disease (see further on) have been excluded.[77] Mucosal biopsies are most often obtained from the rectum or duodenum. Colonoscopy permits one to take biopsies from any part of the colon and sometimes from the terminal ileum. From the point of view of obtaining adequate tissue for optimal diagnostic yield, however, suction biopsies provide deeper, larger, and less traumatized specimens than samples obtained through endoscopes. Because granulomas can be detected about as frequently in grossly normal-appearing tissue as in obviously diseased mucosa,[7] suction biopsy of the rectum appears to provide a useful diagnostic approach, even in patients without obvious rectal involvement. If binding of lectins to mucins secreted by rectal biopsies proves to be reliably specific for Crohn's disease and ulcerative colitis,[78] this approach may increase the usefulness of rectal biopsy.

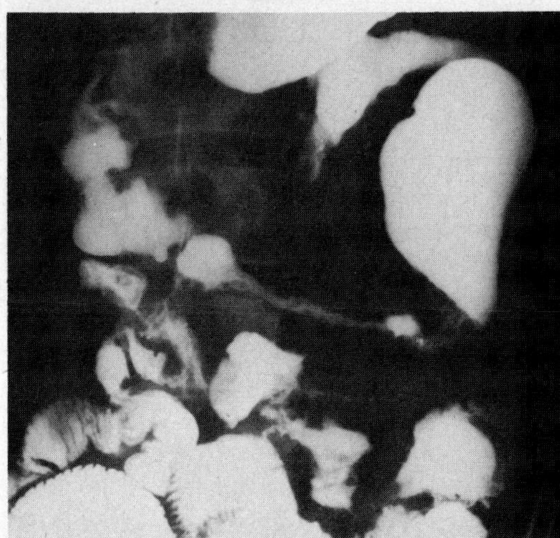

Figure 71–23. Diffuse involvement of segments of duodenum and jejunum with interspersed dilated segments of small bowel. (Courtesy of P. Kramer, M.D.)

DIFFERENTIAL DIAGNOSIS

The list of illnesses that potentially could be considered in the differential diagnosis of Crohn's disease could, in theory, be virtually endless in view of its remarkably diverse clinical features, complications, and modes of presentation. In practical terms, however, the spectrum of diagnostic possibilities is substantially narrowed depending upon whether the patient's illness begins acutely or insidiously and upon the location of identifiable bowel disease (Table 71–9).

When, as is often the case, the disease begins abruptly with an apparently transient episode of nonbloody diarrhea, abdominal cramps, malaise, and low-grade fever, the physician is likely to pass this initial episode off as *viral gastroenteritis,* particularly if the patient appears to recover promptly. In an adolescent or young adult, however, diarrhea lasting more than a few days, the presence of even mild right lower quadrant tenderness, and a slower than expected return to well-being should alert the physician to the possibility of beginning Crohn's disease and the need for continued careful follow-up. During the early, acute phase of illness, Crohn's disease may also be confused with *appendicitis.* Patients with appendicitis are likely to have less diarrhea, more prominent pain, guarding and tenderness in the right lower quadrant, more marked leukocytosis, and a more rapid course. Nevertheless,

Table 71–9. THE DIFFERENTIAL DIAGNOSIS OF CROHN'S DISEASE

- Involvement of small bowel alone or small bowel and colon
  - Early, acute phase of disease
    - Viral gastroenteritis
    - Appendicitis
    - *Yersinia* enterocolitis
    - *Salmonella* infection
  - Chronic or recurrent phase of disease
    - Giardiasis
    - Amebiasis
    - Intestinal tuberculosis
    - Nongranulomatous ulcerative jejunoileitis
    - Intestinal lymphoma
    - Fungal infections
    - Pseudomembranous enterocolitis
    - Duodenal ulcer disease
- Involvement limited to colon and rectum
  - Ulcerative colitis (after specific microbial causes of acute colitis are excluded)
  - Ischemic colitis
  - Cancer of the colon
  - Diverticulitis

the same clinical features are frequently present in both disorders, and differentiation may be extremely difficult. When abdominal findings worsen or doubt continues, laparotomy should not be delayed. Less harm is done by discovering and ignoring acute ileitis at operation than by delaying necessary surgery for the patient with a gangrenous or perforated appendix (see pp. 1382–1389). Infection with *Yersinia enterocolitica* results in acute ileitis or ileocolitis with symptoms and signs that closely mimic those of an acute episode of Crohn's disease.[78a] Initial evaluation of the patient in this clinical setting should therefore include culturing of stool samples specifically for *Yersinia*.

If the patient presents with chronic or recurrent diarrhea, abdominal pain, fever, and weight loss, other diseases of the intestine must be included in the differential diagnosis. In any patient with prolonged, undiagnosed diarrhea, it is important to exclude the possibility of giardiasis (see pp. 1153–1155). In addition to diarrhea, patients with this infestation often have cramping abdominal pain, weight loss, lactase deficiency, and malabsorption of several nutrients. Fever is unusual, however. The diagnosis can be established by finding trophozoites or cysts of *Giardia lamblia* in fresh stool specimens, samples of rectal mucus, or rectal biopsies. In some cases, however, it may be necessary to examine duodenal aspirates to find the organism.

The clinical features, distribution of bowel disease, and X-ray findings of *amebiasis* may be indistinguishable from those of Crohn's disease. Moreover, when amebiasis is localized to the terminal ileum and cecum causing a chronic intramural lesion (ameboma), it may not be possible to find the parasite in stool specimens, rectal mucus, or biopsies. A serologic diagnosis should be sought, for high antibody titers are extremely helpful (see pp. 1155–1162). Differentiation from Crohn's disease is extremely important because amebiasis may rapidly become fulminant if the patient is treated with immunosuppressive agents for presumed Crohn's disease.

A similar situation exists with respect to *intestinal tuberculosis*: treatments frequently used for Crohn's disease are likely to affect tuberculosis adversely. Although now uncommon in Western industrialized nations, tuberculous involvement of bowel and peritoneum remains a major medical problem in Asia. Both Crohn's disease and intestinal tuberculosis share cardinal features, including diarrhea, abdominal pain, fever, weight loss, and radiologic demonstration of ileocecal involvement, with X-ray findings of intramural swelling, strictures, and fistulas (see pp. 1221–1224). In tuberculosis, skip lesions are rather rare. The presence of pulmonary tuberculosis is obviously helpful in diagnosing intestinal involvement, but in underdeveloped countries, patients often have intestinal tuberculosis without clinically apparent pulmonary disease. The results of a tuberculin skin test cannot be depended upon, because patients with systemic tuberculosis frequently do not respond to the antigen, and the tuberculin skin test is often incidentally positive among patients with Crohn's disease.

When disease diffusely involves the small bowel, Crohn's disease must be distinguished from *nongranulomatous ulcerative jejunoileitis*.[79] Abdominal pain and diarrhea are prominent features of this disorder, and the radiologic appearance of the small bowel may resemble that seen in the diffuse form of Crohn's disease. In nongranulomatous disease, however, weight loss, malabsorption, and hypoproteinemia tend to be much more prominent. Moreover, small bowel biopsy shows a more diffuse lesion with flattened and thickened villi, infiltration of the lamina propria, and mucosal ulcerations (see p. 1325).

Although *lymphoma* involving the small intestine may produce a clinical picture that closely resembles Crohn's disease, symptoms are usually constant in lymphoma, and deterioration is more rapid. The average time from onset of symptoms to exploration being about six to nine months. In patients with lymphoma, palpable abdominal masses tend to be hard rather than firm, well-circumscribed rather than vaguely defined, and usually not tender. Although lymphadenopathy, pulmonary hilar adenopathy, and hepatosplenomegaly all favor a diagnosis of lymphoma, these findings are frequently absent in the diffuse form of small bowel lymphoma that is likely to be confused with Crohn's disease. X-ray examination may be helpful, because the presence of distinct mass lesions within the bowel wall and the absence of true cicatricial narrowing serve to distinguish lymphoma from Crohn's disease. In some cases, rectal biopsy may be helpful by demonstrating granulomas and focal colitis.[80] If it diffusely involves the small intestine, lymphoma often can be diagnosed by small bowel biopsy (see pp. 1550–1553).

Fungal infections of the bowel can produce transmural inflammatory changes with consequent indolent ulceration, fistulas, and abscess cavities that can be confused with Crohn's disease. Aspergillosis, blastomycosis, and other fungal infections cause an insidious and lengthy illness, but unlike the situation in Crohn's disease, prolonged remissions are rare. Furthermore, fungal infections are most likely to develop in patients already debilitated by an underlying disease, particularly one that is being treated by immunosuppressive agents. Cultures of enterocutaneous fistulas for fungi, the finding of typical "sulfur granules," and appropriate skin tests all help to identify the presence of fungal infection (see pp. 392–395).

Because duodenal abnormalities may be seen by X-ray in up to 22 per cent of patients with Crohn's disease,[80a] duodenal ulcer disease, particularly *postbulbar ulcer,* must be differentiated from Crohn's disease. Although the history and course are quite different in these two diseases, the differential diagnosis may be difficult in some cases. Any patient with atypical gastrointestinal symptoms and X-ray findings suggestive of postbulbar ulcer should have a careful diagnostic evaluation for Crohn's disease of the small bowel, including biopsy when indicated.

Pseudomembranous enterocolitis produces ulcerating inflammatory lesions of the colon and, less often, of small bowel together with clinical features that need to be distinguished from Crohn's disease (see pp. 1310–1315). This disorder usually occurs in older or debilitated patients being treated with antibiotics. The characteristic proctoscopic finding of well-circumscribed ulcers covered by thick white "pseudomembranes" is helpful but not always present. *C. difficile* cytotoxin is recovered from the stools of a high proportion of patients with pseudomembranous enterocolitis, and a search for this toxin may be helpful in reaching the correct diagnosis. Although *C. difficile* toxin may be found during symptomatic relapses in patients with chronic inflammatory bowel disease, including Crohn's disease,[81] in one study[82] all afflicted patients had received antibiotics within two months, and it remains uncertain whether any specific relation exists between *C. difficile* toxin and inflammatory bowel disease.[70]

When Crohn's disease is limited to the colon and rectum, *ulcerative colitis* is the disease that causes the most difficulty in terms of differential diagnosis. If the onset of Crohn's colitis is abrupt and the patient presents with acute diarrhea and blood in the stools, the same specific microbial causes of acute colitis must be excluded as are described in the differential diagnosis of ulcerative colitis (see pp. 1310–1315). In particular, these include shigellosis, acute colitis due to *Campylobacter fetus,* and acute amebic dysentery. Bloody diarrhea tends to occur late in the course of Crohn's disease, and patients rarely first present with hematochezia. Instead, the disease characteristically begins insidiously, with nonbloody diarrhea, cramping lower abdominal pain, and low-grade fever. A previous history or the concomitant presence of perianal fistulas and abscesses is much more common in Crohn's disease of the colon than in ulcerative colitis. Also more common in Crohn's colitis is a protracted course of low-grade fever, malaise, weakness, and microcytic anemia due to chronic blood loss. In contrast, patients with ulcerative colitis are much more likely to present initially with an acute illness in which bloody diarrhea predominates and systemic symptoms are much less marked. As can be imagined, however, there is considerable overlap between the modes of presentation in these two diseases. Toxic megacolon as part of a fulminant onset or relapse, for example, is considered characteristic of ulcerative colitis but can certainly occur in patients with documented Crohn's colitis.[83]

Sigmoidoscopic and radiologic findings assist in differentiating ulcerative colitis from Crohn's disease of the colon by documenting the distribution of disease within the colon and also by demonstrating the nature of the colonic lesion. Sigmoidoscopy is useful because the inflammatory lesion extends throughout the rectum in virtually all patients with ulcerative colitis, whereas in Crohn's colitis the rectum appears grossly normal in approximately half the cases. Moreover, the endoscopic appearance is usually quite different in the two disorders. In ulcerative colitis, the mucosa is more or less uniformly involved with a diffuse, friable lesion in which the entire mucosa appears denuded and studded with numerous pinpoint excrescences. In Crohn's colitis, on the other hand, the mucosa appears more thickened, is not usually diffusely friable, and frequently exhibits discrete deep round, linear, or serpiginous ulcerations separated by relatively normal-appearing mucosa. In addition, skip lesions may be seen on endoscopy in Crohn's disease, whereas in ulcerative colitis the disease process is virtually always continuous. Rectal biopsy is frequently useful and should be performed even if the rectum appears grossly normal. Although the finding of crypt abscesses in mucosal biopsies is not at all specific and can certainly occur in Crohn's disease, a lesion that appears to be confined to the mucosa and in which crypt abscesses are prominent is much more characteristic of ulcerative colitis than of Crohn's disease. On the other hand, the finding of discrete granulomas in the lamina propria or muscularis mucosae is a strong indication for a diagnosis of Crohn's disease. As discussed earlier, such granulomas may be found in as many as 30 per cent of patients with Crohn's colitis,[7] even when the rectum does not appear to be grossly involved.

Sparing of the rectum as determined by barium enema is not helpful, because ordinary contrast studies fail to document rectal disease in about 20 per cent of patients with ulcerative colitis. Thus, the question of whether or not the rectum is spared can be settled only by proctosigmoidoscopy. Similarly, segmental involvement of the left colon is observed frequently in both diseases and by itself is not helpful. Segmental involvement of the transverse or ascending colon, on the other hand, occurs in about one third of patients with Crohn's disease and is virtually never seen in patients with ulcerative colitis. The presence of skip lesions in the colon strongly favors a diagnosis of Crohn's colitis, but skip lesions occur in only 20 to 25 per cent of cases of Crohn's colitis (see Table 71–3).

In general, the radiographic appearance of the disease process is less helpful in distinguishing Crohn's disease from ulcerative colitis than is the distribution of lesions. In both conditions, the barium enema may demonstrate shallow or deep ulcers, "collar-button" ulcers, or a cobblestone appearance. Although lesions tend to involve the colon in an asymmetric fashion in Crohn's colitis, eccentric narrowing also occurs in ulcerative colitis, and the symmetry of the lesion is not a reliable differential sign. Moreover, pseudopolyps are considered characteristic of ulcerative colitis but are also radiographically demonstrable in Crohn's disease.[84] Although the X-ray picture of pseudopolyps is indistinguishable in both diseases, linear confluent ulcerations that penetrate deeply into the wall of the colon, sinus tracts, fistulas, and pericolic abscesses all indicate transmural disease and are therefore characteristic of Crohn's disease rather than ulcerative colitis.

It should be emphasized that when the inflammatory process is limited to the colon and rectum, Crohn's disease can be distinguished from ulcerative colitis in only 70 to 75 per cent of patients on the basis of clinical, radiologic, endoscopic, and biopsy findings.[85] In the remaining 25 to 30 per cent, the inflammatory bowel disease must be considered "indeterminate." As

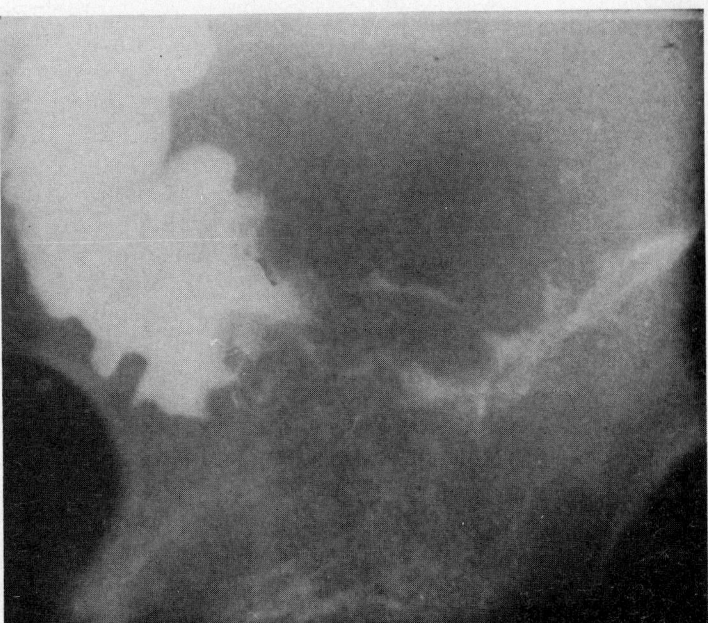

Figure 71–24. A segment of sigmoid colon with narrowing and irregularity. The irregular ulcerated mucosa, the lack of diverticula, and the fistula (parallel to the lumen) aid in differentiating Crohn's colitis from diverticulitis. (Courtesy of H. I. Goldberg, M.D.)

will be discussed in relation to management, difficulties in distinguishing between these two forms of inflammatory bowel disease may play a role in uncertainties concerning the prognosis of patients who require total colectomy for Crohn's disease limited to the colon.

Ischemic bowel disease occasionally causes segmental lesions of the bowel similar to those of Crohn's disease as seen by X-ray and endoscopy, but these techniques are usually capable of distinguishing the two disorders. Moreover, the clinical picture of ischemic colitis (see pp. 1903–1916) is usually quite different from that of Crohn's disease. In ischemic bowel disease, the onset is almost always abrupt and abdominal pain is prominent and precedes the development of diarrhea, which is almost always bloody.

Cancer of the colon may on occasion simulate Crohn's disease, particularly if the lesion infiltrates the bowel wall and is accompanied by secondary ulceration with consequent formation of sinus tracts and fistulas into bowel or bladder. Usually, however, these manifestations of colonic cancer occur late, and almost always some of the X-ray features are suggestive of carcinoma (see pp. 1519–1560). Nevertheless, a localized lesion of the colon—no matter how much it may resemble Crohn's disease by X-ray—should raise the suspicion of colon cancer, particularly in patients whose history is atypical for Crohn's disease. In addition, colon cancer may complicate Crohn's colitis.[54–57] Dysplastic changes occur in the colonic mucosa of patients with Crohn's colitis,[86] but criteria for colonoscopic surveillance remain uncertain.

Diverticulitis is a common disorder that is characterized by cramping pain and tenderness in the left lower quadrant, fever, and leukocytosis (see pp. 1426–1432). X-ray findings of Crohn's disease localized to the sigmoid may be quite similar to those of diverticulitis (Fig. 71–24). However, the presence of diverticula and the absence of disease elsewhere in the colon will strongly favor a diagnosis of diverticulitis. In contrast, deep confluent tracts, ulceration of the mucosa, and thickened folds all point to a diagnosis of Crohn's disease. Despite these differences, however, radiologic distinction between Crohn's disease and diverticulitis may be virtually impossible in some cases. When the issue cannot be resolved on clinical grounds, endoscopic or surgical diagnosis may be necessary.

MANAGEMENT

As is true for all chronic, complicated illnesses of unknown etiology, the management of Crohn's disease varies greatly, depending upon the clinical status of the individual patient. No single therapeutic regimen can be considered "routine" for patients with Crohn's disease; this discussion can only outline general principles that need to be considered in the development of an individual treatment program. In this section, four approaches to management are discussed: (1) general supportive measures, including symptomatic therapy; (2) treatment with anti-inflammatory and immunosuppressive agents directed against the disease process itself; (3) management of the patient's nutritional status, including enteric and parenteral administration of nutrients; and (4) surgical treatment. Although considered separately here, all these components are often simultaneously required for effective management.

Supportive Measures. When symptoms suggesting active disease are present, the patient should be placed at bed rest and treated symptomatically. Diarrhea is often effectively reduced by codeine, Lomotil, or loperamide, with concomitant decrease in abdominal cramps. On occasion, more potent analgesics may be required; in such instances, however, obstruction, bowel perforation, or abscess formation should be suspected and carefully excluded before the patient is given agents that may mask the progression of disease and the need for surgery. Early surgical consultation is certainly warranted when patients do not respond appropriately to standard antidiarrheal agents and mild sedation. In moderately or severely ill patients, it is generally advisable to eliminate all oral intake and maintain the patient with intravenous fluids and nutrients. When symptoms and findings suggest small bowel obstruction, continuous nasogastric suction is usually indicated until edema and spasm of the bowel subside. Particularly important during acute attacks is careful intravenous replacement of fluid and electrolyte losses. When the combination of localized abdominal pain and tenderness, fever, and leukocytosis suggests the possibility of abscess formation, one should initiate broad-spectrum antibiotic coverage specified by the clinical situation, but only after one has obtained appropriate cultures of blood, urine, fistulas, or other possible sources of infection.

The patient with Crohn's disease requires emotional support for this chronic, complicated illness not only during acute attacks but also during periods of quiescence. Particularly important is the early detection and prompt management of depression.[35] Sustained positive interactions between patient and physician are crucial for successful long-term care. Although many consultations with many specialists may be required to manage a complicated case, one physician should be directly and continuously responsible for overall care of the patient. Time-consuming efforts directed at listening sympathetically to the patient's problems and offering helpful advice are essential in management and often yield rewarding results. Psychiatric consultation may occasionally be necessary for specific problems, but successful management requires that continuous emotional support come from a single physician who is directing the patient's overall medical care.

Although many patients and a few physicians pay compulsive attention to diet, there is no evidence that what the patient eats in any way affects the symptoms or course of Crohn's disease, with two notable exceptions: (1) Patients with narrowing of the gut lumen and a propensity for obstructive episodes should certainly avoid substances not readily digested in the upper gastrointestinal tract; and (2) the possibility of lactose intolerance should be considered, since acquired lactase deficiency does occur in some patients with Crohn's disease. Beyond these restrictions in specific clinical situations, the physician should encourage an appetizing, nutritious diet. Obviously, if the patient's experience indicates that certain foods seem to cause symptoms, such foods need not be eaten. In fact, an "exclusion diet" of this sort was significantly more effective than was a fiber-rich diet in treating small numbers of patients with Crohn's disease.[87] On the other hand, many patients with Crohn's disease, like those with other chronic disorders of the gastrointestinal tract, eventually incriminate so many foods as the cause of symptoms that proper nutrition becomes a serious problem. In such cases, the physician must carefully analyze the patient's options concerning diet and provide necessary reassurance and guidance.

Drug Treatment. Perhaps as many as 10 to 20 per cent of patients with Crohn's disease enjoy symptom-free intervals lasting many years and do not require treatment. In most cases, however, prolonged periods of symptomatic active disease or frequent relapses necessitate attempts to treat the disease process itself with anti-inflammatory and immunosuppressive agents. Unfortunately, evaluation of the efficacy of such agents is extremely difficult, given the fluctuating activity and unpredictable long-term course of Crohn's disease. Randomized controlled trials of therapy are therefore necessary.[88] In general, trials have attempted to document whether various agents actually reduce disease activity in symptomatic patients (Table 71–10) or significantly prolong remissions in patients with inactive Crohn's disease (Table 71–11). Effects of treatment have usually been assessed on the basis of changes in quantitative indices of disease activity which have been developed for use in controlled trials.[89, 90] Although important information may ultimately be derived from such trials, they are difficult to perform, always require confirmation, and must be cautiously interpreted before they are generally applied in clinical practice. Patients enlisted in controlled trials are often not as sick as those who receive treatment without randomization. When trials involve relatively small numbers of precisely defined patients, results documenting an effect, even though "statistically significant," may nevertheless be due to chance alone. On the other hand, when studies involve large numbers of cases, results may be difficult to interpret because of the broad spectrum of disease among the patients being studied.

Adrenocortical steroids seem to relieve the symptoms of active Crohn's disease, particularly early in its course. Indeed, in the carefully executed National Cooperative Crohn's Disease Study (NCCDS), prednisone was clearly more effective than placebo in diminishing the activity of the disease process (Fig. 71–25).[91] A large controlled trial conducted in Europe subsequently confirmed these observations.[92] In the latter study, 6-methylprednisolone was clearly superior to placebo in the treatment of acute exacerbations. In one controlled trial involving a relatively small number of subjects,[93] prednisone was about as effective as oral antibiotics in treating exacerbations.

In practice, patients whose active disease process continues despite bed rest and symptomatic measures are usually treated with adrenocortical steroids. Although benefits are not always dramatic and may be difficult to sustain, steroid therapy clearly plays a role in the treatment of symptomatic relapses and is particularly indicated for extraintestinal manifestations.[58] Steroid therapy is best begun with relatively large doses, amounting to the equivalent of 50 to 80 mg of prednisone per day. In more severely ill patients, the steroid should be administered intravenously.

As active disease subsides, oral medication can re-

Table 71–10. DRUG TREATMENT OF ACTIVE CROHN'S DISEASE: RESULTS OF CONTROLLED CLINICAL TRIALS*

Drug (Daily Dose)	Efficacy†	Comments	Reference
Prednisone (0.25–0.75 mg/kg)	+	Less effective in patients already treated with drugs or when disease is limited to colon	91
Prednisolone (0.5 mg/kg)	–	No placebo; found to be as effective as oral antibiotics framycetin and colistin	93
6-Methylprednisolone (48 mg)	+	More effective than sulfasalazine; combination of prednisone and sulfasalazine was most effective	92
Sulfasalazine (1.0 gm/15 kg)	+	Most effective in previously untreated patients; less effective when disease is limited to small bowel	91
(3.0 gm)	±	More effective in unoperated patients	94a
(4–6 gm)	+		95
(3.0 gm)	–	No placebo; compared with metronidazole and found to be about as effective; less effective if disease is limited to small bowel	110
(3.0 gm)	+	Most effective in patients with colitis	92
Sulfasalazine (1.0 gm/15 kg) plus prednisone (0.25–0.75 mg/kg)	–	No placebo; compared with prednisone alone, addition of sulfasalazine had no effect	95a
Azathioprine (2.0 mg/kg)	0		108
(2.5 mg/kg)	0		91
(3.0 mg/kg)	±	Given with corticosteroid	107
6-Mercaptopurine (1.5 mg/kg)	+	Slow response (at least two months) in most cases; given with corticosteroid; steroid "sparing" effect documented	109
Metronidazole (800 mg)	+	Response rate of 57% in one month, 17% in placebo group	111
Metronidazole (800 mg)	–	No placebo; found to be at least as effective as sulfasalazine; less effective if disease is limited to small bowel	110

*Adapted from data reviewed and collated by M. H. Sleisenger.

†Efficacy: + = Significantly more effective than placebo. ± = Improvement, sometimes dramatic, in some cases, but overall results not statistically different from placebo. 0 = Results not significantly different from palcebo. – = Drug compared with another drug rather than with placebo.

Table 71–11. MAINTENANCE OR REMISSIONS IN INACTIVE CROHN'S DISEASE: RESULTS OF CONTROLLED CLINICAL TRIALS*

Drug (Daily Dose)	Efficacy†	Comments	Reference
Prednisone (0.25 mg/kg)	0		91
(7.5 mg)	0		103
6-Methylprednisolone (12 mg)	0		92
Sulfasalazine (1.0 gm/15 kg)	0		91
(3.0 gm)	0		111a
Sulfasalazine (1.0 mg/15 kg) plus prednisone (0.25–0.75 mg/kg)	–	No more effective than prednisone alone; did not reduce steroid requirement	95a
Azathioprine (2.0 mg/kg)	+	Some (15 of 51) patients also received prednisone and/or sulfasalazine	104
(2.0 mg/kg)	+	Given with corticosteroids; steroid "sparing" effect	111
(2.0 mg/kg)	+	Given with corticosteroids; steroid "sparing" effect	106
(1.5 mg/kg)	0		91

*Adapted from data reviewed and collated by M. H. Sleisenger.

†Efficacy: + = Significantly more effective than placebo. 0 = Not significantly different from placebo. – = Compared with another drug rather than with placebo.

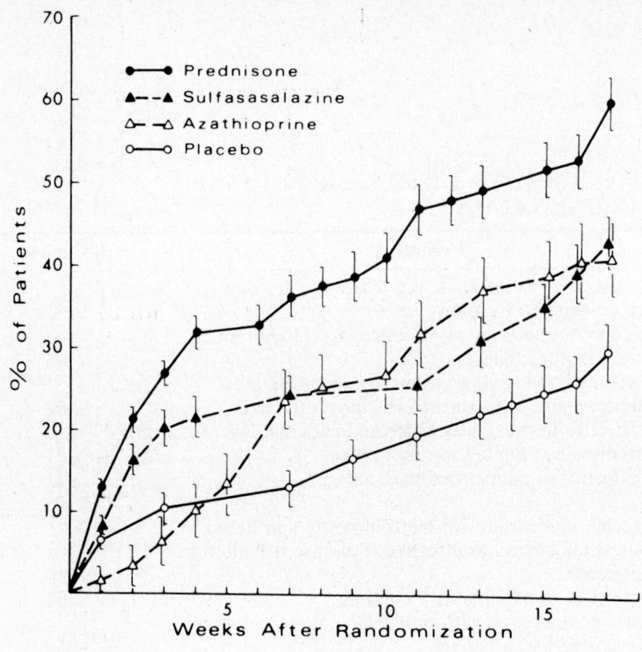

Figure 71–25. Response to different treatments in patients with active symptomatic Crohn's disease as determined by the Crohn's disease activity index (CDAI). Decrease in the CDAI was significantly greater in patients treated with sulfasalazine or prednisone than in those receiving a placebo. There was no statistically significant difference between azathioprine-treated and placebo-treated patients. (Reprinted with permission from: National Cooperative Crohn's Disease Study: results of drug treatment, by Summers, R. W., Switz, D. M., Sessions, J. T., et al. Gastroenterology *77*:847–869. Copyright 1979 by The American Gastroenterological Association.)

place parenteral therapy and the dose can be gradually reduced to the minimal level needed to suppress signs of inflammation. The amount necessary for maintenance varies from patient to patient. Unfortunately, long-term steroid therapy is associated with a high rate of unacceptable side effects,[94] and there is no evidence that frequency of recurrence or long-term outcome is altered by maintenance steroid therapy (Fig. 71–26).[91, 92] The physician should therefore withdraw steroids gradually over a period of several weeks to a few months, with the goal of ultimately eliminating this agent. However, this objective cannot always be achieved, and many patients become symptomatic when the dose of prednisone is reduced below 5 to 15 mg per day. Because this "steroid dependence" occurs frequently, the decision to treat with steroids should be made only after other less potent alternatives for management prove impractical or ineffective.

Sulfasalazine has also been used frequently for patients with symptomatic Crohn's disease. In large trials, sulfasalazine was more effective than placebo[91, 92, 95] but less effective than 6-methylprednisolone in one of these studies.[92] Sulfasalazine appears to be more effective in patients with colonic disease than in those with involvement limited to the small bowel.[91, 95] Unacceptable side effects from sulfasalazine occur less often than from prednisone.[94] Therefore, it seems worth while to treat patients during the active phase of the disease with 3

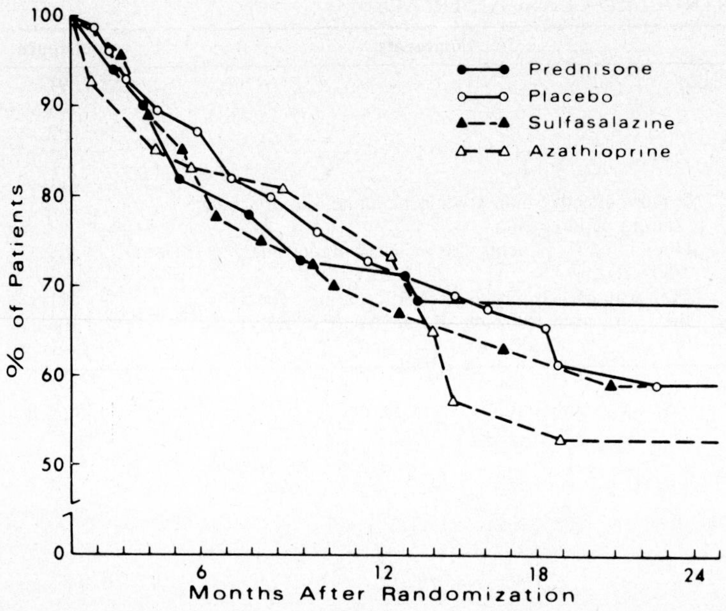

Figure 71–26. Percentage of patients in remission when maintained on different treatments. Relapse was defined as withdrawal from the study because of (1) increase in the CDAI greater than 100 points to a level of higher than 150 for two weeks; (2) need for operation; (3) development of fistula; (4) persistent fever for two weeks; or (5) worsening barium enemas. There was no statistically significant difference between any of the treatments and placebo. (Reprinted with permission from: National Cooperative Crohn's Disease Study: results of drug treatment, by Summers, R. W., Switz, D. M., Sessions, J. T., et al. Gastroenterology *77*:847–869. Copyright 1979 by The American Gastroenterological Association.)

to 4 gm of sulfasalazine daily before beginning a patient on steroid therapy, particularly in persons who are only mildly or moderately symptomatic. Patients with Crohn's disease are frequently treated between attacks with 1 to 2.5 gm of sulfasalazine daily. When examined in controlled trials, however, this agent was no more effective than placebo in preventing recurrences (see Fig. 71–26).[91, 92] Sulfasalazine, when added to prednisone, appears to be no more effective[91] or slightly more effective[92] than prednisone alone in suppressing an acute attack.

Although sulfasalazine appears to be effective in active Crohn's disease and the frequency of severe side effects is less than that observed with prednisone, the drug should not be used at higher doses or for longer periods than are necessary. As is the case with prednisone, the goal of management should be gradual withdrawal of the drug. In addition to causing skin rashes, platelet dysfunction, and occasional bone marrow suppression, sulfasalazine can decrease sperm counts and cause infertility in males.[94] Because this drug competes with folate for receptor sites and impairs absorption of folate (see pp. 1046–1048), patients treated with sulfasalazine should regularly receive folic acid supplements.

Sulfasalazine is split by colonic bacteria into sulfapyridine and 5-aminosalicylic acid (5-ASA). The weight of present evidence suggests that 5-ASA is the active constituent of sulfasalazine.[96] Whether the formation of the active metabolite within the colon is responsible for its apparently greater efficacy in patients with Crohn's colitis[91, 92] remains to be determined. Also still unclear is whether 5-ASA exerts its beneficial effects by acting upon prostaglandin metabolism in intestinal tissue.[29] In any case, the Crohn's disease activity index was significantly lowered in 72 per cent of patients treated with a slow release form of 5-ASA.[97] As another indication of its anti-inflammatory activity, this agent decreased fecal excretion of granulocytes that had been labeled with indium-111 and injected into patients with Crohn's disease.[98] A related agent, disodium azodisalicylate, which is split by colon bacteria to yield active salicylate, is currently being tested for its effects in patients with active disease.[99]

When active Crohn's disease persists or progresses despite treatment with sulfasalazine, prednisone, and resective surgery, patients are sometimes treated with more potent immunosuppressive agents, such as azathioprine or its metabolite 6-mercaptopurine.[100] Opinions differ concerning the role of these agents in the management of Crohn's disease.[101, 102] On the one hand, reports continue to suggest that azathioprine or 6-mercaptopurine suppresses intestinal symptoms, reduces requirements for steroids, and promotes the healing of fistulas in patients whose treatment with steroids and surgery has failed.[103] Moreover, in one controlled trial,[104] the frequency of recurrence of active disease was significantly reduced in patients maintained on azathioprine for one year. Similar results were obtained in trials involving smaller numbers of patients, all of whom also received corticosteroids.[105, 106] In these trials, it was possible to reduce the dose of steroids in azathioprine-treated patients. On the other hand, both azathioprine and 6-mercaptopurine are toxic agents, and one death due to azathioprine-induced pancytopenia was reported in one of these trials.[104] Even during relatively short-term (four months) treatment with azathioprine, side effects were considerable.[94] Because neither prednisone nor sulfasalazine effectively maintains remissions in patients with Crohn's disease,[91, 92] it seems reasonable to continue the search for safer long-term maintenance therapy with other immunosuppressive or anti-inflammatory agents, particularly if a "steroid-sparing" effect can be achieved.

With respect to the use of these agents to treat exacerbations, azathioprine has not proved statistically more effective than placebo in improving symptomatic patients in some studies.[91, 107, 108] However, in one controlled trial,[109] 6-mercaptopurine decreased symptoms, healed fistulas, and reduced steroid requirements more effectively than did placebo. The necessity of long-term treatment was emphasized in an open trial of azathioiprine and 6-mercaptopurine.[103] In many instances, more than two months of treatment is required before improvement becomes apparent.[103, 109]

Because of serious side effects and lack of a consensus about benefits, azathioprine or 6-mercaptopurine should be considered as a therapeutic option only in those patients with persistent severe disease that has not responded to treatment with sulfasalazine, corticosteroids, and resective therapy or in those patients in whom reduction in steroid dosage is badly needed but otherwise unachievable. Physicians should continue to administer these agents only in the setting of carefully monitored trials designed to provide objective assessments of their efficacy.

Other agents have been evaluated for efficacy in Crohn's disease. Metronidazole, 800 mg daily, is at least as effective as sulfasalazine[110] and more effective than placebo[111] in improving symptoms and diminishing disease activity in patients with active Crohn's disease. When larger doses (20 mg per kg) of metronidazole are given, dramatic healing of perineal Crohn's disease has also been observed.[112] However, peripheral neuropathy, which may be irreversible, occurs frequently with these high doses,[113] and perineal disease promptly returns or worsens when the dose of metronidazole is reduced to more tolerable levels.[114]

Given reports about a possible etiologic role for mycobacteria in Crohn's disease, a controlled trial of treatment with rifampin and ethambutol[115] was of considerable interest. Short-term treatment in a small number of patients, however, yielded no evidence of efficacy, and a large-scale trial does not seem warranted at present.

Randomized controlled trials in small numbers of patients have failed to demonstrate that manipulating immunologic mechanisms has any beneficial effect.[14] These include treatment with oral cromoglycate, levamisole, oral BCG, and transfer factor.

Nutritional Considerations (see also pp. 1983–2027).

Maintenance of adequate nutrition is often difficult for patients with extensive Crohn's disease, particularly for those who have been subjected to extensive small bowel resection (see pp. 1106–1112). Specific replacement of vitamin D, calcium, vitamin K, folic acid, iron, and other nutrients that may be poorly absorbed by patients with Crohn's disease is indicated whenever there is clinical or laboratory evidence of deficiency of these substances. In the absence of vitamin A deficiency, however, treatment with this nutrient appears to have no clinical benefit.[116] Parenteral vitamin B_{12} should be administered to all patients with abnormal Schilling tests following ileal resection. In patients with bile salt deficiency resulting from extensive disease or resection of the terminal ileum, substitution of medium-chain triglycerides (MCT) for long-chain triglycerides in the diet diminishes steatorrhea and increases assimilation of calories. Many patients benefit from commercially available forms of MCT. These preparations often contain considerable quantities of lactose, however, and may be poorly tolerated by patients who are lactase-deficient because of diseased or resected small bowel.

Because the bile salt concentration in the proximal intestine is greatest at the time of the first meal of the day, it is probably best to recommend that larger quantities of fat be taken at breakfast than at other meals. When diarrhea results from excessive quantities of bile salts entering the colon rather than from impaired absorption of fat, administration of cholestyramine or aluminum hydroxide will bind intraluminal bile salts and reduce their deleterious effects. Such binding may, however, further deplete the bile salt pool and thus make steatorrhea worse (see pp. 1106–1112).

Patients afflicted with extensive, symptomatic Crohn's disease usually require an artificial nutritional program that "rests" the bowel, allows fistulas to heal, induces positive nitrogen balance, and even causes weight gain. Total parenteral nutrition is capable of successfully maintaining patients for several years.[117] By receiving infusions at night, patients can carry on normal activities during the day even though they require total parenteral nutrition.[118] Aggressive nutritional programs are particularly important for preventing or reversing growth retardation and delayed sexual maturation.[65, 66] Many patients respond well to enteral programs in which they receive an elemental diet containing only monosaccharides, amino acids, and minerals supplemented by vitamins and essential fatty acids. In a small number of subjects this approach has been effective in managing episodes of active inflammation.[119] On the other hand, a low-residue diet had no long-term advantage when compared with a normal diet in one randomized trial.[120]

Although modern methods of effectively delivering nutrients to patients severely ill with Crohn's disease unquestionably improve nutritional status, relieve symptoms, heal fistulas, and make it possible to treat perirectal disease effectively, artificial parenteral or enteral feeding systems have little effect on the long-term course of severe Crohn's disease. Too often progressive symptoms and troublesome complications recur soon after patients resume a normal diet. In assessing the benefits of total parenteral nutrition, the physician must constantly keep in mind the risks of pneumothorax, infection, electrolyte disorders, unanticipated specific nutritional deficiencies, pancreatitis,[121] or the development of still poorly understood painful bone lesions.[122]

Surgical Treatment. In view of the previously discussed high rate of recurrence of Crohn's disease following resection of diseased bowel,[43–45] resective therapy for patients with uncomplicated Crohn's disease is warranted only in unusual circumstances; operative therapy should be reserved for complications of the disease or for unequivocal failure to respond to optimal medical treatment. The optimal time for surgery and the kind of operation vary considerably with the major sites of involvement and with the nature of the complication.[123]

When disease of the small bowel progresses to the point that the patient is incapacitated by frequently recurrent or sustained bowel obstruction, the usual recourse is primary resection or bypass of the diseased bowel. If bypass is necessary, most clinicians would agree that the diseased bowel should be excluded from the stream of intestinal contents.[124] Although bypass may occasionally be the only surgical option, reports of persistent or reactivated disease, perforation, or even carcinoma in bypassed segments of bowel tend to argue for primary resection whenever feasible. Another option, which should currently be considered investigational, is operative dilatation of strictures.[125] This approach avoids debilitating resections and may prove useful in cases of relatively inactive disease in which one or more stable strictures are causing recurrent episodes of obstruction. In cases of active disease, though, early recurrences are likely. When the duodenum is involved with Crohn's disease, bypass rather than resection is preferred, and gastrojejunostomy with vagotomy is the procedure of choice.[126]

If acute Crohn's disease is discovered during laparotomy for suspected appendicitis, no resection or bypass procedure is indicated, because the course of acute enteritis is usually self-limited and many of these patients do not develop chronic Crohn's disease. If there is no inflammatory involvement at the base of the appendix or in the cecum, the appendix may be removed at the time of laparotomy. If the patient subsequently has recurrent attacks, appendectomy at the time of operative diagnosis of Crohn's disease will have resolved the vexing problem of differentiating Crohn's disease from appendicitis. In general, fistula formation or perforation will not occur following appendectomy if the appendix and cecum are normal. Subsequent fistulas nearly always emanate from diseased small bowel rather than from the site of appendectomy.

When an inflammatory mass is present together with fistulas, sinus tracts, or other evidence of extramural penetration, surgery needs to be considered. In many instances, treatment with steroids may be attempted first, but the physician should proceed cautiously and must recognize the risk of an enlarging abscess, perforation, or spreading peritonitis. Whether or not surgery is required when fistulous tracts have formed depends entirely upon the individual clinical situation. Rarely, fistulas disappear completely when the active phase of the disease subsides, either spontaneously or in response to parenteral alimentation or steroid therapy. Usually, however, the draining fistulous tract, particularly if it drains into rectum or vagina, persists and causes disabling symptoms. Under these circumstances, surgery is necessary. Simple local removal of the fistulous tract or fissure, without simultaneous extirpation of diseased bowel, does not usually prove satisfactory and may lead to further fistula formation and progression of the disease. Because of the hazards of prolonged urinary tract infection, prompt surgical attention is indicated for enterovesicular fistulas.

An indication for immediate surgery is the presence of free perforation into the abdominal cavity.[63] Although rare, this complication can occur in either acute or chronic Crohn's disease. Even though the peritoneal cavity is contaminated, the involved intestine should be resected in preference to attempting mere closure of the perforation.

The most uncertain and controversial aspect of surgery for Crohn's disease relates to operative treatment when the disease process is limited to the colon.[123] Some of this uncertainty results from the difficulties, already discussed, in distinguishing ulcerative colitis from Crohn's disease. Further, the most common indication for surgery in Crohn's colitis is medical intractability,[45] an indication more difficult to assess than intestinal obstruction, which is the usual indication for surgery in Crohn's disease involving the small bowel. Investigators also continue to disagree about the frequency with which inflammatory disease develops in previously uninvolved small bowel following colonic resection for Crohn's colitis. Clearly, some cases of "recurrence" turn out to be late postoperative complications unrelated to the Crohn's disease itself.[127]

When the rectum has apparently been spared in patients with Crohn's colitis, surgical options include total colectomy with permanent ileostomy, subtotal colectomy with primary ileorectal anastomosis, or subtotal colectomy with temporary ileostomy and subsequent ileorectal anastomosis. On the basis of currently available information, opinions vary concerning which procedure should be performed in which patient.[123] In one recent investigation,[128] preoperative measurement of rectal capacity served to predict successful ileorectal anastomosis in this setting. Although primary ileorectal anastomosis is being performed with increasing frequency, recurrent anastomotic disease can be particularly troublesome. Surgeons for the most part still prefer ileostomy and prolonged observation of the rectal stump before performing the anastomosis. On the other hand, proctitis can occasionally develop following diversion of bowel contents.[129] This superficial inflammatory process disappears with reanastomosis and must be distinguished from Crohn's disease itself before anastomosis is attempted.

PROGNOSIS

The manifestations and complications of Crohn's disease are so diverse that its management requires a thorough knowledge of gastroenterology, general internal medicine, clinical nutrition, and the principles of gastrointestinal surgery. For the patient with Crohn's disease, the outlook in some respects seems bleak. Asymptomatic intervals can be rudely interrupted by exacerbations of disease activity at any time. Symptomatic episodes are often discouragingly long, troublesome, and debilitating. For at least one half of patients, the indolent inflammatory process will at one time or another lead to complications that require surgery. Surgical extirpation of involved bowel is ultimately followed by recurrent disease in the vast majority of cases. Extensive clinical investigations have failed to uncover the cause or causes of Crohn's disease, and there is no cure.

Despite this grim picture, the future of the patient with Crohn's disease should not be painted as hopeless. The completely unpredictable course of the disease means that some patients, perhaps 10 to 20 per cent, will lead completely symptom-free lives after one or two attacks.[40] Given the serious nature of the disorder and its complications, surprisingly few patients die as a direct result of Crohn's disease.[51] Although medical and surgical therapy can neither cure the disease nor predictably ameliorate its course, sulfasalazine and corticosteroids can suppress exacerbations of the inflammatory process and make patients feel better (see Table 71–10), while modern surgery safely and effectively treats complications. Moreover, results of controlled trials document the tendency for spontaneous improvement by showing that a substantial proportion of patients in the placebo-treated group do quite well.[130] Recent advances in nutritional therapy make it possible to sustain even severely afflicted patients through prolonged periods of active disease. With proper medical supervision, the majority of patients adjust remarkably well to their chronic illness, cope with its exacerbations and complications, and manage to lead productive lives.[131]

References

1. Lockhart-Mummery, H., and Morson, B. Crohn's disease (regional enteritis) of the large intestine and its distinction from ulcerative colitis. Gut *1*:87, 1960.
2. Crohn, B. B. Granulomatous diseases of the large and small bowel. A historical survey. Gastroenterology *52*:767, 1967.
3. Whitehead, R. Pathology of Crohn's disease. *In* Kirsner, J. B., and Shorter, R. G. (eds.): Inflammatory Bowel Disease. Ed. 2. Philadelphia, Lea & Febiger, 1980, pp. 296–310.
4. Chong, S. K., Blackshaw, A. J., Boyle, S., Williams, C. B., and Walker-Smith, J. A. Histological diagnosis of chronic inflammatory bowel disease in childhood. Gut *26*:55–59, 1985.
5. Dvorak, A. M., and Silen, W. Differentiation between Crohn's

disease and other inflammatory conditions by electron microscopy. Ann. Surg. *201*:53–63, 1985.
6. Margulis, A. B., Goldberg, H. I., Lawson, T. L., and Montgomery, C. K. The overlapping spectrum of ulcerative and granulomatous colitis: A roentgenographic-pathologic study. Am. J. Roentgenol. *113*:325, 1971.
7. Surawicz, C. M., Meisel, J. L., Ylvisaker, T., Saunders, D. R., and Rubin, C. E. Rectal biopsy in the diagnosis of Crohn's disease: Value of multiple biopsies and serial sectioning. Gastroenterology *80*:66, 1981.
8. Mendeloff, A. I. The epidemiology of idiopathic inflammatory bowel disease. *In* Kirsner, J. B., and Shorter, R. G. (eds.): Inflammatory Bowel Disease. Ed. 2. Philadelphia, Lea & Febiger, 1980, pp. 5–23.
9. Goldman, C. D., Kodner, I. J., Fry, R. D., and McDermott, R. P. Clinical and operative experience with non-Caucasian patients with Crohn's disease. Dis. Colon Rectum *29*:317, 1986.
10. Serlin, S. M., Benkof, K. J., Kazlow, P., et al. Occurrence of Crohn's disease in twins. J. Clin. Gastroenterol. *8*:290–294, 1986.
11. Whorwell, P. J., Eade, O. E., Hossenbocus, A., and Bamforth, J. Crohn's disease in a husband and wife. Lancet *2*:186, 1978.
12. Mayberry, J. F., and Rhodes, J. Epidemiological aspects of Crohn's disease: A review of the literature. Gut *25*:886–899, 1984.
13. Sonnenberg, A. Geographic variation in the incidence of and mortality from inflammatory bowel disease. Dis. Colon Rectum *29*:854, 1986.
14. Kirsner, J. B., and Shorter, R. G. Recent developments in "nonspecific" inflammatory bowel disease. N. Engl. J. Med. *306*:775, 1982.
15. Crohn, B. B., Ginzburg, L., and Oppenheimer, G. D. Regional ileitis. A pathologic and clinical entity. JAMA *99*:1323, 1932.
16. Burnham, W. R., Lennard-Jones, J. E., Stanford, J. L., and Bird, R. G. Mycobacteria as a possible cause of inflammatory bowel disease. Lancet *2*:693, 1978.
17. Chiodini, R. J., Van Kruinengen, H. J., Thayer, W. R., Merkel, R. S., and Coutu, J. A. Possible role of mycobacteria in inflammatory bowel disease. Dig. Dis. Sci. *29*:1073, 1984.
17a. Chiodini, R. J., Van Kruinengen, H. J., Thayer, W. R., Coutu, J. A., and Merkel, R. S. Mycobacterial spheroplasts isolated from patients with Crohn's disease (abstract). Gastroenterology *88*:1348, 1985.
18. Graham, D. Y., Markesich, D. C., and Yoshimura, H. H. Mycobacteria and inflammatory bowel disease. Results of culture. Gastroenterology *92*:436, 1987.
19. Orr, M. M. Experimental intestinal granulomas. Proc. R. Soc. Med. *68*:14, 1975.
20. Parent, K., and Mitchell, P. Cell wall defective variants of pseudomonas-like (Group Va) bacteria in Crohn's disease. Gastroenterology *75*:368, 1978.
21. Cave, D. R., Mitchell, D. N., and Brooke, B. N. Experimental animal studies of the etiology and pathogenesis of Crohn's disease. Gastroenterology *69*:618, 1975.
22. Rozen, P., Zonis, J., Yekutiel, P., and Gilat, T. Crohn's disease in the Jewish population of Tel-Aviv Yafo. Gastroenterology *76*:25, 1979.
23. Gitnick, G. L., Rosen, V. J., Arthur, M. S., and Hertweck, S. A. Evidence for the isolation of a new virus from ulcerative colitis patients: Comparison with virus derived from Crohn's disease. Dig. Dis. Sci. *24*:609, 1979.
24. Miller, D. S., Keighley, A., and Smith, P. G. A case control method for seeking evidence of contagion in Crohn's disease. Gastroenterology *71*:385, 1976.
25. Sedlack, R. E., Whisnant, J., and Elveback, L. R. Incidence of Crohn's disease in Olmsted County, Minnesota. J. Epidemiol. *112*:759, 1980.
26. Elson, C. O., Kagnoff, M. F., Fiocchi, C., Befus, A. D., and Targan, S. Intestinal immunity and inflammation: Recent progress. Gastroenterology *91*:746–768, 1986.
27. Meuret, G., Bitzi, A., and Hammer, B. Macrophage turnover in Crohn's disease and ulcerative colitis. Gastroenterology *74*:501, 1978.
28. Krause, U., Michaelsson, G., and Juhlin, L. Skin reactivity and phagocytic function of neutrophil leucocytes in Crohn's disease and ulcerative colitis. Scand. J. Gastroenterol. *13*:71, 1978.
29. Donowitz, M. Arachidonic acid metabolites and their role in inflammatory bowel disease. Gastroenterology *88*:580, 1985.
30. Schwartz, S. E., Siegelbaum, S. P., Fazio, T. L., Hubbell, B. S., and Henry, J. B. Regional enteritis: Evidence for genetic transmission by HLA typing. Ann. Intern. Med. *93*:424, 1980.
31. Eade, O. E., Moulton, C., MacPherson, B. R., St. Andre-Ukena, S., Albertini, R. J., and Beeken, W. L. Discordant HLA haplotype segregation in familial Crohn's disease. Gastroenterology *79*:271, 1980.
32. Biemond, I., Bunham, W. R., D'Amaro, J., and Langman, M. J. S. HLA-A and HLA-B antigen in inflammatory bowel disease. Gut *27*:934, 1986.
33. Monk, M., Mendeloff, A. I., Siegel, C. I., and Lilienfeld, A. An epidemiological study of ulcerative colitis and regional enteritis among adults in Baltimore. III. Psychological and possible stress-precipitating factors. J. Chron. Dis. *22*:565, 1970.
34. McKegney, F. P., Gordon, R. O., and Levine, S. M. A psychosomatic comparison of patients with ulcerative colitis and Crohn's disease. Psychosom. Med. *32*:153, 1970.
35. Helzer, J. E., Chammas, S., Norland, C. C., Stillings, W. A., and Alpers, D. H. A study of the association between Crohn's disease and psychiatric illness. Gastroenterology *86*:324–330, 1984.
36. Thornton, J. R., Emmett, P. M., and Heaton, K. W. Diet and Crohn's disease: Characteristics of the pre-illness diet. Br. Med. J. *2*:762, 1979.
37. Mekhjian, H. S., Switz, D. M., Melnyk, C. S., Rankin, G. B., and Brooks, R. K. Clinical features and natural history of Crohn's disease. Gastroenterology *77*:898, 1979.
38. Farmer, R. G., Whelan, G., and Fazio, V. W. Long-term follow-up of patients with Crohn's disease. Relationship between the clinical pattern and prognosis. Gastroenterology *88*:1818–1825, 1985.
39. Chan, A. T. J., Fleming, C. R., O'Fallon, W. M., and Huizenga, K. A. Estimated versus measured basal energy requirements in patients with Crohn's disease. Gastroenterology *91*:75, 1986.
40. Bergman, L., and Krause, U. Crohn's disease: A long-term study of the clinical course of 186 patients. Scand. J. Gastroenterol. *12*:937, 1977.
41. Brignola, C., Campieri, M., Bazzocchi, G., Farruggia, P., Tragnone, A., and G. A. Lanfranchi. A laboratory index for predicting relapse in asymptomatic patients with Crohn's disease. Gastroenterology *91*:1490, 1986.
42. Korelitz, B. I. An indicator of Crohn's disease activity: A need unfulfilled. J. Clin. Gastroenterol. *8*:220, 1986.
43. Greenstein, A. J., Sachar, D. B., Pasternak, B. S., and Janowitz, H. D. Reoperation and recurrence in Crohn's colitis and entercolitis. N. Engl. J. Med. *293*:685, 1975.
44. Mekhjian, H. S., Switz, D. M., Watts, H. D., Deren, J. J., Katon, R. M., and Beman, F. M. National Cooperative Crohn's Disease Study: Factors determining recurrence after surgery. Gastroenterology *77*:907, 1979.
45. Whelan, G., Farmer, R. G., Fazio, V. W., and Goormastic, M. Recurrence after surgery in Crohn's disease. Relationship to location of disease (clinical patients) and surgical intervention. Gastroenterology *88*:1826, 1985.
46. Rutgeerts, P., Geboes, K., Ventrappen, G., Kerremans, R., Coenegrachts, J. L., and Coremans, G. Natural history of recurrent Crohn's disease at the ileocolonic anastomosis after curative surgery. Gut *25*:665–672, 1984.
47. Farmer, R. G., and Michener, W. M. Prognosis of Crohn's disease with onset in childhood or adolescence. Dig. Dis. Sci. *24*:752, 1979.
48. Donaldson, R. M., Jr. Management of medical problems in pregnancy—inflammatory bowel disease. N. Engl. J. Med. *312*:1616, 1985.
49. Fabricius, P. J., Gyde, S. N., Shouler, P., Allan, R. N.,

Keighley, M. R., and Alexander-Williams, J. Crohn's disease in the elderly. Gut *26*:461, 1985.

50. Foxworthy, D. M., and Wilson, J. A. P. Crohn's disease in the elderly. J. Am. Gerontol. *33*:492, 1985.
51. Mayberry, J. F., Newcombe, R. G., and Rhodes, J. Mortality in Crohn's disease. Q. J. Med. *49*:63, 1980.
52. Farmer, R. G., Hawk, W. A., and Turnbull, R. B., Jr. Indications for surgery in Crohn's disease: Analysis of 500 cases. Gastroenterology *71*:245, 1976.
53. Greenstein, A. J., Mann, D., Sachar, D. B., and Aufses, A. H., Jr. Free perforation in Crohn's disease: I. A survey of 99 cases. Am. J. Gastroenterol. *80*:682–689, 1985.
54. Hamilton, S. R. Colorectal carcinoma in patients with Crohn's disease. Gastroenterology *89*:398–407, 1985.
55. Allan, D. C., Hughes, D. F., and Calvert, C. H. Carcinoma in Crohn's disease of the colon. Dis. Colon Rectum *29*:760, 1986.
56. Gyde, S. N., Prior, P., Macartney, J. C., Thompson, H., Waterhouse, J. A. H., and Allan, R. N. Malignancy in Crohn's disease. Gut *21*:1024, 1980.
57. Greenstein, A. J., Sachar, D. B., Smith, H., Janowitz, H. D., and Aufses, A. H. Patterns of neoplasia in Crohn's disease and ulcerative colitis. Cancer *46*:403, 1980.
58. Greenstein, A. J., Janowitz, H. D., and Sachar, D. B. The extraintestinal complications of Crohn's disease and ulcerative colitis: A study of 700 patients. Medicine *55*:401, 1976.
59. Rankin, G. B., Watts, H. D., Melnyk, C. S., and Kelley, M. L., Jr. National Cooperative Crohn's Disease Study: Extraintestinal manifestations and perianal complications. Gastroenterology *77*:914, 1979.
60. Hylander, E., Jarnum, S., and Frandsen, I. Urolithiasis and hyperoxaluria in chronic inflammatory bowel disease. Scand. J. Gastroenterol. *14*:475, 1979.
61. Talbot, R. W., Heppell, J., Dozors, R. R., and Beart, R. W., Jr. Vascular complications of inflammatory bowel disease. Mayo Clin. Proc. *61*:140–145, 1986.
62. Edwards, R. L., Levine, J. B., Green, R., Duffy, M., Mathews, E., Brande, W., and Rickles, F. Activation of blood coagulation in Crohn's disease. Gastroenterology *92*:329, 1987.
63. Lesko, S. M., Kaufman, D. W., Rosenberg, L., Helmrid, S. P., Miller, D. R., Stolley, P. D., and Shapiro, S. Evidence for an increased risk of Crohn's disease in oral contraceptive users. Gastroenterology *89*:1046, 1985.
64. Sitrin, M. D., Rosenberg, I. H., Chawla, K., Meredith, S., Sellin, J., Rabb, J. M., Coe, F., Kirsner, J. B., and Kraft, S. C. Clinical conference: Nutritional and metabolic complications in a patient with Crohn's disease and ileal resection. Gastroenterology *78*:1069, 1980.
65. Morin, C. L., Roulet, M., Roy, C. C., and Weber, A. Continuous elemental enteral alimentation in children with Crohn's disease and growth failure. Gastroenterology *79*:1205, 1980.
66. Kirschner, B. S., Klich, J. R., Kalman, S. S., DeFavaro, M. V., and Rosenberg, I. H. Reversal of growth retardation in Crohn's disease with therapy emphasizing oral nutritional restitution. Gastroenterology *80*:10, 1981.
67. Mock, D. M. Growth retardation in chronic inflammatory bowel disease. Gastroenterology *91*:1019, 1986.
68. Kirschner, B. S., and Sutton, M. M. Somatomedin-C levels in growth impaired children and adolescents with chronic inflammatory bowel disease. Gastroenterology *91*:830, 1986.
69. Surawicz, C. M. Diagnosing colitis: Biopsy is best. Gastroenterology *92*:538, 1987.
70. Bartlett, J. G. *Clostridium difficile* and inflammatory bowel disease. Gastroenterology *80*:863, 1981.
71. Laufer, I., Mullens, J., and Hamilton, J. Correlation of endoscopy and double-contrast radiography in the early stages of ulcerative and granulomatous colitis. Radiology *118*:1, 1976.
72. Goldberg, H. I., Caruthers, S. B., Nelson, J. A., and Singleton, J. W. Radiographic findings of the National Cooperative Crohn's Disease Study. Gastroenterology *77*:925, 1979.
73. Stein, D. T., Gray, G. M., Gregory, P. B., et al. Location and activity of ulcerative colitis and Crohn's disease by indium-111 leukocyte scan. A prospective comparison study. Gastroenterology *84*:388–393, 1984.
74. Saverymuttu, S. H., Camilleri, M., Rees, H., Lavender, J. P., Hodgson, H. J., and Chadwick, V. S. Indium-111–granulocyte scanning in the assessment of disease extent and disease activity in inflammatory bowel disease. A comparison with colonoscopy, histology, and fecal indium-111–granulocyte excretion. Gastroenterology *90*:1121, 1986.
75. Pullman, W., Hanna, R., Sullivan, P., Booth, J. A., Lomas, F., and Doe, W. F. Technetium-99 in autologous phagocyte scanning: A new imaging technique for inflammatory bowel disease. Br. Med. J. *293*:171, 1986.
76. Dawson, D. J., Khan, A. N., Miller, V., Ratcliffe, J. F., and Shreeve, D. R. Detection of inflammatory bowel disease in adults and children: Evaluation of a new isotopic technique. Br. Med. J. *291*:1227, 1985.
77. Hill, R. B., Kent, T. H., and Hansen, R. N. Clinical usefulness of rectal biopsy in Crohn's disease. Gastroenterology *77*:938, 1979.
78. Jacobs, L. R., and Huber, P. W. Regional distribution and alterations of lectin binding to colorectal mucin in mucosal biopsies from controls and subjects with inflammatory bowel diseases. J. Clin. Invest. *75*:112, 1985.

78a. Vantrappen, G., Ponette, E., Geboes, K., and Bertrand, P. Yersinia enteritis and enterocolitis: Gastroenterological aspects. Gastroenterology *72*:220, 1977.

79. Jeffries, G. H., Steinberg, H., and Sleisenger, M. H. Chronic ulcerative non-granulomatous jejunitis. Am. J. Med. *44*:47, 1968.
80. Hyams, J. S., Goldman, H., and Katz, A. J. Differentiating small bowel Crohn's disease from lymphoma. Role of rectal biopsy. Gastroenterology *79*:340, 1980.

80a. Sanders, M. G., and Schimmel, E. M. The relationship between granulomatous bowel disease and duodenal ulcer. Am. J. Dig. Dis. *17*:1100, 1972.

81. Trnka, Y. M., and LaMont, J. T. Association of *Clostridium difficile* toxin with symptomatic relapse of chronic inflammatory bowel disease. Gastroenterology *80*:693, 1981.
82. Meyers, S., Mayer, L., Bottone, E., Desmond, E., and Janowitz, H. D. Occurrence of *Clostridium difficile* toxin during the course of inflammatory bowel disease. Gastroenterology *80*:697, 1981.
83. Grieco, M. B., Bordan, D. L., Geiss, A. C., and Beil, A. R., Jr. Toxic megacolon complicating Crohn's colitis. Ann. Surg. *191*:75, 1980.
84. Freeman, A. H., Berridge, F. R., Dick, A. P., Gleeson, J. A., and Zeegan, R. Pseudopolyposis in Crohn's disease. Br. J. Radiol. *51*:782, 1978.
85. Schacter, H., and Kirsner, J. Definitions of inflammatory bowel disease of unknown etiology. Gastroenterology *68*:591, 1975.
86. Simpson, S., Traube, J., and Riddell, R. H. The histologic appearance of dysplasia (precarcinomatous change) in Crohn's disease of the large and small intestine. Gastroenterology *81*:492, 1981.
87. Jones, V. A., Dickinson, R. J., Workman, E., Wilson, A. J., Freeman, A. H., and Hunter, J. O. Crohn's disease: Maintenance of remission by diet. Lancet *2*:177, 1985.
88. Sack, D. M., and Peppercorn, M. A. Drug therapy of inflammatory bowel disease. Pharmacotherapy *3*:158, 1983.
89. Best, W. R., Becktel, J. M., Singleton, J. W., and Kern, F., Jr. Development of a Crohn's disease activity index. Gastroenterology *70*:439, 1976.
90. Van Hees, P. A. M., Van Elteren, P. H., Van Lier, H. J. J., and Van Tongeren, J. H. M. An index of inflammatory activity in patients with Crohn's disease. Gut *21*:279, 1980.
91. Summers, R. W., Switz, D. M., Sessions, J. T., Becktel, J. M., Best, W. R., Kern, F., Jr., and Singleton, J. W. National Cooperative Crohn's Disease Study: Results of drug treatment. Gastroenterology *77*:847, 1979.
92. Malchow, H., Ewe, K., Brandes, J. W., Goebell, H., Ehns, H., Sommer, H., and Jesdinsky, H. European cooperative Crohn's disease study (ECCDS): Results of drug treatment. Gastroenterology *86*:249–266, 1984.
93. Saverymuttu, S., Hodgson, H. J. F., and Chadwick, V. S. Alternative strategies in Crohn's disease. Controlled trial comparing prednisolone with an elemental diet plus non-absorbable antibiotics in active Crohn's disease. Gut *26*:994–998, 1985.

94. Singleton, J. W., Law, D. H., Kelley, M. L., Jr., Mekhjian, H. S., and Sturdevant, R. A. L. National Cooperative Crohn's Disease Study: Adverse reactions to study drugs. Gastroenterology *77*:870, 1979.

94a. Anthonisen, P., Barany, F., Folkenborg, O., Holtz, A., Jarnum, S., Dristensen, M., Riis, P., Walan, A., and Worning, H. The clinical effect of salazosulphapyridine (Salazopyrin r) in Crohn's disease. A controlled double-blind study. Scand. J. Gastroenterol. *9*:549, 1974.

95. Van Hees, P. A. M., Van Lier, H. J. J., Van Elteren, P. H., Driessen, W. M. M., Van Hogezand, R. A., Ten Velde, G. P. M., Bekker, J. H., and Van Tongeren, J. H. M. Effect of sulphasalazine in patients with active Crohn's disease: A controlled double-blind study. Gut *22*:404, 1981.

95a. Singleton, J. W., Summers, R. W., Kern, F., Jr., Becktel, J. M., Best, W. R., Hansen, R. N., and Winship, D. H. A trial of sulfasalazine as adjunctive therapy in Crohn's disease. Gastroenterology *77*:887, 1979.

96. Peppercorn, M. A. Sulfasalazine. Pharmacology, clinical use, toxicity, and related new drug development. Ann. Intern. Med. *101*:377, 1984.

97. Rasmussen, S. N., Binder, V., Maier, K., et al. Treatment of Crohn's disease with peroral 5-aminosalicylic acid. Gastroenterology *85*:1350, 1983.

98. Saverymuttu, S. H., Gupta, S., Keshavarzian, A., Donovan, B., and Hodsson, H. J. Effect of a slow-release 5-aminosalicylic acid preparation on disease activity in Crohn's disease. Digestion *33*:89, 1986.

99. Van Hogezand, R. A., Van Hees, P. A., Zwanenburg, B., Van Rossum, J. M., and Van Tongeren, J. H. Disposition of disodium azodisalicylate in healthy subjects. A possible new drug for inflammatory bowel disease. Gastroenterology *88*:717, 1985.

100. Sleisenger, M. H. How should we treat Crohn's disease? N. Engl. J. Med. *302*:1024, 1980.

101. Korelitz, B. I., and Present, D. H. Shortcomings of the National Crohn's Disease Study: The exclusion of azathioprine without adequate trial. Gastroenterology *80*:193, 1981.

102. Lennard-Jones, J. E., and Singleton, J. W. The azathioprine controversy. Dig. Dis. Sci. *26*:364, 1981.

103. Nyman, M., Hansson, I., and Eriksson, S. Long-term immunosuppressive treatment in Crohn's disease. Scand. J. Gastroenterol. *20*:1197, 1985.

104. O'Donoghue, D. P., Dawson, A. M., Powell-Tuck, J., Bowen, R. I., and Lennard-Jones, J. E. Double-blind withdrawal trial of azathioprine as maintenance treatment for Crohn's disease. Lancet *2*:955, 1978.

105. Willoughby, J. M. T., Kumar Parveen, J., Beckett, J., and Dawson, A. M. Controlled trial of azathioprine in Crohn's disease. Lancet *2*:944, 1971.

106. Rosenberg, J. L., Levin, B., Wall, A. J., and Kirsner, J. B. A controlled trial of azathioprine in Crohn's disease. Dig. Dis. Sci. *20*:721, 1975.

107. Klein, M., Binder, H. J., Mitchell, M., Aaronson, R., and Spiro, H. Treatment of Crohn's disease with azathioprine: A controlled evaluation. Gastroenterology *66*:916, 1974.

108. Rhodes, J., Bainton, D., Beck, P., and Campbell, H. Controlled trial of azathioprine in Crohn's disease. Lancet *2*:1273, 1971.

109. Present, D. H., Korelitz, B. I., Wisch, N., Glass, J. I., Sachar, D. B., and Pasternak, B. S. Treatment of Crohn's disease with 6-mercaptopurine: A long-term randomized double-blind study. N. Engl. J. Med. *302*:981, 1980.

110. Ursing, B., Alm, T., Barany, F., Bergelin, I., Ganrot-Norlin, K., Hoevels, J., Huitfeldt, B., Jarnerot, G., Krause, U., Krook, A., Nordle, O., and Rosen, A. A comparative study of metronidazole and sulfasalazine for active Crohn's disease. The cooperative Crohn's disease study in Sweden (CCDSS). Gastroenterology *83*:550, 1982.

111. Keighley, M. R. Infection and the use of antibiotics in Crohn's disease. Can. J. Surg. *27*:438, 1984.

111a. Lennard-Jones, J. E. Sulphasalazine in asymptomatic Crohn's disease. A multicentre trial. Gut *18*:69, 1977.

112. Bernstein, L. H., Frank, M. S., Brandt, L. J., and Boley, S. J. Healing of perineal Crohn's disease with metronidazole. Gastroenterology *79*:357, 1980.

113. Duffy, L. F., Fredrik, D., Fisher, S. E., Selman, J., et al. Peripheral neuropathy in Crohn's disease patients treated with metronidazole. Gastroenterology *88*:681, 1985.

114. Brandt, L. J., Bernstein, L. S., Boley, S. J., and Frank, M. S. Metronidazole therapy for perineal Crohn's disease: A follow-up study. Gastroenterology *83*:383, 1982.

115. Shaffer, J. L., Hughes, S., Linaker, B. D., Baker, R. D., and Turnberg, L. A. Controlled trial of rifampin and ethambutol in Crohn's disease. Gut *25*:203, 1984.

116. Wright, J. P., Mee, A. S., Parfitt, A., Marks, I. N., Burns, D. G., Sherman, M., et al. Vitamin A therapy in patients with Crohn's disease. Gastroenterology *88*:512, 1985.

117. Jeejeebhoy, K. N., Langer, B., Tsallas, R. C., Chu, R. C., Kuksis, A., and Anderson, G. H. Total parenteral nutrition at home: Studies in patients. Gastroenterology *71*:943, 1976.

118. Matuchansky, C., Morichau-Beauchant, M., Druart, F., and Tapin, J. Cyclic (nocturnal) total parenteral nutrition in hospitalized adult patients with severe digestive diseases. Report of a prospective study. Gastroenterology *81*:433, 1981.

119. O'Morain, C., Segal, A. W., and Levi, A. J. Elemental diet as primary treatment of acute Crohn's disease. A controlled trial. Br. Med. J. *288*:1859, 1984.

120. Levenstein, S., Prantera, C., Luzi, C., and D'Ubaldi, A. Low residue or normal diet in Crohn's disease: A prospective controlled study in Italian patients. Gut *26*:989–993, 1985.

121. Lashner, B. A., Kirsner, J. B., and Hanauer, S. B. Acute pancreatitis associated with high concentrations of lipid emulsion during total parenteral nutritional therapy for Crohn's disease. Gastroenterology *90*:1039, 1986.

122. Shapiro, S. C., Rothstein, F. C., Newman, A. J., Fletcher, B., and Halpin, T. C., Jr. Multifocal osteonecrosis in adolescents with Crohn's disease: A complication of therapy? J. Pediatr. Gastroenterol. Nutr. *4*:502, 1985.

123. Glotzer, D. J. Operation in inflammatory bowel disease: Indications and type. Clin. Gastroenterol. *9*:371, 1980.

124. Harper, P. H., Lee, E. C., Kettlewell, M. G., Bennett, M. K., and Jewell, D. P. Role of the faecal stream in the maintenance of Crohn's colitis. Gut *26*:279, 1985.

125. Kendall, G. P. N., Hawley, R. P., Nichols, J. R., and Lennard-Jones, J. E. Strictureplasty. A good operation for small bowel Crohn's disease. Dis. Colon Rectum *29*:312, 1986.

126. Murray, J. J., Schoctz, D. J., Jr., Nugent, F. W., Collier, J. A., and Veidenheimer, M. C. Surgical management of Crohn's disease involving the duodenum. Am. J. Surg. *147*:58, 1984.

127. Nugent, W., Fromm, D., and Silen, W. Pseudo-Crohn's disease. Am. J. Surg. *137*:566, 1979.

128. Weaver, R. M., and Keighley, M. R. B. Measurement of rectal capacity in assessment of patients for colectomy and ileorectal anastomosis in Crohn's colitis. Dis. Colon Rectum *29*:443, 1986.

129. Korelitz, B. I., Cheskin, L. J., Sohn, N., and Sommers, S. C. Proctitis after fecal diversion in Crohn's disease and its elimination with reanastomosis: Implications for surgical management. Gastroenterology *87*:710, 1984.

130. Meyers, S., and Janowitz, H. D. Natural history of Crohn's disease. An analytic review of the placebo lesson. Gastroenterology *87*:1189, 1984.

131. Meyers, S., Walfish, J. S., Sachar, D. B., Greenstein, A. J., Hill, A. G., and Janowitz, H. D. Quality of life after surgery for Crohn's disease: A psychosocial survey. Gastroenterology *78*:1, 1980.

Benign Neoplasms and Vascular Malformations of the Large and Small Intestine

72

DENNIS R. SINAR
THOMAS F. O'BRIEN, JR.

GENERAL CONSIDERATIONS

Considering its length, total cellular mass, and diversity of structural elements, the small intestine is relatively resistant to the development of neoplasms. Multiple factors are thought to reduce the incidence of small intestinal neoplasia. These factors include a short contact time between potential carcinogens and the mucosa due to rapid transit of intestinal contents through the small intestine, a well-developed immune system mediated principally by IgA secretion, few bacterial flora for breakdown of substrates to potential carcinogens, the presence of mucosal enzymes such as benzopyrene hydroxylase for detoxification of luminal contents, a liquefied chyme that reduces mechanical trauma, and an alkaline pH. In addition, it is felt that the small intestinal stem cell, the undifferentiated cell type likely to be susceptible to neoplastic changes, is well protected deep within the crypts. Rapid differentiation of stem cells to mature nonproliferative columnar and goblet cells may protect against potential cellular regulation defects which may lead to neoplasia. In humans, the loss and replacement of 1 gm of small intestinal mucosal cells every 16 minutes may account for the low incidence of carcinoma of the small intestine.[1]

Nevertheless, benign and malignant growths develop in all histologic components and either heterotopic or hamartomatous tissue may give rise to tumors in the small intestine.

Neoplasms of the small intestine account for 1 to 5 per cent of all gastrointestinal tumors. The higher figure is usually obtained from reports that include autopsy material because many small intestinal neoplasms are asymptomatic and remain undiscovered during life. Intermittent symptoms, with asymptomatic intervals lasting for weeks, are frequently described by patients with tumors in the distal small intestine. Delay in the diagnosis of small intestinal tumors is due to the relative rarity of the lesions, the vague nature of early symptoms in the absence of gross hemorrhage, the paucity of physical findings, and the relative inaccessibility of many of the lesions to routine diagnostic techniques.

BENIGN TUMORS OF THE SMALL INTESTINE

Adenomas, leiomyomas, and *lipomas* are the three most frequently discovered primary benign tumors of the small intestine. *Hamartomas, fibromas, angiomas,* and *neurogenic tumors* are much less common. As a general rule, benign tumors are least common in the duodenum and increase in frequency toward the ileum. Benign tumors often remain asymptomatic and are usually found incidentally during surgery or at postmortem examination. When tumors are symptomatic, the clinical picture is determined by the gross structural characteristics of the neoplasm and by the distance from the pylorus, and less significantly by the histologic type. Benign tumors arising in the relatively fixed duodenum often produce nausea, vomiting, and early postprandial distress, while polypoid tumors arising beyond the ligament of Treitz are more likely to produce *intussusception* and intermittent *intestinal obstruction.* Among primary small bowel tumors, the benign lesions are scattered throughout the small intestine with somewhat more of a proximal distribution. This finding is in contrast with malignant tumors of the small intestine which are distributed according to histologic type, with *adenocarcinomas* more proximal, *sarcomas* in the jejunum or ileum, and *carcinoid* lesions at all levels with an increased incidence in the ileum (see pp. 1519–1570).[2]

Although primary benign tumors are seen in all age groups, the peak incidence is in the seventh decade. There are also differences in clinical symptoms between benign and malignant lesions. Benign lesions present with occult gastrointestinal bleeding in 38 per cent of patients, and with pain, nausea, and vomiting in 23 per cent of patients. This symptom complex is similar to that seen with malignant small intestinal lesions except that pain is more common in malignant lesions and occurs in 42 per cent of patients. The median duration of symptoms before diagnosis in benign lesions is six months, a figure comparable among clinical reviews.[3]

Etiology

The etiology of isolated benign small intestinal tumors is unknown. No particular dietary, chemical, or toxic process has been clearly identified as pathogenic. Hereditary factors cannot be implicated in most patients, but adenomas of the small intestine may occasionally be present in patients with genetic varieties of colon polyposis syndromes such as Gardner's syndrome or familial polyposis (see pp. 1501–1507). With the exception of *villous adenomas,* there seems to be no propensity for malignant degeneration of benign small intestinal tumors. However, about 70 per cent of patients with benign small intestinal tumors have associated benign and malignant tumors in extraintestinal sites, and almost one quarter of these patients have a nonintestinal malignant neoplasm.[4] The frequent association of small intestinal tumors with separate primary neoplastic lesions further implies a malfunction of an immune mechanism for tumor surveillance (see above).

Pathology

Adenoma. Three types of adenoma are found in the small intestine: *Brunner's gland adenomas, islet cell adenomas,* and *papillary-polypoid adenomas.* Brunner's gland adenomas are distinguished from the more common nodular hyperplasia of the duodenum because they are true polypoid tumors which may be pedunculated. It is important to recognize that Brunner's gland adenomas may not be diagnosed by routine endoscopic biopsies because of the submucosal location and histologic similarity to normal Brunner's glands.[5] An increased incidence of circumscribed nodular hyperplasia of Brunner's glands in the duodenum has been described in uremic patients.[6] Islet cell adenomas may represent either a heterotypic development or a pancreatic metastasis (see pp. 1884–1890).

Adenomas account for about 25 per cent of all benign small intestinal tumors. They are usually asymptomatic and are generally discovered incidentally during surgery or at autopsy. Symptomatic patients, usually 30 to 60 years of age, may have bleeding or intermittent obstruction due to intussusception. Proximity of the adenoma to the ampulla of Vater may produce recurrent pancreatitis.

Small intestinal adenomas are most common in the ileum. Their gross and microscopic appearance is similar to adenomas occurring in the large intestine, with *tubular, villous,* and *mixed* (*tubulovillous*) patterns (see pp. 1483–1495 and 1547–1549). Small intestinal villous adenomas are rare. Most villous adenomas arise in the duodenum, and 27 per cent will demonstrate invasive changes, particularly those that are larger than 4 cm.[7]

Leiomyoma. Clinically, leiomyomas are the most important primary tumors of the small intestine. Although they are less common than adenomas, they are the most common symptomatic nonmalignant tumors Leiomyomas are found at all levels of the small intestine, but are most common in the jejunum. Grossly, they may appear as submucosal or subserosal growths with either a major intraluminal or extraluminal component. Dumbbell-shaped lesions with both components are also encountered. At surgery, leiomyomas are grossly similar to leiomyosarcomas, and are best distinguished by histologic appearance.[8] Central necrosis and ulceration of the overlying mucosal surface produces bleeding in the majority of symptomatic patients (Fig. 72–1). Gross luminal *obstruction* and *intussusception* are uncommon, but lesions with large exophytic components may cause a *volvulus.* Leiomyomas occur with equal frequency in both sexes, and most are discovered in later life, either incidentally at surgery, or in the workup of occult bleeding. The radiographic finding of a smooth, ovoid intralumenal filling defect with an intact overlying mucosa is highly suggestive of a leiomyoma. Because of the macroscopic similarity to leiomyosarcoma, each lesion should be surgically resected.

Lipoma. Lipomas account for 8 to 20 per cent of benign small intestinal tumors; third in frequency.[9] They are present in all segments of the small or large intestine, although 65 to 75 per cent are colonic. Small intestinal lipomas are most often single lesions located in the distal ileum or ileocecal valve (Fig. 72–2), but in 10 to 15 per cent of patients the tumors are multiple. On the average, they are 4 cm in diameter and remain submucosal or intramural. Less than one third of lipomas discovered at surgery or at autopsy are symptomatic. Symptoms may be due to *intussusception, obstruction* by large lesions, or *bleeding* from superficial ulceration of the overlying mucosa. The striking radiolucency on X-ray and the endoscopic and radiographic deformability are helpful diagnostic clues. Asymptomatic lipomas discovered incidentally need not be removed because there is no malignant potential.

Hamartomas. Polypoid hamartomas of the small intestine are usually associated with the Peutz-Jeghers syndrome and are discussed on pages 1507 to 1509.

Neurogenic Tumors. Rarely, primary benign tumors may arise from neural elements, including nerve sheath cells (*neurilemomas*), sympathetic ganglia (*ganglioneuromas*), and neural connective tissue (*neurofibromas*). Ganglioneuromas and neurofibromas are present in 25 per cent of patients with *von Recklinghausen's disease* and can be numerous in these patients.[10] The lesions can produce abdominal pain, melena, and intussusception by the same mechanisms as other benign small intestinal tumors. The clinical considerations in the workup of a suspected isolated small intestinal tumor must be expanded to include multiple potential duodenal and small intestinal tumors in these patients. Multiple bleeding tumors should be considered when interpreting nuclear bleeding scans, which may seem conflicting with multiple positive sites. Neurogenic tumors may also be an integral feature of multiple endocrine adenomatosis (see pp. 491–494).

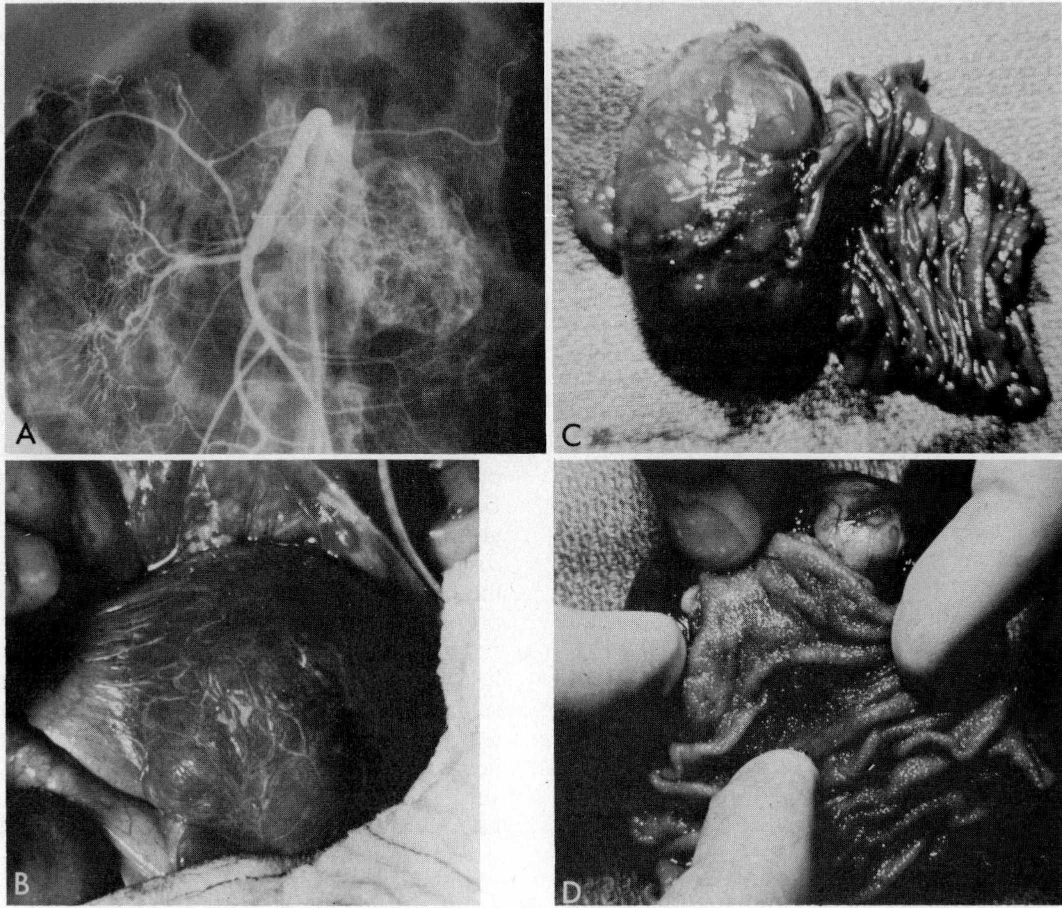

Figure 72–1. Asymptomatic leiomyoma of the small intestine that bled massively on three occasions in one year. *A*, Mesenteric arteriogram, demonstrating a large vascular mass on the left. *B*, Specimen at operation. *C*, Gross specimen, showing large extraluminal component. *D*, Ulceration of small intraluminal component.

Clinical Picture

The incidence of benign small intestinal tumors is the same in men and women. They are discovered most commonly in persons between 50 and 80 years of age and the symptoms are generally mild and intermittent. The patient may have transient *colicky abdominal pain,* or may have more severe pain that progresses to *intestinal obstruction.* Constitutional symptoms such as anorexia, malaise, fever, and weight loss are uncom-

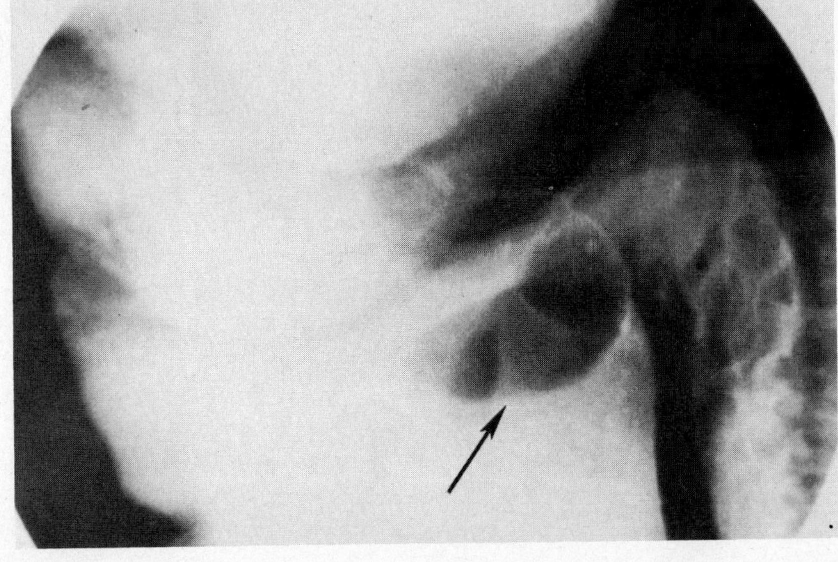

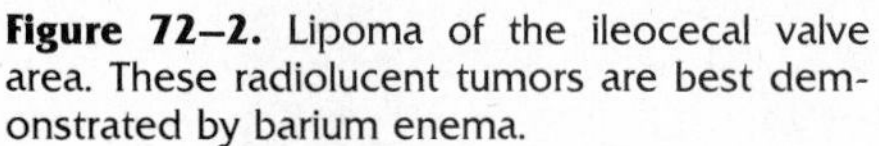
Figure 72–2. Lipoma of the ileocecal valve area. These radiolucent tumors are best demonstrated by barium enema.

mon. *Occult bleeding* can occur over many years, or *acute bleeding* can occur with life-threatening hemorrhage. Bleeding may occur as the slowly expanding tumor compresses and erodes the overlying mucosa. A benign tumor is rarely palpable on physical examination.

Diagnosis

Various roentgenologic techniques are used in the diagnosis of benign small intestinal tumors, and the diagnostic study of choice depends on the suspected level of the lesion and the probable histologic type. Unfortunately, routine barium small intestinal radiographs often fail to demonstrate benign tumors of the small intestine, but will occasionally demonstrate a localized intussusception (Fig. 72–3). For tumors close to the ligament of Treitz, hypotonic duodenography can differentiate between infiltrative and inflammatory lesions of the duodenum.

Selective barium studies of the small intestine either by prograde enteroclysis or by retrograde barium infusion through an incompetent ileocecal valve may identify small intestinal tumors missed by a standard small intestinal barium examination. In enteroclysis the small intestine is rapidly filled with barium under pressure to produce distention. The advantage of the technique is identification of focal lesions such as benign tumors, metastatic lesions, and short segment involvement with Crohn's disease. Enteroclysis is not considered to be a screening examination because of the increased procedure time compared with the standard small bowel series.[11] In 45 patients with surgically proved lesions of the small bowel, enteroclysis detected 48 lesions missed by standard small bowel radiographs. The majority of the lesions were in the ileum.[12]

Gastrointestinal contrast agents such as ferric ammonium citrate may be useful in delineating the intestinal wall thickness in magnetic resonance scanning.[13] This may improve diagnostic discrimination in the gastrointestinal tract between malignant infiltrative lesions and more benign localized or encapsulated lesions. Visceral angiography with selective catheterization of the celiac and mesenteric arteries is often useful in identifying benign vascular tumors and other lesions such as angiodysplasia (see below). Angiography may also establish the general location of one or more bleeding lesions within the small intestine (see pp. 1903–1932). Positive angiograms may show bleeding from a polypoid lesion with overlying ulcerated mucosa or an abnormal blood supply in nonbleeding lesions. Benign tumors are invariably fed by a branch of the gastroduodenal or superior mesenteric artery. When a so-called parasitic blood supply from the renal or lumbar arteries is present, a malignant lesion is most probable.

The development of more sophisticated fiberoptic instruments designed for use in the long and tortuous small intestine may offer improved diagnostic capability for intraluminal lesions. The instruments under development present new problems for the endoscopist such as a longer examination time, decreased patient tolerance, and movement of the enteroscope with each peristaltic contraction, making therapeutic endoscopy more challenging.[14] Prior to a lengthy enteroscopic evaluation, the location of a focal lesion should be determined by enteroclysis or angiography.

Surgical laparotomy remains an important diagnostic as well as therapeutic maneuver for symptomatic patients.

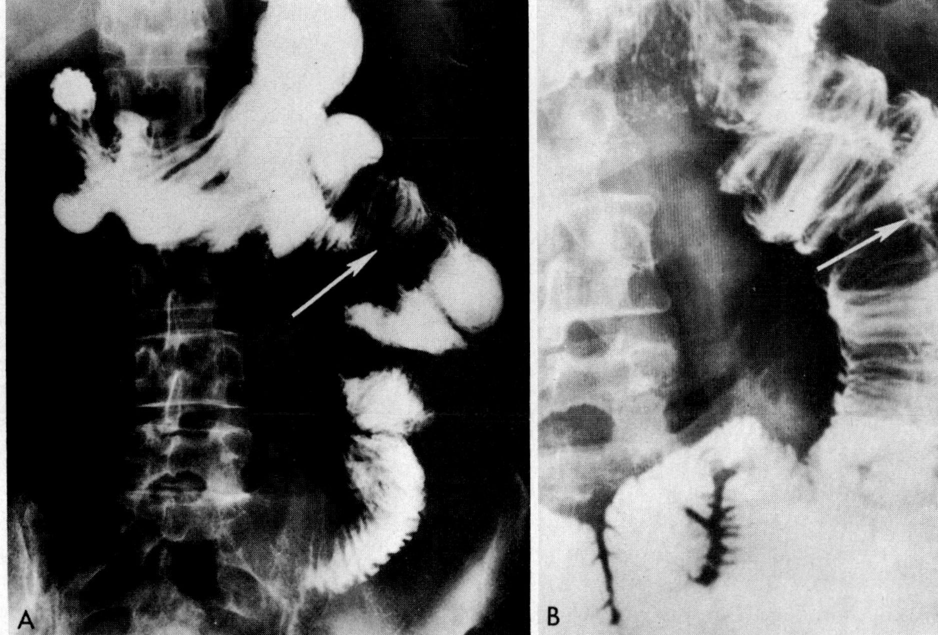

Figure 72–3. *A*, Intussusception in the proximal jejunum produced by a benign adenoma. *B*, Intussusception, close-up view. Note the typical coiled-spring appearance produced by the intussusceptum *(arrow)* within the intussuscipiens.

Treatment

Surgical excision is the treatment of choice for virtually all symptomatic primary, benign small intestinal tumors. Endoscopic polypectomy in the duodenum is a more difficult procedure than the more routine colonoscopic polypectomy.[15] Special methods are under development for polypectomy in the more mobile small intestine.[14]

PSEUDOTUMOR

Pseudotumors are lesions which simulate common benign and malignant neoplasms. Intestinal pseudotumors, like benign neoplasms, are often found incidentally at surgery, but may also produce clinical symptoms by obstruction or intussusception. Surgical excision and histologic examination are usually required for definitive diagnosis.

Inflammatory Pseudotumors (Fibroid Polyps). Approximately two thirds of patients with inflammatory pseudotumors are symptomatic. These lesions are usually composed of multiple cell types including fibroblasts, blood vessel elements, and various leukocytes (lymphocytes, eosinophils, plasma cells, and polymorphonuclear leukocytes). A single cell type, usually the fibroblast, may predominate. An association has not been made between inflammatory pseudotumor and noxious stimulant exposure, or with any systemic disease.[16] Ileal pseudopolyps in patients with Crohn's disease may produce occult GI blood loss and anemia.[17]

Helminthic Pseudotumors. Invasion of the gut wall by *nematodes* of the Strongyloidea group may result in the formation of a mass lesion that is clinically indistinguishable from a primary tumor of the small intestine. The process has been described principally in native Africans (Uganda), but has also affected nonnatives who have spent time in the tropics. The region of the ileocecal junction is most often involved, and the disease may resemble carcinoma, tuberculosis, or Crohn's disease. Although theoretically treatable by appropriate anthelmintic drugs, the lesions are often identified and resected during diagnostic laparotomy, especially in nonendemic areas.

Endometrioma. *Intestinal endometriosis* is predominantly a subserosal process. Transmural involvement of the small intestine by endometriosis occurs less frequently and less severely than subserosal involvement. Symptomatic GI tract involvement is rare, but patients may present with polypoid lesions in the ileum that simulate primary tumors, or with small intestinal obstruction due to transmural scarring and adhesion formation.[18] Characteristically, the patients are premenopausal women approaching 40 years of age. If pelvic endometriosis is present on physical examination, intestinal endometriosis should be considered in the evaluation of middle-aged women if symptoms occur or become more severe with the onset of menses (see pp. 1592–1595).

Amyloidosis. Amyloidosis involving the small intestine has produced a radiographic appearance that mimics polypoid tumors (see pp. 509–510).

VASCULAR MALFORMATIONS OF THE SMALL AND LARGE INTESTINE

Angiodysplasia (Colonic Ectasia)

General Characteristics. The term *angiodysplasia* has become synonymous with localized *arteriovenous malformations* (AVM) that occur predominantly in the cecum and ascending colon. Angiodysplasia is not associated with vascular lesions of the skin, central nervous system, or lungs and is not a familial disorder. With the refinement of specialized angiographic techniques, vascular ectasias of the small intestine, cecum, and colon have been identified in an increasing number of elderly patients.[19, 20] Angiodysplasia can be subdivided into two broad types: those lesions that occur throughout the GI tract in patients younger than 50 years of age, and those lesions exclusively in the cecum and right colon in patients older than 50 years of age. The pathologic features of colonic ectasias in patients over 50 years old have been studied by Boley and associates, who distinguish angiodysplasia from congenital or neoplastic vascular GI tract abnormalities. Their theory is that angiodysplasia is a degenerative lesion of submucosal veins that occurs in a significant portion of the population over 50 years of age. Ectasia of normal vascular structures may be produced by chronic low-grade venous obstruction at the site of penetration of circular and longitudinal muscle.[21] Histologically, the earliest lesion consists of dilated submucosal veins, while late lesions consist of dilated and distorted veins, venules, or capillaries with a thinly lined epithelium and little or no vascular smooth muscle. Other authors feel that apart from size and tortuosity, the vessels in angiodysplasia resemble normal veins, venules, and capillaries. Colonic telangiectasias of any type, including those of *hereditary hemorrhagic telangiectasia* (see below), are not distinguishable from angiodysplasia on histologic grounds.[19]

An unusual but distinctive endoscopic finding in vascular ectasia of the gastric antrum deserves mention. The "watermelon stomach" is described as a radiating pattern of tortuous vessels on longitudinal folds, with the vessels radiating from the pylorus toward the antrum; a picture similar to the stripes on a watermelon. Microscopically the lesion is characterized by hyperplastic antral glands, dilated mucosal capillaries, and dilated submucosal venous channels. The few reported cases have been mainly in elderly patients with iron deficiency anemia due to GI tract blood loss and achlorhydria. The majority of patients have been successfully treated by antrectomy.[22–24]

Clinical Picture. The prevalence of *angiodysplasia* is difficult to determine, but has been estimated at between 1.4 and 2 per cent of patients older than 50 years of age. In angiodysplasia, clinically significant gastrointestinal hemorrhage usually affects patients between 45 and 85 years of age (mean age, 60 years). The bleeding site is most commonly the right colon, although small intestinal angiodysplasia is not uncommon.[20] The percentage of black patients is very low, about 1.8 per cent, but there is no gender predilection for the angiodysplastic process.[25] Many patients present with a history of multiple acute or chronic bleeding episodes, negative barium studies, and unrewarding diagnostic laparotomies. Some patients present with continued bleeding after "blind" resections of stomach or right or left colon. In some individuals the presence of concomitant gastrointestinal disease as a potential source of bleeding obscures the diagnosis.

Up to 15 to 25 per cent of patients with angiodysplasia have significant aortic stenosis.[25] Patients with aortic stenosis and bleeding angiodysplastic lesions are older (mean age, 72 years) and often have recurrent bleeding with long delays in the diagnosis. A literature review notes that 21 of 22 patients had a specific association between bleeding from colonic angiodysplasia and critical aortic stenosis.[26] In a small subset of these patients, bleeding from angiodysplastic lesions has not recurred after aortic valve replacement.[26] On the other hand, about 1 per cent of patients admitted with aortic stenosis had concomitant gastrointestinal hemorrhage.[27] Hemodynamic studies done in two of these patients to explore possible causes for the association between colonic angiodysplasia and aortic stenosis showed that an abnormal peripheral pulse pattern in patients with aortic stenosis was transmitted to the ileocolic artery, a finding not seen in control patients. This suggests an association between colonic vascular ectasia and the abnormal arterial pulse wave in patients with aortic stenosis.

Patients with *chronic renal failure* on *dialysis* may have a higher incidence of bleeding from angiodysplastic lesions located primarily in the stomach and duodenum.[28–30] This has been proposed as an explanation for the significant GI blood loss (6.3 ml per day) previously described in patients with chronic renal failure on dialysis using chromium-labeled red blood cell studies.[31] The increased incidence of Brunner's gland hyperplasia in uremic patients is an additional cause for upper GI tract bleeding in patients with chronic renal failure[5] (see pp. 512–514).

In addition, patients with genetic and acquired *von Willebrand's* disease have vascular ectasias throughout the upper and lower GI tract which may produce clinically significant bleeding.[32] The characteristic pattern is continued bleeding for many years before a diagnosis is established. Patients generally continue to bleed from the gastrointestinal tract in spite of treatment with cryoprecipitate. An association between angiodysplasia and von Willebrand's disease may involve a common endothelial cell disorder or a defect of connective tissue.[33]

Diagnosis. The diagnosis of angiodysplasia should be considered in all cases of obscure gastrointestinal hemorrhage without a positive family history of similar bleeding episodes. Selective mesenteric angiography with enhancement magnification has been the most sensitive test in establishing the diagnosis. Positive findings include an early filling vein which is generally visualized four to five seconds after injection (Fig. 72–4), a localized blush, capillary stain, or vascular tuft usually located at the termination of a branch of the ileocolic artery, and a slowly draining vein which remains visualized after other mesenteric veins have emptied.[21] Intraluminal extravasation of contrast is not seen in the absence of significant bleeding. Lesions are usually located within the lateral (antimesenteric) wall.

The diagnosis often can be made by flexible sigmoidoscopy, or by colonoscopy (see pp. 1575–1576). The lesions are often multiple and appear as 4 to 8 mm flat or slightly raised red submucosal collections of blood. The edges are scalloped, and a prominent draining vein may be visible. Comparison studies estimated the sensitivity of colonoscopy in relation to angiography as 81 per cent when adjusted for the segments of colon examined. The positive predictive value of colonoscopy was 90 per cent compared to subsequent confirmable tests.[34, 35] Colonoscopy offers the diagnostic advantage of detecting other lesions (*polyps* and *diverticula*) which may bleed in the same population and the therapeutic advantage of coagulation and destruction of the lesion.

Other authors have improved the diagnostic yield in actively bleeding patients by nuclear scanning after injection of tracer-tagged red blood cells to localize the source of bleeding to the upper GI tract, small intestine, or colon.[36, 37] In a group of patients with continued bleeding and consistently negative studies, elective small bowel endoscopy or intraoperative panendoscopy of the small intestine and colon may be helpful diagnostic and therapeutic maneuvers. The lesions may not be visible from the serosal surface, and intraoperative enteroscopy allows transillumination of the intestinal wall to more easily locate vascular lesions.

Treatment. In those instances when angiodysplastic lesions are clustered in the right colon, treatment has included endoscopic application of a heater probe, a BICAP unit, or laser energy to coagulate the lesion.[38] The intent is to heat the lesion to the submucosal level to coagulate the small central submucosal artery, but to avoid a full-thickness burn in the thin-walled cecum. Clinical trials with the argon and Nd:YAG laser generally include all varieties of angiodysplasia and telangiectasia in the upper and lower GI tract. Results show significant lowering of blood transfusion requirements, and fewer rebleeding episodes in patients with colonic lesions.[39] In another report, angiodysplasia of the colon was successfully treated in 82 per cent of the 49 patients followed up to 18 months after laser treatment.[40] All patients with vascular ectasias associated with *von Willebrand's disease* rebled after laser therapy in one study.[40] Whether the benefit to the patient of endoscopic treatment of angiodysplasia outweighs the effort, expense, and risk has not been determined. In a small number of patients with renal failure and bleeding from GI tract angiodysplasia, Bronner and associates have been able to decrease monthly transfusion

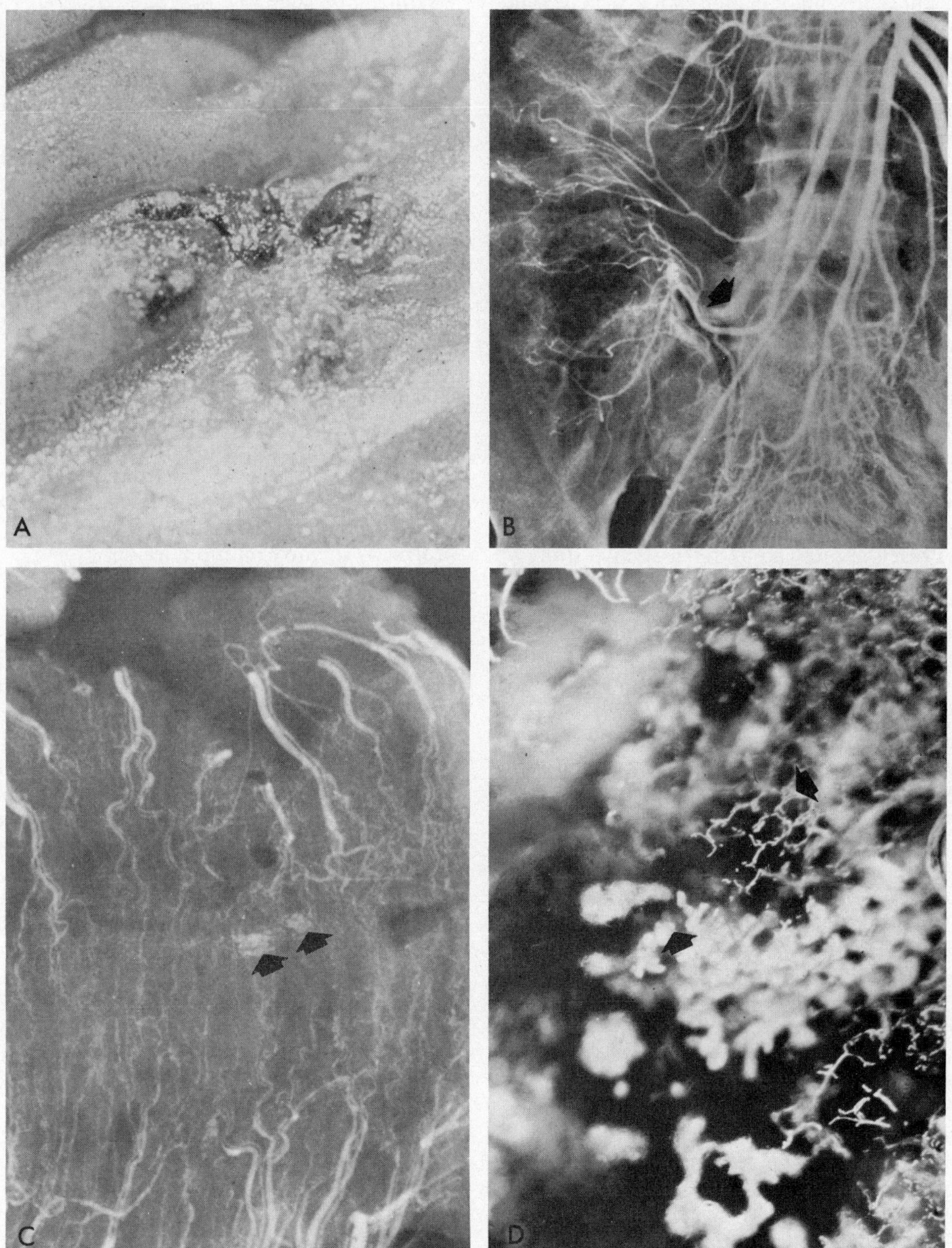

Figure 72–4. Angiodysplasia. *A,* Close-up mucosal surface resected specimen. *B,* Note early draining vein *(arrow)* during arterial phase of mesenteric arteriogram. *C,* Radiographic contrast study of resected specimen. Note that ectatic vessels are located on the antimesenteric surface. *D,* Silicone injection specimen. Note difference between delicate and normal vasculature *(upper arrow)* and dilated structures in area of dysplasia *(lower arrow).*

requirements with oral estrogen therapy.[41] In other patients, generous resection of right colon has been the preferred treatment.

In long-term follow-up of patients with cecal or right colonic angiodysplasia who were treated by right hemicolectomy, 63 per cent remained free of bleeding with follow-up of six months to seven years. The remaining 37 per cent of patients have had recurrent intestinal bleeding.[25]

Telangiectasia

General Characteristics. Telangiectasias of the small and large intestine may be either hereditary or acquired. Most clinical interest has been in *hereditary hemorrhagic telangiectasia* (*Osler-Weber-Rendu disease,* or HHT) because of the limited treatment options in these patients. The classic features include repeated epistaxis in childhood, chronic gastrointestinal bleeding, and a family history of the disorder. Telangiectasias may be characteristically seen on the palms and soles of the feet, on the skin and the buccal mucosa, and in the nail beds.

Clinical Presentation. Careful retrospective study of the clinical manifestations of hereditary hemorrhagic telangiectasia (HHT) in many symptomatic patients shows that there is no correlation between the location of skin lesions and the incidence of GI bleeding. In 20 per cent of patients with HHT, *pulmonary arteriovenous fistulas* were demonstrable by standard chest X-rays with no symptoms or signs of pulmonary disease. Patients with HHT can develop *passive congestion* of the *liver* (30 per cent), *hepatic telangiectasia* (30 per cent),[42, 43] and *iron overload* (50 per cent). Clinically significant lesions were also found in the cardiovascular system and in the central nervous system. Epistaxis was the most common clinical presentation, with onset during the first decade. In contrast, GI bleeding was present at some time in 44 per cent of patients, with the age of onset in the fifth decade or later. This late onset of GI bleeding may be enhanced by other degenerative vascular ectasias that are often present in patients greater than 50 years old (see above).

The reported incidence of bleeding ranges from 13 to 44 per cent.[41, 44] The discrepancy in bleeding rates may be explained by the inclusion in the series with the lower incidence of asymptomatic family members and a higher percentage of young persons.[44] Both studies support the increased incidence of duodenal ulcer in HHT; 6 to 9 per cent of all HHT patients had a duodenal ulcer, and 14 to 19 per cent of bleeding HHT patients had a duodenal ulcer.[41, 44]

Intestinal telangiectasia has been associated with *Turner's syndrome* and with disorders of collagen synthesis.[45] Patients with scleroderma and the CREST syndrome (*c*alcinosis, *R*aynaud's phenomenon, *e*sophageal dysmotility, *s*clerodactyly, and *t*elangiectasia) may have gastric telangiectasia as one of several potential sources of GI blood loss[46] (see pp. 505–506). These lesions are indistinguishable from the telangiectasia of HHT described above. Problems with a differential diagnosis between CREST and other telangiectasia syndromes can generally be resolved with serologic testing.[47]

Diagnosis. Childhood epistaxis and a family history of bleeding should increase the clinical suspicion for *hereditary hemorrhagic telangiectasia.* Acquired telangiectasia should be considered in patients with the appropriate disease entity.

The diagnosis of telangiectasia is often made by endoscopy. Barium studies are usually negative owing to the small size and mucosal location of the lesions. Angiography is occasionally useful in identifying visceral telangiectasias in patients with negative endoscopic studies.[42] Some authors have localized and stained small lesions prior to surgery by injection of methylene blue during angiography.[48] Nuclear scanning after injection of tagged red blood cells may help localize a slowly bleeding lesion. Small intestinal endoscopy or intraoperative endoscopy can be used to make the diagnosis and to coagulate the lesions (see above). In assessing the accuracy of various tests to diagnose obscure small intestinal hemorrhage, multiple tests, including laparotomy, were often needed to correctly identify multiple lesions.[49]

Treatment. Treatment of telangiectasias of the GI tract is frustrating. In endoscopic studies of the effect of coagulation, patients with lesions of the upper GI tract frequently rebleed after therapy with laser (argon or Nd:YAG). Gastric lesions tend to be larger, and often rebleed for several weeks after laser treatment.[39] Patients with HHT are often excluded from endoscopic treatment because of the number of lesions (> 100). Patients with HHT who are eventually treated have significant rebleeding after laser therapy, and some of the patients require surgical removal of the bleeding site for control of bleeding.

Patients with telangiectasias of the upper GI tract have been successfully treated with endoscopic injection of denatured ethanol as a sclerosing solution with disappearance of the telangiectasias on follow-up endoscopic examination.[50] Epistaxis from hereditary hemorrhagic telangiectasia has been successfully treated with the Nd:YAG laser and with oral estrogens,[51] and a limited number of cases of gastrointestinal bleeding have been treated with oral estrogens.[52] Similarly, patients with the upper gastrointestinal tract lesions of HHT have been treated with H_2 blockers to minimize transfusion requirements.[53]

Surgical resection may provide a temporary decrease in transfusion requirements, but the large number of lesions and the distribution of lesions throughout the GI tract makes extensive resection less appealing.

Hemangiomas

General Characteristics. Hemangiomas are much less common than the small intestinal and colonic vascular malformations described above. Histologically, the lesions are large, blood-filled sinuses with an endothelial lining and a small amount of connective tissue, and are classified as capillary, cavernous, or mixed lesions. In the GI tract the lesions are usually cavernous rather than capillary, and are usually single rather than multiple. Hemangiomas probably arise from the submucosal vascular plexus.

Kaposi's sarcoma is a multicentric neoplastic vascular proliferation of tumors with endothelium-lined channels, vascular spaces, and intermixed spindle cells (see p. 1244).

Clinical Presentation. Hemangiomas are clinically important because of their propensity for *bleeding,* and the majority of patients with intestinal hemangiomas eventually experience painless gastrointestinal bleeding. Patients can present with either acute life-threatening bleeding or occult bleeding with severe anemia of several years' duration. The distribution of lesions in children is approximately equal between small intestine and colon. The most common type of tumor is a diffuse expansive hemangioma with the rectum as the most common site of origin (40 per cent of cases). Tumors range from 1 cm in size to larger masses that encircle the intestinal wall. It is impressive that 72 per cent of the children over five years of age have bleeding, anemia, and ill health for five to 15 years before a diagnosis is established.[54]

Cutaneous hemangiomas may occur in up to 50 per cent of patients with intestinal hemangiomas. Hemangiomas which have a significant extraluminal component can bleed either into the abdominal cavity or into the retroperitoneal space.

Patients with the *blue rubber bleb nevus syndrome* and *Maffucci's syndrome* have cavernous hemangiomas in the GI tract which can produce massive bleeding.[55] Children and young adults with *Klippel-Trenaunay-Weber syndrome* can have mixed and cavernous hemangiomas of the gastrointestinal tract with GI tract bleeding.[44]

Patients with the *acquired immunodeficiency syndrome* (AIDS) can have gastrointestinal involvement with Kaposi's sarcoma in up to 50 per cent of patients. The duodenum is the most common site of involvement, but lesions may be scattered throughout the gastrointestinal tract. Patients with GI tract involvement may be asymptomatic, or may present with abdominal pain, bowel obstruction, or GI bleeding[56, 57] (see pp. 1233–1257).

Diagnosis. At least 31 per cent of children have abdominal phleboliths on radiographic examinations due to thrombosis and clot organization within the hemangioma.[54] Barium examinations, including enteroclysis, may detect a polypoid or diffuse hemangioma in the intestinal wall. Barium studies may also aid in the diagnosis in the presence of an intramural or retroperitoneal bleed. Up to 29 per cent of lesions may be detected by rigid sigmoidoscopy in children, a yield that would likely improve with current endoscopic techniques.

Radiographic abnormalities seen in early gastrointestinal involvement with *Kaposi's sarcoma* are nodularity and thickened folds. The endoscopic appearance of the lesions at this stage is characteristic, but superficial endoscopic biopsies may not reach the lesion in the submucosa.[56] The lesions may range from maculopapular reddish purple blebs with central ulcerations to smaller "flea-bite" erythematous areas with or without coalescence (Color Fig. 72–5, p. xli). Diagnosis is generally made by large endoscopic biopsy.[57] Later mucosal infiltration produces a radiologic pattern similar to lymphoma.

Selective angiography is often the most helpful diagnostic test in patients with hemangioma. Angiography can establish the diagnosis even in the absence of significant active bleeding due to the abnormal collection of vessels.

Treatment. Treatment is surgical excision of the

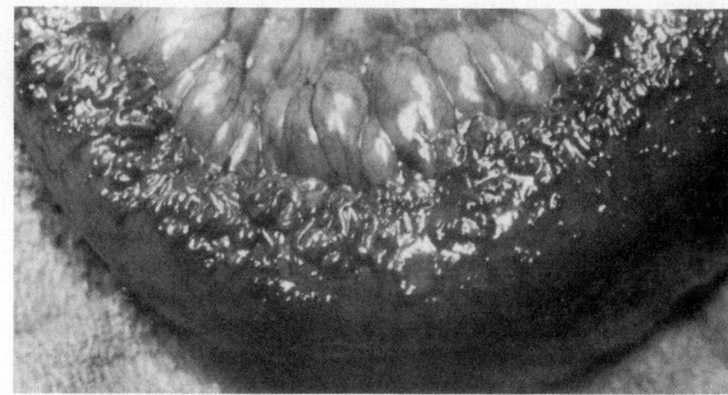

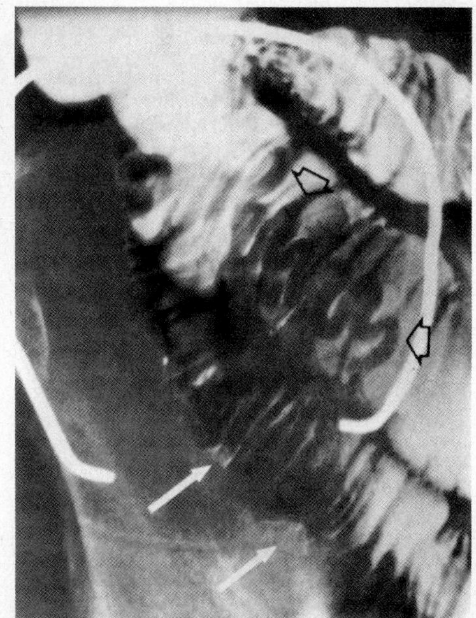

Figure 72–6. *A,* Intraoperative photograph showing extensive varices along the serosal surface of distal ileum. *B,* Spot film of the distal ileum showing small intestinal varices as intraluminal filling defects *(open arrows).* Serosal metastases are seen in an adjacent area of ileum *(white arrows).* (From Radin, D. R. Small bowel varices. Gastrointest. Radiol. *11*:183, 1986. Used with permission.)

lesions by segmental or wedge resection. It is important that an endoscopist recognize the highly vascular nature of this malformation before attempting coagulation and destruction by therapeutic endoscopy. The extent of the vascular network should be confirmed by selective arteriography to determine whether therapeutic endoscopy (heater probe, laser) may be of benefit. None of the reviews describes the treatment of a sufficient number of hemangiomas to address efficacy of one method over another.

Mesenteric Varices

Mesenteric varices are a rare, acquired form of vascular malformation.[58] Patients with this disorder may be subgrouped under an earlier classification scheme as intestinal phlebectasias. The patient with mesenteric varices will typically have signs of hepatic cirrhosis and will present with massive GI tract bleeding without an identifiable source of blood loss after upper endoscopy. The lesions are non-neoplastic venous varicosities with a normal endothelial lining. Varices may develop in large adhesions at the site of previous abdominal surgery. Mesenteric varices may also be the cause of bleeding in the vicinity of an ileostomy or colostomy when there is underlying portal hypertension. Small intestinal varices can present in a patient without portal hypertension but with mesenteric venous occlusion by metastatic tumor (Fig. 72–6).[59] Mesenteric angiography is the diagnostic test of choice.

References

1. Potten, C. S. Clonogenic, stem and carcinogen-target cells in small intestine. Scand. J. Gastroenterol. *104*:3, 1984.
2. Barclay, T. H. C., and Schapira, D. V. Malignant tumors of the small intestine. Cancer *5*:878, 1983.
3. Zollinger, R. M., Sternfeld, W. C., and Schreiber, H. Primary neoplasms of the small intestine. Am. J. Surg. *151*:654, 1986.
4. Alexander, J. W., and Altemeier, W. A. Association of primary neoplasms of the small intestine with other neoplastic growths. Ann. Surg. *167*:958, 1968.
5. Kehl, O., Buhler, H., Stamm, B., and Amman, R. W. Endoscopic removal of a large, obstructing and bleeding duodenal Brunner's gland adenoma. Endoscopy *17*:231, 1985.
6. Paimela, H., Tallgren, L. G., Stenman, S., Numers, H., and Scheinin, T. M. Multiple duodenal polyps in uremia: A little known clinical entity. Gut *25*:259, 1984.
7. Kutin, N. D., Ranson, J. H. C., Gouge, T. H., and Localio, S. A. Villous tumors of the duodenum. Ann. Surg. *181*:164, 1975.
8. O'Rourke, M. G. E., and Lancashire, R. P. The operating room diagnosis of small bowel tumors. Aust. N.Z. J. Surg. *56*:247, 1986.
9. Mayo, C. W., Pagtalunan, R. J. G., and Brown, D. J. Lipoma of the alimentary tract. Surgery *53*:598, 1963.
10. Mirovsky, Y., Schachner, E., Morag, B., and Orda, R. Intestinal neurofibromatosis: Multiple complications in a single case. Isr. J. Med. Sci. *21*:750, 1985.
11. Ott, D. J., Chen, Y. M., Gelfand, D. W., Van Swearingen, F., and Munitz, H. A. Detailed per-oral small bowel examination vs. enteroclysis. Radiology *155*:29, 1985.
12. Maglinte, D. D. T., Hall, R., and Miller, R. E. Detection of surgical lesions by enteroclysis. Am. J. Surg. *147*:225, 1984.
13. Wesbey, G. E., Brasch, R. C., Goldberg, H. I., Engelstad, B. L., and Moss, A. A. Dilute oral iron solutions as gastrointestinal contrast agents for magnetic resonance imaging: Initial clinical experience. Magnetic Resonance Imaging *3*:57, 1985.
14. Tada, M., and Kawai, K. Small bowel endoscopy. Scand. J. Gastroenterol. *102*:39, 1984.
15. Hochter, W., Weingart, J., Seib, H. J., and Ottenjann, R. Duodenalpolypen. Dtsch. Med. Wochenschr. *109*:1183, 1984.
16. LiVolsi, V. A., and Perzin, K. H. Inflammatory pseudopolyps (inflammatory fibrous polyps) of the small intestine: A clinicopathologic study. Am. J. Dig. Dis. *20*:325, 1975.
17. Manning, R. J., and Lewis, C. Inflammatory ileal polyps in Crohn's disease presenting as refractory iron deficiency anemia. Gastrointest. Endosc. *32*:122, 1986.
18. Afdhal, N. H., Doyle, J. S., Gaffney, E., Smith, J., and Heffernan, S. Acute small bowel obstruction secondary to endometriosis: Two case reports and a review of the literature. Irish Med. J. *77*:141, 1984.
19. Pounder, D. J., Rowland, R., Pieterse, A. S., Freeman, R., and Hunter, R. Angiodysplasias of the colon. J. Clin. Pathol. *35*:824, 1982.
20. Duray, P. H., Marcal, J. M., LiVolsi, V. A., Fisher, R., Scholhamer, C., and Brand, M. H. Small intestinal angiodysplasia in the elderly. J. Clin. Gastroenterol. *6*:311, 1984.
21. Boley, S. J., Sammartano, R., Adams, A., DiBiase, A., Kleinhaus, S., and Sprayregen, S. On the nature and etiology of vascular ectasias of the colon: Degenerative lesions of aging. Gastroenterology *72*:650, 1977.
22. Rider, J. A., Klotz, A. P., and Kirsner, J. B. Gastritis with veno-capillary ectasia as a source of massive gastric hemorrhage. Gastroenterology *24*:118, 1953.
23. Jabbari, M., Cherry, R., Lough, J. O., Daly, D. S., Kinnear, D. G., and Goresky, C. A. Gastric antral vascular ectasia: The watermelon stomach. Gastroenterology *87*:1165, 1984.
24. Rawlinson, W. D., Barr, G. D., and Lin, B. P. Antral vascular ectasia—the "watermelon" stomach. Med. J. Aust. *144*:709, 1986.
25. Meyer, C. T., Troncale, F. J., Galloway, S., and Sheahan, D. G. Arteriovenous malformations of the bowel: An analysis of 22 cases and a review of the literature. Medicine *60*:36, 1981.
26. Cappell, M. S., and Lebwohl, O. Cessation of recurrent bleeding from gastrointestinal angiodysplasias after aortic valve replacement. Ann. Intern. Med. *105*:54, 1986.
27. Greenstein, R. J., McElhinney, A. J., Reuben, D., and Greenstein, A. J. Colonic vascular ectasias and aortic stenosis: Coincidence or causal relationship? Am. J. Surg. *151*:347, 1986.
28. Dave, P. B., Romeu, J., Antonelli, A., and Eiser, A. R. Gastrointestinal telangiectasias: A source of bleeding in patients receiving hemodialysis. Arch. Intern. Med. *144*:1781, 1984.
29. Zuckerman, G. R., Cornette, G. L., Clouse, R. E., and Harter, H. R. Upper gastrointestinal bleeding in patients with chronic renal failure. Ann. Intern. Med. *102*:588, 1985.
30. Blackstone, M. O. Angiodysplasia and gastrointestinal bleeding in chronic renal failure. Ann. Intern. Med. *103*:805, 1985.
31. Rosenblatt, S. G., Drake, S., and Fadem, S. Gastrointestinal blood loss in patients with chronic renal failure. Am. J. Kidney Dis. *1*:232, 1982.
32. Duray, P. H., Marcal, J. M., LiVolsi, V. A., Fisher, R., Scholhamer, C., and Brand, M. H. Gastrointestinal angiodysplasia: A possible component of von Willebrand's disease. Hum. Pathol. *15*:539, 1984.
33. Hanna, W., McCarroll, D., Lin, D., Chua, W., McDonald, T. P., Chen, J., Congdon, C., and Lange, R. D. A study of a Caucasian family with variant von Willebrand's disease in association with vascular telangiectasia and hemoglobinopathy. Thromb. Hemost. *30*:275, 1984.
34. Richter, J. M., Hedberg, S. E., Athanasoulis, C. A., and Shapiro, R. H. Angiodysplasia, clinical presentation and colonoscopic diagnosis. Dig. Dis. Sci. *29*:481, 1984.
35. Salem, R. R., Wood, C. B., Rees, H. C., Kheshavarzian, A., Hemingway, A. P., and Allison, D. J. A comparison of colonoscopy and selective visceral angiography in the diagnosis of colonic angiodysplasia. Ann. R. Coll. Surg. Engl. *67*:225, 1985.
36. Vyberg, M., Miskowiak, J., Nielson, S. L., Fahrenkrug, L., and Tomsen, H. S. Cecal angiodysplasia localized by ^{99m}technetium blood-pool scan. Cardiovasc. Intervent. Radiol. *9*:28, 1986.
37. Front, D., Israel, O., Groshar, D., and Weininger, J. Techne-

tium-99m–labeled red blood cell imaging. Semin. Nucl. Med. *14*:226, 1984.
38. Jensen, D., and Bown, S. Gastrointestinal angiomata: Diagnosis and treatment with laser therapy and other endoscopic modalities. *In* Fleisher, D., Jensen, D. and Bright-Asare, P. (eds.): Therapeutic Laser Endoscopy in Gastrointestinal Disease. The Hague, Martinus Nijhoff Publishers, 1983, p. 151.
39. Cello, J. P., and Grendell, J. H. Endoscopic laser treatment for gastrointestinal vascular ectasias. Ann. Intern. Med. *104*:352, 1986.
40. Rutgeerts, P., Van Gompel, F., Geboes, K., Vantrappen, G., Broeckaert, L., and Coremans, G. Long term results of treatment of vascular malformations of the gastrointestinal tract by Neodymium Yag laser photocoagulation. Gut *26*:586, 1985.
41. Bronner, M. H., Pate, M. B., Cunningham, J. T., and Marsh, W. H. Estrogen-progesterone therapy for bleeding gastrointestinal telangiectasias in chronic renal failure. Ann. Intern. Med. *105*:371, 1986.
42. Reilly, P. J., and Nostrant, T. T. Clinical manifestations of hereditary hemorrhagic telangiectasia. Am. J. Gastroenterol. *79*:363, 1984.
43. Solis-Herruzo, J. A., Garcia-Cabezudo, J., Santalla-Pecina, F., Duran-Aguado, A., and Olmedo-Camacho, J. Laparoscopic findings in hereditary hemorrhagic telangiectasia (Osler-Weber-Rendu disease). Endoscopy *16*:137, 1984.
44. Smith, R. C., Bartholomew, L. G., and Cain, J. C. Hereditary hemorrhagic telangiectasia and gastrointestinal hemorrhage. Gastroenterology *44*:1, 1963.
45. Camilleri, M., Chadwick, V. S., and Hodgson, H. J. Vascular anomalies of the gastrointestinal tract. Hepatogastroenterology *31*:149, 1984.
46. Rosenkrans, P. C., deRooy, D. J., Bosman, F. T., Eulderink, F., and Cats, A. Gastrointestinal telangiectasia as a cause of severe blood loss in systemic sclerosis. Endoscopy *12*:200, 1980.
47. Pitlik, S. D., Chitkara, R., Tafreshi, M., and Giron, J. A. Hereditary hemorrhagic telangiectasia versus CREST syndrome: Can serology aid diagnosis? J. Am. Acad. Dermatol. *10*:192, 1984.
48. Athanasoulis, C. A., Moncure, A. C., Greenfield, A. J., Ryan, J. A., and Dobson, T. F. Intraoperative localization of small bowel bleeding sites with combined use of angiographic methods and methylene blue injection. Surgery *87*:77, 1980.
49. Thompson, J. N., Hemingway, A. P., McPherson, G. A. D., Rees, H. C., Allison, D. J., and Spencer, J. Obscure gastrointestinal hemorrhage of small-bowel origin. Br. Med. J. *2*:1663, 1984.
50. Sugawa, C., Fujita, Y., Ikeda, T., and Walt, A. J. Endoscopic hemostasis of bleeding of the upper gastrointestinal tract by local injection of ninety-eight per cent dehydrated ethanol. Surg. Gynecol. Obstet. *162*:159, 1986.
51. Shapshay, S. M., and Oliver, P. Treatment of hereditary hemorrhagic telangiectasia by Nd-YAG laser photocoagulation. Laryngoscope *94*:1554, 1984.
52. McGee, R. R. Estrogen-progesterone therapy for gastrointestinal bleeding in hereditary hemorrhagic telangiectasia. South. Med. J. *72*:1503, 1979.
53. Kueh, Y. K., and LaBrooy, S. Hereditary hemorrhagic telangiectasia: the use of H_2 receptor antagonists in symptomatic gastric telangiectasia. Ann. Acad. Med. Singapore. *14*:682, 1985.
54. Abrahamson, J., and Shandling, B. Intestinal hemangiomata in childhood and a syndrome for diagnosis: A collective review. J. Pediatr. Surg. *8*:487, 1973.
55. Baker, A. L., Kahn, P. C., Binder, S. C., and Patterson, J. F. Gastrointestinal bleeding due to blue rubber bleb nevus syndrome. A case diagnosed by angiography. Gastroenterology *61*:530, 1971.
56. Wall, S. D., Friedman, S. L., and Margulis, A. R. Gastrointestinal Kaposi's sarcoma in AIDS: Radiographic manifestations. J. Clin. Gastroenterol. *6*:165, 1984.
57. Ell, C., Matek, W., Gramatzke, M., Kaduk, B., and Demling, L. Endoscopic findings in a case of Kaposi's sarcoma with involvement of the large and small bowel. Endoscopy *17*:161, 1985.
58. Ricci, R. L., Lee, K. R., and Greenberger, N. J. Chronic gastrointestinal bleeding from ileal varices after total proctocolectomy for ulcerative colitis: Correction by mesocaval shunt. Gastroenterology *78*:1053, 1980.
59. Radin, D. R., Siskind, B. N., Alpert, S., and Bernstein, R. G. Small-bowel varices due to mesenteric metastasis. Gastrointest. Radiol. *11*:183, 1986.

73

Radiation Enteritis and Colitis

DAVID L. EARNEST
JERRY S. TRIER

In 1897, two years after Wilhelm Roentgen discovered X-rays, Walsh reported a person working with the new form of energy who developed crampy abdominal pain and diarrhea during regular X-ray exposure and whose symptoms stopped when the abdomen was shielded by lead.[1] In 1917, the first clinical report appeared of a patient who developed severe intestinal injury following radiation therapy for a malignant disease.[2] In 1930, "factitial proctitis" was described in a group of patients undergoing pelvic radiation.[3] Since then, there have been numerous reports of radiation damage to the small intestine, colon, and rectum that have documented the serious complications this potentially curative treatment for cancer can induce. In the early years of radiation therapy, the amount of radiation that could be delivered to a patient by external beam orthovoltage equipment was limited by hyperemia and the induced burn of the overlying skin. The advent of newer supervoltaged techniques utilizing much higher energy waves made it possible to give larger and more effective doses of X-ray without skin injury, but with more risk of injury to the intestine. The addition of an internally placed radiation source permitted delivery of sufficient total radiation to abdominopelvic tumors either to improve the response rate dramatically or to produce a cure. In view of improved efficacy of radiation therapy there has been a progressive increase in its use as part of the overall treatment plan for a variety of malignant tumors. It is now estimated that almost half of cancer patients will receive some form of X-ray treatment.[4] In recent years, radiation therapy has often been combined with surgery and some form of chemotherapy, both of which may lower the threshold for radiation-induced intestinal injury, as will be discussed subsequently.

INCIDENCE

Many series of patients reported in the 1960s and 1970s with radiation enteritis following X-ray therapy for abdominopelvic malignancy had undergone radiation therapy utilizing techniques employed during the preceding 15 years. Transient early symptoms of altered intestinal function were frequent, but usually dissipated. In one study, all of 11 patients receiving pelvic radiation therapy had an abnormality of rectal mucosa, as indicated by biopsy, that resolved one month after therapy.[5] In other similar studies, reversible abnormalities of small intestinal mucosa were also found.[6, 7] The incidence of late complications of radiation enteritis varied between 2.5 and 25 per cent.[8–11] More recent evaluation suggests that the incidence of significant late complications may be less, especially when modern computerized techniques for delivery of therapeutic radiation are utilized.[12] However, other authors report no significant change or even an increase in this complication.[13] In view of the absence of controlled prospective studies, the exact incidence of radiation-induced injury to the intestine remains unknown. It is likely that the majority of patients who experience minimal injury remain clinically asymptomatic. Nevertheless, physicians who treat patients who have undergone radiation therapy will not infrequently encounter some whose X-ray therapy may have eradicated the cancer but also led to a slowly progressive iatrogenic disorder, radiation enterocolitis. These patients present with diarrhea, tenesmus, abdominal pain, intestinal hemorrhage, obstruction and perforation, fistula formation, and malabsorption. The morbidity can be substantial and the effects of radiation damage to the intestine may be fatal. Indeed, the price paid for extension of life by the radiation therapy–induced control of the tumor may seem high in view of the complications resulting from radiation injury to the intestine. This chapter will discuss pathophysiology, pathology, clinical manifestations, diagnosis, and treatment of radiation enteritis and colitis.

PATHOPHYSIOLOGY

Current radiation therapy utilizes short-wavelength, high-frequency X-rays or gamma rays that carry enough energy to produce ionization in body tissues that absorb them. Ionization refers to the production of atoms or molecules with an electrical charge sufficient to cause injury to living cells. The units of measure for ionizing radiation employed in clinical therapy are the rad and the Gray. One rad equals the dose of radiation that results in absorption of 100 ergs of energy per gram in the medium of interest, usually tissue. The rad thus measures quantity. To express the intensity of energy delivered or absorbed, a dose rate must also be specified. The Gray is the international unit for radiation energy and utilizes metric equivalents. One Gray corresponds to 100 rads. Since most clinical publications use rads to report radiation doses, we will use rads in this chapter.

Cellular Response to Radiation

The mechanism by which ionizing radiation injures or kills tissue has been extensively studied, especially in cells grown in culture.[14, 15] Radiation may produce overt injury with immediate cell death or, alternatively, loss of the ability of the cell to sustain reproduction or division.[16, 17] Cellular DNA, located in the nucleus, appears to be the target of greatest importance.[18] In cells that survive, the radiation energy may also induce alterations in cell membrane systems and in specific molecules causing abnormal cell function or an altered genetic program. The number of cells that survive radiation exposure is an exponential function of the radiation dose (Fig. 73–1*A*).[17, 18] Even at low radiation dosages, each increment in dose leads to a decrease in the number of surviving cells. This type of dose response curve shows that one hit of ionizing radiation may be all that is required for inactivation of a small, definable number of cells.

Cell survival is also critically affected by radiation dose rate, that is, administration of a specific total dose over a short or long exposure time. Rapid delivery of the total required dose is usually more harmful to cells than is slower delivery over a prolonged period or in many small separate doses known as fractions. It is notable that at a low radiation dose (Fig. 73–1*A*), the initial portion of the cell survival curve is nonlinear and demonstrates a threshold or shoulder region. This probably reflects the requirement for more than one ionization event to inactivate most cells, or shows the ability of some cells to effectively repair minimal levels of injury.[16–18] The resistance of a cell to radiation dose rate probably relates to its ability to effect concomitant repair of sublethal injury during a prolonged slow

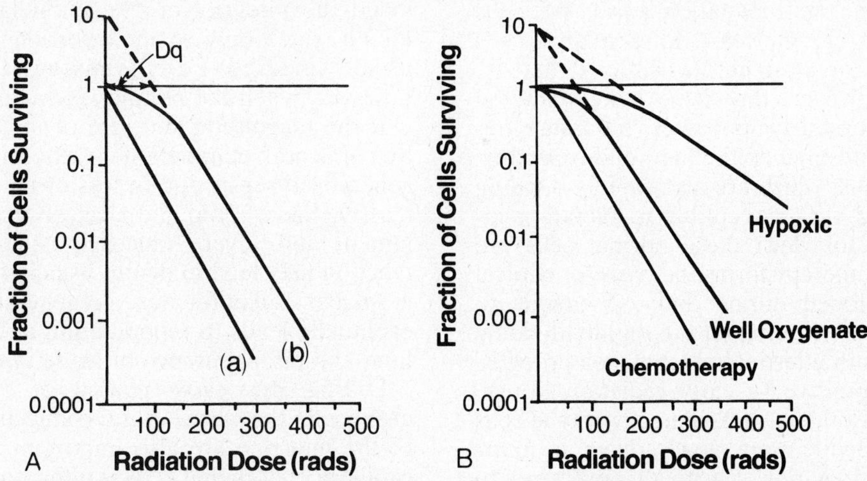

Figure 73–1. *A*, Typical cell survival curve in response to radiation exposure. Densely ionizing radiation, line (a), can produce cell death from each radiation hit. Less dense radiation, line (b), produces sublethal damage at low radiation doses. This results in a shoulder on the cell survival curve reflecting cell repair. Radiation doses below the quasi-threshold (Dq) for cell death kill few cells, whereas radiation doses above the Dq kill more cells per unit dose. *B*, Illustration of how tissue oxygenation and chemotherapy modify the cell survival curve. Hypoxia makes cells more resistant to the killing effects of radiation. Oxygenation makes them more sensitive. Certain forms of chemotherapy impair cell regeneration and thus produce a more narrow shoulder on the cell survival curve, reflecting increased cell death.

exposure time or rapid repair immediately after the radiation exposure when short fractionated doses are used.[16–18]

One of the most important factors governing response of a cell to X-radiation is the stage in the cell cycle when the radiation exposure occurs.[19] In a proliferating cell population, the cell cycle can be divided into four stages. Following mitosis (M), there is a rest interval known as the first gap (G1). This is followed by the S phase, during which new DNA is synthesized. A second interval or gap (G2) occurs after completion of DNA synthesis and prior to mitosis. During mitosis the cell divides to produce two cells from one. Cells are most sensitive to injury by ionizing radiation during mitosis. Resistance to radiation injury increases progressively during G1, reaching a peak in late S phase, and then rapidly declines during G2 prior to mitosis.[17–20] Since only a fraction of the total population of proliferating cells in a tissue is in the same stage of cell proliferation at any one instant, only some of the dividing cells die after a single substantial but sublethal dose of radiation. Subsequent recruitment of noncycling stem cells into actively proliferating cells affects radiation tolerance of a tissue in a manner that depends on future time fractionation of the radiation dose. Studies assessing intestinal mucosal regeneration and repair by stem cells following fractionated radiation have confirmed the importance of a rest period between radiation doses to permit regrowth of normal epithelium from the stem cells.[18, 20]

Other factors that may significantly modify the susceptibility of a cell to radiation injury include the degree of tissue oxygenation, the effect of administered drugs, and the level of endogenous radioprotectant substances.[16–18] For example, molecular oxygen potentiates many of the harmful effects of ionizing radiation on cells (Fig. 73–1*B*), possibly by increasing production of free radicals.[17, 18] Hypoxic tissue is less sensitive to the effects of ionizing radiation than is well-oxygenated tissue. Accordingly, poorly perfused tumor tissue may be less responsive to X-ray treatment than the more normal surrounding tissue. Attempts to enhance oxygen tension in cancer tissue by utilizing hyperbaric techniques have increased tumor killing by normal radiation dosages. Unfortunately, in some instances there is also increased damage to adjacent normal tissue. Various chemotherapeutic drugs can cause direct injury to intestinal epithelium, increase cellular sensitivity to radiation injury, and interfere with important reparative processes. These drugs include adriamycin, bleomycin, 5-fluorouracil, and actinomycin D.[16, 22–24] Exposure of cells to these drugs in culture results in a more narrow shoulder on the radiation dose/cell survival curve, reflecting drug impairment of cell repair mechanisms, and a steeper slope to the curve, reflecting increased cell killing per unit of radiation dose (Fig. 73–1*B*). On the other hand, some chemicals within cells, as, for example, sulfhydryl agents, tend to protect them from the effects of ionizing radiation.[18, 19, 25] When present in adequate concentrations, they may provide a substrate for oxidation by free radicals. The exact mechanism for their radioprotectant effect is, however, unknown. A number of newer radioprotectant agents, such as 2-mercaptopropionyl and ethyl phosphorathionic acid (WR-2721), have recently been tested and may potentially be clinically useful.[25–27]

Tissue Response to Radiation

When a tissue is exposed to ionizing radiation, all cells impacted by the energy will sustain an effect. There is often a moderate degree of variability in the response of different types of cells in the tissue to radiation, especially in regard to cell death. In general, inhibition of DNA synthesis is greatest in rapidly dividing cells. Radiation therapy takes advantage of the principle that the most radiation-responsive cells in a treatment field are the least differentiated cells and those with the greatest mitotic activity, that is, malignant cells. However, the tissue being radiated may also include normal lymphocytes, immature hematopoietic cells, intestinal epithelium, and reproductive system germ cells, which are also rapidly dividing cell populations and very susceptible to radiation injury.[17] The degree to which these normal cells are injured by radiation therapy forms the basis for clinical complications developed during and subsequent to radiation treatment. For example, the rapidly dividing crypt epithelial cells in intestinal mucosa (see pp. 992–1002) are very responsive to early radiation injury, whereas vascular endothelial and connective tissue cells in intestinal tissue divide more slowly, have an intermediate degree of radiation sensitivity, and tend to manifest the effect of radiation injury at a later date.[17] Thus, the intestine contains cells with varying responsiveness to radiation. This may produce a biphasic tissue response and clinical picture. The early symptoms of radiation injury result primarily from alterations in epithelial cell function; the later symptoms are due primarily to abnormalities in vascular and connective tissue components.

Cell renewal studies with tritiated thymidine have shown that normal intestinal mucosa is populated by a proliferating pool of undifferentiated cells located in the intestinal crypts that complete cell division about every 24 hours. Many progeny cells so produced lose the ability to divide, undergo dramatic internal reconstruction, express enzymatic and metabolic activity similar to surface epithelial cells, and are pushed up toward the villous tips or colon surface maturing during this migration. Complete replacement of surface epithelial cells from the proliferative cell zone in the crypts requires four to six days in the small intestine, colon, and rectum.[28] In the steady state, extrusion of senescent cells from the mucosal surface is balanced by cell replication in the crypt base. Ionizing radiation preferentially damages proliferating cells in the crypts and leads to interference with renewal of the surface epithelium.

Within hours after a single significant radiation exposure, there is a change in exposed intestinal crypt cells that progresses to cell death and loss from the crypt walls. The impaired repopulation of surface cells from crypt epithelial progenitor cells leads to a number of significant morphologic changes, especially in the small intestine. These include retraction of villous core cells, spreading out of enlarged villous epithelial cells in an attempt to protect greater areas of basement membrane, prolonged retention of epithelial cells on villi, formation of a cell syncytium at the villous tips, and a reduction in villous height.[6, 7, 29] Severe interference with cell replication thus leads to an inadequate amount of epithelium to provide coverage of the surface. This results in significant alteration in epithelial cell function and possibly to ulceration. In the usual situation when the X-ray dose rate is satisfactory, these changes, while substantial, rarely cause symptoms provided the integrity of the epithelial barrier is maintained, since only a small portion of the intestine is usually involved. Early symptoms are more common, however, when the rectum is irradiated.

If the magnitude and rate of radiation dose is such that mucosal denudation is extensive, there may be generalized sepsis due to loss of the epithelial barrier, massive loss of fluid and electrolytes into the intestinal lumen, and severe mucosal bleeding.[17] This severe reaction may lead to death, usually from sepsis.[30] With a smaller radiation dose, regeneration in the crypts eventually leads to repopulation of the surface epithelium and disappearance of acute symptoms.

During the early phases of radiation therapy, changes in the vascular and connective tissue elements of the intestine are also important.[17, 29, 31] Swelling of capillary endothelial cells is often quite prominent. An alteration in permeability of capillary and lymphatic walls is suggested by the presence of interstitial edema. The acute vasculopathy may coincide in time with the period of maximum epithelial cell damage. Any mucosal ischemia resulting from these vascular changes can certainly potentiate the deleterious effects of radiation on the epithelium. Generally, the acute vascular changes resolve, at least in part, but may recur and become progressive over weeks, months, or years after the acute epithelial change has resolved. Eventually, the progressive vascular and connective tissue changes can lead to obliterative endarteritis and endophlebitis, producing intestinal ischemia and contributing to new or more extensive mucosal injury, ulceration, and necrosis.[32] If mucosal integrity is lost owing to the compromised blood supply, intestinal bacteria may invade the necrotic tissue, increase local damage, and cause generalized sepsis. Extensive fibrosis may develop, causing formation of strictures, disorientation and disruption of the mucosal surface, and impairment of normal intestinal motility. These fibrotic changes are usually progressive and result from ischemia caused by the irradiation-induced vasculopathy.[32] The end result can be a chronically inflamed, thickened, ulcerated, and fibrotic bowel with marked impairment of mucosal function.

Radiation Dosage and Clinical Injury

Although some patients develop significant intestinal radiation injury following total dosages below 4000 rads, the incidence of serious injury rises sharply when the dose exceeds 5000 rads. Current guidelines for radiation tolerance of various segments of the gastrointestinal tract are based on the evaluation of Rubin and Casarette.[33] These authors define the "minimal tolerance" radiation dosage (TD 5/5) of the intestine as that at which 1 to 5 per cent of patients would be expected to manifest chronic radiation bowel damage within five years after therapy. The "maximum tolerance" radiation dose (TD 50/5) is that at which 25 to 50 per cent of patients will develop intestinal damage within five years. These bracketing radiation dose values for the various segments of the gastrointestinal tract are: esophagus, 6000 to 7500 rads; stomach, 4500 to 5000 rads; small intestine, 4500 to 6500 rads; colon, 4500 to 6000 rads; and rectum, 5500 to 8000 rads.

Unfortunately, these doses of radiation are all near to those required for a significant effect on many tumors. Thus, there may be only a narrow or no real margin of safety between the dose of radiation required to effect tumor control and the dose that produces a harmful effect on the intestinal tract. Moreover, it is often difficult to determine exactly how many rads of radiation were truly delivered to areas of the intestine, even during modern computer-directed therapy. Other factors that influence whether persisting radiation injury to the intestine will develop include the dose rate and fractionation schedule used, the part of the intestine irradiated, and the presence or absence of apparent predisposing factors.[34, 35] These include previous abdominopelvic surgery or pelvic inflammatory disease, which might produce adhesions immobilizing loops of small intestine in the field of radiation, hypertension, diabetes mellitus (i.e., coexisting vascular disease), and concomitant or previous chemotherapy, as discussed previously.

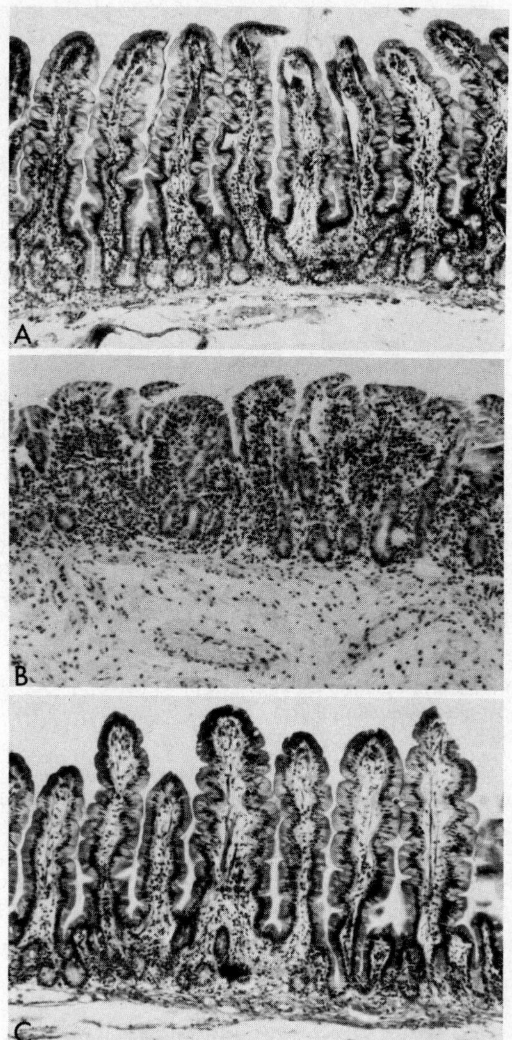

Figure 73–2. Three biopsies from the duodenojejunal junction of a patient undergoing abdominal X-ray therapy. *A,* Before treatment, the villous architecture is normal. *B,* After 3300 rads of X-ray therapy, the villi are shortened, there is increased infiltration of the lamina propria with inflammatory cells, and submucosal edema is present. *C,* Twelve days after cessation of therapy, villous architecture has returned to normal. Hematoxylin and eosin stain, × 75. (From Trier, J. S., and Browning, T. H. Reproduced from the Journal of Clinical Investigation 1966, *45*:194, by copyright permission of The American Society for Clinical Investigation.)

PATHOLOGY

The gross pathologic changes induced in the intestine by radiation therapy can be conveniently divided into acute, subacute, and chronic forms.[17, 29, 31, 36] Acute changes, occurring during and immediately after irradiation, involve abnormal epithelial cell proliferation and maturation associated with a decrease in crypt cell mitosis, as discussed previously. In the small bowel, this characteristically leads to villous shortening and a marked decrease in mucosal thickness (Fig. 73–2). In addition, hyperemia, edema formation, and extensive inflammatory cell infiltration of the mucosa occur. Crypt abscesses, consisting of acute inflammatory cells, eosinophils,[5] and sloughed epithelial cells, may be present (Fig. 73–3). If the radiation dose rate is high or the exposure time is prolonged, the mucosa may ulcerate owing to inadequate epithelial regeneration. Such ulceration may be diffuse or localized, depending upon the area and extent of exposure.

Later, during the subacute period, which begins 2 to 12 months after radiation therapy, the intestinal mucosa has regenerated and healed to a variable extent. However, during this period the endothelial cells of the small arterioles in the submucosa may undergo progressive swelling, detachment from their basement membrane, and, ultimately, degeneration.[29, 36] Fibrin plugs that form in the lumen can lead to thrombosis. In some instances, recanalization occurs (Fig. 73–4). Large foam cells are seen beneath the intima. These cells are considered by some to be diagnostic of radiation vascular injury in man.[17] The submucosa becomes thickened and fibrotic and often contains large, bizarre-appearing fibroblasts (Fig. 73–5).[17, 29, 36] The end result of the obliterative arteriolar changes is progressive ischemia. Vascular damage and ischemic fibrosis are progressive, though often at different rates, and are not reversible.[32] In the subacute period the circulation to the bowel is often adequate. With the onset of other medical conditions that may significantly affect the vasculature, such as hypertension, diabetes mellitus, generalized atherosclerosis, or coronary insufficiency and heart failure, the splanchnic circulation may become progressively compromised. Then, areas of microvascular insufficiency resulting from radiation vasculitis can acquire dangerous significance.[10]

Pathologic changes in the subacute and late stages of radiation enterocolitis tend to blend and are usually insidious in their development. Major complications

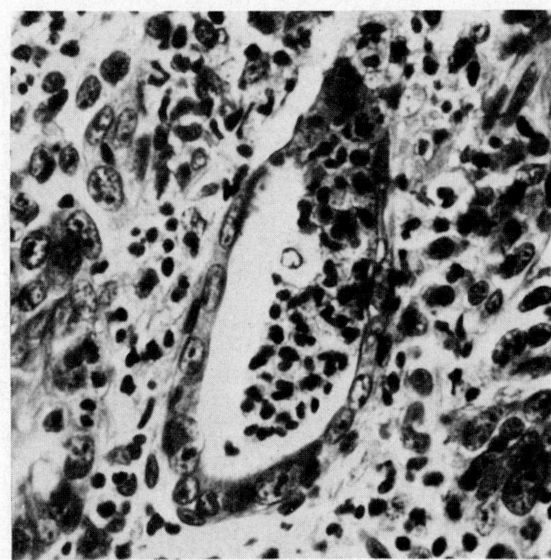

Figure 73–3. A crypt abscess in a biopsy of small bowel exposed to 3300 rads X-ray. The surrounding epithelial cells are flattened and contain megaloblastic nuclei. The crypt abscess is composed primarily of polymorphonuclear leukocytes, which are also seen in the lamina propria. Eosinophils may be prominent. Hematoxylin and eosin stain, × 500. (From Trier, J. S., and Browning, T. H. Reproduced from the Journal of Clinical Investigation 1966, *45*:194, by copyright permission of The American Society for Clinical Investigation.)

or damage from ischemia usually occurs early in the epithelium and submucosa, whereas the serosa is involved late. The muscularis propria may exhibit some focal areas of fibrosis or be involved by deep fissures or penetrating ulcers. The serosa develops a diffuse hyaline change and contains radiation fibroblasts, telangiectasia of smaller vessels, and ischemic changes in larger vessels. The result is often opaque, grayish, and thickened tissue enveloping the intestinal wall. Severe adhesions may develop between loops of intestine, and ischemic necrosis in areas so affected may lead to formation of fistulous tracts between adjacent bowel loops. Ischemic ulceration is particularly prone to develop in the sigmoid colon and rectum (Fig. 73–5).

Abscess and fistula formation may occur, with sinus tracts connecting the involved bowel with the vagina, bladder, or ileum. Inflammation and progressive fibrosis can lead to stricture formation producing partial or complete intestinal obstruction (Fig. 73–6). Carcinoma of the intestine can be a late complication; however, this consequence is uncommon.[37]

CLINICAL MANIFESTATIONS

The clinical setting in which one might encounter symptomatic radiation enterocolitis is in a patient with an intra-abdominal, most often pelvic, malignancy who either has just begun or may have completed radiation therapy. In those persons who develop late radiation symptoms, the total dose usually exceeded 4000 rads. Thus, symptoms may appear early during therapy, shortly after therapy has been completed, or months to many years after treatment has ended.

Early Symptoms

Gastrointestinal symptoms can develop during the first or second week of radiation therapy. Nausea and vomiting often occur early, but the cause is not clear. Nausea probably originates from a central nervous system response to any major dose of irradiation, as indicated by the fact that it also occurs when the gastrointestinal tract is not directly exposed to X-ray, such as during irradiation of the chest or neck. Nausea usually can be effectively controlled by treatment with phenothiazines or dopamine antagonists such as metoclopramide or domperidone.[38] However, use of modern dose rate and fractionation programs has tended to minimize the occurrence of these early radiation symptoms.[39] Later during treatment, the patient whose intestine is within the field of irradiation may experience diarrhea or constipation. This is most often seen in patients having pelvic irradiation. They may develop

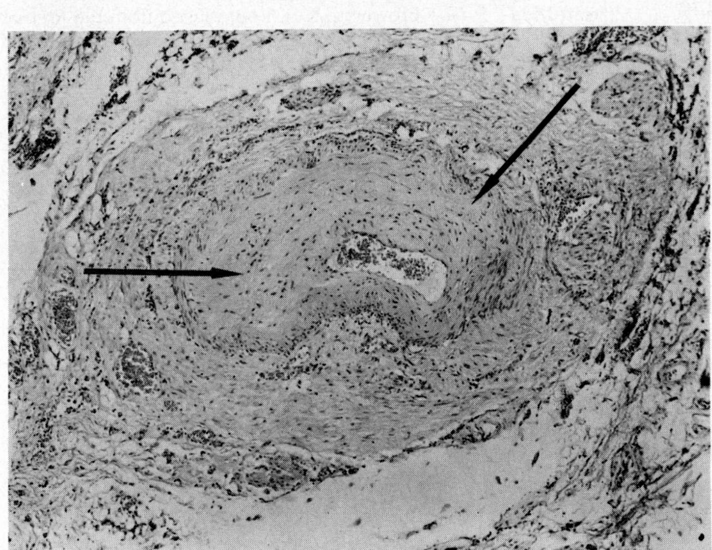

Figure 73–4. Characteristic radiation-induced change in a small submucosal arteriole. There is marked thickening of the vessel wall *(arrows)* and hydropic change of the subintimal cells. Luminal occlusion, thrombosis, and recanalization may occur. This progressive vascular lesion leads to tissue ischemia. Hematoxylin and eosin stain, × 100.

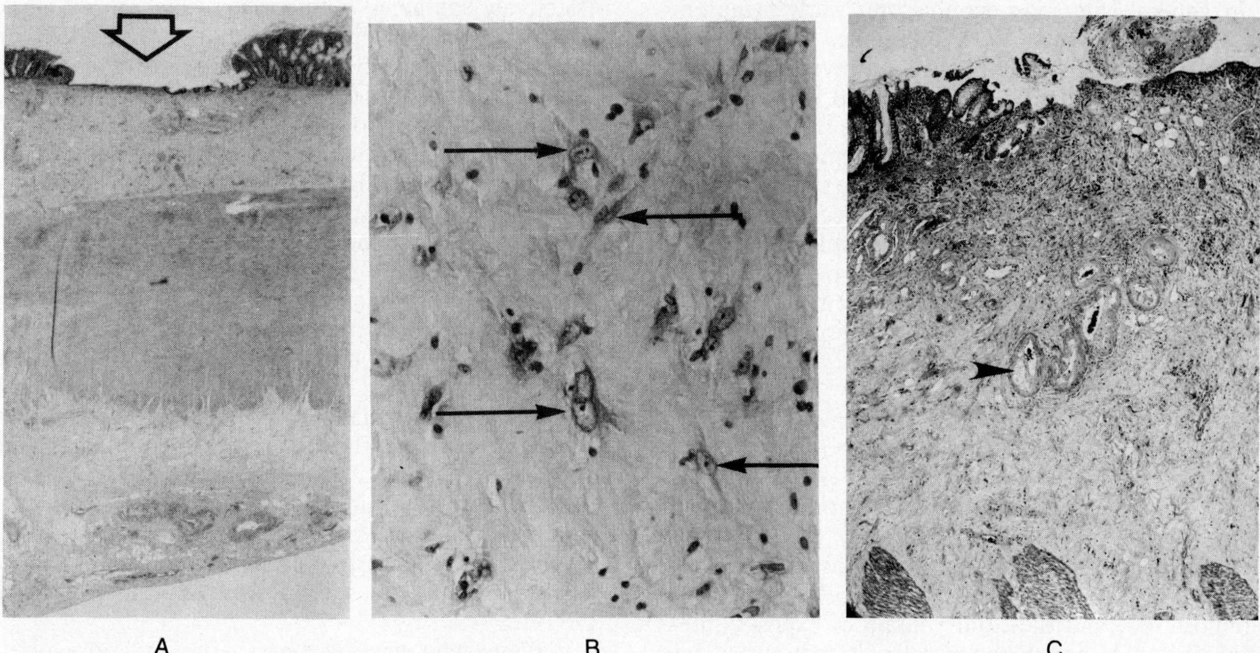

Figure 73–5. *A,* Full-thickness section (× 13) of sigmoid colon from a patient six years after radiation therapy for carcinoma of the cervix. There is mucosal ulceration *(arrow),* thickening and scarring in both submucosa and serosa, and narrowing of the lumen of arterioles, especially in the subserosa. *B,* A high-power (× 250) view of the subserosa showing the characteristic large, bizarre radiation fibroblasts *(arrows). C,* Section from a similar patient with a radiation-induced colon ulceration. The ulcer surface (upper right) is covered by granulation tissue. There are residual and regenerating glands in the upper left quadrant. The submucosa is greatly thickened and contains clusters of thick-walled, small arteries *(arrowhead)* with mural aggregates of lipid-filled histiocytes. The resultant arteriolar narrowing causes progressive ischemia. (*C,* courtesy of David C. White, M.D.)

an acute radiation proctocolitis manifested by tenesmus, diarrhea, and a mucoid rectal discharge. Rectal bleeding can also occur, especially if there is mucosal ulceration.[40] In many respects, the onset and clinical picture of early radiation colitis resembles that of acute idiopathic ulcerative proctitis or colitis.

Sigmoidoscopy during this acute period demonstrates a dusky, edematous, and inflamed mucosa with edema obscuring the normally visible vascular pattern. Friability is not marked and ulceration is infrequent in this early stage. However, as the cumulative dose of radiation increases, or if a high dose rate is used, mucosal ulceration and friability may occur (Color Fig. 73–7, p. xli). This is generally accompanied by marked tenesmus and by significant rectal bleeding. In such patients, sigmoidoscopy then demonstrates a hyperemic and occasionally necrotic mucosa with patchy areas of superficial ulceration.

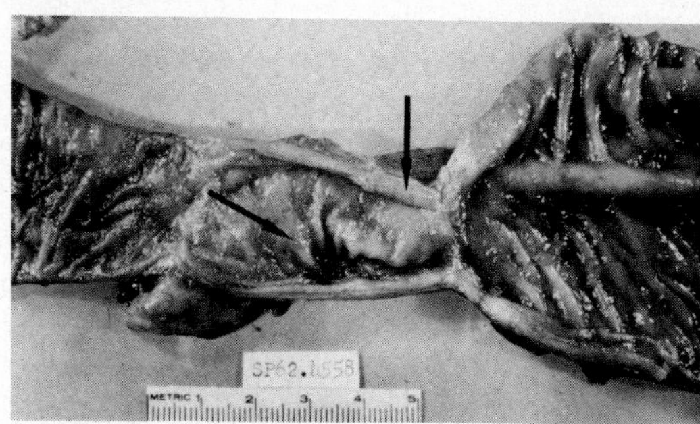

Figure 73–6. Narrow stricture of the ileum *(arrows)* one year after radiation therapy for carcinoma of the urinary bladder. The patient presented with symptomatic small bowel obstruction.

Involvement of the small intestine by the acute radiation response may produce abdominal cramping, nausea, and watery diarrhea. However, many patients remain asymptomatic even when significant mucosal lesions are present.[6] Radiation damage of ileal mucosa reduces bile acid reabsorption, which, in turn, causes diarrhea by inhibiting colonic water absorption.[41] Owing to depletion and impaired maturation of villous absorptive cells, brush border enzyme activity is reduced.[42] Breath tests have demonstrated malabsorption of lactose, trioctanoin, and cholylglycine. Absorption of D-xylose and vitamin B_{12} can be impaired. Fat malabsorption may be present but is usually not severe during the acute period of injury.[43, 44] Evidence for these various mucosal absorptive defects has recently been reviewed.[23, 40] Thus, reversible alterations of many aspects of small intestinal absorptive function can accompany acute radiation enteropathy. However, nutritionally significant impairment of absorption is rare.

In general, the most troublesome early symptoms for the patient are nausea, tenesmus, and diarrhea. These symptoms usually resolve shortly after completion of radiation treatment or respond to a reduction in daily dose rate or frequency of dose fraction administration that allows crypt cell repopulation of the epithelial surface. The absence of acute symptoms does not indicate protection against late occurrence of radiation-induced changes in the bowel.[45] While the severity of early symptoms correlates poorly with risk for developing late radiation damage, the occurrence of any early symptoms does signal an increased risk that late sequelae may develop.[46]

Late Symptoms

The complications of chronic radiation damage to the intestine and the symptoms they produce are a complex problem. The major predisposing factors appear to be the radiation dose rate, the total dose administered, and the total volume of exposed intestinal tissue. Although the onset of symptoms of late radiation injury is generally insidious, the clinical manifestations tend to progress relentlessly. Patients may develop symptoms as early as a few months or as late as many years after treatment is completed. The interval from the time of radiation to that of required surgery for intestinal complications ranges from 3 months to 31 years.[10, 40, 47] The variability of this latent period emphasizes the importance of the past medical history in evaluating patients with intestinal symptoms who have had radiation treatment for an abdominopelvic neoplasm. The overall frequency of late bowel injury following radiation has been estimated to be at least 10 per cent, especially when the rectum has been irradiated.[8, 10, 46, 48, 49]

The most common symptom experienced by patients with late small intestinal radiation damage is colicky abdominal pain due to partial small bowel obstruction. Nausea, vomiting, and symptoms from varying degrees of malabsorption may also be present. Symptoms that result from partial small bowel obstruction often begin in a subacute manner but may progress to complete obstruction. Obstruction usually is caused by a localized stricture but may be due to impaired motility in segments of intestine with interruption of normal peristalsis. In the latter circumstance, multiple segments of intestine may be involved simultaneously. Physical examination will demonstrate signs of bowel obstruction and occasionally a palpable mass due to inflammation in the intestine and mesentery. Fistulas may develop between the intestine and other pelvic and abdominal organs. The onset of a feculent vaginal discharge, pneumaturia, or rapid passage of undigested food in diarrheal stool should suggest the possibility of this complication. Clinical evidence for formation of a rectovaginal fistula is usually preceded by symptoms of proctitis. Abscesses are usually located in the pelvis and produce signs of sepsis. If such abscesses are not effectively contained by omentum, generalized peritonitis can develop. Free perforations of the involved ileum and colon, although uncommon, can also be the cause of acute peritonitis. Rarely, massive intestinal bleeding may develop from ileal or colonic ulcerations.

If the small intestine, particularly the ileum, is extensively involved, signs and symptoms of malabsorption may be prominent[43, 44] (see pp. 263–282). Therefore, patients with known radiation involvement of the small intestine who have a history of recent unexplained weight loss should have intestinal absorptive function evaluated by such indicators as stool fat, vitamin B_{12} absorption, malabsorption of bile salts, and D-xylose absorption. Malabsorption of bile salts may contribute to both diarrhea and steatorrhea. If a small bowel stricture or functional obstruction has developed, the resulting stasis may predispose to bacterial overgrowth in the lumen of the proximal small intestine. Enterocolonic fistulas, if present, may also lead to massive bacterial overgrowth and result in severe steatorrhea and malabsorption of vitamin B_{12} (see pp. 1289–1297).

Patients who have chronic radiation injury of the rectum will have symptoms of proctitis, including tenesmus and a mucoid rectal discharge that may be bloody. Occasionally, constipation may be prominent. A persisting decrease in stool caliber warrants early evaluation for colonic or rectal stricture or for recurrence of tumor. At sigmoidoscopy, the mucosa may appear granular and friable. Multiple telangiectasias are characteristic and are usually most prominent around ulcerated or necrotic areas of mucosa (Color Fig. 73–7, p. xli). Discrete ulceration of the rectal mucosa occurs in approximately 10 per cent of cases and is often located on the anterior rectal wall 4 to 8 cm from the anus.[10, 47] The ulcer may vary considerably in size and is frequently oriented transversely. Occasionally, the ulcer may have a neoplastic appearance. Rectal strictures tend to be located higher than ulcerations, usually 8 to 12 cm above the anal verge.[10] Biopsy of an ulcer or a strictured area may be helpful but should be performed with care because severe bleeding and perforation of the necrotic bowel may occur.

RADIOLOGIC AND ENDOSCOPIC EXAMINATIONS

During the early phase of radiation enteritis, plain films of the abdomen may show an ileus if small intestinal involvement is present. Barium studies of the small intestine, rarely performed during this phase, show mucosal edema and dilated, hypotonic loops of intestine.[50, 51] Both the intestinal wall and mesentery become quite edematous during the subacute stage of radiation injury. If severe, the edema may cause separation of intestinal loops, lead to thickening and straightening of mucosal folds, and impart a spiked

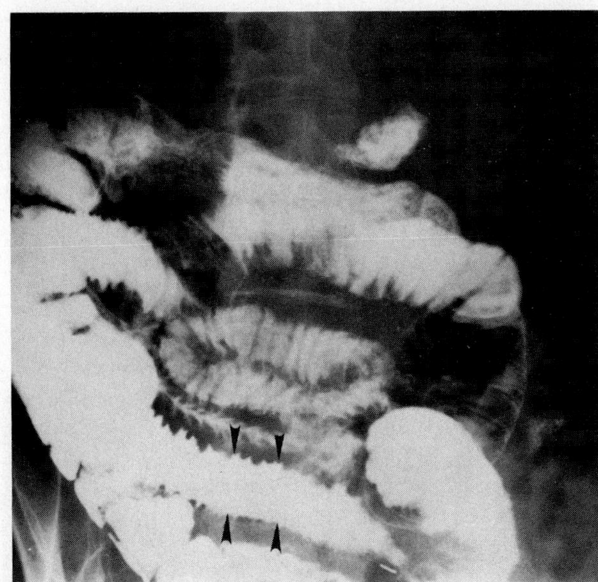

Figure 73–8. In early radiation injury of the small intestine, edema may cause separation of intestinal loops, lead to thickening and straightening of mucosal folds, and impart a spiked appearance *(arrowheads)* to the mucosa.

appearance to the mucosa (Fig. 73–8). Barium contrast studies of the rectum during the acute phase often demonstrate severe spasm. Rarely, an isolated ulcer may be present on the anterior rectal wall. If edema of the surrounding mucosa is present, the radiographic changes may suggest carcinoma. Thumbprint-like indentations of the barium column by edematous mucosa may lead to the mistaken diagnosis of a primary ischemic process.[40] When more diffuse mucosal ulceration occurs, fine spiculations of the rectocolonic mucosa may be seen (Fig. 73–9). When haustral markings are also lost, the radiologic picture may resemble other superficial acute ulcerating mucosal diseases, such as ulcerative colitis.

In late or chronic radiation enterocolitis, barium studies of the small intestine may show mucosal edema, separation of the intestinal loops, and excessive secretions in the intestinal lumen. Progressive fibrosis can lead to a narrowed, fixed, tubular, and poorly distensible intestinal segment or segments in which mucosal markings may be absent. The appearance may also closely resemble the radiologic features of intestinal Crohn's disease or an ischemic stricture.[50] Functional small bowel obstruction may be evident in the absence of mechanical narrowing of the bowel lumen owing to impaired motility. A simple barium contrast infusion technique is useful to demonstrate subtle changes induced by irradiation treatment.[52]

Radiologic changes in the rectosigmoid colon area often show narrowed, straightened, and ahaustral segments that may be indistinguishable from those of chronic ulcerative colitis or Crohn's colitis. A focal collection of barium in the anterior rectal wall may suggest ulceration, but the presence of fistulas to pelvic organs should also be suspected. Fibrosis of the colon or the rectum may result in both long and short areas of luminal narrowing that are smooth and symmetric and have tapered edges (Fig. 73–10). However, short strictures with overhanging margins indistinguishable from carcinoma have also been reported.[50, 51] Occasionally, a stricture may represent invasion of the intestinal wall by recurrent extraintestinal neoplasm. If recurrent cancer can be excluded, the history of previous radiation therapy and the absence of other radiologic changes of idiopathic inflammatory bowel disease suggest radiation damage as the cause of the observed X-ray changes.

Some help in the differential diagnosis of nonspecific barium X-ray findings in radiation enterocolitis may come from mesenteric angiography, computed tomography, and colonoscopy. Since arteriolar damage with ischemic change is the pathologic process that leads to stricture formation, it is not surprising that abnormal-

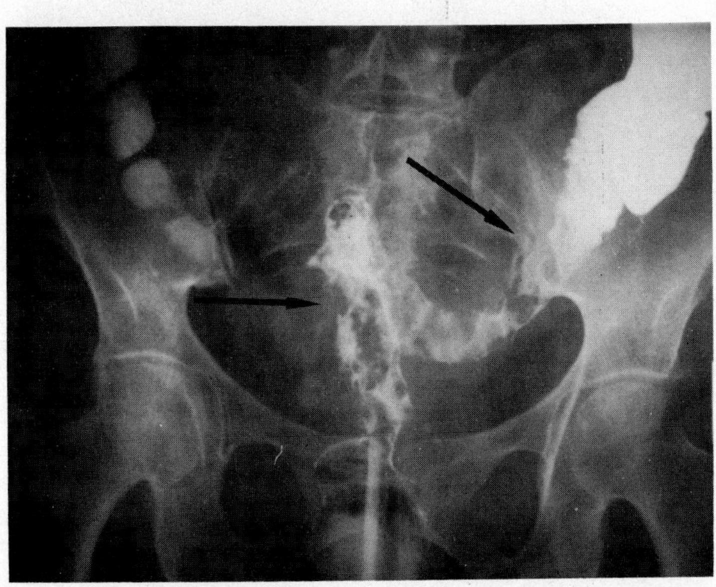

Figure 73–9. Severe radiologic abnormalities of the rectosigmoid colon are present on this barium enema performed two months after the patient underwent radiation therapy for cervical carcinoma. Subacute radiation injury of the colon may present radiologically as edematous, occasionally ulcerated mucosa, with asymmetric areas of narrowing suggestive of granulomatous colitis or recurrent tumor *(arrows).*

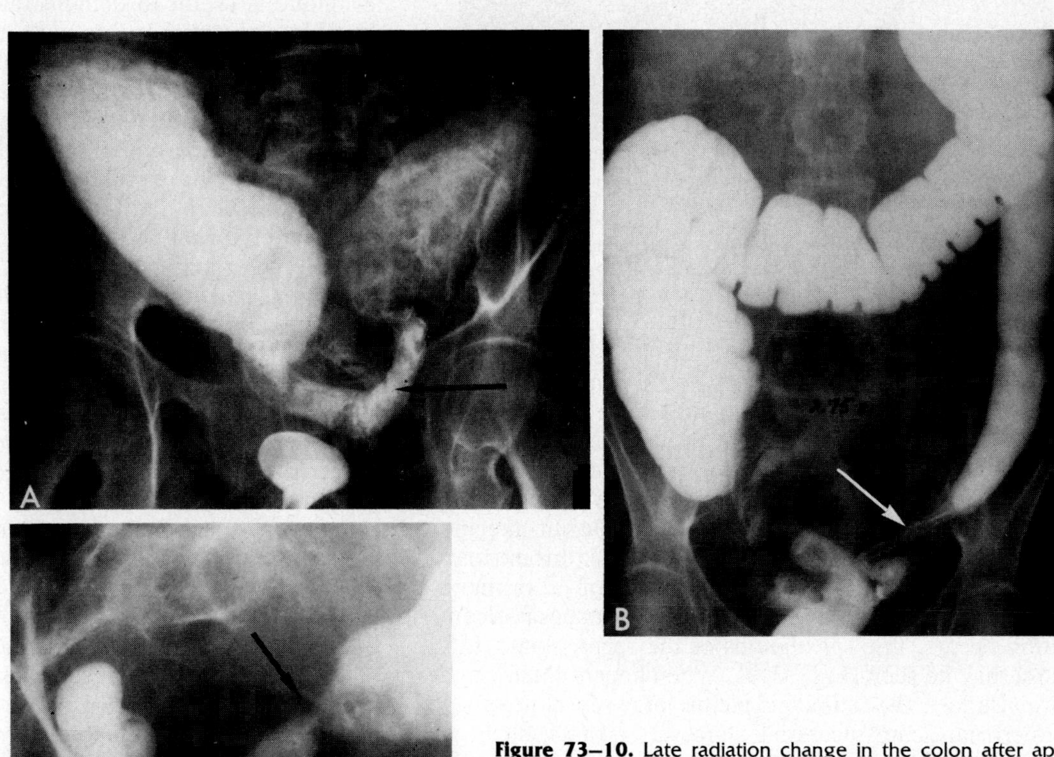

Figure 73–10. Late radiation change in the colon after approximately 5500 rads. *A,* Long stricture of rectum and sigmoid colon with symmetric concentric luminal narrowing. There is dilatation of the colon proximal to the stricture. *B,* The mucosal pattern is generally intact throughout this long radiation stricture of the descending and proximal sigmoid colon. *C,* A short postradiation stricture, such as this one in the proximal sigmoid colon, may be difficult to differentiate radiologically from malignancy.

ities in the smaller branches of the mesenteric vasculature are often present on an angiographic study.[53, 54] A CT scan may demonstrate recurrent tumor or nonspecific changes such as widening of the presacral space and thickening of the perirectal fibrous tissue, findings also present in perirectal abscess and ulcerative colitis.[55] Colonoscopy is useful for evaluating lesions beyond the reach of the sigmoidoscope. Mucosal changes in acute and chronic radiation injury, as viewed colonoscopically in more proximal colon, are similar to those seen at sigmoidoscopy (Color Fig. 73–7, p. xli). Depending upon the stage of radiation change, the findings include edema, granularity and friability, pale opaque mucosa, and prominent submucosal telangiectatic vessels.[56, 57] Because the true safety of colonoscopy in the different stages of radiation colitis has yet to be defined, the colonoscopist should be cautious during the examination.

MANAGEMENT

Modern radiation therapy techniques directed at minimizing complications include careful planning, detailed calculation of radiation dose, and proper dosing techniques. Measurement of radiation delivered to the pelvic organs by use of various types of radiation-sensitive probes has largely been replaced by computer-generated dosage calculations. Also, the treatment procedure is computer-managed and involves controlled variations in dose delivery ports and beam focus combined with changes in patient position, all directed at minimizing radiation exposure of normal tissues.[58, 59] Proposed methods to minimize the incidence of radiation enteropathy have been reviewed and include use of antibiotics, suppression of mucosal prostaglandins with aspirin, neutralization of pancreatic secretions, and the feeding of elemental diets during therapy.[31, 60] The true clinical value of these remains unknown. Pretreatment localization of the position of small intestinal loops in the pelvis by barium X-rays may aid in planning of dosimetry and body positioning during therapy to move the small bowel up out of the pelvis. Construction of special omental or synthetic mesh slings to keep the small intestine out of the pelvis or placing a temporary displacing device in the pelvis for the same purpose during any preradiation therapy surgery may also minimize subsequent injury to the intestine.[61, 62] Nevertheless, careful monitoring of the dose rate and its delivery in small fractions at definitely specified intervals remains the most reliable way to reduce intestinal complications. The use of radioprotectant chemicals during radiation therapy is promising conceptually, but more clinical experience is needed.

During the acute radiation reaction, a decrease in dose of as little as 10 per cent may significantly reduce symptoms. Conservative measures will usually suffice to treat any mild diarrhea and discomfort of proctitis and sigmoiditis. Sedation, antispasmodics, agents that increase stool bulk (such as the hydrophilic mucilloids), local analgesics, warm sitz baths, adequate nutrition, and careful general surveillance are the principal components of therapy at this stage. If watery diarrhea becomes a problem, bile salt malabsorption may be the cause, and treatment with cholestyramine (4 to 12 gm per day) may give dramatic improvement.[63] In the rare circumstance in which early radiation reaction is severe, especially in children, it has been suggested that use of an elemental diet free of gluten, cow's milk protein, and lactose may also have a beneficial effect.[64] Patients who are already malnourished and become more anorectic during radiation therapy may benefit from an elemental diet or from parenteral hyperalimentation before and during X-ray treatment.[23, 65] However, there is little evidence that supplemental oral nutrition during radiotherapy specifically modifies the primary radiation damage process.[66]

Symptoms of rectal urgency, frequency, incontinence of feces, and bleeding may occur weeks, months, or years after the radiation therapy. Such symptoms are usually due to mucosal injury, but may result in part from abnormal function of the internal anal sphincter caused by radiation damage to the myenteric plexus.[67] Treatment of symptomatic radiation proctitis is often initiated with steroid retention enemas. However, data documenting the efficacy of this approach are lacking. Oral salicylazosulfapyridine (Azulfidine) therapy has also been used, but a documented beneficial effect has been reported in only a small number of patients.[68] The active ingredient, 5-aminosalicylic acid (5-ASA), is now available in an enema preparation. It is possible that 5-ASA enema treatment may produce more favorable results than those observed with oral Azulfidine in the past.

Rectal bleeding is usually not severe, but occasionally may require administration of oral or parenteral iron or transfusion of whole blood. Recent reports suggest that control of minor bleeding can often be achieved endoscopically by use of Nd-YAG laser cauterization.[69] Other less expensive forms of cauterization including fulguration and application of 10 per cent silver nitrate might be tried, but they have not been systematically evaluated. There is also a single case report in which irrigation of the rectum with a 3.6 per cent formalin solution controlled acute bleeding and prevented its recurrence during the subsequent 14 months of observation.[70] This therapy was based on the observation that formalin treatment has been shown to control bleeding in intractable hemorrhagic cystitis. Rarely, a patient bleeds massively and unrelentingly. In such patients, if control of bleeding by topical cautery methods is not successful, a direct surgical approach is indicated, with ligation of the bleeding site if it can be localized. A colostomy or ileostomy to divert the fecal stream may be required, but generally does not stop chronic blood loss.

As the disease progresses, symptomatic strictures or fistulas may develop. Manual dilation of painful low anorectal strictures may improve symptoms of obstruction dramatically. However, care must be taken in dilating long and well-established strictures, since the bowel may be perforated during the dilation and this complication may not be immediately apparent. Mild symptoms of partial sigmoid or rectal obstruction are often temporarily helped by oral administration of mineral oil. Progression of a stricture to significant obstruction, regardless of its location in the large or small intestine, usually necessitates surgery. Partial small bowel obstruction should be managed nonoperatively for as long as possible.

A surgical approach to intestinal complications of radiation injury to the bowel leads to increased morbidity in some patients and thus should be reserved for definite indications.[60, 71, 72] Extensive surgery to remove suspected adhesions or to straighten kinked bowel should be avoided. The vascular supply of the intestine is already compromised by radiation change, and healing may be severely impaired. The perforation rate at surgery is high, and progressive ischemic necrosis may develop in the remaining adjacent bowel segments. Fistulous tracts usually require surgical treatment. Management has been divided into three phases: (1) stabilization of the patient with fluid, electrolytes, and nutritional repletion; (2) definition of the fistula by X-ray contrast studies; and (3) definitive operative therapy.[73] Total parenteral nutrition may be a useful initial treatment, but usually does not lead to permanent closure of the fistula.[74] Occasionally, rectovaginal fistulas close either spontaneously or after diversion of the fecal stream by a transverse colostomy. On the other hand, enterovesical, rectovesical, most enterocolic, and some rectosigmoid fistulas must be treated surgically. The results are generally good, but may be influenced by unrecognized radiation damage to the small intestine used in the repair.[75] Intra-abdominal and pelvic abscesses should be drained promptly; free perforations are, of course, a surgical emergency. Presacral sympathectomy has been recommended for severe pelvic pain that is resistant to medical management, but long-term results are uncertain.

For severe strictures or extensive erosive mucosal involvement of the distal colon, a colostomy, preferably placed in the transverse colon near the hepatic flexure, is often helpful as the initial procedure unless a pelvic abscess that requires drainage is present.[76] Such a colostomy may subsequently provide a long, mobile segment for a pull-through operation if resection of the rectum is ultimately necessary. Once a colostomy has been established, its closure is usually not attempted for 6 to 12 months in order to allow adequate time for healing of the defunctionalized bowel. The surgical approach to the radiation-injured bowel is undergoing constant re-evaluation owing to the high-risk nature of operating on such patients. The current surgical literature should be consulted prior to any planned operation, and, if possible, the procedure should be done by an experienced abdominal surgeon or surgical oncologist.[77]

In patients with malabsorption resulting from chronic radiation enteritis, the cause of the malabsorption should be evaluated and specific treatment given, if such is possible. For example, if there is stasis with bacterial overgrowth caused by impaired motility or stricture, broad-spectrum antibiotics should be administered (see pp. 1295–1296). As a last choice, a localized stricture unresponsive to medical treatment or one that causes severe or complete obstruction should be resected. Severe bacterial overgrowth caused by enterocolonic fistulas usually requires early surgery, either resection or bypass. If there is sufficient damage to ileal mucosa to compromise bile salt absorption but no major obstruction exists, administration of cholestyramine may reduce diarrhea by binding malabsorbed bile salts. If malabsorption is evident and surgery is too risky or is not indicated, nutritional supplementation with medium-chain triglycerides or polymeric and monomeric diet preparations may help (see pp. 279–280). Those patients who require hospitalization can experience dramatic improvement during total parenteral nutrition. In some patients there may be sustained improvement once normal oral feeding is reinstituted. In one study of TPN in severe radiation enteritis, concomitant treatment with methylprednisolone appeared to enhance the therapeutic results.[78] Thus, a period of total parenteral nutrition should be considered in patients not responding to other medical therapy in whom surgery is not warranted. Lastly, chronic strictures and localized ulcers must be closely monitored for the small but present risk of a secondary malignancy.

If treatment of the underlying neoplastic process has been successful, if X-ray therapy has been properly administered, and if systemic vascular disease is absent, most patients will not experience persisting or significant morbidity from radiation damage to the intestine. In many instances in which there is evidence of significant colon injury, the small bowel is also affected to some degree. The overall management strategy and prognosis for the patient's bowel-related symptoms will, in large part, be determined by the extent and severity of the damage to the small intestine. The outcome of radiation therapy usually depends on the response of the underlying malignancy. The onset of symptomatic radiation enteritis and colitis, however, may present the physician with yet another complicated therapeutic challenge.

References

1. Walsh, D. Deep tissue traumatism from roentgen ray exposure. Br. Med. J. *2*:272, 1897.
2. Franz, K., and Orth, J. Fall einer Röntgenschadingung. Berl. Klin. Wochenschr. *45*:662, 1917.
3. Buie, L. A., and Malmgren, G. E. Factitial proctitis. Trans. Am. Proctol. Soc. *29*:80, 1930.
4. Kinsella, T. J., and Bloomer, W. D. Tolerance of the intestine to radiation therapy. Surg. Gynecol. Obstet. *151*:273, 1980.
5. Gelfand, M. D., Tepper, M., Katz, L. A., Binder, H. J., Yesner, R., and Floch, M. H. Acute irradiation proctitis in man. Gastroenterology *54*:401, 1968.
6. Trier, J. S., and Browning, T. H. Morphologic response of human small intestine to X-ray exposure. J. Clin. Invest. *45*:194, 1966.
7. Tarpila, S. Morphological and functional response of the human small intestinal mucosa to ionizing radiation. Scand. J. Gastroenterol. (Suppl. 12) *6*:1, 1971.
8. Yudelev, M., Kuten, A., Tatcher, M., Rubinov, R., Karmeli, R., Cohen, Y., and Robinson, E. Correlations of dose and time-

dose-fraction factors (TDF) with treatment results and side effects in cancer of the uterine cervix. Gynecol. Oncol. *23*:310, 1986.

9. Roswit, B., Malsky, S. J., and Reid, C. B. Severe radiation injuries of the stomach, small intestine, colon and rectum. Am. J. Roentgenol. *157*:62, 1963.
10. DeCosse, J. J., Rhodes, R. S., Wentz, W. B., Reagan, J. W., Dwarken, H. J., and Holden, W. D. The natural history and management of radiation-induced injury of the gastrointestinal tract. Ann. Surg. *170*:369, 1969.
11. Dietel, M., and Vasic, V. Major intestinal complications of radiotherapy. Am. J. Gastroenterol. *72*:65, 1979.
12. Morgenstern, L., Hart, M., Luso, D., and Friedman, N. B. Changing aspects of radiation enteropathy. Arch. Surg. *120*:1225, 1985.
13. Allen-Mersh, T. G., Wilson, E. J., Hope-Stone, H. F., Mann, C. V. Has the incidence of radiation-induced bowel damage following treatment of uterine carcinoma changed in the last 20 years? J. R. Soc. Med. *79*:387, 1986.
14. Barendsen, G. W., and Walter, H. M. D. Effects of different ionizing radiations in human cells in tissue culture. Radiat. Res. *18*:106, 1963.
15. Elkind, M. M., and Redpath, J. L. Molecular and cellular biology of radiation lethality. *In* Becker, F. F. (ed.). Cancer: A Comprehensive Treatise. Vol. 6. New York, Plenum, 1977, pp. 51–59.
16. Holahan, E. V., Jr. Cellular radiation biology. *In* Conklin, J. J., and Walker, R. I. (eds.). Military Radiobiology. New York, Academic Press, 1987, pp. 87–110.
17. Anderson, R. E. Radiation injury. *In* Kissane, J. M. (ed.). Anderson's Pathology. St. Louis, C. V. Mosby Co., 1985, pp. 239–277.
18. Painter, R. B. The role of DNA damage and repair in cell killing by ionizing radiation. *In* Meyer, R. E., and Withers, H. R. (eds.). Radiation Biology in Cancer Research. New York, Raven Press, 1980, pp. 59–68.
19. Sinclair, W. K. Cell cycle dependence on the lethal radiation response in mammalian cells. Curr. Top. Radiat. Res. Q. *1*:264, 1972.
20. Hagemann, R. F., Sigvestad, C. P., and Lesher, S. Intestinal crypt survival and total crypt levels of proliferating cellularity following irradiation; fractionated X-ray exposure. Radiat. Res. *47*:149, 1971.
21. Withers, H. R., and Mason, K. A. The kinetics of recovery in irradiated colonic mucosa of the mouse. Cancer *34*:896, 1974.
22. Phillips, T. L., and Fu, K. K. Quantification of combined radiation therapy and chemotherapy effects on critical normal tissue. Cancer *37*:1186, 1976.
23. Kinsella, T. J., Bloomer, W. D. Tolerance of the intestine to radiation therapy. Surg. Gynecol. Obstet. *151*:273, 1980.
24. Shaw, M. T., Spector, M. H., and Ladman, A. J. Effects of cancer, radiotherapy and cytotoxic drugs on intestinal structure and function. Cancer Treatment Rev. *6*:141, 1979.
25. Nagata, H. Studies on sulfhydryl radioprotectors with low toxicities. Tokushima J. Exp. Med. *27*:15, 1980.
26. Ito, H., Meistrich, M. L., Barkley, T. H., Thomas, H. D., Jr., and Milas, L. Protection of acute and late radiation damage of the gastrointestinal tract by WR-2721. Int. J. Radiat. Oncol. Biol. Phys. *12*:211, 1986.
27. France, H. G., Jirtle, R. L., and Mansbach, C. M., II. Intracolonic WR-2721 protection of the rat colon from acute radiation injury. Gastroenterology *91*:644, 1986.
28. MacDonald, W. C., Trier, J. S., and Everett, N. B. Cell proliferation and migration in the stomach, duodenum and rectum of man. Radioautographic studies. Gastroenterology *46*:405, 1964.
29. White, D. C. An atlas of radiation histopathology. Technical Information Center, Office of Public Affairs, U.S. Energy Research and Development Administration, TID-26676, 1975, pp. 141–160.
30. Walker, R. I., and Conklin, J. J. Mechanisms and management of infectious complications of combined injury. *In* Conklin, J. J., and Walker, R. I. (eds.). Military Radiobiology. New York, Academic Press, 1987, pp. 219–230.
31. Berthrong, M., and Fajardo, L. F. Radiation injury in surgical pathology. II. Alimentary tract. Am. J. Pathol. *5*:153, 1981.
32. Hasleton, P. S., Carr, N., and Schofield, P. F. Vascular changes in radiation bowel disease. Histopathology *9*:517, 1985.
33. Rubin, P., and Casarette, G. A direction for clinical radiation pathology. *In* Vaeth, J. N. (ed.). Frontiers of Radiation Therapy and Oncology. Vol. 6. Baltimore, University Park Press, 1972, pp. 1–16.
34. Potish, R. A. Importance of predisposing factors in the development of enteric damage. Am. J. Clin. Oncol. *5*:189, 1982.
35. Potish, R. A. Prediction of radiation-related small bowel damage. Radiology *135*:219, 1980.
36. Ackerman, L. V. The pathology of radiation effect of normal and neoplastic tissue. Am. J. Roentgenol. *114*:447, 1972.
37. Sandler, R. S., and Sandler, D. P. Radiation-induced cancers of the colon and rectum: assessing the risk. Gastroenterology *84*:51, 1983.
38. Gunter-Smith, P. J. Effect of ionizing radiation on gastrointestinal physiology. *In* Conklin, J. J., and Walker, R. I. (eds.). Military Radiobiology. New York, Academic Press, 1987, pp. 135–151.
39. Cassady, J. R., Order, S., Camitter, B., and Marck, A. Modification of gastrointestinal symptoms following irradiation by low dose rate technique. Int. J. Radiat. Oncol. Biol. Phys. *1*:15, 1975.
40. Novak, J. M., Collins, J. T., Donowitz, M., Farman, J., Sheaham, D. G., and Spiro, H. M. Effects of radiation on the human gastrointestinal tract. J. Clin. Gastroenterol. *1*:9, 1979.
41. Stryker, J. A., Mortel, R., and Hepner, G. W. The effect of pelvic irradiation on ileal function. Radiology *124*:213, 1977.
42. Alpers, D. H., Seetharam, B. Pathophysiology of diseases involving intestinal brush border proteins. N. Engl. J. Med. *296*:1047, 1977.
43. Greenberger, N. J., and Isselbacher, K. J. Malabsorption following radiation injury to the gastrointestinal tract. Am. J. Med. *36*:450, 1964.
44. Tankel, H. I., Clark, D. H., and Lee, F. D. Radiation enteritis with malabsorption. Gut *6*:560, 1965.
45. Kline, J. C., Buchler, D. A., Boone, M. L., Peckham, B. M., and Carr, W. F. The relationship of reactions to complications in the radiation therapy of cancer of the cervix. Radiology *105*:413, 1972.
46. Bourne, R. G., Kearsley, J. H., Grove, W. D., and Roberts, S. J. The relationship between early and late gastrointestinal complications of radiation therapy for carcinoma of the cervix. Int. J. Radiat. Oncol. Biol. Phys. *9*:1445, 1983.
47. Galland, R. B., and Spencer, J. The natural history of clinically established radiation enteritis. Lancet *1*:1275, 1985.
48. Strockbine, M. F., Hancock, J. E., and Fletcher, G. H. Complications in 831 patients with squamous cell carcinoma of the intact uterine cervix treated with 3000 rads or more whole pelvis radiation. Am. J. Roentgenol. *108*:293, 1970.
49. Palmer, J. A., and Bush, R. S. Radiation injuries of the bowel associated with carcinoma of the cervix. Surgery *80*:458, 1976.
50. Mason, G. R., Dietrich, P., Friedland, G. W., and Hanks, G. E. The radiological findings in radiation-induced enteritis and colitis. A review of 30 cases. Clin. Radiol. *21*:232, 1970.
51. Rogers, F., and Goldstein, A. M. Roentgen manifestations of radiation to the gastrointestinal tract. Gastrointest. Radiol. *2*:281, 1979.
52. Mendelson, R. M., and Nolan, D. J. The radiological features of chronic radiation enteritis. Clin. Radiol. *36*:141, 1985.
53. Bosniak, M. A., Hardy, M. A., Quint, J., and Ghoessein, N. A. Demonstration of the effect of irradiation on canine bowel using in vivo photographic magnification angiography. Radiology *93*:1361, 1969.
54. Dencker, H., Holmdahl, K. H., Lunderquist, A., Olivecrona, H., and Tylen, U. Mesenteric angiography in patients with radiation injury of the bowel after pelvis irradiation. Am. J. Roentgenol. *114*:476, 1972.
55. Doubleday, L. C., and Bernardino, M. E. CT findings in the perirectal area following radiation therapy. J. Comput. Assist. Tomogr. *4*:634, 1980.
56. Reichelderfer, M., and Morrisey, J. F. Colonoscopy in radiation colitis. Gastrointest. Endosc. *26*:41, 1980.
57. den Hartog, J. F. C., van Haastert, M., Batterman, J. J., and Tytgat, G. N. The endoscopic spectrum of late radiation damage of the rectosigmoid colon. Endoscopy *17*:214, 1985.

58. Levene, M. B., Kijewski, D. K., Chin, L. M., Bjarngard, B. E., and Hellman, S. Computer controlled radiation therapy. Radiology *129*:769, 1978.
59. Stewart, J. R., and Gibbs, F. A., Jr. Presentation of radiation injury: predictability and preventability of complications of radiation therapy. Annu. Rev. Med. *33*:385, 1982.
60. Morgenstern, L., Thompson, R., and Friedman, N. B. The modern enigma of radiation enteropathy: sequelae and solutions. Am. J. Surg. *134*:166, 1977.
61. Green, N. The avoidance of small intestine injury in gynecologic cancer. Int. J. Radiat. Oncol. Biol. Phys. *9*:1385, 1983.
62. Kavanah, M. T., Feldman, M. I., Devereaux, D. F., and Kondi, E. S. New surgical approach to minimize radiation-associated small bowel injury in patients with pelvic malignancy requiring surgery and high-dose irradiation. Cancer *56*:1300, 1985.
63. Heusinkveld, R. S., Manning, M. R., and Aristizabal, S. A. Control of radiation-induced diarrhea with cholestyramine. Radiat. Oncol. Biol. Phys. *4*:687, 1978.
64. Donaldson, S. S., Jundt, S., Ricour, C., Sarrazin, D., Lemerle, J., and Schweisguth, O. Radiation enteritis in children: a retrospective review, clinicopathologic correlation, and dietary management. Cancer *35*:1167, 1975.
65. McArdle, A. H., Reid, E. C., Laplante, M. P., and Freeman, C. R. Prophylaxis against radiation injury. The use of elemental diet prior to and during radiotherapy for invasive bladder cancer and in early postoperative feeding following radical cystectomy and ileal conduit. Arch. Surg. *121*:879, 1986.
66. Brown, M. S., Buchanan, R. B., and Karran, S. J. Clinical observations on the effects of elemental diet supplementation during irradiation. Clin. Radiol. *31*:19, 1980.
67. Varma, J. S., Smith, A. N., and Busuttil, A. Function of the anal sphincters after chronic radiation injury. Gut *27*:528, 1986.
68. Goldstein, F., Khory, J., and Thornton, J. J. Treatment of chronic radiation enteritis and colitis with salicylazosulfapyridine and systemic corticosteroids. Am. J. Gastroenterol. *65*:201, 1976.
69. Ahlquist, D. A., Gostout, C. J., Viggiano, T. R., and Pemberton, J. H. Laser therapy for severe radiation-induced rectal bleeding. Mayo Clin. Proc. *61*:927, 1986.
70. Rubinstein, E., Isben, T., Rasmussen, R. B., Reimer, E., and Sorensen, B. L. Formalin treatment of radiation-induced hemorrhagic proctitis. Am. J. Gastroenterol. *81*:44, 1986.
71. Localio, S. A., Pachter, H. L., and Gouge, T. H. The radiation injured bowel. Surg. Annu. *11*:181, 1979.
72. Schmitt, E. H., III, and Symmonds, R. E. Surgical treatment of radiation induced injuries of the intestine. Surg. Gynecol. Obstet. *153*:896, 1981.
73. Smith, D. J., Pierce, V. K., and Lewis, J. L., Jr. Enteric fistulas encountered on a gynecologic oncology service. Surg. Gynecol. Obstet. *158*:71, 1984.
74. Rose, D., Yarborough, M. F., Canizaro, P. C., and Lowry, S. F. One hundred fourteen fistulas of the gastrointestinal tract treated with total parenteral nutrition. Surg. Gynecol. Obstet. *163*:345, 1986.
75. Bricker, E. M., Kraybill, W. G., and Lopez, M. J. Functional results after postirradiation rectal reconstruction. World J. Surg. *10*:249, 1986.
76. Jao, S. W., Beart, R. W., Jr., and Gunderson, L. L. Surgical treatment of radiation injuries of the colon and rectum. Am. J. Surg. *151*:272, 1986.
77. Harling, H., and Balslev, I. Radical surgical approach to radiation injury of the small bowel. Dis. Colon. Rectum *29*:371, 1986.
78. Loiudice, T. A., and Lang, J. A. Treatment of radiation enteritis: a comparison study. Am. J. Gastroenterol. *78*:481, 1983.

74 Acute Appendicitis

THEODORE R. SCHROCK

GENERAL CONSIDERATIONS

Historical Note

Inflammation in the right lower quadrant was regarded as a disease of the cecum (typhlitis or perityphlitis) until the late nineteenth century.[1] Careful studies at that time revealed perforation of the appendix and an intact cecum in fatal cases of so-called typhlitis, and the term *appendicitis* was introduced. The emphasis subsequently has been on early diagnosis and appendectomy, before perforation can occur.[2]

Incidence

Acute appendicitis is the most common abdominal surgical emergency. Between 7 and 12 per cent of people develop appendicitis at some time of life. The peak incidence is in the second and third decades, but it can occur at any age.[3] The incidence of acute appendicitis is declining;[4] the proportion of persons over age 60 with appendicitis is rising.[5] Appendicitis is 1.3 to 1.6 times more common in males than in females.[3] There is little or no seasonal effect on the incidence.[3]

Anatomy and Function of the Appendix

The vermiform appendix in the newborn is a conical structure that projects from the apex of the cecum for a distance of 4.5 cm.[6] The infrequency of appendicitis in neonates is attributed to the wide appendiceal orifice in this age group. During childhood, the junction between appendix and cecum becomes more distinct and shifts dorsally and to the left.[6] The adult appendix averages 9 to 10 cm in length; it arises from the posteromedial wall of the cecum about 3 cm inferior to the ileocecal valve.[6] Congenital anomalies (agenesis, double appendix) are very rare.

The position of the appendix has clinical implications; it is *retrocecal, retroileal, preileal, subcecal,* or *pelvic* according to one classification.[6] The relative incidence of these positions varies greatly in different studies.[6] In more than 50 per cent of people, the appendix is not fixed in one site and presumably is free to move in response to cecal distention and postural changes, although whether it actually does so has been questioned.[6]

The function of the human appendix is unknown, but the abundance of organized lymphoid tissue suggests an immunologic role.[7] Although the density of IgA and IgM immunocytes is only slightly higher in the appendix than in the colon, the density of IgG immunocytes is much greater in the appendix than in the colon.[7] It is hypothesized that immature lymphocytes migrate from the appendix to lamina propria in distant intestinal sites where they develop into IgA-producing cells.[7] These lymphocytes respond to luminal antigens.[8]

Contrary to an earlier suggestion, there is no convincing evidence of an increased risk of malignant disease of the colon or other organ systems after appendectomy, regardless of the age at which appendectomy is performed.[9]

PATHOLOGY

Acute appendicitis is classified as *simple, gangrenous,* or *perforated* on the basis of the operative findings and the histologic appearance. The inflamed appendix is viable and intact in simple appendicitis. Focal or extensive necrosis of the wall characterizes gangrenous appendicitis, and microscopic perforation often is present. Perforated appendicitis refers to gross disruption or even dissolution of the appendix.

Edema and serosal telangiectasia are prominent in early simple appendicitis. At a later stage, the appendix is tensely distended and discolored, and patches of fibrinous exudate appear on the serosa. Gangrene and gross perforation are unmistakable if present. Inflammation may involve the entire appendix or only the part distal to an obstruction, but inflammation limited to the proximal portion is rare. The mesoappendix is edematous, and contiguous structures become inflamed also. Microscopically, an acute inflammatory exudate of polymorphonuclear leukocytes is found in the lumen and mucosa in the early stages; this infiltrate extends to all layers of the wall as the disease progresses.

PATHOGENESIS

The pathogenesis of acute appendicitis remains controversial. Classically, appendicitis is believed to develop primarily from obstruction of the lumen with secondary bacterial infection. When the long, narrow appendiceal lumen becomes obstructed, the mucosa continues to secrete fluid until the intraluminal pressure reaches 85 cm of water or more. At this point, intraluminal pressure exceeds venous pressure, the appendix becomes hypoxic, the mucosa ulcerates, and bacteria invade into the wall. Infection causes more swelling and more ischemia owing to thrombosis of small intramural vessels. Gangrene and perforation occur in 24 to 36 hours, but the timing is highly variable. Perforation may develop earlier if the appendix is obstructed near its tip than if the obstruction is closer to the base.

The lumen is obstructed by *fecaliths* or viscid *fecal masses* in about 35 per cent of acutely inflamed appendices; other, less common obstructing lesions include *calculi, tumors, parasites,* or *foreign bodies.*[10, 11] Barium is a debatable cause of appendiceal obstruction leading to appendicitis. Fecaliths probably develop more readily in people who consume a diet deficient in fiber and thus have more tenacious stools; this has been offered as an explanation for the frequency of appendicitis in Western populations.[10] The declining incidence of acute appendicitis has been postulated to result from the inclusion of more fiber in the diet,[10, 12] but the importance of dietary fiber is controversial, and alternative explanations for the changing incidence of appendicitis are just as plausible.[13]

At least one third of inflamed appendices have no obstructing lesion in the lumen, however, and the pathogenesis of appendicitis in these patients is not clear.[14] Extrinsic obstructions (bands, strictures, and kinks) are uncommon. The existence of a sphincter that impedes appendiceal emptying has been postulated but remains unproved. Lymphoid hyperplasia in response to viral (e.g., measles) or bacterial (e.g., salmonellosis) infection can obstruct the lumen and initiate appendicitis. There is conflicting evidence regarding variation in the incidence of acute appendicitis during the menstrual cycle.[15, 16]

DIAGNOSIS

Although it is easy to make the diagnosis of acute appendicitis in typical cases, at times it is very difficult to distinguish appendicitis from other diseases. A careful history and thorough physical examination are essential; laboratory tests and radiographic studies are only ancillary measures. The physical examination must be repeated if the diagnosis is not clear initially, but prolongation of these efforts for many hours to achieve absolute certainty is not justified; complications of appendicitis are avoided by prompt diagnosis and treatment.[17]

The most reliable historical feature is the sequence of symptoms described in the next section. Progressively severe symptoms are characteristic of appendicitis, compared with the fluctuating course of some conditions that mimic appendicitis.[18] The single most valuable physical finding is localized tenderness.

Symptoms and Signs

The classic sequence of symptoms in acute appendicitis is as follows: (1) pain; (2) anorexia, nausea, or vomiting; (3) sensitiveness over the appendix; and (4) fever. Not all patients have every one of these symptoms, but when these symptoms occur in some other order, the diagnosis of appendicitis must be questioned.

Pain is the initial symptom in nearly all patients.[2, 17–20] Typically, the patient awakens at night with pain in the epigastrium or periumbilical area; pain can, however, be diffuse in the abdomen or even localized in the right lower quadrant from the onset. The initial pain often is described as colicky, but it usually is not severe, and it may be so vague that the patient believes the problem is just a gastric upset. It reaches a peak of intensity in about four hours and then subsides gradually, only to reappear in the right lower quadrant as a progressively severe ache that is exacerbated by movement. This "shift" of the location of pain is an important clue if it is present. The initial pain is visceral and is referred from the appendix to other sites; the secondary right lower quadrant pain is due to inflammation of periappendiceal tissues. Patients generally seek medical attention 12 to 48 hours after the pain begins, but delays up to several days may occur.

About 95 per cent of patients have anorexia, nausea, or vomiting.[18] The patient vomits only once or twice a few hours after the onset of pain, but anorexia persists even though nausea subsides.[2] A low-grade fever is typical; high fever or shaking chills point either to some other diagnosis or to a complication of appendicitis.

A sensation of constipation and the conviction that a good bowel movement will solve the problem is called the "gas stoppage sensation."[18] This common symptom motivates patients or parents to administer cathartics or enemas, but of course defecation does not bring relief. A few patients have diarrhea during an attack of appendicitis. Testicular pain occurs in some men.

On physical examination, the temperature averages 37.8° C in simple appendicitis.[18] Abdominal tenderness is elicited first by asking the patient to cough; the patient usually can localize the painful spot with one finger. The examiner confirms localized tenderness by gently and systematically palpating the abdomen with one finger. McBurney's point (2 inches from the anterior superior iliac spine on a line drawn from this process through the umbilicus) bears an inconstant relationship to the underlying inflamed appendix, and often the site of maximal tenderness is some distance away. Rebound tenderness is referred to the right lower quadrant. Local hyperesthesia of the skin and muscular rigidity may be present. Bowel sounds are not a useful sign. Pelvic and rectal examinations are normal, or tenderness is detected high on the right side. The psoas sign is elicited by asking the patient to raise the straightened right lower extremity against resistance by the examiner. The obturator sign is sought by passive rotation of the right lower extremity with the patient supine and the right hip and knee flexed. These signs are present when inflammation adjacent to the particular muscle causes pain during movement.

Atypical Appendicitis. The symptoms and signs just described apply to classic appendicitis. Many cases of appendicitis are atypical, however, because of the position of the appendix, the age of the patient, or the presence of associated conditions such as pregnancy.

Retrocecal appendicitis and retroileal appendicitis differ from the classic variety in several ways.[21] The inflamed appendix is shielded from the anterior abdominal wall by the overlying cecum and ileum. The pain, therefore, seems less intense, and there is less discomfort on walking or coughing.[18] The classic shift of pain from epigastrium to right lower quadrant may not occur; indeed, pain may remain so poorly localized that the diagnosis is overlooked entirely. Urinary frequency sometimes results from direct irritation of the ureter. Muscular rigidity is absent, and abdominal tenderness is minimal. The examiner should elicit tenderness by carefully palpating into the right flank with one finger.[18]

Pelvic appendicitis is a treacherous disease.[18] Pain, frequently very severe, is a constant symptom. It begins in the epigastrium but quickly settles in the lower abdomen. Of great importance, pain more often localizes on the *left* than on the right. The urge to urinate and the urge to defecate (gas stoppage sensation) are prominent symptoms. Dysuria and diarrhea may occur. The absence of muscular rigidity and of abdominal tenderness is particularly deceptive. Tenderness must be sought by rectal or pelvic examination, and these maneuvers should be repeated in a few hours if the results are negative initially. Pelvic tenderness is found eventually in these patients.

Obstructive appendicitis is a clinical entity characterized by severe cramping abdominal pain that mimics the colic of small bowel obstruction. Rapid progression to gangrene makes acute mesenteric vascular occlusion the more likely diagnosis in some of these people.[18]

Bizarre forms of appendicitis occur when the cecum is located in the right upper quadrant or on the left side of the abdomen because of malrotation. A very long appendix may extend from a normally placed cecum into other parts of the abdomen and create a confusing picture.

Appendicitis in infants is a diagnostic dilemma for obvious reasons.[22, 23] Pain is difficult to appreciate in the infant, and lethargy, irritability, and anorexia are the earliest symptoms noted by parents. Sedation often is required to detect localized tenderness by abdominal and rectal examination. Perforation of the appendix may be a complication of necrotizing enterocolitis in neonates.

Appendicitis in the elderly is particularly dangerous because the symptoms are vague, the patient often delays seeking medical treatment, and the physician does not entertain the diagnosis.[24–26] Pain often is minimal. Temperature may be elevated only slightly, even in advanced stages of appendicitis. Tenderness is localized to the right lower quadrant in most cases, but the tenderness may be deceptively mild.

Appendicitis in pregnancy does not present a diagnostic problem in the first three or four months, but if it occurs late in gestation, there is a tendency to seek obstetric explanations for the symptoms and signs.[27, 28] Abdominal pain on the right side is the most common symptom, just as in nonpregnant patients. Tenderness is maximal in the usual location in some patients, but in others it is found adjacent to the umbilicus or in the right subcostal area because of cecal displacement by the gravid uterus.

Laboratory Findings

The average leukocyte count varies from 10,000 to 16,000 cells/cu mm in different reports, depending on the stage of the disease. Between 80 and 90 per cent of patients with appendicitis have a leukocyte count greater than 10,000 cells/cu mm.[29] A "shift to the left," with more than 75 per cent neutrophils, is found in about 90 per cent or more of cases.[29] Altogether, 96 per cent of patients have leukocytosis, abnormal differential cell counts, or both.[29] It must be emphasized, however, that a completely normal white blood cell profile does not exclude the diagnosis of appendicitis.

Small numbers of erythrocytes and leukocytes are found in the urine in about one fourth of patients with appendicitis.

Radiographic Findings

Radiographic studies are of value in atypical cases, particularly in the extreme age groups. About 55 per cent of patients with early acute appendicitis have abnormal plain abdominal X-rays.[30] Localized ileus and increased soft tissue density in the right lower quadrant are the most consistent findings. Less commonly seen are appendicoliths, altered right psoas shadow, and abnormal right-flank stripe. A fecalith in the appendiceal region in a patient with possible appendicitis is a highly reliable indicator.[30] Plain films also may show evidence of diseases that mimic appendicitis, such as perforated ulcer and cholecystitis.

Ultrasonography may be helpful in diagnosing appendicitis or conditions that mimic it.[31] Computed tomography (CT scan) identifies abscesses and appendicoliths particularly well.[32] Barium enema X-rays are rarely necessary; nonfilling of the appendix, plus a mass, is strongly suggestive of appendicitis. Intravenous urography helps to differentiate appendicitis from diseases of the urinary tract; CT scan also provides this information.

DIFFERENTIAL DIAGNOSIS

Acute appendicitis should never be lower than second in the differential diagnosis of any acute abdominal problem. Considered here are some of the diseases that are confused with appendicitis in Western countries; the list is different in developing countries and in tropical climates.

Gastroenteritis and Mesenteric Lymphadenitis

Inflammation of the small intestine, the mesenteric lymph nodes, or both is a common disorder that mimics early acute appendicitis and actually may precipitate appendicitis by causing lymphoid hyperplasia. Gastroenteritis may occur at any age, but mesenteric lymphadenitis is limited to children and young adults. Nausea and vomiting precede abdominal pain, in contrast to the sequence in appendicitis.[17, 18] Patients often complain of other symptoms of viral illness, including high fever, headache, pharyngitis, myalgias, and photophobia. The presence or absence of diarrhea has little differential value. The abdominal pain is more generalized and the tenderness is localized less well than in appendicitis.

Although most of these cases are believed to be viral in origin, bacterial infection is responsible for some of them. *Yersinia enterocolitica* and *Yersinia pseudotuberculosis* have been isolated from patients operated on with the diagnosis of appendicitis and found instead to have enteritis or mesenteric lymphadenitis.[33]

Gynecologic Diseases

Acute salpingitis begins in the lower abdomen without the shift of pain characteristic of appendicitis. High fever (>38° C), infrequent vomiting, pain for more than two days, and diffuse bilateral lower abdominal tenderness in a young woman who does not appear ill enough to have perforated appendicitis are other differential points.[34, 35] The cervix is tender, and gram-negative intracellular diplococci are seen in the vaginal discharge in some cases but not in all. Salpingitis caused by *Chlamydia trachomatis* seems especially prone to produce periappendicitis.[36]

Mittelschmerz is pain caused by rupture of an ovarian follicle at the time of ovulation. The typical picture is sudden onset of lower abdominal pain in the middle of the menstrual cycle. Gastrointestinal symptoms are not prominent. The patient does not appear ill, but sharply localized right lower quadrant tenderness sometimes makes it difficult to exclude appendicitis. There may be a mild fever and leukocytosis. Pain and tenderness slowly improve without treatment in the majority of cases.

In *ruptured ectopic pregnancy,* pain also begins suddenly.[37] Some patients rapidly lapse into shock from profuse bleeding. Pelvic tenderness is diffuse. The tubal pregnancy may be palpable on pelvic examination, and culdocentesis returns bloody fluid. *Twisted ovarian cyst* causes sudden pain and simultaneous vomiting. The mass is palpable in most patients, but anesthesia may be required.

Diseases of the Urinary Tract

Ureteral colic typically radiates into the groin and is associated with no muscular rigidity and little direct tenderness.[17] Erythrocytes are present in the urine, but the same may be true in appendicitis. Although an opaque calculus is seen outside the appendiceal region on plain X-ray in a few patients, CT scan and intravenous urography are the most useful diagnostic tests. *Acute pyelonephritis* is a difficult differential problem, especially in girls. High fever (38 to 40° C), sometimes with shaking chills, and maximal tenderness in the costovertebral angle are important features. Marked pyuria, white cell casts, and gross bacteria are characteristic findings on urinalysis.

Other Acute Surgical Diseases

Meckel's diverticulitis can mimic appendicitis so closely that the differentiation is impossible. Associated symptoms of small bowel obstruction, poor localization of pain, and maximal tenderness more medially than usual are clues to this diagnosis.[17, 18]

Other surgical emergencies that simulate appendicitis include sigmoid diverticulitis, perforated peptic ulcer, cholecystitis, intestinal obstruction, cecal diverticulitis and perforated colonic carcinoma.[17, 18, 38] Acute appendicitis can cause small bowel obstruction, and the diagnosis of the problem that precipitated the obstruction may be difficult. Crohn's disease of the appendix is a form of appendicitis that can be indistinguishable from ordinary appendicitis.[39, 40] Neutropenic enterocolitis is a concern in leukemic patients[41] (see pp. 369–377, 502–503, and 1327–1358).

Systemic Diseases

Abdominal pain caused by diaphragmatic irritation from basilar pneumonia may be confused with appendicitis, especially in children. The question of appendicitis arises in some patients with diabetic ketoacidosis, acute porphyria, tabetic crisis, and connective tissue disorders in which, however, pain is usually more diffuse. Diabetes may be diagnosed by elevation of blood and urine glucose and ketones; dark urine with a positive Watson-Schwartz test for porphobilinogen will make the diagnosis of acute intermittent porphyria, and Argyll Robertson pupils and absent deep tendon reflexes will facilitate the diagnosis of tabetic crisis.[17]

DIAGNOSTIC ACCURACY

From 10 to 40 per cent of patients with a preoperative diagnosis of acute appendicitis do not have appendicitis when the abdomen is explored.[2, 19, 20, 42] This error is more common in young women than in any other group.[34, 35, 37] Another acute surgical disease is encountered instead of appendicitis in 4 to 13 per cent of patients who undergo operation; most of these people are elderly. Negative exploration (no acute surgical problem of any kind) occurs in 8 to 26 per cent of operations for suspected appendicitis; gastroenteritis, mesenteric lymphadenitis in children, and gynecologic disorders in young women are the diseases that cause confusion most often.[2, 42] About 5 per cent of patients with appendicitis undergo abdominal exploration with some other preoperative diagnosis; this type of error is more frequent in the older age group.

Another kind of mistake is more serious than any of those mentioned earlier—that is, the failure to diagnose appendicitis before the appendix perforates. There is an inverse correlation between the rate of negative abdominal exploration and the rate of perforation in most reported series, and a direct correlation between the perforation rate and the morbidity and mortality of appendicitis is found in all published reports.[2, 19, 20, 42] Clinical scoring systems and computer-aided models have had mixed success in improving diagnostic accuracy.[43–45] A certain number of negative explorations, therefore, actually are necessary to avoid a high incidence of perforation and its consequences. Negative exploration rates of 20 per cent overall, 10 per cent in men and 30 per cent in women, are probably acceptable. Laparoscopy has the potential for reducing the negative appendectomy rate.[46]

COMPLICATIONS

Perforation

The overall frequency of perforation is 10 to 32 per cent, with most figures in the neighborhood of 20 per cent.[5, 18, 19, 20] The rate of perforation is highest in the extreme age groups. Perforation develops in 93 per cent of children under two years of age, in 55 to 71 per cent of those under six years of age, and in about 35 per cent of all children.[22, 23, 47, 48] From 40 to 75 per cent of patients over 60 years of age have perforation by the time of operation.[5, 24, 25, 26] Perforation within 12 hours of the onset of pain is unusual, but the risk of this complication climbs steeply after 24 hours.

Perforation is recognized preoperatively in 70 per cent of patients.[2, 47, 48] Suggestive clinical features include duration of symptoms beyond 36 hours, fever greater than 38.5° C, toxic appearance, diffuse abdominal tenderness, abdominal mass, and marked leukocytosis or elevated neutrophil count.

Appendiceal perforation leads to peritonitis or abscess formation.

Peritonitis. Spreading or generalized peritonitis causes diffuse abdominal pain and high fever. The patient appears toxic, and the abdomen is distended and diffusely tender.[17, 18] There is free air in the abdomen in a few patients.

Abscess. Localized perforation results in a tender mass in the right lower quadrant. In the early stages, the mass consists of the perforated appendix surrounded by edematous small bowel and omentum (a "phlegmon"). Later, a true abscess containing pus may form. Abscesses may develop elsewhere after perforation, most commonly in the pelvis, where examination discloses a mass anterior to the rectum. Abscesses in the subphrenic space or at other remote sites are consequences of generalized peritonitis.[17, 18]

Pylephlebitis

Pylephlebitis is septic thrombophlebitis of the portal venous system and is characterized by high fever (39 to 40° C), shaking chills, and jaundice.[17, 18] If the other symptoms of appendicitis are not marked, primary disease of the biliary tract may seem more likely. Pylephlebitis (or, at least, portal bacteremia) should be suspected in any patient with appendicitis who has a shaking chill. Vigorous therapy with antibiotics is necessary to avoid formation of hepatic abscesses. Fortunately, pylephlebitis is uncommon today.

TREATMENT

Appendectomy (appendicectomy) is the only acceptable treatment for acute simple appendicitis if adequate facilities and qualified personnel are available. Although appendicitis may resolve without operation, a policy of nonoperative treatment is hazardous because delay leads to perforation in most cases.

Little preparation for operation is necessary in young adults with simple appendicitis. Children require fluid and electrolyte repletion, and elderly patients need evaluation and treatment of associated diseases. Perforation in a patient of any age, on the other hand, demands intensive preparation before operation. Replacement of fluid and electrolyte deficits and correction of acid-base imbalance may take several hours. Systemic antibiotics are essential,[49] and nasogastric suction is a useful adjunct. High fever, particularly in children, must be lowered before anesthesia is induced.

A muscle-splitting incision is made in the right lower quadrant in most cases. The appendix is removed, even if it is normal. In the latter situation, of course, other disease (e.g., Meckel's diverticulitis) must be sought. If the diagnosis is incorrect and the source of the problem cannot be identified or treated through the small incision in the right lower quadrant, the incision is extended or a new one is made elsewhere.

Antibiotics are instilled into the peritoneal cavity in patients with generalized peritonitis, but drains are not used unless there is a well-defined abscess.[18, 48] Gangrenous appendicitis and perforated appendicitis are associated with a high incidence of postoperative wound infection; systemic or topical antibiotics help prevent this complication.[50] Delayed primary closure of the wound is also effective.

Appendectomy is mandatory for perforated appendicitis with spreading or generalized peritonitis. If a mass is palpable in the right lower quadrant, however, initial treatment may be operative or nonoperative.[51–53] Operation resolves the problem promptly in most cases, and proponents believe that overall morbidity is lessened and hospital stay is shortened by this direct approach. Operation for appendiceal abscess can be difficult, however, and there is some risk of spreading a localized infection into other parts of the peritoneal cavity. Expectant management with intravenous fluids and antibiotics is favored by some surgeons for this reason. The mass may resolve completely, or a true abscess may develop and require surgical drainage. From 10 to 30 per cent of patients treated nonoperatively initially must undergo drainage of the abscess within a few days because they fail to respond to conservative management;[51–53] the appendix is excised at the same time, if possible. If the appendix is not removed during the acute episode, elective appendectomy should be performed after an interval of six weeks to three months to prevent recurrent appendicitis, which occurs in 20 per cent of patients.[53]

Minimal care is needed after appendectomy for simple appendicitis; most patients are ready to be discharged from the hospital in three to five days. The postoperative course in perforated cases may be stormy, and operation for drainage of secondary abscesses is common.

PROGNOSIS

The mortality of appendicitis is the mortality of delay. The prognosis of simple appendicitis is excellent. Complications, mostly minor, occur in approximately 10 per cent of patients, and the mortality rate is 0 to 0.3 per cent.[5, 18–20] The outcome of perforated appendicitis is much worse.[54] The morbidity rate is 15 to 60 per cent;[5, 22, 23, 47–49] many of these complications are severe, and hospital stays are lengthy. The overall mortality rate of perforated appendicitis is 1 per cent or less, but death has been reported in up to 15 per cent of elderly patients with perforation.[5, 19, 20, 24, 25]

The overall mortality rate of appendicitis has declined over the years, largely because patients with perforation receive better supportive care, not because the incidence of perforation is lower. Delay by the patient or parents is one reason for perforation, and delay by the physician is another.[54] In one study, 45 per cent of children with perforated appendicitis had been seen by a physician who failed to recognize the disease.[47] Prolonged observation in the hospital and accumulation of vast quantities of laboratory data do not substitute for a careful history, thorough physical examination, and prompt operation in cases of possible appendicitis.

CHRONIC AND RECURRENT APPENDICITIS

Chronic appendicitis is an uncommon but probably authentic clinical and pathologic entity.[55] Recurrent appendicitis is more frequent, and it is not unusual for a patient with typical appendicitis to relate a history of previous similar, but self-limited, episodes.[55, 56] If the appendix is not removed after drainage of an appendiceal abscess, appendicitis can develop again.[53] Recurrence after incomplete appendectomy also occurs.

PROPHYLACTIC AND INCIDENTAL APPENDECTOMY

The risk of developing appendicitis during one's remaining lifetime is about 1 in 5 at birth and 1 in 35 at age 50.[57] The chances of having appendicitis during the next year of life are greatest at ages 15 to 19 years: 1 in 99 for females and 1 in 110 for males.[57] In view of these statistics, elective prophylactic appendectomy in the normal person is not justified; an exception may be made for the individual who plans to live in a remote area without access to medical facilities. Prophylactic appendectomy has been suggested for patients with appendiceal calculi seen on abdominal films, but this policy has not been widely adopted.

Incidental appendectomy during abdominal operation for some other disease is worthwhile if the primary operation is not compromised and if the appendix can be exposed easily,[58, 59] but it is probably unnecessary in elderly patients. Incidental appendectomy does not increase operative morbidity when done in association with gynecologic or certain other operations.[58, 59] The patient must be informed that the appendix was removed.

References

1. Williams, G. R. Presidential address: A history of appendicitis with anecotes illustrating its importance. Ann. Surg. *197*:495, 1983.
2. Berry, J. Jr., and Malt, R. A. Appendicitis near its centenary. Ann. Surg. *200*:567, 1984.
3. Martin, D. L., and Gustafson, T. L. A cluster of true appendicitis cases. Am. J. Surg. *150*:554, 1985.
4. Raguveer-Saran, M. K., and Keddie, N. C. The falling incidence of appendicitis. Br. J. Surg. *67*:681, 1981.
5. Peltokallio, P., and Tykka, H. Evolution of the age distribution and mortality of acute appendicitis. Arch. Surg. *116*:153, 1981.
6. Buschard, K., and Kjaeldgaard, A. Investigation and analysis of the position, fixation, length and embryology of the vermiform appendix. Acta Chir. Scand. *139*:393, 1973.
7. Bjerke, K., Brandtzaeg, P., and Rognum, T. O. Distribution of immunoglobulin producing cells is different in normal human appendix and colon mucosa. Gut *27*:667, 1986.
8. Ohtani, O., Ohtsuka, A., and Owen, R. L. Three-dimensional organization of the lymphatics in the rabbit appendix. Gastroenterology *91*:947, 1986.
9. Moertel, C. G., Nobrega, F. T., Elveback, L. R., and Wentz, J. R. A prospective study of appendectomy and predisposition to cancer. Surg. Gynecol. Obstet. *138*:549, 1974.
10. Jones, B. A., Demetriades, D., Segal, I., and Burkitt, D. P. The prevalence of appendiceal fecaliths in patients with and without appendicitis. Ann. Surg. *202*:80, 1985.
11. Onuigbo, W. L. B. Appendiceal schistosomiasis. Dis. Colon Rectum *28*:397, 1985.
12. Arnbjornsson, E. Acute appendicitis and dietary fiber. Arch. Surg. *118*:868, 1983.
13. Barker, D. J. Acute appendicitis and dietary fibre: An Alternative hypothesis. Br. Med. J. *290*:1125, 1985.
14. Arnbjornsson, E., and Bengmark, S. Role of obstruction in the pathogenesis of acute appendicitis. Am. J. Surg. *147*:390, 1984.
15. Arnbjornsson, E. The influence of oral contraceptives on the frequency of acute appendicitis in different phases of the menstrual cycle. Surg. Gynecol. Obstet. *158*:464, 1984.
16. Robinson, J. A., and Burch, B. H. An assessment of the value of the menstrual history in differentiating acute appendicitis from pelvic inflammatory disease. Surg. Gynecol. Obstet. *159*:149, 1984.
17. Silen, W. Cope's Early Diagnosis of the Acute Abdomen. 15th edition. New York, Oxford University Press, 1979, p. 62.
18. Way, L. W. Appendix. *In* Way, L. W. (ed.). Current Surgical Diagnosis and Treatment. 7th edition. Los Altos, California, Lange Medical Publications, 1985, p. 555.
19. Jess, P. Acute appendicitis: epidemiology, diagnostic accuracy, and complications. Scand. J. Gastroenterol. *18*:161, 1983.
20. Pieper, R., Kager, L., and Nasman, P. Acute appendicitis: a clinical study of 1018 cases of emergency appendectomy. Acta Chir. Scand. *148*:51, 1982.
21. Shperber, Y., Halevy, A., Oland, J., and Orda, R. Familial retrocaecal appendicitis. J. R. Soc. Med. *79*:405, 1986.
22. Harrison, M. W., Lindner, D. J., Campbell, J. R., Campbell, T. J. Acute appendicitis in children: factors affecting morbidity. Am. J. Surg. *147*:605, 1984.
23. Gilbert, S. R., Emmens, R. W., and Putnam, T. C. Appendicitis in children. Surg. Gynecol. Obstet. *161*:261, 1985.
24. Burns, R. P., Cochran, J. L., Russell, W. L., and Bard, R. M. Appendicitis in mature patients. Ann. Surg. *201*:695, 1985.
25. Lau, W. Y., Fan, S. T., Yiu, T. F., Chu, K. W., and Lee, J. M. H. Acute appendicitis in the elderly. Surg. Gynecol. Obstet. *161*:157, 1985.
26. Smithy, W. B., Wexner, S. D., and Dailey, T. H. The diagnosis and treatment of acute appendicitis in the aged. Dis Colon Rectum *29*:171, 1986.
27. Masters, K., Levine, B. A., Gaskill, H. V., and Sirinek, K. R. Diagnosing appendicitis during pregnancy. Am. J. Surg. *148*:768, 1984.
28. Horowitz, M. D., Gomez, G. A., Santiesteban, R., and Burkett, G. Acute appendicitis during pregnancy. Arch. Surg. *120*:1362, 1985.
29. Bower, R. J., Bell, M. J., and Ternberg, J. L. Diagnostic value of the white blood count and neutrophil percentage in the evaluation of abdominal pain in children. Surg. Gynecol. Obstet. *152*:424, 1981.
30. Shimkin, P. M. Commentary. Radiology of acute appendicitis. AJR *130*:1001, 1978.
31. Parulekar, S. S. Ultrasonographic findings in diseases of the appendix. J. Ultrasound Med. *2*:59, 1983.
32. Shin, M. S., and Ho, K. J. Appendicolith: significance in acute appendicitis and demonstration by computed tomography. Dig. Dis. Sci. *30*:184, 1985.
33. Attwood, S. E. A., Cafferkey, M. T., West, A. B., et al. Yersinia infection and acute abdominal pain. Lancet *1*:529, 1987.
34. Bongard, F., Landers, D. V., and Lewis, F. Differential diagnosis of appendicitis and pelvic inflammatory disease. A prospective analysis. Am. J. Surg. *150*:90, 1985.
35. Nakhgevany, K. B., and Clarke, L. E. Acute appendicitis in women of childbearing age. Arch. Surg. *121*:1053, 1986.

36. Mardh, P. -A., and Wolner-Hanssen, P. Periappendicitis and chlamydial salpingitis. Surg. Gynecol. Obstet. *160*:304, 1985.
37. McIntyre-Seltman, K. Gynecological pathology encountered during exploration for appendicitis. Infections in Surgery 5:524, 1986.
38. Bova, J. G., Hopens, T. A., and Goldstein, H. M. Diverticulitis of the right colon. Dig. Dis. Sci. *29*:150, 1984.
39. Fonkalsrud, E. W., Ament, M. E., and Fleisher, D. Management of the appendix in young patients with Crohn's disease. Arch. Surg. *117*:11, 1982.
40. Rawlinson, J., and Hughes, R. G. Acute suppurative appendicitis. A rare associate of Crohn's disease. Dis. Colon Rectum *28*:608, 1985.
41. Brooke, A., Glass, N. R., and Sollinger, H. Neutropenic enterocolitis in adults: review of the literature and assessment of surgical intervention. Am. J. Surg. *149*:405, 1985.
42. Lau, W. -Y., Fan, S. -T., Yiu, T. -F., Chu, K. -W., and Wong, S. -H. Negative findings at appendectomy. Am. J. Surg. *148*:375, 1984.
43. Way, C. W. V., III, Murphy, J. R., Dunn, E. L., and Elerding, S. C. A feasibility study of computer aided diagnosis in appendicitis. Surg. Gynecol. Obstet. *155*:685, 1982.
44. Teicher, I., Landa, B., Cohen, M., Kabnick, L. S., and Wise, L. Scoring system to aid in diagnoses of appendicitis. Ann. Surg. *198*:753, 1985.
45. Edwards, F. H., and Davies, R. S. Use of a Bayesian algorithm in the computer-assisted diagnosis of appendicitis. Surg. Gynecol. Obstet. *158*:219, 1984.
46. Diehl, J. T., Eisenstat, M. S., Gillinov, S., and Rao, D. The role of peritoneoscopy in the diagnosis of acute abdominal conditions. Cleve. Clin. Q. *48*:325, 1981.
47. Savrin, R. A., and Clatworthy, H. W., Jr. Appendiceal rupture: a continuing diagnostic problem. Pediatrics *63*:37, 1979.
48. Schwartz, M. Z., Tapper, D., and Solenberger, R. I. Management of perforated appendicitis in children. The controversy continues. Ann. Surg. *197*:407, 1983.
49. Gill, M. A., Chenella, F. C., Heseltine, P. N. R., Appleman, M. D., Yellin, A. E., Berne, T. V., Feldman, M. J., and Sharon, D. Cost analysis of antibiotics in the management of perforated or gangrenous appendicitis. Am. J. Surg. *151*:200, 1986.
50. Gaffney, P. R. Wound infections in appendicitis: effective prophylaxis. World J. Surg. *8*:287, 1984.
51. Paull, D. L., and Bloom, P. Appendiceal abscess. Arch. Surg. *117*:1017, 1982.
52. Skoubo-Kristensen, E., and Hvid, I. The appendiceal mass. Results of conservative management. Ann. Surg. *196*:584, 1982.
53. Hoffman, J., Lindhard, A., and Jensen, H. -E. Appendix mass: conservative management without interval appendectomy. Am. J. Surg. *148*:379, 1984.
54. Buchman, T. G., and Zuidema, G. D. Reasons for delay of the diagnosis of acute appendicitis. Surg. Gynecol. Obstet. *158*:260, 1984.
55. Crabbe, M. M., Norwood, S. H., Robertson, H. D., and Silva, J. S. Recurrent and chronic appendicitis. Surg. Gynecol. Obstet. *163*:11, 1986.
56. Lee, A. W., Bell, R. M., Griffen, W. O., Jr., and Hagihara, P. F. Recurrent appendiceal colic. Surg. Gynecol. Obstet. *161*:21, 1985.
57. Ludbrook, J., and Spears, G. F. S. The risk of developing appendicitis. Br. J. Surg. *52*:856, 1965.
58. Strom, P. R., Turkleson, M. L., and Stone, H. H. Safety of incidental appendectomy. Am. J. Surg. *145*:819, 1983.
59. Westermann, C., Mann, W. J., Chumas, J., Rochelson, B., and Stone, M. L. Routine appendectomy in extensive gynecologic operations. Surg. Gynecol. Obstet. *162*:307, 1986.

75

Megacolon: Congenital and Acquired

SIDNEY F. PHILLIPS

DEFINITION AND CLASSIFICATION

Megacolon is a descriptive term which, it has been suggested, should be applied when the diameter of the rectosigmoid colon is greater than 6.5 cm.[1] It encompasses clinical circumstances as diverse as Hirschsprung's disease (congenital megacolon), idiopathic megacolon (resulting from chronic constipation of any cause), and toxic megacolon occurring as a complication of the idiopathic inflammatory bowel diseases or specific infections, such as amebiasis or shigellosis.

Congenital megacolon (Hirschsprung's disease) is colonic dilatation resulting from functional obstruction of the rectum in which there is a congenital absence of intramural neural plexuses (aganglionosis) resulting in a "narrowed segment." Acquired megacolon occurs secondary to any of the causes of constipation discussed under that heading (see pp. 1395–1399) and may be assumed to be present when it can be ascertained that colonic dilatation was not present at some earlier examination. Spastic constipation is usually seen in young and middle-aged adults and often accompanies the irritable bowel syndrome (see pp. 1402–1418). In this disorder it is assumed that spastic contraction of intestinal muscle impedes the transit of intestinal contents. Atonic constipation (colonic inertia) is more common at both ends of the aging spectrum, afflicting children and the elderly. It is this form of constipation that is most commonly associated with acquired megacolon, and in children it can be confused with the congenital condition.

A subset of patients acquire megacolon as part of a generalized pseudo-obstruction (see p. 337). They may have a neurologic disorder, albeit often of poorly documented type. Infection with *Trypanosoma cruzi* (Chagas' disease) is best known. Included also in this category are other neuromuscular disorders of uncertain cause, such as variants of the type IIb familial endocrine adenomatosis (Sipple's syndrome), diseases associated with autonomic denervation, and degenerations of muscle (systemic sclerosis, amyloid, and so forth) (see pp. 505–511). When more acute and associated with a specific event (abdominal or orthopedic surgery, spinal cord injuries, serious cardiovascular or other medical problems), the term Ogilvie's syndrome is often applied.

CONGENITAL MEGACOLON (HIRSCHSPRUNG'S DISEASE)

Hirschsprung's disease becomes apparent shortly after birth when the infant passes little meconium and develops a distended colon (Fig. 75–1). Digital examination of the rectum, insertion of a rectal tube, or administration of a small enema may result in a gush of retained fecal material with apparent relief of the symptoms. This respite is short-lived, however; signs of partial obstruction return, with persistent vomiting and distention as the major features. In about 20 per cent of patients diarrhea persists; it is caused by pseudomembranous enterocolitis that develops as a complication of the obstruction.

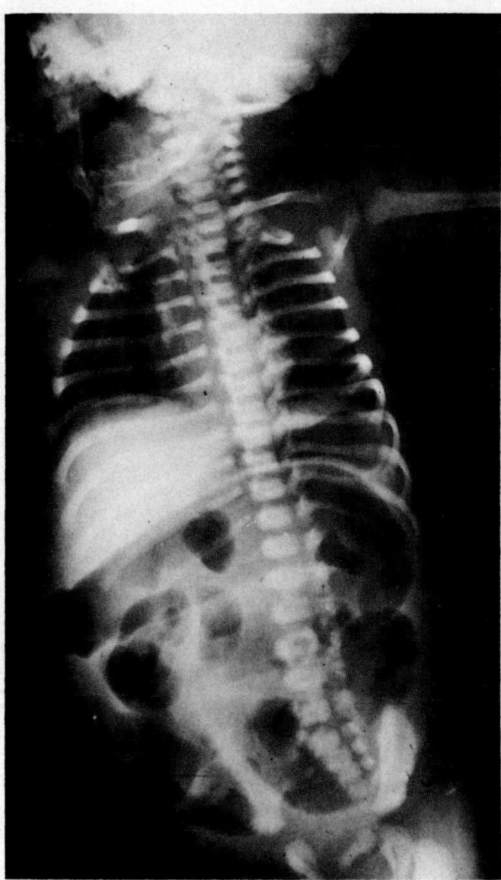

Figure 75–1. Plain film of neonate with colonic distention and retention of meconium caused by aganglionosis of the colon (Hirschsprung's disease). (Courtesy of H. I. Goldberg, M.D.)

Later in life, the presentation is less dramatic and may *not* mimic acute intestinal obstruction. Severe constipation and recurrent fecal impactions are more common. Children occasionally show evidence of anemia, and even malnutrition and hypoproteinemia from protein-losing enteropathy; their resistance to infections can also be impaired. Although most children have major difficulties before the second month of life, very short segment aganglionosis may not cause severe symptoms until after infancy.

Frequency and Genetics

The defect occurs in approximately one of each 5000 live births and is familial.[2, 3] Seventeen of 326 index males and 13 of 88 females had affected siblings, with an overall frequency of 3.6 per cent among siblings of all index cases.[4] The risk for short segment disease was 5 per cent in brothers and 1 per cent in sisters of index cases; for long segment disease, the risk was 10 per cent irrespective of sex.[3] As the disease was highly lethal until the introduction of curative surgery in 1948, accurate assessment of the frequency in offspring of successfully treated patients is incomplete. Initial observations estimate[3] a risk of 2 per cent for offspring of index cases with short segment disease, but a higher risk when the parent's disease involved a long segment. Consanguinity of parents is exceptional, and only three such instances have been reported in a study of 326 patients. The disease is reported as being discordant in dizygotic twins and concordant in monozygotic twins.

Association of congenital aganglionosis of the colon with Down's syndrome is ten times more frequent than would be expected by chance.[4] Approximately 2 per cent of the patients with congenital megacolon have Down's syndrome. Other anomalies reported to be associated with congenital megacolon include hydrocephalus, ventricular septal defect, cystic deformities and agenesis of the kidney, cryptorchidism, diverticulum of the urinary bladder, imperforate anus, Meckel's diverticulum, hypoplastic uterus, polyposis of the colon, ependymoma of the fourth ventricle, and the Laurence-Moon-Biedl-Bardet syndrome. It has been proposed that Hirschsprung's disease is only one feature of more generalized abnormal development of the neural crest.[5]

Pathogenesis and Pathology

Aganglionosis is thought to result from arrest of the caudad migration of cells from the neural crest; these

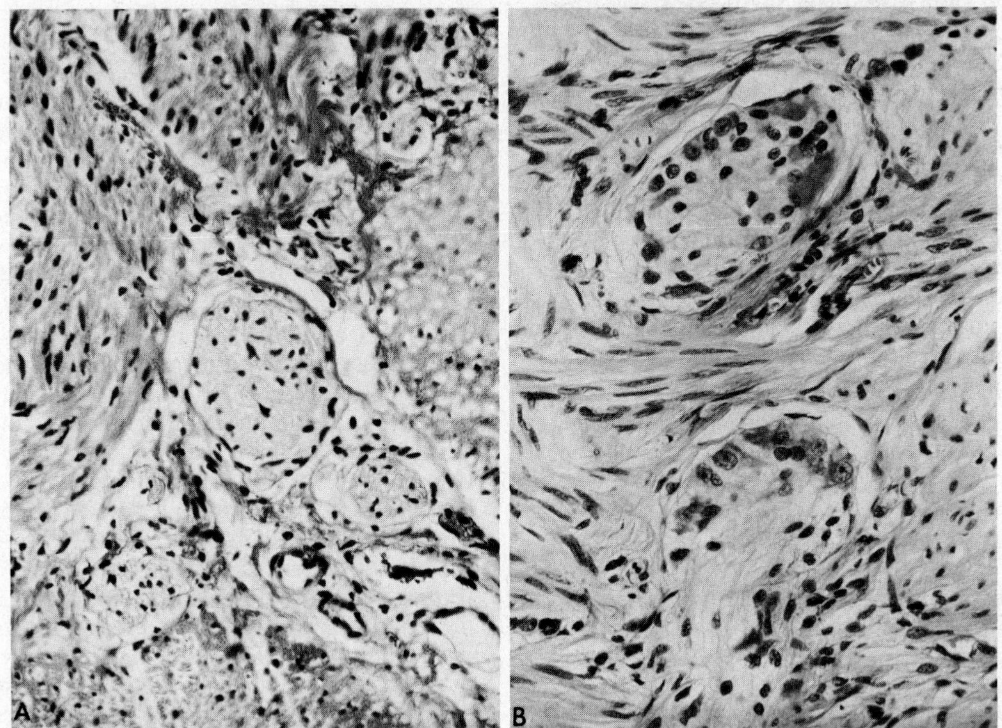

Figure 75–2. *A,* Biopsy of rectum in a patient with Hirschsprung's disease, showing Auerbach's plexus at center with neural elements but absence of ganglion cells. Hematoxylin and eosin stain, × 200. *B,* Normal specimen at same magnification and staining techniques, showing ganglion cells within plexus.

are the cells that are destined to develop as intramural plexuses. However, a separate, caudal origin for ganglion cells is also possible.[6] The aganglionic segment always extends from the internal anal sphincter for a variable distance proximally. In most instances, the aganglionic segment is within the rectum and sigmoid colon; involvement of very short segments, affecting only the region of the anal sphincters, has also been described. The aganglionic segment is permanently contracted, causing dilation proximal to it. A longer aganglionic segment affects less than 20 per cent of individuals. Involvement of the entire colon is infrequent, and reports of aganglionosis extending proximally, throughout the entire small intestine, are rare. Thus, the hallmark of diagnosis (Fig. 75–2) is the absence of ganglion cells from the myenteric and submucosal plexuses, as seen on a full-thickness or suction (mucosal-submucosal) biopsy of the rectum (see p. 1393). Proximal contents fail to enter the unrelaxed, aganglionic segment; although longer aganglionic segments tend to produce more dramatic syndromes, the condition of some patients with short segment disease deteriorates rapidly.

Morphologically, ganglion cells are absent from the narrowed segment and for a variable distance (usually 1 to 5 cm) into the dilated segment. The pattern of nerve fibers is also abnormal, being hypertrophied with abundant, thickened bundles. Specific stains for acetylcholinesterase have been used to highlight the abnormal morphology. Adrenergic denervation of the dilated segment is another prominent but inconsistent finding, as is decreased innervation by peptidergic tissues (containing vasoactive intestinal peptide, substance P, enkephalins, and probably other peptides). Experimentally, an inherited aganglionosis in mice is thought to be mediated by loss of spontaneously active inhibitory neurons. At this time, however, no unifying neurophysiologic defect can be identified.[7]

Pathophysiology

The most characteristic abnormality of aganglionosis is a failure of relaxation of the internal anal sphincter after rectal distention.[8] In health, a rectal inhibitory reflex is demonstrable; transient distention of a balloon in the rectum decreases the intraluminal pressure at the level of the internal sphincter, often accompanied by a reflex contraction of the external sphincter (Fig. 75–3). Although up to 20 per cent of normal children may have a falsely absent reflex, especially if they are premature or of low birth weight, a positive response is strong evidence against Hirschsprung's disease. Resting pressure in the sphincter is normal or slightly elevated in aganglionosis, and in some instances the response of the internal sphincter to rectal distention is an inappropriate contraction.

Another pathophysiologic aspect of colorectal motility in aganglionosis is a failure of the contracted segment to relax after administration of parasympathomimetic agents; by contrast, the innervated or dilated segment was able to relax in aganglionosis (four of six patients) and in most healthy controls.[9]

A third abnormality described recently in Hirsch-

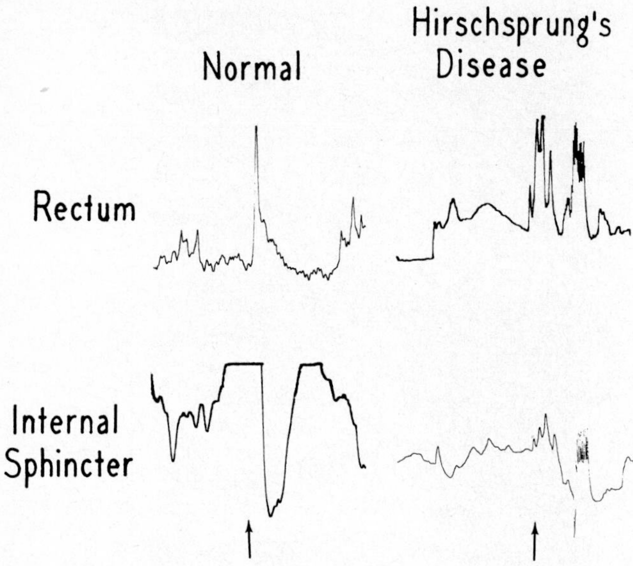

Figure 75–3. Response of rectum and internal sphincter to distention (*arrows*) of rectal balloon in normal control subject and in an infant with Hirschsprung's disease.

sprung's disease is a "stiff" rectal wall. This increased resistance to stretch was noted even in the dilated, uncontracted bowel; moreover, the greater the degree of stiffness, the more severe was the clinical picture.[10] Whether these changes relate to properties of connective or contractile tissues is unknown.

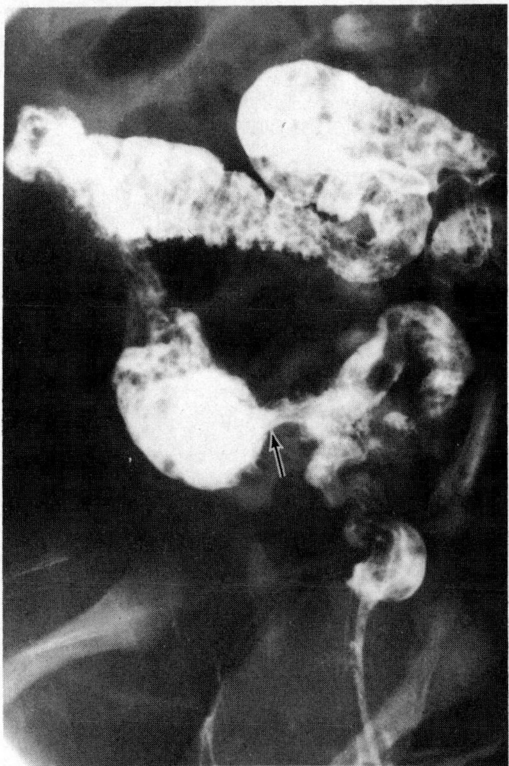

Figure 75–4. Barium enema in 11-month-old child with Hirschsprung's disease, showing transition zone *(arrow)* between dilated proximal and narrowed distal segments.

Clinical Picture

In most instances, regardless of the eventual severity of the clinical picture, the initial passage of meconium is delayed 48 hours or more after birth. One of every four patients with meconium plugs ultimately proves to have congenital megacolon. Vomiting ensues if there is no relief after 48 to 72 hours. Although plain films demonstrate dilated gas- and fluid-filled loops, delineation of small and large bowels is difficult in the newborn, and the films often are not diagnostic (see Fig. 75–1). Digital examination usually reveals no stool in the rectum, but withdrawal of the finger or passage of a rectal tube may lead to a gush of meconium and to decompression. Barium enema may not be diagnostic initially, because sufficient time may not have elapsed in a newborn infant for the characteristic transition zone (narrowed segment), from aganglionic to dilated segments, to develop (Fig. 75–4).

The subsequent clinical course varies. Some infants continue with complete obstruction, do not pass any meconium, and require surgery in the first few weeks of life. In others, there is recurrent, delayed or incomplete obstruction, usually relieved by repeated enemas after the second or third day of life. As a third manifestation, repeated enemas for continuing partial obstruction are suddenly followed by bloody diarrhea heralding the development of fulminant enterocolitis. In addition to neonatal bowel obstruction by a meconium plug and enterocolitis, neonatal perforation of the appendix occurs occasionally. At surgery, an uninflamed but perforated appendix is found, which, on histologic examination, may show diminution or absence of ganglion cells.

The syndrome among older infants and children, especially those with shorter segments of aganglionosis, features persistent abdominal distention, recurrent fecal impaction, and constipation. The picture is that of distal bowel obstruction. Large quantities of inspissated feces collect at the upper border of the aganglionic segment, progressively distending the bowel and slowly obstructing the more proximal portion of the bowel. Stercoral ulcers are caused by pressure of the fecal mass on the bowel wall. Rarely, these ulcers bleed or are associated with malnutrition and protein exudation; occasionally they may perforate. The initial presentation in those instances in which the entire colon is aganglionic is similar to distal aganglionosis, except that the abdomen may not be distended, and barium enema will then reveal a microcolon.

Acute enterocolitis[11, 12] is the most serious complication of Hirschsprung's disease. Ulceration and necrosis begin in the dilated segment and may extend into the small intestine. Perforation, pericolic abscess, and septicemia may follow and, in a more chronic form, anorexia and exudative enteropathy develop. The bowel must be decompressed and placed at rest while fluids and blood are replaced by vein; broad antibiotic coverage is also given. Under these circumstances, most surgeons advise deferring definitive surgery for aganglionosis for at least six months.

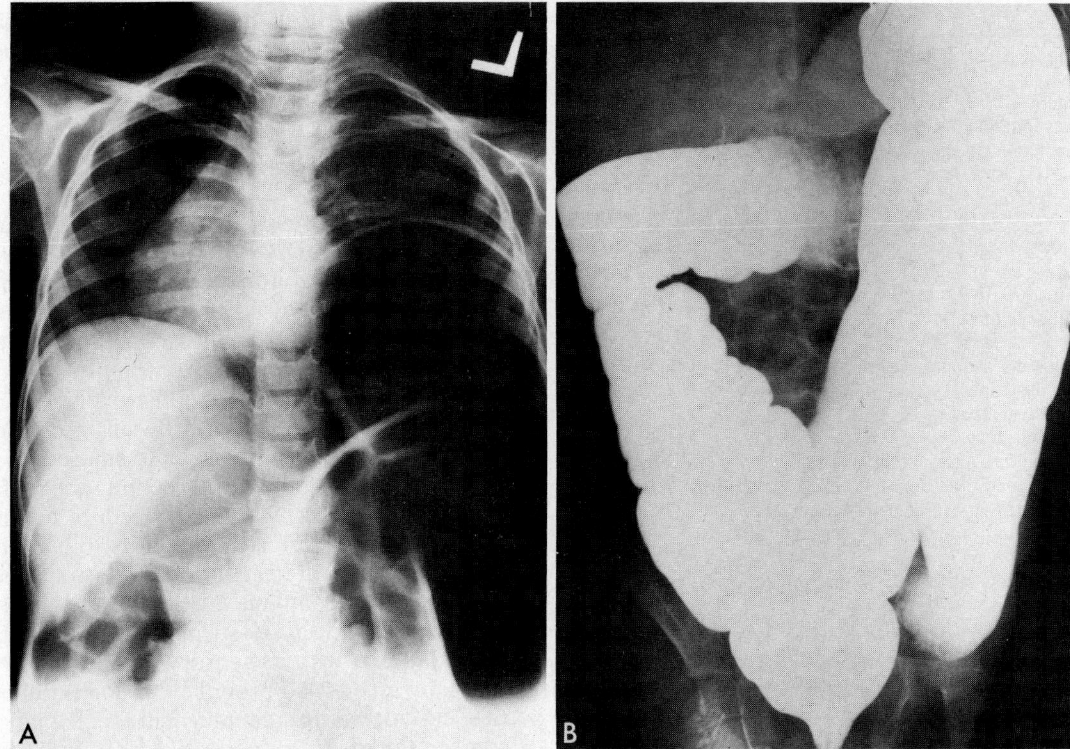

Figure 75–5. *A,* Plain film in seven-year-old boy with acquired megacolon and severe obstipation, showing enormous enlargement of colon with elevation of left hemidiaphragm and mediastinal shift. *B,* Barium enema in same patient, showing marked dilatation of entire colon, including rectal segment.

Differential Diagnosis. Congenital aganglionosis must be distinguished in the neonate from other causes of intestinal obstruction, such as intestinal atresias and imperforate anus. Later, acquired (secondary) megacolon is the major other consideration (Table 75–1 and Fig. 75–5). The diagnosis of congenital aganglionosis usually is not difficult beyond the neonatal period. Obstipation, with infrequent spontaneous passage of stool, dates from infancy, and the rectal examination reveals an empty ampulla. In extreme instances, the abdominal wall is stretched and the venous pattern is prominent; large fecal masses may be palpable over the left colon.

Barium enema X-ray will confirm the diagnosis if the characteristic transition from the narrowed distal rectal or rectosigmoid segment to the more dilated proximal portion of the colon is seen (Fig. 75–4). This finding is usually best demonstrated in a lateral view. However, when the aganglionic segment is very short, a narrowed segment will not be seen radiographically. Among patients with acquired megacolon, dilation extends all the way to the anus, and a transition zone is not seen (Fig. 75–5).

Proctosigmoidoscopy reveals a normal but empty rectum. The dilated proximal bowel, if within range of the endoscope, is easily traversed except for feces in the dilated lumen; occasionally, stercoral ulcers may be noted. The key findings are the empty lower segment and no evidence of organic obstruction.

In doubtful cases, the diagnosis requires a full-thickness biopsy of the rectum. The presence of normal numbers of ganglion cells excludes the diagnosis. Mucosal suction biopsy, satisfactory in many instances, is the initial procedure of choice, because it is performed easily and requires no anesthesia. If the depth of the examination is sufficient to show the presence of ganglia in Meissner's (submucosal) plexus, Hirschsprung's disease is excluded. Absence of ganglion cells in such a specimen does not establish the diagnosis and should be followed by a full-thickness biopsy obtained at least 3 cm proximal to the pectinate line. Diminution or absence of ganglion cells *distal* to this point is difficult to interpret. Careful measurements proximal to the internal sphincter have suggested that myenteric ganglia may be absent in normal infants over a distance of 4 to 5 mm in this segment; none may be seen in the deep submucosal layer for 7 to 10 mm and in the superficial submucosal layer for 10 to 20 mm. Immunohistochemical techniques appear to be helpful in highlighting the morphologic abnormalities, which feature an abundance of hyperplastic axons but absence of ganglion cells. Several approaches, using acetylcholinesterase, neuron-specific enolase, and neural filament antibodies, have been described.[6, 13–16]

Physiologic tests may aid in diagnosis in doubtful cases; these may be crucial when the aganglionic segment is short, less easily detectable by X-ray, and also likely to be missed by biopsy. The most important pathophysiologic test is the response of the anal sphincters to distention of the rectum. In contrast to the response in normal individuals and in patients with acquired megacolon, the internal sphincter in patients

Table 75–1. CAUSES OF MEGACOLON

Congenital Megacolon (Hirschsprung's Disease)
Classic type
Short segment
Ultra-short segment
Total colonic aganglionosis, zonal loss of ganglia and other variants
Acquired Megacolon
Idiopathic
In children
In adults
Acute form (Ogilvie's syndrome)
Psychogenic constipation
Neurologic diseases
Parkinson's disease and central nervous system dysfunction
Myotonic dystrophy
Diabetic neuropathy
Chagas' disease
Other (gangliomatosis, familial autonomic dysfunction)
Intestinal pseudo-obstruction ("neurogenic"forms)
Diseases involving intestinal smooth muscle
Scleroderma and other collagen vascular diseases
Amyloidosis
Intestinal pseudo-obstruction ("myogenic" forms)
Metabolic diseases
Hypothyroidism
Hypokalemia, porphyria
Diabetes mellitus
Pheochromocytoma (with ganglioneuromatosis)
Rectoanal pain
Fissures, abscesses
Mechanical obstruction
Drugs

with congenital aganglionosis fails to relax (or even contracts) after distention of the rectum.

One group[17] compared anorectal manometry and histochemistry of a superficial rectal biopsy (stained for acetylcholinesterase); all nine patients with proven aganglionosis had elevated levels of acetylcholinesterase, and all of 15 controls were normal. In a larger number of subjects studied manometrically, 1 of 18 patients had a falsely present rectal inhibitory reflex and 11 of 104 normals had an absent reflex. When results of the two tests were combined, these authors found that the need for deep rectal biopsy for a positive diagnosis was virtually eliminated. However, other authors maintain that a muscular level biopsy is required to exclude the diagnosis of Hirschsprung's disease. The prenatal diagnosis of colonic obstruction by ultrasonography, with Hirschsprung's disease being high on the list of differential diagnoses, has been reported.[18]

Treatment

Once the diagnosis is established, definitive surgery is the treatment of choice. Preliminary decompression by colostomy is often necessary to relieve obstruction or may be required in infants for whom it is decided to postpone definitive surgery. Patients whose aganglionic segments do not extend above the sigmoid often can undergo decompression preoperatively with regular enemas only. However, serious complications may result from the uncontrolled use of evacuating enemas. Large amounts of plain tap water (greater than 2.0 L) are readily absorbed by the dilated, hypertrophied colon, and serious symptoms of water intoxication may result.[19] The use of hypertonic phosphate enemas is also attended by complications; large quantities of water move into the colon while sodium or phosphate, or both, is absorbed.

Surgical Treatment. The main goals of surgery are to establish regular and spontaneous defecation, to maintain normal continence, and to avoid interference with sexual potency. The surgical procedure should have essentially no mortality and a minimal morbidity. A number of operations have been proposed to remove or to counterbalance the obstructing effect of the aganglionic segment. In the Swenson operation, normally innervated colon is anastomosed to an aganglionic segment of the distal rectum, above the internal sphincter.[20, 21] The Duhamel procedure retains the wall of the distal rectal segment as a blind pouch, and normally innervated colon is anastomosed end-to-side.[22] In the technique of Soave, the mucosa of the aganglionic rectum is stripped off, the surrounding muscular coat with its sensory reflexes is retained, and normally innervated propulsive colon is pulled through this cuff down to the mucocutaneous junction.[23] In some mild cases, associated with aganglionosis of a very short segment, anal myectomy (which is in effect an extended internal anal sphincterotomy) has been successful.[24] The choice of operation (Fig. 75–6) should

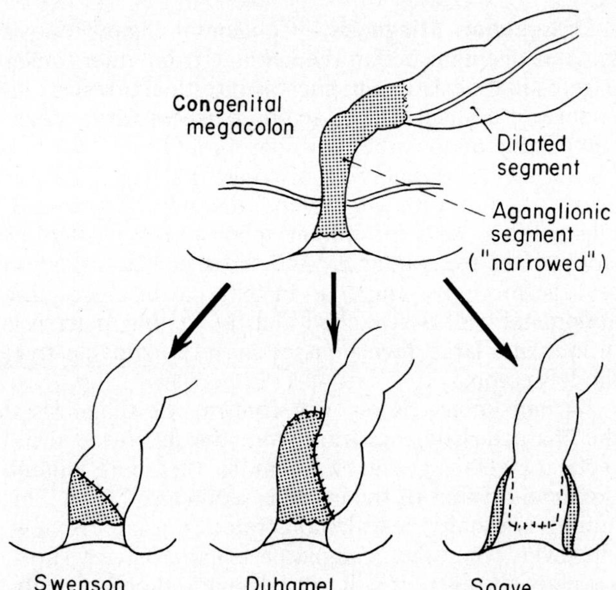

Figure 75–6. The Swenson proçedure includes removal of the distal aganglionic segment to the dentate line posteriorly, leaving a 2.0-cm segment of abnormal bowel anteriorly. Normally innervated colon is pulled down and sutured to the remaining bowel. The Duhamel procedure involves excision of the aganglionic segment above the peritoneal reflection and closure of the distal rectal stump. Normally innervated proximal colon is then anastomosed end-to-side with the posterior aspect of the aganglionic rectal stump. Half the circumference of the new rectal segment is aganglionic, half is normal colon. The Soave procedure is an endorectal mucosal proctectomy with the rectal muscle layer left in place. Normally innervated colon is pulled through the aganglionic cuff and sutured to the dentate line.

be left to an experienced surgeon, who will have good results.[25, 26]

Variants of Congenital Megacolon

The spectrum of Hirschsprung's disease has widened considerably, and patients with a compatible clinical picture may have an ultra-short segment of aganglionosis (involving only the internal anal sphincter, which requires physiologic testing for the diagnosis), patchy or zonal loss of ganglia (ladder pattern), or abnormal or dysplastic neurons.[27, 28] These reports point out the vagaries attendant on superficial, mucosal-submucosal suction biopsies and the difficulties encountered in their histologic interpretation. Indeed, cases of so-called acquired aganglionosis have been reported in which ganglia have been seen retrospectively in tissues removed at an initial operation, but, when clinical failure has led to further surgery, an aganglionic segment is clearly demonstrable. It seems just as likely, however, that the aganglionic segment was missed on the initial biopsies. Furthermore, with greater awareness of the more subtle morphologic and physiologic abnormalities, it is not surprising that previously undiagnosed Hirschsprung's disease is being detected more often in adults.[29] The clinical, physiologic, and morphologic features in adults are usually similar to those of the milder form of the disease that are recognized earlier in life. Thus, congenital megacolon should be subdivided into the classic form, short segment types, ultra-short segments, and other variants (Table 75–1).

ACQUIRED MEGACOLON

The best proof that megacolon in a given patient has an acquired basis is the demonstration that megacolon did not exist on a previous evaluation. Unfortunately, this information usually is not available, and megacolon must be assumed to be acquired if there is no detectable congenital abnormality (aganglionosis, atresia, or stricture) or if symptoms of constipation did not appear in early infancy. Once megacolon is judged to be acquired, it is necessary to establish whether or not an underlying, and possibly treatable, cause exists (Table 75–2).

Table 75–2. DIFFERENTIATING TYPES OF MEGACOLON IN CHILDREN

	Congenital	Acquired
Early history		
Neonatal failure of bowel movement	+	±
Passage of small, hard stools	±	+
Visible straining with bowel movement	−	+
Presence of early enterocolitis	+	−
Later history		
Evidence of voluntary withholding	−	+
Overflow soiling	−	+
Physical and laboratory findings		
Palpable stool at internal sphincter	−	+
Fecal impaction (physical examination and X-ray)	+	+
Dilated colon on barium enema	+	+
Transition zone on X-ray	+	−
Aganglionosis on biopsy	+	−
Abnormal motility responses	+	−
Absent internal sphincter reflex	+	−
Inconsistent response to parasympathomimetic agents	+	−

Idiopathic Megacolon

The terms functional megacolon, psychogenic megacolon, and pseudo-Hirschsprung's disease have been applied to this entity, but the term idiopathic megacolon appears more appropriate, because it makes clear that the cause is not known. It afflicts mainly the young (first and second decades) and the elderly (seventh decade and beyond).

Megacolon in Children. Most cases of megacolon presenting after infancy are associated with "sluggish" colonic activity, for which no clear cause can be determined. Moreover, many patients with this disorder have been on an extensive laxative program for prolonged periods; thus, it is difficult to determine the role that laxatives may have played in the causation and course of the constipation and colonic dilatation. However, many young patients with idiopathic megacolon have a history of constipation beginning during the first month of life. This implies, but does not prove, a physiologic abnormality that was present at birth, perhaps even a functional abnormality of neurons. Moreover, like Hirschsprung's disease, these conditions are more common in boys. Encopresis (fecal incontinence) is the hallmark of idiopathic megacolon and appears in about half the cases, whereas this symptom is absent in Hirschsprung's disease.

There is evidence that a form of megacolon exists in children in whom no neuromuscular abnormality can be demonstrated. It is still uncertain whether or not some of these infants have an ultra-short segment of aganglionic bowel; however, the basis appears to be organic, as (1) the history begins during the first few months of life, (2) the family history is often positive, (3) a congenital syndrome of constipation, abdominal pain, and a specific fingerprint pattern has been reported,[30] and (4) related psychopathology is absent. Thus, just as physical stature and the patterns of striated muscle development can be inherited, variable patterns of colonic motility may also be heritable. This does not negate the psychologic influences of subtle attitudinal factors in certain family constellations (Fig. 75–7).

The major differential diagnosis at this stage is aganglionic megacolon (Table 75–1). Rectosphincteric manometry is at present the most reliable means of establishing this diagnosis and may be the only accurate means of diagnosis in ultra-short segment aganglionosis. The other major diagnostic techniques, full-thickness biopsy and barium enema, are most accurate when a positive finding is present. Histology is more accurate in diagnosing idiopathic megacolon and in ruling out Hirschsprung's disease (i.e., when ganglion cells are present). Barium enema is more accurate in diagnosing

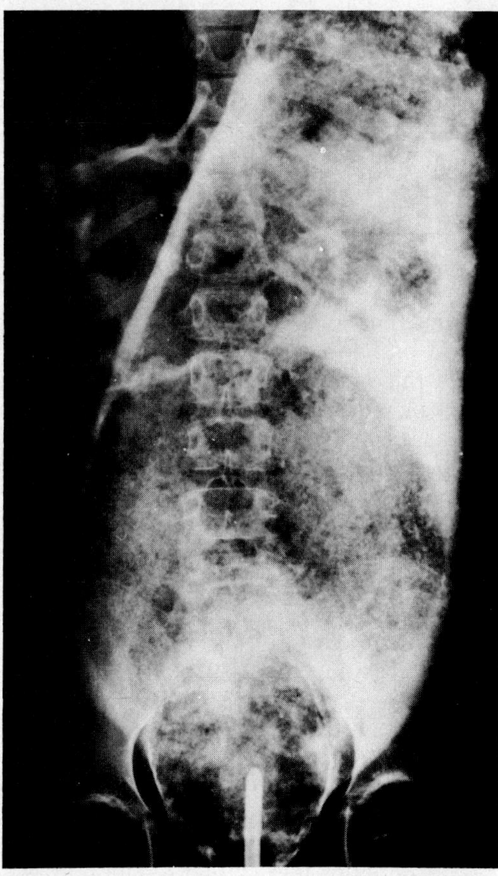

Figure 75–7. Barium enema in a young child with acquired (psychogenic) megacolon. Entire rectum is markedly dilated down to the anal sphincter. (Courtesy of H. I. Goldberg, M.D.)

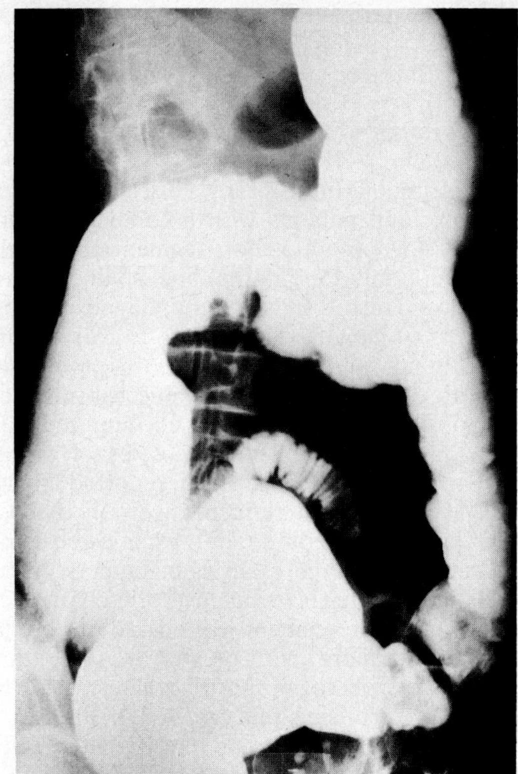

Figure 75–8. Barium enema in patient with lifelong cathartic abuse (cascara sagrada), showing dilated colon with absent haustra simulating ulcerative colitis. (Courtesy of H. I. Goldberg, M.D.)

Hirschsprung's disease and in ruling out idiopathic megacolon (i.e., when a narrowed [aganglionic] segment is revealed by the films).

Megacolon in Adults. In megacolon of the elderly the entire colon appears dilated; stool mixed with air is often seen in the right colon on plain film; and the stool felt in the dilated rectal ampulla often is quite hard. All of these features suggest a different mechanism from the idiopathic megacolon of younger persons. Some younger adults also describe the late onset of constipation. Fecal impaction and overflow incontinence are also more frequent in this group than in those whose constipation begins during infancy and in whom abnormal morphology of the myenteric plexus also suggests aganglionosis.

In these adults it is not known what role laxative abuse,[31] decreased physical activity, and altered dietary habits play in the pathogenesis of their symptoms (Fig. 75–8). Underlying and potentially treatable diseases must be carefully excluded (Table 75–2). Adults whose symptoms begin in infancy occasionally can be diagnosed as having Hirschsprung's disease that was previously missed.[29]

Psychogenic Constipation

Psychogenic constipation is divisible into three types of severe constipation, each of which may be associated with megacolon: pseudo-, neurotic, and psychotic.

Pseudo-Constipation. Pseudo-constipation is quite common, often being based on misconstrued beliefs fostered by advertisements that exalt the virtues of "regularity." As a result, many persons have a misconception that there is a magical number of bowel movements that constitutes normality, usually one per day, although some think that multiple daily stools are necessary. It is sad, indeed, when a patient's misconceptions are responsible for constipation and even megacolon, but it is tragic when these misconceptions cause megacolon in offspring. Some of this group may respond to a simple educational approach and withdrawal of medications but, for others, a comprehensive program of bowel retraining may be necessary.

Neurosis. When megacolon results from faulty habits based on a more deep-seated neurosis, insight therapy may be required. Megacolon may be associated with pseudocyesis or may result from an obsessive-compulsive neurosis. Defecatory urges may be suppressed because of a desire to avoid toilet facilities outside the patient's own home. Neurotic symptoms of this type may require formal psychotherapy.

Psychosis. Constipation is a fairly common occurrence in patients with schizophrenia or severe depression.[32, 33] Many psychopharmacologic agents, including phenothiazines and diazepam (Valium), inhibit gastrointestinal motility either directly or via the central nervous system and may therefore contribute to constipation. When constipation attains serious proportions and produces anorexia, abdominal distention, and fecal impaction, laxatives or enema programs are necessary. Recurrent sigmoid volvulus (usually associated with dolichocolon and a loose redundant mesentery) has been reported in patients institutionalized in mental hospitals. Permanent reduction often requires a surgical approach. Giant megacolon in the insane[32] may present with symptoms of large bowel obstruction, obstipation, abdominal pain, nausea, vomiting, and marked abdominal distention. Bowel sounds are hyperactive; fecal impactions of soft but tenacious stool may be present. Sphincter tone is often diminished. Plain films of the abdomen demonstrate large quantities of fecal material in a colon that is distended throughout its entire length. Enema solutions that are not isotonic can cause water intoxication with acute cardiopulmonary embarrassment and even death. Ganglion cells are present, but the muscular wall may be hypertrophied and the colon is prone to recurrent volvulus. Although it may be treated conservatively with maintenance of decompression, subtotal colectomy with ileoproctostomy may be required.

Long-term use of laxatives, especially colonic stimulants such as anthracine derivatives (senna, cascara, aloes), may cause megacolon (Fig. 75–8), perhaps related to an associated degeneration of ganglion cells of the myenteric plexus owing to chronic use of laxatives.[31] Enemas and mineral oil are possibly less likely to induce megacolon; however, the best form of treatment is prevention. Corrective therapy comprises a program that avoids medications as much as possible and replaces them with an increased intake of dietary fiber.

Intestinal Pseudo-obstruction

Intestinal pseudo-obstruction is yet another term applied to syndromes characterized by dilated, nonpropulsive segments of bowel in the absence of mechanical obstruction. It may be idiopathic or secondary (e.g., to progressive systemic sclerosis), and localized involvement of the colon may lead to megacolon. Whereas a variety of esophageal, gastric, and jejunal motor abnormalities have been detected by manometric techniques in pseudo-obstruction, little is known about colonic motor function in this disorder. Relatives of patients with primary idiopathic pseudo-obstruction may have radiologic or manometric evidence of abnormal motor patterns. In some variants of the syndrome, an autosomal mode of inheritance has been suggested. Evidence exists to suggest that the smooth muscle itself, the intramural nervous elements, or hormonal regulation of contractility might be the pathophysiologic basis.[34–37]

Pseudo-obstruction syndromes can therefore present as generalized hypomotility of esophagus, stomach, and small and large intestines, or, if more prominent in the large bowel, as megacolon. Dilation and delayed transit may be secondary to an underlying disease (see pp. 377–379), or the primary cause may be within the gut (idiopathic intestinal pseudo-obstruction). Of the primary enteropathies, abnormalities have been localized morphologically[36–40] to smooth muscle (intestinal myopathies) or to the enteric nervous system (intestinal neuropathies).

When it is more acute and related clearly to an underlying process, the term Ogilvie's syndrome[41] has also been applied. In a review of 400 cases of acute pseudo-obstruction of the colon,[42] major predisposing causes included trauma and orthopedic surgery, obstetric procedures, pelvic and abdominal surgery, infections, cardiopulmonary disease, metabolic imbalance, cancer, and neurologic disorders (see p. 1398).

Neurologic Disorders

Parkinsonism and Central Nervous System Dysfunction. The frequency of megacolon in patients with Parkinson's disease is unknown, but it is probably higher than 10 per cent. Many of these patients are on drugs (Artane, Kemadrin, and Cogentin) that have some anticholinergic activity. However, there are isolated case reports of patients with parkinsonism who developed megacolon without receiving any medications for their disease. Factors contributing to the colonic dilatation include deficient tone of the abdominal and diaphragmatic muscles, faulty bowel habits, inadequate fluid intake, and inactivity as a result of invalidism. The frequency of minor autonomic disturbances in parkinsonism has prompted speculation that an autonomic imbalance may also play a role.

Other forms of central nervous system dysfunction (e.g., multiple sclerosis) may feature constipation, which can lead to megacolon. Patients with spinal cord lesions require regular enemas or suppositories to produce automatic defecation, to keep the bowel decompressed, and to avoid overflow incontinence.

Myotonic Dystrophy. Myotonic dystrophy affects the colon; rectosphincteric manometry shows a myotonic

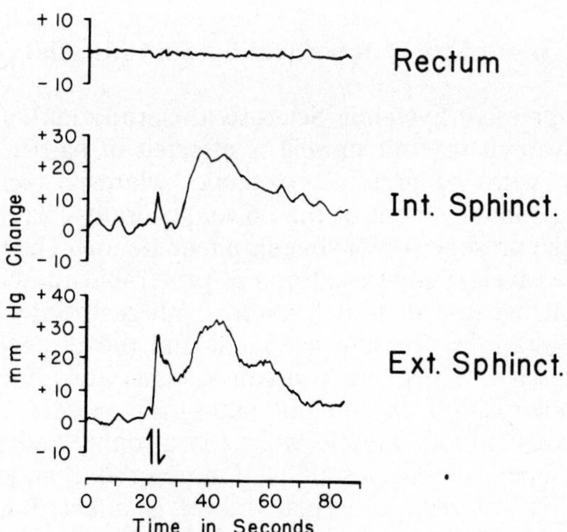

Figure 75–9. Rectosphincteric manometric study in a patient with myotonic dystrophy. Rectal distention *(arrows over time axis)* results in myotonic contraction of high amplitude and prolonged duration in both the internal anal sphincter (smooth muscle) and the external sphincter (striated muscle). (From Harvey, J. C., et al. Am. J. Med. *39*:31, 1965. Used by permission.)

response in both the smooth muscle of the internal anal sphincter and the striated muscle of the external anal sphincter (Fig. 75–9). This is an hereditary disorder transmitted in dominant fashion, characterized early by myotonic contractions of both smooth and striated muscles, and later by muscular weakness and atrophy.

Diabetic Neuropathy. Evidence of a diabetic visceral neuropathy is presumptive when diabetes is complicated by peripheral neuropathy and by orthostatic hypotension. Esophageal motility studies often show diminution of peristaltic contractions in the body of the esophagus. The hallmarks of diabetic visceral neuropathy are gastroparesis and diarrhea, which is often profuse, watery, and nocturnal. They may coexist with megacolon and in some cases with gastric and small bowel dilatation. Unfortunately, instituting good diabetic control does not halt the course of diabetic visceral neuropathy. Its treatment therefore is symptomatic (see pp. 494–500).

Chagas' Disease. Chagas' disease, a disorder seen most commonly in the São Paulo region of Brazil, results from degeneration of the ganglion cells of Auerbach's plexus as a result of trypanosomiasis. The trypanosome, which is transmitted by the bite of the "kissing bug," causes inflammation, atrophy, and fibrosis of the myenteric plexuses of the entire gastrointestinal tract. Megaesophagus and megacolon are common. Contrary to the situation in Hirschsprung's disease, it is the dilated, not the contracted, segment that is aganglionic. For this reason surgical resection is directed toward the dilated portion (the megacolon itself) rather than the normal-appearing segments. Esophageal motility studies suggest that degeneration of 70 per cent or more of ganglion cells must be present before even this very sensitive technique is able to detect an abnormality, and nearly 90 per cent of cells must be damaged before symptoms appear.

Disorders of Intestinal Smooth Muscle

Progressive Systemic Sclerosis (Scleroderma). Gastrointestinal smooth muscle is affected in half of patients with progressive systemic sclerosis (scleroderma); involvement of the bowel generally correlates with the presence of Raynaud's phenomenon. The term progressive systemic sclerosis is preferable to scleroderma, because in some patients with gastrointestinal manifestations the skin is spared and the disorder is progressive. Thus, many organ systems are affected, and sclerosis is an integral pathologic feature. The intestinal smooth muscle is usually atrophic and sclerotic. The esophagus is affected more often than is the small bowel, and the small bowel is affected more often than is the colon (see pp. 505–506).

The classic appearance of the colon on barium enema is pathognomonic for the disease (Fig. 75–10). Large, wide-mouthed pseudodiverticular sacculations (albeit true diverticula, as they are composed of the whole wall thickness) are seen on the inferior margin of the transverse colon and in the descending colon. The internal anal sphincter, composed of smooth muscle, is often involved. Rectosphincteric manometry may be helpful in the differential diagnosis of progressive systemic sclerosis from other collagen vascular disorders, such as dermatomyositis. In the latter, smooth muscle of the internal sphincter is spared, but the striated external sphincter is involved.

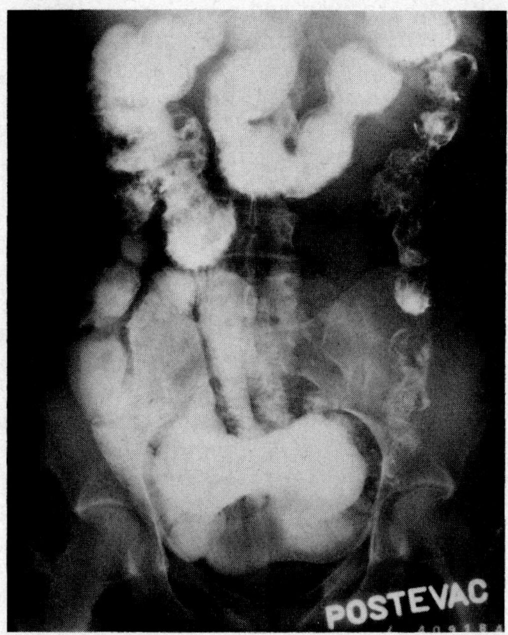

Figure 75–10. Barium enema in a patient with progressive systemic sclerosis, demonstrating wide-mouthed pseudodiverticula characteristic of this disorder.

Amyloidosis. Megacolon may accompany amyloidosis as a result of infiltration of either smooth muscle or nerve. Rectal biopsy establishes the diagnosis and is best performed at a rectal valve with enough underlying submucosa and blood vessels to be stained effectively for deposits of amyloid. Primary amyloidosis may respond to L-phenylalanine mustard therapy, whereas amyloidosis that is secondary to chronic underlying inflammatory disorders is more difficult to treat.

Metabolic Disorders

When megacolon complicates a metabolic disorder, early diagnosis is critical, because most metabolic disturbances are treatable, and the associated megacolon may also respond dramatically. Megacolon is frequently seen with cretinism and may occur at any stage of life with hypothyroidism. Because hypothyroidism may be insidious in adults, the diagnosis of this disorder as the cause of severe constipation is often delayed. Thyroid replacement therapy can be dramatically effective (see pp. 489–490).

The megacolon of hypokalemia is usually an acute dilatation that responds readily to decompression and potassium replacement. Treatment of lead poisoning and porphyria may also alleviate the signs and symptoms of associated megacolon. Megacolon with pheochromocytoma has been associated with neurogangliomatosis.[35]

Toxic Megacolon

Toxic megacolon is a recognized and dramatic complication of ulcerative colitis and Crohn's colitis, which is an acute surgical emergency. Its diagnosis and management are described on pages 1327–1358 and 1435–1477.

Spasm from Painful Anal Conditions

Fissures, perirectal abscesses, and hemorrhoidal pain can lead to spasm of the anal sphincters, causing fecal retention, constipation, and megacolon. These conditions are easily missed in the young, and can create difficulty in differential diagnosis with congenital megacolon. The adult-type history of a burning pain during defecation, pruritus ani, and bright red blood around a hard stool will be absent. The diagnosis must be made by careful inspection and confirmed by anoscopy with a side-viewing anoscope; fissures are often missed when an end-viewing instrument is employed. Treatment is directed toward healing the fissure and retraining the bowel, because treating only one aspect of this symptom complex can lead to perpetuating a vicious circle (see pp. 1579–1581).

Stool softeners and laxatives are helpful and sitz baths are employed whenever possible prior to a bowel movement, to help relax sphincter spasm. Wipettes are employed after bathing, with care taken that the area is kept dry subsequently. Hydrocortisone ointment (0.1 per cent) can be applied locally three times a day. When fissures remain bothersome despite medical management, surgical procedures directed toward relief of spasm of the internal sphincter appear to carry the greatest benefit.

Perirectal abscesses can be exquisitely tender and are best detected by palpation of the tender area, which often presents with fluctuation and sometimes can be felt to be warm. Surgical incision and drainage may be required, with subsequent bowel retraining.

Mechanical Obstruction

Lesions intrinsic to the colon occasionally produce mechanical obstruction of a sufficient degree and duration to result in a chronic megacolon that can be treated medically. Thus, anorectal strictures may result from prior surgery or from inflammatory conditions and may respond to dilation.

Radiation proctitis can appear years after pelvic irradiation and may continue to progress. The proctoscopic appearance of radiation proctitis is that of an atrophic mucosa with telangiectases. Pseudo-obstruction, with degeneration of intramural nerves and muscles, has been seen after radiation ileitis.[43] Topical steroid enemas and cautious dilation may be required. When topical steroids are ineffective, low-dose systemic steroids may be tried. For the mucosal bleeding, laser therapy has been effective[44] (see pp. 1379–1380).

Drugs

Constipation is a major side effect of many drugs. When constipating drugs are administered to frail, elderly patients with poor muscular tone, often taking diets low in bulk, severe constipation and even megacolon can develop. Particular attention must be paid to drugs given for psychiatric conditions, anticholinergics, opiates, and tranquilizers.

TREATMENT OF ACQUIRED MEGACOLON AND PSEUDO-OBSTRUCTION

Treatment of acute, nontoxic megacolon (Ogilvie's syndrome) has been facilitated by the technique of colonoscopic decompression. If colonic dilatation is of only moderate degree, nasointestinal suction, fluid replacement, and cessation of all drugs might suffice. More severe cases (colonic diameter greater than 10 cm) are at risk for colonic perforation and will require colonoscopy, without air insufflation but with suction; 80 per cent of patients treated in this way will respond, although some may require more than one procedure.[45] Addition of a decompression tube passed over an endoscopically placed guide wire appears to help further.[46]

The treatment of chronic acquired megacolon is directed toward the underlying disorder whenever a specific therapy is available. In addition, symptomatic treatment must be planned with the primary goals of using the minimal amount of medication for the shortest possible time. Frequent attempts should be made to wean the patient from medication, by decreasing dosage or by substituting milder drugs. Retraining of the bowels is the goal and dietary or therapeutic supplements of fiber, or both, are the primary means of achieving it. Success cannot be anticipated without education of the patient. In all cases it is important to prevent dependency on laxatives; these only obtund normal defecation and lead to increased constipation. Treatment of chronic pseudo-obstruction is symptomatic, and in advanced cases it is not dramatically successful. Antibiotics might be helpful if bacterial overgrowth of the small intestine is prominent. Standard laxatives may be of benefit in milder cases; the muscle stimulant metoclopramide, which stimulates gastric emptying, has little effect on the lower bowel. A new prokinetic agent (Cisapride), naloxone, and cholinergic medications (Urecholine) yield varying degrees of success.[47, 48] Surgery is to be avoided if at all possible, because patients with this disorder withstand surgery very poorly.

General Goals of Treatment

After initial relief of obstruction by laxatives or enemas, the goal is to keep the bowel decompressed and to establish a routine schedule for voluntary evacuation, preferably in response to the physiologic stimulus of the gastroileocolic response to meals. The technique likely to be most successful begins with enemas after breakfast or supper, if the patient has not been able to evacuate voluntarily. This program has the advantage of rapidly establishing the association of the gastrocolic stimulus and response (see pp. 342–344 and 1408–1410).

Treatment is more difficult in the elderly than in the young. Impacted feces may have to be removed or broken up manually. Enemas of mineral oil soften the mass and make evacuation easier and less painful. An exercise program is designed to conform with the patient's physical capabilities. Leg-raising exercises are effective in strengthening abdominal muscles (see pp. 162–169).

Drug therapy for severe constipation and megacolon in the aged is tricky at best. The ultimate goal of therapy should be its elimination, but this goal is rarely realized. Treatment should begin with the simplest laxative, and the aim is to withdraw all except bulking agents. When stools are hard, wetting agents such as dioctyl sodium sulfosuccinate (Colace, Doxinate) may help. These medications not only affect the physical state of stools, they also stimulate intestinal secretion.[49] Lubricants, such as mineral oil, generally are not advisable for long-term use because of the possibilities of damage to the lungs (aspiration in the elderly) or to the liver (fatty changes), or of anal seepage. In selected patients they may be used for short-term management with gradual withdrawal. Harsh cathartics such as castor oil and the anthracine derivates (senna, cascara, aloes, rhubarb, phenolphthalein, and bisacodyl) are best avoided. Long-term administration of some drugs (including senna and cascara) in high doses may cause degeneration of the ganglion cells in the myenteric plexus[31] and result in resistance to continued therapy.

Suppositories exert their actions several ways: (1) by drawing water into the rectum (e.g., glycerin suppositories), (2) by distending the rectum with carbon dioxide (e.g., Vacuetts), or (3) by local stimulation of smooth muscle or ganglion cells (e.g., bisacodyl- or senna-containing suppositories). The primary value of suppositories is the ability to elicit instantaneous action. This immediate effect can be utilized for bowel training to help re-establish gastroileocolic responses after meals. Patients are instructed to attempt to have a bowel movement within 5 minutes after breakfast or supper. If within 5 minutes they are unsuccessful, they take a suppository or enema (see pp. 353–361 and 1414–1415).

Retraining of the colon's function relies mainly on the provision of enough residue to produce stools of sufficient bulk and of the appropriate consistency to stimulate the desire to evacuate and to facilitate the mechanics of defecation. Low residue, "bland colonic" diets should be avoided and patients should be instructed to broaden their dietary selections to include fresh fruit and vegetables daily. After many years of voluntary or iatrogenic restriction of the diet, patients are often resistant to suggestions that their intake of foods be made more normal. Proprietary bulking agents can be very helpful in these circumstances; they are standardized preparations, often based on psyllium seed (Konsyl, Effersyllium, Metamucil, Fiberall). Resistance to their use may be less than to the advice to increase the intake of fiber. However, key to the use of bulking agents is a clear explanation of how such treatments should be used and of the results that are to be expected. Bulking agents are *not* aperients; they are *not* followed by an immediate evacuation. These agents *must* be used every day, preferably as a supplement to each meal, and the dosage must be determined individually.

Dietary Fiber and Fecal Bulk

The role of dietary fiber in normal human nutrition and of the deficiency of fiber as a cause of disease has received considerable attention. The most consistent effect of fiber, and the one that is least controversial, is an increase in fecal bulk; bulking is accompanied by a moderate reduction in the mouth-to-anus transit time.[50, 51]

There is no satisfactory definition of fiber, and methods for its chemical quantification are not well standardized.[50] Trowell proposed that dietary fiber is "skeletal remains of plant cells that are resistant to digestion by enzymes of man."[52] Operationally, this is an adequate definition. Chemically, the major components of fiber are (1) cellulose; (2) hemicellulose; (3) pectins, each of which is a polysaccharide; and (4) lignin, which is not a carbohydrate but a polymer of substituted phenylpropanes. The amounts of these major constituents and of other, minor constituents of fiber vary greatly among similar foods. They even change in the same item of food at various stages of aging or processing. Thus, definition of normal dietary intakes of fiber or the quantification of supplemental fiber is difficult, except by persons working in specialized research laboratories. Bran and other cereal products have received most attention therapeutically.

The mechanism by which fiber increases fecal bulk is twofold. Although many fiber components are resistant to digestion by mammalian enzymes, fiber varies greatly in its susceptibility to hydrolysis by bacterial enzymes. Cereal grains that have highly lignified components (e.g., bran) are resistant to bacterial digestion; they are thought to increase fecal bulk mainly by physicochemical means (i.e., by acting as "sponges" for water, increasing the weight and the water content of stools.[53] Other components of fiber are more susceptible to bacterial degradation, and their availability to the fecal flora as substrate is thought to represent a major source of carbon for bacterial growth. In these instances, fecal bulk is largely accounted for by an increase in the excretion of bacteria.[54, 55]

Role of Surgery

Operative treatment for acquired megacolon is unusual; occasionally a diverting ileostomy or colostomy might be needed for megacolon, and most large centers have experience with partial resections of the colon for otherwise uncontrollable symptoms.

Attention has focused recently on the various syndromes of constipation (with or without megacolon); regional or total colonic inertia has been separated from disorders of fecal evacuation, which appear to involve primarily the muscles of the anal sphincters or those of the pelvic floor, or both. Novel tests for pathophysiologic defects are being developed, and their wider application will increase the therapeutic options, including the possibility of new surgical approaches[56–59] (see pp. 349–361).

References

1. Preston, D. M., Lennard-Jones, J. E., and Thomas, B. M. Towards a radiologic definition of idiopathic megacolon. Gastrointest. Radiol. *10*:167, 1985.
2. Ehrenpreis, T. Hirschsprung's Disease. Chicago, Year Book Medical Publishers, 1970.
3. Carter, C. O., Evans, K., and Hickman, V. J. Children of those treated surgically for Hirschsprung's disease. J. Med. Genet. *18*:87, 1981.
4. Passarge, E. The genetics of Hirschsprung's disease. Evidence for heterogeneous etiology and a study of sixty-three families. N. Engl. J. Med. *276*:138, 1967.
5. Johnston, M. C., Vig, K. W. L., and Ambrose, L. J. H. Neurocristopathy as a unifying concept: clinical correlations. Adv. Neurol. *29*:97, 1981.
6. Tam, P. K. H. An immunochemical study with neuro-specific-enolase and Substance P of human enteric innervation. The normal developmental pattern and abnormal deviations in Hirschsprung's disease and pyloric stenosis. J. Pediatr. Surg. *21*:227, 1986.
7. Christensen, J. Motility of the colon. *In* Johnson, L. R. (ed.). Physiology of the Gastrointestinal Tract. Vol. 1. 2nd edition. New York, Raven Press, 1987, p. 665.
8. Tobon, F., Rein, N. C. R. W., Talbert, J. L., and Schuster, M. M. Nonsurgical test for the diagnosis of Hirschsprung's disease. N. Engl. J. Med. *278*:188, 1968.
9. Davidson, M., Sleisenger, M. H., Steinberg, H., and Almy, T. P. Studies of distal colonic motility in children. III. The pathologic physiology of congenital megacolon (Hirschsprung's disease). Gastroenterology *29*:803, 1955.
10. Arhan, P., Devroede, G. J., Danis, K., Dornic, C., Faverdin, C., Persoz, B., and Pellerin, D. Viscoelastic properties of the rectal wall in Hirschsprung's disease. J. Clin. Invest. *62*:82, 1978.
11. Bill, A. J., Jr., and Chapman, N. D. The enterocolitis of Hirschsprung's disease. Its natural history and treatment. Am. J. Surg. *103*:70, 1962.
12. Fraser, G. C., and Berry, C. Mortality in neonatal Hirschsprung's disease: with particular reference to enterocolitis. J. Pediatr. Surg. *2*:205, 1967.
13. Ikawa, H., Kim, S. H., Hendren, W. H., and Donahoe, P. K. Acetyl choline-esterase and manometry in the diagnosis of the constipated child. Arch. Surg. *121*:435, 1986.
14. Vinores, S. A., May, E. Neuron-specific enolase as an immunohistochemical tool for the diagnosis of Hirschsprung's disease. Am. J. Surg. Pathol. *9*:281, 1985.
15. Kluck, P., Vanmuisen, G. N. P., Vanderkamp, A. W. M., Tibboel, D., Van Hoorn, W. A., Warnaar, S. O., and Moelnaar, J. A. Hirschsprung's disease studied with monoclonal antineurofilament antibodies on tissue section. Lancet *1*:652, 1984.
16. Scallen, C., Puri, P., and Reen, D. J. Identification of rectal ganglion cells using monoclonal antibodies. J. Pediatr. Surg. *20*:37, 1985.
17. Morikawa, Y., Donahoe, P. K., and Hendren, W. H. Manometry and histochemistry in the diagnosis of Hirschsprung's disease. Pediatrics *63*:865, 1979.
18. Vermesh, J., Mayden, K. L., Confino, E., Giglia, R. V., and Gleicher, N. Prenatal sonographic diagnosis of Hirschsprung's disease. J. Ultrasound Med. *5*:37, 1986.
19. Hiatt, R. B. The pathologic physiology of congenital megacolon. Ann. Surg. *133*:313, 1951.
20. Swenson, O. A new surgical treatment for Hirschsprung's disease. Surgery *28*:371, 1950.
21. Swenson, O. Follow-up on 200 patients treated for Hirschsprung's disease during a ten-year period. Ann. Surg. *146*:706, 1957.
22. Duhamel, B. New operation for treatment of Hirschsprung's disease. Arch. Dis. Child. *35*:38, 1960.
23. Soave, F. Hirschsprung's disease: a new surgical technique. Arch. Dis. Child. *39*:116, 1964.
24. Lynn, H. B., and van Heerden, J. A. Rectal myectomy in Hirschsprung's disease. Arch. Surg. *110*:991, 1975.
25. Nixon, H. H. Hirschsprung's disease: Progress in management and diagnostics. World J. Surg. *9*:189, 1985.
26. Martin, L. W., and Torres, A. M. Hirschsprung's disease. Surg. Clin. North Am. *65*:1171, 1985.
27. McMahon, R. A., Moore, C. C. M., and Cussen, L. J. Hirschsprung's-like syndromes in patients with normal ganglion cells on suction rectal biopsy. J. Pediatr. Surg. *16*:835, 1981.
28. Nixon, H. H., and Lake, B. "Not Hirschsprung's disease"—rare conditions with some similarities. S. Afr. J. Surg. *29*:97, 1982.
29. Barnes, P. R. H., Lennard-Jones, J. E., Hawley, P. R., and Todd, I. P. Hirschsprung's disease and idiopathic megacolon in adults and adolescents. Gut *27*:534, 1986.
30. Gottlieb, S. H., and Schuster, M. M. Dermatoglyphic (fingerprint) evidence for a congenital syndrome of early onset constipation and abdominal pain. Gastroenterology *91*:428, 1986.
31. Smith, B. Effect of irritant purgatives on the myenteric plexus in man and the mouse. Gut *9*:139, 1968.
32. Watkins, G. L., Oliver, G. A., and Rosenberg, B. F. Giant megacolon in the insane. Subtotal colectomy as the method of management. Ann. Surg. *143*:409, 1961.
33. Ehrentheil, O. F., and Wells, E. P. Megacolon in psychotic patients: clinical entity. Gastroenterology *29*:295, 1955.
34. Faulk, D. L., Anuras, S., and Christensen, J. Chronic intestinal pseudo-obstruction. Gastroenterology *74*:922, 1978.
35. Carney, J. A., Go, V. L. W., Sizemore, G. W., and Hayles, A. B. Alimentary tract ganglioneuromatoses: a major component of the syndrome of multiple endocrine neoplasia, type 2b. N. Engl. J. Med. *295*:1287, 1976.
36. Anuras, S., Mitros, F., Soper, R. T., Pringle, K. C., Maves, B. V., Younoszai, M. K., Franken, E. A., and Whitington, P. Chronic intestinal pseudo-obstruction in young children. Gastroenterology *91*:62, 1986.
37. Anuras, S., Mitros, F. A., Milano, A., Kuminsky, R., Decanio, R., and Green, J. B. A familiar visceral myopathy with dilatation of the entire gastrointestinal tract. Gastroenterology *90*:385, 1986.
38. Krishmamurthy, S., Schuffler, M. D., Rohrmann, C. A., and Pope, C. E. Severe idiopathic constipation is associated with a distinctive abnormality of the colonic myenteric plexus. Gastroenterology *88*:26, 1985.
39. Schuffler, M. D., Baird, H. W., Fleming, C. R., Bell, C. E., Bouldin, T. W., Malagelada, J. R., McGill, D. B., LeBauer, S. M., Abrams, M., and Love, J. Intestinal pseudo-obstruction as the presenting manifestation of small cell carcinoma of the lung. Ann. Intern. Med. *98*:129, 1983.
40. Krishmamurthy, S., Schuffler, M. D., Belic, L., and Schweid, A. I. An inflammatory axonopathy of the myenteric plexus producing a rapidly progressive intestinal pseudo-obstruction. Gastroenterology *90*:754, 1986.
41. Ogilvie, H. Large intestinal colic due to sympathetic deprivation: a new clinical syndrome. Br. Med. J. *2*:671, 1948.
42. Vanek, V. W., and Al-Salti, M. Acute pseudo-obstruction of the colon (Ogilvie's syndrome): an analysis of 400 cases. Dis. Colon Rectum *29*:203, 1986.
43. Perino, L. E., Schuffler, M. D., Mehta, S. J., and Everson, G. T. Radiation induced intestinal pseudo-obstruction. Gastroenterology *91*:994, 1986.

44. Ahlquist, D. A., Gostout, C. J., Viggiano, T. R., and Pemberton, J. H. Laser therapy for severe radiation induced rectal bleeding. Mayo Clin. Proc. *61*:927, 1986.
45. Bode, W. E., Beart, R. W., Spencer, R. J., Culp, C. E., Wolff, B. G., and Taylor, B. M. Colonoscopic decompression of acute pseudo-obstruction of the colon. Am. J. Surg. *147*:243, 1984.
46. Lavignolle, A., Jutel, P., Bonhomme, J., Cloarec, D., Cerbelaud, P., Lehur, P. A., Galmiche, J. P., and LeBodic, L. Syndrome d'Ogilvie: resultats de l'exsufflation endoscopique dans une série de 29 cas. Gastroentest. Clin. Biol. *10*:147, 1986.
47. Camilleri, M., Brown, M. L., Malagelada, J.-R. Impaired transit of chyme in chronic intestinal pseudo-obstruction. Correction by Cisapride. Gastroenterology *91*:619, 1986.
48. Schang, J. C., and Devroede, G. Beneficial effects of naloxone in a patient with intestinal pseudo-obstruction. Am. J. Gastroenterol. *80*:407, 1985.
49. Saunders, D. R., Sillery, J., and Rachmilewitz, D. Effect of dioctyl sodium sulfosuccinate on structure and function of rodent and human intestine. Gastroenterology *69*:380, 1975.
50. Spiller, G. A., and Amen, R. J. (eds.). Fiber in Human Nutrition. New York, Plenum Press, 1976.
51. Spiller, G. A., and Kay, R. M. (eds.). Medical Aspects of Dietary Fiber. New York, Plenum Press, 1980.
52. Trowell, H. C. Crude fiber, dietary fiber and atherosclerosis. Atherosclerosis *16*:138, 1972.
53. Eastwood, M. A., Brydon, W. G., and Tadesse, K. Effect of fiber on colon function. *In* Spiller, G. A., and Kay, R. M. (eds.). Medical Aspects of Dietary Fiber. New York, Plenum Press, 1980.
54. Cummings, J. H., and Stephen, A. M. The role of dietary fiber in the human colon. Can. Med. Assoc. J. *123*:1109, 1980.
55. Stephen, A. M., and Cummings, J. H. The microbial contribution to human fecal mass. J. Med. Microbiol. *13*:45, 1980.
56. Read, N. W., Timms, J. M., Barfield, L. J., Connolly, T. C., and Bannister, J. J. Impairment of defecation in young women with severe constipation. Gastroenterology *90*:53, 1986.
57. Shouler, P., and Keighley, M. R. B. Changes in colorectal function in severe idiopathic chronic constipation. Gastroenterology *90*:414, 1986.
58. Preston, D. N., and Lennard-Jones, J. W. Severe chronic constipation of young women: idiopathic slow transit constipation. Gut *27*:41, 1986.
59. Metcalf, A. M., Phillips, S. F., Zinsmeister, A. R., MacCarty, R. L., Beart, R. W., and Wolff, B. G. Simplified assessment of segmental colonic transit. Gastroenterology *92*:40, 1987.

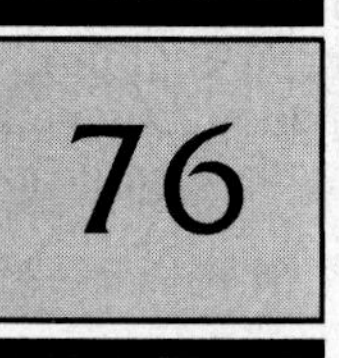

Irritable Bowel Syndrome

MARVIN M. SCHUSTER

The *irritable bowel syndrome* (IBS) is a motor disorder consisting of altered bowel habits, abdominal pain, and the absence of detectable organic pathology. Symptoms are markedly influenced by psychologic factors and stressful life situations. Although diagnosis requires the exclusion of organic diseases, it is confirmed by positive clinical, psychologic, laboratory, and motility findings. Four symptoms that help distinguish IBS from organic disease are (1) visible abdominal distention, (2) relief of abdominal pain by bowel movement, (3) more frequent bowel movements with the onset of pain, and (4) looser stools with onset of pain.

Ninety-one per cent of IBS patients have two or more of these four symptoms, whereas only 30 per cent with organic disease have two or more.[1] Although IBS is a disorder of intestinal motility, the motor dysfunctions recorded in the laboratory correlate only imperfectly with the clinical pattern, and in many instances may be simply exaggerations of normal responses.

IBS is one of the most commonly encountered gastrointestinal disorders, and it is also one of the least understood, in part because it is not a disease but a syndrome composed of a number of conditions with similar manifestations. With new scientific advances, disorders formerly included in this syndrome, such as lactose intolerance causing diarrhea, have been clearly distinguished from IBS. Although other causes will be recognized in the future, it is likely that IBS will remain appropriate for the large proportion of these patients.

Irritable bowel syndrome is the most suitable and accurate term currently available, as it emphasizes that the condition is a motor disorder manifesting irritability, that it is not a single disease but a syndrome, and that many areas of the gut are involved. Many of the other commonly used terms are either inadequate, inaccurate, or both. Nervous colon, unstable colon, and spastic colon are inadequate because they describe only some possible etiologic influences (such as nervous factors) or some signs (e.g., spasticity). Furthermore, they ignore the involvement of areas other than the colon. The terms nervous colitis, spastic colitis, and mucous colitis have two additional faults. They are physiologically incorrect, because inflammation is not present, and they are frightening to the patient because they are easily confused with ulcerative colitis. Therefore, the use of the term "colitis" is to be sharply condemned as both inaccurate and psychologically damaging. Although it may be associated with severe pain and discomfort, IBS does not predispose to other chronic or life-threatening conditions, such as inflammatory bowel disease or cancer, and there is no evidence that it interferes with longevity.

EPIDEMIOLOGY

Although IBS is recognized widely as one of the most commonly encountered gastrointestinal disorders,[2] reliable data on prevalence are not available because the disorder is not reportable, is not fatal (and therefore does not appear on death certificates as a cause of death), and is not well represented in hospital statistics because it rarely requires hospitalization. Nevertheless, IBS was recorded as the primary diagnosis in 96,000 discharges from hospitals in the United States in 1976 and as the secondary diagnosis in an additional 85,000. Another 37,000 hospital discharges that were labeled "psychogenic gastrointestinal disorders" were indistinguishable from IBS. The two groups together utilized hospital beds for 450,000 days and made heavy use of diagnostic facilities.[3] As the vast majority (perhaps as many as 90 per cent) of patients with IBS are never hospitalized for this condition, these statistics underscore the frequent appearance of this disorder. IBS ranks close to the common cold as a leading cause for absenteeism from work due to illness[4]; it is the most common cause for referral to gastroenterologists, constituting 20 to 50 per cent of referred patients. Moreover, surveys of the general population indicate that symptoms that justify the diagnosis of IBS are present in 15 per cent or more of the general population who do not seek medical attention.[5–7]

Female patients outnumber male patients 2:1, and there is a higher incidence among whites than nonwhites and among Jews than non-Jews. The preponderance of women with this diagnosis may reflect patterns of seeking care and referral rather than actual incidence. Symptoms begin before the age of 35 in half of patients, and 40 per cent of patients are 35 to 50 years of age. The disorder is a chronic one, with symptoms that are characteristic for any given patient but vary considerably from patient to patient. The severity may fluctuate and, although remission may last several years, recurrence is the rule.

CLINICAL FEATURES OF IBS

Abdominal pain is generally considered to be an important feature of IBS. As it is assumed (but not proved) that the pain is a result of colonic or intestinal spasm, the disorder is also described as *spastic colon* or *spastic bowel syndrome*.

Painless diarrhea is more likely to be a separate entity than a variant of IBS. Only 2 to 20 per cent of patients with chronically altered bowel habits have painless diarrhea.[8–11] Painless diarrhea is discussed rarely in American and uncommonly in British reports.[12] Although constipation develops slowly and is not recognizable until more than three days have passed between stools, diarrhea appears rapidly and, therefore, may be more easily correlated with emotional and other antecedents; a stressful event can lead to immediately evident diarrhea but not to immediately evident constipation. Therefore, painless diarrhea of this type is called "nervous diarrhea." In addition to being more directly related to specific stressful situations, painless diarrhea also appears to be more isolated and short-lived and more likely to represent a physiologic (rather than pathophysiologic) response to stress. It is a symptom that has been experienced more universally by a healthy population at one time or another under stressful situations and is more likely than the painful form to disappear after stress is removed. However, these features, characteristic of painless diarrhea, are not typical of patients with diarrhea-predominant, painful IBS, whose symptoms are more difficult to relate to immediately preceding stress.

Separation of painless diarrhea from painful irritable bowel syndrome is also based upon physiologic observations of motility recordings, which demonstrate a characteristic response to rectal distention of patients with painful IBS and either diarrhea or constipation—a response not seen in patients with painless diarrhea. In light of the recent recognition that gastrointestinal hormones (e.g., gastrin, VIP) as well as hormones of nongastrointestinal origin (e.g., serotonin from bronchial carcinoid and calcitonin from thyroid medullary carcinomas) can cause painless diarrhea, it is possible that some types of chronic painless diarrhea are a response to such circulating substances.

Altered Bowel Habits

Most patients with irritable bowel syndrome complain of a change in bowel habits beginning in adolescence or early adult life. Only a small number have had lifelong bowel irregularity. The disturbance in bowel function is gradually progressive, eventually developing a characteristic pattern, which for most is one of alternating constipation and diarrhea, with one of these symptoms predominating. The frequency and quality of each symptom, although highly variable from individual to individual, are fairly consistent for a specific patient. The physician's perception of the progressive nature of the disorder may be influenced significantly by a screening bias, as only those patients whose symptoms reach a point of discomfort or disability seek medical attention; the rest accept their symptoms simply as part of their usual living.

Concepts of normal bowel habits not only are extremely variable but also are profoundly influenced by parental and societal attitudes, medical fads, and commercial advertising. The views of an entire generation were molded by radio and, later, television commercials extolling the virtues of regularity, which in the public mind was equated with daily bowel movements. However, the "normal" frequency of defecation ranges widely in the population at large, from three movements per day to three per week[13] (see pp. 331–332).

Patients with constipation predominance may have many days or weeks of constipation interrupted with brief periods of diarrhea. Constipation dating to childhood or adolescence sometimes may be recognized only in retrospect. Some patients report having accepted a weekly bowel movement as a normal pattern until frequency decreased along with progression of other symptoms. Constipation, which at first is episodic, eventually may become continuous and increasingly intractable to laxatives and later to enemas. It is not known whether the increasing laxative requirement results from progression of the underlying disorder or from increasing laxative dependence. Clinical experience suggests that it is the latter. Stools are usually hard, possibly reflecting excessive dehydration due to prolonged retention in the absorbing colon. Often stool caliber is narrow (described as pencil-thin or ribbon-like), presumably because of colonic and rectal spasm. On the other hand, exaggerated haustral contractions, seen on X-ray film and recorded manometrically, can produce scybalous stools described by patients as pellets, marble-like, or small hard balls (Fig. 76–1). Although the number of movements can be documented easily, accounts of consistency and ease of passage are descriptive and depend on the accuracy of the observer.

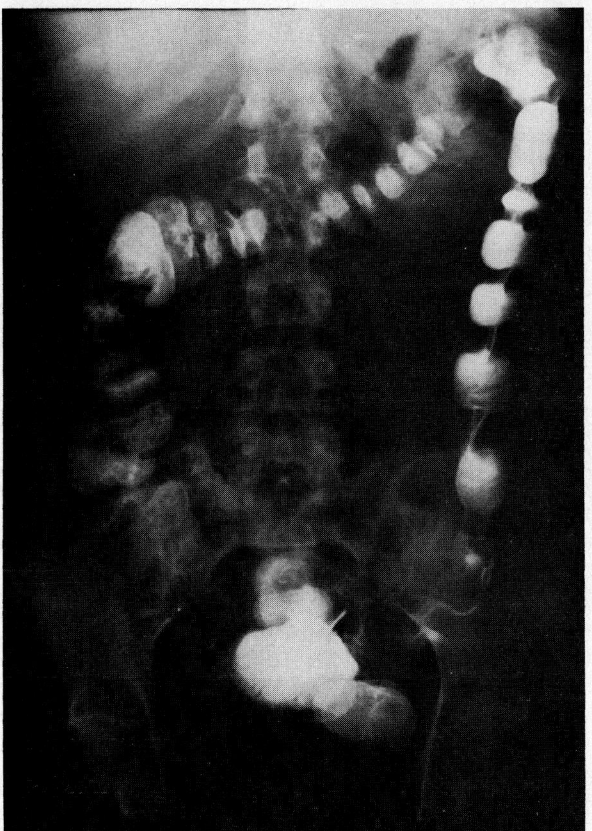

Figure 76–1. Exaggerated haustral contractions on barium enema X-ray in IBS patient with constipation and pain. Patient complained of scybalous stools.

Pain may become more severe with increasing duration and severity of constipation. In half of patients, evacuation leads to relief of pain, but frequently there is a sense of incomplete evacuation leading to repeated attempts at defecation with minimal or no success. Several hours may be devoted to this process before some relief ensues.

Constipation is difficult to define because it has both objective and subjective components. It may be defined objectively as the passage of fewer than three stools per week.[13] The subjective symptom is that of difficult or painful evacuation. Most patients who seek medical attention for constipation complain of both infrequent and difficult passage of stool; pain is viewed as the more troublesome component. Stool consistency (hard stool) is a more variable complaint, and one that is more difficult to evaluate. The best historical evidence of altered bowel habits is a reliable account of a definite change in frequency, consistency, and ease of passage. Because laxatives are usually taken during periods of constipation, it is sometimes difficult to determine whether the diarrheal phase is part of the natural history or is induced by the laxatives. Likewise, in chronic cases, it is difficult to determine whether the constipation has developed naturally in the course of the illness or whether it is a result of repeated and chronic laxative abuse.

Diarrhea attributable to IBS usually consists of small volumes of loose stool. Evacuation is often preceded by extreme urgency or tenesmus, occurring typically in the morning or after meals. The initial movement may be normal in consistency, being rapidly followed by a softer, unformed stool, and then by increasingly loose stools. Abdominal pain preceding the movements is commonly relieved by defecation, albeit sometimes only briefly. Postprandial diarrhea, except in the case of lactose intolerance, correlates with the quantity rather than the type of food; this diarrhea is sometimes explosive, as it consists of a mixture of gas and fluid, and it is usually associated with extreme urgency or pain. The bowel pattern of patients who have diarrhea exclusively, whether or not associated with pain, usually differs from that of patients with alternating constipation and diarrhea in that even the initial stool is liquid and is often passed with explosive urgency.

It is even more difficult to define diarrhea than constipation objectively, as this symptom may refer to both altered frequency and altered consistency of stools. However, the number of stools described as diarrheal (that is, loose, mushy, or watery) sometimes is not more than three per day, the accepted upper limit of normal. Indeed, a single abnormal stool daily may be viewed by the patient as diarrhea. To confirm the existence of diarrhea under these circumstances, the physician must determine that established bowel habit has changed.

Abdominal Pain

Pain is variously described as vague, bloating, crampy, burning, dull, aching, knifelike, sharp, or steady. It may be mild, moderate, or severe and localized or diffuse. Acute episodes of severe, sharp, knifelike pain may be superimposed on a constant or intermittent background of dull aching pain. The pain is more often located in the left lower quadrant than at any other site and more often in the lower abdomen than in the upper. It is experienced more often in several sites than in one site.[14] It usually does not radiate, but when severe it may be associated with low back pain. When asked to indicate the site of pain, patients are likely to use the palm of the hand describing a circular motion rather than the finger to designate a circumscribed point. Rectal pain or tenesmus may be present and ranges from mildly annoying to extremely disturbing. The locus of this pain is also diffuse rather than discrete. Experimental balloon distention demonstrates that trigger areas for production of abdominal pain may be located anywhere in the gut from the esophagus to distal portion of the colon, and one trigger point may induce pain in several sites.[15] Colonic distention reproduces the pain of irritable bowel syndrome in three fourths of patients and reproduces referred pain in one half.[15, 16] This evidence suggests that the pain of IBS is triggered by intraluminal distention.

Because the splenic flexure is the highest part of the colon, intestinal gas tends to rise to this area when the patient is upright. When distal colonic spasm makes it difficult to pass this gas, it may become trapped in the splenic flexure, giving rise to a sense of distention and pain, which can mimic heart pain but, unlike heart pain, is relieved by passing gas. Release of gas is sometimes made easier by lying down and elevating the buttocks from the bed so that the air will rise to the rectum. This symptom complex, sometimes called "splenic flexure syndrome" can be reproduced by distending a balloon in the splenic flexure.[17]

Pain is often precipitated by meals and relieved by defecation. When associated with meals, pain is usually related to the act of eating rather than to a specific type of food. A notable exception is the pain following milk ingestion in patients with IBS who also have lactose intolerance.

Rarely, if ever, does the pain awaken the patient from sleep. This is an important point, and the question concerning awakening must be carefully phrased. For example, depressed patients may experience early morning awakening and subsequently may note pain, so that a depressed patient may report awakening with pain. But careful questioning clarifies that the patient is not awakened *by* the pain. The distinction is critical in helping to distinguish between pain of organic (i.e., demonstrable disease) and nonorganic (i.e., probable motor disorder) causes. In some instances the pain of IBS is so intense that it dominates the patient's life.

Abdominal Distention (Bloating), Belching, and Flatus

Patients with all forms of IBS commonly complain of abdominal distention and increased belching or flatulence, all of which they attribute to increased gas. For some the distention may be so prominent that they are unable to wear their usual belt or garment toward the end of the day. Although some patients with these complaints actually may have larger than normal volume of gas, quantitative measurements reveal that most patients who complain of increased gas, bloating, and flatulence generate a normal amount of intestinal gas.[18] Studies have shown that most IBS patients develop symptoms even with minimal gut distention,[8, 18, 19] suggesting that the basis of their complaints is a decreased tolerance to distention rather than an abnormal quantity of intraluminal gas. The disordered motility that can account for this situation is discussed later in this chapter. Reflux of gas from the lower small intestine into the upper occurs more readily in patients with IBS than in normal subjects[18] and may explain the belching of these patients. Therefore, it appears that the majority of patients with IBS do not have excessive quantities of gas; nor do all patients with excessive gas have IBS. Obviously, however, the small number of IBS patients who do have excessive gas are doubly cursed and most unhappy.

There are three possible sources for intraluminal gas. Air ingestion (aerophagia) has been mistakenly assumed to be the major cause[20] (see pp. 257–263). Production of gas by bacteria seems to be more important, the amount being determined by particular fecal flora that result from exposure (usually to family members) during the first eight years of life. The sugars stachyose and raffinose (present in legumes) are not digested appreciably by humans but are readily handled by colonic flora and therefore contribute to the gas content of the colon. A third mechanism is diminished absorption of intraluminal gas across the colonic membrane into the bloodstream, which may result from rapid transit during diarrhea. The implications for treatment of gas based on these three known causes are discussed on page 1415.

Mucus in the Stool

The amount of mucus produced by patients with irritable bowel syndrome is variable and its pathogenesis obscure. In some instances it goes unnoticed until questions draw attention to it, whereas in others it is prominent enough to cause concern to the patient. Mucus production has been variously attributed to "irritation," muscular spasm, and autonomic stimulation without evidence to support any of these hypotheses. Some of the earliest descriptions of IBS[21] emphasized this as one of the cardinal features of the disorder and incorrectly attributed it to inflammation of the intestine—an error that has been perpetuated, unfortunately, in continued use of inappropriate terminology, such as "mucous colitis."

Upper and Other Gastrointestinal Symptoms

Dyspepsia, heartburn, pyrosis, nausea, and vomiting appear in one fourth to one half of patients.[9, 22] Diminished resting pressure in the lower esophageal sphincter and abnormal contractions in the body of the esophagus have been demonstrated[23] in IBS and may account for some of these symptoms. Another possible mechanism (excessive reflux into the stomach) has been mentioned. These findings are supported by gastroscopic observation of excessive bile reflux into the stomachs of IBS patients when compared with normal subjects.

The frequency of appendectomy varies from 4 per cent[24] to 40 per cent.[9] The high frequency in the latter report raises the question of whether or not the diagnosis of appendicitis was based on symptoms more correctly attributable to irritable bowel syndrome, particularly as 19 of the 20 patients who underwent appendectomy had symptoms persisting for over a month prior to surgery.

Autonomic-Type Symptoms

Dysmenorrhea has been noted in as many as 90 per cent of patients with IBS, urinary frequency in 65 per cent, and dyspareunia in one third.[25] Headaches, usually of the migraine type, may occur with an increased frequency in both children[26] and adults[27] with IBS. Urodynamic studies reveal urinary bladder dysfunction in 50 per cent of IBS patients, compared to 13 per cent of controls,[28] and urinary symptoms are significantly more common in IBS patients than in matched controls.[29] The frequency of these associated symptoms involving autonomically innervated organs has raised the suspicion of a generalized autonomic disturbance that includes the bowel and genitourinary and vascular systems.

Psychologic Features and Stress

Symptoms of IBS appear after or during periods of stress and emotional tension. Patients with IBS report increased frequency of stressful life experiences;[30] moreover, an increased state of arousal may add further to the susceptibility of the patient to these onslaughts. The particular vulnerability of the intestine (rather than skin, bronchi, or vascular system) to stressful conflicts may originate during early life as a result of visceral responses that are learned through social reinforcement (secondary gain).[5] Alternatively, patients with IBS may have an inherited or otherwise acquired abnormal myoelectric and motor abnormality (which will be discussed further under Pathophysiology) that may determine the intestine as the target organ responsive to emotional stress.

Abnormal psychologic features are noted in 70 to 90 per cent of patients with IBS,[10, 24, 31–33] although a recent study disputes this association.[34] The most common are depression, anxiety, and somatization of affect (substitution of somatic complaints for anxiety or depression). Two lines of evidence suggest that psychologic factors are not a result of the disorder, but instead contribute to the onset and exacerbation of symptoms. In 85 per cent of patients, psychologic factors either precede or coincide with the onset of gastrointestinal complaints and in only 15 per cent do the gastrointestinal complaints come first.[33, 35] On the other hand, a study comparing people with IBS who do not seek medical care with those who do concluded that psychopathology is less important as a determinant of IBS than as a determinant of who will consult a physician.[36] Half of patients also note a relationship between emotional stress and exacerbation of symptoms.[10, 24, 33, 35] No specific personality profile seems to be characteristic of this disorder.[5] Depression, although frequently present, usually is not severe, but suicidal tendencies have been reported to be detectable in over 20 per cent of patients.[33]

Although emotional stress can trigger hypermotility in normal subjects as well as in patients with IBS,[35, 37] the threshold seems to be lower in IBS patients. This fact may explain why IBS patients are also more sensitive to mechanical stimulation of the colon with a rectosigmoid balloon.[19] Patients with IBS tend to be more preoccupied with illness than are normal subjects; they report more illness not related to irritable bowel syndrome and more debilitation from these illnesses than does a control group.[5] This suggests that illness behavior persists because it has been supported by social reinforcement, which provides secondary gain. Past history of major illness is also higher in patients with IBS than in normal subjects (or even in patients with ulcerative colitis),[30] which implies that prior illness serves as one of the stresses contributing to the development of IBS, or, perhaps, that IBS patients may be more susceptible to other illnesses. Cancer phobia occurs in as many as half of patients,[25, 33] and needs to be handled as part of the treatment program. Recurrent abdominal pain of childhood is noted more often in children whose parents have functional gastrointestinal disorders,[26, 38, 39] but it is not known whether this relates more to genetic or to environmental factors.

PATHOPHYSIOLOGY

The failure of laboratory studies to show any morphologic, histologic, microbiologic, or biochemical abnormalities in patients with IBS supports the concept that IBS is primarily a disorder of gastrointestinal motility. Therefore, knowledge of the pathophysiology of this syndrome derives from studies of motility and the myoelectric activity that governs motility. Because the small intestine is not as accessible as the colon to manometric and electrical studies, most physiologic information has been accumulated from studying the colon; however, it is likely that other organs of the gastrointestinal tract, particularly the small intestines, participate to some degree in the pathophysiology of IBS. Transit of a meal through the small intestine is shorter in IBS patients with diarrhea and longer in IBS patients with constipation than in normal controls,[40] although one study questions this.[41] Both the pain and the altered bowel habits seen in IBS can be explained on the basis of altered motility, which, in turn, may be a response to emotional states (e.g., anxiety, depression, fear, and hostility),[42] to meals (the gastrocolic response), to neurohumoral agents (e.g., cholinergic, anticholinergic, adrenergic, and adrenergic-blocking substances), to gastrointestinal hormones (e.g., cholecystokinin, glucagon, VIP), to toxins (e.g., staphylococcal, choleraic), to prostaglandins, and to intestinal distention.

Basal Motility

During symptomatic periods, a pattern of hypermotility, consisting of high-amplitude pressure waves, is ten times as common in patients with pain-predominant IBS than in normal subjects, whereas patients with the diarrhea-predominant disorder have normal or lower than normal pressure waves.[35, 43] These observations fit with basic data from recordings of colonic motility of normal subjects and patients with constipation or diarrhea.[44] Such studies have demonstrated that the predominant form of motor activity recorded from the colon consists of segmental contractions, which impede the forward progress of stool and promote mixing, absorption, and dehydration; these appear on barium enema X-ray films as haustral markings, and they account for more than 90 per cent of recorded motor activity. Augmentation of segmenting contraction produces constipation, and inhibition of segmentation produces diarrhea.

These studies have shown also that contractions distributed over a long segment of colon may be accompanied by abdominal pain, analogous to diffuse esophageal spasm and chest pain. Indeed, such high-amplitude contractions over long segments are often recorded in patients with IBS during episodes of crampy abdominal pain.[45, 46] Hypermotility of the small intestine also has been found in association with pain.[47] Radiologic studies demonstrating small bowel hyperactivity under stress support the contention that irritable bowel syndrome can involve gastrointestinal areas other than the colon,[48, 49] a reason to prefer the term irritable bowel to irritable colon. As the heightened pressure appears before the pain, it is likely that spasm produces the pain rather than vice versa.[45]

Effects of Sleep, Emotional Stress, Eating, and Distention

The diminution of motor activity of the colon during sleep[50] may result from a reduction of psychologic and physiologic stimuli affecting this organ and may account for the infrequency with which patients are awakened from sleep by the symptoms of IBS.

Altered motility appears during stressful interviews.[37, 51–55] Specific effects correlate with specific motor responses—hostility with heightened spastic activity and depression with inhibition of motor contractions (Fig. 76–2).[55] However, these emotionally induced responses are not specific for irritable bowel syndrome as they are found in persons not suffering from this disorder as well. Moreover, stressful interviews alter motility to an equal degree in patients with both functional and organic diarrhea as well as those with

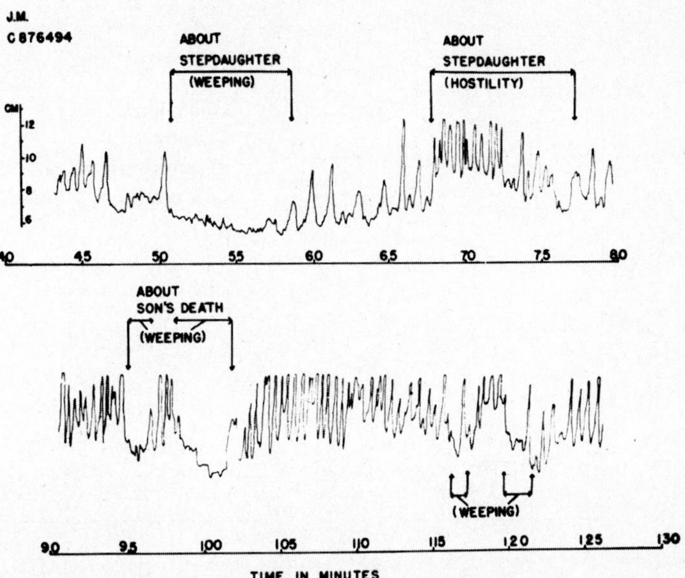

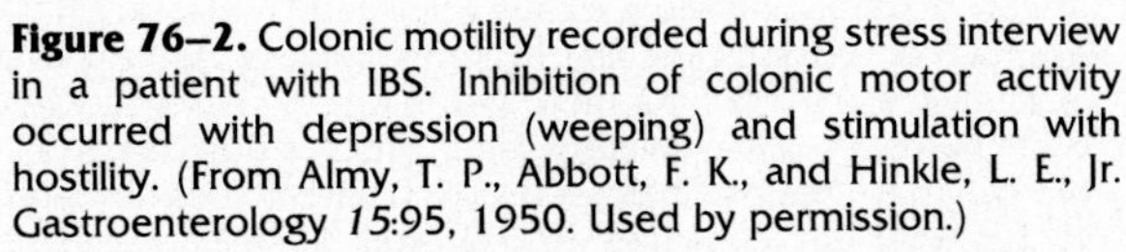
Figure 76–2. Colonic motility recorded during stress interview in a patient with IBS. Inhibition of colonic motor activity occurred with depression (weeping) and stimulation with hostility. (From Almy, T. P., Abbott, F. K., and Hinkle, L. E., Jr. Gastroenterology *15*:95, 1950. Used by permission.)

functional and organic constipation. Thus, although emotional stress perhaps is necessary, it is not sufficient to produce irritable bowel syndrome. Stress may be only one factor contributing to the genesis of IBS or one factor precipitating symptoms in the established syndrome; whether it is a necessary factor remains to be determined. Emotional stress is more potent in altering motility than feeding, but less potent than prostigmine.[35]

In IBS patients, food induces colonic hypermotility,[35, 56–58] generally 50 minutes or more after the start of the meal, and probably accounts for some of the typical postprandial symptoms. This motor pattern, characteristic of IBS, differs from the normal response to meals in two respects. First, augmentation of motility normally appears as soon as eating begins; in IBS this response is blunted (Fig. 76–3). Second, the motor response induced by eating normally quiets within 50 minutes; in IBS the abnormal blunted response not only continues postprandially but also gradually gets stronger. Investigators disagree as to whether food-induced motility is different in patients with diarrhea-predominant IBS as opposed to the constipation-predominant form.[35, 56]

Balloon distention of the rectosigmoid and rectum provides an artificial stimulus that mimics the arrival of stool in this area. This stimulus induces spastic contractions, which are significantly greater in IBS patients than in normal subjects (Fig. 76–4).[19, 59] These more sensitive and quantitative manometric studies confirm radiologic and proctologic observations supporting the clinical suspicion that a spastic motor disturbance underlies this disorder. This demonstration of an exaggerated motor response to colonic distention may explain further the symptoms that are produced in IBS with even small volumes of colonic gas or stool and also may explain some of the postprandial symptoms as the gastroileocolic response to meals empties material into the distal colon, thus distending it. Patients in whom diarrhea predominates have contractions at a faster frequency than those whose problem is constipation.[19] The significance of this finding is not understood.

Effects of Pharmacologic Agents and Hormones

Cholinergic agents, such as prostigmine, are more potent than feeding or emotional stress in producing colonic hyperactivity in both normal individuals and in patients with IBS. The response is more pronounced in patients with IBS and is present during both symptomatic and asymptomatic periods.[27, 35, 43, 60] This exaggerated response is not seen in patients with ulcerative colitis.[61]

Exogenous cholecystokinin infusion produces an increase in colonic motility that is associated with abdominal pain. This response is found more often in patients who complain of postprandial pain than in those who do not, suggesting that cholecystokinin, a gastrointestinal hormone released by meals, may account for some of the postprandial symptoms in patients with irritable bowel syndrome.[62] The ability of fatty meals to induce postprandial hypermotility further implicates cholecystokinin as a possible hormonal mediator of symptoms of IBS.[56]

Altered Myoelectric Activity in IBS

The findings of altered motor activity become even more fascinating when interpreted in light of recent studies that compare myoelectric activity in IBS patients and normal subjects. These investigations discovered a frequency of myoelectric rhythm that appears to characterize IBS patients, although there is some dispute about the interpretation of these findings and the validity of their significance. It has been suggested that this abnormal frequency may serve as a marker for IBS. It is not known currently whether this myoelectric abnormality is congenital or acquired. As

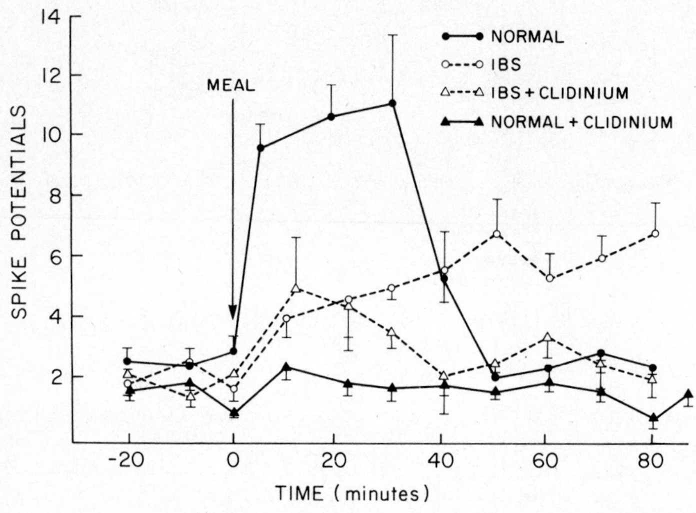

Figure 76–3. Postcibal colonic electrical spike activity in normal individuals and those with IBS before and after administration of an anticholinergic drug (clidinium). Spike activity is a reflection of colonic motility. In normal subjects, spike activity is stimulated rapidly by a meal and returns to baseline within 50 minutes. The anticholinergic agent inhibits postcibal rise. In IBS patients, the postcibal response is blunted, does not return to baseline, but continues to rise after 50 minutes. In IBS subjects, the anticholinergic drug does not affect the early (blunted) rise but inhibits the late response. (From Tucker, H., and Schuster, M. M. Adv. Intern. Med., *27*:183, 1982. Adapted from Snape, W. Gastroenterology *77*:1235, 1979. Used by permission.)

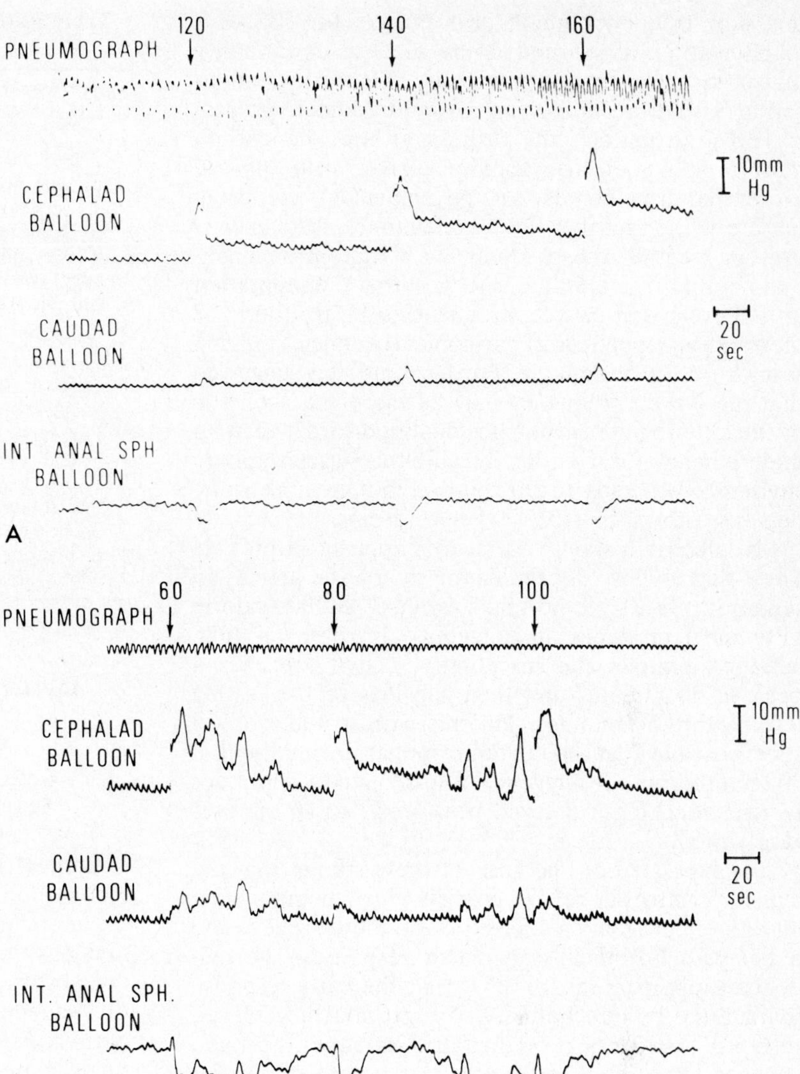

Figure 76–4. Motility response to rectosigmoid distention in normal control subject *(A)* and IBS patient *(B).* Twenty ml of air is instilled into a rectosigmoid balloon (cephalad balloon) every 20 minutes. Cumulative volumes are indicated above pneumograph tracing. The pneumograph monitors respiration and movement. In normal subjects *(A),* distentions induce a brief contraction in the rectosigmoid (cephalad balloon) and rectum (caudad balloon), with rapid return to a steady recording. The internal anal sphincter relaxes with each distention. In IBS patients, distention induces diffuse spastic contractions simultaneously in the rectosigmoid and rectum, associated with internal sphincter relaxations.

motor activity is controlled by underlying myoelectric activity, it is possible that the abnormal myoelectric activity may set the stage for an abnormal motor response of the end organ even when neurohumoral stimulation is normal.

A brief review of some basic principles of intestinal normal myoelectric activity will provide a background to the understanding of altered myoelectric activity in IBS (see pp. 21–52 and 1088–1097).

Smooth muscle cells of the gut act as small electrical oscillators or batteries that produce myoelectric activity in much the same manner as heart muscle produces the electrocardiogram or brain cells produce the electroencephalogram. Two types of electric activity have been recorded—first, a sinusoidal wave that results from depolarization and repolarization, which has been called the *slow wave, basic electric rhythm* (BER), or *electric control activity* (ECA). This wave form is sodium dependent and its predominant rhythmic frequency in the normal distal colon is approximately 6 cycles/minute. The slow wave provides the background and sets the stage for the second form of electric activity, *spike action potentials* or *electric response activity* (ERA), which is superimposed upon the slow waves, usually during the depolarization phase. Short bursts of spike potentials are commonly associated with phasic motor activity and longer bursts with tonic contractions. Spike potentials are calcium dependent.

Few known stimuli affect the frequency of slow waves. Most agents that augment or inhibit motor activity do so by altering spike activity. For example, cholinergic drugs and morphine induce spike activity and muscle contraction.

In contrast to normal subjects, whose predominant myoelectric rhythm frequency is 6 cycles/minute, 40 per cent of patients with IBS have a predominant frequency of 3 cycles/minute.[63, 64] The 3-cycle/minute activity is present in the basal state during both symptomatic and asymptomatic periods and is unaltered by successful treatment, supporting the speculation that this slow frequency might be a marker for IBS or a manifestation of an underlying electric abnormality that predisposes to altered motility. The further implication is that the underlying pathophysiologic process of IBS (and perhaps the pathology) is in the smooth muscle as myoelectric activity derives from muscle rather than from nerves. An unexplained and confusing feature is the fact that the 3-cycle/minute frequency is present whether the predominant symptom is constipation or diarrhea. Studies[65] suggest that the separation into 3-cycle and 6-cycle frequencies is arbitrary, as there exists a spectrum of harmonic frequencies ranging from 2 to 13 cycles/minute. Furthermore, it is suggested that the 3-cycle frequency may be more characteristic of the underlying neurotic personality disorder than an underlying motor disorder, because the 3-cycles/minute rhythm also seems to be more common in neurotic persons without irritable bowel syndrome.

Myoelectric response to feeding appears to provide a test that is more discriminating than basal activity in separating IBS from normal subjects.[56] A 1000-calorie fatty meal produces an immediate increase in spike action potentials and in motility; activity reaches a peak in 30 minutes and then subsides to the fasting level within 50 minutes. Patients with irritable bowel syndrome have an attenuated response during the first 30 minutes, but the incidence of spike activity continues to rise, reaching a delayed peak in 70 to 90 minutes (Fig. 76–3).

It is suggested on the basis of these studies that the classic "gastrocolic reflex" consists of two components: an early neurogenic myoelectric and motor reflex, and a delayed, hormonally mediated response. The evidence supporting this thesis is that the early response is inhibited by anticholinergic drugs, and the delayed response is dependent on the fatty content of the meal; because intraluminal fatty acids are potent stimuli for cholecystokinin release and because this hormone causes colonic contractions, dependence of the delayed response on a hormone seems very likely.[66] The mode of action of cholecystokinin in the gastrocolic response and its role in IBS is unclear, because cholecystokinin functions as both hormone and neurotransmitter. It appears to act via opioid receptors, because its effect is not inhibited by atropine but is inhibited by naloxone.[67, 68] An unexplained finding relates to the different effects of anticholinergics on the two phases of gastrocolic response in normal subjects and IBS patients. Although anticholinergics suppress the initial (presumably neurogenic) phase in normal subjects but not in IBS patients, they inhibit the delayed response in IBS.[69] Slow wave activity is unaffected by feeding and by many agents tested in both normal subjects and IBS patients.

Thus, IBS patients differ from normal subjects in (1) the basal frequency of myoelectric slow waves, (2) the myoelectric and motor response to meals, and (3) the effect of anticholinergic medication on meal induced colonic activity.

Table 76–1. CLINICAL FEATURES OF IRRITABLE BOWEL SYNDROME (IBS)

Supporting the Diagnosis of IBS
1. Lower abdominal pain
   a. Aggravated by meals
   b. Relieved by defecation
   c. More frequent bowel movements with onset of pain
   d. Looser stools with onset of pain
   e. Does not awaken patient
2. Visible abdominal distention
3. Small stools (with constipation or diarrhea)
4. Chronic symptoms consistent in pattern but variable in severity
5. Symptoms worse with periods of stress

Against the Diagnosis of IBS
1. Onset in old age
2. Steady progressive course
3. Frequent awakening by symptoms
4. Fever
5. Weight loss
6. Rectal bleeding from other than fissures or hemorrhoids
7. Steatorrhea
8. Dehydration
9. New symptoms after a long period

DIAGNOSIS, DIFFERENTIAL DIAGNOSIS, AND DIAGNOSTIC TESTS

General Considerations; History, Physical Examination, Routine Laboratory Tests

Clinical Features. The diagnosis of IBS relies on a recognition of positive clinical features as well as on the meticulous exclusion of the many other disorders that have similar manifestations (Table 76–1). This is not always an easy task, and the temptation to utilize this diagnosis as a wastebasket in which to deposit elusive disorders must be resisted. Some of the more reliable positive features are the presence of lower abdominal pain, small stools, and the persistence or recurrence of symptoms that are fairly constant in their pattern but variable in their severity. The intensity of the symptoms is not a differentiating feature and even extremely severe pain, constipation, or vomiting is compatible with the diagnosis. It is acceptable for symptoms to have initially appeared during an intercurrent illness, such as amebiasis or a viral gastroenteritis, and to have persisted in chronic form subsequently.

Further positive support is found in the correlation of onset of symptoms with periods of stress and heightened emotional tension, although it may take time and diligent probing for these features to become apparent. It is neither necessary nor likely that correlations be found with immediately preceding, discrete, stressful events; rather, the focus should be on determining general stressful periods that precede or coincide with symptomatic stages of illness. The "life chart" described by Almy and illustrated in Table 76–2 may be helpful in establishing temporal correlation of stressful periods with symptoms. Clinical features that argue

Table 76–2. LIFE CHART OF L. E., A 36-YEAR-OLD NURSE ANESTHETIST

Age	Life Situation	Bowel Function
13–20	Home, father dead, dominating mother	Irregular constipation, given castor oil
20–23	Nursing training, living near home	Steadily constipated
23–27	Private duty nursing, away from home	Regular, without laxatives
28	Mother ill, died; patient returned home to care for her in terminal illness	Severely constipated
29–30	Returned to private duty nursing	Regular, without laxatives
31–36	Worked as nurse anesthetist	Severely constipated

Comment: This evidence prompted inquiry into the emotional significance of her work as an anesthetist. The patient then revealed that while nursing her mother in her terminal illness, she had had to fight off a recurring desire to give her an overdose of morphine. Her guilt feelings about these thoughts returned painfully whenever she "put a patient to sleep" when she again held "a life in (her) hands."

against the diagnosis are the appearance of the disorder for the first time in old age; a steady, progressive course from time of onset; nocturnal symptoms that frequently awaken the patient; fever; significant weight loss not attributable to associated depression; rectal bleeding; or steatorrheal stools.

Physical Examination. Physical examination may demonstrate a tense, anxious patient (who is often unaware of these features) with autonomic lability, as evidenced by rapid, labile pulse or elevated blood pressure, sweaty palms, abdominal tympany, no evidence of weight loss, and a palpable, tender sigmoid cord. Simple finding of a firm, palpable sigmoid itself is not significant, because firm stool normally may be present in this area, but demonstration of tenderness is a significant finding. As *sigmoidoscopy* is essential to the evaluation of these patients, it may be considered part of the physical examination. Impressive spastic contraction may be seen at sigmoidoscopy and may be strong enough to prevent passage of the instrument beyond 10 to 12 cm. This spasm may contribute to the inordinate amount of pain that accompanies sigmoidoscopy in patients with IBS. Reproduction of symptoms with air insufflation is an additional suggestive finding. Large volumes of mucus, although not commonly encountered on sigmoidoscopy in patients with IBS, can be an additional helpful clue when present. The mucosa should be free of ulcers, bleeding, friability, and masses. Sigmoidoscopy should be performed without an enema preparation as the enema may initiate mucus production and produce enough edema of the mucosa to obscure the normal submucosal tracery of vessels, the presence of which indicates a mucosa of normal thickness without inflammation or edema. Enema preparation for sigmoidoscopy is used only if digital examination prior to the procedure or the examination itself reveals stool obscuring the lumen.

Table 76–3. ROUTINE LABORATORY TESTS IN IBS

Test	Condition Investigated
1. Complete blood count	1. Anemia, inflammation
2. Erythrocyte sedimentation rate	2. Inflammation
3. Differential count	3.
a. Eosinophilia	a. Parasites
b. Monocytosis	b. Tuberculosis
c. Toxic granulation	c. Inflammation
4. Lactose tolerance test or two-week lactose free diet	4. Lactose intolerance
5. Stools for ova and parasites	5. Parasites
6. During sigmoidoscopy	6.
a. Microscopic examination of mucus in warm saline	a. Amebiasis
b. Methylene blue stain of stool for leukocytes	b. Inflammation
c. Occult blood test	c. Inflammation, tumor
7. Sigmoidoscopy or barium enema	7. Structural abnormality

Diagnostic Tests. Because the differential diagnosis is broad, and because IBS is in part a diagnosis of exclusion, certain diagnostic tests should be performed routinely, whereas others are selected on the basis of a specific presenting symptom, particularly diarrhea, constipation, and pain (Tables 76–3 and 76–4). In nearly all patients it is desirable to perform at least the following diagnostic studies, in the order listed:

1. During sigmoidoscopy (without cathartic or enema preparation), mucus or fecal material adherent to the wall is examined immediately on a slide that contains several drops of warm saline solution. This is viewed microscopically for motile amebic trophozoites. Methylene blue stain is used to exclude the presence of leukocytes and mucus. Stool is examined chemically (by techniques such as Hemoccult slide tests) for occult blood, and, if positive, stool is obtained higher (during sigmoidoscopy) within the rectum for repeat examination.

2. A complete blood count and the sedimentation rate are obtained to rule out anemia and inflammation. The differential count is to detect eosinophilia, suggesting parasitosis; monocytosis, suggesting tuberculosis; or vacuolated cells, suggesting inflammation.

3. Three additional stool specimens should be examined for ova and parasites, with the specific request to search for *Giardia*.

4. A trial on a lactose-free diet for two weeks is recommended after the first visit (when organic disease is believed unlikely) in all patients who complain of either distention and bloating (even with constipation)

Table 76–4. LABORATORY FEATURES AGAINST DIAGNOSIS OF IBS

1. Elevated erythrocyte sedimentation rate
2. Leukocytosis
3. Blood, pus, or fat in stool
4. Stool weight greater than 200 gm/day
5. Persistent diarrhea during 48-hour fast (indicates secretory diarrhea)
6. Hypokalemia
7. Manometry failing to show spastic response to rectal distention

or diarrhea. Alternatively, a lactose tolerance test or breath hydrogen test may be performed, but the author's preference (and that of many patients) is for the therapeutic trial on a lactose-free diet (pp. 1997–1998).

5. A double-contrast barium enema or (if this is not available) a routine single-contrast barium enema should be obtained. Exaggerated haustral contractions, particularly in the descending colon, may be seen or, conversely, effacement and absence of normal haustral markings, often with a lumen of narrowed caliber.

6. In the IBS patient who also has dyspepsia, an upper gastrointestinal evaluation should be obtained. If it is normal and dyspepsia persists, an oral cholecystogram or ultrasonography of the gallbladder is indicated.

7. In the patient with either diarrhea or symptoms suggestive of obstruction, a small bowel series should be performed.

Laboratory Tests. Laboratory features weighing *against* irritable bowel syndrome are an elevated sedimentation rate, leukocytosis or blood, pus, or fat in the stool. Stool volumes of over 200 ml/day point to other causes, as does the persistence of diarrhea after a 48-hour fast, because persistent diarrhea and the absence of oral intake imply that the diarrhea is secretory (pp. 290–316). In the author's experience, the absence of spastic responses to rectosigmoid distention during *manometric studies* is substantial evidence against the diagnosis of IBS. On the other hand, the presence of spasm induced under these conditions, although statistically more prominent in IBS patients than in control subjects, is not pathognomonic of this condition.

Special Considerations in Differential Diagnosis

If the appropriate diagnosis does not become apparent as a result of the routine studies just listed, or if it is immediately evident that there are special diagnostic considerations—that is, if pain is a major complaint or physical findings raise questions of organic disease—additional special tests are ordered. Other special considerations must be given patients with severe diarrhea or constipation.

Prominent Pain

The qualities, location, timing, and so on of severe abdominal pain suggest specific diagnoses, (pp. 238–250). For example, gallbladder disease may be investigated by oral cholecystogram or ultrasonography; intestinal obstruction by plain and upright X-ray films of the abdomen; acute intermittent porphyria by appropriate urine tests for porphobilinogen, porphyrins, and delta-aminolevulinic acid; tabes dorsalis by serologic test for syphilis and cerebrospinal fluid examination; angina pectoris by electrocardiogram; pulmonary embolus by lung scans; and lead poisoning by serum lead levels.

Diarrhea

When diarrhea is a major complaint, the following conditions need to be considered, and each requires specific evaluation (pp. 290–316).

Osmotic Diarrhea. One cause of osmotic diarrhea, lactose intolerance, produces symptoms that are indistinguishable from those of IBS (p. 269). Because it is so readily and simply treated, lactose intolerance must be excluded in all patients suspected of having IBS. (Deficiencies of other disaccharidases, particularly sucrase, are very rare causes of diarrhea.) Symptoms of lactase deficiency result from bacterial digestion and fermentation of lactose, which reaches the colon undigested by small intestinal enzymes. This fermentation leads to gaseous bloating and often to diarrhea. Infrequently, constipation instead of diarrhea may occur. The most practical and meaningful test is a two week trial on a lactose-free diet, as this answers the clinical question of whether the patient improves when lactose is excluded from the diet. Hydrogen breath tests and lactose tolerance tests are preferred by some clinicians. As there is no universal agreement on the appropriate quantity of lactose to utilize in the oral tolerance test, and since these tests will not always predict the response to lactose, withdrawal—placing a patient with suspected IBS on a lactose-free diet for two to three weeks—is justified.

A lactose-free diet leads to one of three responses: no response (most patients), implying that lactose plays no role in the symptoms; some improvement in symptoms, especially in bloating and gaseous distention, but not total alleviation of symptoms; this response implies that lactose intolerance may play a contributory role. The third and least frequent response is complete relief of symptoms, suggesting that lactose intolerance is the problem. Abuse of such laxatives as Cephulac or mannitol can cause osmotic diarrhea and bloating. If the patient is not thoroughly queried on this point, the diagnosis will be missed.

Secretory Diarrhea. This type of diarrhea may be induced by surreptitious use of stimulatory laxatives like Ex-Lax that contain phenolphthalein, the presence of which can be demonstrated sometimes by the pink color obtained when the stool is alkalinized with potassium hydroxide. Factitious diarrhea caused by laxatives can sometimes be discovered (especially in a hospital setting) by appropriate search of room and belongings (with the patient's knowledge and consent). Secretory diarrhea resulting from carcinoid tumors is suspected on the basis of associated flushing, shortness of breath, and a pulmonic murmur and is confirmed by serum serotonin levels or elevated urinary 5-HIAA. These tests are best performed during or immediately after an attack (pp. 1560–1570). Gastrinomas or VIP-producing tumors are investigated by measuring serum gastrin or VIP levels, although only a few laboratories measure VIP (p. 303). Medullary carcinoma of the thyroid is suspected usually on the basis of the physical examination. Short bowel syndrome, obviously in patients who have had a significant length of small gut resected, may produce choleretic diarrhea because of decreased bile salt absorption and consequent stimulation of colonic secretion by bile salts (pp. 1106–1112). Demonstration of excessive bile salts in the stool confirms the diagnosis but this is a difficult and little-used test. These patients have malabsorption syndrome as well. Pancreatic insufficiency or malabsorption caused by intestinal disease is suspected on the basis of the history of steatorrhea and demonstration of increased stool fat by Sudan III tests, followed by quantitative three-day stool collection (pp. 300–303).

Inflammatory Conditions Associated with Diarrhea. Confusion of ulcerative colitis with IBS is rare because of the rectal bleeding and striking sigmoidoscopic findings that characterize ulcerative colitis. Endoscopic biopsy usually confirms the diagnosis. However, it has recently been recognized that IBS may be superimposed on ulcerative colitis in remission[70] (and presumably also while active). The recognition of this diagnosis can spare the patient unnecessary use of steroids. Crohn's disease is more likely to present bloating, pain, and diarrhea (or occasionally constipation). It is suspected on the basis of an elevated sedimentation rate, leukocytosis, and fever and is confirmed by barium X-ray studies or endoscopy. Parasitic infestation, particularly giardiasis or amebiasis, may mimic IBS in an otherwise normal subject or precipitate it; that is, symptoms persist after the parasitosis is cured. Indeed, recurrence or reinfection with parasites may often be mistaken for IBS. It is customary to examine three stools for ova and parasites. Certainly this examination should be performed in patients who live in endemic areas, who have traveled recently to places known to be endemic for amebiasis (e.g., Mexico) or giardiasis (e.g., Leningrad and some of the ski areas in Colorado). If there is a strong suspicion of *Giardia* and stool examination is not confirmatory, duodenal aspirate may be helpful, or stools can be examined after purgation. Most bacterial pathogens produce only acute (days) or subacute (weeks) diarrhea and, therefore, generally are not important considerations in the differential diagnosis of chronic diarrhea. *Salmonella* and *Shigella* infections are less common than lactose intolerance or parasitosis but produce similar symptoms; hence, stool cultures are reasonable. *Shigella* is not usually confused with IBS because of the acuteness of the bloody diarrhea of that infection (see pp. 1199–1203).

Endocrinopathy. Diarrhea is seen in Addison's disease, particularly in crisis, which is suspected on the basis of salt craving, muscle weakness, croaky voice, hyponatremia, and elevated BUN. Hyperthyroidism generally results in increased frequency of formed stool rather than watery diarrhea (see pp. 488–489).

Constipation

Constipation may be a side effect of many different drugs, particularly adrenergic, anticholinergic, antihypertensive, and antidepressant drugs that suppress propulsive activity. Lifelong *laxative abuse* may result in laxative dependence, with continuing and worsening constipation as a result of increasing tolerance to the laxative. Factitious constipation may result from use of antidiarrheal agents, such as opiates, diphenoxylate, or anticholinergics. Endocrinopathies, such as hypothyroidism and hypoparathyroidism, can be associated with constipation and are suspected on the basis of their clinical presentation and confirmed by appropriate serum studies. Malignancy of the colon also must be considered in the differential diagnosis of altered bowel habits of either type, particularly if symptoms are of fairly recent onset. Diverticular disease of the colon may present in a fashion similar to that of IBS, painful constipation being present more often than diarrhea. The physical findings in diverticular disease are also similar to those of IBS—namely, a tender sigmoid cord. Diverticula are best demonstrated by barium enema X-rays or colonoscopy (pp. 1419–1434).

TREATMENT

Within the first few visits, a firm diagnosis of IBS can usually be established. The manner in which this is done and the way in which it is explained to the patient can influence indelibly the patient's reaction to the illness, the patient's cooperation and relationship with the physician, and the ultimate response to treatment. It is wise to perform those examinations and tests necessary to resolve the questions that exist in the mind of the patient and the physician and establish the diagnosis firmly. The patient should then be informed that the necessary tests have been performed to rule out organic disease, and that the results have been reassuring in this regard. An incomplete work-up can lead only to the subsequent need for further tests, which then erodes the patient's confidence in both the physician and the diagnosis.

Treatment involves a collaborative effort between patient and physician. There will be recognizable causes for some recurrences, although the reasons for others will not be apparent. This does not mean that causes do not exist; it simply means that they are not known. Every effort should be made to discover them by cooperative exploration.

Psychologic Management

Comfort is often derived from the simple act of applying a name to the disorder. If an inappropriate term (such as colitis) has been employed, it is helpful to explain why the term IBS is preferred. IBS can be described as a disorder involving spastic responses of the intestine to a number of stimuli, including infection and emotional stress. It should be emphasized that the spasm is measurable and the resulting pain real, and that they are influenced by a number of factors that need to be managed to control the spasticity. Treatment entails altering the stressful situations whenever possible, improving the patient's response to stress, or using drugs to suppress spasm. It must be understood that the therapeutic program for IBS, like that for esophagitis, is a comprehensive one, utilizing a number of treatment methods that can provide relief even though (as with many chronic disorders) there is no single magical cure. Explanation of the chronic and recurrent nature of the condition will allay some of the alarm engendered by persistent or recurrent symptoms, which otherwise might raise questions concerning the validity of the diagnosis. Repeated explanation and reassurance may be needed. The patient should be assured that IBS does not lead to more serious underlying disorders, such as colitis or cancer, or in any way shorten the life span. The symptoms can be controlled, although usually not completely or permanently.

Reassurance and *psychologic support* are key factors in dealing with the anxiety and stress. It is particularly important to explore with the patient not only possible precipitating factors but also the patient's reaction to them. In the treatment of IBS, emotional catharsis often is more beneficial than physical catharsis. A caring and steady interest serves not only to uncover important factors, but also is inherently therapeutic. Frequent, although not necessarily prolonged, follow-up visits may initially be required, with gradual reduction becoming possible as rapport is established and the patient develops more effective coping mechanisms. Other techniques, such as relaxation exercises and physical exercise, may be useful adjuncts. Formal psychiatric treatment usually is not required, although a recent study suggests that the combination of medical treatment and short-term behavioral therapy may improve long-term outcome compared with medical treatment alone.

Sedatives, tranquilizers, and *antidepressants* are to be avoided if possible because of potential drug dependence, but these drugs should not be withheld from patients who require them. Patients should clearly understand, however, that drugs are used only as a temporary expedient to dull the edge of anxiety and to make it bearable. Drugs certainly cannot substitute for supportive therapy, insight therapy, or counseling, most of which can be provided adequately and within a reasonable time frame by a trained and interested physician. The goal should be to support the patient, building security to help him or her gradually to overcome stressful situations. In the search for "scientific" (drug) cures, the physician may overlook the patients' inherent strengths which, with help, will permit them to solve their own problems rather than become dependent on drugs to cover them.

Investigation will reveal environmental stresses from time to time, some of which can be managed by eliminating, altering, or avoiding the situation. The physician serves as a catalyst and enabler to assist the patient in discovering these factors, in determining how they influence symptoms, and in arriving at the most satisfactory treatment program. All possible resources should be mobilized, including family members, the clergy, and other health professionals.

It is important to detect and to manage factors that reinforce the illness and to minimize gratification from the illness. To accomplish this, the patient and family can be encouraged to look on IBS as a physical deformity, recognizing the existence of the disability while minimizing it and helping the patient perform at maximum capacity. The patient should be discouraged from talking to others about the disability.

Some evidences of depression have been noted earlier in the chapter. Every effort should be made to determine what specific external factors contribute to the depression and what can be done about them. In addition to purposeful environmental manipulation (such as job changes), *relaxation training* may be provided by behavioral therapists or by use of audiotapes. Antidepressant medication given either in divided doses or as a single dose at night (e.g., amitriptyline, 25 mg four times a day or 25 to 75 mg at bedtime) has been found to be more helpful in treating the symptoms of IBS than have tranquilizing agents.[33] Patients should understand that drugs of this type are used only as a temporary expedient; as soon as possible, drugs should be tapered and discontinued. Psychotherapy may be indicated for severe depression or when significant psychopathology is present. One study of severe IBS has shown short-term psychotherapy combined with medical management to be more effective than medical management alone,[71] whereas another study has shown hypnotically induced relaxation to be more effective than psychotherapy.[72]

Early experimental results suggest that approximately two thirds of patients with irritable bowel syndrome can suppress rectal and rectosigmoid spasm induced by balloon distention using biofeedback (operant conditioning) techniques.[5, 21, 73] It is not known whether suppression of spasm under these experimental conditions will contribute to clinical improvement.

Diet and Drugs

High-fiber diets are widely accepted in treating IBS, especially for patients with constipation. Initially 12 to 16 gm of unprocessed miller's bran as two tablespoons four times a day are prescribed, which is gradually reduced to the optimally effective tolerable dose. Alternatively, the patient may start with smaller doses and gradually increase until the desired effect is achieved. There are no hard data documenting the effectiveness of fiber in IBS; indeed, 15 to 25 per cent of patients complain that a high-fiber diet aggravates symptoms, particularly bloating and distention. These undesirable effects usually disappear spontaneously after two to three weeks but may necessitate diminishing the quantity of fiber or eliminating fiber completely. A meticulous dietary history occasionally may reveal substances (such as coffee, disaccharides, legumes, and cabbage) that aggravate symptoms. Patients should be encouraged to eliminate as a therapeutic trial any foodstuffs that appear to be deleterious. The implicated food subsequently may be reinstituted to determine whether symptoms recur.

Psyllium preparations such as Metamucil, Konsyl,

L. A. Formula, and Mitrolan are logical agents for the treatment of IBS, whether the predominant symptom is constipation or diarrhea, and particularly when there are alternating constipation and diarrhea. Because of their hydrophilic properties, these agents bind water and thus prevent excessive dehydration of stool as well as excess liquidity. Hydrophilic colloids are best prescribed at mealtime so that they mix with the stool as it is being formed. Obese people may benefit from appetite depressant effects if the bulk agents are given before meals; thin people should take the medication after meals. When taken before sleep, bulk agents may result in the usual hard, scybalous stool followed by a gelatinous mass of colloid. There are conflicting reports about the effectiveness of these agents in irritable bowel syndrome.[74, 75] Bulk agents may retard rapid transit.[76, 77] At times, low doses of cholestyramine (half a packet with each meal) have been found to be helpful.[78]

Whenever other antidiarrheal agents or laxatives are required for severe symptoms, the mildest form should be used in the smallest dose and for the shortest time possible, with special recognition of the problems of inducing diarrhea from laxatives or constipation from antidiarrheal agents in patients who have alternating constipation and diarrhea. When diarrhea is severe, frequent small doses of diphenoxylate (Lomotil) (2.5 to 5 mg) every four to six hours can be prescribed, or loperamide (Imodium) (2 mg) every six to eight hours. Loperamide is longer acting than diphenoxylate, thus requiring less frequent administration. These agents are similar in their effect to paregoric, codeine, or deodorized tincture of opium, but are less addictive. The intestines do not become tolerant of the antidiarrheal effect of opiates as does the mind for psychogenic effects, and increasing doses are not required to maintain antidiarrheal potency. The physician should be very suspicious of psychologic or physiologic dependence if increasing doses become necessary. Patients whose social life has been seriously disrupted by diarrhea may derive a sense of security from taking antidiarrheal medication prior to anticipated stressful events. This technique should be viewed as a first step in the management of a difficult situation, with the goal being gradual withdrawal of medicine and substitution of internal support systems.

Antispasmodics (anticholinergics) serve mainly to provide temporary relief for symptoms such as painful cramps related to intestinal spasm. Usually such relief is neither dramatic nor permanent.[79] Antispasmodics are most effective when prescribed in anticipation of predictable pain. For example, postprandial pain is best managed by giving antispasmodics (e.g., dicyclomine [Bentyl], 20 mg; Pro-Banthine, 15 mg; or tincture of belladonna, 10 to 20 drops) 30 to 45 minutes before meals so that effective blood levels will be achieved shortly before the anticipated onset of pain. A fat-free diet empirically may be found to be helpful. In theory, it should be, if cholecystokinin (released by fat) produces altered motility. Because the goal of this treatment is the control of disordered motility and not suppression of secretion, it seems reasonable to use spasmolytic agents like dicyclomine (Bentyl), which have little effect on secretion and which therefore produce fewer undesirable side effects, such as dryness of the mouth. Anticholinergics (e.g., Pro-Banthine, 15 to 30 mg) also may alleviate diarrhea in IBS patients, especially if taken 30 to 45 minutes before meals.

Other Types of Treatment

The management of "excessive gas" is rarely satisfactory, except when there is obvious aerophagia or disaccharidase deficiency. Prominent air swallowing may be managed by biting gently on a pencil or other object to prevent closure of the jaws, thus inhibiting swallowing. Patients are advised to eat slowly, not to chew gum or drink carbonated beverages, and to avoid artificial sweeteners (such as sorbitol), legumes, and foods of the cabbage family. Simethecone, antacids, antibiotics, activated charcoal, pancreatic enzymes, and metoclopramide have all been tried, usually with disappointing results. Physical exercise, curtailment or discontinuation of tobacco, and a heating pad to the abdomen have all been reported to be beneficial and are worth trying. In the author's experience, rare and extreme circumstances may warrant partial colectomy, but thorough psychiatric evaluation is essential before undertaking such a drastic step (see pp. 257–263).

IBS IN CHILDHOOD AND ADOLESCENCE

Unlike lactose intolerance, which was first described in children and is now known to be more common in adults, IBS until recently was rarely recognized in children, even though one third of adult patients trace the onset of symptoms back to childhood.[25] These facts strongly imply underdiagnosis of pediatric IBS. The female preponderance among adults raises the question of whether the adult disorder differs from that of childhood, or whether sexual (hormonal?) factors determine the presentation in different age groups. The following brief comments will address demographic, clinical, and diagnostic differences between children and adults and stress special therapeutic considerations.

Demographic Features

It is estimated that two thirds of referrals to pediatric gastroenterologists are because of functional disturbances.[80] Two types of IBS are recognized. A diarrhea-predominant type is seen in the first three years of life and is referred to as chronic, nonspecific diarrhea.[81] This group includes recurrent painless diarrhea. A pain-predominant type, referred to as recurrent abdominal pain (RAP), appears in the 6 to 18 year age group.[82] An adult pattern of IBS may appear in the older adolescent. Each of these groups may be distinct, or they may overlap.

A high familial incidence has been reported;[83] in 75 per cent of children with IBS, one or both parents or one or more siblings have a functional gastrointestinal disorder. Both types are more common in Jewish than in non-Jewish children and in Caucasians than in non-Caucasians, although this may reflect referral patterns. The 2.3 to 1 female predominance that exists in adults is not found in children. In many reported series, boys outnumber girls, suggesting that more boys outgrow the syndrome or that females have a later onset, or both.[80]

Clinical Features

One of every nine school children has painful episodes once every three months.[84] Children with IBS have normal growth and development, but weight loss may occur because of pain associated with eating. Ninety per cent of children with pain predominance are 5 to 10 years of age. Pain is usually periumbilical in the preteenager but more often in the left lower quadrant in the adolescent. Pain is cramplike in nature, does not radiate, and often is aggravated by eating and alleviated by defecation or passing flatus. There is no association with menstruation. Headache, nausea (usually without vomiting), and excess gas are reported in decreasing order of frequency.

In the diarrhea-predominant group, age of onset is between 6 months and 2 years in 80 to 90 per cent of patients. The painless diarrhea seen in preschool children, particularly under age 3 years, is usually intermittent and occasionally alternates with constipation. The number of stools is fewer than five per day, and the stool is mushy or watery, often containing mucus and undigested food particles. Bright red blood per rectum may indicate anal fissures, which develop from constipation or excessive diarrhea. As with adults, the first stool may be formed and subsequent ones progressively softer or watery. Nocturnal diarrhea is as unusual in children as in adults with functional colonic disorder. Firm, infrequent stools less often than every two days are noted in the pain-predominant group, and older adolescents with IBS frequently report hard pellets with mucus.

Three fourths of school-age children with IBS have a history of onset of symptoms with stress-associated school problems and parental marital problems. As with adults, there is no personality disorder specific for IBS. Physical factors, such as teething, respiratory infections, and acute gastrointestinal infections, may precipitate symptoms that become chronic or recurrent.[80] Specific food intolerance (usually to wheat or milk products) is reported by parents in half of cases, but few children have been shown to be lactose-intolerant.

Diagnosis

In addition to the historical features already discussed, physical examination usually reveals a healthy-appearing child with a palpable sigmoid colon that is tender in half of cases. Rectal examination may show a dilated rectal ampulla filled with hard or soft stool, even though normal bowel habits are claimed. Gynecologic examination is important in postpubertal girls who had delayed menarche or who have been sexually active.

Although sigmoidoscopy is routine in evaluation of adult IBS, it is not recommended in children unless there is appreciable weight loss, arthralgia or arthritis, bleeding, leukocytosis, elevated sedimentation rate, or pus in stool specimens to suggest inflammatory bowel disease. Barium X-ray studies are reserved for similar indications or for failure to respond to treatment. Colonic spasm, so often found on barium enema in adults, is uncommon in children. Instead, the constipation of childhood is more often associated with an atonic colon, the appearance of which may resemble megacolon; but dilatation is rarely as pronounced as in megacolon. Encopresis appears to be less common (and rectal mucus more common) in constipated children with IBS than in constipated children with megacolon. Children with Hirschsprung's disease likewise do not have encopresis, but they, like children with other forms of megacolon, generally develop abdominal pain only as stool builds up between evacuations (see pp. 1390–1395).

Laboratory investigation should include complete blood count, erythrocyte sedimentation rate, stool examination for occult blood, and routine urine analysis. In the diarrhea-predominant form of IBS in children, stools should be examined for white cells, and the pH should be determined.

If the patient is malnourished, sweat electrolyte concentrations, particularly Na^+ and Cl^-, are determined to exclude cystic fibrosis, the most common cause of malabsorption in children.[83] In pain-predominant IBS in children, possible disease of the urinary tract should be investigated thoroughly, as this system is the most common site of organic disease in childhood.

Treatment

Therapeutic principles and practices outlined for adults are equally applicable to children; however, additional consideration are also appropriate. Children have many fears, some rational and some irrational, and these must be recognized and allayed. Much time may be required for the child (and particularly the teenager) to develop confidence in the physician. It is best achieved by *private* discussions with the patient. This approach may help to overcome the child's natural suspicion of authority figures and his or her concept that all adults have the same (i.e., parental) attitudes.

Medications should be prescribed sparingly. Opiates are particularly to be avoided because of the danger of addiction. Palatability of medications and bulk agents is a matter of more immediate concern to children than to adults. Dioctylsodium sulfosuccinate (1 to 4 mg/kg/dose three times daily) may be prescribed in quantities sufficient to produce daily stools. In children even more than in adults, laxative habituation potential is a matter of serious concern. Most important is the establishment of a bowel training program that can be facilitated by utilizing breakfast or supper as a gastrocolic stimulus, asking the child to attempt a movement after this meal on a regular basis. Here a relationship of mutual trust greatly facilitates the physician's program to help the child achieve a more normal bowel habit. The physician also must deal with the parents, who often have unexpressed guilt about the possibility of having transmitted the disorder to the child.

References

1. Manning, A. P., Thompson, W. G., Heaton, K. W., and Morris, A. F. Towards positive diagnosis of the irritable bowel. Br. Med. J. *2*:633, 1978.
2. McHardy, G., Browne, D. C., McHardy, R. J., Welch, G. E., and Ward, S. S. Psychophysiologic gastrointestinal reactions: therapeutic observations. Postgrad. Med. *31*:346, 1962.
3. Mendeloff, A. I. Epidemiology of the irritable bowel syndrome. Practical Gastroenterol. *3*:12, 1979.
4. Almy, T. P. Digestive disease as a national problem. II. A white paper by the American Gastroenterological Association. Gastroenterology *53*:821, 1967.
5. Whitehead, W. E., and Schuster, M. M. Psychological management of the irritable bowel syndrome. Practical Gastroenterol. *3*:32, 1979.
6. Thompson, W. G., and Heaton, K. W. Functional bowel disorders in apparently healthy people. Gastroenterology *79*:283, 1980.
7. Ferguson, A., Sircus, W., and Eastwood, M. Frequency of "functional" gastrointestinal disorders. Lancet *2*:613, 1977.
8. Ritchie, J. Pain in IBS. Practical Gastroenterol. *3*:16, 1979.
9. Keeling, P. W. N., and Fielding, J. F. The irritable bowel syndrome. A review of 50 consecutive cases. J. Irish Coll. Phys. Surg. *4*:91, 1975.
10. Chaudhary, N. A., and Truelove, S. C. The irritable colon syndrome: A study of the clinical features, predisposing causes, and prognosis in 130 cases. Q. J. Med. *31*:307, 1962.
11. Kalser, M. H., Zion, D. E., and Bockus, H. L. Functional diarrhea: an analysis of the clinical and roentgen manifestations. Gastroenterology *31*:629, 1965.
12. Misiewicz, J. J. Clinical features, diagnosis and differential diagnosis of IBS. Practical Gastroenterol. *3*:42, 1979.
13. Connell, A. M., Hilton, C., Irvine, G., Lennard-Jones, J. E., and Misiewicz, J. J. Variation of bowel habit in two population samples. Br. Med. J. *2*:1095, 1965.
14. White, B. V., and Jones, C. M. Mucous colitis: a delineation of the syndrome with certain observations on its mechanism and on the role of emotional tension as a precipitating factor. Ann. Intern. Med. *14*:854, 1940.
15. Moriarty, K. J., and Dawson, A. M. Functional abdominal pain: further evidence that whole gut is affected. Br. J. Med. *284*:1670, 1982.
16. Swarbrick, E. T., Hegarty, J. E., Bat, L., Williams, C. B., and Dawson, A. M. Site of pain from the irritable bowel. Lancet *2*:443, 1980.
17. Machella, T. E., Dworken, H. J., and Biel, F. N. Observation on the splenic flexure syndrome. Ann. Intern. Med. *37*:543, 1952.
18. Lasser, R. B., Bond, J. H., and Levitt, M. D. The role of intestinal gas in functional abdominal pain. N. Engl. J. Med. *293*:524, 1975.
19. Whitehead, W. E., Engel, B. T., and Schuster, M. M. Irritable bowel syndrome. Physiological and psychological differences between diarrhea-predominant and constipation-predominant patients. Dig. Dis. Sci. *25*:404, 1980.
20. Greenbaum, D. S. Intestinal gas in normal subjects and patients with IBS. Practical Gastroenterol. *2*:26, 1979.
21. Da Costa, J. M. Membraneous enteritis. Am. J. Med. Sci. *62*:321, 1871.
22. Watson, W. C., Sullivan, S. N., Corke, M., and Rush, D. Incidence of esophageal symptoms and pain in patients with irritable bowel syndrome. Gut *17*:827, 1976.
23. Whorwell, P. J., Clouter, C., and Smith, C. L. Oesophageal motility in the irritable bowel syndrome. Br. Med. J. *282*:1101, 1981.
24. Waller, S. L., and Misiewicz, J. J. Prognosis in irritable bowel syndrome. Lancet *2*:753, 1969.
25. Fielding, J. F. A year in outpatients with irritable bowel syndrome. Irish J. Med. Sci. *146*:162, 1977.
26. Oster, J. Recurrent abdominal pain, headache and limb pain in children. Pediatrics *50*:429, 1972.
27. Kirsner, J. B., and Palmer, W. L. The irritable colon. Gastroenterology *34*:491, 1958.
28. Whorwell, P. J., Lupton, E. W., Erduran, D., and Wilson, K. Bladder smooth muscle dysfunction in patients with irritable bowel syndrome. Gut *27*:1014, 1986.
29. Whorwell, P. J., McCallum, M., Creed, F. H., and Roberts, C. T. Noncolonic features of irritable bowel syndrome. Gut *27*:37, 1986.
30. Mendeloff, A. I., Monk, M., Siegel, C. I., and Lilienfeld, A. Illness experience and life stress in patients with irritable colon syndrome and with ulcerative colitis. An epidemiologic study of ulcerative and regional enteritis in Baltimore, 1960–1964. N. Engl. J. Med. *282*:14, 1970.
31. Liss, J. L., Alpers, D., and Woodruff, R. A. The irritable colon syndrome and psychiatric illness. Dis. Colon Rectum *34*:151, 1973.
32. Young, S. J., Alpers, D. H., Norland, C. C., and Woodruff, R. A. Psychiatric illness and the irritable bowel syndrome: Practical implications for the primary physician. Gastroenterology *70*:162, 1976.
33. Hislop, I. G. Psychological significance of the irritable colon syndrome. Gut *12*:452, 1971.
34. Welch, G. W., Hillman, L. C., and Pomare, E. W. Psychoneurotic symptomatology in the irritable bowel syndrome: a study of reporters and non-reporters. Br. Med. J. *291*:1382, 1985.
35. Wangle, A. G., and Deller, D. J. Intestinal motility in man: III. Mechanisms of constipation and diarrhea with particular reference to the irritable colon syndrome. Gastroenterology *48*:69, 1965.
36. Whitehead, W. E., Bosmajian, L., Zonderman, A., Costa, P., and Schuster, M. M. Role of psychological symptoms in irritable bowel syndrome: comparison of community and clinic samples. Gastroenterology *94*:A495, 1988.
37. Almy, T. P., and Tulin, M. Alterations in colonic function in man under stress: Experimental production of changes simulating the "irritable colon." Gastroenterology *8*:616, 1947.
38. Stone, R. T., and Barbero, G. J. Recurrent abdominal pain in childhood. Pediatrics *45*:732, 1970.
39. Christensen, M. F., and Mortensen, D. Long-term prognosis in children with recurrent abdominal pain. Arch. Dis. Child. *50*:110, 1965.
40. Cann, P. A., Read, N. W., Brown, C., Hobson, N., and Holdsworth, C. D. Irritable bowel syndrome: relationship of disorders in the transit of a single solid meal to symptom patterns. Gut *24*:405, 1983.
41. Kingham, J. G., Bown, R., Colson, R., and Clark, M. L. Jejunal motility in patients with functional abdominal pain. Gut *25*:375, 1984.
42. Kumar, D., and Wingate, D. L. The irritable bowel syndrome: a paroxysmal motor disorder. Lancet *2*:973, 1985.
43. Chaudhary, N. A., and Truelove, S. C. Human colonic motility: a comparative study of normal subjects, patients with ulcerative colitis and patients with irritable bowel syndrome. Gastroenterology *40*:1, 1961.
44. Connell, A. M. The motility of the pelvic colon. II. Paradoxical motility in diarrhea and constipation. Gut *3*:342, 1962.
45. Connell, A. M., Jones, F. A., and Rowlands, E. N. Motility of the pelvic colon. IV. Abdominal pain associated with colonic hypermotility after meals. Gut *6*:105, 1965.

46. Holdstock, D. J., Misiewicz, J. J., and Waller, S. L. Observations on the mechanisms of abdominal pain. Gut *10*:19, 1969.
47. Horowitz, L., and Farrar, J. T. Intraluminal small intestinal pressure in normal patients and in patients with functional gastrointestinal disorders. Gastroenterology *42*:455, 1962.
48. Goin, L. S. Some factors in the production of unusual small bowel patterns. Radiology *59*:177, 1952.
49. Friedman, J. Roentgen studies of the effects on the small intestines from emotional disturbances. AJR *72*:367, 1954.
50. Adler, H. F., Atkinson, A. J., and Ivy, A. C. A study of the motility of the human colon. An explanation of dysynergia of the colon or irritable colon. Am. J. Dig. Dis. *8*:197, 1941.
51. Almy, T. P., and Tulin, M. Alteration in colonic function in man under stress: Experimental production of changes simulating the "irritable colon." Gastroenterology *8*:616, 1947.
52. Almy, T. P., Kern, F., and Tulin, M. Alterations in colonic function in man under stress. II. Experimental production of sigmoid spasm in healthy persons. Gastroenterology *12*:425, 1949.
53. Almy, T. P., Hinkle, L. E., Berle, B., and Kern, F. Alterations in colonic function in man under stress. III. Experimental production of sigmoid spasm in patients with spastic constipation. Gastroenterology *12*:437, 1949.
54. Almy, T. P., Abbott, F. K., and Hinkle, L. E. Alterations in colonic function in man under stress. IV. Hypomotility of the sigmoid colon, its relationship to the mechanism of functional diarrhea. Gastroenterology *15*:95, 1950.
55. Almy, T. P. Experimental studies on the irritable colon. Am. J. Med. *10*:60, 1951.
56. Sullivan, M., Cohen, S., and Snape, W. J., Jr. Colonic myoelectric activity in irritable bowel syndrome. Effect of eating and anticholinergics. N. Engl. J. Med. *298*:878, 1978.
57. Waller, S. L. The irritable bowel syndrome: clinical and pathophysiological features. Rend. Gastroenterol. *3*:80, 1971.
58. Waller, S. L., Misiewicz, J. J., and Kiley, N. Effect of eating on motility of the pelvic colon in constipation and diarrhea. Gut *13*:805, 1972.
59. Mitra, R., Chura, C., Rajendra, G. R., and Schuster, M. M. Effect of progressive rectal distension in irritable bowel syndrome. Gastroenterology *66*:770, 1974.
60. Atkinson, A. J., Adler, H. G., and Ivy, A. C. Motility of the human colon. The normal pattern, dyskinesia and the effects of drugs. JAMA *121*:646, 1943.
61. Chaudhary, N. A., and Truelove, S. C. Colonic motility: a critical review of methods and results. Am. J. Med. *31*:86, 1961.
62. Harvey, R. F., and Read, A. E. Effect of cholecystokinin on colonic motility and symptoms in patients with irritable bowel syndrome. Lancet *1*:1, 1973.
63. Snape, W. J., Jr., Carlson, G. M., and Cohen, S. Colonic myoelectric activity in the irritable bowel syndrome. Gastroenterology *70*:326, 1976.
64. Taylor, I., Darby, C., and Hammond, P. Comparison of rectosigmoid myoelectrical activity in the irritable colon syndrome during relapses and remissions. Gut *19*:923, 1978.
65. Latimer, P., Sarna, S., Campbell, D., Latimer, M., and Daniel, E. E. Colonic motor and myoelectrical activity. A comparative study of normal subjects, psychoneurotic patients, and patients with irritable bowel syndrome. Gastroenterology *80*:893, 1981.
66. Snape, W. J., Jr., Carlson, G. M., and Cohen, S. Human colonic myoelectric activity in response to prostigmine and the gastrointestinal hormones. Dig. Dis. Sci. *22*:881, 1977.
67. Walsh, J. H., Lamers, C. B., and Valenzuela, J. E. Cholecystokinin-octapeptidelike immunorectivity in human plasma. Gastroenterology *82*:438, 1982.
68. Renny, A., Snape, W. J., Sun, E. A., Landon, R., and Cohen, S. Role of cholecystokinin in the gastrocolonic response to a fat meal. Gastroenterology *85*:17, 1983.
69. Snape, W. J., Wright, S. H., Battle, W. M., and Cohen, S. The gastrocolic response: evidence for a neural mechanism. Gastroenterology *77*:1235, 1979.
70. Isgar, B., Harman, M., Kaye, M. D., and Whorwell, P. J. Symptoms of irritable bowel syndrome in ulcerative colitis in remission. Gut *24*:190, 1983.
71. Svedlund, J., Sjodin, I., Ottosson, J. O., and Dotevall, G. Controlled study of psychotherapy in irritable bowel syndrome. Lancet *2*:589, 1983.
72. Whorwell, P. J., Prior, A., and Faragher, E. B. Controlled trial of hypnotherapy in the treatment of severe refractory irritable-bowel syndrome. Lancet *2*:1232, 1984.
73. Kaufman, N. M., and Schuster, M. M. Colonic motility studies discriminate three types of constipation (Abstract). Gastroenterology *76*:1166, 1979.
74. Longstretch, G. F., Fox, D., Youkeles, L., Forsythe, A. B., and Wolochow, D. A. Psyllium therapy in irritable bowel syndrome. Ann. Intern. Med. *95*:53, 1981.
75. Ritchie, J. A., and Truelove, S. C. Treatment of irritable bowel syndrome with lorazepam hyoscine, butylbromide and ispaghula husk. Br. Med. J. *1*:376, 1979.
76. Harvey, R. F., Heaton, K. W., and Pomera, E. W. Effects of increased dietary fiber on intestinal transit. Lancet *1*:1278, 1973.
77. Payler, D. K., Pomera, E. W., Heaton, R. W., and Harvey, R. F. The effect of wheat bran on intestinal transit. Gut *16*:209, 1975.
78. Shapiro, R. H., Fleizer, W. D., Goldfinger, S. E., and Azerkoff, B. R. Cholestyramine response of idiopathic diarrhea. Gastroenterology *58*:993, 1970.
79. Ivy, K. J. Are anticholinergics of use in the irritable colon syndrome? Gastroenterology *68*:130, 1975.
80. Silverberg, M., Daum, F. IBS in children and adolescents. Practical Gastroenterol. *2*:25, 1979.
81. Cohlan, S. Q. Chronic non-specific diarrhea in infants and children treated with diiodohydroxyquinoline. Pediatrics *18*:424, 1956.
82. Apley, J., and Naish, N. Recurrent abdominal pain: a full survey of 1000 school children. Arch. Dis. Child. *33*:165, 1958.
83. Davidson, M., and Wasserman, R. The irritable colon of childhood (chronic, non-specific diarrhea syndrome). J. Pediatr. *69*:1027, 1966.
84. Apley, J. The Child with Abdominal Pains. 2nd edition. Philadelphia, F. A. Davis, 1964.

77

Diverticular Disease of the Colon

ARTHUR NAITOVE
THOMAS P. ALMY

Diverticular disease of the colon represents the clinical consequences of an acquired deformity of the colon (diverticulosis), its associated physiologic changes, and its complications. The basic abnormality is a pseudodiverticulum, a herniation of the mucosa and the submucosa through the muscular coat of the colon to lie within the serosa. It is extremely common in developed Western societies, in which its prevalence is strikingly correlated with advancing age.[1] Although rarely it is reversible, the deformity is usually asymptomatic. Of all those affected, an estimated 20 per cent develop symptoms and signs of illness; a small minority endure serious or life-threatening complications, and not more than 1 in 10,000 will succumb to the disease.[2]

PREVALENCE AND EPIDEMIOLOGY

The true prevalence of diverticular disease is unknown, as estimates are based on necropsy or radiologic findings in nonrandom population samples. These indicate that it occurs in about 10 per cent of the people in the United States, the United Kingdom, Australia, and other developed countries. It is uncommon before the age of 40 years and increases in frequency from 5 per cent in the fifth decade to 50 per cent or more in the ninth decade. Equally striking has been the increase in its prevalence over time: Although before 1900 it was regarded as a pathologic curiosity, currently it is found in one third to one half of all autopsies of persons over 60 years of age.[3]

Diverticular disease is much less common in other geographic areas than those listed and varies in frequency among different racial and ethnic groups (Table 77–1).[4] It affects about 1 per cent of the population of Asian nations, including Japan.[5] It is found in Ashkenazic more often than in Sephardic Jews.[6] In migrants from low-prevalence areas to westernized communities (Honolulu, Johannesburg),[7, 8] diverticula increase in frequency within ten years.

The incidence and prevalence of diverticulitis and other complications must be estimated from figures based upon very different patient populations. In general, probably 4 to 5 per cent of those who harbor diverticula (20 per cent of those clinically recognized) will develop some complication, 1 to 2 per cent will require hospitalization, and 0.5 per cent will require surgical intervention. As most clinical surveys are based on hospital admissions, the usually reported frequency of complications is much higher.[1]

The hypothesis most often drawn from these observations is that the current high frequency of diverticular disease has resulted from consumption of a diet low in cereal fiber by an aging population.[3] Although in westernized countries in the last century crude cereal grains have been replaced largely by refined carbohydrates, the concurrent effects of many other dietary, environmental, and social changes are difficult to dismiss.

DIVERTICULOSIS

Pathology

The colon is the most common site of diverticulum formation in the digestive tract. As elsewhere, isolated true diverticula, whose walls contain all layers of the intestine, are occasionally found. However, the vast majority of those of clinical significance are pseudodiverticula, or herniations of the mucosa and submucosa through the muscular coats of the colon (Fig. 77–1). They penetrate the clefts between bundles of circular muscle fibers at points where nutrient arteries pass through to the submucosa,[9] and hence nearly all emerge in the serosa in parallel rows between the mesentric and lateral taeniae (Fig. 77–2), varying in number from a few to several hundred and in diameter up to or greater than 1 cm. The close relationship between the herniated sacs and the arteries that invest

Table 77–1. INCIDENCE OF DIVERTICULITIS IN VARIOUS POPULATIONS

Country	Population Served		Diverticulitis *Mean Age*	Diverticulitis *Cases/10⁶/Yr*
Scotland	European	400,000	68	12.88
Nigeria	African	400,000	53	0.17
Singapore	European	15,000	59	5.41
	Chinese	1,014,000	58	0.14
	Malay	190,500	53	0.10
	Indian	111,000	49	0.18
Fiji	European	7,500	60	7.62
	Indian	165,000	51	0.34

Modified from Kyle, J., Adesola, A. D., Tinckler, L. F., and de Beaux, J. Scand. J. Gastroenterol. *2*:77, 1967. Used with permission.

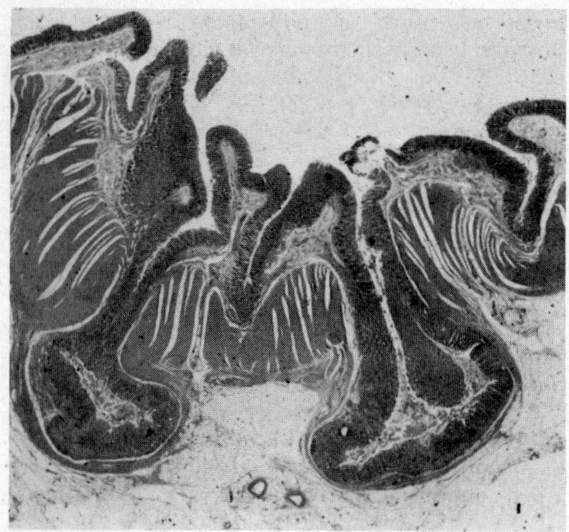

Figure 77–1. Herniation of mucosa of sigmoid colon between thickened folds of circular muscle, forming pseudodiverticula. (From Fleischner, F. G. Diverticular disease of the colon. New observations and revised concepts. Gastroenterology *60*:316–324. © by Williams & Wilkins, 1971.)

the domes and the necks of the diverticula (Fig. 77–3) is considered an important factor in the causation of hemorrhage in patients with uninflamed diverticula.[10] Rarely, diverticula appear on the antimesenteric border, between the lateral taeniae; here the vascular investment is less abundant and the serosal covering is comparatively thin.

The most common site of diverticula is the sigmoid, which is involved in 95 per cent of cases. When more proximal segments are affected, these are invariably in continuity with the involvement of the sigmoid. Over the lifetime of the patient, diverticula may increase in number and size, but only rarely extend to other portions of the colon.[1] Several distinct anatomic patterns are recognized (Table 77–2).

Spastic colon diverticulosis is the most common type in the regions of high prevalence.[11] The wall of the sigmoid and lower descending colon is greatly thickened and its lumen indented by arcuate, overlapping folds of circular muscle, separated by narrow haustra from which the diverticula protrude (Fig. 77–4). Although both the circular muscle and the taeniae appear contracted, the muscle cells are neither hypertrophic nor hyperplastic. Recent findings indicate that the corrugated appearance is due to shortening of the taeniae caused by the excessive deposition of elastin in contracted form.[12] This deformity, often called *myochosis*, so narrows the lumen that muscle contractions can divide the bowel into discontinuous chambers (Fig. 77–5). At times, myochosis has been found on barium enema, at laparotomy, or at autopsy in the absence of grossly recognizable diverticula. This condition has been called the prediverticular state.

Simple massed diverticulosis (Fig. 77–6) denotes the appearance of multiple, usually very numerous pseudodiverticula with little or no thickening of the circular muscle layer, although the colon is shortened to some degree.[11] It accounts for about 30 per cent of cases of diverticulosis in regions of high prevalence. It usually involves both the sigmoid and more proximal portions of the colon and frequently the entire colon.

Right-sided diverticulosis, as distinct from solitary diverticulum of the right colon, is an extremely rare form in Western countries but is the predominant pattern in Asia and in Hawaii.[13, 14] The average age of those affected is lower than with other forms, and the pattern is seen more often in men than in women.

Solitary diverticula, both true and pseudodiverticula, may be found in any portion of the colon, but notably on the right side. Some of those that appear on the antimesenteric border, usually in the sigmoid, may grow in diameter to 6 to 27 cm and be filled with air or exhibit an air-fluid interface. These *giant sigmoid diverticula* vary from one to three in number but are usually associated with other, smaller diverticula. The sacs often lose their epithelial lining and consist only of fibrous tissue lined with granulation tissue, leaving a narrow or occluded orifice.[15]

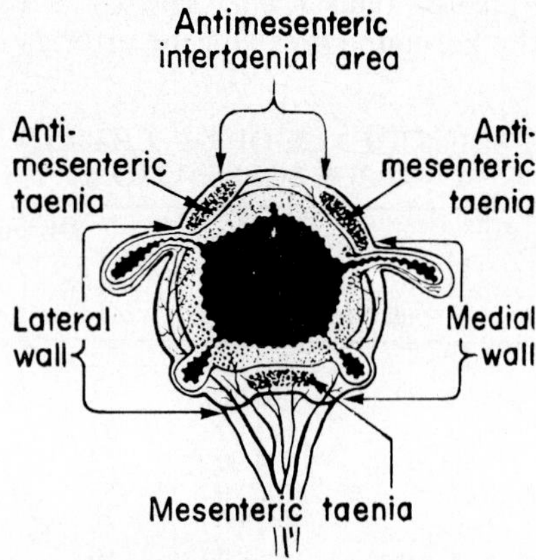

Figure 77–2. Cross-sectional drawing of colon, showing principal points of diverticular formation between mesenteric and antimesenteric taeniae. (From Goligher, J. C. Surgery of the Anus, Rectum and Colon. Ed. 4. London, Baillière Tyndall, 1980, p. 883. Used by permission.)

Pathogenesis

A priori, the herniation of the colonic mucosa appears to require at least two factors: (1) one or more points of diminished resistance of the intestinal wall,

Table 77–2. CLASSIFICATION OF DIVERTICULAR DISEASE OF THE COLON

I. Prediverticular state: Myochosis without gross diverticula
II. Diverticulosis: Multiple pseudodiverticula
    Spastic colon diverticulosis
    Simple massed diverticulosis
    Diverticulosis of the right colon
III. Single diverticulum: True or pseudodiverticulum
    of the cecum or ascending colon
    of the sigmoid—variant: giant sigmoid diverticulum
IV. Diverticulitis: Necrotizing inflammation in one or more diverticula
    with microperforation (local inflammation)
    with macroperforation (manifested by abscess, fistula, peritonitis, fibrosis or obstruction or both)

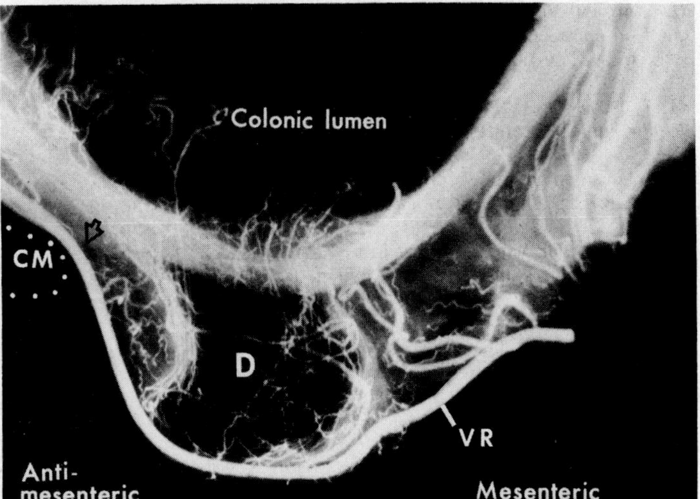

Figure 77–3. Radiograph of a specimen of colon prepared by intra-arterial injection of barium-gelatin. A vas rectum (VR) arches over the dome of the diverticulum (D), then penetrates circular muscle layer (CM) at *arrow.* Neck of diverticulum is surrounded by small vessels of submucosal plexus. (From Meyers, M. A., Alonso, D. R., Gray, G. F., et al. Pathogenesis of bleeding colonic diverticulosis. Gastroenterology *71*:577–583. © by Williams & Wilkins, 1976.)

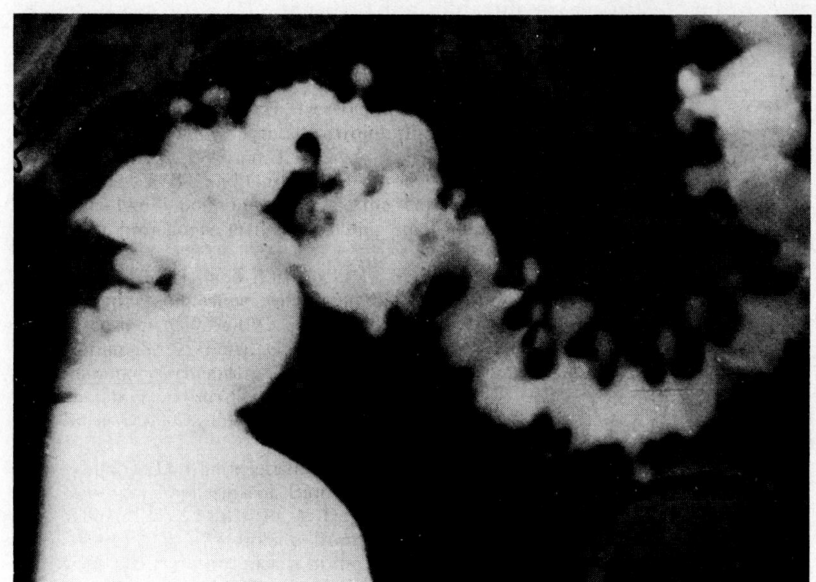

Figure 77–4. Typical findings on barium enema in spastic colon diverticulosis. The lumen is narrowed and corrugated, with narrow haustra from which diverticula protrude.

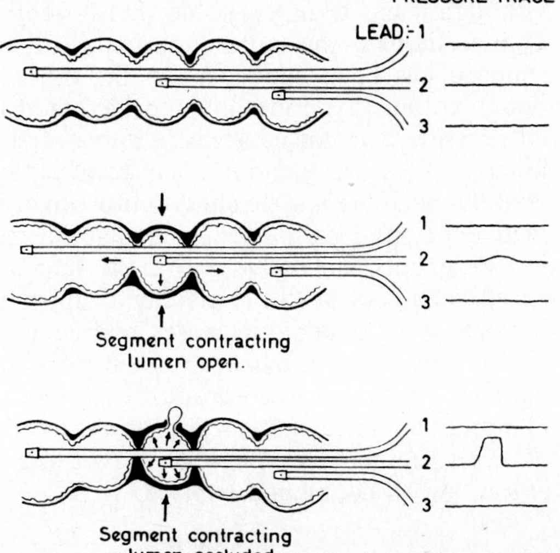

Figure 77–5. Painter's conception of formation of "little bladders" in sigmoid colon with myochosis. Manometric traces from three different sites show that intraluminal pressure rises higher when contractions occlude the lumen and form isolated segments. (From Painter, N. S. Ann. R. Coll. Surg *34*:98, 1964. Used by permission.)

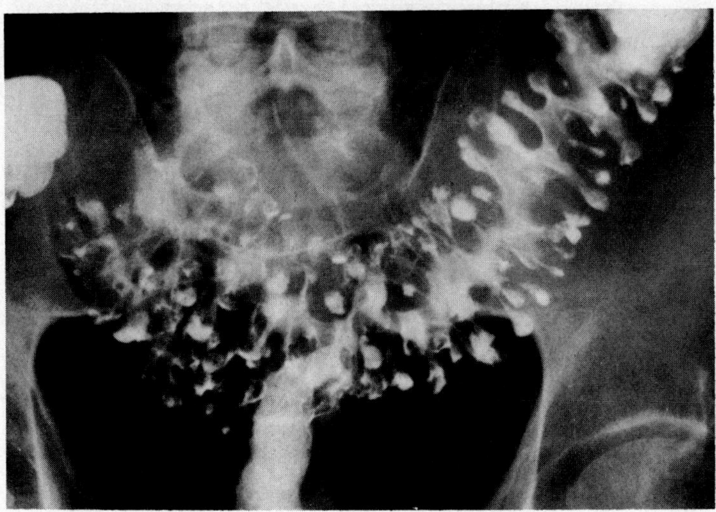

Figure 77–6. Simple massed diverticulosis. Numerous diverticula and a narrowed lumen are present without muscular thickening. (Courtesy of R. Berk, M.D., Southwestern Medical School, Dallas, Texas.)

and (2) a transmural gradient of pressure between the colonic lumen and the peritoneal cavity.[2]

Abnormalities of the Colonic Wall. Clearly, the principal sites of diverticulum formation in the colon are the clefts in the circular muscle layer through which blood vessels reach the submucosa (Fig. 77–2). Despite the increased thickness of its muscular coats, the colonic wall in diverticulosis is reported to have lowered resistance to distention from within,[16] a property that may reflect age-related molecular changes in collagen,[17] but which now appears attributable to progressive deposition of elastin in longitudinal muscle.[12]

The hypothetic importance of changes in the connective tissue of the gut wall is supported by the precocious development of diverticula in young persons with connective tissue disorders, such as Marfan's,[18] Ehlers-Danlos,[19] and the Williams "elfin facies" syndromes.[20] Furthermore, the appearance of wide-mouthed diverticula in the colon affected by systemic sclerosis (scleroderma) may be related to associated changes in tensile strength of the wall.

Motor Abnormalities. The pressure gradient between colonic lumen and peritoneal space is the product of colonic motility or distention by gas, or both. Although it has been suggested that distention due to retained flatus is the more important,[21] no convincing evidence has been adduced. On the other hand, although colonic hypermotility and increased intraluminal pressure are not constant features of diverticular disease,[22] they are found in a subset of patients, most of whom have the muscle abnormality (myochosis) and recurrent colonic pain.[23] When circular muscle contraction interrupts the continuity of the lumen, creating closed chambers or "little bladders," further contraction causes exponential increases of pressure.[24]

This phenomenon has been noted principally in the sigmoid, the narrowest portion of the normal colon. The predominance of this region as a site for formation of diverticula may be attributed in part to a derivation of the law of Young and Laplace:

$$P = kT/R$$

in which intraluminal pressure *(P)* is proportional to the wall tension *(T)* generated by muscle contraction, but inversely proportional to the radius *(R)* of the cylindrical bowel.[25] In accord with this concept, the addition of indigestible fiber to the diet, while increasing the wet weight and the diameter of the stool, has been shown to diminish spontaneous motility and intraluminal pressure in the sigmoid colon.[26] The relationship between the size of the fecal mass and the motility of the colon emerged again in the several attempts to produce an experimental model of diverticulosis in animals. When rats and rabbits were fed diets unnaturally low in vegetable fiber, the most consistent findings were shortening and narrowing of the colon apparently attributable to sustained muscular contraction.[27]

The "fiber hypothesis" is now supported by the finding of an inverse relationship between the dietary concentration of cereal fiber and the prevalence of colonic diverticula, both in a lifespan study of rats[28] and in carefully matched groups of vegetarians and nonvegetarians residing in the city of Oxford, England.[29]

Relationship to the Irritable Bowel Syndrome (IBS). Recognition of the sometimes associated hypermotility of the distal colon has helped sustain a recurring hypothesis that diverticulosis may represent, at least in some persons, a late consequence of the "spastic colon" subtype of IBS. Despite similar symptoms and patterns of colonic motility,[30] the two conditions appear unrelated by reason of their differing natural history and different patterns of myoelectric activity (see pp. 1403–1410).[31, 32] The true causes of the hypermotility seen in spastic colon diverticulosis remain unknown.

Clinical Features

In approximately 80 per cent of those affected, uncomplicated diverticulosis is an asymptomatic condition, recognized during life only at laparotomy or by radiographic signs. In most of the others, diverticula are identifiable many months or years before symptoms occur. In a smaller number, single or even repeated episodes of symptoms may precede by as much as two to five years the first radiologic evidence of diverticula. In such cases myochosis is found, with or without microscopic herniations of mucosa (the prediverticular state).[23] The usual course of symptomatic illness is one of many years of remissions and relapses, the latter measured in days or weeks. If the patient is not treated, the intensity of symptoms is likely to increase over time.[1]

Symptoms. By far the most common symptom is pain, or colic—an often severe, griping pain in the lower abdominal quadrants, more often on the left, which persists with variable intensity over a period of a few hours to several days. The pain is often worse after eating, and temporary partial to complete relief may follow a bowel movement or passage of flatus. In such episodes, the patient may also experience constipation, diarrhea, flatulence, or dyspepsia. The mechanism of pain is believed to be increased tension in the colonic wall, with associated rise in intraluminal pressure. The only other presenting symptom in uncomplicated diverticulosis is painless rectal bleeding; this is discussed in detail later in this chapter.

Physical and Laboratory Findings. On physical examination, a firm and tender loop of sigmoid colon may be felt in the left iliac fossa, while the rest of the abdomen is tympanitic and often distended. There is, nevertheless, no rebound tenderness or other sign of peritoneal inflammation; the body temperature, leukocyte count, and erythrocyte sedimentation rate remain normal. Barium enema usually reveals the diverticula and the extent of shortening, narrowing, and haustral deformity in the distal colon (Fig. 77–4). In some instances, the sacs themselves are better visualized on films taken 24 or 48 hours after a barium meal. Flexible or rigid sigmoidoscopy and colonoscopy are of value chiefly in differential diagnosis, although the muscular folds and the orifices of diverticula may be visible. The risk of perforation, especially if a diverticulum is entered, approaches 1 per cent.[33]

Diagnosis and Differential Diagnosis

Despite the usual absence of physical findings, the diagnosis of diverticular disease comes easily to mind whenever in a Western society an elderly person, usually overweight and often showing signs of atherosclerosis, complains of abdominal pain or profuse rectal bleeding. However, the demonstration of diverticula on X-ray film, usually so easily accomplished, adds only a little to the diagnostic probability because of the high prevalence of diverticulosis among all persons in that age group. Alternate explanations for the symptoms must be weighed with care.

On the one hand, the recurring pain may be due to the irritable bowel syndrome, especially if the episodes began in early or middle life and are strikingly associated with life stress and emotional tension, with neurotic personality features, or with other stress disorders, manifest illness behavior (the "sick role"), or secondary gain (see pp. 1402–1418). On the other hand, the patient may already have diverticulitis; both the local and the systemic signs of this inflammatory process (see p. 1426) may be absent at the beginning of a painful episode, only to appear during repeated observation of the patient. The clinical spectrum of diverticulosis overlaps those of many gynecologic and urologic disorders, of lactose intolerance and other brush border enzyme deficiencies, and of carcinoma of the distal colon and upper rectum. Many other diagnostic pitfalls exist.

Treatment

The treatment of uncomplicated diverticulosis is undertaken to relieve symptoms and to prevent or postpone its complications.

Diet. For many years it was believed that the colon in diverticular disease could be "put at rest" by a diet low in indigestible residue, and that the skins and seeds of fruits and vegetables were harmful. These concepts were never validated by controlled studies and have now been re-examined in the light of the "fiber hypothesis" and the supporting evidence cited earlier. Diets high in vegetable fiber, especially in the celluloses and lignins of whole cereal grains, have been shown in controlled studies not only to increase stool mass and lower the intraluminal pressure in the sigmoid[26] but also to relieve pain and associated symptoms.[34, 35] The best results have been achieved with unprocessed, coarse wheat bran in the maximal amounts tolerated, or at least 10 to 25 gm/day in divided portions with meals, added to porridge, soups, fruit juice, or other liquid or semi-liquid foods. The recommended amounts usually must be reached by slowly raising the level of intake over a period of four to six weeks, during which time the patient's bloating and discomfort actually may increase before improvement is obtained. The same fiber intake may be achieved by eating whole wheat bread (five slices, or 150 gm, daily), various breakfast cereals, or high-fiber crispbread or bran biscuits.[2]

The resulting increase in fecal mass is due only in small part to the passage of the undigested fiber itself, which has increased in volume through the imbibing of water. Indeed, from 50 to 75 per cent of the ingested fiber disappears in passage through the gut, being degraded by colonic flora chiefly to propionate, butyrate, and other organic anions.[36] These exert a mild but persistent osmotic effect, further increasing the water content and the mass of the stool.

Qualitatively similar effects can be obtained at higher cost with other dietary sources of fiber, including potatoes, legumes, salads and other leafy vegetables, bananas, and apples. Much larger quantities are needed than are recommended for bran, chiefly because of their higher content of water. Their effectiveness is not yet demonstrated by controlled trials.

Drugs. A comparatively expensive but usually satisfactory alternative to bran for the purpose of increasing the bulk and water content of the stool is the use of hydrophilic colloid laxatives. These products, including various forms of psyllium, agar, ispaghula, and methylcellulose, have the advantage of being better tolerated than bran in the first weeks of treatment.[37] Favorable clinical impressions have been strengthened somewhat by controlled trials.[38] The amounts used can be tapered as the natural fiber content of the diet is progressively increased. Some clinicians suggest that the fluid bulk provided by the saline laxatives sodium phosphate and magnesium sulfate, as well as lactulose, may be useful in the relief of acutely painful episodes.[39]

Antispasmodics. The effectiveness of agents that might directly inhibit muscular contraction in the affected colon remains in doubt for lack of direct physiologic observation and of controlled therapeutic trials. In Europe, musculotropic agents such as mebeverine and trimebutine, which inhibit normal sigmoid motility, have been shown to give significant symptomatic relief.[40] These are not available in the United States. Atropine and the synthetic quaternary anticholinergic drugs, which clearly inhibit normal motility, have not been proved clinically effective in painful diverticulosis. Prompt relief of this condition has been reported to follow intravenous injection of glucagon, whose role as a smooth muscle relaxant is now familiar to radiologists.[41] The effect can apparently be sustained for one to two days by repeated injections.

Analgesics. When the direct relief of pain is required temporarily, the choice of an analgesic is critical. Morphine has been directly observed to raise intraluminal pressure in the sigmoid colon and to cause marked distention of the diverticula themselves, presumably increasing the risk of perforation.[42] Consequently, the use of any opiate is believed to be contraindicated. Meperidine may be used, nevertheless, in customary doses without incurring this risk and is probably the agent of choice. While pentazocine has been shown to actually reduce sigmoid motility in regular analgesic doses,[43] it may cause confusion, disorientation, and hallucinations in elderly patients.

Antibiotics. There is no rational place for antibiotics in the management of uncomplicated diverticulosis, as necrotizing inflammation is by definition excluded. The difficulties attending the clinical diagnosis of minimal diverticulitis, as well as the recommended therapeutic strategy in view of the natural course of that disease, are discussed fully later (see p. 1426).

DIVERTICULAR BLEEDING

Rectal bleeding of varying significance may be evident in 10 to 30 per cent of patients with diverticular disease; severe blood loss from colonic diverticula is reported to occur in 3 to 5 per cent of those with diverticulosis and is considered to be the most common cause of life-threatening lower gastrointestinal hemorrhage in the elderly.[44–51] These estimates, however, which are based on studies in which the actual bleeding site was not always identified, do not provide assurance in any given instance that bleeding is of diverticular origin. The importance of vascular ectasias (angiodysplasia, arteriovenous malformations) of the right colon as the second most frequent cause of severe lower gastrointestinal hemorrhage in the elderly has become apparent in recent years[50–56] (see p. 1922). A variety of other lesions, including adenomas and carcinomas of the colon, have also been implicated, but these most often are responsible for the passage of small to moderate amounts of blood per rectum.[45] Furthermore, in approximately 10 per cent of patients whose clinical presentation is that of lower intestinal hemorrhage, a lesion in the upper gastrointestinal tract can be responsible for the bleeding.[57, 58] Thus, in any patient it may be necessary to evaluate the entire gastrointestinal tract using a variety of endoscopic and radiologic diagnostic techniques before concluding that rectal bleeding is the consequence of diverticular disease. A more complete discussion of gastrointestinal bleeding is found on pages 397 to 427.

Pathology

In approximately 70 per cent of the instances in which the site of massive diverticular bleeding can be identified, it is located in the right colon.[46, 47, 51, 59–64] The source is usually a single diverticulum, which in 80 per cent of cases is not inflamed.[47, 49, 60] Although the specific bleeding vessel is seldom visualized grossly, the close anatomic relationship of the colonic intramural arterial branches to the herniated diverticular sacs makes their involvement no surprise (Fig. 77–3).[10, 64] Precise microscopic studies have shown the source of bleeding to be a minute rupture of one of these vessels, asymmetrically placed on the wall adjacent to the lumen of the diverticulum.[10, 64] Usually little or no inflammation is evident in the vessel or the juxtaposed, focally eroded wall of the diverticulum. The most significant finding is an eccentric focus of medial thinning, intimal thickening and duplication, and fragmentation of the internal elastic lamina in the wall of the involved artery at the point of its disruption.[64] The pathogenesis of the vascular lesion is unclear, but the evidence indicates that a focus of diverticular inflammation is not responsible. On the other hand, in some instances of less severe chronic or intermittent bleeding attributed to diverticular disease, ulceration and inflammatory changes have been noted in the necks of diverticula.[44]

Clinical Features

Massive diverticular hemorrhage occurs predominantly in patients with otherwise uncomplicated diverticulosis. In a typical case, an elderly person, with no specific previous bowel complaints but with the usual stigmata of one or more of the common degenerative diseases of the aged, suddenly experiences mild lower abdominal cramps and an urge to defecate. Shortly thereafter either a large volume of bright red blood or clots, or both, or a dark red, maroon, or (least commonly) black stool is passed per rectum. Symptoms and signs of hypovolemia may or may not be present. Presumably, in some instances, a steady but relatively slow rate of blood loss from small arteries into a distensible colon allows time for cardiovascular adjustments to be made before the sudden evacuation of a large, bloody stool.

Bleeding may be continuous or intermittent over several days, ceasing spontaneously in about 80 per cent of patients.[47, 48, 50] The chances of a second hemorrhage in the days, weeks, months, or years after an initial episode of bleeding are of the order of 20 to 25 per cent.[47, 48, 52, 56, 61, 62] However, once bleeding recurs, the risk of another recurrent hemorrhage increases to 50 per cent or more.[47, 50, 56]

Diagnosis and Differential Diagnosis

Given the classic onset of sudden, painless, profuse rectal bleeding in an elderly patient, the probability that the hemorrhage is from a colonic diverticulum is high. Testing of the clinical diagnosis begins with an evaluation of whether the bleeding site is in the upper gastrointestinal tract. A nasogastric tube is passed, and stomach contents are aspirated and examined for blood. If none is found, and particularly if the aspirate is bile-stained, it is at least 90 per cent certain that the bleeding site is not proximal to the ligament of Treitz.[57, 58] The chance of error can be further reduced by carrying out esophagogastroduodenoscopy. If these studies are negative, proctosigmoidoscopy should be performed to rule out other nondiverticular causes of bleeding in the lowermost segments of the gut. As is appropriate in any patient who presents with gastrointestinal hemorrhage, blood coagulation studies should be performed. If the results of all of the examinations seeking to localize the bleeding are normal, efforts to locate and define the source of hemorrhage more precisely should be initiated (see pp. 397–427).

If rectal bleeding continues to be severe, angiography should be performed as the first direct approach to the diagnosis. This procedure may identify the source of hemorrhage in 60 to 90 per cent of cases. The majority will be of diverticular origin, and 70 per cent of these are located in the right colon.[46, 51, 59–64] However, as the site may be located elsewhere in the gut, a thorough examination can require arteriographic studies of the superior and inferior mesenteric vessels and the celiac axis, in that order. This sequence is halted only when luminal extravasation of contrast medium localizes a bleeding site, or convincing angiographic signs of vascular malformations, tumors, or other nondiverticular sources are found. The demonstration of a collection of radiopaque material in the colonic lumen, in the absence of other findings in the area, strongly supports the diagnosis of diverticular bleeding, whether in the right or left colon (Fig. 77–7) and whether or not the presence of diverticula has been previously documented. The diagnosis, nevertheless, depends on bleeding being relatively brisk at the time of the study. Concern for this limitation, and for the invasive nature and hazards of arteriography, has prompted some clinicians to advocate prior radionuclide imaging with ^{99m}Tc-labeled sulfur colloid or red blood cells[65–67] (see pp. 411–413). This noninvasive procedure can provide assurance that bleeding is still active and that conditions for successful angiographic demonstration of the bleeding site are present. In addition, it may enhance and simplify the arteriographic search by indicating the approximate location of the bleeding site, thereby serving as a direct guide to selective arterial studies.

When bleeding is severe, barium contrast X-ray studies of the colon and more proximal portions of the gastrointestinal tract should be deferred until angiog-

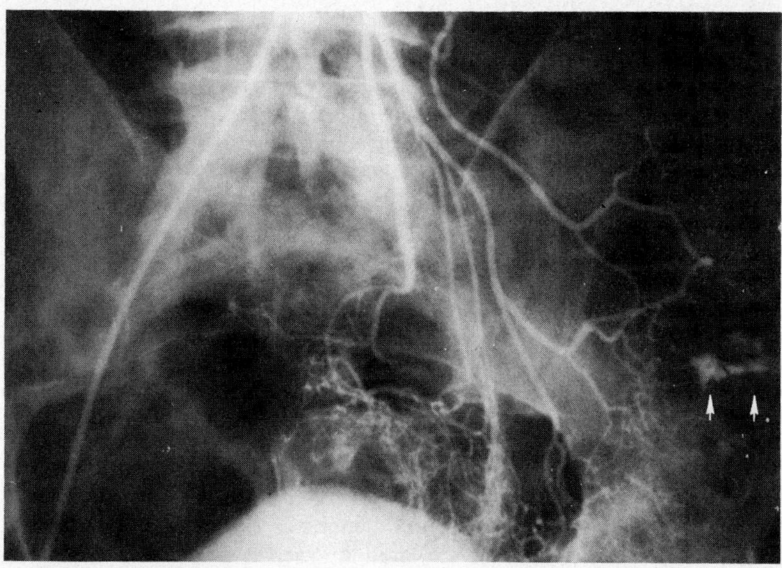

Figure 77–7. Angiographic localization of bleeding from a diverticulum in the descending colon. An inferior mesenteric arteriogram in a patient with severe rectal bleeding. Contrast material is shown collecting in the contiguous lumina of the bleeding diverticulum and colon *(arrows)*.

raphy has been performed. The persistence of barium in the bowel can preclude obtaining meaningful information angiographically for one to seven days thereafter. Furthermore, barium studies cannot identify vascular abnormalities, nor can they disclose which of several lesions demonstrated is the source of bleeding. Colonoscopy has a limited role when hemorrhage is severe, as an adequate examination seldom is feasible when the bowel is filled with blood (see pp. 411–413).

In patients in whom bleeding is minimal or has ceased at the time they are first being evaluated, colonoscopy followed by barium contrast X-ray studies of the colon, upper gastrointestinal tract, and small bowel is performed in the search for a cause. If these efforts are unproductive, elective angiography then can be employed to identify vascular lesions.

The high prevalence of innocent asymptomatic diverticulosis in elderly persons makes it likely that it may coexist with some other disorder that is the true cause of rectal hemorrhage. Now placed at the top of the list in this differential diagnosis is angiodysplasia (vascular ectasia), which also most often is found in the right colon by angiography or colonoscopy.[50–55, 67] Severe rectal bleeding may be an early sign of ulcerative colitis, Crohn's disease of the colon and rectum, and, rarely, colorectal carcinomas and adenomas. Ischemic colitis also can be associated with rectal hemorrhage, but more often presents with severe abdominal pain and characteristic radiographic findings in the colon that aid in the differential diagnosis.

Treatment

In most patients, diverticular bleeding ceases spontaneously during application of familiar conservative medical measures, including restoration of blood volume and red cell mass by transfusion, repair of coagulation defects, intravenous fluids or clear liquid diet, sedation, and bed rest. In those who continue to bleed actively and in whom the source is identified angiographically, selective intra-arterial infusion of vasopressin has been advocated.[46, 51, 55, 61, 62] Starting at 0.2 to 0.3 units/minute, vasopressin is administered continuously in serially decreasing doses over a period of 24 to 36 hours via a catheter placed in the appropriate mesenteric artery at the time of arteriography. Given in this manner, vasopressin can be effective in arresting diverticular hemorrhage, at least temporarily. Although initial success rates of up to 90 per cent have been achieved, rebleeding after cessation of intra-arterial delivery of the agent has been observed up to 50 per cent of the time.[51] Still another technique reported to be of value in such instances is transcatheter arterial embolization of the bleeding vessel, using any of a variety of materials for the purpose.[68] This procedure, however, with its potential to cause bowel infarction, is not widely used.

Emergency surgical treatment of diverticular bleeding becomes a consideration when severe hemorrhage persists or recurs despite adequate medical therapy. According to evidence accumulated in recent years, the choice of operation is determined by what is known about the bleeding site.[50–55, 67] When angiography has identified its location and medical treatment, including selective intra-arterial infusion of vasopressin, has failed, segmental resection of the portion of colon containing the offending diverticulum should be performed. Rebleeding is very infrequent provided that the segment of bowel resected contains the bleeding site that was identified.[50, 51, 55] The presence of other diverticula in the remaining portions of bowel apparently is not a cause for concern. Subtotal colectomy, as advocated in the past,[46, 47, 49] with its higher operative morbidity and more disabling long-term sequelae, currently is reserved as a last resort for those patients with continued severe bleeding in whom the specific bleeding site has not been identified angiographically.[50, 51, 55]

Elective surgery also can be considered in some patients whose bleeding ceases spontaneously or in response to medical management. The decision depends on whether the source of bleeding has been clearly identified, on the estimated operative risk, and on the probability of recurrent hemorrhage.

DIVERTICULITIS

Diverticulitis is the most frequent complication of diverticulosis. Its clinical manifestations are the consequences of peridiverticular extension of inflammation (peridiverticulitis) to the adjacent bowel wall or surrounding tissues. The process can be localized and relatively benign or more extensive and life-threatening. It has been estimated that 10 to 20 per cent of persons known to have colonic diverticula will develop diverticulitis at some time in their lives.[2] In one large series of ambulatory patients, this became clinically evident in 10 per cent of those followed up to 5 years and in 37 per cent of those followed 11 to 18 years.[69] In general, the likelihood of a patient's developing an inflammatory complication of diverticulosis is greater than average if diverticula are numerous, are widely distributed in the colon, appear at an early age, or have been known to be present for a decade or longer.

Pathology

The initial pathologic change in diverticulitis is a focal area of inflammation in the wall of a diverticulum at its apex, rarely its neck, developing in response to the irritating presence of inspissated fecal material.[70, 71] Unlike appendicitis, it is not acute suppuration in the lumen that spreads diffusely to the walls of the sac should a fecalith obstruct its outlet. It is not known whether the initial apical lesion can be symptomatic when it is confined to the wall of the diverticulum. However, the evidence is clear that peridiverticular extension of inflammation from this focus is present when diverticulitis becomes clinically manifest, and that peridiverticulitis results when the intramural process in the apex progresses to cause necrosis, micro- or macroperforation, and fecal contamination of the surrounding tissues.[70,71] Commonly, only one diverticulum is involved. Most often it is located in the sigmoid colon.

Peridiverticulitis usually remains localized, being contained by the appendices epiploicae, pericolonic fat, mesentery, or adjacent organs. With microperforation, a small paracolonic abscess or area of fibrosis can be found (Fig. 77–8). Repeated episodes lead to more extensive phlegmonous and fibrotic reactions in or around the colonic wall that cause segmental narrowing and even obstruction of the bowel. Similar consequences can result from even a single episode of macroperforation. In addition, the larger abscesses formed can burrow longitudinally, along or within the bowel wall, eventually to re-enter the colonic lumen or to rupture into adherent structures. In the latter instance, fistulas can develop between the colon and the bladder, ureter, vagina, small bowel, or external surface of the abdominal wall. Free perforation of a diverticulum into the peritoneal cavity, with associated widespread peritonitis is, fortunately, uncommon.

Clinical Features

When diverticulitis intervenes, pain and fever are the most common presenting symptoms.[72] The pain is frequently acute in onset, persistent, and localized to the left lower quadrant, often with extension into the back. With displacement of a redundant sigmoid colon to the right, or when a right colonic diverticulum is involved, the pain can be suprapubic or in the right lower quadrant. The fever can be accompanied by chills and may be the patient's only complaint. Anorexia, nausea, and vomiting may occur, and changes in bowel habits are common, ranging from diarrhea to constipation. Dysuria and frequency of urination also may be present, indicating involvement of the bladder.

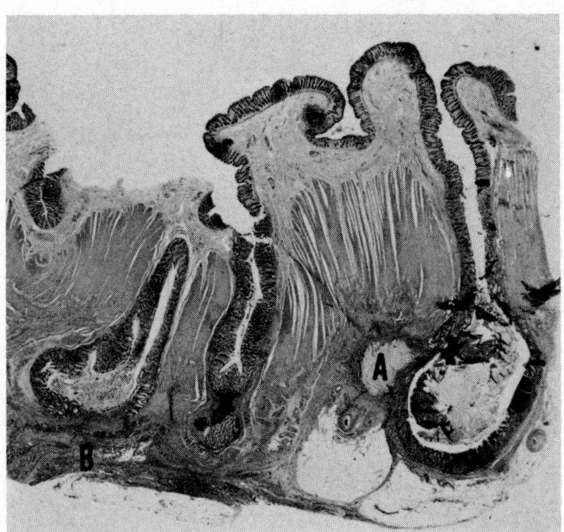

Figure 77–8. A small localized abscess *(A)* is adjacent to a perforated diverticulum. An area of fibrosis *(B)* is seen beneath another diverticulum, the residue of a prior perforation of that diverticulum. (From Fleischner, F. G. Diverticular disease of the colon. New observations and revised concepts. Gastroenterology *60*:316–324. © by Williams & Wilkins, 1971.)

On physical examination, tenderness in the left lower quadrant usually is found. It may be marked and associated with involuntary guarding and other signs of parietal peritoneal inflammation. A tender, sausage-like, fixed mass may be palpable, and the abdomen is often distended and tympanic. Bowel sounds are usually depressed but can be increased with intestinal obstruction, or they may be normal when the inflammatory reaction is mild and well localized. Rectal examination may reveal tenderness, induration, and the presence of a mass in the cul-de-sac.

An almost invariable laboratory finding is an elevated white blood count with a marked predominance of polymorphonuclear leukocytes. The notable exception is the aged patient with acute overwhelming infection in whom the total count may not be high. Urinalysis may disclose the presence of red or white blood cells if there is involvement of the bladder or ureter by the inflammatory process.

Diagnosis

The diagnosis frequently can be made on the basis of the typical findings just described. It is to be remembered, however, that this may not be as true in aged, steroid-dependent, and immunocompromised patients whose clinical responses may be blunted and less typical.

In most instances when the diagnosis of diverticulitis is entertained, the performance of proctosigmoidoscopy early in the work-up is considered. There are those who would argue that unless the diagnosis is in doubt or the patient's response to initial therapy is unsatisfactory, this diagnostic measure can be deferred until after the acute inflammatory stage of the disease has subsided. Others do not subscribe to this conservative approach to diagnosis. Today, proctosigmoidoscopy can be carried out more comfortably, safely, and productively than in the past with the use of a flexible as compared with a rigid sigmoidoscope. This examination, done gently with minimal bowel preparation and little air insufflation, is of value in the differential diagnosis of other disorders (e.g., ulcerative or granulomatous colitis, carcinoma) and in assessing whether the rectum and distal sigmoid are free of diverticular disease should surgical resection and anastomosis become urgent considerations. Although this is not pathognomonic, inability to pass the instrument beyond the rectosigmoid junction owing to fixation, angulation, and tenderness is a consistent finding with acute diverticulitis. Finally, albeit not a primary goal of endoscopic examination in the acute phase of diverticulitis, the visualization of the ostia of diverticula will confirm their presence.

Radiologic evaluation also may be important in the early work-up. Plain supine and erect X-ray films of the abdomen can assess the degree of ileus or intestinal obstruction and reveal the presence of free air in the

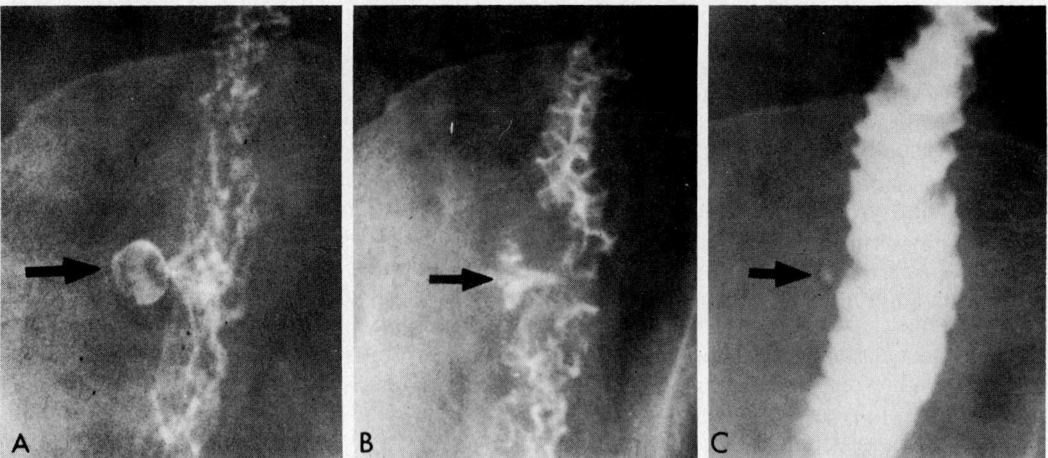

Figure 77–9. A diverticulum is seen in the descending colon *(A)*; eight months later *(B)*, during attack of diverticulitis, barium is demonstrated outside the diverticulum. After recovery *(C)*, a fleck of barium remains. (From Fleischner, F. G. Diverticular disease of the colon. New observations and revised concepts. Gastroenterology *60*:316–324. © by Williams & Wilkins, 1971.)

peritoneal cavity when a diverticular perforation is not contained. Diagnostic use of barium contrast X-ray studies in the presence of acute diverticulitis, on the other hand, is controversial. A number of physicians believe this examination should be deferred, because the increased intraluminal pressure attendant on the introduction of barium may disrupt a localized perforation and cause soilage of the peritoneal cavity with feces and contrast material. Others argue that if it is performed carefully, the risk of complications is minimal and is outweighed by the diagnostic value of the procedure.[73, 74] In any event, all agree that barium enema should be performed at some point in the course of the illness, and if the diagnosis is in doubt, the sooner the better. Evidence of diverticulitis includes the demonstration of barium outside the lumen of the colon or of a diverticulum (Fig. 77–9), a paracolic mass (Fig. 77–10), a fistula leading from the colon, or a segment of narrowed colon in which the normal mucosal pattern is intact. Spasm, irregularity, and thickening of the bowel wall are seen too often in spastic colon diverticulosis to be of help in the diagnosis of diverticulitis. In patients with urinary tract involvement, intravenous pyelography or cystoscopy may also be helpful.

The most recent and impressive addition to the list of radiologic techniques for the diagnosis of acute diverticulitis and its complications is computed tomography (CT).[75, 76] This technique is noninvasive and can be used in septic patients for whom barium contrast X-ray studies are potentially hazardous. It is versatile in identifying diverticula, in recognizing changes in the wall of the colon and pericolic fat that are indicative of diverticulitis, and in identifying related abscesses and fistulas (Fig. 77–11). Undoubtedly, the use of CT as a primary diagnostic tool in diverticular disease will become widespread, being limited only by its cost and availability.

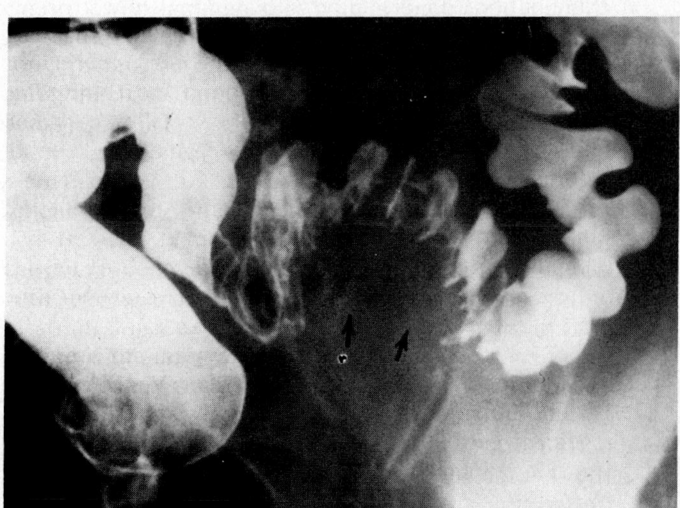

Figure 77–10. A paracolic mass that deforms and displaces the sigmoid lumen is delineated in a patient with diverticulitis and a palpable left lower quadrant mass. (Courtesy of R. Berk, M.D., Southwestern Medical School, Dallas, Texas.)

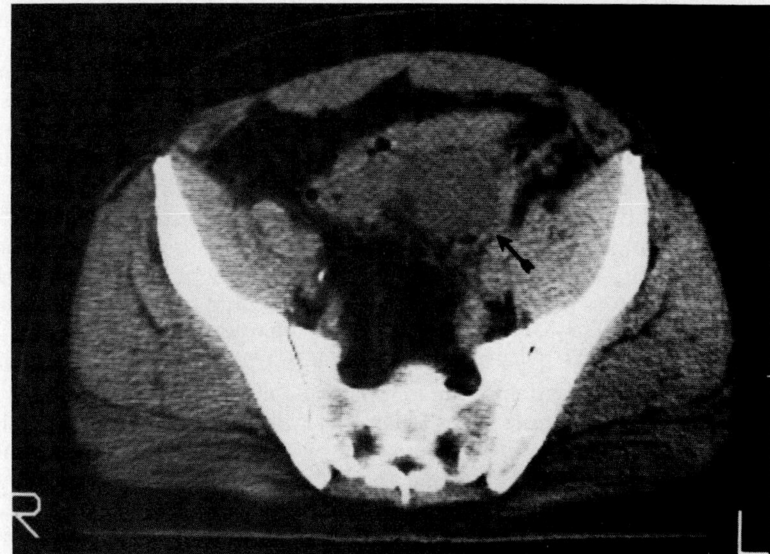

Figure 77–11. CT scan showing air-filled diverticula in a contract segment of sigmoid colon lying just anterior to a paracolic abscess, indicated by a circumscribed area of uniform low density *(arrow).*

Complications

When the inflammatory consequences of diverticular perforation cannot be contained or resolved locally, secondary complications ensue.[77–80] The more common of these, accounting for most of the severe morbidity associated with diverticulitis, are intra-abdominal abscess, fistulas, bowel obstruction, and generalized peritonitis.

Intra-abdominal Abscess. Extensive collections of putrescent pus develop adjacent to the bowel, in the pelvis, under the diaphragm, or elsewhere in the abdominal cavity.[78] The possibility that an abscess has developed is suggested by persistent spiking temperatures and leukocytosis; persistence or recurrence of a tender palpable mass on abdominal, rectal, or vaginal examination; and radiographic evidence of elevation and fixation of the diaphragm. Barium enema showing a mass displacing the colon may reveal its presence (Fig. 77–10), but computed tomography is currently the best means for confirming the diagnosis and following the course of an intra-abdominal abscess (Fig. 77–11).

Fistulas. Direct extension and rupture of an abscess into surrounding structures or, less commonly, direct perforation of an adherent diverticulum can cause a fistula to form.[79] The most common is a colovesical fistula, usually between the sigmoid colon and posterior bladder wall.[77, 79, 80] More apt to occur in men, its presence is indicated by persistent or recurrent urinary tract infection, pneumaturia, and fecaluria. In approximately one third of cases, no history of a prior symptomatic intra-abdominal disorder can be elicited when the patient presents with a colovesical fistula. Proctosigmoidoscopy, barium enema, intravenous pyelography, and cystography are helpful in the diagnosis (Fig. 77–12). Although not uniformly successful in demonstrating the fistula, these methods also are of value in revealing other diseases that underlie it. Cystoscopy should be performed. Even if the fistulous tract is not visualized, a characteristic focal area of inflammation that signifies its presence usually will be

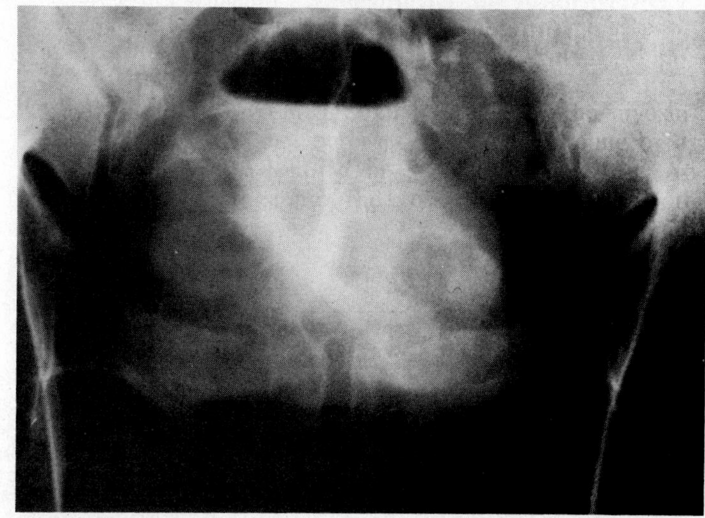

Figure 77–12. An upright film of the bladder made during an intravenous pyelogram performed in a patient with pneumaturia reveals air in the bladder, confirming the presence of a colovesical fistula. (Courtesy of R. Berk, M.D., Southwestern Medical School, Dallas, Texas.)

seen. Coloenteric fistulas frequently are asymptomatic. However, if bacterial overgrowth in the small bowel or bypass of sufficient intestinal absorptive surface results, diarrhea and steatorrhea may be present (pp. 263–282.)

Bowel Obstruction. During an acute episode of diverticulitis, severe peridiverticular inflammation in or about the colonic wall can cause partial or complete obstruction of the large bowel.[78] Ileus and obstruction of the small bowel also can occur when contiguous intestinal loops become involved by the inflammatory process. The signs and symptoms are the same as would be present from any cause of acute obstruction and may be the patient's predominant manifestations. Plain supine and erect abdominal X-ray films and, at times, judicious use of barium contrast studies are helpful in establishing the diagnosis and level of obstruction. Sometimes, more chronic pathologic changes in the wall of the large bowel will cause a partial obstruction after the acute phase has subsided. This may have to be considered in the differential diagnosis of an elderly patient who has an obstructive lesion of the colon.

Generalized Peritonitis. An infrequent complication, generalized peritonitis can be the consequence of an uncontained "free" perforation of a diverticulum or delayed rupture of an intraperitoneal peridiverticular abscess.[78] Such a catastrophe is usually indicated by the sudden onset of diffusely spreading, severe abdominal pain, prostration, signs of septic shock, and board-like rigidity of the abdominal wall. When a diverticulum has perforated freely, radiographic evidence of free intraperitoneal air may be present. This complication can be the first clinical manifestation of diverticular disease and should be considered a possibility in any elderly patient who has generalized peritonitis. The rupture of an abscess, on the other hand, is more likely to be the cause in a patient who is being treated for a clinically severe episode of acute diverticulitis.

Differential Diagnosis

Diverticulosis and Diverticulitis. Clinical features of symptomatic diverticulosis can be difficult to differentiate from those associated with diverticulitis. The lower abdominal pain described by patients with these disorders may be quite similar. In those with *diverticulosis*, findings of a tender, palpable loop of sigmoid and abdominal distention can be misinterpreted as signs of diverticulitis and peridiverticular inflammation. In such instances, a diagnosis of *diverticulitis* can be made with certainty only if fever, leukocytosis, and signs of peritoneal irritation are present. Barium enema and CT also can aid in the diagnosis, if radiologic features peculiar to diverticulitis are present.

Carcinoma of the Colon. Obstruction, perforation, and fistula formation are manifestations of colon carcinoma as well as diverticulitis. Both diseases afflict the same age group and can be present concomitantly in the same patient. The different therapeutic and prognostic implications of the two diseases make a precise diagnosis all the more important. Barium enema studies can be helpful in the differentiation by demonstrating mucosal irregularities and luminal filling defects that are more consistent with carcinoma. However, such radiologic signs can be seen with diverticulitis, making the diagnosis uncertain (Fig. 77–13). At times, with resolution of the acute inflammatory episode, marked improvement or disappearance of the radiologic findings of an intraluminal lesion make it clear that it was not neoplastic. Endoscopic visualization and biopsy of the lesion is the most direct approach to the diagnosis. Current use of the fiberoptic flexible sigmoidoscope or colonoscope has improved the success with which this can be accomplished, as compared with the more limited examination permitted by the rigid sigmoidoscope. In some cases, the diagnosis cannot be made with certainty by any means, and surgical exploration and resection will be necessary to differentiate carcinoma from diverticulitis.

Crohn's Disease of the Colon. Pain, fever, leukocytosis, abdominal tenderness, palpable masses, and fistulas are features of granulomatous colitis (Crohn's disease) making it difficult to distinguish this disease from diverticulitis. Furthermore, both can be present in the same patient. Endoscopic and radiologic features more typical of granulomatous colitis may help to differentiate between the two (i.e., cobblestoning, deep ulcerations of the mucosa, skip lesions, and associated involvement of the small bowel). Mucosal biopsy also may be of value in this situation.

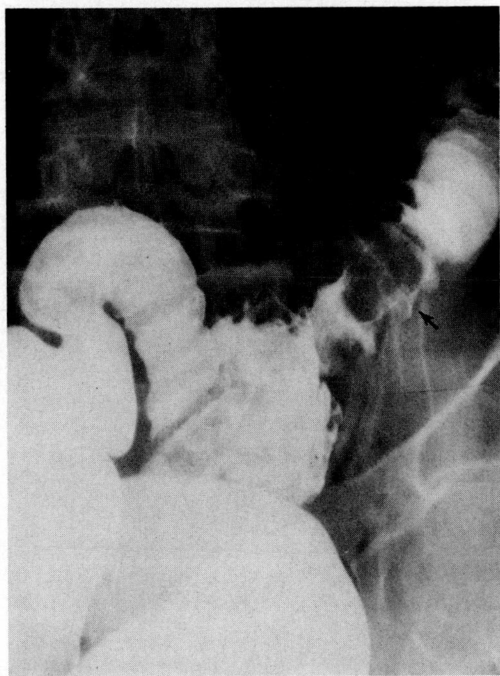

Figure 77–13. An intraluminal filling defect is seen in the sigmoid colon of a patient recovering from an attack of diverticulitis. Radiographically, a tumor could not be excluded. This defect subsequently was found to be a mural abscess secondary to a perforated diverticulum. (Courtesy of R. Berk, M.D., Southwestern Medical School, Dallas, Texas.)

Ulcerative Colitis. Fever, leukocytosis, abdominal pain, and rectal bleeding are features of ulcerative colitis. Usually, the typical mucosal changes of ulcerative colitis, seen in the rectum or more proximal colon by endoscopic examination or barium enema, serve to identify ulcerative colitis. Fortunately, the two diseases rarely coexist in the same patient.

Ischemic Colitis. Stigmata of diffuse atherosclerotic vascular disease are common in the elderly, as is diverticular disease. As such, they are prone to the complications of both. Severe acute abdominal pain and signs of peritonitis with infarction of the bowel can be difficult to distinguish. The characteristic radiographic findings of thumbprinting in the colon sometimes can serve to identify ischemic colitis as the cause. Flexible fiberoptic endoscopic examination for ischemia-related colorectal mucosal changes can also be helpful.

Treatment

The initial therapy of diverticulitis is usually medical. Precise information about the actual success of such management is not available. However, on the basis of experience primarily with patients hospitalized with the diagnosis of diverticulitis, some data have been provided.[1, 69, 81] It has been estimated that 70 to 85 per cent of patients will recover on medical therapy; the remainder will require surgical intervention. Of those with a first episode who are successfully managed medically, up to two thirds will not have subsequent attacks requiring hospitalization, although many in this subset will continue to have symptoms of diverticular disease. Of those patients requiring readmission to hospital for a second attack, approximately 50 and 90 per cent are readmitted within one and five years, respectively.

Medical Therapy. Patients who have pain sufficient to require strong analgesics, fever, leukocytosis, and signs of peritoneal irritation should be admitted to the hospital. Therapeutic efforts are directed at "resting" the bowel, resolving the infection and consequences of inflammation, and preventing or minimizing the severity of secondary complications. The patient should be placed at bed rest and given nothing by mouth, particularly when nausea, vomiting, and abdominal distention are present. If such features are prominent, nasogastric suction should be instituted, long intestinal intubation being reserved only for those in whom signs of small bowel obstruction are evident. Intravenous fluid therapy adequate to the needs for maintaining intravascular volumes, urinary output, electrolyte and acid-base balance, and caloric intake should be started. Laboratory studies, including blood and urine cultures, should be obtained.

Antibiotics usually are indicated in hospitalized patients. The bacterial spectrum involved predictably includes gram-negative aerobic *Escherichia coli* and anaerobic *Bacteroides fragilis*. An aminoglycoside (gentamicin or tobramycin, 5 mg/kg/day) plus clindamycin (1.6 to 2.4 gm/day) given parenterally in divided doses every six hours is an effective therapeutic combination. Alternatively, a single agent, cefoxitin (4.0 to 6.0 gm/day given in divided doses every six hours), is the choice of many clinicians. A host of newer third-generation cephalosporins and beta-lactams (in particular imepenem) are also available. Once started, antibiotic therapy is continued for seven to ten days.

The patient should be carefully followed with frequent examinations of the abdomen and appropriate laboratory and radiologic studies to ascertain whether the therapeutic response is adequate or whether complications are ensuing. In most uncomplicated cases, symptoms and signs will abate in three to four days, and the patient can be placed on a diet and allowed to convalesce. With more severe episodes, it may take eight to ten days before the acute process resolves, at which time deferred diagnostic studies (i.e., barium enema, colonoscopy) can be carried out electively. After the patient's discharge from the hospital, it seems reasonable to prescribe a long-term therapeutic regimen consisting of measures employed in the management of uncomplicated symptomatic diverticulosis (as described earlier).

Surgical Therapy. Urgent surgical intervention during an episode of acute diverticulitis is indicated by the presence of generalized peritonitis from a "free" perforation of a diverticulum or abscess; the persistence, progression, or appearance of an abscess in the face of appropriate antibiotic therapy; persistent high-grade large or small bowel obstruction; and severe persistent urosepsis secondary to colovesical fistula. Although the risks of surgery are considerable in such circumstances, particularly in the elderly patient whose medical status also may be compromised by concomitant cardiovascular, pulmonary, or renal disease, they are less formidable than the risks of continuing with unsuccessful medical management.

The extent of the surgery performed should be the least procedure that can be safely employed effectively to treat the life-threatening circumstance that exists.[82–85] In most instances of free diverticular perforation and peritonitis, optimal emergency management consists of a resection of the leaking bowel segment; using the proximal end of the bowel as an end-colostomy; bringing the distal end up as a mucous fistula or closing and leaving it in the pelvis (Hartmann procedure); and thorough intraperitoneal lavage. Anastomotic reconstitution of bowel continuity in the presence of severe uncontrolled sepsis is fraught with hazard, and it is safer to defer this step until a later date. At times, it is judged that the patient cannot tolerate colonic resection and a lesser operation involving only proximal diverting colostomy and drainage of the fecal soilage is performed. These circumstances may lead to the need for three stages of operative treatment: the initial diversion and drainage, resection of the involved bowel segment, and then colostomy closure.

Multistaged operative procedures also may have to be used in the management of large pelvic abscesses. Drainage and proximal diverting colostomy can be carried out without contaminating the peritoneal cavity at the first operation. Resection of the bowel is done at the second procedure; and if the colostomy is not closed at this stage, a third operation at a later date is required. In contrast, when abscesses are small and well contained in the adjacent colonic mesentery or paracolic fat, resection of the involved bowel and contiguous inflammatory process, as well as primary reanastomosis of the divided colon, can be carried out in one stage.

Surgical treatment of intestinal obstruction secondary to diverticulitis is defined by the location and nature of the process causing the obstruction. Colonic obstruction related to a stricture or intramural inflammatory process frequently requires a two-stage approach. Distention and edema of the bowel wall, plus difficulties in obtaining a satisfactory mechanical bowel preparation preoperatively, make it hazardous to attempt primary anastomosis. Thus, the initial procedure consists of resection of the involved segment of colon, creating an end-colostomy with the proximal cut end of the bowel and fashioning of a Hartmann's pouch or a mucous fistula with the distal end. A one-stage procedure, however, can be elected at the time of operation, provided that the prevailing circumstances make it a reasonable and relatively safe choice. Small bowel obstruction, on the other hand, may not require resection of the involved loop of small intestine. Often it can be freed of its adherence to other intra-abdominal structures, and with correction of angulation and distortion, patency can be restored without removal of a small intestinal segment. Then the surgeon can deal with the involved portion of colon as a separate matter.

The design of surgical therapy in the treatment of a colovesical fistula is to remove the involved sigmoid colonic segment and related fistulous tract. If necessary, this will include a resection of a small portion of the dome of the bladder. Any lesser procedure will not result in a cure. Optimally, this can be carried out as a one-stage procedure. However, should extensive pelvic inflammatory changes increase the risks of injury to the bladder trigone, ureters, or other important structures, it is wiser to consider a two-stage approach. The initial procedure consists of proximal diverting colostomy; at the second operation the sigmoid colon and fistula are resected, the bladder wall is repaired, and intestinal continuity is restored.

The indications for elective surgical treatment are more controversial.[82–84] It is generally agreed that surgery is appropriate (1) in a patient with recurrent disabling attacks of diverticulitis; (2) in the presence of a fistula, particularly a colovesical fistula causing recurrent urinary tract infection; and (3) in the presence of a persistent partial obstruction of the colon when carcinoma cannot be ruled out as a cause. Other indications that have been considered by some surgeons are persistent chronic segmental narrowing of the colon following a bout of diverticulitis, the risks of complete obstruction being high with another episode; urinary symptoms suggesting bladder wall involvement and adherence that could be the setting for formation of a colovesical fistula with the next acute episode; or unusual severity of the first attack in a patient in whom another similar episode is considered a greater risk to life than surgery, particularly in patients under 40 years of age who are more likely to suffer severe recurrent attacks.[86]

At present, most skilled and experienced surgeons will endeavor to carry out a one-stage procedure with primary resection and anastomosis. This is modified to two stages only if the bowel cannot be adequately prepared, if there are technical difficulties in performing the resection or anastomosis, or if some associated medical problem indicates the wisdom of initially doing a lesser operation. Resection, proximal sigmoid colostomy, and either a distal mucous fistula or Hartmann's procedure could be carried out in the first stage, with restoration of colonic continuity and colostomy closure in the second stage. Alternatively, colostomy diversion, per se, could be the initial procedure, and resection and anastomosis the second.

When resections of the colon are carried out as definitive procedures in the treatment of diverticular disease, the distal line of resection optimally should be placed below the level of the lowest diverticulum and the myochotic muscular changes in the wall of the bowel.[87] This usually necessitates its being at the proximal end of the rectum at the level of the peritoneal reflection in the cul-de-sac. As for the proximal line of resection, it need not include *all* segments of the colon-containing diverticula, but it should be placed only at a site free of diverticula above the level at which diverticulitis and peridiverticular changes occurred. The presence of residual diverticula proximally seems to engender no additional risk of episodes of diverticulitis occurring at a subsequent time. In general, after appropriate surgical therapy, the chance of a patient's needing reoperation for recurrent diverticulitis is about 3 per cent.[87]

PREVENTION

It is clear from the foregoing that, although diverticular disease develops in a majority of the aged without impairing their health, it has unpredictable and often catastrophic consequences for a few. To what extent may present conceptions of its pathogenesis be applied to its prevention?

In addition to affording symptomatic relief, the high-fiber diet has been reported in the United Kingdom to reduce the frequency of recurrences and of complications.[88] For lack of controlled trials, the significance of these reports is not clear, and it is equally uncertain whether adherence to such a diet would prevent or postpone the appearance of symptoms or complications in an asymptomatic person. Thus, although the screening of the well population for diverticula is entirely feasible from the point of view of radiation hazard, there is no present justification for campaigns of prevention based on case-finding.[89]

But is *primary* prevention possible? Could a diet higher in vegetable fiber, if adopted by the population as a whole, prevent or postpone the formation of diverticula? This possibility is strongly supported by the finding (previously mentioned) of a much lower frequency among vegetarians than nonvegetarians in the same English community.[29] Such a diet might, according to many current reports, also reduce susceptibility to coronary artery disease, obesity, gallstones, colon cancer, and other diseases. The only clinical condition it is known to exacerbate is volvulus of the sigmoid colon. However, metabolic balance studies have shown that a high-fiber vegetable diet increases fecal losses of calcium, magnesium, and zinc and thus indicates the possibility of depletion of trace elements.[90] In persons with dietary intakes that are otherwise marginal nutritionally, the reduced efficiency of absorption of the end products of protein and carbohydrate digestion—also noted with such diets high in vegetable fiber—might lead to malnutrition.[91]

As the net long-term benefits of such a diet have not yet been demonstrated empirically, there is no present consensus in the scientific community in its favor. Physicians, accustomed as they are to deciding and advising others on the basis of less than complete information, can and should form their own policy with respect to dietary advice to their patients.

References

1. Parks, T. G. Natural history of diverticular disease of the colon. Clin. Gastroenterol. *4*:53, 1975.
2. Almy, T. P., and Howell, D. A. Diverticular disease of the colon. N. Engl. J. Med. *302*:324, 1980.
3. Painter, N. S., and Burkitt, D. P. Diverticular disease of the colon, a 20th century problem. Clin. Gastroenterol. *4*:3, 1975.
4. Kyle, J., Adesola, A. D., Tinckler, L. F., and de Beaux, J. Incidence of diverticulitis. Scand. J. Gastroenterol. *2*:77, 1967.
5. Narasaka, T., Watanabe, H., Yamagata, S., Munakata, A., Tajima, T., and Matatsunaga, F. Statistical analysis of diverticulosis of the colon. Tohoku J. Exp. Med. *115*:271, 1975.
6. Levy, N., Luboshitzki, R., Shiratzki, Y., and Ghivarello, M. Diverticulosis of the colon in Israel. Dis. Colon Rectum *20*:477, 1977.
7. Stemmermann, G. N., and Yatani, R. Diverticulosis and polyps of the large intestine: a necropsy study of Hawaii Japanese. Cancer *31*:1260, 1973.
8. Segal, I., Solomon, A., and Hunt, J. A. Emergence of diverticular disease in the urban South African black. Gastroenterology *72*:215, 1977.
9. Noer, R. J. Hemorrhage as a complication of diverticulitis. Ann. Surg. *141*:674, 1955.
10. Meyers, M. A., Volberg, F., Katzen, B., Alonso, D., and Abbott, G. The angio-architecture of colonic diverticula: significance in bleeding diverticulosis. Radiology *108*:249, 1973.
11. Fleischner, F. G. Diverticular disease of the colon—new observations and revised concepts. Gastroenterology *60*:316, 1971.
12. Whiteway, J., and Morson, B. C. Elastosis in diverticular disease of the sigmoid colon. Gut *26*:258, 1985.
13. Peck, D. A., Labat, R., and Waite, V. C. Diverticular disease of the right colon. Dis. Colon Rectum *11*:49, 1968.
14. Lee, Y.-S. Diverticular disease of the large bowel in Singapore—an autopsy survey. Dis. Colon Rectum *29*:330, 1986.
15. Gallagher, J. J., and Walsh, J. P. Giant diverticula of the sigmoid colon. Arch. Surg. *114*:1078, 1979.
16. Smith, A. N., Shepherd, J., and Eastwood, M. A. Pressure changes after balloon distension of the colon wall in diverticular disease. Gut *22*:841, 1981.
17. Bornstein, P. Disorders of connective tissue function and the aging process: a synthesis and review of current concepts and findings. Mech. Aging Dev. *5*:305, 1976.
18. Cook, J. M. Spontaneous perforation of the colon: report of two cases in a family exhibiting Marfan stigmata. Ohio Med. J. *64*:73, 1968.
19. Beighton, P. H., Murdoch, J. L., and Votteler, T. Gastrointestinal complications of the Ehlers-Danlos syndrome. Gut *10*:1004, 1969.
20. Pleatman, S. I., and Dunbar, J. S. Colon diverticula in Williams' elfin-facies syndrome. Radiology *137*:869, 1980.
21. Wynne-Jones, G. Flatus retention is the major factor in diverticular disease. Lancet *2*:211, 1975.
22. Weinreich, J., and Anderson, D. Intraluminal pressure in the sigmoid colon. II. Patients with sigmoid diverticula and related conditions. Scand. J. Gastroenterol. *11*:581, 1976.
23. Arfwidsson, D., and Dock, N. G. Pathogenesis of multiple diverticula of the sigmoid colon in diverticular disease. Acta Chir. Scand. (Suppl.) *342*:5, 1964.
24. Painter, N. S. The etiology of diverticulosis of the colon with special reference to the action of certain drugs on behavior of the colon. Ann. R. Coll. Surg. *34*:98, 1964.
25. Almy, T. P. Diverticular disease of the colon—the new look. Gastroenterology *49*:109, 1965.
26. Findlay, J. M., Smith, A. N., Mitchell, W. D., Anderson, A. J. B., and Eastwood, M. A. Effects of unprocessed bran on colon function in normal subjects and in diverticular disease. Lancet *1*:146, 1974.
27. Hodgson, J. Animal models in the study of diverticular disease. I. Aetiology and treatment. Clin. Gastroenterol. *4*:201, 1975.
28. Fisher, N., Berry, C. S., Fearn, T., Gregory, J. A., and Hardy, J. Cereal dietary fiber consumption and diverticular disease: a lifespan study in rats. Am. J. Clin. Nutr. *42*:788, 1985.
29. Gear, J. S. S., Ware, A., Fursdon, P., Mann, J. I., Nolan, D. J., Brodribb, A. J. M., and Vessey, M. P. Symptomless diverticular disease and intake of dietary fibre. Lancet *1*:511, 1979.
30. Connell, A. M., Jones, F. A., and Rowlands, E. N. Motility of the pelvic colon. IV. Abdominal pain associated with colonic hypermotility after meals. Gut *6*:105, 1965.
31. Snape, W. J., Jr., Carlson, G. M., and Cohen, S. Colonic myoelectric activity in the irritable bowel syndrome. Gastroenterology *70*:326, 1976.
32. Taylor, I., and Duthie, H. L. Bran tablets and diverticular disease. Br. Med. J. *1*:988, 1976.
33. Geenen, J. E., Schmitt, M. G., and Hogan, W. J. Complications of colonoscopy. Gastroenterology *66*:812, 1974.
34. Brodribb, A. J. Treatment of symptomatic diverticular disease with a high-fiber diet. Lancet *1*:664, 1977.
35. Weinreich, J. Controlled studies with dietary fibre in the therapy of diverticular disease and irritable bowel syndrome. *In* Colon and Nutrition (Proceedings of Falk Symposium #32). Lancaster, England, MTP Press, 1981, p 239.
36. Stephen, A. M., and Cummings, J. H. Water-holding by dietary fibre *in vitro* and its relationship to faecal output in man. Gut *20*:722, 1979.
37. Yang, P., and Banwell, J. G. Dietary fiber—its role in the pathogenesis and treatment of constipation. Practical Gastroenterol. *10*:28, 1986.
38. Ewerth, S., Ahlberg, J., Holmström, B., Persson, U., and Uden, R. Influence on symptoms and transit-time of Vi-Siblin in diverticular disease. Acta Chir. Scand. (Suppl.) *500*:49, 1980.
39. Eastwood, M. A. Medical and dietary management. Clin. Gastroenterol. *4*:85, 1975.
40. Srivastava, G. S., Smith, A. N., and Painter, N. S. Sterculia, bulk-forming agent with smooth-muscle relaxant, versus bran in diverticular disease. Br. Med. J. *1*:315, 1976.
41. Daniel, O., Basu, P. K., and Al-Samarrae, H. M. Use of glucagon in the treatment of acute diverticulitis. Br. Med. J. *3*:720, 1974.
42. Painter, N. S., and Truelove, S. C. The intraluminal pressure patterns in diverticulosis of the colon. Gut *5*:201, 1964.
43. Stanciu, C., and Bennett, J. R. Colonic response to pentazocine. Br. Med. J. *1*:312, 1974.
44. Quinn, W. C. Gross hemorrhage from presumed diverticulosis of the colon. Ann. Surg. *153*:851, 1961.
45. Noer, R. J., Hamilton, J. E., Williams, D. G., and Broughton, D. S. Rectal hemorrhage: moderate and severe. Ann. Surg. *155*:794, 1962.
46. Lewis, E. E., and Schnug, G. E. Importance of angiography in the management of massive hemorrhage from colonic diverticula. Am. J. Surg. *124*:573, 1972.
47. McGuire, H. H., Jr., and Haynes, B. W., Jr. Massive hemor-

rhage from diverticulosis of the colon: guidelines for therapy based on bleeding patterns observed in fifty cases. Ann. Surg. *175*:847, 1972.
48. Behringer, G. E., and Albright, N. L. Diverticular disease of the colon. A frequent cause of massive rectal bleeding. Am. J. Surg. *125*:419, 1973.
49. Gennaro, A. R., and Rosemond, G. P. Colonic diverticula and hemorrhage. Dis. Colon Rectum *16*:409, 1973.
50. Thompson, N. W. Vascular ectasias and colonic diverticula: common causes of lower gastrointestinal hemorrhage in the aged. *In* Fiddian-Green, R. G., and Turcotte, J. G. (eds.). Gastrointestinal Hemorrhage. New York, Grune & Stratton, 1980, p 375.
51. Browder, W., Cerise, E. J., and Litwin, M. S. Impact of emergency angiography in massive lower gastrointestinal bleeding. Ann. Surg. *204*:530, 1986.
52. Baum, S., Athanasoulis, C. A., Waltman, A. C., Galdabini, J., Schapiro, R. H., Warshaw, A. L., and Ottinger, L. W. Angiodysplasia of the right colon: a cause of gastrointestinal bleeding. AJR *129*:789, 1977.
53. Welch, C. E., Athanasoulis, C. A., and Galdabini, J. J. Hemorrhage from the large bowel with special reference to angiodysplasia and diverticula disease. World J. Surg. 2:73, 1978.
54. Boley, S. J., Sammartano, R., Adams, W. A., DiBiase, A., Kleinhaus, S., and Sprayregan, S. On the nature and etiology of vascular ectasias of the colon. Gastroenterology *72*:650, 1977.
55. Boley, S. J., DiBiase, A., and Brandt, L. J. Lower intestinal bleeding in the elderly. Am. J. Surg. *137*:57, 1979.
56. Nath, R. L., Sequeira, J. C., Weitzman, A. F., Birkett, D. H., and Williams, L. F. Lower gastrointestinal bleeding. Am. J. Surg. *141*:478, 1981.
57. Levinson, S. L., Powell, D. W., Callahan, W. T., Jones, J. D., Kinard, H. B., III, Jackson, A. L., Lapis, J. L., and Drossman, D. A. A current approach to rectal bleeding. J. Clin. Gastroenterol. *3*(Suppl. 1):9, 1981.
58. Jensen, D. M., and Machicado, G. A. Emergent colonoscopy in patients with severe lower gastrointestinal bleeding. Gastroenterology *80*:1184, 1981.
59. Casarella, W. J., Kanter, I. E., and Seaman, W. B. Right-sided colonic diverticula as a cause of acute rectal hemorrhage. N. Engl. J. Med. *286*:450, 1972.
60. Eisenberg, H., Laufer, I., and Skillman, J. J. Arteriographic diagnosis and management of suspected colonic diverticula hemorrhage. Gastroenterology *64*:1091, 1973.
61. Baum, S., Rösch, J., Dotter, C. T., Ring, E. J., Athanasoulis, C. A., Waltman, A. C., and Courey, W. R. Selective mesenteric arterial infusions in the management of massive diverticular hemorrhage. N. Engl. J. Med. *288*:1269, 1973.
62. Athanasoulis, C. A., Baum, S., and Rösch, J. Mesenteric arterial infusions of vasopressin for hemorrhage from colonic diverticulosis. Am. J. Surg. *129*:212, 1975.
63. Veidenheimer, M. C. Colonic diverticular disease: management of massive bleeding. Dis. Colon Rectum *18*:568, 1975.
64. Meyers, M. A., Alonso, D. R., Gray, G. F., and Baer, J. W. Pathogenesis of bleeding diverticulosis. Gastroenterology *71*:577, 1976.
65. Alavi, A., Dann, R. W., Baum, S., and Biery, D. N. Scintigraphic detection of acute gastrointestinal bleeding. Radiology *124*:753, 1977.
66. Winzelberg, G. G., Froelich, J. W., McKusick, K. A., Waltman, A. C., Greenfield, A. J., Athanasoulis, C. A., and Strauss, H. W. Radionuclide localization of lower gastrointestinal hemorrhage. Radiology *139*:465, 1981.
67. Boley, S. J., Brandt, L. J., and Frank, M. S. Severe lower intestinal bleeding: diagnosis and treatment. Clin. Gastroenterol. *10*:65, 1981.
68. Goldberger, L. E., and Bookstein, J. J. Transcatheter embolization for treatment of diverticular hemorrhage. Radiology *122*:613, 1977.
69. Horner, J. L. Natural history of diverticulosis of the colon. Am. J. Dig. Dis. *3*:343, 1958.
70. Ming, S. C., and Fleischner, F. G. Diverticulitis of the sigmoid colon: reappraisal of pathology and pathogenesis. Surgery *58*:627, 1965.
71. Morson, B. C. Pathology of diverticular disease of the colon. Clin. Gastroenterol. *4*:37, 1975.
72. Asch, M. J., and Markowitz, A. M. Diverticulosis coli: a surgical appraisal. Surgery *62*:239, 1967.
73. Fleischner, F. G. The question of barium enema as a cause of perforation in diverticulitis. Gastroenterology *1*:290, 1966.
74. Nicholas, G. G., Miller, W. T., Fitts, W. T., and Tondreau, R. L. Diagnosis of diverticulitis of the colon: role of barium enema in defining pericolic inflammation. Ann. Surg. *176*:205, 1972.
75. Hulnick, D. H., Megibow, M. D., Balthazar, E. J., Naidich, D. P., and Bosniak, M. A. Computed tomography in the evaluation of diverticulitis. Radiology *152*:491, 1984.
76. Morris, J., Stellato, T. A., Haaga, J. R., and Lieberman, J. The utility of computed tomography in colonic diverticulitis. Ann. Surg. *204*:128, 1986.
77. Colcock, B. P., and Stahman, F. D. Fistulas complicating diverticular disease of the sigmoid colon. Ann. Surg. *175*:838, 1972.
78. Hughes, L. E. Complications of diverticular disease: inflammation, obstruction and hemorrhage. Clin. Gastroenterol. *4*:147, 1975.
79. Small, W. P., and Smith, A. N. Fistula and conditions associated with diverticular disease of the colon. Clin. Gastroenterol. *4*:171, 1975.
80. King, R. M., Beart, R. W., and McIlrath, D. C. Colovesical and rectovesical fistulas. Arch. Surg. *117*:680, 1982.
81. Larson, D. M., Masters, S. S., and Spiro, H. M. Medical and surgical therapy in diverticular disease—a comparative study. Gastroenterology *71*:734, 1976.
82. Colcock, B. P. Diverticular disease: proven surgical management. Clin. Gastroenterol. *4*:99, 1975.
83. Goligher, J. C. Diverticulosis and diverticulitis of the colon. *In* Goligher, J. C. (ed.). Surgery of the Anus, Rectum and Colon. London, Baillière Tyndall, 1980, p 1076.
84. Rodkey, G. V., and Welch, C. E. Changing patterns in the surgical treatment of diverticular disease. Ann. Surg. *200*:466, 1984.
85. Lambert, M. E., Knox, R. A., Schofield, P. F., and Hancock, B. D. Management of the septic complications of diverticular disease. Br. J. Surg. *73*:576, 1986.
86. Ouriel, K., and Schwartz, S. I. Diverticular disease in the young patient. Surg. Gynecol. Obstet. *156*:1, 1983.
87. Benn, P. L., Wolff, B. G., and Ilstrup, D. M. Level of anastomosis and recurrent colonic diverticulitis. Am. J. Surg. *151*:269, 1986.
88. Hyland, J. M., and Taylor, I. Does a high fibre diet prevent the complications of diverticular disease? Br. J. Surg. *67*:77, 1980.
89. Ardran, G. M., Nolan, D. J., Geer, J. S. S., Fursdon, P. S., and Brodribb, A. J. M. X-ray dose received by patients in a population survey for colonic diverticular disease. Br. J. Radiol. *51*:472, 1978.
90. Ismail-Beigi, F., Reinold, J. G., and Abadi, P. Effects of cellulose added to diets of low and high fiber content upon the metabolism of calcium, magnesium, zinc and phosphorus by man. J. Nutr. *107*:510, 1977.
91. Kelsay, J. L. A review of research on effects of fiber intake on man. Am. J. Clin. Nutr. *31*:142, 1978.

78

Ulcerative Colitis

JOHN P. CELLO
DAVID J. SCHNEIDERMAN

Ulcerative colitis is an inflammatory disease of unknown cause, affecting principally the mucosa of the rectum and left colon but in many instances the entire organ. It is a chronic disease with remissions and exacerbations, characterized by rectal bleeding and diarrhea, appearing principally but not exclusively in youth and early middle age. It is a disease with serious local and systemic complications. Medical therapy can adequately treat the majority of symptomatic flares of disease.

HISTORICAL ASPECTS

Ulcerative colitis was first described by Wilks and Moxon in 1875; it has been recognized with increasing frequency, particularly in the past several decades.[1] Its discovery was undoubtedly delayed by the tendency to believe all diarrheal illnesses to be forms of infectious dysentery. Wilks and Moxon were the first therefore to clearly separate idiopathic ulcerative colitis from colitis caused by bacilli or parasites. Interestingly, for many decades this disorder was considered a disease exclusively of Europe and North America; however, its incidence in South and Central America appears to be rising with its increasing recognition. Ulcerative colitis is being reported with increasing frequency in Japan, India, Thailand, and other countries in the Far East.

With the description of regional enteritis in the early 1930s by Crohn and his colleagues, separation of mucosal ulcerative colitis from transmural Crohn's disease of the intestine appeared relatively clear-cut; the two diseases appeared initially to have distinct pathologic features, and each affected a different organ system. Over the past several decades, a marked overlap has been appreciated not only pathologically but also in anatomic distribution. In many cases (nearly 10 per cent of patients with chronic idiopathic inflammatory bowel disease), resected specimens may show features of both diseases, and in some specimens the findings are completely compatible with either diagnosis. As the cause for both diseases is unknown, the possibility exists that they share a common cause and that pathologic differences reflect variable tissue reactions to the same or similar noxious agent.

EPIDEMIOLOGY

Early studies on the epidemiology of ulcerative colitis suffered from several aspects: population areas were poorly defined; incidence and prevalence rates were derived by comparing patients who had ulcerative colitis with other hospitalized patients instead of with total populations of the area; data were gathered from selected centers; or socioeconomic or ethnic data were not controlled against the normal population of the area. Impressions gained from these older studies were that ulcerative colitis seemed to be more prevalent in higher socioeconomic groups, among persons who have positions of greater responsibility or who have achieved a higher degree of education, and among Jews. The disease was thought to be less common in rural than in urban areas.

More recent studies (Table 78–1) have avoided the deficiencies of the earlier studies.[2–6] Both the Oxford and Copenhagen studies attempted to survey both inpatient and outpatient cases within a well-defined population area, whereas the Baltimore study identified all hospitalized cases (above age 20 years) within Baltimore County. (References for these studies may be found in the article cited in the footnote to Table 78–1.) Incidence rates from all three studies were comparable. Incidence rates were low below age 20 years; highest incidence rates were found in those in the third to sixth decades of life. The Oxford study, moreover, found a bimodal incidence, with peaks in the third and fifth decades. Although the bimodal peak was not seen in the other two studies, both of the latter also noted a relatively high incidence after age 50 years (see p. 1458). As up to 25 per cent of cases of ulcerative colitis may go undiagnosed for more than two years after the onset of symptoms, the higher prevalence noted in the Oxford study may relate to the longer duration of the study, allowing inclusion of some of the cases with delayed diagnosis.

Both the Oxford and Baltimore studies support the earlier impression of higher incidence among Jews. Incidence among nonwhites was considerably lower than among whites in Baltimore. Although these ethnic-racial differences may partly reflect cultural differences in use of medical facilities, their magnitude (twice to four times the incidence in Jews versus non-Jews, four times the incidence in whites versus nonwhites)

Table 78–1. EPIDEMIOLOGIC STUDIES OF ULCERATIVE COLITIS

Area Studied	Years of Study	Incidence (cases/10^5/yr)	Prevalence (cases/10^5 population)
Oxford, England	1951–1960	6.5	79.9
North Tees, England	1971–1977	15.1	99
Copenhagen, Denmark	1961–1967	7.3	44.1
Copenhagen, Denmark	1962–1978	8.1	117
Iceland	1970–1979	7.6	122.2
Marburg, Germany	1962–1975	5.1	48.8
Czechoslovakia	1978	1.3	23.9
Baltimore County, United States	1977–1979	2.9 (white male) 1.3 (white female) 1.9 (black male) 2.9 (black female)	
Tel Aviv–Jafo, Israel	1961–1971	3.7	37.4

Modified from Mayberry, J. F. Gut *26*:969, 1985.

suggests genetic rather than culturally determined differences.

A comprehensive survey of Jews living in Tel Aviv, however, has raised considerable disagreement with older reports.[2] Many previous reports did not encompass all patients within a defined geographic area. Records of both inpatients and outpatients in the Tel Aviv survey revealed an incidence of 3.66 per 100,000 population over a ten-year period. A prevalence rate of 37.4 per 100,000 was established, with a male-to-female ratio of 0.8:1. The incidence and prevalence of the disease among Jews living in Tel Aviv were lower than those reported in the Copenhagen, Oxford, and Baltimore County studies. Of considerable interest is the reported significant difference in prevalence rates between European- and American-born Israelis (51.46 per 10^5 population) and Asian- and African-born Israelis (27.82 per 10^5 population), respectively. These data for European-born Israeli Jews are similar to those reported from Copenhagen and Oxford. Thus, the previously reported increased prevalence of ulcerative colitis among Jews in Europe and America may be due to bias in sampling techniques.

Data obtained from such epidemiologic studies obviously cannot take into consideration subclinical ulcerative colitis. The frequency of asymptomatic ulcerative colitis in the general population has been estimated to be about 4 per 100,000, based upon 50,000 proctoscopies performed for the detection of colonic cancer. Only two cases of asymptomatic ulcerative colitis were found in that series of proctoscopies; however, it was a selected population seeking preventive medical care.[3]

Multiple reports have suggested a negative association between smoking and ulcerative colitis. The Boston Collaborative Drug Surveillance Program noted, among 239 patients with ulcerative colitis and a matched group of hospitalized controls, a substantially reduced risk among current smokers. The risk of ulcerative colitis in current smokers was 0.31 times that in nonsmokers. The risk reduction occurred in every age group and in both men and women.[7] Additional studies are needed both to confirm these reports and to suggest potential mechanisms for the risk reduction.

ETIOLOGY

The cause of ulcerative colitis is not known. For many years it has been postulated that an infectious agent was responsible, but many arguments in favor of an infectious cause have been discarded for lack of scientific evidence. Other workers have formulated genetic, psychosomatic, or immunologic theories of pathogenesis. As yet none of these theories is supported by adequate evidence. The theories are reviewed briefly here.

The infectious theory of the cause of ulcerative colitis remains attractive because of the inflammatory nature of the disease, which in many respects resembles the tissue reaction in the bowel caused by known pathogens (see pp. 1191–1232). Microbiologic search for infectious agents that can consistently be found in ulcerative colitis and that fulfill Koch's postulates has not been successful. There is no good evidence implicating agents such as *Chlamydia*, cytomegalovirus, or *Yersinia* in the pathogenesis of ulcerative colitis.[8, 9] Animal experiments in a few instances have been able to duplicate superficial mucosal colonic ulcerations when rabbits were injected intramurally with 0.2-μm filtrates (small enough to allow passage of only viral particles and L-forms of bacteria) of homogenized human ulcerative colitis tissue.[10]

Viral agents, such as rotavirus and Norwalk agents, which are commonly implicated in acute viral enteritis, cannot be identified serologically as important factors in the flares of inflammatory bowel disease. A cytopathic agent has been extracted from resected colons of patients with ulcerative colitis. This agent was passaged 15 times in tissue culture.[11] Physical and chemical characteristics of the isolated agent suggest a 60-nm RNA virus (Fig. 78–1). Duplication of these results to exclude a noninfectious agent is essential before widespread acceptance of a viral cause can be accepted. Several studies have attempted to associate toxin from

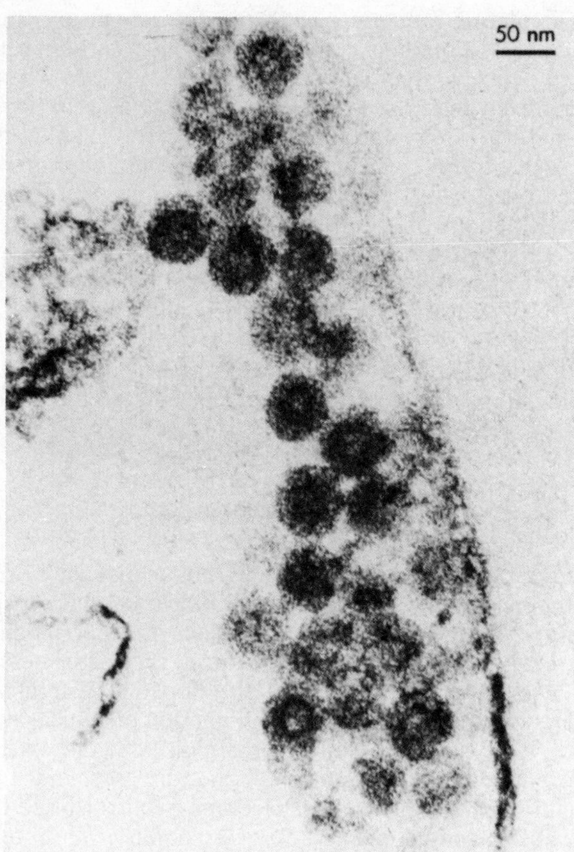

Figure 78–1. Electron microscopic appearance of virus particles isolated in chick embryo tissue culture from an ulcerative colitis patient (× 168,000). (From Gitnick, G. L., Rosen, V. J., Arthur, M. H., and Hertweck, S. A. Dig. Dis. Sci. *24*:617, 1979. Used by permission of Plenum Publishing Corp.)

Clostridium difficile, the agent responsible for many cases of antibiotic-associated pseudomembranous colitis, with the relapses of inflammatory bowel disease.[12–15] Toxin positivity may be correlated with disease activity, although some evidence suggests it may correlate better with prior antibiotic administration rather than disease activity itself.[14, 15]

Data supporting a genetic hypothesis are likewise suggestive but far from complete, owing to retrospective analyses of families and incomplete reporting. As noted, ulcerative colitis has a higher incidence among Jews than non-Jews and a lower incidence among blacks than whites. Additional cases of ulcerative colitis in families of patients with the disease occur with much greater frequency (10 to 15 per cent) than in families of control patients without ulcerative colitis. Some families have had up to six members afflicted. The disease has appeared in monozygotic twins. In Israeli Jews of European origin, HLA phenotypes AW24 and BW35 are associated with ulcerative colitis, with the AW24 phenotype increased in frequency in patients with early-onset ulcerative colitis and moderate-to-severe disease.[16] Confirmation of these results in other patient populations is necessary before they are accepted.

Psychologic determinants in the pathogenesis of ulcerative colitis have been championed for many years. However, most investigators have stressed that psychologic factors, rather than being causative, may merely facilitate the colonic mucosal reaction to another etiologic agent. Until recently, data marshaled to support the psychologic theory have been uncontrolled and anecdotal. More recent controlled studies of psychologic factors in ulcerative colitis have challenged the importance of psychologic influences. An extensive psychiatric evaluation of 34 consecutive patients presenting with ulcerative colitis failed to reveal a higher incidence of psychiatric aberration than in a control population similarly examined.[17] Furthermore, emotionally traumatic events preceding the onset of ulcerative colitis could be identified in fewer than 20 per cent of the cases. In the epidemiologic studies from Baltimore County (Table 78–1), surveys were conducted among patients with ulcerative colitis, normal control subjects, and control patients with irritable colon in an effort to identify psychosocial factors unique to patients with ulcerative colitis.[18, 19] No precipitating stresses (marital discord, indebtedness, overwork, or physical trauma) could be identified as occurring more frequently in the ulcerative colitis patients than in the control population; in general, the social and occupational background of the ulcerative colitis patients resembled that of the normal population. Thus, although psychologic factors may influence onset and course of the disease in some patients, until more convincing facts are available it is fair to state that they are not necessarily a major etiologic factor.

Immunologic mechanisms have been postulated to be the cause of ulcerative colitis or to contribute to the colonic mucosal inflammation and noncolonic manifestations of the disease. Experimentally, rabbits skin-sensitized to dinitrochlorobenzene (DNCB), then receiving intrarectal DNCB, develop an acute distal colonic inflammation similar to human ulcerative colitis.[20] Indeed, repeated instillation of DNCB leads to development of mild ileal, duodenal, and even portal inflammation, further suggesting an immune mechanism. Gut mucosal lymphocytes in patients with ulcerative colitis are markedly increased, both qualitatively on pathologic sections and quantitatively by counting after enzymatic or mechanical dissociation. Cell yields in ulcerative colitis tissue are many times greater than in controls, with over 80 per cent of the cells being small lymphocytes.[21] In control biopsy specimens, mononuclear cell yields averaged $3.6 \pm 0.3 \times 10^6$/gm compared to $11.4 \pm 2.1 \times 10^6$/gm in patients with active ulcerative colitis. Moreover, the percentage of B lymphocytes increased from 15 ± 1 per cent in normals to 43 ± 4 per cent in ulcerative colitis patients.[22]

Spontaneous or antibody-dependent cell-mediated cytotoxicity has been proposed as a mechanism of injury in ulcerative colitis. Nonspecific cell-mediated cytotoxic activity of intestinal mononuclear cells is not increased, however, in ulcerative colitis patients. Markedly decreased natural killer (NK) cell (non-B, non-T cell) cytotoxicity of isolated gut mononuclear cells from ulcerative colitis patients against a myeloid cell line as target cells has been noted.[23] Furthermore, the decreased cytotoxicity was not the result of a decreased absolute number of NK cells. Other studies likewise have demonstrated hyporesponsiveness of ulcerative colitis intestinal and peripheral mononuclear cells to human fibroblastic interferon and mitogenic lectins, suggesting that cell-mediated cytotoxicity is not enhanced in these patients.[24] In addition, bowel mononuclear cells demonstrate decreased secretion of IgA compared with controls, with a higher percentage of the IgA from ulcerative colitis bowel mononuclear cells being monomeric and of the IgA subclass 1 than in normal subjects.[25] Specifically sensitized T cells have, however, been demonstrated to have enhanced cell-mediated cytotoxicity for autologous epithelial cell targets (Fig. 78–2).[26] Thus, intestinal lymphocytes from ulcerative colitis patients may contain T cells or Fc receptor–bearing cells that are specifically sensitized to antigens present in normal gut epithelium.

Abnormalities of the complement system have been noted by some observers in patients with ulcerative colitis. C′3, C3–C9, C4, and CH50 serum levels are normal; however, C′3 and C1q metabolism may be increased.[27, 28]

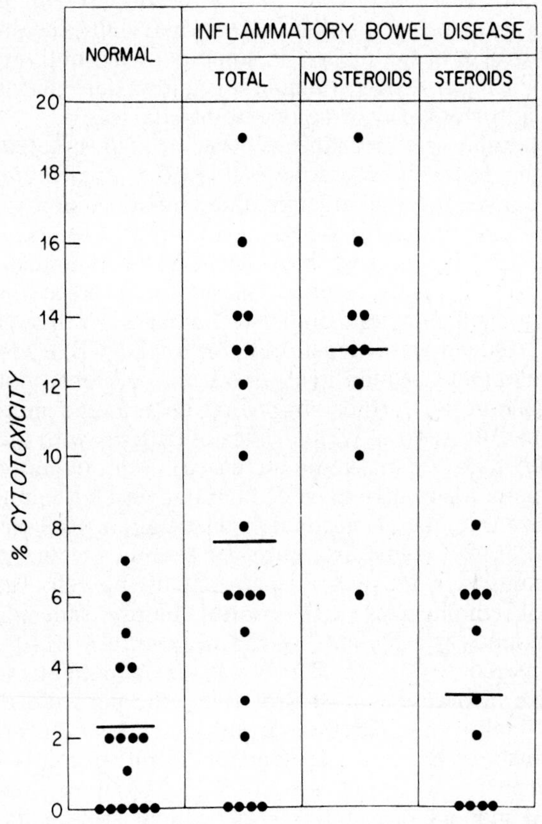

Figure 78–2. Peripheral blood mononuclear cell (PBMC) cytotoxicity for autologous human colonic epithelial cells. PBMC from patients with inflammatory bowel disease produced significantly greater toxicity than PBMC from normal control subjects ($p < 0.01$). (From Kemler, B. J., and Alpert, E. Gut *21*:356, 1980. Used by permission.)

Circulating immune complexes determined by Raji cell and C1q binding assays may be found in the serum of patients with inflammatory bowel disease. These complexes may, however, be the result of *in vitro* formation under certain conditions. The circulating immune complexes may be more common among ulcerative colitis patients with some extraintestinal manifestations of the disease, such as primary sclerosing cholangitis.[29] Skin test anergy has been demonstrated in patients with ulcerative colitis, particularly to DNCB sensitization.[30] In a series of ulcerative colitis patients tested against a panel of five common test antigens, however, no significant difference was noted from control subjects in another survey[31] (see pp. 114–144).

PATHOPHYSIOLOGY

Idiopathic ulcerative colitis is not a distinct histopathologic entity; most of the individual histologic features of the disease may be seen in other inflammations of the colon of known cause, such as bacterial or parasitic. The diagnosis of idiopathic ulcerative colitis, therefore, rests on a combination of clinical and pathologic data; the course of the disease, the extent and anatomic distribution of the disease, and the exclusion of other forms of ulcerating colitis caused by specific infectious agents (*Shigella, Salmonella,* enterotoxigenic *Escherichia coli, Entamoeba histolytica, Campylobacter,* gonococcus). Before embarking on a detailed account of the clinical features of ulcerative colitis, the histopathological findings are outlined and a brief attempt is made to relate these lesions to the clinical and radiographic features of the disease.

Except in rare instances (see p. 1441), ulcerative colitis is an inflammatory disease confined to the mucosa and to a lesser extent to the adjacent submucosa. The deeper layers of muscularis propria and serosa of the colon usually are not involved, and the process does not extend to the regional lymph nodes, except perhaps as a nonspecific reactive hyperplasia.[32] Many pathologists believe that the crypt abscess involving the crypts of Lieberkühn is the primary lesion. In the crypt abscess, polymorphonuclear cells accumulate near the tip of the crypt, and the crypt epithelial cells show degenerative changes. On light microscopy, poor staining or vacuolization may be seen in these epithelial cells, whereas on electron microscopic examination these cells show shortening of epithelial microvilli, dilatation of the endoplasmic reticulum, swelling of the mitochondria, increased numbers of lysosomes, and widening of the intercellular spaces. In crypt abscess, frank necrosis of the crypt epithelium occurs, with extension of the polymorphonuclear infiltrate through the colonic epithelium. In addition to acute superficial crypt abscesses, superficial erosions of the mucosa are noted microscopically in acute ulcerative colitis. These erosions, together with the coalescence of adjacent crypt abscesses, produce the shallow ulcerations of the mucosa down to the lamina propria that are seen at colonoscopy, sigmoidoscopy, and air-contrast barium radiography. Extension of these ulcerations may destroy larger areas of mucosa, leaving islands of intact mucosa surrounded by ulcerations producing pseudopolyps (i.e., the "polyp" is actually more normal intact mucosa that is elevated above the surrounding denuded mucosa). These pseudopolyps seen both endoscopically and radiographically are indicative of more extensive and severe disease. Concomitant with tissue destruction, the reparative process appears. Highly vascular granulation tissue may develop in denuded areas. Collagen is deposited in the lamina propria, but such fibrosis is patchy and usually minimal and is not a prominent feature in ulcerative colitis. With disease of long duration, the muscularis mucosae may hypertrophy.

The aforementioned histopathologic features of ulcerative colitis, although not specific, are helpful in understanding many of the clinical features of the disease, which are discussed in more detail in subsequent paragraphs. The two most prominent and common symptoms of the disease—*hematochezia* and *diarrhea*—relate to extensive colonic mucosal damage. Bleeding results from ulceration, vascular engorgement, and the development of highly vascular, friable granulation tissue; watery diarrhea results when the extensive amount of colonic mucosa, predominantly of the distal portion, is destroyed or damaged, rendering it less capable of sodium and water reabsorption (see pp. 1033–1040).[33] The superficial and distal colonic ulceration also accounts for the extensive amount of white blood cells found in the mucus of patients with ulcerative colitis. The confinement of the pathologic processes to the mucosa and submucosa accounts for the rarity of sharply localized abdominal pain, well-defined peritoneal signs, colonic perforation, and fistula formation; further, symptoms of obstruction are rare even when the disease extends to the adjacent ileum ("backwash ileitis"). Although the colon in ulcerative colitis may stenose or the ulceration may occasionally extend beyond the submucosa, such pathologic developments are uncommon and do not always underlie radiographic foreshortening and narrowing of the colon, loss of haustral markings, and apparent stricture formation. Indeed, these findings are often reversible, because they are due to hypertrophy and spasm of the muscularis mucosae and not fibrosis.[34]

Although ulcerative colitis generally is confined to the mucosa and submucosa, in the more severe forms of the disease, especially in a condition known as toxic megacolon, the disease process may extend through the deeper muscular layers of the colon and even to the serosa. On rare occasions, crypt abscesses penetrate the muscularis propria, often extending along a blood vessel. When the disease extends to the serosa, the colon may perforate. If the inflammatory process arrests short of perforation, healing may result in fibrosis of the deeper layers of the colon. In toxic megacolon, which occurs in 1 to 3 per cent of all cases of ulcerative colitis, ulcers extend deeply, through the mucosa and submucosa, into the muscular layers of the colon. In addition, vasculitis is often seen, along with swelling and irregularity of the vascular endothelium, inflammatory infiltration into the vessel walls, and thrombosis of small arteries. The extension of ulceration into the muscular layers of the colon and its associated infiltration and vasculitis probably account for the apparent loss of colonic motor tone in this condition, producing colonic dilatation. Deep extension of the inflammatory process, together with dilatation of the colon, predisposes these patients to perforation (see p. 1460).

DIAGNOSIS

The diagnosis of ulcerative colitis is usually made on the basis of clinical symptoms and on the demonstration of an abnormal, inflamed colonic mucosa by sigmoidoscopy. Diagnosis may also be supported by barium enema, colonoscopy, negative stool examinations, and colonic mucosal histology. Radiographic examination will often reveal characteristic, although not specific, findings, and rectal biopsy may show crypt abscesses and mucosal inflammation, likewise not specific for ulcerative colitis.

Physical examination is useful in confirming the presence of extracolonic complications (uveitis, aphthous stomatitis, pyoderma gangrenosum, erythema nodosum, arthritis) and in demonstrating the systemic sequelae of severe colitis (tachycardia, fever, dehydration, contracted blood volume). In addition, physical examination can be helpful in detecting the complications of toxic megacolon (abdominal distention and tympany) or colonic perforation (direct and rebound abdominal tenderness). Physical examination may suggest ulcerative colitis rather than Crohn's colitis, with the former associated with less right lower quadrant tenderness and fullness and less extensive perianal disease. Indeed, in uncomplicated mild and moderate forms of the disease the results of physical examination may be normal. As ulcerative colitis is a disease that affects predominantly the colonic mucosa, the most useful methods of establishing a diagnosis involve procedures that assess the integrity of this mucosa. In 90 to 95 per cent of persons with ulcerative colitis, the mucosa of the rectosigmoid colon is diseased[35]; even cases of localized colitis are most commonly localized in the distal part of the colon. Therefore, sigmoidoscopy and biopsy can be used to establish a diagnosis in the majority of patients.

Proctosigmoidoscopy

The normal distal colonic mucosa appears as a smooth, glistening, pink surface that uniformly reflects the endoscopic light from a broad area. Ramifying superficial submucosal blood vessels may be discerned, particularly in the rectum, where a prominent vascular pattern is often noted. The normal colonic mucosa may bleed to a small degree after it has been scraped by the rigid sigmoidoscope, but normally the mucosa beyond the tip of the instrument does not bleed spontaneously; nor will the normal mucosa bleed when it is gently massaged with a cotton swab (i.e., it is not "friable"). The rectosigmoid colon is usually easily distensible, although an occasional normal patient, and more often a patient with irritable bowel syndrome, will evidence a fair amount of spasm limiting the extent of the examination. The margins of the rectal valves are sharply defined (see pp. 1574–1575).

The colonic mucosa in patients with ulcerative colitis is markedly altered in many respects. These mucosal changes in most patients with idiopathic ulcerative colitis are uniform throughout the distal portion of the colon, beginning just inside the anal verge. With submucosal inflammation and edema, the overlying mucosa becomes less translucent so that submucosal vessels may no longer be seen. Subepithelial infiltration and edema as well as microscopic mucosal erosions and crypt abscesses make the normally smooth surface irregular in height and depth. Diffusely and uniformly reflected light from the normally smooth surface, which gives the impression of a glistening membrane, is then replaced by scattered pinpoints of light reflected from these tiny mucosal elevated irregularities; this gives the surface a granular appearance when examined tangentially. As the mucosa becomes much more irregular with more intense inflammation, this fine granularity gives way to coarse granularity, which results in greatly scattered reflected light; as a consequence, most of the reflected light is lost to the eye of the observer, and the mucosa then appears "dry" as opposed to the normal "moist" or glistening surface. If subepithelial and submucosal edema becomes more marked, it may be appreciated by the examiner as blunting of the normally sharply angulated rectal valves. Increased vascularity accompanies inflammation in the submucosa and may be appreciated as "hyperemia" of the mucosa. Because of this increased vascularity and because of erosions that undermine the mucosa in some areas and denude it in others, the mucosa becomes friable; that is, it bleeds easily from many small punctate bleeding sites when gently massaged with a cotton swab or rubbed by a sigmoidoscope or colonoscope. With more intense inflammation, the mucosa may be seen to bleed spontaneously beyond the leading edge of the scope. In the more severe and chronic forms of the disease, areas of ulceration may become visible in the rectosigmoid, although as a rule discrete ulceration is seen less often in the rectosigmoid than in the more proximal areas of the colon in resected specimens. Similarly, with more severe forms of the disease, pseudopolyps can be seen; these are small projections of tissue above the general plane of the surrounding mucosa. They are made up of tags of undermined mucosa or heaped-up granulation tissue, or a combination of these abnormalities. Pseudopolyps are usually shallow in depth, but with more chronic disease they may become accentuated by mild submucosal fibrosis and contracture of the colonic surface surrounding them. In active disease, the walls of the rectosigmoid colon may appear "rigid" or nondistensible. Like contractures seen on barium enema, this feature is related more to spasm of the rectosigmoid than to fibrosis; indeed, with healing this rigidity may disappear. Finally, exudate or "mucopus"—a term that refers to tenacious and discolored (yellow) mucus—may be seen adhering to the mucosa.

These findings vary widely from patient to patient. Thus, in the mildest forms of ulcerative colitis, changes seen at sigmoidoscopy may be very subtle, consisting only of mild friability, granularity, and hyperemia, and sometimes in mild disease the results of sigmoidoscopic examination appear entirely normal. At the other extreme, severe disease floridly displays most of these features that are readily appreciated: The rectosigmoid is spastic to the point that the instrument cannot be passed more than 8 to 10 cm without undue discomfort to the patient; widespread spontaneous mucosal bleeding is present; all light reflex is lost; and pseudopolyps and a few ulcers may be seen (Color Fig. 78–3, p. xlii). It is important to re-emphasize that these sigmoidoscopic features are not specific for ulcerative colitis but, rather, can be seen in a variety of other conditions, particularly in certain colonic infections. Moreover, these features are the same whether the patient is examined using rigid or flexible instruments. Care must be exercised, however, in advancing the flexible sigmoidoscope deeply within the sigmoid colon in patients with severe distal ulcerative disease.

In addition to the variable appearance of these characteristics, it can be readily appreciated that evaluation of many of these features is subjective. Thus it is not surprising that wide observer variation has been documented among experienced examiners regarding the presence or absence of such features as granularity, edema, rigidity, and hyperemia. More uniform agreement is reached over the presence or absence of such features as friability (bleeding on swabbing) or spontaneous bleeding, ramifying blood vessels, and pseudopolyps or ulcers.[36] Despite these difficulties, the overall agreement among observers as to whether the mucosa is normal or abnormal is fairly good, ranging from 70 to 90 per cent.[36, 37]

Nevertheless, the fact that there is observer disagreement at sigmoidoscopy in patients with known ulcerative colitis means that the individual examiner may not always feel certain of his or her findings in any given patient, especially when sigmoidoscopy shows only mild or subtle abnormalities. In such circumstances, rectal biopsy may be useful in clarifying the diagnosis. Rectal biopsy may be done either with a rigid forceps (usually below the peritoneal reflection and preferably along a rectal valve to minimize the dangers of perforation) or with a suction instrument, which minimizes the dangers of perforation and therefore may safely be used higher in the rectosigmoid colon if desired. When sigmoidoscopy is performed with a flexible instrument, a standard biopsy forceps can be used safely anywhere, although the small size of the biopsy forceps may limit the value of the single specimen. Multiple biopsies are therefore essential when the flexible instrument is used.

In patients with small discrete focal ulcerations of the rectum on sigmoidoscopy, the suspicion of amebic disease should be raised. The ideal setting for examining the mucus and stools for amebae is at the time of sigmoidoscopy, when a small amount of mucopus can be suctioned from an ulcerated area and examined directly with warm saline solution under the microscope. Moreover, rectal mucosal biopsy may likewise demonstrate erythrocytophagic amebae within the amorphous eosinophilic debris of an amebic ulceration.[38] In general, no patient should be treated with steroids for ulcerative colitis unless the physician has examined the stools, rectal mucus, or rectal biopsy specimen for the presence of motile trophozoites of *E. histolytica*.

Histology of Ulcerative Colitis

The diagnosis of ulcerative colitis is supported by the presence of appropriate histologic features. Although the colonic crypt abscess may well be the primary and most striking histologic lesion in ulcerative colitis, its finding is *not* specific for idiopathic inflammatory bowel disease.[39] Acute self-limited colitis caused by infectious or even toxic agents (such as toxic compounds in nonmedically administered enemas) will commonly demonstrate features of crypt abscesses. In nonidiopathic ulcerative colitis, the crypt abscesses tend to be more superficial in location; however, even this feature may be noted in some patients with idiopathic ulcerative colitis. Other histologic features may also help differentiate acute self-limited colitis from ulcerative colitis (Fig. 78–4). Distorted crypt architecture with atrophy and horizontal and vertical branching glands is commonly noted in biopsy specimens from patients with ulcerative colitis, although it is uncommon in specimens from patients with acute self-limited colitis. Similarly, the inflammatory cell infiltrate in ulcerative colitis characteristically shows increases in both mononuclear cells and polymorphonuclear cells, as opposed to the predominantly polymorphonuclear cell exudation in acute self-limited colitis. The increase in mononuclear cells in ulcerative colitis also may form basal lymphoid aggregates, rarely encountered in acute self-limited colitis. A villous-like surface mucosa and superficial mucosal erosions are likewise more characteristic of ulcerative colitis. Some features, on the other hand, may be more common histologically in acute self-limited colitis, including normal crypt architecture, superficial giant cells, and superficial crypt abscesses.

In a study of 56 patients with ulcerative colitis, compared with 44 patients with acute self-limited colitis, distorted crypt architecture, mixed lamina propria inflammation, villous surface, crypt atrophy, basal lymphoid aggregates, and surface erosions were independently significantly more common in ulcerative colitis[39] (Table 78–2). In the same study, colonic histologic features also helped distinguish ulcerative colitis from Crohn's colitis, with superficial polymorphonuclear cells, surface erosions, crypt atrophy, distorted crypt architecture, and villous-like surface being more common in colonic biopsy specimens from ulcerative colitis patients than in biopsy specimens from Crohn's colitis patients. Conversely, the presence of granulomas was found in only 5 per cent of ulcerative colitis biopsy specimens, compared to 62 per cent of specimens from patients with Crohn's colitis.

Thus, although not diagnostic for ulcerative colitis, colonic mucosal histologic features can be supportive of the diagnosis and play an important role in approaching the patient with distal colonic inflammation. Colonic biopsies should therefore be routinely performed in evaluating patients with the potential diagnosis of ulcerative colitis.

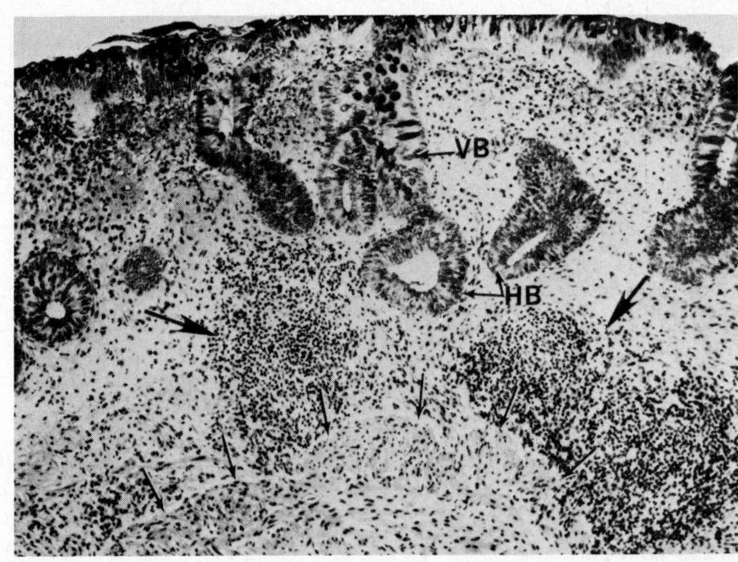

Figure 78–4. Rectal biopsy specimen from a patient with ulcerative colitis showing distorted crypt architectures with both vertical *(arrow VB)* and horizontal *(arrow HB)* branching. Atrophy is noted with shortened, sparse glands and increased space between the base of the crypts and the muscularis mucosae *(small arrows).* Hematoxylin and eosin, Alcian blue, and saffron stains, × 125. (Reprinted with permission from: Rectal biopsy helps to distinguish acute self-limited colitis from idiopathic inflammatory bowel disease, by Surawicz, C. M., and Belic, L. Gastroenterology *86*:104–113. Copyright 1984 by The American Gastroenterological Association.)

Table 78–2. HISTOLOGIC FEATURES DISTINGUISHING ACUTE SELF-LIMITED COLITIS FROM ULCERATIVE COLITIS AND CROHN'S DISEASE, RESPECTIVELY*

	ASLC (44)	UC (56)	ASCL vs. UC p*	CD (26)	ASCL vs. CD p*	UC vs. CD p*
Distorted crypt architecture	0	32	0.00001	7	<0.0005	0.01
Mixed lamina propria inflammation	0	15	0.001	7	<0.001	NS
Villous surface	0	22	0.00001	3	<0.047	<0.011
Granuloma	1†	3†	NS	16	<0.0017	<0.00001
Crypt atrophy	0	16	0.00001	3	<0.048	<0.047
Basal lymphoid aggregates	0	12	0.0011	3	NS	NS
Surface erosions	4	21	0.0011	2	NS	<0.007
Superficial isolated giant cell	7	3	NS	0	NS	NS
Basal isolated giant cell	1	6	NS	3	NS	NS
Polymorphonuclear cells in surface epithelium	9	19	NS	3	NS	<0.04

Reprinted with permission from: Rectal biopsy helps to distinguish acute self-limited colitis from idiopathic inflammatory bowel disease, by Surawicz, C. M., and Belic, L. Gastroenterology *86*(1):104–113. Copyright 1984 by The American Gastroenterological Association.

*Statistics compared ASLC with UC and with CD, and UC with CD, using the Pearson chi-square test.

†The presence of granulomas in three UC cases probably reflects the fact that rectal biopsy information was not used in the clinical categorization of cases.

ASLC, Acute self-limited colitis; CD, Crohn's disease; UC, ulcerative colitis; NS, not significant.

Colonoscopy (see pp. 216–222)

The necessity of routine colonoscopy in the definitive diagnosis of ulcerative colitis is uncertain. There is little doubt that the newer colonoscopes, with lengths to 1.7 meters, dual channels for biopsy and suction, expanded tip deflection capabilities, and improved light sources and optics, have enabled the endoscopist to visualize the entire colon (see pp. 1570–1576). Rarely is this technical capability necessary in diagnosing new cases of ulcerative colitis.[39, 40] Rectal and distal sigmoid mucosa are almost always involved in ulcerative colitis, and a carefully performed sigmoidoscopy, using either rigid or flexible instruments, together with rectal biopsy, usually can make the correct diagnosis when coupled with a high-quality double-contrast barium enema examination (see p. 1445).

In cases of ulcerative colitis in which the rectum is minimally involved and barium enema examination results are normal, colonoscopy can help define the nature and extent of disease. Pancolonoscopy should never be performed, however, in the setting of acute, moderately severe, or severe ulcerative colitis because of the risk of perforation. In quiescent ulcerative colitis, the colonoscopic examination may indeed be technically easier because of shortening of the colon with the reduction in acute angulations at the flexures and in the sigmoid colon. Superficial mucosal changes in early ulcerative colitis as seen through the colonoscope include hyperemia, mucosal friability, a finely granular pattern, and shallow small superficial ulcerations or erosions. These changes are similar to those seen in the rectosigmoid at sigmoidoscopy. Later changes include a coarsely granular appearance, deeper mucosal ulcerations, pseudopolyp formation, and shortening and loss of haustrations.

Colonoscopy is more sensitive than the single-contrast barium enema study in detecting early mucosal changes in ulcerative colitis. Substantial disagreement between colonoscopy and barium enema findings in the evaluation of the extent and severity of disease in ulcerative colitis has been reported. Three of 14 patients with colonoscopically diagnosed ulcerative colitis had completely normal barium enema examinations.[41] Also, substantial underestimation of the extent of disease by barium enema, when compared with colonoscopy and biopsy, has been reported. Fourteen per cent of patients in one series with pancolitis by colonoscopy had normal findings on barium enema examination.[42] The prognostic and therapeutic implications of detecting by colonoscopy these presumably milder forms of ulcerative colitis with normal barium enema studies are unknown.

The double-contrast (or "air contrast") barium enema using high-density barium with good mucosal coating properties is thought by some to be as sensitive as colonoscopy in detecting early changes of ulcerative colitis.[43, 44] The earliest recognizable change in double-contrast enemas is a diffusely granular appearance comparable to that seen by the colonoscopist (see Fig. 78–6*B*).

Even with this major advance in radiography, however, comparisons of colonoscopy and double-contrast barium enema suggest considerable underestimation of disease extent by the latter technique. In two thirds of patients in one survey, greater extent of involvement (averaging an additional one third of colon length) was noted on endoscopy than on double-contrast barium enema study.[45] In addition to determining the extent of involvement in patients with established ulcerative colitis, colonoscopy is also particularly helpful in assessing patients with considerable symptoms of colitis yet minimal changes on sigmoidoscopy and barium enema.

Radiography

Radiographic examination of the colon is an important technique for confirming the diagnosis of ulcerative colitis. A plain film of the abdomen alone may often provide a great deal of information, especially in

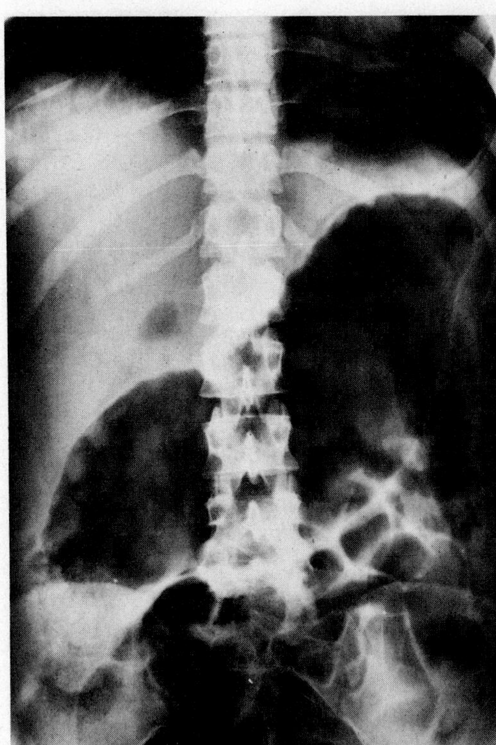

Figure 78–5. Plain film of the abdomen from a patient with ulcerative colitis and toxic megacolon. Note that the air in the colon silhouettes an irregular colonic mucosa.

patients with more severe ulcerative colitis, in whom barium enema examination may be contraindicated. Thus the colon may be more or less filled with air so that on plain film, features such as foreshortening of the colon and loss of haustration may be appreciated. Many times there is sufficient air in a segment of the colon to silhouette the mucosa, revealing an irregular mucosa caused by pseudopolyps, ulcerations, and mucosal tags (Fig. 78–5). Patients suspected of having toxic megacolon (high fever, abdominal tenderness, and distention) may be seen on plain film to have a midtransverse colon dilated with air to a diameter of 6 cm or more; in toxic megacolon, dissection of gas into deep ulcers may produce a double contour appearance of intramural air in the colon.

Barium enema examination may provide information useful in three ways to the clinician.

1. It is at present still the preferable means of diagnosing disease proximal to the sigmoidoscope. From the standpoints of cost, patient safety and tolerance, and clinical convenience, the double-contrast barium enema, not colonoscopy, must be used first in the routine evaluation of the patient suspected of having ulcerative colitis. When sigmoidoscopic examination supports the diagnosis of ulcerative colitis, the barium enema examination is useful in determining whether the disease is localized to the rectum or whether it extends proximally in the colon. If the sigmoidoscopy findings are negative, barium enema is useful in determining whether the patient's symptoms (bleeding or diarrhea, or both) are attributable to ulcerative colitis or to some other disease of the colon (such as tumor, diverticular disease of the colon, ischemic colitis, or Crohn's colitis). As noted, the sensitivity of the standard barium enema technique in detecting superficial mucosal lesions may be enhanced considerably by employing a double-contrast enema[43, 44, 46] (Fig. 78–6).

2. By demonstrating changes consistent with ulcerative colitis, the barium enema examination may strengthen the diagnosis of ulcerative colitis when sigmoidoscopy or rectal biopsy findings are equivocal. Such findings usually pertain to cases of mild ulcerative colitis or more severe ulcerative colitis in remission.

3. Barium enema examination is helpful in distinguishing ulcerative colitis from Crohn's colitis (see pp. 1327–1358) and is still useful in detecting the presence of cancer in the proximal colon in long-standing cases of ulcerative colitis.[4]

It is well to keep these indications clearly in mind

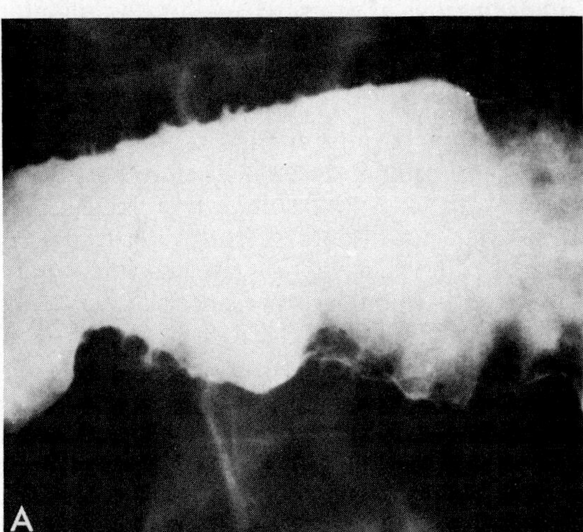

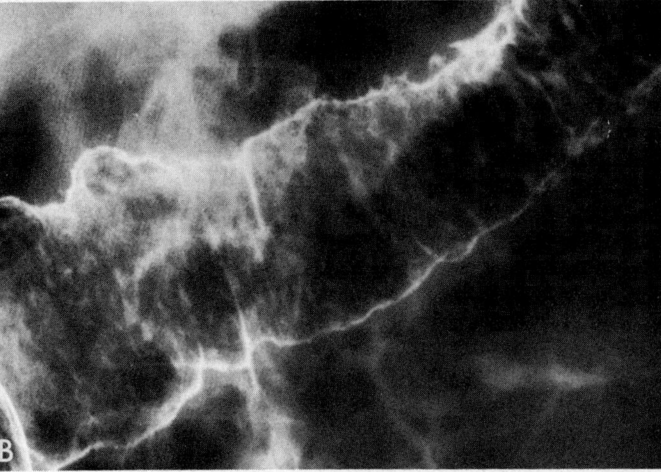

Figure 78–6. Single-contrast *(A)* and double-contrast *(B)* barium enema radiographs in a patient with universal ulcerative colitis. Multiple irregular serrations are noted along the transverse colon, representing shallow mucosal ulcerations. The double-contrast radiograph demonstrated finer details of the shallow ulcerations and diffuse granularity.

when deciding whether to obtain a barium enema examination. This examination is not without some hazard to the patient with ulcerative colitis. A vigorous preparation with irritative cathartics and enemas may exacerbate mild ulcerative colitis or moderate ulcerative colitis in remission and is not necessary. Mild saline cathartics (240 ml of magnesium citrate solution) with a simple tapwater enema or oral nonabsorbable colonic lavage fluid is usually sufficient.[47] In more severe forms of the illness, a barium enema may precipitate either dilation of the colon or perforation; high pressures usually employed to fill the colon with barium may decompensate an already compromised colonic musculature or may cause perforation where inflammation has extended through the muscular walls of the colon. If absolutely necessary, a barium enema examination in patients with acute colitis (without toxic megacolon) may be done with extreme care by the radiologist, using a soft rubber tip and instilling slowly a small amount of barium by gravity flow.[47] Fortunately, in those patients with more severe disease, barium enema examination is not required for routine management of the patient.

Barium enema examination should therefore be performed routinely on all patients with ulcerative colitis, but at an appropriate time. Under no circumstances should a patient with ulcerative colitis be prepared with irritant cathartics; such treatment may worsen the disease.

The radiographic features vary according to the location and state of the disease. Many patients with early ulcerative colitis will have perfectly normal findings on barium enema radiography. This point cannot be emphasized too heavily; diagnosis must rest on the sigmoidoscopic appearance or the rectal biopsy, or both. In some patients with early disease, on the other hand, minute ulcerations along the edge of the bowel may be noted (Fig. 78–6); evidence of mucosal disease may better be seen on the evacuation film, which reveals denudation of the mucosa with disappearance of its reticulated pattern. Double-contrast barium enemas, however, may demonstrate earlier mucosal lesions in ulcerative colitis than those seen by single-contrast techniques. A diffusely granular appearance of the mucosa is seen with high-density barium and air, a technique that delineates mucosal detail better than the standard barium enema study.[44] Much has been made of the loss of haustra, particularly in the left colon in patients with ulcerative colitis. This sign is nonspecific, for it may be seen in a large number of persons; however, when present along with other evidences of colitis, it must be considered as part of the disease.

Usually when haustra have disappeared from the left colon and even the transverse colon, the disease is more advanced and other evidences are noted. These include ulceration of the mucosa with further denudation; the ulcers may be particularly accentuated along the margins, where they assume a "collar button" appearance. The bowel shortens progressively, becomes rigid in appearance, and looks like a narrow tube resembling a pipe (Fig. 78–7).

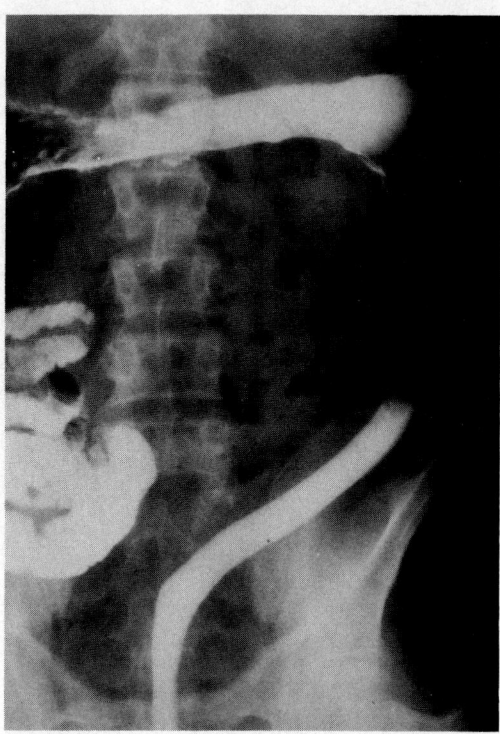

Figure 78–7. Barium enema showing a shortened, narrowed, tubular colon in a patient with chronic ulcerative colitis. (Courtesy of Ruedi F. Thoeni, M.D.)

At variable intervals, pseudopolyps make their appearance. These are radiolucent filling defects that are scattered throughout the bowel but may be localized in certain areas (Fig. 78–8). They may develop in a short period of time. Although they tend to be permanent, they have been noted on occasion to disappear with therapy.

Radiologists pay particular attention to the presacral space, which is increased as the disease progresses owing to inflammation and spasm or fibrosis. Somewhat arbitrarily, a distance greater than 2 cm is considered by the radiologist to be abnormal when associated with other findings of ulcerative colitis on radiography. It is good evidence that the patient has relatively severe inflammatory involvement of the rectum and presacral tissues.

Frequently on barium enema examination an area of narrowing presumed to be a stricture may be found in patients with ulcerative colitis. Histologically, these areas are often not fibrotic strictures but rather represent segments in which there is marked smooth muscle hypertrophy.[34] Although its presence suggests a napkin ring type of carcinoma, if the lesion is present on the left side it generally represents muscle hypertrophy. In some instances it is merely spasm, because it may disappear with the intravenous administration of glucagon or treatment. A full discussion of the comparison between the findings in ulcerative colitis and in Crohn's disease of the colon can be found on page 1446.

During the barium enema study it is important to fill the terminal ileum, because about 10 to 15 per cent of patients with ulcerative colitis who have universal

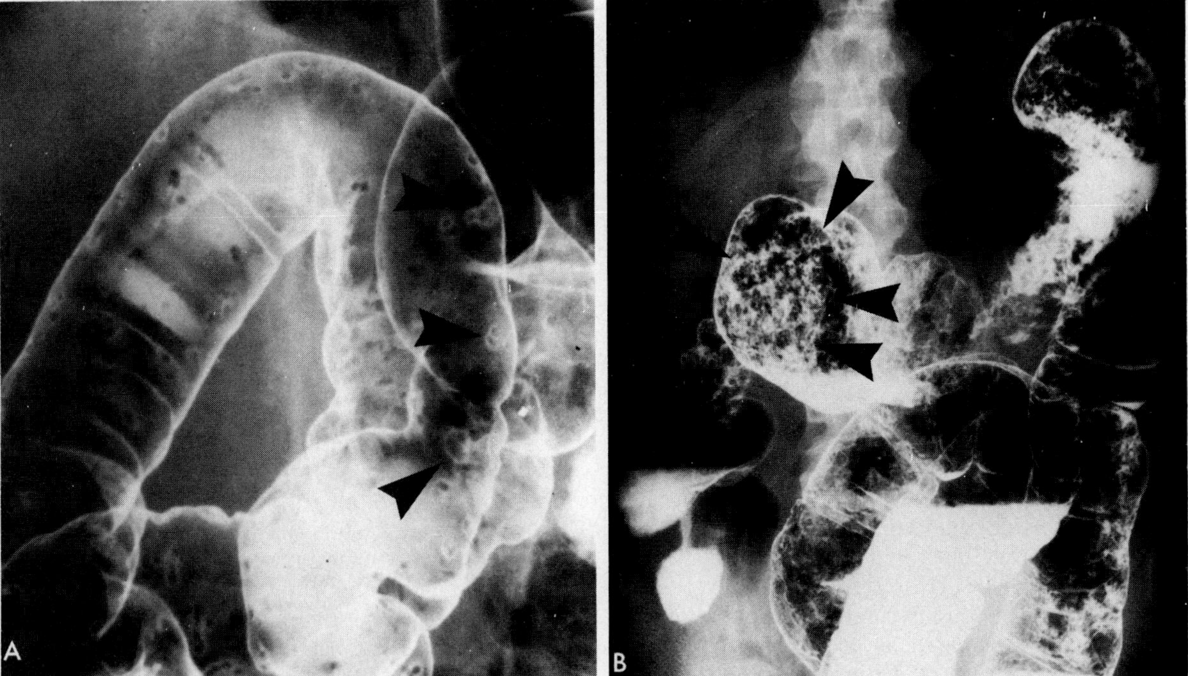

Figure 78–8. Pseudopolyp in ulcerative colitis on double-contrast barium radiography. Pseudopolyps *(arrows)* can range from small (1 to 10 mm) superficial lesions *(A)* to large complex masses throughout the colon *(B)*. (Courtesy of R. Brooke Jeffrey, M.D.)

involvement will also have some superficial inflammation of the ileal mucosa associated with edema and possibly some spasm, giving an abnormal appearance to the terminal ileum on radiography. Often, however, this so-called "backwash ileitis" can be readily distinguished from Crohn's disease of the terminal ileum by barium enema, because the terminal ileum is not visualized owing to involvement of the ileocecal valve in granulomatous disease.

DIFFERENTIAL DIAGNOSIS

As noted, the typical patient with moderately severe ulcerative colitis presents with chronic watery, large-volume diarrhea, lasting weeks rather than days at a time; there is often some lower abdominal cramping and intermittent low-grade fever. Blood is usually noted in the watery stools from time to time. Infectious colitis (particularly that caused by *Shigella, Salmonella,* amebae, or *Campylobacter*) may present with similar symptoms, but these, however, are not commonly chronic. Viral gastroenteritis is a short-lasting, acute illness with upper as well as lower gastrointestinal tract symptoms, not associated with either fecal leukocytes or gross hematochezia (see pp. 1191–1232).

Chronic colonic infections in immunocompromised patients may sometimes mimic ulcerative colitis (see pp. 1242–1257). Chlamydial proctosigmoiditis may produce a month-long illness with tenesmus and mucous diarrhea, and it is associated with a uniformly inflamed distal colon (rarely with inflammation above the rectosigmoid junction). Diagnosis depends on specific lymphogranuloma venereum (LGV) serologies or by appropriate *Chlamydia* cultures of biopsy material. Herpetic proctosigmoiditis may be associated with a prolonged clinical illness characterized by mucous diarrhea. Proctosigmoidoscopic features, although usually demonstrating focal disease, may occasionally be indistinguishable from idiopathic ulcerative colitis. Diagnosis of herpetic proctosigmoiditis can be established by viral cultures of fresh rectal biopsy material. Recently, cytomegalovirus (CMV) colitis has been suggested as a cause of chronic colitis among immunocompromised patients with AIDS. Although it is usually noted clinically to be associated with small bowel disease as well (with its large-volume watery diarrhea, weight loss, and cramping paraumbilical pains), CMV colitis can mimic idiopathic inflammatory bowel disease.[48] In some instances, CMV colitis has a characteristic appearance with focal 2- to 5-mm, raised, hyperemic papules or shallow ulcerations, whereas, in other patients, the colonic mucosa is uniformly eroded, friable, and hyperemic. Once again, diagnosis depends on specific viral cultures and histologic examination of tissue biopsy specimens for CMV. Occasionally, immunocompromised patients will develop a chronic colitis-like illness attributable to *Cryptosporidium* or *Isospora belli*. These infections usually are detected by requesting specific examinations of the stool; however, occasionally they are detected on careful high-power light microscopic examination of the apical cell surface of colonic epithelial cells.

Suffice it to say with the foregoing discussion, the clinician must be vigilant in excluding colonic infections mimicking ulcerative colitis. At the present time in immunocompetent patients with no known or suspected risk factors for human immunodeficiency virus

(HIV), multiple stool cultures for routine enteric pathogens and stools for ova and parasites are sufficient to exclude common enteric pathogens. For patients with *any* risk factors for immunodeficiency (multiple blood transfusions, intravenous drug abuse history, homosexual lifestyle, sexual promiscuity, underlying malignancies, or the use of immunosuppressive agents), extreme care must be used in excluding the atypical bowel infections already mentioned. For these latter patients, in addition to routine stool bacterial cultures and examination of the stool on multiple occasions for common ova and parasites (including *Cryptosporidium* and *Isospora belli*) the authors strongly recommend careful viral and chlamydial cultures of colonic mucosa and histologic examination of colonic mucosa for viral inclusions and parasites.

Irritable bowel syndrome is characterized by a similar course of chronic, intermittent diarrhea with cramps, but in this disorder stools are usually small in volume, and low-grade fever and hematochezia are not features (see pp. 1402–1418). Diverticular disease of the colon may also exhibit intermittent attacks of lower abdominal cramping, diarrhea, and fever. Although hematochezia appears on occasion, the bleeding from colonic diverticulosis is usually of massive proportions and does not tend to be associated with periods of acute diverticulitis (see pp. 1426–1432). Ischemic colitis may present with hematochezia and diarrhea. The course is usually self-limited, although repeated bouts of ischemia may occur over several months (see pp. 1903–1932). Chronic watery diarrhea may result from a variety of small bowel diseases (see pp. 290–316). Ulcerative colitis of moderate severity may be easily differentiated from irritable colon, diverticular disease of the colon, and chronic small bowel diarrhea by proctosigmoidoscopy and barium enema examination, which will demonstrate the diagnostic features of ulcerative colitis in almost all cases of moderate and active disease. Differentiation between ulcerative and Crohn's colitis is discussed on pages 1328 and 1348.

In mild ulcerative colitis, symptoms are more variable. In the patient with recurrent rectal bleeding in the absence of diarrhea, the differential diagnosis includes hemorrhoids, anal fissure, rectal polyp, carcinoma of the rectum, factitious proctitis (mechanical trauma to the rectum resulting from the insertion of foreign objects), Crohn's colitis, and ulcerative colitis. Most of these conditions can be diagnosed by proctosigmoidoscopy. If the ulcerative colitis is the cause of the rectal bleeding, the rectosigmoid mucosa will invariably show generalized friability and usually many of the other changes consistent with ulcerative colitis. Crohn's colitis, however, may not always be distinguishable from ulcerative colitis proctoscopically, although the ulcers of Crohn's disease are larger, deeper, and more discrete (see p. 1348). Factitious colitis caused by trauma or caustic enema administration is usually confined to the rectum; granularity, loss of vascular markings, and pseudopolyps are not seen. Whether or not a lesion is found at sigmoidoscopy that can explain the bleeding, barium enema or pancolonoscopic examination is indicated to detect polyps, carcinoma, or segments involved by Crohn's disease or ulcerative colitis beyond the reach of the sigmoidoscope. Postradiation colitis may also present with bleeding, usually in women after irradiation for carcinoma of the cervix and in men after irradiation for prostatic cancer. In this situation, the diagnosis is made primarily on the basis of history and the distribution of colitis along the colon (see pp. 1373–1379).

Patients with mild ulcerative colitis who do not bleed are misdiagnosed most commonly as having irritable bowel syndrome because they usually suffer from chronic and intermittent low-volume diarrhea with mild lower abdominal cramps but without systemic symptoms. Although results of proctosigmoidoscopic and barium enema examinations are normal in patients with irritable colon, they are usually abnormal in those with mild ulcerative colitis; in mild cases the barium enema results may be normal and the proctosigmoidoscopic examination may show only minimal or equivocally abnormal findings. In this situation, rectal biopsy may be helpful in establishing the correct diagnosis by demonstrating crypt abscesses or a generalized infiltration of both mononuclear and polymorphonuclear leukocytes in the lamina propria.

CLINICAL COURSE

Ulcerative colitis is a disease that is highly variable in severity, clinical course, and ultimate prognosis. The onset of the disease is typically in the second, third, or fourth decade of life, and both onset and subsequent exacerbations may be insidious or abrupt. The symptoms may range from small amounts of rectal bleeding, often mistaken for hemorrhoidal bleeding, to fulminant diarrhea with colonic hemorrhage and hypotension. Most patients (about 60 to 75 per cent) will have intermittent attacks of symptoms, with complete symptomatic remissions between attacks.[49] A smaller number (about 4 to 10 per cent) will have one attack with no subsequent symptoms for up to 15 years after the initial episode; a few patients (5 to 15 per cent) will be troubled by continuous symptoms without any remission.

The severity of the disease, whether in the initial episode or in a subsequent exacerbation, has important therapeutic and prognostic implications. For example, as seen in Table 78–3, most of the immediate deaths

Table 78–3. PERCENTAGE OF PATIENTS DYING FROM AN ACUTE ATTACK OF ULCERATIVE COLITIS

	Severity of Attack		
Years of Study	***Severe***	***Moderate***	***Mild***
1938–1952	33.8%	19.7%	1.5%
1952–1962	26.8%	2.4%	0.4%
1975–1982	2.5%	0%	0%

From Edwards, F. C., and Truelove, S. C. Gut *4*:299, 1964, and Rolny, G. J., and Sandberg-Gertzen, H. Gastroenterology *89*:1005, 1985.

occur in those patients with severe disease, whereas patients with mild disease rarely die. Moreover, as judged by death rates, severe disease has remained refractory to all types of treatment over the last 30 years, but significantly fewer patients with moderate disease now die of ulcerative colitis than previously.

Because of these therapeutic and prognostic implications, it is important for the physician to assess the severity of the disease in every patient. Although in general the intensity of mucosal disease as seen at sigmoidoscopy parallels the severity of the attack, the findings do not always reflect clinical severity accurately, probably because only a small portion of the total colonic mucosa is seen. Likewise, radiographic evaluation does not provide a reliable assessment of the severity or extent of disease. Colonoscopy is superior to radiography in these aspects; however, like the barium enema, it is better employed when patients have mild clinical disease or are recovered from symptoms of moderate or severe disease. The best indices of severity, then, are clinical symptoms and signs. Thus large volumes of diarrhea indicate that the colonic mucosa has been involved to such an extent and degree that sodium and water reabsorption are significantly impaired. Frequent bowel movements, on the other hand, may result from either large volume diarrhea or colonic or rectal irritability. Frequency per se, then, is an unreliable indicator of severity.

A large amount of blood in the stools, a fall in hematocrit, and hypoalbuminemia are all signs of widespread and severe mucosal destruction with its attendant significant loss of blood into the colon. Similarly, sustained high fever, tachycardia, and marked elevation of the erythrocyte sedimentation rate indicate intense or widespread inflammation; however, the degree of elevation of the white blood count does not always correlate well with the extent and severity of disease and symptoms, although counts over 20,000 cells/cu mm usually indicate serious disease. Rapid weight loss resulting from anorexia and increased catabolism (fever, blood loss) has the same implication. Steady abdominal pain and tenderness point to transmural involvement in the severest forms of the disease.

The classification of ulcerative colitis into three categories of severity is purely arbitrary, but, as noted earlier, such classification assumes significance because of its prognostic value. It is possible to define *mild* disease arbitrarily as that associated with fewer than four bowel movements a day and lacking anemia, fever, tachycardia, weight loss, and hypoalbuminemia.[50] *Severe* disease is defined as that associated with more than six stools a day, with considerable colonic bleeding, anemia, hypoalbuminemia, fever, tachycardia, and weight loss. In the next few paragraphs the clinical features of mild, moderate, and severe ulcerative colitis are described briefly, followed by a consideration of diagnostic and therapeutic measures in the disease as a whole. In considering patients with ulcerative colitis, the physician must remember that patients do not necessarily remain in an individual category for life. Thus, patients with clinically mild disease may develop severe exacerbations of ulcerative colitis.

Mild Disease

Mild ulcerative colitis is the most common form of the disease, afflicting about 60 per cent of all patients.[51] It may occur in either of two ways: most commonly (80 per cent of the cases), clinically mild ulcerative colitis is segmental in distribution, usually involving just the distal colon (sigmoid and rectum); less often, clinically mild ulcerative colitis is seen in patients in whom the whole colon is involved with the disease. The age of onset, sex predilection, and familial incidence of ulcerative colitis are the same in mild disease as in the more severe forms of ulcerative colitis. Similarly, the course of the disease—that is, the percentages of patients having only one attack, intermittent attacks, or chronic continuous disease—is the same for mild ulcerative colitis as for the more severe forms. Anorectal complications as well as extracolonic manifestations of ulcerative colitis (arthritis, pyoderma gangrenosum, uveitis, and erythema nodosum) are noted in mild disease as in more severe forms but appear less frequently in patients with proctitis alone than with universal colitis. Sometimes these extraintestinal complications are the chief complaints of the patient, rather than diarrhea or rectal bleeding, and on rare occasions they may be evident long before significant colonic symptoms develop. Because of all of these similarities to the more severe forms of ulcerative colitis, mild ulcerative colitis, even when sharply limited to the rectosigmoid colon, is considered to be the same disease as more severe ulcerative colitis. Indeed, a small number (5 to 15 per cent) of patients with disease limited to the rectosigmoid colon will show ultimate progression of their disease to involve a much larger—if not the entire—length of the colon, with the simultaneous development of more severe diarrhea or bleeding.[52]

By definition, neither colonic bleeding nor diarrhea is severe in mild ulcerative colitis, and systemic signs and symptoms are absent. Occasionally, patients with mild ulcerative colitis may suffer from short episodes of anorexia and fatigue or mild lower abdominal cramps; but most often hospitalization is not required, and the patient may continue his or her usual activities. A patient may present with a small amount of rectal bleeding in the absence of diarrhea and be mistakenly diagnosed as bleeding from hemorrhoids. Alternatively, some patients have frequent stools, generally small in volume, without gross bleeding but with mucus; these patients may be misdiagnosed as having irritable bowel syndrome. In either case, the correct diagnosis may be established by sigmoidoscopy, colonoscopy, or barium enema. As mentioned earlier, a few patients with mild ulcerative colitis may present with anorectal or extracolonic complications of ulcerative colitis in the absence of either diarrhea or colonic bleeding. It is not known how often the patient with mild ulcerative colitis may be asymptomatic or be undiagnosed. Because of the uncertainty of the incidence of undiagnosed mild ulcerative colitis, available figures on incidence, prevalence, and mortality in ulcerative colitis may be somewhat inaccurate.

The immediate mortality in mild ulcerative colitis (that is, in those patients sick enough to be hospitalized or seen as outpatients) is almost nil (Table 78–3). Similarly, patients with mild ulcerative colitis have a long-term prognosis little different from that of a control population. The development of colonic cancer in mild ulcerative colitis, particularly proctosigmoiditis, is much rarer, occurring about one seventh as often as in the more severe forms of the disease.

Moderate Disease

Clinically moderate disease affects about 25 per cent of all patients with ulcerative colitis.[51] In these patients, symptoms are somewhat more intense. During the initial attack or an exacerbation, diarrhea is a major symptom, in contrast to what occurs in the mild category. Stools are frequent, usually numbering four to five per day; they are loose and almost invariably contain blood. Crampy abdominal pain, particularly left lower quadrant, is usually more prominent than in persons with the mild form of the disease, although not incapacitating; often, it may wake the patient at night. Usually cramps are relieved by defecation. Many of these patients will have intermittent low-grade fever of 99° to 100° F. Generally the patient is somewhat tired, fatigues easily, and cannot take part normally in all activities. Appetite is usually maintained, but there may be intervals of anorexia and weight loss. The patient may complain of extracolonic symptoms such as low backache or arthritis. On laboratory testing, there may be anemia (hematocrit rarely less than 30 per cent) and hypoalbuminemia (albumin levels between 3.0 and 3.5 gm/dl).

During the initial attack or an exacerbation of ulcerative colitis, the patient with moderate disease may at any time become more severely ill, developing severe or fulminant colitis characterized by high fever and profuse diarrhea.[53] Rapid deterioration may also be manifested by massive bleeding or rapid and progressive dilation of the colon (toxic megacolon).

Generally, it is this moderate category of patient who most dramatically responds to treatment with corticosteroids or sulfasalazine, or both (see pp. 1450–1452). Indeed, since the advent of steroid treatment, the immediate mortality of this type of ulcerative colitis has fallen significantly (see Table 78–3); however, statistically, the long-term prognosis for this category of patient remains poor. Repeated attacks of equal or greater severity are common, and the risk of ultimately developing cancer is appreciable. Long-term prognosis is discussed in more detail on page 1457.

Severe or Fulminant Ulcerative Colitis

This is the least common form of ulcerative colitis, affecting about 15 per cent of all patients with the disease.[51] Patients with severe ulcerative colitis generally have a relatively sudden onset of symptoms, which rapidly progress to a point at which the patient is dangerously ill. Occasionally, a less severe attack will progress to this stage. Diarrhea is generally profuse, and rectal bleeding is constant. Fever is high, 101° to 103° F or higher; it may be spiking or sustained. The patient complains of tenesmus with frequent passage of bloody and watery stools. Appetite and weight are quickly lost. Weakness is profound, and pallor is striking.

On physical examination, the patient is acutely ill, febrile, dehydrated, and profoundly weak. Often the patient may draw up his or her legs in an effort to relieve abdominal cramps. In extreme instances, he or she may be somewhat obtunded owing to dehydration, fever, and acidosis. The pulse is rapid and blood pressure is low because of decreased extracellular fluid volume; if blood volume is sufficiently depleted as the result of profuse colonic bleeding, the patient may be in shock. Abdominal examination usually reveals a distended tender tympanitic abdomen without evidence of localized or generalized peritonitis. Bowel sounds may be absent. The white blood cell count is markedly elevated, often in excess of 20,000 cells/cu mm and occasionally as high as 50,000 cells/cu mm, with a high percentage of immature polymorphonuclear cells. Anemia is found universally, with hypochromic microcytic red blood cell indices. Anemia usually results from a combination of blood loss, iron deficiency, and marrow suppression; occasionally hemolytic anemia develops as a consequence of severe ulcerative colitis. Hypoalbuminemia is the hallmark of severe ulcerative colitis and results from low protein intake (anorexia), colonic protein loss enteropathy, and decreased albumin synthesis in the debilitated condition. Radiographs of the abdomen usually reveal some gas in the colon, with minimal colonic distention; the radiolucent intraluminal colonic gas may allow visualization of an irregularly thickened colonic mucosa (Fig. 78–5). Occasionally massive colonic distention (toxic megacolon) may be seen on the initial radiographs of the abdomen.

The patient with severe ulcerative colitis remains the most refractory to medical therapy. Death from the acute attack of ulcerative colitis is almost always the result of disease of this degree of severity.

MEDICAL THERAPY

As already stated, in recent years, there has been a dramatic decline in mortality rate from acute attacks of moderately severe ulcerative colitis (Table 78–3). Undoubtedly much of this decrease has resulted from the introduction of corticosteroids in the treatment of this disease in the 1950s; however, other factors have also contributed to this change, including greater understanding of the pathophysiology of ulcerative colitis and clearer criteria for the diagnosis of severe disease. Rational treatment for associated fluid and electrolyte disorders evolved, and blood transfusions became more available and safer. Together, all these factors may account for the declining mortality rate in the medical management of acute moderately severe ulcerative colitis. In addition, there are now better-defined indications for colectomy and improvements in surgical care for those patients not responding to medical management; these are discussed in more detail on pages 1470–1472.

General Measures

Those patients having significant diarrhea (moderate and severe ulcerative colitis), particularly when complicated by fever, are prone to dehydration. Colonic losses of sodium and potassium may result in reduced extracellular fluid volume (sodium and water depletion) and hypokalemia. Patients on large doses of corticosteroids may, in addition, suffer significant renal potassium losses that further contribute to hypokalemia. Fever (increased catabolism), colonic loss of bicarbonate, and decreased extracellular fluid volume that may produce prerenal azotemia together cause metabolic acidosis. Each of these defects should be corrected when it appears. Uncorrected fluid and electrolyte deficits (such as hypokalemia) have been incriminated in the development of toxic megacolon and renal calculi (see p. 1459).

In the more severe forms of chronic ulcerative colitis, blood loss from the colon is the rule, and patients tend to develop iron deficiency anemia. This may be corrected by oral or parenteral iron. Patients severely ill and showing signs of systemic toxicity may have bone marrow suppression in addition to iron deficiency;[54] such patients are prone to hypoalbuminemia from colonic protein losses, low protein intake (anorexia), and systemic illness. In such patients, blood transfusions will be beneficial in restoring hemoglobin concentration and blood volume toward normal.

Dietary management in ulcerative colitis, as in all gastroenterologic disease, enjoys its vogues. Most dietary regimens have assumed either (1) allergy to specific dietary protein or (2) mechanical trauma to the damaged colonic mucosa by high-residue diets. There is no evidence that the latter plays any role in exacerbations of ulcerative colitis. Evidence in favor of allergy to specific food protein stems largely from the clinical impressions that many patients with ulcerative colitis improve on a diet free of cow's milk, an observation documented by a small clinical trial.[55] A few patients with ulcerative colitis have hemagglutinating antibodies to tanned red cells coated with cow's milk proteins; however, normal subjects also have these antibodies, and in patients with ulcerative colitis the titers of such antibodies bear no relation to the state of activity of the disease, the presence or absence of clinical milk sensitivity, or the withdrawal of milk from the diet.[56] Some patients with ulcerative colitis have intestinal lactase deficiency, which could account for the deleterious effects of cow's milk. The frequency of lactase deficiency in ulcerative colitis has not been well studied (usually only by oral tolerance tests) and varies from 8 to 84 per cent of patients, similar to the frequency in the general population.

In general the diet in patients ill with ulcerative colitis should be appealing to the patient to overcome anorexia; should contain adequate protein and calories to compensate for enteric protein losses and increased catabolic rates (fever); and should exclude only those substances (such as milk) that careful history indicates may worsen diarrhea. General dietary restrictions cannot be recommended. Occasionally a trial of a low-residue diet may be indicated in those patients with significant diarrhea.

The use of opiates (or synthetic derivatives) for symptomatic relief of diarrhea in patients with ulcerative colitis is generally contraindicated. Opiates are effective in diarrheas, such as viral enteritis, because they slow the passage of stool through the colon, allowing more time for the absorption by the normal colonic mucosa of excessive amounts of sodium and water delivered to the colon from the small bowel. In the more severe forms of ulcerative colitis, profuse diarrhea usually results from widespread destruction of the colonic mucosa (loss of colonic absorptive capacity); in this situation, opiates generally are not effective. Furthermore, they may contribute to the development of colonic dilatation (toxic megacolon) and worsen anorexia. For similar reasons, anticholinergic drugs generally are not recommended as symptomatic treatment for the diarrhea of ulcerative colitis.

Psychotherapy

Just as it is undocumented that psychologic factors play an important role in the development and recrudescence of ulcerative colitis, it is not clear whether psychotherapy is a useful therapeutic adjunct in most patients with the disease. Usually supportive therapy from an interested and understanding physician and family helps most patients with ulcerative colitis.[57] Those patients with personality disorders or severe psychoneuroses may be helped by formal psychiatric treatment. Although psychotic patients may not derive long-term benefits from psychiatric treatment with respect to their ulcerative colitis, the management of a psychotic patient ill with ulcerative colitis is usually improved by the joint care of psychiatrist and internist, encouraging adequate compliance with a medical treatment program.

Hyperalimentation

Total parenteral nutrition (TPN or parenteral hyperalimentation) may be a valuable adjunct in the treatment of patients with ulcerative colitis. The catabolic state, decreased intake of nutrients, and excessive fluid, electrolyte, protein, and blood loss in the diarrheal stools all contribute to the severe debilitation of many patients with active ulcerative colitis. Restoration of positive nitrogen balance, rehydration, and adequate caloric intake are difficult to achieve in many patients with moderately severe to severe colitis despite the use of low-residue oral intake and supplemental peripheral intravenous fluids.

It is clear that patients with active ulcerative colitis improve subjectively and objectively while maintained on hyperalimentation. The indications include (1) severe dehydration and cachexia with marked fluid and nutrient deficits; (2) excessive diarrhea that has failed to respond to the usual therapeutic measures; or (3) debilitated patients undergoing surgical resection.

The hyperosmolar solution (usually casein hydrolysate or a defined amino acid mixture with glucose, 10 to 20 gm/L) is instilled by a central venous line (usually via the subclavian or internal jugular veins) to avoid the sclerosis of smaller peripheral veins. Meticulous attention must be given to the catheter site. Adequately trained supervisory nursing personnel must ensure the sterility of the puncture wound, and with proper care the catheters can be maintained safely for several weeks if necessary. The absolute inviolateness of the parenteral line is to be observed; the line must not be used for any purpose other than hyperalimentation. Supplementation with electrolytes, vitamins, and trace elements is indicated when total parenteral nutrition is employed for more than two to three weeks.[58]

Hyperalimentation will unquestionably improve the nutritional status and fluid and electrolyte balance of the vast majority of patients with severe ulcerative colitis.[59] In one uncontrolled study of intravenous hyperalimentation, 90 per cent of ulcerative colitis patients who lost an average of 20 pounds before treatment regained their weight while on hyperalimentation. One third of the patients did not require surgery, and 80 per cent of fistulas closed.[59] Although hyperalimentation is valuable adjunctive therapy in patients with ulcerative colitis, there is little evidence from controlled trials that the course of serious ulcerative colitis is altered by the use of hyperalimentation. In one controlled trial, ulcerative colitis patients randomized to bowel rest and intravenous hyperalimentation did no better than those randomized to a normal hospital diet taken ad libitum.[60] Identical rates for surgery and for duration of medical treatment were noted in that study. In another controlled study of bowel rest and hyperalimentation versus food, 60 per cent of both bowel rest and oral diet groups responded to medical therapy and did not require operation.[61] Patients given nothing by mouth, however, noted more rapid decrease in diarrhea. Until further controlled trials are conducted, hyperalimentation should be used primarily to improve the metabolic status of severely ill patients, but not in the unfounded expectation that definitive surgical therapy can be avoided (see pp. 1971–2028 for detailed discussions of nutritional problems in gastrointestinal disorders).

Corticosteroids

Because ulcerative colitis is an inflammatory disease of unknown cause, adrenocorticotropic hormone (ACTH) and cortisone, known anti-inflammatory agents, were tried empirically in the treatment of ulcerative colitis in the 1950s. Controlled clinical trials conducted in England quickly demonstrated that a short course of steroids produced an increased incidence of complete remission in the initial attack or during an acute exacerbation. Follow-up studies on these patients, however, showed that the benefits of the short course of steroids were transitory: by nine months to two years there was no longer a distinction between the course of the treated patients and the control patients, the numbers of symptomatic patients in each group being equal.[50] Other studies indicated that maintenance doses of cortisone (50 mg daily) or prednisolone (15 mg daily) after cortisone-induced remissions were not useful in prolonging the remissions.[62, 63] In the years since these studies were completed, newer and more effective cortisone analogues have become available, and more experience has been gained with modes of administration and dose schedules. Yet, even though it is clear that corticosteroid therapy may induce remission or improvement in the acute attack, the question of the most effective form of maintenance therapy is still open, and the long-term benefits of steroid treatment have not been adequately assessed.

Dosage and routes of administration of corticosteroid therapy vary with the severity and activity of the disease. In patients with mild disease, especially those with disease limited to the distal portion of the colon, rectal instillation of steroids will induce or maintain remission in a high percentage of patients, as judged by controlled clinical trials.[64] Dosages usually employed are 50 to 100 mg of hydrocortisone hemisuccinate or 20 to 40 mg of prednisolone phosphate in water; oil-soluble forms may be given in an oil carrier rectally. Patients should be encouraged to instill the solution in a left decubitus position and remain in this position for at least 30 minutes to achieve maximal topical coverage. When studied using technetium-99m (99^m Tc) sulfur colloid as a marker, a 60-ml volume of hydrocortisone enema solution (containing 100 mg of hydrocortisone) will spread as far proximally as the ascending colon.[65]

The beneficial effects of rectal steroids may be both local and systemic. Though earlier studies using ^{14}C-labeled prednisolone demonstrated only 3 to 4 per cent excretion of metabolites in the urine, recent studies note substantial blood levels after steroid enemas, with up to one half of the rectal drug absorbed systemically (Fig. 78–9).[66] The volume and composition of the fluid vehicle may well influence absorption. In addition, the nature of the steroid compound used may also determine systemic availability, with less prednisolone-metasulfobenzoate being absorbed, compared with prednisolone-21-phosphate.[67]

When given as an enema, tixocortol pivalate, a C-21 thioester corticosteroid with no systemic glucocor-

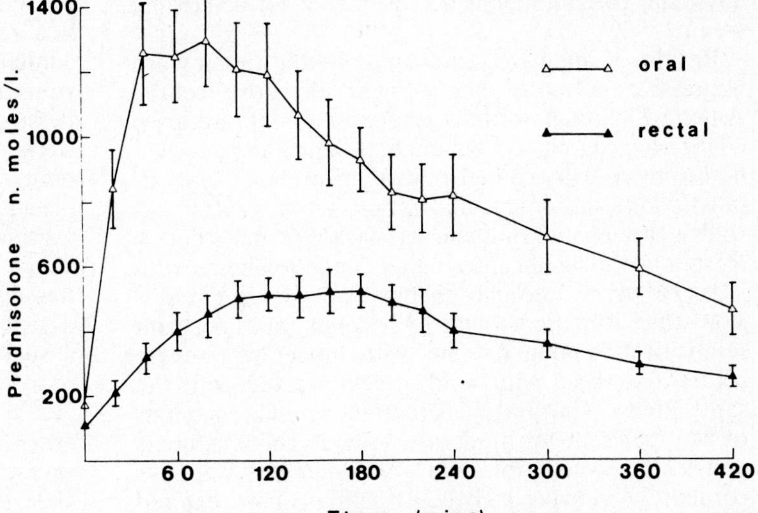

Figure 78–9. Mean plasma concentration (1 nmol/L = 0.36 ng/L) after enema and oral 20 mg prednisolone administration. Mean area under the curve for rectal prednisolone is 44 per cent of oral drug in patients with ulcerative colitis. (From Lee, D. A. H., Taylor, G. M., James, V. T., and Walker, G. Gut *20*:353, 1979. Used by permission.)

ticoid or mineralocorticoid effect, has been demonstrated in limited controlled trials to be at least as effective as hydrocortisone.[68, 69] In a randomized trial compared to hydrocortisone 100 mg in 60 ml diluent, tixocortol pivalate (250 mg in 100 ml diluent once daily) resulted in comparable control of diarrhea and rectal pain together with improved appetite.[69] Furthermore, rectal bleeding was controlled earlier among patients treated with tixocortol pivalate enemas. By the end of 3 weeks' therapy, 50 per cent of tixocortol-treated patients and 40 per cent of hydrocortisone-treated patients were improved. Further studies are needed in evaluating this new rectally administered steroid.

Although inconvenient and messy for many patients, twice daily rectal steroids should be strongly considered for most patients with mild to moderately severe ulcerative proctitis. Steroid enemas or foam should likewise be advised in patients with more proximal disease, especially if systemic steroids and sulfasalazine have not controlled diarrhea. Even though systemic absorption does occur, adrenocortical responsiveness is preserved.[66]

In active pancolonic disease of moderate severity, prednisolone or prednisone should be used in doses of 40 to 60 mg daily. For patients with mild flares of ulcerative colitis not responsive to steroid enemas and sulfasalazine (see p. 1453), prednisone or prednisolone should be used in doses from 20 to 40 mg daily. In patients with coincidental hepatic cirrhosis, conversion of the inactive prednisone to active prednisolone may be affected; thus, prednisolone is preferred in these cirrhotic patients.[70] The pattern of intestinal absorption of prednisolone may be altered in patients with acute colitis with decreased peak total prednisolone concentrations and prolonged half-life in patients versus control subjects. Total drug bioavailability, however, remains unchanged.[71] A single daily dose of prednisone or prednisolone is most convenient for patients and suppresses the adrenal minimally. In one recent study, no significant difference or trend between groups given single dose or multiple (divided) oral steroids could be detected.[72] Thus, for most patients with colitis of moderate severity, oral prednisone or prednisolone can be given once daily. In patients responding promptly to oral steroids, withdrawal should be gradual at rates not exceeding a 5-mg reduction every three to seven days. If no significant improvement appears after two or three weeks of oral steroids, parenteral therapy should be considered.

ACTH is not superior to oral or parenteral steroids.[73] Steroids are preferable to ACTH, particularly over long periods of time, because they may be given orally as well as parenterally, their dosage is regulated more precisely, they do not depend on adrenal responsiveness, and they have fewer and less serious side effects (such as hypertension, diabetes mellitus, weight gain, aseptic necrosis of the femoral head, and hyperpigmentation).[74] Given the wide availability of potent steroids, there is nothing to recommend use of ACTH in ulcerative colitis patients.

In the severely ill patient, prednisolone, 100 mg administered continuously or in divided doses by intravenous infusion over a 24-hour period, is recommended. Equivalent doses of methylprednisolone, betamethasone, or dexamethasone (the latter two are without systemic salt-retaining effect) may likewise be used. The dose is continued for 10 to 14 days, by which time sufficient improvement is usually achieved so that oral prednisolone in high dosage (60 to 100 mg/day) may then be substituted. During this period of intensive corticosteroid therapy, the patient should receive intravenous potassium (40 to 60 mEq/day) to prevent steroid-induced hypokalemia, which may contribute to colonic dilatation. High-dose corticosteroid therapy may mask symptoms and signs of sepsis or colonic perforation; for this reason, the patient must be examined carefully and his or her clinical status appraised several times daily during this therapy. Attention to details of fluid and electrolyte management is imperative for a successful outcome of treatment. If no improvement is produced by this treatment in 10 to 14 days, the patient should be considered for colectomy (see p. 1470).

Results of intensive intravenous steroid therapy are impressive in most patients with ulcerative colitis. Among 70 patients with 79 severe attacks of ulcerative colitis, a program of betamethasone, 3 mg intravenously twice daily (together with intravenous hyperalimentation, antibiotics, and supplementary rectal steroids), achieved remission in 44 (55.7 per cent).[61] Results were significantly better among patients with less extensive ulcerative colitis (88.2 per cent remission) than in patients with total colitis (46.8 per cent remission). Among patients with moderately severe colitis and those with mild attacks treated with the same intensive intravenous program, overall remissions of 86.9 per cent for moderately severe colitis patients and 91.8 per cent for mild attack patients were recorded. Moreover, only 2 of 158 patients expired during the acute flare of colitis when treated with intensive intravenous therapy.

Despite vigorous steroid therapy, some patients, particularly those with severe ulcerative colitis, will require urgent surgical therapy. In the study just cited, among patients experiencing a severe attack of ulcerative colitis, 52.8 per cent of pancolitis patients and 40.7 per cent of all patients with severe colitis required surgery within 3 weeks of instituting intensive intravenous therapy. As would be anticipated, a more favorable response without the need for surgery was recorded among patients experiencing moderately severe or mild attacks of ulcerative colitis. For those patients with moderately severe attacks, only 16 of 54 (29.6 per cent) failed medical therapy and ultimately required surgery whereas only 5 of 38 patients (13.2 per cent) with mild attacks of ulcerative colitis ultimately required surgery.[61]

In case of either medical failure (colectomy) or corticosteroid-induced improvement, signs and symptoms of adrenal insufficiency after withdrawal of corticosteroid therapy must be sought, because adrenal insufficiency is common during withdrawal from high-dose corticosteroids. Another characteristic phenomenon, withdrawal rebound, may be noted in patients with ulcerative colitis who are being weaned from high-dose corticosteroid therapy. In addition to some flare-up in bowel symptoms, patients often complain of fatigability, muscle aches, arthralgias, or arthritis; those patients with associated liver disease are prone to develop an increase in jaundice, and similarly those with uveitis or pyoderma gangrenosum may experience worsening of these complications. Reinstitution of steroid therapy at a higher dose level with a more gradually tapered program is often necessary in these patients to alleviate this syndrome.

Maintenance Therapy

The question of the long-term usefulness of maintenance corticosteroid therapy is unresolved. Existing data suggest that low-dose steroid therapy (10 to 15 mg of prednisone) in the patient in remission will not prevent future exacerbations of ulcerative colitis. For this reason the patient in whom the disease remits completely on treatment should be withdrawn from steroid medication while maintaining sulfasalazine for those patients with recent, active, severe disease. Extreme caution must be exercised in withdrawing patients from high-dose steroids.[75] A fasting morning plasma cortisol level of greater than 10 μg/dl (with the morning dose of steroids withheld) is excellent evidence of recovery of basal adrenocorticoid function. If the disease remains in remission after steroid withdrawal, no further steroid treatment is indicated until a subsequent exacerbation, when treatment may be reinstituted at a level commensurate with the severity of the exacerbation (steroid enemas for mild to moderate exacerbations; oral steroids for moderate to severe relapse). If, on the other hand, the patient experiences only partial amelioration of symptoms on steroid treatment, long-term steroid therapy may be continued until the patient experiences remission. However, the continued use of relatively high doses of oral steroids over a long period of time to maintain the patient relatively free of symptoms is not recommended in view of the potentially serious complications of such treatment (muscle wasting, osteoporosis, growth retardation in children, moon facies, hypertension, diabetes) (Fig. 78–10).

The authors recommend, therefore, that if the patient requires more than 15 mg of oral prednisone daily for more than two, or at the most three, months to keep the colitis or extracolonic complications in control, elective colectomy should be considered as an alternative means of treatment. Lower dose oral steroid therapy, particularly alternate-day steroid use, or steroid enema treatments, may be continued indefinitely at the option of the physician and the patient, because the risk of long-term complications from such treatment is much less. Sometimes the patient may be benefited by the long-term use of steroid enemas together with low-dose oral therapy when only high-dose oral therapy without steroid enemas sufficed to control the disease previously.

Long-Term Effect on Morbidity and Mortality

Whether corticosteroid therapy has altered the long-term morbidity and mortality rates of ulcerative colitis cannot be answered from existing data. Evidence from a large number of clinics indicates that the cumulative mortality rate in ulcerative colitis has been reduced dramatically since the advent of steroid therapy in the 1950s. Some of this reduction has resulted from decreased mortality in the acute attack of moderate disease, in which situation steroids unquestionably increase the chance of temporary remission or improvement. More liberal use of elective colectomy probably accounts for a significant reduction in long-term mortality in those patients not remitting on steroid treatment. Increasing recognition of complications of long-term disease, together with a vast improvement in general medical treatment of patients with ulcerative colitis, has also reduced overall mortality.

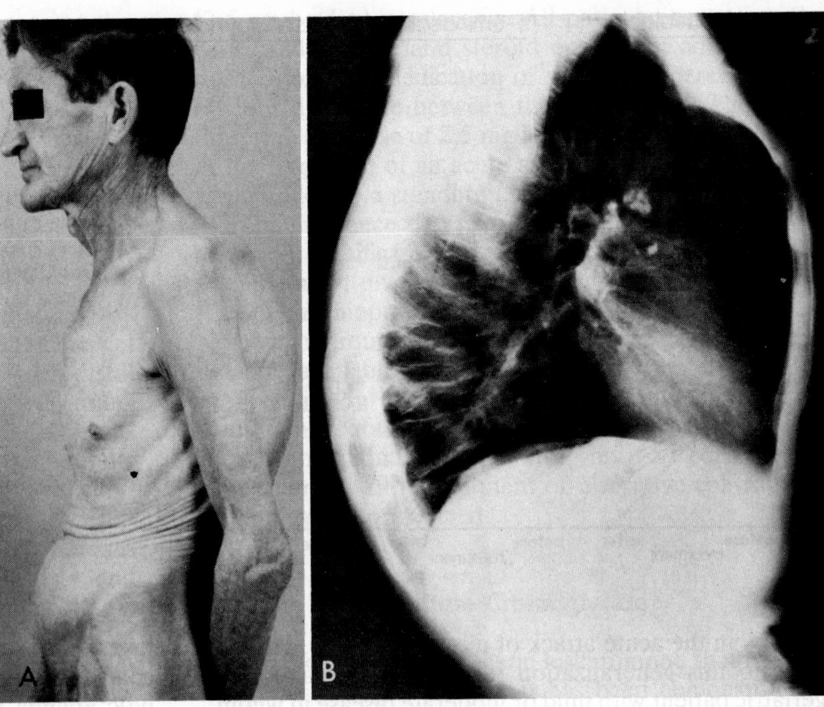

Figure 78–10. *A,* Photograph of a 46-year-old patient with ulcerative colitis treated for six years with corticosteroids. Note kyphosis, muscle wasting, and atrophy of subcutaneous tissues. *B,* Lateral chest film from the same patient, illustrating kyphosis caused by marked vertebral osteoporosis with collapse of several vertebral bodies.

Parenteral Antibiotics for Severe Ulcerative Colitis

Although it is not the subject of extensive controlled clinical trials, broad-spectrum antibiotic coverage is recommended by the authors for those patients with severe attacks of ulcerative colitis treated with intensive intravenous steroids and hyperalimentation. Whereas there is little evidence to suggest that infectious agents are largely responsible for ulcerative colitis, in the acutely ill patient with severe pancolitis, secondary bacterial infection of deeply inflamed colonic mucosa probably is common. In one study of oral vancomycin therapy among 33 patients with severe ulcerative colitis, only 11 per cent of vancomycin-treated patients required surgery, compared with 47 per cent of placebo antibiotic–treated patients.[76] The authors would recommend, however, intravenous rather than oral antibiotics in patients with severe ulcerative colitis. Several combinations of antibiotics would be acceptable; however, the authors would use ampicillin (1.5 to 2.0 gm intravenously every 4 hours), tobramycin (1.0 to 1.5 mg/kg intravenously every 8 hours), and clindamycin (600 mg intravenously every 6 hours) or ampicillin, tobramycin, and metronidazole (500 mg intravenously by continuous infusion every 6 hours).

Sulfasalazine (Salicylazosulfapyridine or Azulfidine)

Sulfasalazine agent was introduced empirically in the treatment of rheumatoid arthritis in the 1940s. Those patients with both arthritis and ulcerative colitis experienced improvement in their colitis as well when given sulfasalazine.

Sulfasalazine is metabolized by colonic flora, releasing sulfapyridine, an absorbable antibiotic, and 5-aminosalicylate. The active compound in colitis is believed to be 5-aminosalicylate. In a six-week trial, 1.5 gm daily of 5-aminosalicylate was equivalent to 3 gm of sulfasalazine in inducing remission of active colitis. Sulfapyridine was ineffective in inducing remission.[77] Aminosalicylate is effective in suppository form for colitis, even though appreciable blood levels cannot be detected when it is administered rectally (Fig. 78–11). The exact mechanism of action of sulfasalazine and 5-aminosalicylate is uncertain. It is unlikely, however, that sulfasalazine's beneficial effect is by inhibiting colonic cyclo-oxygenase, as indomethacin and other nonsteroidal anti-inflammatory agents are of no documented benefit in treating ulcerative colitis. Lipoxygenase product synthesis by colonic mucosa is profoundly altered, however, by sulfasalazine. Thromboxane B_2 and 12- and 15-hydroxyeicosatetraenoic acid (HETE) synthesis are significantly decreased when colonic mucosa is exposed *in vitro* to 1 mM sulfasalazine.[78] 5-Acetylsalicylic acid itself also inhibited overall production of prostaglandins and thromboxane.

Sulfasalazine has limited usefulness in the treatment of an acute attack of ulcerative colitis. Although somewhat effective in attacks of mild left-sided colitis, even in this situation sulfasalazine produces fewer remissions less promptly than do moderate doses of systemic steroids, and it is not clearly superior to steroid enemas.[79, 80] The drug's benefit in more severe forms of ulcerative colitis or in universal colitis has yet to be documented, but it is probable that sulfasalazine is inferior to corticosteroids in the treatment of these forms of the disease. For these reasons the authors use sulfasalazine as an adjunct to corticosteroid therapy, either rectal or systemic, and not as the first line of

inflammatory polyps as they represent heaped-up granulation tissue or swollen, edematous mucosa surrounded by ulcerations. As there is no primary epithelial or glandular alteration, these are neither true polyps nor premalignant lesions. Although more likely to be found in patients with prolonged universal colitis, the most common locations for pseudopolyp formation are the rectosigmoid and descending colon. Once developed, they tend to persist, but on occasion may regress completely when the colitis remits for long periods of time.

Perianal disease includes hemorrhoids (found in 20 per cent of patients), anal fissures (12 per cent), perianal or ischiorectal abscesses (4 to 6 per cent), and rectal prolapse (2 per cent). Although they are not features of ulcerative colitis per se, these lesions frequently appear during periods of active colitis when diarrhea is prominent. Their slightly higher prevalence in patients with pancolitis than with distal colitis probably reflects the more severe diarrhea usually seen in the former. Most perianal disease responds promptly to local anti-inflammatory measures and to control of the underlying colitis. Perirectal abscesses and fistulas generally heal with conservative surgical management—that is, incision and drainage of abscesses and opening of fistulous tracts. On occasion, chronic secondary perianal disease of ulcerative colitis may be so uncomfortable and debilitating when associated with refractory colitis that a colectomy may be required to afford symptomatic relief.

Major Local Complications

Massive Colonic Hemorrhage

Although diffuse oozing of blood from areas of active disease is noted in the majority of patients with ulcerative colitis, massive, life-threatening hemorrhage necessitating rapid and frequent blood transfusions is rare, occurring in fewer than 5 per cent of patients (usually in those with severe colitis). Colonic hemorrhage is not well tolerated in patients already compromised by fever, tachycardia, and extracellular volume depletion. As in all forms of acute hemorrhage, the hematocrit does not always accurately reflect the magnitude of blood loss. Most patients with massive colonic hemorrhage can be managed medically with blood transfusions, as the colonic bleeding usually subsides spontaneously. Occasionally, however, a patient may require emergent colectomy to control bleeding and, rarely, death may result from an exsanguinating hemorrhage.

Colonic Stricture

Colonic strictures complicate ulcerative colitis in 6 to 11 per cent of patients.[117, 119] Although most strictures are asymptomatic and discovered incidentally on digital examination of the rectum, barium enema examination, proctosigmoidoscopy, colonoscopy, or colectomy, abdominal cramping unrelieved by defecation may be a sign of partial colonic obstruction produced by a stricture. The majority of strictures are found in patients with long-standing and extensive colitis, have a predilection for the rectum and transverse colon, and may be multiple.

Although most are histologically benign, strictures may present a difficult clinical problem because they cannot be distinguished readily from colonic cancer. Certain radiographic features on barium enema examination, such as "shelving" and mucosal irregularities along the stricture, suggest carcinoma, but the absence of these findings does not exclude malignancy as the cause of the stricture (Fig. 78–14). Colonoscopy may be helpful in differentiating benign and malignant strictures. Multiple mucosal biopsies (at least eight to ten) and brush cytology specimens should be obtained from the strictured area. The shallowness of the standard colonic biopsy, however, may allow an occasional deeply infiltrating carcinoma to escape detection by these means. In patients with significant focal strictures, colectomy may be required despite negative biopsy findings. Symptomatic strictures with benign histologic features may occasionally be palliated with hydrostatic balloon dilatation under endoscopic or fluoroscopic control.

Toxic Megacolon

Acute dilatation of the colon associated with systemic toxicity is probably the most severe, life-threatening complication of ulcerative colitis. Data from

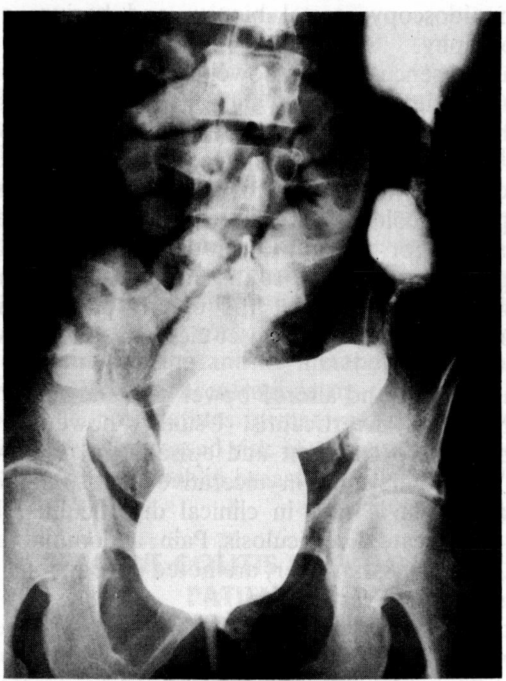

Figure 78–14. Barium enema of a patient with ulcerative colitis of 15 years' duration. The patient had been asymptomatic for ten years and off medication until six weeks prior to this examination. Multiple strictures are evident, and the distal stricture appears smooth in contour, suggesting a benign process. At operation both strictures were found to arise from colonic carcinoma.

large retrospective studies have reported its occurrence in 1.6 to 13 per cent of patients.[117, 120] Although it usually occurs in the fourth decade of life, toxic megacolon may appear at any age. Moreover, it may be the first manifestation of ulcerative colitis or develop in the course of chronic disease. The vast majority of patients demonstrate universal colitis, although toxic megacolon has been reported to complicate disease whose proximal extent is the splenic flexure.

The pathogenesis of toxic megacolon is not well understood. Histologic examination of colons removed at surgery or autopsy from patients with toxic megacolon show extensive deep ulceration and acute inflammation involving all muscle layers, often with extension of the inflammatory process to the serosa. The depth and extent of the inflammatory process in the colon of patients with toxic megacolon are usually more marked than in the resected colon specimens of patients with severe or fulminant ulcerative colitis without colonic dilatation. Presumably, the presence of widespread inflammation involving all layers of the colon in toxic megacolon accounts for both the systemic toxicity (fever, tachycardia, abdominal pain and tenderness, leukocytosis) and the apparent loss of colonic muscular tone, resulting in dilation of the colon. Evidence of inflammation can be found in small arterioles (vasculitis) and myenteric or submucosal nerve plexuses. However, these latter findings are variable, and probably vasculitis and inflammation and destruction of the myenteric or submucosal plexuses are secondary phenomena in this syndrome.

In addition to widespread inflammation and destruction of the colonic musculature, other factors that tend to promote high intraluminal pressures or decrease colonic muscular tone are thought to contribute to colonic dilatation; these include aerophagia, excessive use of opiates or anticholinergic drugs, and hypokalemia. None of these latter factors individually appears to be causative, because several cases of toxic megacolon have been reported in their absence, and many patients with severe colitis receiving opiates or anticholinergics or having hypokalemia do not develop toxic megacolon. The association between barium enema and toxic megacolon is uncertain. Although many patients with toxic megacolon have undergone barium enema examinations, a high proportion of these studies were done several days prior to the development of toxic dilatation of the colon. Nonetheless, the interdiction of barium enema studies in patient who are acutely ill with ulcerative colitis still holds.

It would appear, therefore, that the pathogenesis of the syndrome is best explained by diffuse inflammation and destruction of colonic musculature, perhaps aggravated by other factors. What is not explained is why relatively few patients with ulcerative colitis develop the deep ulcerations beneath the submucosa characteristically seen in toxic megacolon. The syndrome may occasionally complicate other forms of infectious colitis, including amebic colitis, bacillary dysentery, typhoid fever, and pseudomembranous colitis. Crohn's disease of the colon may also evolve into toxic megacolon.

Clinical Picture and Diagnosis. As the name implies, the patient with toxic megacolon usually is severely ill. Fever, abdominal pain and distention, and fatigue are prominent complaints. Occasionally, a patient with active colitis and bloody diarrhea will experience a sudden decrease in frequency of bowel movements on development of a toxic megacolon. The decrease in stool frequency reflects diminished colonic evacuation rather than an improvement in the patient's status. Misinterpretation may be avoided by examination of the patient, which frequently reveals a toxic appearance, with fever, dehydration, tachycardia, diminished bowel sounds, tympany, abdominal distention, and local or diffuse rebound tenderness. Patients receiving corticosteroids may display attenuated signs and symptoms that should not be underestimated by the examining physician.

Leukocytosis (often greater than 20,000 cells/cu mm), anemia, and hypoalbuminemia are common laboratory findings. A plain radiograph of the abdomen will reveal dilatation of the entire colon or limited solely to the transverse colon (Fig. 78–5). Although dilatation of the transverse colon on plain supine abdominal radiography (usually greater than 7 cm in diameter) is the most conspicuous finding, this distention is not indicative of the severity of the disease in this segment of the colon, but rather is determined by the anterior position of the transverse colon. Repositioning the patient prone, for example, redistributes gas to the more posterior descending colon and dramatically decreases gas distention of the transverse colon. Irregular colonic mucosa, occasionally with intramural air silhouetted against the gas in the colon, may also be discerned on flat film. An upright abdominal film may reveal free air under the diaphragm if colonic perforation has already occurred.

Perforation is a common complication of toxic megacolon, occurring most often in the transverse and sigmoid colon. Free perforation may be dramatic in its suddenness, and shock may be irreversible. The presence of perforation has by far the greatest impact on mortality rates in toxic megacolon, regardless of whether the perforation is free or sealed off.[121] The appearance of free colonic perforation may be associated with a marked increase in abdominal distention and obliteration of hepatic percussion dullness by free air. Peritonitis and septicemia closely follow fecal contamination of the intraperitoneal space.

When toxic megacolon is the initial clinical presentation of ulcerative colitis, the diagnosis may be difficult. Toxic megacolon may develop so rapidly that a history of antecedent rectal bleeding and diarrhea is obscured. In this setting, the condition may be confused with acute diverticulitis and pericolic abscess or carcinoma (presenting with lower quadrant pain, fever, and colonic dilatation), ischemic colitis (which occasionally may be associated with colonic dilatation proximal to the vascular insult), or colonic volvulus. The correct diagnosis may be established by a plain film of the abdomen and sigmoidoscopy. Sigmoidoscopy should be carried out despite the severe illness and the obvious discomfort to the patient. It can be done in the left lateral position, in bed if necessary, without colonic preparation. The sigmoidoscope need only be inserted a short distance without air insufflation, for in the vast majority of individuals presenting with toxic megacolon of ulcerative colitis, the rectosigmoid mucosal will reveal findings characteristic of inflammatory bowel disease.

Treatment. Therapy for toxic megacolon can be divided into (1) initial resuscitative and supportive measures and (2) definitive medical or surgical treatment aimed at the underlying necrotic process ongoing in the colon. Although early therapy is generally agreed on, the role of early surgical intervention versus prolonged medical treatment remains somewhat controversial. Careful correction of fluid and electrolyte deficits demands immediate attention as hypovolemia and hypokalemia may be profound on initial presentation, owing to antecedent diarrhea, vomiting, and loss of fluid into the dilated colon. Not uncommonly, 80 to 100 mEq of potassium chloride in the first 24 hours is needed to correct hypokalemia. Blood transfusions should be given when indicated for anemia and hypovolemia in the face of significant colonic bleeding. Prednisolone, 100 to 200 mg (or an equivalent dose of hydrocortisone), should be administered intravenously in divided doses throughout the day. Large doses of corticosteroids are given not only to ameliorate the inflammatory process in the colon but also to avoid relative adrenal insufficiency in patients who have received lower doses of steroids prior to the superimposed stress of toxic megacolon. Nasogastric suction should be instituted in an effort to remove swallowed air and thereby reduce the passage of air and fluid into the colon. A long peroral intestinal tube may further facilitate decompression of bowel gas. Additional decompression of the colon may be gained by repositioning the patient prone for a period of time. This allows gas redistribution to the more posterior descending colon.

Anticholinergic drugs and opiates should be withdrawn if the patient had been receiving them previously. Usually, abdominal pain is not severe enough to require opiate analgesics. In view of the transmural and often serosal inflammation in patients with toxic megacolon, frank perforation is a constant danger. To help contain the consequences of these perforations, intravenous antibiotics are recommended. Broad-spectrum coverage aimed at enteric gram-negative and anaerobic pathogens, as well as the enterococci, should be provided. Several regimens are acceptable: intravenous ampicillin, 1.5 to 2.0 gm every 4 hours, with glutamycin or tobramycin, 1.0 to 1.5 mg/kg every 8 hours, and either clindamycin, 600 mg every 6 hours or metrinidazole, 500 mg every 6 hours, all given intravenously.

The patient's response to treatment must be monitored carefully in an intensive care facility with adequate nursing supervision. Abdominal girth should be measured and recorded two to three times daily, and the physician should examine the patient at frequent intervals to ascertain whether bowel sounds are returning, whether an area of localized tenderness or rebound tenderness has developed, whether signs of perforation are present, and whether cardiovascular complications associated with bacterial sepsis have appeared. In addition, adequacy of fluid and electrolyte repletion must be recorded carefully; in difficult situations, appropriate treatment includes monitoring of central venous pressure and pulmonary wedge pressure, in addition to standard intake and output balance sheets. Frequent radiographs of the abdomen are mandatory during the acute phase.

When clinical or radiographic evidence of colonic perforation is present, or if perforation is strongly suspected, early emergent colectomy with ileostomy is clearly necessary. What is less clear is how to manage the patient whose clinical condition stabilizes or improves with the aforementioned medical regimen. Most of the recent literature includes patients with toxic megacolon complicating both ulcerative colitis and Crohn's colitis but demonstrates a similar outcome in both groups. Roughly 70 to 80 per cent of patients with toxic megacolon will require surgery during their initial hospitalization for documented or suspected perforation or for fulminant colitis.[121, 122] Many surgeons favor early laparotomy because of the formidable mortality rates associated with colonic perforation. Perforation (both free and sealed off) complicates toxic megacolon in approximately 35 per cent of patients. Furthermore, mortality rates approach 40 to 50 per cent in the presence of perforation, regardless of whether they are free or contained. Several authors have noted a considerably decreased incidence of perforation and postoperative mortality by adopting a policy of early surgery for toxic megacolon.[123, 124]

The outlook for patients who initially respond to medical therapy adds additional support for surgical intervention for toxic megacolon. Up to 60 per cent of this subgroup require subsequent hospitalization for fulminant colitis or recurrent toxic megacolon during periods of follow-up lasting up to two years after the initial episode.[121, 122] Unfortunately, there are no discriminating factors that can predict the likelihood of recurrence in a particular patient.

Mortality rates for surgery in patients with toxic megacolon are highest during the first few days after presentation (presumably when the patient is most critically ill) and when operations are delayed for more than a month.[121] The optimum timing of "elective" surgery, therefore, is between one and four weeks after diagnosis—that is, after initial medical management has ameliorated the activity of the necrotizing colitis. Mortality rates during this period are expected to be as low as 5 to 10 per cent.

Subtotal colectomy and ileostomy or proctocolectomy and ileostomy remain the procedures of choice, depending on the overall medical condition of the patient. During surgery and for three to four days postoperatively, the patient should be continued on high-dose corticosteroids to prevent relative adrenal insufficiency. Thereafter, the dose is tapered and the drug may be withdrawn completely by several weeks after surgery if the patient has recovered. At surgery, technical difficulties, as well as the extensively inflamed, dilated, "paper-thin" colonic wall, may result in peritoneal contamination with bacteria; postoperative intra-abdominal abscess formation is common and may be masked by continued administration of corticosteroids. Therefore, it is recommended that antibiotics be given for two weeks after corticosteroids have been discontinued. If a postoperative intra-abdominal abscess develops, it should be treated by surgical or percutaneous drainage; again, in the event of this complication, the patient must be observed carefully for signs of relative adrenal insufficiency.

Colonic Perforation

As noted earlier, the vast majority of colonic perforations complicating ulcerative colitis are associated with toxic megacolon. A small percentage of patients with moderately severe or severe colitis may have perforation, but this complication is not seen in mild disease. In a recent large retrospective series of 613 patients with ulcerative colitis,[125] 29 (4.7 per cent) perforations were reported (Table 78–5). Roughly three fourths of these perforations arose in the setting of toxic megacolon and often were multiple and predominantly in the transverse colon, including the hepatic and splenic flexures. For reasons that are not clear, the risk of perforation seems to be greatest in the initial severe episode of ulcerative colitis.[126]

In severe ulcerative colitis, the colonic inflammatory process may occasionally extend deep into the colonic wall, just as in toxic megacolon. However, unlike the situation in toxic megacolon, generalized transmural extension is uncommon in most patients with severe disease; when present, it is often localized at one point rather than spread extensively along large segments of the colon. Presumably, perforation of the colon in severe colitis arises from such a point of transmural involvement.

Some have claimed that corticosteroid treatment for ulcerative colitis may increase the frequency of perforation by rendering the bowel and surrounding peritoneum less capable of containing transmural inflammation. Available data do not substantiate this notion, however, because the frequency of colonic perforation complicating ulcerative colitis has not increased since the introduction of corticosteroid therapy. However, corticosteroids may mask symptoms and signs of perforation. High intraluminal pressures developed in the colon during barium enema and colonoscopic examinations theoretically would promote perforation through an area of transmural disease. The frequency of perforation in severe disease after barium enema or colonoscopy is not well documented, but prudence would dictate that these procedures be deferred until the patient has recovered from the severe attack. Unfortunately, it is the patient most prone to perforation—a severely ill patient seen for the first time with the initial attack of ulcerative colitis—who makes the physician anxious to diagnose the patient's problem quickly with a barium enema or colonoscopy. Diagnosis, however, can usually be made with gentle proctoscopy and water-soluble contrast medium (Hypaque enema) radiography.

Perforation may be easily diagnosed or strongly suspected in many patients with colitis. Sudden deterioration with increased abdominal pain, tachycardia, fever, increased abdominal girth, and direct and rebound tenderness point to perforation. On occasion, increased colonic bleeding may be noted secondary to disseminated intravascular coagulation resulting from perforation and bacterial sepsis. However, these signs and symptoms may not be present, particularly if the patient is receiving high doses of corticosteroids. In this situation, perforation may be heralded only by a deterioration (i.e., hypotension, tachypnea, tachycardia, or profound diaphoresis) in the patient's status in the absence of abdominal signs. In either case, diagnosis may be confirmed by the demonstration of free air within the abdominal cavity on upright or left lateral decubitus abdominal radiographs. Sometimes serial films must be taken daily before free air in the peritoneal cavity is appreciated.

Without question, the diagnosis of perforation or indeed of strongly suspected perforation necessitates laparotomy. The mortality rate in patients experiencing colonic perforation is extremely high (Table 78–5); overall, perforation accounts for approximately one third of all deaths directly related to ulcerative colitis.[126]

Table 78–5. INCIDENCE AND OUTCOME OF PERFORATIONS COMPLICATING ULCERATIVE COLITIS

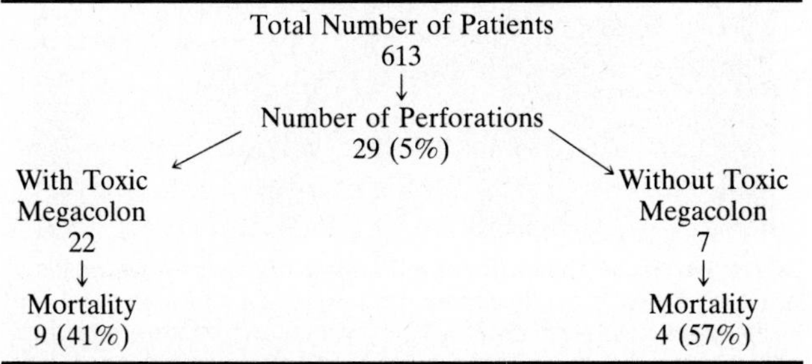

Adapted from Greenstein, A. J., and Aufses, A. H. Surg. Gynecol. Obstet. *160*:63, 1985.

Carcinoma of the Colon

It has been well established that patients with ulcerative colitis are at a higher risk for the development of colorectal carcinoma than is the general population. The frequency of colon cancer in adults with universal colitis has been reported to be 26 times greater and with left-sided colitis, eight to nine times greater than expected in the age- and sex-matched general population.[127] Moreover, colorectal carcinoma accounts for approximately one third of deaths related to ulcerative colitis.[126]

Both in adults and children, the risk for cancer complicating ulcerative colitis is related to two major

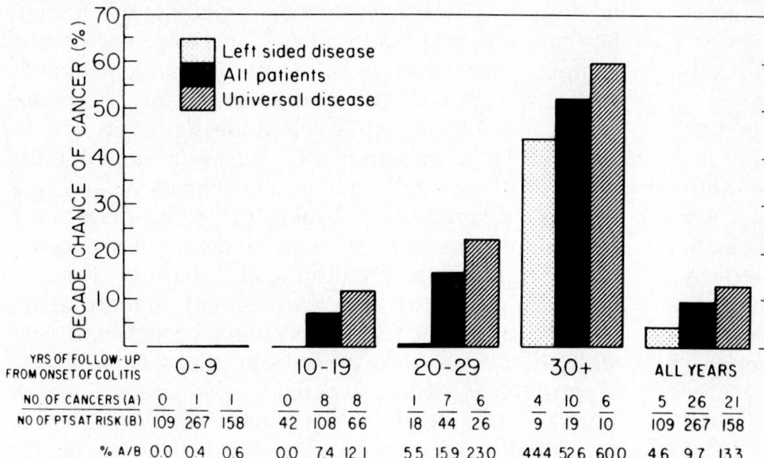

Figure 78–15. Decade incidence of colonic cancer among 158 patients with pancolitis versus 109 patients with left-sided disease, expressed as a proportion of the number of patients at risk in each decade after onset of disease. (From Greenstein, A. J., Sachar, D. B., Smith, H., Pucillo, A., et al. Cancer in universal and left-sided ulcerative colitis: factors determining risk. Gastroenterology 77:290–294. © by Williams & Wilkins, 1979.)

factors—the duration of the colitis and the extent of colonic involvement (Fig. 78–15). In addition, there is some indication that carcinoma arises more frequently (but not exclusively) in patients with chronically active ulcerative colitis than in those with intermittently active or previously active disease.

Duration of Colitis. Actuarial or life table methods of estimating the cumulative risks of cancer in ulcerative colitis indicate that the chance of developing carcinoma rises steadily in all patients with the duration of the colitis.[119, 128] The risk of colorectal cancer in patients with disease lasting less than ten years is minimal in most series,[129, 130] although one study reported that one fifth of the ulcerative colitis patients with cancer had disease for less than one decade.[131] The generally reported low risk for disease activity of less than ten years must be taken cautiously, as the absolute duration of disease activity prior to patient presentation or diagnosis cannot always be estimated accurately. After ten years of ulcerative colitis, the frequency of colorectal cancer rises steeply. Excess risk for patients with disease activity lasting from 10 to 20 years is 23 times that of the general population; after 20 years, the risk is 32 times the cancer risk of the population at large.[131] Although it was once believed that patients developing ulcerative colitis at a younger age were at greater risk for the development of cancer, subsequent reports have demonstrated that cancer risk is directly dependent on the duration of the disease and independent of the age of onset.[130]

Extent of Colonic Involvement. Patients with universal colitis are at highest risk for colorectal carcinoma. Indeed, 75 to 80 per cent of patients who develop cancer have a history of pancolonic involvement.[128, 130] Left-sided colitis still remains a prominent predisposing condition for carcinoma, but in this subgroup, malignancy generally develops a decade later than in patients with universal colitis.[130] Ulcerative proctitis without more proximal involvement probably poses no risk for cancer greater than that in a normal age-matched population.[132]

Characteristics of Colon Cancer in Ulcerative Colitis. Colonic malignancy associated with ulcerative colitis is histologically an adenocarcinoma, displaying a wide spectrum of differentiation. Poorly differentiated glands may be seen in one half of tumors but do not appear to affect patient outcome significantly. Multiple tumors are seen in up to one fourth of patients,[133, 134] a frequency considerably greater than that of synchronous cancers in patients without ulcerative colitis. Carcinomas are, in general, evenly distributed throughout the colon, with approximately one half located proximal to the splenic flexure[135] (Fig. 78–16).

Colorectal cancer arising in ulcerative colitis has

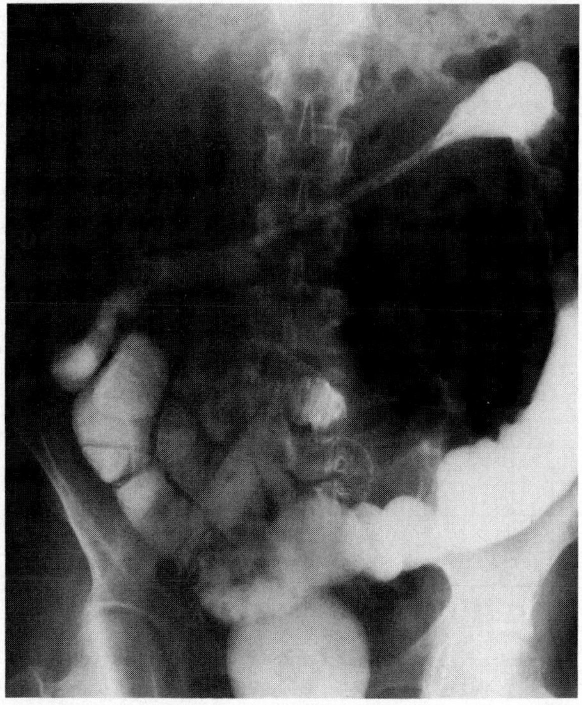

Figure 78–16. Colonic carcinoma arising from ulcerative colitis. A large ulcerating mass occupies the hepatic flexure and distal part of the right colon, which at surgery was found to be adenocarcinoma extending beyond the serosa. The transverse colon is narrowed and no normal haustrations are seen proximal to the sigmoid colon.

been considered previously to be extremely virulent, owing to the flat and infiltrative nature of many of these malignancies. Recently, a more hopeful prognosis has been given by several reports indicating that five-year survival was not significantly different from that of patients developing de novo carcinoma in the absence of ulcerative colitis.[133, 134] These encouraging results must be tempered with the realization that this similarity in survival rates is derived from the data of prospective surveillance programs in patients with colitis, indicating that malignancies in ulcerative colitis are as yet not diagnosed any earlier than in the general population, a reminder that, in part, it is the stage of detecting carcinoma that determines outcome.

Surveillance. Because of the extremely high cumulative risk of cancer in ulcerative colitis, multiple diagnostic techniques have been applied in an attempt to detect patients with early malignant changes. The histologic finding of dysplasia is generally regarded as a precursor or marker for malignancy.[136] Dysplastic changes include nuclear and cellular pleomorphism, loss of nuclear polarity, and marked stratification of nuclei (Fig. 78–17). Unfortunately, similar architectural changes may be seen as part of the normal cellular reparative process of chronic ulcerative colitis and may limit the sensitivity and specificity of dysplasia as a harbinger of malignancy. Furthermore, dysplastic changes may be focal and not visible macroscopically, may regress, and may be absent adjacent to, or remote from, a carcinoma.[137] Rectal dysplasia, once thought to be an accurate predictor of more proximal dysplasia or carcinoma, has proved to be an insensitive marker in two subsequent studies.[138, 139] Proctosigmoidoscopy alone, with or without biopsy, is not a sufficient screening procedure for carcinoma.

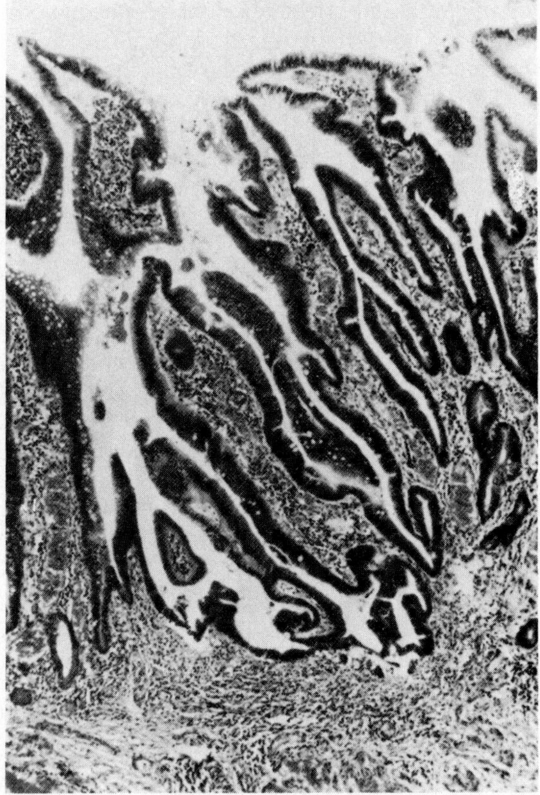

Figure 78–17. Severe epithelial dysplasia with villous changes in a patient with long-standing ulcerative colitis. (From Lennard-Jones, J. E., Morson, B. C., Ritchie, J. K., et al. Cancer in colitis: assessment of the individual risk by clinical and histological criteria. Gastroenterology *73*:1280–1289. © by Williams & Wilkins, 1977.)

Despite these apparent limitations to the use of dysplasia as a marker for colonic malignancy, it remains the best histologic adjunct to surveillance colonoscopy. Foci of dysplasia have been shown to accompany carcinoma in as many as 80 to 90 per cent of cases.[139, 140] A more sensitive indicator for underlying colonic carcinoma than simple dysplasia is the presence of high-grade epithelial dysplasia in a polypoid mass or plaque-like lesion (dysplasia-associated lesion or mass, called DALM), detected on colonoscopy; indeed, one study considers it an indication for proctocolectomy[141] (see also pp. 1529–1531 for a fuller discussion of dysplasia in ulcerative colitis). Although still in the early phases of evaluation, flow-cytometric DNA analysis of colonic biopsies screening for aneuploid cell lines has been suggested as a useful tool for detecting colonic malignancies.[142]

Given the difficulties in interpreting these diagnostic procedures as just described, how should patients with ulcerative colitis be followed to detect curable lesions in patients who have them and to exclude colonic cancer in those free of it? Simply stated, no test or group of diagnostic tests can absolutely guarantee that a patient is free of focal malignancy. The foundation of an adequate screening program rests initially on proper patient education. All patients should be informed of the excess cancer risk shortly after the diagnosis of ulcerative colitis is made. This will help ensure that patients with long-standing disease and especially those whose disease activity is quiescent or intermittent will not be lost to follow-up with a false sense of security that well-controlled or absent symptoms have eliminated any risk for subsequent carcinoma. Additionally, patients must realize that rectal bleeding or weight loss during the high-risk period should not necessarily be mistaken for an exacerbation of colitis and they should not merely begin self-treatment. This may delay consultation with the physician for a possible underlying colonic cancer. Lastly, patients with a colectomy and retained rectum, whether in continuity or defunctionalized, remain at risk for rectal carcinoma[143, 144] and thus require an indefinite period of surveillance of this region.

Colonoscopy has largely supplanted barium enema examination as the screening procedure of choice. The latter may be helpful to delineate colonic strictures not well appreciated by colonoscopy. No formal guidelines exist for the frequency of screening of patients with extensive colitis of less than 8 to 10 years' duration, although full colonoscopy with multiple biopsies every two or three years may suffice. Patients with pancolitis lasting more than 10 years, or with left-sided colitis lasting more than 20 years, should be enrolled in a yearly colonoscopic surveillance program. Multiple sites of each colonic segment should be randomly biopsied and examined histologically. Random biopsies, however, sample only about 0.05 per cent of a 100 cm long colon and, therefore, even the most well-adhered-to surveillance program is subject to sampling error. More stringent inspection with additional biopsies should be applied to strictured areas or raised lesions. Often, pseudopolyps may be difficult to differentiate from neoplastic growths.

The detection of frank carcinoma or dysplasia-associated lesion or mass is a clear indication for proctocolectomy.[141] Flat mucosa demonstrating high- or low-grade dysplasia warrants a shorter interval for subsequent evaluation, usually within six months. Patients with high-grade dysplasia on repeated colonoscopy or multiple areas of high-grade dysplasia on any colonoscopic examination should be strongly considered for total proctocolectomy. Even with close attention, colonic cancer may be detected too late for curative resection (see pp. 1519–1547).

The issue of prophylactic colectomy remains unsettled. Most experts believe that close, careful screening programs, when compared to the operative morbidity and mortality rates of proctocolectomy and the inconveniences of life with an ileostomy, offer a more suitable choice. In the decision to undertake prophylactic colectomy, both the physician and patient must weigh several factors: the risks and inconveniences of chronic colitis and its medical therapy, the need for lifelong screening colonoscopy examinations, the definitive cure of ulcerative colitis and prevention of cancer afforded by surgery, and the adaptation required for life with an ileostomy (see pp. 1477–1482).

Systemic Complications

Liver Disease

The incidence of liver disease in colitis is uncertain. Approximately 7 per cent of patients with ulcerative colitis will have some evidence of liver disease on the basis of clinical and laboratory data[145] (Table 78–6). Minor abnormalities in one or more liver tests (serum alkaline phosphatase, serum alanine or aspartate aminotransferase) are much more common but are not precisely correlated with demonstrable histologic lesions.[146, 147] There are large discrepancies in the reported prevalence of various hepatic lesions in ulcerative colitis as determined by needle biopsy, wedge resection (at laparotomy), or autopsy. Many of these discrepancies are related to patient selection: needle biopsies have been performed most frequently in patients with overt jaundice, hepatomegaly, or abnormal liver tests. Some of the hepatic lesions in ulcerative colitis have a patchy distribution, raising the possibility of sampling error by percutaneous needle biopsy. Surgical biopsy specimens have been taken from patients with more severe or chronic forms of colitis requiring colectomy, and postmortem specimens have obviously come from a highly selected minority of patients with ulcerative colitis.

Table 78–6. SYSTEMIC COMPLICATIONS OF ULCERATIVE COLITIS (202 PATIENTS)

Joint	53 (26%)
Skin	39 (19%)
Liver	15 (7%)
Kidney	11 (5%)
Eye	9 (4%)
Mouth	8 (4%)

Adapted from Greenstein, A. J., Janowitz, H. O., and Sachar, D. B. Medicine 55:401, 1976.

Few patients have been studied over long periods of time by serial biopsies; thus, the natural history of hepatic lesions is not well documented. Until needle biopsy examinations are applied prospectively to large numbers of unselected patients with ulcerative colitis, the prevalence and evolution of liver disease in ulcerative colitis will remain obscure. In spite of these difficulties, it is apparent that several histologic liver abnormalities are seen in patients with ulcerative colitis more frequently than in control populations; these include pericholangitis, sclerosing cholangitis, bile duct carcinoma, fatty infiltration, chronic active hepatitis, and postnecrotic cirrhosis.

The cause of hepatobiliary disease in patients with ulcerative colitis remains unknown. Early theories supporting a cause-and-effect relationship postulated that portal bacteremia originating from denuded, inflamed colonic mucosa resulted in recurrent cholangitis. Because hepatobiliary disease may precede, coincide with, or follow a clinical diagnosis of ulcerative colitis, this theory is not generally accepted.[148] Abnormal or increased concentrations of portal vein bile acids have also been postulated to play a role in the hepatic disease of ulcerative colitis. Total serum bile acid concentrations are normal, however, in patients with ulcerative colitis, unless substantial liver disease is present. Sampling of the inferior mesenteric vein for bile acids in colitis patients undergoing colectomy has also failed to demonstrate a qualitative or quantitative correlation between bile acid levels and the histologic features of liver biopsy specimens taken during the same procedure.[149] It is possible that genetic factors may predispose patients to both ulcerative colitis and hepatobiliary disorders such as sclerosing cholangitis, chronic active hepatitis and bile duct carcinoma. Identical loci (B8, DWR3) of the human leukocyte antigen (HLA) system have been identified in ulcerative colitis patients with these hepatobiliary complications.[150]

Pericholangitis may be found in 35 to 50 per cent of liver specimens obtained from patients with ulcerative colitis.[151, 152] It seems more common in patients with universal or subtotal colitis than in those with disease limited to the distal part of the colon. As the inflammatory changes involve connective tissue surrounding branches of the hepatic artery and portal vein as well as the bile ductules, it is probably more aptly termed "portal triaditis." Portal round cell and eosinophil infiltration, edema, and degenerative changes of the bile ductules predominate. The latter include fibrous thickening and occasionally obliterative cholangitis with the formation of nodular scars and loss of interlobular bile ducts.

Recent studies have suggested that pericholangitis may be part of the histologic and clinical spectrum of sclerosing cholangitis.[152, 153] In support of this concept is the frequent cholangiographic evidence of extrahepatic and intrahepatic biliary stricturing in patients with prior biopsy-proved pericholangitis. Moreover, intrahepatic histologic manifestations of pericholangitis (small-duct primary sclerosing cholangitis) and primary sclerosing cholangitis (large-duct primary sclerosing cholangitis) may be indistinguishable.[154]

Pericholangitis is asymptomatic and jaundice is rare. Mild elevations of serum alkaline phosphatase activity may be seen, but transaminase values generally are normal. Evaluation of the patient with pericholangitis on needle biopsy should include endoscopic retrograde cholangiography to exclude the possibility of concomitant large-duct disease. Medical treatment of underlying colitis is neither indicated for nor effective in ameliorating the histologic expression of pericholangitis or its possible progression to large-duct sclerosing cholangitis. Likewise, colectomy does not appear to alter this hepatobiliary complication.

Primary sclerosing cholangitis (PSC) has become an increasingly recognized complication of ulcerative colitis with the availability of endoscopic retrograde cholangiopancreatography (ERCP). In this disorder, both extrahepatic and intrahepatic bile ducts become severely narrowed and, in some cases, completely obstructed. Patients may present with recurrent attacks of jaundice, right upper quadrant pain, fever, and leukocytosis, with biochemical evidence of cholestasis. Differential diagnosis of obstructing common duct gallstones, tumor, and PSC is usually made only with transhepatic cholangiography, with ERCP, or at laparotomy. Patients with PSC and no prior diagnosis of ulcerative colitis should be evaluated for the presence of colitis as nearly 50 per cent of cases of PSC are associated with inflammatory bowel disease, predominantly ulcerative colitis.[155] PSC does not reliably respond to corticosteroids or other immunosuppressive agents. Pruritus, when present, may be relieved with the bile acid–binding resin cholestyramine. Endoscopic balloon dilation or stenting of focal strictures may provide palliation in patients with repeated bouts of extrahepatic obstruction. Unfortunately, many patients with PSC progress to develop secondary biliary cirrhosis.

Carcinoma of the bile ducts is found more frequently in patients with ulcerative colitis than in the general population, occurring almost exclusively in those with pericholangitis or PSC.[152, 156] Autopsy specimens demonstrate bile duct carcinoma in up to 1.4 per cent of patients with chronic ulcerative colitis.[155] These lesions are frequently multicentric. Diagnosis is difficult and often delayed owing to the similar appearance of preexisting PSC and biliary carcinoma and the lack of easy accessibility to the bile ducts for biopsy.

Fatty infiltration is a common hepatic lesion in ulcerative colitis. The frequency varies widely, being highest in autopsy material and in wedge resections taken at colectomy; however, as many as 40 per cent of needle liver biopsy samples from patients with ulcerative colitis may show fatty changes, either as the sole abnormality or associated with other histologic changes, such as pericholangitis. Fat accumulation is heaviest at the periphery of lobules. Serial biopsies have shown that this lesion is reversible. Although the cause is not known, fat accumulation is assumed to be due to malnutrition and protein depletion resulting from anorexia, diarrhea, and chronic illness. Consistent with this theory is the higher frequency of fatty liver in autopsy material and in patients with low serum albumin concentrations.[151]

The condition is usually asymptomatic, and hepatomegaly may be the sole finding on physical examination. Biochemical liver tests generally are normal or mildly elevated in patients who have fatty infiltration as the only lesion demonstrable on biopsy.[146]

Chronic active hepatitis is detected in 1 to 13 per cent of liver specimens from patients with chronic ulcerative colitis. Its pathogenesis has not been clearly defined but it may represent transfusion-related non-A, non-B viral hepatitis, an autoimmune hepatitis, or a lobular extension of the histologic abnormalities associated with pericholangitis. Frequently, chronic active hepatitis progresses to cirrhosis, which is seen in 3 to 4 per cent of biopsy specimens. Histologically, postnecrotic cirrhosis in patients with ulcerative colitis may present clinically with hepatic failure or with complications of portal hypertension, such as bleeding esophageal varices. Peristomal varices in colectomized patients can present an especially difficult management problem. In general, life expectancy in patients with ulcerative colitis and cirrhosis is shorter than in patients with cirrhosis alone.[146]

With rare exception, medical therapy of ulcerative colitis does not modify the outcome of complicating hepatobiliary disease. Likewise, there is no evidence that proctocolectomy arrests, ameliorates, or reverses liver disease associated with ulcerative colitis.

Hematologic Abnormalities

The most common hematologic defect in ulcerative colitis is an iron deficiency anemia secondary to colonic blood loss. Its severity varies depending on the rate and duration of bleeding. Most patients with mild anemia may be treated with iron supplementation. Oral ferrous sulfate is quite effective, although a few patients will experience nausea, vomiting, abdominal pain, or even a worsening of their diarrhea while taking this medication. Parenteral iron injections may be required in such patients to correct their anemia. During severe episodes of ulcerative colitis, especially those associated with significant colonic hemorrhage, blood transfusions may be necessary.

Some patients with ulcerative colitis may develop hemolytic anemia. Mild hemolytic anemia associated with Heinz bodies on peripheral smear is seen in occasional patients receiving sulfasalazine. This type of hemolysis appears to be drug-related and responds to withdrawal of the medication. An idiopathic Coombs'-positive autoimmune hemolytic anemia has been described in ulcerative colitis.[157] When cirrhosis complicates ulcerative colitis, a megaloblastic anemia may develop.

Leukocytosis is a common finding associated with the more severe varieties of ulcerative colitis. Sometimes this leukocytosis may be marked, with total white cell counts as high as 40,000 to 50,000 cells/cu mm and a predominance of young cell forms. A mild leukocytosis can be expected in patients receiving systemic corticosteroids.

Thrombocytosis may appear in ulcerative colitis, most commonly in those patients having marked leukocytosis. Unlike primary thrombocytosis, however, this condition in ulcerative colitis is not associated with coagulation defects. Immune thrombocytopenia is extremely uncommon.[158]

Deficiencies in coagulation factors may complicate ulcerative colitis. Hypoprothrombinemia is a commonly found defect in moderate or severe ulcerative colitis. Advanced liver disease associated with colitis accounts for some of these cases, but this defect is more common than can be accounted for by hepatic disease alone. Malnutrition (low vitamin K intake, low protein intake) and prolonged antibiotic administration may be responsible in many of these patients. Prolonged prothrombin times in patients with ulcerative colitis can usually be corrected with oral or intramuscular administration of vitamin K. It is important to restore the prothrombin time to normal in such patients, because hypoprothrombinemia may underlie profuse colonic bleeding. In severe ulcerative colitis or after emergency surgery, multiple coagulation defects occasionally arise from disseminated intravascular coagulation. A marked drop in platelet count and fibrinogen concentration with the appearance of fibrin monomers and fibrin split products provides laboratory evidence of this syndrome.

Thromboembolic Disease

A serious and potentially fatal complication of ulcerative colitis is pulmonary embolism resulting from thrombosis of the leg or pelvic veins. These vascular complications most often affect patients with severe active colitis, especially those who have recently undergone colectomy. In a recent study, deep venous thrombosis or pulmonary embolism accounted for 60 per cent of vascular complications in patients with ulcerative colitis.[159] In rare instances, arterial thrombosis and emboli may develop. Occlusion of retinal vessels or even large intracranial vessels may produce devastating visual or neurologic dysfunction.[159, 160]

Significant differences in the hemostatic parameters of patients with ulcerative colitis have been found when compared with normal subjects and hospitalized control patients. In addition to thrombocytosis, increased levels of factor V, factor VIII, and fibrinogen have been demonstrated, together with reductions in the levels of circulating antithrombin III.[159, 161]

Therapy of thromboembolism in ulcerative colitis is complicated by the risks of colonic bleeding during anticoagulation. Heparin is the drug of choice and should be administered by continuous intravenous infusion; the dose must be monitored by measuring the partial thromboplastin time. Repeated pulmonary embolism despite adequate anticoagulation therapy or massive colonic hemorrhage during anticoagulation may necessitate interruption of the inferior vena cava with a percutaneously inserted umbrella or surgical clip. The decision regarding colectomy at the time of caval ligation must be dictated by the clinical course and status of the patient.

Arthritis

Rheumatologic complications of ulcerative colitis may be divided into two main categories: (1) those affecting the peripheral joints and (2) ankylosing spondylitis (Table 78–6). They can be distinguished further by their contrasting relation to the activity of the underlying colitis and the tendency for progression.

The peripheral arthritis, which is not associated with rheumatoid factor (i.e., seronegative arthritis), may be found in 10 to 24 per cent of children and adults with ulcerative colitis during the course of their disease.[145, 162] It usually appears at the same time that bowel symptoms become prominent, although occasionally it may antedate clinically active colitis. Exacerbations of colitis are frequently accompanied by flares of joint disease, although the converse does not appear to be true. Colitic arthritis appears to be migratory, monoarticular or pauciarticular (i.e., involving a few joints), and to affect larger joints more than smaller joints (Table 78–6). There is often synovitis with effusion, and the joint may become swollen, erythematous, and tender. Motion is limited to a varying degree, depending on the extent of involvement. Importantly, it differs markedly from rheumatoid arthritis because the joint cartilages and bony appositions are unaffected and no chronic damage is incurred, particularly ankyloses. This peripheral arthritis usually subsides with control of the symptoms of the colitis.

There is a high incidence of ankylosing spondylitis in patients with ulcerative colitis. It has been estimated that the frequency of such involvement of the spine is perhaps 10 to 20 times greater than in the normal population. Conversely, the incidence of inflammatory bowel disease in patients with ankylosing spondylitis is high. Of interest, the frequency of ankylosing spondylitis among first-degree relatives of patients with ulcerative colitis is also increased. The prevalence of histocompatibility antigen phenotype HLA-B27 is clearly increased in ulcerative colitis patients with ankylosing spondylitis.[163] In general, patients with this phenotype also appear to have a higher percentage of total colonic involvement with ulcerative colitis. Occasionally, the onset of arthritis of the spine antedates bowel symptoms; whether or not the bowel is diseased at this time cannot be ascertained because the colon generally is not investigated in those patients whose colons are asymptomatic.

The progress of spondylitis in these individuals is relatively gradual, but it is inexorable and independent of the activity or extent of the inflammatory bowel disease. Generally, the course of the ankylosing spondylitis in ulcerative colitis is identical to that of the classic form of the disease. It is not only progressive but is also deforming, and it is frequently generalized. The ankylosing spondylitis does not seem to respond to corticosteroids and in many instances, the spinal arthritis progresses despite remissions of colitis or even after colectomy.

The incidence of sacroiliitis is higher than that of ankylosing spondylitis in patients with ulcerative colitis.[164] The disease may be found in many cases only by appropriate radiographs of the pelvis, including oblique views. Many of these patients are asymptomatic. A high percentage of them, especially men, have evidence of associated spondylitis. As with spondylitis in general, serologic tests for rheumatoid factor are negative.

Ocular Lesions

Various ocular abnormalities may arise in approximately 3 to 10 per cent of patients with ulcerative colitis[164, 165] (Table 78–6). The pathogenesis of these lesions is not understood, but their frequent association with peripheral arthritis, erythema nodosum, and aphthous ulcerations of the oral cavity suggests a systemic immune phenomenon. Iritis (uveitis) is the most common lesion seen with ulcerative colitis. In the acute phase, the patient experiences blurred vision, ocular pain, and photophobia. Physical findings include iridospasm, protein flare and cells in the anterior chamber, and keratitic precipitates. The attack may be recurrent and followed by atrophy of the iris, anterior and posterior synechiae, and pigment deposits on the lens. In about half of the cases, the uveitis will be bilateral. Episcleritis is less common. This lesion is characterized by inflammation of the episcleral tissues associated with discomfort but no discharge or infection. It is most commonly bilateral, but it usually involves only a small portion of the episcleral area in each eye. Other lesions seen in ulcerative colitis include superficial keratitis with blepharitis, interstitial keratitis, retinitis, and retrobulbar neuritis, but their infrequent association may reflect coincidence alone.

Dermatologic Disease

About 2 to 4 per cent of patients with ulcerative colitis will develop erythema nodosum, with raised, tender, erythematous swellings measuring 2 to 5 cm in diameter along the extensor surfaces of the arms and especially the legs[145, 166] (Fig. 78–18). As with erythema nodosum in general, this disorder is more common in women than in men with ulcerative colitis. The condition usually appears during an exacerbation of the colitis (particularly pancolitis) and is prone to develop when arthritis also accompanies the bowel disease. Erythema nodosum responds promptly to medical or surgical treatment of the underlying colitis. Occasionally, both arthritis and erythema nodosum may appear just prior to the first attack of overt ulcerative colitis, when bowel symptoms are not as yet prominent; in this situation, the patient may be thought to have rheumatic fever. However, the diagnosis of erythema nodosum should always raise suspicion of chronic inflammatory disease of the bowel, because it is seen in both ulcerative colitis and Crohn's disease of the colon. Erythema nodosum typically occurs as a single episode, recurring in only 20 per cent of patients.

Pyoderma gangrenosum afflicts approximately 2 to 5 per cent of patients with ulcerative colitis. Most

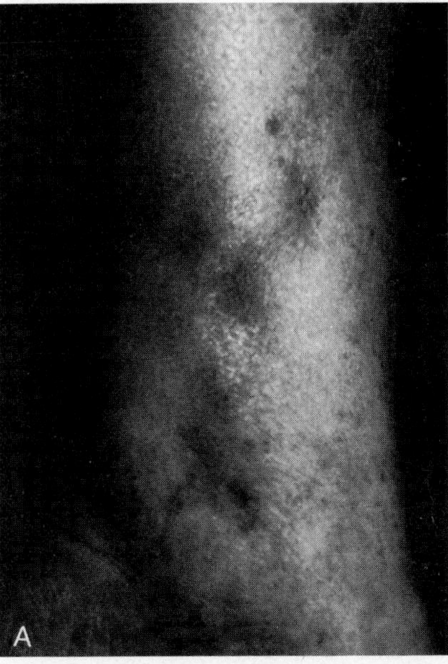

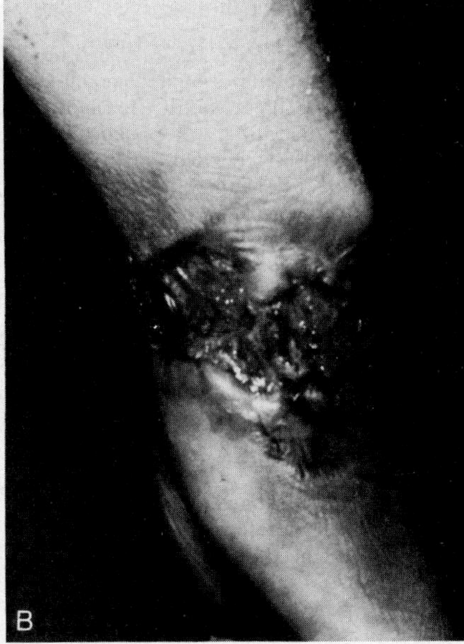

Figure 78–18. *A,* Erythema nodosum affecting the leg of a patient with ulcerative colitis. *B,* Pyoderma gangrenosum in an advanced stage with ulceration and necrosis.

commonly, this condition complicates universal ulcerative colitis, but it has been seen in a few patients with only left-sided disease. The lesion may appear at a site of prior trauma, at the outset resembling a boil or infected hair follicle. As it grows, it collects purulent-appearing material that may drain spontaneously (Fig. 78–18). This material, however, contains few polymorphonuclear cells and is sterile. Eventually, these lesions become gangrenous, resulting in progressive necrosis of the surrounding dermis, with deeply ulcerated areas often involving the underlying soft tissue. When the ulcerations are widespread, the skin disease can be serious and, on rare occasions, fatal.

Almost invariably, these lesions appear during a bout of active colitis; healing of skin lesions will usually follow control of the colitis with corticosteroid therapy. Occasionally, pyoderma gangrenosum requires additional therapy with dapsone or intralesional steroids.[167] Persistent severe pyoderma gangrenosum, involving many areas of the skin and underlying tissues, is an indication for colectomy. In rare instances, even proctocolectomy will not control the skin disease.

Aphthous ulceration of the mouth is a less serious complication of ulcerative colitis and is seen in about 4 per cent of patients. It is most frequent during severe attacks of colitis, but it occasionally appears even during remissions. It may be complicated by candidiasis, for which specific treatment should be given. Uncomplicated aphthous ulcerations may be treated with hydrocortisone mouthwashes.

Other skin lesions seen in ulcerative colitis are usually drug reactions (maculopapular eruptions, urticaria, erythema multiforme). Rarely, a patient with ulcerative colitis may develop a generalized eczematoid maculopapular eruption unrelated to medication but appearing during exacerbations of colitis. Necrotizing cutaneous vasculitis producing digital gangrene has also been reported.[168]

Renal Disease

Two types of renal disease appear to be associated with ulcerative colitis: pyelonephritis and nephrolithiasis or urolithiasis (Table 78–6). The explanation for the former is not clear unless it is related in some way to dehydration and its consequent scanty urine flow with high concentration of solutes and electrolytes.

The increased frequency of nephrolithiasis and urolithiasis (5 per cent) may be explained by dehydration, inactivity of the patient (calcium mobilization), and changes in the composition of the urine, which predispose to stone formation. In some cases, glomerulonephritis has been reported in ulcerative colitis, but it is quite uncommon. Rare persons with severe diarrhea caused by ulcerative colitis or extensive ileostomy drainage containing a high content of potassium may, over a long period of time, develop renal changes secondary to hypokalemia (hypokalemic nephropathy). This lesion is often not reversible and results in slowly progressive renal dysfunction.

SURGERY FOR PATIENTS WITH ULCERATIVE COLITIS

In contrast to surgery for Crohn's disease, removal of the entire colon in ulcerative colitis is always curative for the enteric disease. Colectomy removes the primary focus of disease and eliminates the risk of future local complications, including carcinoma of the colon. Additionally, colonic resection eliminates most extraintestinal complications (with the exception of hepatobiliary disease, ankylosing spondylitis, and rare cases of pyoderma gangrenosum). On the other hand, colectomy carries an operative risk; some patients will require further surgery for both early complications (anastomotic leaks, intraperitoneal abscess) and late sequelae (adhesions, mechanical problems with ileostomy, stomal ileitis); and not all patients will accept an ileostomy. It is obvious, therefore, that colectomy is not indicated in those patients whose disease can be easily controlled by medical therapy. However, it is equally obvious that surgery has an important therapeutic role in ulcerative colitis that responds incompletely to medical management or in which medical therapy has produced significant adverse side effects.

At present, the postoperative mortality rate for an elective one-stage colectomy is extremely low (Table 78–7); even in patients with acute severe disease,

Table 78–7. CAUSES OF DEATH IN 137 PATIENTS WITH ULCERATIVE COLITIS (1930 TO 1966)

Death as a direct outcome of colitis:		
Colonic perforation		16
Postoperative deaths		16
Postoperative peritonitis	10	
Miscellaneous	6	
Fulminant colitis		12
Colonic hemorrhage		1
Malnutrition		1
		46 patients
Death related to colitis:		
Carcinoma of the colon		16
Deaths related to treatment		15
Transfusion		
Incompatibility	3	
Fulminant hepatitis	2	
Congestive heart failure	2	
Drug-related		
Drug reactions	3	
Steroid ulcers	2	
Crystalluria	1	
Anticoagulation bleeding	1	
Other	1	
Suicide		6
Liver disease		5
Bleeding varices	3	
Hepatic failure	2	
Thromboembolism		2
Renal amyloidosis		1
Pyoderma gangrenosum		1
		46 patients
Deaths not related to colitis:		45 patients

From Morowitz, D. A., and Kirsner, J. B. Mortality in ulcerative colitis: 1930 to 1966. Gastroenterology *57*:481–490. © by Williams & Wilkins, 1969.

mortality rate of subtotal colectomy with ileostomy has been reduced to as low as approximately 5 per cent in skilled hands.[169] This improvement in mortality has resulted from many technical advances, including improved anesthesia, better surgical techniques, meticulous bowel preparation, more skillful management of fluid and electrolyte problems or cardiovascular complications, and better selection of antimicrobial agents for postoperative infections.[170] In addition, the declining surgical mortality rate also reflects earlier operative intervention in patients with ulcerative colitis before the patient becomes desperately ill or chronically debilitated.

Indications for Colectomy

There are three general situations in which surgery is undertaken for patients with ulcerative colitis (Table 78–8):

1. A complication arises from which the risk of death is high or for which medical management is known to be ineffective. In this category are suspected or proved colonic perforation, symptomatic colonic stricture, or suspected or documented colonic cancer.

2. The clinical condition of the patient is grave, but medical management may be effective; however, as time elapses without apparent benefit from medical treatment, the chance of successful outcome as a result of medical therapy diminishes. In this category are severe ulcerative colitis, toxic megacolon, and uncontrolled colonic hemorrhage.

3. There is no immediate threat to life, but the cumulative morbidity or mortality rate is high. This would include morbidity from recurrent or intractable moderate or severe colitis, refractory uveitis or pyoderma gangrenosum, ill effects from long-term systemic corticosteroid treatment, growth retardation in pediatric patients, and the ultimate risk of colonic cancer or colitis-related death.

Only indications under the first category are clear. In the second category, there is general agreement as to which patients are at risk of dying but few data indicating how long medical treatment should be continued before being abandoned in favor of surgery. In the third category, cumulative risks or acceptable morbidity rates remain poorly defined.

Acute severe colitis, with or without toxic megacolon, is the form of the disease most often refractory to medical management and most often fatal. Because of this fact, it is recommended that patients with acute severe colitis, uncomplicated by toxic megacolon, undergo surgery if little or no improvement occurs after 7 to 10 days of intensive medical treatment. It must be admitted that the recommended duration of this trial is suggested only as a reasonable period beyond which the chance of remission is small and the continued severe morbidity of the patient increases the risk of surgery. Proponents of even earlier surgical intervention in acute severe colitis claim that perioperative mortality is less after 4 or 5 days of unsuccessful medical therapy than after 10 days.[171] The lack of response to medical therapy in some of these patients is evident early; the question is one of timing definitive surgical treatment optimally. All advocates of early surgery for severe disease—that is, after 5 to 10 days of ineffective medical therapy—also argue that statistically a large number of patients with acute severe colitis will ultimately undergo colectomy for refractory disease. Although this statement may be true, it is difficult to predict the ultimate outcome of the disease in an individual patient on the basis of the severity of a single episode.

Similarly, the authors recommend that patients with toxic megacolon undergo colectomy if their condition does not show improvement within 72 hours of intensive medical therapy. This recommendation is based on survival rates that have been improved by early surgery for toxic megacolon and the awareness that the chance of perforation increases with prolonged colonic dilatation, plus the knowledge that the long-term outlook in patients recovering from toxic megacolon is poor.[120–124]

As definition of uncontrollable colonic hemorrhage in ulcerative colitis is difficult, and because both the severity of bleeding and the tolerance of patients for acute blood loss are highly variable, clearly the decision to operate for bleeding is highly individualized.

Indications for colectomy based on cumulative long-term morbidity are most difficult to outline and depend on the clinical judgment of the physician, the overall adjustment of the patient to the disease, and the patient's attitude toward surgery. The authors can only point out certain general guidelines that they find helpful in making decisions concerning colectomy. First among these are the functional capacity of the patient—that is, how well the patient can carry out his or her chores in the face of continuing disease. Obviously related to this question is the amount of systemic corticosteroids needed to maintain the patient at a reasonable functioning level. Together, these two considerations make the decision for colectomy a joint undertaking. Patients are usually best able to judge whether they can cope with their colonic disease, and

Table 78–8. INDICATIONS FOR COLECTOMY IN ULCERATIVE COLITIS

	Total Number of Patients	Refractory to Medical Therapy	Hemorrhage	Toxic Megacolon or Perforation or Both
Oakley et al. (1985)	277	173 (62%)	11 (4%)	93 (34%)
Beauchamp et al. (1981)	72	47 (65%)	7 (10%)	18 (25%)

Adapted from Oakley, J. R., Lavery, I. C., Fazio, V. W., Jagelman, D. G., Wenkley, F. L., and Easley, K. Dis. Colon Rectum *28*:394, 1985, and Beauchamp G., Beliveau, D., and Archambault, A. Can. J. Surg. *24*:463, 1981.

physicians must decide whether the duration and dosage of corticosteroid needed is a serious hazard. Long-term oral administration of more than 20 mg daily of prednisone to control the colitis at acceptable levels of activity is a cumulative hazard to the patient that may not be justifiable when colectomy is an alternative.

The long-term course of the colitis is also important in deciding on electing colectomy. Regardless of the initial severity of the disease, if the subsequent attacks are mild, the patient may be managed without surgery. On the other hand, continued exacerbations of moderate severity requiring repeated hospitalizations or even one severe episode complicating an otherwise mild series of attacks of colitis may warrant elective colectomy.

The age of the patient is also important. The mortality and especially the long-term morbidity rates in the young patient with ulcerative colitis are forbidding; colectomy should be entertained relatively early as an effective mode of treatment in these patients with active disease. Systemic steroids are less well tolerated by the elderly, whereas colectomy (as in the younger patient) is curative. Conversely, the decision may be more safely deferred in the older patient who requires 10 mg or less of prednisone daily to control the disease.

A potential threat to many patients with ulcerative colitis is the development of colonic cancer. Duration and extent of the disease are the two most important parameters in determining the risk of cancer and are more predictive than the severity. Patients with distal colitis are at little risk. Those with total colonic involvement, and especially with the continuous form of the disease, are at the highest risk. This risk becomes much greater after the first 10 years of the disease (see earlier discussion). Because of this fact, the authors recommend colectomy to adult patients who have universal colitis of more than 10 years' duration when the disease remains active, albeit intermittently. The decision for colectomy in patients in this category who are asymptomatic or who tolerate mild colitis is obviously extremely difficult—in these instances, the risks should be explained to the patient and he or she should be closely involved in the decision-making process.

Surgical Options

The standard surgical procedure for ulcerative colitis is proctocolectomy and ileostomy in one or two stages. In the two-stage procedure, the rectum is not removed initially, and the patient has a functioning ileostomy with a sigmoid mucous fistula or rectal pouch. Proctectomy is performed at the second stage. Although a single-stage proctocolectomy is preferable in elective cases, the rectum should not be removed initially in patients with colonic perforation, toxic megacolon, or other severe underlying diseases.

Small bowel obstruction may follow proctocolectomy in up to 17 per cent of patients as a consequence of adhesions or intestinal volvulus. Although many respond to conservative management, surgical lysis of adhesions or reduction of volvulus is required in 6 to 8 per cent of patients.[172, 173] Local complications at the ileostomy site are uncommon owing to improved operative technique, although occasionally stomal recession or prolapse may require surgical revision. Lastly, stomal leakage may predispose to displacement of the external appliance and local skin irritation.

Whereas proctocolectomy offers definitive cure of ulcerative colitis and its long-term sequelae, several unfortunate drawbacks to this procedure exist. Prolonged perineal wound drainage and infection may occur, and healing may not be complete for up to six months after surgery, especially in women. Up to 20 per cent of patients may require a subsequent hospitalization for perineal wound complications, including abscess formation and persistent sinus tract drainage.[173, 174] Proctectomy may also result in sexual problems for 10 per cent of male patients, from either inability to maintain an erection (owing to presacral nerve damage) or inability to ejaculate or experience orgasm (owing to parasympathetic nerve injury).[175] A few women will experience dyspareunia as a result of excessive scarring from healing of the perineal wound. Infertility in women after proctocolectomy has also been reported and is believed to be due to either retroflexion of the uterus or extrinsic scarring of the fallopian tubes after extensive pelvic inflammation.[176]

In an attempt to avoid the inconvenience of ileostomy and the pelvic complications of proctectomy, some surgeons have advocated abdominal colectomy and ileorectal anastomosis. Major limitations of this approach are the frequent persistence or recurrence of inflammatory proctitis and the risk of cancer in the rectal stump. A cumulative risk of rectal carcinoma of up to 6 per cent has been reported after ileorectal anastomosis and may be greatest in patients whose resected colon shows evidence of cancer or mucosal dysplasia.[177–179]

Proctocolectomy with continent (Kock) ileostomy was developed both as a cure for ulcerative colitis and a means to avoid some of the complications (odor, leakage, skin excoriations) and inconveniences (cosmetic considerations, use of an external appliance) of an ileostomy. In this procedure, two limbs of the terminal ileum are anastomosed side-to-side to serve as a functional reservoir and a nipple valve is exteriorized just above the pubic hairline. Patients intubate the valve with a rubber catheter and drain the stoma three or more times daily, depending upon the size of the reservoir. Although it is effective in 80 to 90 per cent of patients, nipple valve dysfunction or deintussusception with loss of continence may occur in the remainder, often requiring operative revision.[180, 181] Conversion from a standard ileostomy to a continent ileostomy is possible, especially in patients who have undergone proctectomy and thus are not candidates for ileoanal anastomosis (see pp. 1477–1482).

The more recently developed procedure of subtotal colectomy with mucosal proctectomy and ileoanal anastomosis offers several advantages. Diseased colon is removed and the rectal mucosa is stripped, thus eradicating ulcerative colitis and preventing its complications. An ileal reservoir is anastomosed to the denuded rectal stump and anal sphincter function is preserved, thus maintaining continence and avoiding external fecal draining devices. An added benefit of this technique is that the perineal wound closes within two months, as opposed to six months for conventional proctectomy. A number of technical revisions have emerged to diminish stool frequency, maximize continence, and avoid late obstruction of the ileal reservoir.[182, 183] Overall, approximately 80 to 95 per cent of patients undergoing ileoanal anastomosis can distinguish feces from flatus and remain continent during waking hours. Occasional nighttime seepage requires the use of protective pads during sleep. Anastomotic strictures (12 per cent), reservoir ileitis (7 per cent), and sexual dysfunction (0 to 10 per cent) in men remain as imposing complications to this procedure.[184, 185] Patients undergoing this operation must be willing to tolerate indefinitely at least 5 to 6 bowel movements per day.

References

1. Wilks, S., and Moxon, W. Lectures on Pathological Anatomy. 2nd edition. London, J. & A. Churchill, 1875.
2. Gilat, T., Ribak, J., Benaroya, Y., Zemishlany, Z., and Weissman, I. Ulcerative colitis in the Jewish population of Tel-Aviv Jafo. I. Epidemiology. Gastroenterology *66*:335, 1974.
3. Almy, T. P., and Sherlock, P. Genetic aspects of ulcerative colitis and regional enteritis. Gastroenterology *51*:757, 1966.
4. Calkins, B. M., Lilienfeld, A. M., Garland, C. F., and Mendeloff, A. I. Trends in incidence rates of ulcerative colitis and Crohn's disease. Dig. Dis. Sci. *29*:913, 1984.
5. Gilat, T., and Rozen, P. Epidemiology of Crohn's disease and ulcerative colitis: etiologic implications. Isr. J. Med. Sci. *15*:305, 1979.
6. Mayberry, J. F. Some aspects of the epidemiology of ulcerative colitis. Gut *26*:968, 1985.
7. Jick, H., and Walker, A. M. Cigarette smoking and ulcerative colitis. N. Engl. J. Med. *308*:261, 1986.
8. Taylor-Robinson, D., O'Morain, C. A., Thomas, B. J., and Levi, A. J. Low frequency of chlamydial antibodies in patients with Crohn's disease and ulcerative colitis. Lancet *1*:1162, 1979.
9. Swarbrick, E. T., Kingham, J. G. C., Price, H. L., Blackshaw, A. J., Griffiths, P. D., Darougar, S., and Buckell, N. A. *Chlamydia*, cytomegalovirus, and *Yersinia* in inflammatory bowel disease. Lancet *2*:11, 1979.
10. Cave, D., Mitchell, D., and Brooke, B. Evidence of an agent transmissible from ulcerative colitis tissue. Lancet *1*:1311, 1976.
11. Gitnick, G. L., Rosen, V. J., Arthur, M. H., and Hertweck, S. A. Evidence for the isolation of a new virus from ulcerative colitis patients. Dig. Dis. Sci. *24*:609, 1979.
12. LaMont, J. T., and Trnka, Y. M. Therapeutic implications of *Clostridium difficile* toxin during relapse of chronic inflammatory bowel disease. Lancet *1*:381, 1980.
13. Bolton, R. P., Sherriff, R. J., and Read, A. E. *Clostridium difficile* associated diarrhoea: a role in inflammatory bowel disease. Lancet *1*:383, 1980.
14. Trnka, Y. M., and LaMont, J. T. Association of *Clostridium difficile* toxin with symptomatic relapse of chronic inflammatory bowel disease. Gastroenterology *80*:693, 1981.
15. Meyers, S., Mayer, L., Bottone, E., Desmond, E., and Janowitz, H. D. Occurrence of *Clostridium difficile* toxin during the course of inflammatory bowel disease. Gastroenterology *80*:697, 1981.
16. Delpre, G., Kadish, U., Gazit, E., Joshua, H., and Zamir, R. HLA antigens in ulcerative colitis and Crohn's disease in Israel. Gastroenterology *78*:1452, 1980.
17. Feldman, F., Cantor, D., Soll, S., and Bachrach, W. Psychiatric study of a consecutive series of 34 patients with ulcerative colitis. Br. Med. J. *2*:14, 1967.
18. Mendeloff, A. I., Monk, M., Siegel, C. I., and Lilienfield, A. Illness experience and life stresses in patients with irritable colon and with ulcerative colitis. N. Engl. J. Med. *282*:14, 1970.
19. Monk, M., Mendeloff, A. I., Siegel, C. I., and Lilienfield, A. An epidemiological study of ulcerative colitis and regional enteritis among adults in Baltimore. III. Psychological and possible stress-precipitating factors. J. Chron. Dis. *22*:565, 1970.
20. Rabin, B. S., and Rogers, S. J. A cell-mediated immune model of inflammatory bowel disease in the rabbit. Gastroenterology *75*:29, 1978.
21. Fiocchi, C., Battisto, J. R., and Farmer, R. G. Gut mucosal lymphocytes in inflammatory bowel disease-isolation and preliminary functional characterization. Dig. Dis. Sci. *24*:705, 1979.
22. Miyazaki, H., Kawasaki, H., and Hirayama, C. Studies on lymphocyte subpopulations in human colonic biopsy specimens by colonoscopy. Dig. Dis. Sci. *30*:143, 1985.
23. Ginsburg, C. H., Dambrauskas, J. T., Ault, K. A., and Falchuk, Z. M. Impaired natural killer cell activity in patients with inflammatory bowel disease: evidence for a qualitative defect. Gastroenterology *85*:846, 1983.
24. MacDermott, R. P., Bragdon, M. J., Kodner, I. J., and Bertovich, M. J. Deficient cell-mediated cytotoxicity and hyporesponsiveness to interferon and mitogenic lectin activation by inflammatory bowel disease peripheral blood and intestinal mononuclear cells. Gastroenterology *90*:6, 1986.
25. MacDermott, R. P., Nash, G. S., Bertovich, M. J., Mohrman, R. F., Kodner, I. J., Delacroix, D. L., and Vaeman, J. -P. Altered patterns of secretion of monomeric IgA and IgA subclass 1 by intestinal mononuclear cells in inflammatory bowel disease. Gastroenterology *91*:379, 1986.
26. Shorter, R. G., McGill, D. B., and Bahn, R. C. Cytotoxicity of mononuclear cells for autologous colonic epithelial cell in colonic diseases. Gastroenterology *86*:13, 1984.
27. Lake, A. M., Stitzel, A. E., Urmson, J. R., Walker, W. A., and Spitzer, R. E. Complement alterations in inflammatory bowel disease. Gastroenterology *76*:1374, 1979.
28. Potter, B. J., Hodgson, H. J. F., Mee, A. S., and Jewell, D. P. C1q metabolism in ulcerative colitis and Crohn's disease. Gut *20*:1012, 1979.
29. Bodenheimer, H. C., LaRusso, N. F., Thayer, W. R., Charland, C., Staples, P. J., and Ludwig, J. Elevated circulating immune complexes in primary sclerosing cholangitis. Hepatology *3*:150, 1983.
30. Meyers, S., Sachar, D. B., Taub, R. N., and Janowitz, H. D. Significance of anergy to dinitrochlorobenzene (DNCB) in inflammatory bowel disease: Family and postoperative studies. Gut *19*:249, 1978.
31. Thayer, W. R., Fixa, B., Komarkova, O., Charland, B. A., and Field, C. E. Skin test reactivity in inflammatory bowel disease in the United States and Czechoslovakia. Am. J. Dig. Dis. *23*:337, 1978.
32. Mottet, N. K. Histopathologic Spectrum of Regional Enteritis and Ulcerative Colitis. Philadelphia, W. B. Saunders Company, 1971.
33. Harris, J., and Shields, R. Absorption and secretion of water and electrolytes by the intact human colon in diffuse untreated proctocolitis. Gut *11*:27, 1970.
34. Goulston, S. J. M., and McGovern, V. J. The nature of benign strictures in ulcerative colitis. N. Engl. J. Med. *281*:290, 1969.
35. Matts, S. F. The value of rectal biopsy in the diagnosis of ulcerative colitis. Q. J. Med. *30*:393, 1961.
36. Baron, J. H., Connell, A. M., and Lennard-Jones, J. E. Variation between observers in describing mucosal appearances in proctocolitis. Br. Med. J. *1*:89, 1964.
37. Watts, J. M., Thompson, H., and Goligher, J. C. Sigmoidoscopy and cytology in the detection of microscopic disease of the rectal mucosa in ulcerative colitis. Gut 7:288, 1966.
38. Krogstad, D. J., Spencer, H. C., Healy, G. R., Gleason, N. N., Sexton, D. J., and Herron, C. A. Amebiasis: epidemiologic

studies in the United States, 1971–1974. Ann. Intern. Med. *88*:89, 1978.

39. Surawicz, C. M., and Belic, L. Rectal biopsy helps to distinguish acute self-limited colitis from idiopathic inflammatory bowel disease. Gastroenterology *86*:104, 1984.
40. Gomes, P., DuBoulay, C., Smith, C. L., and Holdstock, G. Relationship between disease activity indices and colonoscopic findings in patients with colonic inflammatory bowel disease. Gut *27*:92, 1986.
41. Myren, J., Eie, H., and Serck-Hanssen, A. The diagnosis of colitis by colonoscopy with biopsy and X-ray examination. A blind cooperative study. Scand. J. Gastroenterol. *11*:141, 1976.
42. Loose, H., and Williams, C. Barium enemas versus colonoscopy. Proc. R. Soc. Med. *67*:1033, 1974.
43. Laufer, I., Mullens, J., and Hamilton, J. Correlation of endoscopy and double-contrast radiography in the early stages of ulcerative and granulomatous colitis. Radiology *118*:1, 1976.
44. Laufer, I., and Hamilton, J. The radiologic differentiation between ulcerative and granulomatous colitis. Am. J. Gastroenterol. *66*:259, 1976.
45. Gabrielsson, N., Granqvist, S., Sundelin, P., and Thorgeirsson, T. Extent of inflammatory lesions in ulcerative colitis assessed by radiology, colonoscopy, and endoscopic biopsy. Gastrointest. Radiol. *4*:395, 1979.
46. Faser, G., and Findlay, J. The double contrast enema in ulcerative colitis and Crohn's colitis. Clin. Radiol. *27*:103, 1976.
47. Goldberg, H. The barium enema and toxic megacolon: Cause-effect relationship? Gastroenterology *68*:617, 1975.
48. Meiselman, M. S., Cello, J. P., and Margaretten, W. Cytomegalovirus colitis. Report of the clinical, endoscopic, and pathologic findings in two patients with the acquired immune deficiency syndrome. Gastroenterology *88*:171, 1985.
49. Edward, F. C., and Truelove, S. C. The course and prognosis of ulcerative colitis. II. Long-term prognosis. Gut *4*:309, 1964.
50. Truelove, S. C., and Witts, L. J. Cortisone in ulcerative colitis. Report on therapeutic trial. Br. Med. J. *2*:375, 1954; *2*:1041, 1955.
51. Edwards, F. C., and Truelove, S. C. The course and prognosis of ulcerative colitis. I. Short-term prognosis. Gut *4*:299, 1964.
52. Sparberg, M., Fennessy, J., and Kirsner, J. B. Ulcerative proctitis and mild ulcerative colitis: a study of 220 patients. Medicine *45*:391, 1966.
53. Ritchie, J. K., Powell-Tuck, J., and Lennard-Jones, J. E. Clinical outcome of the first ten years of ulcerative colitis and proctitis. Lancet *1*:1140, 1978.
54. Beal, R. W., Skyring, A. P., McRae, M. B., and Firkin, G. G. The anemia of ulcerative colitis. Gastroenterology *45*:589, 1963.
55. Wright, R., and Truelove, S. C. A controlled therapeutic trial of various diets in ulcerative colitis. Br. Med. J. *2*:138, 1965.
56. Wright, R., and Truelove, S. C. Circulating antibodies to dietary protein in ulcerative colitis. Br. Med. J. *2*:142, 1965.
57. Groen, J., and Bastiaans, J. Psychotherapy of ulcerative colitis. Gastroenterology *17*:344, 1951.
58. Jeejeebhoy, K., Langer, B., Tsallas, G., Chu, R. C., Kuksis, A., and Anderson, G. H. Total parenteral nutrition at home: studies in patients surviving 4 months to 5 years. Gastroenterology *71*:943, 1976.
59. Mullen, J. L., Hargrove, W. C., Dudrick, S. J., Fitts, W. T., and Rosato, E. F. Ten years' experience with intravenous hyperalimentation and inflammatory bowel disease. Ann. Surg. *187*:523, 1978.
60. Dickinson, R. J., Ashton, M. G., Axon, A. T. R., Smith, R. C., Young, C. K., and Hill, G. L. Controlled trial of intravenous hyperalimentation and total bowel rest as an adjunct to the routine therapy of acute colitis. Gastroenterology *79*:1199, 1980.
61. Jarnerot, G., Rolny, P., and Sandberg-Gertzen, H. Intensive intravenous treatment of ulcerative colitis. Gastroenterology *89*:1005, 1985.
62. Truelove, S. C., and Witts, L. J. Cortisone and corticotropin in ulcerative colitis. Br. Med. J. *1*:387, 1959.
63. Lennard-Jones, J. E., Misiewicz, J. J., Connell, A. M., Baron, J. H., and Jones, F. A. Prednisone as maintenance treatment for ulcerative colitis in remission. Lancet *1*:188, 1965.
64. Truelove, S. Treatment of ulcerative colitis with local hydrocortisone hemisuccinate. A report on a controlled therapeutic trial. Br. Med. J. *2*:1072, 1958.
65. Jay, M., Digenis, G. A., Foster, T. S., and Antonow, D. R. Retrograde spreading of hydrocortisone enema in inflammatory bowel disease. Dig. Dis. Sci. *31*:139, 1986.
66. Lee, D. A. H., Taylor, G. M., James, V. H. T., and Walker, G. Plasma prednisolone levels and adrenocortical responsiveness after administration of prednisolone-21-phosphate as a retention enema. Gut *20*:349, 1979.
67. Lee, D. A. H., Taylor, M., James, V. H. T., and Walker, G. Rectally administered prednisolone—evidence for a predominantly local action. Gut *21*:215, 1980.
68. Larochelle, P., Du Souich, P., Bolte, E., Lelorier, J., and Goyer, R. Tixocortol pivalate, a corticosteroid with no systemic glucocorticoid effect after oral, intrarectal, and intranasal application. Clin. Pharmacol. Ther. *33*:343, 1983.
69. Levinson, R. A. Comparative safety and efficacy of tixocortol pivalate enema vs. hydrocortisone enema in the treatment of left-sided ulcerative colitis. *In* Recent Developments in the Therapy of Inflammatory Bowel Disease. Proceedings of a Symposium. Baltimore, Meyerhoff Center for Digestive Disease, at Johns Hopkins, 1986, p. 26.
70. Madsbad, S., Bjerregaard, B., Henriksen, J. H., and Juhl, E. Impaired conversion of prednisone to prednisolone in patients with liver cirrhosis. Gut *21*:52, 1980.
71. Elliott, P. R., Powell-Tuck, J., Gillespie, P. E., Laidlow, J. M., Lennard-Jones, J. E., English, J., Chakraborty, J., and Marks, V. Prednisolone absorption in acute colitis. Gut *21*:49, 1980.
72. Powell-Tuck, J., Bown, R. L., and Lennard-Jones, J. E. A comparison of oral prednisolone given as single or multiple daily doses for active proctocolitis. Scand. J. Gastroenterol. *13*:833, 1978.
73. Kaplan, H., Portnoy, B., Binder, H., Amatruda, T., and Spiro, H. A controlled evaluation of intravenous adrenocorticotropic hormone and hydrocortisone in the treatment of acute colitis. Gastroenterology *69*:91, 1975.
74. Axelrod, L. Glucocorticoid therapy. Medicine *55*:39, 1976.
75. Byyny, R. Withdrawal from glucocorticoid therapy. N. Engl. J. Med. *295*:30, 1976.
76. Dickinson, R. J., O'Connor, H. J., Pinder, I., Hamilton, I., Johnston, D., and Axon, A. T. R. Double-blind controlled trial of oral vancomycin as adjunctive treatment in acute exacerbations of idiopathic colitis. Gut *26*:1380, 1985.
77. Klotz, U., Maier, K., Fischer, C., and Heinkel, K. Therapeutic efficacy of sulfasalazine and its metabolites in patients with ulcerative colitis and Crohn's disease. N. Engl. J. Med. *303*:1499, 1980.
78. Hawkey, C. J., Boughton-Smith, N. K., and Whittle, B. J. R. Modulation of human colonic arachidonic acid metabolism by sulfasalazine. Dig. Dis. Sci. *30*:1161, 1985.
79. Lennard-Jones, J. E., Longmore, A. J., Newell, A. C., Wilson, C. W. F., and Jones, F. A. An assessment of prednisone, salazopyrin, and topical hydrocortisone used as outpatient treatment for ulcerative colitis. Gut. *1*:217, 1960.
80. Truelove, S. C., Watkinson, G., and Draper, G. Comparison of corticosteroid and sulphasalazine therapy in ulcerative colitis. Br. Med. J. *2*:1708, 1962.
81. Lennard-Jones, J. E., Connell, A. M., Baron, J. H., and Jones, F. A. Controlled trial of sulphasalazine in maintenance therapy for ulcerative colitis. Lancet *1*:185, 1965.
82. Dissanayake, A., and Truelove, S. A controlled therapeutic trial of long-term maintenance treatment of ulcerative colitis with sulphasalazine. Gut *14*:818, 1973.
83. Azad Khan, A. K., Howes, D. T., Piris, J., and Truelove, S. C. Optimum dose of sulphasalazine for maintenance treatment in ulcerative colitis. Gut *21*:232, 1980.
84. Taffet, S. L., and Das, K. M. Sulfasalazine—adverse effects and desensitization. Dig. Dis. Sci. *28*:833, 1983.
85. McPhee, M. S., and Greenberger, N. J. Proctocolitis refractory

to conventional therapy: response to 5-aminosalicylic acid (5-ASA) enemas. *In* Recent Developments in the Therapy of Inflammatory Bowel Disease. Proceedings of a Symposium. Baltimore, Meyerhoff Center for Digestive Disease, at Johns Hopkins, 1986, p. 44.

86. Campieri, M., Lanfranchi, G. A., Boschi, S., Brignola, C., Bazzocchi, G., Gionchetti, P., Minguzzi, M. R., Belluzzi, A., and Labo, G. Topical administration of 5-aminosalicylic acid enemas in patients with ulcerative colitis. Studies on rectal absorption and excretion. Gut *26*:400, 1985.
87. Friedman, L. S., Richter, J. M., Kirkham, S. E., DeMonaco, H. J., and May, R. J. 5-Aminosalicylic acid enemas in refractory distal colitis: a randomized, controlled trial. Am. J. Gastroenterol. *81*:412, 1986.
88. Campieri, M., Lanfranchi, G. A., Bertoni, F., Brignola, C., Bazzocchi, G., Minguzzi, M. R., and Labo, G. A double-blind clinical trial to compare the effects of 4-aminosalicylic acid to 5-aminosalicylic acid in topical treatment of ulcerative colitis. Digestion *29*:204, 1984.
89. Selby, W. S., Barr, G. D., Ireland, A., Mason, C. H., and Jewell, D. P. Olsalazine in active ulcerative colitis. Br. Med. J. *291*:1373, 1985.
90. Sandberg-Gertzen, H., Jarnerot, G., and Kraaz, W. Azodisal sodium in the treatment of ulcerative colitis—a study of tolerance and relapse-prevention properties. Gastroenterology *90*:1024, 1986.
91. Jewell, D., and Truelove, S. Azathioprine in ulcerative colitis: final report on a controlled therapeutic trial. Br. Med. J. *4*:627, 1974.
92. Caprilli, R., Carratu, R., and Babbini, M. A double-blind comparison of the effectiveness of azathioprine and sulfasalazine in idiopathic proctocolitis—preliminary report. Am. J. Dig. Dis. *20*:115, 1975.
93. Dronfield, M. W., and Langman, M. J. S. Comparative trial of sulphasalazine and oral sodium cromoglycate in the maintenance of remission in ulcerative colitis. Gut *19*:1136, 1978.
94. Buckell, N. A., Gould, S. R., Day, D. W., Lennard-Jones, J. E., and Edwards, A. M. Controlled trial of disodium cromoglycate in acute persistent ulcerative colitis. Gut *19*:1140, 1978.
95. Willoughby, C. P., Heyworth, M. F., Piris, J., and Truelove, S. C. Comparison of disodium cromoglycate and sulphasalazine as maintenance therapy for ulcerative colitis. Lancet *1*:119, 1979.
96. Lechin, F., van der Dijs, B., Insausti, C. L., Gomez, F., Villa, S., Lechin, A. E., Arocha, L., and Oramas, O. Treatment of ulcerative colitis with clonidine. J. Clin. Pharmacol. *25*:219, 1985.
97. Watts, J. M., deDombal, F. T., Watkinson, G., and Goligher, J. C. Early course of ulcerative colitis. Gut *7*:16, 1966.
98. Jalan, K. N., Prescott, R. J., Sircus, W., Card, W. I., McManns, J. P. A., Falconer, C. W. A., Small, W. P., Smith, A. N., and Bruce, J. An experience with ulcerative colitis. II. Short-term outcome. Gastroenterology *9*:589, 1970.
99. Watts, J. M., deDombal, F. T., and Goligher, J. C. Long-term prognosis of ulcerative colitis. Br. Med. J. *1*:1447, 1966.
100. Jalan, K. N., Prescott, R. J., Sircus, W., Card, W. I., McManns, J. P. A., Falconer, C. W. A., Small, W. P., Smith, A. N., and Bruce, J. An experience with ulcerative colitis. III. Long-term outcome. Gastroenterology *59*:598, 1970.
101. Willoughby, C. P., and Truelove, S. C. Ulcerative colitis and pregnancy. Gut *21*:469, 1980.
102. Webb, M. J., and Sedlack, R. E. Ulcerative colitis in pregnancy. Med. Clin. North Am. *58*:823, 1974.
103. Weeke, E., Binder, V., Olsen, J. H., Riis, P., and Anthonisen, P. The relationship between pregnancy and hemorrhagic proctocolitis. Acta Med. Scand. *180*:179, 1966.
104. Levi, A. J., Fisher, A. M., Hughes, K., and Hendry, W. F. Male infertility due to sulphasalazine. Lancet *2*:276, 1979.
105. Toovey, S., Hudson, E., Hendry, W. F., and Levi, A. J. Sulphasalazine and male infertility: reversibility and possible mechanism. Gut *22*:445, 1981.
106. O'Morain, C., Smethurst, P., Dore, C. J., and Levi, A. J. Reversible male infertility due to sulphasalazine: studies in man and rat. Gut *25*:1078, 1984.
107. Mogadam, M., Dobbins, W. O., Korelitz, B. I., and Ahmed, S. W. Pregnancy in inflammatory bowel disease: effect of sulfasalazine and corticosteroids on fetal outcome. Gastroenterology *80*:72, 1981.
108. Baiocco, P. J., and Korelitz, B. I. The influence of inflammatory bowel disease and its treatment on pregnancy and fetal outcome. J. Clin. Gastroenterol. *6*:211, 1984.
109. DeDombal, F. T., Watts, J. M., Watkinson, G., and Goligher, J. C. Ulcerative colitis and pregnancy. Lancet *2*:599, 1965.
110. McEwan, H. P. Ulcerative colitis and pregnancy. Proc. R. Soc. Med. *65*:279, 1972.
111. McKenzie, S. A., Sellez, J. A., and Agnar, J. E. Secretion of prednisolone into human milk. Arch. Dis. Child. *50*:894, 1975.
112. Azad Khan, A. K., and Truelove, S. C. Placental and mammary transfer of sulphasalazine. Br. Med. J. *2*:1553, 1979.
113. Jarnerot, G., and Into-Malmberg, M. D. Sulfasalazine treatment during breastfeeding. Scand. J. Gastroenterol. *14*:869, 1979.
114. Carr, N., and Schofield, P. F. Inflammatory bowel disease in the older patient. Br. J. Surg. *69*:223, 1982.
115. Gupta, S., Saverymuttu, S. H., Keshavarzian, A., and Hodgson, H. J. F. Is the pattern of inflammatory bowel disease different in the elderly? Age Ageing *14*:366, 1985.
116. Gebbers, J. O., and Otto, H. F. Ulcerative colitis in the elderly. Lancet *2*:714, 1975.
117. Edwards, F. C., and Truelove, S. C. The course and prognosis of ulcerative colitis. III. Complications. Gut *5*:1, 1964.
118. DeDombal, F. T., Watts, M. B., Watkinson, G., and Goligher, J. Incidence and management of anorectal abscess, fistula and fissure in patients with ulcerative colitis. Dis. Colon Rectum *9*:201, 1966.
119. DeDombal, F. T., Watts, J. M., Watkinson, G., Goligher, J. Local complications of ulcerative colitis: stricture, pseudopolyps, and carcinoma of the colon and rectum. Br. Med. J. *1*:1442, 1966.
120. Jalan, K. N., Sircus, W., Card, W. I., Falconer, C. W. A., Bruce, J., Crean, G. P., McManus, J. P. A., Small, W. P., and Smith, A. N. An experience of ulcerative colitis. I. Toxic dilation in 55 cases. Gastroenterology *57*:68, 1969.
121. Greenstein, A. J., Sachar, D. B., Gibas, A., Schrog, T., Heimann, T., Janowitz, D., and Aufses, A. H. Outcome of toxic dilatation in ulcerative and Crohn's colitis. J. Clin. Gastroenterol. *7*:137, 1985.
122. Grant, C. S., and Dozois, R. R. Toxic megacolon: ultimate fate of patients after successful medical management. Am. J. Surg. *147*:106, 1984.
123. Flatmark, A., Fretheim, B., and Gjone, E. Early colectomy in severe ulcerative colitis. Scand. J. Gastroenterol. *10*:427, 1975.
124. Goligher, J. C., Hoffman, D. C., and DeDombal, F. T. Surgical treatment of severe attacks of ulcerative colitis, with special reference to the advantage of early operation. Br. Med. J. *4*:703, 1970.
125. Greenstein, A. J., and Aufses, A. H. Differences in pathogenesis, incidence and outcome of perforation in inflammatory bowel disease. Surg. Gynecol. Obstet. *160*:63, 1985.
126. Morowitz, D. A., and Kirsner, J. B. Mortality in ulcerative colitis: 1930 to 1966. Gastroenterology *57*:481, 1969.
127. Greenstein, A. J., Sachar, D. B., Smith, H., Janowitz, H. D., and Aufses, A. H. A comparison of cancer risk in Crohn's disease and ulcerative colitis. Cancer *48*:2742, 1981.
128. Edwards, F. C., and Truelove, S. C. The course and prognosis of ulcerative colitis. IV. Carcinoma of the colon. Gut *5*:15, 1964.
129. Lennard-Jones, J. E., Morson, B. C., Ritchie, J. C., Shore, D. C., and Williams, C. B. Cancer in colitis: assessment of the individual risk by clinical and histological criteria. Gastroenterology *73*:1280, 1977.
130. Greenstein, A. J., Sachar, D. B., Smith, H., Pucillo, A., Papatislas, A. E., Kreel, I., Geller, S. A., Janowitz, H. D., and Aufses, A. H. Cancer in universal and left-sided ulcerative colitis: factors determining risk. Gastroenterology *77*:290, 1979.
131. Nugent, F. W., Haggitt, R. C., Colcher, H., and Kutteruf, G. C. Malignant potential of chronic ulcerative colitis—preliminary report. Gastroenterology *76*:1, 1979.

132. MacDougall, I. P. M. The cancer risk in ulcerative colitis. Lancet *1*:655, 1964.
133. Gyde, S. N., Prior, P., Thompson, H., Waterhouse, J. A. H., and Allan, R. N. Survival of patients with colorectal cancer complicating ulcerative colitis. Gut *25*:228, 1984.
134. Ritchie, J. K., Hawley, P. R., and Lennard-Jones, J. E. Prognosis of carcinoma in ulcerative colitis. Gut *22*:752, 1981.
135. Slater, G., Greenstein, A. J., Gelernt, I., Kreel, I., Bauer, J., and Aufses, A. H. Distribution of colorectal cancer in patients with and without ulcerative colitis. Am. J. Surg. *149*:780, 1985.
136. Riddell, R. H., Goldman, H., Ransohoff, D. F., Appelman, H. D., Fenoglio, C. M., Haggitt, R. C., Ahren, C., Correa, P., Hamilton, S. R., Morson, B. C., Sommers, S. C., and Yardley, J. H. Dysplasia in inflammatory bowel disease: standardized classification with provisional clinical applications. Hum. Pathol. *14*:931, 1983.
137. Ransohoff, D. F., Riddell, R. H., and Levin, B. Ulcerative colitis and colonic cancer—problems in assessing the diagnostic usefulness of mucosal dysplasia. Dis. Colon Rectum *28*:383, 1985.
138. Riddell, R. H., and Morson, B. C. Value of sigmoidoscopy and biopsy in the detection of carcinoma and premalignant change in ulcerative colitis. Gut *20*:575, 1979.
139. Dobbins, W. O. Current status of the precancer lesion in ulcerative colitis. Gastroenterology *73*:1431, 1977.
140. Rosenstock, E., Farmer, R. G., Petras, R., Sivak, M. V., Rankin, G. B., and Sullivan, B. H. Surveillance for colonic carcinoma in ulcerative colitis. Gastroenterology *89*:1342, 1985.
141. Blackstone, M. O., Riddell, R. H., Rogers, B. H. G., and Levin, B. Dysplasia-associated lesion or mass (DALM) detected by colonoscopy in long-standing ulcerative colitis: an indication for colectomy. Gastroenterology *80*:366, 1981.
142. Hammerberg, C., Slezak, P., and Tribukait, B. Early detection of malignancy in ulcerative colitis. A flow-cytometric DNA study. Cancer *53*:291, 1984.
143. Kurtz, L. M., Flint, G. W., Platt, N., and Wise, L. Carcinoma in the retained rectum after colectomy for ulcerative colitis. Dis. Colon Rectum *23*:346, 1980.
144. Baker, W. N. W., Glass, R. E., Ritchie, J. K., and Aylett, S. O. Cancer of the rectum following ileorectal anastomosis for ulcerative colitis. Br. J. Surg. *65*:862, 1978.
145. Greenstein, A. J., Janowitz, H. O., and Sachar, D. B. The extra-intestinal complications of Crohn's disease and ulcerative colitis: a study of 700 patients. Medicine *55*:401, 1976.
146. Perrett, A. D., Higgins, G., Johnson, H. H., Massarella, G. R., Truelove, S. C., and Wright, R. The liver in ulcerative colitis. Q. J. Med. *40*:211, 1971.
147. Dew, M. J., Thompson, H., and Allan, R. N. The spectrum of hepatic dysfunction on inflammatory bowel disease. Q. J. Med. *48*:113, 1979.
148. Steckman, M., Drossman, D. A., and Lesesne, H. R. Hepatobiliary disease that precedes ulcerative colitis. J. Clin. Gastroenterol. *6*:425, 1984.
149. Holzbach, R. T., Marsh, M. E., Freedman, M. R., Fazio, V. W., Lavery, I. C., and Jagelman, D. A. Portal vein bile acids in patients with severe inflammatory bowel disease. Gut *21*:478, 1980.
150. Christophi, C., and Hughes, E. R. Hepatobiliary disorders in inflammatory bowel disease. Surg. Gynecol. Obstet. *160*:187, 1985.
151. Eade, M. N. Liver disease in ulcerative colitis. I. Analysis in operative liver biopsy in 138 patients having colectomy. Ann. Intern. Med. *72*:475, 1970.
152. Wee, A., and Ludwig, J. Pericholangitis in chronic ulcerative colitis: primary sclerosing cholangitis of the small bile ducts? Ann. Intern. Med. *102*:581, 1985.
153. Sivak, M. V., Farmer, R. G., and Lalli, A. F. Sclerosing cholangitis: its increasing frequency of recognition and association with inflammatory bowel disease. J. Clin. Gastroenterol. *3*:261, 1981.
154. Weisner, R. H., and LaRusso, N. F. Clinicopathologic features of the syndrome of primary sclerosing cholangitis. Gastroenterology *79*:200, 1980.
155. Roberts-Thompson, I. C., Strickland, R. G., and Mackey, I. R. Bile duct carcinoma in chronic ulcerative colitis. Aust. N.Z. J. Med. *3*:264, 1973.
156. Wee, A., Ludwig, J., Coffey, R. J., LaRusso, N. F. and Wiesner, R. H. Hepatobiliary carcinoma associated with primary sclerosing cholangitis and chronic ulcerative colitis. Hum. Pathol. *16*:719, 1985.
157. Altman, A. R., Maltz, C., and Janowitz, H. D. Autoimmune hemolytic anemia in ulcerative colitis. Dig. Dis. Sci. *24*:282, 1979.
158. Dooley, D. P., Mills, G. M., Spiva, D. A. Immune thrombocytopenia and ulcerative colitis. So. Med. J. *79*:1044, 1986.
159. Talbot, R. W., Heppell, J., Dozois, R. R., and Beart, R. W. Vascular complications of inflammatory bowel disease. Mayo Clin. Proc. *61*:140, 1986.
160. Yassinger, S., Adelman, R., Cantor, D., Halsted, C. H., and Bolt, R. J. Association of inflammatory bowel disease and large vascular lesions. Gastroenterology *71*:844, 1976.
161. Lam, A., Borda, I., and Inwood, M. Coagulation studies in ulcerative colitis and Crohn's disease. Gastroenterology *68*:245, 1975.
162. Passo, M. H., Fitzgerald, J. F., and Brandt, K. D. Arthritis associated with inflammatory bowel disease in children. Dig. Dis. Sci. *31*:492, 1986.
163. Mallas, E., MacKintosh, P., Asquith, P., and Cooke, W. T. Histocompatibility antigens in inflammatory bowel disease. Gut *17*:906, 1976.
164. Wright, R., Lumsden, K., Luntz, M. H., Sevel, D., and Truelove, S. C. Abnormalities of the sacro-iliac joints and uveitis in ulcerative colitis. Q. J. Med. *34*:229, 1965.
165. Billison, F. A., DeDombal, F. T., Watkinson, G., and Goligher, J. C. Ocular complications of ulcerative colitis. Gut *8*:102, 1967.
166. Mir-Madjlessi, S. H., Taylor, J. S., and Farmer, R. G. Clinical course of erythema nodosum and pyoderma gangrenosum in chronic ulcerative colitis: a study of 42 patients. Am. J. Gastroenterol. *80*:615, 1985.
167. Goldstein, F., Krain, R., and Thornton, J. J. Intralesional steroid therapy of pyoderma gangrenosum. J. Clin. Gastroenterol. *7*:499, 1985.
168. Chaun, H., Day, J., Dodd, W. A., and Dunn, W. L. Ischemic skin lesions in ulcerative colitis. Can. Med. Assoc. J. *132*:937, 1985.
169. Block, G. E., Moossa, A. R., Simonowitz, D., and Hassan, S. Z. Emergency colectomy for inflammatory bowel disease. Surgery *82*:531, 1977.
170. Ambrose, N. S., Alexander-Williams, J., and Keighly, M. R. B. Audit of sepsis for operations for inflammatory bowel disease. Dis. Colon Rectum *27*:602, 1984.
171. Goligher, J. C., DeDombal, F. T., Graham, R. G., and Watkinson, G. Early surgery in the management of ulcerative colitis. Br. Med. J. *3*:193, 1967.
172. Steinberg, D., Allan, R., Brooke, B., Cooke, W. T., and Alexander-Williams, J. Sequelae of colectomy and ileostomy: comparison between Crohn's colitis and ulcerative colitis. Gastroenterology *68*:33, 1975.
173. Roy, P. H., Sauer, W. G., Beahrs, O. H., and Farrow, G. M. Experience with ileostomies: evaluation of long term rehabilitation in 497 patients. Am. J. Surg. *119*:77, 1970.
174. Hawley, P. R., and Ritchie, J. K. Complications of ileostomy and colostomy following excisional surgery. Clin. Gastroenterol. *2*:403, 1979.
175. Burnham, W. R., Lennard-Jones, J. E., and Brooke, B. N. Sexual problems amongst married ileostomists. Gut *18*:673, 1977.
176. Daly, D. W., and Brooke, B. N. Ileostomy and excision of the large intestine for ulcerative colitis. Lancet *2*:62, 1967.
177. Baker, W. N. W., Glass, R. E., Ritchie, J. K., and Aylett, S. O. Cancer of the rectum following colectomy and ileorectal anastomosis for ulcerative colitis. Br. J. Surg. *65*:862, 1978.
178. Grundfest, S. F., Fazio, V., Weiss, R. A., Jagelman, D., Lavery, I., Weakley, F. L., and Turnbull, R. B. The risk of cancer following colectomy and ileorectal anastomosis for extensive mucosal ulcerative colitis. Ann. Surg. *193*:9, 1981.

179. Oakley, J. R., Jagelman, D. G., Fazio, V. W., Lavery, I. C., Weakly, F. L., Easky, K., and Farmer, R. G. Complications and quality of life after ileorectal anastomosis for ulcerative colitis. Am. J. Surg. *149*:23, 1985.
180. Koch, N. G. Present status of the continent ileostomy. Dis. Colon Rectum *19*:200, 1976.
181. Goldman, S. L., and Rombeau, J. L. The continent ileostomy: a collective review. Dis. Colon Rectum *21*:594, 1978.
182. Stone, M. M., Lewin, K., and Fonkalsrud, E. W. Late obstruction of the lateral ileal reservoir after colectomy and endorectal ileal pullthrough procedures. Surg. Gynecol. Obstet. *162*:411, 1986.
183. Martin, L. W., Torres, A. M., Fischer, J. E. and Alexander, F. The critical level for preservation of continence in the ileoanal anastomosis. J. Pediatr. Surg. *20*:664, 1985.
184. Dozois, R. Restorative proctocolectomy and ileal reservoir. Mayo Clin. Proc. *61*:283, 1986.
185. Fonkalsrud, E. W. Endorectal ileal pullthrough with isoperistaltic ileal reservoir for colitis and polyposis. Ann. Surg. *202*:145, 1985.

79

Conventional and Alternative Ileostomies

SIDNEY F. PHILLIPS

Proctocolectomy and permanent ileostomy will return the majority of patients with ulcerative colitis to excellent health. Many of the former inconveniences and dangers associated with an ileal stoma have now been eliminated by improved surgical techniques, by a wider range of better stomal appliances, and by more effective education of patients.[1]

Between 1930 to 1950 ileostomy and colectomy became established surgical procedures. During this time, the metabolic consequences of ileostomy became more apparent, as did the frequent mechanical complications caused by "ileostomy dysfunction." Better understanding of fluid, electrolyte, and blood replacement provided answers to the first problem; the surgical techniques of Turnbull[2] and Brooke[3] resolved the second. Up until these advances ileostomies were made by withdrawal of the intestine through the abdominal wall, with the serosal surface then being sutured to the skin. Ileostomy dysfunction resulted from the (not unexpected) serositis that follows exposure of ileal serosa to the stomal effluent. However, the mucosa of the ileum should not be susceptible to a similar inflammation, and a solution was therefore conceptually simple. Evert the mucosal surface of the bud, suturing mucosa to skin. Simultaneous development of new ileostomy appliances quickly led to better acceptance by patients and ultimately to the excellent long-term results now expected.[4] Enterostomal therapy was introduced in the 1960s as an additional allied health support, and ileostomy societies have blossomed in most countries, providing a lay component to the total support of treatment.

During the 1960s Kock of Goteborg, Sweden,[5] developed the first effective continent ileostomy. The procedure features an ileal pouch, a nipple valve, and an ileal conduit leading to the cutaneous stoma (Fig. 79–1). Sufficient clinical experience has been accumulated to recommend its use in selected cases of ulcerative colitis and polyposis coli.

Stimulated by patients' acceptance of the "Kock pouch," surgeons have sought other alternatives to the incontinent ileostomy, with its ever-present bag. The ileoanal pull-through operation[6] has been resurrected, this procedure offering the advantages of a normal flow of stool and preservation of the anal sphincters. An important technical modification of the approach has been the addition of an ileal reservoir,[7] several forms of which are advocated by different surgical groups (Fig. 79–2). Attention has also been directed toward mechanical devices for occlusion of traditional end-ileostomies.[8]

PATHOPHYSIOLOGIC CONSEQUENCES OF PROCTOCOLECTOMY

Fecal Outputs After Proctocolectomy. After any ileostomy is made, the colon loses the capacity to reabsorb electrolytes and water. Usually, this creates no major pathophysiologic disturbance, but some important principles should be remembered. A normal colon absorbs at least 1000 ml (1 L) of water and 100 mEq of sodium chloride daily.[9] More important, these amounts can be augmented; when overloaded progressively, the healthy colon absorbs more than 5 L daily.[10] Also, the colon responds to salt depletion by conserving NaCl avidly, but the small intestine lacks the capacity to respond similarly. For example, under

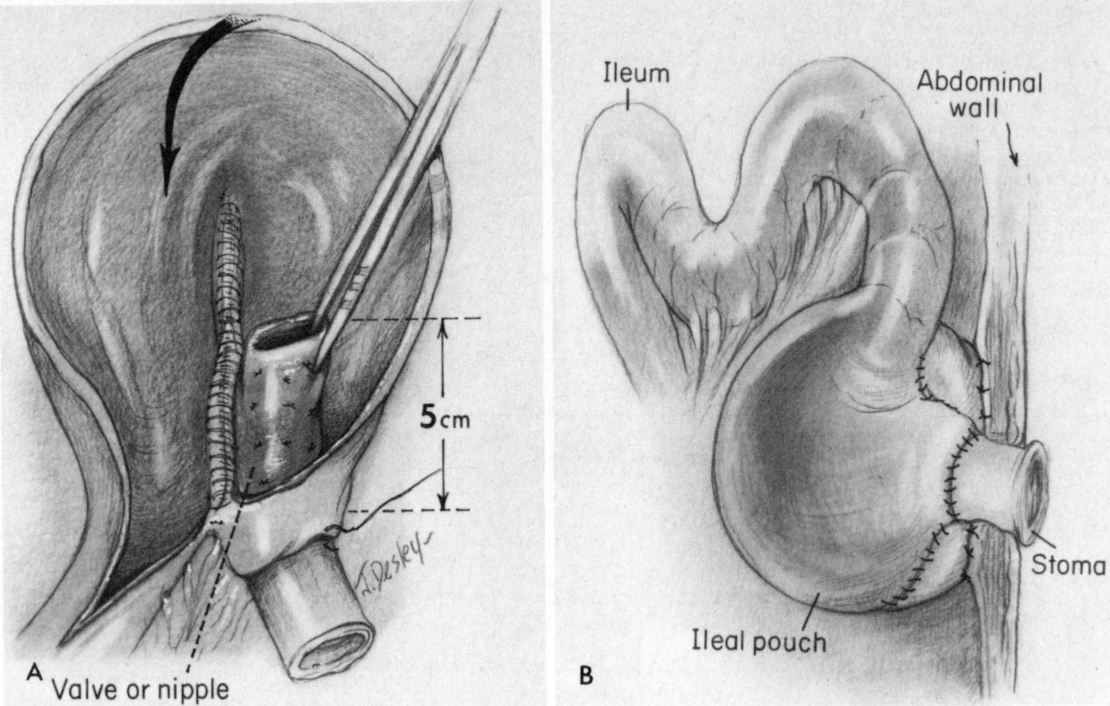

Figure 79–1. The continent ileostomy. *A*, The pouch is formed from a loop of ileum, folded on itself as a U, and sutured along with antimesenteric borders. The limbs are then incised, exposing the mucosa, and the nipple valve is fashioned. The pouch is closed and sutured in the direction of the arrow. *B*, The final anatomy, demonstrating the flush stoma.

conditions of extremely low salt intake, fecal losses of sodium can be reduced to 1 or 2 mEq per day,[11] whereas patients with ileostomies have obligatory losses of sodium of 30 to 40 mEq per day.[12, 13]

Well-functioning conventional ileostomies discharge 300 to 800 gm of material daily; 90 per cent of this is water.[12, 13] Continent ileostomies and ileal pouch–anal anastomoses have similar volumes of effluent.[14] Foods containing much unabsorbable residue increase the total output by increasing the amount of solids discharged. Although many anecdotes are reported as to the effect of certain foods on the volume and consistency of effluents, the response to specific foods varies from patient to patient, and changes are usually minimal.[15] Prunes, which contain a chemical cathartic (diphenylisatin), increase the volumes of output.

Functional Sequelae. When oral intakes of sodium, chloride, and fluid are adequate, patients with ileostomies do not become depleted; however, negative sodium balance may follow periods of diminished oral intake, vomiting, or excess loss in perspiration.[16] In addition, chronic oliguria is to be anticipated,[16, 17] because normal stools contain approximately 100 ml of water, whereas ileostomies lose 500 to 600 ml daily. Ileostomists also have lower Na^+-K^+ ratios in urine owing to compensatory renal conservation of sodium and water. These changes in the composition of urine presumably contribute to the increased frequency of urolithiasis (probably about 5 per cent) in these patients.[18] The stones are predominantly urate or calcium salts.

When ileostomy is accompanied by resection of terminal ileum, abnormalities of bile acid reabsorption (see pp. 144–161) and malabsorption of vitamin B_{12} may result. Steatorrhea and greater daily losses of fluid (1 L/day or more) also may be seen. However, these abnormalities do not occur in the usual circumstances when colectomy is performed for inflammatory disease of the colon or polyposis coli; the ileum, being free of disease, is usually preserved.

Lack of a colon also reduces the exposure of bile acids to the metabolic effects of the fecal flora. After ileostomy, secondary bile acids largely disappear from bile,[19, 20] but no metabolic consequences of significance have been recognized. The flora of ileostomy effluents has quantitative (10^4 to 10^7 organisms/ml) and qualitative characteristics that are intermediate between those of feces and those of normal ileal contents.[21, 22]

Pathophysiologic sequelae are therefore mainly the potential consequences of a salt-losing state; patients should be advised to use salt liberally and to increase their fluid intake, especially at times of stress, particularly in very hot weather and on vigorous exercise. Unfortunately, the limited ability of the small intestine to absorb sodium and water means that stomal volumes will also increase when the oral intake is increased.[13]

OVERALL CLINICAL CONSEQUENCES

After successful surgery, life expectancy is slightly below normal for the first few years owing to complications around the stoma and to intestinal obstruction. A few patients may develop cancer in a retained rectal stump. However, in general, the long-term mortality rate in patients after proctocolectomy and conventional ileostomy is virtually the same as for a matched normal population.[23] Ninety per cent of patients with conventional ileostomies who responded to a survey rated the results of their operation as excellent and claimed little inconvenience.[4] Almost all are able to lead normal lives and enjoy normal sexual relationships. Certain strenuous physical activities are avoided by a minority of patients.

Sufficient time has not passed to allow firm statements to be made on all points relative to ileostomy alternatives. The metabolic consequences of proctocolectomy per se should be no different in these groups, and it is self-evident that those patients in whom the ileostomy alternative achieves excellent results will have a better quality of life; they need not wear a bag constantly. Certain special complications of the newer operations are discussed in the following section.[7, 14, 24]

COMPLICATIONS AND MANAGEMENT OF CONVENTIONAL ILEOSTOMIES

Major long-term complications relate to malfunctioning ileostomies, prestomal ileitis, and irritation of the peristomal skin. If the ileostomy was improperly constructed (with newer techniques this is now a much less frequent problem), the stoma may become obstructed. Obstruction leads to cramping abdominal pain, increased ileal discharge (up to 4 L daily), and fluid and electrolyte depletion. Excessive ileal output arises, at least in part, from increased intestinal secretion as the result of dilatation of the intestine proximal to the obstructed stoma. Stomal obstruction can usually be demonstrated by examining the stoma with the little finger, by endoscopy with a small sigmoidoscope, or by barium enema examination through the stoma. X-rays will reveal a dilated ileum proximal to the point of obstruction. Many of these ileostomies require reconstruction. At operation, ulcerations are often found in the resected terminal ileum; their pathogenesis is unclear but probably relates in some way to the mechanical problem of obstruction.

Prestomal ileitis is a much less common problem.[25] Patients with this syndrome exhibit the features of mechanical obstruction but in addition have signs of systemic toxicity (fever, tachycardia, anemia). The ileum has numerous punched-out ulcers, sometimes extending to the serosa. It is not clear whether prestomal ileitis has a different pathogenesis from the changes that follow simple mechanical obstruction of the stoma. Both may develop in a segment of ileum that was normal histologically at the time of colectomy. "Backwash ileitis" does not seem to predispose the patient to the development of either problem. On the other hand, in patients who have had colectomy and ileostomy for Crohn's disease, subsequent problems with the ileal stoma may arise from spread of transmural granulomatous disease to the new terminal ileum. In some instances, it may be difficult to determine with certainty whether stomal dysfunction is due to mechanical obstruction or to recurrent Crohn's disease.

Most ileostomists can lead a normal life and eat a normal diet;[4] poorly digested foods (nuts, corn, some fruits, lightly cooked vegetables) may obstruct the stoma and should be eaten in moderation, after careful chewing. However, a few patients experience continuing problems of management. These vary in severity, some being minor inconveniences and others being significant drawbacks to the success of the operation. Mechanical difficulties with a malfitting appliance on the stoma may cause excoriation of the skin around the ileostomy or may even erode the stoma to produce a fistula. Occasionally, peristomal abscess and peristomal hernias may develop, and a small number of pregnant women develop prolapse of the stoma. Some patients have unpleasant odors in the ileostomy bag, especially after eating certain foods, such as onions and beans. However, because most odor arises from bacterial action on the contents of the bag, the problem is offset by frequent emptying of the bag and by adding sodium benzoate or chlorine tablets to the bag. Orally administered bismuth subgallate also controls odor,[26] but doubts exist as to whether its long-term use is justified, as questions of toxicity have been raised.[27]

In the handling of these many aspects of postoperative care, trained stomal therapists and lay societies of ileostomists can be most helpful. Education of the patient is best started prior to surgery, when meetings with ileostomists and reference to specialized texts[28–30] can allay many fears and uncertainties.

The United Ostomy Association (2001 W. Beverly Boulevard, Los Angeles, California 90057; telephone 213-413-5510) publishes an excellent series of booklets dealing with all aspects of life for the ileostomist. These materials are of great help also to nursing staffs in the absence of registered enterostomal therapists. The geographic location of therapists can be obtained from the International Association for Enterostomal Therapy (5000 Birch, P.O. Box 2690-175, Newport Beach, California 92660; telephone 714-476-0268).

CONTINENT ILEOSTOMIES

Kock Pouch

Clearly, the major social drawbacks to ileostomy could be largely prevented if a continent stoma were possible. Kock[5] reasoned that a pouch constructed of terminal ileum could store ileal content internally until emptied voluntarily, obviating an external appliance. The pouch would need to hold about 500 ml, so that it would fill only once or twice each day. For continence to be achieved, a valve would be needed to separate the pouch from the exterior. A catheter could then be passed through the stoma, past the valve, and into the pouch, to drain its content.

The first operations were reported in 1969, and the results were promising.[5] A 30-cm segment of ileum provided a pouch of adequate size. However, the valves that were constructed in the early cases were not always successful in providing continence. At the present time, the valve is made by intussuscepting the efferent ileal limb into the pouch for a distance of 3 to 5 cm, and anchoring the intussusceptum in place with nonabsorbable sutures (Fig. 79–1). This approach has been successful, providing continence in the majority of patients. Two surgical groups with much experience have reported their results.[31, 32] In Goteborg, Sweden, 8 per cent of pouches fail ultimately and must be removed.[31] The Mayo Clinic group, which considers Crohn's disease a contraindication for the operation, has a lesser failure rate; once the surgical techniques were well established, fewer than 1 per cent of pouches needed removal.[32] In both series, well over 90 per cent of patients were completely continent for gas and feces (i.e., they never required a bag).

Pouches are made as primary steps at the time of proctocolectomy, even in severely ill patients, and as secondary conversions of conventional stomas. The operation can then be performed in most patients, but those with Crohn's disease should not be considered. Recurrence of disease in the pouch can lead to removal of the pouch, with sacrifice of a considerable length of small intestine. No surgical approach to utilizing the pouch in the restoration of normal anatomy has been developed.

Long-term follow-up (up to 10 years) has shown excellent acceptance by the majority of patients.[31, 32] Most pouches have remained continent, with no skin irritation, no unpleasant odors from the stoma, and no social, sexual, or psychologic disability. Patients have gained weight, returned to good health, and taken up their former employment. A very few patients have required excision of the pouch in the late postoperative period. This has been necessary for (1) persistent incontinence, especially in early cases in which a less effective valve was constructed, (2) excessive fluid loss from the pouch, or (3) recurrent Crohn's disease when the operation was performed unwittingly for Crohn's colitis. In up to one third of all pouches, incontinence develops, usually during the first year. This is due to extrusion of the nipple valve from the pouch. Although new approaches, which secure the valve in place by special sutures, have reduced the overall frequency of valve prolapse, failure of the nipple valve remains an important problem. Risk factors have been examined by the Mayo Clinic group; older, overweight men who had a conventional ileostomy converted to a pouch were most at risk. Young, thin women having a pouch fashioned as a primary procedure had a risk of nipple valve failure rate estimated at less than 10 per cent.[33]

Outputs from the stoma are not significantly different from those from conventional stomas.[24] Absorptions of D-xylose, L-phenylalanine, sodium, chloride, water, and vitamin B_{12} were also similar in pouches and normal intestine.[24] Thus, ileal pouches possess many of the functions of normal ileum. In approximately 25 per cent of patients, however, stomal outputs of water, electrolytes, or fat are increased above values from control patients with conventional ileostomies; absorption of vitamin B_{12} may also be reduced concomitantly.[34] Quantitative recovery of flora from jejunal aspirates suggests that a blind loop syndrome (iatrogenic) might be the cause of malabsorption[22] (see pp. 1289–1297). Fortunately, the degree of malabsorption is usually minimal and of no major clinical significance.

Some patients have these abnormalities in association with acute inflammation in the pouch. "Pouchitis" does not appear to represent regional enteritis in most patients, although in some cases the distinction can be difficult. Bleeding from the pouch and discomfort on distention are common features. The syndrome may be associated with malabsorption (steatorrhea or an abnormal Schilling test) but, even if not, stomal output is usually increased. This and other causes of "stomal diarrhea" need careful evaluation.[14] To be excluded are (1) mechanical obstruction, which may be partial and intermittent, (2) causes of diarrhea unassociated with the operation (lactose intolerance, specific infections), and (3) steatorrhea as a result of associated resection of the ileum and bile acid malabsorption. Only then, in the presence of clinical and endoscopic evidence of superficial inflammation of the pouch, can pouchitis be considered the cause of diarrhea, with or without concomitant malabsorption. Antibiotic therapy with metronidazole has often produced dramatic improvement,[22] although some patients need treatment with corticosteroids or sulfasalazine.

Major dilemmas arise when pouchitis is associated with systemic symptoms, low-grade fever, abdominal pain, anorexia, weight loss, and arthralgias—features that may mimic the original inflammatory bowel disease. The separation from recurrent inflammatory bowel disease can be impossible and, in a few patients, the failure to respond to medical therapy necessitates surgical removal of the pouch, with conversion to a Brooke ileostomy.[24]

Mechanical Occlusion of Ileostomies

Initial experiences with mechanical occlusion of stomas were directed toward colostomies, but magnetic devices were soon applied to ileostomies.[35] The potential for mechanical occlusion was extended when Beahrs and coworkers[36] developed a balloon device to occlude continent ileostomies of patients in whom the nipple valve had failed repeatedly and who were unsuitable candidates for another surgical repair. This experience prompted questions as to whether conventional ileostomies could be occluded by a similar balloon device. Experimental studies in dogs have been successful,[8] and the method has been used cautiously in humans.

Ileoanal Pouch Anastomosis

Total colectomy, mucosal proctectomy, and endorectal ileoanal anastomosis has been revived, and currently is the most exciting alternative to the conventional, or incontinent, ileostomy. The operation is suitable for patients with chronic ulcerative colitis or familial polyposis coli but not for those with Crohn's disease. The operation has several major advantages: (1) all mucosal disease is removed (in contrast to ileorectostomy), (2) the normal route for elimination is maintained (a stoma is not required), (3) the anal sphincters should be undisturbed, and (4) the pelvic dissection, being less extensive, should not endanger innervation of the sexual organs. The general approach was first described by Ravitch and Sabiston[6] in 1947, and the revival was influenced by the success of local resections performed by pediatric surgeons for Hirschsprung's disease. Early approaches[37] used only a straight pull-through whereby the ileum was sutured directly to the anal verge. Although results in children were encouraging,[38] excessive stool frequency and anal seepage were unacceptable to many adult patients. Subsequently, the operative approach was modified to include one of several forms of ileal pouch (Fig. 79–2). The principles are as follows: an abdominal colectomy is performed; the rectoanal mucosa is stripped from the underlying muscular cuff, which is left in place; an ileal pouch is fashioned; and the reservoir is sutured to the anal verge. A diverting ileostomy is required for two to three months until the anastomosis heals completely. At a second operation, the diverting ileostomy is closed.

Several centers have acquired considerable experience, and the Mayo Clinic series is now greater than 500, with the same generally excellent results reported at the last time of major follow-up,[39] when approximately 200 operations were evaluated. Pouches of different configurations are advocated by several groups,[39–41] and surgical techniques are still evolving; differences among the procedures are likely to be minimal.

The major surgical complication is leakage at the anastomosis with pelvic sepsis. In the initial Mayo experience, 11 per cent had a clinical diagnosis of sepsis, but only half required reoperation, and 3 per cent required pouch excision. Strictures at the anastomosis are common, occurring in 10 to 20 per cent of patients, but most respond to simple digital dilation. The metabolic complications of an ileal pouch are similar to those occurring after continent ileostomy. Most patients have no steatorrhea, and fecal outputs are comparable to those from conventional ileostomies.[14, 24] Mean stool frequency is five to six during the day and one at night; most patients soil so infrequently that no special precautions are needed. Diarrhea and pouchitis occur; although the reported frequencies vary widely, a figure of 10 per cent of clinically significant problems is realistic. The features, management, and outcome are similar to pouchitis in continent ileostomies.

Experience thus encourages continued, although selective, use of these alternatives to the incontinent stoma. The current techniques offer a high probability of continence, and patients are pleased with the results. These operations are most attractive to young, unmarried people, who may have great concerns about the social, psychologic, and sexual disadvantages of an incontinent stoma. Younger patients are also more suitable candidates than are elderly persons, in that they are better able to understand and undergo additional operations should these become necessary. However, until the long-term consequences are fully evaluated, these newer operations should be done mainly in centers at which the numbers performed are sufficient to allow careful follow-up.

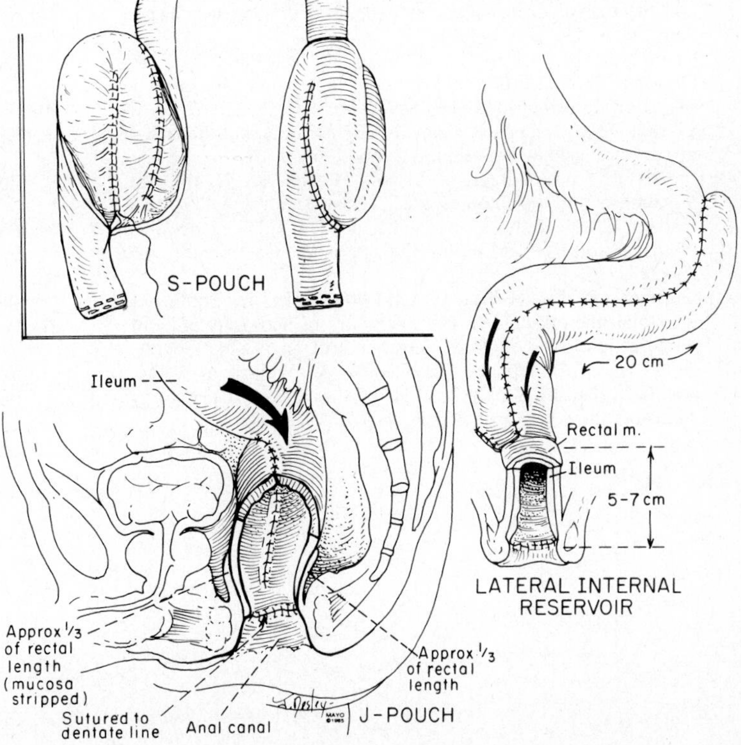

Figure 79–2. Anatomy of the major forms of ileal pouch used for anastomosis to a cuff of anorectal muscle (ileal pouch–anal anastomosis).

References

1. Hill, G. L. Historical introduction. *In* Ileostomy: Surgery, Physiology and Management. New York, Grune & Stratton, 1976, p. 1.
2. Turnbull, R. B. Symposium on ulcerative colitis; management of ileostomy. Am. J. Surg. *86*:617, 1953.
3. Brooke, B. N. Management of ileostomy including its complications. Lancet *2*:102, 1952.
4. Roy, P. H., Sauer, W. G., Beahrs, O. H., and Farrow, G. N. Experience with ileostomies. Evaluation of long-term rehabilitation in 497 patients. Am. J. Surg. *119*:77, 1970.
5. Kock, N. G. Intra-abdominal reservoir in patients with permanent ileostomy. Preliminary observations on a procedure resulting in fecal continence in five ileostomy patients. Arch. Surg. *99*:223, 1969.
6. Ravitch, M. M., and Sabiston, D. C. Anal ileostomy with preservation of the sphincter. Surg. Gynecol. Obstet. *84*:1095, 1947.
7. Dozois, R. R. Alternatives to Conventional Ileostomy. Chicago, Year Book Medical Publishers, 1985.
8. Pemberton, J. H., Kelly, K. A., and Phillips, S. F. Achieving ileostomy continence with an indwelling stomal device. Surgery *90*:336, 1981.
9. Phillips, S. F., and Giller, J. Contribution of the colon to electrolyte and water conservation in man. J. Lab. Clin. Med. *81*:733, 1973.
10. Debongnie, J. C., and Phillips, S. F. Capacity of the human colon to absorb fluid. Gastroenterology *74*:698, 1978.
11. Dole, V. P., Dahle, L. K., Cotzias, G., Eder, H. A., and Krebs, M. E. Dietary treatment of hypertension: clinical and metabolic studies of patients on the rice-fruit diet. J. Clin. Invest. *29*:1189, 1950.
12. Kramer, P. The effect of varying sodium loads on the ileal excreta of human ileostomized subjects. J. Clin. Invest. *45*:1710, 1966.
13. Kanaghinis, T., Lubran, M., and Coghill, N. F. The composition of ileostomy fluid. Gut *4*:322, 1963.
14. Metcalf, A. M., and Phillips, S. F. Ileostomy Diarrhea. Clin. Gastroenterol. *15*:705, 1986.
15. Kramer, P., Kearney, M. S., and Ingelfinger, F. J. The effect of specific foods and water loading on the ileal excreta of ileostomized human subjects. Gastroenterology *42*:535, 1962.
16. Gallagher, N. D., Harrison, D. D., and Skyring, A. P. Fluid and electrolyte disturbances in patients with long established ileostomies. Gut *3*:219, 1962.
17. Clarke, A. M., Chirnside, A., Hill, G. L., Pope, G., and Stewart, M. K. Chronic dehydration and sodium depletion in patients with established ileostomies. Lancet *2*:740, 1967.
18. Clarke, A. M., and McKenzie, R. G. Ileostomy and the risk of urinary uric acid stones. Lancet *2*:395, 1969.
19. Morris, J. S., Low-Beer, T. S., and Heaton, K. W. Bile salt metabolism and the colon. Scand. J. Gastroenterol. *8*:425, 1973.
20. Gadacz, T. R., Kelly, K. A., and Phillips, S. F. The Kock ileal pouch: absorptive and motor characteristics. Gastroenterology *72*:1287, 1977.
21. Gorbach, S. L., Nahas, L., and Weinstein, L. Studies of intestinal microflora. IV. The microflora of ileostomy effluent: a unique microbial etiology. Gastroenterology *53*:874, 1967.
22. Kelly, D. G., Phillips, S. F., Kelly, K. A., Weinstein, W. M., and Gilchrist, M. J. Dysfunction of the continent ileostomy: clinical features and bacterology. Gut *24*:193, 1983.
23. Watts, J. M., de Dombal, F. T., and Goligher, J. C. Long-term complications and prognosis following major surgery for ulcerative colitis. Br. J. Surg. *53*:1014, 1966.
24. Phillips, S. F. Metabolic consequences of a stagnant loop at the end of the small bowel. World J. Surg. *11*:763, 1987.
25. Knill-Jones, R. P., Morson, B., and Williams, R. Prestomal ileitis: clinical and pathological findings in five cases. Q. J. Med. *39*:287, 1970.
26. Sparberg, M. Bismuth subgallate as an effective means for control of ileostomy odor: a double blind study. Gastroenterology *66*:476, 1974.
27. Report from the Australian Drug Evaluation Committee. Adverse effects of bismuth subgallate. Med. J. Aust. *2*:664, 1974.
28. Lenneberg, E., and Rowbotham, J. L. The Ileostomy Patient: A Descriptive Study of 1425 Persons. Springfield, Illinois, Charles C Thomas, 1970.
29. Honesty, H. The Essentials of Abdominal Ostomy Care. New York, Springer Publishing Company, 1972.
30. Sparberg, M. The Ileostomy Case. Springfield, Illinois, Charles C Thomas, 1971.
31. Koch, N. G., Mynvold, H. E., Nilsson, L. O., Philipson, B. N. Continent ileostomy: the Swedish experience. *In* Dozois, R. R. (ed.). Alternatives to Conventional Ileostomy. Chicago, Year Book Medical Publishers, 1985, p. 163.
32. Dozois, R. R., Kelly, K. A., Beart, R. W., and Beahrs, O. H. Continent ileostomy: the Mayo experience. *In* Dozois, R. R. (ed.). Conventional Ileostomy. Chicago, Year Book Medical Publishers, 1985, p. 180.
33. Dozois, R. R., Kelly, K. A., Ilstrup, D., Beart, R. W., and Beahrs, O. W. Factors affecting revision rate after continent ileostomy. Arch. Surg. *116*:610, 1981.
34. Kelly, D. G., Branon, M. E., Phillips, S. F., and Kelly, K. A. Diarrhea after continent ileostomy. Gut *21*:711, 1980.
35. Papachristou, D. M., Claudatou, D., and Fortner, J. G. Continent ileostomy without intestinal reservoir: a new experimental procedure. Surg. Forum *29*:481, 1978.
36. Beahrs, O. W., Bess, M. A., Beart, R. W., and Pemberton, J. H. Indwelling ileostomy valve device. Am. J. Surg. *141*:111, 1981.
37. Stryker, S. J., and Dozois, R. R. The ileoanal anastomosis: historical perspectives. *In* Dozois, R. R. (ed.). Alternatives to Conventional Ileostomy. Chicago, Year Book Medical Publishers, 1985, p. 225.
38. Coran, A. G. Straight endorectal pull-through of the ileum for the management of benign disease of the colon and rectum in children and adults. *In* Dozois, R. R. (ed.). Alternatives to the Conventional Ileostomy. Chicago, Year Book Medical Publishers, 1985, p. 335.
39. Beart, R. W., Jr., Metcalf, A. M., Dozois, R. R., and Kelly, K. A. The J ileal pouch–anal anastomosis: the Mayo Clinic experience. *In* Dozois, R. R. (ed.). Alternatives to the Conventional Ileostomy. Chicago, Year Book Medical Publishers, 1985, p. 384.
40. Rothenberger, D. A., Wong, W. D., Buls, J. G., and Goldberg, S. M. The S ileal pouch–anal anastomosis. *In* Dozois, R. R. (ed.). Alternatives to Conventional Ileostomy. Chicago, Year Book Medical Publishers, 1985, p. 345.
41. Fonkalsrud, E. W. Endorectal ileoanal anastomosis with isoperistaltic ileal reservoir. *In* Dozois, R. R. (ed.). Alternatives to the Conventional Ileostomy. Chicago, Year Book Medical Publishers, 1985, p. 402.

80

Colonic Polyps and the Gastrointestinal Polyposis Syndromes

C. RICHARD BOLAND
STEVEN H. ITZKOWITZ
YOUNG S. KIM

A gastrointestinal polyp is a discrete mass of tissue that protrudes into the lumen of the bowel (Fig. 80–1). Increased interest in polyps has resulted from recent progress in the ability not only to detect polyps with a high degree of sensitivity but also to remove them endoscopically. A polyp may be characterized by its gross morphology, the presence or absence of a stalk, and whether it is one of multiple similar masses elsewhere in the gut. Regardless of these features, specific definition rests on the histologic characteristics.

Because of their protrusion into the lumen of the gut and the stresses of the fecal stream to which they are subject, polyps may cause various symptoms. Thus, they may ulcerate and bleed; abdominal pain may result when a peristaltic wave propels a polyp downstream; large polyps may even obstruct the intestine. However, symptomatic polyps are uncommon; the greatest concern with polyps is their potential to become malignant. Although debate continues, the bulk of evidence supports the hypothesis that most colonic cancers arise within previously benign adenomas. Theoretically, then, all colonic adenomas should be removed. However, colonic polyps are so common in the industrialized world that universal detection and removal is impractical. To manage colonic polyps, therefore, the physician must understand the differences in pathogenesis and natural history of the distinct pathologic categories of these lesions. This approach also facilitates understanding of the polyposis syndromes.

COLONIC POLYPS

Colonic polyps may be divided into two major groups: neoplastic (the adenomas and carcinomas) and non-neoplastic (Table 80–1). The adenomas and carcinomas share a common characteristic—cellular atypia or dysplasia—but they may be subdivided according to the relative contribution of certain microscopic features. The non-neoplastic polyps may be grouped into several distinct categories, including "mucosal polyps," hyperplastic polyps, juvenile polyps, inflammatory polyps, and others.

Submucosal lesions may also impart a polypoid appearance to the overlying mucosa; these will be discussed later in this chapter (p. 1500).

NEOPLASTIC POLYPS (ADENOMATOUS AND MALIGNANT POLYPS)

Histologic Characteristics

Adenomatous polyps are tumors of benign neoplastic epithelium that may be pedunculated, attached by a narrow base to a long stalk, or sessile, attached by a broad base with little or no stalk. The neoplastic nature of adenomas is apparent by histologic examination. Adenomatous epithelium is characterized by abnormal

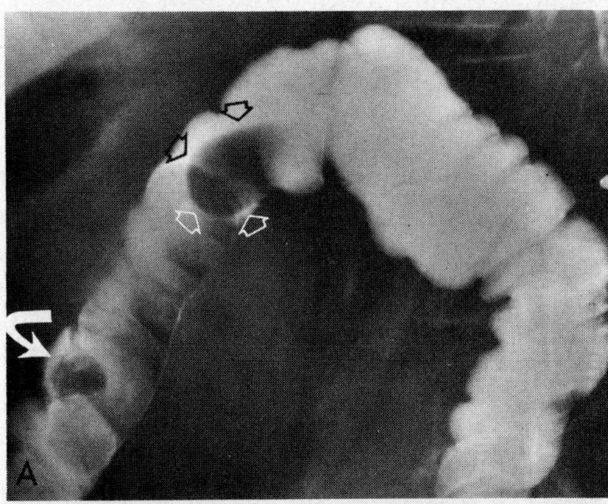

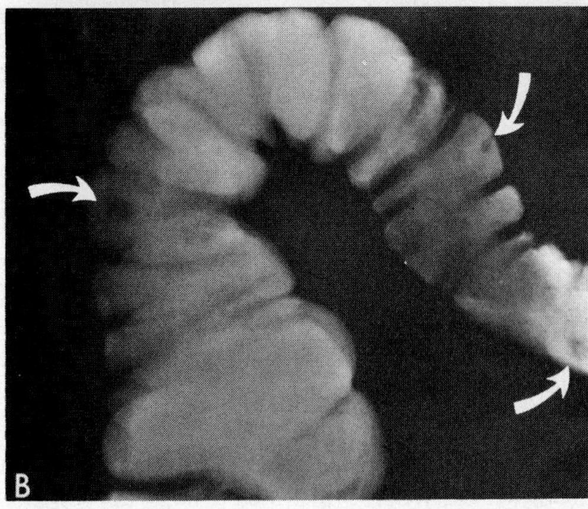

Figure 80–1. This barium enema demonstates several polypoid lesions of the colon (*A*, splenic flexure, *B*, hepatic flexure). The largest polyp *(open arrows)* was a pedunculated lipoma. The other polyps were adenomas; the largest one contained tubular and villous elements and a focus of dysplasia. A total of eight polyps were removed from this patient.

Table 80–1. CLASSIFICATION OF COLORECTAL POLYPS

Colorectal Polyps	Neoplastic Mucosal Lesions	Benign (Adenoma)	Tubular adenoma
			Tubulovillous adenoma
			Villous adenoma
		Malignant (Carcinoma)	Carcinoma *in situ* (intramucosal)
			Invasive carcinoma (through muscularis mucosae)
	Non-neoplastic Mucosal Lesions		Normal epithelium (in a polypoid configuration)
			Hyperplastic polyp (metaplastic polyp)
			Juvenile polyp (retention polyp)
			Peutz-Jeghers polyp
			Inflammatory polyps (pseudopolyps)
			• inflammatory bowel disease
			• in bacterial infections or amebiasis
			• schistosomiasis
			• colitis cystica profunda
	Submucosal Lesions		Pneumatosis cystoides intestinalis
			Lymphoid polyps (benign and malignant)
			Lipomas
			Carcinoids
			Metastatic neoplasms
			Other rare lesions

cellular differentiation and renewal, resulting in hypercellularity of colonic crypts with cells possessing variable amounts of mucin and hyperchromatic, elongated nuclei arranged in a picket-fence pattern. By definition, all colorectal adenomas are dysplastic. These cytologic alterations confer a more basophilic appearance to the adenomatous epithelium by conventional hematoxylin-eosin staining. Although the predominant cell type is an immature goblet cell or columnar cell, adenomas may contain other cell types, such as neuroendocrine cells, Paneth cells, squamous morules, and, rarely, melanocytes. The gland lumina of adenomatous polyps are usually round, in contrast to the serrated appearance of hyperplastic gland lumina (see p. 1495).

The dysplasia (a histologic term) or atypia (a cytologic term) exhibited by all adenomas can be graded subjectively into three categories: mild, moderate, and severe. Some polyps may contain the entire spectrum from mild to severe dysplasia. In all cases, the adenoma is classified according to the most atypical or dysplastic focus within it. Cells exhibiting mild dysplasia have slightly enlarged nuclei, which are uniform in size, elongated, and without prominent nucleoli, but which maintain their basal polarity in the cell (Fig. 80–2*A* and *B*). In contrast, severe dysplasia is characterized by cells with increased nuclear-cytoplasmic ratio wherein the nuclei are pleomorphic, contain prominent nucleoli, and demonstrate pseudostratification, with loss of polarity in relation to the cell basement membrane (Fig. 80–2*D*). Moderate dysplasia has features intermediate between mild and severe dysplasia (Fig. 80–2*C*). In addition to these cytologic abnormalities, architectural alterations accompany the dysplastic progression. Thus, severe dysplasia is marked by a loss of stroma between adenomatous glands, resulting in a "back-to-back" glandular pattern with intraglandular bridging and budding, giving a disorderly, cribriform appearance (Fig. 80–2*D*). The term severe dysplasia is often used synonymously with carcinoma *in situ* to indicate the frankly malignant nature of these cells. Either term is appropriate to describe a focus of cancer within an adenoma that has not extended through the muscularis mucosae. However, if such a focus extends beneath the muscularis mucosae into the submucosa (even in the head of a polyp), this constitutes invasive carcinoma (see p. 1493).

Mild dysplasia may be found in 70 to 80 per cent of adenomatous polyps, moderate dysplasia in 10 to 20 per cent, severe dysplasia (carcinoma *in situ*) in 5 to 10 per cent, and invasive carcinoma in 5 to 7 per cent.[1–3] Severe dysplasia is more common in adenomas that are large, distal, and near a coexisting carcinoma.[4]

Adenomas may also be classified by histologic type. Tubular adenomas are the most common subgroup, characterized by a complex network of branching adenomatous glands (Fig. 80–2). In villous adenomas, the adenomatous glands extend straight down from the surface to the center of the polyp, thereby creating long, finger-like projections (Fig. 80–3). Tubulovillous (villoglandular) adenomas manifest a combination of these two histologic types. A polyp is assigned a histologic type on the basis of its predominant glandular pattern, and, in practice, pure villous adenomas are quite rare. Tubular adenomas account for 65 to 80 per cent of adenomatous polyps, tubulovillous for 15 to 25 per cent, and villous adenomas for 3 to 10 per cent.[1–3] Tubular adenomas are usually small and exhibit mild dysplasia, whereas villous architecture is more often encountered in large adenomas and tends to be associated with more severe degrees of dysplasia (Table 80–2).

The three histopathologic criteria that correlate with

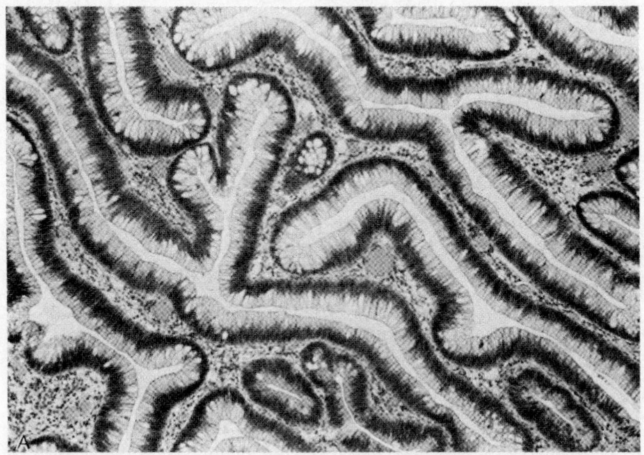

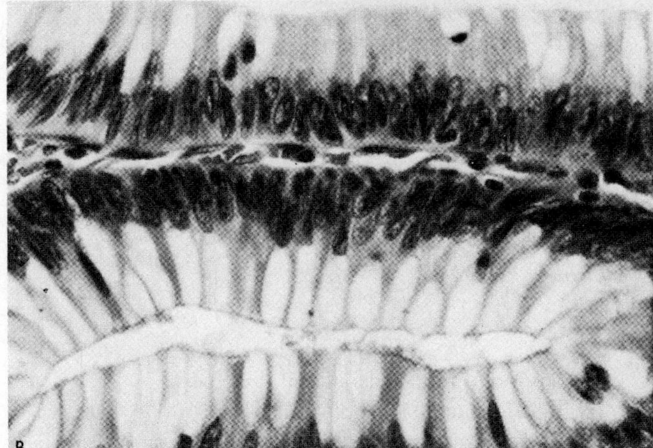

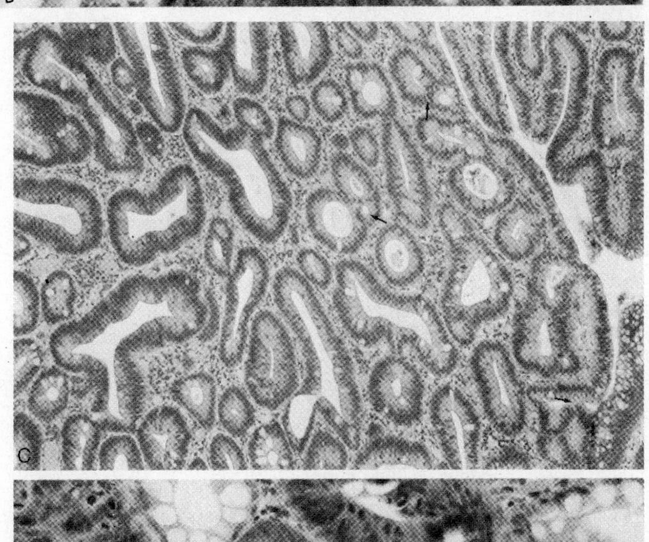

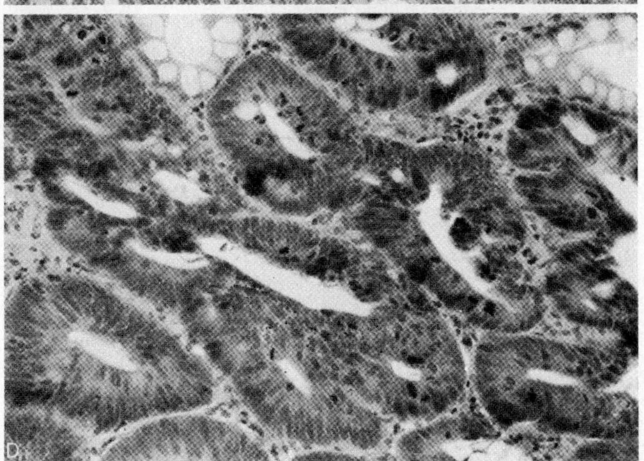

Figure 80–2. Tubular adenoma. *A,* This low-power photomicrograph demonstrates the proliferation of glandular epithelium in a tubular adenoma showing only mild atypia. The nuclei are basally oriented, and a normal cytoplasmic-nuclear ratio is preserved in most of the epithelial cells. *B,* This high-power photomicrograph demonstrates mild degrees of nuclear atypia and crowding, characteristic of adenomatous epithelium. *C,* This low-power photomicrograph of a tubular adenoma demonstrates mild to moderate degrees of atypia in which an increased degree of cellular crowding, larger nuclei, and migration of the nuclei away from their normal basal orientation are seen. Some glands are beginning to show a back-to-back configuration *(arrows). D,* This photomicrograph demonstrates severe atypia in which the cells are more densely packed, the nuclear-cytoplasmic ratio is very high, and rudimentary malignant glands are seen. Foci of severe atypia are equivalent to carcinoma *in situ* (CIS).

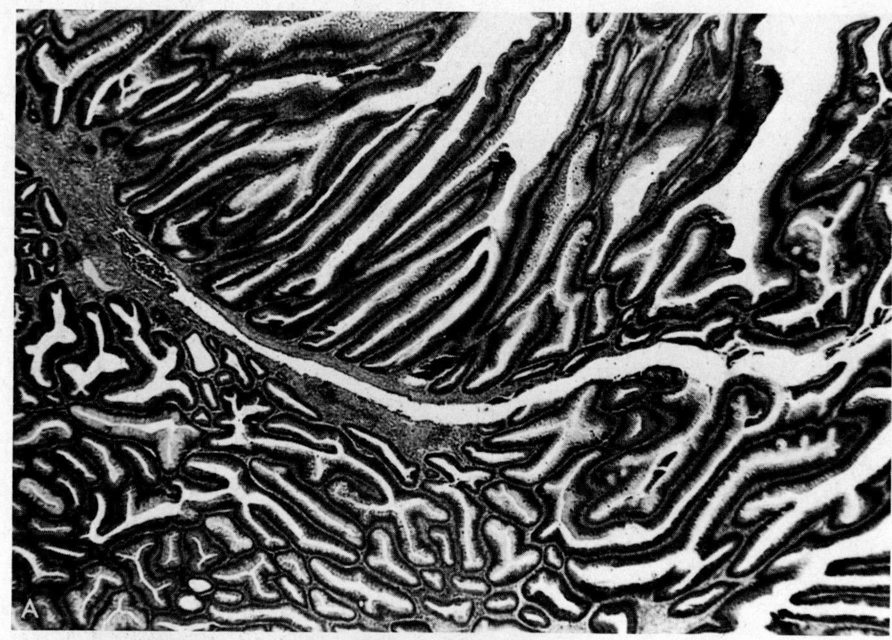

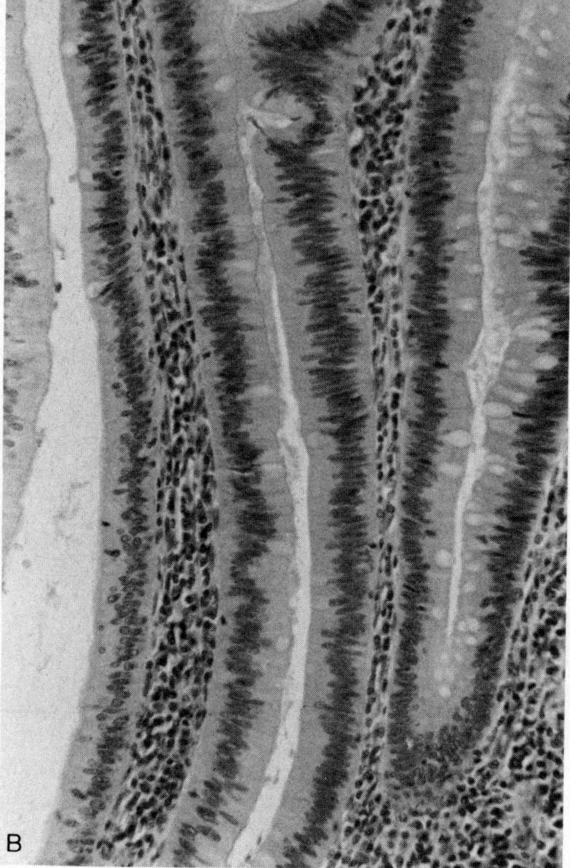

Figure 80–3. Tubulovillous adenoma. *A,* This low-power photomicrograph demonstrates tubular epithelium in the lower half of the field and villous elements in the upper half. *B,* This high-power photomicrograph of a villous frond demonstrates the cellular crowding, nuclear palisading and nuclear pleomorphism characteristic of villous epithelium. These abnormalities are classified as mild to moderate atypia or dysplasia.

Table 80–2. FREQUENCY OF ADENOMAS: RELATIONSHIP OF HISTOLOGIC TYPE TO ADENOMA SIZE AND DEGREE OF DYSPLASIA

Type of Adenoma	Adenoma Size*			Degree of Dysplasia†		
	<1 cm	*1–2 cm*	*>2 cm*	*Mild*	*Moderate*	*Severe*
Tubular	77%	20%	4%	88%	8%	4%
Tubulovillous	25%	47%	29%	58%	26%	16%
Villous	14%	26%	60%	41%	38%	21%

*Adapted from Muto, T., Bussey, H. J. R., and Morson, B. C. Cancer *36*:2251, 1975. Used by permission.

†Adapted from Konishi, F., and Morson, B. C. J. Clin. Pathol. *35*:830, 1982. Used by permission.

malignant potential for an adenomatous polyp are polyp size, histologic type, and degree of dysplasia (Table 80–3). These three parameters are probably highly interactive, and it may be difficult to assign a predominant premalignant role to any one of them. For example, although only 1.3 per cent of all adenomas under 1 cm may harbor a malignancy (Table 80–3), if these small lesions have a predominant villous component or contain a focus of severe dysplasia, the malignancy rate rises to 10 per cent or 27 per cent, respectively (Table 80–4).

Diminutive Polyps

A diminutive polyp is a polyp that measures 5 mm or less in diameter. The original notion that these lesions were almost always non-neoplastic[5, 6] has been challenged in flexible sigmoidoscopy and colonoscopy studies, in which 30 to 50 per cent of diminutive polyps have been found to be adenomatous.[7–10] Compared with hyperplastic diminutive polyps, which are usually located in the sigmoid colon and rectum, adenomatous diminutive polyps may be seen more proximally, particularly in older persons.[7–9] Finding an invasive carcinoma within a diminutive polyp is extremely rare, and fewer than 1 per cent of all diminutive polyps are villous or contain a focus of severe dysplasia.[7, 8, 10, 11]

Table 80–3. MALIGNANT POTENTIAL OF ADENOMATOUS POLYPS

	Total Number	Number with Carcinoma (%)
Adenoma Size		
< 1 cm	1479	19 (1.3)
1–2 cm	580	55 (9.5)
> 2 cm	430	198 (46.0)
Histologic Type		
Tubular	1880	90 (4.8)
Tubulovillous	383	86 (22.5)
Villous	243	99 (40.7)
*Degree of Dysplasia**		
Mild	1734	99 (5.7)
Moderate	549	99 (18.0)
Severe	223	77 (34.5)

Adapted from Muto, T., Bussey, H. J. R., and Morson, B. C. Cancer *36*:2251, 1975. Used by permission.

*This category refers to the most extensive degree of dysplasia *outside* the area of carcinoma within the polyp. However, by convention, because an adenoma is classified according to the most severe grade of dysplasia, if carcinoma is present, it is considered a malignant polyp regardless of the degree of surrounding dysplasia.

Morphogenesis

Adenomatous polyps are thought to arise from a failure in a step (or steps) of the normal process of cellular proliferation and differentiation. Cell kinetic studies of adenomas with labeled DNA precursors have demonstrated a shift of the proliferative compartment from the lower crypt to the upper crypt (see pp. 992–1002 and 1502). Figure 80–4, based on detailed histologic analysis by several investigators, depicts the proposed sequence of events in adenoma morphogenesis.[12] The initial aberration may arise in a single colonic crypt in which the proliferative compartment, instead of being confined to the crypt base, is expanded throughout the entire crypt (so-called unicryptal adenoma). The DNA-synthesizing cells at the surface are not sloughed into the lumen normally and accumulate by downward infolding, interposing themselves between normal pre-existing crypts. New adenomatous glands are then created either by further infolding or by branching. It is hypothesized that the histologic type of adenoma is then determined by the reaction of the underlying mesenchyme (connective tissue and capillaries). Thus, in tubular adenomas, mesenchymal proliferation is minimal, so that epithelial infolding develops against a resistance, tending to limit the overall polyp size. However, in villous adenomas, mesenchymal proliferation accompanies epithelial proliferation, resulting in longer projections and eventually larger polyps.

The Adenoma-Carcinoma Hypothesis

It is now generally accepted that most, if not all, colon cancers originate within previously benign adenomas, and several lines of evidence can be cited to support this hypothesis. First, epidemiologic observations indicate that the adenoma prevalence within a population, as well as the multiplicity of adenomas per person, geographically parallels the prevalence of colon cancer.[13] Indeed, adenoma prevalence increases in migrants from low-risk to high-risk colon cancer regions.

Table 80–4. ADENOMAS CONTAINING INVASIVE CARCINOMA: RELATIONSHIP OF ADENOMA SIZE TO HISTOLOGIC TYPE AND DEGREE OF DYSPLASIA

Adenoma Size	Per Cent with Carcinoma					
	Histologic Type			*Degree of Dysplasia*		
	TUBULAR	TUBULOVILLOUS	VILLOUS	MILD	MODERATE	SEVERE
< 1 cm	1	4	10	0.3	2	27
1–2 cm	10	7	10	3	14	24
> 2 cm	35	46	53	42	50	48

Adapted from Muto, T., Bussey, H. J. R., and Morson, B. C. Cancer *36*:2251, 1975. Used by permission.

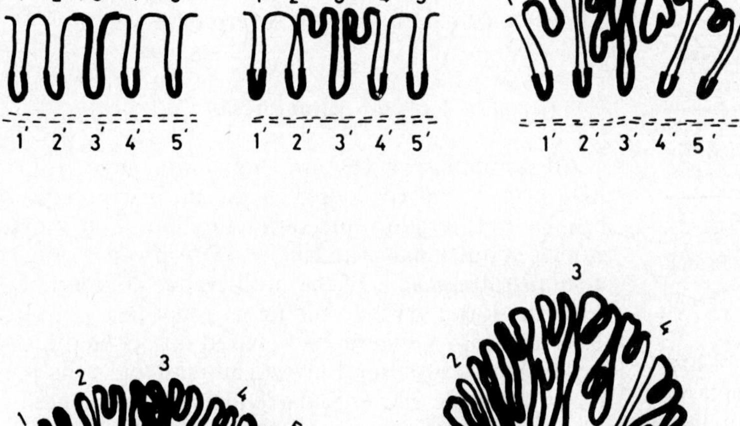

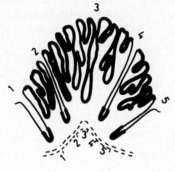

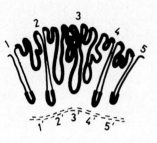

Figure 80–4. Adenoma morphogenesis. Postulated scheme of adenoma morphogenesis in human colorectal mucosa. *Thin lines*: Differentiated epithelium; *thick lines*: proliferative epithelium. Normally, one crypt opening (1–5) corresponds to one crypt base (1′–5′), with the proliferative zone limited to the lower crypt. The earliest lesion is an expansion of the proliferative zone to involve the entire crypt (3–3′). Further proliferation of cells on the surface results in infolding and branching, with adenomatous glands interdigitating between normal crypts. The resistance of the underlying connective tissue and forces from the fecal stream contribute to the final gross polypoid appearance. (Courtesy of A. P. Maskens, M.D.)

The prevalence rates for both adenomatous polyps and cancer increase with age, and analyses of age distribution curves indicate that the development of adenomas precedes that of carcinomas by five to ten years. Also, in the familial polyposis syndromes (see pp. 1501–1511), the appearance of benign adenomas antedates the development of carcinoma by an average of 10 to 12 years.[1] Even with sporadic adenomas, the polyp-to-cancer interval is at least four years[1] and perhaps longer, depending on the degree of dysplasia.[14] Second, clinical studies have demonstrated that removal of rectal polyps by proctosigmoidoscopy prevents the subsequent development of rectal cancer.[15] Third, some pathologic studies describe the frequent presence of remnant adenoma tissue within colon cancers.[16] Small foci of cancer are extremely rare in normal mucosa but are commonly found in adenomas, particularly those that are larger, are more dysplastic, and contain more of a villous component (Tables 80–3 and 80–4). Furthermore, the site distribution within the colon is similar for large adenomas and colon cancers. In addition, adenomatous polyps are found in one third of surgical specimens containing a single colon cancer and in over two thirds of specimens containing more than one simultaneous colon cancer (see p. 1490).

A few exceptions to the adenoma-carcinoma sequence have been described. Although this is rare, colon cancers may develop *de novo* in flat nonadenomatous epithelium.[17, 18] However, it is possible that even these rare cases of *de novo* carcinoma arose within pre-existing adenomatous epithelium that assumed a flat rather than polypoid configuration.[19] In familial nonpolyposis colon cancer syndromes, it has been suggested that cancers may arise without passing through a polyp phase, although recently precursor adenomas have been observed.[20, 21] In rats given the chemical carcinogen dimethylhydrazine, colorectal cancers often develop without an adenoma phase.[22] However, the same carcinogen will induce colorectal adenomas (and carcinomas) in certain strains of mice.[22]

The relative contributions of genetic and environmental factors to the formation of adenomas and their progression to malignancy can only be speculative. Although there is a strong genetic component to the well-defined colonic polyposis and cancer family syndromes, which exhibit a mendelian pattern of inheritance, the vast majority of common (sporadic) adenomas or carcinomas arise in persons not having these syndromes. In the past, this has been interpreted to mean that genetic predisposition plays only a minor role. However, a dominant mode of inheritance for common colonic adenomas and carcinomas has recently been demonstrated in a large pedigree.[23] This finding supports a hypothesis proposed several years ago concerning adenoma causation, which is based mainly on epidemiologic and histopathologic observations.[24] It is postulated that an adenoma-prone genotype is actually extremely common throughout the world. Several environmental factors may then act in concert: one may be responsible for the initial development of adenomas, another may enhance the growth of adenomas that develop, and one or more carcinogens or tumor promoters may finally give rise to cancer.

Molecular Markers of the Adenoma-Carcinoma Sequence

Over the last decade, major advances in scientific technology have provided an opportunity to investigate at the molecular level the pathobiology of polyps, providing experimental support for the adenoma-carcinoma hypothesis. At present, results using a variety of techniques have been mainly descriptive, so it is premature to assign a specific pathophysiologic role to any given molecular alteration. The general approach has been to identify an alteration that distinguishes colon cancer from normal colonic tissue, and then determine how changes in polyps compare with these tissues.

At the genetic level, certain quantitative and qualitative alterations of DNA have been noted in adenomas. Aneuploidy, which may occur in up to half of colorectal cancers and is believed to be a marker of poor prognosis,[25] has been found in approximately 5 to 15 per cent of adenomas, particularly those of larger size, with more villous component, and with greater degrees of dysplasia.[26, 27] Hypomethylation of DNA, an event that is associated with gene activation, has been observed in adenomas and colon cancers but not in normal colonic mucosa.[28] Other studies have found that persons with familial polyposis or sporadic adenomatous polyps have circulating mononuclear leukocytes that are deficient in DNA repair synthesis, suggesting that these patients might be more susceptible to environmental mutagens.[29] Colon cancer tissues, and to a lesser extent, adenomatous polyps, have been examined for the presence of various oncogene products, particularly of the *ras* and *myc* genes; enhanced expression of these products is not characteristic of early colorectal neoplasia (i.e., adenomas).

At the phenotypic level, several antigens have recently been recognized as cancer-associated antigens in the colorectum. Most of them are oncodevelopmental in nature, such as the prototype carcinoembryonic antigen (CEA). The expression of CEA in colonic polyps is quite variable; both adenomatous and hyperplastic polyps may express the antigen, and among adenomatous polyps there is no consistent relationship between CEA expression and either villous morphology or degree of dysplasia.[30] A partial explanation for the inconsistencies in CEA expression is that CEA is actually a family of glycoprotein antigens, and antibodies used by different investigators may be recognizing different cross-reacting epitopes.

Some groups have examined antigens with known immunodeterminant structure using more specific probes, such as monoclonal antibodies and lectins. Indeed, many colon cancer–associated antigens have carbohydrate epitopes that are identical or closely related to blood group substances. For example, certain alterations in the expression of blood group antigens A, B, H(O), and Lewis^b have been observed in the colonocytes of adenomas and cancers but not in hyperplastic polyps or normal mucosa.[31] Furthermore, in persons with sporadic adenomas, a blood group H–recognizing lectin (*Ulex europaeus*-1) binds to adenomatous but not normal epithelium, whereas in patients with familial polyposis, both the adenoma and the normal-appearing flat mucosa bind this lectin.[32] The Lewis^x and Lewis^y antigens have recently been shown to be cancer-associated antigens that are expressed preferentially by adenomatous but not hyperplastic polyps, and their expression directly correlates with adenoma size, villous histology, and severity of dysplasia.[33, 34]

The T antigen, a precursor substance for the MN blood group antigens, is another carbohydrate cancer-associated antigen that is expressed in most adenomas but also in many hyperplastic polyps.[35] However, if staining is performed with a monoclonal antibody instead of peanut lectin, fewer hyperplastic polyps express the T antigen and, in adenomas, antigen expression correlates with polyp size, histologic type, and degree of dysplasia.[36]

Certain enzymes may be useful markers of the polyp-cancer sequence. The activity of ornithine decarboxylase, an enzyme involved in cell proliferation, is elevated in adenomas and even flat mucosa of polyp-prone individuals (see p. 1502). Urokinase, a plasminogen-activator type of protease that may play a role in colon cancer cell invasion, is also expressed by adenomatous tissue.[37] In fact, adenomas exposed to a tumor promoter *in vitro* can be induced to secrete this enzyme in an amount commensurate with their malignant potential.[38] Moreover, an *in vitro* model designed to investigate how a focus of cancer cells invades surrounding adenoma cells has also invoked a role for urokinase.[39]

The foregoing experimental observations are a firm foundation for further investigations into the pathogenesis of colonic malignancy. The challenge ahead will be to determine how multiple genetic and environmental factors interact to regulate these various markers, and to integrate this information with the growing knowledge of the clinical behavior of colonic malignancy and premalignancy.

Epidemiology, Prevalence, and Distribution of Adenomas

The frequency of colonic adenomas varies widely among populations but tends to be higher in populations at greater risk for colon cancer[13] (Table 80–5). Adenoma prevalence correlates positively also with socioeconomic class even in regions of low colon cancer risk, although this may be biased to favor adenoma detection for those who can afford medical care. Age is the single most important independent determinant of adenoma prevalence[40–46] (Table 80–5). Indeed, with advancing age there is a greater likelihood that multiple polyps, adenomas with more severe degrees of dysplasia, and (in some cases) larger adenomas will develop. In general, the development of adenomas is independent of sex. Race, *per se,* is also not an independent determinant; adenomas rarely develop in blacks residing in South Africa, whereas the prevalence rate for those living in New Orleans is comparable to that city's high-risk white population.[13]

The true prevalence rate of adenomatous polyps within an asymptomatic, living population cannot be known with certainty because of inherent practical and ethical considerations. Therefore, data from autopsy series provide the closest approximation. In populations at low risk for colon cancer, adenoma prevalence rates are under 12 per cent (Table 80–5). In most intermediate and high-risk populations, adenomas are found in 30 to 40 per cent of the population, but rates of 50 to 60 per cent have been observed.[40, 42] One half to two thirds of persons over age 65 years in high-risk areas may harbor colonic adenomas.[40–42]

The distribution of adenomas within the colon has also differed depending on the method of investigation. In surgical and colonoscopic studies, adenomas assume a left-sided predominance—a distribution resembling that of colon cancer. In autopsy series, however, adenomas in general are more uniformly distributed throughout the colorectum, although larger adenomas maintain a more distal predilection. These observations suggest that distal adenomas are more likely to come to clinical attention, but the autopsy data are reminders that many presumably asymptomatic adenomas are in the proximal colon—a distribution that becomes accentuated with advanced age.[44–48]

Growth Rate of Polyps

Little is known about adenoma growth rate, primarily because in the endoscopy era polyps are readily removed, thereby interrupting the natural history of their growth. Thus, the limited knowledge about polyp growth rate has been pieced together from studies that have used a variety of approaches. A population distribution study, comparing the mean ages of patients manifesting polyps of different degrees of dysplasia with those of patients who died of colon cancer, estimates that the transition period for polyps with mild dysplasia to malignancy is 11 years, whereas the interval for adenomas with severe dysplasia to become malignant is 3.6 years.[14]

Follow-up observations on patients with unresected adenomas suggest that the progression to malignancy requires five to ten years.[1] Previous serial sigmoidoscopic observations in large numbers of persons with asymptomatic rectal polyps (histology unknown) who agreed to allow the lesions to remain *in situ* unless they reached 1.5 cm had demonstrated slow growth.[49] Thus, after three to five years, only 4 per cent of polyps had increased in size, 70 per cent had remained unchanged, 8 per cent got smaller, and 18 per cent disappeared spontaneously. (The disappearance of polyps by autoamputation occurs more often with juvenile polyps than with adenomatous polyps).[50] Another approach has been to measure adenoma size on serial barium enemas in patients who eventually underwent resections and had histologic confirmation.[51, 52] These data indicate that the vast majority of adenomas, especially tubular adenomas, either do not enlarge or grow very slowly, so that they never become a clinical problem.

Even in the majority of adenomas with growth rates similar to those of colon cancer, doubling times are longer than four to six months. Mathematical models suggest that a diminutive polyp (less than 5 mm) requires two to three years to reach 1 cm in size,[53] and a 1-cm polyp, based on barium enema measurements, requires at least two to five years to become malignant.[54] From all of the foregoing observations, it is fair to conclude that colorectal polyps in general grow very slowly.

Multiple Adenomas and Carcinomas

Knowledge of the frequency with which adenomas coexist with other adenomas or carcinomas is important in clinical practice and for the design of cancer screening and surveillance programs. The term "multiple adenoma" (or carcinoma) simply means two or more neoplasms and should not be confused with the "multiple adenomatosis syndromes" characterized by hundreds of polyps (see p. 1500). An adenoma or carcinoma that is diagnosed at the same time as an index colorectal neoplasm is called a synchronous lesion, but one that is diagnosed at least six months later (a somewhat arbitrary limit) is considered metachronous.

The adenomatous polyp itself is often regarded as a marker of a neoplasm-prone colon.[55] Indeed, 30 to 50 per cent of colons with one adenoma will contain at least one other synchronous adenoma—multiple adenomas being more common in older age groups.[1, 44, 45] The risk of colon cancer rises with the number of

Table 80–5. PREVALENCE OF ADENOMATOUS POLYPS

		Prevalence Rate (%)					
		Males			*Females*		
		Age			Age		
Population	**Colon Cancer Frequency**	20–39	40–59	60+	20–39	40–59	60+
Hawaiian-Japanese	Very high	50	69	64	0	71	58
New Orleans, white	High	0	39	47	0	10	35
New Orleans, black	High	19	26	52	0	27	41
Brazil (São Paulo)	Intermediate	5	14	30	8	14	23
Japan (Akita)	Intermediate	21	31	46	0	8	37
Japan (Miyagi)	Low	1	9	23	4	9	17
Costa Rica (San José)	Low	0	6	13	2	4	9
Colombia (Cali)	Low	2	7	18	2	10	15

From Correa, P. *In* Morson, B. C. (ed.). The Pathogenesis of Colorectal Cancer. Philadelphia, W. B. Saunders Company, 1978. Used by permission.

adenomas present (Table 80–6) and is essentially 100 per cent in individuals with familial polyposis coli.

A synchronous adenoma can be found in 30 per cent of colons harboring a carcinoma[1, 56–58] and in 50 to 85 per cent of those harboring two or more synchronous cancers.[1, 55, 56, 59–61] In the presence of a coexisting carcinoma, an adenoma is more likely to exhibit greater degrees of dysplasia.[4, 62] If the synchronous adenoma is diagnosed preoperatively and is distant from the carcinoma, the surgical approach is adapted to the particular circumstances.[56] Also, the presence of a synchronous adenoma in a patient with colon cancer confers an increased risk for developing a subsequent colon cancer.[1, 57] Similarly, a synchronous adenoma in a patient with a colonic polyp places that individual at greater risk for developing metachronous polyps[63] and cancer.[63, 64]

Conditions Associated with Adenomatous Polyps

An association between adenomatous polyps and atherosclerosis has been documented by necropsy studies,[65, 66] one of which noted a correlation between the degree of atherosclerosis and the multiplicity, size, and degree of dysplasia of adenomas.[66] This suggests that these two conditions of westernized populations share certain risk factors—for example, elevated serum cholesterol levels. However, a cause-and-effect relationship between serum cholesterol concentration and adenomatous polyps has not been elucidated. Serum cholesterol levels in individuals with adenomas were high in one study[67] but normal in another.[68] The association of low cholesterol levels with colon cancer is most likely a metabolic consequence of the malignancy.[68]

In acromegalic patients, the presence and multiplicity of simple skin tags (acrochordons) have been found to correlate with the presence of colonic polyps.[69] This led to further investigations on whether skin tags (usually located on the upper trunk or axillae) could serve as a cutaneous marker of colonic polyps for the general population. Three studies examined symptomatic patients presenting for colonoscopy prospectively for the presence of skin tags in a blinded fashion, and found a significant correlation between the presence of skin tags and adenomatous polyps.[70–72] However, an autopsy study of presumably asymptomatic persons[73] and a colonoscopic study of members of familial polyposis kindreds[74] found no such correlation. Thus, at present, it is premature to conclude that skin tags may be useful markers for polyps in an average-risk, asymptomatic population.

Bacteremia and endocarditis caused by *Streptococcus bovis* have been associated with colorectal carcinoma,[75] adenomatous polyps,[76] and even polyposis coli.[77] The fecal carrier rate of this organism is higher in persons with adenomas or carcinomas than in those with benign colonic diseases or normal controls.[75, 78] It has therefore been suggested that patients with *S. bovis* bacteremia undergo thorough colonic examination to exclude a neoplasm. Recently, *Streptococcus agalactiae* (an organism that is rarely pathogenic in adults) endocarditis was reported in two patients who each had a rectal villous adenoma with foci of carcinoma.[79]

Table 80–6. CORRELATION BETWEEN THE NUMBER OF ADENOMAS AND ASSOCIATED CARCINOMA AT ST. MARK'S HOSPITAL

Number of Adenomas per Patient	Number of Patients	Number of Patients with Carcinoma
1	1331	395 (30%)
2	296	153 (52%)
3	83	47 (57%)
4	40	20 (50%)
5	13	10 (77%)
6–48	25	20 (80%)

From Day, D. W., and Morson, B. C. *In* Morson, B. C. (ed.). The Pathogenesis of Colorectal Cancer. Philadelphia, W. B. Saunders Company, 1978. Used by permission.

Diagnosis and Management

Signs and Symptoms

Most patients with colonic polyps either have no symptoms referable to the gastrointestinal tract or have nonspecific intestinal symptoms. Occult or overt rectal bleeding is the most common presenting symptom that can be attributed to colonic polyps. Histopathologic observations suggest that in contrast to colonic carcinomas, which exhibit considerable surface erosion, the generally less rigid adenomas maintain the integrity of the surface epithelium but may bleed into the polyp stroma.[80] These findings help to explain the clinical impression that bleeding from polyps is often intermittent and does not usually cause anemia.

Other symptoms that may be attributable to colonic polyps are constipation, diarrhea, or flatulence. Constipation or decreased stool caliber is more likely to be caused by bulky lesions in the distal colon. Secretory diarrhea with hypokalemia and dehydration may rarely be associated with a villous adenoma, and prostaglandin production has been implicated in the pathogenesis of the diarrhea associated with adenomas. Large colonic polyps may be associated with cramping lower abdominal pain owing to intermittent intussusception. Unless these symptoms disappear with the removal of the polyp, they must be attributed to other causes.

The actual frequency of bleeding from adenomas is difficult to determine. Fewer than 20 per cent of persons who report frank rectal bleeding will be found to have a significant adenoma (i.e., $\geq$ 1 cm) as the cause.[81] In general, polyps under 1 cm in size do not bleed. This is supported by quantitative measurements of fecal blood loss in people with known adenomas, which indicate that only those with adenomas larger than 1.5 to 2.0 cm lose more than the usual amounts of blood (regardless of the location of the polyp within the colon).[82–84] Likewise, when occult blood loss is detected qualitatively with Hemoccult cards, only 20 to 40 per cent of patients with known adenomas show positive test results,[82–87] and the rates are higher in patients with larger polyps and polyps of the distal large bowel. The advent of more sensitive assays to detect occult blood in stool may improve detection of polyps, although evidence so far indicates that only 40 to 60 per cent of patients with polyps larger than 1 cm exhibit excess amounts of fecal blood.[88]

Detection of Adenomas

As colorectal polyps are usually clinically silent, they are diagnosed either during investigation for symptoms referable to the colon (including unexplained iron-deficiency anemia or weight loss) or in asymptomatic persons being screened for colorectal neoplasia. In either case, the diagnostic work-up usually begins with a digital rectal examination and sigmoidoscopy (see p. 1575). Whenever possible, flexible rather than rigid sigmoidoscopy should be used. In symptomatic patients, the yield for detecting polyps (and cancer) is three times greater with the flexible instrument than with the rigid one,[89] and this diagnostic advantage also applies to asymptomatic patients undergoing screening or surveillance sigmoidoscopy (see p. 1575). The increased yield is due primarily to the fact that 44 to 82 per cent of polyps detected are located beyond the average depth of insertion achieved with the rigid endoscope.[90–92] A shorter (35 cm) flexible sigmoidoscope has been developed for use as a primary screening device for colorectal neoplasia in asymptomatic individuals (see p. 1493). However, even in symptomatic patients this instrument permits detection of more polyps and cancers than the rigid sigmoidoscope[93] and a similar number of polyps and cancers as the 60-cm flexible instrument[94, 95] with excellent patient acceptance.

If a neoplasm is discovered by sigmoidoscopy, the remainder of the large bowel should be visualized either radiographically or endoscopically because finding synchronous neoplasms (reported in about 35 per cent of patients in this situation[96–98]) may influence initial and subsequent management. If a barium enema examination is chosen, the air-contrast rather than single-contrast technique should be used to maximize the detection of small polyps.[99–101] A properly performed air-contrast barium enema examination can have a sensitivity of 85 to 95 per cent for detecting colorectal polyps. However, common sources of error include inadequate cleansing of the colon, which contributes to the 5 to 10 per cent false positive rate, and diagnostic difficulty caused by the presence of diverticulosis or redundant bowel, which results in a 10 per cent false negative rate.

Colonoscopy is usually preferred to air-contrast barium enema examination for adenoma management because it has therapeutic capability and enhanced diagnostic accuracy (pp. 1570–1576). This diagnostic superiority has been demonstrated in studies of patients with known polyps[102, 103] as well as symptomatic patients who have had negative findings on proctosigmoidoscopic and barium enema examinations.[104–106] Despite its reputation as the "gold standard" for adenoma detection, colonoscopy has some limitations, such as the inability to reach the cecum in 10 per cent of cases; potential for missing neoplasms, especially those located at flexures or behind folds; the need for patient sedation; and the often higher cost in comparison to barium enema.

Negative biopsy results of a fraction of a polyp cannot possibly exclude cancer; therefore total excision of a polyp is the only acceptable method of providing an accurate histologic diagnosis. However, for diminutive polyps it can be argued that as the frequency of severe dysplasia or invasive carcinoma is extremely rare (see earlier discussion), small growths could be simply fulgurated without biopsy. Indeed, for small rectosigmoid polyps this approach does not pose any unusual risk for the subsequent development of colon cancer or for survival.[107] The use of the "hot biopsy" forceps on small polyps provides an acceptable compromise in which the top of the polyp is removed while the base is destroyed by electrocautery. More important is the removal and histologic examination of all polyps during the initial colonoscopy, as this is appropriate to the management of these patients.

The role of colonoscopic laser ablation of colorectal adenomas is not yet defined. It appears to be most efficacious and safe for surveillance of the rectal stump in patients with familial polyposis coli who have undergone subtotal colectomy with ileorectal anastomosis.[108] Currently, in all other situations, laser ablation of adenomas should be confined to those lesions that are histologically confirmed in medically frail patients and that cannot be readily removed by usual endoscopic techniques or resected safely via laparotomy.

Screening Methods

For certain groups at high risk for developing colon cancer, such as those with previously treated adenomas or cancer or with a history suggesting a familial colonic cancer syndrome, periodic surveillance of the entire colon by either barium enema examination or, preferably, colonoscopy is indicated. The larger task is identifying premalignant lesions in the thousands of asymptomatic persons at average risk; clearly, less costly, more convenient, and acceptable screening approaches are necessary for this task. The two main approaches to colon cancer screening, namely, fecal occult blood testing and sigmoidoscopy, are discussed in more detail on page 1493. At this point, information on the detection of asymptomatic polyps is given.

Approximately 1 to 3 per cent of asymptomatic adults over age 40 years have a positive test for occult blood with guaiac-impregnated cards.[109] Fewer than half of these persons have a colorectal neoplasm; when found, adenomas outnumber carcinomas by 3:1. Thus, the percentage of all positive guaiac tests attributable to colonic neoplasms (i.e., positive predictive values) are 30 to 35 per cent for adenomas and 8 to 12 per cent for cancer.[110, 111] Despite the predominance of adenomas, 75 per cent of adenomas may be missed unless they are large or located in the distal portion of the colon.[84] Positive test results for occult blood one to two years after a negative search will detect some of these missed polyps.[112] However, because small polyps rarely bleed, sigmoidoscopy should be performed to complement occult blood testing.

Most experience to date for screening asymptomatic persons with sigmoidoscopy has been with the rigid instrument. By this method, polyps (of all histologic types) are detected in approximately 7 per cent of allegedly asymptomatic persons over 40 years old.[113] The removal of polyps through periodic rigid proctosigmoidoscopy decreases the expected number of subsequent rectal cancers by 85 per cent, and those persons who develop carcinoma have earlier stage lesions and better survival rates.[15]

Flexible sigmoidoscopy has now been demonstrated in several studies to be superior to rigid sigmoidoscopy in both symptomatic and asymptomatic populations[89–91, 114] (see also pp. 1537–1540). When used strictly for screening asymptomatic persons over the age of 40 years, the flexible instrument reveals polyps in 10 to 15 per cent.[89, 96, 97, 115] This yield is lower in screens of younger persons[116] and higher in persons with occult bleeding.[117] Most studies with flexible sigmoidoscopy (for any clinical indication) have used the 60-cm instrument. Its efficient use, however, requires more training than is anticipated for the 35-cm flexible sigmoidoscope, which has been developed mainly for screening purposes. Furthermore, it is expected that the shorter flexible instrument will be more readily accepted by both patients and physicians. The only study that has compared the 35-cm and 60-cm endoscopes in a screening setting (albeit by endoscopists) reported comparable sensitivity for detecting polyps within the range of the short instrument.[96] Further trials with the 35-cm endoscope will help to define its role in colon cancer screening.

Management of the Malignant Polyp

The term malignant polyp refers to any polyp containing a focus of carcinoma (Table 80–1). Cancer confined to the mucosa (none in the muscularis mucosae) is carcinoma *in situ* (Fig. 80–5). If it extends into or beyond the muscularis mucosae, it is termed invasive carcinoma. Sometimes, inclusions of benign adenomatous epithelium are found beneath the muscularis mucosae, and care must be taken not to mistake such "pseudocarcinomatous invasion" for true invasive carcinoma. Misplaced benign epithelium is seen more often in larger pedunculated polyps, particularly in the sigmoid colon.[118] Rarely, polyps consist entirely of carcinoma. These so-called polypoid carcinomas are usually considered a subset of malignant polyps, and they most likely represent a previous adenoma that is completely replaced by carcinoma.

The distinction between carcinoma *in situ* and invasive carcinoma is quite important because only the latter has the ability to metastasize. This is because there are virtually no lymphatic channels in the mu-

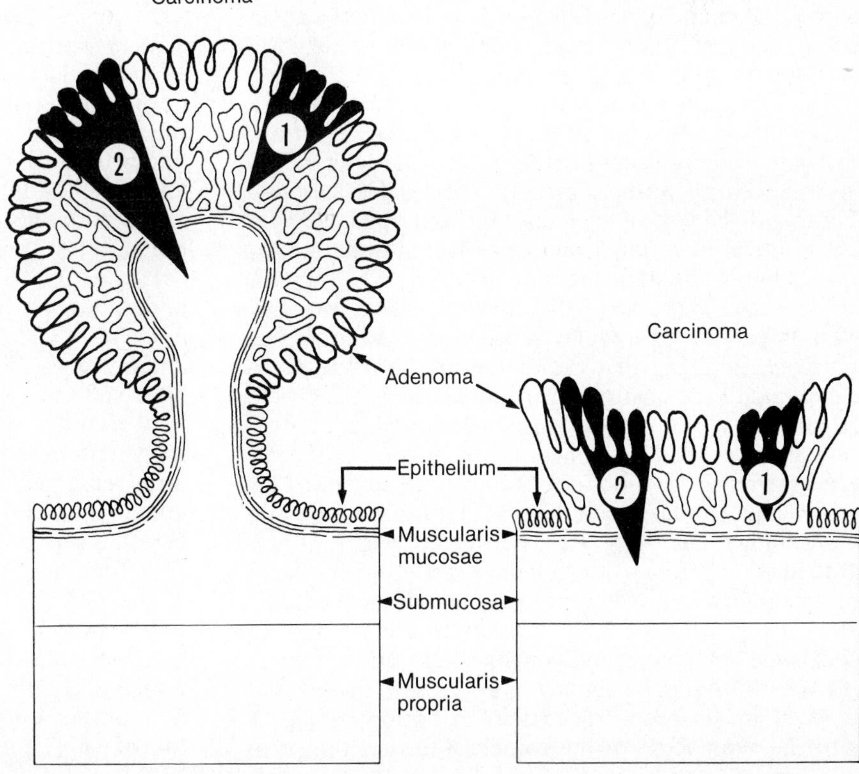

Figure 80–5. Carcinoma *in situ* versus invasive cancer. Carcinoma (shaded dark) is considered intramucosal or carcinoma in situ (as indicated by 1) either in a pedunculated adenoma (on the left) or in a sessile lesion (on the right). This lesion, as a rule, does not metastasize. Cancer in an adenomatous polyp is considered invasive when it breaches the *muscularis mucosae* (as indicated by 2). Invasive cancer in a pedunculated polyp is unlikely to metastasize, but it is managed differently from invasive cancer in a sessile polyp, which requires surgical resection (see text).

cosa.[119] Because the lymphatic plexus essentially begins at the muscularis mucosae, foci of cancer that pass the boundary between mucosa and muscularis mucosae can metastasize. The correct diagnosis will influence both management and prognosis, making proper orientation of tissue for pathologic examination crucial, as well as close communication between endoscopist, surgeon, and pathologist.[120, 121]

The removal of the vast majority of colorectal polyps endoscopically raises two central questions: is endoscopic polypectomy alone adequate therapy for the malignant polyp, and if not, what features of the polyp can predict the presence of residual disease or subsequent recurrence? The answers are vital because on them rests the decision for laparotomy and surgical resection of bowel to complement the polypectomy. Complete endoscopic removal of an adenoma with carcinoma *in situ* represents curative therapy. However, the therapeutic issue becomes much more difficult when polyps contain invasive carcinoma. Although many of these lesions are treated adequately by endoscopic polypectomy, at least 5 to 10 per cent of patients will experience an adverse outcome, defined as residual or metastatic carcinoma noted at subsequent operation or recurrent carcinoma developing during the follow-up period.

Several histopathologic features that might contribute to adverse outcome deserve strong emphasis. These include cancer involving the polypectomy margin; the presence of poorly differentiated (grade III) carcinoma; lymphatic or blood vessel invasion by cancer cells; sessile morphology; deep stalk invasion; and polypoid carcinoma. A strict comparison of studies of this problem is limited by selection bias, retrospective study design, small sample size, frequent coexistence of more than one histopathologic feature within a given polyp, and insufficient length of follow-up, particularly in more recent colonoscopic series.[122]

From these analyses, the following principles have emerged. If cancer involves the margin of resection, the polypectomy is considered inadequate and should be followed by further resection, preferably surgical. The major benefit of such an approach appears to be the removal of residual tumor, as lymph node metastases in this situation are rare in many[123–125] but not all[126] series. There are patients with positive margins who have not undergone subsequent resection but survived, implying that the diathermy burn can sufficiently eradicate microscopic residual disease.[123] Grade III histology (see pp. 1533–1535) and lymphatic invasion are most likely harbingers of an adverse outcome, although each one is rarely found independently of other adverse histopathologic determinants. Sessile morphology has also been correlated with adverse outcome.[126, 127] Invasive carcinoma limited to the head of a pedunculated polyp rarely has nodal metastases[126] and, when present, they are often attributable to coexisting lymphatic invasion or grade III histologic features.[119] As polypectomy may grossly distort the pedicle, it has been argued that extension of cancer into the submucosa of the colonic wall, not the presence or absence of a stalk, is the important criterion of significant invasion.[120, 128] Such extension, more readily achievable in sessile polyps (Fig. 80–5), carries a greater risk of nodal metastasis.[120] Polypoid carcinomas removed by polypectomy have been associated with a surprisingly favorable outcome when not complicated by grade III histologic type, lymphatic invasion, or tumor involving the margins.[120, 123, 126, 129]

Deciding on an optimal plan of management involves weighing the risk of death from residual or recurrent cancer after polypectomy alone against the risk of morbidity and mortality from a surgical attempt to cure residual disease or lymph node metastasis. Following are recommendations for making a decision. If adenoma excision is complete, endoscopic polypectomy alone is adequate therapy for adenomas containing carcinoma *in situ*, pedunculated adenomas harboring well-differentiated or moderately differentiated invasive carcinoma, and probably uncomplicated polypoid carcinomas. Resective surgery is indicated for malignant polyps in which the invasive carcinoma (1) is poorly differentiated (grade III); (2) involves endothelium-lined channels (lymphatics, blood vessels); (3) extends to the margin of resection; or (4) involves the submucosa of the colonic wall (this would include all sessile adenomas). Clearly, the ultimate plan of therapy must be individualized according to each patient's medical condition. However, for most patients with malignant polyps, polypectomy without surgical resection seems adequate, with the caveat that careful postpolypectomy endoscopic surveillance should be incorporated into the patient's health care.

Follow-up after Polypectomy

It is known that patients in whom a colorectal adenoma has been completely excised are likely to develop subsequent neoplasms, but the frequency and time course of this future transformation are poorly understood. Because it is impossible to distinguish among a lesion that is truly metachronous, a missed synchronous lesion, and an actual regrowth of a former polyp, all of these lesions are considered recurrences.

It is estimated that one third of persons who have undergone polypectomy will develop recurrent adenomas.[130–137] The recurrence rate at one year is approximately 5 to 15 per cent,[63, 136–138] although figures as high as 30 to 55 per cent have been reported.[133, 134, 139, 140] Certainly, some of these one-year "recurrences" represent missed synchronous adenomas.[140] In long-term retrospective studies, the cumulative risk of adenoma recurrence five years after polypectomy is 20 per cent, but after 15 years the risk rises to 50 per cent.[63]

Definition of clinical and histopathologic risk factors at the time of index polypectomy might help predict recurrence of polyps and is important in determining optimal intervals for surveillance examinations. Virtually all studies agree that the presence of multiple index adenomas is an important predictor of subsequent adenoma (and carcinoma) recurrence.[11, 63, 131, 132, 136–138, 141] This dictum applies despite negative findings on colonoscopy one year after polypectomy.[134, 140] Other factors that indicate increased risk of recurrence include large polyp size (greater than 1 cm),[135, 137, 138] severe dysplasia,[132, 138, 142] villous structure,[131, 137] and older age.[133, 141] The relative importance of each of these risk factors is uncertain, and results of studies are contradictory. Moreover, surprisingly little attention has been given to aging as a risk for recurrence despite the fact that the frequency and multiplicity of polyps increase with age. Until more data are available, it seems reasonable to divide patients into high- and low-risk categories, as listed in Table 80–7.

The optimal time intervals for colonoscopies of post-polypectomy patients have not been established. Knowledge of the growth rate of polyps, the frequency of missed synchronous adenomas, and the frequency of polyp recurrence leads to the following recommendations: (1) On the basis of findings at index polypectomy, patients should be assigned to either a low-risk or a high-risk category (Table 80–7); (2) after polypectomy, patients should undergo a colonoscopy within one year (perhaps at 6 to 12 months for high-risk patients) to detect missed synchronous lesions; (3) if results of this second examination are negative, colonoscopy should be performed every three to five years for low-risk individuals and every two years for the high-risk group. However, if the second examination reveals additional neoplasms, further examinations should be performed at yearly intervals to achieve an adenoma-free colon, at which point future examinations will be performed at the three- to five-year or two-year intervals. In all patients, fecal occult blood testing should be performed in the intervals between colonoscopies and, if results are positive, lead to immediate investigation.

This program of surveillance is based on limited knowledge about growth rates and recurrence rates of polyps, which comes primarily from retrospective studies with relatively short follow-up periods; hence, the foregoing recommendations may be too cautious. For example, an argument can be made for deferring or deleting the colonoscopy one year after removal of a solitary diminutive tubular adenoma. The understanding of adenoma prevalence and incidence will be greatly enhanced by results of large-scale prospective colonoscopic studies, such as the ongoing National Polyp Study[143] and the St. Mark's Neoplastic Follow-up Study.[135] When these data become available, both assignments of risk of future cancer and recommendations for surveillance will be based more accurately.

Table 80–7. RISK FACTORS FOR ADENOMA RECURRENCE

Low Risk	High Risk
Solitary adenoma	Multiple adenomas
Size <1 cm	Size ≥1 cm
Mild, moderate dysplasia	Severe dysplasia (carcinoma *in situ*)
Pedunculated	Sessile tubulovillous or villous
	Invasive carcinoma

NON-NEOPLASTIC POLYPS

Pathologically, all neoplastic polyps are part of an identifiable spectrum, but non-neoplastic polyps fall pathologically into several distinct and unrelated groups, including mucosal polyps, hyperplastic polyps, juvenile polyps, Peutz-Jeghers polyps, inflammatory polyps (secondary to numerous inflammatory lesions), and many different submucosal lesions (see Table 80–1).

Mucosal Polyps

Frequently an excrescence or mammillation of tissue is present in the colon that histologically is normal mucosa. In this instance, the submucosa has elevated the normal tissue overlying it. These lesions may be termed mucosal polyps, and their presence has no clinical significance. Mucosal polyps are almost always small and may constitute 8 to 20 per cent of the material recovered in a collection of colonoscopic biopsies. Colonic polyps less than 5 mm that were removed two years after their initial detection had neither grown nor become neoplastic.[144]

Hyperplastic Polyps

The commonest non-neoplastic polyp in the colon is the hyperplastic polyp, referred to by some pathologists as metaplastic polyps. These lesions have been reported to constitute as many as 29 per cent of the polyps found by magnifying glass in colons at autopsy.[44] However, as these lesions are small and are more common in the distal portion of the colon and rectum, their reported prevalence will be greater in studies that detect very small lesions or that are limited to the rectum.

Histologic Characteristics

Hyperplastic polyps are tiny, usually sessile lesions that are grossly indistinguishable from small adenomatous polyps. Microscopically, the colonic crypts have become elongated and the epithelium has assumed a characteristic papillary configuration (Fig. 80–6). The epithelium is made up of well-differentiated goblet and absorptive cells, and cytologic atypia is not seen. Mitoses and DNA synthesis are found at the base of the crypts, and orderly cell maturation is preserved.[6, 145] The epithelial cell and attendant pericryptal sheath fibroblast make up an epithelial-mesenchymal unit that migrates up the colonic crypt. In contrast to adenomatous polyps, in which the epithelium and fibroblast appear to be immature, this tissue is better differentiated, and abundant collagen is synthesized in the basement membrane.[146] It is thought that the migration of epithelial cells up the colonic crypt is slow, and that hyperplastic polyps develop from the failure of mature cells to detach normally.[147, 148] Hyperplastic polyps are usually small; the average size is less than 5 mm and

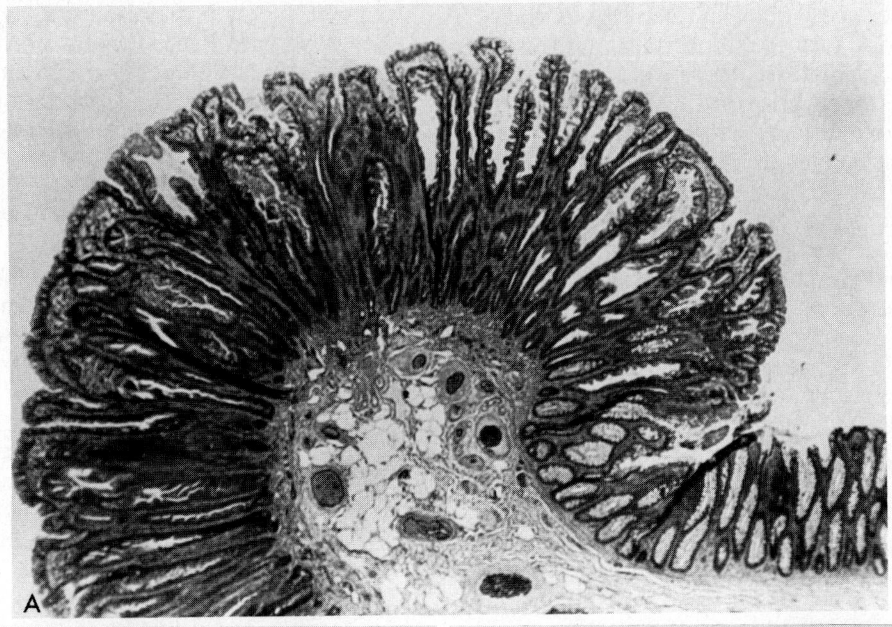

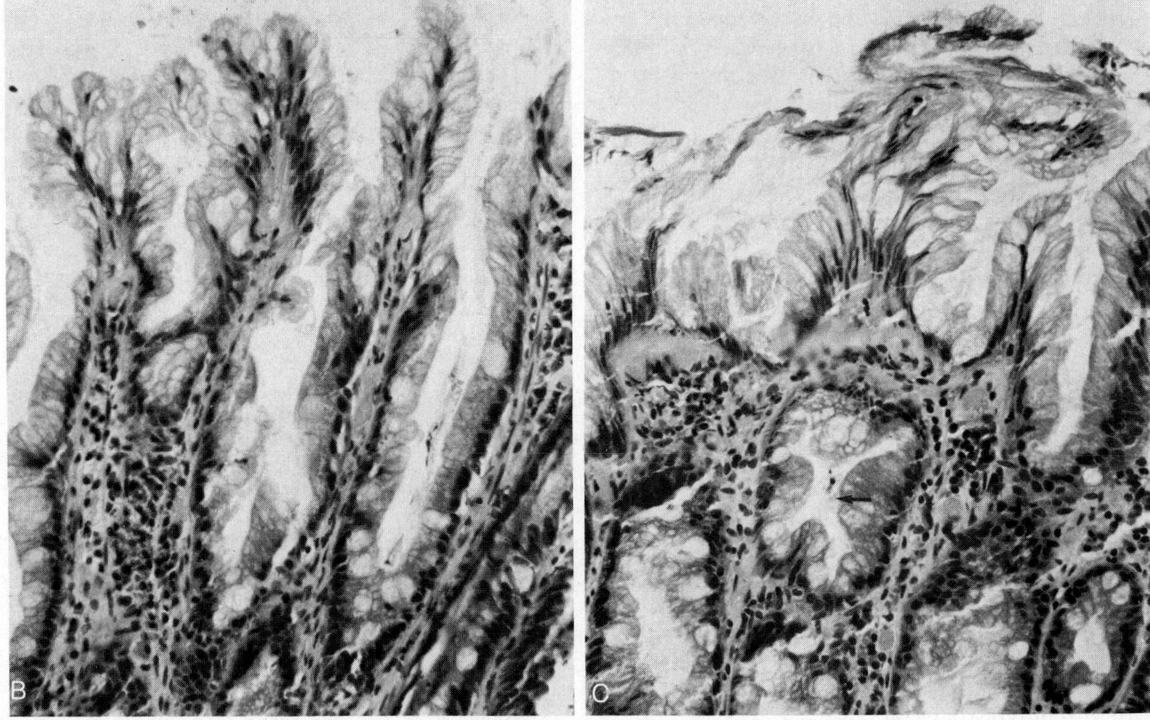

Figure 80–6. Hyperplastic polyp. *A*, Low-power photomicrograph of a hyperplastic polyp, demonstrating the typical serrated surface of the polyp. *B*, This high-power photomicrograph demonstrates the papillary fronds of a hyperplastic polyp, consisting of elongated epithelial cells containing generous amounts of mucus. The nuclei retain their basal orientation and demonstrate no atypia. *C*, This photomicrograph demonstrates the characteristic "starfish" appearance of hyperplastic glands cut in cross section (see *arrow*). Again, the orderly appearance of the nuclei, the generous cytoplasmic-nuclear ratio, and the abundance of secreted mucus at the surface of the polyp *(top)* can be readily appreciated.

only rarely greater than 10 mm, although giant hyperplastic polyps have been reported.[149]

Mixed hyperplastic-adenomatous polyps are not rare, constituting about 13 per cent of hyperplastic polyps,[150] and even foci of dysplasia and carcinoma may occasionally be found.[151, 152] Hyperplastic polyps and neoplastic lesions tend to appear in the same colons, suggesting that the two may be pathogenetically related. In addition, a variety of tumor markers (see pp. 1488–1489) are expressed in both hyperplastic polyps and neoplastic lesions of the colon.[35, 153, 154]

Epidemiology and Distribution of Hyperplastic Polyps

Although autopsy studies have reported that hyperplastic polyps are the most common colorectal polyps,[5, 6, 40, 155] more recent studies indicate that their frequency depends largely on the age and geographic distribution of the study population and on the method used to examine the colons.[43, 44, 47, 144, 156] Using a hand lens to scrutinize the colon at autopsy increases the detection of very small lesions, and hence, the relative proportion of hyperplastic polyps.[5] Sigmoidoscopic studies, which focus upon the distal colon and rectum, will also find more hyperplastic polyps. Colonoscopic studies selecting patients with pre-existing neoplastic lesions may increase the relative proportion of adenomas reported. The prevalence and multiplicity of hyperplastic polyps increases with age,[40, 44] and remarkably, 90 per cent of rectums resected for cancer contain hyperplastic polyps. In addition, more than 90 per cent of rectal polyps less than 3 mm in diameter are hyperplastic polyps.[6] The regional distribution of hyperplastic polyps based on autopsy series indicates a distal predominance,[40, 44–46, 156] with some studies noting a proximal shift with older age. It is fair to conclude that hyperplastic polyps make up the majority of tiny polyps in the distal colon and rectum, are epidemiologically associated with adenomas, are present near colorectal cancers, and are more common in elderly patients.[40, 46] Furthermore, they are most unlikely to give rise to a cancer. Thus, although hyperplastic polyps are not premalignant, they serve as markers of an increased risk of colorectal cancer.

Management

Hyperplastic polyps remain small, are usually sessile, and rarely give rise to symptoms. Inasmuch as they are very unlikely to give rise to cancer, little is gained by removing these polyps. However, because they cannot be distinguished from neoplastic polyps by gross examination, they are usually removed during surveillance for neoplastic lesions. The natural history of hyperplastic polyps is to remain small or to regress. The presence of hyperplastic polyps in the distal colon is not an alarming finding, particularly in the elderly patient. Their association with neoplastic lesions should alert the clinician to the possibility of an associated neoplasm, but follow-up colonoscopy is not necessary because of isolated hyperplastic polyps.

Juvenile Polyps

Juvenile polyps are mucosal tumors that consist primarily of an excess of lamina propria and dilated cystic glands, rather than an overabundance of epithelial cells, as seen in adenomatous and hyperplastic polyps. Juvenile polyps appear not to be neoplastic and are properly classified as hamartomas. The appearance of the distended, mucus-filled glands, inflammatory cells, and edematous lamina propria has prompted some observers to call these retention polyps. Juvenile polyps appear to be acquired lesions, as they are rarely seen in the first year of life and are most frequent from ages 1 to 7. They usually slough or regress spontaneously but are found occasionally in adults.[157] Juvenile polyps more often are single than multiple, usually are pedunculated, and tend to range in size from 3 mm to 2 cm (Fig. 80–7). Nearly three fourths of the lesions in one large study were found in the rectum. The stroma contains a generous vascular supply, which explains the considerable blood loss suffered by some patients. Because these polyps tend to be rectal and develop a stalk, they may prolapse during defecation. Juvenile polyps have no malignant potential when single, and they tend not to recur. Because of the high likelihood of bleeding and prolapse, removal of juvenile polyps is suggested. When they are multiple (i.e., in juvenile polyposis), the risk of developing cancer is present, apparently because of the adenomatous epithelium present in some juvenile polyps. This is discussed in more detail in the section on familial juvenile polyposis on pages 1509 and 1510.

Peutz-Jeghers Polyps

The Peutz-Jeghers polyp is a unique hamartomatous lesion characterized by prominent branching bands of smooth muscle within the lamina propria. This type of polyp is rarely found in the colon in the absence of generalized polyposis; it is discussed further on pages 1507 to 1509.

Inflammatory Polyps (Pseudopolyps)

Inflammatory polyps are found in the regenerative and healing phases of inflammation. They are formed by full-thickness ulceration of epithelium followed by a regenerative process that leaves the mucosa in bizarre polypoid configurations. The lesions may be large and solitary, mimicking a neoplastic mass. Mucosal bridges may be formed across the lumen. Multiple lesions are frequently seen that may mimic a polyposis syndrome (Fig. 80–8). The term pseudopolyp is often used to distinguish them from neoplastic lesions, but, by definition, these are true polyps. Histologically, inflammation and exuberant granulation tissue may be seen in the early postinflammatory period, but later the polyp may histologically resemble entirely normal mucosa.

Any form of severe colitis, including inflammatory

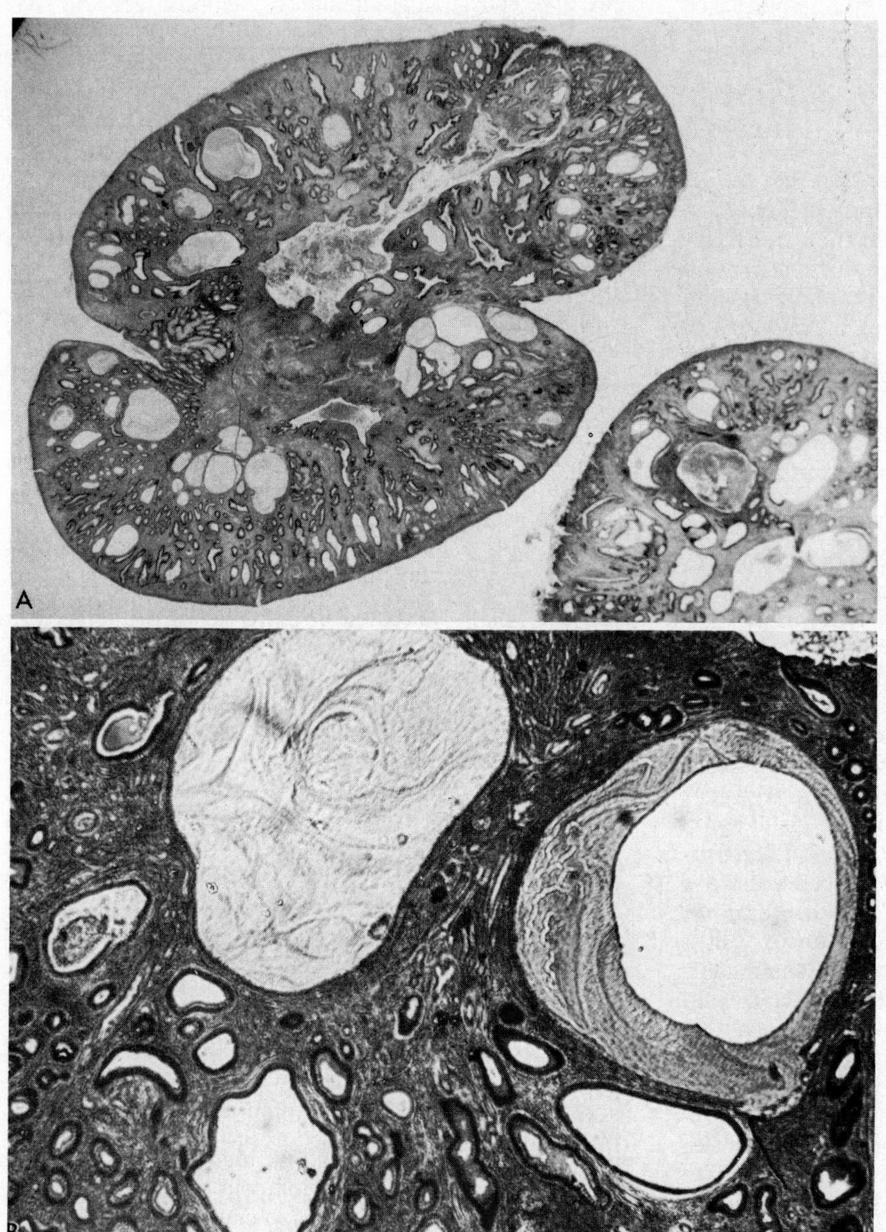

Figure 80–7. Juvenile polyp. *A,* This low-power photomicrograph demonstrates the dilated, mucus-filled glands and the extensive edema and inflammatory reaction in the lamina propria. *B,* This high-power view of a juvenile polyp demonstrates that in contrast to the adenomatous and hyperplastic polyps, the (darker) epithelial cells compose a relatively minor proportion of the total mass of the polyp, the majority of which consists of dilated glands and an expanded lamina propria.

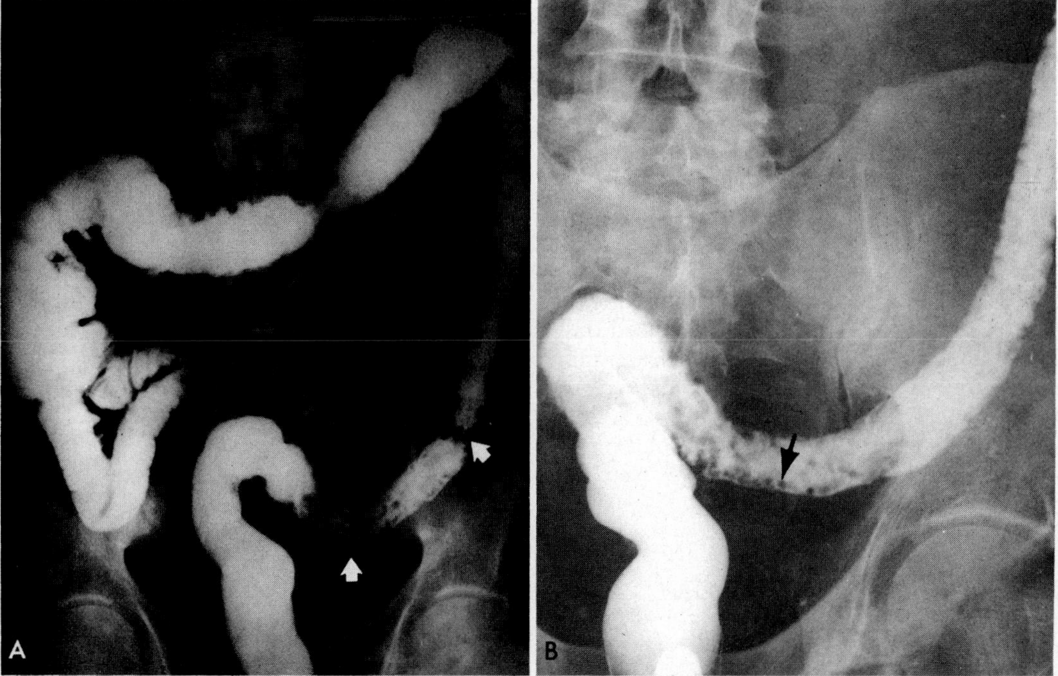

Figure 80–8. Pseudopolyps. *A,* This barium enema from a patient with ulcerative colitis demonstrates numerous inflammatory polyps ("pseudopolyps"). From the barium enema it can be concluded only that many polyps are present, and a colonoscopic biopsy is required to identify the nature of the lesion. The associated mucosal abnormalities seen at colonoscopic examination will assist in the proper identification of pseudopolyps; however, the physician must not overlook the possibility of a neoplastic lesion occurring in this setting. *B,* This spot film of the rectosigmoid region demonstrates the presence of multiple pseudopolyps in the sigmoid colon.

bowel disease,[158] amebic colitis,[159] or bacterial dysentery, may give rise to inflammatory polyps. In chronic schistosomiasis, multiple inflammatory polyps that contain granulation tissue, eggs, or adult worms are commonly seen.[160] The significance of these lesions, which have no intrinsic neoplastic potential, is that they often appear in diseased colons that are at high risk for developing colon cancer (ulcerative colitis, schistosomiasis), and therefore they must be distinguished from neoplastic lesions.

Rare cases of multiple and recurrent inflammatory gastrointestinal polyps producing pain and obstruction have been reported on a sporadic, and more recently, a familial, basis.[161] These lesions are found primarily in the ileum, may be very large, and may even cause intussusception.

Colitis Cystica Profunda

Colitis cystica profunda is a rare lesion, consisting of dilated, mucus-filled glands in the submucosa, which may form solitary or multiple polyps. The lesion typically is a solitary polyp less than 3 cm in size and is found most often in the rectum in the setting of chronic inflammation. Prior surgical procedures and ulcerative proctitis have been linked to the pathogenesis of this abnormality. The involved epithelium shows no evidence of dysplasia. The primary significance of this lesion is that it must be recognized and distinguished from colloid carcinoma, which may look similar histologically, because a mistaken diagnosis of colloid carcinoma could lead to inappropriate radical surgery.[162, 163] The lesion is presumably due to the displacement of normal colonic glands beneath the epithelium during the healing of a surgical wound or inflammation. Rarely, the lesions may become large or recurrent and can produce colonic obstruction.[164] It has been suggested that the pathologic picture and clinical presentation of colitis cystica profunda are similar to those of the so-called "solitary" rectal ulcer, and that both may be produced by rectal prolapse[163] (see pp. 1600–1605).

Pneumatosis Cystoides Intestinalis

Multiple air-filled cysts are frequently encountered within the submucosa of the colon (and small intestine) and may produce a polypoid appearance. The diagnosis of pneumatosis cystoides intestinalis (PCI) may be made on full-thickness pathologic sections or by the characteristic X-ray or endoscopic appearance of the intramural gas-filled cysts. This condition may produce symptoms suggestive of colitis, but it may also be associated with vague symptoms or be essentially asymptomatic.[165]

Two forms of PCI have been recognized. PCI may be associated with a fulminant mucosal process, such as inflammatory or ischemic bowel disease in adults, or necrotizing enterocolitis in children. In this setting, it is thought that the cysts result from invasion of the submucosa by gas-forming bacteria, which is commonly fatal.[166] In the adult, however, PCI is more typically a chronic or even incidental finding, and it may even be associated with an asymptomatic pneumoperitoneum. PCI is associated with chronic obstructive pulmonary disease and may be seen in patients with scleroderma. The genesis of the gas-filled cysts is incompletely understood, but it has been demonstrated that gas within the bowel lumen diffuses into the cysts, which may contribute to their maintenance. Oxygen therapy results in the resolution of these cysts,[167–169] but the pathophysiologic basis of this response is by no means clear. The natural history of PCI can be deduced only from a small number of cases, but the disease may persist for months.[165, 167] A single course of oxygen therapy (in surprisingly modest doses—often as low as 5 to 6 L O_2/minute) provides a long resolution of symptoms. Antibiotics are of no benefit[170] (see pp. 1595–1600).

OTHER SUBMUCOSAL LESIONS

Lesions beneath the colonic mucosa may elevate the overlying epithelium to produce a polypoid appearance. Colonoscopic biopsy of these polyps reveals normal mucosa.

Lymphoid tissue is present throughout the colon, and hypertrophied follicles may be mistaken for a pathologic mucosal process. Benign lymphoid polyps may even grow large enough to produce symptoms (pain, bleeding) or may become pedunculated. Multiple benign lymphoid polyps may be found as normal variants in children in particular (Fig. 80–9), and a malignant lymphoma may present with multiple polypoid lesions.[171] The importance of benign lymphoid polyps is in their difficult distinction from the malignant lymphoid lesions.

The colon is the most common gastrointestinal site for lipomas, which tend to be solitary (but may be multiple) submucosal lesions. They usually are asymptomatic and are detected incidentally. The low density of fat may give the lesion a characteristic radiographic appearance, and the soft, deformable nature of the lesion is helpful to the colonoscopist. Colonic lipomas are most frequent in the right colon and tend to occur on or near the ileocecal valve.[172] Removal of these lesions is usually unnecessary.

Important lesions such as carcinoids, metastatic neoplasms (especially melanoma), and other rare malignancies may produce submucosal lesions without distinctive identifying characteristics. Other submucosal lesions may be detected incidentally as curiosities, including fibromas, neurofibromas, leiomyomas, hemangiomas, and endometriosis (see pp. 1359–1369).

POLYPS AT URETEROSIGMOIDOSTOMY SITES

Patients who have undergone a previous urinary diversion procedure with implantation of the ureters into the sigmoid colon are at particularly high risk to develop neoplastic lesions at the ureterosigmoidostomy sites.[173, 174] The most important lesions are adenomatous polyps and carcinomas, which have been found after latent periods of 2 to 38 years, with mean latent periods of 20 and 26 years for adenomas and carcinomas, respectively.[174] Lesions resembling juvenile polyps and inflammatory polyps have also been reported at ureterosigmoidostomy sites.[175] It appears that at least 29 per cent of such patients develop colonic neoplasms, usually close to the stoma, after this procedure.[174] It has been suggested that these lesions are produced by the generation of *N*-nitrosamines from urinary amines in the presence of the fecal flora.[176] In view of the extremely high frequency of neoplasia in this setting, these patients must undergo lifelong colonoscopic surveillance in keeping with the long latent period between the implantation of the ureters and the subsequent development of colonic neoplasia.

THE POLYPOSIS SYNDROMES

Although the gastrointestinal polyposis syndromes were described over a century ago, only recently have

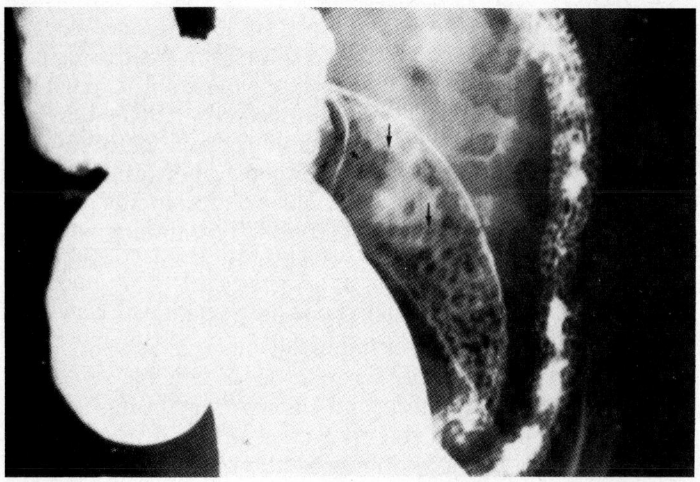

Figure 80–9. Lymphoid polyps. This spot film of the sigmoid colon demonstrates diffuse lymphoid hyperplasia throughout the colon of a child. Exuberant lymphoid hyperplasia may be a normal variant in some children; a malignant lymphoma may also rarely present a similar X-ray picture. At close examination of the radiograph, these polyps often display characteristic umbilication.

the clinical features, heredity, pathology, and natural history of these disorders been categorized.[177] Some of the traditional literature attempted to subdivide the polyposis syndromes according to diverse yet characteristic clinical features. Information regarding the pathology, natural history, and cellular biology of these disorders has permitted a more rational classification of certain of these syndromes and indicates that the familial adenomatous polyposis syndromes are all variable expressions of a single disease process.

Classification

The polyposis syndromes may be classified first into familial and nonfamilial groups. The familial polyposis syndromes are all inherited as autosomal dominant diseases. The nonfamilial polyposes are a heterogeneous collection of syndromes linked only by the presence of multiple gastrointestinal polyps. The familial polyposis syndromes may be subdivided into two major groups depending on whether the polyps are adenomas or hamartomas. It is critical to identify the polyposis syndrome properly, as carcinomas generally do not evolve from hamartomas, whereas the very high frequency of malignant change is the primary problem in the adenomatosis syndromes.

The Inherited Adenomatous Polyposis Syndromes

The inherited adenomatous polyposis syndromes include several entities that are characterized by the development of hundreds of adenomatous polyps in the colon. The various syndromes are distinguished by the presence or absence of other related features (Table 80–8).

Table 80–8. FAMILIAL ADENOMATOUS POLYPOSIS SYNDROMES: CLINICAL CHARACTERISTICS

Syndrome	Location of Polyps	Extraintestinal Abnormalities
Familial polyposis coli	Primarily colonic adenomas; also ileal, duodenal, ampullary, and antral adenomas Fundic gland hyperplasia Lymphoid polyps of terminal ileum	Osteomas of the mandible; dental abnormalities
Gardner's syndrome	Colonic, small intestinal, ampullary, and gastric adenomas Fundic gland hyperplasia Lymphoid aggregates of terminal ileum	Osteomas of the mandible, skull, and long bones; epidermoid and sebaceous cysts; lipomas; fibromas; desmoid tumors; thyroid and adrenal tumors Hypertrophy of pigmented retinal epithelium
Turcot's syndrome	Colonic adenomas	Malignant gliomas and other brain tumors

Familial Polyposis Coli

Clinical Characteristics. Familial polyposis coli (FPC) is a disease in which the defect is inherited as an autosomal dominant trait; however, the abnormal gene has not been identified. Recently, genetic linkage analysis localized the gene for FPC to the long arm of chromosome 5, but the exact identity and function of the gene are not yet known.[177a] It is characterized by the progressive development of hundreds to thousands of adenomatous polyps in the large intestine. If the colon is not removed, the development of colon cancer is inevitable. A patient who inherits the gene for FPC is usually asymptomatic until after puberty, at which time polyps may begin to appear in some patients; rarely, however, polyps appear in the first decade of life. In the largest series of FPC cases, the average age at onset of polyps was 25 years, but symptoms did not appear until 33 years. The average age for the diagnosis of adenomas was 36 years, for cancer 39 years, and for death from cancer 42 years. Ninety per cent of FPC cases have been identified by age 50 years.[178] Approximately 20 per cent of cases have a negative prior family history and may represent new mutations.

Younger patients initially have a small number of polyps, but the number increases progressively until the colon becomes studded with lesions throughout its length (Figs. 80–10 and 80–11). All varieties of adenomatous polyps may be seen, including tubular adenomas, tubulovillous adenomas, and villous adenomas. The initial macroscopic lesions may be one or a small number of tiny polyps; eventually, the colon will develop thousands of polyps. The number of macroscopic polyps in a colectomy specimen averages 1000. Histologic examination of the colon reveals numerous microscopic adenomas as well, the smallest of which may involve a single colonic crypt. The size and number of polyps correspond to the latent period between the onset of clinical disease and the time of colectomy, so that tumors tend to be larger in the symptomatic propositus cases than in asymptomatic, usually younger, relatives discovered by screening. In all cases, the vast majority of polyps are tiny (less than 5 mm). Individually, these polyps are identical to adenomatous polyps found in the general population.

Colorectal cancer should be considered an inevitable consequence in the natural history of FPC, appearing approximately 10 to 15 years after the onset of the polyposis. Colorectal cancer is found in 79 per cent of the index cases of FPC but in only 9 per cent of asymptomatic relatives screened for the disease. Therefore, diligent surveillance of the relatives of FPC patients is the key to the prevention of cancer. The cancers have the same pathologic grades of malignancy and the same distribution within the colon as is seen in the general population, except that multiple simultaneous cancers are much more frequent (48 per cent of cases).[178]

A variety of extracolonic lesions previously assumed to be characteristic of Gardner's syndrome are now recognized in many cases of FPC. In fact, families with polyposis cannot always be categorized exclusively as

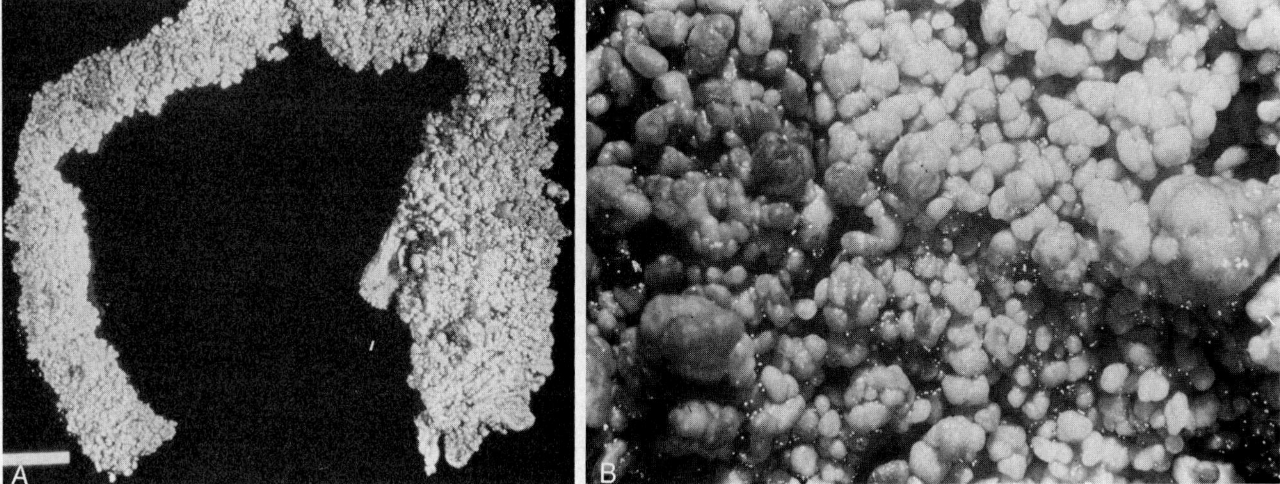

Figure 80–10. Familial polyposis coli. *A*, Patients with familial polyposis have multiple adenomatous polyps often carpeting the colon, as demonstrated in this specimen. *B*, This close-up of an excised specimen of colon demonstrates the presence of innumerable polyps of varying shapes and sizes. The polyps are all adenomas and may contain villous elements or carcinoma. Obviously, a total colectomy is the only reasonable management in this situation. (Courtesy of Stanley R. Hamilton, M.D., and Gordon D. Luk, M.D.)

having purely FPC or Gardner's syndrome. Certain extracolonic manifestations are seen in most FPC patients, whereas others seem to segregate in certain FPC families. When carefully sought, mandibular osteomas can be seen in up to 90 per cent of patients with FPC.[179, 180] Orthopantomography of the mandible is a simple and noninvasive means that may be used to screen for early carriers of the FPC gene; however, it is critical to distinguish nonspecific sclerotic lesions in the mandible from true osteomas. Mandibular osteomas in FPC tend to be multiple throughout the mandible, whereas nonspecific sclerotic bony lesions are usually single and are located close to a diseased tooth (see Fig. 80–14*B*).

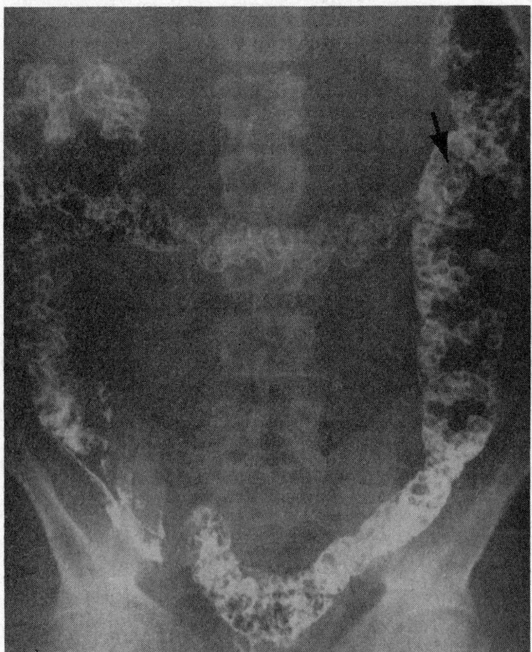

Figure 80–11. Familial polyposis coli. This barium enema of a patient with familial polyposis demonstrates the diffuse studding of the large bowel with the polyps, as seen in Figure 80–10. Note the variation in size and shape of the polyps. This radiograph is consistent with any of the multiple adenomatous polyposis syndromes.

Polyps may also be seen in the upper gastrointestinal tract in FPC.[181] Adenomatous polyps may be found in the gastric antrum, duodenum, periampullary region, and ileum.[182] In addition to the adenomatous polyps, polypoid lymphoid aggregates may be seen in the terminal ileum of patients with FPC, and fundic gland polyposis may occur in the proximal stomach of FPC patients.[183] Fundic gland polyposis consists of multiple small hyperplastic gastric glands that appear not to grow in size or undergo adenomatous or carcinomatous transformation.[184] In addition, adenomatous changes have been reported in the papilla of Vater in 50 per cent of FPC patients.[185] Over half of FPC patients have gastric lesions of some variety, including microcarcinoids in addition to the aforementioned lesions.[186] Gastric carcinoma has been reported in FPC but is actually quite rare in this setting in the United States.

Metabolic and Cellular Abnormalities in FPC (Table 80–9, Fig. 80–12). The familial transmission of FPC indicates that a genetic mechanism must be responsible for abnormal growth of gastrointestinal epithelium. In the normal colon, the proliferative compartment is limited to the lower half of the crypts of Lieberkühn. The new cells migrate to the upper half of the crypt, where they differentiate, and new DNA synthesis is repressed. In adenomatous polyps, DNA synthesis is seen throughout the glandular crypts, indicating a failure of the normal repression of DNA synthesis, consistent with the neoplastic nature of the lesion. However, in normal-appearing colonic mucosa from FPC patients, a similar defect in normal cell differentiation is seen throughout the colonic crypt, indicating that the flat epithelium behaves like neoplastic tissue.[187]

Ornithine decarboxylase is the rate-limiting enzyme in polyamine biosynthesis, which is essential for intes-

Table 80–9. CELLULAR AND METABOLIC ABNORMALITIES IN THE ADENOMATOUS POLYPOSIS SYNDROMES

Colonic Epithelium
Inappropriate proliferation in the upper colonic crypt[187]
Increased ornithine decarboxylase activity[188]
Abnormal response to tumor promoter[197]
Increased tetraploidy in cultured colonic fibroblasts (Gardner's syndrome)[200]
Abnormal mucins[32, 204, 205]
Skin Fibroblasts in Culture
Loss of contact inhibitions[189]
Decreased serum requirements for growth[189]
Elevated production of plasminogen activator[189]
Disordered actin cables[190]
Increased susceptibility to transforming virus,[189] irradiation,[191] and chemical carcinogens[192–193]
Abnormal response to tumor promoters[194–196]
Increased tetraploidy in mixed fibroblast-epithelial cell cultures[198]
Chromosomal instability[199, 202] and heterochromatin inversions[201]
Increased methionine dependence[203]
Fecal Studies[206, 207]
Abnormal flora
Abnormal degradation of fecal steroids (cholesterol and bile acids)

tinal mucosal proliferation. The activity of this enzyme is increased in colonic adenomas. A significant increase in ornithine decarboxylase activity is also seen in the flat colonic mucosa of patients with FPC compared with controls, again indicating an abnormality in the control of mucosal proliferation in these colons. An increase in the activity of this enzyme is seen in some at-risk but unaffected first-degree relatives of patients with FPC, suggesting that this abnormality may antedate the onset of polyposis and be useful as a screening tool.[188]

Fibroblasts from skin biopsies of patients with FPC have been maintained in monolayer culture, permitting the study of their growth. Cultured skin fibroblasts from the normal-appearing skin of FPC patients demonstrate a loss of the normal contact inhibition, a reduction in the serum requirements for growth, increased production of plasminogen activator, and an abnormality in the actin cable array, indicating that these mesenchymally derived cells also have disordered control of growth.[189, 190] These fibroblasts are 100- to 1000-fold more susceptible to transformation by murine sarcoma virus than control fibroblasts.[189] Similarly, these fibroblasts are more susceptible than control cells to damage by X-ray and ultraviolet light irradiation[191] and to the effects of chemical carcinogens.[192, 193] Culture of these cells in the presence of a phorbol ester, a tumor promoter, produces an unusual response compared to normal skin fibroblasts. FPC fibroblasts are more resistant to the toxic effects of the tumor promoter, to which they respond with increased cloning efficiency, enhanced growth, and the ability to grow in

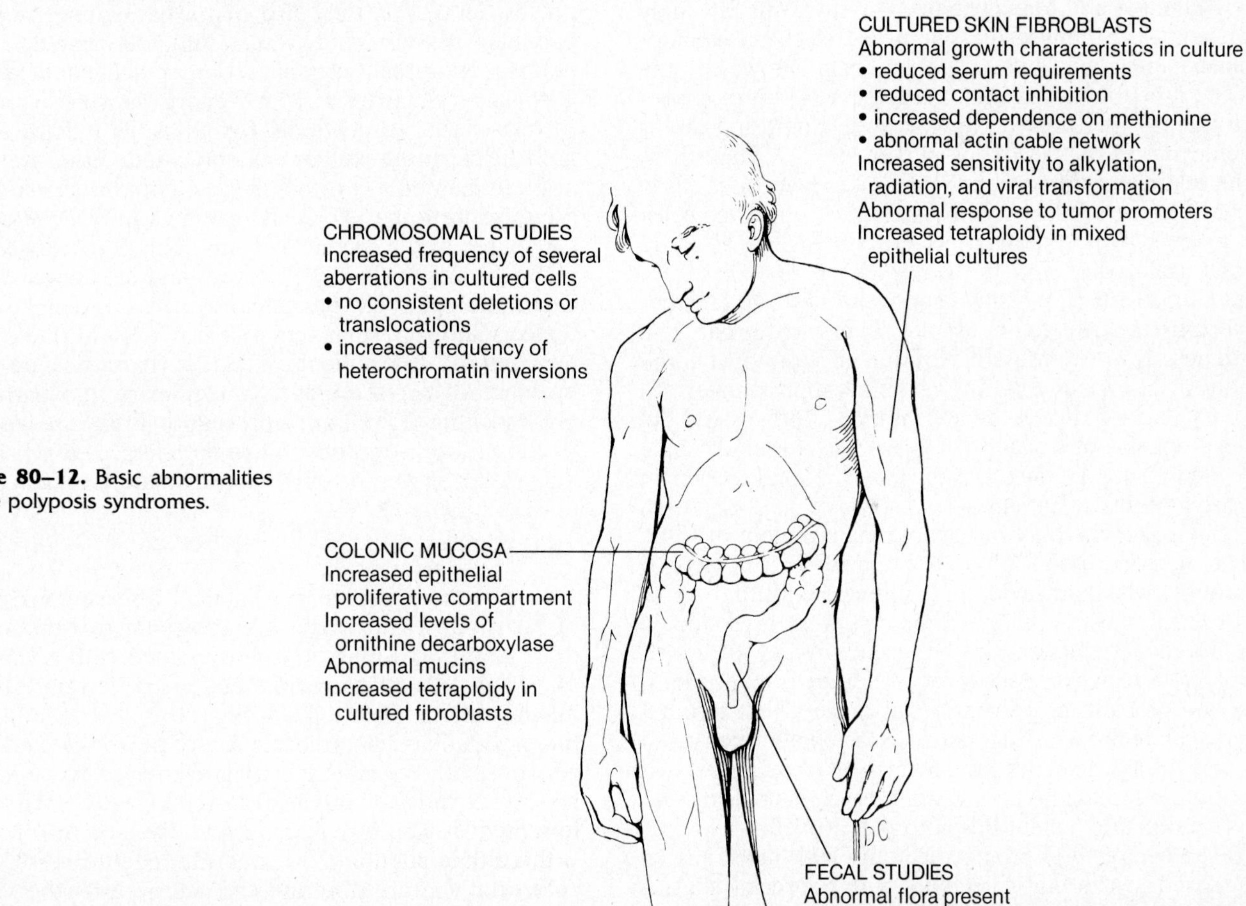
CULTURED SKIN FIBROBLASTS
Abnormal growth characteristics in culture
• reduced serum requirements
• reduced contact inhibition
• increased dependence on methionine
• abnormal actin cable network
Increased sensitivity to alkylation, radiation, and viral transformation
Abnormal response to tumor promoters
Increased tetraploidy in mixed epithelial cultures
CHROMOSOMAL STUDIES
Increased frequency of several aberrations in cultured cells
• no consistent deletions or translocations
• increased frequency of heterochromatin inversions
COLONIC MUCOSA
Increased epithelial proliferative compartment
Increased levels of ornithine decarboxylase
Abnormal mucins
Increased tetraploidy in cultured fibroblasts
FECAL STUDIES
Abnormal flora present
• decreased degradation of cholesterol
DC

Figure 80–12. Basic abnormalities in the polyposis syndromes.

semi-solid medium.[194–196] Primary cultures of colonic epithelial cells from FPC patients also show enhanced DNA synthesis in response to tumor promoter.

Early-passage skin fibroblast cultures from patients with FPC show an increase in all classes of chromosome aberrations compared with control cells.[198, 199] A similar type of chromosomal instability is also found in cultured colonic fibroblasts and lymphocytes from these patients.[199, 200] Chromosomes from cultured skin fibroblasts of FPC patients have a significantly higher than normal frequency of partial and total heterochromatin inversions on chromosome number 9.[201] In addition, chromosomes from cultured skin fibroblasts of FPC patients are significantly more susceptible to damage after exposure to chemical carcinogen.[202]

Abnormalities of mucin structure are also seen throughout the colons of patients with FPC, including increased expression of sialomucins[204] and mucins binding *Ulex europaeus*-1 lectin[32] and peanut lectin.[205]

It has been suggested that the fecal flora may be abnormal in FPC patients, resulting in the production of carcinogenic compounds. Stool from FPC patients contains lower levels of the anaerobic flora capable of dehydrogenating the steroid nucleus, resulting in increased excretion of undegraded cholesterol and other fecal bile acids.[206, 207] However, the stool from FPC patients does not appear to contain unusual carcinogens, and the precise role of the altered colonic flora in this disease is still unclear.

Diagnosis and Management. Patients with FPC may present with nonspecific symptoms, such as hematochezia, diarrhea, and abdominal pain. However, the key to the diagnosis and management of this disease is to identify the presymptomatic individual, and this is achieved by the assiduous pursuit of the diagnosis in the relatives of affected patients. The diagnosis is easily made or excluded by colonoscopy or an air-contrast barium enema examination. The presence of more than 100 polyps and the confirmation that these are adenomas establishes the diagnosis of FPC, and further work-up of the colon usually is not required. The studies from St. Mark's Hospital in London on the natural history of FPC suggests that approximately 10 years elapse between the appearance of polyps and the development of cancer;[178] however, it is not advisable to delay surgery once the diagnosis is made, even in presymptomatic patients.

Surgery is the only reasonable management of FPC. The administration of ascorbic acid (3 gm/day) to patients who had undergone subtotal colectomy with ileorectal anastomosis has been reported to produce a temporary reduction in the total number of rectal polyps.[208] However, this form of therapy is inadequate, in and of itself, to prevent rectal cancer. Nonsteroidal anti-inflammatory drugs have occasionally been used in an attempt to reduce the formation of rectal polyps, but the scientific basis of this approach is unclear, and its therapeutic benefit has not been proved.

The use of total proctocolectomy with ileostomy as opposed to subtotal colectomy with ileorectal anastomosis is a decision that must be made on an individual basis. The former operation is clearly the most effective in terms of eliminating the possibility of recurrent rectal carcinoma; however, it is unacceptable to some patients. The success of the latter operation, of course, depends on prevention of future carcinoma in the rectal segment. The subset of patients with adenomatous polyposis coli for whom rectal preservationis ideal are those with relatively few rectal polyps, as they tend not to develop rectal carcinoma subsequently.[209] This group of patients is older (with a median age of 58 years) and often has negative family history for polyposis. Subtotal colectomy in younger persons (median age of 35 years) with many rectal polyps, on the other hand, is risky. In contrast to the older patients, for whom the operation is successful, about one fifth of this group will develop cancer in 5 to 23 years. Of those who are followed for more than 20 years, about three fifths will develop carcinoma in the rectal stump despite semi-annual sigmoidoscopic surveillance and fulguration of polyps. The prognosis in patients who develop rectal cancers is dismal, the five-year disease-free survival rate being about 25 per cent.[209]

These data provide a strong case for total proctocolectomy with ileostomy for FPC patients who have rectal polyps. In spite of this ominous warning, some physicians have advocated rectum-sparing operations and have achieved a reasonable degree of success.[210–212] Internists at one large clinic agree that a subtotal colectomy is safe for those whose rectums are free of polyps. However, they also spare the rectum in those patients with rectal polyps, carefully following them to perform additional surgery as soon as malignant change is found.[210] A British group reports satisfaction with rectum-sparing procedures for all patients with FPC and, furthermore, fulgurates only adenomas 5 mm or more in diameter at three- to six-month intervals. This group reports that 11 of 173 patients have developed carcinoma in the rectum, but that only 3 of 11 died of rectal cancer.[211] Investigators at another large clinic also support the use of colectomy with ileorectal anastomosis and report an actuarial survivorship rate of 88 per cent of 133 patients after 20 years, despite the presence of rectal polyps.[212] It appears that patients may elect the more limited procedure if they are willing to comply with rigorous follow-up and accept a risk of malignancy in the rectum of approximately 10 per cent.

Gardner's Syndrome

Gardner's syndrome is a familial disease consisting of gastrointestinal polyposis and osteomas of the mandible, skull, and long bones, associated with a variety of benign soft tissue tumors and other extraintestinal manifestations (Table 80–8, Fig. 80–13). The colon is the predominant but not sole site of polyposis, and the genetic, pathologic, and clinical characteristics of this disease include all of the features of FPC. Both are inherited as autosomal dominant diseases that begin with colonic adenomatosis and ultimately progress to colorectal cancer. Both are characterized by the same abnormalities of epithelial cell proliferation in the

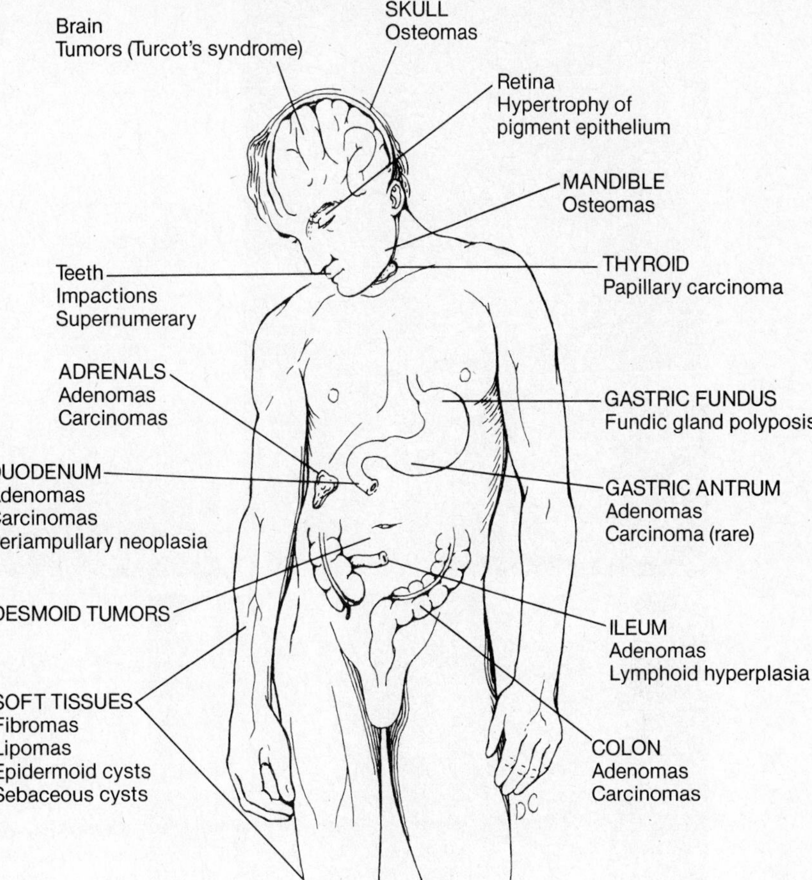

Figure 80–13. Schematic representation of Gardner's syndrome. The primary features consist of a triad of colonic polyposis, bone tumors (particularly in the skull and mandible), and soft tissue tumors. The organs and tissues principally involved are shown in capitals; other structures with associated findings are given in lower case.

colon, and both demonstrate abnormal growth characteristics in cultured skin fibroblasts (Table 80–9, Fig. 80–12).

An additional abnormality in cultured dermal biopsies was initially reported in Gardner's syndrome but has subsequently been found also in some patients with FPC. Mixed fibroblast-epithelial cell cultures of normal-appearing skin from patients with polyposis show an increase in incorporation of ^{3}H-thymidine and increased tetraploidy based upon metaphase preparations and flow cytometry.[198] Increased tetraploidy is seen in cultured colonic fibroblasts from patients with Gardner's syndrome as well.[200] Gardner's syndrome is considered by many investigators to be a form of FPC that includes a variety of additional inherited extraintestinal manifestations.

The small intestine is subject to neoplastic growth in Gardner's syndrome. The duodenum, and in particular the periampullary region, may develop adenomatous polyps, and the frequency of carcinoma in this region may be as high as 12 per cent.[213] Jejunal and ileal polyps are less common, and small intestinal carcinoma outside the duodenum is rare. Lymphoid hyperplasia is present in Gardner's syndrome and can be distinguished from adenomatous polyps only by biopsy.

The stomach also has multiple polyps in Gardner's syndrome, including adenomas, fundic gland hyperplasia, and microcarcinoids.[186] Gastric carcinoma has been reported to complicate Gardner's syndrome in Japan, but it is rare in the Western world.

The extracolonic manifestations of Gardner's syndrome include osteomas of the mandible, skull, and long bones; exostoses; epidermoid cysts, including sebaceous cysts; fibromas; lipomas; mesenteric fibromatosis and desmoid tumors (in the presence or absence of prior surgery); various dental abnormalities (including mandibular cysts, impacted teeth, and supernumerary teeth); and rarely, neoplasms of the thyroid and adrenal glands (Fig. 80–14).

Hypertrophy of the pigmented retinal epithelium has been reported in some families with Gardner's syndrome.[214] Over 90 per cent of affected persons have pigmented ocular fundus lesions (versus 4.8 per cent of controls), which are likely to be multiple (63.4 per cent have four or more lesions) and are bilateral in 86.5 per cent of those affected. Pigmented ocular fundic lesions are found in approximately half of the unaffected but at-risk first-degree relatives and have been identified in infants as young as three months old, suggesting that they are probably congenital. The presence of multiple, bilateral lesions appears to be a reliable marker for gene carriage in Gardner's syndrome.[215]

Confusion between Gardner's syndrome and FPC has resulted from the variable inheritance or penetrance of the extraintestinal features of Gardner's syndrome. Certain extraintestinal features are ex-

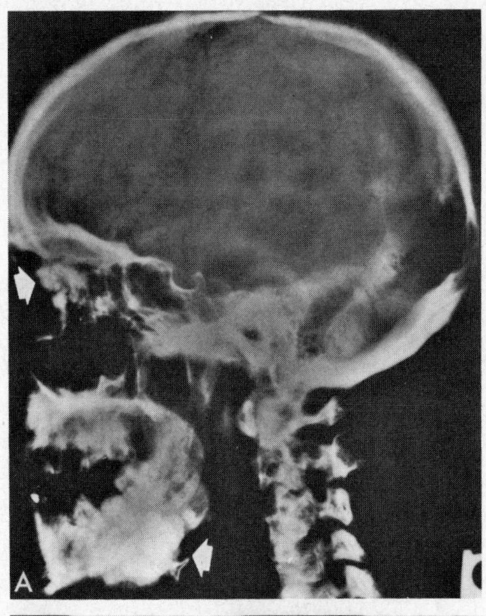

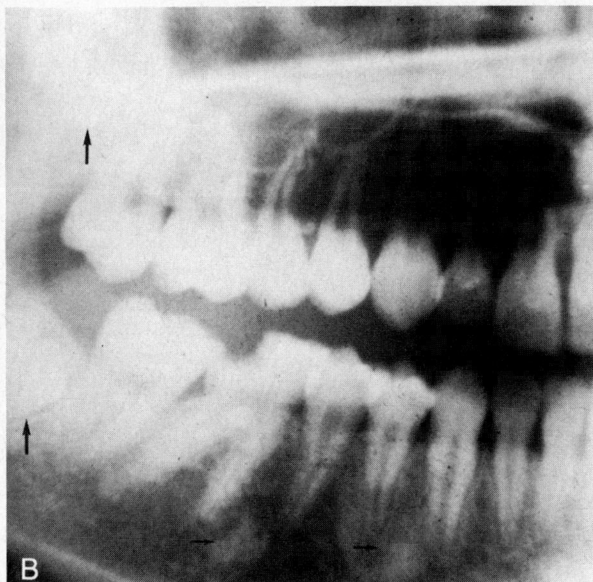

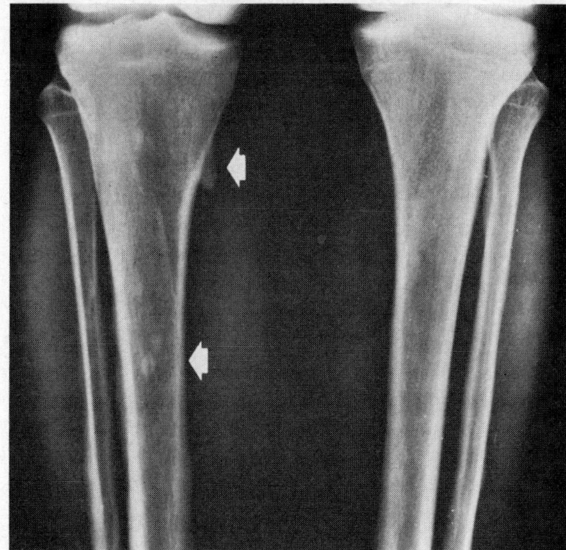

Figure 80–14. Stigmata of Gardner's syndrome. *A,* Multiple osteomas are apparent in the skull of this patient with documented colonic polyposis. Supernumerary and impacted teeth are also visible on this X-ray. The mandible contains numerous osteomas. *B,* This X-ray of the jaw demonstrates two impacted teeth *(larger vertical arrows),* and at least two mandibular osteomas *(smaller horizontal arrows).* The osteomas characteristic of Gardner's syndrome may be distinguished from ordinary sclerotic lesions of the jaw when they are multiple (as demonstrated here) and not contiguous with the root of the tooth. (Courtesy of Stefan Levin, D.D.S., and Gordon D. Luk, M.D.) *C,* Tibial osteomas and osteosclerosis are apparent in this patient with Gardner's syndrome *(arrows).*

pressed more prominently in some families with Gardner's syndrome. Within a single family, the disease may express itself variably in different individuals, including skipped generations and even discordance in identical twins. Some extraintestinal manifestations may appear in the absence of polyposis coli.

The foregoing observations make it difficult to argue that FPC and Gardner's syndrome are completely distinct entities. Occult osteomas of the mandible may be found in 90 per cent of FPC patients without other stigmata of Gardner's syndrome.[179] Most FPC patients are found to have duodenal adenomas when they are specifically sought.[216] These observations, coupled with the overlapping abnormalities in colonic epithelial cell proliferation, cultured skin fibroblasts, chromosomal fragility, and so forth, make a strong argument that FPC and Gardner's syndrome are variable expressions of a single disease that is characterized by a generalized abnormality of epithelial and fibroblast cell growth and has a variable association with a multiplicity of clinical manifestations. It is not yet clear whether one or more genes participate in the variable expression of the disease spectrum.[217]

Desmoid Tumors. A particularly serious complication of the polyposis syndromes (FPC and Gardner's syndrome) is the development of diffuse mesenteric fibromatosis, also called desmoid tumors. Commonly, these are progressive growths of mesenteric fibroblasts occurring after laparotomy, but they may occasionally appear spontaneously. They cause gastrointestinal obstruction, vascular obstruction, involvement of the ureters, and ultimately, death. Additional operative procedures are of no avail in this condition. Desmoid tumors complicate the course of nearly one fifth of patients with Gardner's syndrome and rank second, after metastatic carcinoma, among lethal complications of the disease.[218] They may, however, respond to radiation when localized and accessible.[219] Unfortunately, most tumors are in the mesentery in these patients, making radiation therapy impractical. Some encouraging results may follow administration of agents such as nonsteroidal anti-inflammatory drugs,[220] an antiestrogen drug,[221] and progesterone.[222] None of these methods is uniformly effective, but neither is surgery. The relationship between the abnormal growth of skin fibroblasts in culture and the behavior of fibroblasts in desmoid tumors in patients with familial colonic polyposis is fascinating, but explanations for it are still quite speculative.

Turcot's Syndrome (Glioma-Polyposis)

The association of familial colonic polyposis with malignant brain tumors has given rise to the term Turcot's syndrome.[223, 224] The initial reports of this entity described pairs of affected siblings whose parents did not have polyposis, suggesting an autosomal recessive mode of inheritance.[224] However, none of these afflicted individuals has borne progeny to test the mode of inheritance. Moreover, brain tumors are well-known features of FPC and Gardner's syndrome.[225–227] At present there is insufficient evidence to prove that they are inherited in an autosomally dominant fashion in the polyposis syndromes, and it appears that brain tumors are part of the extraintestinal manifestations of FPC and Gardner's syndrome.

Other Familial Adenomatous Polyposis Syndromes

Patients with the familial adenomatous polyposis syndromes typically have 100 to 5000 colonic adenomas. Some patients without familial polyposis develop recurrent adenomatous polyps of the colon, but rarely do they have more than 50 adenomas. Other familial syndromes in which a high incidence of colonic cancer is associated with a small number of colonic adenomas, such as Muir's and Torre's syndromes, are probably part of the spectrum of nonpolyposis familial colonic cancer[177] and should not be confused with FPC or Gardner's syndrome. Also, a tendency to develop adenomatous polyps and colorectal cancer appears to occur on a familial basis in the absence of polyposis.[23] The relationship between the adenomatous polyposis syndromes and the familial predisposition to develop a few adenomatous polyps and colon cancer is not understood.

Table 80–10. FAMILIAL HAMARTOMATOUS POLYPOSIS SYNDROMES

Syndrome	Pathology	Location	Other Manifestations
Peutz-Jeghers syndrome	Hamartomas with bands of smooth muscle in the lamina propria	Small intestine; also stomach and colon	Pigmented lesions of the mouth, hands, and feet; ovarian sex cord tumors (5–12%); gastrointestinal cancers (2–3%)
Juvenile polyposis	Juvenile polyps; also, adenomatous and hyperplastic polyps	Colonic; also small intestine and stomach	Colon cancer in some families
Neurofibromatosis	Neurofibromas	Stomach and small intestine	Generalized neurofibromatosis
Cowden's syndrome (multiple hamartoma syndrome)	Hamartomas	Stomach and colon	Trichilemmomas and papillomas; breast cancer; multiple other hamartomas
Basal cell nevus syndrome	Hamartomas	Colon	Multiple basal cell carcinomas

Familial Hamartomatous Polyposis Syndromes

There are five discrete familial syndromes that are characterized by multiple hamartomatous polyps of the gastrointestinal tract. These include the Peutz-Jeghers syndrome, juvenile polyposis, von Recklinghausen's syndrome, Cowden's syndrome, and basal cell nevus syndrome (Table 80–10).

Peutz-Jeghers Syndrome

Peutz in 1921 and Jeghers in 1949 described the familial syndrome consisting of mucocutaneous pigmentation and gastrointestinal polyposis that now bears their names. Peutz-Jeghers syndrome appears to be inherited as a single pleiotropic autosomal dominant gene with variable, incomplete penetrance.

Pathology. The gastrointestinal polyps in Peutz-Jeghers syndrome are hamartomas in which glandular epithelium is supported by an arborizing framework of well-developed smooth muscle that is contiguous with the muscularis mucosae (Fig. 80–15). The smooth muscle bands fan out into the head of the polyp and become progressively thinner as they project toward the surface of the polyp. Unlike the case with the juvenile polyp, the lamina propria appears normal, and the characteristic architecture of the lesion appears to derive chiefly from the abnormal smooth muscle tissue. These polyps almost always are multiple, and their distinctive appearance, in association with the extraintestinal manifestations, makes Peutz-Jeghers syndrome easily identifiable.

Clinical Features (Fig. 80–16). Early in infancy the characteristic mucocutaneous pigmentation of the Peutz-Jeghers syndrome may be noted. The melanin deposits are found most commonly around the mouth, nose, lips, buccal mucosa, hands, and feet, and they may also be present in the perianal and genital regions (Fig. 80–17). The macular lesions are brown to greenish-black, are glabrous, and, except for the buccal pigmentation, tend to fade at puberty. The clinician must distinguish these melanin deposits from ordinary freckles. Freckles are sparse near the nostrils and

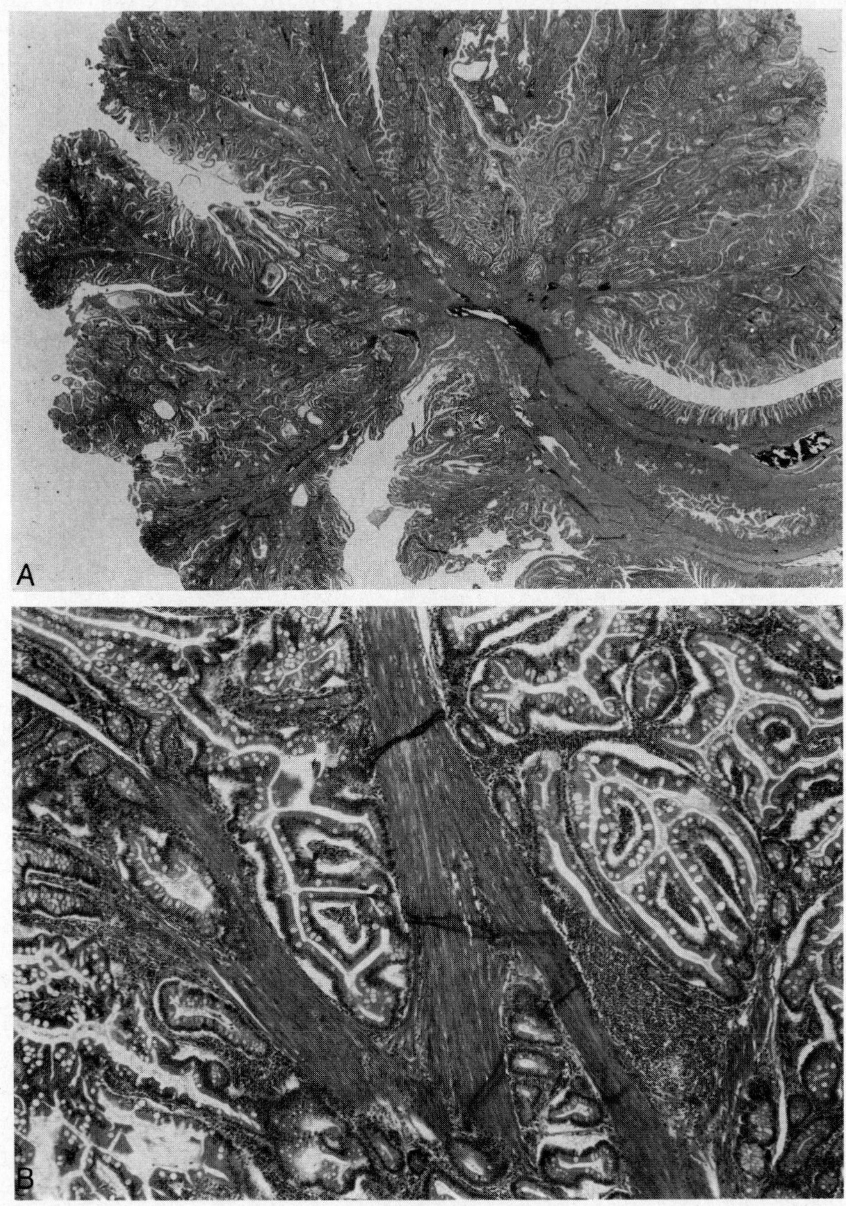

Figure 80–15. Peutz-Jeghers polyp. *A*, Low-power photomicrograph of a Peutz-Jeghers polyp of the small intestine. The central core, containing broad bands of smooth muscle not seen in other gastrointestinal polyps, arborizes and gives rise to the characteristic architecture of the lesion. *B*, A high-power view of the Peutz-Jeghers polyp in *A*. Note the branching bands of smooth muscle surrounded by small intestinal glandular epithelium.

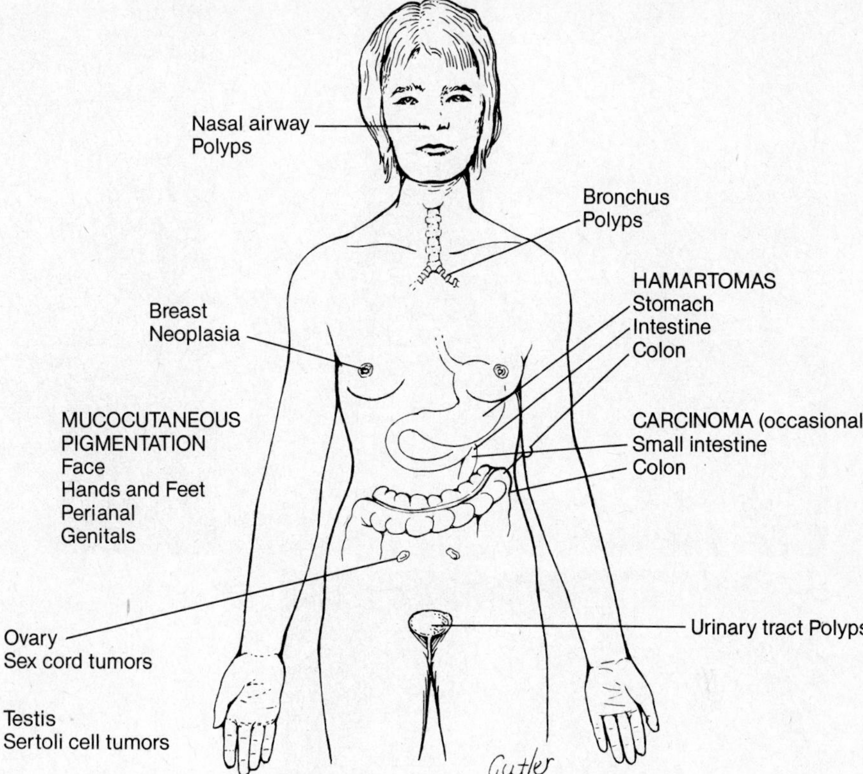

Figure 80–16. Schematic representation of Peutz-Jeghers syndrome. Mucocutaneous pigmentation and benign gastrointestinal polyposis (capitals) are the primary feature of the syndrome. The secondary features of the syndrome are indicated in lower case.

mouth, are absent at birth (but may occur in infancy), and never appear on the buccal mucosa. The presence of this pigmentation should alert the clinician to this syndrome, but the skin lesions and intestinal lesions occasionally are inherited separately.

Peutz-Jeghers polyps are not true neoplasms but may increase in size progressively and cause small intestinal obstruction or intussusception. The polyps may be found in the stomach, small intestine, or colon, but they tend to be most prominent in the small intestine. Acute upper gastrointestinal bleeding and chronic fecal blood loss may complicate the disease.

Carcinoma of the colon and duodenum has been reported in patients with Peutz-Jeghers syndrome.[228, 229] However, the frequency has been reported to be 2 to 3 per cent, which, depending on the period of surveillance, may not represent an increase over the predicted rate of colonic cancer. However, the reports of small intestinal carcinoma are more disturbing, and these appear to arise from foci of adenomatous epithelium that may develop within the Peutz-Jeghers polyps.[229] The colonic polyps should be removed for histologic examination. The relative inaccessibility of small intestinal polyps and the unpredictability of neoplastic complications make a routine surveillance program for small intestinal cancer a difficult problem.

Ovarian cysts and distinctive ovarian sex cord tumors are seen in 5 to 12 per cent of female patients with Peutz-Jeghers syndrome,[230] and endocrinologically active Sertoli cell testicular tumors have been reported in boys.[231] Occasionally, bladder and nasal polyps have been reported with this syndrome. Breast cancer has been reported in association with the Peutz-Jeghers syndrome, but it is not yet evident that the frequency of this common cancer is increased.

Juvenile Polyposis

Juvenile polyps are distinctive hamartomas that usually are solitary and occur principally in the rectums of children and occasionally in an adult. They are smooth and are covered by normal colonic epithelium. Juvenile polyposis typically occurs in families; however, new mutations in patients with a negative family history have also been reported.[232] At least three different varieties of familial juvenile polyposis have been recorded: familial juvenile polyposis coli (limited to the colon),[233] familial juvenile polyposis of the stomach,[234] and generalized juvenile polyposis (involving the entire gastrointestinal tract).[235] These different familial pictures may actually be multiple manifestations of a single pleiotropic gene similar to familial adenomatous polyposis.

The clinical presentations of juvenile polyposis and familial adenomatous polyposis syndromes differ. Juvenile polyps produce symptoms in childhood, whereas the adenomatosis syndromes rarely present before puberty and typically become evident in early adult life.[235] Juvenile polyposis typically causes gastrointestinal bleeding, intussusception, and obstruction.

It now seems to be clear that the risk of colon cancer is increased in familial juvenile polyposis.[236] Although

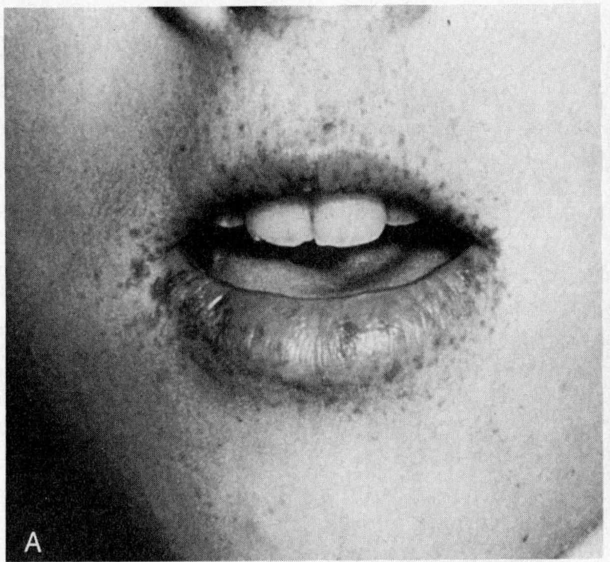

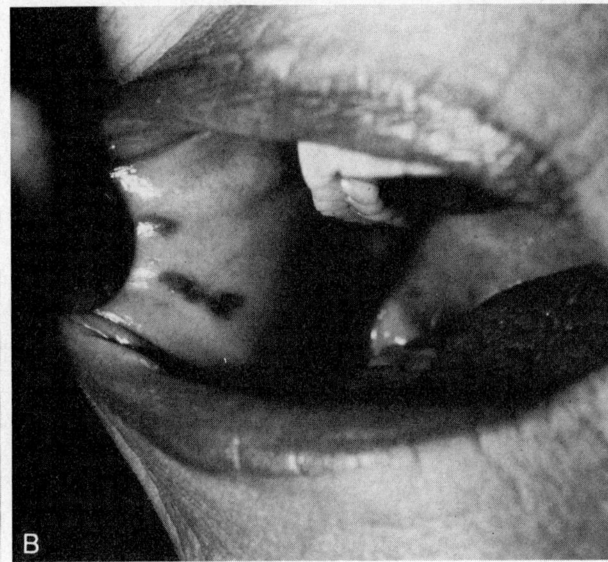

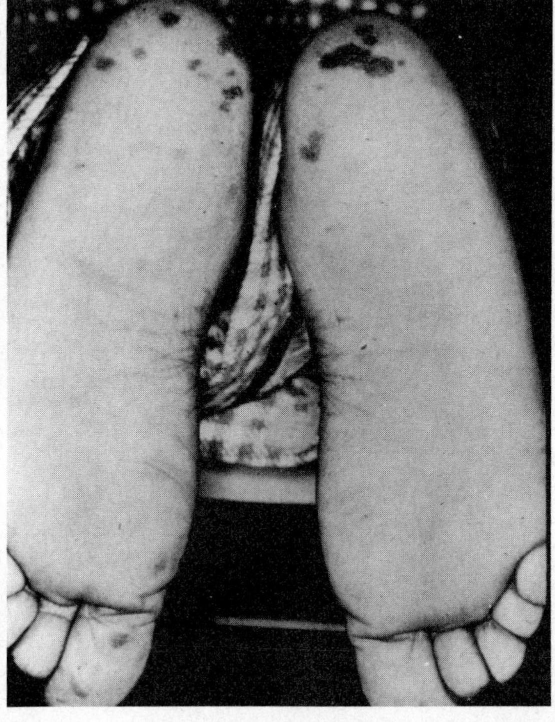

Figure 80–17. Peutz-Jeghers syndrome. *A*, Mucocutaneous pigmentation characteristic of Peutz-Jeghers syndrome. The "freckles" are seen around the lips, and cross the vermilion border. *B*, The pigmentation may also be seen on the buccal mucosa. *C*, Cutaneous pigmentation may also be found on the hands, fingers, palms, nostrils, and feet, as demonstrated here. The cutaneous pigmentation may fade with age, whereas the mucocutaneous pigmentation persists.

the juvenile polyps per se are not neoplastic, the synchronous adenomatous polyps and mixed juvenile-adenomatous polyps of these patients may give rise to cancer.[232, 233, 236, 237]

In general, juvenile polyps should be removed because of their tendency to bleed and obstruct. Family history must be defined in patients with multiple juvenile polyps to determine the sites of involvement and the history of neoplastic lesions. Synchronous adenomatous polyps or mixed juvenile-adenomatous polyps are possibly premalignant and must certainly be excised. To date, there have been no reports of upper gastrointestinal tract carcinoma attributable to this group of syndromes.

Neurofibromatosis

Neurofibromatosis, or von Recklinghausen's syndrome, may involve the upper digestive tract with multiple submucosal neurofibromas that may cause dyspepsia, abdominal pain, or hemorrhage.[238] Severe, uncontrolled symptoms may require surgical excision in a few selected cases.

Other Familial Hamartomatous Polyposis Syndromes

Although reported in only a very small number of families, other inherited diseases have been associated with multiple gastrointestinal hamartomas. One is Cowden's syndrome, or the multiple hamartoma syndrome, which consists of multiple orocutaneous hamartomas, fibrocystic disease and cancer of the breast, nontoxic goiter, thyroid cancer, and hamartomatous polyps of the stomach, small intestine, and colon.[239] The colorectal polyps in Cowden's disease are distinctive lesions characterized by disorganization and proliferation of the muscularis mucosae with nearly normal overlying colonic epithelium.[240] The disease appears to be inherited in an autosomal dominant mode. Gastrointestinal symptoms and colorectal cancer appear to be uncommon in association with this syndrome. The hallmark of the disease is the presence of multiple facial trichilemmomas, which arise from follicular epithelium and typically occur around the eyes, nose, and mouth. Ganglioneuromatosis of the colon and glycogenic acanthosis of the esophagus have been reported in association with Cowden's disease.[241] Excess circulating epidermal growth factor does not appear to play a role in the genesis of this disease. The underlying biologic lesion in this disease is completely unknown. The major complication is breast cancer.

The basal cell nevus syndrome has also been associated with multiple gastric hamartomatous polyps;[242] however, several kindreds have been reported without mention of gastrointestinal lesions.

Multiple and recurrent inflammatory "fibroid polyps" have been reported in a family.[161] These lesions, histologically distinct from juvenile polyps, may cause gastrointestinal obstruction, with symptoms beginning in adult life.

Table 80–11. NONFAMILIAL MULTIPLE POLYPOSIS SYNDROMES

Cronkhite-Canada syndrome
Inflammatory polyposis (pseudopolyps)
Lymphoid polyposis
Benign lymphoid polyposis
Malignant lymphoma
Others
Lipomatous polyposis
Hyperplastic polyposis
Pneumatosis cystoides intestinalis

Nonfamilial Gastrointestinal Polyposis Syndromes

Multiple gastrointestinal polyps are occasionally seen on a nonfamilial basis (Table 80–11).

Cronkhite-Canada Syndrome
(Figs. 80–18 and 80–19)

In 1955 Cronkhite and Canada reported the first examples of an acquired, nonfamilial syndrome that now bears their names.[243] It is characterized by the presence of diffuse gastrointestinal polyposis, dystrophic changes in the fingernails, alopecia, cutaneous hyperpigmentation, diarrhea, weight loss, abdominal pain, and complications of malnutrition.[244] Patients are typically middle-aged (average, 62 years) and present with a progressive illness consisting of chronic diarrhea and protein-losing enteropathy with the associated integumentary abnormalities (see pp. 283–290). The

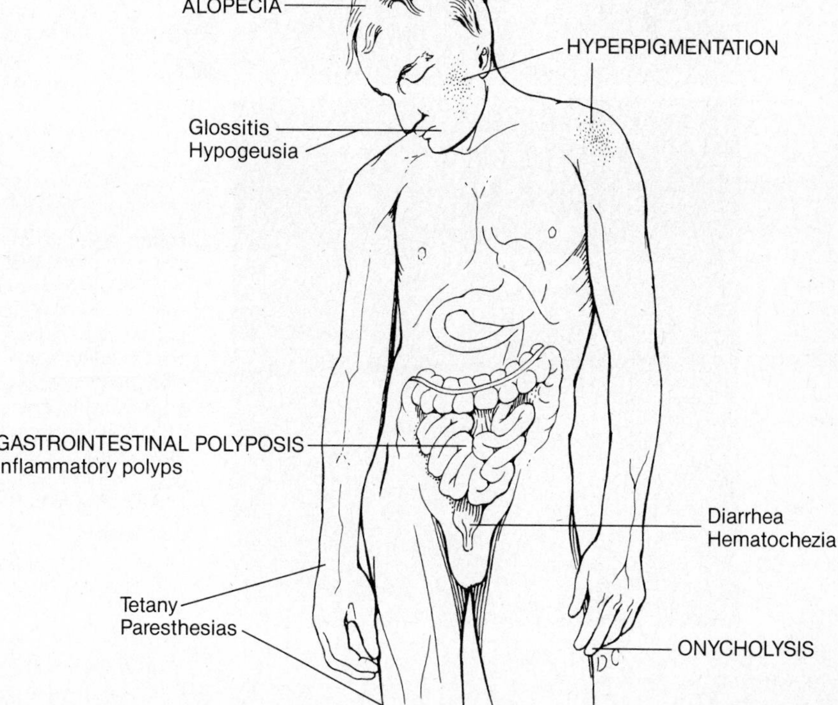

Figure 80–18. Schematic representation of Cronkhite-Canada syndrome. Acquired gastrointestinal polyposis presenting with diarrhea and weight loss and associated with the integumentary change illustrated here are characteristic of the Cronkhite-Canada syndrome. These polyps are histologically similar to juvenile (retention) polyps.

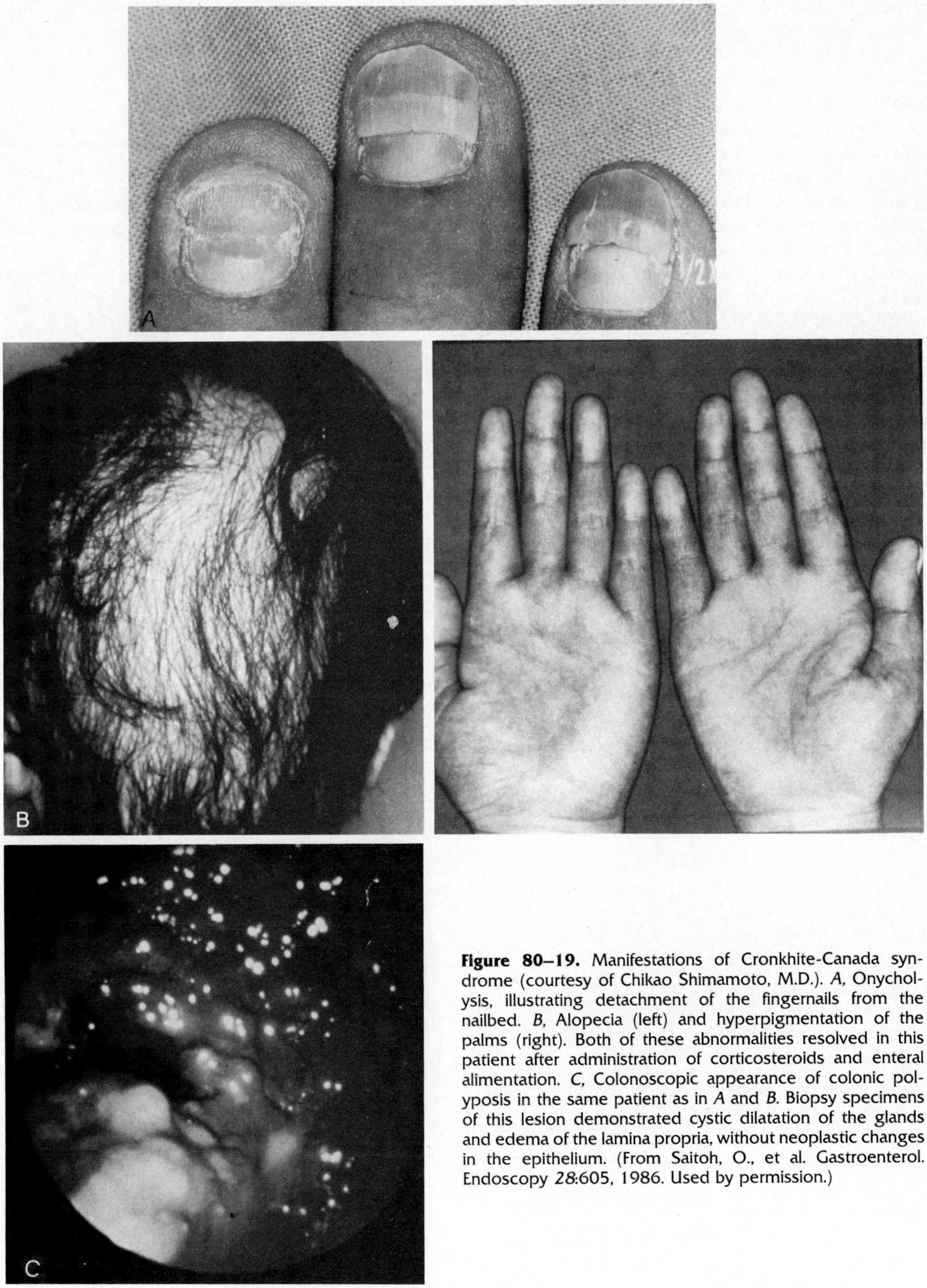

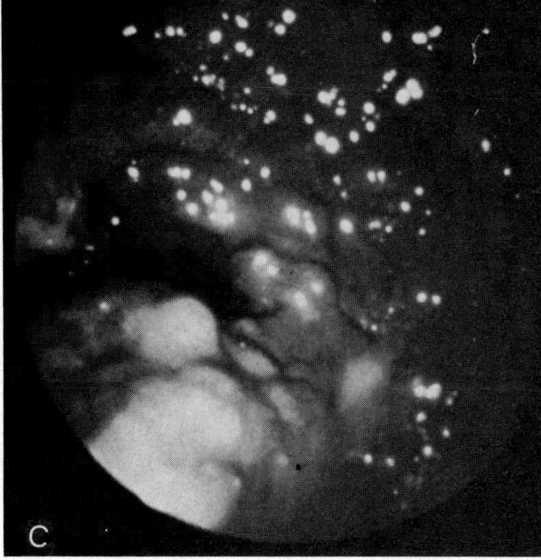

Figure 80–19. Manifestations of Cronkhite-Canada syndrome (courtesy of Chikao Shimamoto, M.D.). *A,* Onycholysis, illustrating detachment of the fingernails from the nailbed. *B,* Alopecia (left) and hyperpigmentation of the palms (right). Both of these abnormalities resolved in this patient after administration of corticosteroids and enteral alimentation. *C,* Colonoscopic appearance of colonic polyposis in the same patient as in *A* and *B.* Biopsy specimens of this lesion demonstrated cystic dilatation of the glands and edema of the lamina propria, without neoplastic changes in the epithelium. (From Saitoh, O., et al. Gastroenterol. Endoscopy *28*:605, 1986. Used by permission.)

diarrhea is attributable primarily to diffuse mucosal injury in the small intestine but may be complicated by bacterial overgrowth. Gastrointestinal polyps are found in 52 to 96 per cent of patients from the stomach to the rectum.[244] In spite of some confusion in the early literature on this subject, these polyps are hamartomas similar to the juvenile (retention) type. As is the case with juvenile polyps, there may be foci of adenomatous epithelium, which may confer a risk of carcinoma. Although adenomatous epithelium has been reported in these polyps and carcinoma has been reported to complicate this syndrome, malignant degeneration is the exception rather than the rule in this disease.[245]

The malabsorption syndrome is progressive in most patients, and the prognosis is poor as there is no specific therapy (see pp. 000–000). It has been suggested that complete symptomatic remission may occasionally be achieved with the appropriate supportive management.[244] In some cases, a variety of medical and surgical measures have been employed, making it difficult to identify the essential therapeutic factor(s). Corticosteroids, anabolic steroids, antibiotics, and surgical resections have been tried in many of these patients, in whom remissions have been reported. Despite this, aggressive nutritional support appears to be the most important factor influencing a favorable outcome. Enteral feeding (if possible) or parenteral feeding (if necessary) with sources of calories, nitrogen, and lipids, in addition to appropriate fluids, electrolytes, vitamins, and minerals, has resulted in complete symptomatic remissions with resolution of all of the ectodermal aberrations.[244] Antibiotics may be beneficial when bacterial overgrowth contributes to the malabsorption. Although corticosteroids have been used in some of the cases of symptomatic remission, the evidence to support their use is weak. Surgical therapy offers less and is risky in malnourished patients. One case of complete remission has been reported in a patient managed only with the enteral administration of a nutritionally balanced complete liquid diet.[246] Attention should be paid to the possibility of secondary lactose or other disaccharide intolerance in patients with diffuse small intestinal disease. Specific management awaits a better understanding of this perplexing syndrome.

Miscellaneous Nonfamilial Polyposes

As mentioned previously, the differential diagnosis of multiple gastrointestinal polyps includes inflammatory polyps (pseudopolyps), lymphoid polyps (benign and malignant), and other rare lesions, such as multiple lipomas, multiple hyperplastic polyps, and pneumatosis cystoides intestinalis. None of these appears to have a familial basis, nor is any associated with an increased risk of cancer.

References

1. Muto, T., Bussey, H. J. R., and Morson, B. C. The evolution of cancer of the colon and rectum. Cancer *36*:2251, 1975.
2. Shinya, H., and Wolff, W. I. Morphology, anatomic distribution and cancer potential of colonic polyps. Ann. Surg. *190*:679, 1979.
3. Konishi, F., and Morson, B. C. Pathology of colorectal adenomas: a colonoscopic survey. J. Clin. Pathol. *35*:830, 1982.
4. Ekelund, G., and Lindstrom, C. Histopathological analysis of benign polyps in patients with carcinoma of the colon and rectum. Gut *15*:654, 1974.
5. Arthur, J. F. Structure and significance of metaplastic nodules in the rectal mucosa. J. Clin. Pathol. *21*:735, 1968.
6. Lane, N., Kaplan, H., and Pascal, R. R. Minute adenomatous and hyperplastic polyps of the colon: divergent patterns of epithelial growth with specific associated mesenchymal changes. Gastroenterology *60*:537, 1971.
7. Granqvist, S., Gabrielsson, N., and Sundelin, P. Diminutive colonic polyps—clinical significance and management. Endoscopy *1*:36, 1979.
8. Tedesco, F. J., Hendrix, J. C., Pickens, C. A., Brady, P. G., and Mills, L. R. Diminutive polyps: histopathology, spatial distribution, and clinical significance. Gastrointest. Endosc. *28*:1, 1982.
9. Ryan, M. E., Parent, K., Wyman, J. B., Nunez, J. F., Kirchner, J. P., Rhodes, R. A., and Norfleet, R. G. Significance of diminutive colorectal polyps in 3281 flexible sigmoidoscopic examinations. Gastrointest. Endosc. *31*:149, 1985.
10. Gottlieb, L. S., Winawer, S. J., Sternberg, S., Magrath, C., Diaz, B., Zauber, A., and O'Brien, M. National Polyp Study (NPS): the diminutive colonic polyp. Gastrointest. Endosc. *30*:143, 1984.
11. Matek, W., Guggenmoos-Holzmann, I., and Demling, L. Follow-up of patients with colorectal adenomas. Endoscopy *17*:175, 1985.
12. Maskens, A. P. Histogenesis of adenomatous polyps in the human large intestine. Gastroenterology *77*:1245, 1979.
13. Correa, P. Epidemiology of polyps and cancer. *In* Morson, B. C. (ed.). The Pathogenesis of Colorectal Cancer. Philadelphia, W. B. Saunders Company, 1978, p. 126.
14. Kozuka, S., Nogaki, M., Ozeki, T., and Masumori, S. Premalignancy of the mucosal polyp in the large intestine. II. Estimation of the periods required for malignant transformation of mucosal polyps. Dis. Colon Rectum *18*:494, 1975.
15. Gilbertsen, V. A., and Nelms, J. M. The prevention of invasive cancer of the rectum. Cancer *41*:1137, 1978.
16. Morson, B. C. Factors influencing the prognosis of early cancer of the rectum. Proc. R. Soc. Med. *59*:607, 1966.
17. Shamsuddin, A. M. Microscopic intraepithelial neoplasia in large bowel mucosa. Hum. Pathol. *13*:510, 1982.
18. Spjut, H. J., Frankel, N. B., and Appel, M. F. The small carcinoma of the large bowel. Am. J. Surg. Pathol. *3*:39, 1979.
19. Muto, T., Kamiya, J., Sawada, T., Konishi, F., Sugihara, K., Kubota, Y., Adachi, M., Agawa, S., Saito, Y., Morioka, T., and Tanprayoon, T. Small "flat adenoma" of the large bowel with special reference to its clinicopathologic features. Dis. Colon Rectum *28*:847, 1985.
20. Love, R. R. Adenomas are precursor lesions for malignant growth in nonpolyposis hereditary carcinoma of the colon and rectum. Surg. Gynecol. Obstet. *162*:8, 1986.
21. Mecklin, J.-P., Sipponen, P., and Jarvinen, H. Histopathology of colorectal carcinomas and adenomas in cancer family syndrome. Dis. Colon Rectum *29*:849, 1986.
22. Maskens, A. P., and Dujardin-Loits, R.-M. Experimental adenomas and carcinomas of the large intestine behave as distinct entities: most carcinomas arise de novo in flat mucosa. Cancer *47*:81, 1981.
23. Burt, R. W., Bishop, D. T., Cannon, L. A., Dowdle, M. A., Lee, R. G., and Skolnick, M. H. Dominant inheritance of adenomatous colonic polyps and colorectal cancer. N. Engl. J. Med. *312*:1540, 1985.
24. Hill, M. Etiology of the adenoma-carcinoma sequence. *In* Morson, B. C. (ed.). The Pathogenesis of Colorectal Cancer. Philadelphia, W. B. Saunders Company, 1978, p. 153.
25. Wolley, R. C., Schreiber, K., Koss, L. S., Karas, M., and Sherman, A. DNA distribution in human colon carcinomas and its relationship to clinical behavior. J. Natl. Cancer Inst. *69*:15, 1982.
26. Quirke, P., Fozard, J. B. J., Dixon, M. F., Dyson, J. E. D.,

Giles, G. R., and Bird, C. C. DNA aneuploidy in colorectal adenomas. Br. J. Cancer *53*:477, 1986.

27. Goh, H. S., and Jass, J. R. DNA content and the adenoma-carcinoma sequence in the colorectum. J. Clin. Pathol. *39*:387, 1986.
28. Goelz, S. E., Vogelstein, B., Hamilton, S. R., and Feinberg, A. P. Hypomethylation of DNA from benign and malignant human colon neoplasms. Science *228*:187, 1985.
29. Pero, R. W., Ritchie, M., Winawer, S. J., Markowitz, M. M., and Miller, D. G. Unscheduled DNA synthesis in mononuclear leukocytes from patients with colorectal polyps. Cancer Res. *45*:3388, 1985.
30. Giordano, G. G., and Rossiello, R. Immunohistochemical approach to the characterization of colorectal adenomas. *In* Fenoglio-Preiser, C. M., and Rossini, F. P. (eds.). Adenomas and Adenomas Containing Carcinoma of the Large Bowel. Advances in Diagnosis and Therapy. New York, Raven Press, 1985, p. 39.
31. Itzkowitz, S. H., Yuan, M., Ferrell, L. D., Palekar, A., and Kim, Y. S. Cancer-associated alterations of blood group antigen expression in human colorectal polyps. Cancer Res. *46*:5976, 1986.
32. Yonezawa, S., Nakamura, T., Tanaka, S., Maruta, K., Nishi, M., and Sato, E. Binding of *Ulex europaeus* agglutinin-1 in polyposis coli: comparative study with solitary adenoma in the sigmoid colon and rectum. J. Natl. Cancer Inst. *71*:19, 1983.
33. Yuan, M., Itzkowitz, S. H., Ferrell, L. D., Fukushi, Y., Palekar, A., Hakomori, S., and Kim, Y. S. Expression of Lewis^x and sialylated Lewis^x antigens in human colorectal polyps. J. Natl. Cancer Inst. *78*:479, 1987.
34. Kim, Y. S., Yuan, M., Itzkowitz, S. H., Sun, Q., Kaizu, T., Palekar, A., Trump, B. F., and Hakomori, S. Expression of Le^y and extended Le^y blood group–related antigens in human malignant, premalignant, and nonmalignant colonic tissues. Cancer Res. *46*:5985, 1986.
35. Boland, C. R., Montgomery, C. K., and Kim, Y. S. A cancer-associated mucin alteration in benign colonic polyps. Gastroenterology *82*:664, 1982.
36. Yuan, M., Itzkowitz, S. H., Boland, C. R., Kim, Y. D., Tomita, J. T., Palekar, A., Bennington, J. L., Trump, B. F., and Kim, Y. S. Comparison of T-antigen expression in normal, premalignant, and malignant human colonic tissue using lectin and antibody immunohistochemistry. Cancer Res. *46*:4841, 1986.
37. Kohga, S., Harvey, S. R., Weaver, R. M., and Markus, G. Localization of plasminogen activators in human colon cancer by immunoperoxidase staining. Cancer Res. *45*:1787, 1985.
38. Friedman, E., Urmacher, C., and Winawer, S. A model for human colon carcinoma evolution based on the differential response of cultured preneoplastic premalignant and malignant cells to 12-O-tetradecanoylphorbol-13-acetate. Cancer Res. *44*:1568, 1984.
39. Friedman, E. A., and Winawer, S. J. Invasion of epithelial monolayer cultured from colonic adenomas by carcinoma cells is enhanced by the secreted protease, plasminogen activator. Gastroenterology *88*:1388, 1985.
40. Stemmermann, G. N., and Yatani, R. Diverticulosis and polyps of the large intestine: a necropsy study of Hawaii Japanese. Cancer *31*:1260, 1973.
41. Sato, E., Ouchi, A., Sasano, N., and Ishidate, T. Polyps and diverticulosis of large bowel in autopsy population of Akita prefecture, compared with Miyagi. Cancer *37*:1316, 1976.
42. Rickert, R. R., Auerbach, O., Garfinkel, L., Hammond, E. C., and Frasca, J. M. Adenomatous lesions of the large bowel: an autopsy survey. Cancer *43*:1847, 1979.
43. Coode, P. E., Chan, K. W., and Chan, Y. T. Polyps and diverticula of the large intestine: a necropsy survey in Hong Kong. Gut *26*:1045, 1985.
44. Vatn, M. H., and Stalsberg, H. The prevalence of polyps of the large intestine in Oslo: an autopsy study. Cancer *49*:819, 1982.
45. Eide, T. J., and Stalsberg, H. Polyps of the large intestine in northern Norway. Cancer *42*:2839, 1978.
46. Clark, J. C., Collan, Y., Eide, T. J., Esteve, J., Ewen, S., Gibbs, N. M., Jensen, O. M., Koskela, E., MacLennan, R., Simpson, J. G., Stalsberg, H., and Zaridze, D. G. Prevalence of polyps in an autopsy series from areas with varying incidence of large-bowel cancer. Int. J. Cancer *36*:179, 1985.
47. Granqvist, S. Distribution of polyps in the large bowel in relation to age: a colonoscopic study. Scand. J. Gastroenterol. *16*:1025, 1981.
48. Eide, T. J. The age-, sex-, and site-specific occurrence of adenomas and carcinoma of the large intestine within a defined population. Scand. J. Gastroenterol. *21*:1083, 1986.
49. Knoernschild, H. E. Growth rate and malignant potential of colonic polyps: early results. Surg. Forum *14*:137, 1963.
50. Paul, R. E., Jr., Gherardi, G. J., and Miller, H. H. Autoamputation of benign and malignant polyps: report of two cases. Dis. Colon Rectum *17*:331, 1974.
51. Welin, S., Youker, J., and Spratt, J. S., Jr. The rates and patterns of growth of 375 tumors of the large intestine and rectum observed serially by double contrast enema study (Malmo technique). AJR *90*:673, 1963.
52. Tada, M., Misaki, F., and Kawai, K. Growth rates of colorectal carcinoma and adenoma by roentgenologic follow-up observations. Gastroenterol. Japon. *19*:550, 1984.
53. Carroll, R. L. A., and Klein, M. How often should patients be sigmoidoscoped? A mathematical perspective. Prev. Med. *9*:741, 1980.
54. Figiel, L. S., Figiel, S. J., and Wieterson, F. K. Roentgenologic observation of growth rates of colonic polyps and carcinoma. Acta Radiol. Diagn. *3*:417, 1965.
55. Copeland, E. M., Jones, R. S., and Miller, L. D. Multiple colon neoplasms. Arch. Surg. *98*:141, 1969.
56. Pagana, T. J., Ledesma, E. J., Mittelman, A., and Nava, H. R. The use of colonoscopy in the study of synchronous colorectal neoplasms. Cancer *53*:356, 1984.
57. Chu, D. Z. J., Giacco, G., Martin, R. G., and Guinee, V. F. The significance of synchronous carcinoma and polyps in the colon and rectum. Cancer *57*:445, 1986.
58. Langevin, J. M., and Nivatvongs, S. The true incidence of synchronous cancer of the large bowel: a prospective study. Am. J. Surg. *147*:330, 1984.
59. Reilly, J. C., Rusin, L. C., and Theuerkauf, F. J., Jr. Colonoscopy: its role in cancer of the colon and rectum. Dis. Colon Rectum *25*:532, 1982.
60. Greenstein, A. J., Heimann, T. M., Sachar, D. B., Slater, G., and Aufses, A. H., Jr. A comparison of multiple synchronous colorectal cancer in ulcerative colitis, familial polyposis coli, and de novo cancer. Ann. Surg. *203*:123, 1986.
61. Lasser, A. Synchronous primary adenocarcinomas of the colon and rectum. Dis. Colon Rectum *21*:20, 1978.
62. Mughal, S., Filipe, M. I., and Jass, J. R. A comparative ultrastructural study of hyperplastic and adenomatous polyps, incidental and in association with colorectal cancer. Cancer *48*:2746, 1981.
63. Morson, B. C., and Bussey, H. J. R. Magnitude of risk for cancer in patients with colorectal adenomas. Br. J. Surg. *72*(Suppl.):S23, 1985.
64. Lotfi, A. M., Spencer, R. J., Ilstrup, D. M., and Melton, J., III. Colorectal polyps and the risk of subsequent carcinoma. Mayo Clin. Proc. *61*:337, 1986.
65. Correa, P., Strong, J. P., Johnson, W. D., Pizzolato, P., and Haenszel, W. Atherosclerosis and polyps of the colon. Quantification of precursors of coronary heart disease and colon cancer. J. Chron. Dis. *35*:313, 1982.
66. Stemmermann, G. N., Heilbrun, L. K., Nomura, A., Yano, K., and Hayashi, T. Adenomatous polyps and atherosclerosis: an autopsy study of Japanese men in Hawaii. Int. J. Cancer *38*:789, 1986.
67. Mannes, G. A., Maier, A., Thieme, C., Wiebecke, B., and Paumgartner, G. Relation between the frequency of colorectal adenoma and the serum cholesterol level. N. Engl. J. Med. *315*:1634, 1986.
68. Neugut, A. I., Johnsen, C. M., and Fink, D. J. Serum cholesterol levels in adenomatous polyps and cancer of the colon. JAMA *255*:365, 1986.
69. Klein, I., Parveen, G., Gavaler, J. S., and VanThiel, D. H. Colonic polyps in patients with acromegaly. Ann. Intern. Med. *97*:27, 1982.

70. Leavitt, J., Klein, I., Kendricks, F., Gavaler, J., and VanThiel, D. H. Skin tags: a cutaneous marker for colonic polyps. Ann. Intern. Med. *98*:928, 1983.
71. Kune, G. A., Gooey, J., Penfold, C., and Sali, A. Association between colorectal polyps and skin tags. Lancet *2*:1062, 1985.
72. Chobanian, S. J., VanNess, M. M., Winters, C., Jr., and Cattau, E. L., Jr. Skin tags as a marker for adenomatous polyps of the colon. Ann. Intern. Med. *103*:892, 1985.
73. Dalton, A. D. A., and Coghill, S. B. No association between skin tags and colorectal adenomas. Lancet *1*:1332, 1985.
74. Luk, G. D., and the Colon Neoplasia Work Group. Colonic polyps and acrochordons (skin tags) do not correlate in familial colonic polyposis kindreds. Ann. Intern. Med. *104*:209, 1986.
75. Klein, R. S., Recco, R. A., Catalano, M. T., Edberg, S. C., Casey, J. I., and Steigbigel, N. H. Association of *Streptococcus bovis* with carcinoma of the colon. N. Engl. J. Med. *297*:800, 1977.
76. Klein, R. S., Catalano, M. T., Edberg, S. C., Casey, J. I., and Steigbigel, N. H. *Streptococcus bovis* septicemia and carcinoma of the colon. Ann. Intern. Med. *91*:560, 1979.
77. Marshall, J. B., and Gerhardt, D. C. Polyposis coli presenting with *Streptococcus bovis* endocarditis. Am. J. Gastroenterol. *75*:314, 1981.
78. Burns, C. A., McCaughey, R., and Lauter, C. B. The association of *Streptococcus bovis* fecal carriage and colon neoplasia: possible relationship with polyps and their premalignant potential. Am. J. Gastroenterol. *80*:42, 1985.
79. Wiseman, A., Rene, P., and Crelinsten, G. L. *Streptococcus agalactiae* endocarditis: an association with villous adenomas of the large intestine. Ann. Intern. Med. *103*:893, 1985.
80. Sobin, L. H. The histopathology of bleeding from polyps and carcinomas of the large intestine. Cancer *55*:577, 1985.
81. Silman, A. J., Mitchell, P., Nicholls, R. J., Macrae, F. A., Leicester, R. J., Bartram, C. I., Simmons, M. J., Campbell, P. D. J., Hearn, C. E. D., and Constable, P. J. Self-reported dark red bleeding as a marker comparable with occult blood testing in screening for large bowel neoplasms. Br. J. Surg. *70*:721, 1983.
82. Macrae, F., and St. John, D. J. B. Relationship between patterns of bleeding and Hemoccult sensitivity in patients with colorectal cancers or adenomas. Gastroenterology *82*:891, 1982.
83. Dybdahl, J. H., Daae, L. N. W., Larsen, S., and Myren, J. Occult faecal blood loss determined by a ^{51}Cr method and chemical tests in patients referred for colonoscopy. Scand. J. Gastroenterol. *19*:245, 1984.
84. Herzog, P., Holtermuller, K., Preiss, J., Fischer, J., Ewe, K., Schreiber, H., and Berres, M. Fecal blood loss in patients with colonic polyps: a comparison of measurements with ^{51}chromium-labeled erythrocytes and with the Haemoccult test. Gastroenterology *83*:957, 1982.
85. Crowley, M. L., Freeman, L. D., Mottet, M. D., Strong, R. M., Sweeney, B. F., Brower, R. A., Sharma, S. P., and Anderson, D. S. Sensitivity of guaiac-impregnated cards for the detection of colorectal neoplasia. J. Clin. Gastroenterol. *5*:127, 1983.
86. Gabrielsson, N., Granqvist, S., and Nilsson, B. Guaiac tests for detection of occult faecal blood loss in patients with endoscopically verified colonic polyps. Scand. J. Gastroenterol. *20*:978, 1985.
87. Norfleet, R. G. Effect of diet on fecal occult blood testing in patients with colorectal polyps. Dig. Dis. Sci. *31*:498, 1986.
88. Ahlquist, D. A., McGill, D. B., Schwartz, S., Taylor, W. F., and Owen, R. A. Fecal blood levels in health and disease: a study using HemoQuant. N. Engl. J. Med. *312*:1422, 1985.
89. Marks, G., Boggs, H. W., Castro, A. F., Gathright, J. B., Ray, J. E., and Salvati, E. Sigmoidoscopic examinations with rigid and flexible fiberoptic sigmoidoscopes in the surgeon's office: a comparative prospective study of effectiveness in 1,012 cases. Dis. Colon Rectum *22*:162, 1979.
90. Bohlman, T. W., Katon, R. M., Lipshutz, G. R., McCool, M. F., Smith, F. W., and Melnyk, C. S. Fiberoptic pansigmoidoscopy: an evaluation and comparison with rigid sigmoidoscopy. Gastroenterology 72:644, 1977.
91. Winnan, G., Berci, G., Panish, J., Talbot, T. M., Overholt, B. F., and McCallum, R. W. Superiority of the flexible to the rigid sigmoidoscope in routine proctosigmoidoscopy. N. Engl. J. Med. *302*:1011, 1980.
92. McCallum, R. W., Meyer, C. T., Marignani, P., Cane, E., and Contino, C. Flexible sigmoidoscopy: diagnostic yield in 1015 patients. Am. J. Gastroenterol. *79*:433, 1984.
93. Grobe, J. L., Kozarek, R. A., and Sanowski, R. A. Flexible versus rigid sigmoidoscopy: a comparison using an inexpensive 35-cm flexible proctosigmoidoscope. Am. J. Gastroenterol. *78*:569, 1983.
94. Zucker, G. M., Madura, M. J., Chmiel, J. S., and Olinger, E. J. The advantages of the 30-cm flexible sigmoidoscope over the 60-cm flexible sigmoidoscope. Gastrointest. Endosc. *30*:59, 1984.
95. Sarles, H. E., Jr., Sanowski, R. A., Haynes, W. C., and Bellapravalu, S. The long and short of flexible sigmoidoscopy: does it matter? Am. J. Gastroenterol. *81*:369, 1986.
96. Dubow, R. A., Katon, R. M., Benner, K. G., vanDijk, C. M., Koval, G., and Smith, F. W. Short (35-cm) versus long (60-cm) flexible sigmoidoscopy. A comparison of findings and tolerance in asymptomatic patients screened for colorectal neoplasia. Gastrointest. Endosc. *31*:305, 1985.
97. Rumans, M. C., Benner, K. G., Keeffe, E. B., Custis, J. M., Lockwood, D. R., and Craner, G. E. Screening flexible sigmoidoscopy by primary care physicians: effectiveness and costs in patients negative for fecal occult blood. West. J. Med. *144*:756, 1986.
98. Warden, M. J., Petrelli, N. J., Herrera, L., and Mittelman, A. The role of colonoscopy and flexible sigmoidoscopy in screening for colorectal carcinoma. Dis. Colon Rectum *30*:52, 1987.
99. Ott, D. J., Chen, Y. M., Gelfand, D. W., Wu, W. C., and Munitz, H. A. Single-contrast vs double-contrast barium enema in the detection of colonic polyps. AJR *146*:993, 1986.
100. deRoos, A., Hermans, J., Shaw, P. C., and Kroon, H. Colon polyps and carcinomas: prospective comparison of the single- and double-contrast examination in the same patients. Radiology *154*:11, 1985.
101. Williams, C. B., Hunt, R. H., Loose, H., Riddell, R. H., Sakai, Y., and Swarbrick, E. T. Colonoscopy in the management of colon polyps. Br. J. Surg. *61*:673, 1974.
102. Thoeni, R. F., and Menuck, L. Comparison of barium enema and colonoscopy in the detection of small colonic polyps. Radiology *124*:631, 1977.
103. Williams, C. B., Macrae, F. A., and Bartrum, C. I. A prospective study of diagnostic methods in adenoma follow-up. Endoscopy *14*:74, 1982.
104. Tedesco, F. J., Waye, J. D., Raskin, J. B., Morris, S. J., and Greenwald, R. A. Colonoscopic evaluation of rectal bleeding: a study of 304 patients. Ann. Intern. Med. *89*:907, 1978.
105. Swarbrick, E. T., Fevre, D. I., Hunt, R. H., Thomas, B. M., and Williams, C. B. Colonoscopy for unexplained rectal bleeding. Br. Med. J. *2*:1685, 1978.
106. Aldridge, M. C., and Sim, A. J. W. Colonoscopy findings in symptomatic patients without X-ray evidence of colonic neoplasms. Lancet *2*:833, 1986.
107. Spencer, R. J., Melton, L. J., III, Ready, R. L., and Ilstrup, D. M. Treatment of small colorectal polyps: a population-based study of the risk of subsequent carcinoma. Mayo Clin. Proc. *59*:305, 1984.
108. Mathus-Vliegen, E. M. H., and Tytgat, G. N. J. Nd:YAG laser photocoagulation in colorectal adenoma. Gastroenterology *90*:1865, 1986.
109. Simon, J. B. Occult blood screening for colorectal carcinoma: a critical review. Gastroenterology *88*:820, 1985.
110. Winawer, S. J., Andrews, M., Flehinger, B., Sherlock, P., Schottenfeld, D., and Miller, D. G. Progress report on controlled trial of fecal occult blood testing for the detection of colorectal neoplasia. Cancer *45*:2959, 1980.
111. Gilbertsen, V. A., McHugh, R., Schuman, L., and Williams, S. E. The earlier detection of colorectal cancers: a preliminary report of the results of the occult blood study. Cancer *45*:2899, 1980.

112. Hardcastle, J. D., Armitage, N. C., Chamberlain, J., Amar, S. S., James, P. D., and Balfour, T. W. Fecal occult blood screening for colorectal cancer in the general population: results of a controlled trial. Cancer *58*:397, 1986.
113. Moertel, C. G., Hill, J. R., and Dockerty, M. B. The routine proctoscopic examination: a second look. Mayo Clin. Proc. *41*:368, 1966.
114. Winawer, S. J., Leidner, S. D., Boyle, C., and Kurtz, R. C. Comparison of flexible sigmoidoscopy with other diagnostic techniques in the diagnosis of recto-colon neoplasia. Dig. Dis. Sci. *24*:277, 1979.
115. Bat, L., Pines, A., Ron, E., Niv, Y., Arditi, E., and Shemesh, E. A community-based program of colorectal screening in an asymptomatic population: evaluation of screening tests and compliance. Am. J. Gastroenterol. *81*:647, 1986.
116. Demers, R. Y., Stawick, L. E., and Demers, P. Relative sensitivity of the fecal occult blood test and flexible sigmoidoscopy in detecting polyps. Prev. Med. *14*:55, 1985.
117. Yarborough, G. W., and Waisbren, B. A. The benefits of systematic fiberoptic flexible sigmoidoscopy. Arch. Intern. Med. *145*:95, 1985.
118. Qizilbash, A. H., Meghji, M., and Castelli, M. Pseudocarcinomatous invasion in adenomas of the colon and rectum. Dis. Colon Rectum *23*:529, 1980.
119. Fenoglio, C. M., Kaye, G. I., and Lane, N. Distribution of human colonic lymphatics in normal, hyperplastic and adenomatous tissue. Gastroenterology *64*:51, 1973.
120. Haggitt, R. C., Glotzbach, R. E., Soffer, E. E., and Wruble, L. D. Prognostic factors in colorectal carcinoma arising in adenomas: implications for lesions removed by endoscopic polypectomy. Gastroenterology *89*:328, 1985.
121. Riddell, R. H. Hands off "cancerous" large bowel polyps. Gastroenterology *89*:432, 1985.
122. Wilcox, G. M., Anderson, P. B., and Colacchio, T. A. Early invasive carcinoma in colonic polyps: a review of the literature with emphasis on the assessment of the risk of metastasis. Cancer *57*:160, 1986.
123. Morson, B. C., Whiteway, J. E., Jones, E. A., Macrae, F. A., and Williams, C. B. Histopathology and prognosis of malignant colorectal polyps treated by endoscopic polypectomy. Gut *25*:437, 1984.
124. Wolff, W. I., and Shinya, H. Definitive treatment of "malignant" polyps of the colon. Ann. Surg. *182*:516, 1975.
125. Lipper, S., Kahn, L. B., and Ackerman, L. V. The significance of microscopic invasive cancer in endoscopically removed polyps of the large bowel. Cancer *52*:1691, 1983.
126. Cooper, H. S. Surgical pathology of endoscopically removed malignant polyps of the colon and rectum. Am. J. Surg. Pathol. *7*:613, 1983.
127. Coutsoftides, T., Sivak, M. V., Jr., Benjamin, S. P., and Jagelman, D. Colonoscopy and the management of polyps containing invasive carcinoma. Ann. Surg. *188*:638, 1978.
128. Morson, B. C., Bussey, H. J. R., and Samoorian, S. Policy of local excision for early cancer of the colorectum. Gut *18*:1045, 1977.
129. Cranley, J. P., Petras, R. E., Carey, W. D., Paradis, K., and Sivak, M. V. When is endoscopic polypectomy adequate therapy for colonic polyps containing invasive carcinoma? Gastroenterology *91*:419, 1986.
130. Brahme, F., Ekelund, G. R., Norden, J. G., and Wenckert, A. Metachronous colorectal polyps: comparison of development of colorectal polyps and carcinomas in persons with and without histories of polyps. Dis. Colon Rectum *17*:166, 1974.
131. Henry, L. G., Condon, R. E., Schulte, W. J., Aprahamian, C., and DeCosse, J. J. Risk of recurrence of colon polyps. Ann. Surg. *182*:511, 1975.
132. Macrae, F. A., and Williams, C. B. A prospective colonoscopic follow-up study of 500 adenoma patients with multivariate analysis to predict risk of subsequent colorectal tumours. Gastrointest. Endosc. *28*:138, 1982.
133. Neugut, A. I., Johnsen, C. M., Forde, K. A., and Treat, M. R. Recurrence rates for colorectal polyps. Cancer *55*:1586, 1985.
134. Wegener, M., Borsch, G., and Schmidt, G. Colorectal adenomas: distribution, incidence of malignant transformation, and rate of recurrence. Dis. Colon Rectum *29*:383, 1986.
135. Williams, C. B., and Macrae, F. A. The St. Mark's neoplastic polyp follow-up study. Front. Gastrointest. Res. *10*:226, 1986.
136. Kirsner, J. B., Rider, J. A., Moeller, H. C., Palmer, W. L., and Gold, S. S. Polyps of the colon and rectum: statistical analysis of a long term follow-up study. Gastroenterology *39*:178, 1960.
137. Kronborg, O., Hage, E., Adamsen, S., and Deichgraeber, E. Follow-up after colorectal polypectomy: II. Repeated examinations of the colon every 6 months after removal of sessile adenomas and adenomas with the highest degree of dysplasia. Scand. J. Gastroenterol. *18*:1095, 1983.
138. Deyhle, P. Results of endoscopic polypectomy in the gastrointestinal tract. Endoscopy *12*(Suppl.):35, 1980.
139. Fowler, D. L., and Hedberg, S. E. Followup colonoscopy after polypectomy. Gastrointest. Endosc. *26*:67, 1980.
140. Waye, J. D., and Braunfeld, S. Surveillance intervals after colonoscopic polypectomy. Endoscopy *14*:79, 1981.
141. Williams, C. B. The logic and logistics of colon polyp follow-up. *In* Glass, G. B. J., and Sherlock, P. (eds.). Progress in Gastroenterology. Vol. 4. New York, Grune & Stratton, 1983, p. 513.
142. O'Brien, M., Winawer, S. J., Gottlieb, L. S., Diaz, B., Zauber, A., and Sternberg, S. Analysis of multiple determinants of significant dysplasia in colorectal adenomas. Gastrointest. Endosc. *31*:148, 1985.
143. Winawer, S. J., Ritchie, M. T., Diaz, B. J., Gottlieb, L. S., Stewart, E. T., Zauber, A., Herbert, E., and Bond, J. The National Polyp Study: aims and organization. Front. Gastrointest. Res. *10*:216, 1986.
144. Hoff, G., Foerster, A., Vatn, M. H., Sauer, J., and Larsen, S. Epidemiology of polyps in the rectum and colon. Recovery and evaluation of unresected polyps two years after detection. Scand. J. Gastroenterol. *21*:853, 1986.
145. Fenoglio, C. M., Richart, R. M., and Kaye, G. I. Comparative electron-microscopic features of normal, hyperplastic and adenomatous human colonic epithelium. Gastroenterology *69*:100, 1975.
146. Kaye, G. I., Pascal, R. P., and Lane, N. The colonic pericryptal fibroblast sheath: replication, migration, and cytodifferentiation of a mesenchymal cell system in adult tissue. Gastroenterology *60*:515, 1971.
147. Hayashi, T., Yatani, R., Apostol, J., and Stemmermann, G. N. Pathogenesis of hyperplastic polyps of the colon: a hypothesis based upon ultrastructural and *in vitro* cell kinetics. Gastroenterology *66*:347, 1974.
148. Kaye, G. I., Fenoglio, C. M., Pascal, R. P., and Lane, N. Comparative electron microscopic features of normal, hyperplastic and adenomatous human colonic epithelium. Variations in cellular structure relative to the process of epithelial cell differentiation. Gastroenterology *64*:926, 1973.
149. Sumner, H. W., Wasserman, H. W., and McClain, C. J. Giant hyperplastic polyposis of the colon. Dig. Dis. Sci. *26*:85, 1981.
150. Estrada, R. G., and Spjut, H. J. Hyperplastic polyps of the large bowel. Am. J. Surg. Pathol. *4*:127, 1980.
151. Cooper, H. S., Patchefsky, A. S., and Marks, G. Adenomatous and carcinomatous changes within hyperplastic colonic epithelium. Dis. Colon Rectum *27*:152, 1979.
152. Franzin, G., and Novelli, P. Adenocarcinoma occurring in a hyperplastic (metaplastic) polyp of the colon. Endoscopy *14*:28, 1982.
153. Jass, J. R. Relation between metaplastic polyp and carcinoma of the colorectum. Lancet *1*:28, 1983.
154. Jass, J. R., Filipe, M. I., Abbas, S., Falcon, C. A., Wilson, Y., and Lovell, D. A morphologic and histochemical study of metaplastic polyps of the colorectum. Cancer *53*:510, 1984.
155. Correa, P., Strong, J. P., Reif, A., and Johnson, W. D. The epidemiology of colorectal polyps. Cancer *39*:2258, 1977.
156. Williams, A. R., Balasooriya, B. A. W., and Day, D. W. Polyps and cancer of the large bowel: a necropsy study in Liverpool. Gut *23*:835, 1982.

157. Roth, S. I., and Helwig, E. B. Juvenile polyps of the colon and rectum. Cancer *16*:468, 1963.
158. Teague, R. H., and Read, A. E. Polyposis in ulcerative colitis. Gut *16*:792, 1975.
159. Berkowitz, D., and Bernstein, L. H. Colonic pseudopolyps in association with amebic colitis. Gastroenterology *68*:786, 1975.
160. Nebel, O. T., El Masry, N. A., Castell, D. O., Farid, Z., Fornes, M. F., and Sparks, H. A. Schistosomal disease of the colon: a reversible form of polyposis. Gastroenterology *67*:939, 1974.
161. Anthony, P. P., Morris, D. S., and Vowles, K. D. J. Multiple and recurrent inflammatory fibroid polyps in three generations of a Devon family: a new syndrome. Gut *25*:854, 1984.
162. Wayte, D. M., and Helwig, E. B. Colitis cystica profunda. Am. J. Clin. Pathol. *48*:159, 1967.
163. Levine, D. S. "Solitary" rectal ulcer syndrome. Are "solitary" rectal ulcer syndrome and "localized" colitis cystica profunda analogous syndromes caused by rectal prolapse? Gastroenterology *92*:243, 1987.
164. Bentley, E., Chandrasoma, P., Cohen, H., Radin, R., and Ray, M. Colitis cystica profunda presenting with complete intestinal obstruction and recurrence. Gastroenterology *89*:1157, 1985.
165. Shallal, J. A., van Heerden, J. A., Bartholomew, L. G., and Cain, J. C. Pneumatosis cystoides intestinalis. Mayo Clin. Proc. *49*:180, 1974.
166. Smith, B. H., and Welter, L. H. Pneumatosis intestinalis. Am. J. Clin. Pathol. *48*:455, 1967.
167. Born, A., Inouye, T., and Diamant, N. Pneumatosis coli. Case report documenting time from X-ray appearance to onset of symptoms. Dig. Dis. Sci. *26*:855, 1981.
168. Miralbes, M., Hinojosa, J., Alonso, J., and Berenguer, J. Oxygen therapy in pneumatosis coli. What is the minimum oxygen requirement? Dis. Colon Rectum *26*:458, 1983.
169. Holt, S., Gilmour, H. M., Buist, T. A., Marwick, K., and Heading, R. C. High flow oxygen therapy for pneumatosis coli. Gut *20*:493, 1979.
170. Read, N. W., Al-janabi, M. N., and Cann, P. A. Is raised breath hydrogen related to the pathogenesis of pneumatosis coli? Gut *25*:839, 1984.
171. Fernandes, B. J., Amato, D., and Goldfinger, M. Diffuse lymphomatous polyposis of the gastrointestinal tract. Gastroenterology *88*:1267, 1985.
172. DeBeer, R. A., and Shinya, H. Colonic lipoma. Gastrointest. Endosc. *22*:90, 1975.
173. Haney, M. J., and McGarity, N. C. Ureterosigmoidostomy and neoplasms of the colon. Arch. Surg. *103*:69, 1971.
174. Stewart, M., Macrae, F. A., and Williams, C. B. Neoplasia and ureterosigmoidostomy: a colonoscopic survey. Br. J. Surg. *69*:414, 1982.
175. Ali, M. H., Satti, M. B., and Al-nafussi, A. Multiple benign colonic polyps at the site of ureterosigmoidostomy. Cancer *53*:1006, 1984.
176. Stewart, M., Hill, M. J., Pugh, R. C. B., and Williams, J. P. The role of *N*-nitrosamine in carcinogenesis at the ureterocolic anastomosis. Br. J. Urology *53*:115, 1981.
177. Boland, C. R. Familial colonic cancer syndromes. West. J. Med. *138*:351, 1983.
177a. Bodmer, W. F., Bailey, C. J., Bodmer, J., Bussey, H. J. R., Ellis, A., Gorman, P., Lucibello, F. C., Murday, V. A., Rider, S. H., Scambler, P., Sheer, D., Solomon, E., and Spurr, N. K. Nature *328*:614, 1987.
178. Bussey, H. J. R. Familial Polyposis Coli. Baltimore, Johns Hopkins University Press, 1975.
179. Utsunomiya, J., and Nakamura, T. The occult osteomatous changes in the mandible in patients with familial polyposis coli. Br. J. Surg. *62*:45, 1975.
180. Bülow, S., Søndergaard, J. O., Witt, I., Larsen, E., and Tetens, G. Mandibular osteomas in familial polyposis coli. Dis. Colon Rectum *27*:105, 1984.
181. Jarvinen, H., Nyberg, M., and Peltokallio, P. Upper gastrointestinal tract polyps in familial adenomatosis coli. Gut *24*:333, 1983.
182. Tonelli, F., Nardi, F., Bechi, P., Taddei, G., Gozzo, P., and Romagnoli, P. Extracolonic polyps in familial polyposis coli and Gardner's syndrome. Dis. Colon Rectum *28*:664, 1985.
183. Burt, R. W., Berenson, M. M., Lee, R. G., Tolman, K. G., Freston, J. W., and Gardner, E. J. Upper gastrointestinal polyps in Gardner's syndrome. Gastroenterology *86*:295, 1984.
184. Iida, M., Yao, T., Itoh, H., Watanabe, H., Kohrogi, N., Shigematsu, A., Iwashıta, A., and Fujishima, M. Natural history of fundic gland polyposis in patients with familial polyposis coli/Gardner's syndrome. Gastroenterology *89*:1021, 1985.
185. Iida, M., Yao, T., Itoh, H., Ohsato, K., and Watanabe, H. Endoscopic features of adenoma of the duodenal papilla in familial polyposis of the colon. Gastrointest. Endosc. *27*:6, 1981.
186. Watanabe, H., Enjoji, M., Yao, T., and Ohsato, K. Gastric lesions in familial adenomatosis coli. Hum. Pathol. *9*:269, 1978.
187. Deschner, E. E., and Lipkin, M. Proliferative patterns in colonic mucosa in familial polyposis. Cancer *35*:413, 1975.
188. Luk, G. D., and Baylin, S. B. Ornithine decarboxylase as a biologic marker in familial colonic polyposis. N. Engl. J. Med. *311*:80, 1984.
189. Kopelovich, L. Phenotypic markers in human skin fibroblasts as possible diagnostic indices of hereditary adenomatosis of the colon and rectum. Cancer *40*:2534, 1977.
190. Kopelovich, L., Conlon, S., and Pollack, R. Defective organization of actin in cultured skin fibroblasts from patients with inherited adenocarcinoma. Proc. Natl. Acad. Sci. USA *74*:3019, 1977.
191. Kinsella, T. J., Little, J. B., Nove, J., Weichselbaum, R. R., Li, F. P., Meyer, R. J., Marchetto, D. J., and Patterson, W. B. Heterogeneous response to X-ray and ultraviolet light irradiations of cultured skin fibroblasts in two families with Gardner's syndrome. J. Natl. Cancer Inst. *68*:697, 1982.
192. Barfnecht, T. R., and Little, J. B. Abnormal sensitivity of skin fibroblasts from familial polyposis patients to DNA alkylating agents. Cancer Res. *42*:1249, 1982.
193. Miyaki, M., Akamatsu, N., Ono, T., Tonomura, A., and Utsunomiya, J. Morphologic transformation and chromosomal changes induced by chemical carcinogens in skin fibroblasts from patients with familial adenomatosis coli. J. Natl. Cancer Inst. *68*:563, 1982.
194. Kopelovich, L., Bias, N. E., and Helson, L. Tumour promoter alone induces neoplastic transformation of fibroblasts from humans genetically predisposed to cancer. Nature *282*:619, 1979.
195. Rider, S. H., Mazzullo, H. A., Davis, M. B., and Delhanty, J. D. A. Familial polyposis coli: growth characteristics of karyotypically variable cultured fibroblasts, response to epidermal growth factor and the tumour promoter 12-O-tetradecanoyl-phorbol-13-acetate. J. Med. Genet. *23*:131, 1986.
196. Gainer, H. S., Schor, S., and Kinsella, A. R. Susceptibility of skin fibroblasts from individual genetically predisposed to cancer to transformation by the tumour promoter 12-0-tetradecanoyl-phorbol-13-acetate. Int. J. Cancer *34*:349, 1984.
197. Friedman, E., Gillin, S., and Lipkin, M. 12-O-tetradecanoylphorbol-13-acetate stimulation of DNA synthesis in cultured preneoplastic familial polyposis colonic epithelial cells but not in normal colonic epithelial cells. Cancer Res. *44*:4078, 1984.
198. Danes, B. S., and Deschner, E. E. Detection of in vitro tetraploidy in heritable colon cancer syndromes. Confirmation by three different assays. Cancer *54*:1353, 1984.
199. Delhanty, J. D. A., Davis, M. B., and Wood, J. Chromosome instability in lymphocytes, fibroblasts, and colon epithelial-like cells from patients with familial polyposis coli. Cancer Genet. Cytogenet. *8*:27, 1983.
200. Danes, B. S. Increased in vitro tetraploidy: tissue specific within the heritable colorectal cancer syndromes with polyposis coli. Cancer *41*:2330, 1978.
201. Heim, S., Berger, R., Bernheim, A., and Mitelman, F. Constitutional C-band pattern in patients with adenomatosis of the colon and rectum. Cancer Genet. Cytogenet. *18*:31, 1985.
202. Heim, S., Johansen, S. G., Kolnig, A. M., and Strombeck, B.

Increased levels of spontaneous and mutagen-induced chromosome aberrations in skin fibroblasts from patients with adenomatosis of the colon and rectum. Cancer Genet. Cytogenet. *17*:333, 1985.
203. Mikol, Y. B., and Lipkin, M. Methionine dependence in skin fibroblasts of humans affected with familial colon cancer or Gardner's syndrome. J. Natl. Cancer Inst. *72*:19, 1984.
204. Filipe, M. I., Mughal, S., and Bussey, H. J. Patterns of mucus secretion in the colonic epithelium in familial polyposis. Invest. Cell Pathol. *3*:329, 1980.
205. Sams, J. S., Lynch, H. T., Burt, R. W., and Boland, C. R. Abnormalities in lectin binding profiles in familial colon cancer and familial polyposis coli. Gastroenterology *88*:1568, 1985.
206. Bone, E., Drasar, B. S., and Hill, M. J. Gut bacteria and their metabolic activity in familial polyposis. Lancet *1*:117, 1975.
207. Lipkin, M., Reddy, B. S., Weisburger, J., and Schechter, L. Nondegradation of fecal cholesterol in subjects at high risk for cancer of the large intestine. J. Clin. Invest. *67*:304, 1981.
208. Bussey, H. J. R., DeCosse, J. J., Deschner, E. E., Eyers, A. A., Lesser, M. L., Morson, B. C., Ritchie, S. M., Thomson, J. P., and Wadsworth, J. A randomized trial of ascorbic acid in polyposis coli. Cancer *50*:1434, 1982.
209. Moertel, C. G., Hill, J. R., and Adson, M. A. Management of multiple polyposis of the large intestine. Cancer *28*:160, 1971.
210. Harvey, J. C., Quan, S. H. Q., and Stearns, W. W. Management of familial polyposis with preservation of the rectum. Surgery *84*:476, 1978.
211. Bussey, H. J. R., Eyers, A. A., Ritchie, S. M., and Thompson, P. S. The rectum in adenomatous polyposis: the St. Mark's policy. Br. J. Surg. *72*:S29, 1985.
212. Sarre, R., Jagelman, D. G., Beck, G. J., McGannon, E., Fazio, V. W., Weakley, F. L., and Lavery, I. C. Colectomy with ileorectal anastomosis for familial adenomatous polyposis: the risk of rectal cancer. Surgery *101*:20, 1987.
213. Bussey, H. J. R. Extracolonic lesions associated with polyposis coli. Proc. R. Soc. Med. *65*:294, 1972.
214. Blair, N. P., and Trempe, C. L. Hypertrophy of the retinal pigment epithelium associated with Gardner's syndrome. Am. J. Ophthalmol. *90*:661, 1980.
215. Traboulski, E. I., Krush, A. J., Gardner, E. J., Booker, S. V., Offerhaus, G. J. A., Yardley, J. H., Hamilton, S. R., Luk, G. D., Giardiello, F. M., Welch, S. B., Hughes, J. P., and Maumenee, I. H. Prevalence and importance of pigmented ocular fundus lesions in Gardner's syndrome. N. Engl. J. Med. *316*:661, 1987.
216. Yao, T., Iida, M., Ohsato, K., Watanabe, H., and Omae, T. Duodenal lesions in familial polyposis of the colon. Gastroenterology *73*:1086, 1977.
217. Cohen, S. B. Familial polyposis coli and its extracolonic manifestations. J. Med. Genet. *19*:193, 1982.
218. Richards, R. C., Rogers, S. W., and Gardner, E. J. Spontaneous mesenteric fibromatosis in Gardner's syndrome. Cancer *47*:597, 1981.
219. Kiel, K. D., and Suit, H. D. Radiation therapy in the treatment of aggressive fibromatoses (desmoid tumors). Cancer *54*:2051, 1984.
220. Jones, I. T., Jagelman, D. G., Fazio, V. W., Lavery, I. C., Weakley, F. L., and McGannon, E. Desmoid tumors in familial polyposis coli. Ann. Surg. *204*:94, 1986.
221. Kinzbrunner, B., Ritter, S., Domingo, J., and Rosenthal, C. J. Remission of rapidly growing desmoid tumors after Tamoxifen therapy. Cancer *52*:2201, 1983.
222. Lanari, A. Effect of progesterone on desmoid tumors (aggressive fibromatosis). N. Engl. J. Med. *309*:1523, 1983.
223. Turcot, J., Despres, J. P., and St. Pierre, T. Malignant tumors of the central nervous system associated with familial polyposis of the colon. Report of two cases. Dis. Colon Rectum *2*:465, 1959.
224. Baughman, F. A., List, C. F., Williams, J. R., Muldoon, J. P., Segarra, J. M., and Volkel, J. S. The glioma-polyposis syndrome. N. Engl. J. Med. *281*:1345, 1969.
225. Binder, M. K., Zablen, M. A., Fleischer, D. E., Sue, D. Y., Dwyer, R. M., and Hanelin, L. Colon polyps, sebaceous cysts, gastric polyps and malignant brain tumor in a family. Am. J. Dig. Dis. *23*:460, 1978.
226. Itoh, H., Ohsato, K., Yao, T., Iida, M., and Watanabe, H. Turcot's syndrome and its mode of inheritance. Gut *20*:414, 1979.
227. Lewis, J. H., Ginsberg, A. L., and Toomey, K. E. Turcot's syndrome. Evidence for autosomal dominant inheritance. Cancer *51*:524, 1983.
228. Burdick, D., and Prior, J. T. Peutz-Jeghers syndrome. A clinicopathologic study of a large family with a 27-year follow-up. Cancer *50*:2139, 1982.
229. Perzin, K. H., and Bridge, M. F. Adenomatous and carcinomatous changes in hamartomatous polyps of the small intestine (Peutz-Jeghers syndrome). Cancer *49*:971, 1982.
230. Scully, R. E. Sex cord tumor with annular tubules. A distinctive ovarian tumor of the Peutz-Jeghers syndrome. Cancer *25*:1107, 1970.
231. Wilson, D. M., Pitts, W. C., Hintz, R. L., and Rosenfeld, R. G. Testicular tumors with Peutz-Jeghers syndrome. Cancer *57*:2238, 1986.
232. Beacham, C. H., Shields, H. M., Raffensperger, E. C., and Enterline, H. T. Juvenile and adenomatous gastrointestinal polyposis. Am. J. Dig. Dis. *23*:1137, 1978.
233. Grotsky, H. W., Rickert, R. R., Smith, W. D., and Newsome, J. F. Familial juvenile polyposis coli. A clinical and pathologic study of a large kindred. Gastroenterology *82*:494, 1982.
234. Watanabe, A., Nagashima, H., Motoi, M., and Ogawa, K. Familial juvenile polyposis of the stomach. Gastroenterology *77*:148, 1979.
235. Sachatello, C. R., Pickren, J. W., and Grace, J. T. Generalized juvenile gastrointestinal polyposis. A hereditary syndrome. Gastroenterology *58*:699, 1970.
236. Stemper, T. J., Kent, T. H., and Summers, R. W. Juvenile polyposis and gastrointestinal carcinoma. A study of a kindred. Ann. Intern. Med. *83*:639, 1975.
237. Goodman, Z. D., Yardley, J. H., and Milligan, F. D. Pathogenesis of colonic polyps in multiple juvenile polyposis. Cancer *43*:1906, 1979.
238. Rutgeerts, P., Hendricks, H., Geboes, K., Ponette, E., Broeckaert, L., and Vantrappen, G. Involvement of the upper digestive tract by systematic neurofibromatosis. Gastrointest. Endosc. *27*:22, 1981.
239. Weinstock, J. V., and Kawanishi, H. Gastrointestinal polyposis with orocutaneous hamartomas (Cowden's disease). Gastroenterology *74*:890, 1978.
240. Carlson, G. J., Nivatvongs, S., and Snover, D. C. Colorectal polyps in Cowden's disease (multiple hamartoma syndrome). Am. J. Surg. Pathol. *8*:763, 1984.
241. Lashner, B. A., Riddell, R. H., and Winans, C. S. Ganglioneuromatosis of the colon and extensive glycogenic acanthosis in Cowden's disease. Dig. Dis. Sci. *31*:213, 1986.
242. Schwartz, R. A. Basal cell nevus syndrome and gastrointestinal polyposis. N. Engl. J. Med. *299*:49, 1978.
243. Cronkhite, L. W., and Canada, W. J. Generalized gastrointestinal polyposis: an unusual syndrome of polyposis, pigmentation, alopecia and onychotrophia. N. Engl. J. Med. *252*:1011, 1955.
244. Daniel, E. S., Ludwig, S. L., Lewin, K. J., Ruprecht, R. M., Rajacich, G. M., and Schwabe, A. D. The Cronkhite-Canada syndrome. An analysis of the pathologic features and therapy in 55 patients. Medicine *61*:293, 1982.
245. Katayama, Y., Kimura, M., and Konn, M. Cronkhite-Canada syndrome associated with a rectal cancer and adenomatous changes in colonic polyps. Am. J. Surg. Pathol. *9*:65, 1985.
246. Russell, D. M., Bhathal, P. S., and St. John, D. J. B. Complete remission in Cronkhite-Canada syndrome. Gastroenterology *85*:180, 1983.

Malignant Neoplasms of the Large and Small Intestine

81

ROBERT S. BRESALIER
YOUNG S. KIM

Cancer of the colon and rectum (colorectal cancer) is a major cause of cancer-associated morbidity and mortality in North America, Europe, and other regions with similar life styles and dietary habits. The second most common cancer overall (excluding nonmelanoma skin cancer) in the United States, colorectal cancer currently constitutes 14 per cent of newly diagnosed cancer cases in men and 16 per cent in women. In 1987 there will be 145,000 new cases in this country and 60,000 related deaths.[1] Survival rates have changed little during the past 20 years. Approximately 6 per cent of the American population will eventually develop colon or rectal cancer, and 6 million Americans who are alive today will die of this disease. Globally, it is the third most common cancer in males and fourth most common cancer in females. Countries where colorectal cancer mortality was low prior to 1950 have experienced substantial increases.

Chapter 80 dealt in detail with the principal premalignant colonic lesion, the adenomatous polyp. In this chapter we will examine what is known about the factors that contribute to the development of colorectal cancer, its predisposing conditions, biology, natural history, clinical presentation, diagnosis, and management. Current concepts and recent advances will be stressed. Cancers of the small intestine will also be discussed in this chapter. New cases of small intestinal cancer will number approximately 2500 in the U.S. in 1987. The pathology, natural history, diagnosis, and management of these lesions will be described.

MALIGNANT NEOPLASMS OF THE LARGE INTESTINE

Descriptive Epidemiology and Epidemiologic Patterns

The frequency of colorectal cancer varies remarkably between different populations[2–5] (Fig. 81–1). Incidence rates are highest in the Westernized countries of North America, Australia, and New Zealand, intermediate in areas of Europe, and low in regions of Asia, South America, and especially sub-Saharan Africa. Internationally, a 60-fold difference exists in colon cancer incidence in males between areas with the lowest and highest rates[4] (Table 81–1), with an 18-fold variation for rectal cancer (cancer within 11 cm of the anus).

Although the incidences of colon and rectal cancer overall are roughly parallel, the incidence of colon cancer varies geographically more than that of rectal cancer. High ratios of colon to rectal cancer prevail in high-risk areas such as North America, while ratios below unity are often found in low-risk Asian and African populations. Females show a steeper rise in the incidence of colon cancer for each unit increase in the incidence of rectal cancer. Although part of the regional variation in the ratios of colon to rectal cancer may arise from local practices in classifying rectosigmoid tumors, these differences nonetheless suggest that colon and rectal cancer have related, but not identical etiologies.

In the United States the incidence of colorectal cancer also varies regionally; the highest rates for both males and females are consistently reported from Connecticut, and the lowest rates from Utah. In general, rates in the Southern and Western United States (except the San Francisco Bay area) are lower than the U.S. average, while the highest rates are in the Northeast and North Central states. Colorectal cancer inci-

Table 81–1. AGE-STANDARDIZED INCIDENCE OF COLORECTAL CANCER IN REGIONS WITH THE HIGHEST AND LOWEST RATES

Males		Females	
Colon			
Dakar, Senegal	0.6	Dakar, Senegal	0.7
Poona, India	3.1	Israel (non-Jews)	1.8
Bombay, India	3.5	Poona, India	2.8
Cali, Colombia	4.5	Singapore (Malays)	3.3
Connecticut, USA	32.3	San Francisco, USA (Japanese)	27.4
New York, USA	31.4	New Zealand (non-Maori)	26.9
Los Angeles, USA (Chinese)	31.3	Connecticut, USA	26.4
(Japanese)	30.8	New York, USA	26.3
Rectum			
Dakar, Senegal	1.5	Dakar, Senegal	1.0
Israel (non-Jews)	3.1	Israel (non-Jews)	1.5
Cali, Colombia	3.4	Cali, Colombia	2.3
Northwest Canada	22.6	Netherlands Antilles	7.6
Los Angeles, USA (Japanese)	21.7	Neuchatel, Switzerland	13.4
Hawaii, USA (Japanese)	21.4	Israel (US or European Jewish immigrants)	13.4
Bas-Rhin, France	21.0	Israel (all Jews)	11.9

Incidence per 100,000 population. Data from Waterhouse et al.[2]
The average incidence world-wide for cancer of the colon is 16.6 per 100,000 in males and 14.7 in females. For rectal cancer the world-wide average is 11.9 in males and 7.7 in females.

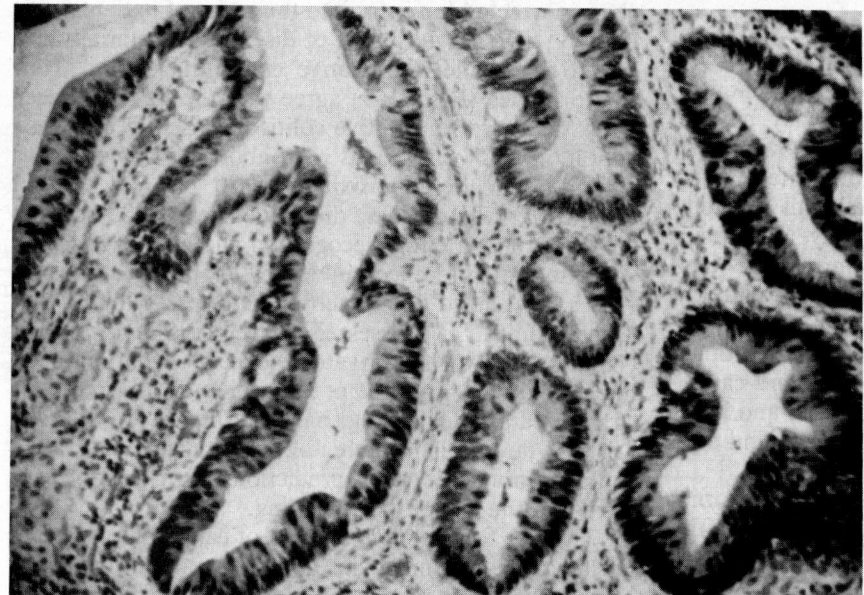

Figure 81–10. High-grade dysplasia in the setting of ulcerative colitis. Goblet cells are decreased. Glands are branched, irregular, and crowded together. Cell nuclei are hyperchromatic and occur at different levels, producing a pseudopalisading or "picket fence" appearance.

The risk for colorectal carcinoma in patients with Crohn's colitis or ileocolitis has been reported to be four to twenty times that in the general population.[103, 104] Cancers arise in a younger age group in the patients than in the general population.[104] Many of these cancers are mucinous carcinomas, and may be present in surgically bypassed or strictured segments of colon. The distribution of tumors in the colon is no different than in the general population.

It is thought that carcinomas do not develop *de novo* from normal mucosa, but from mucosa that has undergone a sequence of morphologic changes that culminate in invasive carcinoma. As with precancerous adenomas, dysplasia is a precursor to carcinoma in inflammatory bowel disease. Dysplasia includes abnormalities in crypt architecture and cytologic detail (Figs. 81–10 and 81–11). Epithelial crypts are reduced in number, irregularly branched, and crowded together ("back to back glands"). Cell nuclei may be enlarged and hyperchromatic, have increased mitoses, and be located at different levels in the cell producing a "picket fence" appearance (pseudostratification). Dysplasia is often classified by grade into mild or low-grade and severe or high-grade dysplasia.

Retrospective analyses report that 90 per cent of resected colons from patients with ulcerative colitis and cancer will contain dysplastic mucosa somewhere in the colon, and 30 per cent of patients with severe rectal or colonic dysplasia on resection or biopsy have coexistent carcinoma.[94, 105, 106] Colonoscopic studies Suggest that 25 per cent of colons that demonstrate severe (high grade) dysplasia on biopsy harbor a car-

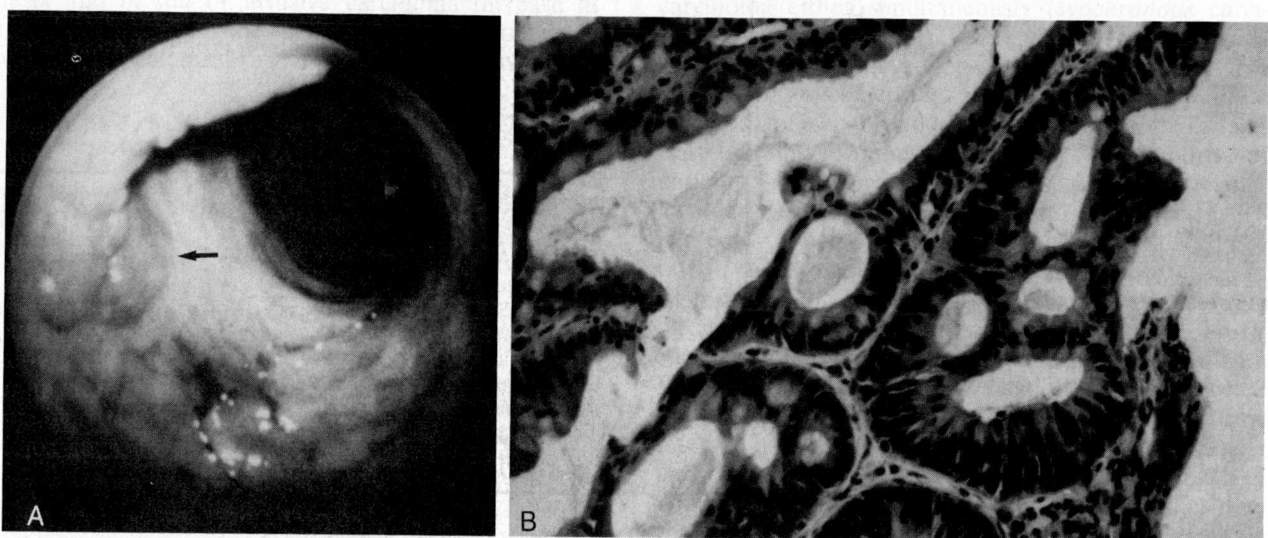

Figure 81–11. Plaque-like "dysplasia associated mass lesions" in a patient with longstanding ulcerative colitis. *A*, Lesions as seen through the colonoscope *(arrow)*. *B*, Biopsy revealing high-grade dysplasia.

cinoma.[95, 107–109] The incidence of dysplasia correlates positively with duration of colitis. Dysplasia is often patchy, and may be present in the colon despite absence from the rectum.

Since the lack of uniformity of the definition of dysplasia may make interpretation of such data difficult, a multidisciplinary "Inflammatory Bowel Disease–Dysplasia–Morphology Study Group" has developed a standardized classification for dysplasia arising in the setting of inflammatory bowel disease.[110] Several large prospective studies are under way to determine the true risk of cancer in patients with colonic dysplasia and ulcerative colitis, as well as the impact of screening programs for dysplasia (see pp. 1537–1542 for discussion of screening for cancer in high-risk groups).[107, 111] The risk of cancer appears highest in those with high-grade dysplasia, and in whom dysplasia arises in visible plaques or masses (dysplasia-associated mass lesions) (Fig. 81–11).[108, 109] Many investigators believe that patients with ulcerative colitis longer than 10 years should have colonoscopy with multiple mucosal biopsies annually to identify areas of dysplasia, and some advocate colectomy in those with severe dysplasia or dysplasia-associated mass lesions.[110] Since the significance of low-grade or moderate dysplasia is less clear, immediate resection is not recommended for patients with these levels of dysplasia.

Both dysplasia and an increased risk of colon carcinoma have been reported in patients with Crohn's disease.[112, 113] As in ulcerative colitis, dysplasia appears in diseased colonic segments, and its presence correlates with duration of disease.

Other Associated Disease States

Diverting bile to the lower small intestine, either surgically or by feeding cholestyramine, increases the yield of proximal colonic tumors in carcinogen-treated animals. Since cholecystectomy in man could analogously lead to an increased delivery of secondary bile acids to the proximal bowel, the possibility of an increase in colon cancer following cholecystectomy has been raised. The clinical evidence for such an association, however, is contradictory. An increased proliferative activity has been demonstrated in the distal colonic mucosa of cholecystectomized patients,[114] and an increased frequency of tubular adenomas has been found in patients greater than 60 years of age with a postcholecystectomy interval greater than 10 years,[115] but an increased risk of colonic cancer in these patients has both been supported[116, 117] and refuted.[118, 119] A Swedish population-based cohort study[119] has now followed a large group of patients for 14 to 17 years after operation and failed to show an association between cholecystectomy and cancer.

An association between Barrett's esophagus and colon cancer has been suggested.[120] This observation requires additional confirmation,[121] and the basis for the possible association remains obscure.

Tumor Pathology, Natural History, and Staging

Gross Features

The gross morphologic features of adenocarcinoma in the large bowel depend on their location. Carcinomas of the proximal colon, particularly those of the cecum and ascending colon, tend to be large and bulky, often outgrowing their blood supply and undergoing necrosis.[122] This polypoid configuration may also be found elsewhere in the colon and rectum. In the more distal colon and rectum tumors more frequently involve a greater circumference of the bowel, producing an annular constriction or "napkin-ring" appearance (Fig. 81–12). The fibrous stroma of these tumors accounts

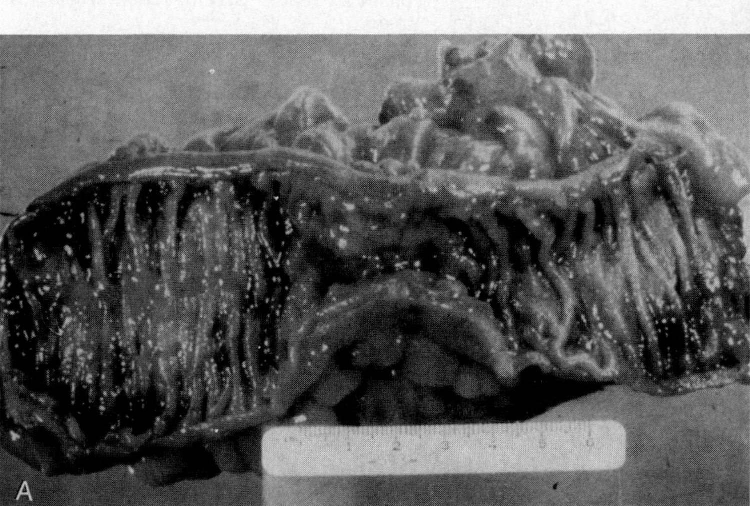

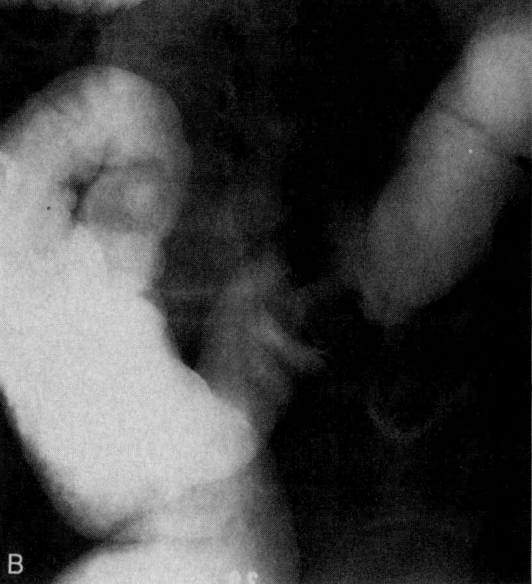

Figure 81–12. Carcinoma of the sigmoid colon. *A,* Surgical specimen demonstrates annular constriction or "napkin ring" appearance. *B,* Lesion seen on full column barium enema.

for constriction and narrowing of the bowel lumen, while the circular arrangement of colonic lymphatics is responsible for their annular growth. These tumors may also become ulcerated. Occasionally tumors will have a flatter appearance with predominantly intramural spread. The latter are most frequently seen in the setting of inflammatory bowel disease. The morphologic features of these carcinomas have clinical, diagnostic, and prognostic implications (see p. 1542).

Histology

Carcinomas of the large bowel are predominantly adenocarcinomas which form moderately to well differentiated glands and secrete variable amounts of mucin (Fig. 81–13*A*). Mucin, a large molecular weight glycoprotein, is the major secreted product of both normal and neoplastic glands of the colon, and may be seen best with histochemical stains such as periodic acid–Schiff (PAS) stain (Fig. 81–13*B*). In poorly differentiated tumors gland formation and mucin production are present, but less prominent. "Signet-ring" cells, in which a large vacuole of mucin displaces the nucleus to one side, are a feature of some tumors. In approximately 15 per cent of tumors large lakes of mucin contain scattered collections of tumor cells (Fig. 81–14). These *mucinous* or *colloid carcinomas*[123] occur most frequently in patients with hereditary non-polyposis-related carcinomas, in the setting of ulcerative colitis, and in patients in which carcinomas occur at an early age. *Scirrous carcinomas*[124] are uncommon and are characterized by sparse gland formation with marked desmoplasia and fibrous tissue surrounding glandular structures. Cancers other than adenocarcinomas compose less than 5 per cent of malignant tumors of the large bowel. Tumors arising at the

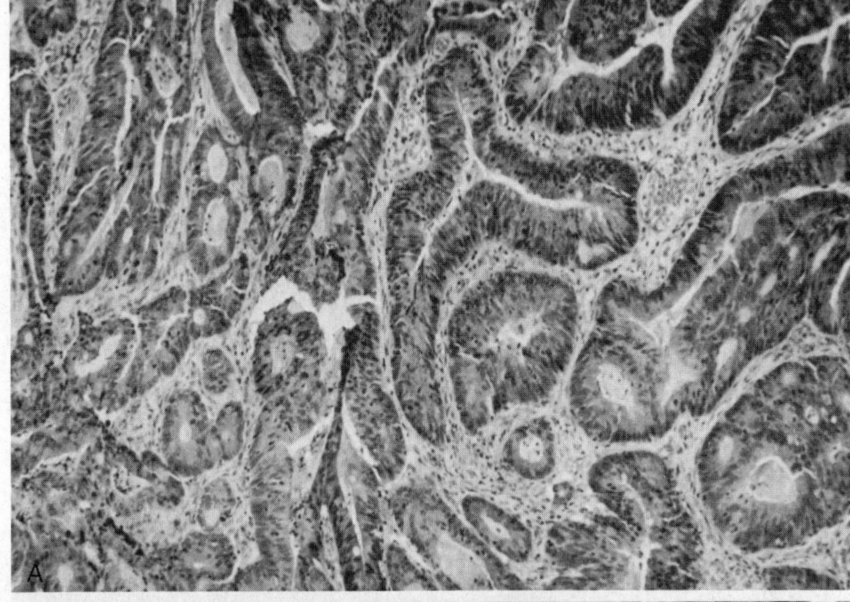

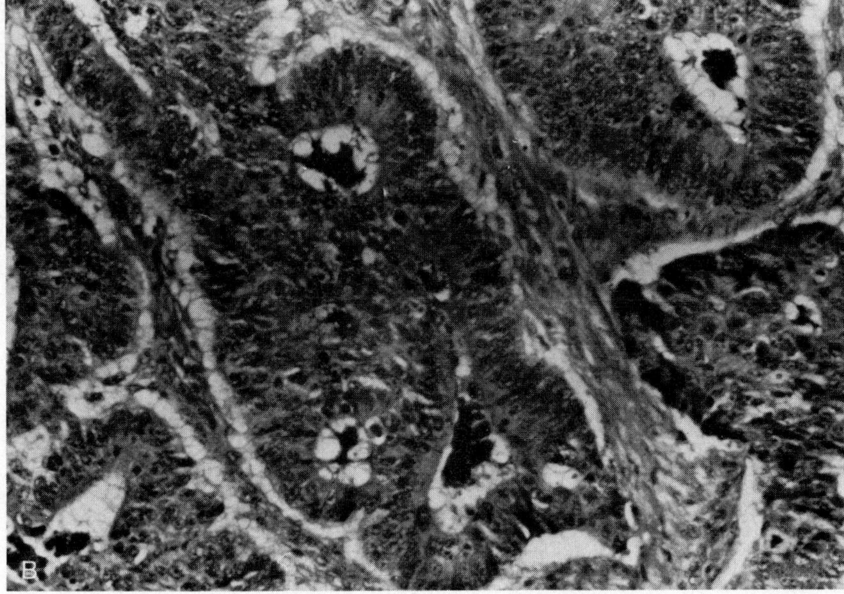

Figure 81–13. *A*, Well-differentiated adenocarcinoma of the colon. Histologic section stained with hematoxylin and eosin demonstrates crowded neoplastic glands containing variable amounts of mucin. *B*, Section stained with periodic acid–Schiff method better demonstrates mucin (dark material) in gland lumens.

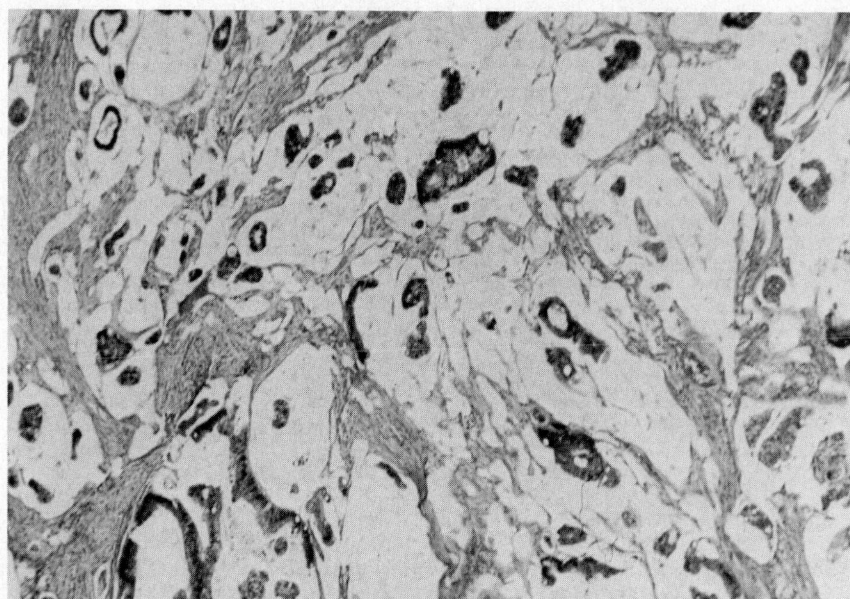

Figure 81–14. Colloid carcinoma of the colon with scattered "nests" of tumor cells floating in "lakes" of mucin.

anorectal junction include squamous cell carcinomas, cloacogenic or transitional cell carcinomas, and melanocarcinomas. Primary lymphomas and carcinoid tumors of the large bowel compose less than 0.1 per cent of all large bowel neoplasms (see p. 1545).

Natural History and Staging

Colorectal cancers begin as intramucosal epithelial lesions usually arising in adenomatous polyps or glands. As cancers grow they become invasive, penetrating the muscularis mucosae of the bowel and invading lymphatic and vascular channels to involve regional lymph nodes, adjacent structures, and distant sites. Adenocarcinomas of the colon and rectum grow at variable rates, but appear to have long periods of silent growth before producing bowel symptoms. The mean doubling time of colon cancers determined radiographically in one study was 620 days.[125] Patterns of spread depend upon the anatomy of the individual bowel segment as well as its lymphatic and vascular supply.

Cancers of the rectum advance locally by progressive penetration of the bowel wall.[126] Extension of the primary tumor intramurally parallel to the long axis of the bowel is most often limited,[127–129] and lymphatic and hematogenous spread are unusual prior to penetration of the muscularis mucosae. An exception appears to be the case of poorly differentiated tumors, which may metastasize lymphatically or hematogenously prior to bowel penetration. Since the rectum is relatively immobile and lacks a serosal covering, rectal cancers tend to spread contiguously to progressively involve local structures. Because of the dual blood supply of the lower one third of the rectum, tumors arising here may metastasize hematogenously to the liver via the superior hemorrhoidal vein and portal system, or to the lungs by way of the middle hemorrhoidal vein and inferior vena cava. The upper and middle thirds of the rectum drain into the portal system, and tumors in these segments first spread hematogenously to the liver. Occasionally lumbar and thoracic vertebral metastases may occur as the result of hematogenous spread via portal-vertebral communications (Batson's vertebral venous plexuses).

Colonic cancers also invade transmurally to penetrate the bowel wall and involve regional lymphatics and then distant nodes. (The lymphatic drainage generally parallels the arterial supply to a given bowel segment.) The liver is the most common site of hematogenous spread from colonic tumors which occurs via the portal venous system. Pulmonary metastases from colon cancer result, in general, from hepatic metastases.

Based on observations of what he felt to be an orderly progression of local-regional invasion by rectal cancers, Cuthbert Dukes proposed a classification in 1929[130] which has since been modified numerous times in attempts to heighten its prognostic value for cancers of both the rectum and colon (Table 81–6). The most commonly employed modification of Dukes' system is that of Astler and Coller.[122] This classification uses the following designations: A, tumors limited to the mucosa; B1, tumors extending into, but not through the muscularis propria; B2, tumors penetrating the bowel wall but without lymph node involvement; and C, tumors with regional lymph node involvement by tumor. Stage C tumors are further divided into those in which the primary tumor is limited to the bowel wall (C1) and those in which the tumor penetrates the bowel wall (C2). In the system proposed by the Gastrointestinal Tumor Study Group,[131] C1 lesions are those in which one to four regional lymph nodes contain tumor, and C2 lesions are those in which more than four lymph nodes contain tumor. Another modification by Turnbull adds a D category to account for distant metastases.[132]

Table 81–6. DUKES' CLASSIFICATION FOR CARCINOMA OF THE RECTUM AND ITS MODIFICATIONS FOR COLORECTAL CARCINOMA

Stage	Dukes, 1932 (Rectum)	Gabriel, Dukes, Bussey, 1935 (Rectum)	Kirklin et al., 1949 (Rectum & sigmoid)	Astler-Coller, 1954 (Rectum & colon)	Turnbull et al., 1967 (Colon)	Modified Astler-Coller (Gunderson & Sosin, 1974) (Rectum & colon)	GITSG, 1975 (Rectum & colon)
A	Limited to bowel wall	Limited to bowel wall	Limited to mucosa	Limited to mucosa	Limited to mucosa	Limited to mucosa	Limited to mucosa
B	Through bowel wall	Through bowel wall	—	—	Tumor extension into pericolic fat	—	—
B1	—	—	Into muscularis propria	Into muscularis propria	—	Into muscularis propria	Into muscularis propria
B2	—	—	Through muscularis propria	Through muscularis propria (and serosa)	—	Through serosa m = microscopic m+g = gross	Through serosa
B3	—	—	—	—	—	Adherent to or invading adjacent structures	—
C	Regional nodal metastases	—	Regional nodal metastases	—	Regional nodal metastases	—	—
C1	—	Regional nodal metastases near primary lesion	—	Same as B1 plus regional nodal metastases	—	Same as B1 plus regional nodal metastases	1–4 regional nodes positive
C2	—	Proximal node involved at point of ligation	—	Same as B2 plus regional nodal metastases	—	Same as B2 plus regional nodal metastases	>4 regional nodes positive
C3	—	—	—	—	—	Same as B3 plus regional nodal metastases	—
D	—	—	—	—	Distant metastases (liver, lung, bone) or due to parietal or adjacent organ invasion	—	—

In an attempt to provide a uniform and orderly classification for colorectal cancers the American Joint Committee (AJC) for Cancer Staging and End Results Reporting, and the International Union Against Cancer (UICC) have each proposed a TNM classification for colorectal cancer.[133, 134] These systems classify the extent of the primary tumor (T), the status of regional lymph nodes (N), and the presence or absence of distant metastases (M). Cases are assigned the highest value of TNM that describes the full extent of disease and are grouped into five stages (Table 81–7).

Prognostic Indicators

Clinical and pathologic variables that may affect the prognosis of patients with colorectal cancer are outlined in Table 81–8. These variables are important in predicting clinical outcome and in designing optimum strategies for treatment and follow-up. Their identification has led to a progressive modification of the staging classifications for colorectal cancer. The roles

Table 81–7. STAGE CLASSIFICATION AND GROUPING—AMERICAN JOINT COMMITTEE CANCER 1978, 1981

Stage 0
- Carcinoma *in situ*
- TIS N0 M0

Stage I
- 1A Tumor confined to mucosa or submucosa T1 N0 M0
- 1B Tumor involves muscularis propria but not beyond T2 N0 M0

Stage II
- Involvement of all layers of bowel wall with invasion of immediately adjacent structures
- T3 N0 M0

Stage III
- Any degree of bowel wall with regional node metastasis
- Any T N1–3 M0
- Extends beyond contiguous tissue or immediately adjacent organs with no regional lymph node metastasis
- T4 N0 M0

Stage IV
- Any invasion of bowel wall with or without regional lymph node metastasis but with evidence of distant metastasis
- Any T Any N M1

From American Joint Committee for Cancer Staging and End Results Reporting.[133]

Table 81–8. PATHOLOGIC AND CLINICAL FEATURES THAT MAY AFFECT PROGNOSIS IN PATIENTS WITH COLORECTAL CANCER

Pathologic Features	Effect on Prognosis
Surgical-pathologic stage	
Depth of bowel wall penetration	Increased penetration diminishes prognosis
Number of regional lymph nodes involved by tumor	1–4 nodes better than >4 nodes
Tumor histology	
Degree of differentiation	Well differentiated better than poorly differentiated
Mucinous (colloid) or signet-cell histology	Diminished prognosis
Scirrhous histology	Diminished prognosis
Venous invasion	Diminished prognosis
Lymphatic invasion	Diminished prognosis
Perineural invasion	Diminished prognosis
Local inflammatory and immunologic reaction	Improved prognosis
Tumor size	No effect in most studies
Tumor morphology	Polypoid/exophytic better than ulcerating/infiltrating
Tumor DNA content	Increased DNA content (aneuploidy) diminishes prognosis
Clinical Features	
Diagnosis in asymptomatic patients	?Improved prognosis
Duration of symptoms	No demonstrated effect
Rectal bleeding as presenting symptom	Improved prognosis
Bowel obstruction	Diminished prognosis
Bowel perforation	Diminished prognosis
Tumor location	?Colon better than rectum ?Left colon better than right colon
Age less than 30	Diminished prognosis
Preoperative serum CEA	Diminished prognosis with high CEA level
Distant metastases	Markedly diminished prognosis

of histologic differentiation, tumor size, location, configuration, degree of invasion, and lymph node status must be evaluated based on the prospective analysis of patients undergoing curative resections for colorectal cancer.

Surgical-Pathologic Stage of the Primary Tumor

The depth of transmural tumor penetration of the bowel wall and the extent of regional lymph node spread are important in determining prognosis[122, 126, 129–132, 134–139] (Fig. 81–15). Further, the degree of bowel wall penetration affects prognosis independent of lymph node status.[135–137] One study that uses Astler and Coller's modification of Dukes' classification demonstrates a significant difference in 5-year survival in patients without nodal metastases which correlates with degree of penetration of the bowel wall.[135] Patients with B1 lesions had a 5-year survival of 65 per cent, compared with 43 per cent for those with B2 lesions. Similarly if lymph nodes contained metastases but the muscularis mucosae was not penetrated (C1), the five-year survival rate was 53 per cent, dropping to 15 per cent if penetration of the bowel wall was complete (C2). Survival rates for Dukes' A lesions range from 70 to 100 per cent with a mean of about 80 per cent.

Degree of tumor penetration correlates with the number of positive nodes[136] as well as with the incidence of local recurrence after surgical resection.[131, 137, 138] The incidence of local failure for Dukes' A rectal lesions is 8 per cent; Dukes' B, 31 per cent; and Dukes' C, 50 per cent.[137] The number of involved regional lymph nodes also appears to correlate independently with outcome[131, 139, 140] (Fig. 81–15*B*). The National Surgical Adjuvant Project for Breast and Bowel Cancer (NSABP)[139] reports a significant difference in postresection survival for colorectal cancer in favor of patients with one to four positive nodes compared with those having more than four nodes involved by tumor, independent of degree of tumor penetration. The Gastrointestinal Tumor Study Group (GITSG)[131] similarly finds that at a median of 5.5 years after surgery, disease recurs in 35 per cent of patients with one to four positive nodes versus 61 per cent of patients with more than four positive nodes.

Tumor Morphology and Histology

The TNM classification (Table 81–7) for human carcinomas is based in part on the observation that, for most cancers, tumor size correlates with local and distant spread and, hence, with prognosis. Numerous studies suggest that colorectal cancer is an exception, and that size of the primary tumor *per se* does not correlate with prognosis.[129, 136, 141–143] The NASBP trial, for example, shows no correlation between the longest diameter of the primary tumor and the status of regional lymph nodes for Dukes' B and C colon or rectal cancers.[143] While the degree of bowel wall penetration in Dukes' C rectal cancers corresponds to tumor size, the number of positive nodes within the C1 and C2 patient subsets does not.[136] The GITSG study, on the other hand, finds a relationship between maximum tumor dimension, adjusted for stage and morphology, and survival.[144] These divergent findings may be related, in part, to methods of measurement and criteria used in determining tumor size. Patients with exophytic or polypoid tumors appear to have a better prognosis than patients with ulcerating or infiltrating tumors.[144]

Tumor prognosis correlates with histologic grade, poor differentiation conferring a worse prognosis than a high degree of differentiation.[130, 137, 140–147] A comparison of poorly versus well differentiated tumors showed the relative risk for survival to be 1.68 in favor of well differentiated cancers.[144] Since no uniform system of grading tumors exists, comparison between studies is difficult. Mucinous[123] and scirrhous[124] carcinomas appear to be biologically more aggressive, and patients with these tumors have a decreased survival compared with those having other adenocarcinomas. Signet-ring carcinomas have been reported to present at an advanced stage and to be highly invasive tumors.[148, 149]

Venous invasion by colorectal cancer correlates with

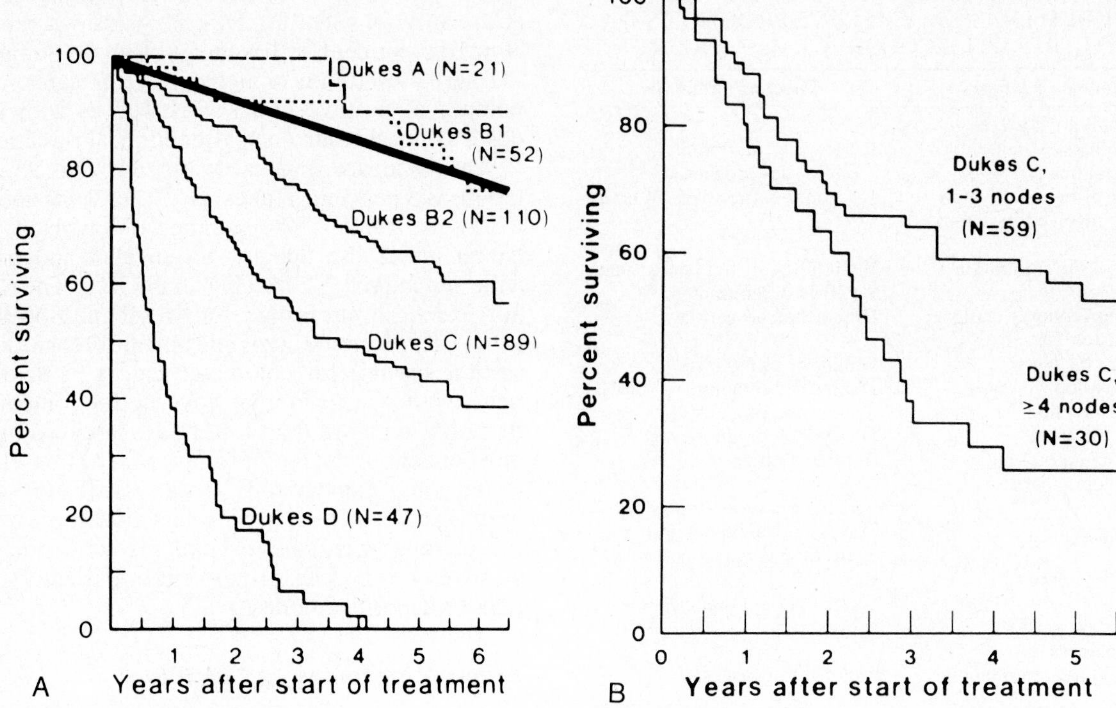

Figure 81–15. *A*, Survival probabilities according to stage of disease in patients undergoing potentially curative surgery for colorectal cancer. Expected survival among age- and sex-matched general population is indicated by heavy line. *B*, Survival probabilities according to number of nodes involved in patients with stage C colorectal carcinoma. (From Moertel, C. G., O'Fallon, J. R., Go, V. L., et al. Cancer *58*:603, 1986. Used by permission.)

local recurrence after resection, visceral metastases, and decreased survival in most studies[137, 147, 150, 151] but may not be of independent prognostic value for tumors confined to the bowel wall.[152] Lymphatic invasion is associated with decreased survival,[141] but it is unclear whether this variable is independent of depth of tumor invasion and regional nodal metastasis. Perineural invasion is also linked to increased local recurrence and decreased survival,[153] but the data are limited.

The amount of inflammatory response[141] and lymphocytic infiltration[154] in and around a cancer may be related to outcome, with increased inflammation and immunologic reaction conferring a better prognosis, but once again the data are limited.

The prognosis of patients with colorectal cancer may be related to the DNA content of the primary tumor,[57, 58, 155, 156] since patients with nondiploid or aneuploid tumors have a decreased survival compared with those having cells with a normal or diploid DNA content. The value of flow cytometric measurements of the DNA content of tumor cells in assessing clinical prognosis and planning treatment remains to be determined.

Clinical Features

While screening programs for colorectal cancer suggest that tumors diagnosed in asymptomatic patients are less advanced (see p. 1537),[157–159] assessment of the impact of early diagnosis on survival in asymptomatic individuals awaits the results of prospective randomized controlled studies. Duration of symptoms may not correlate directly with prognosis,[135, 160, 161] and some presenting symptoms such as rectal bleeding may be associated with better rates of survival.[163]

Bowel obstruction or perforation has been linked with a poor prognosis.[162–166] Patients who present with obstructing lesions may not be candidates for curative surgery, and have a higher operative morbidity and mortality. Recurrence following "curative" surgery in patients presenting with obstruction or perforation is also higher.

The location of the primary tumor may influence outcome. According to one study, tumors of the rectosigmoid and rectum have the worst prognosis, and tumors of the left colon (transverse and descending colon) and sigmoid colon the best.[163] On the other hand, another study finds tumor location to be of insignificant prognostic importance.[165] Disease-free survival at three years has been found to be 2 to 14 per cent higher following surgery for tumors of the left than of the right colon.[163, 165] Acceptance of the data from such studies is reduced by selection since these patients may not be representative of the general population with colorectal cancer. Many but not all studies suggest a survival advantage in patients with colonic versus rectal cancers.

One to 3 per cent of colorectal carcinomas arise in patients less than 30 years of age, 11 per cent of whom have a predisposing condition such as familial polyposis or ulcerative colitis. The incidence of nonpolyposis familial colon cancers in this group is unknown. The prognosis is worse than for older patients with this disease, and is particularly poor in the pediatric age group.[167–170] Poor prognosis may be related to the high number of more advanced cancers at diagnosis, poorly differentiated cancers, and mucinous adenocarcinomas in these patients.

Outcome is related to the preoperative serum *carcinoembryonic antigen* (CEA) level.[140, 171, 172] Tumor recurrence is higher and the estimated mean time to recurrence is shorter in patients with Dukes' B and C cancers who have high preoperative CEA levels.[171] The preoperative CEA level may be of prognostic value only in patients with Dukes' C colorectal cancers with four or more involved lymph nodes, but may not be indicative of survival in patients with Dukes' A and B lesions or Dukes' C lesions with less than four nodes involved.[173]

Approximately one fourth of patients with colorectal cancer will have clinical evidence of hematogenous spread when initially seen, and 50 per cent will eventually develop metastases to distant sites, the most common being the liver. These metastases confer a very poor prognosis at all times in the clinical course. The most important determinant of duration of survival for patients presenting with liver metastases is the extent of hepatic involvement by tumor[173] (see p. 1543).

Clinical Picture

Adenocarcinomas of the colon and rectum grow slowly and may be present for as long as five years before symptoms appear (see p. 1533). However, those with asymptomatic disease will often have occult blood loss from their tumors, and the bleeding rate increases with tumor size and degree of ulceration.

Symptoms depend to some extent on the location of the primary tumor.[174] Cancers of the proximal colon usually attain a larger size than those of the left colon and rectum before becoming symptomatic. Constitutional symptoms (fatigue, shortness of breath, angina) due to microcytic hypochromic anemia may be the principal manner of presentation of right colonic tumors. Less commonly, blood from right colonic cancers is admixed with stool, appearing as mahogany feces. As a tumor grows it produces vague abdominal discomfort or presents as a palpable mass. Obstruction is uncommon because of the large diameters of the cecum and ascending colon.

The left colon has a narrower lumen than the proximal colon, and cancers of the descending and sigmoid colon often involve the bowel circumferentially and cause obstructive symptoms. Patients may present with colicky abdominal pain, particularly after meals, and a change in their bowel habits. Constipation may alternate with an increased frequency of defecation, as small amounts of retained stool move beyond the obstructing lesion. Hemotochezia is more often present with distal than proximal lesions, and bright red blood passed per rectum or coating the surface of the stool is common with cancers of the left colon and rectum. Rectal cancers also cause obstruction and changes in bowel habits, including constipation, diarrhea, and tenesmus. Rectal cancers may invade locally to involve the bladder, vaginal wall, or surrounding nerves resulting in perineal or sacral pain, but this is a late occurrence.

Symptomatic patients with colorectal cancer are often misdiagnosed. Symptoms are ascribed to benign diseases such as diverticular disease (abdominal pain, bleeding, change in stool caliber), irritable bowel syndrome (abdominal pain, change in bowel habits), or hemorrhoids (rectal bleeding). Colorectal carcinoma should be considered in patients presenting with hypochromic microcytic anemia or frank hematochezia and rectal bleeding, especially in persons over 40 years of age. Too often anemia in the elderly is ascribed to "chronic disease," only to be diagnosed later as an advanced colorectal cancer. Abdominal pain in any form also merits evaluation for cancer in this age group. Large bowel cancer affects younger patients, particularly those with inflammatory bowel disease or a strong family history for colorectal and other cancers. Judicious evaluation of younger patients for colorectal cancer is therefore warranted when suggested by history and clinical presentation.

Diagnosis and Screening

Diagnosis When Colorectal Cancer Is Suspected

When colorectal cancer is suspected because of clinical signs and symptoms or when screening suggests the possibility of a large bowel tumor (see below), prompt diagnostic evaluation should be undertaken endoscopically or radiographically (Fig. 81–16). Colonoscopy is 12 per cent more accurate than air contrast barium enema, especially in detecting small lesions such as adenomas (see pp. 1492–1493).[175–178] If colonoscopy is unavailable, technically difficult, or refused by the patient, an air contrast barium enema should be performed following sigmoidoscopy. Air contrast exams are more accurate than full-column barium enemas not only for diagnosing cancers but for detecting small adenomas which are often present as synchronous lesions.[177–182] Neoplasms in the rectum and sigmoid are sometimes difficult to diagnose radiologically, and rectosigmoidoscopy should be used as a complement to double-contrast enemas.[175, 177, 183] Flexible fiberoptic sigmoidoscopy is superior to rigid sigmoidoscopy.[177, 178, 184]

If a carcinoma is detected radiographically or by sigmoidoscopy, a full colonoscopic examination should be done because of the high incidence of synchronous lesions, and the possible effect of the colonoscopic findings or the surgical plan.[88, 185] Up to half of patients with proven cancers of the colon and rectum may harbor additional lesions, and in almost 10 per cent the operative plan will require modification as the result of preoperative colonoscopy.[185]

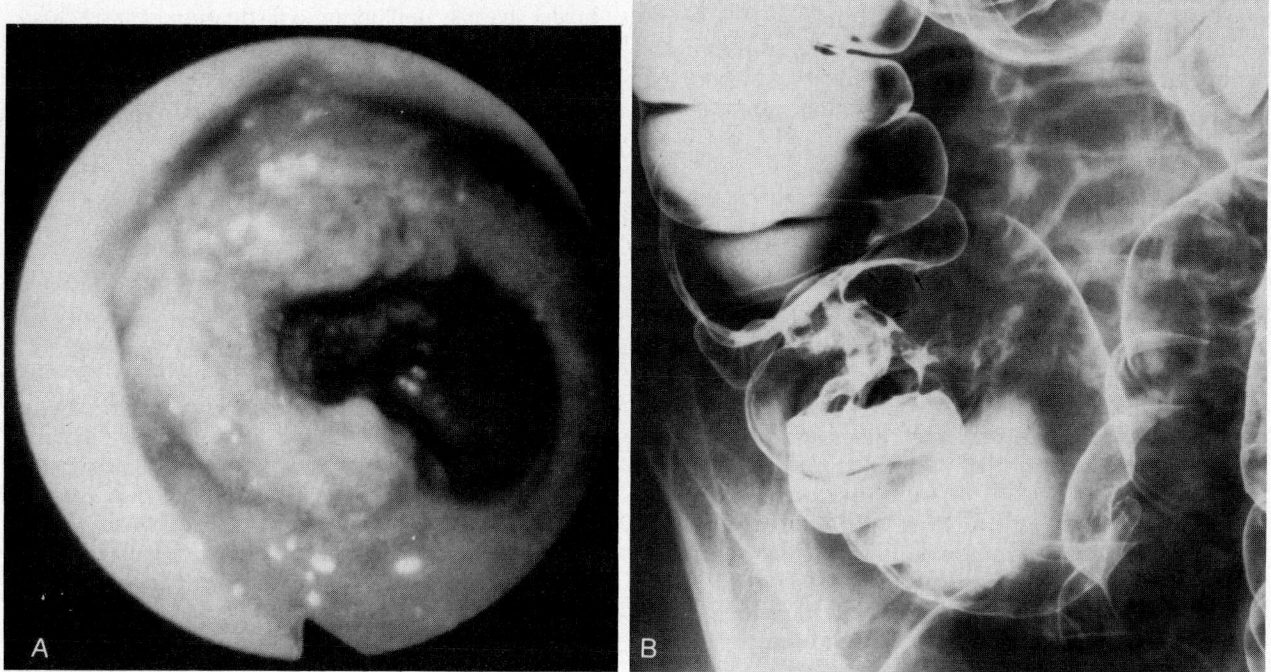

Figure 81–16. Carcinoma of the cecum as seen by *(A)* colonoscopy and *(B)* air contrast barium enema *(arrows).*

Principles of Screening

Cancer prevention may be categorized as primary or secondary. *Primary* prevention concerns the ability to identify genetic, biologic, and environmental factors that are etiologic or pathogenetic and to alter their effects on carcinogenesis (see p. 1521). Although several areas of study have been identified that may lead to primary prevention of large bowel cancer, available data do not yet provide a basis for primary preventive measures.

The goal of *secondary* prevention is to identify existing preneoplastic and early neoplastic lesions, symptomatic and asymptomatic, and treat them in a thorough and expeditious manner. The implicit but unproven assumption is that early detection improves prognosis. In symptomatic patients it is important to minimize the delay in diagnosis. When the clinical setting suggests a colorectal malignancy (e.g., iron deficiency anemia in an elderly patient), a prompt diagnostic evaluation should be undertaken. This approach pertains to individual patients and small groups in daily practice and is known as *case finding. Screening* pertains to large populations. Screening a symptomatic population for any disease is worthwhile if (1) the disease represents a major health problem; (2) effective therapy is available if the disease is found; (3) a "good" screening test is available that is readily acceptable by the patients and physicians, and (4) the screening test is cost-effective. Colorectal cancer fulfills conditions (1) and (2) since it represents a major health problem, and localized lesions are curable by surgical resection. The challenges are conditions (3) and (4); that is, to develop an effective, easily administered, and cost-effective screening test for this disease. The American Cancer Society currently recommends that all individuals over 40 years of age have yearly digital rectal examinations, that individuals over 50 have their stool tested yearly for occult blood and have sigmoidoscopy performed every three to five years after two negative initial examinations one year apart. A recent survey indicates that while most physicians agree with these guidelines, many do not follow them with all patients.[186]

The use of screening modalities for the detection of adenomatous polyps in the colon has been discussed on pages 1492 to 1493. Table 81–9 presents some of the characteristics of tests used in diagnosing and screening for colorectal adenomas as well as carcinomas.

Screening Techniques

Fecal Occult Blood Testing. The testing of stool for the presence of occult blood as an indication of colorectal cancer is a concept originally described by Van Deen in 1864 and popularized by Greegor in 1967.[187] The most widely used tests are qualitative chromagen tests, which rely on the oxidative conversion of a colorless compound to a colored one in the presence of the pseudoperoxidase activity of hemoglobin. Early tests utilizing orthotoluidine, benzidine, or the bench guaiac test produced too many false positive reactions to be clinically practical for screening. More recently, standardized tests employing guaiac-impregnated paper and developing solutions (hydrogen peroxide in denatured alcohol) have been widely studied and utilized clinically (e.g., Hemoccult, Hemoccult II). These

Table 81–9. PROCEDURES FOR DIAGNOSING AND SCREENING FOR COLORECTAL POLYPS AND CANCERS

Proportion of adenomatous polyps and cancers that can be detected by various instruments:	
Rigid sigmoidoscope	30%
35-cm flexible sigmoidoscope	40%
60-cm flexible sigmoidoscope	55%
Colonoscope	95%
Air-contrast barium enema	92%
Single-column barium enema	85%
Random false negative rates:	
FOBT*	40%
Sigmoidoscopies†	15%
Colonoscopy	5%
Air-contrast barium enema	15%
Single-column barium enema	30%
Random false positive rates:	
FOBT	2%
Air-contrast barium enema	3.5%
Single-column barium enema	3%
Charges for each procedure:	
FOBT	$ 5.00
Rigid sigmoidoscopy	$ 70.00
35-cm flexible sigmoidoscopy	$100.00
60-cm flexible sigmoidoscopy	$135.00
Colonoscopy	$500.00
Air-contrast barium enema	$200.00
Single-column barium enema	$150.00
Charges for work-up for a person with a false positive FOBT:	$800.00

Data from Eddy et al.[178]

*FOBT, fecal occult blood test.

†Rigid sigmoidoscopy may miss two to three times as many lesions as flexible sigmoidoscopy in examining the same bowel segment.[207]

are commercially available, convenient, and inexpensive. Their effectiveness in detecting occult blood in the stool depends, however, on the degree of fecal hydration (increases sensitivity), amount of hemoglobin degradation (decreases sensitivity owing to storage or the action of fecal flora), and the absence of interfering substances that enhance (iron preparations) or inhibit (e.g., ascorbic acid) oxidation of the indicator dye.[188, 189] Any food containing pseudoperoxidase or peroxidase activity such as nonhuman hemoglobin in rare red meat and uncooked fruits and vegetables[190] can produce a positive reaction. Red meat and peroxidase-containing foods (broccoli, turnips, cauliflower, radish, cantaloupe) should therefore be avoided for three days prior to and during testing.[191] Although a drop of water added to the slide prior to development (rehydration) increases sensitivity, this is not recommended for screening average-risk populations (too many false positive tests). The advantages and limitations of fecal occult blood testing with the Hemoccult-type slide guaiac tests are outlined in Table 81–10, and recommendations concerning proper performance of these tests in Table 81–11.

Colorectal cancers and adenomas bleed intermittently, and detection of fecal occult blood by Hemoccult depends on the degree of blood loss.[192] In general, 2 ml of blood in the stool is necessary to produce a positive test. Sampling multiple stool specimens is therefore likely to result in fewer false negative evaluations. Sampling one specimen yields a 50 per cent false negative rate, which falls progressively as more stools are sampled. Two samples of each of three consecutive (daily) stools should therefore be tested. Location of the lesion also affects the ability to detect a cancer by Hemoccult (Table 81–12). Right-sided cancers produce fewer false negative tests, presumably owing to greater blood loss. A potential "blind spot" of the Hemoccult test is in detecting cancers of the transverse colon and descending colon.

Numerous studies, many of them uncontrolled, have examined the potential benefit of fecal occult blood testing for detecting colorectal neoplasms in large populations.[193–199] Compliance has been in the range of 50 to 70 per cent, although elderly patients who are at

Table 81–10. ADVANTAGES AND LIMITATIONS OF THE GUAIAC-IMPREGNATED SLIDE TEST FOR FECAL OCCULT BLOOD TESTING

Advantages
- Readily available
- Convenient
- Inexpensive
- Good patient compliance in motivated groups

Disadvantages
- Depends on degree of fecal hydration
- Affected by storage (hemoglobin degradation)
- Affected by tumor location

False Positive Tests
- Exogenous peroxidase activity
  - Red meat (nonhuman hemoglobin)
  - Uncooked fruits and vegetables (vegetable peroxidase)
- Any source of gastrointestinal blood loss (epistaxis, gingival bleeding, upper GI tract pathology, hemorrhoids, etc.)
- Medications
  - Iron supplements
  - Topical iodine
  - Aspirin, nonsteroidal anti-inflammatory agents (induce upper GI bleeding)

False Negative Tests
- Storage of slides
- Ascorbic acid (vitamin C)
- Improper sampling/developing
- Lesion not bleeding at time of stool collection
- Degradation of hemoglobin by colonic bacteria

Table 81–11. PROPER PERFORMANCE OF THE SLIDE GUAIAC TEST FOR OCCULT FECAL BLOOD

1. For three days before and during testing, patients should avoid:
   a. Rare red meat
   b. Peroxidase-containing vegetables/fruits (e.g., broccoli, turnip, cantaloupe, cauliflower, radish)
   c. The following medications:
      - Iron supplements
      - Vitamin C
      - Aspirin
      - Nonsteroidal anti-inflammatory drugs
2. Two samples of each of three consecutive stools should be tested. (It is proper to sample areas of obvious blood.)
3. Slides should be developed within 4–6 days.
4. Slides should not be rehydrated prior to developing (for average-risk screening).
   If rehydrated, red meat must have been avoided (otherwise, too many false positives).

Table 81–12. COLORECTAL CANCER: RATE OF BLOOD LOSS AND DETECTABILITY BY HEMOCCULT

Location	Mean Daily Blood Loss*	False Negative Hemoccult	
		Standard	*Rehydrated*
Ascending colon and cecum	9.3 ml	17%	4%
Transverse and descending colon	1.5 ml	46%	46%
Sigmoid colon	1.9 ml	36%	3%
Rectum	1.8 ml	31%	7%
Overall		31%	9%

Data from Macrae, F., and St. John, D. J. B. Gastroenterology *82*:891, 1982.

*Determined by injecting ^{51}Cr-labeled erythrocytes intravenously and measuring fecal excretion of label. Normal stool contains less than 1 ml of blood per day.

substantial risk for colon cancer development have tended to be less compliant. The overall positivity rate ranges from 2 to 6 per cent of those tested, with the predictive value (the proportion of positive tests actually due to the disease) for adenomas being about 20 per cent and for cancers 5 per cent. The majority of studies report that a large percentage of cancers detected are Dukes' A and B lesions. Two large controlled studies of Hemoccult testing of asymptomatic patients in the general population are under way in the United States,[193, 194] and one has recently been reported from Great Britain.[199] These studies cite a 2 to 4 per cent rate of test positivity, a predictive value for adenomas of 29 to 36 per cent and carcinomas of 8 to 12 per cent. Sixty-five to 94 per cent of cancers in the tested groups were Dukes' A and B, versus 33 to 50 per cent in the control groups. It would appear then that screening for occult blood is effective in detecting early stage cancers, but it is yet to be determined whether screening decreases mortality from colorectal cancer. Mortality data are not yet available from controlled studies, and existing data cannot be interpreted in terms of survival benefit because of the various biases inherent in the screening process.[198]

Methods that may decrease the false positive rates of fecal occult blood testing are currently being developed and compared for efficacy with Hemoccult-type slide tests. Vegetable peroxidase inhibitors and immunologic tests for human hemoglobin[200] have been described. A quantitative assay for fecal blood (HemoQuant) based on the fluorescence of heme-derived porphyrins[201] is commercially available. This test is very sensitive for determining fecal blood; is not affected by hydration, iron, or ascorbic acid; and measures both total hemoglobin and that converted in the intestine to breakdown products by colonic bacteria (intestinally converted fraction).[202] Although HemoQuant appears to be a very sensitive and specific assay for fecal hemoglobin, its predictive value for disease remains to be determined. In one recent study[202] HemoQuant detected an abnormal amount of blood in stool samples for 97 per cent of patients with colon cancer and 3 per cent of normal subjects; however, patients and controls were not studied under the same conditions. Upper gastrointestinal bleeding from aspirin alone or in combination with alcohol has been shown to cause a significant number of positive tests with HemoQuant.[203]

Proctosigmoidoscopy. The benefit of proctosigmoidoscopy in screening programs for colorectal cancer is suggested by several uncontrolled studies using the rigid proctosigmoidoscope.[204–206] These studies indicate that proctosigmoidoscopy in asymptomatic average-risk persons might detect early-stage cancers,[204] and that detection and removal of adenomas could result in a lower than expected frequency of rectosigmoid cancers in the screened population[194, 206] (see pp. 1483–1495). Several studies have demonstrated the superiority of flexible fiberoptic sigmoidoscopes in detecting lesions when compared with rigid instruments.[177, 178, 184, 207, 208] The 60-cm flexible scope used in most comparisons can examine 2.5 times more bowel, detects at least two to three times more adenomas and carcinomas, and has greater patient acceptance than rigid instruments. The 60-cm flexible scope is therefore the instrument of choice in experienced hands, but its use requires a good deal of training. A 35-cm flexible instrument has recently been introduced which may require less training and should provide a good alternative for screening by the primary care physician.[209]

CEA and Serologic Tumor Markers. A great deal of effort has been spent in search of serologic markers that would enable the early detection and diagnosis of colorectal cancer. A variety of proteins, glycoproteins, and cellular and humoral substances have been studied as potential tumor markers, but none has been found to be specific for colorectal cancer.[63] The most widely studied marker, CEA, may be useful in the preoperative staging and postoperative follow-up of patients with large bowel cancer,[140, 172, 210, 211] but has a low predictive value for diagnosis in asymptomatic patients.[211, 212] The test's relatively low sensitivity and specificity combine to make it unsuitable for screening large asymptomatic populations. Its lack of sensitivity in detecting early colorectal cancer makes CEA determination especially poor for screening. The sensitivity for detecting Dukes' A and B lesions is only 36 per cent, compared with 74 per cent for Dukes' C and 83 per cent for Dukes' D disease when 2.5 mg/ml is used as the upper limits of normal. Several new carbohydrate antigens are being examined and hold some promise in terms of specificity for preneoplastic and early neoplastic lesions in the colon.[61, 63] Their effectiveness for screening, however, remains to be determined.

Approach to Screening

Screening and case finding approaches are different for patients in average-risk (over age 40 years) and high-risk groups. The latter includes patients with longstanding ulcerative colitis, prior colorectal cancer, prior adenomas, female genital cancer, familial polyposis or Gardner's syndrome, and familial colon cancer.

Average-Risk Group. Patients registered in a health care system should be categorized according to risk so that appropriate screening can be added to other aspects of medical evaluation. Relative risk should be assessed by family and personal history questionnaires. Screening should include annual digital rectal examinations and testing of stool for occult blood for those over 40 years of age, and proctosigmoidoscopy once every three to five years, beginning between the ages of 40 and 50 years. Rigid sigmoidoscopy should be used only if flexible fiberoptic sigmoidoscopy (with a 35-cm or 60-cm instrument) by a skilled physician is unavailable. A diagnostic work-up is indicated for patients with a positive fecal occult blood test (Fig. 81–17). Colonoscopy is the diagnostic modality of choice if available. If not, an air contrast barium enema combined with flexible proctosigmoidoscopy should be performed (see above).

Screening should be accompanied by programs to educate patients and heighten physicians' awareness of the concepts and technology involved in screening, diagnosis, treatment, and follow-up. Public misconceptions that colorectal cancer is an incurable disease and that surgical intervention invariably leads to an impaired lifestyle with a colostomy need to be discredited.

High-Risk Groups

Familial Polyposis and Familial Cancer. Patients with a family history of familial polyposis, or Gardner's syndrome, should have flexible sigmoidoscopy at least annually, beginning at puberty. Female patients with a history of genital or breast cancer should have yearly fecal occult blood testing and sigmoidoscopy every three years following diagnosis (see pp. 1501–1507).

Patients with a family history of site-specific colon cancer or the cancer family syndrome must be examined colonoscopically beginning at age 20, since one cannot rely only on fecal occult blood testing in these very-high-risk patients. A reasonable follow-up approach would be a fecal occult blood test annually and colonoscopy every three to five years (Fig. 81–18). The search would be primarily for the scattered adenomas that precede carcinomas in these syndromes, and detection by colonoscopy is more sensitive than radiography. The number of patients with familial colon cancer is not known but probably is greater than is currently appreciated. The approach to patients with a suggestive family history—for example, one first-degree relative with colon cancer and one first-degree relative with breast cancer—is not established. Whether these patients should be monitored in the same way as average-risk patients or be screened more rigorously[178] remains to be determined.

Prior Adenoma or Colon Cancer. The suggested follow-up of patients after diagnosis and removal of an adenomatous polyp is detailed on pages 1494 to 1495. Patients who have had a large bowel cancer resected should have colonoscopy performed at six months to one year following surgery, followed by yearly colonoscopy on two occasions (Fig. 81–19). If the results are negative, colonoscopy should then be performed every three years. This should be combined with yearly fecal occult blood testing. Serum CEA levels should be measured at regular intervals (three times at six-month intervals, then five times at yearly intervals) since postoperative CEA determinations may be cost-effective for detecting recurrent cancers.[213] How long an asymptomatic patient who has had multiple negative

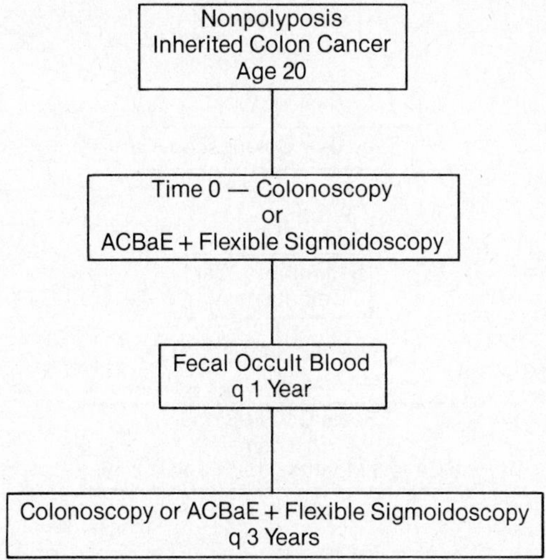

Figure 81–18. Algorithm for surveillance of patients with a family history of nonpolyposis inherited colon cancer.

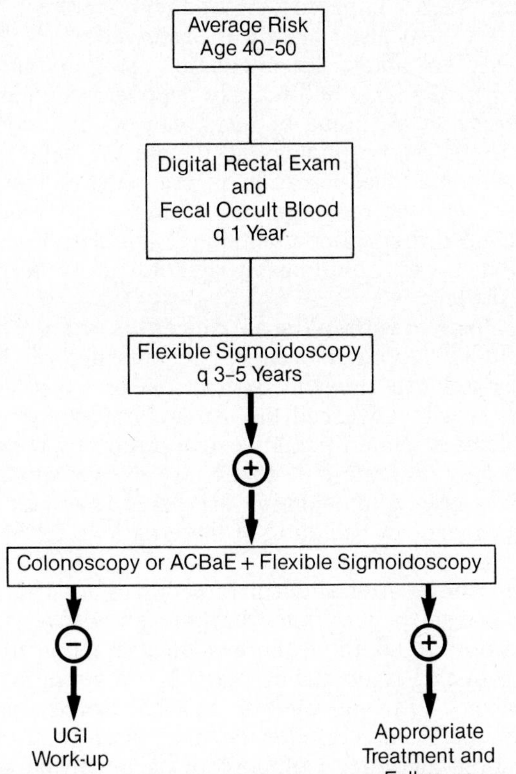

Figure 81–17. Algorithm for surveillance of average-risk patients in the general population. ACBaE, air contrast barium enema.

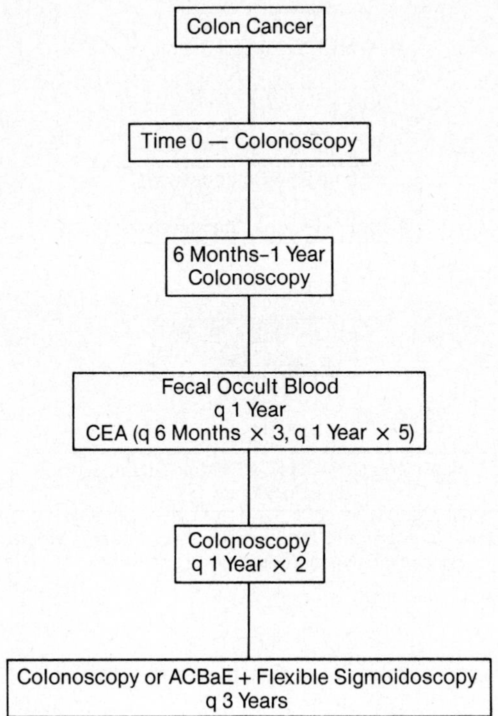

Figure 81–19. Algorithm for surveillance of patients who have had a colorectal cancer resected.

examinations should be tested by various modalities is at present unclear. It should be noted that the above recommendations are to some extent "educated guesses" and that firmer conclusions await the results of prospective trials.[214]

Inflammatory Bowel Disease. The appropriate surveillance schedule for patients with inflammatory bowel disease remains to be determined, and is being examined in long-term prospective studies[107, 111] (see pp. 1435–1477). Colonoscopy combined with mucosal biopsy may be effective in detecting preneoplastic and early neoplastic lesions in patients with ulcerative colitis. The current recommendation is yearly colonoscopy in patients who have had universal colitis for seven years or left-sided ulcerative colitis for 15 years.[110] Biopsies should be taken throughout the colon at 10-cm intervals, with special attention to areas that suggest a dysplasia-associated lesion (see p. 1531). Patients with Crohn's disease of the colon should be evaluated endoscopically as dictated by symptoms, and special attention should be paid to strictured areas. If dysplasia is high-grade or associated with a macroscopic lesion, consideration should be given to colectomy. A histologic diagnosis of low-grade dysplasia merits endoscopic follow-up at short intervals such as three to six months, as does an "indeterminate" reading due to active inflammation.[110]

Treatment

Surgery

Surgical resection is the treatment of choice for most patients with colorectal cancer. Preoperative colonoscopy should be performed if possible to rule out synchronous lesions, and a preoperative measurement of serum CEA should be obtained to aid in staging and postoperative follow-up. Computerized tomography is not indicated as a routine preoperative staging procedure.[215] CT can be valuable, however, for the evaluation of focal hepatic metastases if partial hepatectomy or regional hepatic artery infusion of chemotherapeutic agents is contemplated (see p. 1543). CT is also useful in the postoperative detection of pelvic recurrence in patients with rectosigmoid tumors.

The goal of surgery is a wide resection of the involved segment of bowel together with removal of its lymphatic drainage (Fig. 81–20). The extent of colonic resection is determined by the blood supply and distribution of regional lymph nodes. The resection should include a segment of colon at least 5 cm on either side of the tumor, although wider margins are often included because of obligatory ligation of the arterial blood supply. Extensive "super radical" colonic and lymph node resection does not increase survival over segmental resection.[216–218]

The approach toward rectal cancers depends on location of the lesion. For lesions of the rectosigmoid and upper rectum a low anterior resection can be performed through an abdominal incision and primary anastomosis accomplished. Even for low rectal lesions a sphincter-saving resection can be performed if a distal margin of at least 2 cm of normal bowel can be resected below the lesion, facilitated by new end-to-end stapling devices. Increased recurrence or attenuated survival does not attend sphincter-saving resections for rectal cancer when compared with abdominoperineal resection if a 2-cm distal margin is preserved.[128, 129, 219] The inability to obtain an adequate distal margin, the presence of a large bulky tumor deep within the pelvis, extensive local spread of rectal cancer, and a poorly differentiated morphology all dictate the need for an abdominoperineal resection of the rectum. Here the distal sigmoid, rectosigmoid, rectum, and anus are removed through a combined abdominal and perineal approach, and a permanent sigmoid colostomy is established.

In a patient with colorectal cancer the primary tumor should be resected, even in the presence of distant metastases, to prevent obstruction or bleeding. In patients with advanced disease and multiple medical problems repeated palliative fulguration of rectal tumors may be preferable to surgery. Newer modalities such as laser photoablation are being tested as alternative means of palliation in these patients.[220, 221]

Postsurgical Follow-up. The incidence of recurrent colon cancer after surgical resection is high in those with serosal penetration or lymph node involvement by tumor. In addition, the incidence of metachronous (subsequent) colorectal cancer is 1.1 to 4.7 per cent.[84, 89] It is not clear how often or by what means a patient should be evaluated following an apparently successful resection for cure. Colonoscopy is beneficial in the detection and removal of synchronous and metachronous adenomatous polyps in this high-risk group (Fig. 81–19).[213] History and physical examination combined

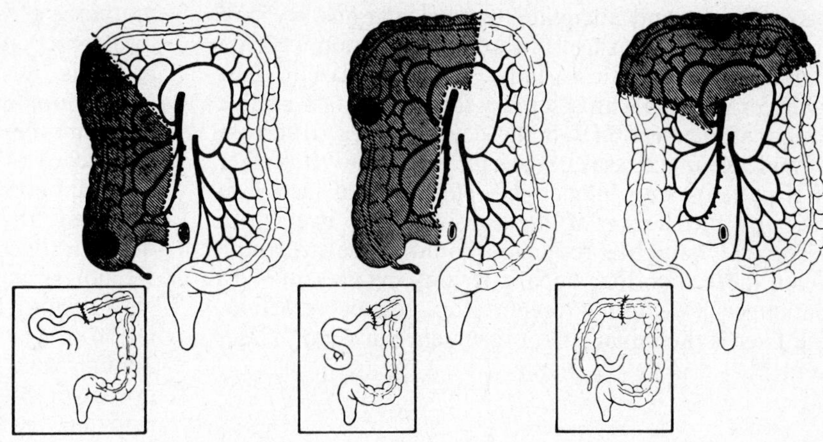

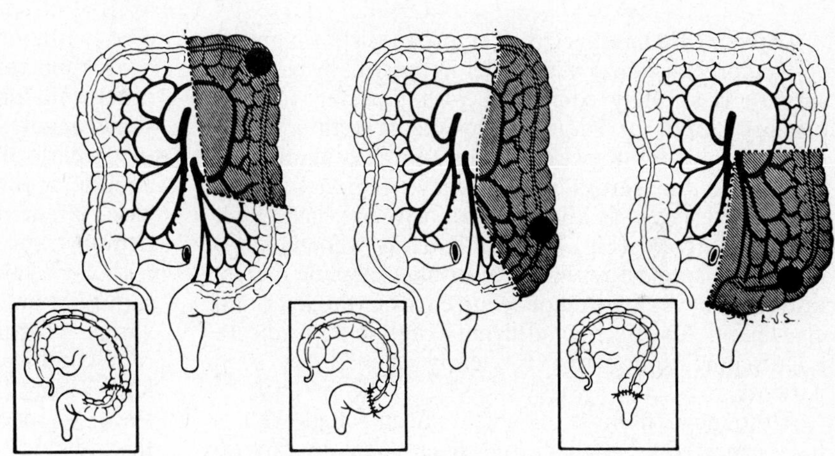

Figure 81–20. Extent of surgical resection for cancer of the colon at various sites. (From Schrock, T. R. Large intestine. *In* Way, L. W. [ed.]. Current Surgical Diagnosis and Treatment. New York, Lange Medical Publishers, 1983. Used by permission.)

with CEA determinations at regular intervals may provide the highest cost-effective benefit for detecting recurrent cancers.[213] The sensitivity for detecting early recurrences is about 61 per cent for either CT or CEA,[213] but CT can be especially useful in examining the pelvis for recurrence after resection of rectosigmoid tumors.

Serial CEA determinations have been used to direct "second look" surgical procedures.[211, 222–224] Measuring CEA levels at least every two months for the first two years after resection and then every four months for the next three years will yield a small percentage of patients (about 5 per cent) for whom CEA-directed second-look operations for recurrent carcinoma may be indicated.[222] Survival following second-look procedures is high when surgeons have specialized training in oncologic surgery,[222] but other surgeons have had more limited success and long-term survival data are lacking.

Surgical Resection of Hepatic Metastases. The most common site of distant metastases from colorectal cancer is the liver. Synchronous metastases to the liver are evident at initial presentation in 10 to 25 per cent of patients with large bowel cancer, and 40 to 70 per cent of those whose cancers disseminate will have hepatic involvement.[225, 226] Seventy to 80 per cent of hepatic metastases appear within two years following primary resection.[226, 227] The uniformly poor prognosis in patients with untreated hepatic metastases[173, 225, 230] underlies an aggressive approach. Candidates for resection of hepatic lesions are those in whom the primary tumor has been resected with curative intent and in whom there is no evidence of extrahepatic disease. The extent of liver involvement that is deemed resectable varies from tumor involving one lobe of the liver to focal disease in multiple lobes. The percentage of "resectable" liver metastases therefore varies in different series ranging from 4.5 to 11 per cent (5 to 6 per cent in most series).[226] Modern techniques of anatomic dissection and hemostasis have resulted in improved operative survival,[227, 228] with an operative mortality of about 2 per cent in highly trained hands. Overall five-year survival rates range from 20 to 34 per cent in selected patients. The literature is difficult to interpret, however, because no uniform staging system is used, and prospective controls are lacking. Further, reported two- and three-year survival rates may not be valid, since recent data suggest that patients with unresected hepatic metastases may live longer than previously reported.[173] Median survival rates for patients with unresected solitary and multiple unilobar lesions are 21 and 15 months, respectively, and more than 20 per cent of patients with unresected solitary liver lesions live at least three years.[173] Long-term survival in patients who undergo surgical resection of hepatic metatases depends on the absence of extrahepatic disease and adequate surgical margins.[173, 229, 230] In some series the stage of the primary lesion is also a significant prognostic variable.[173, 227, 228] It is not clear whether patients with a solitary focus of metastasis live longer after resection than those who undergo resection of multiple metastases in the same lobe.[173, 227] It is clear that patients with bilobar metastases are at increased risk for recurrence of metastasis in the liver after resection,[229] and that resection should not be attempted when more than four hepatic lesions are present.[230] In patients whose tumor recurs after hepatic resection, the liver is the initial site of recurrence in about 35 per cent.[229]

Chemotherapy

Adjuvant Chemotherapy. The prognosis for patients with colorectal cancer who undergo potentially curative surgery is strongly correlated with the stage of the primary tumor at surgery. Despite resection of all macroscopic tumor, patients whose primary tumor has penetrated the serosa or who have regional lymph node metastases at the time of surgery have high recurrence rates (Fig. 81–15). Patients who undergo aggressive surgical resection of isolated hepatic metastases also have high tumor recurrences in the liver and elsewhere. An effective adjuvant program to eradicate microscopic tumor foci is clearly needed for such patients.

Although a number of small uncontrolled studies have reported a benefit for adjuvant chemotherapy in patients so treated compared with historical controls, prospectively randomized clinical trials of adjuvant chemotherapy have met with limited success.[131, 231–233] A large multicenter trial prospectively assigned patients with modified Dukes' B2, C1, or C2 colon carcinoma to receive adjuvant postsurgical chemotherapy with fluorouracil (5-FU) and methyl-CCNU (semustine), immunotherapy with bacillus Calmette-Guérin (BCG), combination chemotherapy and immunotherapy, or close follow-up only.[134] No significant differences in recurrence or survival rates among the four groups were noted after a median follow-up of 5.5 years. This study demonstrates the importance of using concurrent controls, since recurrence and mortality rates were lower in all groups than anticipated from historical controls. 5-Fluorouracil might have been more effective if given in optimal dosage; the addition of semustine necessitated a suboptimal amount of 5-FU and contributed to the toxicity of the regimen. Other trials of adjuvant chemotherapy for colon cancer have been equally disappointing, although most show a modest, statistically nonsignificant benefit for 5-FU therapy.

Results of a long-term prospectively randomized trial that evaluated the efficacy of combined adjuvant therapy in patients with modified Dukes' B2 and C rectal cancer following curative surgery are more encouraging.[234] The recurrence rate is lower and the time to recurrence significantly prolonged in those who receive combined radiotherapy (4000 to 4500 rads) and chemotherapy (5-FU plus semustine) than in those treated by surgery alone. Survival for the combined therapy group is only marginally improved, but the study of larger numbers of patients may strengthen these data.

Chemotherapy of Advanced Disease. Existing systemic chemotherapy for disseminated colorectal cancer is disappointing, with only modest proven efficacy reported for the fluoropyrimidines (5-FU, 5′-fluorodeoxyuridine), the nitrosoureas, and mitomycin C. 5-Fluorouracil inhibits DNA synthesis by interacting with thymidylate synthetase and inhibiting the methylation of deoxyuridylic to thymidylic acid. It has been administered as an oral agent, intravenously in bolus doses, or by continuous intravenous infusion and is associated with a response rate of approximately 20 per cent in most studies. Responses are often short-lived (four to five months) and have not been associated with long-term survival. Similar response rates have been reported for the nitrosoureas (10 to 15 per cent) and mitomycin C (12 to 16 per cent) given as single agents. Although small pilot studies often report the superiority of various combinations of chemotherapeutic agents for the management of metastatic disease, larger multicenter phase III trials have failed to demonstrate stastistically significant benefit compared with 5-FU alone.[235] Toxicity to 5-FU includes myelosuppression, vomiting, diarrhea, and stomatitis and varies according to dose and mode of administration.

A combination of 5-FU and high-dose intravenous leucovorin (tetrahydrofolate) is being investigated since leucovorin potentiates the binding of 5-FU to thymidylate synthetase, and the combination may be more effective than 5-FU alone.[236] Methotrexate added to 5-FU with or without leucovorin is not uniformly superior to 5-FU alone, and toxicity is greater.

Selective infusion of chemotherapeutic agents into the hepatic arterial system may be employed to treat hepatic metastases. This method delivers more concentrated drug into the tumor capillary bed than is achievable by conventional means.[237–243] The infusion catheter is usually implanted into the common hepatic artery via the gastroduodenal artery at laparotomy. The development of implantable infusion pumps has led to increasing use of such therapy in major centers. Fluorinated pyrimidines such as 5-FU and floxuridine (FUdR) have high hepatic extraction (80 to 95 per cent), and it is felt that high concentrations of these drugs can be delivered by direct hepatic arterial infusion with low systemic toxicity. Floxuridine has received the most attention. Continuous hepatic arterial infusion of this drug to treat hepatic metastases from colorectal cancer in patients not previously treated may achieve response rates of 54 to 83 per cent.[237–240] Criteria for response vary, however, and it is still unclear whether there will be an impact on survival. Complications of the procedure, which include arterial occlusion, local infection, and catheter leak, occur in a small number of patients. Morbidity of treatment consists of gastrointestinal tract inflammation and ulceration, elevations in bilirubin and transaminases, and biliary sclerosis, all of which may be substantial.[242, 243]

Immunotargeted Therapy

Recent advances in immunology, molecular biology and imaging have led to the development of radiolabeled monoclonal antibodies that can be used in the detection of metastatic lesions from colorectal cancer (radioimmunodetection).[63, 244, 245] These same antibodies can be linked to cytotoxic agents such as the A subunit of the plant toxin ricin, the toxin A chain of diphtheria, or chemotherapeutic agents for immunotargeted therapy.[63] Most patients treated thus far with such therapy have had advanced disease, and further studies utilizing these agents in adjuvant therapy are needed.

Radiation Therapy

Patients with rectal cancers whose lesions have penetrated the bowel wall or who have regional lymph nodes involved by tumor are at high risk for local recurrence following resection of their primary tumor. The incidence of local recurrence is 40 to 50 per cent in this group. Radiation therapy is used preoperatively[246–249] or postoperatively[250–253] to decrease local recurrence in those with high-risk rectal and rectosigmoid cancers (Dukes' B2 and C lesions), or in a combined preoperative-postoperative "sandwich approach."[254, 255] It is also used to convert unresectable large tumors and those fixed to pelvic organs to resectable lesions.[256] Radiation therapy may occasionally be useful for palliation of bleeding and pain due to advanced rectal disease. The possible advantages of radiation therapy must be balanced against its potential complications of radiation proctitis and small bowel damage (see pp. 1369–1382).

Preoperative radiation reduces local recurrence in patients with rectal and rectosigmoid cancers, but there is no convincing evidence that it improves survival. Although a large retrospective report suggests improved survival for those with Dukes' C rectal lesions who receive preoperative treatment,[246] two randomized controlled trials by the Veterans Administration show conflicting results.[248, 249] The initial study[248] demonstrates a 13 per cent increase in five-year survival for patients who receive low-dose (2000 to 2500 rads) pelvic irradiation prior to abdominoperineal resection of rectal cancer. Further analysis suggests, however, that these results are partially the result of the randomization of a high proportion of patients with lymph node metastases to the control group. A second study[249] shows no difference in five-year survival (50 per cent) between those who received over 3000 rads prior to abdominoperineal resection and those who did not. Since preoperative radiation delays surgery and prevents adequate pathologic staging, postoperative radiotherapy may be preferable.

Postoperative radiotherapy is generally restricted to patients at high risk for local recurrence of rectal cancer (penetration of the bowel wall, positive lymph nodes). Patients receive 4500 to 5500 rads over five to six weeks. Prospective but nonrandomized series show a substantial reduction in local recurrence for those receiving postoperative radiotherapy (6 to 8 per cent for those receiving radiation versus 40 to 50 per cent for those receiving surgery alone).[250–252] Distant metastases remain a problem however, and it is not yet clear if survival is substantially altered. A randomized European multicenter study[253] suggests increased survival for patients with Dukes' C (but not Dukes' B) rectal cancers who receive postoperative radiation, but long-term follow-up is lacking. Combined postoperative radiotherapy and chemotherapy may be most promising (see p. 1544).

Low-dose preoperative radiation (500 rads 24 hours prior to surgery) plus postoperative radiation has been used in high-risk patients.[254, 255] Whether this approach is superior to postoperative radiation alone remains to be determined.

Other Malignant Large Bowel Tumors

Malignant tumors other than adenocarcinomas rarely originate in the large bowel. These include lymphomas, malignant carcinoid tumors, and leiomyosarcomas. In addition, lymphomas, leiomyosarcomas, malignant melanomas, and cancers of the breast, ovary, prostate, lung, and stomach can be metastatic to the colon.

Large Bowel Lymphoma

Primary lymphomas of the large bowel are rare, representing approximately 0.5 and 0.2 per cent, respectively, of all colonic and rectal malignancies.[257–260] Colorectal lymphoma accounts for 10 to 20 per cent of primary gastrointestinal lymphomas.[261–263] The cecum is the commonest site of primary lymphoma of the large bowel, followed by the rectum. These tumors occur in all age groups, but are most common in the age group 50 to 70. Most are non-Hodgkin's lymphomas having a "diffuse" histologic pattern.

Primary lymphoma of the large bowel may develop in association with longstanding ulcerative colitis,[264, 265] or as a complication of immunosuppressive therapy,[266] ureterosigmoidostomy,[267] or radiation therapy.[268] An increased incidence of rectal lymphoma has also been reported in homosexual men.[269, 270] A few patients have been described with both primary lymphomas and carcinomas of the large bowel.

The symptoms produced by primary large bowel lymphomas are similar to those from carcinomas, and depend on the location of the lesion. The most common symptoms of colonic lymphoma are crampy abdominal pain, weight loss, and a change in bowel habit.[271] Bleeding and diarrhea are common with rectal lymphomas.[259]

Barium enemas are abnormal in the majority of cases of large bowel lymphoma, but are not pathognomonic for this disease. Five different patterns have been described[272] and reflect the varied macroscopic appearances of the tumors. These include (1) mass lesions with extensive mucosal destruction (Fig. 81–21), (2) large lobulated masses, (3) mucosal nodularity resembling the pseudopolyposis of inflammatory bowel

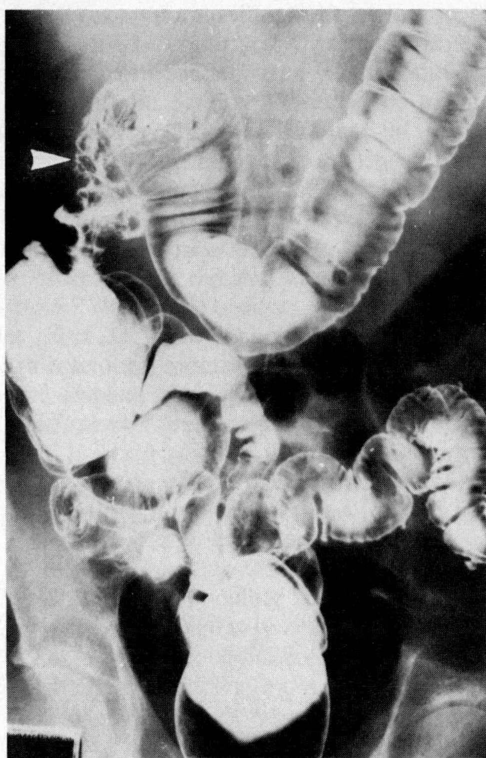

Figure 81–21. Barium enema demonstrating extensive mucosal destruction from a primary lymphoma of the right colon *(arrowhead).*

disease, (4) infiltrative forms appearing as a rigid bowel segment or an annular stricture, and (5) bulky extracolonic masses. Fiberoptic sigmoidoscopy and colonoscopy with biopsy help establish the histologic diagnosis.

Surgery should be performed, if possible, and is often combined with radiation therapy and systemic chemotherapy. The optimum combination of treatment modalities is currently unclear.[257] Five-year survival is about 35 per cent[258, 262] overall, although higher survival rates may be expected if localized disease can be resected.[271]

Lymphoma may involve the large bowel secondarily as part of widespread systemic disease, and carries a grave prognosis. In this case colonic involvement is often multicentric.

Malignant Carcinoid Tumors

Carcinoid tumors arise from enterochromaffin or enterochromaffin-like cells that are present in the gastrointestinal tract, ovaries, and lungs (see also pp. 1549 and 1560–1570). Over 90 per cent of carcinoids originate in the gastrointestinal tract with the most common sites in order of frequency being the appendix, terminal ileum, rectum, and the remainder of the colon. Gastroduodenal and pancreatic carcinoids are infrequent. Carcinoid tumors can be divided according to embryonic origin into groups with characteristic clinical histochemical and biochemical features[273] (Table 81–13). These tumors secrete a variety of substances, including 5-hydroxytryptophan, serotonin (5-hydroxytryptamine), histamine, catecholamines, kinins, prostaglandins, substance P, and motilin, that are responsible for the carcinoid syndrome (see pp. 1560–1570). The syndrome usually indicates the presence of hepatic metastases, although it is seen in less than 50 per cent of patients with metastatic tumors. Associated malignancies are seen in up to 45 per cent of patients with carcinoids, the most common being adenocarcinoma of the colon.[274]

Table 81–13. CHARACTERISTICS OF CARCINOID TUMORS BASED ON EMBRYONIC ORIGIN

	Foregut	Midgut	Hindgut
	Bronchus, Pancreas, Stomach	***Ovary, Intestine***	***Rectum***
Argentaffin and diazo reaction	Negative	Positive	Negative
Carcinoid syndrome	Frequent	Frequent	Absent
Tumor 5-HT	Low	High	Absent
Urine 5-HIAA	High	High	Normal
5-HTP secretion	Frequent	Rare	Absent
Histamine secretion	Present	Absent	Absent
Bone and skin metastases	Frequent	Rare	Frequent

5-HT, 5-hydroxytryptamine (serotonin); 5-HIAA, 5-hydroxyindoleacetic acid; 5-HTP, 5-hydroxytryptophan.

The typical pathologic appearance is that of small submucosal nodules with intact overlying mucosa. Large tumors can become polypoid, annular, and intraluminal. Carcinoids are composed of uniform small round cells with hyperchromatic nuclei and granular cytoplasm arranged in a variety of histologic patterns (insular, trabecular, glandular, undifferentiated, and mixed), which may have prognostic significance[275] (Fig. 81–22). The diagnosis of malignant carcinoid tumors rests on the extent of invasion into and beyond the wall of the organ involved and on the presence of metastases. Metastasis is related to size (more likely if the primary tumor is over 2 cm) and degree of invasion.

The appendix is the most common site of carcinoid tumors, accounting for 30 to 40 per cent of cases.[276–280] These tumors are often asymptomatic, but may present as acute appendicitis or chronic right lower quadrant pain. Tumors less than 2 cm in size and without invasion of the cecum can be treated by simple appendectomy.[276, 277, 281, 282] Larger and invasive tumors require a right hemicolectomy. Five-year survival approaches 99 per cent.[278] A rare histologic subtype with features of both carcinoid and adenocarcinoma is more aggressive.[283]

Rectal carcinoids represent approximately 10 to 15 per cent of carcinoid tumors and about 1 per cent of rectal malignancies.[278, 284–286] Common symptoms include pain, bleeding, and constipation.[285] There is a high rate of synchronous rectal carcinomas and other associated malignancies. Approximately 15 per cent of rectal carcinoids metastasize, but the carcinoid syndrome is extremely rare. Treatment consists of simple surgical excision for tumors less than 2 cm in size, and abdominoperineal or low anterior resection for larger tumors, or where muscular invasion is demonstrated.[286] Five-year survival approaches 80 per cent.

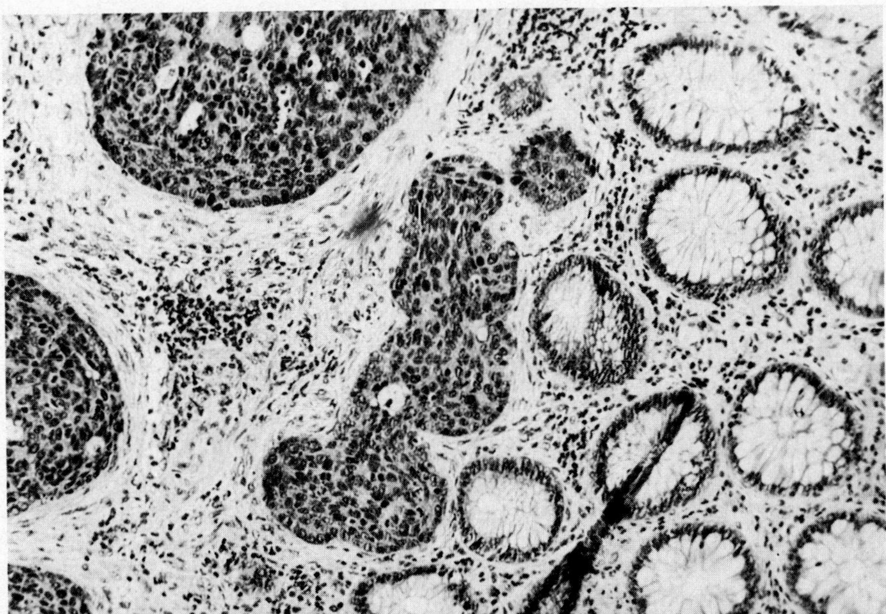

Figure 81–22. Nests of invasive carcinoid are seen below the muscularis mucosa (Hematoxylin and eosin stain, × 170). (Courtesy of Steven I. Hajdu, M.D., Department of Pathology, Memorial Sloan-Kettering Cancer Center, New York.)

Carcinoids of the cecum, right colon, and left colon account for less than 10 per cent of carcinoid tumors, but have the highest malignant potential.[282, 287] These large tumors present with signs and symptoms similar to adenocarcinomas, and frequently have metastasized when diagnosed. Treatment consists of wide surgical resections like those for carcinomas. Surgical excision of hepatic metastases may provide symptomatic relief in patients with the carcinoid syndrome.[288]

Cytotoxic agents that have been used in treating patients with malignant carcinoids with metastases include 5-FU, streptozotocin, L-phenylalanine mustard (L-PAM), cyclophosphamide, doxorubicin (Adriamycin), and DTIC, singly or in combination.[289] The combination of 5-FU plus streptozotocin produces responses (but not cures) in about one third of patients.[290] Such therapy is indicated only for patients with unresectable metastases who experience significant symptoms or disability or who have rapidly advancing disease. Cytotoxic chemotherapy may precipitate an acute exacerbation of symptoms in these patients. The possible roles of radiotherapy[291] and hormonal therapy[292] need to be clarified.

MALIGNANT NEOPLASMS OF THE SMALL INTESTINE

Tumors of the small intestine are rare, accounting for only 5 per cent of benign and malignant gastrointestinal neoplasms (see pp. 1359–1363) and 1 per cent of malignant G.I. cancers.[293] There will be approximately 2500 new small bowel cancers in the United States in 1987.[1] Adenocarcinomas, carcinoids, lymphomas, and sarcomas are the most common small bowel malignancies. Table 81–14 lists the distribution of malignant tumors in the small intestine compiled from several series.[262, 294–300] Since carcinoids may be benign or malignant, and are difficult to classify on the basis of histology alone, malignant carcinoids may be overrepresented in the series.

The small intestine may also be involved secondarily by direct extension from other intra-abdominal tumors (colon, stomach, pancreas) and retroperitoneal tumors (kidney and retroperitoneal lymph node metastases), or by hematogenous spread from malignant melanoma and carcinomas of the breast, lung, esophagus, and ovary.

Adenocarcinoma

Adenocarcinomas account for approximately half of malignant small bowel tumors.[294–301] The duodenum is the most common site, followed by the jejunum, with the lowest incidence in the ileum (Table 81–14). Approximately two thirds of duodenal adenocarcinomas are in the region of the ampulla of Vater. Jejunal adenocarcinomas tend to be proximal lesions, with the majority arising within 100 cm of the ligament of Treitz, while ileal lesions are distal, arising in proximity to the

Table 81–14. DISTRIBUTION OF MALIGNANT NEOPLASMS IN THE SMALL INTESTINE

Tumor	Percentage by Region			Percentage of Total by Tumor Type
	Duodenum	*Jejunum*	*Ileum*	
Adenocarcinoma	40	38	22	45
Carcinoid	6	10	84	34
Sarcoma	10	36	54	18
Lymphoma	5	47	48	3
Percentage of total by region	22	28	50	

Compiled from references 262 and 294 to 300.

ileocecal valve. These cancers are unusual prior to age 30, with a peak incidence in the sixth and seventh decades. There is a slight male predominance. The descriptive epidemiology of small bowel adenocarcinoma parallels that of colon carcinoma, with a higher incidence in Western countries.

Etiology and Risk Factors

Little is known about the etiology of small bowel adenocarcinomas. Unlike colorectal cancers, small bowel adenocarcinomas are uncommon. It has been postulated that the small intestinal mucosa is protected from exposure to noxious substances by the liquidity and rapid transit of its contents.[302, 303] Other potential protective mechanisms include its alkalinity, high concentration of secretory immunoglobulin, low bacterial population, and the presence of small intestinal hydroxylases[304] which may inactivate potential carcinogens.[303]

An increased incidence of small intestinal adenomas and adenocarcinomas is associated with familial polyposis and Gardner's syndrome.[305–307] The majority are periampullary carcinomas of the duodenum, although ileal adenomas have also been reported.[308] A 2 per cent incidence of small bowel adenocarcinoma has been reported in patients with the Peutz-Jeghers syndrome.[309] These malignancies probably arise in coexisting adenomas and not in the hamartomas associated with this syndrome.

Crohn's disease of the small intestine carries an increased risk for the development of adenocarcinomas.[310, 311] Cancers are most common in the terminal ileum and in surgically bypassed segments of small bowel.

Pathology

Small bowel adenocarcinomas tend to be infiltrative, annular lesions resembling carcinomas of the distal colon (Fig. 81–23), although polypoid masses are also seen. These cancers arise in the glands of the small intestinal crypts and are moderately or well differentiated mucin-producing tumors. Regional lymph nodes and the liver are the most common sites of metastasis.

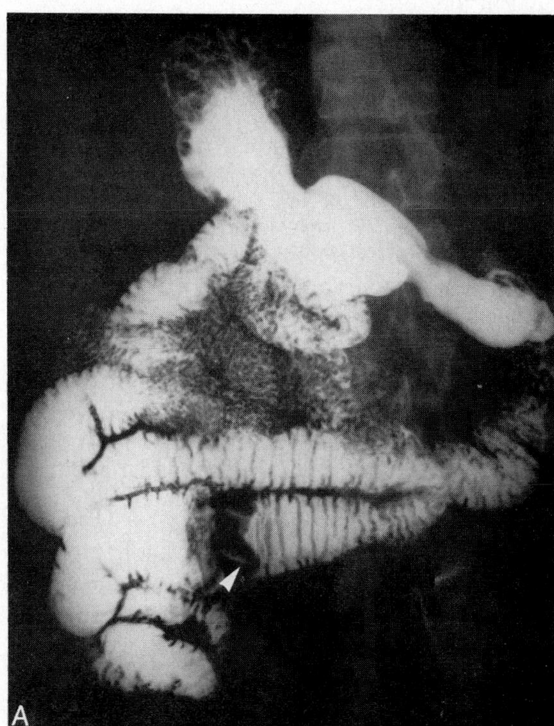

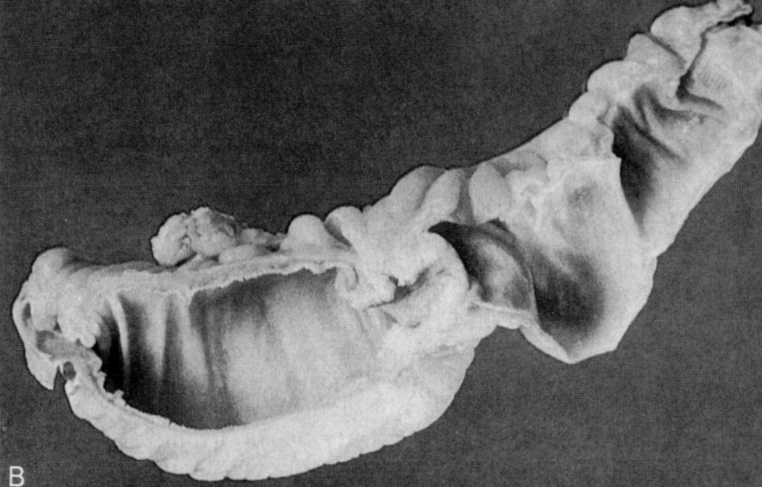

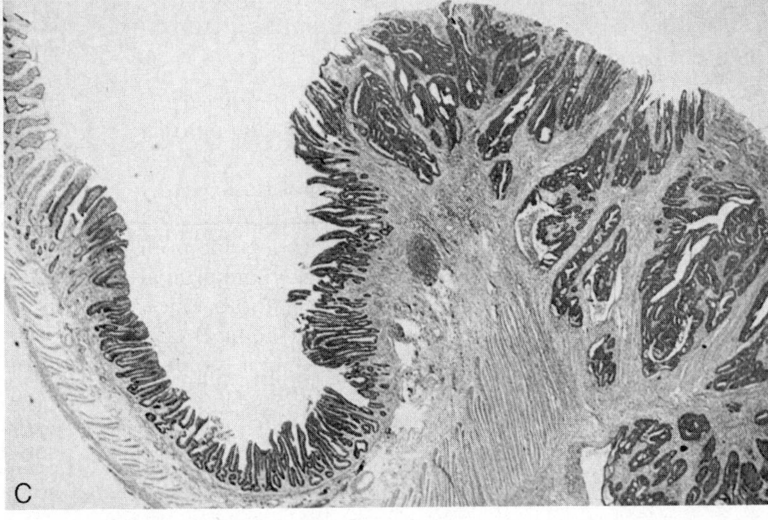

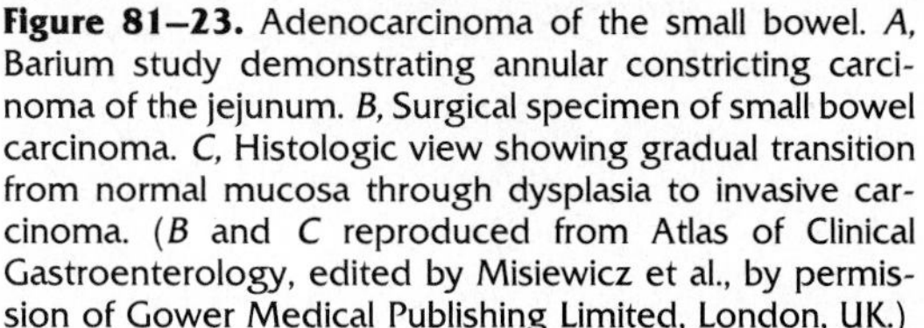
Figure 81–23. Adenocarcinoma of the small bowel. *A*, Barium study demonstrating annular constricting carcinoma of the jejunum. *B*, Surgical specimen of small bowel carcinoma. *C*, Histologic view showing gradual transition from normal mucosa through dysplasia to invasive carcinoma. (*B* and *C* reproduced from Atlas of Clinical Gastroenterology, edited by Misiewicz et al., by permission of Gower Medical Publishing Limited, London, UK.)

Clinical Features

The clinical features of small bowel adenocarcinomas depend upon their location. Duodenal carcinomas present with iron deficiency anemia, epigastric pain, and obstructive jaundice. Carcinomas of the jejunum produce small bowel obstruction with crampy mid-abdominal pain, distention, weight loss, and fatigue. Chronic occult blood loss and iron deficiency anemia are again common. Ileal carcinomas present with crampy lower abdominal pain, iron deficiency anemia, weakness, and weight loss. Some patients may have a palpable abdominal mass.

Diagnosis

The typical clinical picture of crampy abdominal pain and weight loss is the best clue to diagnosis of adenocarcinoma of the small intestine. An abdominal mass may be palpable in up to a third of patients with jejunal or ileal lesions. Occult blood in the stool, iron deficiency anemia, and hypoproteinemia are nonspecific but helpful findings.

Barium studies of the small bowel show typical constricting "apple core" lesions with destruction of the mucosa and shouldering of the margins (Fig. 81–23*A*). Barium enema with ileal reflux may be helpful in defining distal lesions, and enteroclysis (barium administered after intubation of the small bowel) is useful in defining jejunal and ileal tumors.[312] Upper endoscopy with brushings and biopsies may diagnose duodenal lesions, and colonoscopy with intubation of the terminal ileum can occasionally detect very distal carcinomas. Diagnostic ultrasound can demonstrate biliary obstruction if jaundice is present, and CT of the abdomen may reveal a duodenal mass. Endoscopic retrograde cholangiopancreatography (ERCP) can help differentiate periampullary tumors from other causes of obstructive jaundice.

Treatment

Surgical resection is the treatment of choice for adenocarcinomas of the small intestine. Duodenal carcinomas are treated by pancreaticoduodenal resection (Whipple's procedure). Such radical resection has resulted in five-year survival rates of 20 to 30 per cent.[313, 314] Carcinomas of the jejunum and ileum should be widely resected together with the supporting mesentery and lymph node drainage. Radical resection for ileal lesions often requires a right colectomy owing to sacrifice of the blood supply to the right colon during mesenteric resection. Five-year survival rates for jejunal and ileal carcinomas average 20 and 10 per cent, respectively. Patients with extensive disease or metastases should undergo palliative segmental bowel resection or bypass to relieve and prevent obstruction.

Radiation therapy for the treatment of small bowel adenocarcinomas has been disappointing and the amount of radiation that can be delivered to this area without significant side effects is limited. Intraoperative radiotherapy may provide some benefit with less risk to normal tissues.[315] The benefit of chemotherapy has also been limited. The principal agents used have been 5-FU, the nitrosoureas, mitomycin C, and doxorubicin, alone or in combination.

Carcinoid Tumors

See also pages 1546 to 1547 and 1560 to 1570.

The small intestine is the second most common site of gastrointestinal carcinoid tumors; the majority of small intestinal carcinoids arise in the ileum.[274] Ileal carcinoids are often multiple, frequently metastasize, and produce the carcinoid syndrome in approximately 40 per cent of cases. These tumors are associated with other malignant neoplasms in almost half of cases.[274, 316]

Histologically small intestinal carcinoids resemble those found elsewhere in the bowel and are composed of nests of uniform small round cells producing submucosal nodules (Fig. 81–22). Ileal carcinoids also produce a desmoplastic reaction leading to fibrosis and small bowel obstruction. Even small ileal tumors can be invasive and produce metastases. Duodenal carcinoids are less aggressive.[317]

Clinically these tumors produce symptoms of intermittent intestinal obstruction (crampy abdominal pain, vomiting), weight loss, and upper gastrointestinal bleeding (melena, hematochezia). The carcinoid syndrome described on pages 1560 to 1570 (vasomotor disturbances, intestinal hypermotility, bronchoconstriction) almost always denotes the presence of hepatic metastases.

Treatment consists of wide surgical resection including the adjacent mesentery.[282, 318] Distal ileal lesions require right colectomy to adequately remove their lymphatic drainage. Since small bowel carcinoids are often multicentric, the remainder of the intestine should be carefully examined. Overall five-year survival is 50 to 60 per cent,[278, 318] dropping to 20 to 35 per cent if liver metastases are present.

Sarcomas

Sarcomas are malignant tumors of mesodermal origin and include leiomyosarcomas (derived from smooth muscle), fibrosarcomas (connective tissue), liposarcomas (lipoblasts), angiosarcomas (vascular elements), and neurofibrosarcomas (neural elements). Leiomyosarcomas (Fig. 81–24) are the most common small intestinal sarcoma, accounting for about 20 per cent of malignant tumors in the organ.[294–300] These tumors have a peak incidence in the fifth to seventh decades with a slight male predominance. Small intestinal sarcomas arise most frequently in the ileum, followed by the jejunum, with a low frequency in the duodenum.

Most sarcomas grow slowly, frequently becoming very large tumors which eventually outgrow their blood supply and develop ischemic necrosis and central ulceration. They typically develop in the submucosa, grow toward the serosal surface, and extend outside

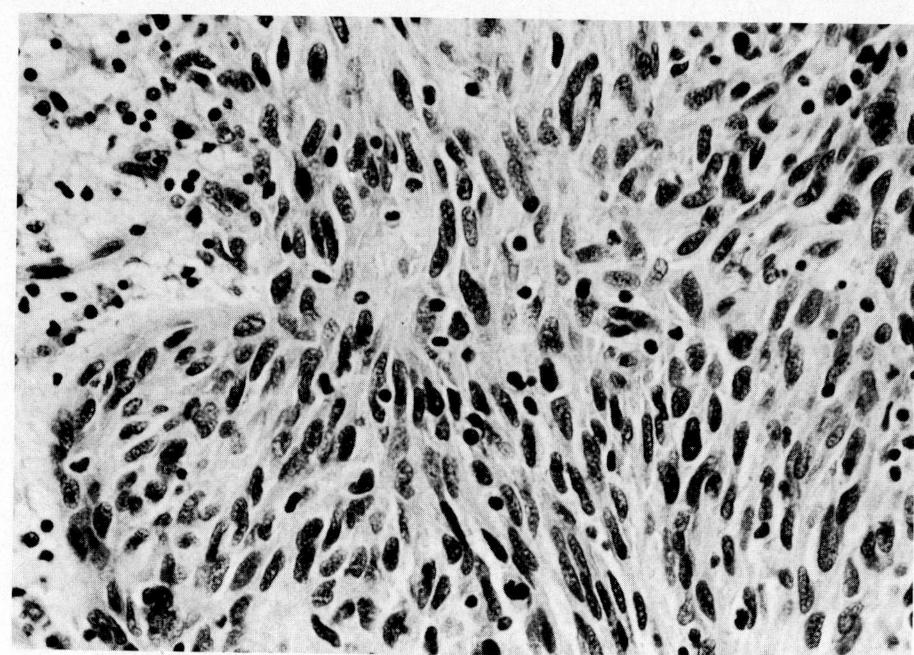

Figure 81–24. Well-differentiated leiomyosarcoma. (Hematoxylin and eosin stain, × 370). (Courtesy of Steven I. Hajdu, M.D., Department of Pathology, Memorial Sloan-Kettering Cancer Center, New York.)

the bowel wall to involve adjacent structures. Lymph node metastases are rare. Hematogenous spread to the liver and lungs is a late event.

Clinical Picture and Diagnosis

The main symptoms of small intestinal sarcomas are crampy abdominal pain, gastrointestinal hemorrhage, nausea and vomiting, and weight loss.[294, 296, 319, 320] Bleeding from leiomyosarcomas is usually chronic, but may be sudden and massive. Angiosarcomas are highly vascular and often present with acute hemorrhage. A palpable mass is present in more than half of patients who present with leiomyosarcomas.

The diagnosis of a small intestinal sarcoma can be suspected from a barium radiograph that demonstrates a large mass with central necrosis displacing other uninvolved loops of bowel. Computerized tomography is helpful in identifying the extent of local tumor invasion and the presence of metastases. Although duodenal lesions may be reached by upper endoscopy, biopsy is often unrevealing because of the submucosal nature of the tumors. Arteriography may reveal a large vascular mass with a tumor blush.

Treatment

Treatment consists of surgical excision of the primary tumor and areas of local tumor spread. Lymph node metastases are rare, and extensive lymph node dissection is unnecessary. Five-year survival rates range from 20 per cent to 50 per cent,[294, 296, 300, 319] with higher survival rates reported following resection of localized disease. High five-year survival rates are in part due to the slow growth of these tumors, and do not necessarily represent cures. Isolated pulmonary metastases may be resectable in some patients.

Radiation therapy may be useful as an adjunct to surgery or in palliating unresectable disease. Combination chemotherapy with doxorubicin, cyclophosphamide, vincristine, and imidazole carboxamide has produced responses (but not cures) in 65 per cent of patients with metastatic disease.[321] The role of adjuvant chemotherapy for this disease is unclear.

Lymphoma

Primary small intestinal lymphomas are a heterogeneous group of tumors originating from the lymphoid cells of the mucosa and submucosa of the small bowel.[322, 323] The small intestine may also become secondarily involved by systemic lymphoma. In Western countries primary lymphomas of the small intestine are often localized to one segment of small bowel, while in underdeveloped countries they are characterized by involvement of long sections of the upper small intestine.

Epidemiology, Etiology, and Risk Factors

Primary small intestinal lymphoma is an uncommon disease of unknown etiology in Western countries. There is a bimodal age distribution with peak incidences below the age of 10 and in the fifth and sixth decades, with a slight male predominance.

The term *immunoproliferative small intestinal disease* (also called Mediterranean abdominal lymphoma and Middle Eastern lymphoma) refers to a group of lymphomas endemic to the Middle East, North Africa, and other Third World regions.[322–325] The disease predominantly affects people in low socioeconomic groups in areas of poor sanitation who have a high incidence of enteric bacterial and parasitic infections during childhood. The peak incidence of this disease is in the second and third decades, with an equal sex distribution. A subgroup of patients is notable for a high incidence of alpha heavy chain paraproteinemia.[322, 325–327] It has been suggested that repeated antigenic stimulation of small intestinal plasma cells and lymphocytes by enteric pathogens leads to cell mutation and malignant transformation in these patients.[322] A predominance of certain HLA types also raises the question of genetic susceptibility.

There is an increased incidence of malignancy, particularly small intestinal lymphoma, in patients with celiac sprue (gluten enteropathy).[328–332] The cumulative risk is 11 to 14 per cent and increases with disease duration.[328, 329] In about two thirds of patients celiac disease precedes the diagnosis of lymphoma, in 19 per cent the two conditions are diagnosed simultaneously, and in 15 per cent celiac disease develops subsequent to the diagnosis of malignancy.[332] It has been postulated that chronic epithelial damage in celiac disease leads to an increased susceptibility to both carcinogens and cell mutation. It is unclear whether adherence to a gluten-free diet decreases the risk of malignancy (see pp. 1134–1152).

Small intestinal lymphoma has been reported in association with a variety of immunodeficiency syndromes,[322] including the acquired immunodeficiency syndromes (AIDS).[333] (See pp. 1233–1257.)

Pathology

Western small bowel lymphoma may arise at any level of the small intestine, but the ileum is by far the most common site. The tumor is generally localized to one bowel segment, although multiple lesions are seen in about 20 per cent of patients. These tumors arise in the lymphoid follicles of the submucosa and expand to invade the mucosa and serosa. They may appear as diffusely infiltrating and constricting lesions, or as nodular and polypoid masses. Involvement of the adjacent mesentery and lymph nodes is common. The majority are non-Hodgkin's lymphomas. In adults approximately 60 per cent are diffuse large cell ("histiocytic") lymphomas, 25 per cent lymphocytic, and the rest mixed.[322] Nearly all are of B cell origin. Small intestinal lymphomas complicating celiac sprue have been thought to be of histiocytic origin,[332] although recent data suggest that they may be derived from T cells.[331]

The lymphomas of immunoproliferative small intestinal disease affect long segments of the proximal bowel. These tumors begin as diffuse mucosal infiltrates which eventually evolve to nodular lesions involving the entire thickness of the intestine. Tumor often involves contiguous lymph nodes, and in an advanced stage may invade adjacent organs.

Clinical Presentation

Patients with primary small intestinal lymphoma present with signs and symptoms of small bowel obstruction (abdominal pain, nausea, vomiting), weight loss, altered bowel habits, and symptoms of anemia. Occult bleeding is common from ulcerated lesions. Intussusception may occur in children with ileocecal masses. Perforation has been reported in a number of cases, and may be increased by cytotoxic agents. Fever usually indicates the presence of systemic lymphoma, infection, or perforation. Patients with diffuse mucosal involvement by lymphoma (Fig. 81–25) may present with malabsorption (see pp. 263–282). Malignancy should be suspected in patients with celiac sprue whose symptoms increase despite adherence to a gluten-free diet.

Common symptoms in patients with immunoproliferative small intestinal disease include abdominal pain, diarrhea, and fever. Clubbing of the fingers and toes is a feature in one half to three quarters of the patients.

Diagnosis and Treatment

The diagnosis of small intestinal lymphoma is suggested by barium radiographs which show infiltration and thickening of the bowel wall with mucosal ulceration. When the mucosa is diffusely involved, the radiologic appearance may resemble that of celiac sprue, but more often is characterized by thickened mucosal folds. Segmental constriction of the bowel with luminal compromise is a feature of localized disease. Computerized tomography is helpful in determining the extent of disease. Small bowel biopsy may be useful when duodenal disease is present, and has a high yield in diagnosing immunoproliferative small intestinal disease. Serum immunoelectrophoresis may detect alpha heavy chain paraproteinemia in these patients.

There is some controversy regarding the optimum therapy for small intestinal lymphoma. While some have advocated extensive resection of involved segments and lymph nodes, with or without radiotherapy,[263, 322] others suggest more limited resections be done.[322, 327] Therapy depends on the extent of disease and tumor histology. Patients with nonbulky localized tumors are likely to be cured by surgery plus whole abdominal radiation.[327] A minority of patients with small lesions limited to the intestinal wall may be cured by surgery alone. In fact cure rates as high as 70 per cent have been reported in patients with localized disease treated with radical surgery alone, or radiotherapy alone in doses of 3500 to 4000 rads. Most studies report 5-year survival rates of 40 to 50 per cent[263, 322, 326] for patients with resectable disease. The placing of radiopaque clips at sites of possible residual tumor at surgery facilitates localization if postoperative radiotherapy is contemplated.

There is now a trend at some institutions to replace radiotherapy with chemotherapy after surgery, since the dose of radiation that can safely be delivered to the abdomen is limited, radiotherapy will delay chemotherapy in patients who are understaged and have disseminated disease, and chemotherapy probably is as effective as radiotherapy for control of local disease.[327] Patients with large bulky lesions or extensive

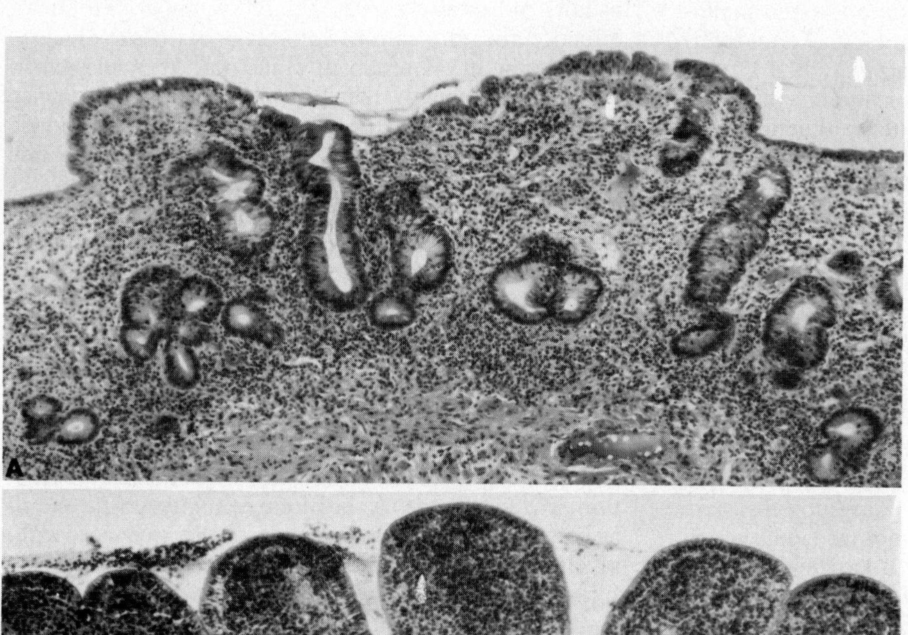

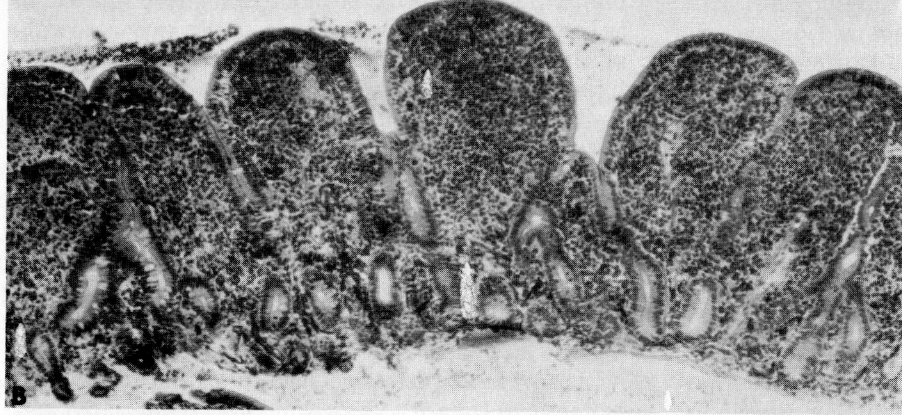

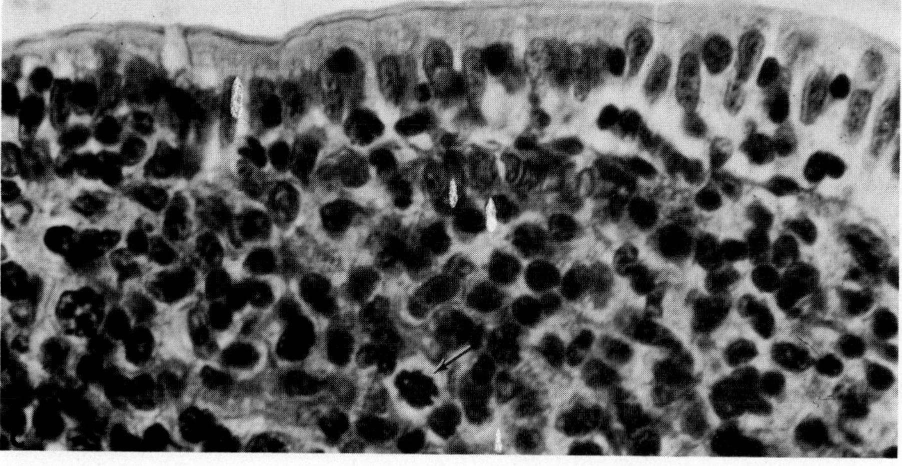

Figure 81–25. Proximal jejunal biopsies from two patients with intestinal malabsorption caused by diffuse involvement of the small intestine with lymphoma.

A, In this specimen, the absorptive surface is flat and villi are absent. However, in contrast to celiac sprue, the crypts of Lieberkühn are reduced in number and their architecture is disorganized. Occasional cells in the lamina propria showed cytologic evidence of lymphoma at high magnification. × 100.

B, Jejunal biopsy specimen from another patient with malabsorption caused by diffuse lymphoma of the small intestine. Although villi are present in this biopsy specimen, they are markedly distorted by an expanded, tremendously cellular lamina propria. × 90.

C, Higher magnification of a portion of the biopsy shown in *B.* The pleomorphic appearance of the cells in the lamina propria is evident, and they are clearly malignant in their morphologic features. The arrow indicates a mitotic figure. Unlike untreated celiac sprue, the villous epithelial cells are not markedly altered except that they are infiltrated by malignant cells. Their striated border is well preserved, and there is little vacuolization of their cytoplasm. × 624.

disease should be treated with chemotherapy similar to that used for systemic lymphomas. Current combination regimens for non-Hodgkin's lymphomas usually include cyclophosphamide, doxorubicin, vincristine, and prednisone. Other drugs that have been useful include bleomycin, CCNU, procarbazine, and methotrexate in high dose with leucovorin rescue. Local bowel resection should probably be performed even if combination chemotherapy is planned because of the potential risk of bowel perforation after cytotoxic therapy. The use of aggressive chemotherapy has resulted in a substantial improvement in cure rates for disseminated non-Hodgkin's lymphomas in adults,[334, 335] and undifferentiated lymphomas in children.[336]

References

1. Silverberg, E., and I ubera, J. Cancer statistics, 1987. CA *37*:2, 1987.
2. Waterhouse, J. A. H., Muir, C. S., Shanmugaratam, K., and Powel, J. Cancer Incidence in Five Continents. Vol. 4, IARC Publ. No. 42, Lyon International Agency for Research on Cancer, 1982.
3. Haenszel, W., and Correa, P. Epidemiology of large bowel cancer. *In* Correa, P., and Haenszel, W. (eds.). Epidemiology of the Digestive Tract. The Hague, Martinaus Nijhoff, 1982, pp. 85–126.
4. Boyle, P., Zaridze, D. G., and Smans, M. Descriptive epidemiology of colorectal cancer. Int. J. Cancer *361*:9, 1985.
5. Ziegler, R. G., Devesa, S. S., and Fraumeni, J. Epidemiologic patterns of colorectal cancer. *In* Devita, V. T., Jr., Hellman, S., and Rosenberg, S. A. (eds.). Important Advances in Oncology 1986. Philadelphia, J. B. Lippincott Co., 1986, pp. 209–231.
6. Haenszel, W. Migrant studies. *In* Schottenfeld, D., and Fraumeni, J. F., Jr., (eds.). Cancer Epidemiology and Prevention. Philadelphia, W. B. Saunders Co., 1982, pp. 194–207.
7. Haenszel, W., and Kurihara, M. Studies of Japanese immigrants. I. Mortality from cancer and other diseases among Japanese in the United States. JNCI *40*:43, 1968.
8. McMichael, A. J., McCall, M. G., Hartshorne, J. M., and Woodings, T. L. Patterns of gastrointestinal cancer in European immigrants to Australia: the role of dietary change. Int. J. Cancer *25*:431, 1980.
9. Snyder, D. N., Heston, J. F., Meigs, J. W., and Flannery, J. T. Changes in site distribution of colorectal carcinoma in Connecticut, 1940–1973. Am. J. Dig. Dis. *22*:791, 1977.
10. Mamazza, J., and Gordon, P. H. The changing distribution of large intestinal cancer. Dis. Colon Rectum *25*:558, 1982.
11. Netscher, D. T., and Larson, G. M. Colon cancer: the left to right shift and its implications. Surg. Gastroenterol. *2*:13, 1983.
12. Zaridze, D. G. Environmental etiology of large bowel cancer. JNCI *70*:389, 1983.
13. Armstrong, B., and Doll, R. Environmental factors and cancer incidence and mortality in different countries, with special reference to dietary practices. Int. J. Cancer *15*:617, 1975.
14. Phillips, R. L. Role of life-style and dietary habits in risk of cancer among Seventh Day Adventists. Cancer Res. *35*:3513, 1975.
15. Weisburger, J. H., Reddy, B. S., and Newell, G. R. Potential for personal modification of risk for developing colon cancer. Cancer Detect. Prev. *8*:399, 1985.
16. Dales, L. G., Friedman, G. D., Wry, H. K., Grossman, S., and Williams, S. R. A case-control study of relationships of diet and other traits to colorectal cancer in American blacks. Am. J. Epidemiol. *109*:132, 1979.
17. Rozen, P., Hellerstein, S., and Horwitz, C. The low incidence of colorectal cancer in a "high risk" population. Its correlation with dietary habits. Cancer *48*:2692, 1981.
18. Tornberg, S. A., Holm, L. E., Carstensen, J. M., and Eklund, G. A. Risks of cancer of the colon and rectum in relation to serum cholesterol and beta-lipoprotein. N. Engl. J. Med. *315*:1629, 1986.
19. Reddy, B. S. Dietary fat and its relationship to large bowel cancer. Cancer Res. *41*:3700, 1981.
20. Reddy, B. S., Tanaka, T., and Simi, B. Effect of different levels of dietary trans fat or corn oil on azoxymethane-induced colon carcinogenesis in F 344 rats. JNCI *75*:792, 1985.
21. Reddy, B. S., and Marayama, H. Effect of dietary fish oil on azoxymethane-induced colon carcinogenesis in male F344 rats. Cancer Res. *46*:3367, 1986.
22. Reddy, B. S., and Wynder, E. L. Large bowel carcinogenesis: fecal constitutents of populations with diverse incidence rates of colon cancer. JNCI *50*:1437, 1973.
23. Reddy, B. S., Hedges, A. R., Laakso, K., and Wynder, E. L. Metabolic epidemiology of large bowel cancer: fecal bulk and constituents of high-risk North American and low-risk Finnish populations. Cancer *42*:2832, 1978.
24. Hill, M. J., Drasar, B. S., Williams, R. E. O., Meade, T. W., Cox, A. G., Simpson, J. E. P., and Morson, B. C. Fecal bile acids and clostridia in patients with cancer of the large bowel. Lancet *1*:535, 1975.
25. Reddy, B. S., Watanabe, K., Weisburger, J. H., and Wynder, E. L. Promoting effect of bile acids in colon carcinogenesis in germ-free and conventional F 344 rats. Cancer Res. *37*:3238, 1977.
26. International Agency for Research on Cancer, Intestinal Microecology Group. Dietary fibre, transit time, faecal bacteria, steroids and colon cancer in two Scandinavian populations. Lancet *2*:207, 1977.
27. Jensan, O. M., MacLennan, R., and Wahrendorf, J. (on behalf of the IARC Large Bowel Cancer Group). Diet, bowel function, fecal characteristics and large bowel cancer in Denmark and Finland. Nutr. Cancer *4*:5, 1982.
28. Bingham, S., Williams, D. R., Dole, T. S., and James, W. P. Dietary fibre and regional large bowel mortality in Britain. Br. J. Cancer *40*:456, 1979.
29. Modan, B., Barrel, V., Lubin, F., Modan, M., Greenberg, P. A., and Grahm, S. Low fiber intake as an etiologic factors in cancer of the colon. JNCI *55*:15, 1975.
30. Greenwald, P., and Lanza, L. Role of dietary fiber in prevention of cancer. *In* De Vita, V. T., Jr., Hellman, S., and Rosenberg, S. A. Important Advances in Oncology, 1986. Philadelphia, J. B. Lippincott Co., 1986, pp. 37–54.
31. Reddy, B. S., Sharma, C., Simi, B., Engle, A. S. W., Laakso, K., Puska, P., and Korpela, R. Metabolic epidemiology of colon cancer: effect of dietary fiber on fecal mutagens and bile acids in healthy subjects. Cancer Res. *47*:644, 1987.
32. Freeman, H. J., Spiller, G. A., and Kim, Y. S. A double-blind study of differing cellulose and pectin fiber diets on 1,2-dimethylhydrazine–induced rat intestinal neoplasia. Cancer Res. *40*:2661, 1980.
33. Freeman, H. J., Spiller, G. A., Kim, Y. S. Effect of high hemicellulose corn bran in 1,2-dimethylhydrazine–induced rat intestinal neoplasia. Carcinogenesis (Lond.) *5*:261, 1984.
34. Freeman, H. J. Effects of differing purified cellulose, pectin and hemicellulose fiber diets or fecal enzymes in 1,2-dimethylhydrazine–induced rat colon carcinogenesis. Cancer Res. *46*:5529, 1986.
35. Kritchevsky, D. Diet, nutrition and cancer. The role of fiber. Cancer *58*:1830, 1986.
36. Bruce, W. R., Varghese, A. J., Furrer, R., and Land, P. C. A mutagen in the feces of normal humans. *In* Hiatt, H. H., and Winsten, J. A. (eds.). Origins of Human Cancer. Cold Spring Harbor, New York, Cold Spring Harbor Laboratory, 1977, pp. 1641–1646.
37. Reddy, B. S., Sharma, C., Darby, L., Laakso, K., and Wynder, E. L. Metabolic epidemiology of large bowel cancer. Fecal mutagens in high- and low-risk populations for colon cancer. Mut. Res. *72*:511, 1980.
38. Mower, H. F., Itchinotsubo, D., Wang, L. W., Mandel, M., Stemmerman, G., Norman, A., Heilbrun, L., Kaniyama, S., and Shimada, A. Fecal mutagens in two Japanese populations with different colon cancer risks. Cancer Res. *42*:1164, 1982.

39. Gupta, I., Baptista, J., Bruce, W. R., Che, C. T., Furrer, R., Gingerich, J. S., Grey, A. A., Marai, L., Yates, P., and Krepinski, J. J. Structures of fecapentaenes, the mutagens of bacterial origin isolated from human feces. Biochemistry *22*:241, 1983.
40. Pollack, E. S., Nomura, A., Heibrun, L. K., Stemmerman, G. N., and Green, S. B. Prospective study of alcohol consumption and cancer. N. Engl. J. Med. *310*:617, 1984.
41. Palmer, S. Dietary considerations for risk reduction. Cancer *58*:1949, 1986.
42. Weisburger, J. H., Reddy, B. S., and Newell, G. R. Potential for personal modification of risk for developing colon cancer. Cancer Detect. Prev. *8*:399, 1985.
43. Garland, C., Shekelle, R. B., Barnett-Conner, E., Criqui, M., Rossof, A. H., and Pau, O. Dietary vitamin D and calcium and risk of colorectal cancer: a 19-year prospective study in men. Lancet *1*:307, 1985.
44. Bird, R. P., Schneider, R., Stump, D., and Bruce, W. R. Effects of dietary calcium and cholic acid on the proliferative indices of murine colonic epithelium. Carcinogenesis *7*:1657, 1986.
45. Lipkin, M., and Newmark, H. Effect of added dietary calcium on colonic epithelial cell proliferation in subjects at high risk for familial colonic cancer. N. Engl. J. Med. *313*:1381, 1985.
46. Buset, M., Lipkin, M., Winawer, S., Swaroup, S., and Friedman, E. Inhibition of human colonic epithelial cell proliferation *in vivo* and *in vitro* by calcium. Cancer Res. *46*:5426, 1986.
47. Lipkin, M., Blattner, W. E., Fraumeni, J. F., Jr., Lynch, H. T., Deschner, E., and Winawer, S. Tritiated thymidrine (ϕ_p,ϕ_h) labeling distribution as a marker for hereditary predisposition to colon cancer. Cancer Res. *43*:1899, 1983.
48. Lipkin, M., Blattner, W. A., Gardner, E. J., Burt, R. W., Lynch, H., Deschner, E., Winawer, S., and Fraumeni, J. F., Jr. Classification and risk assessment of individuals with familial polyposis, Gardner's syndrome, and familial nonpolyposis colon cancer from ^{3}H thymidine labeling patterns in colonic epithelial cells. Cancer Res. *44*:4201, 1984.
49. Lipkin, M., Uehara, K., Winawer, S., Sanchez, A., Burt, R. W., Lynch, H., Blattner, W. A., and Fraumeni, J. F., Jr. Seventh Day Adventist vegetarians have a quiescent proliferative activity in colonic mucosa. Cancer Letters *26*:139, 1985.
50. Luk, G. D., and Baylin, S. B. Ornithine decarboxylase as a biologic marker in familial colonic polyposis. N. Engl. J. Med. *311*:80, 1984.
51. Luk, G. D., Hamilton, S. R., Yang, P., Smith, P. A., O'-Ceallaigh, D., McAvinchey, D., and Hyland, J. Kinetic changes in mucosal ornithine decarboxylase activity during azoxymethane-induced colonic carcinogenesis in the rat. Cancer Res. *46*:4449, 1986.
52. Der, C. J., and Cooper, G. M. Altered gene products are associated with activation of cellular ras^K genes in human lung and colon carcinomas. Cell *32*:201, 1982.
53. McCoy, M. S., Toole, J. J., Cunningham, J. M., Chang, E. H., Lowy, D. R., and Weinberg, R. A. Characterization of a human colon/lung carcinoma oncogene. Nature *302*:79, 1983.
54. Alitalo, K., Wingvist, R., Lin, C. C., De la Chapelle, A., Schwab, M., and Bishop, J. M. Aberrant expression of an amplified C-myb oncogene in two cell lines from a colon carcinoma. Proc. Natl. Acad. Sci. USA *81*:4534, 1984.
55. Alexander, R. J., Buxbaum, J. N., and Raicht, R. F. Oncogene alterations in primary human colon tumors. Gastroenterology *91*:1503, 1986.
56. Thor, A., Hand, P. H., Wunderlich, D., Caruso, A., Muraro, R., and Schlom, J. Monoclonal antibodies define differential ras gene expression in malignant and benign diseases. Nature (Lond.) *311*:562, 1984.
57. Wolley, R. C., Schreiber, K., Koss, L. G., Karas, M., and Sherman, A. DNA distribution in human colon carcinomas and its relationship to clinical behavior. JNCI *69*:15, 1982.
58. Kokal, W., Sheibani, K., Terz, J., and Harada, J. R. Tumor DNA content in the prognosis of colorectal carcinoma. JAMA *255*:3123, 1986.
59. Boland, C. R., Montgomery, C. K., and Kim, Y. S. Alterations in colonic mucin occurring with cellular differentiation and malignant transformation. Proc. Natl. Acad. Sci. USA *79*:2051, 1982.
60. Shioda, Y., Brown, W. R., and Ahnen, D. J. Serial observations of colonic carcinogenesis in the rat. Premalignant mucosa binds *Ulex europeus* agglutinin. Gastroenterology *92*:1, 1987.
61. Itzkowitz, S. H., and Kim, Y. S. New carbohydrate tumor markers. Gastroenterology *90*:491, 1986.
62. Bresalier, R. S., Boland, C. R., and Kim, Y. S. Characteristics of colorectal carcinoma cells with high metastatic potential. Gastroenterology *87*:115, 1984.
63. Bresalier, R. S., Boland, C. R., Itzkowitz, S. H., and Kim, Y. S. Basic gastrointestinal oncology. *In* Kern, F., Jr., and Blum, A. L. (eds.). The Gastroenterology Annual/2. Amsterdam, Elsevier/North Holland, 1985, pp. 271–319.
64. Lynch, P. M., Lynch, H. T., and Lynch, J. F. Hereditary nonpolyposis colon cancer: epidemiologic and clinical features. *In* Lynch, P. M., and Lynch, H. T. (eds.). Colon Cancer Genetics. New York, Van Nostrand Reinhold Co., 1985, pp. 52–98.
65. Lynch, H. T., Kimberling, W., Albano, W. A., Lynch, S. F., Biscone, K., Schuelke, G. S., Sandberg, A. A., Lipkin, M., Deschner, E. E., Mikol, Y. B., Elston, R. C., Bailey-Wilson, J. E., and Danes, B. S. Hereditary nonpolyposis colorectal cancer (Lynch syndromes I and II). I. Clinical description of resource. Cancer *56*:934, 1985.
66. Boland, C. R. Familial colonic cancer syndromes—medical staff conference, University of California, San Francisco. West. J. Med. *129*:351, 1983.
67. Mecklin, J. P., Sipponen, P., and Jarvinen, H. J. Histopathology of colorectal carcinomas and adenomas in cancer family syndrome. Dis. Colon Rectum *29*:849, 1986.
68. Mecklin, J. P., Jarvinen, H. J., and Peltokallio, P. Cancer family syndrome. Genetic analysis of 22 Finnish kindreds. Gastroenterology *90*:328, 1986.
69. Lynch, H. T., Kimberling, W., Albano, W. A., Lynch, S. F., Biscone, K., Schuelke, G. S., Sandberg, A. A., Lipkin, M., Deschner, E. E., Mikol, Y. B., Elston, R. C., Bailey-Wilson, J. E., and Danes, B. S. Hereditary nonpolyposis colorectal cancer (Lynch syndromes I and II). II. Biomarker studies. Cancer *56*:939, 1985.
70. Markowitz, J. F., Aiges, H. W., Cunningham-Rundles, S., Kahn, E., Teichberg, S., Fisher, S. E., and Daum, F. Cancer family syndrome: marker studies. Gastroenterology *91*:581, 1986.
71. Burt, R. A., Bishop, D. T., Cannon, L. A., Dowdle, M. A. S., Lee, R. S. G., and Skolnick, M. H. Dominant inheritance of adenomatous polyps and colorectal cancer. N. Engl. J. Med. *312*:1540, 1985.
72. Lovett, E. Familial factors in the etiology of carcinoma of the large bowel. J. Roy. Soc. Med. *67*:21, 1974.
73. Macklin, M. Inheritance of cancer of the stomach and large intestine in man. JNCI *24*:551, 1960.
74. Woolf, C. M., Richards, R. C., and Gardner, E. J. Occasional discrete polyps of the colon and rectum showing an inherited tendency in a kindred. Cancer *8*:403, 1955.
75. Brahme, F., Ekelund, G., Norden, J. G., and Wenkert, A. Metachronous colorectal polyps. Comparison of development of colorectal polyps and carcinomas in persons with and without histories of polyps. Dis. Colon Rectum *117*:166, 1974.
76. Bussey, H. J. R. Multiple adenomas and carcinomas. *In* Morson, B. C. (ed.). The Pathogenesis of Colorectal Cancer. Philadelphia, W. B. Saunders Co., 1978, p. 72.
77. Muto, T., Bussey, H. T. R., and Morson, B. C. The evolution of cancer of the colon and rectum. Cancer *36*:2251, 1975.
78. Shinya, H., and Wolff, W. I. Morphology, anatomic distribution and cancer potential of colonic polyps. An analysis of 7,000 polyps endoscopically removed. Ann. Surg. *190*:679, 1979.
79. Jass, J. R., and Morson, B. C. Epithelial dysplasia in the gastrointestinal tract. *In* Glass, G. B. J., and Sherlock, P. (eds.). Progress in Gastroenterology. Volume IV. New York, Grune and Stratton, 1983, pp. 345–371.
80. Rickert, R. R., Auerbach, O., Garfinkle, L., Hammond, E. C., and Frasca, J. M. Adenomatous lesions of the large bowel. An autopsy study. Cancer *43*:1847, 1979.
81. Eide, T. J., and Stalsberg, H. Polyps of the large intestine in northern Norway. Cancer *42*:2839, 1978.
82. Williams, A. R., Balasooriya, B. A. W., and Day, D. W.

Polyps and cancer of the large bowel: a necropsy study in Liverpool. Gut *23*:835, 1982.

83. Eide, T. J. Risk of colorectal cancer in adenoma-bearing individuals within a defined population. Int. J. Cancer *38*:173, 1986.
84. Lockhart-Mummery, H. E., and Heald, R. J. Metachronous cancer of the large intestine. Dis. Colon Rectum *15*:261, 1972.
85. Ekelund, G., and Pihl, B. Multiple carcinomas of the colon and rectum. Cancer *33*:1630, 1974.
86. Heald, R. J., Bussey, H. J. R. Clinical experience at St. Marks Hospital with multiple synchronous cancers of the colon and rectum. Dis. Colon Rectum *18*:6, 1975.
87. Langevin, J. M., and Nivatvongs, S. The true incidence of synchronous cancer of the large bowel. A prospective study. Am. J. Surg. *147*:330, 1984.
88. Pagana, T. J., Ledesma, E. J., Mittelman, A., and Nava, H. R. The use of colonoscopy in the study of synchronous colorectal neoplasms. Cancer *55*:356, 1984.
89. Kaibara, N., Koga, S., and Jinnai, D. Synchronous and metachronous malignancies of the colon and rectum in Japan with special reference to a coexisting early cancer. Cancer *54*:1870, 1984.
90. Anderson, D. E. An inherited form of large bowel cancer. Muir's syndrome. Cancer *45*:1103, 1980.
91. Cochet, B., Carvel, J., Desbaillets, L., and Widgren, S. Peutz-Jeghers syndrome associated with gastrointestinal carcinoma. Gut *20*:169, 1979.
92. Stemper, T. J., Kent, T. H., and Summers, R. W. Juvenile polyposis and gastrointestinal carcinoma. A study of a kindred. Ann. Intern. Med. *83*:639, 1975.
93. Farmer, R. G., Hawk, W. A., and Turnbull, R. B., Jr. Carcinoma associated with mucosal ulcerative colitis and with transmural colitis and enteritis (Crohn's disease). Cancer *28*:289, 1971.
94. Lennard-Jones, J. E., Morson, B. C., Ritchie, J. K., Shove, D. C., and Williams, C. B. Cancer in colitis: assessment of the individual risk by clinical and histologic criteria. Gastroenterology *73*:1280, 1977.
95. Nugent, F. W., Haggitt, R. C., Colcher, H., and Kutteruf, G. C. Malignant potential of chronic ulcerative colitis. Gastroenterology *76*:1, 1979.
96. Sachar, D. B., and Greenstein, A. J. Cancer in ulcerative colitis: good news and bad news. Ann. Intern. Med. *95*:642, 1981.
97. Sackett, D. L., and Whelen, C. Cancer in ulcerative colitis: scientific requirements for study of prognosis. Gastroenterology *78*:1632, 1980.
98. Devroede, G. J., Taylor, W. F., Saur, W. G., Jackman, R. J., and Stickler, G. B. Cancer risk and life expectancy of children with ulcerative colitis. N. Engl. J. Med. *285*:17, 1971.
99. Greenstein, A. J., Sachar, D. B., Smith, H., Pucillo, A., Papatestas, A. E., Kreel, I., Geller, S. A., Janowitz, H. D., and Aufses, A. H., Jr. Cancer in universal and left-sided ulcerative colitis: factors determining risk. Gastroenterology *77*:290, 1979.
100. Katska, I., Brody, R. S., Morris, E. L., and Katz, S. Assessment of colorectal cancer risk in patients with ulcerative colitis: experience from a private practice. Gastroenterology *85*:22, 1983.
101. Lennard-Jones, J. E., Ritchie, J. K., Morson, B. C., and Williams, C. B. Cancer surveillance in ulcerative colitis. Experience over 15 years. Lancet *2*:149, 1983.
102. Gyde, S., Prior, P., Thompson, H., Waterhouse, J. A. H., and Allan, R. N. Survival of patients with colorectal cancer complicating ulcerative colitis. Gut *25*:228, 1984.
103. Thompson, E. H., Clayden, G., and Price, A. B. Cancer in Crohn's disease—an occult malignancy. Histopathology *7*:265, 1983.
104. Hamilton, S. R. Colorectal carcinoma in patients with Crohn's disease. Gastroenterology *80*:318, 1985.
105. Dobbins, W. O. Current status of the precancer lesion in ulcerative colitis. Gastroenterology *73*:1431, 1977.
106. Kewenter, J., Hulten, L., and Ahren, C. The occurrence of severe epithelial dysplasia and its bearing of treatment of long-standing ulcerative colitis. Ann. Surg. *195*:209, 1982.
107. Lennard-Jones, J. E., Morson, B. C., Ritchie, J. K., and Williams, C. B. Cancer surveillance in ulcerative colitis. Experience over 15 years. Lancet *2*:149, 1983.
108. Blackstone, M. O., Riddel, R. H., Rodgers, B. H. G., and Levin, B. Dysplasia-associated lesion or mass (DALM) detected by colonoscopy in long-standing ulcerative colitis: an indication for surgery. Gastroenterology *80*:366, 1981.
109. Rosenstock, E., Farmer, R. G., Petras, R., Sivak, M. V., Jr., Rankin, G. B., and Sullivan, B. Surveillance for colonic carcinoma in ulcerative colitis. Gastroenterology *89*:1342, 1985.
110. Riddell, R. H., Goldman, H., Ransohoff, D. F., Appelman, H. D., Fenoglio, C., Haggitt, R. C., Ahren, C., Correa, P., Hamilton, S. R., Morson, B. C., Sonners, S. C., and Yardley, J. H. Dysplasias in inflammatory bowel disease: standardized classification with provisional clinical application. Hum. Pathol. *11*:14, 1983.
111. Nugent, F. W., and Haggitt, R. C. Results of a long-term prospective surveillance program for dysplasia in ulcerative colitis. Gastroenterology *86*:1197, 1984.
112. Simpson, S., Traube, J., and Riddel, R. H. The histological appearance of dysplasia (precarcinomatous change) in Crohn's disease of the small and large intestine. Gastroenterology *81*:492, 1981.
113. Warren, R., and Barwick, K. W. Crohn's colitis with carcinoma and dysplasia. Report of a case and review of 100 small and large resections for Crohn's disease to detect incidence of dysplasia. Am. J. Surg. Pathol. *7*:151, 1983.
114. Bandettini, L., Filipponi, F., and Romagnoli, P. Increase of the mitotic index of colonic mucosa after cholecystectomy. Cancer *58*:685, 1986.
115. Mannes, A. G., Weinzierl, M., Stellaard, F., Thiene, C., Wiebecke, B., and Paumgartner, G. Adenomas of the large intestine after cholecystectomy. Gut *25*:863, 1984.
116. Vernick, L. J., and Kuller, L. H. A case-control study of cholecystectomy and right-sided colon cancer: the influence of alternative data sources and different interview participation proportions on odds ratio estimates. Am. J. Epidemiol. *116*:86, 1982.
117. Alley, P. G., and Lee, S. P. The increased risk of proximal colonic cancer after cholecystectomy. Dis. Colon Rectum *26*:522, 1983.
118. Blanco, D., Ross, D. K., Paganini-Hill, A., and Henderson, B. E. Cholecystectomy and colonic cancer. Dis. Colon Rectum *27*:290, 1984.
119. Adanik, H. O., Meirik, O., Gustavsson, S., Nyren, O., and Krusemu, U. B. Colorectal cancer after cholecystectomy: absence of risk increase within 11–14 years. Gastroenterology *85*:859, 1983.
120. Sontag, S. J., Schnell, T., Chejfec, G. T., Stanley, M. M., Chintam, R., Wanner, J., Schnell, T. G., O'Connel, S., Bert, W., Nemchausky, B., and Moreni, B. Barrett's esophagus and colonic tumors. Lancet *1*:946, 1985.
121. Tripp, M. R., Sampliner, R. E., Kogan, F. J., and Morgan, T. R. Colorectal neoplasms and Barrett's esophagus. Am. J. Gastroenterol. *81*:1063, 1986.
122. Astler, V. B., and Coller, F. A. The prognostic significance of direct extension of carcinoma of the colon and rectum. Ann. Surg. *139*:846, 1954.
123. Symonds, D. A., and Vickery, A. L. Mucinous carcinomas of the colon and rectum. Cancer *37*:1891, 1976.
124. Woolan, G. L., Jackman, R. J., Ramirez, R. J., Beahrs, O. H., and Dockerty, M. B. Scirrhous carcinoma of the lower intestine. Surg. Gynecol. Obstet. *121*:753, 1965.
125. Welin, S., Youker, J., and Spratt, J. S. The rates and patterns of growth of 375 tumors of the large intestine and rectum observed serially by double contrast enema study (Malbo technique). AJR *90*:673, 1963.
126. Dukes, C. E. Cancer of the rectum. An analysis of 1000 cases. J. Pathol. Bacteriol. *50*:527, 1940.
127. Grinnel, R. S. Distal intramural spread of carcinoma of the rectum and rectosigmoid. Surg. Gynecol. Obstet. *99*:421, 1954.
128. Williams, N. S. The rationale for preservation of the anal sphincter in patients with low rectal cancer. Br. J. Surg. *71*:575, 1984.
129. Wolmark, N., and Fisher, B. An analysis of survival and

treatment failure following abdominoperineal and sphincter-saving resection in Dukes' B and C rectal carcinoma. Ann. Surg. *204*:480, 1986.
130. Dukes, C. E. The classification of cancer of the rectum. J. Pathol. *35*:323, 1932.
131. Gastrointestinal Tumor Study Group. Adjuvent therapy of colon cancer—results of a prospectively randomized trial. N. Engl. J. Med. *310*:737, 1984.
132. Turnbull, R. B., Kyle, K., Watson, F. B., and Spratt, J. Cancer of the colon. Influence of the no-touch isolation technique on survival rates. Ann. Surg. *166*:420, 1967.
133. American Joint Committee for Cancer Staging and End Results Reporting: Manual for Staging of Cancer 1978. Chicago, National Cancer Institute, 1978.
134. Beahrs, O. H. Colorectal cancer staging as a prognostic feature. Cancer *50*:2615, 1982.
135. Copeland, E. M., Miller, L. D., and Jones, R. S. Prognostic factors in carcinoma of the colon and rectum. Am. J. Surg. *116*:875, 1968.
136. Wollmark, N., Fisher, E. R., Wieand, S., and Fisher, B. The relationship of depth of penetration and tumor size to the number of positive nodes in Dukes' C colorectal cancer. Cancer *53*:2707, 1984.
137. Rich, T., Gunderson, L. L., Lew, R., Galdibini, J. J., Cohen, A. M., and Donaldson, G. Patterns of recurrences after potentially curable surgery. Cancer *52*:1317, 1983.
138. Heiman, T. M., Szporn, A., Bolnick, K., and Aufses, A. H., Jr. Local recurrence following surgical treatment of rectal cancer. Comparison of anterior and abdominoperineal resection. Dis. Colon Rectum *29*:862, 1986.
139. Wolmark, N., Fisher, B., and Wieand, H. S. The prognostic value of the modifications of the Dukes' C class of colorectal cancer. Ann. Surg. *203*:115, 1986.
140. Moertel, C. G., O'Fallon, J. R., Go, V. L., O'Connel, M. J., and Grenville, S. T. The preoperative carcinoembryonic antigen test in the diagnosis, staging, and prognosis of colorectal cancer. Cancer *58*:603, 1986.
141. Spratt, J. S., and Spjut, H. J. Prevalence and prognosis of individual clinical and pathologic variables associated with colorectal carcinoma. Cancer *20*:1976, 1967.
142. McSherry, C. K., Cornell, G. N., and Glen, F. Carcinoma of the colon and rectum. Ann. Surg. *119*:502, 1969.
143. Wolmark, N., Cruz, I., Redmond, C. K., and Fisher, B. Tumor size and regional lymnph node metastasis in colorectal cancer. Cancer *51*:1315, 1983.
144. Steinberg, S. M., Barwick, K. W., and Stablein, D. M. Importance of tumor pathology and morphology in patients with surgically resected colon cancer. Cancer *58*:1340, 1986.
145. Rankin, F. W., and Broders, A. C. Factors influencing prognosis in carcinoma of the rectum. Surg. Gynecol. Obstet. *46*:660, 1928.
146. Grinnel, R. S. The grading and prognosis of carcinoma of the colon and rectum. Ann. Surg. *109*:500, 1939.
147. Freedman, L. S., Macaskill, P., and Smith, A. N. Multivariate analysis of prognostic factors for operable rectal cancer. Lancet *1*:733, 1984.
148. Almagro, V. A. Primary signet-ring carcinoma of the colon. Cancer *52*:1453, 1983.
149. Giacchero, A., Aste, H., Baracchini, P., Conio, M., Fulceri, E., Lapertosa, G., and Tanzi, R. Primary signet-ring carcinoma of the large bowel. Cancer *56*:2723, 1985.
150. Grinnel, R. S. The lymphatic and venous spread of carcinoma of the rectum. Ann. Surg. *116*:200, 1942.
151. Grinnell, R. S. Lymphatic metastases of carcinoma of the colon and rectum. Ann. Surg. *131*:494, 1950.
152. Khankhanian, N., Mavligit, G. M., Russel, W. O., and Schimek, M. Prognostic significance of vascular invasion in colorectal cancer of Dukes' B class. Cancer *39*:1195, 1977.
153. Seefeld, P. H., and Bargen, J. A. The spread of carcinoma of the rectum: invasion of lymphatics, veins, and nerves. Ann. Surg. *118*:76, 1943.
154. Zhou, X. G., Yu, B. M., and Shen, Y. X. Surgical treatment and late results in 1226 cases of colorectal cancer. Dis. Colon Rectum *26*:250, 1983.
155. Armitage, N. C., Robins, R. A., Evans, D. F., Turner, D. R., Baldwin, R. W., and Hardcastle, J. D. The influence of tumor cell DNA abnormalities on survival in colorectal cancer. Br. J. Surg. *72*:828, 1985.
156. Banner, B. F., Tomas-De La Vega, J. E., Roseman, D. L., and Coon, J. S. Should flow cytometric DNA analysis precede definitive surgery for colon carcinoma? Ann. Surg. *202*:740, 1985.
157. Gilbertson, V. A., and Nelms, J. M. The prevention of invasive cancer of the rectum. Cancer *41*:1137, 1978.
158. Hardcastle, J. D., Armitage, N. C., Chamberl, J., James, P. D., and Balfour, T. W. Fecal occult blood screening for colorectal cancer in the general population. Results of a controlled trial. Cancer *58*:397, 1986.
159. Elliot, M. S., Levenstein, J. H., and Wright, J. P. Faecal occult blood testing in the detection of colorectal cancer. Br. J. Surg. *71*:785, 1984.
160. Welch, C. E., and Burke, J. F. Carcinoma of the colon and rectum. N. Engl. J. Med. *266*:211, 1962.
161. McDermott, F. T., Hughes, S., Pihl, E., Milne, B. J., and Price, A. B. Prognosis in relation to symptom duration in colon cancer. Br. J. Surg. *68*:846, 1981.
162. Glenn, F., and McSherry, C. K. Obstruction and perforation in colorectal cancer. Ann. Surg. *173*:983, 1971.
163. Wollmark, N., Wieand, H. S., Rockette, H. E., Fisher, B., Glass, A., Lawrence, W., Lerner, H., Cruz, A. B., Volk, I. T., Shibata, H., Evans, J., and Prayer, D. The prognostic significance of tumor location and bowel obstruction in Dukes' B and C colorectal cancer. Ann. Surg. *198*:743, 1983.
164. Phillips, R. K. S., Hittinger, R., Blesovsky, L., Fry, J. J., and Fielding, L. P. Local recurrence following 'curative' surgery for large bowel cancer. I. The overall picture. Br. J. Surg. *71*:12, 1984.
165. Steiberg, S. M., Barlin, J. S., Kaplan, R. S., and Stablein, D. M. Prognostic indicators of colon tumors. Cancer *57*:1866, 1986.
166. Willet, C., Tepper, J. E., Cohen, A., Orlow, E., and Welch, C. Obstructive and perforative colonic carcinoma: pattern of failure. J. Clin. Oncol. *3*:379, 1985.
167. Recio, P., and Bussey, H. J. R. The pathology and prognosis of carcinoma of the rectum in the young. Proc. R. Soc. London *58*:789, 1965.
168. Anderson, A., and Bergdahl, L. Carcinoma of the colon in children: a report of six new cases and a review of the literature. J. Pediatr. Surg. *11*:967, 1976.
169. Enker, W., Paloyan, E., and Kirsner, J. Carcinoma of the colon in the adolescent. A report of survival and analysis of the literature. Am. J. Surg. *133*:737, 1977.
170. Bhaskar, N. R., Pratt, C. B., Fleming, I. D., Dilwar, R. A., Green, A. A., and Austin, B. A. Colon carcinoma in children and adolescents. A review of 30 cases. Cancer *55*:1322, 1985.
171. Wanebo, H., Rao, B., Pinsky, C. M., Hoffman, R. G., Stearns, M., Schwartz, M. K., and Oettger, H. F. Preoperative carcinoembryonic antigen level as a prognostic indicator in colorectal cancer. N. Engl. J. Med. *299*:448, 1978.
172. Goslin, R., Steele, G., and MacIntyre, J. The use of preoperative plasma CEA levels for the stratification of patients after curative resection of colorectal cancers. Ann. Surg. *192*:747, 1980.
173. Wagner, J. S., Adson, M. A., Van Heerden, J. A., Adson, M. H., and Ilstrup, D. M. The natural history of hepatic metastases from colorectal cancer. A comparison with resective treatment. Ann. Surg. *199*:502, 1984.
174. Postlethwait, R. W. Malignant tumors of the colon and rectum. Ann. Surg. *129*:34, 1949.
175. Fork, F. T. Double contrast enema and colonoscopy in polyp detection. Gut *22*:971, 1981.
176. Hogan, W. J., Steward, E. T., Geenen, J. E., Dodds, W. J., Bjork, J. T., and Leinicke, J. A. A prospective comparison of the accuracy of colonoscopy versus air-barium contrast exam for detection of colonic polypoid lesions. Gastrointest. Endosc. *23*:230, 1977.
177. Stroehlein, J. R., Goulston, K., and Hunt, R. H. Diagnostic approach to evaluating the cause of a positive fecal occult blood test. CA *34*:148, 1984.
178. Eddy, D. M., Nugent, F. W., Eddy, J. F., Coller, J., Gilbert-

son, V., Gottlieb, L. S., Rice, R., Sherlock, P., and Winawer, S. Screening for colorectal cancer in a high-risk population. Results of a mathematical model. Gastroenterology *92*:682, 1987.

179. Maxfield, R. G., and Maxfield, C. M. Colonoscopy as a primary diagnostic procedure in chronic gastrointestinal bleeding. Arch. Surg. *121*:401, 1986.
180. Dodd, G. D. The radiologic diagnosis of carcinoma of the colon in gastrointestinal cancer. *In* Stroehlein, J. R., and Rumsdahl, M. M. (eds.). Gastrointestinal Cancer. New York, Raven Press, 1981, pp. 327–344.
181. Ott, D. J., Chen, Y. M., Gelfand, D. W., Wu, W. C., and Munitz, H. A. Single-contrast vs. double-contrast barium enema in detection of colonic polyps. AJR *146*:993, 1986.
182. DeRoos, A., Hermans, J., Shaw, P. C., and Kroon, H. Colon polyps and carcinomas: prospective comparison of the single- and double-contrast examination in the same patients. Radiology *154*:11, 1985.
183. Jensen, J., Kewenter, J., Haglind, E., Lycke, G., Svensson, C., and Ahren, C. Diagnostic accuracy of double-contrast enema and rectosigmoidoscopy in connection with faecal occult blood testing for detection of rectosigmoid neoplasms. Br. J. Surg. *73*:961, 1986.
184. Crespi, M., Weissman, G. S., Gilbertson, V. A., Winawer, S. J., and Sherlock, P. The role of proctosigmoidoscopy in screening for colorectal neoplasia. CA *34*:159, 1984.
185. Weber, C. A., Deveney, K. E., Pellegrini, C. A., and Way, L. W. Routine colonoscopy in the management of colorectal carcinoma. Am. J. Surg. *152*:87, 1986.
186. American Cancer Society. Survey of physician's attitudes and practices in early cancer detection. CA *35*:197, 1985.
187. Greegor, D. H. Diagnosis of large bowel cancer in the asymptomatic patient. JAMA *201*:943, 1967.
188. Gnauck, R., Macrae, F. A., and Fleisher, M. How to perform the fecal occult blood test. CA *34*:134, 1984.
189. Lifton, L. J., and Kreiger, J. False-positive stool occult blood tests caused by iron preparations. Gastroenterology *83*:860, 1982.
190. Caligiore, P., Macrae, F. A., St. John, J. B., Rayner, J., Legge, J. W. Peroxidase levels in food: relevance to colorectal cancer screening. Am. J. Clin. Nutr. *35*:1487, 1982.
191. Macrae, F. A., St. John, J. B., Caligiore, P., Taylor, L. S., and Legge, J. W. Optimal dietary conditions for Hemoccult testing. Gastroenterology *82*:899, 1982.
192. Macrae, F., and St. John, D. J. B. Relationship between patterns of bleeding and Hemoccult sensitivity in patients with colorectal cancers or adenomas. Gastroenterology *82*:891, 1982.
193. Winawer, S., Andrews, M. N. A., Flehinger, B., Sherlock, P. K., Schohenfeld, D., and Miller, D. G. Progress report on controlled trial of fecal occult blood testing for detection of colorectal neoplasia. Cancer *45*:2959, 1980.
194. Gilbertson, V. A., McHugh, R., Schuman, L., Williams, S. E. The early detection of colorectal cancers. A preliminary report of the results of the occult blood study. Cancer *45*:2899, 1980.
195. Winchester, D. P., Shull, J. H., Scanlon, E. F., Murrell, S. V., Smeltzer, C., Vrba, P., Iden, M., Streelman, D. H., Magpayo, R., Dow, J. W., and Sylvester, J. A mass screening program for colorectal cancer using chemical testing for occult blood in the stool. Cancer *45*:2955, 1980.
196. Elliot, M. S., Levenstein, J. H., and Wright, J. P. Faecal occult blood testing in the detection of colorectal cancer. Br. J. Surg. *71*:785, 1984.
197. Winawer, S. J., Porok, P., Macrae, F., and Bralow, S. P. Surveillance and early diagnosis of colorectal cancer. Cancer Detec. Prev. *8*:3763, 1985.
198. Simon, J. B. Occult blood screening for colorectal carcinoma: a critical review. Gastroenterology *88*:820, 1985.
199. Hardcastle, J. D., Armitage, N. C., Chamberlain, J., James, P. D., and Balfour, T. W. Fecal occult blood screening for colorectal cancer in the general population. Results of a controlled trial. Cancer *58*:397, 1986.
200. Sasito, H., Tsuchida, S., Nakaji, S., Kakizaki, R., Alisawas, T., Munakata, A., and Yoshida, Y. An immunologic test for fecal occult blood by counter immunoelectrophoresis. Cancer *56*:1549, 1985.
201. Ahlquist, D. A., McGill, D. B., Schwartz, S., Taylor, W. F., Ellerson, M., and Owen, R. A. HemoQuant, a new quantitative assay for fecal hemoglobin. Ann. Intern. Med. *101*:297, 1984.
202. Ahlquist, D. A., McGill, D. B., Schwartz, S., Taylor, W. F., and Owen, R. A. Fecal blood levels in health and disease. A study using HemoQuant. N. Engl. J. Med. *312*:1422, 1985.
203. Fleming, J. L., Ahlquist, D. A., McGill, D. B., Zinsmeister, A. R., and Schwartz, S. Influence of aspirin and ethanol on fecal blood levels as determined by using the HemoQuant assay. Mayo Clin. Proc. *62*:159, 1987.
204. Hertz, R. E., Deddish, M. R., and Day, E. Value of periodic examination in detecting cancer of the rectum and colon. Postgrad. Med. *27*:2901, 1960.
205. Dales, L. G., Friedman, D. G., and Ramcharan, S. Multiphasic checkup evaluation study. 3. Outpatient clinic utilization, and mortality experience after seven years. Prev. Med. *2*:221, 1973.
206. Gilbertson, V. A., Nelma, J. M. The prevention of invasive cancer of the rectum. Cancer *41*:1137, 1978.
207. Bohlman, T. W., Katon, R. M., Lipshutz, G. R., McCool, M. F., Smith, F. W., and Melnyk, C. S. Fiberoptic pansigmoidoscopy. An evaluation and comparison with rigid sigmoidoscopy. Gastroenterology *72*:644, 1977.
208. Winnan, G., Beci, G., Panish, J., Talbot, T. M., Overhold, B. F., and McCullum, R. W. Superiority of the flexible to the rigid sigmoidoscope in routine proctosigmoidoscopy. N. Engl. J. Med. *302*:1011, 1980.
209. Dubow, R. A., Kator, R. M., Benner, K. G., Van Dijk, C. M., Koval, G. T., and Smith, F. W. Short (35 cm) versus long (60 cm) flexible sigmoidoscopy: a comparison of findings and tolerance in asymptomatic patients screened for colorectal neoplasia. Gastrointest. Endosc. *31*:305, 1985.
210. Rognum, T. O. A new approach in carcinoembryonic antigen–guided follow-up of large-bowel carcinoma patients. Scand. J. Gastroenterol. *21*:641, 1986.
211. Fletcher, R. H. Carcinoembryonic antigen. Ann. Intern. Med. *104*:66, 1986.
212. Williams, R. R., McIntire, K. R., and Waldmann, T. A. Tumor-associated antigen levels (carcinoembryonic antigen, human chorionic gonadotropin and alpha-fetoprotein) antedating the diagnosis of cancer in the Framingham Study. JNCI *58*:1547, 1977.
213. Deveney, K. E., and Way, L. W. Follow-up of patients with colorectal cancer. Am. J. Surg. *148*:717, 1984.
214. Winawer, S., Ritchie, M. T., Diaz, B. J., Gottlieb, L. S., Stewart, E. T., Zauber, A., Herbert, E., and Band, J. The National Polyp Study: aims and organization. Front. Gastrointest. Res. *10*:216, 1986.
215. Thompson, W. M., and Halvorsen, R. A. Computed tomographic staging of gastrointestinal malignancies. Part II. The small bowel, colon, and rectum. Invest. Radiol. *22*:96, 1987.
216. Rosi, P. A., Cahill, W. J., and Care, J. A ten-year study of hemicolectomy in the treatment of carcinoma of the left half of the colon. Surg. Gynecol. Obstet. *114*:15, 1962.
217. Dwight, R. W., Higgins, G. A., and Keehn, R. J. Factors influencing survival after resection in cancer of the colon and rectum. Am. J. Surg. *117*:512, 1969.
218. Grinnell, R. S. Results of ligation of inferior mesenteric artery at the aorta in resections of carcinoma of the descending and sigmoid colon and rectum. Surg. Gynecol. Obstet. *120*:1031, 1965.
219. Heimann, T. M., Szporn, A., Bolnick, K., and Aufses, A. H., Jr. Local recurrence following surgical treatment of rectal cancer. Comparison of anterior and abdominoperineal resection. Dis. Colon Rectum *29*:862, 1986.
220. Russin, D. J., Kaplan, S. R., and Barkin, J. S. Neodymium-YAG laser. A new palliative tool in the treatment of colorectal cancer. Arch. Surg. *121*:1399, 1986.
221. Brown, S. G., Mattenson, K., Hawes, R., Swain, C. P., Clark, C. G., and Boulas, P. B. Endoscopic treatment of inoperable colorectal cancers with the Nd YAG laser. Br. J. Surg. *73*:949, 1986.
222. Minton, J. P., Hoehn, H., Gerber, D. M., Horsley, J. S., Connolly, D. P., Salwan, F., Fletcher, W. S., Cruz, A. B., Gatchell, F. G., Oviedo, M., Meyer, K. K., Leffall, L. D.,

Berk, R. S., Stewart, P. A., and Kurucz, S. E. Results of a 400-patient carcinoembryonic antigen second-look colorectal cancer study. Cancer *55*:1284, 1985.

223. Hine, K. R., and Dykes, P. W. Serum CEA in postoperative surveillance of colorectal carcinoma. Br. J. Cancer *49*:689, 1984.

224. Rognum, T. O. A new approach in carcinoembryonic antigen–guided follow-up of large bowel carcinoma patients. Scand. J. Gastroenterol. *21*:641, 1986.

225. Daly, J. M., and Kemeny, N. Therapy of colorectal hepatic metastases. *In* De Vita, V. T., Jr., Hellman, S., and Rosenberg, S. A. (eds.). Important Advances in Oncology 1986. Philadelphia, J. B. Lippincott Company, 1986, pp. 251–268.

226. Ridge, J. A., and Daly, J. M. Treatment of colorectal hepatic metatases. Surg. Gynecol. Obstet. *161*:597, 1985.

227. Butler, J., Attiyeh, F. F., and Daly, J. M. Hepatic resection for metastases of the colon and rectum. Surg. Gynecol. Obstet. *102*:109, 1986.

228. Fortner, J. G., Silva, J. J., Golbey, R. B., Cox, E. B., and Maclean, B. J. Multivariate analysis of a personal series of 247 consecutive patients with liver metastases from colorectal cancer. I. Treatment by hepatic resection. Ann. Surg. *199*:306, 1984.

229. Hughes, K., Simon, R., Songhorabodi, S., Adson, M. A., Ilstrup, D. M., Fortner, J. G., Maclean, B. J., Foster, J., Daly, J. M., Fitzherbert, D., Sugarbaker, P., Iwatsuki, S., Starzl, T., Ranning, K. P., Longmire, W. P., Jr., O'Toole, K., Petrelli, N. J., Herrera, L., Cady, B., McDermott, W., Nims, T., Enker, W. E., Coppa, G. F., Blumgart, L. H., Bradpiece, H., Urist, M., Aldiete, J. S., Schlog, P., Hohenberger, P., Steele, G., Jr., Hodgson, W. J., Hardy, T. G., Harbora, D., McPherson, T. A., Lim, C., Dillon, D., Itapp, R., Ripepi, P., Villella, E., Rossi, R. L., Remine, S. G., Oster, M., Connolly, D. P., Abrams, J., Aljurf, A., Hobbs, K. E. F., Li, M. K. W., Howard, T., and Lee, E. Resection of the liver for colorectal carcinoma metastases: a multi-institutional study of patterns of recurrence. Surgery *100*:278, 1986.

230. Ekberg, H., Tranberg, K. -G., Andersson, R., Lundstedt, C., Hagerstrand, I Ranstan, J., and Bengmark, S. Determinants of survival in liver resection for colorectal secondaries. Br. J. Surg. *73*:727, 1986.

231. Higgins, G. A., Jr., Humphrey, E., Juler, G. L., LeVeen, H. H., McCaughan, J., and Keehn, R. J. Adjuvant chemotherapy in the surgical treatment of large bowel cancer. Cancer *38*:1461, 1976.

232. Higgins, G. A., Donaldson, R. C., Humphrey, E. W., Rodges, L. S., and Shields, T. W. Update of Veterans Administration Surgical Oncology Group trials. Surg. Clin. North Am. *61*:1311, 1981.

233. Grage, T. B., and Moss, S. E. Adjuvant chemotherapy in cancer of the colon and rectum. Demonstration of effectiveness of prolonged 5-FU chemotherapy in a prospectively controlled randomized trial. Surg. Clin. North Am. *61*:1321, 1981.

234. Gastrointestinal Tumor Study Group. Prolongation of the disease-free interval in surgically treated rectal carcinoma. N. Engl. J. Med. *312*:1465, 1985.

235. Engstrom, P. F., MacIntyre, J. M., Douglas, H. O., Muggia, F., and Mittelman, A. Combination chemotherapy of advanced colorectal cancer utilizing 5-fluorouracil, semustine, dacarbazine, vincristine, and hydroxyurea. Cancer *49*:1555, 1982.

236. Petrelli, N., Herrera, L., Stulc, J., Burke, P., Rustum, Y., and Mittelman, A. A Phase III study of 5-fluorouracil (5-FU) versus 5-FU + methotrexate (MTX) versus 5-FU + high dose leucovorin (CF) in metastatic colorectal adenocarcinoma. (Abstract.) Proc. Am. Soc. Clin. Oncol. *5*:78, 1986.

237. Stagg, R. J., Lewis, B. J., Friedman, M. A., and Ignoffo, R. J. Hepatic arterial chemotherapy for colorectal cancer metastatic to the liver. Ann. Intern. Med. *100*:736, 1984.

238. Ensminger, W., Niederhuber, J., and Gyves, J. Effective control of liver metastases from colon cancer with an implanted system for hepatic arterial chemotherapy. Proc. Am. Soc. Clin. Oncol. *1*:94, 1982.

239. Balch, C. M., Urist, M. M., and McGregor, M. L. Continuous regional chemotherapy for metastatic colorectal cancer using a totally implantable infusion pump. Am. J. Surg. *145*:285, 1983.

240. Keneny, N., Daly, J. M., Oderman, P., and Shike, M. Hepatic infusion chemotherapy for metastatic colorectal carcinoma, results, and complications. Proc. Am. Soc. Clin. Oncol. *2*:123, 1982.

241. Patt, Y. Z., Boddie, A. W., Jr., Charnsangavej, C., Ajani, A., Wallace, S., Soski, M., Claghorn, L., and Mavligit, G. M. Hepatic arterial infusion with floxuridine and cisplatin: overriding importance of antitumor effect versus degree of tumor burden as determinants of survival among patients with colorectal cancer. J. Clin. Oncol. *4*:1356, 1986.

242. Daly, J. M., Keneny, N., Oderman, P., and Botet, J. Long-term hepatic arterial infusion chemotherapy: anatomic considerations, operative technique, and treatment morbidity. Arch. Surg. *119*:1984, 1984.

243. Anderson, S. D., Holley, H. C., Berland, L. L., Van Dyke, J. A., and Stanley, R. J. Causes of jaundice during hepatic artery infusion chemotherapy. Radiology *161*:439, 1986.

244. Colcher, D., Esteban, J. M., Carrasquillo, J. A., Sugarbaker, P., Reynolds, J. C., Bryant, G., Larson, S. M., and Schlom, J. Quantitative analysis of selected radiolabelled monoclonal antibody localization in metastatic lesions of colorectal cancer patients. Cancer Res. *47*:1185, 1987.

245. Esteban, J. M., Colcher, D., Carrasquillo, J. A., Bryant, G., Thor, A., Reynolds, J. C., Larson, S. M., and Schlom, J. Quantitative and qualitative aspects of radiolocalization in colon cancer patients of intravenously administered MAb B72.3. Int. J. Cancer *39*:50, 1987.

246. Quan, S. H. Q., Deddish, M. R., and Stearns, M. W. The effect of preoperative roentgen therapy upon the 10- and 5-year results of the surgical treatment of cancer of the rectum. Surg. Gynecol. Obstet. *111*:507, 1960.

247. Stearns, M. W., Deddish, M. R., and Quan, S. H. Q. Preoperative irradiation for cancer of the rectum and rectosigmoid. Preliminary review of recent experience (1957–1962). Dis. Colon Rectum *11*:281, 1968.

248. Roswit, B., Higgins, G. A., and Keehn, R. J. Preoperative irradiation for carcinoma of the rectum and rectosigmoid colon. Report of a national Veterans Administration randomized study. Cancer *35*:1597, 1975.

249. Higgins, G. A., Humphrey, E. W., Dwight, R. W., Roswit, B., Lee, L. E., Jr., and Keehn, R. J. Preoperative radiation and surgery for cancer of the rectum. Veterans Administration Surgical Oncology Group Trial II. Cancer *58*:352, 1986.

250. Gunderson, L. L. Radiation therapy of colorectal carcinoma. *In* Thatcher, N. (ed.). Digestive Cancer 9. XII International Cancer Congress Proceedings. New York, Pergamon Press, 1979, pp. 29–38.

251. Romsdahl, M., and Withers, H. R. Radiotherapy combined with curative surgery. Arch. Surg. *113*:446, 1978.

252. Allee, P. E., Gunderson, L. L., Munzenrider, J. E. Postoperative radiation therapy for residual colorectal carcinoma. ASTR Proceedings. Int. J. Radiat. Oncol. Biol. Phys. *7*:1208, 1981.

253. Balslev, I. B., Pedersen, M., Teglbjaerg, P. S., Hanberg-Soerensen, F., Bone, J., Jacobsen, N. O., Overgaard, J., Sell, A., Bertelsen, K., Hage, E., Fenger, L., Kronborg, O., Hansen, L., Hoestrup, H., and Noergaard-Pedersen, B. Postoperative radiotherapy in Dukes B and C carcinoma of the rectum and rectosigmoid. A randomized multicenter study. Cancer *58*:22, 1986.

254. Gunderson, L. L., Dosoretz, D. E., Hedberg, S. E., Blitzer, P. H., Rodkey, G., Hoskins, B., Shipley, W. U., and Cohen, A. C. Low-dose preoperative irradiation, surgery, and elective postoperative radiation therapy for resectable rectum and rectosigmoid carcinoma. Cancer *52*:446, 1983.

255. Mohiuddin, M., Marks, G. L., Kramer, S., and Pajak, T. Adjuvant radiation therapy for rectal cancer. Int. J. Radiat. Oncol. Biol. Phys. *10*:997, 1984.

256. Mella, O., Dahl, O., Horn, A., Morild, I., and Odland, G. Radiotherapy and resection for apparently inoperable rectal adenocarcinoma. Dis. Colon Rectum *27*:663, 1984.

257. Richards, M. A. Lymphoma of the colon and rectum. Postgrad. Med. J. *62*:615, 1986.
258. Jinnai, D., Iwasa, Z., and Wastanuki, T. Malignant lymphoma of the large intestine: operative results in Japan. Jpn. J. Surg. *13*:331, 1983.
259. Perry, P. M., Cross, R. S. M., and Morson, B. L. Primary malignant lymphoma of the rectum (22 cases). Proc. R. Soc. Med. *65*:72, 1972.
260. Devine, R. M., Beart, R. W., and Wolff, B. G. Malignant lymphoma of the rectum. Dis. Colon Rectum *29*:821, 1986.
261. Dragosics, B., Bauer, P., and Radaasziewicz, T. Primary gastrointestinal non-Hodgkins' lymphomas. Cancer *55*:1060, 1985.
262. Loehr, W., Mujahed, Z., Zah, F. D., Gray, G., and Thorbjarnarson, B. Primary lymphoma of the gastrointestinal tract: a review of 100 cases. Ann. Surg. *170*:232, 1969.
263. Weingrad, D. N., DeCosse, J. J., Sherlock, P., Straus, D., Lieberman, P. H., and Filippa, D. A. Primary gastrointestinal lymphoma: a 30-year review. Cancer *49*:1258, 1982.
264. Wagonfeld, J. B., Platz, C. E., Fishman, F. L., Sibley, R. K., and Kirsner, J. B. Multicentric colonic lymphomas complicating ulcerative colitis. Am. J. Dig. Dis. *22*:502, 1977.
265. Bartolo, D., Goepel, J. R., and Parsons, M. A. Rectal malignant lymphoma in chronic ulcerative colitis. Gut *23*:164, 1982.
266. Marshak, R. H., Lindner, A. E., and Maklansky, D. Lymphoreticular disorders of the gastrointestinal tract: roentgenographic features. Gastrointest. Radiol. *4*:103, 1979.
267. Ghanem, A. N., and Perry, K. C. Malignant lymphoma as a complication of ureterosigmoidostomy. Br. J. Surg. *72*:559, 1985.
268. Sibly, T. F., Keane, R. M., Lever, T. V., and Southwood, W. F. Rectal lymphoma in radiation injured bowel. Br. J. Surg. *72*:879, 1985.
269. Burkes, R. L., Meyer, P. R., Parkash, S., Parker, J. W., Rasheed, S., and Levine, A. M. Rectal lymphoma in homosexual men. Arch. Intern. Med. *146*:913, 1986.
270. Lee, M. H., Waxman, M., and Gillooley, J. F. Primary malignant lymphoma of the anorectum in homosexual men. Dis. Colon Rectum *29*:413, 1986.
271. Wychulis, A. R., Beahrs, O. H., and Woolner, L. B. Malignant lymphoma of the colon. Arch. Surg. *93*:215, 1966.
272. O'Connell, D. J., and Thompson, A. J. Lymphoma of the colon: the spectrum of radiologic changes. Gastrointest. Radiol. *2*:377, 1978.
273. Williams, E. D., and Sandler, M. The classification of carcinoid tumors. Lancet *1*:238, 1963.
274. Peck, J. J., Shields, A. B., Boyden, A. M., Dworkin, L. A., and Nadal, J. W. Carcinoid tumors of the ileum. Am. J. Surg. *146*:124, 1983.
275. Johnson, L. A., Lavin, P., Moertel, C. G., Weiland, L., Dayal, Y., Doos, W. G., Geller, S. A., Cooper, H. S., Nime, F., Masse, S., Simson, I. W., Sumner, H., Folsch, E., and Engstrom, P. Carcinoids: the association of histologic growth pattern and survival. Cancer *51*:882, 1983.
276. Moertel, C. G., Dockerty, M. B., and Judd, E. S. Carcinoid tumors of the vermiform appendix. Cancer *21*:270, 1968.
277. Morgan, J. G., Marks, C., and Hearn, D. Carcinoid tumors of the gastrointestinal tract. Ann. Surg. *180*:720, 1974.
278. Goodwin, J. D. Carcinoid tumors. An analysis of 2837 cases. Cancer *36*:560, 1975.
279. Syracuse, D. C., Perzin, K. H., Price, J. B., Wiedel, P. D., and Mesa-Tejada, R. Carcinoid tumors of the appendix. Ann. Surg. *190*:58, 1979.
280. Thirlby, R. C., Kasper, C. S., and Jones, R. C. Metastatic carcinoid of the appendix. Dis. Colon Rectum *27*:42, 1984.
281. Kirkegaard, P., Hjortrup, A., Halse, C., Luke, M., and Christiansen, J. Long-term results of surgery for carcinoid tumors of the gastrointestinal tract. Acta Chir. Scand. *147*:693, 1981.
282. McFadden, D., and Jaffe, B. M. Surgical approaches to endocrine-producing tumors of the gastrointestinal tract. *In* Cohen, S., and Soloway, R. D. (eds.). Hormone-Producing Tumors of the Gastrointestinal Tract. New York, Churchill Livingstone, 1985, pp. 139–157.
283. Edmonds, P., Merino, M. J., Li Volsi, V. A., and Duray, P. H. Adenocarcinoid (mucinous carcinoid) of the appendix. Gastroenterology *86*:302, 1984.
284. Caldarola, V. T., Jackman, R. J., Moertel, C. G., Dockerty, M. B. Carcinoid tumors of the rectum. Am. J. Surg. *107*:844, 1964.
285. Orloff, M. J. Carcinoid tumors of the rectum. Cancer *28*:175, 1971.
286. Naunheim, K. S., Zeitels, J., Kaplan, E. L., Sugimoto, J., Shen, K.-L., Lee, C.-H., Strauss, F. H. Rectal carcinoid tumors—treatment and prognosis. Surgery *94*:670, 1983.
287. Berardi, R. S. Carcinoid tumors of the colon (exclusive of rectum). Dis. Colon Rectum *15*:P383, 1972.
288. Martin, J. K., Moertel, C. G., Adson, M. A., and Schutl, A. J. Surgical treatment of functioning metastatic carcinoid tumors. Arch. Surg. *1128*:537, 1983.
289. Haller, D. G. Chemotherapeutic management of endocrine-producing tumors of the gastrointestinal tract. *In* Cohen, S., and Soloway, R. D. (eds.). Hormone-Producing Tumors of the Gastrointestinal Tract. New York, Churchill Livingstone, 1985, pp. 129–137.
290. Moertel, C. G., and Hanley, J. A. Combination chemotherapy trials for metastatic carcinoid tumor and the malignant carcinoid syndrome. Can. Clin. Trials *2*:327, 1979.
291. Keane, T. J., Rider, W. D., Harwood, A. R., Thomas, G. M., and Cummings, B. J. Whole abdominal radiation in the management of metastatic gastrointestinal carcinoid tumor. Int. J. Radiat. Oncol. Biol. Phys. *7*:1519, 1981.
292. Stathopoulas, G. P., Karvountzis, G. G., and Yiotis, J. Tamoxifen in carcinoid syndrome. N. Engl. J. Med. *305*:52, 1981.
293. Ebert, P. A., and Zuidema, G. D. Primary tumors of the small intestine. Arch. Surg. *91*:452, 1965.
294. Wilson, J. M., Melvin, D. B., Gray, G. F., and Thorbjarnarson, B. Primary malignancies of the small bowel: a report of 96 cases and a review of the literature. Ann. Surg. *180*:175, 1974.
295. Silberman, H., Crichlow, R. W., and Caplan, H. S. Neoplasms of the small bowel. Ann. Surg. *180*:157, 1974.
296. Rich, J. D. Malignant tumors of the intestine: review of 37 cases. Am. Surg. *43*:445, 1977.
297. Freund, H., Lavi, A., Pfeffermann, R., and Durst, A. L. Primary neoplasms of the small bowel. Am. J. Surg. *135*:757, 1978.
298. Sagar, G. F. Primary malignant tumors of the small intestine. A 22-year experience with 30 patients. Am. J. Surg. *135*:601, 1979.
299. Barclay, T. H. C., and Schapira, D. V. Malignant tumors of the small intestine. Cancer *51*:878, 1983.
300. Martin, R. G. Malignant tumors of the small intestine. Surg. Clin. North Am. *66*:779, 1986.
301. Williamson, R. C., Welch, C. E., and Malt, R. A. Adenocarcinoma and lymphoma of the small intestine: distribution and etiologic associations. Ann. Surg. *197*:172, 1983.
302. Lowenfeld, A. B. Why are small bowel tumours so rare? Lancet *1*:24, 1973.
303. Lightdale, C. J., Koepfell, T. C., and Sherlock, P. Small intestinal cancer. *In* Schottenfeld, D., and Fraumeni, J. (eds.). Cancer Epidemiology and Prevention. Philadelphia, W. B. Saunders Co., 1982, pp. 692–702.
304. Wattenberg, L. W. Studies of polycyclic hydrocarbon hydroxylases of the intestine possibly related to cancer: effect of diet on benzpyrene hydroxylase activity. Cancer *28*:99, 1971.
305. Jones, T. R., and Nance, F. C. Periampullary malignancy in Gardner's syndrome. Ann. Surg. *185*:565, 1977.
306. Burt, R. W., Berensen, M. M., Lee, R. G., Tolman, K. G., Freston, J. W., and Gardner, E. J. Upper gastrointestinal polyps in Gardner's syndrome. Gastroenterology *86*:295, 1984.
307. Guyton, D., and Schreiber, H. Intestinal polyposis and periampullary carcinoma—changing concepts. J. Surg. Oncol. *29*:158, 1985.
308. Hamilton, S. R., Bussey, H. J. R., Mendelsohn, G., Diamond, M. P., Pavlides, G., Hutcheon, D., Harbison, M., Shermeta, D., Morson, B. C., and Yardley, J. H. Ileal adenomas after colectomy in nine patients with adenomatous polyposis coli/Gardner's syndrome. Gastroenterology *77*:1252, 1979.

309. Reid, J. D. Intestinal carcinoma in the Peutz-Jeghers syndrome. JAMA *229*:833, 1974.
310. Lightdale, C. J., Sternberg, S. S., Posner, G., and Sherlock, P. Carcinoma complicating Crohn's disease: report of seven cases and review of the literature. Am. J. Med. *590*:262, 1975.
311. Collier, P. E., Turowski, P., and Diamond, D. Small intestinal adenocarcinoma complicating regional enteritis. Cancer *55*:516, 1985.
312. Maglinte, D. D. T., Elmore, M. F., Chernish, S. M., Miller, R. E., Lehman, G., Bishop, R., Blitz, G., Kohne, J., Isenberg, M. T. Enteroclysis in the diagnosis of unexplained gastrointestinal bleeding. Dis. Colon Rectum *28*:403, 1985.
313. Jones, B. A., Langer, B., Taylor, B. R., and Girotti, M. Periampullary tumors: which ones should be resected? Am. J. Surg. *149*:46, 1985.
314. Tarazi, R. Y., Hermann, R. E., Vogt, D. P., Hoerr, S. O., Esselstyn, C. B., Cooperman, A. M., Steiger, E., and Grunfest, S. Results of surgical treatment of periampullary tumors: a thirty-five year experience. Surgery *100*:716, 1986.
315. Abe, M., Takahashi, M., and Yabumoto, E. Clinical experiences with intraoperative radiotherapy of locally advanced cancers. Cancer *45*:40, 1980.
316. Moertel, C. G., Sauer, W. G., Dockerty, M. B., and Baggenstoss, A. H. Life history of the carcinoid tumor of the small intestine. Cancer *14*:901, 1961.
317. Lasson, A., Alwmark, A., Nobin, A., and Sundler, F. Endocrine tumors of the duodenum. Clinical characteristics and hormone content. Ann. Surg. *177*:393, 1983.
318. Strodel, W., Talpos, G., Eckhauser, F., and Thompson, N. Surgical therapy for small bowel carcinoid tumors. Arch. Surg. *118*:391, 1983.
319. Herbsman, H., Wetstein, L., Rosen, Y., Orces, H., Alfonso, A. E., Iyer, S. K., and Gardner, B. Tumors of the small intestine. Curr. Probl. Surg. *17*:3, 1980.
320. Starr, G. F., and Dockerty, M. B. Leiomyomas and leiomyosarcomas of the small intestine. Cancer *8*:101, 1955.
321. Gottlieb, J. A. Combination chemotherapy for metastatic sarcoma. Cancer Chemother. Rep. *58*:265, 1974.
322. Al-Mondhiry, H. Primary lymphomas of the intestine: East-West contrast. Am. J. Hematol. *22*:89, 1986.
323. Al-Bahrani, Z. R., Al-Mondhiry, H., Bakir, H., and Al-Saleem, T. Clinical and pathologic subtypes of primary intestinal lymphoma. Experience with 132 patients over a 14-year period. Cancer *52*:1666, 1983.
324. Salem, P. A., Nassar, V. H., Shahid, M. J., Hajj, A. A., Alami, S. Y., Balikian, J. B., and Salem, A. A. "Mediterranean abdominal lymphoma" or immunoproliferative small intestinal disease. I. Clinical aspects. Cancer *40*:2941, 1977.
325. Khojasteh, A., Haghshenass, M., and Haghighi, P. Immunoproliferative small intestinal disease. A "Third-World lesion." N. Engl. J. Med. *308*:1401, 1983.
326. Al-Bahrani, Z., Al-Saleem, T., Al-Mondhiry, H., Bakir, F., Yahia, H., Taha, I., and King, J. Alpha-heavy chain disease (report of 18 cases from Iraq). Gut *19*:627, 1978.
327. Rambaud, J. C. Small intestinal lymphomas and alpha-chain disease. Clin. Gastroenterol. *12*:743, 1983.
328. Harris, O. D., Cooke, W. T., Thompson, H., and Waterhouse, J. A. H. Malignancy in adult celiac disease. Am. J. Med. *42*:899, 1967.
329. Holmes, G. K. T., Stokes, P. L., Sorahan, T. M., Prior, P., Waterhouse, S. A. H., and Cooke, W. T. Coeliac disease, gluten-free diet and malignancy. Gut *17*:612, 1976.
330. Selby, W., and Gallagher, N. D. Malignancy in a 19-year experience of adult coeliac disease. Dig. Dis. Sci. *24*:684, 1979.
331. Isaacson, P. G., O'Connor, N. T. J., Spencer, J. O., Bevan, D. H., Connolly, C. E., Kirkham, N., Pollock, D. J., Wainscoat, J. S., Stein, H., and Mason, D. Y. Malignant histiocytes of the intestine: a T-cell lymphoma. Lancet *2*:688, 1985.
332. Swinson, C. M., Slavin, G., Coles, E. C., and Booth, C. C. Coeliac disease and malignancy. Lancet *1*:111, 1983.
333. Collier, P. E. Small bowel lymphoma associated with AIDS. J. Surg. Oncol. *32*:131, 1986.
334. Elias, L., Portlock, C. S., and Rosenberg, S. A. Combination chemotherapy of diffuse histiocytic lymphoma with cyclophosphamide, Adriamycin, vincristine, and prednisone (CHOP). Cancer *42*:1705, 1978.
335. Klimo, P., and Connors, J. M. MACOP-B chemotherapy for the treatment of large cell lymphoma. Ann. Intern. Med. *102*:596, 1985.
336. Magarth, I. T., Janus, C., Edwards, B. K., Spiegel, R., Jaffe, E. S., Berard, C. W., Milianskas, J., Morris, K., and Barnwell, R. An effective therapy for both undifferentiated (including Burkitt's) lymphomas and lymphoblastic lymphomas in children and young adults. Blood *63*:1102, 1984.

82

The Carcinoid Syndrome

O. DHODANAND KOWLESSAR

The carcinoid syndrome is rare. Its unique and often bizarre clinical, biochemical, and pharmacologic features have brought together the skills of basic scientists and physicians to produce advances of basic biologic significance. The biochemistry and pharmacologic action of substances synthesized, secreted, and released by carcinoid tumors and their metastases have been translated into therapeutic benefits for the patients whose illnesses have been responsible for such intensive investigation.

Most carcinoid tumors arise from the enterochromaffin (EC) or enterochromaffin-like (ECL) cells, with characteristic clinical, histochemical, and biochemical features that are dependent upon their sites of origin.

The enterochromaffin cell belongs to a larger family that shares the features of *a*mine content, *p*recursor *u*ptake, and *d*ecarboxylation; hence, the mnemonic name APUD.[1] Over 90 per cent of carcinoid tumors originate in the gastrointestinal tract; they constitute 1.5 per cent of gastrointestinal neoplasms. The most frequent enteral sites are the appendix, terminal ileum, and rectum. The colon, stomach, duodenum, and Meckel's diverticulum are less frequently involved. Although rare, carcinoid tumors have been reported to develop in the biliary tract and pancreatic duct, as gonadal teratomas, and, most recently, in the esophagus and thymus. Bronchial carcinoids, originating from the enterochromaffin cells in the epithelium of the bronchial tree, are reported with increasing frequency.

Carcinoid tumors secrete a variety of potential humoral agents in relation to their site of origin. The similarity of the clinical and biochemical features of many of the lesions producing the carcinoid syndrome suggests that these tumors may be derived from stem cells of similar embryologic anlagen with pluripotential endocrine function. Furthermore, the tendency of these tumors to produce ectopic hormones may depend on the state of derepression of their cellular genetic material.

The complex of symptoms and signs that compose the carcinoid spectrum includes diarrhea, abdominal cramps, borborygmi, episodic flushing, telangiectasia, cyanosis, pellagra-like skin lesions, bronchospasm with wheezing and asthma-like attacks, dyspnea, and murmurs of valvular lesions of the heart. These signs and symptoms, in turn, result in part from increased production of a variety of substances with pharmacologic and physiologic actions represented principally by 5-hydroxytryptamine (serotonin), 5-hydroxytryptophan (5-HTP), kinin peptides, histamine, catecholamines, and prostaglandins. Insulin, adrenocorticotropic hormone (ACTH), melanophore-stimulating hormone (MSH), glucagon, gastrin, parathormone, vasoactive intestinal peptide (VIP), gastric-inhibiting polypeptide (GIP), ACTH-releasing factor (CRF), calcitonin, vasopressin (ADH), substance P, neuropeptide K, neurokinin A (substance K), motilin, methionine enkephalin, and beta-endorphin have also been secreted excessively in this syndrome (see below).

Table 82–1. PRINCIPAL MANIFESTATIONS OF THE CARCINOID SYNDROME

1. Vasomotor disturbances—cutaneous flushes, "cyanosis," telangiectasias
2. Hepatomegaly—large nodular liver
3. Intestinal hypermotility—borborygmi, cramps, diarrhea, vomiting, nausea
4. Bronchoconstriction—cough, dyspnea, wheezing
5. Cardiac involvement—endocardial fibrosis with valvular deformity
6. Absence of hypertension—incidence no greater than in general population
7. Prolonged clinical course—patients survive years longer than those with other tumors with metastases
8. Edema and ascites
9. Arthralgias and localized edema
10. Hyperpigmentation
11. Pellagra

CLINICAL PICTURE OF THE CARCINOID SYNDROME

Symptoms

A summary of the principal manifestations is given in Table 82–1. The earliest clinical manifestations of the classic carcinoid syndrome are episodic. Patients may complain of palpitations, swelling of the face, recurrent attacks of mild to explosive diarrhea, abdominal pain, and tenesmus. The abdominal pain may arise from intestinal obstruction, hepatic metastases, intestinal necrosis, increased intestinal motility, or peptic ulcer.[2] Later in the course, patients will experience episodes of tenseness, weakness, and nausea. Eventually, the *classic vasomotor episodes* appear, comprising repeated episodes of cyanotic, tricolored, or bright red flushes over the face, upper extremities, and chest. Almost one third of the patients do not suffer flushing episodes or the episodes are so insignificant that they are overlooked. They can be brought on or aggravated by anger, tension, active exercise, and the ingestion of alcohol and certain foods such as cheese and salty bacon. The administration of pentagastrin and beta-adrenoreceptor agonists (epinephrine) can induce episodes of vasodilatation[3] (thus, the caveat that these drugs should be avoided or used cautiously in these patients). The flushes may be repetitive during the day, lasting for minutes, and are usually associated with perspiration, a feeling of warmth, palpitation, and tremulousness. On occasion, they are associated with conjunctival injection or increased lacrimation and salivation (bronchial carcinoid). With severe flushing, the patient may experience striking hypotension, increased respiratory rate, wheezing, borborygmi, and diarrhea. During episodes of prolonged flushing, periorbital and facial edema may appear and the patient may become oliguric. Rarely, intense generalized pruritus and pressure-induced orange blotching of the skin occurs. In far advanced disease, these manifestations may become chronic in addition to being episodic.

Physical Examination

In this situation the patient is usually cachectic from severe weight loss. Funduscopic examination of the eye may reveal pigment clumping in the region of the macula, exudative punched-out lesions, pigment deposits, and colloid degeneration.[4] The skin of the face, trunk, and arms may show bluish-red discoloration, with associated telangiectasia. Pellagra and scleroderma-like changes have also been described. The characteristic auscultatory finding of the heart is a precordial murmur of valvular pulmonic stenosis. Congestive changes of right-sided heart failure appear: pleural effusion, hepatic congestion, ascites, and edema of the legs. The distention of the superficial jugular veins associated with a pulsatile liver suggests tricuspid regurgitation. If there is evidence of mitral or aortic valvular disease, one should suspect an atrial septal defect with right-to-left shunt, a bronchial carcinoid, or acquired or congenital valvular defects unrelated to the carcinoid tumor.[5] Evidence of high cardiac output at rest has been reported in patients with flushing and has been attributed to the release of a vasodilator substance (possibly bradykinin) by the tumor or to excessive flow in the metastatic tumors.

Abdominal examination may reveal the signs of ascites, striking hyperactive bowel sounds, and an enlarged, firm, and nodular liver. Occasionally, an epigastric or right lower quadrant mass may be felt. Systolic bruits may be heard in the left upper quadrant secondary to involvement of the splenic artery by carcinoid tumors of the pancreas. Occasionally, a friction rub may be heard over the liver secondary to necrosis of metastatic lesions in the liver. The joints of the fingers may show changes of arthritis. Early in the disease, one may note brawny edema and resultant disabling stiffness of the legs. Peripheral edema secondary to heart failure and hypoproteinemia is a late manifestation. Plastic induration of the penis (Peyronie's disease) has been described in two patients with carcinoid syndrome.[6] Tumor-associated myasthenia may accompany the syndrome.

The physical findings associated with acromegaly, Cushing's syndrome, and pluriglandular adenomatosis have been described in association with the carcinoid spectrum on rare occasions. The signs, symptoms, and physical findings of the malabsorption syndrome are present in some patients with the carcinoid syndrome[7] (see pp. 263–282).

PATHOPHYSIOLOGIC FEATURES OF CARCINOID TUMORS

Role of Neuroendocrine Cells

Endocrine-type cells are present in the gastrointestinal tract, adenohypophysis, thymus, thyroid, lung, and urogenital tract. Pearse demonstrated that these widely distributed cells are capable of amine precursor uptake and decarboxylation (APUD).[1]

Although the endocrine cells in the gut were initially recognized because of their amine storage capacity, current evidence suggests that the predominant secretory products of normal and neoplastic enteric cells are peptides. The embryologic, cytochemical, and functional capabilities of the neuroendocrine cells of the foregut are interrelated; when these cells become hyperplastic or neoplastic, they can produce bizarre clinical pictures. Diagnosis of the underlying tissue pathology is now made more readily by analysis of peptide amines or measurement of neuron-specific enolase[8] or of common antigens (including chromogranin)[9] by monoclonal antibodies, than by conventional histologic methods.

Secretory Products

Serotonin

Although carcinoid tumors differ widely in their ability to produce or store 5-hydroxytryptamine (5-HT), the excessive production of this substance and its metabolite, 5-hydroxyindoleacetic acid (5-HIAA), remains their most characteristic chemical abnormality. Normally, 99 per cent of dietary tryptophan is available for the formation of niacin and protein. In patients with a large mass of carcinoid tumor, more than half the tryptophan intake is hydroxylated by tryptophan hydroxylase to 5-HT which has a high affinity for aromatic L-amino acid decarboxylase, converting 5-HTP to 5-HT (Fig. 82–1). Serotonin is the most active pharmacologic indole produced by the tumor. It may be metabolized by monoamine oxidase in the tumor (in which case it will have little pharmacologic effect) or in the blood, after release from the tumor, to 5-HIAA, which is excreted in the urine as the free acid primarily, although small amounts may be conjugated to the o-sulfate ester before excretion. Characteristically, patients with the carcinoid syndrome have expansion of the serotonin pool size,[10] a striking increase in blood and platelet concentration of serotonin, and elevations of 5-HIAA in the urine.

The physiologic effects of serotonin are diverse. It may mediate the diarrhea and possibly the malabsorption, intestinal hypermotility, abdominal cramps, nausea, and vomiting observed in patients with the carcinoid syndrome.[10] Both the tone and the motility of the human jejunum are increased with infusions of serotonin.[11] It has been suggested that the stimulation of peristalsis by serotonin results from a reduction of the threshold of intraluminal pressure required to elicit the peristaltic reflex, with a resultant increase in both the frequency of contraction and the volume of fluid transported.[12] Serotonin or bradykinin or both may be responsible for the extensive fibrosis frequently observed within the heart and on the peritoneal surface in the carcinoid syndrome. Serotonin produces marked stimulation of cellular growth and fiber production when introduced into fibroblast tissue culture. The

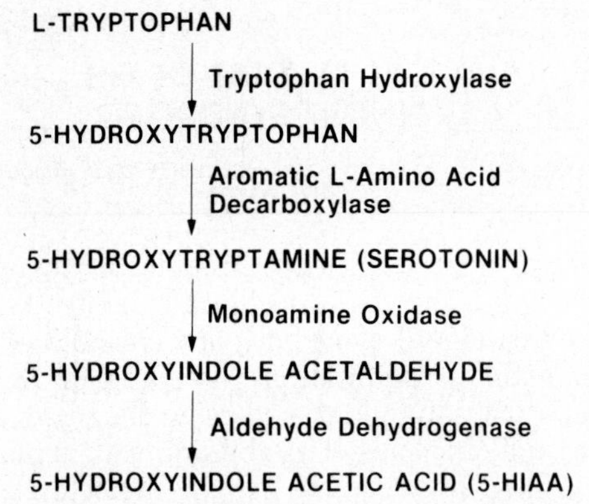

Figure 82–1. Tryptophan metabolic pathway in the carcinoid spectrum.

serotonin antagonist, methysergide, occasionally causes extensive retroperitoneal fibrosis with ureteral obstruction, and its long-term administration has been associated with endocardial and valvular lesions indistinguishable from those of patients with carcinoid syndrome.[13] Serotonin can produce bronchoconstriction in the isolated lung, but correlation of the release of serotonin with bronchoconstriction and wheezing is lacking at present. The edema seen in some patients may represent a direct effect of serotonin promoting sodium retention via the renal tubule, or possibly to secondary aldosteronism. Serotonin reduces renal blood flow in the carcinoid syndrome, and this diminution may stimulate the release of aldosterone from the adrenal cortex.

Histamine, Catecholamines, Kinins, Prostaglandins

Other amines have been found in the urine of carcinoid patients. Some patients with gastric carcinoid have frequent and consistent elevations of histamine, which is inconsistently elevated in those with ileal tumors. Increased 5-HTP excretion is often seen in patients with gastric and bronchial carcinoids, who lack the enzyme aromatic L-amino acid decarboxylase and therefore are unable to decarboxylate 5-HTP effectively. Although catecholamines and their metabolities have been elevated in the urine of some patients with the carcinoid syndrome, this abnormality is unusual and to date has not been correlated with specific symptoms or origins of the tumors.

Formerly *serotonin* (5-HT) was thought to be primarily responsible for the carcinoid flush. There is now considerable evidence that serotonin is not the sole mediator. Intravenous injection of 5-HT does not reproduce the characteristic spontaneous attacks of flushing in carcinoid patients, nor is there a correlation between the levels of free plasma 5-HT and flushing episodes. Although the infusion of epinephrine or norepinephrine provokes typical flushing attacks, it is not often accompanied by increased levels of 5-HT in blood obtained from either the brachial artery or the hepatic vein. Metastatic carcinoid tumors do not always cause the syndrome even in the presence of elevations of urinary 5-HIAA. It is currently held that the flush in any given patient with the carcinoid syndrome is caused by a variety of biologically active substances, among which are lysyl-bradykinin, bradykinin, prostaglandins, and calcitonin. Thus, the combination of flush-promoting substances can vary from patient to patient according to a design that reflects the number and variety of cells of origin.

Lysyl-bradykinin and *bradykinin* are produced by the enzymatic action of kallikrein on an alpha-2-globulin substrate kininogen. When synthetic bradykinin is infused rapidly into patients with the carcinoid syndrome, the flush produced is similar to the spontaneous flushes. Higher levels of bradykinin are present in the hepatic venous blood of some patients during spontaneous and epinephrine-induced flushes. The enzyme kallikrein has been extracted from the carcinoid tumors of patients with flushing and has been localized in a carcinoid tumor by immunofluorescent techniques.

Epinephrine, sympathetic discharge, and ethanol ingestion, which are flush-provoking stimuli, are capable of liberating kallikrein from the tumor. Once liberated, kallikrein splits lysyl-bradykinin from kininogen. The lysyl-bradykinin is rapidly converted to bradykinin by a plasma aminopeptidase, after which it is rapidly broken down to inactive smaller peptides and amino acids.[14] Besides the ability of lysyl-bradykinin and bradykinin to induce flushing, these polypeptides are capable of producing profound vasodilatation, tachycardia, systemic hypotension, and edema as well as increased salivation, lacrimation, and cardiac output. They may also promote fibrosis and play a contributory role in the asthma-like attacks from which patients with the carcinoid syndrome may suffer.

A group of vasodilator peptides of the *tachykinin family* have recently been identified in ileal carcinoid tumors and are released during flushing attacks.[15] The family of tachykinins include substance P, neuropeptide K (NPK), neurokinin A (NKA), neurokinin B (NKB), and eledoisin-like peptides. NPK is found in highest concentration in the plasma and tumor tissue and is capable of inducing long-lasting bronchoconstriction and vasodilatation.

Prostaglandins, which are structural derivatives of prostanoic acid, are widely distributed in human tissues. They exert multiple pharmacologic actions on many organ systems, including the gastrointestinal system. Prostaglandin $F_2\alpha$ ($PGF_2\alpha$) was found in a bronchial carcinoid, and an unidentified hydroxy fatty acid, most likely a prostaglandin, was also found in two ileal carcinoids,[16] thus raising the possibility that prostaglandins may be related to the diarrhea, flushing, and other symptoms associated with the carcinoid syndrome. Modestly increased levels of $PGF_2\alpha$ have been found in two patients with the carcinoid syndrome.[17] However, levels are not increased in most patients, and the magnitude of the elevation in those with high values did not correlate with the symptoms of the carcinoid syndrome. Other prostaglandins may play a role in the carcinoid syndrome, especially since elevated levels of PGE have been found in two patients with the carcinoid syndrome.[18] A patient with carcinoid syndrome improved clinically on Ketanserin, a 5-hydroxytryptamine receptor antagonist, with a fall in the elevated jejunal luminal levels of PGE_2.[19] Thus, diarrhea could be related to a primary mediator stimulating local prostaglandin synthesis.[20]

DIAGNOSIS

The diagnosis of carcinoid tumors is ultimately made by study of tissue obtained by liver biopsy or at exploratory laparotomy. It is strongly suggested by findings of X-ray studies or ultrasonography, computed tomography (CT), or even endoscopy (in the case of esophageal, gastric, duodenal, or rectal tumors). These techniques are carried out because of specific symptoms such as cramping pain of obstruction, cough, or rectal bleeding, or by the patient's having developed the classic clinical carcinoid syndrome. A high index of suspicion in patients with unexplained intermittent diarrhea, telangiectasia over the face, episodic flushing, wheezing, or psychosis will suggest the diagnosis of metastatic carcinoid. Isolated hepatomegaly or unilateral wheezing may give a clue to the underlying pathologic process.

Routine clinical laboratory tests are rarely helpful. Liver function tests may reveal only a modest elevation of the alkaline phosphatase and gamma glutamyl transpeptidase with normal serum bilirubin. As the disease progresses, hypoproteinemia and hypoalbuminemia will develop. Occult malabosrption of fat, although rare, can be revealed by a 72-hour quantitative measurement of stool fat. Roentgenographic examination of the chest may demonstrate a carcinoid lesion or metastases to the lung. Pleural biopsy may reveal the characteristic histologic features of the carcinoid tumor. Upper gastrointestinal series can reveal polypoid lesions of the esophagus, stomach, duodenum, and jejunum. Endoscopy plays a valuable role in the diagnosis of primary esophageal, gastric, duodenal, and rectal carcinoids. Biopsy under direct vision will establish the diagnosis. It should be recognized that 40 per cent of patients with carcinoid tumors have a history of synchronous or metachronous neoplasms, and these lesions should be sought. Multiple lesions in the ileum should arouse suspicion of carcinoid. Narrowing of the intestinal lumen secondary to tumor mass and adjacent fibrous tissue reaction, with associated kinking and buckling of the small intestine and mesentery in the region of the tumor, have been described (Fig. 82–2). The polypoid tumor may also act as the leading point of an intussusception.

Computed tomography portrays the gastrointestinal tract, mesentery, lymph nodes, and the liver in a single non-invasive examination. The diagnosis of an ileal carcinoid is suggested by the presence of a well-defined, low-density right lower quadrant mass with either a stellate or a concentrated pattern of mesenteric neurovascular bundles[21] (Fig. 82–3). Additionally, the presence of a soft tissue, solid mass with surrounding fat density strongly suggests carcinoid.[22] Retroperitoneal masses and lymph nodes, liver metastasis, ascites, fibrosis, and thickening can also be revealed by CT scan. A liver biopsy, with the sample taken under ultrasonic guidance, will reveal tumor with the histologic characteristics of carcinoid. If CT scan can identify the lesions and the urinary 5-HIAA is elevated, selective celiac and superior mesenteric arteriography may not be necessary. If performed it may reveal any of the following findings in ileal carcinoids: a stellate pattern, narrowing of the deep mesenteric branches, poor to moderate accumulation of contrast medium, and nonvisualization of veins. The metastases to the liver are highly vascular with accumulated contrast material.[23] When the hepatic arteriogram is negative in the presence of significant evidence for the carcinoid syndrome, the injection of epinephrine markedly enhances the tumor staining of the primary lesions and their hepatic metastases.[24] The angiographic findings in a nonmetastatic gastric carcinoid reveal intense accumulation of contrast material in the tumor, with identification of several larger veins draining the area of the tumor. The arteries are regular, of normal caliber, and without any stellate pattern.[25]

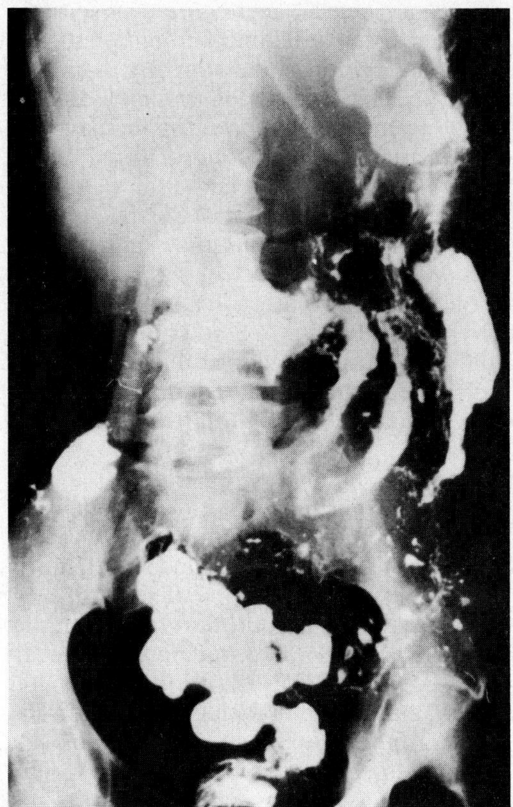

Figure 82–2. Four-hour roentgenogram of a small bowel series in a patient with a malignant ileal carcinoid, showing rigid loops of ileum and mucosal irregularities. (From Kowlessar, O. D., et al. Am. J. Med. *27*:673, 1959.)

Special Studies

The biochemical hallmark of the majority of patients with the carcinoid syndrome is the increased excretion of 5-HIAA. A positive qualitative test suggests a urinary excretion greater than 30 mg per 24-hour period. Since some carcinoids (e.g., gastric) do not produce enough serotonin to elevate urinary 5-HIAA above 15 mg, it is essential to perform the quantitative test. Urinary excretion of 5-HIAA in the range of 9 to 25 mg per 24-hour period has been described in patients with untreated celiac disease, tropical sprue, and Whipple's disease. The urinary levels of 5-HIAA in patients with classic carcinoid syndrome vary widely, from 60 to 1000 mg per 24 hours. False positive increases in urinary 5-HIAA occur with medications containing glyceryl guaiacolate, acetanilid, mephenesin, and methocarbamol.[26] Methenamine mandelate (Mande-

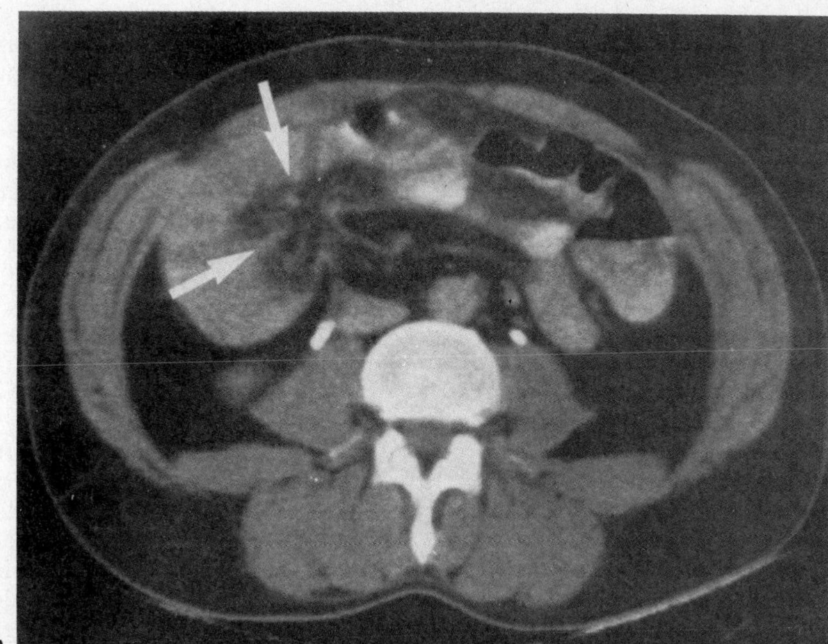

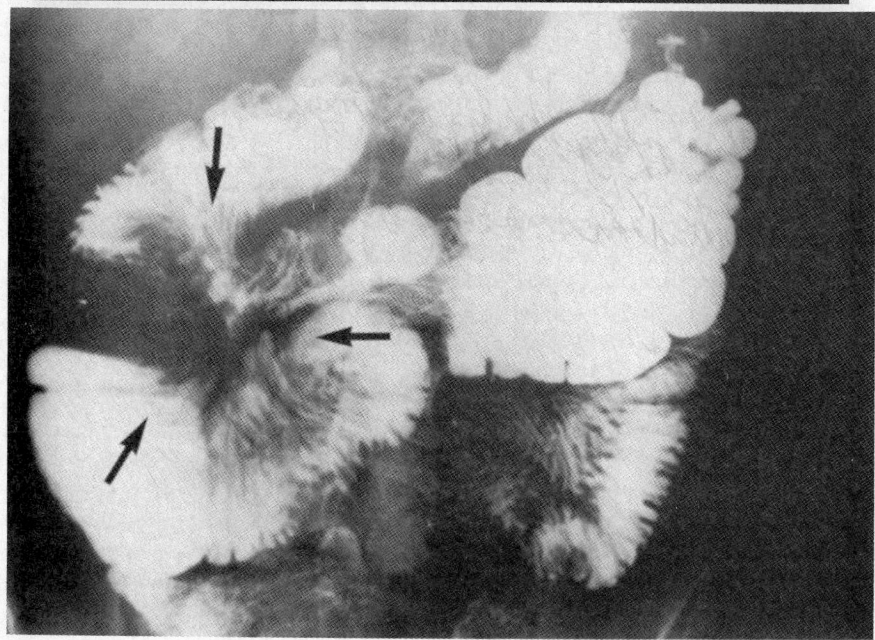

Figure 82–3. Carcinoid showing mesenteric changes. *A,* CT scan through mid-abdomen shows dilated loops of ileum with neurovascular markings in a stellate configuration *(arrows). B,* Small bowel roentgenogram demonstrates angulation with kinked loops, and partial obstruction with separation of involved small intestine *(arrows).* (Reproduced by permission from: Hulnick, D. H. Small intestine. *In* Megibow, A. J., and Balthazar, E. J. (eds.). Computed Tomography of the Gastrointestinal Tract. St. Louis, 1986, The C. V. Mosby Co.)

lamine) and phenothiazine derivatives with N-substituted aliphatic groups, such as promethazine hydrochloride (Phenergan), promazine hydrochloride (Sparine), prochlorperazine (Compazine), and chlorpromazine (Thorazine), may cause false negative tests for 5-HIAA.[26] Foods rich in serotonin, such as plantains, bananas, pineapples, walnuts, hickory nuts, avocados, tomatoes, eggplants, red plums, and kiwi fruit[27] should be excluded from the diet. Gastric and bronchial carcinoids secrete 5-HTP, which is converted to 5-HT in the kidney. In such cases, urinary 5-HTP and histamine are increased above the normal limits of 1.5 mg and 100 μg per 24 hours, respectively.

Determination of the 5-HT content of fasting whole blood extracts by reverse-phase high performance liquid chromatography will confirm the diagnosis in those rare patients with the syndrome and normal urinary excretion of 5-HIAA. The mean concentration of serotonin in normal subjects is 215 ± 58 ng/ml (range 71 to 310), while for patients with the carcinoid syndrome the range is 790 to 4500 ng/dl.[28] Measurements of bradykinin, tumor-kallikrein, NPK, and substance P released into the peripheral circulation are available in some research laboratories.

In view of the known production of ectopic hormones by carcinoid tumors derived from the pancreas, bronchus, and other organs, determinations of 17-hydroxysteroids and ketosteroids, adrenocorticotropic hormone, melanocyte-stimulating hormone, insulin, gastrin, glucagon, and other hormones should be performed when the clinical picture suggests overproduction of these substances. In a similar vein, it should be kept in mind that a number of pluriglandular adenomatoses have been seen in conjunction with carcinoid tumors arising from organs of the embryonic foregut. The associated tumors are diverse and have included parathyroid adenomas, pancreatic tumors producing Zollinger-Ellison syndrome, and acromegaly (see pp. 491 and 1896).

Provocative testing to elicit flushing with alcohol, calcium, pentagastrin, or 5 μg of epinephrine is probably not indicated, since it may produce serious side effects.

DIFFERENTIAL DIAGNOSIS

The differential diagnosis of carcinoid tumors without metastases is dependent on the location of the tumor. Bronchial carcinoids must be differentiated from other solitary lung lesions, especially carcinoma. Other polypoid lesions of the stomach and small intestine will enter into the differential diagnosis. Similarly, in patients with right lower quadrant pain, other considerations will have to be taken into account, especially acute appendicitis and Crohn's disease. Indeed, on X-ray carcinoid tumors may resemble Crohn's disease (Fig. 82–2). Of note, the coexistence of Crohn's disease and the carcinoid tumor has been described.[29] Colonic carcinoids with associated bleeding or obstruction must be differentiated from carcinomas, lymphomas, and leiomyomas in these areas.

Other clinical syndromes characterized by flushing, such as menopause, cirrhosis, and idiopathic flushing, can be differentiated by measuring urinary 5-HIAA and by the epinephrine test, which give uniformly negative results in these patients. In some patients with systemic mastocytosis, the differentiation from the carcinoid syndrome may be difficult. Flushing, hepatomegaly, diarrhea, and, occasionally, steatorrhea and either osteoblastic or osteolytic bone lesions occur in both diseases. However, both urinary 5-HIAA and the epinephrine provocative test are uniformly negative in systemic mastocytosis (see p. 509).

PATHOLOGY

In general, the carcinoid syndrome is associated only with carcinoid tumors with extensive metastases to the liver. Patients with tumors of ovarian origin, namely ovarian teratomas, or some bronchial carcinoids whose products are introduced directly into the general circulation may have the carcinoid syndrome without metastases to the liver or other organs. The most common primary tumor associated with the carcinoid syndrome arises in the small bowel, especially in the terminal third of the ileum. Primary tumors arising from the stomach, pancreatoduodenal region, common bile ducts, appendix, Meckel's diverticulum, colon, rectum, ovaries, and pulmonary bronchial tree have all been associated with the carcinoid syndrome.

Usually, primary tumors are small, asymptomatic, rarely demonstrable by roentgenograms, and are incidental findings on surgical exploration or at autopsy. Metastases in the lymph nodes and liver tend to rapidly outstrip the primary tumor in growth. After metastasis to the liver, the tumor can spread to lung, bone, skin, and almost all parenchymal organs. The sclerosing metastases in the bowel wall and the extensive metastases to the mesenteric lymph nodes, with their tendency to sclerose and coalesce, lead to significant shortening of the mesentery, thereby impairing the blood supply to the bowel. This cicatrization causes loops of small bowel to become narrowed, kinked, and fixed in a central retroperitoneal point (Fig. 82–2). Dense, proliferative fibrosis involves the peritoneal and pleural surfaces, as well as the endocardium of the right side of the heart and its valves. Lesser degrees of fibrosis of the left side of the heart occur in patients with long-standing carcinoid syndrome, in contradistinction to its earlier occurrence in patients with primary bronchial carcinoids and in persons with an atrial septal defect with a right-to-left intracardiac shunt. It is of note that extensive retroperitoneal and pelvic fibrosis may result in ureteral obstruction and can mimic retroperitoneal fibrosis.

Carcinoid tumors arising from the ileum, appendix, and ascending colon have the histologic appearance of dense nests of cells with small, dark oval nuclei with uniform size and shape and a moderate amount of pale, faintly granular cytoplasm. Histochemically they exhibit an argentaffin reaction in which the cells convert a silver salt to metallic silver. Bronchial, gastric, and pancreatic carcinoids have a trabecular architecture and contain argyrophilic rather than argentaffin granules. Confirmation of the pathology of the tumor can be obtained with immunoperoxidase stains for serotonin, chromogranin, neuron-specific enolase, and PGP 9.5. Chromogranin, a constituent of the secretory granules of peptide-producing endocrine cells, and neuron-specific enolase, a neuronal form of the glycolytic enzyme enolase, were present in 100 per cent of lung carcinoids.[30]

CARCINOID VARIANTS

Bronchial Carcinoids

These tumors produce the most striking clinical features of any of the variants of the carcinoid syndrome (Table 82–2). Characteristically, the flushes are a livid red and the flushing attacks are more prolonged and severe, lasting for as long as three to four days. The flushes are frequently associated with or preceded by disorientation, tremulousness of the hands, severe anxiety, temperature elevations, periorbital and facial edema, increased salivation and lacrimation, rhinorrhea, and diaphoresis. Nausea, vomiting, explosive diarrhea, and wheezing, which are commonly encoun-

Table 82–2. DISTINCTIVE CLINICAL FEATURES OF BRONCHIAL CARCINOIDS WITH CARCINOID SYNDROME

1. Severe and prolonged flushes of high intensity
2. Facial edema
3. Anxiety, tremulousness, and agitation
4. Lacrimation, sweating, and salivation
5. Nausea and vomiting; explosive diarrhea
6. Fever
7. Tachycardia; hypotension
8. Oliguria; sodium retention and potassium loss
9. Left-sided heart lesions

tered during the flushing episodes, are usually absent between flushes. Likewise, the flushes may be associated with severe hypotension, oliguria, and, in the presence of left-sided cardiac lesions, pulmonary edema. Other unusual features include left-sided cardiac lesions, increased incidence of Cushing's syndrome, multiple endocrine neoplasia (MEN) syndrome, acromegaly, and metastases to bone, which are frequently osteoblastic in nature. In contrast to other forms of the carcinoid syndrome, these patients have a tendency to be hypertensive. Similarly, headaches are prominent, and in time patients may develop marked enlargement of lacrimal, parotid, and submaxillary and submandibular salivary glands. Patients who survive the disease for several years may show thickening, hardening, and creasing of the face and forehead with associated rhinophyma.

Biochemically, the tumors appear to produce large amounts of 5-HTP as well as 5-HT.[31] Patients with asymptomatic pulmonary "coin" lesions discovered during routine roentgenograms of the chest should be screened with quantitative urinary excretion of 5-HIAA.

Gastric Carcinoid Tumors

The syndrome associated with primary tumors of gastric origin is distinctive from other carcinoid syndromes in both clinical and biochemical features (Table 82–3). The flush begins with a *bright red, patchy erythema* with sharply delineated serpentine borders. The patches tend to coalesce as the flush intensifies. Certain highly spiced foods and cheeses tend to aggravate and precipitate the flushes. Increased production of large amounts of histamine may contribute to the peculiar geographic distribution of the flushes. The excessive production of histamine may be responsible in part for the increased production of hydrochloric acid and the concomitant increase of peptic ulcers seen in some of these patients.

In association with the fairly consistent histaminuria, the pattern of urinary excretion of tryptophan metabolites appears to be distinct from that of other carcinoid patients. The tumor usually lacks aromatic L-amino acid decarboxylase and consequently releases 5-HTP rather than 5-HT into the blood. A portion of the released 5-HTP is decarboxylated in the kidney with a resultant increase in urinary serotonin; 5-HIAA may not be increased above 15 mg per 24 hours. Patients with gastric carcinoid tumors are less likely to have diarrhea and cardiac lesions.[14] Of note, gastric carcinoids have been described in association with pernicious anemia. The high serum gastrin levels, as found in pernicious anemia, have been reported to cause hyperplasia and neoplasia of enterochromaffin-like cells and a causal relationship between pernicious anemia, atropic gastritis, and carcinoid tumors is postulated. A recent report suggests that these lesions represent gastric endocrine hyperplasia and not true neoplasia and that the terms microcarcinoid or carcinoid tumors should therefore be avoided.[32] There are no reports of the carcinoid syndrome secondary to the hyperplasia seen in pernicious anemia.

Other Tumors with Typical Features of the Carcinoid Syndrome

Medullary carcinoma of the thyroid characteristically produces calcitonin but can produce increased quantities of prostaglandins and serotonin. In patients with very large primary tumors or with extensive metastases, flushing and multiple watery bowel movements may be common complaints. Rarely, high values of urinary 5-HIAA have been found, but generally the values are normal or only slightly increased. There has been no reported involvement of the endocardium or peritoneum with extensive fibrosis (see pp. 492–493).

Ovarian teratomas have been associated with the classic carcinoid syndrome, including the extensive fibrosis of the endocardium and the peritoneal surfaces in the absence of hepatic metastases. It is proposed that the active substances released from the tumors drain directly into the general circulation. *Oat-cell carcinomas* of the bronchus producing the carcinoid syndrome have been described. *Tumors of the common bile duct or pancreatic islets* may produce biochemical and clinical features of the carcinoid syndrome. They tend to produce both 5-HTP and serotonin.

NATURAL HISTORY

The natural history of carcinoid tumors varies with the location of the lesion. Metastases are infrequent in

Table 82–3. DISTINCTIVE CLINICAL FEATURES OF GASTRIC CARCINOID WITH CARCINOID SYNDROME

1. Flushes begin with bright red, patchy erythema with sharply delineated serpentine borders
2. Patches tend to coalesce as blush intensifies
3. Highly spiced foods and cheeses aggravate and precipitate flushes
4. Increased 5-hydroxytryptophan in blood
5. Increased urinary excretion of histamine, 5-hydroxytryptophan, 5-hydroxytryptamine
6. Less likely to have diarrhea and cardiac lesions

carcinoids of the appendix but are common in extra-appendiceal carcinoids. Intra-abdominal carcinoids spread in a progressive, stepwise pattern, initially involving the muscle coats by direct invasion, and then involving the regional lymph nodes and the liver. These tumors tend to be less aggressive than adenocarcinomas, and survival of five to ten years or longer is not uncommon, even after metastasis to the liver. Bronchial carcinoids tend to be more aggressive, with earlier metastases to liver, bone, skin, and brain. The morbidity from these tumors appears to be directly related to the pharmacologically active substances secreted by the tumors. Congestive heart failure, shock, fluid and electrolyte disturbances, intestinal obstruction, and the sequelae of metastases eventually lead to death in these patients.

TREATMENT

Surgical

Patients with the carcinoid syndrome cannot be cured by surgery except in the rare instances in which a primary ovarian or bronchial tumor is responsible for the symptoms. The surgical removal of ileal or other gastrointestinal primary tumors with secondary metastases may be indicated if the primary lesion is large or is responsible for mechanical obstruction. However, it should be recognized that a significant amount of small bowel may have to be removed, resulting in increase in diarrhea, steatorrhea, fluid and electrolyte imbalance, and weight loss. In some instances, it may be more judicious for the surgeon to create one or several enteroenterostomies to bypass areas of intestinal obstruction rather than to attempt massive resection. Partial hepatic resection has been advocated in patients with slow-growing hepatic metastases who have significant symptoms and in whom the metastases are confined to a single hepatic lobe. Removal of hepatic metastases has been recommended in patients with unbearable abdominal pain secondary to necrosis of hepatic metastases.[2]

The risk of complications of surgery in patients with the carcinoid syndrome is high. The complications include the susceptibility to adhesion formation, the sequelae of short bowel syndrome (see pp. 1106–1112), and the danger that anesthesia or surgical manipulation of the tumor may induce a crisis of carcinoid symptoms, mainly hypotension and severe bronchial constriction. Release of vasoactive substances can be minimized by the preoperative use of promethazine hydrochloride, avoidance of atropine, prophylactic administration of corticosteroids, and administration of diazepam and thiopentone as inducing agents and dimethyltubocurarine hydrochloride as the muscle relaxant.[33] Aprotinin (Trasylol), epsilon-aminocaproic acid (Amicar), and Iniprol (CY66), a group of proteinase and peptidase inhibitors, have been recommended for the control of bradykininogenic signs during anesthesia.[34] Naturally occurring somatostatin is useful in correcting hypotension and flushing during anesthesia.[35] However, a longer-acting analogue of somatostatin (SMS 201-995, Sandoz), an experimental agent in a dose of 50.0 μg intravenously, followed by another 50 μg given 15 seconds later, is highly effective and should be available for emergency use in patients with the carcinoid syndrome who are undergoing surgery.[36]

Hepatic arterial ligation or ligation with prior infusion of cytotoxic agents has been tried with varying degrees of success. Encouraging results have been obtained with the injection of yttrium microspheres into the hepatic artery as well as with embolization of hepatic metastases via a percutaneous transfemoral arterial route using steerable catheters. With adequate pharmacologic cover this latter technique is safe, effective, and relatively painless.

Medical

The medical therapy of patients who are symptomatic from the various substances elaborated by the tumor and metastases can be divided conveniently into the following categories.

Serotonin Antagonists. Methysergide maleate (Sansert) is given in a dose of 6 to 24 mg per day orally. It irregularly controls flushes, asthmatic attacks, and diarrhea. It is more effective than cyproheptadine against the diarrhea. The side effects of this drug are hypotension, syncope, lassitude, and development of resistance. Unfortunately, severe complications, including fluid retention and the development of fibrotic lesions of the retroperitoneal area, heart valves, and other tissues, restrict the use of this drug. Cyproheptadine (Periactin) can be given in a dose of 6 to 30 mg per day orally. For relief of acute attacks, 50 to 75 mg in 100 to 200 ml saline infused over one to two hours may be beneficial. It is as effective as methysergide but seems to control flush better. The side effects are similar to those of methysergide but, since it does not cause serious fibrosis, cyproheptadine is the preferred drug.

Other Drugs. A number of drugs are useful for relief of symptoms. These include:

1. Combination of H_1 and H_2 receptor antagonists, diphenhydramine hydrochloride, 50 mg orally every six hours, and cimetidine, 300 mg every six hours, produced blockade of the flush associated with a gastric carcinoid and elevated histamine excretion.[28]
2. *Corticosteroids* (prednisone), in doses of 15 to 40 mg per day, may dramatically benefit the patients with bronchial carcinoids and the carcinoid syndrome; otherwise, corticosteroids are usually ineffective.
3. *Prochlorperazine*, in doses of 10 mg three to four times daily, is occasionally helpful in controlling the flush.
4. *Phenoxybenzamine*, 10 to 30 mg daily, may diminish flushing by preventing kallikrein release.
5. *Methyldopa* (Aldomet), 250 to 500 mg every six to eight hours, has been useful in reducing the diarrhea in patients with the gastric carcinoid syndrome.
6. *Somatostatin* administered intravenously has been shown to suppress flushing, hypotension, bronchial constriction, and watery diarrhea in patients with car-

cinoid syndrome. Somatostatin may reduce diarrhea by inhibiting the effect of tumor amines on intestinal mucosa, reducing gastric inhibitory polypeptide, or reducing intestinal motility.[37] Recently SMS 201-995, an analogue of somatostatin, self-administered by subcutaneous injection at a dose of 150 μg three times daily, has been shown to be highly effective in relieving the flushing and diarrhea associated with the syndrome.[38] Steatorrhea,[39] hyperglycemia, cholelithiasis, and tachyphylaxis, which are associated with its use, may pose potential problems.[40]

7. *Cholestyramine* (Questran), 4 to 8 gm orally every six hours, will improve patients with bile salt–induced diarrhea secondary to ileal resection. If steatorrhea is also present, medium-chain triglycerides should be substituted for long-chain triglycerides.

Chemotherapy. It seems prudent to delay initiation of chemotherapy in the early metastatic stage of the disease, because the course is often indolent. Objective responses have been observed in patients with far advanced carcinoid syndrome with combinations of 5-fluorouracil (5-FU) and streptozotocin (STZ), STZ and cyclophosphamide (CTX), 5-FU and doxorubicin (DOX) and CTX and STZ, and STZ plus DOX.[41] Leukocyte interferon has also been used to treat symptoms.[42]

Radiation. Whole abdominal radiation (2000 to 2500 rad) improved survival in patients with metastatic gastrointestinal carcinoid tumor but was ineffective in patients with carcinoid syndrome.[43]

Supportive Measures. A nutritious diet, containing 70 gm of protein and high in fat (except if significant small bowel has been resected) and calories, with vitamin supplementation, especially niacin, is recommended. Milk, cheeses, eggs, and citrus fruits may initiate episodes of flushing and diarrhea and thus should be avoided. A high fluid intake to ensure a proper state of hydration is advised. In the event of cardiac failure, the patient should be given digoxin and diuretics. Some success has been achieved with valve replacement in patients with refractory heart failure. Implantation of a mechanical, rather than a tissue valve prosthesis might be preferable.[44] For patients with severe intractable diarrhea, one may have to resort to diphenoxylate (Lomotil), 5 to 10 mg every three to four hours; loperamide hydrochloride (Imodium), 4 to 16 mg daily; or deodorized tincture of opium, 10 to 20 drops in water every four to six hours, alone or in conjunction with one of the antiserotonin agents. Ketanserin A[19] and recently ICS 205-930[45] are serotonin antagonist, whose actions are predominantly on the (5-HT–M) receptor and not on the (5-HI-D) receptor. These experimental drugs caused profound improvement by decreasing the frequency and the volume of the diarrhea in patients with the carcinoid syndrome.

PROGNOSIS

Despite metastasis of the tumor, supportive and symptomatic treatment is extremely important. It should be kept in mind that patients with ileal carcinoids with metastases have lived as long as 23 years, and some have lived for 10 or more years after the syndrome appeared. On the other hand, patients with bronchial carcinoids, oat-cell carcinoma, and anaplastic pancreatic carcinoma with the carcinoid syndrome have a much poorer prognosis.

References

1. Pearse, A. G. E., and Takor, T. T. Neuroendocrine embryology and the APUD concept. Clin. Endocrinol. *5*(Suppl.):229S, 1976.
2. Grahame-Smith, D. G. The Carcinoid Syndrome. London, William Heinemann Medical Books, 1972, p. 73.
3. Frölich, J. C., Bloomgarden, Z. T., Oates, J. A., McGuigan, J. E., and Rabinowitz, D. The carcinoid flush. Provocation by pentagastrin and inhibition by somatostatin. N. Engl. J. Med. *299*:1055, 1978.
4. Wong, V. G., and Melmon, K. L. Ophthalmic manifestations of the carcinoid flush. N. Engl. J. Med. *277*:406, 1967.
5. Ross, E. M., and Roberts, W. C. The carcinoid syndrome: comparison of 21 necropsy subjects with carcinoid heart disease to 15 necropsy subjects without carcinoid heart disease. Am. J. Med. *79*:339, 1985.
6. Bivens, C. H., Marecek, R. L., and Feldman, J. M. Peyronie's disease—a presenting complaint of the carcinoid syndrome. N. Engl. J. Med. *289*:844, 1973.
7. Kowlessar, O. D., Law, D. H., and Sleisenger, M. H. Malabsorption syndrome associated with metastatic carcinoid tumor. Am. J. Med. *39*:568, 1965.
8. Bishop, A. E., Polak, J. M., Facer, P., Ferri, G. L., Marangos, P. J., and Pearse, A. G. E. Neuron specific enolase: a common marker for the endocrine cells and innervation of the gut and pancreas. Gastroenterology *83*:903, 1982.
9. Lloyd, R. V., and Wilson, B. S. Specific endocrine tissue marker defined by a monoclonal antibody. Science *222*:628, 1983.
10. Sjoerdsma, A., Weissbach, H., Terry, L. L., and Udenfriend, S. Further observations on patients with malignant carcinoid. Am. J. Med. *23*:5, 1957.
11. Haverback, G. J., and Davidson, J. D. Serotonin and the gastrointestinal tract. Gastroenterology *35*:570, 1958.
12. Bullbring, E., and Lin, R. C. Y. The effect of intraluminal application of 5-hydroxytryptamine and 5-hydroxytryptophan on peristalsis; the local production of 5-HT and its release in relation to intraluminal pressure and propulsive activity. J. Physiol. *40*:381, 1958.
13. Graham, J. R. Cardiac and pulmonary fibrosis during methysergide therapy for headache. Am. J. Med. *254*:23, 1967.
14. Oates, J. A., and Butler, C. Pharmacologic and endocrine aspects of carcinoid syndrome. Adv. Pharmacol. *5*:109, 1967.
15. Theodorsson-Norheim, E., Norheim, I., Öberg, K., Brodin, E., Lundberg, J. M., Tatemotok, K., and Lindgren, P. G. Neuropeptide K: a major tachykinin in plasma and tumor tissues from carcinoid patients. Biochem. Biophys. Res. Commun. *131*:77, 1985.
16. Sandler, M., Karmin, S. M., and Williams, E. D. Prostaglandins in amine-peptide–secreting tumors. Lancet *2*:1053, 1968.
17. Feldman, J. M., Plonk, J. W., and Cornette, J. C. Serum prostaglandin $F_2\alpha$ concentration in the carcinoid syndrome. Prostaglandins *7*:501, 1974.
18. Jaffe, B. M., Behrman, H. R., and Parker, C. W. Radioimmunoassay measurement of prostaglandin E, A and F in human plasma. J. Clin. Invest. *52*:398, 1973.
19. Antonsen, S., Hansen, M. G. J., Bukhare, K., Rask-Madsen, J. Influence of a new selective $5HT_2$ receptor antagonist (Ketanserin) on jejunal PGE_2 release and ion secretion due to malignant carcinoid syndrome. Gut *23A*:887, 1982.
20. Hawkey, C. J., and Rampton, D. S. Prostaglandins and the gastrointestinal mucosa: are they important in its function, disease, or treatment? Gastroenterology *89*:1162, 1985.
21. Hulnick, D. H. Small intestine. *In* Megibow, A. J., and Balthazar, E. J. (eds.). Computed Tomography of the Gastrointestinal Tract. St. Louis, C. V. Mosby Co., 1986, pp. 257–259.

22. Siegel, R. S., Kuhns, L. R., Borlaza, G. S., McCormick, T. L., and Simmons, J. L. Computed tomography and angiography in ileal carcinoid and retractile mesenteritis. Radiology *134*:437, 1980.
23. Reuter, S. R., and Joijsen, E. Angiographic findings in two ileal carcinoid tumors. Radiology *87*:836, 1966.
24. Goldstein, H. M., and Miller, M. Angiographic evaluation of carcinoid tumors of the small intestine: the value of epinephrine. Radiology *115*:23, 1975.
25. Andersen, J. B., Madsen, B., and Skjoldborg, H. Angiography in a case of carcinoid tumor in the stomach. Br. J. Radiol. *44*:218, 1971.
26. Pedersen, A. T., Batsakis, J. G., Vanselow, N. A., and McLean, J. A. False-positive tests for urinary 5-hydroxyindoleacetic acid. Error in laboratory determinations caused by glycerylguaiacolate. JAMA *211*:1184, 1970.
27. Feldman, J. M., and Lee, E. M. Serotonin content of foods: effect on urinary excretion of 5-hydroxyindoleacetic acid. Am. J. Clin. Nutr. *42*:639, 1985.
28. Richter, G., Stöckmann, F., Conlon, J. M., and Creutzfeldt, W. Serotonin release into blood after food and pentagastrin. Studies in healthy subjects and in patients with metastatic carcinoid tumors. Gastroenterology *91*:612, 1986.
29. Brown, G. A., Kollin, J., and Rajan, R. K. The coexistence of carcinoid tumor and Crohn's disease. J. Clin. Gastroenterol. *8*:286, 1986.
30. Said, J. W., Vimadalal, S., Nash, G., Shintaku, I. P., Heusser, R. C., Sassoon, A. F., and Lloyd, R. V. Immunoreactive neuron-specific enolase, bombesin, and chromogranin as markers for neuroendocrine lung tumors. Hum. Pathol. *16*:236, 1985.
31. Melmon, K. L., Sjoerdsma, A., and Mason, D. T. Distinctive clinical and therapeutic aspects of the syndrome associated with bronchial carcinoid tumors. Am. J. Med. *39*:568, 1965.
32. Rode, J., Dhillon, A. P., Papadaki, L., Strockbrugger, R., Thompson, R. J., Moss, E., and Cotton, P. Pernicious anemia and mucosal endocrine cell proliferation of the non-antral stomach. Gut *27*:789, 1986.
33. Patel, K. D., and Dalal, F. Y. Anesthetic management of a patient with carcinoid tumor undergoing myocardial revascularization. Can. Anaesth. Soc. J. *27*:260, 1980.
34. Déry, R. Theoretical and clinical considerations in anesthesia for secreting carcinoid tumors. Can. Anaesth. Soc. J. *18*:245, 1971.
35. Thulin, L., Samnegård, H., Tydén, G., Long, D., and Efendić, S. Efficacy of somatostatin in a patient with carcinoid syndrome. Lancet *2*:43, 1978.
36. Krols, L., K., Martin, J. K., Marsh, H. M., and Moertel, C. G. Rapid reversal of carcinoid crisis with a somatostatin analogue. N. Engl. J. Med. *313*:1229, 1985.
37. Dharmasathaphorn, K., Sherwin, R. S., Cataland, S., Jaffe, B., and Dobbins, J. Somatostatin inhibits diarrhea in the carcinoid syndrome. Ann. Intern. Med. *92*:68, 1980.
38. Krols, L. K., Moertel, C. G., O'Connell, M. J., Schutt, A. J., Rubin, J., and Hahn, R. G. Treatment of the malignant carcinoid syndrome. Evaluation of a long acting somatostatin analogue. N. Engl. J. Med. *315*:663, 1986.
39. Richter, G., Stöckmann, F., Lembcke, B., Conlon, J. M., and Creutzfeldt, W. Short term administration of the somatostatin analogue SMS 201-995 in patients with carcinoid tumors. Scand. J. Gastroenterol. *21*(Suppl. 119):193, 1986.
40. Oates, J. A. The carcinoid syndrome. N. Engl. J. Med. *315*:702, 1986.
41. Krols, L. K. Metastatic carcinoid tumors and the carcinoid syndrome. A selective review of chemotherapy and hormonal therapy. Am. J. Med. *81*(Suppl. 6B):49, 1986.
42. Öberg, K., Funa, K., and Alm, G. Effects of leukocyte interferon on clinical symptoms and hormone levels in patients with mid-gut carcinoid tumors and carcinoid syndrome. N. Engl. J. Med. *309*:129, 1983.
43. Samlowski, W. E., Eyre, H. J., and Sause, W. T. Evaluation of the response of unresectable carcinoid tumors to radiotherapy. Int. J. Radiat. Oncol. Biol. Phys. *12*:301, 1986.
44. Schoen, F. J., Hausner, R. J., Howell, J. F., Beazley, H. L., and Titus, J. L. Porcine heterograft replacement in carcinoid heart disease. J. Thorac. Cardiovasc. Surg. *85*:100, 1981.
45. Coupe, M., Anderson, J., Barnard, M., Alstead, E., Bloom, S. R., and Hodgson, H. J. F. New serotonin antagonist (α5HT-M receptor) blocks diarrhea in carcinoid syndrome. Gut *27*:A1243, 1986.

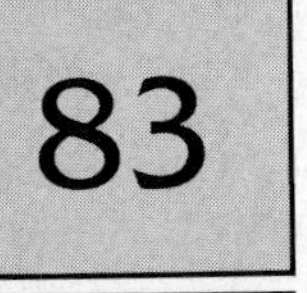

83 Examination of the Anorectum, Rigid Sigmoidoscopy, Flexible Sigmoidoscopy, and Diseases of the Anorectum

THEODORE R. SCHROCK

ANATOMY

The anal canal is derived from the proctodeum (ectoderm), and the rectum originates from the hindgut (entoderm). The anal canal fuses with the rectum over a zone several centimeters in width, and together these structures constitute the anorectum[1, 2] (Fig. 83–1).

The anal canal is 4 cm long,[3] pointed toward the umbilicus, and collapsed in the resting state. The anal verge (anal orifice) is marked by corrugated skin; clinicians describe the location of anorectal lesions in terms of the distance above this landmark. The pectinate (dentate) line lies 2 cm above the anal verge (Fig. 83–2). Anal papillae, tiny bits of projecting tissue, give the appearance of a serrated fringe to this structure. At the pectinate line, transverse flaps of epithelium

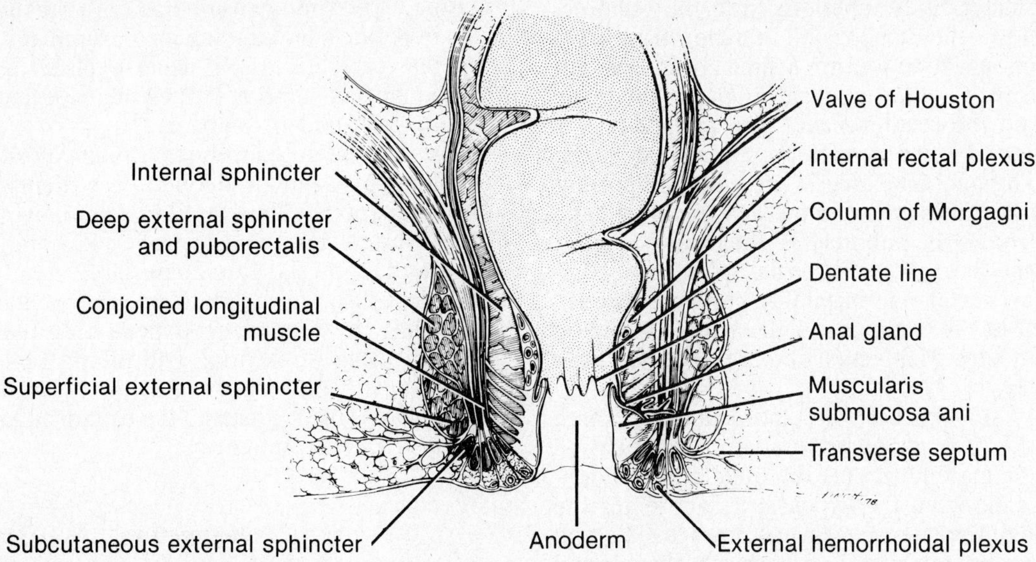

Figure 83–1. The anorectum. (From Goldberg, S. M., Gordon, P. H., and Nivatvongs, S. Essentials of Anorectal Surgery. Philadelphia, J. B. Lippincott Company, 1980. Used by permission.)

(anal valves) overlie anal crypts with their mouths facing upward toward the fecal stream. A primitive anal gland or duct extends from the base of each crypt into the underlying muscle. The columns of Morgagni are longitudinal gatherings of mucosa above the pectinate line.

The lower 2 cm of the anal canal are lined by thin, pale, stratified squamous epithelium (anoderm), which is devoid of hair follicles, sweat glands, and sebaceous glands. Cuboidal cells are found in a 1-cm band proximal to the pectinate line; this epithelium is sometimes called "transitional." The typical red, glistening columnar mucosa of the rectum begins above the transitional zone.

The internal anal sphincter is the thickened lower portion of the circular smooth muscle layer of the gut. It ends inferiorly with a well-defined rounded edge just inside the anal orifice. The internal sphincter is involuntary and can be divided partially with little consequence; complete severance impairs continence in some individuals. Some fibers of the conjoined longitudinal muscle outside the internal sphincter fan out and attach to skin, causing the corrugated effect at the anal verge.

The external anal sphincter is a continuous sheet of striated muscle surrounding the anal canal.[1, 2] A sulcus (intersphincteric groove) is easily palpable between the internal and external sphincters at the anal orifice. The

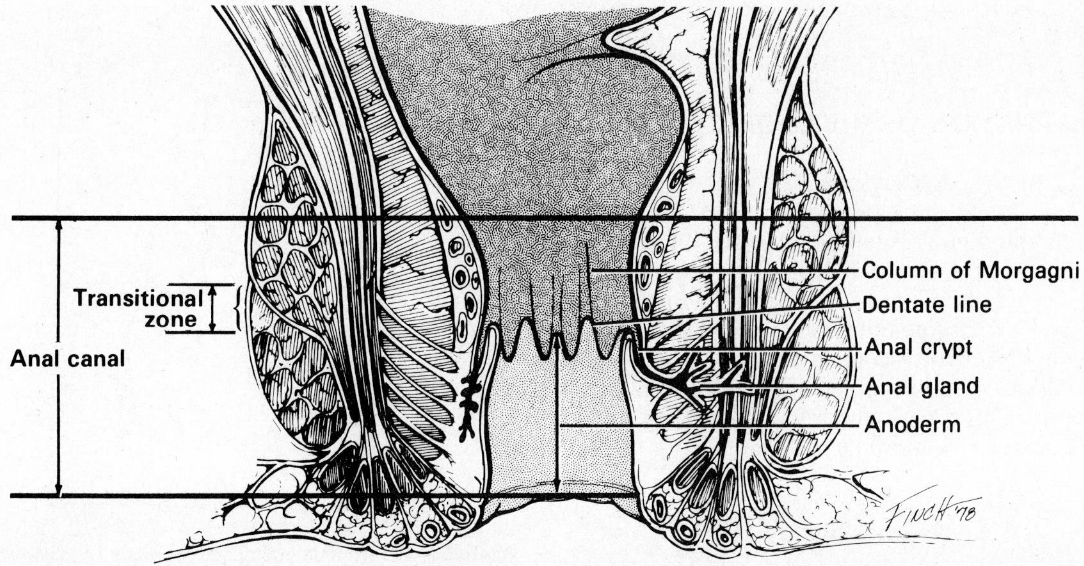

Figure 83–2. The lining of the anal canal. (From Goldberg, S. M., Gordon, P. H., and Nivatvongs, S. Essentials of Anorectal Surgery. Philadelphia, J. B. Lippincott Company, 1980. Used by permission.)

external sphincter fuses superiorly with the puborectalis portion of the levator ani muscle; these two muscles function as one to form a sling around the gut and pull it forward, thus creating an angle where the anal canal and the rectum meet.[4] The puborectalis is prominent laterally and posteriorly, but it is deficient anteriorly. The anorectal ring is the vitally important musculature at the junction of the anal canal and the rectum; it includes the puborectalis sling and the upper portions of the internal and external sphincters. Division of the anorectal ring inevitably produces incontinence. Potential tissue spaces in the anorectal region are important sites of infection and are discussed later in this chapter.

Arterial blood reaches the anorectum by three routes: (1) the superior hemorrhoidal, a continuation of the inferior mesenteric; (2) the middle hemorrhoidals, which arise from the hypogastrics and enter the rectum through the lateral ligaments on each side; and (3) the inferior hemorrhoidals, branches of the internal pudendals. Venous blood drains upward to the portal vein by way of the superior hemorrhoidal and inferior mesenteric veins, or it passes directly into the systemic circulation through the middle and inferior hemorrhoidal veins (see pp. 1903–1932). Hematogenous metastases from neoplasms low in the anorectum can occur through either or both routes. Lymphatics above the pectinate line accompany the blood vessels to the inferior mesenteric and periaortic nodes. Lymph from the lower anal canal empties into the inguinal lymph nodes. Inguinal lymphadenopathy is seen in patients with inflammatory or malignant anal diseases.

Somatic innervation of the anoderm and perianal skin accounts for the extreme sensitivity of this area to painful stimuli. The upper portions of the anal canal and the rectum are supplied by autonomic nerves and are relatively insensitive to pain. Motor nerves to the internal sphincter are autonomic, but the voluntarily contracting external sphincter and levator ani muscles are somatically innervated by branches from the inferior hemorrhoidal and fourth sacral nerves (see Fig. 2–12, p. 34).

EXAMINATION OF THE ANORECTUM

Indications

Inspection and digital examination of the anorectum should be incorporated into all complete physical examinations in adults. Thorough evaluation, including anoscopy and proctosigmoidoscopy, is mandatory in patients with anorectal or colonic complaints. Parts of the examination may be deferred briefly for specific reasons (e.g., severe anal tenderness), but they must be completed when circumstances permit.

Preparation

The physician establishes rapport by taking the history and performing other parts of the physical examination first. Apprehension and embarrassment are the rule in patients undergoing anal examination, and they are reassured if the physician explains each step in simple language and describes the expected sensations before they suddenly appear.

The left lateral decubitus (Sims') position is well tolerated by aged or debilitated patients, and some examiners prefer Sims' position routinely[1] (Fig. 83–3). The inverted (knee-chest, prone jackknife) position is also used; a special examining table greatly facilitates the procedure. The patient's sense of vulnerability is minimized by draping to expose only the perineum. Good lighting is essential, and the instruments should be arranged within easy reach. An assistant, usually a nurse, hands instruments to the examiner and reassures and instructs the patient.

Inspection

Retraction of the buttocks with the fingers of both hands exposes the perineum. Many patients contract the buttock musculature from fear and, perhaps, as an effort to preserve a vestige of privacy. If the buttocks are large, this reaction precludes a view of the anus. Reassurance and patience are rewarded by relaxation of the buttock muscles, and examination proceeds.

Table 83–1 lists abnormal findings on inspection. The buttocks, sacrococcygeal region, vulva or base of the scrotum, and upper thighs should be examined

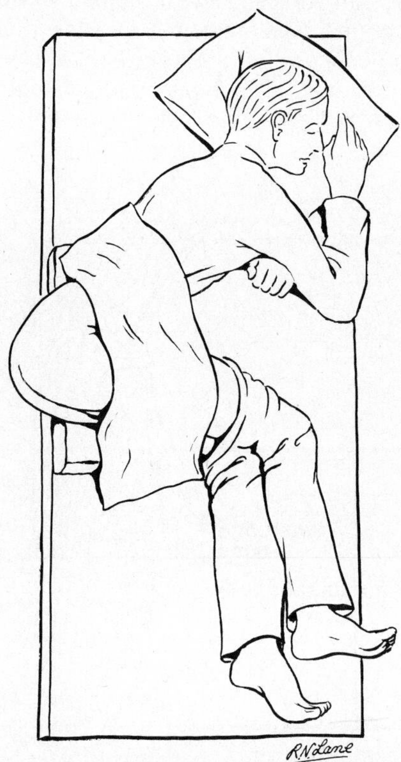

Figure 83–3. The left lateral decubitus (Sims') position for anorectal examination. Elevation of the left hip on a small sandbag is important. (From Goligher, J. C. Surgery of the Anus, Rectum and Colon. 5th ed. London, Bailliere Tindall, 1984. Used by permission.)

Table 83–1. PERIANAL AND ANAL ABNORMALITIES DETECTABLE ON INSPECTION

Perianal
Asymmetry (congenital, scar, tumor, abscess)
Dermatologic disease—primary or specific
Dermatologic change—secondary (erythema, edema, excoriation, lichenification)
Feces, mucus, pus
Neoplasm, wart, cyst
Fistula or sinus opening
Anal
Anal verge (deformity, scarring, gaping)
Skin tag
Neoplasm, wart
Fissure
Hemorrhoids (thrombosed external, prolapsing)
Prolapsing lesion (hemorrhoid, papilla, polyp, procidentia)

before attention is focused on the perianal area. Asymmetrical contour of the perineum has many causes, but they should not be difficult to differentiate. Primary or specific dermatologic disorders generally affect skin elsewhere too; secondary changes are seen in patients with chronic pruritus ani or acute inflammation. Feces or mucus on perianal skin may reflect incontinence, poor hygiene, or conditions that make cleansing difficult or painful. Pus most often drains from a fistula or sinus.

The contour of the anal verge is examined and lesions noted. Then the anal orifice is everted by traction on both sides; gauze squares help obtain purchase without slipping (Fig. 83–4). The lower anal canal can be inspected in this way, sometimes up to the pectinate line, and a variety of abnormalities are exposed to view. The location of anal lesions around the circumference should be described anatomically; reference to the face of a clock is confusing because it depends on the patient's position.

Palpation

The gloved but unlubricated index finger is used to palpate the sacrococcygeal, perineal, and perianal tissues for tenderness, masses, and induration. The firm cord of a fistula tract may be traced, and pus may be expressed from the secondary opening. Lubricant is then applied liberally to the anus, and perianal palpation is repeated; induration and masses often are best appreciated by gliding the finger across the lubricated skin. The fingertip is placed at the anal orifice and slowly inserted. Most adults and children accommodate the index finger; infants and those adults with anal stenosis or painful anal lesions are examined more comfortably with the small finger. Reassurance and gentle pressure overcome the sphincteric contraction in anxious patients. If a tender lesion is present, pressure should be applied to the opposite wall; anesthetic ointment may be necessary.

The intersphincteric groove is palpable circumferentially just inside the orifice; abscesses sometimes are present at this site. The tone of the sphincters and the caliber of the anal canal are noted as the finger is inserted. *Fissures, fistula tracts, abscesses,* and *carcinomas* are detected in the lower anal canal. *Hypertrophied papillae* or *fistula openings* may be felt at the pectinate line. *Internal hemorrhoids* are not palpable unless they are thrombosed.

After sweeping the finger circumferentially around the lower anal canal, the finger is inserted its full length and the same circumferential motion is used to feel for masses and tenderness in the rectum and the adjacent organs. The average index finger is about 10 cm long, with an effective insertion of 7.5 cm;[1, 2] the depth of penetration also varies with the size of the buttocks. More mucosa is brought into position for examination if the patient strains. Particular attention is directed to the posterior rectal wall above the anorectal ring. Soft, velvety *villous tumors*, hard, centrally ulcerated *cancers* with rolled edges, and *pedunculated polyps* are among the intrinsic abnormalities sought. Stool in the rectum is deformable, in contrast to other rectal masses. Tumors and abscesses may be found posterior or lateral to the rectum. The mucosa in inflammatory bowel disease is gritty.

The anorectal ring is prominent laterally and posteriorly. The patient is instructed to contract this muscle, and the strength of the contraction is noted. Spasm and tenderness are felt in the levator and coccygeus muscles in some patients with rectal pain. Sacrotuberous ligaments are firm cords extending from the sacrum to the ischial tuberosities on both sides.

The anterior peritoneal reflection is situated about 7 cm from the anal verge in women and 8 to 10 cm in men; masses in the cul-de-sac are usually within reach.[1] The cervix is the most common rectal "tumor" and can be mistaken for a pathologic lesion by the unwary; vaginal tampons are easily palpable. Digital rectal examination is the most efficient screening test for prostatic cancer.[5] Benign prostatic enlargement is a firm nodularity involving the gland diffusely. Early prostatic cancer is a small, stony hard nodule at the edge of the gland. The seminal vesicles lie above the prostate anterior to the tough fascia of Denonvilliers.[4]

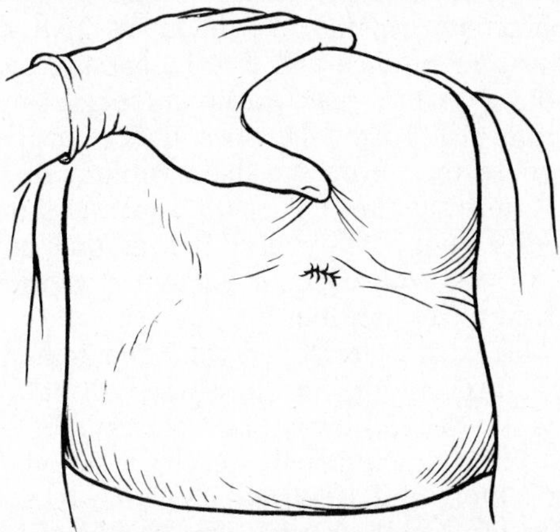

Figure 83–4. Lateral traction permits inspection inside the anal verge. (From Goligher, J. C. Surgery of the Anus, Rectum and Colon. 5th ed. London, Bailliere Tindall, 1984. Used by permission.)

The seminal vesicles are soft and difficult to palpate rectally.

The coccyx is grasped and moved with a thumb on the perineum and a finger in the rectum. The rectovaginal septum is palpated bidigitally. Bimanual examination with the patient in the lithotomy position is useful, but in men it is required only in special situations.

The exact position of lesions is noted with respect to the anal verge, anorectal ring, coccyx, ischial tuberosities, rectovaginal septum, and prostate and seminal vesicles. Size, degree of circumferential involvement, and fixation are important also.

The examining finger should be inspected for blood, pus, mucus, and feces after it is withdrawn. Tests for occult blood are misleading in these circumstances. If fecal occult blood testing is indicated, specimens should be collected by the patient following an established protocol.

Anoscopy

The anal canal can be inspected in its entirety only by anoscopy. Proctosigmoidoscopy, rigid or flexible—even with retroflexion—is inadequate for this task. Anoscopes (proctoscopes) are tubular metal or plastic instruments with straight or beveled tips. The beveled type is best for most purposes because it affords a side view of a good length of the anal canal. The adult anoscope is about 7 cm long and has a diameter of 2 cm at the tip. Smaller instruments are available. Some anoscopes contain a built-in fiberoptic lighting system, and others require external illumination. Various types of specula, retractors, probes, and hooks are used to examine the anal canal also.

With the patient in the same position as before, the left hand exposes the anus, and the anoscope is held in the right hand with the thumb pressed against the obturator so that it does not slip out as the anoscope is inserted. Lubricant is applied to the instrument and transferred to the anus. The anoscope is introduced with slow gentle pressure in the longitudinal axis of the anal canal, that is, pointed toward the umbilicus. The sphincters grip the instrument at first, but they relax with reassurance and instructions to bear down. When the anoscope reaches the anorectal ring, about 3 cm from the orifice, the tip is deflected posteriorly to negotiate the anorectal angle without discomfort, and it is inserted the full length until the flange rests against the anus. At or just before this point, the handle of the anoscope is rotated posteriorly and transferred to the left hand.

The obturator is removed, and the lumen of the rectum is inspected for masses. Material that obscures the view is swabbed away. The presence of blood or pus and the character of the feces are noted. Normal mucosa is pink, and a delicate network of submucosal vessels is visible; thickened, granular friable mucosa with obliterated submucosal vascular pattern indicates proctitis. Material for cultures and biopsies of lesions in the lower rectum can be obtained.

The anoscope is withdrawn to the pectinate line, where the papillae and crypts are inspected and fistula openings are sought. Hemorrhoids arise above the pectinate line and bulge into the lumen when the patient strains. Fissures and other lesions are evident in the anoderm below the pectinate line. If the anoscope is beveled, the obturator is reinserted carefully and the instrument is rotated 90 degrees to bring another quadrant into view. The entire circumference should be inspected.

RIGID PROCTOSIGMOIDOSCOPY

Indications

Proctosigmoidoscopy (examination of the rectum and sigmoid colon) is an important step in the evaluation of the lower tract. Flexible sigmoidoscopy is performed in most circumstances, but rigid proctosigmoidoscopy is still preferred in certain situations[6] (Table 83–2). The presence of anal or rectal symptoms suggests that rigid examination be performed preceding flexible sigmoidoscopy. Exact location of the height of a rectal cancer above the anal verge is crucial to making therapeutic decisions, and this distance can be measured most accurately with the rigid instrument. Only the rectum need be examined to diagnose most cases of infectious proctitis, obtain a rectal biopsy, or monitor response of colitis to systemic treatment. Avoidance of contamination of expensive flexible instruments in patients with suspected transmissible disease may be possible if rigid proctosigmoidoscopy will suffice.

There are no absolute contraindications to rigid proctosigmoidoscopy.

Technique

Rigid proctosigmoidoscopes are tubular metal or plastic instruments, 25 cm long and between 11 and 19 mm in diameter.[1, 2, 7] They are equipped with distal fiberoptic lighting, a magnifying lens, and a connection for insufflation of air. Other necessary equipment includes biopsy and grasping forceps, suction tubing, swabs, and culture materials.

Some examiners perform proctosigmoidoscopy without preparation so that blood, pus, and mucus will not be washed away. Also, enemas may cause mucosal edema and erythema, and the profuse liquid secretions can be troublesome in patients who received an irritant

Table 83–2. INDICATIONS FOR RIGID PROCTOSIGMOIDOSCOPY

Preceding flexible sigmoidoscopy
Locate position of rectal cancer
Rectal biopsy
Monitor activity of colitis
Evaluate infectious proctitis
Rectal polypectomy
Avoid contamination of flexible scope

enema just before examination. Other endoscopists routinely have their patients prepared with a phospha-soda (Fleet) enema. Certainly, an enema is necessary if the rectum is impacted with stool or if the field is obscured by feces despite swabbing and suction.

Premedication is seldom required. Topical anesthetic lubricant is helpful in some patients with painful anal lesions.

The patient remains in the same position as for anoscopy. The lubricated instrument is held in the right hand with the obturator firmly in place. The proctosigmoidoscope is inserted in the same manner as the anoscope, deflecting the tip posteriorly at the anorectal ring (Fig. 83–5). The obturator is withdrawn when 5 to 10 cm has been inserted, and the proctosigmoidoscope is advanced with the lumen in view at all times. Insufflation of air is helpful, but it increases discomfort and should be used sparingly. The left hand steadies the instrument against the perineum, so that if the patient jumps suddenly a length of the scope will not enter abruptly.

The rectosigmoid junction is about 12 to 15 cm from the anus; it appears to be a cul-de-sac, because the lumen bends forward sharply and to the left. This turn is straightened out with anterior pressure on the tip, and the sigmoid colon is entered (Fig. 83–5). It is important to avoid inserting more instrument without advancing the tip, causing discomfort and risking perforation. Success often depends upon reassurance of the patient during the procedure. The average depth of insertion is 16 to 20 cm;[8] only one third of female and one half of male patients can be examined for a depth greater than 20 cm.[8]

The lumen of the bowel is carefully examined as the instrument is withdrawn. The tip is swept circumferentially to see the entire wall; this is especially important in the rectal ampulla, where the capacious lumen may hide large masses. The rectal valves of Houston, two on the left and one on the right, should be ironed out so that lesions on their superior surfaces are not overlooked. The source of blood should be identified, if possible; many times, blood comes from some point above the reach of the instrument. *Neoplasms* and *mucosal inflammation* are noted, and the distance from the anal verge is recorded.

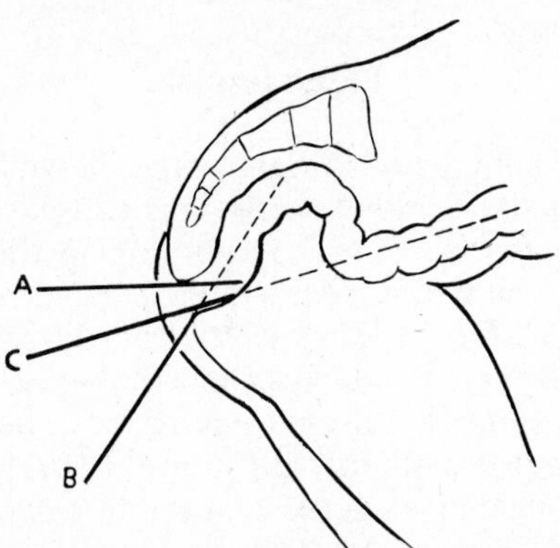

Figure 83–5. Changes in axis of instrument during rigid proctosigmoidoscopy. *A*, Initial insertion toward umbilicus. *B*, Deflection posteriorly after sphincters are passed. *C*, Negotiation of the rectosigmoid junction. (From Goligher, J. C. Surgery of the Anus, Rectum and Colon. 5th ed. London, Bailliere Tindall, 1984. Used by permission.)

Table 83–3. INDICATIONS FOR FLEXIBLE SIGMOIDOSCOPY

Screening for neoplasms
Rectal bleeding:
Chronic gross bleeding
Radiographic lesion in sigmoid
Suspected colitis, normal rectum
Complicated sigmoid diverticular disease

Biopsy specimens of neoplasms or the mucosa are obtained most easily with angled forceps (see p. 1624). The safest place to take a specimen for biopsy is the posterior rectal wall; the anterior wall above 7 to 10 cm is a hazardous site, because it is above the peritoneal reflection and perforation is a risk. Bleeding from biopsy sites usually stops by applying pressure with a swab. It may be necessary to soak the swab in dilute epinephrine solution.

Small mucosal lesions can be electrically fulgurated, and polypectomy can be carried out with an electrocautery snare. The technique is similar to that of colonoscopic polypectomy, although the snares are shorter and the outer sheath is rigid. Complications of rigid proctosigmoidoscopy are discussed in Chapter 13.

FLEXIBLE SIGMOIDOSCOPY

The earliest flexible colonoscopes were short instruments capable of reaching only the rectum and sigmoid colon in most patients. Short instruments gave way to longer ones as the advantages of examining the entire colon became apparent. Short instruments were later reintroduced as flexible sigmoidoscopes. These instruments are 30 to 65 cm long, have a large-caliber suction channel and full control of tip direction, and permit torquing of the shaft by rotating the head of the instrument.[8] Fiberoptic viewing systems predominate in flexible sigmoidoscopy, but videoendoscopes probably will become the standard eventually.

Indications

Indications for flexible sigmoidoscopy are listed in Table 83–3.[6, 8, 9] Flexible sigmoidoscopy is superior to rigid proctosigmoidoscopy for screening of presumably normal populations for colon cancer or polyps because the flexible instrument examines more intestinal length.[8, 10, 11] Neoplastic lesions, mostly benign polyps, are found in about 10 per cent of flexible sigmoidoscopy procedures at an average cost of $1168 per patient with a neoplasm and $10,119 per patient with a malignant lesion.[12] This yield is two to six times greater than the yield of rigid proctosigmoidoscopy.[8, 9, 11, 12] Patient acceptance of flexible sigmoidoscopy is at least equal to that of rigid proctosigmoidoscopy, time required for examination is 5 to 6 minutes for rigid and 8 to 15 minutes for flexible, and complication rates are about the same[8] (see pp. 216–222). Costs of equipment and cleaning are substantially higher for flexible endoscopy.

Flexible sigmoidoscopes are manufactured in 30 to 35 cm and 60 to 65 cm lengths. The shorter instruments are more easily mastered, but the longer ones allow inspection of more colonic mucosa. Opinion varies over the optimal length.[8, 13–15] Perhaps non-endoscopists should use the 30 to 35 cm scopes, at least initially; endoscopists and others who become skilled with the short instruments will find the 60 to 65 cm sigmoidoscopes advantageous.

Flexible sigmoidoscopy detects only two thirds of polyps and two thirds of cancers of the colorectum, and fully 50 per cent of colon cancers located beyond the reach of the rigid colonoscope cannot be detected by the flexible sigmoidoscope either.[16] Total colonoscopy is indicated instead of or in addition to flexible sigmoidoscopy in circumstances listed in Table 83–4. Redundant procedures, such as flexible sigmoidoscopy followed by colonoscopy, can be avoided by careful planning.

Technique

Preparation for flexible sigmoidoscopy ordinarily consists of one or two phosphasoda (Fleet) enemas. The procedure is done in the office or clinic, usually with no sedation or anesthesia. The left lateral decubitus position is preferred by most endoscopists, but the prone jackknife position can also be used. The technique of advancement takes advantage of torque, which can be applied to the shaft and tip from the head of the instrument. Counterclockwise torque tends to cause a loop of the sigmoid colon, and clockwise rotation of the head applies torque that tends to straighten the sigmoid colon. These maneuvers are described in other texts on endoscopy.[6–8] Advancement of the tip of the instrument to the descending colon should be possible with the 60-cm instrument in 80 per cent of patients.[8]

If a neoplastic lesion is encountered, a biopsy should be taken, but polypectomy should not be done in most instances. There are two reasons for this restriction: (1) The preparation is inadequate for safe polypectomy; and (2) total colonoscopy is required for every patient with a polyp of the rectum or sigmoid colon, and polypectomy is best deferred until the time of colonoscopy.

Complications are described on pages 216 to 222.

Table 83–4. INDICATIONS FOR TOTAL COLONOSCOPY

Surveillance for neoplasms:
Previous polyps or cancer
Inflammatory bowel disease
Familial colon cancer syndromes
Rectal bleeding:
Occult blood
Acute severe hemorrhage
Radiographic lesion above sigmoid
Mapping of inflammatory bowel disease
Right-sided diverticular disease
Miscellaneous (volvulus, megacolon)

HEMORRHOIDS

Hemorrhoids are masses of vascular tissue in the anal canal. *Hemorrhoid* means bleeding, and *pile* means ball; despite the etymologic difference, these terms are used interchangeably by clinicians and the lay public.[1]

Internal hemorrhoids arise from the superior (internal) hemorrhoidal vascular plexuses above the pectinate line; they are covered by mucosa (Fig. 83–1). *External hemorrhoids* are dilatations of the inferior (external) hemorrhoidal plexuses; they lie below the pectinate line and are covered by anoderm and perianal skin. Symptoms rarely are attributable to external hemorrhoids alone. Because the two plexuses anastomose freely, many patients have a combination of both types (interoexternal or mixed hemorrhoids) (Color Fig. 83–6, p. xlii).

Small internal hemorrhoids that project a short way into the anal canal are called "first-degree." If they prolapse with defecation but reduce spontaneously, they are "second-degree." "Third-degree" hemorrhoids must be reduced manually, and "fourth-degree" hemorrhoids are irreducible.[1, 7, 17] Internal hemorrhoids occur in three primary positions around the anal circumference: right anterior, right posterior, and left lateral (Color Fig. 83–6, p. xlii). Smaller secondary (accessory) hemorrhoids can develop in the left posterior and left anterior sites.

Internal hemorrhoids are normal structures present at birth.[18, 19] Symptoms arising from hemorrhoids are more common with advancing age; 5 per cent of people in Western countries are symptomatic, but the prevalence of symptoms reaches 50 per cent after age 50.[1, 17] Men are afflicted more commonly than women.[17]

Pathogenesis

Traditionally hemorrhoids were believed to be varicosities of the hemorrhoidal veins caused by elevated portal venous pressure.[20] According to this view, because the superior hemorrhoidal veins contain no valves, pressure in them is chronically raised by the upright posture of humans, and the veins dilate. The rarity of hemorrhoids in quadrupeds, hemorrhoidal enlargement in patients with portal hypertension, and the high incidence of the disease in pregnancy were thought to support this concept.

Other observations do not fit with the notion that hemorrhoids are merely venous dilatations in response to pressure changes. Hemorrhoids often appear early in pregnancy, before the uterus is large enough to exert effects on pressure in the abdomen or in the pelvic veins; hormonal factors are probably important.[17] There is also the inescapable fact that hemorrhoidal bleeding is not the dark blood one would expect from congested veins; it is bright red—arterial—suggesting some sort of arteriovenous communication in hemorrhoids.[18]

Finally, although rectal varices can develop in patients with portal hypertension, the incidence of hemorrhoids is not increased.[20] Rectal varices arise several centimeters above the pectinate line, well proximal to the location of internal hemorrhoids (Fig. 83–1). Massive rectal bleeding in patients with portal hypertension often reflects coagulopathy.[20]

The most widely accepted concept today is that internal hemorrhoids are normal vascular *cushions* containing a rich arteriovenous network.[19] They are present at birth in three discrete masses, and they help plug the anus and thus contribute to continence.[18, 21] These vascular cushions project into the lumen, where they are subjected to downward pressure during defecation. The muscular fibers that anchor the cushions become attenuated, the hemorrhoids slide, they become congested and bleed, and eventually they prolapse.[18, 21] Although high anal sphincter pressures have been reported in patients with hemorrhoids, the importance of this observation is unclear; high pressures may be secondary to the presence of hemorrhoids, not contributory to their formation.[22]

Diagnosis

Bleeding is one cardinal symptom of hemorrhoids, and *prolapse* is the other. Blood appears as a bright red streak or spot on the toilet tissue or on the surface of the stool. Later, it may spurt at the height of straining or may drip from the anus for a few minutes after the stool has been expelled. Chronic blood loss may cause iron deficiency anemia.[1] When prolapse develops, the patient senses a mass protruding from the anus during defecation; it slips back spontaneously at first, but later it must be reduced manually, and still later it protrudes with walking, coughing, or other exertion. Eventually, the prolapsed tissue is irreducible. *Mucoid discharge* stains the underclothing when the hemorrhoids prolapse permanently. Mucous drainage irritates perianal skin and causes pruritus or discomfort. Pain is not a symptom of hemorrhoids unless they are complicated by thrombosis; most patients who complain of pain have another, coincidental anorectal lesion.

On examination, external hemorrhoids are visible in the subcutaneous tissue. Prolapsed internal hemorrhoids are separated by radial grooves, and moist red mucosa covers the upper portions of the masses (Color Fig. 83–6, p. xlii). Digital rectal examination allows evaluation of the tone of the sphincters—often increased in young men with hemorrhoids. First- and second-degree uncomplicated internal hemorrhoids are not palpable, and anoscopy is necessary to make the diagnosis. The hemorrhoids bulge into the lumen and may follow the instrument to the outside if the patient strains. Proctosigmoidoscopy or flexible sigmoidoscopy is required to detect neoplastic or inflammatory disease that may be responsible for the symptoms. Colonoscopy or barium enema X-rays may also be necessary. It is important that rectal bleeding not be attributed to hemorrhoids until other, more serious disease is excluded.

The differential diagnosis is not difficult. Mucosal prolapse, procidentia, anal skin tags, and thrombosed external hemorrhoids are discussed below. A hypertrophied anal papilla may prolapse; it is a whitish fibrous polypoid structure with a slender base at the pectinate line.

Complications

Prolapsed hemorrhoids can become acutely incarcerated from thrombosis and inflammation, causing severe pain that makes it difficult to sit or defecate (Color Fig. 83–7, p. xlii). This condition is sometimes called strangulated hemorrhoids.[7] One or all of the hemorrhoids may be affected. Pain results from edema of the sensitive external portions. Ulceration and secondary infection may supervene. Hepatic abscesses established by septic emboli from hemorrhoids are extremely rare.[1]

Treatment

Various methods of treatment of symptomatic hemorrhoids and the rationale for each are listed in Table 83–5. If current concepts of pathogenesis described above are correct, hemorrhoidal symptoms are preventable to some extent by avoidance of excessive downward pressure on the anal cushions. When symptoms develop, they should be treated by simple fixation methods to avoid further enlargement and prolapse of the hemorrhoids.[23] The value of methods of sphincter modification is controversial. Excision is reserved for symptomatic hemorrhoids that do not respond to fixation.

Table 83–5. TREATMENT OF INTERNAL HEMORRHOIDS

Rationale	Method
Reduce downward pressure	Diet, bulk agents Avoid prolonged sitting at stool

Fixation of cushions to underlying sphincter	Sclerosing injections
	Rubber band ligation
	Photocoagulation:
	  Infrared
	  Laser
	Electrocoagulation
	  Bipolar
	  Direct current
	Cryotherapy

Reduce sphincter pressure	Internal sphincterotomy Manual dilatation
Excision of hemorrhoids	Hemorrhoidectomy

Measures to Reduce Downward Pressure. Small symptomatic hemorrhoids should be treated with a high-fiber diet, with or without bulk agents in addition to food. The patient should respond to the urge to defecate as soon as possible, and prolonged sitting at stool should be avoided. Prolapse should be reduced by gentle pressure. Ointments and suppositories containing anesthetics, astringents, and emollients have limited value.

Fixation Methods. The common goal of these procedures is promotion of fibrosis between the hemorrhoidal cushions and the underlying internal sphincter to prevent sliding, congestion, and prolapse.

Sclerosing Injections. Injection of sclerosing solutions (e.g., 5 per cent phenol in vegetable oil) is effective for small bleeding internal hemorrhoids.[17, 23] The solution is injected submucosally into the loose areolar tissue of the hemorrhoid above the pectinate line to produce fibrosis and fixation.[1] The method is simple, painless, and inexpensive. Uncommon complications include slough of the overlying mucosa, infections, and reaction to the injected material.[24] Injections are successful in nearly all patients with first-degree hemorrhoids, and about 75 per cent of patients with second degree hemorrhoids have good results.[23] Third- and fourth-degree prolapsing hemorrhoids do not respond well to this method.

Rubber Band Ligation. Placement of rubber bands over the base of the hemorrhoid with a special apparatus causes necrosis and slough of the tissue in about seven days; ulceration and fibrosis tether the mucosa with the anal canal to prevent sliding. The hemorrhoid must be ligated at least 0.5 cm above the pectinate line; lower application is severely painful. This method is also simple, inexpensive, and painless if properly performed. Good results are obtained in 75 to 80 per cent of patients with first- or second-degree hemorrhoids and in about 65 per cent of those with third-degree hemorrhoids.[25] Fourth-degree prolapse is not suitable for rubber band ligation. Reports of fatal sepsis after rubber band ligation have caused some surgeons to abandon this method.[26] Others continue to use rubber band ligation, but the appearance of a triad of anal pain, urinary retention, and fever after banding calls for prompt, aggressive intervention.[27]

Photocoagulation. Infrared photocoagulation is relatively new.[28] Infrared light from a bulb is transmitted through a conducting system to a probe that is applied to the internal hemorrhoid. A white spot results from a thermal burn at the point of application. The therapeutic benefit derives from fibrosis. The method seems simple and uncomplicated, and discomfort is mild and transient. Equipment for infrared photocoagulation is more costly than that needed for injections or banding. Relief of hemorrhoidal symptoms is similar to the outcome of injections and banding.[29]

Laser photocoagulation can be used as a method of fixation. Strictures can result from excessive enthusiasm. High costs of equipment limit wide adoption of lasers for the treatment of hemorrhoids, since other equally effective methods are much cheaper.

Electrocoagulation. Thermal injury inflicted with a bipolar probe is a new fixation method.[30] Direct current applied to hemorrhoids through a needle-tipped probe probably acts as still another way to promote fibrosis.[31]

Cryosurgery. Application of a metal probe cooled by liquid nitrogen or carbon dioxide freezes hemorrhoids and probably acts as a fixation procedure rather than an excisional one. Imprecise control of the depth of destruction, postoperative pain, and prolonged profuse drainage are disadvantages. Cryotherapy has few proponents.[32]

Methods to Reduce Sphincter Pressure. The importance of elevated internal sphincter pressure in the pathogenesis of hemorrhoids is controversial, and therefore the value of methods to reduce sphincter pressure is open to question.[22]

Internal Sphincterotomy. Partial division of the internal sphincter lowers sphincter pressures and seems to relieve symptoms.[33] Few surgeons perform sphincterotomy, however, unless a fissure coexists.

Manual Dilatation. Vigorous stretching of the anus under anesthesia divulses the internal sphincter to an unpredictable extent. Although good results have been reported, the method has few proponents because of the possibility of permanent severe damage to the sphincters.[17]

Hemorrhoidectomy. Surgical excision of the three hemorrhoidal masses by a variety of techniques has the virtue of removing all redundant tissue, including the external components.[1, 2, 7, 17, 34] Disadvantages are pain, expense, length of hospitalization, and time lost from work. Postoperative complications, mainly anal stenosis, are uncommon following expert hemorrhoidectomy with careful follow-up. The value of hemorrhoidectomy depends on the objectives of treatment. Bleeding can be eliminated by most of the other methods, but only surgical excision removes the redundant tissue and external components. Recurrences are unusual.

Special Considerations. Acutely prolapsed, inflamed, thrombosed hemorrhoids can be treated by bed rest, cold compresses, analgesics, and bulk laxatives. Injection of a mixture of anesthetic and hyaluronidase often permits prompt reduction with immediate relief of pain.[17]

Hemorrhoids in pregnancy are best treated medically unless complications develop. Symptomatic hemorrhoids can be treated safely by fixation methods in patients with ulcerative colitis; Crohn's disease of the anorectum is a contraindication to any of the operative techniques.

THROMBOSED EXTERNAL HEMORRHOID

Thrombosed external hemorrhoid is a blood clot within subcutaneous hemorrhoidal veins. It occurs mainly in young adults as the result of heavy lifting, childbirth, straining to defecate, or other vigorous activity. A painful lump appears suddenly at the anus. Pain is constant, is aggravated by sitting and defecation, reaches peak intensity in two or three days, and disappears in about a week.[17] Bleeding from ulceration overlying the clot is sometimes noticed.

One or more tender, bluish, spherical masses, varying from a few millimeters to several centimeters in diameter, are present at the anal verge (Color Fig. 83–8, p. xlii). The overlying skin is tense and edematous; sometimes the skin is thin and ulcerated with partial extrusion of the clot. Thrombosed external hemorrhoids should not be confused with prolapsed, thrombosed (strangulated) internal hemorrhoids (Color Fig. 83–7, p. xlii). In the latter condition, reddish mucosa covers part of the mass; in thrombosed external hemorrhoid, the pectinate line is distinctly separate from the mass, and the rectal mucosa is still higher in the anal canal.

Analgesics, warm sitz baths, stool softeners, and topical emollients to minimize friction on walking should suffice if pain already has begun to wane. The lesion belongs in an external position and should not be forced into the anal canal. If the patient is seen within a day or two of the onset, speedy resolution is obtained by excising the thrombosed veins under local anesthesia. If clot has partially extruded, it may be simpler to evacuate the remaining clotted veins, but a skin tag may be left after resolution of inflammation. Recurrence at other sites is frequent, and, if the thrombosed veins are not excised, thrombosis may recur at the same site.

ANAL SKIN TAGS

Single or multiple tags of excess anal or perianal tissue of varying sizes are ubiquitous in the population. Idiopathic skin tags are pliable, soft, and covered by normal skin.[1] They may be residua of resolved thrombosed external hemorrhoids, pregnancy, or anal operations, but in many patients no apparent cause can be found. No treatment is indicated unless the tags interfere with hygiene; in that event, they can be excised. Secondary skin tags are related to other anorectal lesions. The sentinel pile associated with active fissure is edematous; it softens when the fissure heals. Perianal dermatitis causes thickened, edematous infected rugae. Secondary skin tags require treatment of the underlying disease.

ANAL FISSURE

Anal fissure (fissure-in-ano, anal ulcer) is a longitudinal elliptical or rounded defect in the anoderm, extending part or all of the way from the anal verge to the pectinate line. Fissures occur at any age but are most common in young and middle-aged adults. The posterior midline is the site of 98 per cent of fissures in men and 90 per cent of fissures in women.[1] The remainder are in the anterior midline. Fissures in other positions suggest underlying diseases such as Crohn's disease or carcinoma.

Most anal fissures are caused by the trauma of passing a large firm stool. Loss of elasticity of the anal canal due to scarring from previous anal surgery may predispose to fissure formation. Anal stenosis from other causes (e.g., chronic diarrheal diseases or laxative abuse) likewise makes injury from scybalous stools more likely.[2]

The predilection for the posterior midline is related to several factors.[1] Because of the configuration of the external sphincter, the posterior midline is deficient in muscular support. The acute angulation at the anorectal junction causes the fecal mass to impinge on the posterior area first, and therefore the anal canal is stretched more posteriorly than anteriorly.[35] The posterior crypt is very large, and chronic inflammation in the crypt tethers the anoderm to the underlying muscle and prevents it from gliding with passage of stool. Deficient muscular support posteriorly may play a role too.[1]

Acute fissures are merely tears, and many of them heal promptly. It is believed that fissures become chronic in patients with elevated resting anal pressures.[35, 36] Spasm of the internal sphincter during and immediately after defecation may not be as important as excessive basal tone.[36] Adherence of the edges of the fissure and ischemia of the anoderm from elevated sphincter pressure may account for pain and failure to heal.[1, 36]

Chronic fissure has a characteristic triad: (1) the fissure itself; (2) a hypertrophied anal papilla at the upper end of the fissure; and (3) a sentinel pile or tag at the lower end of the fissure at the anal verge (Fig. 83–9). The latter two features reflect edema and fibrosis of adjacent tissues.

Diagnosis

Pain is the chief symptom of anal fissure. A severe tearing or burning sensation, attributed to local irritation of the fissure, occurs with evacuation and subsides

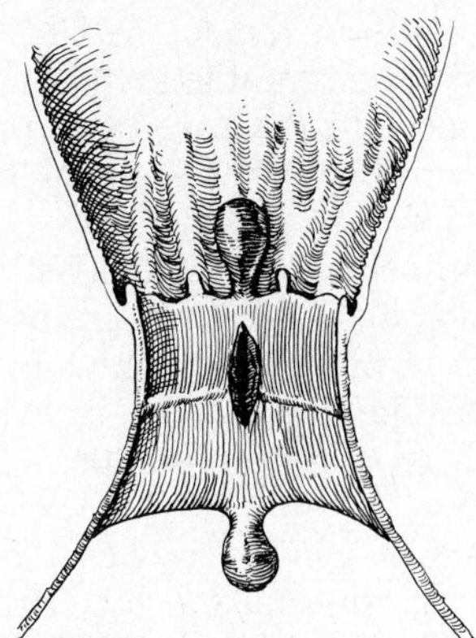

Figure 83–9. Diagram of the anorectum showing the fissure triad. (From Birnbaum, W. Anorectum. *In* Dunphy, J. E., and Way, L. W. [eds.]. Current Surgical Diagnosis and Treatment. Ed. 5. Los Altos, California, Lange Medical Publications; 1981. Used by permission.)

after a few minutes. Some patients also have another type of pain; it is a less severe gnawing discomfort that begins after a latent period of an hour and lasts for two to four hours. The secondary pain may be due to sphincter spasm, ischemia, or other mechanisms. The pain of fissure is so severe that patients fear defecation and may suppress the urge for days. A few spots of bright red blood on the toilet tissue, a mass at the anus (sentinel pile), discharge, and pruritus are other symptoms.

Fissures are extremely tender, and examination must be gentle. Many patients cannot tolerate digital rectal examination unless topical anesthetic is applied to the fissure. Fortunately, the diagnosis can be made by external inspection. An acute fissure is a superficial tear with a reddish base that bleeds easily. If the fissure is chronic, a sentinel pile may be evident as a swollen tag of skin at the anal verge, and gentle eversion of the anus reveals the fissure with the white transverse fibers of the internal sphincter exposed in the base. Digital rectal examination confirms the induration, tenderness, and sphincter spasm, and the hypertrophied anal papilla is palpable in some cases. It may be necessary to defer digital rectal, anoscopic, and proctosigmoidoscopic examinations.

Large or multiple fissures or lesions off the midline should raise the question of inflammatory bowel disease. Carcinoma, tuberculosis, syphilis, and other infectious diseases can cause fissures or ulcers in atypical sites. Immune-deficient patients have ulcers with necrotic margins and surrounding cellulitis.

Treatment

The aim of treatment is easier passage of stools, by changing stool consistency or by performing some procedure to allow the anal canal to dilate more easily during defecation.[35]

General Measures. Acute fissures may heal in four to eight weeks on a conservative regimen of bulk agents, sitz baths, and emollient suppositories.[17] Insertion of a small anal dilator coated with anesthetic lubricant, first by the physician and then by the patient, gives short-term improvement in 50 per cent of patients.[36] Injection of anesthetic followed by sodium tetradecyl sulfate into the base of the fissure brought relief of pain in 80 per cent of patients in a recent study.[37]

Surgical Treatment. Chronic anal fissures with a fully developed triad are unlikely to respond to medical treatment. The common denominator of the three surgical methods described below is division or disruption of the internal sphincter to improve anal stretching during defecation.

Excision (fissurectomy) removes the sentinel pile, the fissure, the crypt, and the hypertrophied papilla, and the lower portion of the internal sphincter is divided in the base of the fissure.[38] The wound may heal slowly, and some patients are left with a "keyhole" deformity of the anal verge that permits leakage of mucus and feces. Excision has been largely abandoned in favor of lateral sphincterotomy.[39]

Lateral subcutaneous sphincterotomy is performed under local or general anesthesia. The internal sphincter is divided up to the pectinate line through a tiny incision in the lateral position. The hypertrophied papilla and the sentinel tag may be excised, but the fissure is ignored; it heals in a few weeks. The long-term cure rate exceeds 95 per cent.[17] Minor defects in continence occur in up to 15 per cent of patients after sphincterotomy.[40] This technique is the treatment of choice for chronic fissure.

Manual dilatation of the anus consists of forceful stretching under anesthesia. The internal sphincter is probably divulsed in successful dilatations. Recurrent fissures as well as the risk of incontinence from uncontrolled tearing has relegated manual dilatation to a minor role in the view of most surgeons.[41]

ANORECTAL ABSCESS

Anorectal abscesses are infections of the tissue spaces in and adjacent to the anorectum. Patients with Crohn's disease, hematologic disorders, or other immune-deficient states are particularly susceptible to development of anorectal abscesses.[17] Infection arises in an anal fissure, prolapsed internal hemorrhoid, superficial skin lesion, or traumatic injury in a few people. In most patients, however, the infection apparently begins in an anal crypt, tracks along the anal ducts through the internal sphincter, and then spreads in various directions.[1, 2, 42] Some patients may develop abscesses through another, as yet unidentified, mechanism.[1]

Anorectal abscesses are classified according to their location in the anatomic spaces (Fig. 83–10). Perianal abscess, the most common, is just beneath the perianal skin.[43] Ischiorectal abscesses lie in the ischiorectal fossa. Intersphincteric abscesses are deep to the internal sphincter. Supralevator abscesses are found above the levators ani and below the pelvic peritoneum. Abscesses sometimes involve multiple compartments simultaneously.

Extension of the abscess is the most common complication. It usually is due to delayed diagnosis and treatment, but some necrotizing infections spread rapidly without regard for tissue planes (Fournier's gangrene[44]). Promptly treated abscesses heal, although 25 to 60 per cent of patients go on to develop anorectal fistulas.[17, 45, 46] Abscesses in immune-deficient patients can be lethal.

Diagnosis

Clinical findings depend upon the location and size of the abscess. Throbbing, constant pain exacerbated by sitting or walking is typical of superficial abscesses. Deeper abscesses may be insidious in onset, often with symptoms high in the rectum or even in the lower

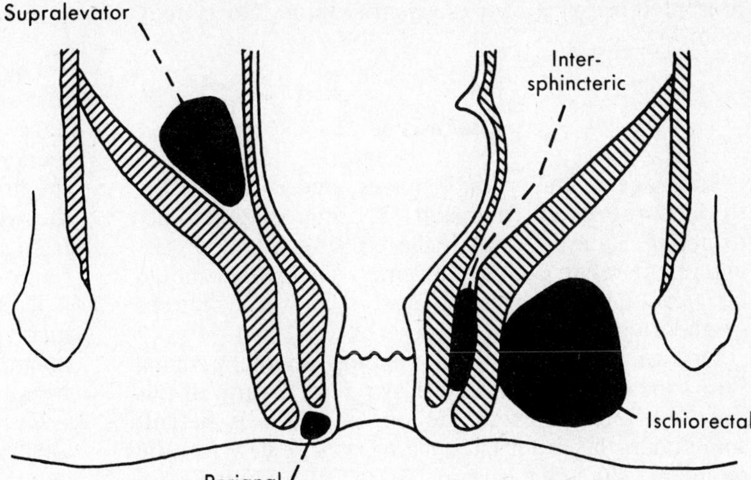

Figure 83–10. Classification of anorectal abscesses. (From Gordon, P. H. Management of anorectal abscesses and fistulous disease. *In* Kodner, I. J., Fry, R. D., and Roe, J. P. Colon, Rectal and Anal Surgery. St. Louis, 1986, The C. V. Mosby Co.)

abdomen.[1] Pain eases if the abscess ruptures and drains spontaneously. Fever is common with large abscesses.

An indurated, tender mass with overlying erythema displaces the anus in cases of superficial abscess. A deep abscess is not evident externally, but digital rectal examination identifies a tender mass in one of the anatomic spaces.

The differential diagnosis includes pilonidal sinus, hidradenitis suppurativa, carcinoma, Bartholin gland abscess, and various other rare conditions.[2]

Treatment

Prompt surgical drainage is the treatment for anorectal abscess. It is incorrect to assume that an abscess is not ready to drain because it is not fluctuant. With very rare exceptions (e.g., in immune-deficient patients), all these painful, tender masses in the anorectal anatomic spaces contain pus whether they are fluctuant or not. To defer drainage, with or without antibiotics, invites extension of the abscess, sometimes with catastrophic consequences.

Fistula tracts associated with abscesses may be incised when the abscess is drained if the anatomy is clear and the surgeon is experienced. Horseshoe abscesses require special care.[47] After drainage, the cavity is allowed to heal from its depths; premature closure of the skin over a persistent deep cavity must be avoided. Proctosigmoidoscopy, barium enema, and small bowel X-rays should be carried out in patients with diarrhea or other symptoms that suggest inflammatory bowel disease, particularly Crohn's disease.[17] Often, anorectal abscess is the presenting problem in such individuals (see pp. 1327–1346).

ANORECTAL FISTULAS

An *anorectal fistula* is a hollow fibrous tract lined by granulation tissue. It has an opening (primary or internal) inside the anal canal or rectum and one or more orifices (secondary or external) in the perianal skin. An anorectal sinus is similar but is blind at one end.

The primary opening is in a crypt at the pectinate line in most cases. The pathogenesis is believed to involve infection in a crypt, extension to form an abscess, rupture or surgical drainage of the abscess, and preservation of a tract as the abscess cavity heals.[1, 42, 43] Other fistulas develop from trauma, fissures, tuberculosis, Crohn's disease, carcinoma, radiation therapy, and chlamydial infections. Fistulas from the colon, small bowel, or urethra can exit through the perineum and mimic anorectal fistulas.

Goodsall's rule is a guide to classification of fistulas (Fig. 83–11). An imaginary line is drawn transversely through the center of the anus. Secondary openings anterior to this line arise from primary openings located radially in the anal canal. If the secondary opening is posterior to the transverse line, the fistula tract is curved, and the primary orifice is in the posterior midline.[17] Firm knowledge of the detailed classification

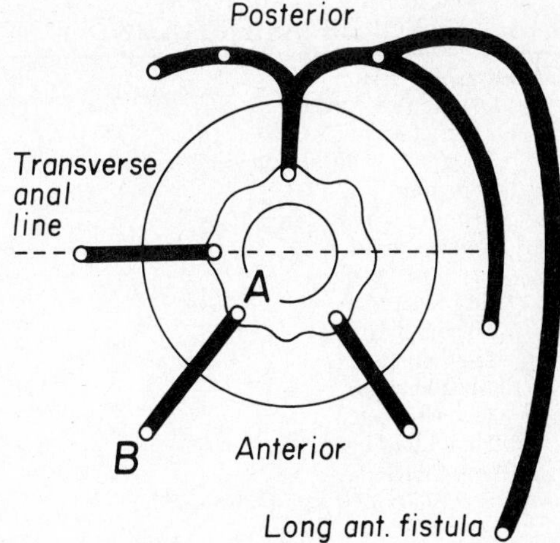

Figure 83–11. Goodsall's rule indicates the usual relationship of primary *(A)* and secondary *(B)* fistula orifices. The long anterior fistula is an exception to the rule. (From Schrock, T. R. *In* Fromm, D. [ed.]. Gastrointestinal Surgery. New York, Churchill Livingstone, 1985. Used by permission.)

presented in Table 83–6 is essential to operative treatment.[17, 43]

Diagnosis

Drainage of pus, blood, mucus, and, occasionally, stool is the chief complaint. Pruritus is sometimes troubling. Pain develops if the tract seals temporarily and relents when drainage resumes. The patient should be questioned for a history of abscess and for symptoms of underlying intestinal disease.

One or more secondary openings on the perianal skin appear as raised, reddish papules. A drop of pus can be expressed from the opening if it is patent; sometimes the external opening has sealed for the moment. The tract is palpable as an indurated cord from the secondary orifice toward the anus. Digital rectal examination helps determine the course of the tract.

Anoscopy reveals the primary opening, usually in a crypt, and a hooked probe can be inserted to confirm it. Probing of the tract externally is helpful at times but must be done cautiously. The relationship of the fistula to the anorectal ring is of paramount importance and is best evaluated in the unanesthetized patient. Proctosigmoidoscopy must be done routinely. Barium enema and X-rays of the upper gastrointestinal tract are indicated in selected patients. Fistulography is performed if the fistula is suspected to arise from the colon, small bowel, or urethra, but findings from this procedure can be very misleading.[48]

Hidradenitis suppurativa, pilonidal disease, and infected sebaceous cysts or Bartholin's glands mimic anorectal fistulas. There is no communication with the anal canal in these conditions, and the location and appearance of the lesions are characteristic. Complex fistulas should raise the suspicion of Crohn's disease (Color Fig. 83–12, p. xliii).[49]

Table 83–6. CLASSIFICATION OF ANORECTAL FISTULAS

Intersphincteric
Simple (low) tract
High blind tract
High tract with opening into lower rectum
Without a perineal opening
Pelvic extension
From pelvic disease
Transphincteric
Uncomplicated
High blind tract
Suprasphincteric
Uncomplicated
High blind tract
Extrasphincteric
Secondary to a transphincteric anal fistula
Due to trauma
Due to specific anorectal disease
Due to pelvic inflammation

After Parks, A. G., Gordon, P. H., and Hardcastle, J. D. Br. J. Surg. *63*:1, 1976.

Treatment

Untreated fistulas may cause systemic infection, and rare examples of carcinoma arising in chronic fistulas have been reported.[2] Surgical treatment is recommended, because few fistulas heal spontaneously. If the fistula is low, the overlying soft tissues are incised, the tract is curetted, and the defect is allowed to heal from its depths (fistulotomy).[2, 17, 42, 43, 50] High fistulas require special treatment.[51]

Definitive procedures for fistulas should not be performed in the presence of active anorectal inflammatory disease.[17] Failure of wound healing is the major complication in this setting.

Recurrent fistula after surgical treatment can be attributed to an overlooked primary opening, inadequate exposure of the tracts, or failure to ensure healing from the base outward.[42, 43] It may also be due to continuing inflammatory bowel disease, particularly Crohn's disease. Minor degrees of soiling or incontinence occur after treatment of fistulas. Gross incontinence is unusual but must be mentioned as a possibility to the patient.

RECTOVAGINAL FISTULA

Rectovaginal fistulas result most commonly from perineal injury during childbirth.[1] Crohn's disease (Color Fig. 83–12; p. xliii), carcinoma, radiation therapy, and other causes may be found.[52] Passage of flatus and sometimes feces through the vagina is unmistakable to the patient. Rectal fecal incontinence is present also if sphincter damage coexists. The fistula usually is evident on examination; most arise at the pectinate line and emerge through the distal vagina. Fistulotomy is *not* performed. Repair techniques are successful without the need for a preliminary colostomy in uncomplicated cases.[53]

PRURITUS ANI

Pruritus ani is itching of the perianal skin. It is a symptom, not a diagnosis, and the causes are many and varied.[7, 54] Leakage of stool onto perianal skin is the common denominator of most causes.[54] One etiologic classification is as follows:

1. *Anorectal diseases:* Fistulas, sinuses, fissures, skin tags, condylomata acuminata, hidradenitis suppurativa, and neoplasms can cause itching. Hemorrhoids do not produce pruritus unless they interfere with hygiene.
2. *Dermatologic diseases:* Psoriasis, seborrheic dermatitis, atopic eczema, lichen planus, and other skin disorders cause pruritus.[2]
3. *Contact dermatitis:* Topical application of ointments, deodorants, powders, soaps, suppositories, and the like can result in itching. Proprietary remedies used for the treatment of pruritus can make it worse.
4. *Infections:* Fungi, notably *Candida*, may cause itching, but because the organisms grow secondarily

on moist warm surfaces, the etiologic relationship is difficult to prove. Bacterial infection similarly may be the consequence of scratching rather than the primary cause of the itch.

5. *Parasites:* Pinworms, trichomonads, scabies, and pediculosis cause pruritus.

6. *Oral antibiotics:* Tetracyclines, erythromycins, and lincomycin are associated with pruritus ani, perhaps because of overgrowth of *Candida*, but more likely stemming from the frequent, loose, irritating stools that develop in many people who ingest these drugs.[1, 2, 54]

7. *Systemic disease:* Diabetes mellitus and liver disease may cause perianal itching.

8. *Hygiene:* Poor hygiene or excessively zealous hygiene leads to pruritus. Frequent applications of soap, an alkaline irritant, and vigorous rubbing are important factors.[54]

9. *Warmth and moisture:* Tight clothing, hot climate, obesity, and vigorous exercise promote perianal warmth and perspiration.

10. *Dietary:* Beverages such as coffee, tea, cola, milk, beer, and wine have been associated with pruritus, and foods (tomatoes, citrus fruits, chocolate, and others) also have been implicated.[2, 7, 54]

11. *Psychogenic:* Anxiety and perhaps the erogenous nature of the perianal skin are psychologic factors related to development of pruritus or the failure to cure it in some people.

12. *Idiopathic:* In many patients, pruritus is categorized as idiopathic because no specific cause can be identified. Soiling is the likely mechanism, however, in most of these patients.[54]

Diagnosis

Pruritus ani may affect only one part of the perianal area initially; in severe cases, it often spreads to involve the entire perineum and vulva or scrotum. Itching is worse at night, regardless of the cause, and the relief obtained by scratching is only transient. The physician should inquire about bowel habits, hygienic practices, antibiotics, topical medications, types of clothing, dietary associations, pruritus elsewhere, and so on, to explore the list of possible causes.

Examination may disclose no abnormality whatsoever, especially in early cases. Erythema and edema of the skin is a common finding, and in chronic pruritus the perianal skin is moist, macerated, lichenified, fissured, and excoriated. Anorectal diseases that cause pruritus are listed above; these conditions should be apparent on examination.

Dermatologic diseases should be kept in mind as the anus is inspected, and biopsy should be performed if there is any question about the diagnosis. *Psoriasis* is the most commonly overlooked dermatologic cause of pruritus ani.[7] Typical psoriatic lesions are red plaques with shiny scales; the adjacent buttocks, the elbows, the knees, and the scalp should be examined. *Seborrheic dermatitis* in the perianal area often is associated with characteristic seborrhea on the scalp, face, and trunk. *Atopic eczema* usually involves the flexor surfaces of the elbows and knees as well as the anal skin. The lesions of *lichen planus* are violaceous flattened papules; lichen planus also ordinarily affects multiple sites. *Contact dermatitis* is suspected from the history.

Candidiasis and other fungal infections are diagnosed by mixing scrapings with 10 per cent potassium hydroxide solution, warming it, and examining the preparation microscopically. As mentioned above, it is difficult to prove that fungi are the primary cause of pruritus.

In *scabies,* the characteristic lesions are present also between the fingers and on the volar surfaces of the wrists. *Pediculosis pubis* is diagnosed when nits or the lice themselves are seen. *Pinworms (Enterobius vermicularis)* are seen occasionally on proctoscopy, and the eggs are detected by having the patient press transparent adhesive tape to the anal skin on awakening in the morning and then placing the tape on a glass slide for examination.

Treatment

The treatment is based upon a careful history and physical examination to determine the cause of pruritus in the individual patient. Specific therapy is used for systemic, dermatologic, malignant, anorectal, fungal, or parasitic disease. The majority of patients have none of these problems, however, and a more general program must be outlined.[2, 54]

All current antibiotics and topical agents must be stopped. Diet is modified if certain foods or beverages are contributory. Laxatives are discontinued, and a hygroscopic (bulk) agent is prescribed, together with reduced intake of liquids, if stools are loose. Tight underclothing, elastic girdles, and heavy bedclothing should be avoided; boxer shorts are preferable to the jockey type in men. Cleansing after defecation is best accomplished with moist cotton followed by gentle drying with a soft cloth or a hair dryer.[2, 54] Nonmedicated talcum powder is useful to combat moisture. Calamine lotion or other preparation with a weakly acidic pH is applied instead in more severe cases. Refractory patients benefit from 1 per cent hydrocortisone cream applied sparingly four times daily.[54] Patients are counseled to keep this medication at the bedside and to rub a bit of the cream into the skin instead of scratching when nocturnal itching occurs. Reassurance is essential in all cases, and sedatives or antihistamines may be needed in exceptional cases.[2]

The prognosis of pruritus ani is good, although a few patients seem refractory to all treatment. Surgical procedures of various kinds have been advocated, but patients who might benefit from these drastic measures are rare indeed.

ANAL STENOSIS

The anal canal may be stenosed congenitally, but more often the problem is an acquired subepithelial annular narrowing.[17] Anorectal operations, diarrheal diseases, inflammatory conditions (e.g., fissure), and habitual use of laxatives, especially mineral oil, are common causes of acquired anal stenosis. Chlamydial infections and malignancy must be excluded. Patients complain of small-caliber stools, difficult and incomplete evacuation, and pain and bleeding if the unyielding anoderm tears. Treatment with dietary bulk agents and graded anal dilatations suffices in many people. If this fails, operation is required.[55]

SEXUALLY TRANSMITTED DISEASES

Sexually transmitted diseases of the anorectum are discussed very briefly here and in more detail on pages 1242 to 1280. Homosexually active men have a high incidence of anorectal, colonic, and enteric infections.[56] The term "gay bowel syndrome" refers to a list of conditions, mostly sexually transmitted infections, that occur in this population.[57] Polymicrobial involvement is common; perhaps 40 per cent of asymptomatic homosexual men harbor transmissible pathogens.[58, 59]

Condylomata Acuminata

Condylomata acuminata (singular: condyloma acuminatum) are warts caused by human papillomaviruses, usually types 6 and 11.[60] Condylomata can occur on the perianal skin of people who have no anal sexual contact, but inoculation of the virus into the anal canal is believed to require sexual intercourse. Condylomata also may affect the penis, vulva, or vagina. Genital and oral condylomata are probably caused by identical viruses.

Condylomata are small discrete excrescences initially. They gradually enlarge to form confluent exophytic masses on the perianal skin and in the anal canal.[2] They may extend above the pectinate line for 1 cm or so but rarely involve the rectum above that level. Pruritus, bleeding, and difficulty with hygiene are common symptoms.

Small external lesions are treated by topical application of 25 per cent podophyllin in tincture of benzoin. Podophyllin ulcerates normal skin, and for this reason it is unwise to apply the material to warts within the anal canal. The patient should bathe to remove the podophyllin six to eight hours after treatment.[2] Topical bichloracetic acid may be effective in the anal canal. Surgical excision or destruction by laser photocoagulation or cryotherapy can be used for large or recurrent lesions and for warts in the anal canal.[7, 17] Intralesional injection of human leukocyte interferon alpha-2b was effective for genital warts in a recent study, and experimental work with other interferons is underway.[60]

There is an association between papillomavirus and squamous cell carcinoma of the cervix, vulva, and anus.[61, 62] If cancer is suspected, biopsy should be obtained before podophyllin is applied, because this drug causes cytologic changes mimicking malignancy.

Giant condyloma acuminatum (Buschke-Lowenstein tumor) is a locally aggressive but histologically benign variant of this disease. It requires wide excision.[7]

Gonococcal Proctitis

Gonococcal proctitis involves the mucosa of the upper anal canal and the rectum; the anoderm-lined lower portion is spared. Pain, frequent defecation, and bloody purulent discharge are the symptoms. Proctoscopy reveals injected, edematous, friable mucosa with minute erosions and ulcerations; thick pus sometimes exudes from the crypts. Cultures should be obtained on modified Thayer-Martin medium, but treatment may be warranted even if cultures are negative (see p. 1264).[7]

Syphilis

The primary lesion of anorectal syphilis is an ulcer that resembles an anal fissure. Symptoms are mild, and the lesion heals in three to four weeks. Secondary lesions are multiple plaques with a wet odorous discharge. The diagnosis is based on suspicion and investigation with darkfield examination and serologic tests.

Chlamydia Trachomatis Proctitis

Chlamydia trachomatis is the most common sexually transmitted bacterial pathogen in the United States.[63] Lymphogranuloma venereum (LGV) is proctitis caused by three immunotypes of this organism.[64] It may resemble Crohn's disease because of the formation of granulomas, strictures, and abscesses. Non-LGV immunotypes may cause asymptomatic infection or very mild inflammation.[64] Tetracycline (500 mg four times a day for two to three weeks) is the treatment in most cases.

Other Diseases

Chancroid forms anorectal papules that rupture and ulcerate.[7] The lesions of granuloma inguinale are progressively enlarging papulovesicles or granulating ulcers. Herpes simplex of the HSV-1 or HSV-2 variety produces typical vesicles or ulcers in the anal canal or perianal skin.[65] *Entamoeba histolytica* is found commonly in stools of homosexual men, but it is probably commensal and not a pathogen in most instances.[66, 67] Many other enteric diseases are transmitted by anorectal sexual contact.[56, 57]

RECTAL FOREIGN BODIES AND RECTAL TRAUMA

A wide array of foreign objects are introduced into the anus by accident, for erotic purposes, for concealment, for self-treatment, or by assault.[68–71] Thermometers, enema catheters, vibrators, bottles, phallic objects, and even fists are used. If the anus is torn during insertion or by attempts to extract the object, pain and bleeding occur. Complications may include perforation of the rectum or the colon as well as obstruction and pararectal infections. Rarely, foreign bodies enter the rectum by ingestion or by erosion from adjacent viscera.[17]

Not all patients volunteer the information that a foreign body was inserted, and the unwary physician may make an erroneous diagnosis of fissure or bleeding hemorrhoids. Foreign objects can be palpated in most instances, but anteroposterior and lateral radiographs are required to document the size, shape, and position of the object.

Removal of foreign bodies is difficult, because the sphincters tighten, trapping the slippery object in the rectal ampulla where it is difficult to grasp. Although general suggestions can be made, the removal of foreign bodies from the rectum must be individualized, and much depends on ingenuity in devising methods for especially difficult situations.[17, 69, 70] Small foreign objects can be removed using an anoscope or sigmoidoscope without anesthesia. Larger objects require local or even regional or general anesthesia.[69, 70] The lithotomy position is preferable to the prone jackknife position, because a hand can be placed on the abdomen to increase intra-abdominal pressure in a supine patient.

Under anesthesia, the anus is gently dilated, and an attempt is made to grasp the foreign body. If the object cannot be grasped or palpated and the radiographs suggest that it resides in the rectum, pressure by the operator's hand on the patient's abdomen or the Valsalva maneuver by the patient may move the object within reach. An object that can be palpated but not extracted requires one of various special techniques. If the caliber of the foreign body is not large, it can be extracted through the anus without dividing the sphincters. Obstetric forceps, a Foley balloon catheter passed above the foreign object, grasping instruments such as a wrench or pliers, and other ingenious techniques have all been used to good advantage in this situation. If a flexible endoscope can be negotiated to a point proximal to the object, insufflation of air may break the suction effect of glass jars or bottles and thus facilitate removal. Laparotomy is required in some patients.

After the object is extracted, proctosigmoidoscopy should be done to search for retained objects and rectal injury.[69] Perforation of the colon or rectum, of course, requires prompt operative intervention.[17, 68–70]

HIDRADENITIS SUPPURATIVA

Hidradenitis suppurativa is a chronic, indolent inflammatory disease of the apocrine glands in the axillae, breasts, groins, genitalia, and anal areas of adults.[72] Recurrent abscesses, chronic draining sinuses, and indurated, scarred skin and subcutaneous tissues are typical. The appearance can be distinguished fairly easily from complex anorectal fistulas. Wide excision and coverage with split-thickness skin grafts or full-thickness flaps often are necessary.

PILONIDAL DISEASE

Pilonidal disease is acquired in the gluteal cleft. Most authorities believe that penetration of hair beneath the skin is the primary event, but enlargement of hair follicles has been proposed as the initial problem.[73] One or several openings are seen in the midline over the sacral region. Hair is present in the sinus tracts and often protrudes from the openings. Pilonidal disease is differentiated from anorectal fistula by its appearance and location, the absence of tracts leading to the anus, and the lack of a primary opening in the anorectum. Treatment consists of incision and evacuation of hair and granulation tissue, avoiding new incisions in the midline, if possible.[73] Refractory cases may require excision and coverage with full-thickness flaps of various kinds. Carcinoma has been reported to occur in chronic pilonidal sinuses.

DISORDERS OF THE PELVIC FLOOR

Recent research has led to the concept of disorders of the pelvic floor, a group of conditions arising wholly or in part from abnormal structure or function of the levators ani and anal sphincter muscles.[74] Table 83–7 is one list of these conditions. The inclusion of hemorrhoids is arguable (see above). Anal fissure was discussed separately above. Constipation is discussed on pages 331 to 368 and will not be described here. Fecal incontinence is discussed on pages 317 to 331, but additional comments are made below.

Anal Incontinence

The causes of anal incontinence are many (Table 83–8). The clinician should determine the severity of incontinence. Partial incontinence is occasional loss of flatus or loose stool; major incontinence is deficient control of stool of normal consistency.[74] A detailed history may reveal the cause or at least provide clues.

Examination may disclose soiling of the skin; scars,

Table 83–7. DISORDERS OF THE PELVIC FLOOR

Hemorrhoids
Anal incontinence
Solitary rectal ulcer syndrome
Descending perineum syndrome
Rectal prolapse
Anal fissure
Constipation
Chronic anal pain syndromes

Table 83–8. CAUSES OF ANAL INCONTINENCE

Normal Sphincters and Pelvic Floor
- Diarrhea
- Fistula

Abnormal Function of Sphincters and/or Pelvic Floor
- Partial incontinence
  - Deficient internal sphincter
    - Trauma
    - Rectal prolapse
    - Third-degree hemorrhoids
  - Fecal impaction
    - Elderly
    - Neurologic disorders
  - Minor external sphincter and pelvic floor denervation
- Major incontinence
  - Congenital anomalies
  - Trauma
  - Complete rectal prolapse
  - Rectal carcinoma
  - Anorectal infection
  - Idiopathic
  - Drug intoxication
  - Neurologic
  - Upper motor neuron
    - Cerebral
    - Spinal
  - Lower motor neuron

Modified from Henry, M. M., and Swash, M. (eds.). Coloproctology and the Pelvic Floor. Pathophysiology and Management. Boston, Butterworths, 1985.

deformity, and gaping of the anus are present in some patients. Absence of the cutaneous anal reflex suggests a neurologic lesion.[74] Anal tone, structural integrity of sphincters, and ability to contract are noted on digital rectal examination. Proctosigmoidoscopy and abdominal examination are required. Special investigations include anorectal manometry and electromyography.[74–77]

The underlying systemic or intestinal disorder, if any, is treated. Loose stools are managed with bulk fiber and constipating agents. Elderly patients who soil because of fecal impaction may need regular laxatives or enemas.[74, 78] Electrical stimulators have been generally unsuccessful.[74] Biofeedback may succeed in patients with organic neuromuscular sensory or motor impairment of sphincter function.[74, 79]

Surgical intervention (sphincteroplasty) is successful for repair of traumatically disrupted sphincters.[17, 80–82] Severe injuries with loss of sphincter substance may require gracilis or gluteus muscle transposition.[7, 74] Selected patients with incontinence but structurally intact sphincters benefit from postanal repair.[74, 83]

Solitary Rectal Ulcer Syndrome

Solitary rectal ulcer syndrome is a chronic benign condition characterized by anal pain, passage of blood and mucus per rectum, and excessive straining to defecate.[74, 84] It affects mainly young adults, women more commonly than men.[74] The syndrome probably has multiple causes, but rectal mucosal prolapse is a common denominator in many cases.[74, 84–86] Excessive straining to defecate can force the anterior rectal mucosa downward, causing damage by ischemia or direct trauma.[74]

Patients have rectal bleeding with no diagnostic pattern.[74] Anal pain is also variable in frequency and severity.[84] Patients describe the defecation disorder as constipation, diarrhea, straining, or a sensation of anal blockage.[74, 87] On digital rectal examination, the anterior rectal mucosa 6 to 10 cm above the anal verge is indurated, and inspection by proctosigmoidoscopy may disclose a shallow ulcer with a zone of surrounding inflammation.[74, 84, 85] An ulcer is not always present, but the mucosa is abnormal in appearance and to the touch. True rectal prolapse is found in up to 60 per cent of patients.[88]

Biopsies confirm the diagnosis. Colitis cystica profunda is a complication of the syndrome in which glands are seen in the submucosa[74, 87] (see pp. 1603–1605). Carcinoma has been diagnosed erroneously in these cases.[74] Anorectal manometric studies and defecography may be helpful.[84–87]

Solitary rectal ulcer syndrome rarely is complicated by severe hemorrhage, and malignant degeneration is unknown, but current methods of therapy are disappointing and patients generally live with the condition. Medical treatment is directed toward avoidance of straining to defecate. Education of the patient, bulk agents, and witch hazel suppositories may help.[74] Surgical treatment of mucosal prolapse gives unsatisfactory results. Patients with true rectal prolapse benefit from posterior proctopexy.[88] Radical excision of the rectum is virtually never necessary.[74]

Descending Perineum Syndrome

Abnormal descent of the anal canal below a line joining the pubic symphysis and the tip of the coccyx results in effacement of the anorectal angle and anterior rectal mucosal prolapse as described above for solitary ulcer syndrome.[74] Patients with descending perineum syndrome, mostly women, complain of a sense of incomplete evacuation and a constant desire to defecate because they are, in effect, attempting to evacuate their own rectal mucosa. Overt mucosal or hemorrhoidal prolapse may occur with prolonged straining, and fecal incontinence may develop from chronic stretching of the pudendal nerves.[74, 89]

The diagnosis may be made if the patient strains and the plane of the perineum balloons downward below a line connecting the ischial tuberosities.[74] Treatment measures include education, bulk agents, and local excision or fixation of the prolapsing mucosa. Unfortunately, the condition frequently is resistant to these manipulations.

Rectal Prolapse

Rectal prolapse is protrusion of some or all layers of the rectal wall through the anus.[1, 2, 74] Partial prolapse is protrusion of the mucosa alone. Complete rectal prolapse (procidentia) is sometimes categorized as follows:[74]

First degree: protrusion of the full thickness of the rectum, including the mucocutaneous junction.

Second degree: complete prolapse without involvement of the mucocutaneous junction.

Third degree: concealed or internal prolapse in which the rectum intussuscepts but does not present through the anus.

The incidence of procidentia is sixfold higher in women than in men.[2] Prolapse occurs in infants, becomes uncommon in childhood and early adulthood, and appears with increasing frequency after age 40. Many patients are in the very advanced age groups.

Prolapse usually is a transient phenomenon in infants.[90] The absence of an angle at the anorectal junction, so that the rectum and anal canal form a straight tube, is probably responsible.[1] The problem corrects itself with growth and development. In adults, prolapse tends to persist and worsen. Surgical and other traumatic injuries are causative in a few patients. Laxity of the pelvic musculature as a result of aging or neurologic diseases may contribute to procidentia in some patients. Structural or physiologic abnormalities of the rectum itself may be present, and excessive straining at stool probably plays a role in at least 50 per cent of cases. The pathology anatomy involves a complex set of abnormalities that include diastasis of the levator ani, an abnormally deep cul-de-sac, redundancy of the sigmoid colon, a patulous anal sphincter, and loss of the horizontal position of the rectum as well as its sacral attachments.[74]

Diagnosis

In children, prolapse during defecation, sometimes with passage of blood or mucus, is noted by the mother. Adults have two types of symptoms: the prolapse itself and the associated impairment of continence. A mass protrudes with defecation and reduces spontaneously initially, but eventually it prolapses with standing and is difficult to reduce. Mucous discharge and bleeding from irritation of the exposed mucosa are common. Incontinence may be partial or complete. Patients with large prolapse do not experience the normal urge to defecate; by straining vigorously, small fecal pellets are passed several times a day and may fall from the rectum with ambulation.[1] Laxatives produce liquid stools that are uncontrollable. Symptoms of internal rectal prolapse (intussusception) seem identical to the symptoms of descending perineum syndrome: excessive straining to defecate, often with little result, and a sense of incomplete evacuation.[91–93]

It is important to perform examination with the patient squatting; some prolapses can be demonstrated or their full extent appreciated only in this position. Mucosal prolapse is a small symmetric projection 2 to 4 cm long. Radial folds are apparent, and palpation between finger and thumb reveals only two layers of mucosa. The sphincters are normal in children and usually lax in adults with mucosal prolapse.

Long-standing procidentia nearly always is associated with lax sphincters and a gaping anal orifice as the buttocks are retracted.[94] The integrity of the sphincters and the ability of the patient to contract them should be assessed. Procidentia protrudes as much as 12 cm from the anus.[1] The mucosal folds are concentric, and the lumen points posteriorly because of the presence of small bowel and omentum in the pouch of Douglas on the anterior wall. Palpation confirms the large mass of tissue anteriorly, and two thicknesses of rectal wall are palpable elsewhere around the circumference.

Proctosigmoidoscopy may show mucosal erythema in the prolapsing segment. A barium enema radiograph should be obtained to exclude associated neoplasia and to determine the length and redundancy of the sigmoid colon. Radiographs of the spine and pelvis may be needed if a neurologic abnormality is suspected. If available, manometric and electromyographic studies and defecography can be useful.[91, 93, 94]

Treatment

Prolapse in children is treated conservatively.[90] Correction of constipation, instruction not to strain for prolonged periods, defecation in a recumbent position, and strapping the buttocks together between bowel movements are useful measures.[1] Operative correction is necessary only in children with mental retardation, neurologic diseases, or incarcerated procidentia.

Mucosal prolapse in adults is managed by fixation or excision as described in the discussion of hemorrhoids (see p. 1578).

Procidentia, however, requires surgical correction as soon as the diagnosis is made.[95] Persistent prolapse further weakens the sphincters and makes restoration of normal function difficult or impossible.[94] Aged and infirm patients are treated by encircling the sphincters with a strip of polypropylene (Marlex) mesh, silicone rubber, or Silastic in a sheet or rod[17, 96] (Thiersch procedure). This simple operation requires only two tiny incisions in the perineum. Erosion and infection are troublesome complications.

Various perineal reconstructions are available, but they have been largely supplanted by transabdominal posterior proctopexy with or without sigmoid resection. In posterior proctopexy, the rectum is mobilized and fixed to the sacrum with sutures or a sling of Teflon or Marlex mesh or polyvinyl (Ivalon) sponge.[2, 17, 74] This operation, sometimes called the Ripstein procedure, is successful in 90 per cent or more of cases and is well tolerated by all but the poorest-risk patients.[2, 17, 74, 97] Resection of the sigmoid colon is added if the colon is very redundant and if the patient is in excellent condition.[95] Persistent incontinence despite permanent reduction of the prolapse mars the results in 40 to 50 per cent of elderly patients. Operative procedures to strengthen the attenuated sphincters may be tried, but results are often disappointing.

Chronic Anal Pain Syndromes

Anal or perianal pain usually has an obvious cause such as abscess or fissure. Perianal pain without an apparent cause can be disabling. Table 83–9 lists features of four perianal pain syndromes.[74] Descending perineum syndrome was discussed above.

Proctalgia Fugax (Levator Syndrome)

Proctalgia fugax is episodic rectal pain of varying severity. Some authorities prefer the term *levator syndrome* to explain that spasm of the levator muscles is the cause of pain, but it is not entirely clear that levator spasm is responsible for all cases of functional rectal discomfort.[98] Pain may result from contractions of the sigmoid colon, implying that proctalgia fugax is a variant of the irritable bowel syndrome.[74] Most patients with proctalgia fugax have a normal examination except for spasm and tenderness of the levator ani and coccygeus muscles.

Warm baths, diathermy, and massage of the involved levator muscle may be helpful. High voltage electrogalvanic stimulation of the levator ani by means of an intra-anal probe gave good to excellent results in 90 per cent of patients in one series.[98]

Coccygodynia

Coccygodynia is throbbing or aching pain in the coccygeal region. Organic causes include fracture of the coccyx and traumatic arthritis of the sacrococcygeal joint.[2] Functional coccygodynia has no definable cause, although prolonged sitting on soft surfaces has been implicated.[2]

Examination discloses pain with motion of the coccyx, sometimes associated with spasm and tenderness of the adjacent muscles. Conservative treatment (bed rest, warm baths) may suffice. Local anesthetic injections are helpful in some cases. Occasional patients with organic coccygodynia benefit from coccygectomy.

Chronic Idiopathic Anal Pain

This syndrome has features that overlap with the others.[74] Pelvic floor muscular spasm does not seem to be a factor. The cause is obscure and treatment disappointing.[74]

MALIGNANT TUMORS OF THE ANUS

Epidermoid Carcinoma

Epidermoid carcinomas of the anus constitute about 2 per cent of cancers of the large bowel.[99, 100] Although various histologic types are described (e.g., squamous cell, basal cell, basaloid squamous, cloacogenic), the histologic pattern is relatively unimportant to the clinician.[99, 101, 102] Management depends on the location of the tumor, the depth of invasion, and the presence or absence of metastases.[99–102] These tumors extend directly into sphincters, perianal tissues, vagina, and prostate. They metastasize upward through lymphatics of the rectum as well as downward to lymph nodes in the groin. Hematogenous spread occurs by way of the portal system, the systemic veins, or both, depending on the location of the lesion. Predisposing causes include chronic inflammation (fissure, fistula, venereal disease) and irradiation. Epidermoid cancer is more common in women; the mean age of onset is in the sixth decade. Recently, however, an association between male homosexual behavior and anal carcinoma has been reported.[61, 62] Condylomata acuminata may become malignant[103] (see p. 1271).

Bleeding, pain, and a mass are the usual symptoms; pruritus, drainage, and change in bowel habits also occur. The size and exact location of the tumor and

Table 83–9. CHRONIC PERIANAL PAIN SYNDROMES

Syndrome	Age of Onset	Sex Predominance	Nature of Pain	Site	Time of Onset	Aggravating Factors	Relieving Factors	Associated Features
Proctalgia fugax	Young adults	M	Sudden, crescendo, lasts minutes, stops spontaneously	Upper anal canal, constant site	Mostly at night	Anxiety	Stretching anus, flexing thighs	Tense introspective personality; irritable bowel syndrome
Coccygodynia	Adults	F	Continuous vague ache with exacerbations	Lower sacrum, perineum and anal canal, thighs, and coccyx	Any time, more during the day	Sitting posture?, defecation?, trauma to coccyx	—	Tender spots in sacrococcygeal region, levator muscle spasm
Descending perineum syndrome	Any age?	F	Constant heavy dull perineal ache, some with brief sharp pain	Perineum and anal canal	Usually late in the day	Standing, walking, after defecation	Lying down	Irregular bowel habit, straining at stool
Chronic idiopathic anal pain	50s	F	Continuous dull throbbing, burning likened to a ball in the anal canal, intermittent or continuous	Mid-anal canal, well localized, may be unilateral; radiates to abdomen, thighs, sacrum, vagina	Any time, usually late in the day	Sitting	Lying down	Pelvic or spinal surgery, myelography, perineal descent

Modified from Henry, M. M., and Swash, M. (eds.). Coloproctology and the Pelvic Floor. Pathophysiology and Management. Boston, Butterworths, 1985.

the depth of invasion should be determined (Color Fig. 83–13, p. xliii). The presence of metastases should be noted. Nearly a third of epidermoid cancers are mistakenly diagnosed as benign lesions until biopsy proves otherwise.

Small lesions in the perianal skin and in the anoderm well below the pectinate line are treated by local excision or irradiation if they do not infiltrate the sphincters or the rectovaginal septum. For large invasive tumors and for those that involve the pectinate line, excellent results are often achieved from radiation therapy with or without chemotherapy (usually mitomycin C and 5-fluorouracil) followed by appropriate surgery; abdominoperineal resection is not required if the tumor responds dramatically.[99, 103–105] Inguinal metastases are treated by radiation therapy or lymph node dissection. Overall five-year survival rates of 60 per cent are expected.[100, 102, 104, 105]

Other Tumors

Malignant melanoma is a rare pigmented or amelanotic lesion that may resemble a thrombosed hemorrhoid or mucosal polyp. It causes trivial symptoms, metastasizes early, and is highly lethal.[106] The treatment is wide local excision or abdominoperineal resection.[106] *Mucinous adenocarcinoma* arises in the anal glands and causes recurrent anorectal fistulas. Abdominoperineal resection is necessary for this rare tumor. Anogenital *Bowen's disease* is a chronic squamous cell carcinoma in situ. Pruritus ani is the usual symptom. Macular, fissured, or ulcerated lesions should be biopsied to establish the diagnosis (Color Fig. 83–14, p. xliii). Wide excision or laser photocoagulation is advised, because Bowen's disease can progress to invasive cancer. There is no evidence to substantiate the earlier claim that Bowen's disease presages the development of internal malignancy (i.e., involving cervix, ovary, lung, breast, stomach, or other organs).[107] Extramammary *Paget's disease* is an intraepithelial mucinous adenocarcinoma, which probably arises in the subepidermal apocrine glands and involves the epidermis secondarily.[108] Grossly it resembles many other dermatologic lesions, and the diagnosis is made by biopsy. Wide excision is the treatment of choice.[108] It tends to recur locally, and it is capable of metastasis.

References

1. Goligher, J. C. Surgery of the Anus, Rectum and Colon. 5th ed. London, Bailliere Tindall, 1984.
2. Goldberg, S. M., Gordon, P. H., and Nivatvongs, S. Essentials of Anorectal Surgery. Philadelphia, J. B. Lippincott Co., 1980.
3. Nivatvongs, S., Stern, H. S., and Fryd, D. S. The length of the anal canal. Dis. Colon Rectum *24*:600, 1981.
4. Huber, A., von Hochstetter, A., and Allgöwer, M. Anatomy of the pelvic floor for translevatoric-transsphincteric operations. Am. Surg. *53*:247, 1987.
5. Guinan, P., Bush, I., Ray, V., et al: The accuracy of the rectal examination in the diagnosis of prostate carcinoma. N. Engl. J. Med. *303*:499, 1980.
6. Marks, G., Eisenstat, T. E., and Borenstein, B. D. Flexible fiberoptic sigmoidoscopy. *In* Dent, T. L., Strodel, W. E., Turcotte, J. G., and Harper, M. L. (eds.). Surgical Endoscopy. Chicago, Year Book, 1985, pp. 219–231.
7. Carman, M. L. Colon and Rectal Surgery. Philadelphia, J. B. Lippincott Co., 1984.
8. Katon, R. M., Keeffe, E. B., and Melnyk, C. S. Flexible Sigmoidoscopy. Orlando, Grune and Stratton, 1985.
9. Hogan, W. J. Flexible sigmoidoscopy versus colonoscopy—when to use which instrument. Gastrointest. Endosc. *29*:126, 1982.
10. Crespi, M., Weissman, G. S., Gilbertsen, V. A., Winawer, S. J., and Sherlock, P. The role of proctosigmoidoscopy in screening for colorectal neoplasia. CA *34*:158, 1984.
11. Wilking, N., Petrelli, N. J., Herrera-Ornelas, L., Walsh, D., and Mittelman, A. A comparison of the 25-cm rigid proctosigmoidoscopy with the 65-cm flexible endoscope in the screening of patients for colorectal carcinoma. Cancer *57*:669, 1986.
12. Rumans, M. C., Benner, K. G., Keeffe, E. B., et al. Screening flexible sigmoidoscopy by primary care physicians. Effectiveness and costs in patients negative for fecal occult blood. West. J. Med. *144*:756, 1986.
13. Dubow, R. A., Katon, R. M., Benner, K. G., et al. Short (35-cm) versus long (60-cm) flexible sigmoidoscopy: a comparison of findings and tolerance in asymptomatic patients screened for colorectal neoplasia. Gastrointest. Endosc. *31*:305, 1985.
14. Lehman, G. A., Hawes, R., Roth, B., and Hast, J. A study of optimal length of flexible fiberoptic sigmoidoscopes for initial endoscopic training. Dis. Colon Rectum *29*:878, 1986.
15. Weissman, G. S., Winawer, S. J., Baldwin, M. P., et al. Multicenter evaluation of training of non-endoscopists in 30-cm flexible sigmoidoscopy. CA *37*:26, 1987.
16. Tedesco, F., Waye, J., and Avella, J. Diagnostic implications of the spatial distribution of colonic mass lesions (polyps and cancers): a prospective colonoscopic study. Gastrointest. Endosc. *26*:95, 1980.
17. Schrock, T. R. Benign and malignant disease of the anorectum. *In* Fromm, D. (ed.). Gastrointestinal Surgery. New York, Churchill Livingstone, 1985, pp. 599–629.
18. Thomson, W. H. F. The nature of haemorrhoids. Br. J. Surg. *62*:542, 1975.
19. Haas, P. A., Fox, T. A., Jr., Haas, G. P. The pathogenesis of hemorrhoids. Dis. Colon Rectum *27*:442, 1984.
20. Bernstein, W. C. What are hemorrhoids and what is their relationship to the portal venous system? (Guest editorial.) Dis. Colon Rectum *26*:829, 1983.
21. Gibbons, C. P., Bannister, J. J., Trowbridge, E. A., and Read, N. W. The role of anal cushions in maintaining continence. Lancet *1*:886, 1986.
22. El-Gendi, M. A., and Abdel-Baky, N. Anorectal pressure in patients with symptomatic hemorrhoids. Dis. Colon Rectum *29*:388, 1986.
23. MacLeod, J. H. Rational approach to treatment of hemorrhoids based on a theory of etiology. Arch. Surg. *118*:29, 1983.
24. Ribbans, W. J., and Radcliffe, A. G. Retroperitoneal abscess following sclerotherapy for hemorrhoids. Dis. Colon Rectum *28*:188, 1985.
25. Sim, A. J. W., Murie, J. A., and Mackensie, I. Three year follow-up study on the treatment of first and second degree hemorrhoids by sclerosant injection or rubber band ligation. Surg. Gynecol. Obstet. *157*:534, 1983.
26. Russell, T. R., and Donohue, J. H. Hemorrhoidal banding. A warning. Dis. Colon Rectum *28*:291, 1985.
27. Shemesh, E., Kodner, I. J., Fry, R. D., and Newfeld, D. M. Severe complication of rubber band ligation of internal hemorrhoids. Dis. Colon Rectum *30*:199, 1987.
28. Leicester, R. J., Mitchells, R. J., and Mann, C. V. Infrared coagulation: a new treatment for hemorrhoids. Dis. Colon Rectum *24*:602, 1981.
29. Ambrose, N. S., Morris, D., Alexander-Williams, J., and Keighley, M. R. B. A randomized trial of photocoagulation or injection therapy for the treatment of first- and second-degree hemorrhoids. Dis. Colon Rectum *28*:238, 1985.
30. O'Connor, J. J. Bipolar electrocoagulation of hemorrhoids. A new technique. Presented to meeting of Society of American Gastrointestinal Endoscopic Surgeons, Washington, D.C., April 24, 1987.

31. Norman, D. A., Newton, R., and Nicholas, G. V. Management of hemorrhoidal disease: an effective, safe, and painless outpatient approach using D.C. current. Gastrointest. Endosc. *33*:176, 1987.
32. MacLeod, J. H. In defense of cryotherapy for hemorrhoids. A modified method. Dis. Colon Rectum *25*:332, 1982.
33. Schouten, W. R., and Van Vroonhoven, T. J. Lateral internal sphincterotomy in the treatment of hemorrhoids. A clinical and manometric study. Dis. Colon Rectum *29*:896, 1986.
34. Mazier, W. P., and Halleran, D. R. Excisional hemorrhoidectomy. *In* Kodner, I. J., Fry, R. D., Roe, J. P. (eds.). Colon, Rectal and Anal Surgery, St. Louis, C. V. Mosby Co., 1985, pp. 3–14.
35. Motson, R. W., and Clifton, M. A. Pathogenesis and treatment of anal fissure. *In* Henry, M. M., and Swash, M. (eds.): Coloproctology and the Pelvic Floor. Pathophysiology and Management. Boston, Butterworths, 1985, pp. 340–349.
36. Gibbons, C. P., and Read, N. W. Anal hypertonia in fissures: cause or effect. Br. J. Surg. *73*:443, 1986.
37. Antebi, A., Schwartz, P., and Gilon, E. Sclerotherapy for the treatment of fissure in ano. Surg. Gynecol. Obstet. *160*:201, 1985.
38. Bode, W. E., Colp, C. E., Spencer, R. J., and Beart, R. W., Jr. Fissurectomy with superficial midline sphincterotomy. A viable alternative for the surgical correction of chronic fissure/ulcer-in-ano. Dis. Colon Rectum *27*:93, 1984.
39. Hsu, T.-C., and Mackeigan, J. M. Surgical treatment of chronic anal fissure. A retrospective study of 1753 cases. Dis. Colon Rectum *27*:475, 1984.
40. Walker, W. A., Rothenberger, D. A., and Goldberg, S. M. Morbidity of internal sphincterotomy for anal fissure and stenosis. Dis. Colon Rectum *28*:832, 1985.
41. Jensen, S. L., Lund, F., Nielsen, O. V., and Tange, G. Lateral subcutaneous sphincterotomy versus anal dilatation in the treatment of fissure in ano in outpatients: a prospective randomized study. Br. Med. J. *289*:528, 1984.
42. Hanley, P. H. Treatment of anorectal abscess fistula. *In* Ferrari, B. T., Ray, J. E., and Gathright, J. B. Complications of Colon and Rectal Surgery. Prevention and Management. Philadelphia, W. B. Saunders Co., 1985, pp. 101–125.
43. Gordon, P. H. Management of anorectal abscesses and fistulous disease. *In* Kodner, I. J., Fry, R. D., and Roe, J. P. (eds.). Colon, Rectal and Anal Surgery. Current Techniques and Controversies. St. Louis, C. V. Mosby Co., 1985, pp. 91–107.
44. Carroll, P. R., Cattolica, E. V., Turzan, C. W., and McAninch, J. W. Necrotizing soft-tissue infections of the perineum and genitalia. Etiology and early reconstruction. West. J. Med. *144*:174, 1986.
45. Henrichsen, S., and Christiansen, J. Incidence of fistula-in-ano complicating anorectal sepsis: a prospective study. Br. J. Surg. *73*:371, 1986.
46. Ramanujam, P., Prasad, M. L., and Abcarian, H. Perianal abscesses and fistulas: a study of 1023 patients. Dis. Colon Rectum *27*:593, 1984.
47. Held, D., Khubchandani, I., Sheets, J., et al. Management of anorectal horseshoe abscess and fistula. Dis. Colon Rectum *29*:793, 1986.
48. Kuijpers, H. C., and Schulpen, T. Fistulography for fistula-in-ano. Is it useful? Dis. Colon Rectum *28*:103, 1985.
49. Wolff, B. G., Culp, C. E., Beart, R. W., Jr., et al. Anorectal Crohn's disease. A long-term perspective. Dis. Colon Rectum *28*:709, 1985.
50. Vasilevsky, C.-A., and Gordon, P. H. Results of treatment of fistula-in-ano. Dis. Colon Rectum *28*:225, 1984.
51. Christensen, A., Nilas, L., Christiansen, J. Treatment of transsphincteric anal fistulas by the seton technique. Dis. Colon Rectum *29*:454, 1986.
52. Cuthbertson, A. M. Resection and pull-through for rectovaginal fistula. World J. Surg. *10*:228, 1986.
53. Hoexter, B., Labow, S. B., and Moseson, M. D. Transanal rectovaginal fistula repair. Dis. Colon Rectum *28*:572, 1985.
54. Smith, L. E., Henrichs, D., and McCullah, R. D. Prospective studies on the etiology and treatment of pruritus ani. Dis. Colon Rectum *25*:358, 1982.
55. Milsom, J. W., and Mazier, W. P. Classification and management of postsurgical anal stenosis. Surg. Gynecol. Obstet. *163*:60, 1986.
56. Rompalo, A. M., and Stamm, W. E. Anorectal and enteric infections in homosexual men. West. J. Med. *142*:647, 1985.
57. Weller, I. V. D. The gay bowel. Gut *26*:869, 1985.
58. Quinn, T. C., Stamm, W. E., and Goodell, S. E. The polymicrobial origin of intestinal infections in homosexual men. N. Engl. J. Med. *309*:576, 1983.
59. Surawicz, C. M., Goodell, S. E., and Quinn, T. C. Spectrum of rectal biopsy abnormalities in homosexual men with intestinal symptoms. Gastroenterology *91*:651, 1986.
60. Eron, L. J., Judson, F., Tucker, S., et al. Interferon therapy for condylomata acuminata. N. Engl. J. Med. *315*:1059, 1986.
61. Nash, G., Allen, W., and Nash, S. Atypical lesions of the anal mucosa in homosexual men. JAMA *256*:873, 1986.
62. Gal, A. A., Meyer, P. R., and Taylor, C. R. Papillomavirus antigens in anorectal condyloma and carcinoma in homosexual men. JAMA *257*:337, 1987.
63. Washington, A. E., Johnson, R. E., and Sanders, L. L., Jr. *Chlamydia trachomatis* infections in the United States. What are they costing us? JAMA *257*:2070, 1987.
64. Klotz, S. A., Drutz, D. J., Tam, M. R., and Reed, K. H. Hemorrhagic proctitis due to lymphogranuloma venereum serogroup L2. Diagnosis by fluorescent monoclonal antibody. N. Engl. J. Med. *308*:1563, 1983.
65. Goodell, S. E., Quinn, T. C., Mkrtichian, E., et al. Herpes simplex virus proctitis in homosexual men. Clinical, sigmoidoscopic, and histopathological features. N. Engl. J. Med. *308*:868, 1983.
66. Goldmeier, D., Price, A. B., Billington, O., et al. Is *Entamoeba histolytica* in homosexual men a pathogen? Lancet *1*:641, 1986.
67. Allason-Jones, E., Mindel, A., Sargeaunt, P., and Williams, P. *Entamoeba histolytica* as a commensal intestinal parasite in homosexual men. N. Engl. J. Med. *315*:353, 1986.
68. Barone, J. E., Yee, J., and Nealon, T. F., Jr. Management of foreign bodies and trauma of the rectum. Surg. Gynecol. Obstet. *156*:453, 1983.
69. Kingsley, A. N., and Abcarian, H. Colorectal foreign bodies. Management update. Dis. Colon Rectum *28*:941, 1985.
70. Busch, D. B., and Starling, J. R. Rectal foreign bodies: case reports and a comprehensive review of the world's literature. Surgery *100*:512, 1986.
71. Bush, R., and Owen, W. Trauma and other noninfectious problems in homosexual men. Med. Clin. North Am. *70*:549, 1986.
72. Culp, C. E. Chronic hidradenitis suppurativa of the anal canal. A surgical skin disease. Dis. Colon Rectum *26*:669, 1983.
73. Bascom, J. Pilonidal disease: long-term results of follicle removal. Dis. Colon Rectum *26*:800, 1983.
74. Henry, M. M., Swash, M. (eds.): Coloproctology and the Pelvic Floor. Pathophysiology and Management. Boston, Butterworths, 1985, pp. 193–392.
75. Snooks, S. J., Henry, M. M., and Swash, M. Anorectal incontinence and rectal prolapse: differential assessment of the innervation to puborectalis and external sphincter muscles. Gut *26*:470, 1985.
76. Lahr, C. J., Rothenberger, D. A., Jensen, L. L., and Goldberg, S. M. Balloon topography. A simple method of evaluating anal function. Dis. Colon Rectum *29*:1, 1986.
77. Roe, A. M., Bartolo, D. C. C., and Mortensen, N. J. M. New method for assessment of anal sensation in various anorectal disorders. Br. J. Surg. *73*:310, 1986.

78. Read, N. W., Abouzekry, L. Why do patients with faecal impaction have faecal incontinence? Gut *27*:283, 1986.
79. Buser, W. D., Miner, P. B., Jr. Delayed rectal sensation with fecal incontinence. Successful treatment using anorectal manometry. Gastroenterology *91*:1186, 1986.
80. Christiansen, J., and Pedersen, I. K.: Traumatic anal incontinence. Results of surgical repair. Dis. Colon Rectum *30*:189, 1987.
81. Corman, M. L. Anal incontinence following obstetrical injury. Dis. Colon Rectum *28*:86, 1985.
82. Browning, G. G. P., Motson, R. W. Anal sphincter injury. Management and results of Parks sphincter repair. Ann. Surg. *199*:351, 1984.
83. Keighley, M. R. B. Postanal repair for fecal incontinence. J. Roy. Soc. Med. *77*:285, 1984.
84. Snooks, R. J., Nicholls, R. J, Henry, M. M., and Swash, M. Electrophysiological and manometric assessment of the pelvic floor in the solitary rectal ulcer syndrome. Br. J. Surg. *72*:131, 1985.
85. Womack, N. R., Williams, N. S., Mist, J. H. H., and Morrison, J. F. Anorectal function in the solitary rectal ulcer syndrome. Dis. Colon Rectum *30*:319, 1987.
86. Pescatori, M., Maria, G., Mattana, C., Vulpio, C., and Vecchio, F. Clinical picture and pelvic floor physiology in the solitary rectal ulcer syndrome. Dis. Colon Rectum *28*:862, 1985.
87. Kuijpers, H. C., Schreve, R. H., and Hoedemakers, H. T. C. Diagnosis of functional disorders of defecation causing the solitary rectal ulcer syndrome. Dis. Colon Rectum *29*:126, 1986.
88. Nichells, R. J., and Simson, J. N. L. Anteroposterior rectopexy in the treatment of solitary rectal ulcer syndrome without overt rectal prolapse. Br. J. Surg. *73*:222, 1986.
89. Womack, N. R., Morrison, J. F. B., and Williams, N. S. The role of pelvic floor denervation in the aetiology of idiopathic faecal incontinence. Br. J. Surg. *73*:404, 1986.
90. Corman, M. L. Rectal prolapse in children. Dis. Colon Rectum *28*:535, 1985.
91. Bartolo, D. C. C., Roe, A. M., Virjee, J., and Mortensen, N. J. M. Evacuation proctography in obstructed defaecation and rectal intussusception. Br. J. Surg. *72*:S111, 1985.
92. Johansson, C., Ihre, T., and Ahlbäck, S. O. Disturbances in the defecation mechanism with special reference to intussusception of the rectum (internal procidentia). Dis. Colon Rectum *28*:920, 1985.
93. Berman, I. R., Manning, D. H., and Dudley-Wright, K. Anatomic specificity in the diagnosis and treatment of internal rectal prolapse. Dis. Colon Rectum *28*:816, 1985.
94. Hiltunen, K.-M. Matikainen, M., Auvinen, O., and Hietanen, P. Clinical and manometric evaluation of anal sphincter function in patients with rectal prolapse. Am. J. Surg. *151*:489, 1986.
95. Watts, J. D., Rothenberger, D. A., Buls, J. G., Goldberg, S. M., and Nivatvongs, S. The management of procidentia—30 years' experience. Dis. Colon Rectum *28*:96, 1985.
96. Earnshaw, J. J., and Hopkinson, B. R. Late results of silicone rubber perianal suture for rectal prolapse. Dis. Colon Rectum *30*:86, 1987.
97. Holström, B., Broden, G., and Dolk, A. Results of the Ripstein operation in the treatment of rectal prolapse and internal rectal procidentia. Dis. Colon Rectum *29*:845, 1986.
98. Nicosia, J. F., and Abcarian, H. Levator syndrome. A treatment that works. Dis. Colon Rectum *28*:406, 1985.
99. Greenall, M. J., Quan, S. H. Q., Stearns, M. W., et al. Epidermoid cancer of the anal margin. Am. J. Surg. *149*:95, 1985.
100. Clark, J., Petrelli, N., Herrera, L., and Mittelman, A. Epidermoid carcinoma of the anal canal. Cancer *57*:400, 1986.
101. Pyper, P. C., and Parks, T. G. The results of surgery for epidermoid carcinoma of the anus. Br. J. Surg. *72*:712, 1985.
102. Salmon, R. J., Zafrani, B., Labib, A., et al. Prognosis of cloacogenic and squamous cancers of the anal canal. Dis. Colon Rectum *29*:336, 1986.
103. Butler, T. W., Gefter, J., Kieto, D., et al. Squamous-cell carcinoma of the anus in condyloma acuminatum. Dis. Colon Rectum *30*:293, 1987.
104. Smith, D. E., Muff, N. S., and Shetabi, H. Combined preoperative neoadjuvant radiotherapy and chemotherapy for anal and rectal cancer. Am. J. Surg. *151*:577, 1986.
105. Meeker, W. R., Jr., Sickle-Santanello, B. J., Philpott, G., et al. Combined chemotherapy, radiation, and surgery for epithelial cancer of the anal canal. Cancer *57*:525, 1986.
106. Ward, M. W. N., Romano, G., and Nicholls, R. J. The surgical treatment of anorectal malignant melanoma. Br. J. Surg. *73*:68, 1986.
107. Arbesman, H., and Ransohoff, D. F. Is Bowen's disease a predictor of the development of internal malignancy? JAMA *257*:516, 1987.
108. Beck, D. E., and Fazio, V. W. Perianal Paget's disease. Dis. Colon Rectum *30*:263, 1987.

84

Other Diseases of the Colon and Rectum

DAVID L. EARNEST
DAVID J. SCHNEIDERMAN

Certain diseases of the colon that cannot conveniently be classified with other inflammatory, vascular, motor, or malignant conditions are discussed in this chapter. Some of these diseases are uncommon, and are frequently perplexing to diagnose since they may arise in submucosal or serosal spaces. Furthermore, treatment may be difficult or unsatisfactory, since a precise etiology often cannot be determined.

INTESTINAL ENDOMETRIOSIS

Endometrial glandular and stromal invasion of the myometrium is referred to as *adenomyosis*. The presence of ectopic endometrial tissue in sites beyond the myometrium defines *endometriosis*, and includes foci involving the gastrointestinal tract. It is estimated that endometriosis affects approximately 15 per cent of menstruating women, and that in up to one half of pelvic explorations, endometriosis will be diagnosed.[1] Intestinal involvement, however, is much less frequently detected and causes considerably less morbidity than that affecting the female reproductive organs. The largest studies report enteric involvement in 12 to 37 per cent of patients with endometriosis, most commonly affecting the rectosigmoid, and less often spreading to the terminal ileum, appendix, and cecum.[1, 2]

Pathogenesis

Of the several theories put forth to explain the etiology of endometriosis, the most widely supported is that of retrograde menstruation, with reflux of viable endometrial tissue through the fallopian tubes and subsequent implantation and growth on pelvic viscera and peritoneum.[3] Although this proposal is in accord with the predominantly pelvic distribution of heterotopic foci, extrapelvic and distant implants are considered to arise via hematogenous or lymphatic dissemination from the basal endometrium. A less widely held theory invokes endometrial metaplasia of multipotential peritoneal mesothelial cells and is thought to explain the rare cases of endometriosis in males and women devoid of endometrium.[4] Lastly, there also appears to be a genetic predisposition toward the development of endometriosis, with a clustering of cases among siblings that exceeds the prevalence in non–blood relatives. Such genetic factors may include hereditary immunologic defects, in that animals with spontaneous endometriosis have demonstrated impaired cell-mediated immunologic responses to autologous endometrial tissue.[5, 6]

Pathophysiology

As stated earlier, enteric endometrial implants most frequently involve those portions of the gastrointestinal tract in closest proximity to the pelvis. Hence, it is uncommon for ectopic foci to be discovered proximal to the terminal ileum, although scattered reports of jejunal or gastric involvement have surfaced. Heterotopic endometrium generally adheres to the serosal surface of the intestine and may invade the subserosa. Such implants, like the uterine endometrial lining, are subject to ovarian hormonal influence. At the termination of the menstrual cycle, endometrial engorgement and sloughing cause hemorrhage, often associated with pain. An intense inflammatory response to the free fibrogenic iron follows which promotes the formation of dense adhesions that may ultimately obscure the primary focus and lead to intestinal kinking, stricture, or obstruction. Cyclic repetition results in dissection of the process through the subserosa and the muscularis to the submucosa. The advancing endometriosis does not usually invade the mucosa. Although uncommon, malignant transformation of ectopic endometrial foci can occur, and adenocarcinoma has been reported to evolve within a colonic implant.[7]

Clinical Picture

Since endometriosis is a disease of the reproductive period, with a peak incidence between the ages of 30 and 40 years, it does not affect females prior to menarche, and those with symptoms after menopause have usually suffered an antecedent fibrotic process or use exogenous estrogens.

The severity of bowel symptoms does not often correlate with the extent of involvement. Small endometriomas in the intestinal wall may produce no symptoms and may be incidentally discovered at laparotomy. Patients with rectosigmoid implants, which account for 72 to 95 per cent of enteric involvement,[1, 2] may experience abdominal pain, tenesmus, constipation or diarrhea, or low backache. Contrary to common belief, symptoms may not always fluctuate in accordance with hormonal changes. If there is a partial luminal obstruction, progressive constipation and a reduction in stool caliber may be associated with worsening lower abdominal pain and rectal discomfort. Hematochezia may rarely accompany colonic endometriosis from mucosal penetration of implants or ischemia related to the pericolonic fibrosis.[8] However, since rectal bleeding is infrequently associated with this disorder, the clinician should diligently search for other diagnostic possibilities.

More proximal colonic involvement is usually asymptomatic unless obstruction develops. The cecum or appendix is seeded with endometrial implants in approximately 3 per cent of patients with intestinal endometriosis. An acute appendicitis-like syndrome caused by an obstructing endometrioma has been reported, as has intussusception with an appendiceal implant serving as the lead point.[9, 10]

Endometriosis of the small intestine is usually an incidental finding during abdominal surgery. Most commonly, the terminal ileum is the site of heterotopic implantation. Lesions, usually single, tend to be limited to the serosa, and unless adhesions develop or deeper layers of the bowel are penetrated, generally remain asymptomatic. When symptoms arise, they are, in general, subacute and consist of postprandial cramping, abdominal pain, nausea, and vomiting. Ileal obstruction may result from luminal encroachment of an enlarging endometrioma with true stricturing, or kinking and buckling of the small bowel from surrounding dense fibrous adhesions.[11–13] An extremely rare but potentially catastrophic complication of intestinal endometriosis is the erosion or rupture of an implant into a large blood vessel resulting in hemoperitoneum.[14] Such a dramatic presentation is often indistinguishable from other causes of an acute abdomen, and the precise diagnosis is generally not discerned until surgical intervention has been carried out.

Diagnosis

Evaluation should begin with a complete pelvic examination, including combined rectovaginal palpation. The finding of tender nodules and irregular induration in the cul-de-sac, especially when palpating anteriorly in the rectum, is strong evidence of endometriosis. Since the character of the lesions often changes during the menstrual cycle, a pelvic examination should be done before, and again after, menstruation. When a mass is palpable in a free portion of the sigmoid and not within the cul-de-sac, the diagnosis of endometriosis is much less certain.

At sigmoidoscopy or colonoscopy, the mucosa is usually intact, but may be puckered over a firm, indurated, and occasionally bluish submucosal mass. The indurated area may be quite tender, in contrast to a carcinomatous mass, which characteristically is painless. If a stricture is present and endometriosis is suspected, a repeat endoscopic visualization 10 to 14 days later may demonstrate a noticeable increase in luminal size resulting from the cyclic sloughing of the endometrial tissue. Mucosal biopsy is often not diagnostic, since endometriosis is usually located in deeper layers of the intestine.[8] Laparoscopy is helpful in that both pelvic and abdominal endometriosis can be directly visualized and biopsied. The diagnostic value of this procedure may be reduced, however, by extensive adhesions.

Air-contrast radiographs of the colon are usually not diagnostic. Intramural endometriosis may present as a submucosal polypoid mass or an irregular narrowing of the lumen from surrounding fibrosis.[12, 15] The mucosa, with rare exception, appears undisturbed. Differential diagnosis of these radiologic findings include carcinoma; diverticulitis; chronic inflammatory diseases with stricture, such as ulcerative colitis and Crohn's colitis; benign intramural tumors and polyps; and pelvic or mesenteric tumors and cysts. Radiologic features that favor endometriosis are (1) an intact mucosa, (2) a long lesion or area of constriction, (3) tapered margins suggestive of an intramural lesion rather than the acutely angulated overhanging margins of a mucosal lesion, and (4) the absence of ulceration within a mass (Fig. 84–1).

After complete evaluation, if uncertainty remains about the nature of a constricting rectosigmoid mass, and if it persistently enlarges and involves the cul-de-sac area, a direct needle biopsy should be attempted, even though the diagnosis of endometriosis seems certain. Primary adenocarcinoma of the rectovaginal septum arising from endometrial tissue has been reported.[16]

When periumbilical right lower quadrant cramping abdominal pain is present in a patient with endometriosis of the ovary and cul-de-sac, one should suspect endometriosis of the small intestine. A small bowel barium radiograph should be taken just before or during the menstrual period to improve diagnostic yield. When there is fixation of the cecum and terminal ileum by adhesions, the picture may be compatible with that of a partial small bowel obstruction. In some cases, a pattern suggesting disordered intestinal motility with segmentation of the barium in the distal small bowel may be all that is seen. General abdominal haziness may suggest ascites, a rare complication of endometriosis.[17]

Treatment

The therapeutic approach to symptomatic intestinal endometriosis should probably be undertaken in conjunction with a gynecologist. Treatment must be individualized and take into account the severity of symptoms, the patient's age, and her desire for future pregnancies. The main treatment options include intestinal surgery, hormonal therapy, and castration.

Surgical resection is obviously indicated for profound rectal bleeding, complete or acute bowel obstruction,

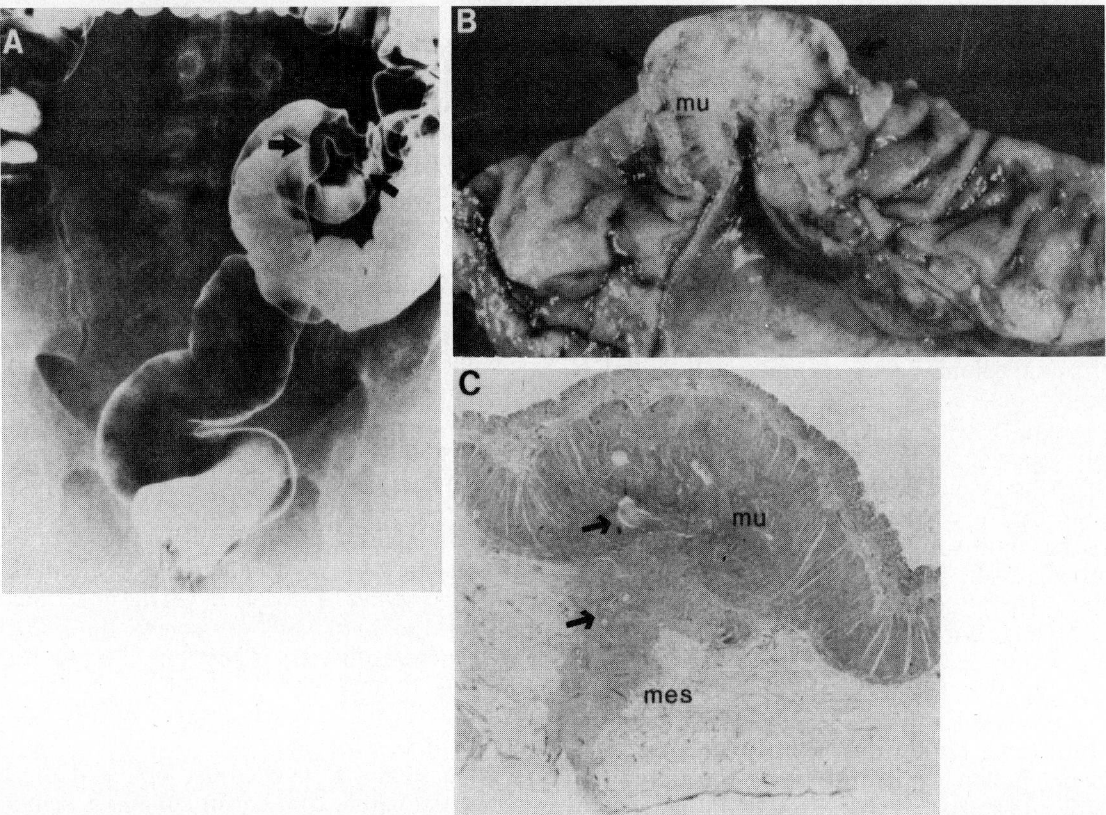

Figure 84–1. Endometriosis of the sigmoid colon. *A,* Air-contrast barium radiograph demonstrating intramural filling defect *(arrows)* in sigmoid colon. *B,* Gross resected specimen of intramural endometrioma *(arrows)* within thickened muscular layers (mu), underlying attenuated but intact colonic mucosa. *C,* Endometrial glandular *(arrows)* and stromal elements within hypertrophied muscular layer (mu) and mesentery (mes). Hematoxylin and eosin stain, × 5 (reduced 30 per cent). (From Croom, R. D., III, Donovan, M. L., and Schwesinger, W. H. Am. J. Surg. *148*:660, 1984. Used by permission.)

hemoperitoneum, and intussusception. The role for surgery is less clear when symptoms are subacute and not life-threatening. In many cases, the initial diagnosis of endometriosis is not made preoperatively. Often, small implants may be dissected without entering the intestinal lumen.[18] Histologic evaluation using frozen sections should be carried out during surgery, since carcinoma is the most serious differential diagnosis. Large constricting adenofibromuscular lesions require resection. In selected cases, intraoperative or laparoscopic excision or ablation of endometrial implants or lysis of adhesions may be accomplished with laser phototherapy, although current information is limited with regard to efficacy of this modality.[19, 20]

Medical treatment of endometriosis is based upon the well-founded premise that growth and recession of ectopic endometrium is governed by ovarian hormones. Since lesions regress during pregnancy and after menopause, exogenous agents administered to induce anovulatory states have produced dramatic and long-lasting improvement. Low-dose estrogen-progestin compounds (usually prescribed as oral contraceptives) produce a pseudopregnancy state which results in a decidual reaction in, followed by necrosis and resolution of, endometrial implants.[21] During the decidual phase, however, symptoms may initially worsen before lesions resolve. Likewise, long-acting parenteral medroxyprogesterone acetate (Depo-Provera), a potent progestin and gonadotropin inhibitor, induces anovulation and a persistent decidual reaction. Despite its efficacy, this agent produces a prolonged anovulatory state after discontinuation and should not be used in women desiring pregnancy within 1 to 2 years.

Danazol is currently the most widely used medication for endometriosis. A potent pituitary gonadotropin inhibitory agent, danazol suppresses ovarian function by inhibiting release of follicle-stimulating hormone (FSH) and luteinizing hormone (LH). The drug appears to have a high degree of efficacy with only moderate side effects and may be the treatment of choice in patients not requiring surgery.[22]

Unless bowel symptoms are promptly relieved by any of the aforementioned medical regimens, surgery should be strongly considered. Overall, it is generally believed that intestinal lesions severe enough to produce symptoms will be unlikely to remit with hormonal therapy. This may be explained by the persistence of a fibrotic scar, despite the disappearance of the endometrial tissue.

Lastly, castration by surgical excision may lead to regression of intestinal endometriosis, but should be reserved for the older woman in whom total abdominal hysterectomy is performed, or for the younger female in whom other therapies have failed and who is incapacitated by the disease.

PNEUMATOSIS CYSTOIDES INTESTINALIS

Pneumatosis cystoides intestinalis is an uncommon disorder characterized by multiple gas-filled cysts in the wall of the large and small intestine. The stomach, mesentery, and omentum may also be involved. In the majority of cases, pneumatosis intestinalis is an unexpected finding on plain abdominal or barium X-ray. However, a variety of symptoms have been attributed to the cysts, and the condition has been described in association with a number of gastrointestinal and pulmonary diseases.

Etiology and Pathogenesis

Most patients with pneumatosis cystoides intestinalis have either pulmonary or pyloroduodenal obstructive disease, or have had recent intestinal surgery, especially jejunoileal bypass.[23–27] Other patients have developed colonic pneumatosis after the trauma of gastrointestinal endoscopy, mucosal biopsy, or polypectomy. Disorders involving the gastrointestinal tract with which pneumatosis cystoides intestinalis has been reported are listed in Table 84–1.[28] Approximately 20 per cent of patients with intestinal pneumatosis have acute or chronic obstructive pulmonary disease and have air cysts mainly in the small bowel.[24–27, 29, 30]

The exact cause of pneumatosis cystoides intestinalis remains unknown. Three general mechanisms have been proposed. The mechanical theory suggests that gas from ruptured pulmonary blebs or from the bowel lumen adjacent to an obstructing pyloric ulcer, a surgical intestinal anastomosis, a mucosal biopsy site, or the like dissects under pressure along tissue spaces to the intestinal wall, mesentery, or omental location. In animal studies, air injected into the mediastinum has been shown to dissect down beside the aorta and eventually along the mesenteric vascular tree to the intestine, producing a picture similar to that of pneumatosis cystoides intestinalis.[27] The mechanical theory is also supported by cases of pneumatosis coli that developed shortly after mucosal disruption by endoscopy or surgery.

Another possible explanation is tissue invasion by bacteria. In newborns or premature infants, pneumatosis intestinalis is most often seen associated with severe necrotizing enterocolitis.[30] Experimentally, injection of gas-producing bacteria into the intestinal wall of germ-free rats produces a picture similar to pneumatosis cystoides intestinalis.[31] Also, in patients with intestinal ischemia, invasion of the intestinal wall by intraluminal bacteria can lead to intramural collections of air (Fig. 84–2) (see pp. 1903–1932). In this situation, gas may also be seen in the portal and mesenteric veins and, when present, is considered a poor prognostic sign.[32–34] Cyst rupture in such a patient is equivalent to intestinal perforation with the associated risk of peritonitis. However, in the majority of cases of pneumatosis cystoides intestinalis not related to infection, cyst rupture does not produce peritonitis. This observation strongly argues against bacterial invasion of the bowel wall as a cause for cyst formation.

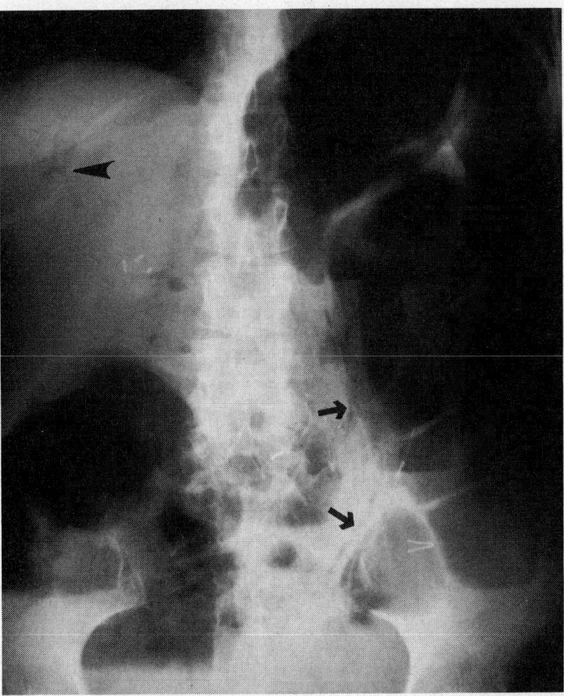

Figure 84–2. Plain abdominal X-ray of a patient with severe intestinal ischemia, pneumatosis intestinalis, and collections of gas in tissue spaces and the portal vein. Areas of pneumatosis *(arrows)* in the intestine wall caused by bacterial invasion often have a linear configuration. Gas in the portal vein *(arrowhead)* extends toward the periphery of the liver and usually signifies an infectious cause for the pneumatosis intestinalis.

Table 84–1. GASTROINTESTINAL CONDITIONS ASSOCIATED WITH PNEUMATOSIS CYSTOIDES INTESTINALIS

Peptic ulcer disease
Intestinal obstruction
Postsurgical bowel anastomosis
Jejunoileal bypass for obesity
Mesenteric vascular occlusion
Acute necrotizing enterocolitis
Chronic inflammatory disease (e.g., regional enteritis, ulcerative colitis)
Perforated diverticulum (small intestine, sigmoid)
Appendicitis
Collagen vascular disorders (scleroderma, dermatomyositis, lupus erythematosus)
Diabetic enteropathy
Cystic fibrosis of pancreas
Whipple's disease
Abdominal trauma
Volvulus of stomach and sigmoid colon
Ingestion of caustic agents
Intestinal parasites and tuberculosis
Intestinal lymphosarcoma, leukemia, Hodgkin's disease
Following sigmoidoscopy and colonoscopy

Moreover, in patients with pneumatosis coli, culture of the cysts and adjacent intestine demonstrated neither unusual bacterial flora nor a significant change in organisms following resolution of the cysts in response to oxygen treatment.[35]

The third mechanism, the biochemical theory, postulates that excessive gas produced by bacterial fermentation of carbohydrate in the intestinal lumen is absorbed and trapped in the intestinal wall. In support of this mechanism are reports documenting (1) large concentrations of hydrogen in cyst gas; (2) increased breath hydrogen excretion, indicating carbohydrate malabsorption; and (3) resolution of the cysts during consumption of an elemental diet that reduces the amount of carbohydrate reaching colonic bacteria.[36–38] Except for variable amounts of hydrogen and methane, analysis of gas in the cysts has demonstrated a composition similar to that of atmospheric air: 70 to 90 per cent nitrogen, 3 to 20 per cent oxygen, and 0.3 to 15 per cent carbon dioxide.[39, 40] Despite the initial source of the gas that led to cyst formation, gas in the intestinal lumen diffuses into the cysts and is probably responsible, at least in part, for persistence or enlargement of the spaces.[36–38]

Pathology of Gas Cysts

The cysts may vary in size from a few millimeters to several centimeters and often give the appearance of multiple lymphangiomas or sessile polyps (Fig. 84–3). The cysts may be single but more commonly occur in clusters and can be either subserosal or submucosal in location. The muscle layers of the intestine are less commonly involved. On cross section, the cystic area has a honeycomb appearance without direct communication with the bowel lumen (Fig. 84–4) and may resemble massively dilated lymphatic channels. The cysts are often lined by endothelial cells that coalesce and form giant cells.[24] Some cysts are lined by simple cuboidal epithelium. In this situation, giant cells are usually absent. Connective tissue around the cysts usually demonstrates inflammatory changes, occasionally with granuloma.[24] A progressive fibrotic reaction may develop, which may ultimately obliterate the cysts and cause rigidity of the intestinal wall.

Clinical Picture

Pneumatosis cystoides intestinalis has been divided into a primary or idiopathic form (about 15 per cent) in the absence of known gastrointestinal disease or a secondary type (about 85 per cent) in which any of a wide variety of associated gastrointestinal, pulmonary, or other conditions are present.[24, 25] The colon is more commonly involved in the primary form, whereas the small intestine is mainly involved in the secondary one.[26] A clinical classification based on the presence or absence of coexisting pulmonary disease has also been suggested.[26]

Pneumatosis cystoides intestinalis is usually discovered during fiberoptic sigmoidoscopy or X-ray examination of the abdomen or intestine. Although there are no symptoms consistently caused by the pneumatosis, patients with primarily colonic involvement may complain of lower abdominal cramping pain, rectal bleeding with mucoid discharge, tenesmus, and recurrent diarrhea. Several patients with pneumatosis have been reported to have mild steatorrhea.[41, 42] However, in these reports it is unclear whether pneumatosis *per se* caused malabsorption (see pp. 263–282).

Rarely, intestinal obstruction may develop either from very large cysts or from adhesions, volvulus, and intussusception (see pp. 369–377). Pneumatosis with intestinal ischemia is an ominous development, as discussed earlier. Pneumatosis coli with or without perforation should be suspected in patients who develop abdominal pain, tenesmus, or rectal discomfort after sigmoidoscopy. Pneumatosis should also be considered in otherwise healthy patients with vague abdominal complaints who are found on X-ray examination to have free air beneath the diaphragm and no other evidence of a perforated viscus.

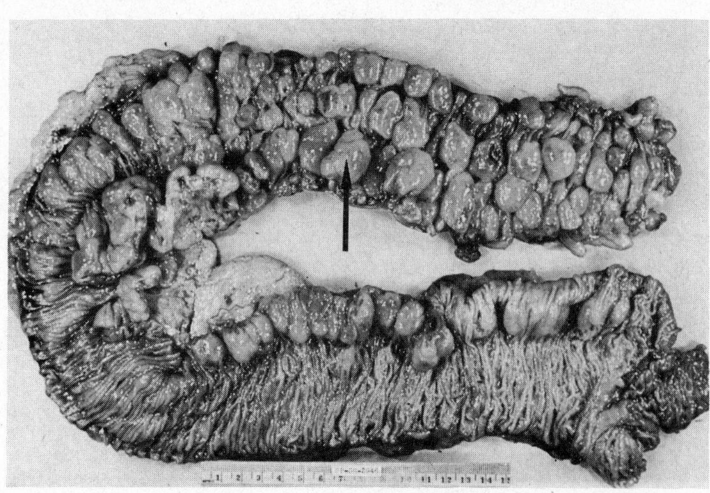

Figure 84–3. Pneumatosis cystoides intestinalis of the small bowel. The gross appearance may suggest lymphangiomas or polyps. Involvement of the rectosigmoid may be diagnosed sigmoidoscopically. The cysts collapse, usually without sequelae, if biopsied.

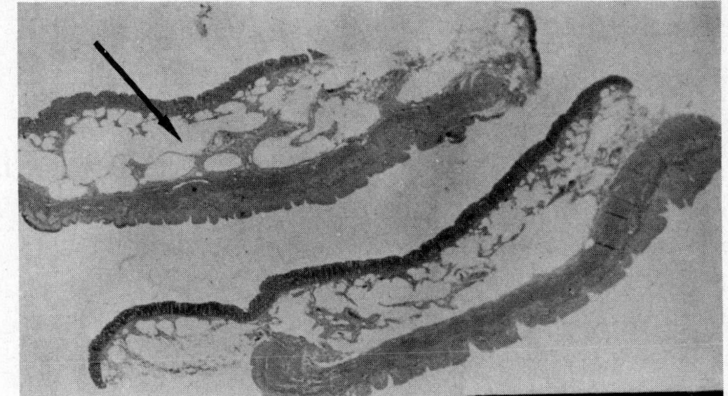

Figure 84–4. A cross section of colon with pneumatosis cystoides intestinalis shows the honeycomb-like air spaces *(arrow)* suggestive of dilated lymphatics. Hematoxylin and eosin stain, × 5.

Diagnosis and Differential Diagnosis

General physical examination usually gives no specific information suggestive of intestinal pneumatosis. Large cysts may cause palpable, nontender, and movable abdominal masses. Firm, grape-like masses may also be felt in the rectal wall during digital examination. When the rectum or colon is involved, pneumatosis may be diagnosed or its presence confirmed by sigmoidoscopy or colonoscopy.[43–45] The cysts appear as pale or bluish, rounded, soft masses protruding into the lumen and are often mistaken for sessile polyps (Color Fig. 84–5, p. xliii). Biopsy will help establish the correct diagnosis, because puncture of the tense cyst wall, which is usually innocuous, will collapse the "polyp," often with a popping sound.

X-ray findings contribute most to the correct diagnosis. Plain films of the abdomen will show localized collections of gas in a scattered and often linear fashion or clustered in segments along the intestinal wall.[46, 47] Occasionally, gas may be seen between the layers of mesentery. Gas in the portal system has been reported with benign jejunal pneumatosis.[25] However, portal vein gas usually reflects ischemia, necrosis, and infection in the bowel wall (Fig. 84–2). Painless rupture of pulmonary alveoli can lead to a wide variety of soft tissue gas collections that can be confused with pneumatosis intestinalis. Also, pneumoperitoneum may be suggested when a single cyst is very large.[32] Computed tomography is reported to permit detection of intramural gas cysts prior to their visualization by other radiologic methods and thus may be useful in differentiating benign pneumatosis from that consequent to infarction of the intestine.[33]

Barium X-ray examination of the small or large bowel is often employed to evaluate for pneumatosis cystoides intestinalis as a cause of unexplained collections of gas in the abdomen. The radiograph can be striking in appearance.[32, 46–48] Small radiolucent spaces are seen to line the intestine wall and indent the barium column (Fig. 84–6). The cysts may have a bubbly appearance. The base of the filling defect caused by the cyst is wide in contrast to that usually produced by polyps, and the margin is smooth, unlike that of carcinoma. The pneumatosis is usually segmental in distribution; skip areas are common. The rectum is rarely involved. The disease is more common in the left colon than in the right. The length of the cystic abnormality in both small and large intestine can vary from inches to several feet.[47]

The cysts may appear to partially obstruct the intestinal lumen. Significant dilatation of the more proximal intestine, however, is rare. The differential diagnosis of the radiologic changes should not be difficult. Enterogenous cysts generally are single, whereas pneumatosis is usually characterized by multiple cysts. In lymphosarcoma, the nodules do not contain gas (see pp. 1545–1546). Colitis cystica profunda may occur proximal to the transverse colon, but, in contrast to pneumatosis, the rectum is usually involved (see p. 1603). *Ischemia* can produce a similar but reversible thumbprint-like deformity (see pp. 1903–1916). Invasion of the intestinal wall by gas-forming organisms is a rare complication of ischemic necrosis, and clinical signs of sepsis are usually present. Ulcerative colitis, Crohn's colitis, and ischemic bowel disease may cause polypoid mucosal irregularities on barium enema, but these filling defects do not have the marked lucency of air cysts when outlined by barium in the adjacent intestine (see pp. 1342–1343 and 1443–1445). This great lucency of the cysts also helps to differentiate constriction of the lumen by the cysts from that by carcinoma (see p. 1537). The most likely mistake is the confusion of localized colonic pneumatosis with polyposis of the colon (see pp. 1483–1518). However, in adults, gas cysts in the colon are frequently subserosal, whereas in polyposis the filling defects are entirely within the intestinal lumen. Colonoscopy should be used to help resolve the wide range of differential possibilities that the X-ray findings may raise.

Treatment

The majority of patients with intestinal pneumatosis require no specific treatment except that indicated for the underlying or primary disease. The intestinal wall gas collections usually resolve spontaneously. The

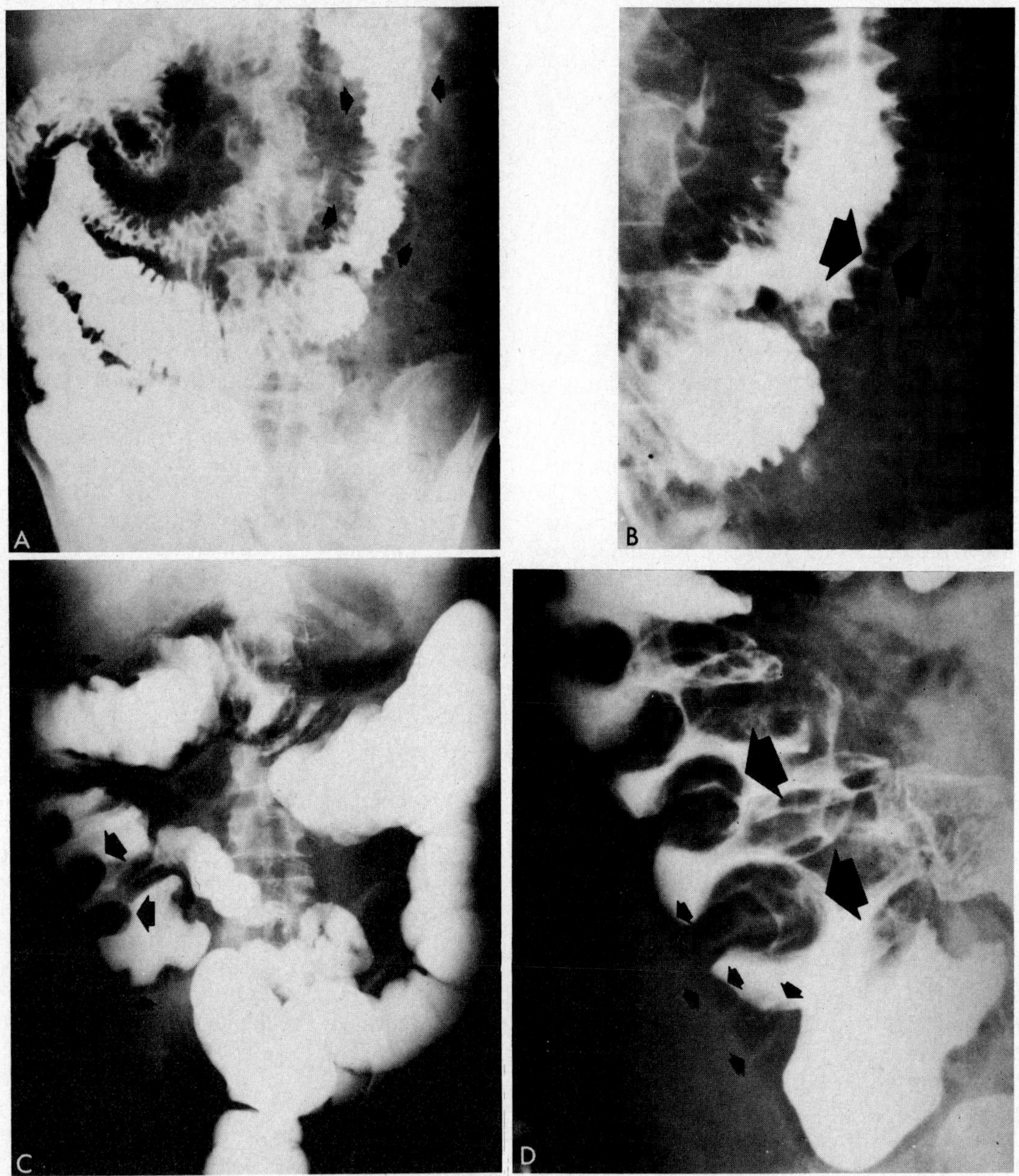

Figure 84–6. Barium contrast X-rays from patients with pneumatosis cystoides intestinalis. The arrows outline the air in the bowel wall. *A*, Extensive pneumatosis of the small intestine. *B*, Close-up view of the segment shown by arrows in *A* demonstrates the spiculated mucosal pattern produced by the air cysts. *C*, Pneumatosis producing large polypoid filling defects *(arrows)* in the right colon. *D*, Close-up view of right colon shows "thumbprint" pattern caused by large air cysts.

Illustration continued on opposite page

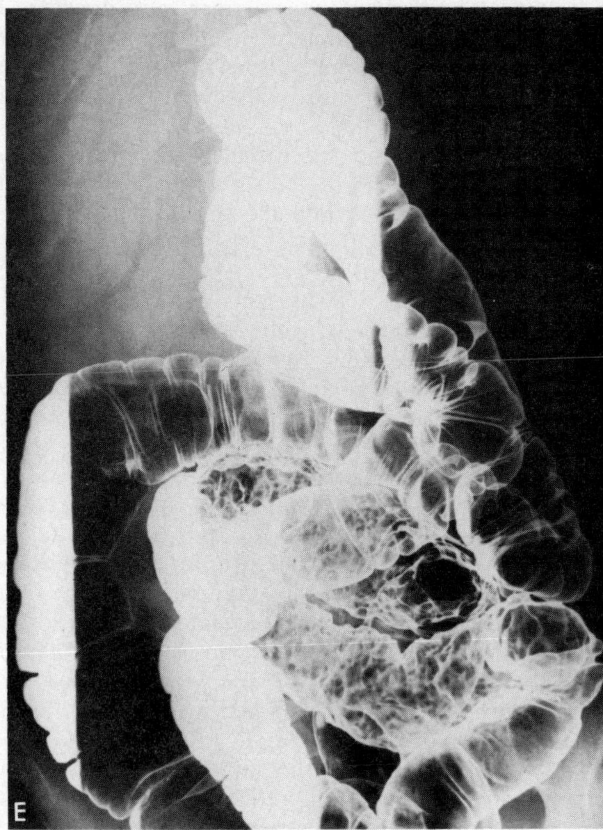

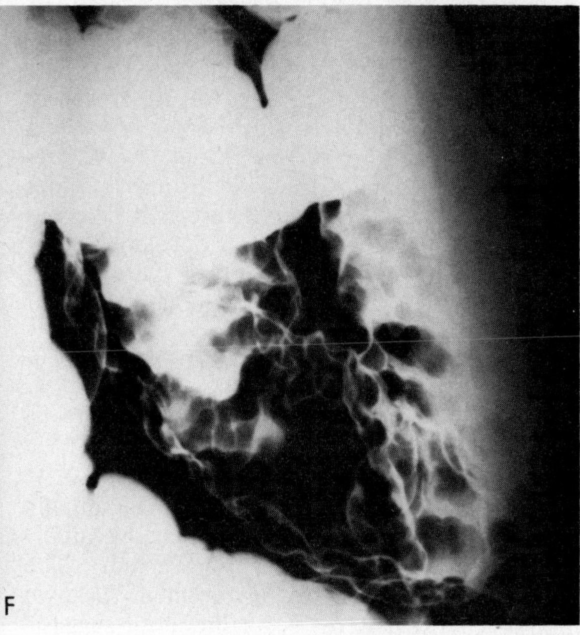

Figure 84–6 *(Continued). E,* Extensive pneumatosis of descending colon. *F,* Close-up view of *E,* showing extensive disruption of the mucosal pattern by the air cysts.

value of a correct diagnosis lies mainly in preventing unnecessary abdominal surgery. Symptomatic pneumatosis intestinalis usually involves the left colon. Therapy for this must be individualized, depending upon symptoms and any apparent underlying cause. Severe tenesmus, bleeding, lower abdominal pain, and symptomatic intestinal obstruction are the problems that may necessitate hospitalization and specific treatment.

Medical treatment of pneumatosis intestinalis is based on the premise that persistence of gas-filled cysts in the intestinal wall implies that the gas in the cysts is replenished at a rate equal to or exceeding the rate at which the cyst gas is absorbed into surrounding tissues.[36] Diffusion of gas across intestinal tissue, into and out of the cysts, depends upon a number of factors including partial pressures of gases in the intestinal lumen, in the cystic spaces, and in capillary blood. Since the cyst gas is composed mainly of nitrogen, treatment has been directed at reducing available nitrogen in atmospheric air. Of note, a few patients with pneumatosis intestinalis have been reported to have increased excretion of hydrogen in breath.[37] Therefore, attempts to decrease intestinal production of hydrogen from malabsorbed carbohydrate may also be important in treatment.

Prolonged breathing of oxygen at high concentrations reduces the partial pressure of other gases, especially nitrogen, in venous blood and thereby promotes diffusion of gas from the cysts into surrounding tissue. Sufficient oxygen can be administered by a tent, a face mask, or a nasal catheter.[34, 49–51] Oxygen concentration in the inspired air should be at least 60 to 70 per cent.[35] Hyperbaric oxygen also has been used successfully.[52] For optimal results, arterial oxygen tension should be regularly monitored to assure a PaO_2 in the range of 200 mm Hg or greater is achieved. Oxygen should be administered continuously overnight and during as much of the day as possible with only short breaks (30 to 60 minutes every 8 hours) in therapy.[35, 49, 51, 53]

During treatment, one should monitor for evidence of oxygen toxicity with daily measurement of vital capacity, blood gas determination, and chest X-ray. A decrease in pulmonary vital capacity may be the most clinically useful early indicator of oxygen toxicity.[35, 55] However, there has been little or no evidence of significant lung injury in patients with pneumatosis intestinalis successfully treated with oxygen. The cysts may disappear by the end of one week.

Occasionally, the cysts reappear after successful oxygen treatment.[35, 56] A second course of oxygen may be tried or, alternatively, attempts may be made to reduce bacterial conversion of dietary carbohydrate to hydrogen. Various reports note resolution of pneumatosis following both antibiotic treatment with metronidazole and feeding of only an elemental diet.[37, 56–58] More experience is necessary before antibiotics can be recommended as initial therapy, since worsening of pneumatosis coli during metronidazole treatment has also been noted.[59]

Surgery may become necessary for the severely symptomatic patient who does not respond to medical treatment. Unfortunately, surgery is not always successful, and the pneumatosis intestinalis may become even more extensive after surgical resection.[60] In the past, less than 5 per cent of patients developed complications necessitating resection.[61] This figure should now be even lower with the use of modern medical treatment.

NONSPECIFIC OR SOLITARY ULCERS OF THE COLON AND RECTUM

Nonspecific ulceration of the colon was initially described as a single process that could involve different segments of the large intestine and rectum.[62] The relative frequency of segmental involvement is shown in Table 84–2.[63] Review of recent literature suggests that this entity can be divided into separate clinical syndromes, depending upon the location of the ulceration. Whereas acute pain, bleeding, and perforation tend to characterize nonspecific ulceration in more proximal colonic locations, the lesions in the rectosigmoid may be asymptomatic, are often accompanied by colitis cystica profunda, and are frustratingly resistant to therapy. This variability in clinical course may reflect different pathogeneses in addition to anatomic variations in colonic and rectal segments. The differences in proposed pathogenesis, clinical presentation, histologic characteristics, and management for nonspecific ulceration occurring in different colorectal locations will be discussed below.

Etiology

Nonspecific cecal ulcers are usually located near the ileocecal valve on the antimesenteric wall. Theories regarding their pathogenesis have been reviewed in detail with the conclusion that the etiology in most cases remains an enigma.[64, 65] Nonspecific ulcerations in the ascending, transverse, and sigmoid colon are histologically similar to the cecal ulcer, and general concepts regarding pathogenesis are also the same.[66–68] They are to be differentiated from the acute ischemic or infectious colonic ulcerations of immunosuppressed patients, especially those with renal failure or transplantation.

Table 84–2. SITES OF NONSPECIFIC COLONIC ULCERS

Site	Per Cent of Cases
Cecum	45
Ascending colon	20
Hepatic flexure	1
Transverse colon	5
Splenic flexure	5
Descending colon	3
Sigmoid	16
Rectum	5

In contrast to nonspecific ulceration in the colon, solitary ulcer of the rectum is a different and better-defined entity.[69–70] While the age range of reported patients is large (10 to 83 years), the majority are young, aged 20 to 35 years, with a slight female predominance.[69, 71, 72] The most common location for solitary rectal ulcer is on the anterior rectal wall 6 to 12 cm above the anus. Some patients also have been reported with histologic changes of *colitis cystica profunda* in adjacent mucosa, raising the possibility that the ulceration developed over or within a pre-existing cystic process[69, 73] (see pp. 1603–1605). However, recent evaluation suggests that both solitary rectal ulcer and colitis cystica profunda are part of the same syndrome.[73] They appear to be different manifestations of the response of the rectal mucosa to chronic trauma and/or possibly ischemia associated with disordered function of the puborectalis muscle and prolapse of rectal mucosa.[69, 73, 74, 76]

Much interest has developed in the possibility that an abnormality in puborectalis muscle function, demonstrated in patients with solitary ulcer of the rectum, traumatizes the mucosa, predisposing it to ulceration.[69, 74–76] Failure of the puborectalis to relax completely during defecation theoretically creates a localized high-pressure zone by its "flap valve" effect which, in turn, could promote trauma, pressure-related ischemia, and, possibly, local prolapse of the rectal wall mucosa.[74–77] Electromyographic evaluations have demonstrated an abnormality in puborectalis muscle function in the majority of patients with solitary rectal ulcer.[76, 78, 79] An abnormality in rectal motility has also been demonstrated by use of a functional balloon proctogram or by a specialized barium enema examination known as defecography.[80] Failure of the puborectalis muscle to relax causes persistence of an acute anorectal angle, which in turn impairs passage of barium from the rectum and, presumably, also feces (Fig. 84–7). Accordingly, persistent contraction of the puborectalis muscle keeps the anal canal closed and leads to severe straining which, in turn, forces the mucosa of the anterior rectal wall against or into the anal canal. This trauma presumably causes stress on and possibly ischemia of the mucosa, leading to prolapse and ultimately the solitary rectal ulcer syndrome.[81] Whether localized mucosal trauma also plays a role in the pathogenesis of solitary ulcers elsewhere in the colon is unknown.

Since rectal prolapse can be demonstrated in almost 90 per cent of patients with solitary rectal ulcer, a strong argument has been made that it is important etiologically and must be considered in planning therapy.[82] Self-induced trauma by digital attempts to remove hard stool from the rectum has also been suggested as a cause.[83, 84] Since prolonged straining at stool is a very common symptom in patients with rectal ulcer and probably prompts digital anal manipulation, it is

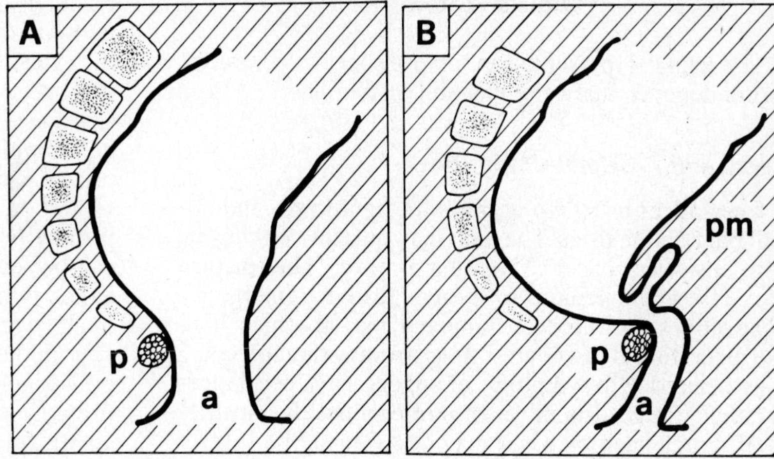

Figure 84–7. Diagrams made from a barium enema functional proctogram in a patient with the solitary rectal ulcer syndrome. *A,* Pattern with normal defecation. The puborectalis muscle (p) relaxes and moves posteriorly, allowing the anorectal channel to straighten. With relaxation of the anal sphincter muscles (a), material in the rectum can be easily passed. *B,* Conditions present in many patients with solitary rectal ulcer syndrome. The puborectalis muscle (p) remains contracted and the recto-anal angle of approximately 90 degrees is maintained, making passage of rectal contents difficult. Continued straining against the puborectalis muscle sling can induce prolapse (pm) of the anterior rectal mucosa. (From Castagnone, D., Rangi, T., Velio, P., et al. Eur. J. Radiol. *4*:110, 1984. Used by permission.)

tempting to believe that some abnormality in the defecatory mechanism is the central defect in this disorder. Occasionally other factors, such as chemical irritation, as has recently been reported with rectal suppositories containing ergotamine tartrate,[85] should also be considered.

Pathology

Nonspecific ulceration of the colon is usually single or solitary, but more than one ulcer may be present. In the cecum and the ascending, transverse, and sigmoid colon, the ulcer is usually located on the antimesenteric wall, in contrast to a diverticulum, which tends to occur along the mesenteric border, especially in the proximal colon.

The ulceration can vary from 5 mm to 5 cm in size. The edges are usually slightly raised and edematous, and the margin is sharply demarcated from the surrounding normal mucosa (Fig. 84–8). If the ulcer is chronic, some increase in connective tissue with fibrotic scarring and contracture may be evident. There may also be considerable inflammatory response with enough cellular reaction to produce a pseudotumor lesion.

Microscopically, there is nothing unusual about the ulcer. The base is covered by a layer of necrotic granulation tissue plus lymphocytes, plasma cells, and fibroblasts. Regenerative activity is evident in adjacent mucosa. Walls of small blood vessels near the ulcer may appear thickened and demonstrate thrombosis and recanalization.[86] If the ulcer extends transmurally, causing perforation, the expected changes of peritonitis will also be present.

In contrast, the histologic picture of nonspecific ulcer of the rectum is different and also characteristic.[69, 75, 86] The specific feature is obliteration of the lamina propria in the region of the ulcer by fibroblasts and by muscular fibers derived from the muscularis mucosae. These stream up between the mucosal crypts, directed at right angles to the hypertrophied muscularis mucosae, and spread the crypts apart. Connective tissue stains demonstrate the characteristic fibrosis, which is a sensitive marker for correct histologic diagnosis of solitary rectal ulcer. Similar but less characteristic histologic changes can be seen in a variety of other conditions.[75] A pre-ulcer phase has been described and is recognized macroscopically by an area of polypoid, hypertrophic, or hyperemic mucosa, which on biopsy has the histologic features described above.[84]

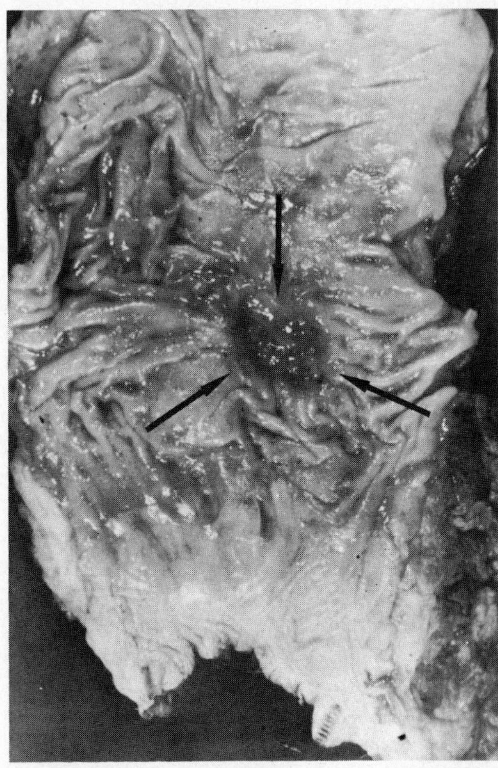

Figure 84–8. Solitary or nonspecific ulcer of the sigmoid colon. Note sharp demarcation of the mucosal ulceration from the surrounding normal tissue *(arrows).*

Clinical Features

The clinical presentation of nonspecific colorectal ulcers depends upon the location of the ulcer.

Cecal and Proximal Colon Ulcer

Cecal ulcer usually presents with right lower abdominal pain and nausea. The pain may be acute or chronic with insidious onset. Vomiting is rare. This picture plus fever and leukocytosis may lead to emergency laparotomy for suspected appendicitis, at which time the ulceration is discovered. If gastrointestinal bleeding is associated with symptoms of appendicitis, cecal ulcer should be placed high on the differential diagnosis.[64, 65] Although such bleeding may occasionally be severe, large amounts of gross blood in the stool are more characteristic of distal colon ulcerations. The clinical picture is obviously affected by the appearance of complications, especially perforation with diffuse peritonitis and localized abscess. A cecal ulcer should be included in the differential diagnosis for symptoms suggesting appendicitis, pelvic inflammatory disease, ovarian disease, Crohn's disease, and tuberculous enteritis. A palpable, tender, right lower quadrant abdominal mass is often present in the latter two conditions and not in uncomplicated cecal ulcer.

Nonspecific ulcer in the colonic flexures, transverse colon, and descending colon usually causes vague, but occasionally severe, abdominal pain with an altered bowel pattern, especially diarrhea. Perforation with peritonitis is a common complication.

Sigmoid Ulcer

The sigmoid colon is the second most common site of nonspecific ulcer, and a correct diagnosis is seldom made prior to surgery. The most frequent symptom is constipation.[68] Chronic lower abdominal pain may be present, but severe or acute pain is not common except with perforation. Recurrent rectal bleeding, however, is frequent. Thus, rectal bleeding with coexisting left lower quadrant abdominal pain is the combination of symptoms that should always raise suspicion of this entity. Since the ulcer is often beyond the reach of the rigid or short fiberoptic sigmoidoscope, a bloody flux coming from the proximal colon in the presence of normal rectal mucosa is the usual finding. Accordingly, a long sigmoidoscope or colonoscope should be used for diagnosis. A barium enema may demonstrate the ulcer but be incorrectly interpreted as diverticulitis, the main differential possibility. Unfortunately, there is a high incidence of bowel perforation with nonspecific ulcer of the sigmoid colon, and often the diagnosis becomes evident only at the time of surgery.

Rectal Ulcer

The most common symptom of a solitary ulcer of the rectum is bleeding, usually consisting of small amounts of fresh blood passed with stool. Blood loss rarely is severe enough to require transfusion. The patient also may pass excessive mucus and complain of tenesmus, symptoms suggesting the possibility of ulcerative colitis or proctitis. A sensation of anal obstruction and a history of frequent straining at stool are common. The necessity for digital manipulation to effect evaluation of the rectum is often reported. However, at least one half of reported patients have normal bowel movements. Pain is usually minimal but can be severe and, when present, tends to be localized to the perineum, the sacral area, or the left iliac fossa. Such pain is frequently described as dull, boring, continuous, and unchanged by defecation. As noted, nonspecific rectal ulcer may be related to isolated prolapse of mucosa on the anterior rectal wall (see p. 1600), and therefore evidence for prolapse should be sought. In contrast to the relatively acute picture of nonspecific ulcers elsewhere in the colon, nonspecific ulcer of the rectum may be asymptomatic and persist unchanged for years.[66, 70]

Diagnosis

Except when located in the rectum, nonspecific ulcer of the colon is usually diagnosed at laparotomy. Symptoms and physical findings are not specific, and full evaluation may be delayed until perforation with peritonitis has developed. Colonoscopy is clearly the most useful test if the diagnosis is suspected.[64, 65, 67, 87]

In solitary rectal ulcer, a digital examination of the rectum may demonstrate an area of induration that can antedate the actual ulceration. In contrast to malignant rectal ulceration, there should be no fixation of the bowel wall to adjacent structures. The correct diagnosis should be suspected from findings at sigmoidoscopy (Color Fig. 84–9, p. xliii). A shallow ulcer, up to 5 cm in size with flat edges and clearly demarcated from normal mucosa by a thin line of hyperemia, is usually seen 6 to 10 cm from the anal margin on the anterior rectal wall. The ulcer may have an irregular outline or may be round or even linear. The base can be white, gray, or yellow and is said to look like "wash leather."[86] The surrounding mucosa may have a slightly nodular appearance. A pre-ulcer, hyperemic, or "granular" phase can antedate the actual crater. Because of its flat margin, the ulcer can be difficult to biopsy. Nevertheless, biopsy must be done to exclude malignancy.

Abnormalities in a barium enema X-ray produced by a solitary ulcer of the colon are quite variable and include an ulcer defect, a nodular swelling caused by edema around the ulcer without the ulcer itself necessarily being seen, a large inflammatory mass simulating carcinoma, and the appearance of a diverticulum, especially if located in the cecum.[64, 65, 87] Colonic motility may be increased adjacent to the ulcer, and localized spasm or actual fibrotic changes may produce a strictured appearance.[67] Since the barium enema may even suggest bowel perforation, the findings of such examinations are nonspecific, provoking an extensive differential diagnosis that can be resolved only by colonoscopy and histologic examination of appropriately taken biopsies.

X-ray is likewise not helpful in the diagnosis of a rectal ulcer.[66, 69, 87] Cancer is often the leading differential possibility, especially if a mass is present. Endoscopic biopsy and possibly surgery will be required to establish the diagnosis.

Treatment

Except when the ulcer is located in the rectum, the conventional management for nonspecific ulcer of the colon has been surgical excision. Clearly, laparotomy is necessary if perforation is present and may be needed if bleeding cannot be controlled. However, if the diagnosis of nonspecific ulcer is suspected, an endoscopy, tissue culture, biopsy, and brush cytologic examination of the ulcer should be performed, because the patient with nonspecific ulcer can recover uneventfully without surgery.[64, 65, 70]

Nonspecific ulcer of the rectum can remain remarkably static for years.[66, 71, 86] Its extreme chronicity is matched by an equal resistance to treatment. Many forms of therapy, including local electrocautery, caustic agents, antibiotics, sulfasalazine, steroid retention enemas, and partial excisional biopsy have failed to alter the course of the disease and should not be used.[71]

Since perforation of rectal ulcers is rare and symptoms may be mild and intermittent, treatment with hydrophilic mucilloids, stool softeners, local analgesics, glycerine suppositories, and monitoring by periodic examinations seems warranted unless excessive bleeding or discomfort forces a more invasive approach such as surgical resection or bypass. Asymptomatic ulcers are best observed since they may spontaneously resolve, even after many years.[71, 86]

If a history of frequent straining at stool or self-digitation to remove hard stool is present, one should consider evaluation for pelvic muscle dysfunction by electromyography or functional defecography, if available. The patient should also be evaluated for the presence of localized rectal prolapse. If rectal prolapse is present and symptoms are very troublesome, surgical repair of the prolapse, even without excision of the ulceration, will usually lead to resolution of the ulceration and associated colitis cystica profunda.[88, 89] Surgery directed toward correction of pelvic muscle dysfunction in patients without demonstrable rectal mucosal prolapse has an uncertain outcome. Resection or bypass of the rectum also cures the problem, but is rarely indicated.

COLITIS CYSTICA PROFUNDA

Benign, mucus-filled lesions of the colon are of two main types. Colitis cystica superficialis is quite rare and has been described mainly in persons with pellagra, even in the absence of typical skin lesions, and in some adults with celiac disease.[90–92] It is characterized by small cysts located superficial to the muscularis mucosae which appear grossly as thousands of minute gray blebs on the mucosal surface. The condition itself has no recognized clinical significance and presumably resolves after successful treatment of the underlying disease.

The second and more common condition producing benign mucus-filled cysts in the colon wall is colitis cystica profunda. Here, the cysts are large in size, located below the muscularis mucosae, and often present clinically as an ulcerating lesion or mass in the rectosigmoid colon which must be differentiated from invasive adenocarcinoma.

Pathology

Three forms of colitis cystica profunda have been described. The most common is localized to the rectum, is also called proctitis cystica profunda, and has been proposed to be part of the solitary rectal ulcer syndrome.[69, 74, 83, 89] A segmental form and the very rare diffuse type involve more extensive areas of proximal large intestine.[93, 94] In all three forms, the intestinal wall is thickened by the submucosal cysts, which vary from 0.1 to 3.0 cm in diameter. Incision into and compression of the cystic area usually produces a thick, gelatinous material. The overlying mucosa may appear normal or may be hyperemic, edematous, ulcerated, or even contain a small umbilication.

Microscopically, the cysts lie below the muscularis mucosae, may even penetrate into the muscularis propria, and contain a basophilic-staining mucoid material. The mucous lakes can have no discernible epithelium or may be lined by colonic epithelium showing varying degrees of pressure atrophy and atypia. While there are no changes in the epithelial cell nuclei to suggest neoplasia, it is this picture of aberrant gland-forming colonic epithelium with acellular mucous lakes that can lead to misdiagnosis of a mucus-producing carcinoma (Fig. 84–10*B*). Communication between the cyst and bowel lumen can occasionally be found by serial sections (Fig. 84–10*A*).[90, 93, 95] The surrounding connective tissue often shows histologic changes of chronic inflammation and fibrosis, especially when colitis cystica profunda occurs as part of the solitary rectal ulcer syndrome. In this situation, there is extensive replacement of the lamina propria around the cysts by fibroblasts arranged at right angles to the muscularis mucosa. The condition must also be differentiated from giant inflammatory polyps which occur with inflammatory bowel disease.[96, 97]

Pathogenesis

Three specific mechanisms have been proposed as causing colitis cystica profunda: (1) congenitally ectopic mucosa, (2) herniation of epithelium into the submu-

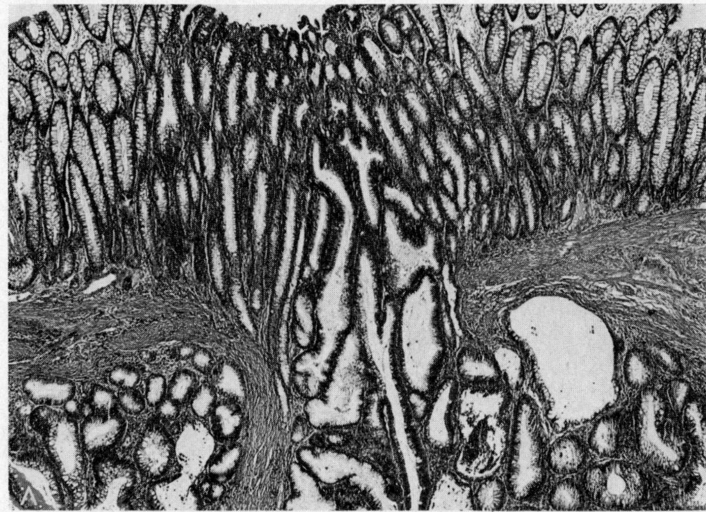

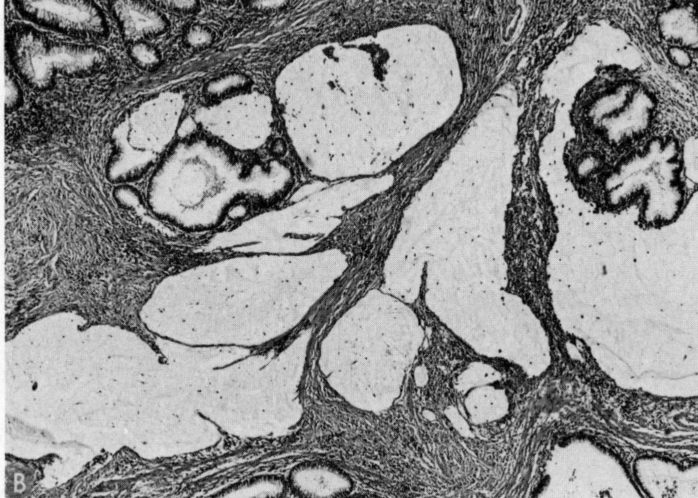

Figure 84–10. *A,* Biopsy of the polypoid sigmoid mass shown in Figure 84–12. Communication between the submucosal cysts and the bowel lumen through a defect in the muscularis mucosae may occasionally be demonstrated by serial sections. Hematoxylin and eosin stain, × 345. (From Fechner, R. R.: Dis. Colon Rectum *10*:359, 1967. Used by permission.) *B,* Pools of mucin without epithelial lining as well as epithelium lined cysts are present in the submucosa. Although the cyst epithelium is benign, this appearance has occasionally resulted in misdiagnosis of mucus-producing carcinoma. Hematoxylin and eosin stain, × 64.

cosa secondary to a "weakness" in the muscularis mucosae, and (3) a postinflammatory or post-traumatic change.[90, 92, 95]

The complete absence of submucosal cysts in autopsy reports of infants and children has been considered evidence against a congenital defect and in favor of an acquired abnormality.[93] There is no specific evidence to support the herniation theory. In many early cases the patients have a history of severe dysentery, and follicular ulcers are occasionally present. Conceptually, a necrotizing mucosal lesion could extend into a submucosal lymphoid follicle. During subsequent healing, downgrowth of colonic epithelium into the sloughed area could produce a narrow-mouthed epithelium-lined submucosal space. However, arguing against an inflammatory cause is the absence of a compatible history in many cases and the infrequent association of colitis cystica profunda with chronic ulcerative colitis.

The localized form, most commonly found in the rectum, probably develops as an aberrant process of mucosal repair occurring in response to chronic trauma and possibly ischemia consequent to prolapse and muscular compression of the rectal mucosa. Clearly documented rectal prolapse has been reported in 54 per cent of patients with localized rectal colitis cystica profunda.[89]

Clinical Picture and Diagnosis

The majority of reported cases are in young adults, although the age ranges from 4 to 68 years.[92] The prevalence is slightly greater in women. The most frequent presenting symptoms are mild diarrhea, tenesmus, cramping lower abdominal pain, and passage of blood and mucus in stool. Rectal or sacral pain may also be present as well as difficulty with defecation accompanied by a sense of rectal fullness, tenesmus, and the presence of rectal prolapse. Some cases have been described following an episode of severe bacillary dysentery[95] or with idiopathic ulcerative proctitis and colitis,[90, 98] but also without any preceding diarrheal illness.[99, 100] One unusual case involved multiple segments of the colon, caused obstructive symptoms, and recurred after surgical resection.[101] Cysts may also be

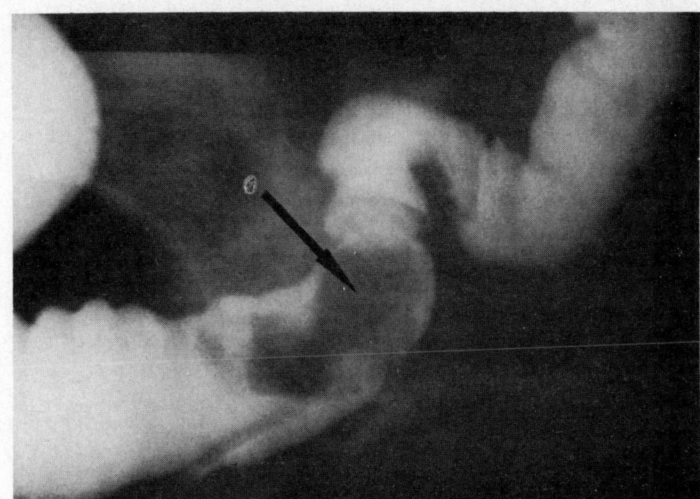

Figure 84–12. Barium enema examination in colitis cystica profunda may disclose small nodular irregularities of bowel wall or large space-occupying lesions, as shown here. (From Fechner, R. F. Dis. Colon Rectum *10*:359, 1967.)

part of the colonic strictures that complicate radiation colitis[102] or may even appear at colostomy sites.[103] However, most commonly colitis cystica profunda is a disease of the rectum, associated with rectal prolapse and a solitary rectal ulcer[73, 89] (see p. 1602).

Rectal examination may demonstrate one or more smooth, rubbery-firm masses that are easily movable and do not adhere to either the overlying mucosa or the surrounding tissue. The cystic area is usually in the anterior rectal wall within 12 cm of the anal verge, but may be in the ascending, transverse, and descending colon.[98, 104] Varying degrees of rectal prolapse may also be evident. At endoscopy, the cysts may have a sessile, plaque-like, or polypoid appearance and are covered by mucosa that may be normal, edematous, congested, umbilicated, or even ulcerated (Color Fig. 84–11, p. xliv). Bulky or fibrotic lesions can produce luminal obstruction.[100] The differential diagnosis is extensive and usually includes adenocarcinoma or lymphoma, benign adenomatous polyps, villous adenoma, submucosal lipoma, neurofibroma, inflammatory pseudopolyps of ulcerative and Crohn's colitis, polypoid granulomatous reaction of schistosomiasis and pneumatosis cystoides intestinalis, and endometriosis of the bowel. Barium enema will show changes varying from only an irregularity in the intestinal wall to large nodular masses with apparent ulceration (Fig. 84–12).[104–106] Similar X-ray changes have also been reported in patients with obliterative arteriosclerosis and focal colonic mucosal necrosis.[107, 108] The difficulty of the extensive differential diagnosis is best resolved by biopsy at sigmoidoscopy or colonoscopy. For rectal lesions, a forceps biopsy instrument and rigid sigmoidoscope should be used. Small mucosal pinch biopsy specimens taken at fiberoptic endoscopy are usually inadequate for diagnosis. Definitive diagnosis may require surgical excision.

Management

A correct preoperative diagnosis may help to avoid inappropriate or radical surgery for suspected cancer. An excisional biopsy is usually adequate therapy for small, movable submucosal cysts. Segmental resection is indicated for large bulky lesions, especially those producing intestinal obstruction or causing iron deficiency from chronic blood loss or hypokalemia and hypoalbuminemia from excessive secretion of colonic mucus.[109] It is most important to determine if rectal prolapse is present as a precipitating cause (see pp. 1586–1587). If symptoms require surgery, then repair of the prolapse should be included in any operation; otherwise, the process is likely to recur.[89] Since carcinoma of the colon does not develop, a conservative course of observation should be followed for small lesions with mild symptoms and not associated with symptomatic rectal prolapse.[110]

NONSPECIFIC ULCERATIVE PROCTITIS

Hematochezia, mucopurulent rectal discharge, and tenesmus due to inflammation of the rectal mucosa may be clearly demarcated on proctosigmoidoscopic examination by normal-appearing more proximal mucosa. When no particular inciting etiology can be elicited, the disorder is termed nonspecific ulcerative proctitis, a variant of diffuse ulcerative colitis characterized by a more favorable clinical course and more benign prognosis.

Approximately 25 to 30 per cent of patients presenting with ulcerative colitis will demonstrate disease limited to the rectum. Both the pediatric and elderly populations can be affected, although the majority of patients present between the ages of 20 and 40 years.[111–114]

Clinical Picture

Typically, patients with ulcerative proctitis present with rectal bleeding which may be persistent, but seldom severe. Alterations in bowel habits are common and are usually reported as increased frequency of small-volume stools, often associated with mucoid or mucosanguinous discharge. Fecal urgency and tenesmus are common, and may relate to an altered sensory response to rectal distention.[115] Although vague abdominal discomfort is occasionally present, severe pain is rare. Systemic symptoms such as fever, malaise, and weight loss are usually absent.

Diagnosis

The diagnosis of nonspecific ulcerative proctitis is one of exclusion. The differential diagnosis includes many infectious causes; therefore, it is most imperative to exclude any potential infectious etiology prior to introducing therapy, since topical corticosteroids may allow localized infection to disseminate widely.

The initial approach to the evaluation is based on a thorough history, with particular attention to duration of illness, recent travel, sexual activity, medications, prior pelvic irradiation, and the presence of previous similar episodes (see pp. 1191–1232 and 1435–1477). In general, acute proctitis is infectious in nature and, depending on the patient's overall clinical condition, therapy may be postponed pending the results of stool examination for ova and parasites and culture for enteric pathogens. If infection with *Campylobacter* species is suspected, a special selective culture medium must be utilized. Stool toxin assay and culture for *Clostridium difficile* may be warranted if the clinical setting suggests pseudomembranous colitis (see pp. 1191–1232 and 1307–1320).

If the aforementioned examinations are unrevealing, or if the illness is more protracted, proctosigmoidoscopy is indicated. The avoidance of a bowel preparation is advised, since purging enemas may remove mucosal exudate and induce mucosal edema and hyperemia.[116] Characteristically, the inflammatory process begins at the dentate line and may extend 15 to 20 cm proximally. The rectal mucosa may appear diffusely erythematous and friable, with touch bleeding. Underlying submucosal vascular networks are generally obscured by edema, hyperemia, or mucosanguinous exudate. Although the mucosa assumes an irregular or granular appearance, discrete ulcerations are rarely seen. The important endoscopic finding that suggests the diagnosis of ulcerative proctitis is a sharp line of demarcation between the distal inflammatory process and the proximal normal rectal or lower sigmoid mucosa.

Biopsy of the rectal mucosa will show changes indistinguishable from those found in diffuse ulcerative colitis and may further distinguish this entity from acute self-limited colitis. Findings more suggestive of idiopathic inflammatory bowel disease include distorted crypt architecture or crypt atrophy, infiltration of neutrophils and round cells (especially plasma cells) into the lamina propria, basal lymphoid aggregates or giant cells, and separation of crypts resulting in a villous-appearing surface. The presence of crypt abscesses is not necessarily specific for ulcerative proctitis[117, 118] (see pp. 1327–1358 and 1435–1477).

In the acute setting, there is no diagnostic or therapeutic advantage to visualization of the more proximal colon when a clear proximal margin of disease has been demonstrated on proctosigmoidoscopy. Later in the course, air-contrast barium radiography of the colon or colonoscopy can be undertaken to exclude the skip lesions of Crohn's colitis. Whereas barium enema is more likely to visualize the terminal ileum, colonoscopy will better allow direct colonic mucosal examination and biopsy. In one study, histologic inflammatory changes were demonstrated underlying grossly normal proximal colon in nearly 60 per cent of patients with idiopathic proctitis and appeared to correlate with a more severe clinical course and poor response to therapy.[119]

Differential Diagnosis

In the patient presenting with the abrupt onset of symptoms suggesting proctitis, it may be extremely difficult to distinguish idiopathic proctitis from the numerous disease processes that may mimic its clinical picture and proctosigmoidoscopic appearance (Table 84–3). Infection is probably the most common cause of proctitis or proctosigmoiditis, and much of the recent emphasis on infectious proctitis stems from studies of its frequency and polymicrobial nature in homosexual men[120–123] (see pp. 1257–1274).

A systematic approach to the patient limits the number of viable possibilities. Many of the historical features that may aid in the differentiation have been mentioned above. On physical examination, the perianal region should be carefully inspected for the presence of fistulas, perirectal abscesses, ulcerations, strictures, and vesicles that are suggestive of anorectal

Table 84–3. DIFFERENTIAL DIAGNOSIS OF NONSPECIFIC ULCERATIVE PROCTITIS

Crohn's disease	Traumatic proctitis
Common infectious causes	Foreign bodies
Amebiasis	Chemical proctitis
Shigellosis	Enemas and suppositories
Salmonellosis	Solitary ulcer syndrome
Campylobacter colitis	Miscellaneous rare causes
Rare infectious causes	Vasculitis
Tuberculosis	Connective tissue disease
Fungal infections	Amyloidosis
Schistosomiasis	Hemolytic-uremic syndrome
Balantidiasis	Behçet's syndrome
Cytomegalovirus infections	Gold-induced enterocolitis
Venereal diseases	Chronic lymphocytic leukemia
Anorectal gonorrhea	Lymphoma
Chlamydial proctitis (LGV and non-LGV)	Following diversion of the fecal stream
Anorectal syphilis	Immunodeficiency diseases
Anorectal herpes simplex infection	Graft-versus-host disease
Antibiotic-associated pseudomembranous colitis	Lipid proctitis
Radiation proctitis	
Ischemic proctitis	

Adapted from Marshall, J. B., and Butt, J. H. J. Clin. Gastroenterol. *4*:321, 1982.

gonorrhea, non–lymphogranuloma venereum (non-LGV) Chlamydia, primary syphilis, or herpes simplex. The latter may also be associated with urinary retention, constipation, and sacral paresthesias.

Proctosigmoidoscopy may further narrow the etiologic spectrum. Discrete ulcerations, vesicles, or mucosal inflammatory changes are, in general, limited to the rectum in these aforementioned disorders. Conversely, chlamydial involvement with LGV serotypes, shigellosis, salmonellosis, and *Campylobacter* species and *Clostridium difficile* infections usually display more diffuse mucosal involvement extending into the sigmoid and descending colon. Furthermore, the rectum is often spared in pseudomembranous colitis (see pp. 1191–1232 and 1307–1320). Cytomegaloviral and amebic colitis are characteristically widespread throughout the colon and may grossly appear as focal ulcerations or diffuse erythema and friability. Histologic examination and culture of mucosal abnormalities may likely identify the causative agent, as will, in some instances, gram stain of the mucopurulent discharge (for gonococci), darkfield examination (for perianal syphilis), and fluorescent antibody testing (for herpesvirus and cytomegalovirus). Finally, serologic studies may be useful in the diagnosis of amebic, syphilitic, and LGV proctitis (see pp. 1159, 1266, and 1268).

Nonspecific causes of proctitis may also be discerned by proctosigmoidoscopy. Mucosal thinning and submucosal telangiectasias are suggestive of radiation proctitis, but diffuse mucosal breakdown and friability may make radiation-induced changes difficult to distinguish from either idiopathic or ischemic proctocolitis (see pp. 1369–1382, 1439–1446, and 1903–1916). Rectal ischemia alone (without more proximal involvement) is uncommon, however, owing to the dual blood supply to this region. Differentiating Crohn's disease of the rectum from nonspecific ulcerative proctitis may be somewhat easier if external (perianal) manifestations of the former are present, or if proctoscopy discloses aphthoid ulcerations or cobblestoning so typical of Crohn's disease. Frequently, however, microscopic examination of the involved mucosa, barium radiography of the more proximal colon (and terminal ileum), and prospective evaluation of the subsequent clinical course may be necessary to be fully confident of either diagnosis (see pp. 1341–1349).

Course of the Disease

Overall, nonspecific proctitis follows a benign course and serious sequelae are uncommon. Seventy-five per cent of patients will experience intermittent symptomatic relapses characterized by rectal bleeding, fecal urgency and frequency, and tenesmus.[124] Most relapses occur within one year of clinical remission and, in general, respond well to conservative medical measures. The remaining 25 per cent of patients with proctitis will have either complete remission or extension of their disease proximally (10 to 15 per cent). Extension into the sigmoid or descending colon alone is more common than the development of universal colitis, and the full extent of disease is usually reached within five years of initial diagnosis. Those with onset of proctitis prior to the age of 21 years are at a substantially higher risk for proximal spread than are middle-aged or older individuals.[112–114, 124, 125]

Except for occasional local problems (fissures, hemorrhoids), the common complications of extensive ulcerative colitis (e.g., toxic megacolon) rarely affect patients with nonspecific proctitis. Likewise, iritis, arthritis, and other extraintestinal features are absent and the risk of colorectal malignancy is not increased. Overall, life expectancy is not altered in patients with well-defined ulcerative proctitis.[112, 126, 127]

Treatment

Therapy should be aimed primarily at ameliorating symptoms and at lessening the degree of inflammation of the rectal mucosa. Unfortunately, gross mucosal appearance may not accurately reflect the patient's clinical condition, since many patients with ulcerative proctitis in clinical remission display endoscopic evidence of active disease.[124] Thus, the physician may concentrate on therapy that achieves clinical, rather than macroscopic or microscopic, remission.

Since the disease process is limited to the terminal 15 to 20 cm of large bowel, topical therapy in the form of hydrocortisone retention enemas or foam usually ameliorates symptoms in about 75 per cent of patients.[113, 128] The active component of sulfasalazine, 5-aminosalicylic acid (5-ASA), appears to be as effective as hydrocortisone when given as a retention enema.[129–131] This preparation may supplant topical hydrocortisone as the agent of choice in patients with distal colitis or proctitis, thus eliminating the potential side effects arising from the absorption either of the sulfa moiety in orally administered sulfasalazine or of topically applied corticosteroids. Also, Tixocortol pivalate, a rapidly metabolized, non-mineralocorticoid, non-glucocorticoid steroid preparation, is being investigated as a topical anti-inflammatory agent. It does not suppress the pituitary-adrenal axis and apparently exhibits no steroid toxicity.

Since the majority of patients benefit from topical therapy, systemic treatment is reserved for individuals with severe refractory proctitis or those unable to self-administer the rectal preparations. In these instances, oral sulfasalazine may be useful to induce and maintain clinical remission.[124, 126] Since this agent is associated with intolerable side effects in up to one fifth of patients, a slow release, orally administered 5-ASA compound, devoid of the sulfapyridine component, is being investigated currently.[132, 133] However, its effect on nonspecific ulcerative proctitis is yet unknown. Systemic steroids are infrequently needed to control symptoms of proctitis, but should be considered for patients with hematochezia, fecal urgency, and tenesmus refractory to the aforementioned drugs.

DIVERSION COLITIS

Diversion colitis is inflammation in an excluded colonic segment, usually a Hartman's pouch, which resolves following reanastomosis of the intestine.[134] Approximately 31 cases have been reported in the English-language literature;[134–139] 13 of these were in otherwise healthy persons who had a fecal diversion procedure for perforated sigmoid diverticulitis,[134, 138–140] and 18 were in patients who had Crohn's disease in intestine proximal to the diversion[135, 136] (see pp. 1327–1358 and 1426–1432).

In some patients, diversion colitis causes severe symptoms. In others, it is only an incidental endoscopic finding. Symptomatic patients typically complain of tenesmus, anorectal pain, and a purulent or bloody rectal discharge. The onset of symptoms is from one month to 22 years after fecal diversion.[139, 140] While the inflammatory process is usually limited to the rectum, sparing of the distal segment has been described.[134] Endoscopic findings include erythema, friability, and granularity of the rectal mucosa with occasionally nodular inflammatory polyps and aphthous ulcerations. Biopsy of the mucosa demonstrates acute inflammation within the lamina propria with epithelial regeneration, crypt abscesses, focal edema, ulcerations, and an increase in the number of lymphoid follicles. Microgranulomas have also been reported in cases of diversion colitis in patients with Crohn's disease.[136] The abnormal appearance and histologic changes in the mucosa can return to normal within two weeks after reanastomosis of the intestine.[140]

The pathogenesis of diversion colitis is unknown. Proposed hypotheses include prolonged contact of the mucosa with toxic luminal contents, an alteration in the bacterial flora, and loss of normal luminal nutrients.[134, 138, 139] There is no evidence at present for the emergence of a harmful strain of bacteria, fungus, or virus causing an infection in the excluded intestine.

Results of medical treatment have been reported in only a small number of cases.[134–140] Corticosteroid enemas as well as oral steroids may or may not be effective.[134–138] Likewise, metronidazole may or may not benefit the patient.[141] Further reported experience with medical treatment is required before the prognosis for nonsurgical management can be assessed. Patients who have severe, persisting symptoms and who can tolerate additional intestinal surgery should have intestinal continuity re-established, if possible.

NEUTROPENIC TYPHLITIS

Typhlitis is a term derived from the Greek "typhlon," meaning blind sac and referring to inflammation of the cecum. More specifically, typhlitis is a necrotizing cecitis that is associated with neutropenic states and was originally described at autopsy of leukemic children dying while undergoing chemotherapy.[142] Since the inflammatory process often extends into the terminal ileum, appendix, and ascending colon, more descriptive names such as *neutropenic enterocolitis, necrotizing enterocolitis*, and *ileocecal syndrome* have been coined. Although earlier reports associate it with hematologic malignancies in children, typhlitis also affects adults receiving immunosuppressive therapy for malignancy[143–145] or organ transplants[146] and those with aplastic anemia,[147] cyclic neutropenia,[148] and drug-induced neutropenia unrelated to malignancy.[149]

Typhlitis is a devastating disease. Mortality rates range between 5 and 100 per cent, and average 40 to 50 per cent.[144, 145, 150–152] Most deaths are attributable to cecal perforation, bowel necrosis, and sepsis. This disorder is not rare. In immunocompromised children, typhlitis accounts for 11 per cent of acute abdominal operations and has been reported in 26 per cent of childhood leukemics followed prospectively.[145, 153]

Pathogenesis

Typhlitis is a necrotizing cecitis often extending both proximal and distal to the cecum. Although the precise etiology is still somewhat unclear, profound neutropenia appears to be a universal predisposing factor and thereby explains the common association of aggressive chemotherapy and necrotizing enterocolitis. The process begins as mucosal ulceration, perhaps induced by cytotoxic chemotherapeutic agents. Support for this assumption comes from the frequent association of stomatitis, necrotizing pharyngitis, and colitis in leukemics undergoing treatment.[147, 154] There appears to be no particular agent or chemotherapeutic regimen that is associated with this disease. Although initial epithelial damage has been attributed to the effects of cytotoxic drugs, these agents cannot be incriminated in the rare patient with aplastic anemia or cyclic neutropenia who develops necrotizing enterocolitis.

Bacterial invasion of the denuded mucosa further disrupts the integrity of the bowel wall and ultimately may produce transmural penetration, infarction, perforation, and peritonitis. Such perforations are poorly contained owing to the paucity of inflammatory reaction. Mucosal and submucosal necrosis may involve the subjacent vasculature and produce subtle or profuse intramural or intraluminal hemorrhage, as well as provide a portal of entry into the circulation for bacterial and fungal pathogens. As stated earlier, the necrotizing process may extend along and through the mucosal epithelial surface of the proximal colon and, less commonly, the terminal small bowel. Leukemic infiltrates are inconsistently found in the area of involved intestine.[155–157]

Gross examination of the involved region may disclose bowel wall thickening, discrete or confluent mucosal ulceration, intramural edema, hemorrhage, and necrosis. Histologically, necrosis, edema, and hemorrhage are seen. Abundant bacteria are present within the bowel wall with a striking lack of lymphoid inflammatory cells and virtually complete absence of neutrophils.

The marked proclivity of necrotizing enterocolitis

for the cecum remains unexplained. Its large size and distensibility may permit a relative stasis of fecal contents and bacterial overgrowth which may normally coexist without incident in immunocompetent hosts.[147] Cecal hypomotility and bacterial pooling may also be promoted by the effect of exogenous agents, such as is seen with the neurotoxicity of the vinca alkaloids.[158]

Clinical Picture

Although typhlitis is often initially discovered at laparotomy or autopsy, the clinical setting and patient presentation may alert the physician to consider this diagnosis. The vast majority of patients will be receiving antineoplastic drugs, immunosuppressed, and profoundly granulocytopenic (less than 1000 cells/mm^3). Typhlitis is more common during induction therapy than during maintenance or consolidation.[150] In general, symptoms begin at the height of bone marrow suppression, that is, 1 to 2 weeks into therapy. Right lower quadrant abdominal pain, either intermittently cramping or consistently dull in nature, is present in nearly all patients. Watery diarrhea (in 40 to 80 per cent of patients) or grossly bloody diarrhea (25 to 45 per cent) commonly accompanies the abdominal pain. Nausea and vomiting may also be prominent symptoms. Fever, rigors, and shock may appear as results of septicemia or colonic perforation. The time course and severity of illness varies and a subacute or prolonged course is more amenable to medical therapy as the bone marrow recovers.[145, 150]

Physical findings in the abdomen are also variable depending on the severity of the disease and the presence of complications. Abdominal distention and tympany may reflect an adynamic ileus, as may the absence of bowel sounds. Tenderness to palpation is often most marked in the right lower quadrant. Diffuse direct and rebound tenderness suggest colonic perforation and peritonitis (see pp. 238–257). Oral or pharyngeal mucositis may be a harbinger of similar changes in the colon. Despite their immunocompromised state, affected patients usually have normal febrile responses.

Diagnosis

Attention and consideration given to the possibility of necrotizing enterocolitis is the most important aspect of diagnosis. The primary differential diagnosis is pseudomembranous or antibiotic-induced colitis, which, like typhlitis, may present with abdominal pain, fever, and watery or bloody diarrhea (see pp. 1307–1320). Neutropenia, however, is not a feature of this disorder. Patients with both illnesses are likely to be receiving broad-spectrum antibiotics, which may add to the diagnostic confusion. Stool specimens cultured or assayed for toxin of *Clostridium difficile* will help to differentiate these two processes. Another diagnostic consideration may be acute colonic pseudo-obstruction, which is discussed on pages 1620 to 1622. While this condition may occur in patients with neutropenia, acute pseudo-obstruction is often painless and is usually not accompanied by bloody diarrhea. Other less likely diagnostic possibilities include ischemic colitis, appendicitis, small bowel obstruction, concomitant Crohn's disease or ulcerative colitis, or infectious colitis from an opportunistic pathogen, such as cytomegalovirus or *Candida*.

Additional studies may help to make the diagnosis. Plain abdominal radiographs may be normal or demonstrate one of the following abnormalities: (1) cecal, ascending colon, or small bowel dilation, (2) diminished or absent gas shadows in the right lower quadrant (due to an atonic and fluid-filled colon), (3) thumbprinting of the ascending colon (suggestive of submucosal edema or hemorrhage), (4) intramural air shadows, or (5) lower abdominal soft tissue mass displacing small bowel[142, 159] (Fig. 84–13).

Single-contrast radiography of the colon will likely display colonic mucosal irregularities and ulcerations and may show thumbprinting. The radiologist involved must be forewarned of the possibility of a transmural process so that high-pressure instillation will be avoided and the use of water-soluble contrast considered. Cecal perforation has been reported following barium enema in this disease.[157] Abdominal computed tomography and ultrasound have been utilized to evaluate pericolic soft tissue masses and to possibly exclude intussusception or appendicitis. These noninvasive imaging modalities may be preferable to contrast enemas if an impending perforation is considered likely.[160, 161]

Colonoscopy or flexible sigmoidoscopy is relatively contraindicated in the presence of neutropenia and thrombocytopenia. Furthermore, air insufflation may accelerate perforation. Overall, there is little to be gained by the use of these procedures with the exception of: (1) gentle proctosigmoidoscopy to exclude pseudomembranous colitis or idiopathic inflammatory bowel disease, or (2) gentle colonoscopy to evaluate a prolonged (longer than 10 to 14 days) course of intermittent hematochezia during or after bone marrow recovery or to decompress the cecum and colon if intestinal diameter greater than 12 cm suggests acute pseudo-obstruction (see p. 1620).

Treatment

Clinical recognition of the early signs of necrotizing enterocolitis in the appropriate setting of neutropenia is essential in view of the high mortality in this disease. Unfortunately, diagnosis at autopsy is not rare. Intravenous fluids to maintain euvolemia and renal perfusion, bowel rest, nasogastric suction, and parenteral broad-spectrum antibiotics are the essentials of therapy for typhlitis without perforation and peritonitis. Antibiotic coverage should include agents bacteriocidal to enteric gram-negative and anaerobic organisms. If pseudomembranous colitis cannot be immediately excluded, vancomycin may be included in the regimen. Anticholinergic medications, particularly antidiarrheal agents, should be avoided and narcotics should be used

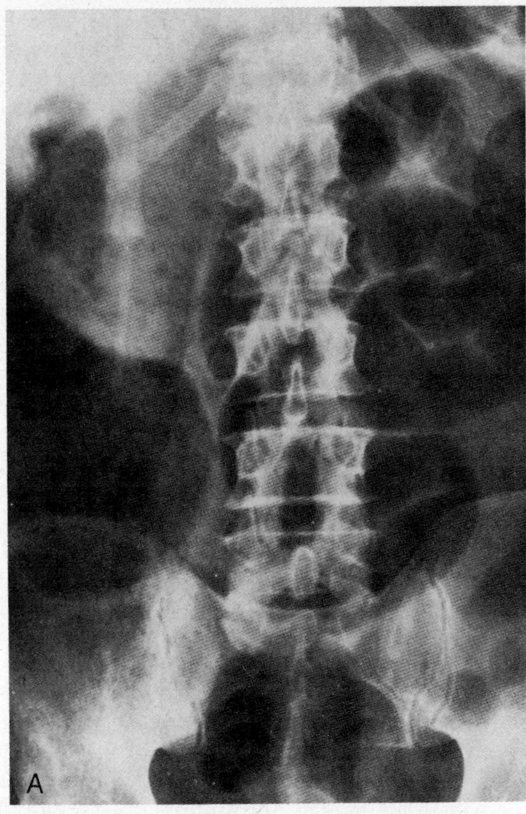

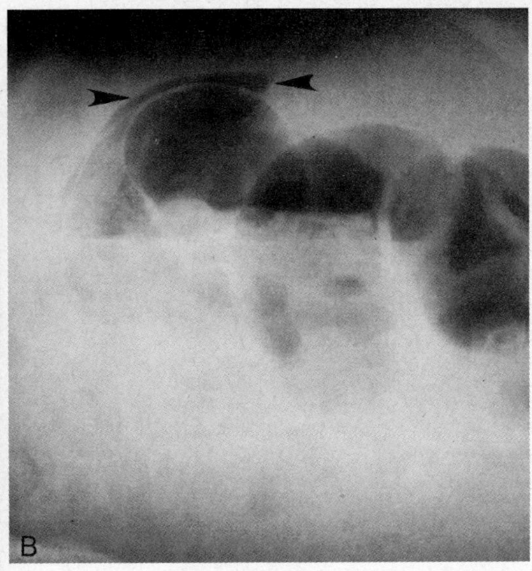

Figure 84–13. Plain abdominal radiographic features of neutropenic typhlitis. *A*, Mottled right lower quadrant mass in the region of the cecum displacing dilated small intestinal loops. (From Taylor, A. J., Dodds, W. J., Gonyo, J. E., and Komorowski, R. A. Gastrointest. Radiol. *10*:363–369, 1985. Used by permission.) *B*, Left lateral decubitus radiograph demonstrating intraluminal air-fluid interface and free peritoneal air *(arrows)* resulting from a cecal perforation. (From Hunter, T. B., and Bjelland, J. C. Gastrointestinal complications of leukemia and its treatment. AJR *142*:513–518. © by the American Roentgen Ray Society, 1984.)

sparingly, since they may cause distention or even ileus, confusing the clinical picture. Continuous observation in an intensive care unit is strongly advised with frequent abdominal examinations by the physician.

Persistent but not life-threatening ileocolonic hemorrhage can be managed with erythrocyte and platelet transfusions as needed. In rare instances, arteriographic embolization has been carried out to arrest ongoing bleeding.[150, 162] Granulocyte transfusions have been advocated by some, but their efficacy remains to be established.[144, 163]

The role of surgery in suspected typhlitis or enterocolitis is somewhat controversial. Clearly, documentation or strong suspicion of a cecal perforation, massive rectal bleeding, fulminant and unrelenting sepsis with severe localized abdominal tenderness, and abscess formation are indications for emergent or urgent surgical intervention. What is less certain is the need for exploration and resection in patients with more protracted illnesses, in whom symptoms persist for several days without evidence of frank perforation or life-threatening hemorrhage. Although there are proponents of early, aggressive surgery in all patients with suspected typhlitis,[164, 165] the recent trend is toward a more conservative approach with meticulous medical management during the period of bone marrow recovery and rapid surgical intervention if the clinical condition deteriorates.[145, 150]

At surgery, care must be taken to resect the entire segment of diseased bowel, since normal appearing serosal surfaces may betray the presence of ongoing mucosal breakdown and necrosis. In general, depending upon the extent of involvement, right hemicolectomy or total abdominal colectomy is preferable to segmental resection. Furthermore, a two-stage procedure, rather than a primary ileocolonic anastomosis, is recommended in such immunocompromised patients.

Finally, in patients successfully treated medically, further chemotherapy should be postponed until complete healing is documented, in light of reports of recurrent episodes of clinical typhlitis on reinstitution of therapy.[145, 150]

COLLAGENOUS COLITIS

In 1976, Lindstrom described a middle-aged woman with chronic diarrhea who had grossly normal rectal mucosa, but microscopically had a heavy deposit of collagenous material beneath the surface epithelium.[166] Since then, almost 70 similar cases have been reported and recently reviewed, confirming the existence of this entity, collagenous colitis.[167–175]

The etiology of collagenous colitis is unknown. It was initially postulated that the dense subepithelial matrix contained immune complexes, but this hypothesis has not been confirmed.[166, 167] Ultrastructural studies have shown the material to be fibrils that immunologically react as collagen and procollagen type III.[167] An inflammatory origin has also been postulated as well as an autoimmune process affecting mesenchymal connective tissue in the pericryptal sheath.[173] The presence of acute inflammatory changes in the epithelium as well as the response of the disease to anti-inflammatory drugs in certain patients (as discussed below) make an abnormal response to some type of inflammation an attractive hypothesis.

Clinical Features

The disease most commonly affects women in the sixth decade of life (mean age 54 years; range 23 to 86 years). The most frequent presenting symptom is watery diarrhea, up to 2 liters daily, that may have been present from weeks to a few years in duration. Vague or colicky abdominal pain is also common. Nausea, vomiting, minimal weight loss, and excessive fecal mucus are occasionally present. The stool does not contain blood but, in early stages of the disease, may have scant numbers of leukocytes. To date, there are no reports of enteric pathogens being cultured from stool or mucosal biopsy specimens and no abnormal organisms have been seen in the mucosa by electron microscopy.[176] There is no convincing evidence to link the condition to idiopathic ulcerative or Crohn's colitis.[167]

A close association has recently been made between collagenous colitis and microscopic colitis, another idiopathic cause of chronic nonbloody diarrhea reported in a similar patient group. This entity, described in 1980, is also characterized by grossly normal colon mucosa which on biopsy demonstrates superficial inflammatory changes with neutrophils present in the surface epithelium and lamina propria.[177–179] While a change in the subepithelial collagen table was not initially noted in biopsy specimens from patients with microscopic colitis, a more recent evaluation reports both increased subepithelial collagen and many other histologic similarities to collagenous colitis.[179] Thus, current information suggests that microscopic colitis and collagenous colitis are either closely related or possibly different stages in evolution of the same process. Indeed, acute inflammatory changes have been described in colon mucosa early in the course of the disease in a few patients with typical collagenous colitis.[173, 180–182]

Studies show no consistent associated changes in small intestinal, gastric, and pancreatic function.[167, 170, 171, 173] The main symptom is diarrhea with stool volumes ranging from 500 to 2000 ml daily. There has been no evidence for a circulating secretagogue or increased levels of hormones which stimulate net intestinal water secretion[167] (see pp. 308–309). The few studies of colonic handling of electrolytes and water suggest there is net fluid secretion by colonic mucosa[172, 182] (see pp. 1030–1040). Similar findings have been reported in patients with microscopic colitis.[178] Presumably, secretion of electrolytes by the uninvolved colon crypt cells and resulting movement of water into the lumen is not impaired, while damage to the surface epithelial cells plus the barrier-like layer of collagen impairs normal ion and water absorption. Colon permeability is not altered.[172] The net result is persistence of excess fluid volume in the colon and diarrhea. Malabsorption of bile salts has been found in some of the patients, possibly augmenting net colonic secretion.[173] The cause for mild degrees of small intestinal malabsorption described in some patients is unknown. Biopsy of the jejunum and ileum have demonstrated normal histology without evidence for collagenous sprue[166, 174] (see pp. 1133–1152).

Barium X-ray studies of the small intestine and colon are usually normal and examination of the colon by fiberoptic endoscopy is reported as also being normal with the occasional exception of some edema and areas of patchy hyperemia.[167, 173, 176] The significance of these minimal changes is unclear since such can result from laxatives and enemas used for endoscopy preparation. The diagnosis of collagenous colitis is made from tissue obtained at biopsy of the colon or rectum.

Pathology

The hallmark of collagenous colitis is a thickened layer of collagen that forms an acellular band of varying diameter just beneath the epithelium (Fig. 84–14). The subepithelial layer or table of collagen below the epithelial cells is produced by a self-renewing population of mesenchymal cells or fibroblasts that also form a sheath around the colonic crypts and migrate and differentiate in a pattern similar to the overlying epithelium, suggesting a role for this sheath in main-

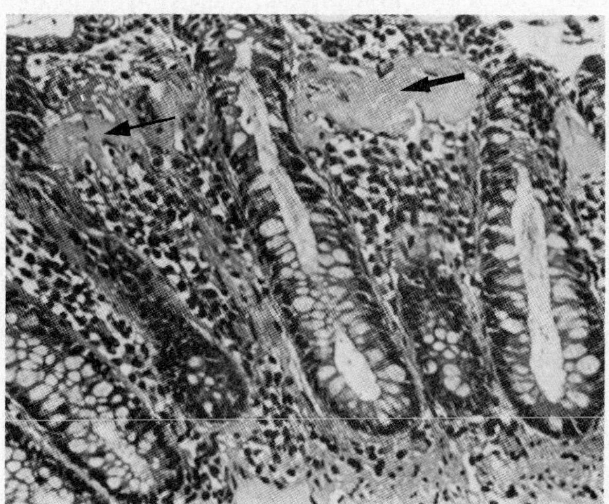

Figure 84–14. Mucosal biopsy from a patient with collagenous colitis. The major abnormality is a 50 to 60 μm thick layer of presumed collagen below the surface epithelium (*arrows*). Hematoxylin and eosin stain, × 200. (From Teglbjaerg, P. S., and Thaysen, E. H. Gastroenterology *82*:561, 1982.) (Reprinted with permission from: Collagenous colitis: an ultrastructural study of a case, by Teglbjaerg, P. S., and Thaysen, E. H. Gastroenterology *82*[3]:561–563. Copyright 1982 by The American Gastroenterological Association.)

tenance of normal mucosal function.[183, 184] An abnormality in the function of this mesenchymal connective tissue system has been postulated to be present in collagenous colitis.[182, 185] Recent ultrastructural studies in patients with collagenous colitis have demonstrated extensive changes in the pericryptal fibroblast sheath.[186] In addition to a thickened layer of collagen, the fibroblasts in the sheath appear to be transformed to cells resembling myofibroblasts, the proliferating cells in granulation tissue that secrete collagen.[187] The cause for a change in connective tissue cell type in the intestinal subepithelial area is unknown as well as its pathogenesis and relationship to inflammation. There is no evidence for similar thickening of the subepithelial collagen table in other inflammatory disorders of the colon.[188] In normal persons, the band of subepithelial cell collagen varies in thickness between approximately 2 and 6 microns.[171, 173, 188] In persons with various colon diseases, it is generally less than 10 microns in thickness. Patients having a collagen table greater than 15 microns usually have associated diarrhea.[188] In patients with collagenous colitis, the width of the collagen table has generally been greater than 15 microns, varies somewhat in depth between different segments of the colon, tends to be thicker in colon proximal to the rectum, and can reach a diameter of at least 100 microns in thickness.[167, 173]

Treatment and Prognosis

Both collagenous and microscopic colitis can undergo spontaneous resolution as well as follow a waxing and waning course.[169, 171, 178, 180, 189–192] This fact makes evaluation of treatment results in individual or small numbers of patients difficult. Standard antidiarrheal drugs, such as loperamide, may reduce the volume of stool, and hydrophilic mucilloid compounds can give increased form to the bowel movement.[193] Dehydration can become a clinical problem. When stool volume is large, close attention should be given to overall water balance, especially if other serious medical conditions are also present.

Experience with drugs in treatment of this disease is not extensive, despite the tremendous and rapid change in our concepts about the nature and treatment of collagenous colitis over the past 5 years. A number of authors have reported marked improvement and even complete resolution of symptoms during oral treatment with sulfasalazine (2 to 3 gm daily).[169, 182, 190, 191] Unfortunately, a number of other patients with collagenous colitis have not responded as well or at all to sulfasalazine treatment.[182, 185, 193] Oral treatment with 5-aminosalicylic acid, the presumed active component of sulfasalazine, has also been reported to induce a remission or cure.[16] In single case reports, a beneficial effect has been noted from treatment with metronidazole and with quinacrine.[189, 190, 192] Again, these agents have not been found effective by others. Patients who do not respond to symptomatic antidiarrheal therapy or to sulfasalazine may have a good response from systemic or topical corticosteroids.[166, 173] In some of the patients who have responded best clinically to sulfasalazine and corticosteroid treatment, the thickness of the subepithelial collagen table progressively decreased toward normal. Thus, an evaluation in subsequent colorectal biopsy specimens for whether this collagen barrier is actually decreased by treatment may provide the best way to judge effectiveness of the treatment and to evaluate prognosis for a lasting resolution of symptoms.

MALAKOPLAKIA

Malakoplakia is a rare chronic inflammatory process that most commonly involves the urinary tract.[194] However, it has also been reported in a wide variety of other organs, including the rectum, colon, ileum, and stomach.[194, 195] The term *malakoplakia* is derived from the Greek, meaning soft plaque, and was introduced by von Hansemann to describe the gross appearance of the lesion in the urinary bladder.[196] Cases of gastrointestinal malakoplakia have involved mainly the rectosigmoid and proximal colon, with occurrence in other intestinal segments being generally an incidental finding. There is a slight female predominance in reported cases and an age range from 6 to 88 years with a bimodal distribution toward children and middle-aged adults. Of importance is the frequent coexistence of gastrointestinal malakoplakia with a malignant neoplasm, especially of the colon.[195] Malnutrition, immune suppression, and chronic infection are other preceding factors. Malakoplakia has been reported in one case of chronic ulcerative colitis.[197]

Clinical Picture and Diagnosis

The most frequent symptoms include fever, abdominal pain, diarrhea, and rectal bleeding. The clinical presentations of gastrointestinal malakoplakia depend to some extent on degree of involvement of the colon. Types of distribution include:

1. Isolated sessile or polypoid masses in the rectosigmoid colon. The mucosa overlying the polypoid lesions may appear normal or ulcerated. Involvement of the mesenteric lymph nodes may produce narrowing of the intestinal lumen suggestive of a malignant stricture.
2. Diffuse involvement of the entire colon, with the gross appearance varying from soft, grayish-tan confluent lesions with serpiginous borders to confluent superficial ulcerations.
3. A mass-like lesion.

The process may also extend to the retroperitoneum with abscess formation. Symptoms range from fever and hematochezia in (1) and (2) to fever and abdominal pain with tenderness in (3). The patient may also have gastric malakoplakia with tannish-yellow, irregular, partially ulcerated mucosal plaques.[195]

Malakoplakia of the gastrointestinal tract is usually not suspected clinically. Sigmoidoscopy may show only changes characteristic of the associated neoplasm. Grossly, areas containing malakoplakia are soft, usually tan-gray in color, and have an irregular margin with central depressed areas.[197] The overlying mucosa may be intact. The area of malakoplakia may have a reddish-tan granular appearance and may be covered with necrotic material. No endoscopic photographs of gastrointestinal tract involvement with malakoplakia have been published to date. Barium X-ray is generally not helpful except for demonstrating changes of an associated malignancy, although nonspecific polypoid mucosal lesions and/or a stricture from isolated malakoplakia may be present. Correct diagnosis usually results from examination of biopsy material that contains the Michaelis-Gutmann inclusion bodies discussed below. These inclusion-filled histiocytes may be confused with Whipple's disease, fungal disease, reticulum cell sarcoma, and ceroid-like colonic histiocytes.[198, 199]

Pathology and Pathogenesis

The frequent presence of *Escherichia coli* and other coliform organisms in the urologic form of the disease led to their incrimination as the etiologic agent. However, considering the frequency of *E. coli* urinary tract infections and the rarity of malakoplakia, a direct causal relationship is unlikely. Moreover, *E. coli* organisms have not been consistently associated with malakoplakia outside the urinary tract.

The most distinctive and diagnostic histologic feature of malakoplakia is the presence of concentrically laminated, round or oval, dark inclusion bodies located in the cytoplasm of histiocytes known as von Hansemann cells (Fig. 84–15). These inclusions are called Michaelis-Gutmann bodies, after the authors who originally described the disease. Characteristically, these bodies are periodic acid–Schiff stain positive, are composed of a glycolipid matrix, probably from a specific microorganism, and are coated by a layer of calcium and iron.[194, 200–203] Agents other than bacteria that undergo histiocytic phagocytosis may also induce a similar reaction.[200]

The cause of the abnormal macrophage response to ingested bacteria is unknown. Postulated explanations include an immunologic abnormality affecting cellular digestion, a lack of lysosomal enzymes necessary for complete bacterial degradation, or a resistant strain of bacteria.[200, 201, 203] In patients with gastrointestinal malakoplakia, levels of cyclic GMP in monocytes may be reduced to a degree that could result in diminished release of lysosomal enzymes and subsequent degradation of ingested bacteria.[204, 205] Indeed, the mononuclear cells have decreased *E. coli* bacteriocidal activity. The abnormality may be corrected both *in vitro* and *in vivo* by cholinergic agonists, coincident with clinical improvement.[204, 205] These cellular findings and the response to cholinergic treatment resemble those in patients with the Chediak-Higashi syndrome.[206]

Treatment

The overall rarity of malakoplakia regardless of location has prevented meaningful evaluation of any form of treatment. Although malakoplakia of the urinary bladder has been successfully treated with streptomycin, para-aminosalicyclic acid, and isoniazid, this treatment has not been successful in polypoid malakoplakia of the colon.[207] Trimethoprim-sulfamethoxazole, ascorbic acid, and bethanechol have also been successfully employed in treating malakoplakia of the urinary bladder. Trimethoprim enters the phagocyte and helps with direct killing of bacteria. Cholinergic agents and ascorbic acid increase the intracellular cyclic GMP/AMP ratio, favoring increased monocyte bacteriocidal function. As noted, cholinergic agents have been successful in treating colonic malakoplakia, mainly in children.[204, 205] Many adult patients with gastrointestinal malakoplakia have had malignancy, a systematic debilitating disease, or evidence of severe immunologic dysfunction.[200, 201] Therefore, any patient with biopsy-proved malakoplakia should have full general medical evaluation. If no specific abnormality is

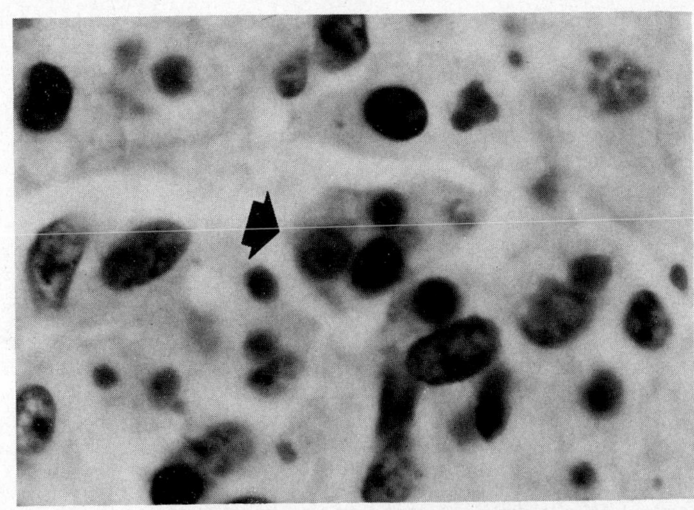

Figure 84–15. Sheets of large pale histiocytes containing Michaelis-Gutmann bodies characterize the histologic change in malakoplakia. High-power view of one of these histiocytes *(arrow)* containing the dark, concentrically laminated Michaelis-Gutmann bodies. Hematoxylin and eosin stain, × 2000. (Courtesy of R. L. Goldman, M.D., Mount Zion Hospital, San Francisco.)

found, localized intestinal malakoplakia can be treated by excisional biopsy or fulguration. For more diffuse gastrointestinal involvement, a trial of antituberculous therapy, antibiotics, and/or cholinergic drugs may be considered, but with limited expectation for a favorable result.[204]

MELANOSIS COLI, CATHARTIC COLON, AND SOAP OR CHEMICAL COLITIS

"Irritant" purgatives have been incriminated as the causative factor in at least three colonic abnormalities: melanosis coli, cathartic colon, and soap or chemical colitis. Because the clinical picture for each is quite different, they are discussed separately.

Melanosis Coli

Melanosis coli was first reported over 150 years ago by Cruveilhier, who described a patient with chronic diarrhea in whom "the inner surface of the large intestine was as black as Chinese ink."[208] Rudolf Virchow later microscopically demonstrated the black pigment in the colon of an autopsy case and termed the condition melanosis coli.[209] Since then, large numbers of patients with the condition have been reported.[210–215] Our current concept is that melanosis coli is a benign condition found in some persons who use cathartics of the anthracene type, including cascara sagrada, senna, aloe, rhubarb, and frangula. Approximately three fourths of patients with melanosis use these laxatives.[216] The shortest time observed for appearance of melanosis coli in patients taking a cascara preparation is 4 months and the longest 13 months (mean, 9 months).[212] In almost all instances, the melanosis is completely reversible over 9 to 12 months after the offending drug is stopped. The age of reported patients varies, but in general the condition occurs in older adults.

Melanosis coli has also been reported in patients with carcinoma of the colon;[210] the mechanism is unknown and it is uncertain how many of these persons may have actually abused laxatives. Stasis of intestinal contents is not likely to contribute to the appearance of melanosis coli.[216] The incidence of bowel carcinoma in patients with known melanosis coli is very low.

Melanosis pigment may be distributed over the entire colon, but occurs mainly in the cecum and rectum.[210, 211] When associated with a partially obstructing colonic carcinoma, the pigmentation is most intense proximal to the tumor, and when related to laxative abuse is darkest just inside the anal sphincter and less so higher in the sigmoid colon.

A pigment similar to that in melanosis coli has been found in the appendix, in mesenteric lymph nodes, in the terminal ileum, and in the liver.[214, 217, 218] A melanosis coli–like dark pigment that may be lipofuscin has been reported in the esophagus in association with esophagitis.[219] Melanosis of the duodenum due to accumulation of true melanin has also been described.[220]

The diagnosis of melanosis coli is usually made at sigmoidoscopy. Various picturesque descriptions have been applied to the gross appearance. It has been compared to tiger or crocodile skin, a toad's back, and a cross-section of nutmeg.[211] The gross coloration varies from light brown or buff to very dark brown or black. The darker areas are divided into a polyhedral design by fine striae of lighter color (Color Fig. 84–16, p. xliv). The unpigmented reticular areas result from variation in degree of pigment deposition. Submucosal lymphoid follicles are not pigmented and therefore appear as light dots on the dark surface.[214] Areas containing inflammatory change or regenerating epithelium may also not be pigmented. It is important to remember that mucosa containing carcinoma or adenomatous and hyperplastic polyps also does not contain melanosis pigment and may have a striking pink appearance against a dark background.[210, 214, 215] Therefore, biopsy of isolated areas lacking pigmentation should be performed to exclude neoplasia.

Microscopic evaluation of melanosis tissue demonstrates that the epithelial cells are normal. Occasionally, the submucosa may be thickened and edematous and contain plasma cells. The main finding is an increased number of large mononuclear cells or macrophages in the lamina propria, many of which contain the brownish-black melanosis pigment (Fig. 84–17). These macrophages are mainly located between the crypts. Pigment-laden cells can also be found microscopically in the absence of gross melanosis.

Histologic grades of melanosis have been defined varying from grade 1, with few cells containing pigment granules, to grade 4, in which the pigmented cells are extensive and found below the muscularis mucosae, in lymph vessels, and in regional lymph nodes.[213] There is no known clinical significance to this classification except for descriptive purposes.

Attempts to characterize the pigment of melanosis coli have contributed little more than to confirm that it gives many of the reactions for both melanin and lipofuscin.[207, 221] An origin from degenerating mitochondria, endoplasmic reticulum, glycogen, and abnormal lysosomes has been suggested.[221, 222]

Special staining techniques have demonstrated both loss in number and abnormal enzymatic activities of neurons in the submucosal plexus of some patients with melanosis coli.[222, 223] While these changes have been attributed to the excessive use of anthraquinone laxatives, more recent studies have documented similar neuronal changes in patients with idiopathic constipation without melanosis coli or abuse of laxative drugs.[224] Such observations raise questions about whether anthraquinone compounds actually cause nerve damage or whether their use is instead simply an epiphenomenon in persons with primary neurogenic impairment of colon function who seek symptomatic relief from these drugs. However, since the myenteric plexus and associated neurons have been closely studied in only a small number of patients, it remains possible that a spectrum of colonic changes can be induced by anthracene-type laxatives, leading to pigment accumulation or to altered neural function or to

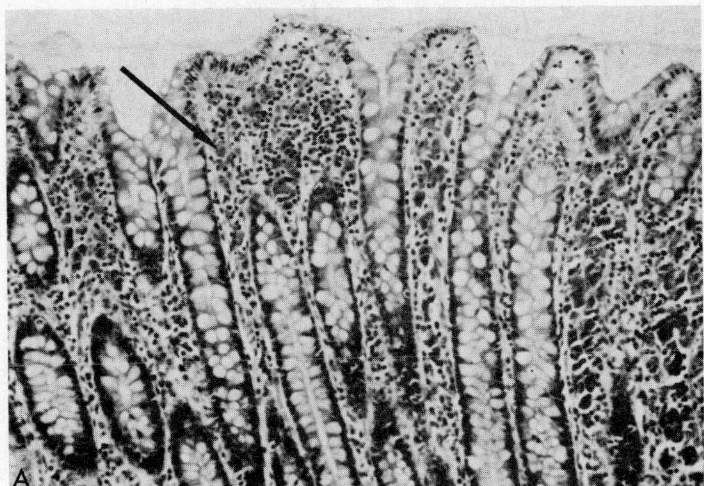

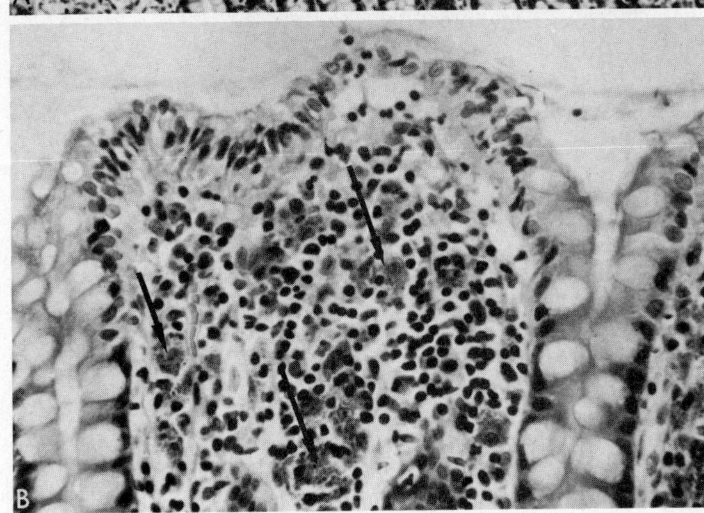

Figure 84–17. *A*, Rectal biopsy from a patient with melanosis coli. The dark mucosal coloration is due to pigment granules in large submucosal macrophages *(arrow)*. Hematoxylin and eosin stain, × 250. *B*, A higher magnification of the area shown by the arrow in *A*. × 500.

both. The discovery of melanosis coli in a patient should prompt questioning about laxative use and colon function. In the absence of a history of anthracene laxative abuse, the finding of melanosis coli warrants further evaluation for an occult colonic malignancy.

Cathartic Colon

In 1943, attention was first drawn to the fact that chronic laxative abuse could produce severe radiologic abnormalities of the colon.[225, 226] The subsequent four decades have witnessed validation of this fact, but have contributed little to our understanding of the pathogenesis.[227, 228] The exact functional significance of cathartic colon is unknown, and the entity remains for the most part a radiologic diagnosis.

Almost all reported cases are in women who have taken "irritant" laxatives for a period of at least 15 years.[226] Nonspecific abdominal complaints led by chronic constipation, vague bloating discomfort, and ill-defined lower abdominal pain are the usual symptoms. Of importance is the absence of fever, recurrent diarrhea, or the passage of mucus or blood in the stool suggesting inflammatory bowel disease.

Diagnosis

Endoscopic findings are usually normal, although the mucosa may be edematous but never friable. If the laxative preparation contained cascara, melanosis coli may be present. The diagnosis, therefore, is radiologic.

In early or mild cases, only the terminal ileum and cecum are involved. The ileocecal valve becomes flattened and gaping with changes similar to those seen in ulcerative colitis[229, 230] (Fig. 84–18). The terminal ileum may also become tubular, slightly narrowed, and without a normal mucosal pattern. The severity of the terminal ileal abnormality tends to correlate with that of the colon. In severely and chronically symptomatic patients, a plain film of the abdomen may show a tubular outline of these gas-filled intestinal segments. The cecum may appear shortened and possibly conical. Later, the more distal ascending colon also becomes tubular with diminished or completely absent haustrations. The hepatic flexure may not be definable as the colon sweeps toward the left upper quadrant of the abdomen. The mucosal pattern is linear or smooth, especially in constricted segments, and ulcers are absent. In most cases, the colonic X-ray changes extend no further than the mid-transverse colon, although the abnormality can reach the lower descending colon.[226]

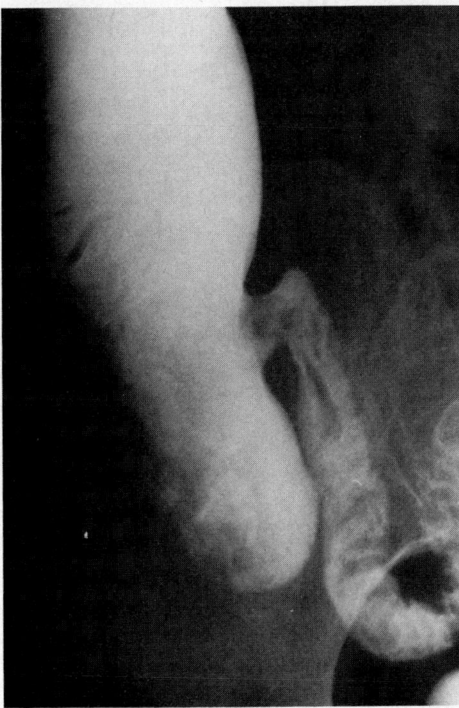

Figure 84–18. This close-up view of the cecum and proximal ascending colon demonstrates a rounded, ahaustral cecum and proximal colon with a gaping, atrophic-appearing ileocecal valve characteristic of cathartic colon. (From Campbell, W. L. Dis. Colon Rectum *26*:445, 1983. Used by permission.)

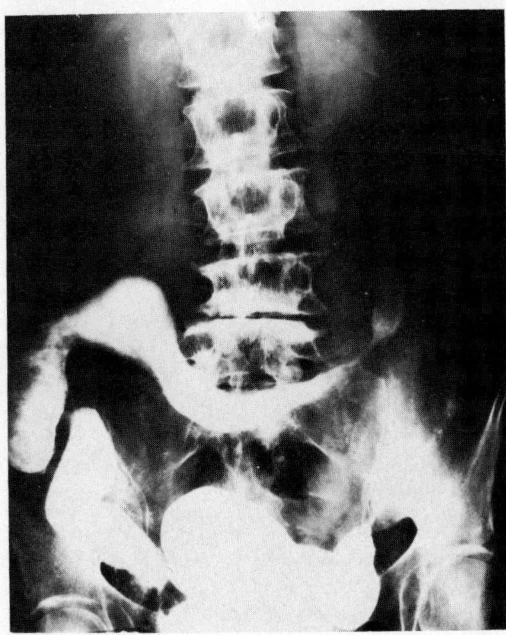

Figure 84–19. Barium enema examination of a patient with severe cathartic colon. The bowel appears shortened with long, tapered areas of narrowing. Haustrations and normal mucosal pattern are absent. The terminal ileum is also dilated. At fluoroscopy the colon distended normally. The barium enema findings may be strikingly similar to those of advanced ulcerative colitis if only part of the roentgenograms are reviewed.

Although segments of the colon appear tonic, no rigidity is present. Inconstant and bizarre areas of apparent constriction with long, tapering margins may be seen (Fig. 84–19). At fluoroscopy, however, normal distensibility is evident, including the areas of contraction. Evacuation of barium is often incomplete. The radiologic differential diagnosis includes chronic ulcerative colitis, Crohn's colitis, and amebic colitis.[226, 227]

Pathology and Pathogenesis

Reported descriptions of the involved bowel at laparotomy vary greatly. The bowel may be thin and have poor tone. The transverse colon is often pendulous, and the sigmoid may be dilated.[231] In contrast, there may be thickening of the terminal ileum and cecum or no gross pathology.[225, 226] Reports of detailed histopathologic examination of resected or postmortem tissue specimens are rare. In one extensively studied case, the mucosa was dark brown, suggesting melanosis coli, the submucosa was infiltrated by excessive fat, and the muscular layers were atrophic. Silver impregnation stain of the myenteric plexus demonstrated abnormalities similar to those in experimental animals given senna.[232]

Activated senna appears to produce colonic contraction by contact stimulation of the submucosal or Meissner's plexus, which, in turn, stimulates the deeper intermuscular myenteric plexus.[233] Therefore, it is possible that prolonged use of a cathartic may induce an abnormality in neural pathways regulating colonic motor activity and lead to the observed pathologic and functional changes. In support of this is the observation that patients with cathartic colon have loss of colonic myenteric neurons and replacement of associated ganglia by Schwann cells.[234] More recent studies suggest that some patients with severe idiopathic constipation without history of cathartic abuse also have a significant derangement of the colonic myenteric plexus.[224] Clearly, more information is needed to determine if the pathologic changes described in cathartic colon are the same as those in idiopathic constipation. The possibility certainly exists that cathartic colon is merely a radiologic description of a previously unrecognized primary neuromuscular disorder of the intestine. However, the reported complete reversibility of the X-ray changes of cathartic colon suggests that an acquired laxative-induced change may indeed be present.[230]

Treatment

The use of irritant laxatives must be discontinued. Other side effects of laxative abuse, such as fluid and electrolyte abnormalities, must be corrected.[235, 236] The underlying problem of constipation should be managed aggressively (see pp. 353–361), but without use of irritant laxatives. The radiologic abnormality may be improved after only one month and in some cases has normalized completely.[225, 227, 230]

Soap or Chemical Colitis

Soap colitis is an acute inflammatory reaction of the colon that develops within hours after the administration of a "cleansing" soapsuds enema.[237–242] Acute colitis has also been reported after rectal instillation of other chemicals including hydrogen peroxide, herbal medications, vinegar, potassium permanganate, and sodium diatrizoate (Hypaque).[243–246] The colonic response to exposure to these substances probably results from a hypertonic, a detergent, or a direct toxic effect on the mucosa. The severity of the reaction depends on the type and concentration of the administered solution, the contact time with the mucosa, and the presence or absence of an underlying colonic disease. The desired result is secretion of water and mucus by the colon mucosa and stimulation of muscular contractions leading to evacuation of colon contents.

Clinical Picture and Diagnosis

The clinical response can vary from the intended secretion of water and mucus and evacuation with slight discomfort to severe abdominal cramps, distention, mucorrhea, serosanguinous diarrhea, hypovolemia, and acute hemoconcentration resulting from severe mucosal damage and rapid transudation of fluid into the colon. Mucosal damage may lead also to sepsis from microorganisms penetrating the disrupted mucosa and to hypokalemia from massive loss of mucus. On physical examination, the transverse and descending colon may be tender to palpation. More serious adverse reactions include anaphylaxis, rectal gangrene, acute hemorrhagic colitis, acute renal failure, and death.[239–242]

Sigmoidoscopy performed shortly after irritant enemas usually demonstrates only hyperemia of rectal mucosa and excessive mucus production. More severe reactions can produce severe edema, hemorrhagic necrosis, ulceration, pseudomembrane formation, and even gangrene of the rectal wall.[239–246] In contrast to soap colitis, which may involve the intestine as proximal as the transverse colon, hydrogen peroxide colitis usually involves only the distal rectosigmoid colon (Color Fig. 84–20, p. xliv).

Barium enema X-ray examination is often uncomfortable for the patient whose colon has been "prepared" with a soap-containing enema. When the mucosa has been badly injured, the X-ray may show marked spasm, abnormal massive propulsive movements, and submucosal edema.[241, 242]

Treatment

Treatment consists of close observation, careful intravenous replacement of fluid and electrolytes, and administration of broad-spectrum antibiotics. Use of corticosteroid therapy has not been reported. Most patients recover completely from this frightening, painful, and serious iatrogenic illness in 4 to 6 weeks.[237, 243]

FECAL IMPACTION AND STERCORAL ULCER

Incomplete evacuation of feces may lead to the formation of a large, firm, immovable mass of stool in the rectum, a fecal impaction. The rectosigmoid colon becomes dilated and the firm, irregular mass (*fecaloma* or *stercoroma*) is not plastic enough to be expelled through the disproportionately small anal canal by the patient's often weak defecatory effort. A smaller, rounded, hard mass of stool that cannot be expelled is called a *stercolith* or *enterolith*; a *scybalum* is a mass composed of small, rounded fecal particles.[247]

Predisposing Conditions

Fecal impactions are most common in children who have psychogenic problems or undiagnosed megacolon, in elderly debilitated or sedentary persons, in narcotic addicts, in persons with spinal cord injury, and in patients taking large doses of tranquilizers. The frequency of impaction is highest among institutionalized geriatric patients and those in mental hospitals.[248] Patients who are inactive for long periods (e.g., with myocardial infarction or orthopedic problems) tend to develop fecal impaction if mild laxatives are not given for constipation (see pp. 359–361). Gentle rectal examination is not harmful in these patients and should be routinely done to make an early diagnosis of impaction or occult, enteric bleeding.[249] Anal diseases that cause painful defecation, such as hemorrhoids, fissures, and cryptitis, may lead to stool retention. Chronic dehydration can also result in firm, dry stool that is difficult to expel. Bismuth, barium, and kaolin can form a hard nidus around which a fecaloma develops. Elderly patients with a history of constipation are especially at risk for development of a colonic "concretion" after barium examination of the upper digestive tract. Obstipation and impaction are also common in patients with megacolon (see pp. 1389–1402).

Clinical Picture

Multiple small fecaliths may cause lower abdominal pain. These are discrete, smooth, often faceted "stones" that have radiopaque calcific laminations.[250] They usually are proximal to an area of stricture in the colon or the terminal ileum and are thought to result from stasis. These "stones" are not expelled with the fecal stream and may remain in place for years. Mucosal ulceration and bowel obstruction are the most common complications. A small fecalith may obstruct the appendix and predispose to appendicitis. Since these masses are usually visible on plain X-ray film of the abdomen, their presence should be excluded in patients with lower abdominal pain.

A fecal impaction is composed of firm, compacted stool. Seventy per cent of fecal impactions are in the rectum, 20 per cent in the sigmoid flexure, and 10 per cent in the more proximal colon, including the cecum.[251] Symptoms of fecal impaction are usually nonspecific. Vague abdominal discomfort is noted, especially after meals. Uncommonly, a sensation of rectal fullness and tenesmus or colicky lower abdominal pain may be present. Weight loss resulting from voluntary decrease in food intake occurs. Nausea and vomiting may appear, and dehydration is frequent. Headache and a general sense of illness are common.[247]

Paradoxically, the patient may complain of uncontrolled passage of small amounts of water and semiformed stool. This symptom represents an "overflow" phenomenon around a large impaction. As liquid stool from the proximal colon is forced around the impacted mass, it elevates the mass like a ball valve and a small amount of fluid escapes, thus preventing complete obstruction.[253] Soft semiformed stool can also be passed. This paradoxical situation is common in elderly bedridden patients. Too often, its significance is missed to the extent that the patient may be treated with constipating drugs for "diarrhea" or fecal incontinence.

On physical examination, a large, firm mass of stool is usually palpable in the left lower quadrant. Bimanual abdominorectal examination can be done in both males and females to facilitate the diagnosis of fecal impaction. The impaction may not be located in the rectal ampulla but lodged in the sigmoid colon above the examining finger and feel like a smooth but irregular mass in the intestinal wall. Pressure on the mass with the examining finger can produce a persisting indentation, helping to differentiate stool from tumor. A variety of unusual physical findings have been described for large fecalomas but are nonspecific.[247] Sigmoidoscopy will usually clarify the nature of the rectosigmoid mass, and X-rays should be diagnostic (Fig. 84–21). A specific ultrasound picture for fecal impaction has also been described.[252] Unfortunately, despite such tests, fecalomas have been confused with colonic malignancy.[254]

Complications, Including Stercoral Ulcer

Interesting but uncommon complications or accompaniments of fecal impaction have been summarized.[255] More common complications include urinary tract obstruction, spontaneous perforation of the colon, and stercoral ulceration. Others include hernia, recurrent volvulus, megacolon, rectal prolapse, dystocia, and intestinal obstruction.

Marked enlargement of the rectosigmoid colon resulting from fecal impaction can produce urinary tract obstruction by compression of the ureters near the ureterovesical junction and, by elevation of the bladder, cause marked angulation of the urethra.[256] Intracystic voiding pressure eventually becomes incapable of overcoming the increased urethral outflow resistance, and hydroureter and hydronephrosis result. Recurrent urinary tract infection without an obvious cause, especially in young girls, should alert one to the possibility of chronic fecal impaction.[255, 256]

Spontaneous perforation of the colon may occur with a large fecal impaction.[257] The patient's history is typical, with constipation almost invariably present.[258] The onset is acute, often after straining. A few hours of left lower abdominal pain precede shock and physical findings of a perforated viscus. At laparotomy, the peritoneal fluid has a foul smell and contains small pieces of stool. A small colonic tear is usually found on the antimesenteric border at the rectosigmoid junction. The diagnosis should be suspected in a patient with an unexplained acute abdomen in whom rectal examination demonstrates fecal impaction. The only treatment is early surgery. Mortality is high, exceeding 30 per cent.[258]

Stercoral ulcers have been called decubitus ulcers of the colon and are thought to result from pressure necrosis of the mucosa induced by a large, firm fecal impaction. The true incidence of this lesion is unknown. One carefully done prospective study reported stercoral ulcers in 4.6 per cent of 175 consecutive adult autopsies, with the average age of those having such ulcers being 68.6 years.[259]

Stercoral ulcers are most often confined to the rectum and sigmoid colon, although the transverse colon may be affected.[259] Ulcer size varies remarkably. The margin is usually irregular or geographic, conforming to the surface of the adjacent fecal mass. Characteristically, the ulcer base is dark with yellow-gray to greenish-purple discoloration. Thinning and stretching of the bowel wall are evident, with depression of the ulcer surface margins below adjacent mucosa. Perforation usually is in the area where thinning is maximal.

Microscopic examination shows denuding of the mucosa and ischemic pressure necrosis of deeper layers. Characteristically, there is minimal inflammatory change with few polymorphonuclear leukocytes.[259] Bacteria line the necrotic surface but do not invade the adjacent bowel wall. Vascular changes are not striking, although thrombi may be present in the small compressed vessels. Suppurative peritonitis usually follows perforation.

Stercoral ulceration of the colon may be asymptomatic for long periods. It may bleed chronically or hemorrhage severely and the bleeding may be noted as long as three to seven days after rectal disimpaction.[260] Perforation with peritonitis is among the most serious sequelae. Treatment for this complication is obviously surgical. The prognosis is poor, and the outcome is directly affected by the speed of correct diagnosis and treatment.[261, 262] For uncomplicated stercoral ulcer, treatment is careful removal of the fecal mass and improved management of constipation. The ulcerated bowel is fragile and may perforate during attempts to relieve the impaction.

Treatment of Fecal Impaction

Treatment should begin with partial removal of the fecal mass by a physician or nurse. An anesthetic (e.g., 5 per cent lidocaine ointment) can be applied to the anal canal a few minutes before the procedure to

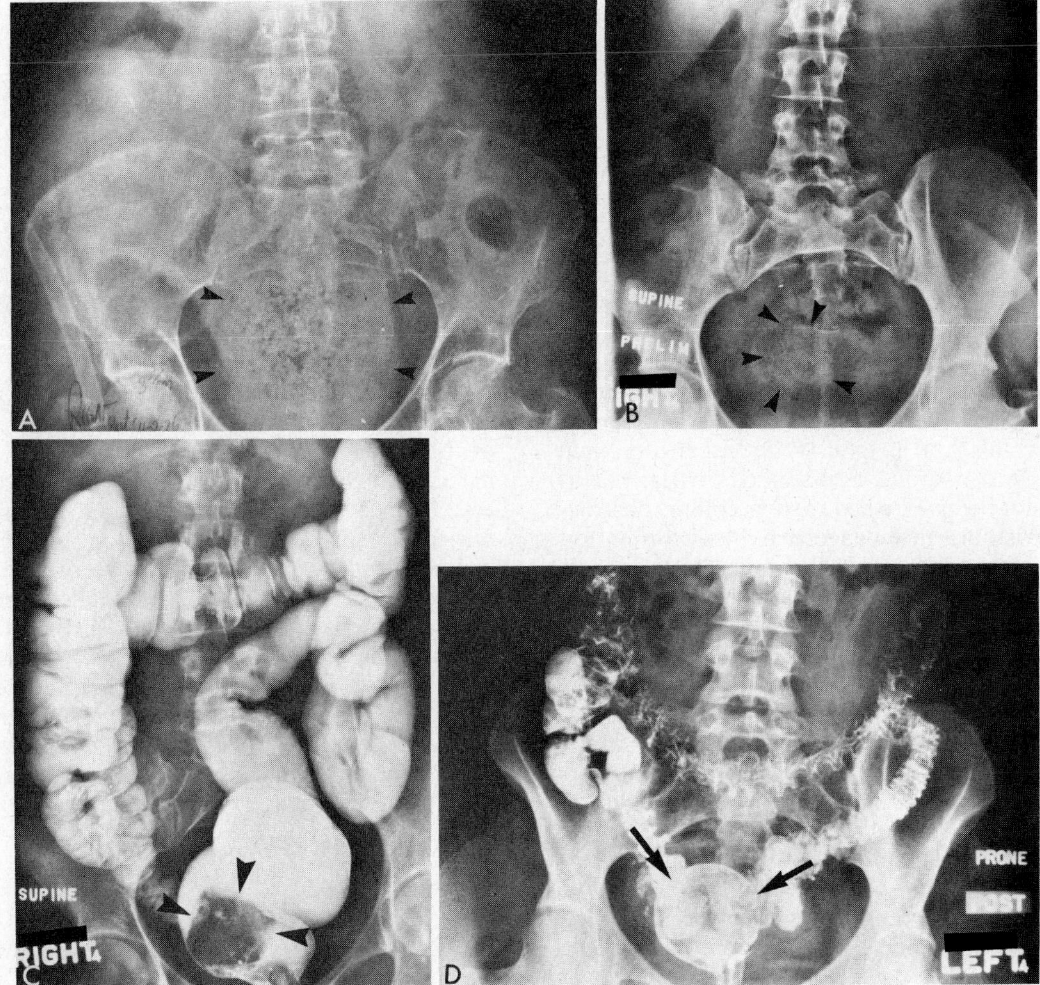

Figure 84–21. *A,* A 70-year-old woman was hospitalized with a history of frequent small volume liquid stools, dehydration, and failure to respond to constipating drugs. X-ray showed typical findings of a large rectal fecal impaction—namely, a soft tissue density *(arrows)* containing irregular small lucent areas produced by pockets of gas in the fecal mass.

B, KUB X-ray of a 36-year-old woman who had extensive hospital evaluation for a pelvic mass associated with lower abdominal discomfort. The mass was shown by ultrasound to be compatible with a 7.5-cm solid tumor. A circumscribed mottled appearance similar to that in *A* was eventually noted on plain X-ray in the area of the mass. *C,* Barium enema demonstrated an intraluminal mass without evident mucosal attachment. *D,* Postevacuation X-ray demonstrated that the rounded barium-coated mass would not pass through the anus. Sigmoidoscopy confirmed the pelvic mass to be a large firm bolus of feces.

alleviate discomfort. A low-lying impaction should first be broken up using one or two fingers in the anus and as much stool as possible removed manually. Frequently, the anal sphincter will relax and dilate as the procedure is carried out. Systemic sedation and analgesia may be necessary. More proximal and firm sigmoid masses can be broken up through a sigmoidoscope. One of the most effective techniques utilizes a dental irrigating unit (Water Pik) to deliver a pulsating stream of water against the stool. This is accomplished by passing the irrigating tube through the biopsy channel of a fiberoptic sigmoidoscope and directing the water jet into the fecal mass under direct vision. The disrupted and solubilized stool can then be removed by suction. Care must be taken not to damage the intestinal wall. Complications of the disimpaction procedure include sepsis, hypotension, perforation, and bleeding.

Once the large mass of feces has been softened and partially removed, warm water or saline enemas may be given as well as mineral oil orally. An enema containing 15 to 20 per cent water-soluble X-ray contrast material may further fragment the stool bolus and relieve the impaction.[263] Enemas containing 0.5 ounce of 1 per cent dioctyl sodium sulfosuccinate in 4 ounces of water may also be helpful.[264] Hydrogen peroxide enemas can be dangerous, as discussed earlier. Lactulose should not be given when there is colonic obstruction, even by stool, since dangerous colonic distention can be produced by gas liberated from bacterial fermentation of the poorly absorbed carbohydrate. Papain and cellulase preparations may disperse nondigestible cellulose and nitrogenous waste products in stool. Warm oil enemas are unnecessary and may be dangerous, causing burns of heat-insensitive colonic mucosa. A recent study in 45 elderly patients with fecal impaction found a very effective approach was to give 2 liters daily (for two days) of an oral electrolyte solution containing a poorly absorbable solution of polyethylene glycol (Golytely).[265] Dilatation of the anus under anesthesia can be necessary for some patients who have painful anal disease or other medical problems and cannot tolerate mechanical disimpaction. In extreme cases, laparotomy has been necessary for removal of the fecal mass.[251, 266]

Fecal impaction most frequently complicates other illness and may itself create serious problems in clinical management. Preventive therapy consists of monitoring the frequency of bowel movements, a periodic examination of the rectum, administration of hydrophilic mucilloids or stool-wetting agents, mild laxatives, and, if necessary, periodic enemas. Treatment of chronic constipation and fecal impaction in the elderly has recently been reviewed[267] and is also discussed on pages 167 and 168. Patient groups at high risk for impaction and its complications are those receiving constipating drugs (including antidepressants); those who are bedridden or who have neurologic disorders; and those who are elderly, debilitated, or psychotic. Awareness of the subtlety of symptoms of fecal impaction and the willingness to perform an early rectal examination are important in preventing development of a serious problem.

Table 84–4. CONDITIONS ASSOCIATED WITH ACUTE COLONIC PSEUDO-OBSTRUCTION

Trauma (nonoperative)
Surgery (gynecologic, orthopedic, urologic)
Inflammatory processes (pancreatitis, cholecystitis)
Infections
Malignancy
Radiation therapy
Drugs (narcotics, antidepressants, clonidine, anticholinergics)
Cardiovascular disease
Neurologic disease
Respiratory failure
Metabolic disease (electrolyte and acid/base imbalance, diabetes, hypothyroidism, alcoholism, uremia)

Data from Vanek, V. W., and Al-Salti, M. Dis. Colon Rectum *29*:203, 1986.

ACUTE COLONIC PSEUDO-OBSTRUCTION (OGILVIE'S SYNDROME)

In 1948, Ogilvie reported two patients with metastatic cancer who developed acute, massive dilatation of the cecum and right colon in the absence of more distal colonic obstruction or an inflammatory process.[268] Since then, this entity—acute colonic pseudo-obstruction or nontoxic megacolon, also called Ogilvie's syndrome—has been widely recognized as a fairly common and potentially serious development in patients who have just undergone surgery or who are already quite ill from other causes.[269–273] It is important to recognize and treat acute colonic pseudo-obstruction, since the process can lead to colonic perforation, peritonitis, and death. Conditions associated with development of Ogilvie's syndrome are listed in Table 84–4. (See also pp. 377–379.)

Clinical Picture

Acute colonic pseudo-obstruction is characterized by massive dilatation of the cecum and right colon with the distention usually ending abruptly by the splenic flexure. Dilated loops of distal small intestine are also present in at least half of reported cases, and air-fluid levels are not uncommon.[272] Painless abdominal distention is the most frequent early presentation. Abdominal symptoms are often minimal, but two thirds of patients have nausea and vomiting. However, this is usually much less severe in mechanical intestinal obstruction.[269, 272, 273] While cessation of bowel movements is frequent, almost half of the patients continue to pass flatus and even experience diarrhea.[274] More than 80 per cent eventually develop abdominal pain, which is neither severe nor colicky in nature.[272, 273, 275–277]

The most dramatic physical finding is severe abdominal distention. Mild rebound tenderness can be present when the colon is very dilated. However, physical findings suggestive of peritonitis are not present in uncomplicated cases. Bowel sounds may be normal, hyperactive, or even high-pitched; uncommonly, they are absent.[273] A low-grade fever is common. Laboratory tests may show an abnormality in electrolytes such as hypokalemia or hypercalcemia. A slightly elevated blood leukocyte count is common, but if it is very high, intestinal ischemia should be suspected.[274–276] Evolution of the process into the clinical picture of a quiet abdomen, increased fever, and progressive elevation in blood leukocyte count should raise major concern that perforation of the colon has occurred.

Diagnosis

The most useful diagnostic test is a plain X-ray of the abdomen, which will demonstrate segmental dilatation of the proximal colon suggesting distal colonic obstruction.[272, 273, 275] Additional differential diagnostic possibilites raised by X-ray findings include fecal impaction, cecal or sigmoid volvulus, ischemic bowel, typhilitis, gastric dilatation, adhesions, or mechanical obstruction from any cause, including carcinoma. In contrast to acute mechanical obstruction, the dilated colon of acute pseudo-obstruction has well-defined colonic septa, preserved haustral markings, and less prominent air/fluid levels.

The most impressive change is the degree of colon dilatation. According to LaPlace's law, the pressure required to stretch the walls of the colon decreases in inverse proportion to its diameter. Thus, at a large diameter, small increments in intraluminal gas or fluid that increase intraluminal volume will markedly increase the tension on the wall. The bursting point will be exceeded earliest in that part of the colon with the greatest diameter, usually the cecum.[278] Progressive dilatation leads to mucosal ischemia, longitudinal splitting of the serosa and tenia, and eventually perforation of the mucosa. The normal diameter of the cecum is 9 cm or less.[279] A cecal diameter of 9 to 12 cm usually raises concern about impending perforation.[275, 279–281] In one recent study, a cecal diameter greater than 14 cm was accompanied by perforation or severe ischemia in 23 per cent of cases.[273] Most patients with acute colonic pseudo-obstruction are already seriously ill, and development of a perforated colon requiring laparotomy has generally led to at least a twofold increase in mortality.[273, 276, 282, 283]

Pathogenesis

The cause of acute pseudo-obstruction of the colon is unknown. The wide variety of clinical conditions with which it occurs suggests a systemic process. Ogilvie's first cases occurred in the setting of metastatic tumor to the celia plexus, which led him to postulate that interruption of sympathetic innervation to the colon was a causative factor.[268] Others have advanced hypotheses focused primarily on disruption of sacral innervation to the distal colon, suggesting that such denervation causes functional obstruction of the distal intestine as is seen in Hirschsprung's disease.[284–286] However, intestinal ganglia in the distal colon wall are normal.[287] Thus, the pathogenesis remains obscure but may be related to a temporary or reversible alteration in function of the autonomic nervous system, the cause of which is unknown.

Treatment

Once the diagnosis is made, initial treatment consists of correcting any metabolic, electrolyte, and fluid abnormalities, discontinuing any narcotic or anticholinergic drugs, withholding oral intake, and instituting nasogastric suction. A rectal tube can help with decompression if the distal colon is also distended. The patient should not be allowed to remain constantly supine, but should periodically lie on either side or on the abdomen. Enemas can be used but with much care, as they can precipitate bowel perforation.[273] Oral laxatives are generally not helpful, and lactulose may be dangerous since it increases intraluminal gas. A search should be made for an infectious process and any indicated treatment begun.[272, 274, 275, 277, 282, 288] Drugs that potentially stimulate colon motility, such as Prostigmin, Urecholine, and metoclopramide, or that inhibit opiate receptors, such as naloxone, can be tried, but without strong expectation of a significant effect.[289]

The diameter of the distended colon should be monitored by abdominal X-ray every 12 hours. As long as cecal dilatation is not massive (less than 12 cm) and there are no clinical signs of colon perforation, conservative treatment can be tried for 48 to 72 hours.[273, 276, 282] If colon diameter increases to greater than 12 to 14 cm or the condition does not resolve, the colon should be decompressed. The currently accepted options are by surgery or by colonoscopy. Colonoscopy can be both diagnostic and therapeutic and, as a nonoperative approach, has great appeal. Colonoscopic decompression of acute colonic megacolon was first described in 1977.[280] Since then, multiple reports have documented a high success rate (80 to 90 per cent) for initial decompression by colonoscopy.[273, 276, 284, 285] Standard colon cleansing procedures prior to colonoscopy are not appropriate in patients with Ogilvie's syndrome. Fortunately, colon contents, especially in the proximal colon, are often liquid in character. Any firm stool in the distal colon can be removed if necessary by small-volume saline enemas.[276, 287] The procedure may occasionally be difficult and it should be recognized that adequate decompression can usually be achieved if only the hepatic flexure is reached.[287] The morbidity reported with colonoscopy in this setting is low, but may reach 2 per cent.[271, 273]

Unfortunately, after successful decompression, cecal dilatation recurs in 20 to 30 per cent of cases.[288, 289] Repeat colonoscopy can again deflate the cecum, but recurrence rates after a second endoscopy tend to be even higher.[273] To avoid recurrence, a suction tube can be placed in the cecum at the time of the initial

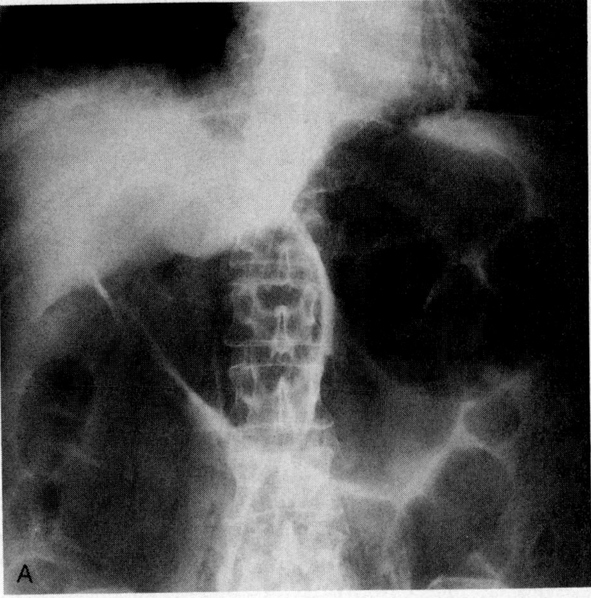

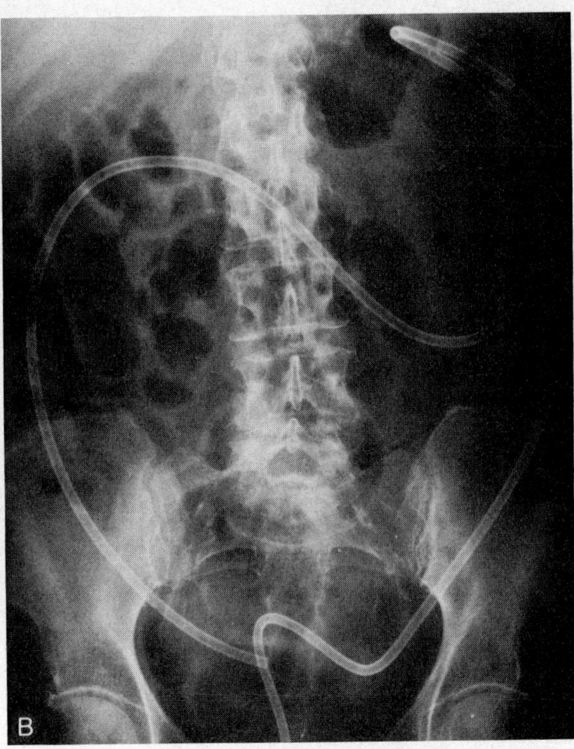

Figure 84–22. Severely ill patient with acute colonic pseudo-obstruction (Ogilvie's syndrome). *A,* Massive dilatation of cecum, ascending colon, and transverse colon raised concern about impending colon perforation. Patient failed to respond to conservative medical treatment and underwent successful colonoscopic decompression of dilated colon. *B,* A radiopaque suction tube was passed into the cecum over a guidewire which was inserted during colonoscopy and removed after the tube was in proper position. Decompression of the colon was maintained by the suction tube. Gas-filled structures are small intestine and stomach. The process resolved completely over three days.

colonoscopy[273, 289] (Fig. 84–22). Our recent experience has shown that placement of such a tube in the distended colon segment is a useful way to maintain decompression. The tube is allowed to pass as colon function returns, or is withdrawn in a few days. No study has reported major complications with endoscopic decompression in patients with acute colonic pseudo-obstruction.

Surgical treatment is indicated in the patient in whom colon distention does not resolve after initial medical management and in whom colonoscopy cannot be performed or is not successful. In the absence of ischemia or intestinal perforation, a simple cecostomy can usually be performed with use of local anesthesia.[284] Unfortunately, more extensive laparotomy may be required in some cases and is generally associated with a much higher mortality rate, especially in comparison with nonoperative treatment.[273, 281] Recently, direct percutaneous methods of cecal decompression have been described, but more experience is needed before such can be recommended, especially in view of the apparent safety and efficacy of colonoscopic decompression.[290, 291] With appropriate treatment, acute colonic pseudo-obstruction usually resolves without sequelae in 3 to 6 days.[272, 273, 282, 285, 287, 292]

HEMORRHAGIC COLITIS

Escherichia coli serotype 0157:H7 has recently been described as a cause of acute hemorrhagic colitis and bloody diarrhea. Since the initial reports of two geographically distinct epidemic outbreaks in 1982, at least 100 clustered or sporadic cases have surfaced.[293–297] Although evidence of its pathogenicity is new, *E. coli* 0157:H7 has been incriminated as the cause of bloody diarrhea in 15 per cent of patients.[294, 296] Despite the inexplicability of some cases, ingestion of partially cooked hamburger meat and untreated water have been cited as point sources in several outbreaks (see pp. 1196–1198).[293, 297, 298]

Clinical Picture

Both adults and children may be infected with this organism, although, in general, deaths have occurred in the elderly population. Typically, the incubation period is four to eight days.[293, 297] Patients initially complain of abdominal cramping and watery diarrhea. The latter is usually replaced in one to two days with gross bloody diarrhea. Nausea and vomiting frequently accompany the illness and account in part for the profound dehydration seen in many patients. High fever is uncommon, and patients are normally euthermic or display mild temperature elevations.

Hospitalization is frequently necessary in light of the marked hypovolemia and blood loss. Such patients appear acutely ill with signs of dehydration and abdominal distress. The abdomen may be distended and tender to direct palpation, especially in the right lower quadrant. Guarding is common, but rebound tenderness or other peritoneal findings are rarely elicited. Digital rectal examination will confirm the presence of blood.

Pathogenesis

The precise mechanism by which *E. coli* 0157:H7 produces hemorrhagic colitis remains uncertain. Although not enteroinvasive, this serotype has been shown to adhere via fimbria to epithelial cell surfaces and produce a cytotoxin similar to that of *Shigella dysenteriae*.[299, 300] Small intestinal colonization may account for the prodromal watery diarrhea, but direct cytotoxic effects on the colon are responsible for mucosal edema, friability, ulceration, and hemorrhage. In general, the cecum, proximal ascending colon, and transverse colon are most affected, with considerably lesser damage incurred by the more distal colon.

Diagnosis

The approach to the patient with bloody diarrhea always begins with investigation for an infectious etiology. To this end, the stool should be examined for fecal leukocytes, ova, and parasites, as well as cultured for enteric pathogens, with special media for *Campylobacter* and *Clostridium difficile* (see pp. 1191–1232).

It is especially important to remember that current microbiologic techniques identify *E. coli* as "normal enteric flora." Therefore, the laboratory must be alerted to the possibility of the serotype 0157:H7 as an etiologic agent. Since most (95 per cent) *E. coli*, with the notable exception of the 0157:H7 serotype, ferment sorbitol, the absence of this reaction within sorbitol-containing MacConkey medium provides a presumptive diagnosis.[301] Thereafter, serotyping will properly confirm the presence of *E. coli* 0157:H7 within the isolated colonies. Culture positivity is greatest when fresh stool specimens are plated within 4 to 6 days into the clinical course, since the organism is rapidly cleared from the bowel.[295, 297]

Plain abdominal radiographs may reveal dilated right colonic or proximal transverse colonic shadows with sparing of the descending and sigmoid colons. Thumbprinting may be seen on plain film or during barium contrast radiography. The latter frequently demonstrates edema and spasm of the right colon. Colonoscopy, usually reserved for culture-negative cases, again emphasizes the right-sided predominance for colitic changes, with edema, friability, and diffuse ulcerations from the cecum to the proximal transverse colon and relative sparing of the descending colon and rectosigmoid.

Differential Diagnosis

The clinical presentation of the *E. coli* 0157:H7 hemorrhagic colitis is not dissimilar from infectious colitis caused by common pathogens such as *Shigella, Campylobacter, Salmonella*, and *Yersinia*. Fever and pancolonic involvement, however, commonly associated with these organisms, is usually absent or mild in hemorrhagic colitis. A history of recent antibiotic use should raise the possibility of pseudomembranous colitis (see pp. 1307–1320).

Since there is a predilection for the right colon, culture-negative hemorrhagic colitis must be distinguished from Crohn's disease of the colon and ischemic colitis. Although mucosal biopsies may be suggestive of one of these disorders, careful examination of the subsequent clinical course will usually provide the most helpful diagnostic clues.

Clinical Course and Treatment

E. coli 0157:H7 hemorrhagic colitis usually runs a self-limited course over 5 to 10 days. Symptoms may be so severe, however, as to require hospitalization for volume repletion and red cell transfusions. Such patients may also require nasogastric suction to decompress an associated small intestinal ileus. Complete bowel rest should be instituted until diarrheal symptoms resolve. Although this *E. coli* serotype is sensitive *in vitro* to all antibiotics providing gram-negative coverage, such treatment is of unproven efficacy in shortening the duration or attenuating the severity of a given episode.[295, 297]

Although most patients recover without sequelae following supportive treatment, several cases of hemolytic-uremic syndrome have accompanied or followed an episode of hemorrhagic colitis.[295, 298, 302] This triad of thrombocytopenia, nephropathy, and microangiopathic hemolytic anemia has been seen in both children and adults and has responded to high-dose corticosteroids, supportive transfusions, and, on occasion, hemodialysis. This complication has also been reported in association with other enteric pathogens such as *Shigella, Salmonella, Yersinia*, and *Campylobacter*.[298]

Finally, the recognition and diagnosis of *E. coli* 0157:H7 hemorrhagic colitis should raise awareness of the possibility of a cluster outbreak. Suspicion of such an epidemic should be evaluated in conjunction with local health authorities.

BIOPSY OF THE RECTUM AND COLON

Biopsy of the rectum and colon is often essential for the diagnosis of some of the miscellaneous diseases discussed in this chapter, or one of the more common inflammatory or neoplastic disorders presented elsewhere in this text. Prior to the endoscopic procedure, one should assure adequate blood coagulation and determine whether prophylactic antibiotics are needed to decrease the risk of endocarditis or infection of a prosthetic joint that might result from any induced bacteremia.

Methods

Today, most colorectal biopsy samples are taken through a fiberoptic endoscope and include mainly intestinal mucosa. These small pinch or avulsion biopsies usually do not provide significant amounts of the submucosa. In certain conditions in which submucosa is needed for diagnosis, such as Hirschsprung's disease, in which an evaluation for submucosal ganglia is required, or suspected vasculitis or amyloid, in which larger submucosal vessels must be inspected, one should use either a jumbo forceps in a large biopsy-channel fiberoptic instrument or, preferably, a cutting or punch-type forceps with a rigid sigmoidoscope. Alternatively, the multipurpose suction biopsy tube can be utilized and may be especially useful for random biopsy of the submucosa above the peritoneal reflection, since perforation of the colon with this instrument does not occur. An excellent description of this biopsy technique has been published.[303, 304] Biopsy specimens taken with grasp or punch forceps should be restricted to rectal valves or mucosal areas below the peritoneal reflection (12 to 15 cm from the anus), owing to the definite risk of causing a perforation when sampling the sigmoid colon above this level.

The main advantages of taking biopsy specimens through a fiberoptic endoscope are the ability to sample the entire colon and to precisely target the area of interest. Also, multiple specimens are easily obtained, which can increase the diagnostic yield. Small sessile polyps can be excised by use of electrocautery biopsy forceps. This procedure yields undamaged tissue for histologic review without excess bleeding. There is some increased risk of perforation with use of the hot biopsy instruments in the right colon and cecum, where the wall of the colon is thin.[305] Pedunculated masses can be removed in whole or piecemeal fashion by snare electrocautery. A portion of the stalk should always be included to allow examination for invasive tumor if a malignancy is found.

Interpretation

To facilitate the most accurate interpretation of tissue specimens, the intestinal location of the biopsy specimens must be clearly defined, and labeled separate containers must be used for tissue from different biopsy sites. Preferably, mucosal specimens should be oriented prior to fixation. The tissue should be mounted mucosal-side-up on a monofilament mesh or a piece of filter paper or gelfoam sponge. A method for best accomplishing proper orientation has been described in detail by Pera and associates.[306] A large pedunculated polyp removed by snare electrocautery can be submitted without special handling. Tissue processing of small pedunculated polyps is enhanced by placing a small-gauge needle through the distal tip of the stalk prior to fixation. This prevents excessive retraction of the stalk and facilitates bisecting and orienting the polyp along its longitudinal axis such that serial sections demonstrate both polyp head and stalk. Multiple sections should be made of all specimens and these thoroughly examined (Fig. 84–23). Diagnostic pathology, such as small granulomas and Crohn's disease or invasion of a polyp stalk by tumor, may otherwise be missed.[307, 308]

It is most desirable for the clinician to review the biopsy tissue with the pathologist. Several excellent monographs and texts can be consulted for useful discussions of the interpretation of colorectal biopsies in both normal and pathologic states.[183, 309–311] Discussions with the pathologist about potential clinical disorders may suggest the need for special stains to facilitate a correct diagnosis.[312]

Clinical Applications

The ability to perform biopsy of the lining of the entire colon afforded by fiberoptic endoscopy provides a powerful tool that facilitates the diagnosis and management of a variety of disorders primarily involving the colon or affecting it as part of a systemic illness, such as amyloid. It should be remembered that significant and potentially diagnostic abnormalities may be present in tissue obtained by colorectal biopsy, despite a normal endoscopic appearance of the mucosa.[307, 310, 313] The disparity between the normal appearance of mucosa at colonoscopy and the distinctly abnormal histology in patients with severe diarrhea from collagenous colitis, discussed on page 1610, is an excellent example. Also, patients with ulcerative or Crohn's colitis can have significant histologic abnormalities in mucosa that appears grossly normal.[314] Accordingly, a biopsy of mucosa from the rectum or sigmoid colon should be obtained in patients with unexplained chronic diarrhea.

Biopsy documentation of normal mucosa in the sigmoid and more proximal colon in a patient with acute proctitis may help in differentiating between variants of similar disorders, such as idiopathic ulcerative colitis and proctitis.[314] Histologic changes may also be useful in differentiating between acute self-limited infectious colitis and idiopathic ulcerative colitis.[117, 118, 315] Patients with chronic ulcerative colitis, especially those whose disease has been present for more than 10 years, should have mucosal biopsy done searching for evidence of high-grade dysplasia, which, if present, would raise concern about a coexisting malignancy.[316] Homosexually active men can have a variety of related causes for acute inflammation in the anorectal area. Mucosal biopsy has been shown to be an important adjunct to cultures and smears of rectal mucosa in detecting an infectious process in these patients.[121, 123] Additionally, mucosal biopsy of the rectum in such patients may demonstrate focal crypt epithelial cell degeneration or apoptosis, which has been described as a characteristic pathologic feature in acquired immunodeficiency syndrome (AIDS).[317]

In schistosomiasis, the eggs of *S. mansoni* and *S. japonicum* can be identified in a squash preparation of the mucosal specimen. One half of the biopsy tissue is placed in saline for a few minutes and then pressed

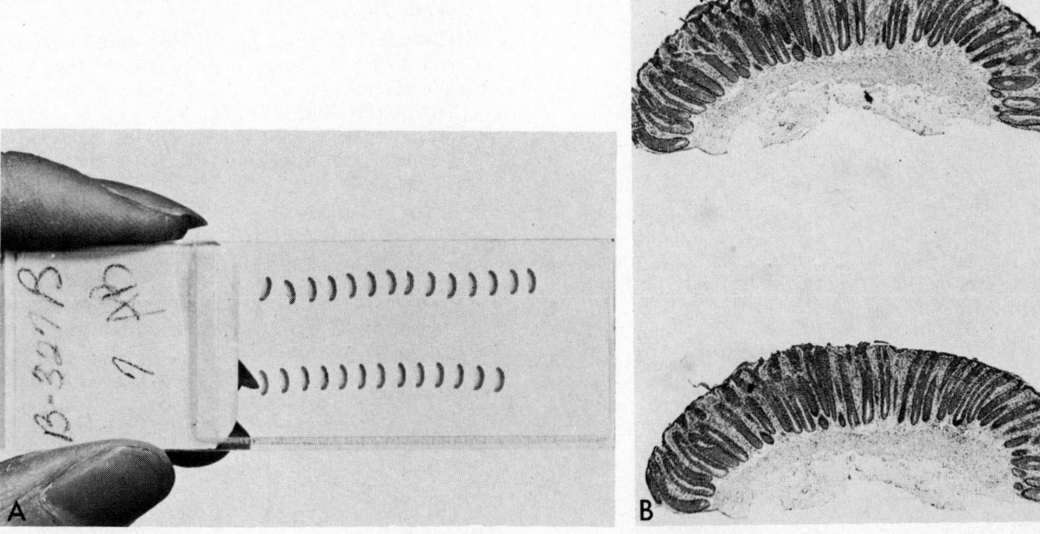

Figure 84–23. *A*, Multiple sections made perpendicular to the mucosa of a properly oriented biopsy specimen can be mounted on the same slide for review. *B*, If staining is adequate, a properly oriented, sectioned, and mounted specimen will provide optimal material for interpretation. The crypts should be long and parallel and should end perpendicular to the muscularis mucosae. Improper mounting and tangential sectioning will produce an artifact similar to that at the right side of this biopsy specimen.

between a glass slide and coverslip before microscopic examination under low magnification. This is the preferred method for demonstrating the ova, because viability can also be assessed.[318] If amebiasis is suspected, prior to the mucosal biopsy mucus from the ulcer should be aspirated using a thin glass or metal tube or obtained by scraping the ulcer with a long-handled spatula through a rigid sigmoidoscope. Alternatively, mucus may be obtained with a biopsy forceps through a fiberoptic instrument. The mucus should then be examined for the parasites. Cotton swabs should not be used to obtain the specimen, since recovery of amebas is reduced. Also, enemas that might remove exudate containing the parasites should not be given. A biopsy of the ulcer should be taken. Special stains for amebas will occasionally demonstrate the parasite invading tissue or present in clumps of adherent exudate, even when repeated stool examinations are negative.[319]

Rectal biopsy may also show evidence of various systemic diseases. For example, a Congo red stain will demonstrate the characteristic green birefringence if amyloid deposits are present in walls of small arterioles in the submucosa and muscularis mucosae (see page 509). However, renal and gastric mucosal biopsies are superior to rectal biopsy in demonstrating evidence of *amyloidosis*.[320, 321] Diagnosis of *Hirschprung's disease* can be made by a punch forceps or cutting forceps biopsy of rectal valves or by a suction biopsy taken at least 3 cm above the pectinate line. Occasionally, jumbo biopsy forceps may also obtain enough submucosa to facilitate this diagnosis. Serial sections of the specimens should be made to ascertain the absence of ganglion cells and the presence of hypertrophied and disorganized nonmyelinated nerve fibers in the submucosa.[322] In patients with *cystic fibrosis*, rectal biopsy often demonstrates widely dilated and gaping mucosal crypts packed with mucus and with prominent goblet cells. However, these changes are not pathognomonic.[323] In *Whipple's disease*, periodic acid–Schiff (PAS)-positive macrophages are present in the lamina propria of the intestine. However, rectal biopsy is not as valuable or as specific as small bowel biopsy in diagnosing Whipple's disease, since typical cases have been described without PAS-positive macrophages in the rectum. In addition, PAS-positive histiocytes are frequently seen in rectal biopsies from patients without Whipple's disease.[324]

The value of rectal biopsy in the diagnosis of various storage diseases has been emphasized.[324, 325] This is especially true for Tay-Sachs disease, in which diagnostic ganglion cell abnormalities may readily be seen in the rectal mucosal specimen.[326] Other systemic diseases can produce abnormalities in rectal tissue, including focal arteritis in patients with rheumatoid arthritis, absence of plasma cells in the lamina propria in some patients with agammaglobulinemia, and cells with nuclear inclusion bodies in specimens from patients with cytomegalovirus disease. Evidence for anorectal tuberculosis, histoplasmosis, gonorrhea, syphilis and granulomatous fibrosis with lymphogranuloma venereum can be found in rectal biopsy specimens (see pp. 1257–1274). Histologic changes characteristic of radiation damage to the colon, which can be seen in rectal biopsy specimens, are discussed on pages 1369 to 1382.

While colonoscopy permits visualization of the entire inner surface of the colon, mucosal biopsy offers the opportunity for a specific diagnosis and a firm basis for therapy. More frequent use of endoscopic biopsy of the rectum and colon should, therefore, facilitate our understanding and treatment of common disorders as well as the unusual miscellaneous diseases of the colon discussed in this chapter.

References

1. Williams, T. J., and Pratt, J. H. Endometriosis in 1,000 consecutive celiotomies: incidence and management. Am. J. Obstet. Gynecol. *129*:245, 1977.
2. McAfee, C. H., and Greer, H. K. Intestinal endometriosis: a report of 29 cases and a review of the literature. J. Obstet. Gyneacol. Brit. Emp. *67*:539, 1960.
3. Sampson, J. A. The development of the implantation theory for the origin of peritoneal endometriosis. Am. J. Obstet. Gynecol. *40*:549, 1940.
4. Gruenwald, P. Origin of endometriosis from the mesenchyme of coelomic walls. Am. J. Obstet. Gynecol. *44*:470, 1942.
5. Simpson, J. L., Elias, S., Malinak, L. R., and Buttram, V. C., Jr. Heritable aspects of endometriosis. I. Genetic studies. Am. J. Obstet. Gynecol. *137*:327, 1980.
6. Dmowski, W. P., Steele, R. W., and Baker, G. F. Deficient cellular immunity in endometriosis. Am. J. Obstet. Gynecol. *141*:377, 1981.
7. Fox, H., and Buckley, C. H. Current concepts of endometriosis. Clin. Obstet. Gynecol. *11*:279, 1984.
8. Meyers, W. C., Kelvin, F. M., and Jones, R. S. Diagnosis and treatment of colonic endometriosis. Arch. Surg. *114*:169, 1979.
9. Heupel, H. W., Reece, R. L., and Pincus, M. Stromal endometrioma mimicking acute appendicitis. Minn. Med. *53*:153, 1970.
10. Martin, L. F. W., Tidman, M. K., and Jamieson, M. A. Appendiceal intussusception and endometriosis. J. Can. Assoc. Radiol. *31*:276, 1980.
11. Martimbeau, P. W., Pratt, J. H., and Gaffey, T. A. Small bowel obstruction secondary to endometriosis. Mayo Clin. Proc. *50*:239, 1975.
12. Croom, R. D., Donovan, M. L., and Schwesinger, W. H. Intestinal endometriosis. Am. J. Surg., *148*:660, 1984.
13. Agha, F. P., Elta, G., and Abrams, G. D. Ileal endometriosis causing acute small bowel obstruction. Mt. Sinai J. Med. *53*:497, 1986.
14. Carmichael, J. L., and Williams, D. B. Hemoperitoneum from erosion of ectopic endometrial tissue. South. Med. J. *65*:371, 1972.
15. Spjut, H. J., and Perkins, D. E. Endometriosis of the sigmoid colon and rectum. Am. J. Roentgenol. *82*:1070, 1959.
16. Beyoung, E. E., and Gamble, C. N. Primary adenocarcinoma of the rectovaginal septum arising from endometriosis. Cancer *24*:597, 1969.
17. Bernstein, J. S., Perlow, V., and Brenner, J. J. Massive ascites due to endometriosis. Am. J. Dig. Dis. *6*:1, 1961.
18. Gray, L. A. Endometriosis of the bowel: role of bowel resection, superficial excision and oophorectomy in treatment. Ann. Surg. *177*:580, 1973.
19. Keye, W. R., and Dixon, J. Photocoagulation of endometriosis with the argon laser. Obstet. Gynecol. *62*:383, 1983.
20. Martin, D. C. CO_2 laser laparoscopy for endometriosis associated with infertility. J. Reproduct. Med. *31*:1089, 1986.
21. Andrews, W. C. Medical versus surgical treatment of endometriosis. Clin. Obstet. Gynecol. *23*:917, 1980.
22. Lauersen, N. H., Wilson, K. H., and Birnbaum, S. Danazol: an antigonadotropic agent in the treatment of pelvic endometriosis. Am. J. Obstet. Gynecol. *123*:742, 1975.
23. Feinberg, S. B., Schwartz, M. Z., Clifford, S., Buchwald, H., and Varco, R. L. Significance of pneumatosis cystoides intestinalis after jejunoileal bypass. Am. J. Surg. *133*:149, 1977.
24. Koss, L. G. Abdominal gas cysts (pneumatosis cystosis cystoides intestinorum hominis). Arch. Pathol. *53*:523, 1952.
25. Seaman, W. B., Fleming, R. J., and Baker, D. H. Pneumatosis-intestinalis of the small bowel. Semin. Roentgenol. *1*:234, 1966.
26. Gruenberg, J. C., Grodsinsky, C., and Ponka, J. L. Pneumatosis intestinalis: a clinical classification. Dis. Colon Rectum *22*:5, 1979.
27. Keyting, W. S., McCarver, R. R., Kovarik, J. L., and Daywitt, A. L. Pneumatosis intestinalis: a new concept. Radiology *76*:733, 1961.
28. Ghahremani, G. G., Port, R. B., and Beachley, M. C. Pneumatosis coli in Crohn's disease. Am. J. Dig. Dis. *19*:315, 1974.
29. Doub, H. P., and Shea, J. J. Pneumatosis cystoides intestinalis. JAMA *172*:1238, 1960.
30. Stevenson, D. K., Graham, C. B., and Stevenson, J. K. Neonatal necrotizing enterocolitis: 100 new cases. Adv. Pediatr. *27*:319, 1980.
31. Yale, C. E., Balish, E., Wu, J. P. The bacterial etiology of pneumatosis cystoides intestinalis. Arch. Surg. *109*:89, 1974.
32. Nelson, S. W. Extraluminal gas collections due to diseases of the gastrointestinal tract. AJR *115*:225, 1972.
33. Hutchins, W. W., Gore, R. M., and Foley, M. J. CT demonstration of pneumatosis intestinalis from bowel infarction. Comput. Radiol. *7*:283, 1983.
34. Scott, J. R., Miller, W. T., Urso, M., and Stadalnik, R. C. Acute mesenteric infarction. AJR *113*:269, 1971.
35. Holt, S., Gilmour, H. M., Buist, T. A. S., Marwick, K., Heading, R. C. High flow oxygen therapy for pneumatosis coli. Gut *20*:493, 1979.
36. Forgacs, P., Wright, P. H., and Wyatt, A. P. Treatment of intestinal gas cysts by oxygen breathing. Lancet *1*:579, 1973.
37. VanDerLinden, W., and Marsell, R. Pneumatosis cystoides coli associated with high H_2 excretion. Scand. J. Gastroenterol. *14*:173, 1979.
38. Gillon, J., Tadesse, K., Logan, R. F. A., Holt, S., and Sircus, W. Breath hydrogen in pneumatosis cystoides intestinalis. Gut *20*:1008, 1979.
39. McGregor, J. K., and McKinnon, D. A. Intestinal interstitial emphysema. Gastroenterology *35*:206, 1958.
40. Lee, S. P., Coverdale, H. A., and Nicholson, G. I. Oxygen therapy for pneumatosis coli: a report of two cases and a review. Aust. N.Z. J. Med. *7*:44, 1977.
41. Yunich, A. M., and Fredkin, N. F. Fatal sprue (malabsorption) syndrome secondary to extensive pneumatosis cystoides intestinalis. Gastroenterology *35*:212, 1958.
42. Merhoff, W. E., Hirschfield, J. S., and Kern, F. Small intestinal scleroderma with malabsorption and pneumatosis cystoides intestinalis. JAMA *204*:854, 1968.
43. Bass, D. B., and Schuster, M. M. Proctoscopic diagnosis of pneumatosis cystoides coli. Gastrointest. Endosc. *16*:164, 1970.
44. Varano, V. J., and Bonnano, C. Colonoscopic findings in pneumatosis cystoides intestinalis. Am. J. Gastroenterol. *59*:353, 1973.
45. Forde, K. A., Whitlock, R. T., and Seaman, W. B. Pneumatosis cystoides intestinalis. Report of a case with colonoscopic findings of inflammatory bowel disease. Am. J. Gastroenterol. *68*:188, 1977.
46. Lerner, H. H., and Gazin, A. L. Pneumatosis intestinalis. Its roentgenologic diagnosis. AJR *56*:464, 1946.
47. Marshak, R. H., Lindner, A. E., and Maklansky, D.: Pneumatosis cystoides coli. Gastrointest. Radiol. *2*:85, 1977.
48. Elliot, G. B., and Elliot, K. A. The roentgenologic pathology of so-called pneumatosis cystoides intestinalis. AJR *89*:720, 1963.
49. Simon, N. M., Nyman, K. E., Divertic, M. B., Rovelstad, R. A., and King, J. E. Pneumatosis cystoides intestinalis. Treatment with oxygen via close fitting mask. JAMA *231*:1354, 1954.
50. Greenburg, J. A., Batra, S. K., and Priest, R. J. Treatment of pneumatosis cystoides intestinalis with oxygen. Arch. Surg. *112*:62, 1977.
51. Down, R. H. L., and Castleden, W. M. Oxygen therapy for pneumatosis coli. Br. Med. J. *1*:493, 1975.
52. Masterson, J. S., Fratken, L. B., Osler, T. R., and Trapp, W. G. Treatment of pneumatosis cystoides intestinalis with hyperbaric oxygen. Ann. Surg. *187*:245, 1978.
53. Lee, S. P., Coverdale, H. A., and Nicholson, G. I. Oxygen therapy for pneumatosis coli: a report of two cases and a review. Aust. N.Z. J. Med. *7*:44, 1977.
54. Clark, J. M., and Lambersten, C. J. Rate of development of pulmonary O_2 toxicity in man during O_2 breathing at 2.0 ata. J. Appl. Physiol. *30*:739, 1971.
55. Gruenberg, J. C., Batra, S. K., and Priest, R. J. Treatment of pneumatosis intestinalis with oxygen. Arch. Surg. *112*:62, 1977.

56. VanDerLinden, W., and Hoflin, F. Pneumatosis cystoides coli recurs after oxygen treatment. A clue to the pathogenesis? Eur. Surg. Res. *10*:225, 1978.
57. Holt, S., Stewart, I. C., Heading, R. C., and Macpherson, A. I. S. Resolution of primary pneumatosis coli. J. R. Coll. Surg. Edinb. *23*:297, 1978.
58. Ellis, B. W. Symptomatic treatment of primary pneumatosis coli with metronidazole. Br. Med. J. *1*:763, 1980.
59. Gillon, J., Logan, R. F. A., Sircus, W., and Heading, R. C. Symptomatic treatment of primary pneumatosis coli with metronidazole. Br. Med. J. *1*:1087, 1980.
60. Witkowski, L. J., Pontius, G. V., and Anderson, R. E. Gas cysts of the intestine. Surgery *37*:959, 1955.
61. Andrade, S., and Andrade, V. H. Intestinal pneumatosis. Presentation of five cases. Am. J. Proctol. *19*:39, 1955.
62. Cruveilhier, J. Un beau cas de cicatrisation d'un ulcere de l'intestine gaele datant d'une douzine d'armees. Bull. Soc. Anat. 7:1, 1832.
63. Mahoney, T. J., Burbick, M. P., and Hitchcock, C. R. Nonspecific ulcers of the colon. Dis. Colon Rectum *21*:623, 1978.
64. Blundell, C. R., and Earnest, D. L. Idiopathic cecal ulcer. Diagnosis by colonoscopy followed by nonoperative management. Dig. Dis. Sci. *23*:494, 1980.
65. Shallman, R. W., Keuhner, M., Williams, G. H. Y., Sajjad, S., and Sautter, R. Benign cecal ulcers. Spectrum of disease and selective management. Dis. Colon Rectum *28*:732, 1985.
66. Barlow, D. Simple ulcer of the cecum, colon and rectum. Br. J. Surg. *28*:575, 1941.
67. Brock, A. L., Reynolds, J. D. H., and Wood, W. G. Nonspecific ulcers of the colon: a case presentation of ulceration of the transverse colon. J. Clin. Gastroenterol. *1*:241, 1979.
68. Yates, J. N., and Clausen, E. G. Simple nonspecific ulcers of the sigmoid colon. Arch. Surg. *81*:535, 1960.
69. Rutter, K. R. P., and Riddell, R. H. The solitary ulcer syndrome of the rectum. Clin. Gastroenterol. *4*:505, 1981.
70. Thompson, G., Clark, A., Handyside, J., and Gillespie, G. Solitary ulcer of the rectum—or is it? A report of six cases. Br. J. Surg. *68*:21, 1981.
71. Kennedy, D. K., Hughes, E. S. R., and Masterson, J. P. The natural history of benign ulcer of the rectum. Surg. Gynecol. Obstet. *144*:718, 1977.
72. Ford, M. J., Anderson, J. R., Gilmore, H. M., Holt, S., Sircus, W., and Harding, R. C. Clinical spectrum of "solitary ulcer" of the rectum. Gastroenterology *84*:1533, 1983.
73. Levine, D. S. "Solitary" rectal ulcer syndrome. Are "solitary" rectal ulcer syndrome and "localized" colitis cystica profunda analogous syndromes caused by rectal prolapse? Gastroenterology *92*:243, 1987.
74. Rutter, K. R. P. Electromyographic changes in certain pelvic floor abnormalities. Proc. R. Soc. Med. *67*:53, 1974.
75. Snooks, S. N., Nicholls, R. J., Henry, M. M., and Swash, M. Electrophysiological and manometric assessment of the pelvic floor in the solitary rectal ulcer syndrome. Br. J. Surg., *72*:131, 1985.
76. Rutter, K. R. P., and Riddell, R. H. The solitary ulcer syndrome of the rectum. Clin. Gastroenterol. *4*:505, 1975.
77. Parks, A. G., Porter, N. H., and Hardcastle, J. The syndrome of the descending perineum. Proc. R. Soc. Med. *59*:477, 1966.
78. Rutter, K. R. P. Electromyographic changes in certain pelvic floor abnormalities. Proc. R. Soc. Med. *67*:53, 1974.
79. Rutter, K. R. P. Solitary rectal ulcer syndrome. Proc. R. Soc. Med. *68*:22, 1975.
80. Kuipers, H. C., Schreve, R. H., Hodemakers, H. T. C. Diagnosis of functional disorders of defecation causing the solitary rectal ulcer syndrome. Dis. Colon Rectum *29*:126, 1986.
81. Pescatori, M., Maria, C., Mattana, C., Vulpio, C., and Vecchio, F. Clinical picture and pelvic floor physiology in the solitary rectal ulcer syndrome. Dis. Colon Rectum *28*:862, 1985.
82. Schweiger, M., and Alexander-Williams, J. Solitary ulcer syndrome of the rectum. Its association with occult rectal prolapse. Lancet *1*:170, 1977.
83. Martin, C. J., Parks, T. G., and Biggart, J. D. Solitary ulcer syndrome in Northern Ireland, 1971–1980. Br. J. Surg. *68*:744, 1981.
84. Thompson, H., and Hall, D. Solitary rectal ulcer: always a self-induced condition? Br. J. Surg. *67*:784, 1980.
85. Eckardt, V. F., Kanzler, G., and Remmele, W. Anorectal ergotism: another cause of solitary rectal ulcers. Gastroenterology *91*:1123, 1986.
86. Madigan, M. R., and Morson, B. C. Solitary ulcer of the rectum. Gut *10*:871, 1969.
87. Castagnone, D., Rangi, T., Velio, P., Bianchi, P., and Polli, E. F. Radiologic features of the solitary rectal ulcer syndrome. Eur. J. Radiol. *4*:110, 1984.
88. Klighley, M. R. B., Shoulder, P. Clinical and manometric features of the solitary rectal ulcer syndrome. Dis. Colon Rectum *27*:507, 1984.
89. Stuart, M. Proctitis cystica profunda—evidence, etiology, and treatment. Dis. Colon Rectum *27*:153, 1984.
90. Goddall, H. B., Sinclair, I. S. R. Colitis cystica profunda. J. Pathol. Bacteriol. *73*:33, 1957.
91. Denton, J. The pathology of pellagra. Am. J. Trop. Med. *5*:173, 1966.
92. Epstein, S. E., Ascari, W. A., Ablow, R. C., Seaman, W. B., and Lattis, R. Colitis cystica profunda. Am. J. Clin. Pathol. *45*:186, 1966.
93. Wayte, D. M., and Helwig, E. B. Colitis cystica profunda. Am. J. Clin. Pathol. *48*:159, 1967.
94. Herman, A. H., and Nasbeth, D. C. Colitis cystica profunda: localized, segmental, and diffuse. Arch. Surg. *106*:337, 1973.
95. Manson-Bahr, P., and Gregg, A. L. The surgical treatment of chronic bacillary dysentery. Br. J. Surg. *13*:701, 1926.
96. Schneider, R., Dickersin, G. R., and Patterson, J. F. Localized giant pseudopolyposis. A complication of granulomatous colitis. Am. J. Dig. Dis. *18*:265, 1973.
97. Aftalion, B., and Lipper, S. Enteritis cystica profunda associated with Crohn's disease. Arch. Pathol. Lab. Med. *108*:532, 1984.
98. Magidson, J. G., and Lewin, K. J. Diffuse colitis cystica profunda. Report of a case. Am. J. Surg. Pathol. *5*:393, 1981.
99. Tedesco, F. J., Sumner, H. W., and Kassens, W. D. Colitis cystica profunda. Am. J. Gastroenterol. *65*:339, 1976.
100. Farman, J., Dallemand, S., Robinson, T., and Koehane, M. F. Colitis cystica profunda: an unusual solitary tumor. Dis. Colon Rectum *17*:565, 1974.
101. Bentley, E., Chandrasoma, P., Cohen, H., Radin, R., and Ray, M. Colitis cystica profunda: presenting with complete intestinal obstruction and recurrence. Gastroenterology *89*:1157, 1985.
102. Gardiner, G. W., McAuliffe, N., and Murray, D. Colitis cystica profunda occurring in a radiation-induced colonic stricture. Hum. Pathol. *15*:295, 1984.
103. Rosen, J., Villant, J. G., and Yermakon, V. Submucosal mucous cysts at a colostomy site. Dis. Colon Rectum *19*:453, 1976.
104. Barner, J. L. Colitis cystica profunda. Radiology *89*:435, 1967.
105. Salzman, E. W., and Castleman, B. Rectal lesion associated with diarrhea and hypoproteinemia. Case records, Massachusetts General Hospital. N. Engl. J. Med. *275*:608, 1966.
106. Rosengren, J. E., Hildell, J., Lindstrom, C. G., and Leander, L. Localized colitis cystica profunda. Gastrointest. Radiol. *7*:79, 1982.
107. Brock, D. R., and Suckow, E. E. Obliterative arteriolosclerosis of the colon with focal mucosal necrosis. Gastroenterology *44*:190, 1963.
108. Sternlieb, I. Brock-Suckow polyposis of the colon (obliterative arteriolosclerosis of the colon?). Gastroenterology, *44*:193, 1964.
109. Crane, C. W. Observations on sodium and potassium content of mucus from the large intestine. Gut *6*:439, 1965.
110. Martin, J. K., Jr., Culp, C. E., and Weiland, L. H. Colitis cystica profunda. Dis. Colon Rectum *23*:488, 1980.
111. Edwards, F. C., and Truelove, S. C. The course and prognosis of ulcerative colitis. Gut *4*:299, 1963.
112. Ritchie, J. K., Powell-Tuck, J., and Lennard-Jones, J. E. Clinical outcome of the first ten years of ulcerative colitis and proctitis. Lancet *1*:1140, 1978.
113. Farmer, R. G. Long-term prognosis for patients with ulcerative proctosigmoiditis (ulcerative colitis confined to the rectum and sigmoid colon). J. Clin. Gastroenterol. *1*:47, 1979.

114. Mir-Madjlessi, S. H., Michener, W. M., and Farmer, R. G. Course and prognosis of idiopathic ulcerative proctosigmoiditis in young patients. J. Pediatr. Gastroenterol. Nutr. *5*:570, 1986.
115. Farthing, J. J. G., and Lennard-Jones, S. E. Sensibility of the rectum to distention and anorectal distention reflex in ulcerative colitis. Gut *19*:64, 1978.
116. Meisel, J. L., Bergman, D., Graney, D., Saunders, D. R., and Rubin, C. E. Human rectal mucosa: proctoscopic and morphologic changes caused by laxatives. Gastroenterology *72*:1274, 1977.
117. Surawicz, C. M., and Belic, L. Rectal biopsy helps to distinguish acute self-limited colitis from idiopathic inflammatory bowel disease. Gastroenterology *86*:104, 1984.
118. Nostrant, T. T., Kumar, N. B., and Appelman, H. D. Histopathology differentiates acute self-limited colitis from ulcerative colitis. Gastroenterology *92*:318, 1987.
119. Das, K. M., Morecki, R., Nair, P., and Berkowitz, J. M. Idiopathic proctitis. I. The morphology of proximal colonic mucosa and its clinical significance. Am. J. Dig. Dis. *22*:524, 1977.
120. Quinn, T. C., Corey, L., Chaffee, R. G., Schuffler, M. D., Brancato, F. P., and Holmes, K. K. The etiology of anorectal infections in homosexual men. Am. J. Med. *71*:395, 1981.
121. Surawicz, C. M., Goodell, S. E., Quinn, T. C., Roberts, P. L., Corey, L., Holmes, K. K., Schuffler, M. D., and Stamm, W. E. Spectrum of rectal biopsy abnormalities in homosexual men with intestinal symptoms. Gastroenterology *91*:651, 1986.
122. Quinn, T. C. Clinical approach to intestinal infections in homosexual men. Med. Clin. North Am. *70*:611, 1986.
123. Quinn, T. C., Stamm, W. E., Goodell, S. E., Mkrtichian, E., Benedetti, J., Corey, L., Schuffler, M. D., and Holmes, K. K. The polymicrobial origin of intestinal infections in homosexual men. N. Engl. J. Med. *309*:576, 1983.
124. Myers, A., Humphreys, D. M., and Cox, E. V. A ten year followup of haemorrhagic proctitis. Postgrad. Med. J. *52*:224, 1976.
125. Powell-Tuck, J., Ritchie, J. K., and Lennard-Jones, J. E. The prognosis of idiopathic proctitis. Scand. J. Gastroenterol. *12*:727, 1977.
126. Nugent, F. W., Veidenheimer, M. C., Zuberi, S., and Garabedian, M. M. Clinical course of ulcerative proctosigmoiditis. Am. J. Dig. Dis. *15*:321, 1970.
127. Mir-Madjlessi, S. H., Farmer, R. G., Easley, K. A., and Beck, G. J. Colorectal and extracolonic malignancy in ulcerative colitis. Cancer *58*:1569, 1986.
128. Truelove, S. C. Treatment of ulcerative colitis with local hydrocortisone. Br. Med. J. *2*:1267, 1956.
129. Palmer, K. R., Goepel, J. R., and Hodsworth, C. D. Sulphasalazine retention enemas in ulcerative colitis: a double blind trial. Br. Med. J. *282*:1571, 1981.
130. Barber, G. B., Lee, D. E., Antonioli, D. A., and Peppercorn, M. A. Refractory distal ulcerative colitis responsive to 5-aminosalicylate enemas. Am. J. Gastroenterol. *80*:612, 1985.
131. Sutherland, L. R., Martin, F., Greer, S., Robinson, M., Greenberger, N., Saibil, F., Martin, T., Sparr, J., Prokipchuk, E., and Borgen, L. 5-Aminosalicylic acid enema in the treatment of distal ulcerative colitis, proctosigmoiditis, and proctitis. Gastroenterology *92*:1894, 1987.
132. Dew, M. J., Harries, A. D., Evans, N., Evans, B. K., and Rhodes, J. Maintenance of remission in ulcerative colitis with 5-amino salicylic acid in high doses by mouth. Br. Med. J. *287*:23, 1983.
133. Selby, W. S., Barr, G. D., Ireland, A., Mason, C. H., and Jewell, D. P. Olsalazine in active ulcerative colitis. Br. Med. J. *291*:1373, 1985.
134. Glotzer, D. J., Glick, M. E., and Goldman, H. Proctitis and colitis following diversion of the fecal stream. Gastroenterology *80*:438, 1981.
135. Korelitz, B. I., Cheskin, L. J., Sohn, N., and Sommers, S. C. Proctitis after fecal diversion in Crohn's disease and its elimination with reanastomosis: implications for surgical management. Gastroenterology *87*:710, 1984.
136. Korelitz, B. I., Cheskin, L. J., Sohn, N., and Sommers, S. C. The fate of the rectal segment after diversion of the fecal stream in Crohn's disease: its implications for surgical management. J. Clin. Gastroenterol. *7*:37, 1985.
137. Lusk, L. B., Reichen, J., and Levine, J. S. Aphthous ulceration in diversion colitis. Gastroenterology *87*:1171, 1984.
138. Bosshardt, R. T., and Abel, M. E. Proctitis following fecal diversion. Dis. Colon Rectum *27*:605, 1984.
139. Ona, F. V., and Boger, J. N. Rectal bleeding due to diversion colitis. Am. J. Gastroenterol. *80*:40, 1985.
140. Winter, V. J., Greiner, L., and Schubert, G. E. Kolitis im funktionslosen Rektosigmoid nach Anlegen eines endstandigen Anus praeternaturalis. Z. Gastroenterologie *21*:27, 1983.
141. Tripp, M. R. Personal communication.
142. Wagner, M., Rosenberg, H., Fernbach, D., and Singleton, E. Typhlitis: a complication of leukemia in childhood. AJR *109*:341, 1970.
143. Ikard, R. W. Neutropenic typhlitis in adults. Arch. Surg. *116*:943, 1981.
144. Kunkel, J. M., and Rosenthal, D. Management of the ileocecal syndrome. Dis. Colon Rectum *19*:196, 1986.
145. Moir, C. R., Scudamore, C. H., and Benny, W. B. Typhlitis: selective surgical management. Am. J. Surg. *151*:563, 1986.
146. Matolo, N. M., Garfinkle, S. E., and Wolfman, E. F. Intestinal necrosis and perforation in patients receiving immunosuppressive drugs. Am. J. Surg. *132*:753, 1976.
147. Dosik, G. M., Luna, M., Valdivieso, M., McCredie, K. B., Gehen, E. A., Gil-Extremera, B., Smith, T. L., and Bodey, G. P. Necrotizing colitis in patients with cancer. Am. J. Med. *67*:646, 1979.
148. Geelhoed, G. W., Kane, M. A., Dale, D. C., and Wells, S. A. Colon ulceration and perforation in cyclic neutropenia. J. Pediatr. Surg. *8*:379, 1973
149. Ryan, M. E., and Morrissey, J. F. Typhlitis complicating methimazole-induced agranulocytosis. Gastrointest. Endosc. *29*:299, 1983.
150. Shamberger, R. C., Weinstein, H. J., Delorey, M. J., and Levy, R. H. The medical and surgical management of typhlitis in children with acute nonlymphocytic (myelogenous) leukemia. Cancer *57*:603, 1986.
151. Taylor, A. J., Dodds, W. J., Gonyo, J. E., and Komorowski, R. A. Typhlitis in adults. Gastrointest. Radiol. *10*:363, 1985.
152. Moir, D. H., and Bale, P. M. Necropsy findings in childhood leukemia, emphasizing neutropenic enterocolitis and cerebral calcification. Pathology *8*:247, 1976.
153. Schaller, R. T., and Schaller, J. F. The acute abdomen in the immunologically compromised child. J. Pediatr. Surg. *18*:937, 1983.
154. Weinstein, H. J., Mayer, R. J., Rosenthal, D. S., Camitta, B. M., Coral, F. S., Nathan, D. G., and Frei, E., III. Treatment of acute myelogenous leukemia in children and adults. N. Engl. J. Med. *303*:473, 1980.
155. Sherman, N. J., and Woolley, M. M. The ileocecal syndrome in acute childhood leukemia. Arch. Surg. *107*:39, 1973.
156. Dworkin, B., Winawer, S. J., and Lightdale, C. J. Typhlitis: report of a case with long term survival and a review of the recent literature. Dig. Dis. Sci. *26*:1032, 1981.
157. Steinberg, D., Gold, J., and Brodin, A. Necrotizing enterocolitis in leukemia. Arch. Intern. Med. *131*:538, 1973.
158. Sandler, S. G., Tobin, W., and Henderson, E. S. Vincristine-induced neuropathy. Neurology *19*:367, 1969.
159. Abramson, S. J., Berdon, W. E., and Baker, D. H. Childhood typhlitis: its increasing association with myelogenous leukemia. Radiology *146*:61, 1983.
160. Adams, G. W., Rauch, R. F., Kelvin, F. M., Silverman, P. M., and Korobkin, M. CT detection of typhlitis. J. Comput. Assist. Tomogr. *9*:363, 1985.
161. McNamara, M. J., Chalmers, A. G., Morgan, M., and Smith, S. E. W. Typhlitis in acute childhood leukaemia: radiological features. Clin. Radiol. *37*:83, 1986.
162. Meyerovitz, M. F., and Fellows, K. E. Typhlitis: a cause of gastrointestinal hemorrhage in children. AJR *143*:833, 1984.
163. Herzig, R. H., Herzig, G. P., Graw, R. G., Bull, M. I., and Ray, K. K. Successful granulocyte transfusion therapy for gram-negative septicemia. N. Engl. J. Med. *296*:701, 1977.
164. Lehman, J. A., and Armitage, J. O. Surgical interventions in complications of acute leukemia. Postgrad. Med. *68*:89, 1980.
165. Exelby, P. R., Ghandchi, A., Lansigan, N., and Schwartz, I. Management of the acute abdomen in children with leukemia. Cancer *35*:826, 1975.

166. Lindstrom, C. G. "Collagenous colitis" with watery diarrhea—a new entity? Pathol. Eur. *11*:87, 1976.
167. Rains, H., Rogers, A. I., and Ghandur-Mnaymneh, L. Collagenous colitis. Ann. Intern. Med. *196*:108, 1987.
168. Nielsen, V. T., and Vetner, M. Collagenous colitis. Histopathology *4*:83, 1980.
169. Wang, K. H., Perrault, J., Carpenter, H. A., Schroeder, K. W., and Tremaine, W. J. Collagenous colitis: a clinicopathologic correlation. Mayo Clin. Proc. *62*:665, 1987.
170. Teglbjaerg, P. S., and Thaysen, E. H. Collagenous colitis: an ultrastructural study of a case. Gastroenterology *82*:561, 1982.
171. Van den Dord, J. J., Begoes, K., and Desmet, V. J. Collagenous colitis: an abnormal collagen table? Two new cases and review of the literature. Am. J. Gastroenterol. *77*:377, 1982.
172. Rask-Madsen, J., Grove, O., Hansen, M. G. J., Bukhave, K., Scient, C., and Henrik-Nielsen, R. Colonic transport of water and electrolytes in a patient with secretory diarrhea due to collagenous colitis. Dig. Dis. Sci. *28*:1141, 1983.
173. Giardiello, F. M., Bayless, T. M., Jessurun, J., Hamilton, S. R., and Yardley, J. H. Collagenous colitis: physiologic and histopathologic studies in seven patients. Ann. Intern. Med. *106*:46, 1987.
174. Palmer, K. R., Berry, H., Wheeler, P. J., Williams, C. B., Fairclough, P., Marson, B. C., and Silk, D. B. A. Collagenous colitis—a relapsing and remitting disease. Gut *27*:578, 1986.
175. Kingham, J. G. C., Levison, D. A., Morson, B. C., and Dawson, A. M. Collagenous colitis. Gut *27*:570, 1986.
176. Flejou, J. F., Grimand, J. A., Molas, G., Baviera, E., and Potet, F. Collagenous colitis: ultrastructural study and collagen immunotyping of four cases. Arch. Pathol. Lab. Med. *108*:977, 1984.
177. Read, N. W., Krejs, G. J., Read, M. G., Santa Ana, C. A., Morowski, S. G., and Fordtran, J. S. Chronic diarrhea of unknown origin. Gastroenterology *78*:264, 1980.
178. Bo-Linn, G. W., Vandrell, D. D., Lee, E., and Fordtran, J. S. An evaluation of the significance of microscopic colitis in patients with chronic diarrhea. J. Clin. Invest. *75*:1559, 1985.
179. Jessurun, J., Yardley, J. H., Giardiello, F. M., Hamilton, S. R., and Bayless, T. M. Chronic colitis with thickening of the subepithelial collagen layer (collagenous colitis): histopathologic findings in 15 patients. Hum. Pathol., *18*:839, 1987.
180. Teglbjaerg, P. S., Thayson, E. H., and Jensen, H. H. Development of collagenous colitis in sequential biopsy specimens. Gastroenterology *87*:703, 1984.
181. Farah, D. A., Mills, P. R., Lee, F. D., McLay, A., and Russell, R. I. Collagenous colitis: possible response to sulfasalazine and local steroid therapy. Gastroenterology *88*:792, 1985.
182. Loo, F. D., Wood, C. M., Soergel, K. H., Komorowski, R. A., Cheung, H., Gay, S., and Gay, R. E. Abnormal collagen deposition and ion transport in collagenous colitis. (Abstract.) Gastroenterology *88*:1481, 1985.
183. Eidelman, S., and Lagunoff, D. The morphology of the normal human rectal biopsy. Hum. Pathol. *3*:389, 1972.
184. Keye, G. I., Lane, N., and Pascel, R. P. Colonic pericryptal fibroblast sheath: replication, migration, and cytodifferentiation of a mesenchymal system in adult tissue. II. Fine structural aspects in normal rabbit and human colon. Gastroenterology *54*:852, 1968.
185. Nielson, V. T., Vetner, M., and Harslof, E. Collagenous colitis. Histopathology *4*:83, 1980.
186. Hwang, W. S., Kelly, J. K., Shaffer, E. A., and Hershfield, N. B. Collagenous colitis: a disease of the pericryptal fibroblast sheath? J. Pathol. *149*:33, 1986.
187. Gabbiani, G., Louis, M. L., Barley, A. J., Bazin, S., and Dulanay, A. Collagen and myofibroblasts of granulation tissue. A chemical, ultrastructural and immunologic study. Virchows Arch. Cell. Pathol. *21*:133, 1976.
188. Gledhill, A., and Cole, F. M. Significance of basement membrane thickening in the human colon. Gut *25*:1085, 1985.
189. Pieterse, A. S., Hecker, R., and Rowland, R. Collagenous colitis: a distinctive and potentially reversible disorder. J. Clin. Pathol. *35*:338, 1982.
190. Weidner, N., Smith, J., and Pattee, B. Sulfasalazine in treatment of collagenous colitis: case report and review of the literature. Am. J. Med. *77*:162, 1984.
191. Debongnie, J. C., DeGalocsy, C., Cahlolesseur, M. O., and Haot, J. Collagenous colitis: a transient condition? Report of two cases. Dis. Colon Rectum *27*:672, 1984.
192. Morgensen, A. M., Olsen, J. H., and Gudmend-Hoyer, E. Collagenous colitis. Acta Med. Scand. *216*:535, 1984.
193. Fausa, O., Foerster, A., and Hovig, T. Collagenous colitis: a clinical, histological and ultrastructural study. Scand. J. Gastroenterol. *20*(Suppl. 107):8, 1985.
194. McClure, J. Malakoplakia. J. Pathol. *140*:275, 1983.
195. McClure, J. Malakoplakia of the gastrointestinal tract. Postgrad. Med. J. *57*:95, 1981.
196. von Hansemann, D. Ueber Malakoplakia der Harnblase. Arch. Pathol. Anat. *173*:302, 1903.
197. Mackay, E. H. Malakoplakia in ulcerative colitis. Arch. Pathol. Lab. Med. *102*:140, 1978.
198. Sansui, I. D., and Tio, F. O. Gastrointestinal malakoplakia. Am. J. Gastroenterol. *62*:356, 1974.
199. Fisher, E. R., and Hellstrom, H. R. Ceroid-like colonic histiocytosis. Am. J. Clin. Pathol. *42*:581, 1964.
200. Lou, T. Y., and Tepitz, C. Malakoplakia: pathogenesis and ultrastructural morphogenesis—a problem of altered macrophage (phagolysosomal) response. Hum. Pathol. *5*:191, 1974.
201. Lewin, K. J., Harrel, G. S., Lee, A. S., and Crowley, L. G. Malakoplakia—an electromicroscopic study. Demonstration of bacilliform organisms in malakoplakia macrophages. Gastroenterology *66*:28, 1974.
202. Sencer, O., Sencer, H., Uluoglu, O., Torunoglu, M., and Tatlicioglu, E. Malakoplakia of the skin. Arch. Pathol. Lab. Med., *103*:446, 1979.
203. Lewin, K. J., Fair, W. R., Steigbigel, R. T., Winberg, C. D., and Droller, M. J. Clinical and laboratory studies into pathogenesis of malakoplakia. J. Clin. Pathol. *29*:354, 1976.
204. Abdou, N. I., Naeombejara, C., Sagawa, A., Ragland, C., Stechschulte, D. J., Nilsson, U., Gourley, W., Watenabe, I., Lindsey, N., and Allen, M. Malakoplakia: evidence for monocyte lysosomal abnormality correctable by cholinergic agonists in vitro and in vivo. N. Engl. J. Med. *297*:1413, 1917.
205. Webb, M., Pincott, J. R., Marshall, W. C., Spitz, L., Harvey, B. A. M., and Soothill, J. F. Hypoglobulinemia and malakoplakia: response to bethanechol. Eur. J. Pediatr. *145*:297, 1986.
206. Oliver, J. M. Impaired microtubule function correctable by cyclic GMP and cholinergic agonists in the Chediak-Higashi syndrome. Am. J. Pathol. *85*:395, 1976.
207. Ganzales-Angulo, A., Corral, E., Garcia-Torres, R., and Quijano, M. Malakoplakia of the colon. Gastroenterology *48*:383, 1965.
208. Cruveilhier, J. Cancer avec malanose. *In* Bailliere, J. B. (ed.). Anatomie Pathologique du Corps Humain. Paris, 1829, p. 6.
209. Virchow, R. Die pathologischen Pigmente. Virchow Arch. Pathol. Anat. *1*:379, 1931.
210. Stewart, N. J., and Hickman, E. M. Observations on melanosis coli. J. Pathol. Bacteriol. *34*:61, 1931.
211. Bockus, H. L., Willard, J. H., and Bank, J. Melanosis coli. JAMA *101*:1, 1933.
212. Speare, G. S. Melanosis coli. Experimental observations on its production and elimination in 23 cases. Am. J. Surg. *82*:631, 1951.
213. Wittoesch, J. H., Jackman, R. J., and McDonald, J. R. Melanosis coli: general review and study of 887 cases. Dis. Colon Rectum *1*:172, 1958.
214. Roden, B. Melanosis coli. A pathological study: its experimental production in monkeys. J. Med. Sci. *6*:654, 1940.
215. Morgenstern, L., Shemen, L., Allen, W., Amodeo, P., and Michel, S. L. Melanosis coli. Changes in appearance when associated with colonic neoplasm. Arch. Surg. *118*:62, 1983.
216. Bodiale, D., Marcheggiano, A., Pallone, F., Paoluzi, P., Bausano, G., Iamoni, C., Materia, E., Anzimi, F., and Corrazziari, T. A. E. Melanosis of the rectum in patients with chronic constipation. Dis. Colon Rectum *23*:241, 1985.
217. Won, K. H., and Ramchand, S. Melanosis of the ileum. Case report and electron microscopic study. Am. J. Dig. Dis. *15*:57, 1940.
218. Dublier, L. D., and Burkhart, R. C.: Melanosis coli with liver involvement. J. Ky. Med. Assoc. *73*:143, 1975.
219 Andrejauskas, G. Rare case of esophagitis with melanosis. Medicine *18*:13, 1937.

220. Bisordi, W. M., and Kleinman, M. S. Melanosis duodeni. Gastrointest. Endosc. *23*:37, 1976.
221. Ghadially, F. N., and Parry, E. W. An electron microscope and histochemical study of melanosis coli. J. Pathol. Bacteriol. *92*:313, 1966.
222. Steer, H. W., and Colin-Jones, D. G. Melanosis coli: studies of toxic effects of irritant purgatives, J. Pathol. *115*:199, 1975.
223. Smith, B. Pathologic changes in the colon produced by anthraquinone purgatives. Dis. Colon Rectum *16*:445, 1973.
224. Krishnamurthy, S., Schuffler, M. D., Rorhmann, C. A., and Pope, C. E., II. Severe idiopathic constipation is associated with a distinctive abnormality of the colonic myenteric plexus. Gastroenterology *88*:26, 1985.
225. Heilbrun, N. Roentgen evidence suggesting enterocolitis associated with prolonged cathartic abuse. Radiology *41*:486, 1943.
226. Heilbrun, N., and Berstein, C. Roentgen abnormalities of the large and small intestine associated with prolonged cathartic ingestion. Radiology *65*:549, 1955.
227. Plum, G. E., Weber, H. M., and Sauer, W. G. Prolonged cathartic abuse resulting in roentgen evidence suggestive of enterocolitis. AJR *83*:919, 1960.
228. Ziter, F. M. Cathartic colon. N.Y. State J. Med. *67*:546, 1967.
229. Margulis, A. R., Goldberg, H. I., Lawson, T. L., Montgomery, C. K., Rambo, O. N., Noona, C. D., and Amberg, J. R. The overlapping spectrum of ulcerative and granulomatous colitis: a roentgenographic pathologic study. AJR *113*:325, 1971.
230. Campbell, W. L. Cathartic colon: reversibility of roentgen changes. Dis. Colon Rectum *23*:445, 1983.
231. Smith, B. Pathology of cathartic colon. Proc. R. Soc. Med. *65*:288, 1972.
232. Smith, B. Effect of irritant purgative on the myenteric plexus in man and the mouse. Gut *9*:139, 1968.
233. Hardcastle, J. D., and Wilkins, J. L. The action of sennosides and related compounds on human colon and rectum. Gut *11*:1038, 1970.
234. Smith, B. Pathologic changes in the colon produced by anthraquinone purgatives. Dis. Colon Rectum *13*:455, 1973.
235. Fleischer, N., Brown, H., Graham, D. Y., and Delena, S. Chronic laxative-induced hyperaldosteronism and hypokalemia simulating Bartter's syndrome. Ann. Intern. Med. *70*:791, 1969.
236. Sladen, G. E. Effect of chronic purgative abuse. Proc. R. Soc. Med. *65*:288, 1972.
237. Hardin, R. D., and Tedesco, F. J. Colitis after Hibiclens enema. J. Clin. Gastroenterol. *8*:572, 1986.
238. Kim, S. K., Cho, C., and Levinson, E. M. Caustic colitis due to detergent enema. AJR *134*:397, 1980.
239. Smith, D. Severe anaphylactic reaction after a soap enema. Br. Med. J. *4*:215, 1967.
240. Bendit, M. Gangrene of the rectum as complication of an enema. Br. Med. J. *1*:664, 1945.
241. Kirchner, S. G., Buckspan, G. S., O'Neill, J. A., Page, D. L., and Burk, H. Detergent enema: a cause of caustic colitis. Pediatr. Radiol. *6*:141, 1971.
242. Pike, B. F., Phillippi, P. J., and Lawson, E. H. Soap colitis. N. Engl. J. Med. *285*:217, 1971.
243. Meyer, C. T., Brand, M., DeLuca, V. A., and Spiro, H. M. Hydrogen peroxide colitis: a report of three patients. J. Clin. Gastroenterol. *3*:31, 1981.
244. Sheehan, J. F., and Byrnjolfsson, G. Ulcerative colitis following hydrogen peroxide enema. Case report and experimental production with transient emphysema of colonic wall and gas embolism. Lab. Invest. *9*:150, 1960.
245. Creteur, V., Douglas, D., Golanti, M., and Margales, A. R. Inflammatory colonic changes produced by contrast material. Radiology *147*:77, 1983.
246. Segal, I., Ou Tim, L., Hamilton, D. G., Lawson, H. H., Solomon, A., Kalk, F., and Cooke, S. A. R. Ritual-enema–induced colitis. Dis. Colon Rectum *22*:195, 1979.
247. Abella, M. E., and Fernandez, A. T. Large fecalomas, Dis. Colon Rectum *10*:401, 1967.
248. Smith, C. W., and Evans, P. R. Bowel motility, a problem in institutionalized geriatric cases. Geriatrics *16*:189, 1961.
249. Earnest, D. L., and Fletcher, G. F. Danger of rectal examination in patients with acute myocardial infarction—fact or fiction? N. Engl. J. Med. *281*:238, 1969.
250. Harland, D. A case of multiple calculi in the large intestine with a review of the subject of intestinal calculi. Br. J. Surg. *41*:209, 1953.
251. Kaufman, S. A., and Karlin, H. Fecaloma of the sigmoid flexure. Dis. Colon Rectum *9*:133, 1966.
252. Derchi, L. E., Musante, F., Giggi, E., Cicio, G. R., and Oliva, L. Sonographic appearance of a fecal mass. J. Ultrasound Med. *4*:573, 1985.
253. Suckling, P. V. The ball-valve rectum due to impacted feces. Lancet *2*:1147, 1962.
254. Cid, A. A., Pietruk, T., Bidari, C. Z., and Ehrinpreis, M. Cecal fecaloma mimicking colonic neoplasm. Dig. Dis. Sci. *26*:1134, 1981.
255. Lal, S., and Brown, G. N. Some unusual complications of fecal impaction. Am. J. Proctol. *18*:226, 1967.
256. Ravich, L., Lerman, T. H., and Schell, N. B. Urinary retention due to fecal impaction. N.Y. State J. Med. *63*:3289, 1963.
257. Grundill, W. L., and Klonpje, J. Spontaneous rupture and stercoral perforation of the colon. S. Afr. Med. J. *69*:203, 1986.
258. Huttunen, R., Heikkinen, E., and Larmi, T. K. I. Stercoraceous and idiopathic perforations of the colon. Surg. Gynecol. Obstet. *140*:756, 1975.
259. Grinvalsky, H. T., and Bowerman, C. I. Stercoraceous ulcers of the colon. Relatively neglected medical and surgical problem. JAMA *171*:1941, 1959.
260. Naderi, M., and Bookstein, J. J. Rectal bleeding secondary to fecal disimpaction: angiographic diagnosis and treatment. Radiology *126*:387, 1978.
261. Hakami, M., Mosavy, S. H., and Tadauon, A. Stercoral perforation of the sigmoid colon: report of two cases. Dis. Colon Rectum *18*:512, 1975.
262. Gekas, P., and Schuster, M. M. Stercoral perforation of the colon: case report and review of the literature. Gastroenterology *80*:1054, 1981.
263. Culp, W. C. Relief of severe fecal impactions with water soluble contrast enemas. Radiology *115*:9, 1975.
264. Klein, H. C. Fecaloma treated with dioctyl sodium sulfosuccinate. Am. J. Dig. Dis. *2*:37, 1957.
265. Puxty, J. A., and Fox, R. A. Golytely: a new approach to fecal impaction in old age. Age Ageing *15*:182, 1982.
266. Engelberg, M., Nudelman, I., and Korzets, Z. Giant fecaloma with dolichomegasigma. Am. J. Proctol. *33*:9, 1982.
267. Earnest, D. L., and MacGregor, I. L. Therapy for gastrointestinal disease. *In* Conrad, K. A., and Bressler, R. (eds.). Drug Therapy for the Elderly. St. Louis, C. V. Mosby Co., 1982, p. 189.
268. Ogilvie, H. Large-intestine colic due to sympathetic deprivation. Br. Med. J. *2*:671, 1948.
269. Villar, H. V., and Norton, L. W. Massive cecal dilatation: pseudo-obstruction versus cecal volvulus? Am. J. Surg. *137*:170, 1979.
270. Snape, W. J., Jr. Pseudo-obstruction and other obstructive disorders. Clin. Gastroenterol. *11*:593, 1982.
271. Golladay, E. S., and Byrne, W. J. Intestinal pseudo-obstruction. Surg. Gynecol. Obstet. *153*:257, 1981.
272. Nanni, G., Barbini, A., Luchetti, P., Nanni, G., Ronconi, P., and Castagneto, M. Ogilvie's syndrome (acute colonic pseudo-obstruction): review of the literature (October 1948 to March 1980) and report of four additional cases. Dis. Colon Rectum *25*:157, 1982.
273. Vanek, V. W., and Al-Salti, M. Acute pseudo-obstruction of the colon (Ogilvie's syndrome): an analysis of 400 cases. Dis. Colon Rectum *29*:203, 1986.
274. Anuras, S., Shirazi, S. S. Colonic pseudo-obstruction. Am. J. Gastroenterol. *79*:525, 1984.
275. Ravo, B., Pollane, M., and Ger, R. Pseudo-obstruction of the colon following cesarean section: a review. Dis. Colon Rectum *26*:503, 1983.
276. Bode, W. E., Beart, R. W., Jr., Spencer, R. J., Culp, C. E., Wolff, B. G., and Taylor, B. M. Colonoscopic decompression for acute pseudo-obstruction of the colon (Ogilvie's syndrome): report of 22 cases and review of the literature. Am. J. Surg. *147*:243, 1984.
277. Clayman, R. V., Reddy, P., and Nivatvongs, S. Acute pseudo-

obstruction of the colon: a serious consequence of urologic surgery. J. Urol. *126*:415, 1981.

278. Kozarek, R. A., Earnest, D. L., Silverstein, M. E., and Smith, R. G. Air pressure–induced colon injury during diagnostic colonoscopy. Gastroenterology *78*:51, 1980.
279. Lowman, R. M., and Davis, L. An evaluation of cecal size in impending perforation of the cecum. Surg. Gynecol. Obstet. *102*:711, 1959.
280. Kukura, J. S., and Dent, T. L. Colonoscopic decompression of massive nonobstructive cecal dilation. Arch. Surg. *112*:512, 1977.
281. Choo, Y. C. Case reports: ileus of the colon with cecal dilatation and perforation. Obstet. Gynecol. *54*:241, 1979.
282. Lopez, M. J., Memula, N., Doss, L. L., and Johnston, W. D. Pseudo-obstruction of the colon during pelvic radiotherapy. Dis. Colon Rectum *24*:201, 1981.
283. Attiyeh, F. F., and Knapper, W. H. Pseudo-obstruction of the colon (Ogilvie's syndrome). Dis. Colon Rectum *23*:106, 1980.
284. Groff, W. Colonoscopic decompression and intubation of the cecum for Ogilvie's syndrome. Dis. Colon Rectum *26*:503, 1983.
285. Nivatvongs, S., Vermeulen, F. D., and Fang, D. T. Colonoscopic decompression of acute pseudo-obstruction of the colon. Ann. Surg. *196*:598, 1982.
286. Spira, I. A., and Wolff, W. I. Gangrene and spontaneous perforation of the cecum as a complication of pseudo-obstruction of the colon: report of three cases and speculation as to etiology. Dis. Colon Rectum *19*:557, 1976.
287. Strodel, W. E., Nostrant, T. T., Eckhauser, F. E., and Dent, T. L. Therapeutic and diagnostic colonoscopy in nonobstructive colonic dilatation. Ann. Surg. *197*:416, 1983.
288. Bernton, E., Myers, R., and Reyna, T. Pseudo-obstruction of the colon. Curr. Surg. *40*:30, 1983.
289. Messmer, J. M., Wolper, J. C., and Loewe, C. J. Endoscopic-assisted tube placement for decompression of acute colonic pseudo-obstruction. Endoscopy *16*:135, 1984.
290. Crass, J. R., Simmons, R. L., Frick, M. P., and Maile, C. W. Percutaneous decompression of the colon using CT guidance in Ogilvie's syndrome. AJR *144*:475, 1985.
291. Ponsky, J. L., and Aszodi, A. Percutaneous endoscopic cecostomy: a new approach to non-obstructive colonic dilatation. Gastrointest. Endosc. *31*:157, 1985.
292. Sloyer, A., Panella, V., Demas, B., Shike, M., Lightdale, C. J., Winawer, S. J., and Kurtz, R. C. Colonic pseudo-obstruction in cancer patients. Gastroenterology *90*:1638, 1986.
293. Riley, L. W., Remis, R. S., Helgerson, S. D., McGee, H. B., Wells, J. G., Davis, B. R., Herbert, R. J., Olcott, E. S., Johnson, L. M., Hargrett, N. T., Blake, P. A., and Cohen, M. L. Hemorrhagic colitis associated with a rare *Escherichia coli* serotype. N. Engl. J. Med. *308*:681, 1983.
294. Pai, C. H., Gordon, R., Sims, H. V., and Bryan, L. E. Sporadic cases of hemorrhagic colitis associated with *Escherichia coli* 0157:H7. Ann. Intern. Med. *101*:738, 1984.
295. Remis, R. S., MacDonald, K. L., Riley, L. W., Puhr, N. D., Wells, J. G., Davis, B. R., Blake, P. A., and Cohen, M. L. Sporadic cases of hemorrhagic colitis associated with *Escherichia coli* 0157:H7. Ann. Intern. Med. *101*:624, 1984.
296. Ratnam, S., and March, S. B. Sporadic occurrence of hemorrhagic colitis associated with *Escherichia coli* 0157:H7 in Newfoundland. Can. Med. Assoc. J. *134*:43, 1986.
297. Ryan, C. A, Tauxe, R. V., Hosek, G. W., Wells, J. G., Stoesz, P. A., McFadden, H. W., Jr., Smith, P. W., Wright, G. F., and Blake, P. A. *Escherichia coli* 0157:H7 diarrhea in a nursing home: clinical, epidemiological and pathological findings. J. Infect. Dis. *154*:631, 1986.
298. Neill, M. A., Agosti, J., and Rosen, H. Hemorrhagic colitis with *Escherichia coli* 0157:H7 preceding adult hemolytic uremic syndrome. Arch. Intern. Med. *145*:2215, 1985.
299. Karch, H., Heesemann, J., Laufs, R., O'Brien, A. D., Tackett, C. O., and Levine, M. M. A plasmid of enterohemorrhagic *Escherichia coli* 0157:H7 is required for expression of a new fimbrial antigen and for adhesion to epithelial cells. Infect. Immun. *55*:455, 1987.
300. O'Brien, A. D., Newland, J. W., Miller, S. F., Holmes, R. K., Smith, H. W., and Formal, S. B. Shiga-like toxin-converting phages from *Escherichia coli* strains that cause hemorrhagic colitis or infantile diarrhea. Science *226*:694, 1984.
301. March, S. B., and Ratnam, S. Sorbitol–MacConkey medium for detection of *Escherichia coli* 0157:H7 associated with hemorrhagic colitis. J. Clin. Microbiol. *23*:869, 1986.
302. Karmali, M. A., Petric, M., Lim, C., Fleming, P. C., Arbus, G. S., and Lior, H. The association between idiopathic hemolytic uremic syndrome and infection by verotoxin-producing *Escherichia coli*. J. Infect. Dis. *151*:775, 1985.
303. Brandborg, L. L., Rubin, C. E., and Quinton, W. E. A multipurpose instrument for suction biopsy of the esophagus, stomach, small bowel and colon. Gastroenterology *37*:1, 1959.
304. Flick, A. L., Quinton, W. E., and Rubin, C. E. A peroral hydraulic biopsy tube for multiple sampling of any level of the gastrointestinal tract. Gastroenterology *40*:120, 1961.
305. Wadas, D. D., and Sanowski, R. A. Complications of the "hot biopsy" forceps (HBF) technique: is too hot or too long too dangerous? Gastrointest. Endosc. *32*:180, 1986.
306. Pera, D. R., Weinstein, W. M., and Rubin, C. E. Small intestinal biopsy. Hum. Pathol. *6*:157, 1975.
307. Surawicz, C. M., Meisel, J. L., Ylvisaker, T., Saunders, D. R., and Rubin, C. E. Rectal biopsy in the diagnosis of Crohn's disease: value of multiple biopsies and serial sectioning. Gastroenterology *81*:66, 1981.
308. Blundell, C. R., and Earnest, D. L. A caution concerning conservative management of colonic polyps containing invasive carcinoma. Gastrointest. Endosc. *26*:54, 1980.
309. Whitehead, R. Mucosal Biopsy of the Gastrointestinal Tract. 3rd ed. Philadelphia, W. B. Saunders Co., 1985.
310. Goldman, H., and Antonioli, D. A. Mucosal biopsy of the rectum, colon and distal ileum. Hum. Pathol. *13*:981, 1982.
311. Shamshuddin, A. M., Phelps, P. C., and Trump, B. F. Human large intestinal epithelium: light microscopy, histochemistry and ultrastructure. Hum. Pathol. *13*:790, 1982.
312. Weinstein, W. M., and Hill, T. A. Gastrointestinal mucosal biopsy. *In* Berk, J. E. (ed.). Bockus Gastroenterology. 4th ed. Philadelphia, W. B. Saunders Co., 1985, p. 626.
313. Dickinson, R. J., Gilmoer, H. M., and McClelland, B. B. L. Rectal biopsy in patients presenting to an infectious disease unit with diarrheal disease. Gut *20*:141, 1979.
314. Sparberg, M., Fennessy, J., and Kirsner, J. B. Ulcerative proctitis and mild ulcerative colitis. A study of 220 patients. Medicine *45*:391, 1966.
315. Anand, B. S., Malhotra, V., Bhattacharya, S. K., Datta, P., Datta, D., Sen, D., Bhattacharya, M. K., Mukherjee, P. P., and Pal, S. C. Rectal histology in acute bacillary dysentery. Gastroenterology *90*:654, 1986.
316. Dobbins, W. O., III. Dysplasia and malignancy in inflammatory bowel disease. Ann. Rev. Med. *35*:33, 1984.
317. Kotler, D. P., Weaver, S. C., and Terzakis, J. A. Ultrastructural features of epithelial cell degeneration in rectal crypts of patients with AIDS. Am. J. Surg. Pathol. *10*:531, 1986.
318. Spingarn, C. L., Edelman, M. H., Gold, T., Yarnis, H., and Turell, R. Value of rectal biopsies in the diagnosis and treatment of *Schistosoma mansoni* infection. N. Engl. J. Med. *256*:290, 1957.
319. Juniper, R., Stelle, V. W., and Chester, C. L. Rectal biopsy in the diagnosis of amebic colitis. South. Med. J. *51*:545, 1958.
320. Blum, A., and Sohar, E. The diagnosis of amyloidosis. Lancet *1*:721, 1962.
321. Yamada, M., Hatekeyama, S., and Tsukagoshi, H. Gastrointestinal amyloid in AL (primary or myeloma)–associated and AA (secondary) amyloidosis and diagnostic value of gastric biopsy. Hum. Pathol. *16*:1206, 1985.
322. Dobbins, W. O., III, and Bill, A. H. Diagnosis of Hirschsprung's disease excluded by rectal suction biopsy. N. Engl. J. Med. *272*:990, 1965.
323. Parkins, R. A., Eidelman, S., Rubin, C. E., Dobbins, W. O., III, and Phelps, P. C. The diagnosis of cystic fibrosis by rectal suction biopsy. Lancet *2*:851, 1963.
324. Gear, E. V., and Dobbins, W. O., III: Rectal biopsy. A review of its diagnostic usefulness. Gastroenterology *55*:522, 1968.
325. Britt, E. M., and Berry, C. L. Value of rectal biopsy in paediatric neurology: report of 165 biopsies. Br. Med. J. *2*:400, 1967.
326. Bodian, M., and Lake, B. O. The rectal approach to neuropathology. Br. J. Surg. *50*:702, 1963.

VI

THE BILIARY TRACT: ANATOMY, PHYSIOLOGY, AND DISEASE

85

Embryology and Anatomy

M. MICHAEL THALER

The common origin of the liver, biliary tract, duodenum, and pancreas from the primitive foregut determines their intimate relationships in the fully differentiated state. Atretic anomalies of the bile ducts occur relatively often, are manifested after birth, and are usually lethal unless correction can be achieved by surgical anastomosis or replacement of the liver.

The hepatic diverticulum, an outcropping of the primitive foregut capped by a cluster of differentiating liver cells (hepatoblasts), appears between the third and fourth weeks of gestation near the yolk stalk (Fig. 85–1*A*). This is the primordium of the liver, bile ducts, gallbladder, and primitive ventral pancreas.[1, 2] At five weeks, three distinct buds can be recognized on the original diverticulum: the large cranial bud gives rise to the liver, the caudal bud becomes the gallbladder, and the small basal segment develops into the ventral pancreas (Fig. 85–1*B* and *C*). Hepatoblasts forming the cranial bud invade the septum transversum and differentiate into cords of liver cells and biliary epithelium. Hepatic sinusoids arise from the interlacing of liver cords with remnants of the umbilical and vitelline veins in the septum. Kupffer cells, fibrous supporting cells, and hemopoietic elements originate from the mesenchymal tissue of the septum.

Canaliculi appear initially in the six-week embryo as small ridges lined with microvilli on the surface of adjoining hepatoblasts.[2, 3] These primitive channels expand into ductules, coursing between hepatoblasts clustered at the fibrous limiting plate supporting the terminal branches of the portal vein (Fig. 85–2). Ductules (cholangioles; ducts of Herring) enlarge with the network of epithelium-lined bile ducts which travel with the interlobular tributaries of the portal vein (Fig. 85–3). The interlobular bile ducts represent the final diversions of the left and right lobar ducts. The coordination between the intrahepatic biliary passages and the network of portal vein branches is lost in the hilar region where the main lobar ducts continue outside the liver as the corresponding hepatic ducts, merging into the common hepatic bile duct. The common bile duct arises at the junction of the common hepatic bile duct and the cystic duct. The length and course of the cystic duct, and its site of anastomosis with the hepatic duct, are extremely variable.

The caudal bud transforms into the gallbladder, which elongates to form the cystic duct at five to six weeks' gestation (Fig. 85–1*D*). Initially, the gallbladder and the hepatic ducts are hollow structures, but proliferation of the epithelial lining temporarily converts them into solid cords. Recanalization occurs by vacuolization of the epithelial cells. The common bile duct reacquires a lumen during the seventh week, followed by the cystic duct, which expands at its distal end to form the definitive gallbladder.

The gallbladder is a distensible sac measuring 3 by 1.5 inches, with a normal capacity of 30 to 50 ml, positioned between the right and left hepatic lobes. The absorptive surface of the gallbladder mucosa is augmented by numerous prominent folds (Fig. 85–4) and by columnar mucosal cells (Fig. 85–5) which carpet the submucosal, muscularis, and serosal layers. The wall of the gallbladder is invested with sheets of smooth muscle arranged in an interlocking pattern of longitudinal and spiral fibers.

The extrahepatic biliary passages and the gallbladder form a dynamic, hormonally regulated apparatus for controlled delivery of bile from the liver to the digestive tract (Fig. 85–6). The common bile duct is approximately 3 inches long. The duct runs distally along the right edge of the lesser omentum, behind the duodenum, between the pancreas and the inferior vena cava, terminating as an intramural structure (papilla of Vater) on the left side of the duodenum, where it unites with the major pancreatic duct (Fig. 85–7). The intrapapillary segment of the common duct has been called the ampulla of Vater. The sphincter of Oddi is a complex of smooth muscle fibers that invests the intraduodenal portion of the common bile duct, the pancreatic duct in 80 per cent of individuals, and the ampulla. The sphincter regulates bile secretion into the intestine, inhibits entry of bile into the pancreatic duct, and prevents reflux of intestinal contents into the ducts. The common bile duct and the hepatic ducts are invested with smooth muscle fibers whose role in biliary dynamics is uncertain.

Fetuses begin to produce bile after the first trimester. Fetal bile is secreted into the intestine at minimal rates, coloring the meconium.[4] At birth, the bile acid pool is less than half its relative size in adults, and is continuously recycled enterohepatically to maintain the critical micellar concentration of bile acids required for efficient absorption of milk fat and lipid-soluble vitamins.[5] The clearance of bile acids from plasma is also delayed, especially in premature infants, resulting in a marked tendency toward cholestasis in early infancy. For these reasons, parenchymal disease or biliary malformations which interfere with hepatic uptake and

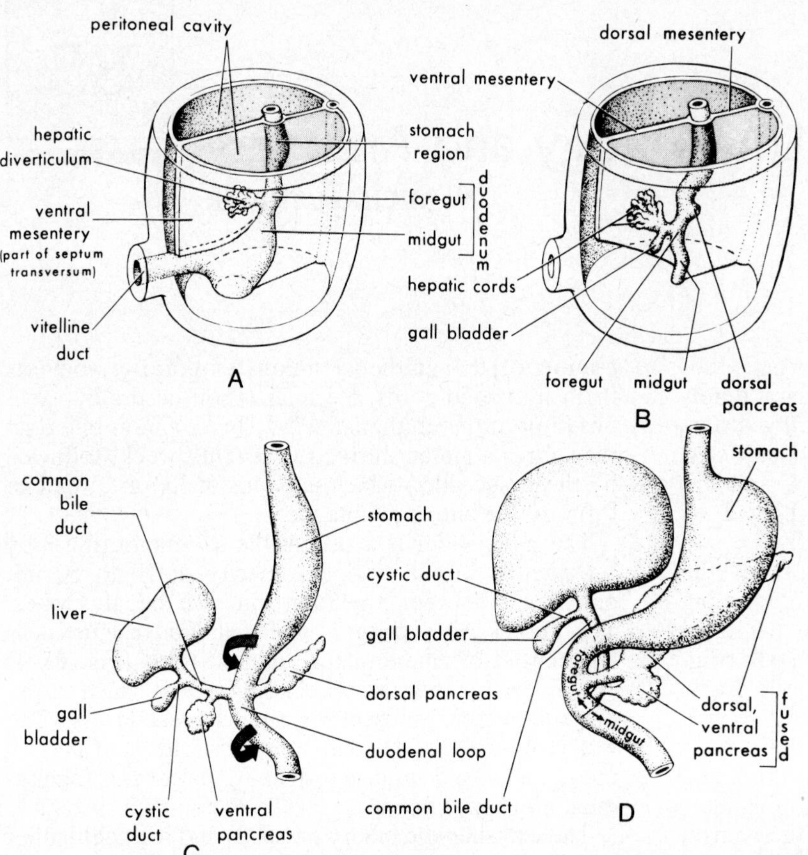

Figure 85–1. Stages in the embryologic development of the liver, gallbladder, extrahepatic bile ducts, pancreas, and duodenum. *A,* four weeks; *B,* and *C,* five weeks; *D,* six weeks. (From Moore, K. L., The Developing Human. Philadelphia, W. B. Saunders Co., 1973.)

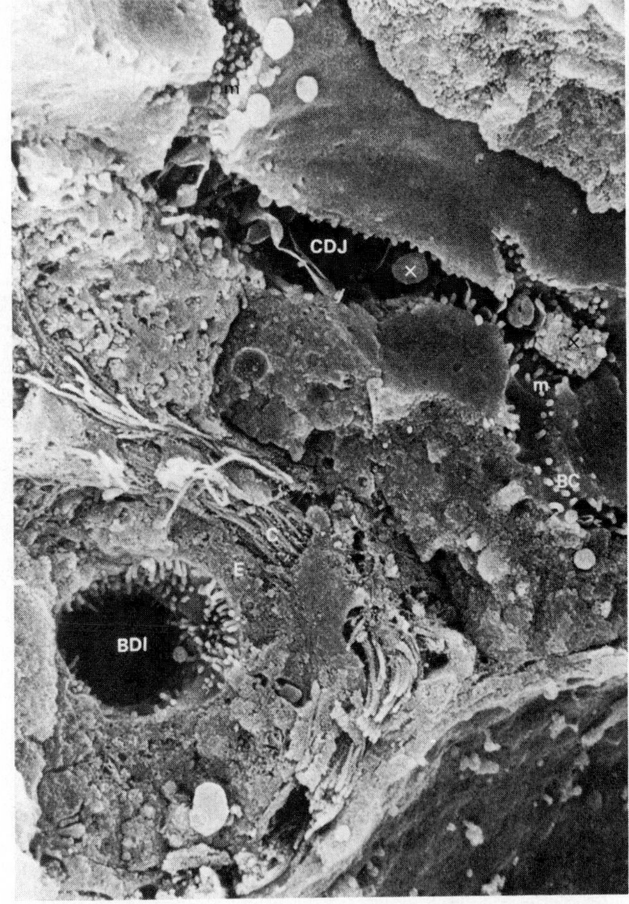

Figure 85–2. Scanning electron micrograph of a periportal zone illustrating relationships among hepatocytes, bile canaliculi, ductules, and interlobular bile ducts. BC, Bile canaliculus coursing between hepatocytes; CDJ, canaliculo-ductular junction; BDI, interlobular bile duct; E, biliary epithelial cell; C, supportive connective tissue; m, canalicular microvilli; X, amorphous material in the canaliculo-ductular junction (× 10,000). (From Motta, P., Muto, M., and Fujita, T. The Liver. An Atlas of Scanning Electron Microscopy. Tokyo, Igaku-Shoin, 1978.)

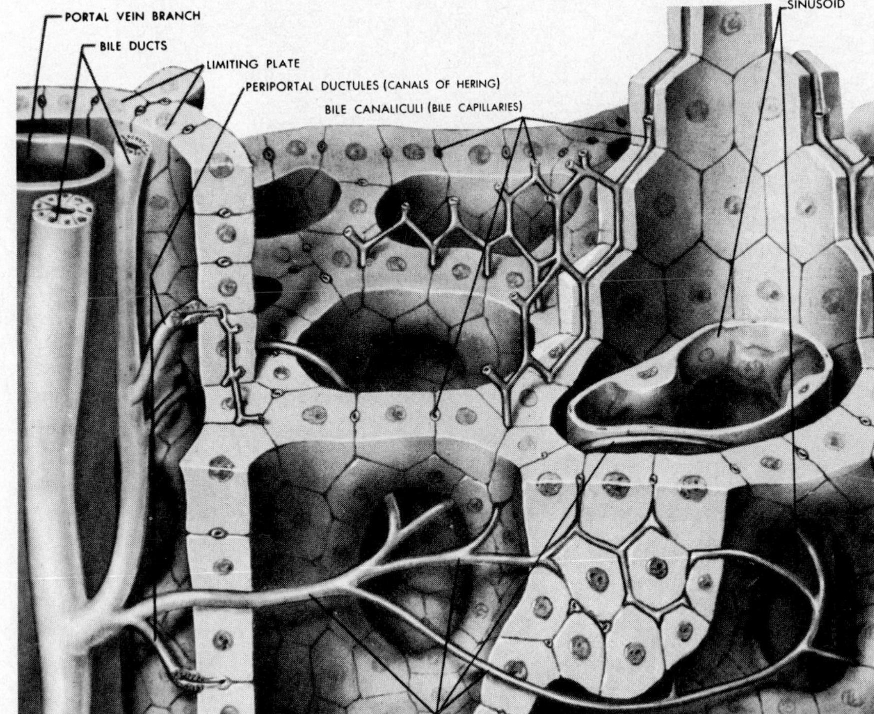

Figure 85–3. Three-dimensional schema of the intrahepatic biliary system. (After Hans Elias. Courtesy of the Ciba Pharmaceutical Company.)

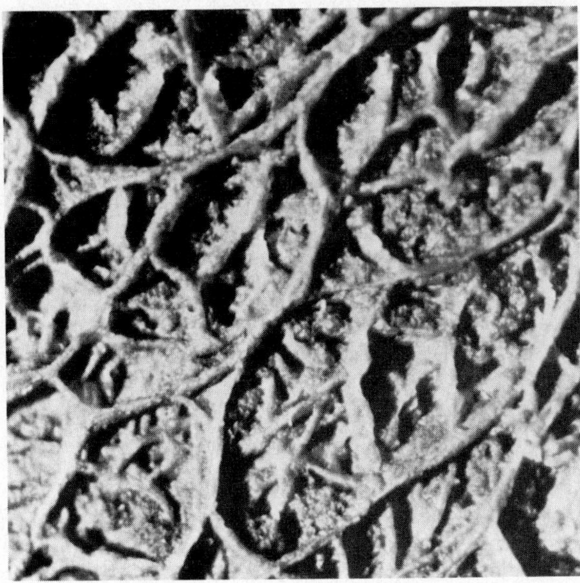

Figure 85–4. Gross appearance of the internal gallbladder surface, demonstrating extensive folds and ridges. (From Elias, H. Die Gallenwege. Boehringer, Ingelheim, 1970.)

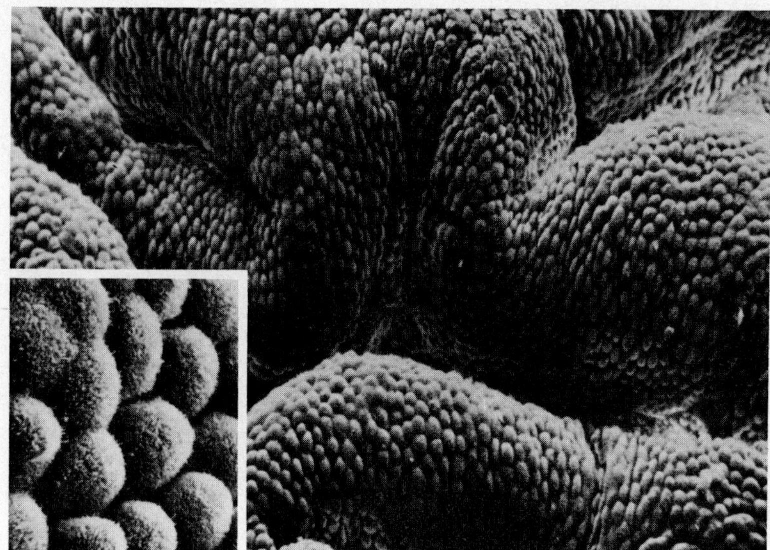

Figure 85–5. Scanning electron micrograph of gallbladder mucosa, showing bulging cell surfaces (× 520). Inset is a higher magnification of individual cell surfaces covered with microvilli (× 3200). (Courtesy of John Mueller, M.D., and Albert L. Jones, M.D., University of California, San Francisco.)

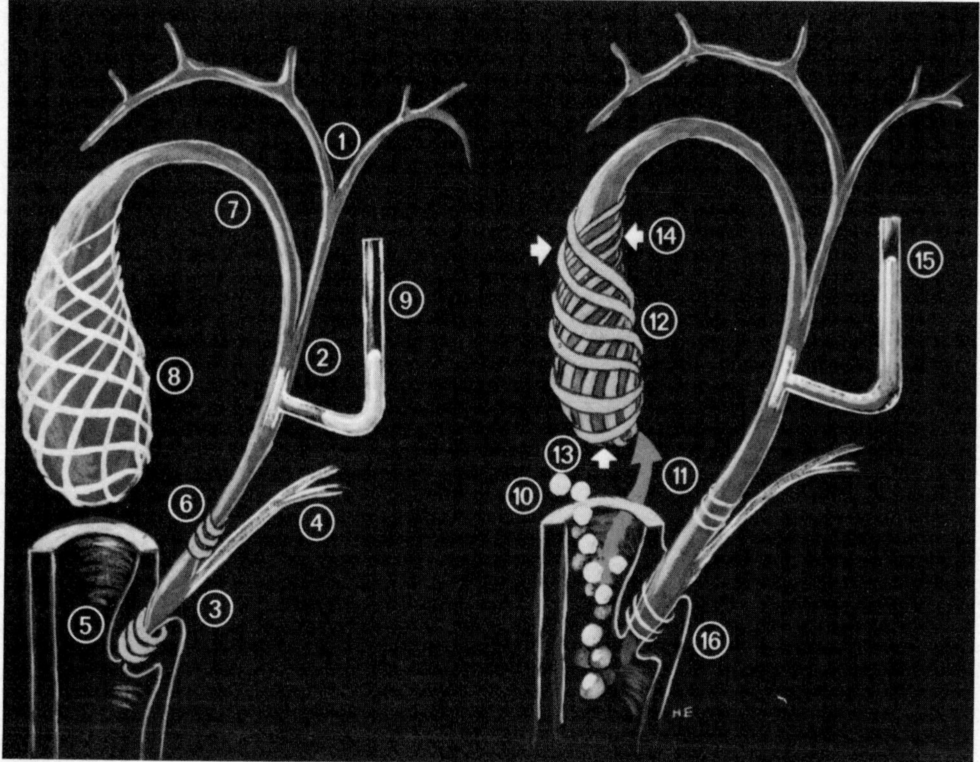

Figure 85–6. The extrahepatic biliary apparatus. Bile formed in the liver flows through the hepatic duct (1) into the common bile duct (2). Bile is mixed in the papilla of Vater (3) with pancreatic juice delivered by the pancreatic duct (4). When the intraduodenal (5) and/or the choledochal (6) arms of the sphincter of Oddi are closed, bile is routed through the cystic duct (7) into the gallbladder (8). The sphincter of Oddi (5 and 6) is closed when the bile pressure is low (9). Entry of fat or amino acids (10) in the upper duodenum triggers release of cholecystokinin (11), causing the gallbladder musculature (12) to contract. As a result, the fundus (13) is raised and the body of the gallbladder is constricted (14). The pressure in the entire system increases (15), the sphincter of Oddi opens (16), and bile enters the duodenum. (From Elias, H., Pauly, J. E., and Burns, E. R. Histology and Human Microanatomy. 4th Ed. New York, John Wiley & Sons, 1978.)

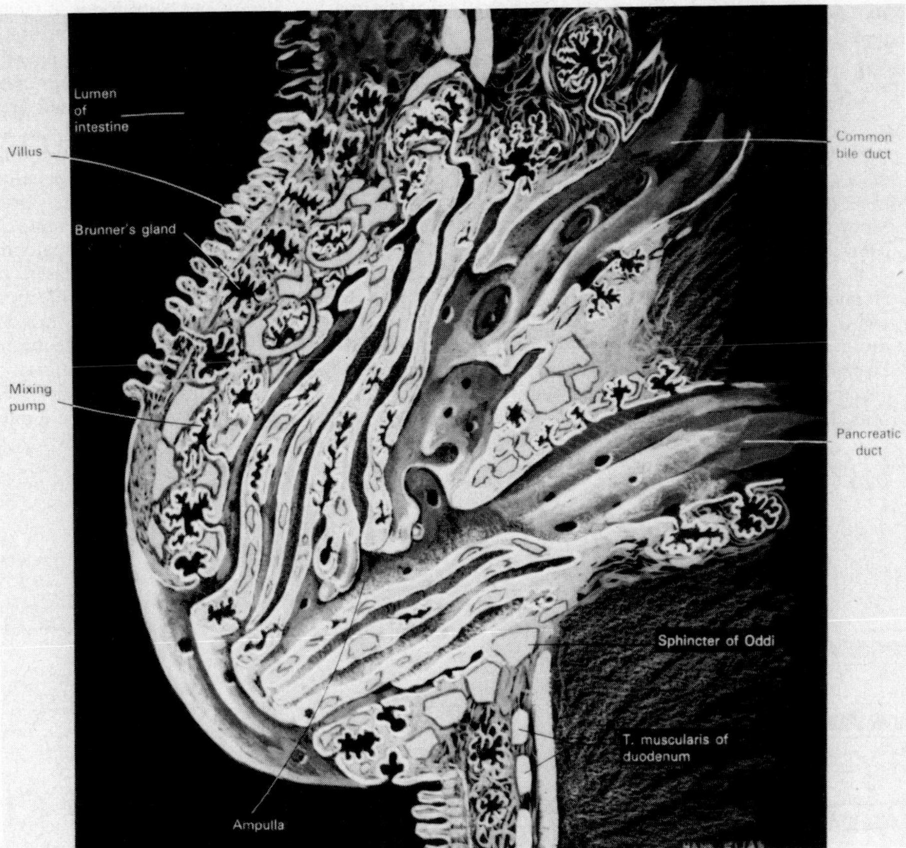

Figure 85–7. Detailed reconstruction of the papilla of Vater, showing junction of the common bile duct and the pancreatic duct in the ampulla and their investment by the smooth muscle of the spincter of Oddi. (From Elias, H. Die Gallenwege. Boehringer, Ingelheim, 1970.)

transport of bile acids in early infancy are usually associated with severe inhibition or cessation of bile flow.

NEONATAL BILIARY ABNORMALITIES

Information about the structural and functional development of the biliary apparatus in humans is helpful in clarifying morphologic defects involving bile ducts and their clinical manifestations in early infancy. Unfortunately, the processes which interfere with organogenesis remain obscure. Biliary malformations do not follow recognizable patterns of genetic inheritance and are not observed in stillborn or aborted fetuses, even in cases with obvious dysmorphisms of other organs, yet they constitute the main cause of persistent cholestasis in infants.[6] Atresia of the extrahepatic bile ducts alone is responsible for approximately half of all patients with infantile cholestasis. Other biliary malformations include intrahepatic bile duct hypoplasia, paucity of interlobular bile ducts, choledochal cyst, congenital hepatic fibrosis, congenital dilatation of the lobar intrahepatic bile ducts (Caroli's disease), and polycystic liver disease.

The lack of genetic or developmental evidence explaining the evolution of biliary malformations leaves room for the possibility that the spectrum of parenchymal and biliary lesions encountered in early infancy may be caused by pathogenic factors such as viruses, drugs or toxins transmitted by the mother. These agents may interfere with recanalization of the main biliary passages during embryonic development; acquired later in gestation or after birth, the same pathogens may induce cholangitis or neonatal hepatitis. Newborns with subsequently confirmed atretic bile ducts occasionally remain free of jaundice and their stools often contain pigment for several weeks prior to the appearance of cholestatic manifestations. In such cases, the postnatal evolution of intrahepatic bile duct hypoplasia or complete sclerosis of the extrahepatic bile ducts can be documented with serial liver biopsies, showing early pericholangitis and gradual development of biliary excretory deficiency.[7, 8] These clinicopathologic observations suggest that certain instances of extrahepatic biliary atresia and many (perhaps most) hypoplastic lesions of the interlobular bile ducts represent sequelae of infectious or inflammatory (immunogenic?) processes.

Recent reports have implicated reovirus type 3 in the pathogenesis of extrahepatic biliary atresia and neonatal hepatitis.[9] Prevalence of reovirus 3–specific serum antibodies was reported initially in infants with biliary atresia and, subsequently, in those with neonatal hepatitis.[10] These observations were not confirmed in similar studies by others.[11] A definitive resolution of this intriguing possibility awaits direct demonstration of virus or virus-specific antigens in tissues removed from infants with biliary atresia at hepatoportoenterostomy or liver transplantation, or in liver biopsy specimens from infants with various liver disorders.

References

1. Moore, K. L. The Developing Human. Clinically Oriented Embryology. Philadelphia, W. B. Saunders Co., 1973.
2. Williams, P. L., Wendell-Smith, C. P., and Treadgold, S. Basic Human Embryology. 2nd ed. Philadelphia, J. B. Lippincott Co., 1969.
3. Motta, P., Muto, M., and Fujita, T. The Liver. An Atlas of Scanning Electron Microscopy. Tokyo, Igaku-Shoin, 1978.
4. Thaler, M. M. Liver function and maturation in the neonatal period. *In* Leventhal, E. (ed.): Textbook of Gastroenterology and Nutrition in Infancy. Vol. I. Gastrointestinal Development and Perinatal Nutrition. New York, Raven Press, 1981.
5. Watkins, J. B., and Perman, J. A. Bile acid metabolism in infants and children. Clin. Gastroenterol. *6*:201, 1977.
6. Silverman, A., and Roy, C. C. Pediatric Clinical Gastroenterology. 3rd ed. St. Louis, C. V. Mosby Co., 1983.
7. Thaler, M. M. Cryptogenic liver disease in young infants. *In* Popper, H., and Schaffner, F. (eds.): Progress in Liver Diseases. Vol. 5. New York, Grune & Stratton, 1976, pp. 476–493.
8. Kahn, E. I., Daum, F., Markowitz, J., et al. Arteriohepatic dysplasia. II. Hepatobiliary morphology. Histology *3*:77, 1983.
9. Morecki, R., Glaser, J. H., Cho, S., et al. Biliary atresia and reovirus type 3 infection. N. Engl. J. Med. *307*:481, 1982.
10. Glaser, J. H., Morescki, R., and Balistreri, W. F. Does liver injury predispose to infection with reo 3 virus? Hepatology *3*:877, 1983 (abstract).
11. Dussoix, E., Hadchouel, M., Tandieu, M., et al. Biliary atresia and reovirus type 3 infection. N. Engl. J. Med. *310*:658, 1984.

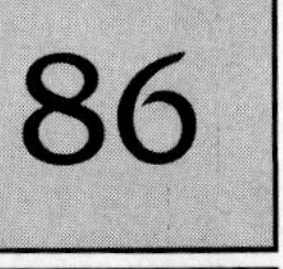

86 Biliary Disease in Infancy and Childhood

M. MICHAEL THALER

DIAGNOSTIC EVALUATION OF BILIARY DISEASE IN INFANTS AND CHILDREN

Biliary malformations, inherited metabolic defects, certain infections, and idiopathic parenchymal disorders (e.g., "giant cell" hepatitis) present with cholestatic jaundice in early infancy. The uniformly nonspecific clinical and biochemical manifestations of these heterogeneous disorders dictate an empirical approach to diagnosis. The scheme outlined in Figure 86–1 separates the causes of conjugated hyperbilirubinemia in infants into relatively uncommon yet clearly identifiable disorders and the more frequently encountered cryptogenic cholestatic "syndromes." The latter are operationally subdivided into *intrahepatic* (parenchymal or ductile) and *extrahepatic* (ductile) categories.

The clinically detectable causes of infantile cholestatic liver disease include heritable metabolic conditions such as alpha$_1$-antitrypsin deficiency, galactosemia, tyrosinosis and cystic fibrosis, and hepatitides due to perinatal infections with cytomegalovirus, hepatitis B virus, herpesvirus, and *Treponema pallidum*. These conditions account for fewer than 20 per cent of all infants with persistent cholestasis. In the order listed, the metabolic disorders can be identified using measurements of serum alpha$_1$-antitrypsin and Pi phenotyping, urinary and plasma amino acid screens, urinary galactose measurements, red blood cell UDP-galactose transferase assays, and sweat chloride determinations. The congenital or postnatal infections may be diagnosed with appropriate viral cultures and antigen or antibody assays.

Approximately 80 per cent of infants with cholestatic jaundice remain undiagnosed after the metabolic and infectious entities are ruled out. This large group includes, in nearly equal proportion, cases of idiopathic intrahepatic cholestasis due to neonatal hepatitis or intrahepatic biliary hypoplasia, and obstructive lesions of the major extrahepatic biliary passages. As previously indicated, most infants with idiopathic or cryptogenic liver disease present with severe cholestasis.[1, 2] Standard liver function tests are nondiscriminatory, except in intrahepatic biliary disease, which often manifests relatively marked elevations in serum alkaline phosphatase, serum cholesterol, and triglycerides, a pattern resembling that observed in primary biliary cirrhosis.[3, 4] The presence of bile in stools provides useful evidence against biliary atresia, except in the slowly evolving cases described in the preceding chapter. Continuity of bile flow from the liver to the intestine may also be demonstrable by visual inspection of duodenal secretions for yellow pigment (bilirubin).

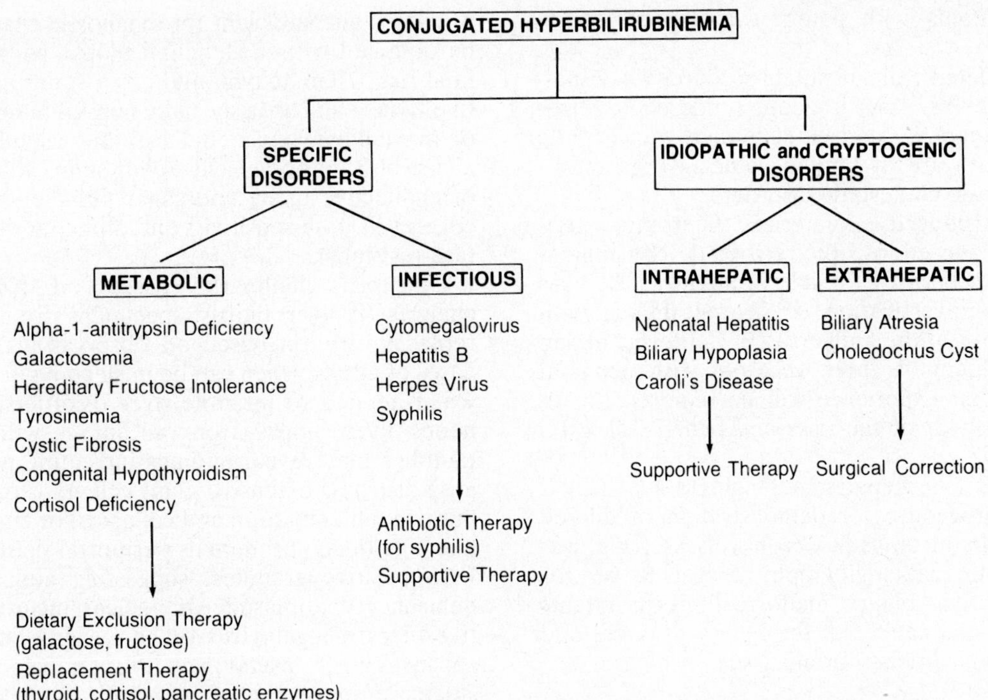

Figure 86–1. Differential diagnosis of conjugated hyperbilirubinemia in young infants. The idiopathic and cryptogenic disorders listed in the right column occur in eight of ten infants with cholestatic jaundice.

Aspiration of duodenal juice for this purpose is routinely performed in Japan[5] and has been described in the American literature.[6] A simpler procedure utilizing an impregnable string introduced into the upper duodenum has been recently reported.[7]

The jaundiced infant with acholic stools represents a difficult diagnostic challenge. Until recently, such babies were invariably subjected to exploratory laparotomy in an effort to delineate the extrahepatic biliary tree. Percutaneous liver biopsies, echography, and radionuclide scanning in young infants are now diagnostic tools with which the distinction between intrahepatic and extrahepatic disease can be established in almost every instance of infantile cholestasis without recourse to exploratory surgery.

Ultrasonic scans are particularly useful in visualization of choledochal cysts or grossly dilated bile ducts. High intensity nuclear imaging with N-substituted iminodiacetates (IDA) labeled with technetium-99m detects bile flow even in the presence of severe cholestasis, but the exact nature of the underlying lesion (i.e., parenchymal disease, intrahepatic biliary hypoplasia, or extrahepatic biliary atresia) is generally not identified. The presence of radioactive label in the subhepatic region rules out extrahepatic biliary atresia, whereas absence of radioactivity from the abdominal region is consistent with severe cholestasis of either intrahepatic or extrahepatic origin (Fig. 86–2). Pretreatment with phenobarbital to stimulate bile flow enhances the probability that radiolabeled bile will be detected in the

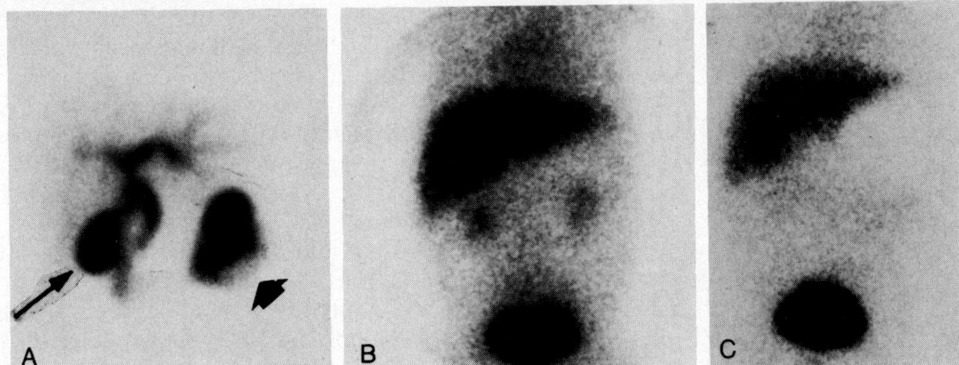

Figure 86–2. High intensity scintigrams employing ^{99}Tc-labeled HIDA for visualization of the extrahepatic biliary passages. *A,* Neonatal hepatitis. The major intrahepatic bile ducts and the entire extrahepatic biliary tree are clearly visualized. The gallbladder *(thin arrow)* and upper intestine *(thick arrow)* contain most of the label at 45 minutes after injection of radioactive imminodiacetate derivative. *B,* Extrahepatic biliary atresia. The liver, kidneys, and urinary bladder are clearly labeled, but biliary structures and intestinal region are not visualized at 45 minutes after injection of radioactive label. *C,* Extrahepatic biliary atresia. The same patient four hours after injection of label. No visualization of biliary structures or intestinal region. (Courtesy of R. S. Hattner, M.D., Nuclear Medicine Division, University of California, San Francisco.)

intestine of infants with patent extrahepatic biliary passages.[8]

The most effective diagnostic procedures for visualization of the biliary tract in adults (endoscopic retrograde cholangiography and percutaneous transhepatic cholangiography) are of limited value in the investigation of infantile cholestatic disorders.

Recently introduced miniaturized fiberoptic endoscopes have made endoscopic retrograde cholangiography (ERC) technically feasible in infants. ERC was helpful in the investigation of several infants with severe cholestasis at the University of California in San Francisco, including a three-week-old with neonatal hepatitis. Further experience will be required for an accurate assessment of the risks and benefits of ERC in early infancy.

Percutaneous transhepatic cholangiography (TC) is an excellent procedure for demonstration of dilated intrahepatic bile ducts, as in Caroli's disease (Fig. 86–3). Transhepatic cholangiography is not useful for detection of other biliary malformations in infants owing to the small caliber of the biliary passages and constriction by cicatricial fibrous tissue.

Liver Biopsy

The percutaneous liver biopsy is a valuable diagnostic tool in infants with persistent cholestasis.[9, 10] A core of liver tissue sufficient for diagnostic examination can be obtained with a Menghini biopsy needle with minimal risk. Hematoxylin and eosin stains and a connective tissue stain are especially helpful in outlining areas of maximal involvement. Another useful stain is the alcian blue–periodic acid–Schiff stain, allowing display of connective tissue and sugar polymers, such as glycogen (diastase-sensitive) and alpha$_1$-antitrypsin (diastase-resistant).

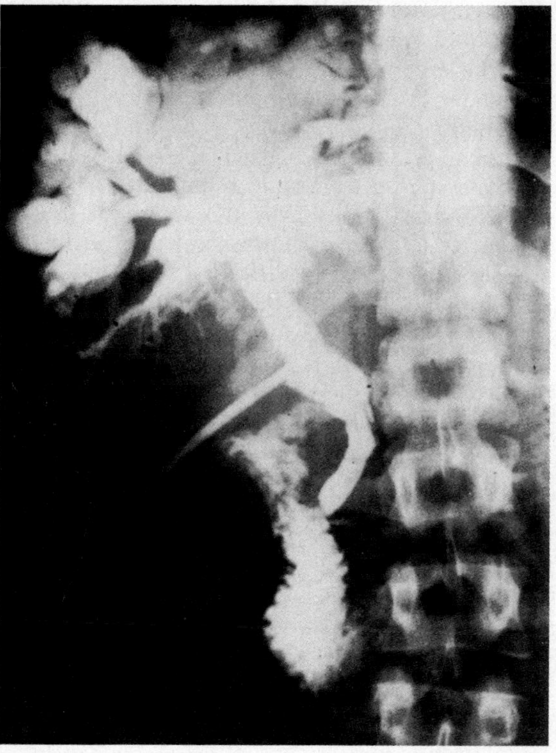

Figure 86–3. Cystic dilatation of the extrahepatic bile ducts (Caroli's disease). Percutaneous transhepatic cholangiogram showing saccular dilatations of intrahepatic bile ducts and enlargement of extrahepatic passages. (From Berk, R. N., Ferrucci, J. T., Jr., and Leopold, G. R. Radiology of the Gallbladder and Bile Ducts. Philadelphia, W. B. Saunders Co., 1983.)

Diagnostic hallmarks based on histopathologic changes in liver biopsy specimens from infants are replacing criteria based on observations in liver diseases of adults which can be misleading or inconclusive when applied to infantile liver disorders. A percutaneous liver biopsy from an infant with cholestatic jaundice may reveal findings indicating neonatal hepatitis, such as extensive giant cell transformation with minimal inflammation and collapsed or empty interlobular bile ducts; prominent periportal diastase-resistant PAS positive granules, suggesting alpha$_1$-antitrypsin deficiency; cytoplasmic or nuclear inclusions, suggestive of cytomegalovirus or herpesvirus infections, respectively; or pseudoglandular transformation and steatosis, suggestive of metabolic disorders (galactosemia, hereditary fructose intolerance, tyrosinosis). Inspection of portal zone structures may reveal hypoplasia, paucity, cystic malformation, or atresia of the interlobular bile ducts or changes characteristic of extrahepatic biliary obstruction, such as prominent portal zones containing proliferating bile ducts and copious peri- and interportal collagen deposits. Perhaps the most useful histologic criterion of the eventual outcome of cholestatic liver disease in early infancy is the presence or absence of significant inflammatory elements surrounding the interlobular bile ducts (pericholangitis). In neonatal hepatitis and intrahepatic biliary hypoplasia, the presence of pericholangitis indicates an evolution toward chronic liver disease due to extensive damage to terminal and interlobular biliary structures. Consequently, resolution of the disease process or progression toward chronic liver disease can be monitored with appropriately timed serial liver biopsies. Finally, intercurrent complications, such as cholangitis following repair of biliary malformations, can be evaluated with microscopic analysis and cultures of tissue obtained by percutaneous liver biopsy.

The combination of percutaneous liver biopsy, echography, and radionuclide scanning permits characterization of the underlying lesion in infantile cholestasis with an accuracy comparable to operative cholangiography.[2, 11] A liver biopsy is necessary in all cases of persistent idiopathic cholestatic liver disease in infants, because nearly complete biliary excretory function fails occasionally in neonatal hepatitis and intrahepatic biliary hypoplasia.[10, 12] In neonatal hepatitis, the "obstructive" phase generally persists for approximately three weeks.[13] During this period, hepatitis cannot be distinguished from extrahepatic biliary atresia by means of functional indices such as radionuclide scans of the abdominal region. Operative cholangiography with surgical exploration of the porta hepatis may also fail to demonstrate patency of threadlike (hypoplastic?) extrahepatic biliary passages when bile flow is completely or nearly completely inhibited.[14] The histologic appearance of tissue obtained by percutaneous liver biopsy correctly identifies extrahepatic and intrahepatic types of cholestasis in 80 to 95 per cent of such severely affected patients.[9]

Operative Cholangiography

Operative cholangiography through a limited incision is indicated in infants in whom the percutaneous liver biopsy and phenobarbital-stimulated radionuclide scan are consistent with extrahepatic biliary obstruction. Demonstration of continuity of the biliary system from the major intrahepatic ducts to the duodenum rules out extrahepatic biliary atresia. When a perioperative cholangiogram cannot be performed owing to a malformed or shrunken gallbladder, the incision is extended and the porta hepatis is carefully explored. Choledochal cysts or bile-containing remnants of the biliary system are anastomosed to the jejunum (Fig. 86–4). If extrahepatic ducts are absent, or only fibrous remnants are found, a hepatic portoenterostomy (Kasai procedure)[15] is performed (Fig. 86–5).

CLINICAL CONDITIONS ASSOCIATED WITH BILIARY MALFORMATIONS

Atresias and Hypoplasias

Extrahepatic Biliary Atresia

With the exception of nonpatency of a single branch of the hepatic duct, or absence of the gallbladder and cystic duct, structural discontinuity of any portion of the extrahepatic biliary duct system results in permanent interruption of bile flow to the intestine. Conjugated hyperbilirubinemia, pale stools, dark urine, and hepatomegaly are noted soon after birth. Splenomegaly develops in most patients.

The diagnosis of extrahepatic biliary obstruction can usually be made with the aid of percutaneous biopsy (Fig. 86–6) and phenobarbital-enhanced radionuclide scans of the abdomen (see Fig. 86–2). Surgical correction by Roux-en-Y choledochojejunostomy or hepatoportoenterostomy is attempted in all cases, but the success rate is well below 50 per cent. Infants with untreated or unsuccessfully repaired extrahepatic biliary malformations eventually develop portal hypertension, ascites, or gastrointestinal hemorrhage. Supportive measures are aimed at prevention of these complications and at maintenance of adequate nutrition. Dietary supplements of medium-chain triglycerides and fat-soluble vitamins (especially K, D, and E) are helpful in counteracting the effects of malabsorption. Low-sodium diets and antidiuretics temporarily retard the progression of ascites. Survival rarely extends beyond two years.

Surgical Repair. The treatment for extrahepatic biliary atresia is anastomosis of a functioning portion of the biliary drainage system to a segment of the upper small intestine. Direct bile duct–to–bowel anastomoses (Roux-en-Y) can be performed in approximately 20 per cent of patients with malformed extrahepatic bile ducts, but bile flow ceases in four of five within one year after surgery.[2, 16] The disparity between attempted and successful repairs of potentially correctable malformations is often attributed to advanced liver damage caused by postponement of the operation beyond two months of age. However, unsatisfactory surgical results may also reflect the intractable perinatal sclerosing process discussed in the preceding chapter. Consistent with the latter possibility is the lack of correlation between the histologic appearance of the liver at the time of attempted surgical repair and age of the patient or long-term outcome of choledochojejunostomy.[17, 18] Hepatocellular damage, as distinct from fibrosis and ductile proliferation, progresses relatively slowly during the first year in infants with biliary atresia, and periportal fibrous tissue and proliferation of pseudoducts begin to regress after restoration of bile flow (Fig. 86–7). Thus, it is likely that advancing sclerosis of both extrahepatic and intrahepatic biliary passages may be responsible for the gradual cessation of bile flow in the majority of infants with potentially correctable types of atresia. Ascending cholangitis may contribute to the failures.

Absence of bile-containing structures in the porta hepatis is noted in the majority of infants with extra-

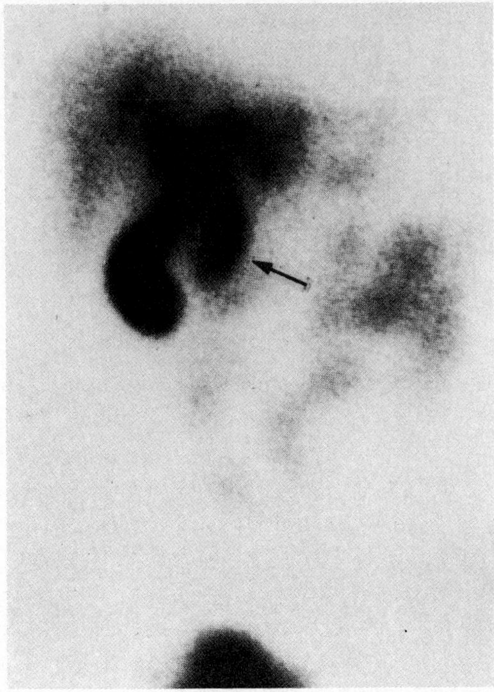

Figure 86–4. High intensity scintigram showing functioning anastomosis between a choledochal cyst *(arrow)* and the jeunum, indicated by the presence of label in the intestinal region.

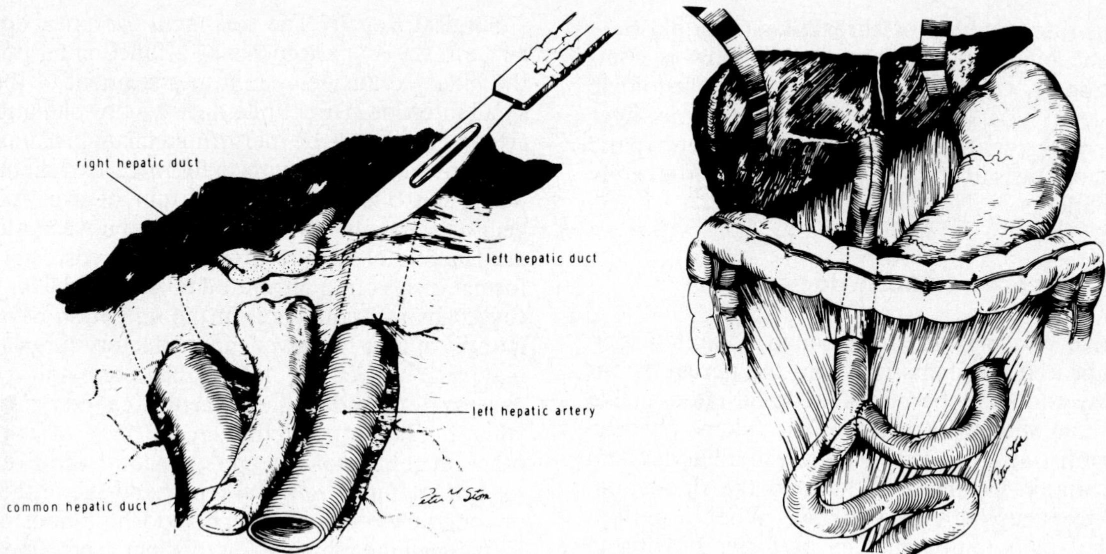

Figure 86–5. Hepatic portoenterostomy (Kasai procedure). *Left panel:* View of the porta hepatis in extrahepatic biliary atresia, showing transsection of solid fibrous cords which have replaced both hepatic bile ducts and the common hepatic duct. *Right panel:* Hepatic portoenterostomy. (From Altman, R. P. Pediatr. Ann. *6*:87, 1977. Used by permission.)

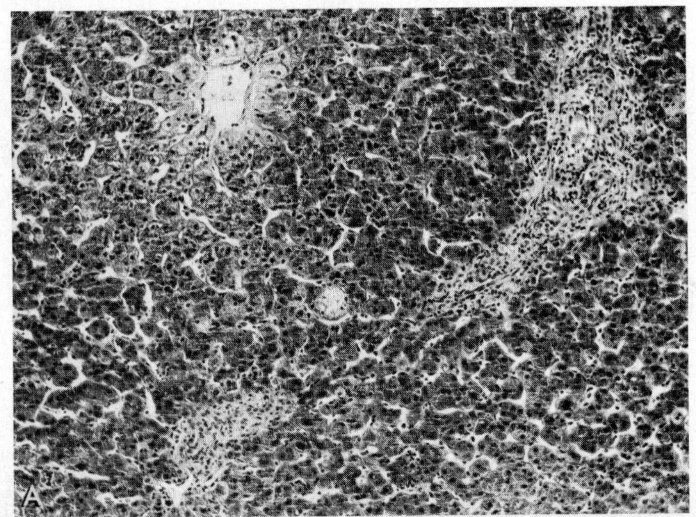

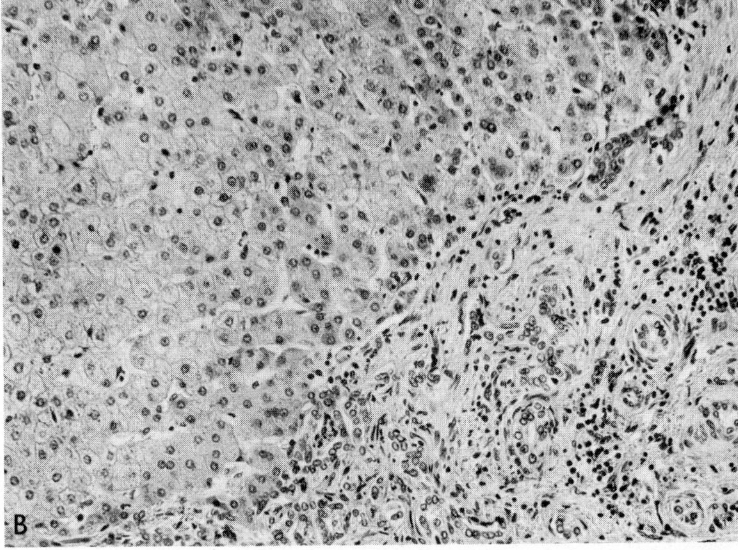

Figure 86–6. Extrahepatic biliary atresia. *A,* Appearance of hepatic parenchyma early in the course. Islands of fibrous tissue are confined to portal areas, in which proliferating interlobular bile ducts are the most prominent feature. The lobular architecture and sinusoid pattern are well preserved. (Masson's trichrome stain, × 180.) *B,* Higher magnification of periportal region (lower right) showing sharply demarcated fibrous tissue, proliferating atypical bile ducts, and inflammatory cells. Occasional parenchymal cells containing inspissated bile. Hepatic cells are otherwise unremarkable. (Hematoxylin and eosin stain, × 250.)

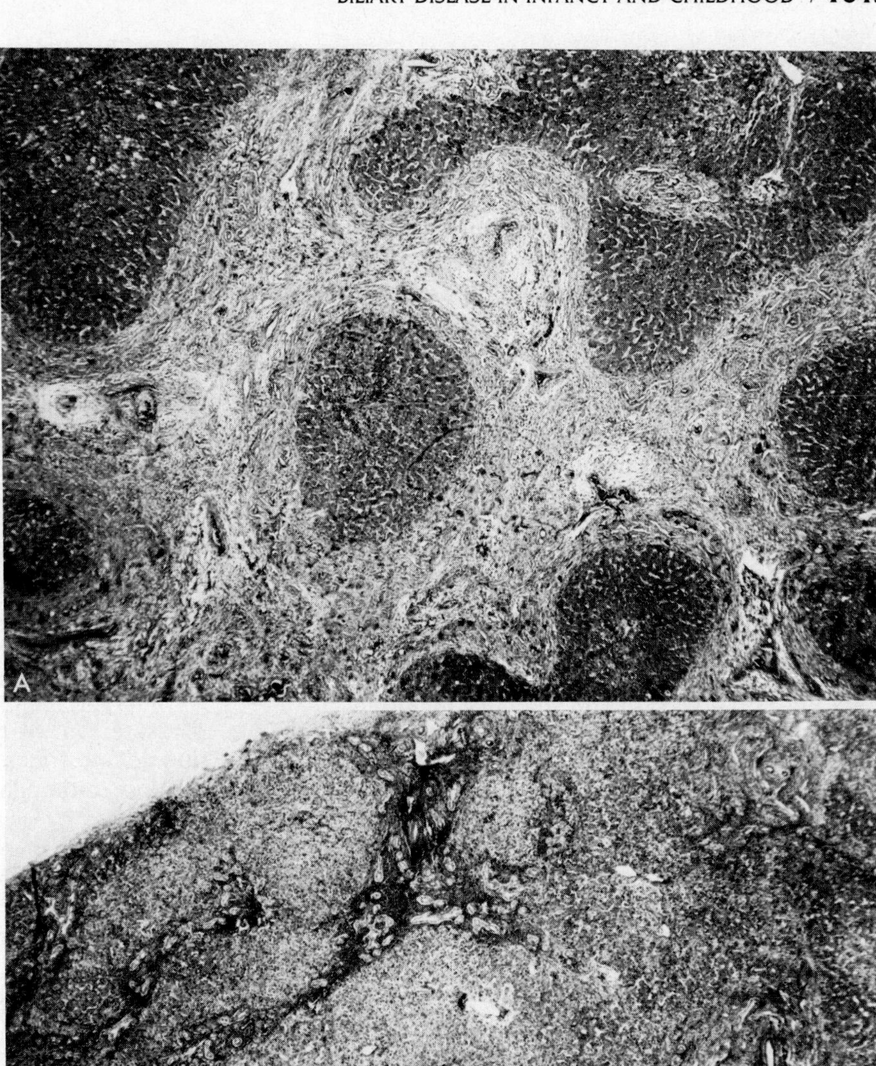

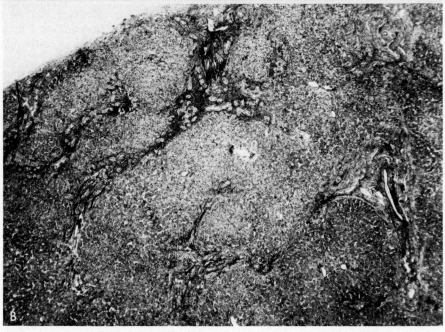

Figure 86–7. Extrahepatic biliary atresia. *A*, Appearance of hepatic parenchyma at two months of age, when a dilated, bile-containing left hepatic duct was anastomosed with the upper small intestine. Broad bands of collagen containing proliferating bile ducts surround islets of viable parenchyma. Note absence of inflammatory cells. (Masson's trichrome stain, × 80.) *B*, Liver biopsy from the same patient at 18 years of age, when a shunting procedure for portal hypertension was performed. A striking decrease in fibrous tissue and excellent preservation of the parenchyma are evident by comparison with *A*. (Masson's trichrome stain, × 80.)

hepatic biliary atresia, eliminating the possibility of a direct bile duct–to–bowel anastomosis. Based on investigations of the most distal intrahepatic portion of the major bile ducts (right and left lobar bile ducts in the quadrate lobe of the liver), Kasai and coworkers[15] suggested that drainage of bile may be achieved in patients with so-called inoperable atresia (i.e., atresia of both hepatic bile ducts) by truncation of the quadrate lobe and anastomosis of the exposed patent ducts to the upper small intestine (Fig. 86–5). Hepatic portoenterostomy temporarily restores bile flow in a majority of infants with sclerosed or absent extrahepatic bile ducts. The eventual outcome is most favorable when the operation is performed by two months of age.[19–21] The requirement for operation under two months of age increases the risk of inadvertent transection of "hypoplastic" but functional structures,[22, 23] especially by inexperienced operators, because operative cholangiography and visual inspection may fail to detect the thin, collapsed, yet patent bile ducts associated with the acute phase of neonatal hepatitis and other hepatocellular cholestatic diseases, such as alpha$_1$-antitrypsin deficiency. Accurate preoperative diagnosis minimizes the possibility of iatrogenic damage to the extrahepatic bile ducts in infants with intrahepatic cholestasis.

As with atresias repaired by choledochojejunostomy, restoration of bile flow by hepatoportoenterostomy results in a remarkable diminution of fibrotic and proliferative changes.[19] Successful outcome of the Kasai procedure correlates with the luminal diameter of biliary structures at the site of transection in the porta hepatis.[24] Because gradual resolution of the critical shutdown phase in parenchymal cholestasis usually begins between two and three months of age,[11, 12] the possibility exists that the cures achieved with this operation in younger infants may reflect cases with transiently or permanently "hypoplastic" bile ducts, whereas operations which fail to establish bile flow may represent those with authentic atretic lesions, in whom the previously mentioned sclerosis of the major intra- and extrahepatic bile ducts progresses to completion. Thus, paradoxically, the Kasai operation, designed specifically for relief of such "inoperable" variants, may achieve its purpose only if executed prior to permanent closure of both major bile ducts at the porta hepatis. Whether early intervention arrests the transformation of inflamed hypoplastic bile ducts into solid fibrous cords is one of the most important unanswered questions concerning the surgical treatment of cholestatic liver disease in early infancy.

The reported five-year survival of patients with biliary atresia corrected by the Kasai operation varies from 20 to 45 per cent.[19–21] The majority develop cholangitis, progress to cirrhosis, portal hypertension, and gastrointestinal hemorrhage and become candidates for liver transplantation. Nevertheless, the results of hepatoportoenterostomy represent an improvement over the absolute mortality rate in unoperated patients.

Intrahepatic Biliary Hypoplasia of the Interlobular Bile Ducts; Paucity of Intrahepatic Bile Ducts

The pathogenesis of these lesions is unclear, but they may represent the intrahepatic locus of the sclerosing process implicated in the pathogenesis of extrahepatic biliary atresia. Certain cases begin with a clinical and histologic picture indistinguishable from idiopathic neonatal hepatitis with pericholangitis. As the disease progresses, the parenchyma reverts to a nearly normal appearance, while the interlobular bile ducts decrease in number until few, or none, are identifiable in liver biopsies (Fig. 86–8). In others, paucity of intrahepatic bile ducts and the absence of pericholangitis may be observed soon after birth. Evidence of parenchymal disease is confined to intracanalicular bile plugs, occasional giant cells, and isolated hepatocytes containing inspissated bile. The unremarkable appearance of parenchyma, coupled with a striking absence of periportal ductular structures, stands in marked contrast to the proliferating ductules and periportal fibrosis of extrahepatic biliary obstruction (compare Figs. 86–7 and 86–8). A third group of cases is characterized by heavy formations of scar tissue in the portal triads, surrounded by "pseudoducts" and inflammatory cells, with constricted terminal branches of the portal vein and hepatic artery, and atretic interlobular bile ducts (Fig. 86–9).

A syndrome known as arteriohepatic dysplasia, or Watson-Alagille syndrome, has been described in infants and children with hepatic ductular hypoplasia, cardiac anomalies (mainly pulmonary artery stenosis), characteristic facies (prominent forehead, mild hypertelorism, micrognathia), anterior vertebral arch defects, and retarded physical development (Fig. 86–10).[25, 26] Multisystem involvement suggests a teratogenic agent acting during the organogenesis phase of fetal development, somewhat analogous to changes produced by rubella virus infection during the first trimester. In most instances, initial liver biopsies reveal a periportal inflammatory process with progressive destruction of the interlobular bile ducts. When the inflammation subsides, the hepatic lobule reveals paucity of intrahepatic bile ducts, often associated with hypoplasia of extrahepatic biliary passages (Fig. 86–11).

The extent of biliary excretory deficiency varies considerably among patients but is seldom complete. Measurement of the 72-hour rose bengal fecal excretion demonstrates greater than 5 per cent excretion of the dose, although excretory failure may also be nearly complete.[12, 27]

Cholestatic jaundice develops during the first month of life in most instances. Characteristic findings are rapidly rising serum cholesterol and triglyceride concentrations and serum alkaline phosphatase values ranging from five to 20 times normal. Xanthomas eventually develop over extensor surfaces, in palmar creases, or embedded in scratch marks, but may extend over larger areas (Fig. 86–12). Generalized arteriosclerotic changes and fatty deposits in the heart, kidneys, and pancreas appear later in the course. A characteristic central nervous system lesion has been described in children with intrahepatic biliary hypoplasia; i.e., areflexia, inability to walk, and weakness of upward gaze. It is associated with vitamin E deficiency due to malabsorption.[28, 29]

Severe pruritus, steatorrhea, and a bleeding tendency are the most common clinical problems encountered in children with intrahepatic biliary atresia. Treatment includes low-fat, high-protein diets, supplemented with medium-chain triglycerides, and fat-soluble vitamins, including vitamins K and E. Cholestyramine feedings usually improve pruritus and may improve the results of liver function tests in cases with partial rather than complete biliary deficiency (hypoplasia versus atresia). Treatment with phenobarbital in daily doses of 5 to 10 mg/kg may eliminate or reduce pruritus, decrease the serum bilirubin concentration, and reduce xanthoma formation in children in whom cholestyramine therapy is relatively unsuccessful.[30] The phenobarbital effect includes enhancement of bile flow, improved biliary excretion of bile salts and bilirubin, and rapid reduction of the extrahepatic bile salt pool.[31] Occasional patients may benefit from concurrent cho-

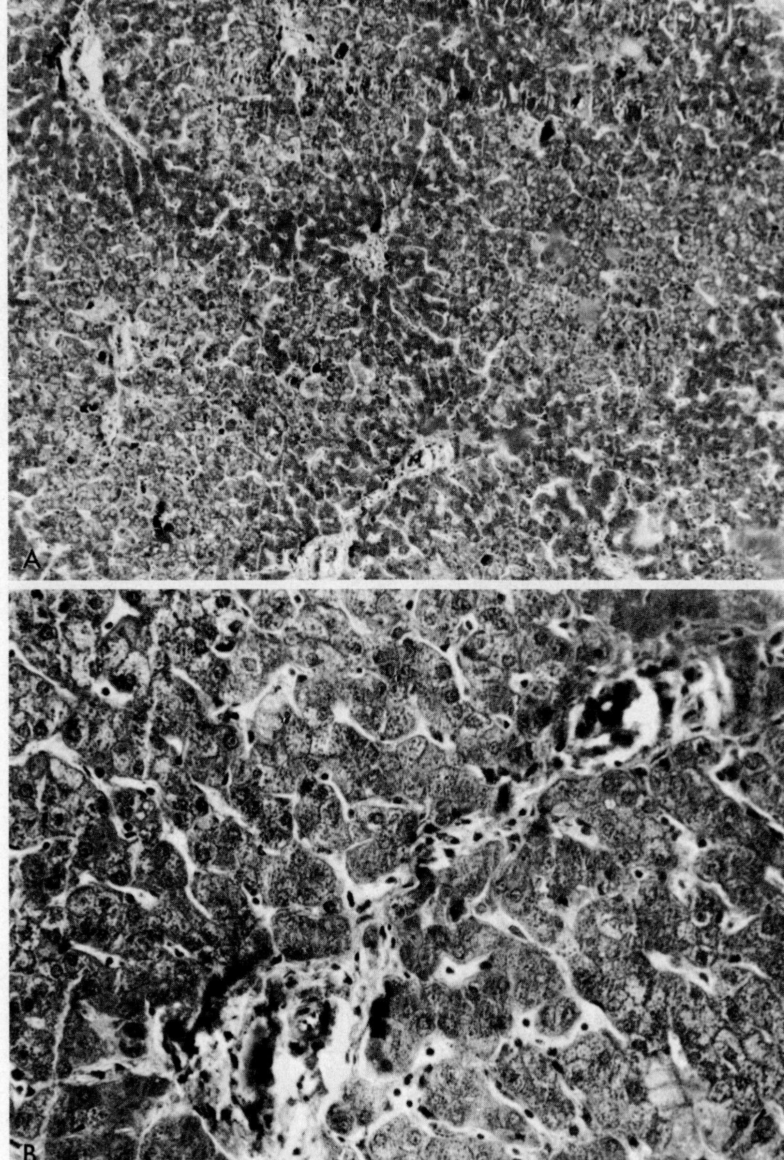

Figure 86–8. Intrahepatic bile duct hypoplasia. *A*, severe canalicular cholestasis and absence of recognizable interlobular bile ducts in portal areas are the most prominent features in liver biopsies. Note absence of fibrous and inflammatory elements. (Masson's trichrome stain, × 80.) *B*, Higher magnification of portal area in lower center of *A*. Branches of hepatic artery and portal vein and dilated lymphatic channels are clearly visible; bile ducts are absent. (× 300.)

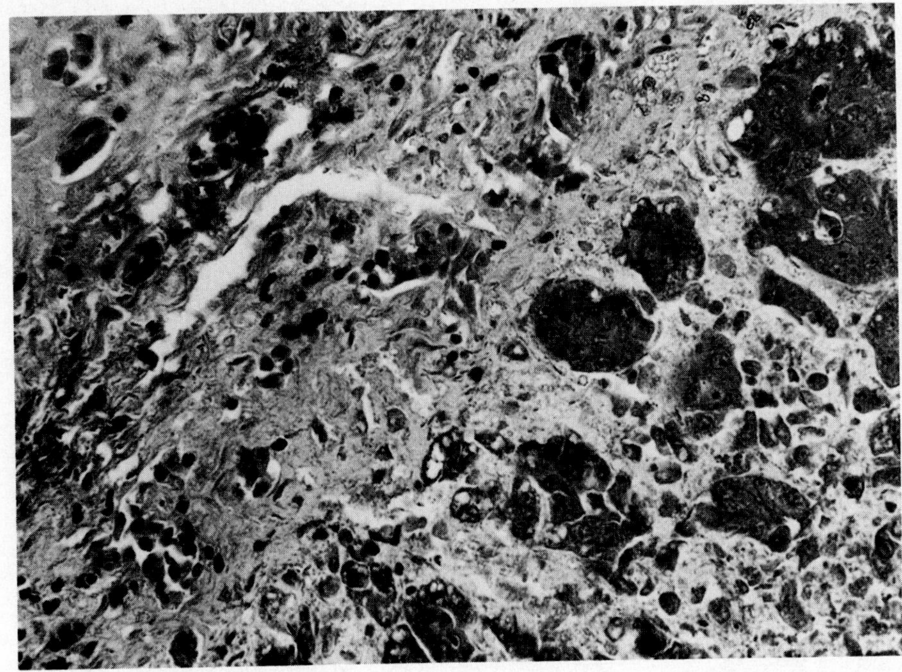

Figure 86–9. Intrahepatic biliary hypoplasia. Extensive scarring of the portal area, with an atretic bile duct surrounded by darkly staining inflammatory cells (upper left corner) and multiple pseudoductile structures containing bile plugs, arranged at the periphery of the portal area (lower right). (Masson's trichrome stain, × 250.)

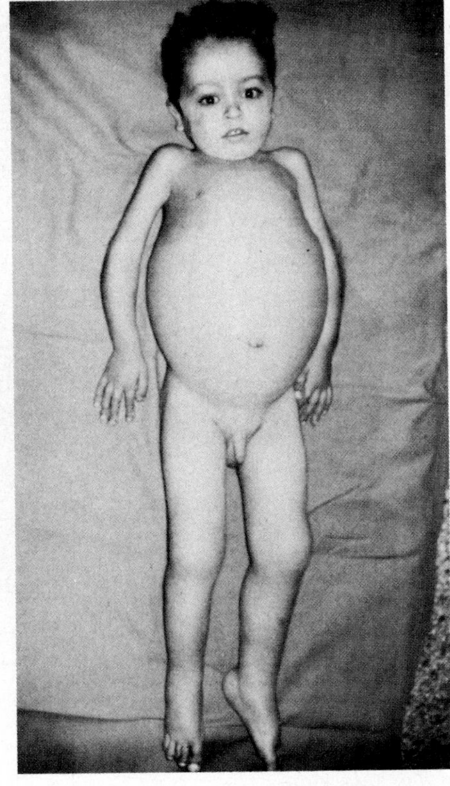

Figure 86–10. Intrahepatic biliary hypoplasia (syndromatic type). A five-year-old boy with characteristic facies (prominent forehead, hypertelor, receding chin). This patient also had pulmonary artery dysplasia and anterior vertebral arch defects. Ascites, clubbing of fingers and toes, and growth retardation indicate an unusually severe form of the syndrome.

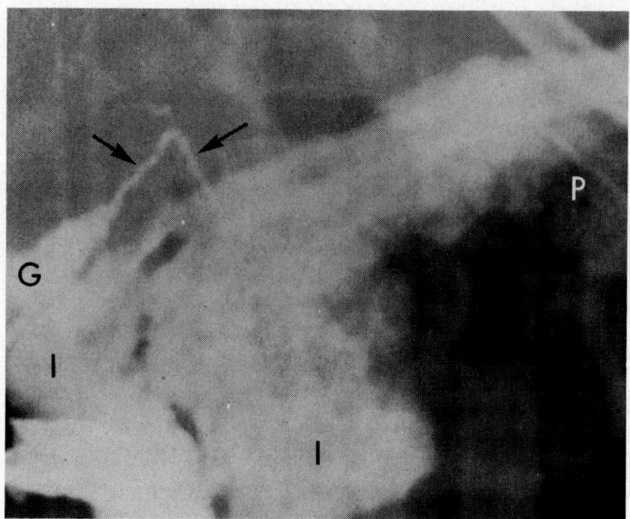

Figure 86–11. Paucity of intrahepatic bile ducts. Operative cholangiogram, showing shrunken gallbladder (G) and hypoplastic extrahepatic bile ducts *(arrows)*. Note opacification of pancreas and pancreatic duct (P) and large collection of dye in the upper intestine (I).

lestyramine and phenobarbital therapy to prevent intestinal reabsorption of biliary components. These measures have improved the well-being of children with intrahepatic biliary atresia, and survival has been prolonged beyond the five to ten years formerly expected. As a result, manifestations due to malabsorption of vitamin E (areflexia, inability to walk, weakness of upward gaze) are increasingly evident in the older children and may require therapy with up to 1000 IU daily orally or intramuscular injections to maintain serum vitamin E levels in the normal range.[29]

Cystic Malformations

As with atresia and hypoplasia, cystic malformations may arise from interference with morphogenetic events in the first trimester or from distortions produced by inflammatory or toxic processes later in gestation or after birth. In either eventuality, bile flow through malformed passages may be sluggish or impeded, causing jaundice, pruritus, cholangitis, gallstone formation, and cirrhosis. Other malformations, characterized by cysts not in direct continuity with the biliary system, may cause minimal or no interference with bile flow. Patients with these malformations remain relatively asymptomatic. A schematic representation of cystic hepatobiliary anomalies, arranged according to predominant clinical pattern (presence or absence of cholestasis, association with renal anomalies, course, and prognosis) is shown in Figure 86–13.

The clinical manifestations of these anomalies depend mainly on their location along the biliary tree: dilatations of the major extrahepatic (choledochal cyst) or intrahepatic (Caroli's disease) bile ducts are associated with bile stasis and progressive liver disease, whereas patchy lesions involving only the terminal interlobular bile ducts (congenital hepatic fibrosis) or noncommunicating parenchymal cysts (polycystic liver disease) produce little disturbance of bile flow. These differences in anatomic distribution and consequent clinical manifestations obscure the possibility that all cystic malformations of the bile ducts may be etiologically related. Thus, an identical insult at different stages in organogenesis or at different loci may result in choledochal cysts, dilatations of the major intrahepatic bile ducts (Caroli's disease), congenital hepatic fibrosis, polycystic liver and kidney disease, or combinations of these anomalies. Each of these malformations has been observed in association with the others, or with cystic anomalies of the kidneys. For example, Caroli's disease, a rare disorder characterized by dilatations of the major branches of the lobar bile ducts, often displays the typical lesions of congenital hepatic fibrosis at the microscopic level and choledochal cysts or dilatations of the extrahepatic bile ducts at the gross level (see Fig. 86–3). Because individual case reports frequently focus on isolated aspects of this spectrum, considerable confusion persists in this area of liver disease.

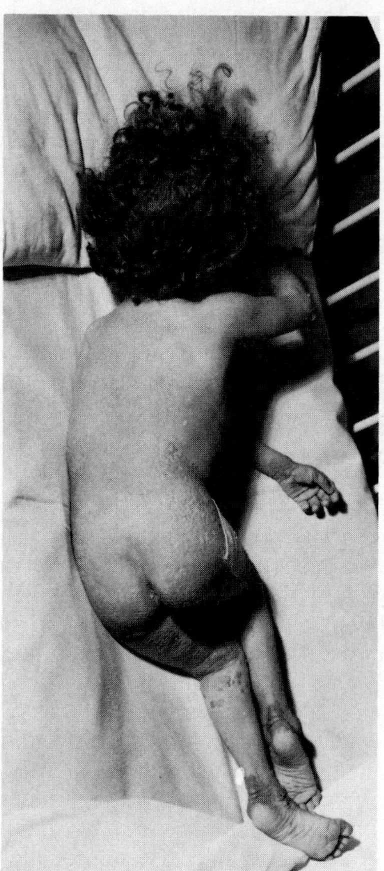

Figure 86–12. Intrahepatic biliary hypoplasia. Extensive xanthomas over the buttocks, knees, ankles, wrists, and elbows of a child with Watson-Alagille syndrome.

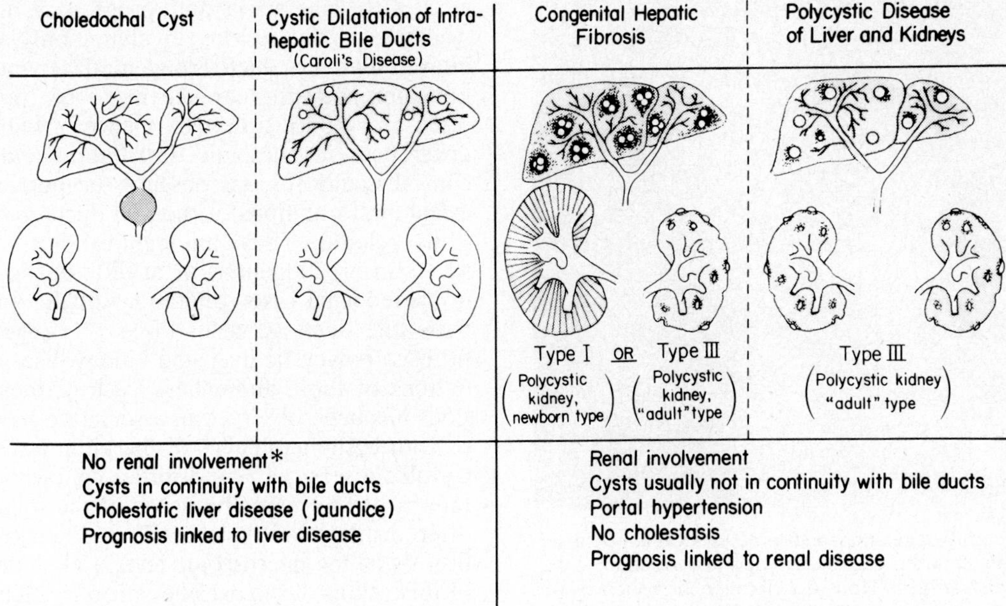

Figure 86–13. Spectrum of cystic lesions involving the bile ducts. Choledochal cysts and cystic dilatations of the major intrahepatic bile ducts (Caroli's disease) are in continuity with the main biliary passages and are not usually associated with renal malformations (the asterisk indicates that renal tubular ectasia has been repeatedly reported in Caroli's disease but is extremely rare in association with choledochal cyst). Patients with these anomalies have chronic liver disease, which determines the prognosis. In contrast, the lesions of congenital hepatic fibrosis and polycystic disease of liver and kidney are not in direct communication with the main biliary passages. They are characterized by heavy deposits of fibrous tissue (more prominent in congenital hepatic fibrosis, denoted by dark stippled areas surrounding small cysts) and by association with cystic renal malformations. Patients with these anomalies usually have well preserved liver functions. Apart from portal hypertension in congenital hepatic fibrosis, prognosis is linked most frequently with renal dysfunction. Polycystic kidneys types I and III are classified according to Potter. Respectively, they represent medullary ("sponge") kidneys and polycystic kidneys of the adult as seen in infants.

Choledochal Cyst

This abnormality of the bile duct wall occurs most frequently as an expansion of the common bile duct (Fig. 86–14). Diverticulum of the common bile duct and choledochocele of the intraduodenal portion of the common duct are relatively rare. Dilatation of the entire intrahepatic and extrahepatic biliary system has been reported in Japanese patients, among whom choledochal cysts occur relatively frequently.[32]

Cholangitis usually develops in infancy or childhood, but it may be delayed for two or three decades. The diagnosis should be suspected in a patient presenting with signs and symptoms consistent with intermittent biliary obstruction and cholangitis. Occasionally, the patient may present with classical acute pancreatitis. Ultrasonography is the procedure of choice for detection of choledochal cysts, especially in infants who rarely manifest the classic triad of jaundice, pain, and abdominal mass. The diagnosis may also become apparent when a liver biopsy shows changes characteristic of extrahepatic biliary obstruction, while stools or duodenal fluid are intermittently pigmented, excluding extrahepatic biliary atresia. The recommended treatment is Roux-en-Y choledochocystojejunostomy with cholecystotomy, or primary excision of the cyst.

Long-term complications in children operated on for choledochal cyst include ascending cholangitis, stricture at the site of anastomosis, residual biliary tract disease, cirrhosis, intestinal obstruction caused by adhesions, and steatorrhea attributed to distal displacement of bile drainage.[33] Patients with choledochal cysts who are not treated surgically suffer from recurrent bouts of cholecystitis and cholelithiasis. Complete excision, if possible, is strongly recommended because unexcised cysts tend to develop cancer during adulthood.

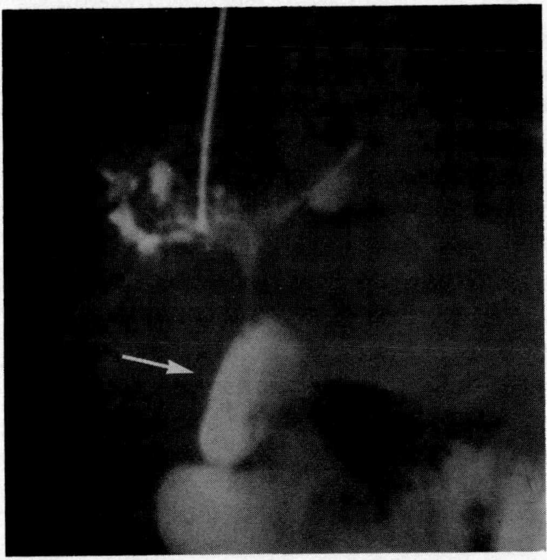

Figure 86–14. Choledochal cyst. Transhepatic cholangiogram in a seven-month-old infant. (Courtesy of H. Goldberg, M.D., Department of Radiology, University of California, San Francisco.)

Cystic Dilatation of the Major Intrahepatic Bile Ducts (Caroli's Disease)

This disease is characterized by "berry-like" cysts lined with normal cuboidal epithelium in continuity with the primary branches of the main intrahepatic bile ducts[34] (Fig. 86–3). Caroli's disease has been associated with cystic disease of the kidneys. Among cystic malformations of the biliary tree, Caroli's disease occupies an intermediate position between choledochal cysts or enlargement of the extrahepatic bile ducts and the microscopic dilatations observed in congenital hepatic fibrosis. It is not surprising, therefore, that the disease has been reported in association with both. Nevertheless, most cases of Caroli's disease are sufficiently distinct in course and treatment to justify separate classification. Cholangitis, cholelithiasis, and liver abscesses are commonly present, caused by bile stasis. Cramping abdominal pain and fever may develop at any time after birth. However, the average age at onset is 22 years. Symptoms subside temporarily after passage of calculi and control of infection, but invariably recur until the anomaly is finally suggested by ultrasonography or computed tomography (Fig. 86–15) and established by percutaneous transhepatic cholangiography or operative cholangiography.[35] A liver biopsy may reveal associated congenital hepatic fibrosis, while intravenous pyelography may (rarely) demonstrate the presence of renal tubular ectasia. Liver function is generally unimpaired, and cirrhosis or portal hypertension does not develop. Temporary palliation can be achieved by surgical removal of stones and relief of biliary obstruction. After cholangitis becomes established, liver abscesses and septicemia contribute to an extremely grave prognosis.

Congenital Hepatic Fibrosis

Congenital hepatic fibrosis is a developmental anomaly characterized by disordered terminal interlobular bile ducts, which form multiple macroscopic and microscopic cysts embedded within wide bands of fibrous tissue[36] (Fig. 86–16*A*). Renal cysts, detectable by ultrasonography, are present in 50 to 75 per cent of patients with congenital hepatic fibrosis.

The origin of these malformations is unknown, but the ultrastructural appearance of the liver in congenital hepatic fibrosis (Fig. 86–16*B*) suggests a disorder in the distribution of connective tissue supporting interlobular bile ducts in the embryonic liver and collecting tubules of the embryonic nephron, resulting in cystic malformations of these hollow structures.[37] The disease is usually discovered in late childhood, when hepatosplenomegaly is noted, or when gastrointestinal bleeding due to portal hypertension supervenes. Thrombocytopenia due to hypersplenism may be severe, while liver function tests are usually normal or modestly disturbed.

In contrast to Caroli's disease, portal hypertension may develop relatively early in congenital hepatic fibrosis and may progress to a fatal termination by bleeding esophageal varices. Rarely, the cystic structures communicate with bile ductules in sufficient numbers to cause interference with bile flow. Such cases are indistinguishable from Caroli's disease.

LIVER TRANSPLANTATION

Liver transplantation has greatly improved the five-year survival rate of children with biliary atresia since the advent of cyclosporin A in 1981.[38] Infants and children presently account for approximately 50 per cent of all recipients of liver implants in the nearly 40 centers operating in the United States and Canada (Fig. 86–17).

The main indications for liver transplantation in the pediatric population, abstracted from current reports, are extrahepatic biliary atresia (44 per cent), inherited metabolic diseases (23 per cent), bile duct hypoplasia (9 per cent), chronic active hepatitis (8 per cent), familial idiopathic cirrhosis (7 per cent), fulminant hepatitis (2 per cent), and miscellaneous disorders (7 per cent).

Long-term survival following orthotopic liver transplantation appears to be more favorable in pediatric patients.[39] Follow-up data from Children's Hospital in Pittsburgh indicate that 75 to 80 per cent of children receiving transplants since 1981 were alive in 1985, compared with approximately 50 per cent of adults (Fig. 86–18). Mortality rate in pediatric recipients appears to be minimal after the first six months, and quality of life is excellent, with a few notable exceptions. Second and third transplants were required in nearly one quarter of all recipients.[40]

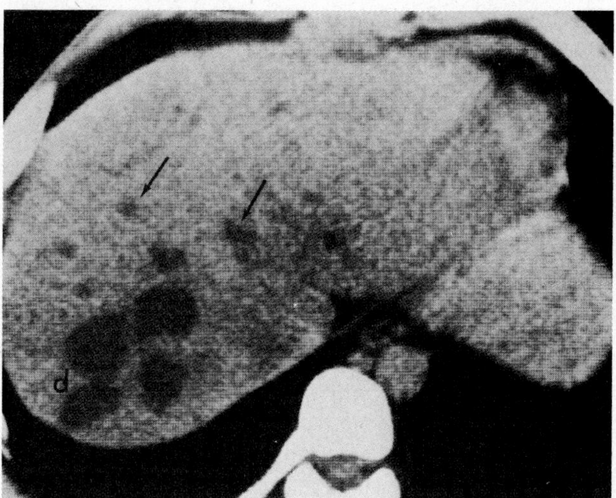

Figure 86–15. Cystic dilatation of the intrahepatic bile ducts (Caroli's disease). Computed tomography reveals large low-density defects in the right hepatic lobe, communicating with smaller branching structures characteristic of dilated bile ducts *(arrows).* (From Berk, R. N., Ferrucci, J. T., Jr., and Leopold, G. R. Radiology of the Gallbladder and Bile Ducts. Philadelphia, W. B. Saunders Co., 1983.)

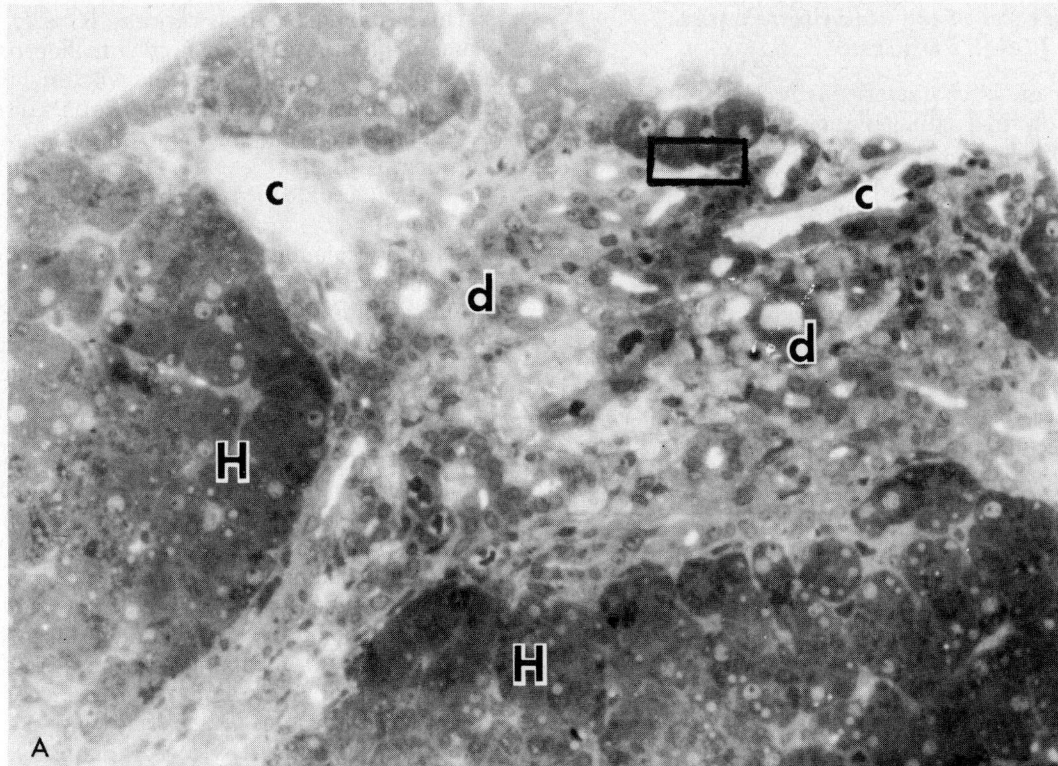

Figure 86–16. Congenital hepatic fibrosis. *A*, Light micrograph of liver tissue embedded in plastic. Normal arrangement and appearance of hepatocytes (H). Proliferating and dilated bile ducts (d), and larger cystic spaces (c) embedded in matrix of fibrous tissue. (× 250.) *B*, Area enclosed in black border in *A* examined with electron microscope, showing arrangement of hepatocyte (H), collagen (C), and ductile cells (B). Hepatocyte displays normal mitochondria, smooth and rough endoplasmic reticulum, and glycogen granules. Bile duct cells contain sparse cytoplasmic structures, and their luminal surfaces are covered by microvilli. Electron-dense "tight" junctions link ductile cells (arrow points to tangenially cut cell junction). (× 14,200.) (From Thaler, M. M., and Ogata, E. S., Goodman, J. R., et al. Am. J. Dis. Child. *126*:374, 1973. Copyright 1973, American Medical Association. Used by permission.)

Illustration continued on opposite page

Causes of post-transplantation mortality and morbidity rates include acute and chronic graft rejection, infection, vascular complications leading to massive hepatic infarction, and cerebrovascular accidents. Transplant recipients are managed with permanent immunosuppression using cyclosporin A and corticosteroids, close monitoring of nutritional status, and avoidance of exposure to communicable diseases.

BILIARY DISEASE IN CHILDHOOD AND ADOLESCENCE

Biliary disease in children is most commonly a continuation of disease processes established in early infancy. Diseases of the biliary system that originate in the pediatric population after the first two years of life are relatively rare. The gallbladder is the usual focus of involvement in such cases.

Acute Cholecystitis

Acute inflammation of the gallbladder in children is usually idiopathic. The common acute viral diseases of childhood, such as gastroenteritis and upper respiratory infections, have been associated with cholecystitis. Rarely, parasitic infestation with *Giardia lamblia* or *Ascaris*, typhoid fever, shigellosis, or streptococcal infections can be documented by means of cultures of bile or fluid recovered from the gallbladder at laparotomy. Gallstones are much less common than in adults with cholecystitis. For example, children represented a bare 0.13 per cent of all instances of cholelithiasis at the Mayo Clinic.[41] A survey of 620 consecutive cholecystectomies performed for calculous cholecystitis included 33 (5.3 per cent) patients under 21; all were females between 16 and 20 years of age, with the exception of one 10-year-old.[42] Gallstones in this group of patients were associated with pregnancy in 84 per cent, suggesting a close relationship between childbearing and calculous cholecystitis in adolescent girls (see p. 1677).

The clinical features of cholecystitis in children are similar to those in adults. Right upper quadrant pain and guarding, nausea, and vomiting occur in most cases. Jaundice develops in approximately one fourth of patients and may suggest the correct diagnosis. Despite this relatively clear-cut clinical picture, the fact that the diagnosis is usually made at exploratory laparotomy probably reflects the rarity of gallbladder disease in children. Operative cholangiography may reveal the presence of gallstones in the common duct or

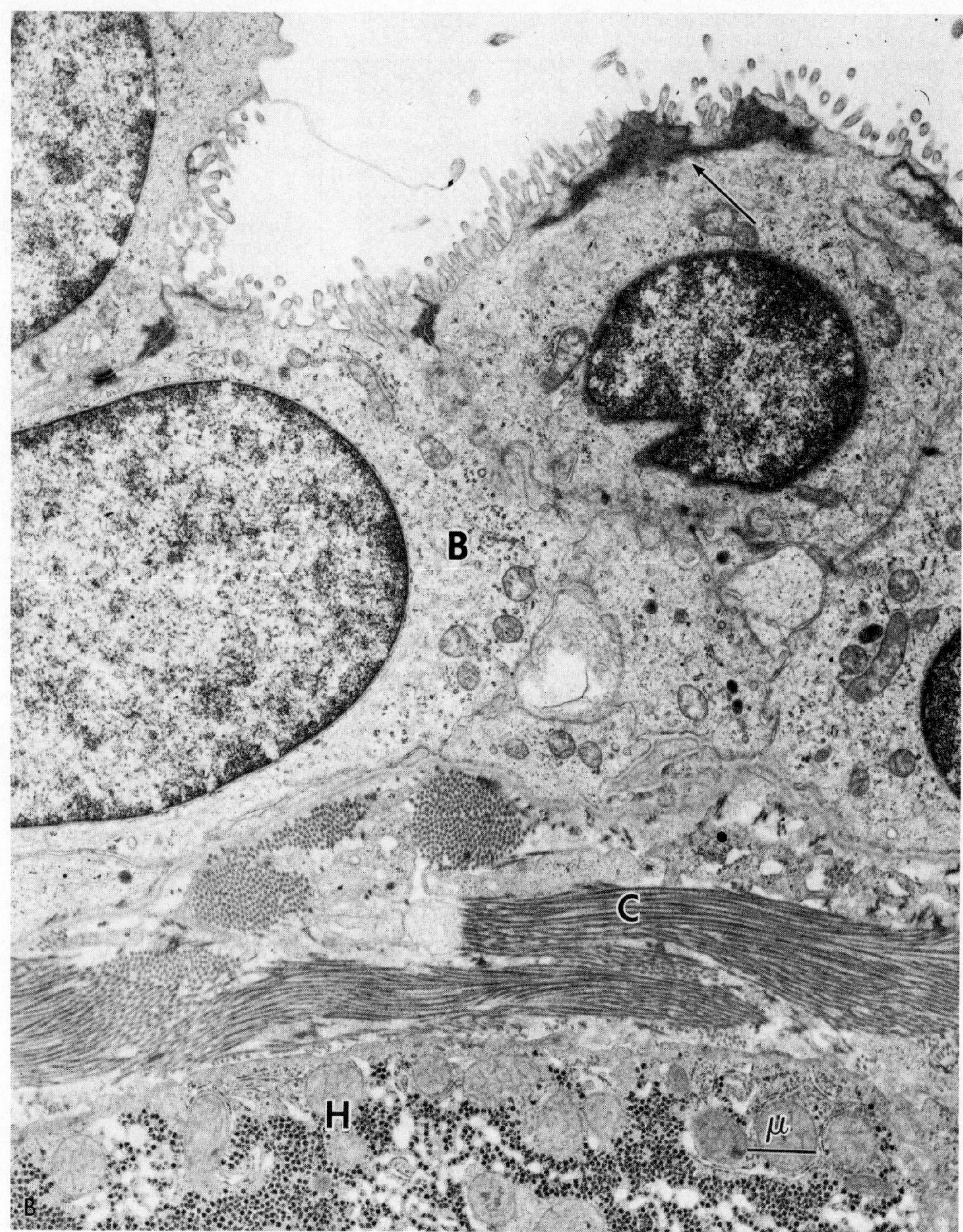

Figure 86–16 *Continued*

gallbladder. Cholecystectomy is generally performed in those with cholelithiasis (see p. 1699).

Cholelithiasis

Cholelithiasis in children is confined to the gallbladder in over 90 per cent of cases. Pigmented and cholesterol stones are found with approximately equal frequency. Pigmented gallstones occur in children with hemolytic diseases, the most common being congenital spherocytosis in Caucasians and sickle cell anemia in blacks. Other hemolytic conditions associated with cholelithiasis include the thalassemias, red blood cell enzymopathies, Wilson's disease, and erythroblastosis fetalis in newborn infants. As for most cases of childhood cholecystitis, the cause of cholecystitis associated with stones is unclear in nearly half of the patients. Obesity and a family history of gallbladder disease are present in a small number.[43] An emerging cause of gallstones in infants is prolonged total parenteral nutrition, especially after extensive ileal resection.[44] Silent stones have also been recently reported in children

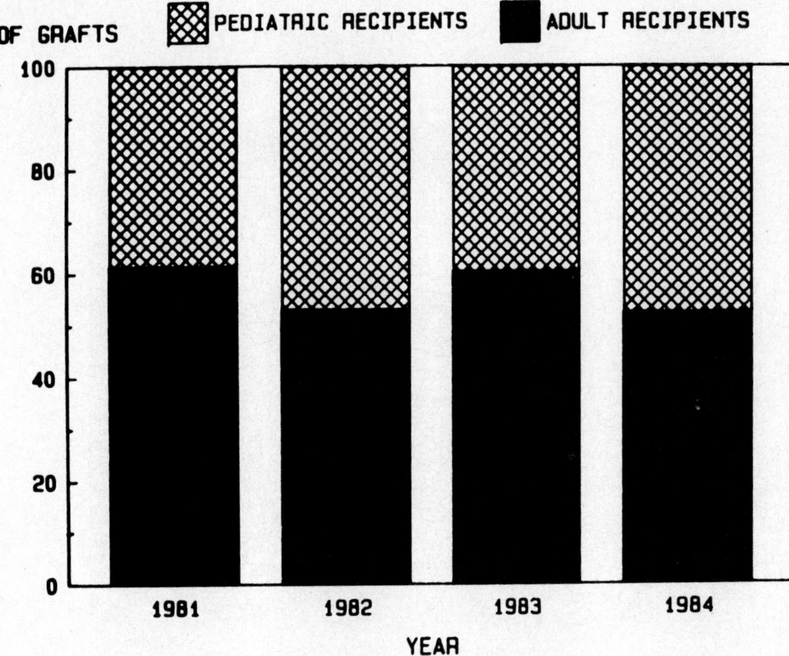

Figure 86–17. Orthotopic liver transplantation. Pediatric recipients at the University of Pittsburgh constituted approximately half of all liver transplant recipients, 1981–1984. (From Starzl, T. E., and Iwatsuki, S., Shaw, E. W., Jr., et al. Semin. Liver Dis. 5:334, 1985. Used by permission.)

with IgA deficiency, suggesting that this immunoglobulin may play a role in protection of the biliary passages.[45] Cholelithiasis may also intervene as a complication of biliary malformations, cystic fibrosis, pancreatitis, portal hypertension, neonatal sepsis, and chronic gastrointestinal infections (see pp. 1668–1714).

Idiopathic cholelithiasis over the age of 10 is noted predominantly in females. Thus, constitutional factors that predispose adult females to biliary disease appear to operate occasionally in childhood. The treatment of cholelithiasis includes measures directed toward the underlying disease and, when indicated, cholecystectomy. Dissolution of gallstones with bile acids or solvents has not been reported in children (see pp. 1678–1680).

Acute Hydrops of the Gallbladder

This idiopathic distention of the gallbladder is independent of obvious obstructive or inflammatory disease. Gallstones are not found. In contrast to cholelithiasis, a predominance of males is apparent among the reported cases, which range in onset from early infancy to adolescence.[46] Noncalculous distention of the gallbladder has been recently recognized as a complication of Kawasaki disease (mucocutaneous lymph node syndrome).[47]

Generalized abdominal tenderness, pain which may be colicky or continuous, and a mass in the right upper quadrant are the typical clinical features. Ultrasonography reveals a massive echo-free gallbladder and

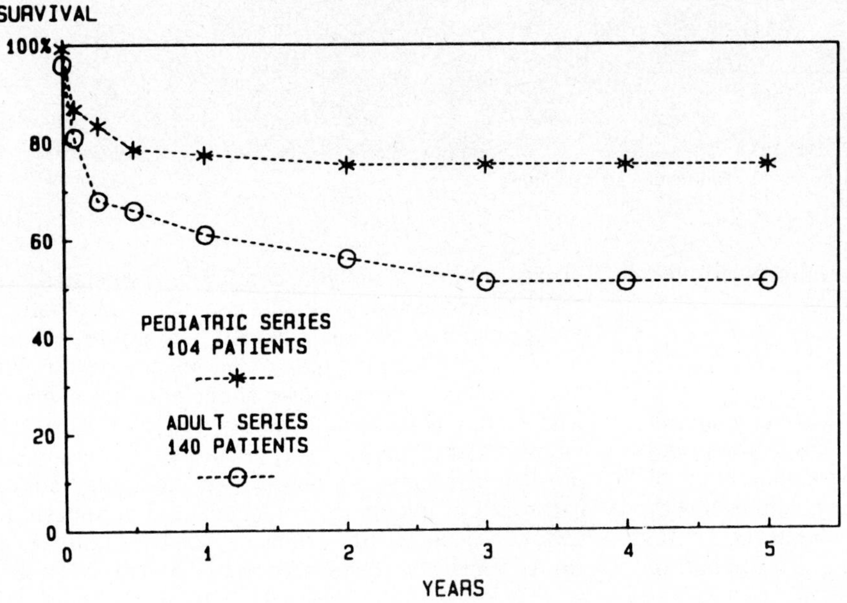

Figure 86–18. Orthotopic liver transplantation. Five-year follow-up experience with liver transplantation at the University of Pittsburgh, 1981–1985. Pediatric recipients have 75 to 80 per cent survival rates, with a minimal mortality rate after the first six postoperative months. In adult recipients, survival declines to approximately 50 per cent during the first three years, with a minimal mortality rate thereafter. (From Starzl, T. E., Iwatski, S., Shaw, E. W., Jr., et al. Semin. Liver Dis. 5:334, 1985. Used by permission.)

normal bile ducts. Surgery reveals an edematous gallbladder and, in most instances, hypertrophied mesenteric lymph nodes. The bile is sterile, and drainage of the gallbladder is usually followed by full recovery. If surgery is avoided, spontaneous resolution of the hydrops is noted within two to five weeks.

References

1. Thaler, M. M., and Gellis, S. S. Studies in neonatal hepatitis and biliary atresia. Am. J. Dis. Child. *116*:280, 1968.
2. Mowat, A. P., Psacharopoulos, H. T., and Williams, R. Extrahepatic biliary atresia versus neonatal hepatitis. Review of 137 prospectively investigated infants. Arch. Dis. Child. *51*:763, 1976.
3. Thaler, M. M. Jaundice in the newborn: Algorithmic diagnosis of conjugated and unconjugated hyperbilirubinemia. JAMA *237*:58, 1977.
4. Silverman, A., and Roy, C. C. Pediatric Clinical Gastroenterology. 3rd Ed. St. Louis, C. V. Mosby Co., 1983.
5. Sakurai, M., and Shiraki, K. Quantitative diagnosis of biliary atresia and neonatal hepatitis. *In* Japanese Medical Research Foundation (ed.): Cholestasis in Infancy. Pathogenesis, Diagnosis and Treatment. Tokyo, Tokyo University Press, 1980, p. 293.
6. Greene, H. L., Herlinek, G. L., Moran, R., and O'Neill, J. A diagnostic approach to prolonged obstructive jaundice by 24-hour collection of duodenal fluid. J. Pediatr. *95*:412, 1979.
7. Rosenthal, P., Liebman, W. P., Sinatra, F. R., et al. String test in the evaluation of cholestatic jaundice in infancy. J. Pediatr. *107*:253, 1985.
8. Majd, M., Reba, R. C., and Altman, R. P. Hepatobiliary scintigraphy with ^{99m}Tc-PIPIDA in the evaluation of neonatal jaundice. Pediatrics *67*:140, 1981.
9. Brough, A. J., and Bernstein, J. Liver biopsy in the diagnosis of infantile obstructive jaundice. Pediatrics *45*:519, 1969.
10. Thaler, M. M. Cryptogenic liver disease in young infants. *In* Popper, H., and Schaffner, F. (eds.): Progress in Liver Diseases. Vol. 5. New York, Grune & Stratton, 1976, pp. 476–493.
11. Kimura, S. The early diagnosis of biliary atresia. Progr. Pediatr. Surg. *6*:91, 1974.
12. Thaler, M. M. Biliary excretory function and excretory patterns in infantile cryptogenic cholestasis. *In* Goresky, C. A., and Fisher, M. M. (eds.): Jaundice. New York, Plenum Press, 1975, pp. 313–324.
13. Thaler, M. M., and Gellis, S. S., II. The effect of diagnostic laparotomy on long-term prognosis of neonatal hepatitis. J. Dis. Child. *116*:262, 1968.
14. Kahn, E. I., Daum, F., Markowitz, J., et al. Arteriohepatic dysplasia. II. Hepatobiliary morphology. Hepatology *3*:77, 1983.
15. Kasai, M., Kimura, S., Asukura, Y., et al. Surgical treatment of biliary atresia. J. Pediatr. Surg. *3*:665, 1968.
16. Danks, D. M., Campbell, P. E., Clarke, A. M., Jones, P. G., and Solomon, J. R. Extrahepatic biliary atresia. The frequency of potentially operable cases. Am. J. Dis. Child. *128*:684, 1974.
17. Krovetz, L. J. Congenital biliary atresia. II. Analysis of the therapeutic problem. Surgery *47*:468, 1960.
18. Thaler, M. M., and Gellis, S. S., III. Progression and regression of cirrhosis in biliary atresia. Am. J. Dis. Child. *116*:271, 1968.
19. Kasai, M., Watanabe, I., and Ohi, R. Follow-up studies of long-term survivors after hepatic portoenterostomy for "non-correctable" biliary atresia. J. Pediatr. Surg. *10*:173, 1975.
20. Altman, R. P. The portoenterostomy procedure for biliary atresia. Ann. Surg. *188*:351, 1978.
21. Alagille, D. Extrahepatic biliary atresia. Hepatology *4*(suppl.):75, 1984.
22. Altman, R. P., and Chandra, R. Biliary hypoplasia consequent to alpha-1-antitrypsin deficiency. Surg. Forum *37*:377, 1976.
23. Markowitz, J., Daum, F., Kahn, E. I., et al. Arteriohepatic dysplasia. I. Pitfalls in diagnosis and management. Hepatology *3*:74, 1983.
24. Chandra, R. S., and Altman, R. P. Ductal remnants in extrahepatic biliary atresia. J. Pediatr. *93*:196, 1978.
25. Watson, G. M., and Miller, V. Arteriohepatic dysplasia: Familial pulmonary arterial stenosis with neonatal liver disease. Arch. Dis. Child. *48*:459, 1973.
26. Alagille, D., Odievre, M., Gautier, M., and Domergues, J. P. Hepatic ductular hypoplasia associated with characteristic facies, vertebral malformations, retarded physical, mental and sexual development, and cardiac murmur. J. Pediatr. *86*:63, 1975.
27. Thaler, M. M. Effect of phenobarbital on hepatic transport and excretion of ^{131}I-rose bengal in children with cholestasis. Pediatr. Res. *6*:100, 1972.
28. Rosenblum, J. L., Keating, J. P., Prensky, A. P., and Nelson, J. S. A progressive disabling neurologic syndrome in children with chronic liver disease: A possible result of vitamin E deficiency. N. Engl. J. Med. *304*:503, 1981.
29. Guggenheim, M. A., Jackson, V., Lilly, J., et al. Vitamin E deficiency and neurologic disease in children with cholestasis: A prospective study. J. Pediatr. *102*:577, 1982.
30. Stiehl, A., Thaler, M. M., and Admirand, W. H. The effects of phenobarbital on bile salts and bilirubin in patients with intra- and extrahepatic cholestasis. N. Engl. J. Med. *286*:858, 1972.
31. Stiehl, A., Thaler, M. M., and Admirand, W. H. Effect of phenobarbital on the kinetics of bile salts in cholestasis due to intrahepatic biliary atresia. Pediatrics *51*:992, 1973.
32. Kobayashi, A., and Obbe, Y. Choledochal cyst in infancy and childhood. Analysis of 16 cases. Arch. Dis. Child. *52*:121, 1977.
33. Trout, H. H., and Longmire, W. P., Jr. Long-term follow-up study of patients with congenital cystic dilatation of the common bile duct. Am. J. Surg. *121*:68, 1971.
34. Caroli, J., and Corcos, V. La dilatation congenitale des voies biliaires intrahepatiques. Rev. Medicochir. Mal. Foie *39*:1, 1964.
35. Hermansen, M. C., Starshak, R. J., and Werlin, S. L. Caroli disease: The diagnostic approach. J. Pediatr. *94*:879, 1979.
36. Kerr, N. S., Harrison, C. V., Sherlock, S., and Walker, R. M. Congenital hepatic fibrosis. Q. J. Med. *30*:91, 1961.
37. Thaler, M. M., Ogata, E. S., Goodman, J. R., et al. Congenital fibrosis and polycystic disease of liver and kidneys. Am. J. Dis. Child. *126*:374, 1973.
38. Gartner, J. C., Jr., Zitelli, B. J., Malatack, J. J., et al. Orthotopic liver transplantation in children: Two-year experience with 47 patients. Pediatrics *74*:140, 1984.
39. Starzl, T. E., Iwatsuki, S., Shaw, B. W., Jr., et al. Immunosuppression and other non-surgical factors in the improved results of liver transplantation. *In* Berk, P. (ed.). Seminars in Liver Disease. Vol. 5. New York, Thieme, Inc., 1985, p. 334.
40. Busuttil, R. W. Liver transplantation today. Arch. Intern. Med. *104*:377, 1986.
41. Brenner, R. W., and Stewart, C. F. Cholecystitis in children. Rev. Surg. *21*:327, 1964.
42. Calabrese, C., and Perlman, D. M. Gallbladder disease below the age of 21 years. Surgery *70*:413, 1971.
43. Hagberg, B., Svennerholm, L., and Thoren, L. Cholelithiasis in childhood. A follow-up study with special reference to heredity, constitutional factors and serum lipids. Acta Chir. Scand. *123*:307, 1962.
44. Whitington, P. F., and Black, D. D. Cholelithiasis in premature infants treated with parenteral nutrition and furosemide. J. Pediatr. *97*:647, 1980.
45. Danon, Y. L., Dinari, G., Gartz, B. -Z., et al. Cholelithiasis in children with immunoglobulin A deficiency. A new gastroenterologic syndrome. J. Pediatr. Gastroenterol. Nutr. *2*:663, 1983.
46. Bloom, R. A., and Swain, V. A. J. Non-calculous distension of the gallbladder in childhood. Arch. Dis. Child. *41*:503, 1966.
47. Slovis, T. L., Hight, D. W., Philippart, A. I., and Dubois, R. S. Sonography in the diagnosis and management of hydrops of the gallbladder in children with mucocutaneous lymph node syndrome. Pediatrics *65*:789, 1980.

87 Bile Formation and Gallbladder and Bile Duct Function

BRUCE F. SCHARSCHMIDT

Bile is a complex fluid isosmotic with plasma that consists of water, inorganic electrolytes, and organic solutes such as bile acids, cholesterol, phospholipid, and bilirubin (Table 87–1). Primary bile is formed in the canaliculus, and it results from active transport of solutes by hepatocytes followed by passive water flow.[1–3] In terms of their absolute amounts and osmotic activity, bile acids and inorganic electrolytes are the predominant biliary solutes and are therefore major determinants of canalicular bile formation. In the first section of this chapter, current information regarding the microanatomy of the primary bile secretory unit, as well as transport by the hepatocyte of bile acids, electrolytes, and other solutes, will be summarized. For additional information regarding the hepatic transport mechanisms involved in the formation of canalicular bile, the reader is referred to recent comprehensive reviews.[1–4]

Prior to delivery to the duodenum, canalicular bile is stored and modified in the gallbladder and bile ducts. These modifications, which are potentially important in gallstone formation, are described in the second section of this chapter. An overview of canalicular bile formation and its modification in the gallbladder and bile ducts is depicted in Figure 87–1.

Bile formation plays an exceedingly important role in the body economy. It is essential for excretion of certain endogenous waste products such as bilirubin as well as for excretion of immunoglobulin A and many drugs and toxins. It is required for normal intestinal lipid absorption, and because biliary excretion and conversion to bile acids represent the principal modes of cholesterol excretion and catabolism, bile formation plays a pivotal role in body cholesterol balance. Information regarding the regulation of bile formation and the pathogenesis of bile secretory failure, i.e., cholestasis, is therefore important and is the subject of the last two sections of this chapter.

CANALICULAR BILE FORMATION

Microanatomy of the Bile Secretory Apparatus

Hepatocytes are arranged in anastamosing single cell thick plates, as shown schematically in Figure 87–2.[2, 5] Plates are bathed on either side by sinusoidal blood. Sinusoidal plasma has free access to the space of Disse and the hepatocyte plasma membrane via fenestrae in the sinusoidal lining cells.[5, 6] This nearly unique microvascular anatomy helps explain the facility with which the liver transports tightly protein-bound substances such as bilirubin and secretes albumin, lipoproteins, and other large molecules. Like other epithelial cells, the hepatocyte is a polarized cell. That is, its plasma membrane consists of distinct areas. The sinusoidal membrane, that portion of the plasma membrane bordering the space of Disse, accounts for about 37 per cent of the total cell surface.[7] Bidirectional exchange of substances across this membrane is facilitated both by the fenestrations in the sinusoidal lining cells, which permit direct contact with plasma, and by the presence of microvilli, which increase surface area. The relatively flat lateral membrane borders the intercellular space and accounts for about 50 per cent of the cell surface.[7] The canalicular membrane, which consists of many irregularly spaced microvilli and is the "business end" of the hepatocyte with respect to bile secretion, accounts for only about 13 per cent of the total cell surface.[7, 8] It is demarcated from the lateral membrane by the junctional complex, and the canalicular membranes of two or, rarely, three adjacent hepatocytes joined by junctional complexes circumscribe the canalicular space. As is true for other transporting epithelia, the net secretion of fluid and solutes into the canaliculus is mediated by plasma membrane–associ-

Table 87–1. COMPOSITION OF HEPATIC BILE*

Component	Concentration (m*M*)
Inorganic electrolytes	
Na^+	140–165
K^+	2.7–6.7
Cl^-	77–117
HCO_3^-	12–55
Mg^{2+}	1.5–3.0
Organic anions	
Bilirubin	1–2
Bile acids	3–45
Lipids	
Cholesterol	100–320 (mg/dl)
Lecithin	140–810 (mg/dl)
Proteins, peptides, and amino acids	
Glutathione	3–5
Amino acids (predominantly glutamic acid, aspartic acid, and glycine)	1–2.5

*Values from human, rat, and rabbit hepatic bile as summarized in references 2 and 4. Additional components not listed include heavy metals (Cu, Mn, Fe, Zn), trace amounts of many plasma proteins, secretory component, enzymes derived from hepatic lysosomes and plasma membranes, vitamins, porphyrins, and CEA.

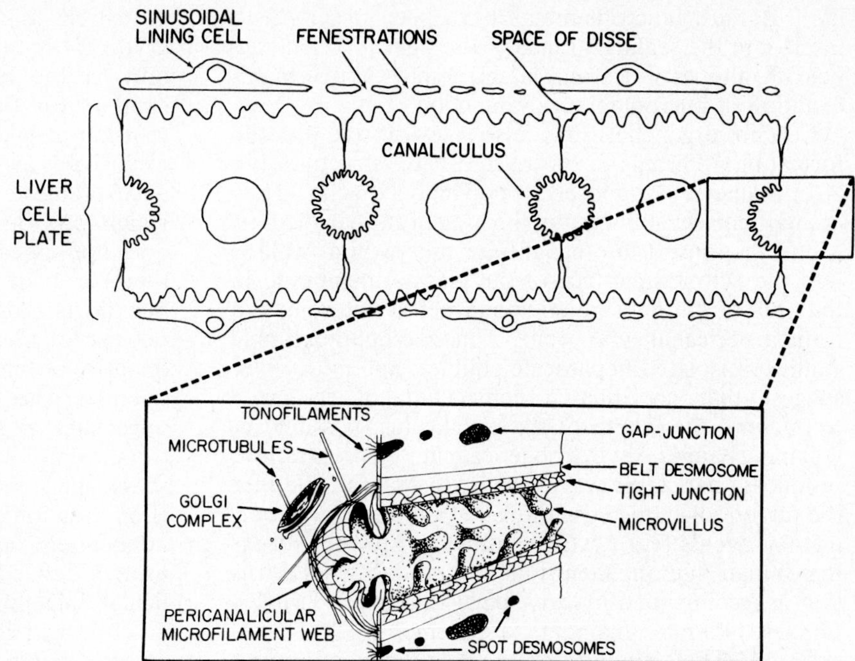

Figure 87–1. Schematic illustration of a liver cell plate. The single-cell-thick liver plate (top panel) is separated from the sinusoidal blood on either side by sinusoidal lining cells. These lining cells have large fenestrations in the cytoplasm which allow free access of plasma to Disse's space. Each hepatocyte surface membrane consists of three distinct areas: the sinusoidal surface, the lateral surface, and the canalicular surface. The bottom panel is an enlargement of the hemicanaliculus shown above. The canalicular membranes of adjacent hepatocytes are joined by tight junctions, shown here *en face,* which seal the canalicular space from the lateral intercellular space and sinusoidal space. The belt desmosomes adjacent to the tight junction help to hold the cells together and serve as a site of attachment of pericanalicular microfilaments. Spot desmosomes can be thought of as "spot welds" between adjacent liver cells. They also help to hold cells together, and are the sites of insertion of intracellular tonofilaments, which transmit passive forces to the membrane surface. Gap junctions allow direct passage of certain molecules between the cytoplasms of adjacent cells. The Golgi complex, microtubules, and microfilaments are characteristically found in the pericanalicular area and may play a role in bile secretion. (From Scharschmidt, B. F. *In* Zakim, D., and Boyer, T. (eds.): Hepatology. Philadelphia, W. B. Saunders Co., 1982.)

ated transport systems asymmetrically distributed to the basolateral and canalicular membrane domains (see below).

Adjacent hepatocytes are joined by junctional complexes, which consist of several discrete structures including the belt desmosome and the tight junction. The belt desmosome forms a continuous band which, like the spot desmosome is probably important primarily in cell-to-cell adhesion.[9] The tight junction forms the principal barrier to free movement of molecules along the intercellular space from blood to bile.[10–12] The tight junction is a continuous band of anastomosing strands. Each strand consists of proteins protruding from the juxtaposed plasma membranes that interlock in a zipper-like arrangement and thus seal the intercellular space. The permeability or "tightness" of the tight junction increases with the number of strands that compose it.[9] Compared with other epithelia, hepatic tight junctions possess an intermediate number of sealing strands.[13] Moreover, the number of strands which line the lateral borders of the bile canaliculus may vary from one to eight, suggesting regional variability in the permeability barrier.[11] There is also evidence that the tight junction of hepatocytes is less permeable to anions than cations,[14] a property which presumably aids in canalicular retention of negatively charged bile acids. Bile formation may be impaired under certain conditions in which the permeability of the tight junction is increased. For example, elimination of perfusate calcium decreases bile formation by isolated rat liver, and this decrease may be mediated by an increase in tight junction permeabil-

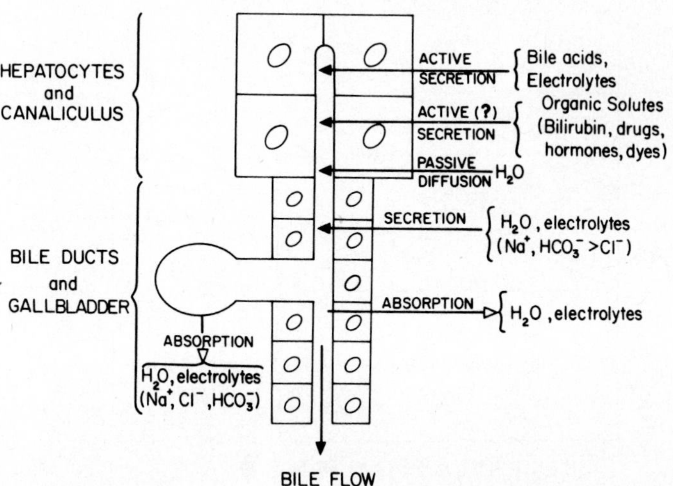

Figure 87–2. Overview of bile formation. Bile formation begins in the canaliculus with active transport of certain inorganic electrolytes and bile acids. Other organic constituents such as bilirubin, phospholipid, and cholesterol also enter bile at the canaliculus. Canalicular bile is subsequently concentrated in the gallbladder by isotonic absorption of water, sodium, chloride, and bicarbonate and further modified in the bile ducts before entering the duodenum. (From Scharschmidt, B. F. *In* Zakim, D., and Boyer, T. (eds.): Hepatology. Philadelphia, W. B. Saunders Co., 1982.)

ity.[15] Because microfilaments have been observed to insert into the sealing strands of the tight junction (see below), altered junctional integrity may be one manifestation of microfilament dysfunction.

Certain organelles may also play a role in bile formation. Microfilaments are contractile structures (70 Å in diameter) composed of polymerized actin. They are particularly abundant in the area of the canaliculus, where they insert into canalicular microvilli as well as into the cytoplasmic face of the plasma membrane in the area of the tight junction and belt desmosomes to form a pericanalicular web.[16] Cinemicrophotographic studies of isolated hepatocyte couplets and intact liver suggest that coordinated contraction of this web throughout the length of the canaliculus, possibly involving changes in cytosolic calcium concentration, produce a peristaltic wave which "massages" bile into the larger collecting structures.[17–19] Conversely, experimental agents (e.g., cytochalasins) and possibly drugs that impair microfilament function produce cholestasis that is accompanied by canalicular dilatation.[20] Microtubules, like microfilaments, are elements of the cytoskeleton. They are noncontractile tubular structures composed of polymerized tubulin, and as in the case of microfilaments, experimental toxins such as colchicine that impair microtubule function have been found also to decrease bile acid–stimulated bile flow and biliary lipid output,[21, 22] albumin and lipoprotein secretion,[23] and the transcellular vesicular transport from blood to bile of fluid phase markers (see below) and immunoglobulin A.[24, 25] Lysosomes appear to discharge their contents, at least in part, into bile.[26] The Golgi complex and other vesicular structures have been demonstrated to be present in greater than normal amounts in pericanalicular cytoplasm under conditions of increased bile secretion. These findings as well as others summarized below indicate that vesicles mediate the transport of certain solutes from blood to bile.

Measurement of Canalicular Bile Formation

Like the measurement of glomerular filtration rate with inulin, canalicular bile formation is commonly measured using metabolically inert solutes, such as erythritol or mannitol, which are assumed to enter bile only at the level of the canaliculus. The principal support for this assumption is the observation that infusion of bile acids, which are believed to enter bile exclusively at the canaliculus, increases biliary clearance of these markers, whereas infusion of secretin, which acts on ducts and ductules, does not.[1–4] This does not appear to be true in all species, however, and there is evidence that these markers may penetrate bile ducts. Although these observations suggest that the use of these inert markers may overestimate the quantity of bile secreted by hepatocytes as opposed to ductules, the magnitude of this error in humans is uncertain, and alternative approaches to measuring canalicular bile production are not available. Using these markers, bile acid–dependent bile formation (that fraction of canalicular bile formation which is "dependent" upon the biliary output of bile acids) is usually defined by the slope of the line relating canalicular bile flow (*y*-axis) to bile acid output (*x*-axis), and bile acid–independent bile formation (that fraction of canalicular bile formation not directly attributable to bile acids and presumably attributable to the active secretion of inorganic electrolytes and/or other solutes) is determined by extrapolating this line to zero bile acid output (*y*-intercept) (Fig. 87–3).

Hepatocyte Transport Mechanisms

The hepatocyte possesses a variety of primary and secondary active transport systems which are asymmetrically distributed between the sinusoidal-lateral and canalicular plasma membranes. *Na^+,K^+-ATPase* has been localized cytochemically to the sinusoidal and lateral plasma membrane in rat hepatocytes,[27, 28] a location analogous to that in virtually all other epithelial cells. Although immunofluorescence studies utilizing polyclonal and monoclonal antibodies against the α subunit of canine or rat kidney Na^+,K^+-ATPase have shown staining of canalicular as well as sinusoidal plasma membranes of canine and rat hepatocytes,[29] a number of issues, including antibody specificity, remain

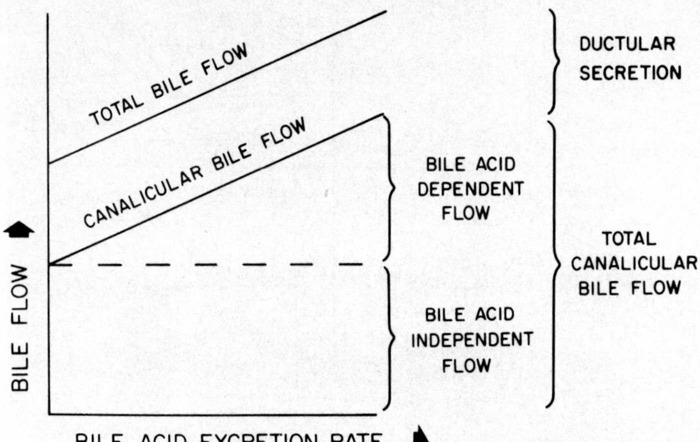

Figure 87–3. Schematic representation of the components of bile flow. Total bile flow consists of ductular secretion, bile acid–independent canalicular secretion, and a bile acid–dependent canalicular secretion which varies directly with bile acid input. In patients with T-tubes, these three components have been estimated to be about 180 ml/day, 225 ml/day, and 200 ml/day, respectively. Bile acid–independent canalicular secretion is defined operationally as the y intercept obtained by extrapolating the line relating canalicular bile flow and bile acid output to zero bile acid output. Although ductular secretion and bile acid–independent canalicular bile formation are depicted as constant, this is probably not true *in vivo.* (From Scharschmidt, B. F. *In* Zakim, D., and Boyer, T. (eds.): Hepatology. Philadelphia, W. B. Saunders Co., 1982.)

to be answered before the apparently disparate results using histochemical and immunofluorescent techniques can be reconciled. For this discussion, functional Na^+,K^+-ATPase pump units are assumed to be sinusoidal-lateral in location.

The factors that regulate or affect Na^+,K^+-ATPase function are potentially of considerable importance to bile formation, yet are not fully understood. Enhanced sodium-coupled uptake of bile acids or amino acids is associated with an increase in Na^+,K^+-ATPase–mediated cation pumping and presumably represents a compensatory mechanism designed to preserve electrochemical driving forces.[30] By contrast, chlorpromazine and ethinyl estradiol have been shown to decrease Na^+,K^+-ATPase activity in both isolated membranes and intact cells, possibly via a direct effect on the composition or physical properties of surrounding plasma membrane lipids.[31–34] The possible pathophysiologic importance of these effects is discussed further below.

The electrogenic pumping of Na^+,K^+-ATPase, in conjunction with the associated conductance of the plasma membrane to K^+ ions,[35] appears to account for the electrical potential difference across the hepatocyte plasma membrane, which is about 35 mV (interior negative) for liver *in situ.*[36] This membrane potential is not fixed, but rather varies considerably in response to a number of stimuli such as fasting (depolarization),[36, 37] exposure to glucagon and cAMP (hyperpolarization),[36] and partial hepatectomy (hyperpolarization).[37]

Sodium-coupled "secondary active" transport mechanisms driven by the electrochemical sodium gradient produced to Na^+,K^+-ATPase accounts for the transport of a wide variety of solutes into and out of hepatocytes as well as epithelial cells.[38] A number of these sodium-coupled solute transport processes have been identified in the sinusoidal-lateral membrane of liver cells and are depicted in Figure 87–4. The role of some of those transporters on the sinusoidal-lateral as well as canalicular membranes, which are believed to play a role in canalicular bile formation, will be discussed further below.

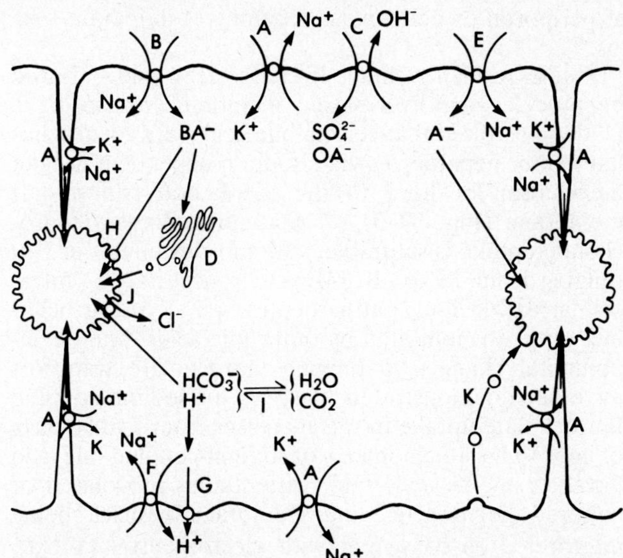

Figure 87–4. Hepatocyte ion transport mechanisms. This figure depicts transport mechanisms possibly important in canalicular bile formation. Na^+,K^+-ATPase (A) has been localized histochemically (see text for discussion of controversy in this area) to the sinusoidal-lateral aspect of the plasma membrane, and the electrochemical Na^+ gradient created by this pump drives a variety of sodium-coupled transport systems (e.g., B, F). Uptake of conjugated trihydroxy bile acids (BA^-) is mediated by such a Na^+-coupled mechanism (B), and exit of bile acids from the cell is mediated by a carrier (H) and driven by the electrical gradient between cytoplasm and canaliculus. Bile acids may interact with cellular membranes (D), and it is possible that such interaction is an early event in mixed micelle or lipid vesicle formation. Biliary HCO_3^- secretion may be driven by sinusoidal-lateral Na^+/H^+ exchange (F) or ATP-dependent H^+ transport (G), in conjunction with hydration of CO_2 by carbonic anhydrase (I) and canalicular HCO_3^-/Cl^- exchange (J). A versatile sinusoidal-lateral antiporter (C) which couples efflux of OH^- to the uptake of SO_4^{2-}, as well as certain organic anions (OA^-) (e.g., BSP) and bile acids (cholate), may also participate in blood-to-bile transport. Na^+-coupled uptake (E) of inorganic anions (A^-) such as Cl^- has also been postulated to play a role in bile formation but is not supported by current data. Finally, a transcellular vesicular pathway (K) mediates the biliary secretion of certain ligands (e.g., IgA) and fluid phase markers. Although certain transport mechanisms are, because of space limitations, depicted as present on only one side of the cell, transport systems present on one sinusoidal-lateral membrane are also present on the other; such is also the case for the canalicular membrane.

Bile Acid Secretion

In all mammals thus far studied, including humans, a positive linear relationship exists between canalicular bile flow and bile acid output.[1–4] This finding plus the observation that bile acid concentration in canalicular bile exceeds that in portal blood by up to 1000-fold indicates that bile acids are actively secreted by the hepatocyte. That portion of bile formation related to bile acid output; i.e., bile acid–dependent bile formation (Fig. 87–3) or, perhaps more correctly, bile acid–stimulated bile formation, has been estimated to be approximately 200 ml per day in humans, or approximately one half of canalicular bile flow.[39]

Bile acids are extracted from portal blood very efficiently by the normal liver, accounting for the fact that mean fasting bile acid concentration in portal blood greatly exceeds that in systemic plasma.[40] Blood in the sinusoid flows from the portal tract to the central vein, and periportal hepatocytes are therefore exposed first to incoming bile acids. Because of the efficient and progressive removal of bile acids by hepatocytes thus arranged in series, there exists a lobular bile acid concentration gradient in sinusoidal blood, with high bile acid concentrations occurring periportally and low concentrations pericentrally.[41, 42] The predominant role of periportal hepatocytes in bile acid transport appears to reflect their strategic position at the "headwaters" of the sinusoid rather than intrinsic differences between periportal and pericentral cells. Such intrinsic differences, however, certainly do exist and have implications that extend far beyond bile acid transport and help explain, for example, the selective susceptibility of periportal or pericentral hepatocytes to certain toxins.[42]

Studies utilizing intact liver, isolated and cultured hepatocytes, and liver plasma membrane vesicles have all demonstrated that certain bile acids (e.g., taurocholate) enter hepatocytes via a sodium-dependent uptake mechanism localized to the basolateral (sinusoidal) membrane (Fig. 87–3).[43–47] Sodium-dependent taurocholate uptake is saturable, with most estimates of Km ranging from 15 to 50 μM, and concentrative (intracelluar:extracellular ratio of up to 50:1).[45, 46] Taurocholate uptake is inhibited by other bile acids, and developmental changes in hepatic taurocholate transport have been demonstrated; the V_{max} for sodium-coupled taurocholate uptake in rats increases from 7 to 56 days of age.[48] The stoichiometry of sodium-coupled bile acid uptake remains uncertain, with studies in isolated or cultured hepatocytes and membrane vesicles being interpreted as consistent with electroneutral (1 Na^+ per taurocholate molecule) as well as electrogenic (>1 Na^+ per taurocholate molecule) transport.[43–46] Recent studies of the relationship between membrane potential and taurocholate uptake by isolated hepatocytes and rat liver *in vivo* suggest that hepatic uptake of taurocholate is electrogenic.[36, 49]

There exists considerable heterogeneity among physiologic bile acids with respect to their dependence on sodium coupling for hepatic uptake.[46] Hydrophobic unconjugated di- and monohydroxy bile acids enter isolated or cultured hepatocytes more rapidly than do conjugated trihydroxy bile acids such as taurocholate, and much of their uptake is nonsaturable and sodium-independent, suggesting that hydrophobic bile acids readily penetrate or cross the membrane bilayer without benefit of a specialized sodium-coupled carrier system. These findings do not necessarily indicate that di- and monohydroxy acids are unsuitable substrates for the sodium-coupled carrier; indeed, many of these hydrophobic bile acids competitively inhibit sodium-copuled taurocholate transport,[50] indicating considerable affinity for the carrier. It is interesting that these characteristics are very similar to those of bile acid transport in the distal ileum, suggesting that fundamentally similar transport mechanisms are responsible for bile acid transport at both the hepatic and intestinal "poles" of the enterohepatic circulation. In addition to the saturable, Na^+-dependent mechanism for taurocholate uptake described above, kinetic studies in intact cells[45] as well as observations in basolateral plasma membranes suggest the existence of a second saturable Na^+-independent system, which may represent an anion exchange mechanism that couples the transport of OH^- to a variety of anions, including bile acids, other organic anions, and sulfate.[51]

As compared with uptake, the intracellular transport and canalicular secretion of bile acids are less well understood.[1–4] Certain characteristics (existence of an apparent maximal secretory rate from hepatocytes and competition between different bile acids for secretion) of bile acid transport *in vivo* are consistent with the presence of a carrier-mediated, rate-limiting mechanism for bile acid secretion across the canalicular membrane.[1] Studies with canalicular membrane vesicles have further demonstrated saturable, electrical potential–sensitive, sodium-independent taurocholate transport, which exhibits trans-stimulation.[47, 52] Collectively, these studies indicate the presence of a canalicular "carrier" for bile acids. They further suggest that the membrane potential (cell interior ~ 30 to 40 mV negative relative to blood and probably canaliculus; see above) represents an important driving force for bile acid secretion.

Recent progress has been made in identifying the plasma membrane bile acid carriers. Bile acid–binding proteins of 48,000 and 54,000 daltons in the basolateral membrane have been identified and are postulated to mediate Na^+-dependent and Na^+-independent bile acid uptake, respectively,[53, 54] and a 100,000 dalton bile acid–binding protein in the canalicular membrane has been identified which appears to be a candidate for the canalicular transporter.[55] Isolation and purification of these proteins will ultimately permit the exploration of factors which regulate their synthesis *in vivo*.

Lipid Secretion

The major biliary lipids are nonesterified cholesterol and the phospholipid phosphatidylcholine (lecithin). Lecithin is poorly water soluble, and cholesterol is virtually insoluble in water, yet both exist in solution in bile in the form of mixed micelles and vesicles (see pp. 144–161 and 1668–1676). Biliary output of both cholesterol and phospholipid increases curvilinearly with bile acid output.[56] At low rates of bile acid output (fasting), there is apparent supersaturation of the micellar phase, and vesicles may be the predominant form of cholesterol carrier.[57] The importance of the molar ratios of bile acid, phospholipid, and cholesterol and the presence in bile of mixed micelles as well as vesicles in the pathogenesis of cholesterol stone formation are discussed on pages 1672 to 1675 and elsewhere.[57]

Knowledge regarding the origin of biliary lipid and the nature of the "coupling" between lipid and bile acid excretion, while crucial to understanding cholesterol stone formation, is as yet incomplete. Animal studies suggest the existence of a hepatic subpool of newly synthesized lecithin destined for biliary excretion,[58] as well as of a labile pool of free cholesterol, the size of which depends upon relative rates of cholesterol synthesis and esterification, which contributes importantly to biliary cholesterol secretion.[59] Although the cellular location of these kinetically defined precursor pools and the mechanisms for transport to the canalicular membrane of cholesterol and phospholipid and assembly into mixed micelles are currently uncertain, it is tempting to postulate that bile acids, which are surface-active agents known to interact with biologic membranes *in vitro*,[60] also interact with membranes *in vivo* and that solubilization of membrane lipids by bile acids, perhaps to form vesicles, represents an early event in bile acid–lipid coupling and biliary lipid secretion.

Inorganic Electrolyte Secretion

Sodium, potassium, chloride, and bicarbonate concentrations in hepatic bile are similar to those in plasma, and these inorganic electrolytes account for most of bile osmolality. Secretion of these electrolytes therefore presumably contributes to that fraction of canalicular bile that is not directly dependent upon bile acid excretion—i.e., the bile acid–independent fraction (Fig. 87–3). The cellular mechanism(s) reponsible for bile acid–independent bile flow and inorganic electrolyte secretion are poorly understood, and concepts regarding this process have undergone considerable evolution. It was initially proposed that bile acid–independent bile flow was directly attributable to the activity of Na^+,K^+-ATPase, which was postulated to reside on the canalicular membrane (see above). This formulation was based on the observations that inhibitors of Na^+,K^+-ATPase such as ouabain also appeared to inhibit bile formation in intact animals and the perfused liver and that certain drugs or hormones which increased (e.g., phenobarbital, taurocholate, thyroid hormone) or decreased (e.g., ethinyl estradiol, rose bengal, chlorpromazine) hepatic Na^+,K^+-ATPase activity produced apparently parallel changes in bile acid–independent bile flow.[4] Subsequently, each of the observations upon which this hypothesis rested has been questioned or refuted, and other mechanisms for bile acid–independent bile flow have been explored.

Na^+-K^+-Cl^- cotransport localized to the sinusoidal-lateral membrane would mediate intracellular accumulation of Cl^- above electrochemical equilibrium and, in conjunction with an asymmetric distribution of Cl^- conductance pathways or carriers, net canalicular Cl^- secretion (Fig. 87–4). However, studies in cultured hepatocytes have not provided evidence of coupling between the uptake of Na^+ and Cl^-, bile acid–independent bile flow by perfused rat liver is minimally altered when Cl^- is replaced by certain other permeant anions, and recent studies suggest that Cl^- is passively distributed across the hepatocyte plasma membrane.[61–63]

In contrast to Cl^-, there is a moderate amount of evidence that active HCO_3^- secretion is important in bile formation, including the following: (1) removal of HCO_3^- from the perfusate of the isolated rat liver decreased bile acid–independent bile flow,[64, 65] (2) the increase in bile flow produced by certain bile acid–independent choleretics (e.g., secretin, salicylates) appears to be at least partly attributable to selective enhancement of canalicular HCO_3^- secretion,[66] and (3) ursodeoxycholic acid and some other nonphysiologic bile acids elicit a dramatic (three- to fivefold) increase in bile flow or "hypercholeresis," which is accompanied by a selective increase in biliary HCO_3^- concentration to two to three times that in plasma.[67, 68] Collectively, these findings suggest the presence of an hepatic mechanism for active HCO_3^- secretion. The latter observation further suggests that the increase in bile flow produced by certain bile acids is attributable, at least in part, to stimulation of active HCO_3^- secretion (hence the term "bile acid–stimulated" bile flow).

Active HCO_3^- transport by other epithelia as well as liver is currently believed to result from the active transport of H^+ (or OH^-) ions. Active secretion of HCO_3^- by hepatocytes could result from the operation of basolateral Na^+-H^+ exchange in conjunction with a canalicular mechanism(s) for HCO_3^- secretion (Cl^-/HCO_3^- exchange being one candidate) (Fig. 87–4). A role for Na^+-H^+ exchange in the choleresis produced by certain bile acids is supported by the finding that experimental maneuvers known to inhibit Na^+-H^+ exchange in other epithelia (amiloride, removal of Na^+) effectively uncouple the biliary output of ursodeoxycholic or taurocholic acid from the associated increase in bile flow.[69] The observation that basal HCO_3^- secretion by isolated rat liver is minimally affected by removal of perfusate sodium or exposure to amiloride[65, 69, 70] also raises the possibility that a Na^+-independent mechanism for H^+ transport, perhaps the same H^+-translocating ATPase identified in endocytic vesicles,[71] may be present also on the hepatocyte plasma membrane and may play a role in biliary HCO_3^- secretion analogous to the role of a similar H^+-ATPase in acid-alkali transport by turtle bladder and distal nephron.[72]

Finally, it has been proposed that the increase in HCO_3^- secretion produced by ursodeoxycholic acid and certain other bile acids may be mediated via an intrahepatic recycling mechanism whereby unconjugated bile acids are protonated in and reabsorbed from the biliary tree, thereby generating biliary HCO_3^-, and recycled to the hepatocytes via the periductular plexus for resecretion.[68, 73] The mechanism(s) responsible for bile acid–independent bile flow and for biliary HCO_3^- secretion represent active areas of investigation. Moreover, the possible importance of HCO_3^- transport in bile acid–stimulated or bile acid–dependent bile formation suggests that fundamentally similar transport mechanisms may be operative in both bile acid–dependent and bile acid–independent bile flow.

Secretion of Bilirubin and Other Organic Solutes

Although bilirubin and other organic substances (excluding bile acids) account for less than 3 per cent of total biliary solutes by weight, hepatic bilirubin transport remains an area of intense interest and study. This is because bilirubin transport serves as a model for transport of certain other organic anions, including drugs and dyes (e.g., sulfobromophthalein), and also because hyperbilirubinemia leading to jaundice is perhaps the most obvious manifestation of cholestasis. Metabolism and hepatic transport of bilirubin are discussed on pages 454 to 467. The liver also exhibits transport mechanisms for neutral (e.g., cardiac glycosides) and cationic (e.g., meperidine) organic compounds. The cellular mechanisms responsible for the transport of these various organic solutes are not fully understood but almost certainly involve the participation of two or more functionally distinct basolateral carrier mechanisms.[74]

Protein Secretion

Protein represents a minor component of bile, with concentrations in mammalian bile ranging up to 300 mg/dl. Some proteins, including lysosomal acid hydrolases,[26] liver plasma membrane enzymes,[26, 75] and enzymes from other organelles and cytoplasm presumably originate in hepatocytes or ductular cells. Serum proteins such as albumin, hemopexin, and certain globulins are also present in small amounts.[75] In contrast to these proteins whose presence in bile may simply reflect "leakage" or cellular extrusion, dimeric IgA is rapidly and efficiently transported into bile via a receptor-mediated vesicular transport mechanism, with secretory component acting as the IgA receptor at the basolateral membrane.[25, 75, 76] The physiologic implications of IgA transport are as yet unknown, but it seems likely to play an important role in host defense against enteric pathogens (see pp. 121–124).

In addition to enzymes and plasma proteins, certain amino acids (particularly aspartic acid, glutamic acid, and glycine) and glutathione appear in bile in appreciable quantities (0.5 to 5.0 m*M*).[77, 78] Recent findings indicate that glutathione, which is transported across the canalicular membrane by a carrier-mediated electrogenic system,[79] is hydrolyzed in the biliary tree by gamma glutamyltranspeptidase into its constituent amino acids, which are then reabsorbed by canalicular transport mechanisms.[77, 78] Biliary glutathione secretion may account for up to 50 per cent of total hepatic glutathione turnover and has been postulated to represent a driving force for bile formation.[78]

Transport by Vesicles

Recently it has been demonstrated that, in addition to IgA, hepatocytes transport a variety of inert, water-soluble, nonreceptor-bound solutes from blood to bile via a transcellular vesicular transport mechanism (Fig. 87–4).[80–82] Included among these solutes, often called fluid phase markers, are solutes such as sucrose which are often used to measure canalicular bile formation (Fig. 87–3) and larger markers such as horseradish peroxidase and dextran. The existence of this pathway indicates that the concentration of solutes such as sucrose in bile relative to plasma cannot be taken as a simple index of the integrity of the tight junction (which has frequently been done based on the assumption that such markers move predominantly via a paracellular route) and may provide a mechanism for the transport to bile of small amounts of a variety of plasma proteins as summarized above. It also appears that transport to bile represents but a minor pathway for fluid phase markers internalized via endocytosis, with most such markers being transported to lysosomes or returned to the plasma membrane, presumably in the process of plasma membrane recycling.[83] The mechanisms whereby fluid phase markers such as sucrose or ligands such as IgA are directed to bile versus lysosomes are currently unknown.

THE BILE COLLECTING SYSTEM AND REGULATION OF BILE FLOW

The Bile Ducts

After leaving the canaliculus, bile flows in order through the following structures: canals of Hering (conduits in the hepatic parenchyma bounded by hepatocyte and ductular cells), ductules (parenchymal structures bounded by poorly developed lining cells), interlobular ducts (recognizable on histologic section by their location within portal tracts), septal ducts, right and left lobar ducts, and the common hepatic duct. These structures plus the gallbladder constitute the bile collecting system. During passage through the collecting system, canalicular bile is modified in a fashion analogous to that of glomerular urine passing through the renal tubules. Unlike glomerular urine, however, the composition of canalicular bile is not precisely known. Modifications in the bile ducts and ductules, such as net fluid absorption or secretion, must therefore be assessed indirectly using markers of canalicular bile formation such as erythritol or mannitol (see above).

Secretin increases bile flow in many species, including humans[39] and subhuman primates.[84] Studies in experimental animals indicate that bile ductular epithelium is capable of actively secreting fluid containing a high bicarbonate concentration.[85–87] Thus, secretin, and possibly other hormones such as cholecystokinin and gastrin,[88–90] probably increase bile flow in humans, at least in part, by stimulating ductular secretion of a bicarbonate-rich fluid. In cholecystectomized patients with indwelling T-tubes, ductular secretion is estimated to account for about one third of the total bile flow of 600 ml per day.[39] Under experimental conditions in which ductular secretion is blocked, bile duct epithelium also appears capable of net fluid absorption in dogs and primates.[84, 91] It is uncertain, however, whether net fluid absorption occurs under physiologic conditions in humans.

Sphincter of Oddi

The sphincter of Oddi has received considerable attention recently, since endoscopic sphincterotomy is now being widely performed and there is increasing evidence that sphincter dysfunction may produce symptoms in some patients.[92–94] Manometric studies in humans suggest that the sphincter corresponds functionally to a short (4 to 6 mm) zone with a basal or resting pressure that is 5 to 10 mm Hg greater than common bile duct pressure. This presumably accounts for the fact that common bile duct pressure is usually about 10 mm Hg greater than duodenal pressure. Phasic, high-pressure contractions occur within the sphincter several times per minute. Most of these contractions appear to be peristaltic and antegrade, that is, toward the duodenum. The frequency and amplitude of these phasic contractions, as well as basal pressure, are decreased by cholecystokinin and are increased by morphine.[95, 96]

The terms "papillary stenosis," "biliary spasm," and "papillary dysfunction" are among those applied to patients, typically female and post cholecystectomy, who exhibit a constellation of findings which may include episodic pain, intermittent mild elevation of liver function tests, and delayed drainage of dye from the bile ducts after retrograde cholangiography (see pp. 1729–1730).[92] Accumulating evidence based on manometric studies shows that such patients represent a heterogeneous group, some of whom have fixed stenosis, some of whom have identifiable sphincter dysfunction (including elevated resting pressures, abnormal phasic contractions, and/or abnormal response to hormones), and some of whom have no identifiable abnormalities.[92–100] Moreover, preliminary reports suggest that manometry may be useful in identifying patients most likely to show a favorable response to sphincterotomy.[101] Clearly, the wider use of manometric techniques will better define the types and consequences of sphincter dysfunction and the utility of sphincterotomy or pharmacologic approaches to management.

The Gallbladder

The gallbladder stores and concentrates hepatic bile during the fasting state. Gallbladder filling is presumably facilitated by tonic contraction of the ampullary sphincter, which maintains a positive pressure in the common hepatic duct (see above). During fasting, about one-half of hepatic bile is sequestered in the gallbladder, the remainder passing directly into the duodenum. The gallbladder does not, however, simply fill passively and continuously during fasting. Rather, periods of filling appear to be punctuated by brief periods of partial emptying of concentrated bile and aspiration of dilute bile in a "bellows-like" fashion.[102] Both hormonal and cholinergic mechanisms appear to be involved in gallbladder emptying. Although cholecystokinin has traditionally been regarded as the principal hormone stimulating gallbladder contraction, preliminary studies suggest that a humoral substance other than cholecystokinin—perhaps motilin[103]—may also be an important physiologic regulator. Recent ultrasonographic techniques which permit continuous study of gallbladder function *in vivo* indicate that sham feeding results in gallbladder contraction which is inhibited by atropine, suggesting a role for cholinergic pathways in gallbladder contraction and that atropine as well as somatostatin decreases gallbladder contraction after a test meal or sham feeding.[104]

The human gallbladder, which has a capacity of about 40 ml, would be rapidly filled with bile (about 600 ml produced per day) were it not for its remarkable absorptive capacity. Within four hours, up to 90 per cent of the water present in hepatic bile can be removed as an isotonic solution composed primarily of sodium, bicarbonate, and chloride (Fig. 87–5).[105] This action results in the formation of "gallbladder bile" having a very high concentration of sodium, bile acids (sometimes exceeding 200 mEq/L), potassium, and calcium, and having low concentrations (5 to 10 mEq/L) of chloride and bicarbonate compared with hepatic bile.[105, 106] This reabsorptive process has been intensively studied, and appears to be largely a result of neutral sodium-coupled chloride transport.[107, 108] As described above, this mechanism involves a presumably "mechanical" coupling of chloride and sodium influx across the luminal membrane of the mucosal cells (possibly in conjunction with K^+), such that energetically "downhill" sodium movement drives "uphill" chloride transport.[107, 108] In addition to its predominant absorptive function, animal studies suggest that the gallbladder may also exhibit net fluid secretion in the postprandial state.[109] The existence or importance of gallbladder secretion in humans has not yet been studied.

In contrast to absorption of water and electrolytes, relatively little absorption of organic constituents of bile occurs in the gallbladder. Conjugation of bilirubin, bile acids, and exogenous substances such as iopanoic acid greatly decreases their lipid solubility and presumably inhibits their absorption.[110] In contrast, unconju-

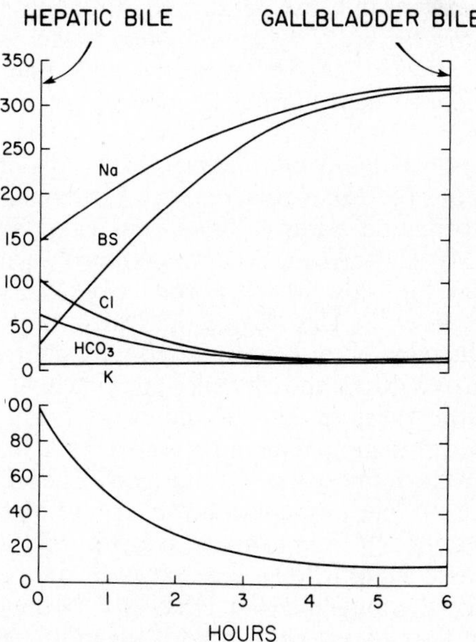

Figure 87–5. Conversion of hepatic bile (left vertical areas) into gallbladder bile (right vertical areas) by the resorptive action of the gallbladder. The upper panel depicts the concentration of inorganic electrolytes in millimoles per liter; the bottom panel depicts gallbladder volume. (From Makhlouf, G. M. Viewpoints Dig. Dis. *11*:1, 1979. Used by permission.)

gated bilirubin and bile acids, which are normally present in minimal amounts in hepatic bile, are absorbed much more readily in the gallbladder.[110, 111]

Regulation of Bile Flow

Bile flow is at its nadir during prolonged fasting. Bile acids are largely sequestered in the gallbladder, thus minimizing flux of bile acids through the enterohepatic circulation and hence bile acid–dependent canalicular bile formation. With entry of food into the duodenum, hormonal and possibly neural stimulation of gallbladder contraction causes release of concentrated gallbladder bile, thus priming the enterohepatic circulation with a bolus of bile acids that subsequently stimulates bile acid–dependent bile formation following their reabsorption in the gut. At the same time, secretin and possibly other hormones stimulate ductular secretion, further increasing bile flow. During the digestive process, the bile acid pool may undergo enterohepatic circulation two to three times (see pp. 150–155).

In contrast to bile acid–dependent bile flow, gallbladder contraction and bile ductular secretion, all of which are regulated largely by events that occur with feeding and fasting, relatively little is known regarding the normal regulation of bile acid–independent bile formation. Corticosteroids and thyroid hormone have been shown to stimulate bile acid–independent canalicular bile formation in animals, and estrogens have been shown to have the opposite effect.[1, 2, 4, 33] Secretin, which is known to stimulate secretion by ducts and ductules, may also stimulate bile acid–independent secretion at the level of the canaliculus.[66] Like secretin, glucose and insulin also appear to stimulate secretin by hepatocytes,[112, 113] whereas somatostatin has the opposite effect.[114, 115] The presence and quantitative significance of such hormonal effects in humans are uncertain.

The intracellular events and possible second messengers responsible for mediating such hormonal effects on bile formation are also largely unknown. Dibutyrl cyclic AMP (DBcAMP) has been shown to increase canalicular bile flow in the portal vein–perfused isolated rat liver.[116] The degree to which hepatocytes and/or ductular cells contribute to this choleresis is unknown. If ducts and ductules are inactive in this preparation, these findings would suggest that cAMP may play a role in mediating the hepatocellular effects of certain hormones such as glucagon. The effects of DBcAMP on bile formation, however, are highly species-dependent.[116, 117] In humans, secretin-induced choleresis is associated with an increase in biliary secretion of cAMP; theophylline and DBcAMP both increase total bile flow two- to threefold.[114] Secretin also produces a choleresis in the baboon that is associated with an increase in the cAMP content of bile duct tissue.[118] These observations suggest that cAMP helps mediate the choleretic effect of secretin on the bile ducts in primates; less is known about the possible role of cAMP in mediating changes in hepatocellular secretion in humans. The possible roles of cytosolic Ca^{2+}-calmodulin and protein phosphorylation in regulating canalicular bile formation are largely unexplored in any animal species.

BILE SECRETORY FAILURE

Cholestasis is the general term used to denote impaired bile formation. Cholestasis is usually manifested clinically by accumulation in the blood of substances such as bilirubin that are normally excreted in bile. The pathophysiology of hyperbilirubinemia, differentiation between intra- and extrahepatic obstruction, and clinical approach to the patient with cholestasis are discussed in detail on pages 454 to 467. The purpose of this section is to develop selected concepts introduced earlier as they relate to cellular mechanisms of intrahepatic cholestasis.

Several cellular structures and functions have now been identified as being particularly important to the process of canalicular bile formation. Plasma membrane carriers are responsible for the uptake or excretion of many biliary solutes, and plasma membrane–associated enzymes such as Na^+,K^+-ATPase appear to provide the driving force that energizes transport of bile acids and perhaps other substances. The strategic location of the tight junction assigns it a crucial role in bile formation, and strong circumstantial evidence suggests a role for microfilaments and microtubules in solute transport.

A number of agents known to cause clinical cholestasis have now been shown to affect one or another of these cellular structures and functions. Chlorpromazine, a drug known to cause a "cholestatic hepatitis" in about 1 per cent of patients and asymptomatic alkaline phosphatase elevation in up to one half of patients,[119] is a particularly well-studied example. Animal experiments have shown that chlorpromazine and its metabolites (1) alter the morphology[120] of hepatocyte membranes as well as the physical properties of plasma membrane lipids,[32] (2) inhibit plasma membrane–associated Mg^{2+}-ATPase and Na^+,K^+-ATPase, both in isolated plasma membranes and intact hepatocytes at concentrations similar to those which alter the physical properties of membrane lipids,[32, 43, 121] (3) inhibit the sodium-coupled transport of amino acids and bile acids,[34] (4) form insoluble complexes with bile acids that might precipitate intracellularly or in canaliculi,[122] and (5) alter *in vitro* polymerization of actin to form microfilaments.[123] Although these effects of chlorpromazine and its metabolites do not explain all features of cholestasis in humans due to this agent (e.g., eosinophilia or rash), they help account for the cholestasis observed upon administration of chlorpromazine to animals as well as the subtle abnormalities observed in many patients taking the drug.

Other cholestatic agents also have been shown to alter these cellular structures critical to bile formation. Estrogens, which are probably responsible for cholestasis related to pregnancy and the use of oral contraceptives, alter the activity of Na^+,K^+-ATPase in liver plasma membranes and the physical properties of plasma membrane lipids.[33, 124] Moreover, agents which inhibit or reverse the effects of estrogens on plasma membranes have also been shown to reverse the cholestasis observed in animals exposed to estrogen[124] and have, in preliminary trials, been shown to improve biochemical abnormalities and reduce itching in woman with cholestasis of pregnancy.[125]

Monohydroxy bile acids such as taurolithocholate, which cause cholestasis in experimental animals, produce striking morphologic alteration of the canalicular membrane[126–128] as well as changes in membrane lipid content and enzymatic activity.[129] Even the tri- and dihydroxy bile acids which predominate in normal bile can alter the enzymatic activity and physical properties of membrane lipids and thus might contribute to hepatic injury under cholestatic conditions.[60] *Norethandrelone,* an anabolic steroid that causes cholestasis in humans, produces changes in rat liver similar to those seen following cytochalasin B administration, including loss of microfilament structure in the pericanalicular region and detachment of microfilaments from isolated plasma membranes.[129] Collectively, these observations reflect growing insight into the pathogenesis of bile secretory failure which may ultimately be turned to therapeutic advantage.

References

1. Van Dyke, R. W., Lake, J. R., and Scharschmidt, B. F. Cellular mechanisms of hepatic fluid and electrolyte transport. *In* Forte, J. B. (ed.): Salivary, Pancreatic, Gastric and Hepatobiliary Secretion. Handbook of Physiology. Bethesda, MD, American Physiological Society, 1986.
2. Boyer, J. L. Mechanisms of bile secretion and hepatic transport. *In* Andreoli, T. E., Hofmann, J. F., Fanestel, D. D., and Schultz, S. G. (eds.): Physiology of Membrane Disorders. New York, Plenum Medical Book Co., 1986, pp. 609–636.
3. Scharschmidt, B. F., and Van Dyke, R. W. Mechanisms of hepatic electrolyte transport. Gastroenterology *85*:1199, 1983.
4. Scharschmidt, B. F. Bile formation and cholestasis, metabolism and enterohepatic circulation of bile acids, gallstone formation. *In* Zakim, D., and Boyer, T. (eds.): Hepatology. Philadelphia, W. B. Saunders Co., 1982.
5. Jones, A. L., Schmucker, D. L., Renston, R. H., and Murakami, T. The architecture of bile secretion. Dig. Dis. Sci. *25*:609, 1980.
6. Motta, P. A scanning electronmicroscopic study of the rat liver sinusoid. Endothelial and Kupffer cells. Cell Tissue Res. *164*:371, 1975.
7. Weibel, E. R., Staubli, W., Gnagi, H. R., and Hess, F. A. Correlated morphometric and biochemical studies on the liver cell, I. Morphometric model, stereologic methods, and normal morphometric data for rat liver. J. Cell Biol. *42*:68, 1969.
8. Blouin, A., Bolender, R. P., and Weibel, E. R. Distribution of organelles and membranes between hepatocytes and nonhepatocyes in the rat liver parenchyma: A sterological study. J. Cell Biol. *72*:441, 1977.
9. Staehin, A. L., and Hull, B. E. Junctions between living cells. Sci. Am. *238*(5):140, 1978.
10. Boyer, J. L. Tight junctions in normal and cholestatic liver: Does the paracellular pathway have functional significance? Hepatology *3*:614, 1983.
11. Lagarde, S., Elias, E., Wade, J. B., and Boyer, J. L. Structural heterogeneity of hepatocyte "tight junctions": A quantitative analysis. Hepatology *1*:193, 1981.
12. Easter, D. W., Wade, J. B., Boyer, J. L. Structural integrity of hepatocyte tight junctions. J. Cell Biol. *96*:745, 1983.
13. Friend, D. S., and Gilula, N. B. Variations in tight and gap junctions in mammalian tissues. J. Cell Biol. *53*:758, 1972.
14. Bradley, S. E., and Herz, R. Perselectivity of biliary canalicular membrane in rats: Clearance probe analysis. Am. J. Physiol. *235*:E570, 1978.
15. Reichen, J., Berr, F., and Le, M. Calcium deprivation increases biliary permeability and leads to failure to translocate bile acids in the perfused rat liver. Hepatology *3*:834, 1983 (abstract).
16. Oda, M., Price, V. M., Fisher, M. M., and Phillips, M. J. Ultrastructure of bile canaliculi, with special reference to the surface coat and the pericanalicular web. Lab. Invest. *31*:314, 1974.
17. Oshio, C., and Phillips, M. J. Contractility of the bile canaliculi: Implication for liver function. Science *212*:1041, 1981.
18. Smith, C. R., Osho, C., Miyauri, M., Katz, H., and Philips, M. J. Coordination of the contractile activity of bile canaliculi: Evidence from spontaneous contractions in vitro. Lab. Invest. *53*:270, 1985.
19. Watanabe, S., Smith, C. R., and Phillips, M. J. Coordination of the contractile activity of bile canaliculi: Evidence from calcium microinjection of triplet hepatocytes. Lab. Invest. *53*:275, 1985.
20. Elias, E., Hruban, Z., Wade, J. B., and Boyer, J. L. Phalloidin-induced cholestasis: A microfilament-mediated change in junctional complex permeability. Proc. Natl. Acad. Sci. USA *77*:2229, 1980.
21. Dubin, M., Maurice, M., Feldman, G., and Erlinger, S. Influence of colchicine and phalloidin on bile secretion and hepatic ultrastructure in the rat. Gastroenterology *79*:646, 1980.
22. Gregory, D. H., Vlahcevic, Z. R., Prugh, M. F., and Swell, L. Mechanisms of secretion of biliary lipids: Role of a microtubular system in hepatocellular transport of lipids in the rat. Gastroenterology *74*:93, 1978.
23. Redman, C. M., Banerjee, D., Howell, K., and Palade, G. E. Colchicine inhibition of plasma protein release from rat hepatocytes. J. Cell Biol. *66*:42, 1975.
24. Lake, J., George, P., Licko, V., and Scharschmidt, B. F. Vesicular transport of fluid phase markers (FPM) and ligands by liver: Effects of colchicine and chloroquine. Clin. Res. *33*:322A, 1985 (abstract).
25. Goldman, I. S., Jones, A. L., Hradek, G. T., Huling, S. Hepatocyte handling of immunoglobulin A in the rat: The role of microtubules. Gastroenterology *85*:130, 1983.
26. La Russo, N. F., and Fowler, S. Acid hydrolases in rat bile: Hepatocyte exocytosis of lysosomal protein. Gastroenterology *A32*:1230, 1977 (abstract).
27. Blitzer, B. L., and Boyer, J. L. Cytochemical localization of Na^+,K^+-ATPase in the rat hepatocyte. J. Clin. Invest. *62*:1104, 1978.
28. Latham, P. S., and Kashgarian, M. The ultrastructural localization of transport ATPase in the rat liver at non-bile canalicular plasma membranes. Gastroenterology *76*:988, 1979.
29. Leffert, H. L., Schenk, D. B., Hubert, J. J., Skelly, H., Schumacher, M., Ariyasu, R., Ellisman, M., Koch, K. S., and Keller, G. A. Hepatic (Na^+,K^+)-ATPase: A current view of its structure, function and localization in rat liver as revealed by studies with monoclonal antibodies. Hepatology *5*:501, 1985.
30. Van Dyke, R. W., and Scharschmidt, B. F. (Na,K)-ATPase–mediated cation pumping in cultured rat hepatocytes. J. Biol. Chem. *258*:12912, 1983.
31. Berr, F., Simon, F. R., and Reichen, J. Ethynylestradiol impairs bile salt uptake and Na-K pump function of rat hepatocytes. Am. J. Physiol. *247*:G437, 1984.
32. Keeffe, E. B., Blankenship, N. M., and Scharschmidt, B. F. Alteration of rat liver plasma membrane fluidity and ATPase activity by chlorpromazine hydrochloride and its metabolites. Gastroenterology *79*:222, 1980.
33. Keeffe, E. B., Scharschmidt, B. F., Blankenship, N. M., and Ockner, R. K. Studies of relationships among bile flow, liver plasma membrane Na,K-ATPase microviscosity in the rat. J. Clin. Invest. *64*:1590, 1979.
34. Van Dyke, R. W., Wong, M. A., and Scharschmidt, B. F. Chlorpromazine (CPZ) inhibits Na,K-ATPase cation pumping

and raises intracellular sodium content in cultured rat hepatocytes. Hepatology *3*:869, 1983 (abstract).

35. Graf, J., Henderson, R., Krumpholz, B., and Boyer, J. L. Ionic dependence of intracellular (IC) and canalicular (C) electric potentials (PD) and effects of sodium pump activity in isolated rat hepatocyte couplets (IRHC). Hepatology *5*:1031, 1985 (abstract).
36. Fitz, J. G., and Scharschmidt, B. F. Regulation of transmembrane potential of rat hepatocytes *in situ*. Am. J. Physiol. *252*:G56, 1987.
37. Paloheimo, M., Linkola, J., Lempinen, M., and Folke, M. Time-courses of hepatocellular hyperpolarization and cyclic adenosine 3′,5′-monophosphate accumulation after partial hepatectomy in the rat. Gastroenterology *87*:639, 1984.
38. Aronson, P. S. Electrochemical driving forces for secondary active transport: Energetics and kinetics of Na^+-H^+ exchange and Na^+-glucose cotransport. *In* Blaustein, M. P., and Lieberman, M. (eds.): Electrogenic Transport: Fundamental Principles and Physiological Implications. New York, Raven Press, 1984, p. 49.
39. Boyer, J. L., and Bloomer, J. R. Canalicular bile secretion in man: Studies utilizing the biliary clearance of [^{14}C] mannitol. J. Clin. Invest. *54*:773, 1974.
40. Lindblad, L., Lundholm, K., and Scherston, T. Bile acid concentrations in systemic and portal serum in presumably normal men and in cholestatic and cirrhotic conditions. Scand. J. Gastroenterol. *12*:395, 1977.
41. Jones, A. L., Hradek, G. T., Renston, R. H., Wong, K. Y., Karlanganis, G., and Paumgartner, G. Autoradiographic evidence for a hepatic lobular concentration gradient of a bile acid derivative. Am. J. Physiol. *238*:G233, 1980.
42. Gumucio, J. J., and Miller, D. L. Functional implications of liver cell heterogeneity. Gastroenterology *80*:393, 1981.
43. Duffy, M. C., Blitzer, B. L., and Boyer, J. L. Direct determination of the driving forces for taurocholate uptake into rat liver plasma membrane vesicles. J. Clin. Invest. *72*:1470, 1983.
44. Inoue, M., Kinne, R., Trau, T., and Arias, I. M. Taurocholate transport by rat liver sinusoidal membrane vesicles: Evidence of sodium cotransport. Hepatology *2*:572, 1982.
45. Scharschmidt, B. F., and Stephens, J. F. Transport of sodium, chloride and taurocholate by cultured rat hepatocytes. Proc. Natl. Acad. Sci. U.S.A. *78*:986, 1981.
46. Van Dyke, R. W., Stephens, J. E., and Scharschmidt, B. F. Bile acid transport in cultured rat hepatocytes. Am. J. Physiol. *243*:G484, 1982.
47. Meier, P. J., Meier-Abt, A. S., Barrett, C., and Boyer, J. L. Mechanisms of taurocholate transport in canalicular and basolateral rat liver plasma membrane vesicles. Evidence for an electrogenic canalicular organic anion carrier. J. Biol. Chem. *259*:10614, 1984.
48. Suchy, F. J., Courchene, S. M., and Blitzer, B. L. Taurocholate transport by basolateral plasma membrane vesicles isolated from developing rat liver. Am. J. Physiol. *248*:G648, 1985.
49. Edmundson, J. W., Miller, B. A., and Lumeng, L. Effect of glucagon on hepatic taurocholate uptake: Relationship to membrane potential. Am. J. Physiol. *249*:G427, 1985.
50. Hardison, W. G. M., Bellentani, S., Heasley, V., and Shellhamer, D. Specificity of an Na^+-dependent taurocholate transport site in isolated rat hepatocytes. Am. J. Physiol. *246*:G477, 1984.
51. Hugentobler, G., and Meier, P. J. Multispecific anion exchange in basolateral (sinusoidal) rat liver plasma membrane vesicles. Am. J. Physiol. *251*:G656, 1986.
52. Inoue, M., Kinne, R., Trau, T., and Arias, I. M. Taurocholate transport by rat liver canalicular membrane vesicles. Evidence for the presence of an Na^+-independent transport system. J. Clin. Invest. *73*:659, 1984.
53. Kramer, W., Bickel, U., Buscher, H., -P., Gerok, W., and Kurz, G. Bile-salt–binding polypeptides in plasma membranes of hepatocytes revealed by photoaffinity labelling. Eur. J. Biochem. *129*:13, 1982.
54. Von Dippe, P., Drain, P., and Levy, D. Synthesis and transport characteristics of photoaffinity probes for the hepatocyte bile acid transport system. J. Biol. Chem. *258*:8890, 1983.
55. Meier, P. J., Ruitz, S., Fricken, G., and Landmann, L. Identical bile acid transport systems are present in apical membranes of liver, ileum, and kidney epithelial cells. Hepatology *6*:1134, 1986.
56. Wagner, C. I., Trotman, B. W., and Soloway, R. D. Kinetic analysis of biliary lipid excretion in man and dog. J. Clin. Invest. *57*:473, 1976.
57. Sömjen, G. J., and Gilat, T. Changing concepts of cholesterol solubility in bile. Gastroenterology *91*:772, 1986.
58. Gregory, D. H., Vlahcevic, Z. R., Schatzki, P., and Swell, L. Mechanism of secretion of biliary lipids. I. Role of bile canalicular and microsomal membranes in the synthesis and transport of biliary lecithin and cholesterol. J. Clin. Invest. *55*:105, 1975.
59. Stone, B. G., Erickson, S. K., and Cooper, A. D. Regulation of rat biliary cholesterol secretion by agents that alter intrahepatic cholesterol metabolism: Evidence for a distinct biliary precursor pool. J. Clin. Invest. *76*:1773, 1985.
60. Scharschmidt, B. F., Keeffe, E. B., Vessey, D. A., Blankenship, N. M., and Ockner, R. K. In vitro effect of bile salts on rat liver plasma membrane lipid fluidity and ATPase activity. Hepatology *1*:137, 1981.
61. Anwer, M. S., and Hegner, D. Role of inorganic electrolytes in bile acid–independent canalicular bile formation. Am. J. Physiol. *244*:G116, 1983.
62. Scharschmidt, B. F., Van Dyke, R. W., and Stephens, J. E. Chloride transport by intact rat liver and cultured rat hepatocytes. Am. J. Physiol. *242*:G628, 1982.
63. Fitz, J. G., and Scharschmidt, B. F. Intracellular chloride activity in intact rat liver: relationship to membrane potential and bile flow. Am. J. Physiol. *252*:G699, 1987.
64. Hardison, W. G. M., and Wood, C. A. Importance of bicarbonate in bile salt-independent fraction of bile flow. Am. J. Physiol. *235*:E158, 1978.
65. Van Dyke, R. W., Stephens, J. E., and Scharschmidt, B. F. Effect of ion substitution on bile acid–dependent and bile acid–independent bile formation by the isolated perfused rat liver. J. Clin. Invest. *70*:505, 1982.
66. Barnhart, J. L., and Combes, B. Erythritol and mannitol clearances with taurocholate and secretin-induced choleresis. Am. J. Physiol. *234*:E146, 1978.
67. Dumont, M., Erlinger, S., and Uchman, S. Hypercholeresis induced by ursodeoxycholic acid and 7-ketolithocholic acid in the rat: Possible role of bicarbonate transport. Gastroenterology *79*:82, 1980.
68. Yoon, Y. B., Hagey, L. R., Hofmann, A. F., Gurantz, D., Michelotti, E. L., and Steinbach, J. H. Effect of side chain shortening on the physiological properties of bile acids: Hepatic transport and effect on biliary secretion of 23-nor ursodeoxycholate in rodents. Gastroenterology *90*:837, 1986.
69. Lake, J., Van Dyke, R. W., and Scharschmidt, B. F. Effects of Na^+ replacement and amiloride on ursodeoxycholic acid-stimulated choleresis and biliary bicarbonate secretion. Am. J. Physiol. *252*:G163, 1987.
70. Renner, E., Lake, J. R., Cragoe, E., Van Dyke, R. W., and Scharschmidt, B. F. Ursodeoxycholic acid (UDCA) choleresis: Relationship to biliary HCO_3^- secretion and further evidence of a role for Na^+/H^+ exchange. Hepatology *5*:1011, 1985 (abstract).
71. Van Dyke, R. W., Steer, C. J., and Scharschmidt, B. F. Clathrin-coated vesicles from rat liver: Enzymatic profile and characterization of ATP-dependent proton transport. Proc. Natl. Acad. Sci. USA *81*:3108, 1984.
72. Gluck, S., and Al-Awqati, Q. An electrogenic proton-translocating adenosine triphosphatase from bovine kidney medulla. J. Clin. Invest. *73*:1704, 1984.
73. Lake, J. R., Scharschmidt, B. F., Hagey, L., Gurantz, D., and Hofmann, A. Inhibition of ursodeoxycholic acid (UDCA)-induced hypercholeresis by Na^+ replacement of amiloride (AM) is associated with replacement of unconjugated UDCA by UDCA glucuronides in bile. Hepatology *5*:1010, 1986.
74. Meijer, D. Drug detoxification transport and excretion in the biliary system. *In* Forte, J. B. (ed.): Salivary, Pancreatic, Gastric and Hepatobiliary Secretion. Handbook of Physiology. Bethesda, MD, American Physiological Society, 1986.

75. Mullock, B. M., Dobrata, M., and Hinton, R. H. Sources of the proteins of rat bile. Biochim. Biophys. Acta *543*:497, 1978.
76. Renston, R. H., Jones, A. L., Christiansen, W. D., and Hradek, G. T. Evidence for a vesicular transport mechanism in hepatocytes for biliary secretion of immunoglobulin A. Science *208*:1276, 1980.
77. Ballatori, N., Moseley, R. H., and Boyer, J. L. Sodium-gradient-dependent L-glutamate transport is localized to the canalicular domain of liver plasma membranes. J. Biol. Chem. *261*:6216, 1986.
78. Ballatori, N., Jacob, R., and Boyer, J. L. Intrabiliary glutathione hydrolysis: A source of glutamate in bile. J. Biol. Chem. *261*:7860, 1986.
79. Inoue, M., Kinne, R., Tran, T., and Arias, I. M. The mechanism of biliary secretion of reduced glutathione—Analysis of transport process in isolated rat-liver canalicular membrane vesicles. Eur. J. Biochem. *134*:467, 1983.
80. Lake, J. R., Licko, V., Van Dyke, R. W., and Scharschmidt, B. F. Biliary secretion of fluid-phase markers by the isolated perfused rat liver: Role of transcellular vesicular transport. J. Clin. Invest. *76*:676, 1985.
81. Lowe, P. J., Kam, K. S., Barnwell, S. G., Sharma, R. J., and Coleman, R. Transcytosis and paracellular movements of horseradish peroxidase across liver parenchymal tissue from blood to bile: Effects of α-naphthylisocyanate and colchicine. Biochem. J. *229*:529, 1985.
82. Lake, J., George, P., Licko, V., and Scharschmidt, B. F. Vesicular transport of fluid phase markers (FPM) and ligands by liver: Effects of colchicine and chloroquine. Clin. Res. *33*:322A, 1985 (abstract).
83. Scharschmidt, B. F., Lake, J. R., Licko, V., and Van Dyke, R. W. Fluid phase endocytosis by cultured rat hepatocytes: Implications for plasma turnover and vesicular trafficking of fluid phase markers. Proc. Natl. Acad. Sci. USA *83*:9488, 1986.
84. Strasberg, S. M., Ilson, R. G., Siminovitch, K. A., Brenner, D., and Palaheimo, J. E. Analysis of the components of bile flow in the Rhesus monkey. Am. J. Physiol. *228*:115, 1975.
85. Chenderovitch, J. Secretory function of the rabbit common bile duct. Am. J. Physiol. *223*:695, 1973.
86. Nahrwold, D. L., and Shariatzedeh, A. N. Role of the common bile duct in formation of bile and in gastrin-induced choleresis. Surgery *70*:147, 1971.
87. Hardison, W. G. M., and Norman, J. C. Electrolyte composition of the secretin fraction of bile from the perfused pig liver. Am. J. Physiol. *214*:758, 1968.
88. Jones, R. S., and Grossman, M. I. Choleretic effects of cholecystokinin, gastrin II, and caerulin in the dog. Am. J. Physiol. *219*:1014, 1970.
89. Thulin, L. The choleretic effects in dogs of the synthetic C-terminal octapeptide of cholecystokinin and of two peptide mixtures, G-1 and G-2, derived from upper hog intestine. Acta Clin. Scand. *139*:641, 1973.
90. Gardiner, B. N., and Small, D. M. Simultaneous measurement of the pancreatic and biliary response to CCK and secretin. Primate biliary physiology XIII. Gastroenterology *70*:403, 1976.
91. Wheeler, H. O., Ross, E. D., and Bradley, S. E. Canalicular bile production in dogs. Am. J. Physiol. *214*:866, 1968.
92. Burnett, D. A. Taking the pressure off the sphincter of Oddi. Gastroenterology *87*:971, 1984.
93. Carr-Locke, D. L., and Gregg, J. A. Endoscopic manometry of pancreatic and biliary sphincter zones in man. Dig. Dis. Sci. *26*:7, 1981.
94. Csendes, A., Kruse, A., Finch-Jensen, P., Oster, J. M., Ornshold, J., and Amdrup, E. Pressure measurements in the biliary and pancreatic duct systems in controls and in patients with gallstones, previous cholecystectomy, or common bile duct stones. Gastroenterology 77:1203, 1979.
95. Toouli, J., Hogan, W. J., Geenen, J. E., Doods, W. J., and Arndorfer, R. C. Action of cholecystokinin-octapeptide on sphincter of Oddi basal pressure and phasic wave activity in humans. Surgery *92*:497, 1982.
96. Venu, R., Toouli, J., Hogan, W. J., Helm, J., Dodds, W. J., and Arndorfer, R. C. Effect of morphine on motor activity of the human sphincter of Oddi. Gastroenterology *84*:1342, 1983 (abstract).
97. Bar-Meir, S., Geenen, J. E., Hogan, W. J., Dodds, W. J., Stewart, E. T., and Arndorfer, R. C. Biliary and pancreatic duct pressures measured by ERCP manometry in patients with suspected papillary stenosis. Dig. Dis. Sci. *24*:209, 1979.
98. Funch-Jensen, P., Kruse, A., Csendes, A., Oster, M. J., and Amdrup, E. Biliary manometry in patients with post-cholecystectomy syndrome. Acta Chir. Scand. *148*:267, 1982.
99. Meshkinpour, H., Mollot, M., Eckerling, G. B., and Bookman, I. Bile duct dyskinesia: A clinical and manometric study. Gastroenterology *87*:759, 1984.
100. Hogan, W., Geenen, J., Dodds, W., Toouli, J., Venu, R., and Helm, J. Paradoxical motor response to cholecystokinin (CCK-OP) in patients with suspected sphincter of Oddi dysfunction. Gastroenterology *82*:1085, 1983 (abstract).
101. Geenen, J., Hogan, W., Toouli, J., Dodds, W., and Venu, R. A prospective randomized study of the efficacy of endoscopic sphincterotomy for patients with presumptive sphincter of Oddi dysfunction. Gastroenterology *86*:1086, 1984 (abstract).
102. Lanzini, A., Jazrawi, R. P., and Northfield, T. C. Simultaneous quantitative measurements of absolute gallbladder storage and emptying during fasting and eating in humans. Gastroenterology *92*:852, 1987.
103. Bloom, S. R., Adrian, T. E., Mitchenere, P., Sagor, G. R., and Cristofides, N. D. Motilin-induced gall bladder contraction—a new mechanism. Gastroenterology *80*:1113, 1981.
104. Fisher, R. S., Rock, E., and Malmud, L. S. Gallbladder emptying response to sham feeding in humans. Gastroenterology *90*:1854, 1986.
105. Makhlouf, G. M. Transport and motor functions of the gallbladder. Viewpts. Dig. Dis. *11*(3):1, 1979.
106. Wheeler, H. O. Concentrating function of the gallbladder. Am. J. Med. *51*:588, 1971.
107. Frizzell, R. A., Field, M., and Schultz, S. G. Sodium-coupled chloride transport by epithelial tissues. Am. J. Physiol. *236*:F1, 1979.
108. Duffy, M. E., Turnheim, K., Frizzell, R. A., and Schulz, S. G. Intracellular chloride activities in rabbit gallbladder: Direct evidence for the role of the sodium-gradient in energizing "uphill" chloride transport. J. Memb. Biol. *42*:229, 1978.
109. Svanvik, J., Allen, B., Pelligrini, C., Bernhoft, R., and Way, L. Variations in concentrating function of the gallbladder in conscious monkey. Gastroenterology *86*:919, 1984.
110. Ostrow, J. D. Absorption of bile pigments by the gallbladder. J. Clin. Invest. *46*:2035, 1967.
111. Ostrow, J. D. Absorption by the gallbladder of bile salts, sulfobromophthalein and iodipamide. J. Lab. Clin. Med. *74*:482, 1969.
112. Garberoglio, C. A., Richter, H. M., Henarejos, A., Moossa, A. R., and Baker, A. L. Pharmacological and physiological doses of insulin and determinants of bile flow in dogs. Am. J. Physiol. *245*:G157, 1983.
113. Strasberg, S. M., Petrunka, C. N., Ilson, R. G., and Paloheimo, J. E. Characteristics of inert solute clearance by the monkey liver. Gastroenterology *67*:259, 1979.
114. Meyers, W. C., Hanks, J. B., and Jones, R. S. Inhibition of basal and meal-stimulated choleresis by somatostatin. Surgery *86*:301, 1979.
115. Ricci, G. I., and Fevery, J. Quantitative aspects of the effect of somatostatin on bile flow in the rat. Biochem. Soc. Trans. *8*:53, 1980.
116. Thomsen, O. Ø. Mechanism and regulation of hepatic bile production: With special reference to the bile acid–independent canalicular bile production. Scand. J. Gastroenterol. *19*(suppl. 97):1, 1984.
117. Kaminski, D. L., Brown, W. H., and Deshpandi, Y. G. Effect of glucagon on bile cAMP secretion. Am. J. Physiol. *238*:G119, 1980.
118. Levine, R. A., and Hale, R. C. Cyclic AMP in secretin choleresis: Evidence for a regulatory role in man and baboons but not in dogs. Gastroenterology *70*:537, 1976.

119. Ishak, K. G., and Irey, N. S. Hepatic injury associated with the phenothiazines. Clinicopathologic and follow-up study of 36 patients. Arch. Pathol. *93*:283, 1972.
120. Hruban, Z., Tavaloni, N., Reed, J. S., et al. Ultrastructural changes during cholestasis induced by chlorpromazine in the isolated perfused rat liver. Virchows Arch. (Zellpath) *26*:289, 1978.
121. Samuels, A. M., and Carey, M. C. Effects of chlorpromazine and metabolites on Mg- and Na,K-ATPase of rat liver plasma membranes. Gastroenterology *74*:1183, 1978.
122. Carey, M. C., Hirom, P. C., and Small, D. M. A study of the physicochemical interactions between biliary lipids and chlorpromazine hydrochloride. Biochem. J. *153*:519, 1976.
123. Elias, E., and Boyer, J. L. Chlorpromazine and its metabolites alter polymerization and gelation of actin. Science *206*:1404, 1979.
124. Davis, R. A., Kern, F., Jr., Showalter, R., Sutherland, E., Sinensky, M., and Simon, F. R. Alterations of hepatic Na^+,K^+-ATPase and bile flow by estrogen: Effects of liver surface membrane lipid structure and function. Proc. Natl. Acad. Sci. *75*:4130, 1978.
125. Frezza, M., Pozzato, G., Chiesa, L., Stramentinoli, G., and Di Padova, C. Reversal of intrahepatic cholestasis of pregnancy in woman after high dose S-adenosyl-L-methionine administration. Hepatology *4*:274, 1984.
126. Miyai, K., Mayr, W. W., and Richardson, A. L. Acute cholestasis induced by lithocholic acid in the rat—a freeze fracture replica and thin section study. Lab. Invest. *32*:527, 1975.
127. Layden, T. J., Schwartz, J., and Boyer, J. L. Scanning electron microscopy of the rat liver—studies of the effect of taurolithocholate and other models of cholestasis. Gastroenterology *69*:724, 1975.
128. Kakis, G., and Yousef, I. M. Mechanism of cholic acid protection in lithocholate-induced intrahepatic cholestasis in rats. Gastroenterology *78*(6):1402, 1980.
129. Phillips, M. J., Oda, M., and Fumatsu, K. Evidence for microfilament involvement in norethandrolone-induced intrahepatic cholestasis. Am. J. Pathol. *93*:729, 1978.

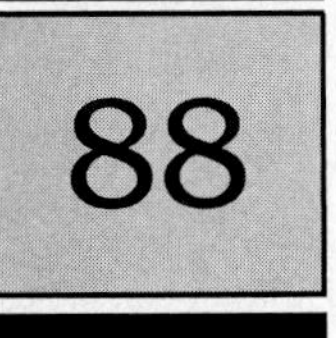

Pathogenesis and Medical Treatment of Gallstones

R. THOMAS HOLZBACH

BACKGROUND

The era of major advances in clinical and basic research on both pathogenesis and treatment of gallstones began about 20 years ago with application of the principles of physical chemistry toward an improved understanding of cholesterol solubilization and transport. The major clinical experimental outcome was the reasonably accurate definition of cholesterol saturation and supersaturation. Supersaturation, the indispensible prerequisite to cholesterol crystallization and precipitation, is the key discovery of this initial advance.

Toward the end of this period the serendipitous discovery that certain, but not most, bile salts when given orally to humans would reduce cholesterol secretion in bile, and thereby reduce its level of saturation, led to treatment of gallstones by resolubilization of gallstone cholesterol, often with partial or complete dissolution. Feeding bile salts was the first nonsurgical treatment for cholesterol gallstones; however, the mechanism by which these agents reduce biliary cholesterol remains unclear. This medical option provoked a desire to gain better insight into the epidemiology and natural history of the clinical disease, and the information gained in these areas has had a major impact on decision making regarding therapy.

Another major technologic advance during this period was the advent of real-time ultrasonography. Its sensitive detection of gallstone disease facilitates prevalence studies in selected populations, and in addition, it is very valuable in studies of human gallbladder motility.

The third great advance has come from investigations of cholesterol crystal nucleation, the initial step in gallstone formation. Almost as important as supersaturation in the pathogenesis of cholesterol gallstones are the factors which promote and inhibit cholesterol crystal nucleation and the balance between them. Discussion of supersaturation and nucleation will occupy a large segment of this chapter's review of the pathogenesis of cholelithiasis.

A recent conceptual advance defines cholesterol solubility in relation to vesicles, hitherto unidentified particles shaped like hollow spheres. The role of vesicles in the transport of cholesterol in bile has clarified a number of issues regarding cholesterol solubility. More important, aggregation of these vesicles may be the initiating step in cholesterol crystal nucleation, with nucleation-promoting and -inhibiting factors likely mediating their effects through interaction with vesicles (see p. 1672).

Thus, the unfolding of the factors important in the pathogenesis of gallstones explains not only the early enthusiasm for medical treatment but also its shortcomings, and hence, the interest in other nonsurgical approaches, such as lithotripsy. Progress has also been made in understanding the pathogenesis of the less common pigment stones. It is slow, however, because of the complex physical chemistry at play in their pathogenesis. To set the stage for an exploration of pathogenesis of all stones, let us first consider their chemical natures.

Gallstone Morphology

With rare exception, human gallstones are morphologically and chemically classified into two categories, i.e., cholesterol stones and pigment stones. Each of these larger groups in turn has two subdivisions. In the case of pigment stones, the main categories are now termed black and brown pigment stones (details of the comparative chemical compositions of pigment stones are considered below). In Western countries pigment stones account for only about 10 per cent of gallstones; the remaining 90 per cent morphologically and chemically are cholesterol stones, either pure (90 per cent cholesterol) or mixed (50 per cent cholesterol). An illustration of typical examples of a pure cholesterol gallstone and of black and brown pigment stones for comparison is given in Figure 88–1.

Of the cholesterol gallstone types, pure stones are less common. These are, as seen in Figure 88–1, generally large (>2.5 cm), pale whitish yellow, and often solitary. The more common mixed cholesterol stones, usually multiple, are also pale yellow and on cross section show a laminated or crystalline structure with a distinct dark central nucleus. Their size spans an intermediate range (0.5 to 2.5 cm) between the larger, solitary, pure cholesterol stones and the smaller pigment stones (<5 mm in diameter). Two characteristics of multiple mixed stones often can be observed: First, closely packed stones of nearly similar size are smooth and faceted upon their contiguous surfaces. Second, occasionally more than one apparent generation can be identified; the position of stones and their uniformity of size reflect different periods of formation.

Pathogenesis of Supersaturated Bile and Cholesterol Cholelithiasis

Underlying Predisposition in Humans. A number of factors underlie the finding of cholesterol-containing stones in the gallbladder. Among these are the virtual insolubility of free cholesterol, the role of the gallbladder in storing aqueous bile, and the strong influence of the liver on amount of cholesterol itself and its water-soluble conversion product, the bile salts excreted into the biliary tract. The crucial factors that directly affect cholesterol solubility in bile include a detergent-based solubilizing system for cholesterol in bile in the form of the abundant biliary lipids, bile salts, and lecithin (phospholipid) secreted by the liver (see pp. 1656–1662). The combination of these lipids with cholesterol in at least two aggregated particulate forms is responsible for the enormously greater apparent solubility of cholesterol in an aqueous system (bile) than could otherwise be possible. In addition, of all

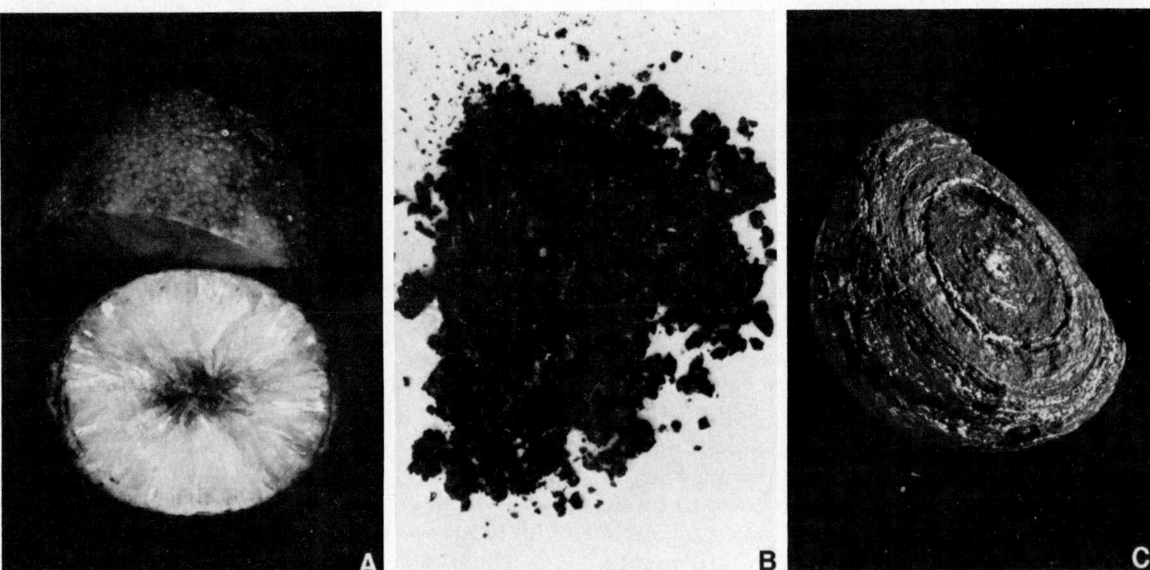

Figure 88–1. Various representative types of gallstones as indicated by both morphologic features and chemical composition. *A*, Large solitary "pure" cholesterol stone with pigmented center and whitish radiating crystalline highlights when sectioned. *B*, Features of "black" pigmented stones that are heterogeneously small and comparatively amorphous. *C*, Features of the rarer form of "brown" pigment stone with typical lamination.

animal species humans alone secrete sufficiently high amounts of cholesterol in bile to exceed the solubilization saturation limit, biliary cholesterol supersaturation, the physical-chemical state in which cholesterol gallstones spontaneously form.

It is reasonable to believe that the pathogenesis proceeds sequentially, beginning with one or more metabolic or disease-related defects in the secretion of biliary lipids, resulting in cholesterol supersaturation (or excessive supersaturation) of bile. At a later and crucial stage, cholesterol is no longer soluble in the supersaturated system, and perhaps by aggregation of transport vesicles, it progressively forms crystal nucleates in the gallbladder. The resulting crystals grow and cluster with each other and with other bile constituents—e.g., mucin, bilirubin, calcium—to form recognizable stones. At the most fundamental level, however, the defects in bile which initiate nucleation and culminate in cholelithiasis remain incompletely understood.

Defects in Biliary Lipid Secretion. The two metabolic or disease-related defects in biliary lipid secretion that produce cholesterol supersaturation of bile are, respectively, *increased cholesterol synthesis* leading to biliary cholesterol hypersecretion and *decreased bile salt secretion.* These defects occasionally combine. Although lecithin is as important as bile salts in solubilizing cholesterol, its secretion is closely linked to secretion of bile salts; in fact, an isolated secretory defect of lecithin has never been identified. Simultaneous cholesterol secretion rates are much less closely linked to bile salt secretion, especially at low flow rates, and, therefore, an unrelated defect in cholesterol secretion is more clearly and commonly discernible.

A summary of the relationship of these secretory defects of bile to specific metabolic states or diseases is given in Table 88–1. Well-documented examples of conditions related to increased cholesterol synthesis leading to biliary cholesterol hypersecretion as the primary or sole metabolic defect include the following: obesity, specific nonobese Caucasians, aging, oral contraceptive steroids in women, and pregnancy.[1–17] Decrease in biliary bile salt secretion due to a putative regulatory defect in bile salt synthesis seen in phenotypically normal nonobese healthy persons[5, 6, 18] can be a secondary consequence of excessive alimentary bile salt loss caused, for example, by ileal disease or resection (see pp. 152–155). The existence of a combination of increased cholesterol secretion and bile salt deficiency has been demonstrated only in a population of obese Amerindian females with gallstones.[19]

Although the majority of these defects in Table 88–1 are primarily genetic in origin, and are poorly understood, the correlation between biliary cholesterol hypersecretion and aging is intriguing for two reasons. It could help explain the increased incidence of gallstones in older persons, and suggests some unknown acquired or environmental factor that over time contributes to biliary cholesterol hypersecretion.[10, 11] Information on the mechanisms by which female hormones cause biliary cholesterol hypersecretion is also incomplete. The

Table 88–1. MECHANISTIC DEFECTS AND RELATED STATES OR DISEASES ASSOCIATED WITH SUPERSATURATED BILE AND CHOLESTEROL GALLSTONE FORMATION

Defects	Related States or Diseases
Biliary cholesterol hypersecretion	Obesity, specific nonobese Caucasian populations, e.g., European and Chilean patients, aging, contraceptive steroids and pregnancy in women, familial hyperlipoproteinemia (types IV and IIb), reduced serum HDL, hypolipidemic therapy (e.g., clofibrate, colestipol, and cholestyramine), diabetes mellitus, marked dietary weight reduction, acute high calorie intake, chronic polyunsaturated fat diet
Biliary bile salt hyposecretion	a. *Abnormally hypersensitive bile salt feedback mechanism—unknown cause,* presumably racial-genetic in apparently normal patients with cholelithiasis b. *Impaired bile salt synthesis*—cerebrotendinous xanthomatosis, congenital 12 α-hydroxylase deficiency, and chronic cholestatic liver diseases, e.g., primary biliary cirrhosis, primary sclerosing cholangitis, etc. c. *Abnormal intestinal bile salt loss*—major ileal disease, resection or bypass, cystic fibrosis with pancreatic insufficiency, primary bile salt malabsorption
Combined defects of cholesterol hypersecretion and bile salt hyposecretion	a. Racial-genetic (associated with massive obesity) in American Indians b. Nonobese Caucasians of diverse groups having no known predisposing factors
Impaired gallbladder function with incomplete emptying and stasis	Last trimester pregnancy, total parenteral nutrition, chronic idiopathic and acalculous cholecystitis, contraceptive steroids in women, unknown causes, e.g., (?) defective neuroendocrine responsiveness

best available evidence, however, suggests that estrogens induce an increase in dietary cholesterol uptake by the liver via chylomicron remnants.[16] In addition, cholesterol stored in the liver is predominantly in its esterified form. The progestin component of female hormones (or oral contraceptives) converts the esterified (storage) form of liver cholesterol to the free form, thus facilitating its mobilization and potential availability for secretion in bile.[16, 17]

The existence of biliary acid hyposecretion attributable to a solitary genetic regulatory defect in nonobese Caucasians has recently been questioned but not disproved. The problem arises from use of dissimilar biliary lipid output measurements resulting from use of two dissimilar intraduodenal perfusion formulas for stimulation of bile flow and cycling rate of the enterohepatic circulation. Many such measurements have been made using a perfusion formula containing 40 per cent of calories as fat.[1–3, 8, 13, 17, 19, 20] Other, more recent, studies have instead used a mixed amino acid solution.[4–7, 9, 11, 12, 14] A recent comparative study of healthy subjects utilizing both of these two perfusion formulas found that with 40 per cent fat perfusion, gallbladder emptying was more complete, intestinal transit more rapid, and secretion rates of all lipids were greater with a reduction in the molar concentration for cholesterol. The conclusions drawn from these results were the following: first, bile acid secretion rates were lower during amino acid infusion because enterohepatic cycling of the bile acid pool was lower compared to that with fat infusion. Also, the lower molar percentage of cholesterol secretion in bile during fat infusion is compatible with the known hyperbolic relationship of cholesterol secretion to bile acid secretion (see p. 1673). The significance of this study lies in the demonstration that if either gallbladder function or intestinal transit differs between groups of study subjects (including healthy control subjects), differences in biliary lipid secretion might be due to an altered enterohepatic cycling rate and not to a primary abnormality of hepatic secretion.[21] To underscore this point, functional gallbladder impairment secondary to gallstone disease has been shown to reduce bile acid pool size, increase enterohepatic cycling, and reduce saturation of cholesterol in bile, an effect similar to that of cholecystectomy[5, 18, 22] (see pp. 152–155).

Relevance of the Regulation of Biliary Cholesterol Secretion to Pathogenesis

The Role of the Liver. About 50 per cent of the total endogenous synthesis of cholesterol is accounted for by the liver.[23] Only about 20 per cent of *biliary* cholesterol, however, is newly synthesized in the liver, and about 80 per cent of it is preformed.[24–26] Much of this preformed cholesterol had been made in the liver, exported to peripheral tissues, and then recycled back to the liver in the form of lipoproteins.[27] This pool is only slightly augmented by minor contributions of cholesterol from other organs. It constitutes the preformed hepatic cholesterol secreted into bile.

Despite daily variability of the body's cholesterol intake and excretion, the liver (as well as all other organs) maintains a sterol balance. A simplified summary of this balance of input and output fluxes affecting sterol balance for the liver cell itself is depicted in Figure 88–2. Each of the major input and output pathways is subject to extremely close metabolic regulation, resulting in little or no net accumulation of cholesterol in the liver. Hence, any increase in delivery of cholesterol to the liver is accompanied by a balanced and reciprocal suppression of the rate of cholesterol synthesis. It is unimportant whether the increased input is from dietary cholesterol or via the various lipoprotein pathways originating in peripheral extrahepatic tissues. Because of this reciprocal adaptive response in sterol synthesis in the liver cell, the rate of bile acid synthesis and secretion, biliary cholesterol secretion, and LDL-receptor synthesis change little, if at all.[28–40]

Conversely, if sterol is lost excessively via the bile acid pathway in certain clinical situations, the rate of cholesterol synthesis increases. Because liver cells store cholesterol in its esterified state (Fig. 88–2), there must be an as yet unidentified feedback response mechanism sensitive to the magnitude of this pool of esterified cholesterol. As a result of these feedback regulations, the cellular subcompartment of sterol from which biliary cholesterol is mobilized remains essentially constant in the steady state. In the steady state, the amount of cholesterol in the liver cell pool(s) that can be mobilized into bile by a specific bile acid is constant.[41, 42] This implies that this intracellular sterol pool(s) must

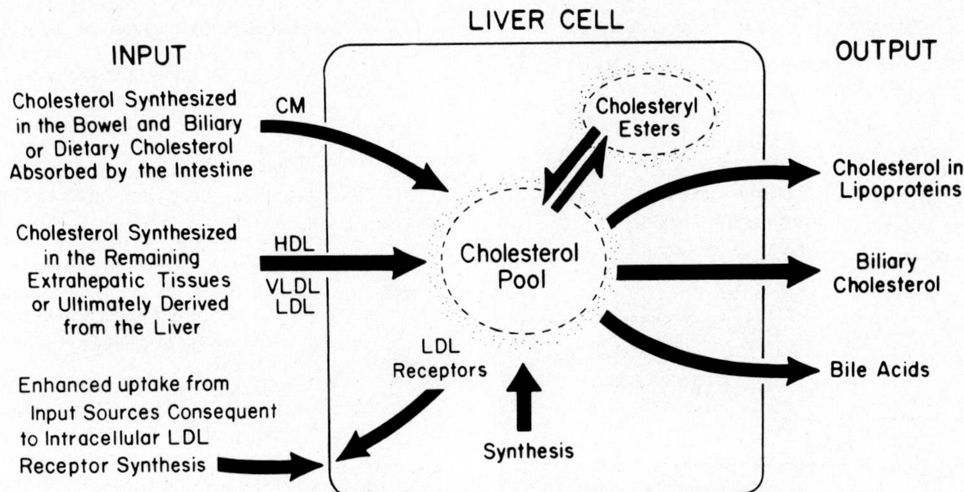

Figure 88–2. Cholesterol balance across the liver. Major sources for cholesterol entering the hepatocyte and the major pathways for the disposition of sterol from the liver are summarized. (Modified from Turley, S. D., and Dietschy, J. M. Cholesterol metabolism and excretion. *In* Arias, I. M., Popper, H., Schacter, D., and Shafritz, D. A. [eds.] The Liver: Biology and Pathobiology. New York, Raven Press, 1982, p. 479. Used by permission.)

be either identical to the pool(s) regulating inputs from both synthesis and receptor-dependent cholesterol uptake or at least in close equilibrium with them.

In light of these exquisitely fine-tuned regulatory controls of secretory output of cholesterol in bile, how does one explain the occurrence of biliary cholesterol hypersecretion? Preliminary studies in animals have recently shown that certain exogenous substances, i.e., drugs, such as mevinolin (new designation, Mevacor), are capable of reversibly inhibiting certain of the regulatory pathways, markedly reducing the liver cell cholesterol pool(s) from which biliary cholesterol is mobilized. Upon acute withdrawal from such an agent, an induced temporary imbalance occurs, resulting in a transient excessively high rate of hepatic cholesterol synthesis and overexpansion of the cholesterol pool(s). This is then accompanied by a marked hypersecretion of biliary cholesterol as an extraordinary compensatory response to help maintain liver cell cholesterol homeostasis (Dietschy, J. M., personal communication). The induced imbalance with resulting biliary cholesterol hypersecretion can be either acute or chronic. Such a defect in normal regulatory pathways must, for example, account for the very high levels of hepatic cholesterol found in a group of Chilean women with biliary cholesterol hypersecretion compared with men from a similar population. The sex difference remained consistent whether or not patients in the two groups had cholesterol gallstone disease.[43]

To summarize, increased biliary secretion of cholesterol does not seem to be due to increased liver cell accumulation of cholesterol from any of the input pathways because of reciprocal regulatory responses maintaining an intracellular homeostatic sterol balance through one of the several alternate pathways[44] (Fig. 88–2). An imbalance or disturbance in these regulatory mechanisms and pathways may result from genetic, environmental (xenobiotic exposure), hormonal, or other factors that lead to uncompensated liver cell accumulation of cholesterol. In consequence, hypersecretion of biliary cholesterol may be the abnormal compensatory response. Let us now look at factors which keep cholesterol in solution.

Roles of Secretion of Bile Salts and Other Biliary Lipids

Participation by Vesicles in Cholesterol Solubilization. Until recently, the conventional assumption has been that cholesterol in bile is entirely solubilized by bile salt and lecithin mixed micelles. As a consequence of this theoretical construct, phase-equilibrium diagrams and derivative lipid molar ratios have been devised to describe and define the solubility of cholesterol in either artificial or native biles of defined lipid composition, an example of which is given in Figure 88–3.[45–47] The resultant definition has been termed a cholesterol saturation (or less accurately, a "lithogenic") index. The prevailing view that essentially all cholesterol in bile is solubilized and transported by micelles, however, has recently undergone a drastic reappraisal based upon independent findings from several groups.[48–59] These studies have shown that com-

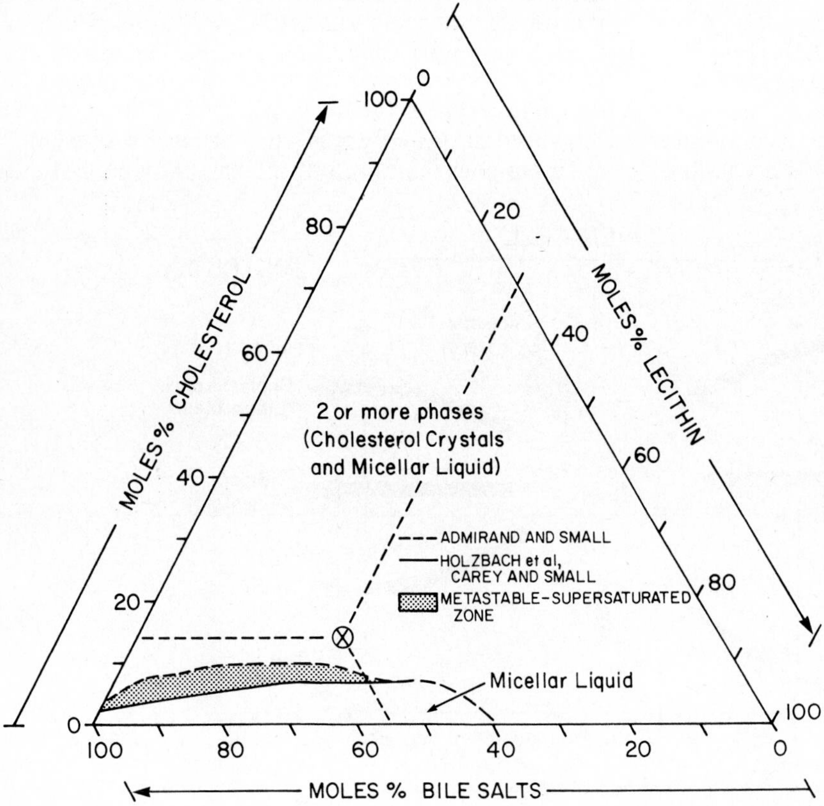

Figure 88–3. Determination of cholesterol saturation index (CSI). Tricoordinate phase diagram for representing by a single intersecting point ⊗ the relative concentrations of cholesterol, lecithin, and bile salt in bile. In this scheme, the relative concentration of each lipid is expressed as a percentage of the sum of the molar concentrations of all three. This manipulation permits representation of the relations between three constituents in two dimensions, the water content being invariant at, say, 90 per cent (10 per cent W/V solids).

In this figure, for example, at the point ⊗ the relative concentration of bile salt from its coordinate is 55 per cent (indicating 55 per cent of the sum of all three lipids), whereas that for lecithin is 30 per cent, and that for cholesterol is 15 per cent. The range of concentrations found consistent with a clear aqueous micellar solution is limited to a small region at the lower left. A solution having the composition represented by the point, on the other hand, would initially be visually turbid and contain precipitated forms of cholesterol crystals in addition to bile salt mixed micelles.

Lastly, a solution represented by a point falling in the shaded area below the dashed line would be unstable (i.e., metastable-supersaturated), meaning that by prediction it would be initially clear (micellar). Within a short time, however, vesicles and various precipitated forms of cholesterol crystals would form, and such a solution would then be visually turbid, similar to all solutions above the dashed line.

paratively abundant phospholipid *vesicles* participate in the solubilizing and transporting of cholesterol in both artificial and native bile (Fig. 88–4). The actual amount or proportion of cholesterol solubilized and transported in these *in vitro* and *in vivo* solutions has been found to vary considerably depending primarily upon physiologic circumstances that affect both differences in lipid composition and in degree of dilution.[53–55] Among other findings, for example, variations in the bile salt flow rate have been shown to alter the distribution of cholesterol transport between biliary micelles and vesicles. Thus, at low bile salt flow rates as observed in the fasting state, compared with the postprandial state, there is a shift toward a greater proportion of total cholesterol in the system being transported in vesicles.[56, 57] In addition, vesicles experimentally isolated from dilute hepatic bile in the presence of artificially raised bile salt concentrations, i.e., stimulated secretion, have been found to dissolve upon equilibration, so that the estimated vesicular contribution to cholesterol transport will appear to have become reduced.[57] These results indirectly suggest that biliary vesicles may actually be a mode of exocytotic lipid secretion by hepatocytes, but the details regarding this at present are far from certain.

Coordinate Secretion. Relatively few patients with cholesterol gallstones have diminished bile salt secretion resulting from clinical situations, e.g., extensive intestinal, especially ileal, inflammatory disease or surgical resection or bypass of a long (> 100 cm) segment of terminal ileum. The vast majority with cholesterol gallstones and diminished bile salt secretion have no obvious explanation for their defective homeostatic regulatory mechanism. This defect is found predominantly in nonobese caucasian patients who have significant reductions in bile acid pool size combined with

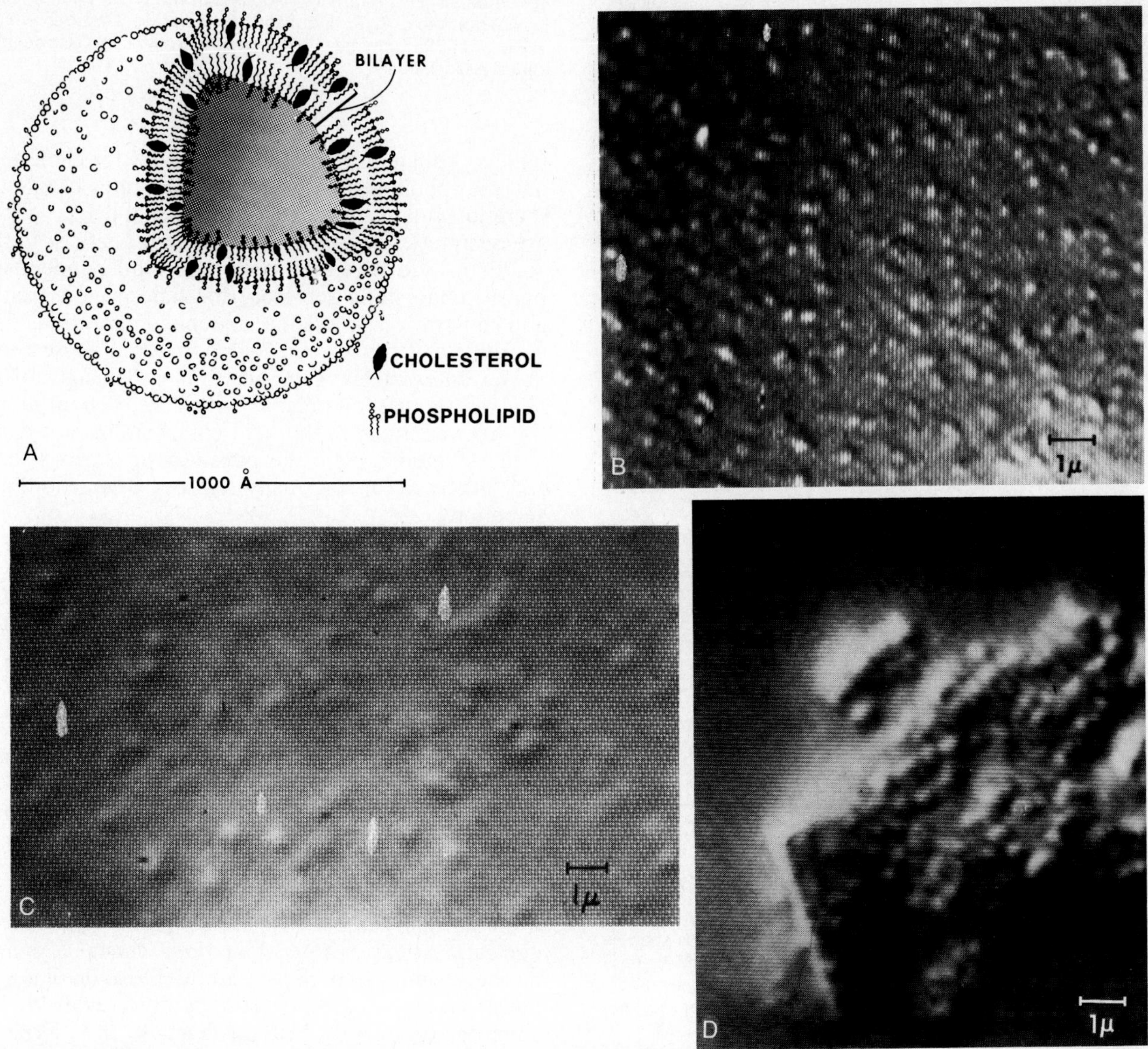

Figure 88–4. Biliary unilamellar vesicles composed of phospholipid (lecithin) and cholesterol. *A*, Schematic view; *B*, vesicles in supersaturated model bile solution; *C*, vesicles in normal human bile; and *D*, aggregated vesicles adherent to cholesterol crystal in a gallstone-associated human bile. (*B*, *C*, and *D* are from author's unpublished observations using video-enhanced microscopy.)

at least a moderate reduction in bile acid enterohepatic circulation (EHC) cycling rate[5, 6, 18, 60] (see pp. 150–155). No evidence exists in these patients for either an impairment of bile acid synthesis rates or impaired intestinal absorption. Thus, it has been believed that the most likely explanation is a complex two-component regulatory defect resulting in inappropriate feedback control of *de novo* bile acid synthesis.[5] The first regulatory defect somehow allows a reduction in bile acid pool size. A normal response to the "sensing" of this reduced bile acid pool size should be derepression (and therefore stimulation) of synthesis with a compensatory increase in the rate of bile acid production by increased activity of the rate-limiting enzyme, hepatic microsomal 7α-hydroxylase.[61] This compensatory mechanism is somehow blunted, and very likely comprises the second regulatory defect in nonobese caucasian cholesterol gallstone patients. This two-component regulatory mechanism is responsible for maintaining an adequate bile salt output in some normal subjects in whom the bile salt pool is low by increasing their bile salt enterohepatic cycling frequency sufficient to maintain a normal bile salt output.

Within the spectrum of high and low ranges of bile salt secretory rate, a tight linkage or coordinate secretion has been observed with lecithin (phospholipid) as well as cholesterol secretory rates (Fig. 88–5).[62] In this typical plot of coordinate secretory rates, both lecithin and cholesterol can be seen to approach a secretory maximum (asymptote) as bile salt secretion increases. A reasonable deduction is that there must be some as yet unidentified but effective rate-limiting step in secretion for lecithin and cholesterol. Figure 88–5 also shows that at high rates of bile salt secretion, there is tight coordination of the secretory rates for cholesterol and phospholipid. In contrast, at low rates of bile salt secretion relatively more cholesterol and less lecithin are secreted. This difference in coordinate secretion could be due to either completely independent and poorly understood secretory mechanisms for lecithin and cholesterol, or to some undefined alteration of the coordinate secretory phenomenon for their secretion at low rates of bile salt secretion.[63–66] In light of the new information on biliary vesicles (see below), it may be that variations in the lipid composition of secreted vesicles could explain the presently mysterious secretory processes operationally referred to as coordinate secretion.

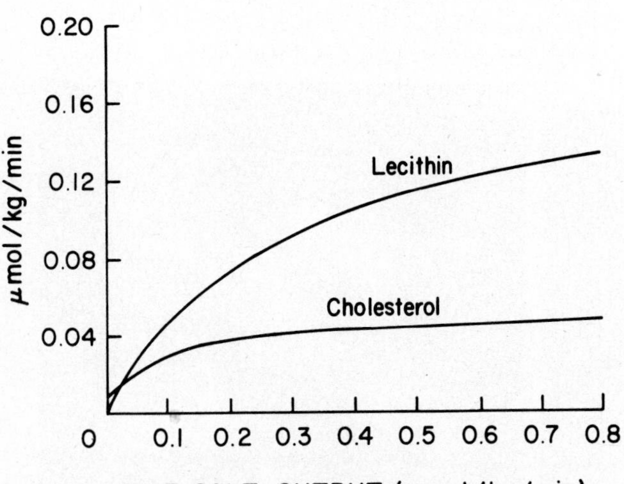

Figure 88–5. Relation of biliary salt secretory output rate to that for biliary cholesterol and lecithin. A hyperbolic relation is seen as the secretory rate for the two biliary lipids (cholesterol and lecithin) approaches a maximum with increasing rates of bile salt secretion. At low rates of bile salt secretion (i.e., below 0.16 μmol per kilogram of body weight per minute), as frequently observed after an overnight fast, relatively more cholesterol and less lecithin are secreted, resulting in biliary cholesterol supersaturation. (Adapted from human data of Wagner, C. I., Trotman, B. W., and Soloway, R. D. J. Clin. Invest. 57:473, 1976. Used by permission.)

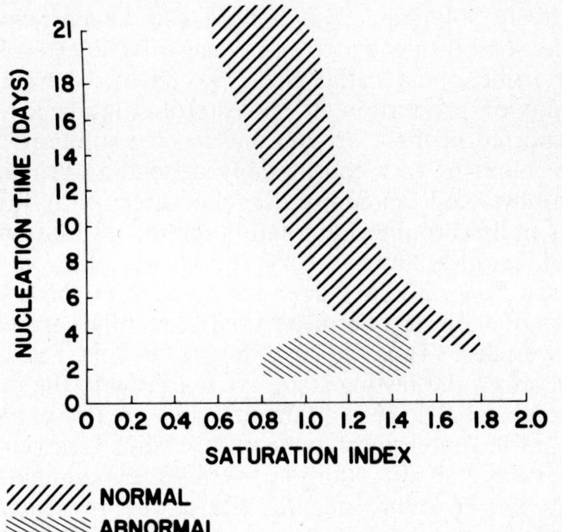

Figure 88–6. Nucleation time as a function of cholesterol saturation index for bile in patients with cholesterol gallstone (abnormal) and in control subjects (normal). (Modified from human data of Holan, K. R., Holzbach, R. T., Hermann, R. E., et al. Gastroenterology 72:611, 1979. Copyright 1979 by The American Gastroenterological Association.)

Regardless, stones must begin as tiny crystals of cholesterol. Supersaturation of bile with cholesterol *per se* is insufficient to explain cholelithiasis. What influences crystal formation, also called nucleation, therefore, is important to consider.

Cholesterol Crystal Nucleation in Bile

Nucleation of cholesterol monohydrate crystals is an essential antecedent to gallstone formation. It is now generally agreed that nucleation is much more rapid in gallbladder bile from patients with cholesterol cholelithiasis (abnormal) than it does in gallbladder bile from normal subjects.[67–71] Indeed, this difference in nucleation time or rate of *de novo* crystal formation has been shown to permit clearer delineation of normal bile from abnormal bile than any other available biochemical or physical criteria (Fig. 88–6).[67] Evidence now available supports the view that the difference in nucleation time between normal and abnormal subjects is explicable on the basis of the operation of two separate, uncharacterized nucleating factors having opposing functional properties, i.e., "inhibiting" and "promoting." These influences can be demonstrated under appropriate conditions.[72–74]

It now seems clear in gallstone disease that a potent nucleation-promoting agent is present.[74] It is not yet clear, however, whether the concentration of inhibiting agent(s) in bile of patients with gallstones is reduced or even absent.[72–74] Likewise, it is unknown whether bile in normal subjects (who surely have the nucleation-inhibiting agents) also has promoting agent(s), albeit in small quantities. Most important, we do not know whether the disease process "turns on" secretion of the promoting factors, or whether the disease process itself is largely a consequence of an increased secretion of the promoting substance. The coexistence of crystallization promoting and inhibiting factors is not a unique event. Rather, it is an ubiquitous biological phenomenon in which small amounts of protein are an adequate matrix for crystallization, the first step in the formation of kidney stones, bone, dental enamel, and possibly ice crystal formation prevented by antifreeze proteins.[75–80] The cascade of factors regulating blood coagulation provides a classical model of the balance of promoting and inhibiting activities which prevents crystallization. The mechanism(s) whereby these proteins exert their effects may well differ considerably, however, from those in bile. This is because they affect ionic electrolyte solutions rather than predominantly colloidal micellar solutions and because their effects are more probably on inhibition of crystal growth, rather than upon crystal nucleation *per se*.

Vesicles, cholesterol carriers, may also help our understanding of cholesterol crystal nucleation. Perhaps the presence of vesicles in bile may account for the frequently observed and hitherto unexplained degree of metastable supersaturation and prolonged duration of stability of cholesterol solubilized in supersaturated human bile. For example, hepatic bile, despite marked cholesterol supersaturation, is resistant to cholesterol crystal nucleation.[69] Perhaps crystals don't appear in supersaturated samples because they contain an abundance of phospholipid vesicles that may transport proportionately more cholesterol than do the bile salt mixed lipid micelles. Further, vesicles in a dilute system such as hepatic bile are relatively unsaturated in cholesterol.[55] This latter finding may be of key importance in understanding the stability and comparative amount of total cholesterol than can be transported in dilute solutions such as those which are artificially made or found in canalicular and hepatic bile. In bile supersaturated with cholesterol, by contrast, isolated vesicles are comparatively cholesterol-rich and the solutions are more prone to nucleation.[55] Increased bile salt/phospholipid ratios and ionized calcium have also been shown to reduce vesicular stability.[53] Recently, both *in vitro,* i.e., model bile solutions, and *in vivo,* i.e., native bile, studies have suggested that vesicle aggregation may be the underlying physical phenomenon of cholesterol nucleation.[54, 55] Although evidence exists that the nucleation-inhibiting factor is most likely a protein, controversy exists whether the nucleation-promoting factor is either primarily a protein, or a lattice-like matrix formed of mucin glycoprotein, complexed with calcium bilirubinate or possibly even both.[73, 74, 81–87]

Role of the Gallbladder in Cholesterol Gallstone Formation

During overnight fasting in humans, approximately 50 to 60 per cent of the total bile acid pool and associated biliary lipids are stored in the gallbladder.[88, 89] Studies of cholesterol and of other biliary lipids in gallbladder bile of patients with cholesterol gallstone disease show the ability of the gallbladder to disturb the coordinate output of bile salts and of biliary lipids significantly[90, 91] (see pp. 144–161). Thus, the degree of cholesterol saturation is heightened and availability of bile salts is diminished by sequestration of bile acids in the gallbladder during fasting, although this effect is mitigated in many persons by direct flow of bile from hepatic ducts to the common duct. In others, this bypass is insufficient and most of the lipid sequesters in the gallbladder with marked increases in biliary cholesterol saturation during fasting. Acute depletion of the bile acid pool also increases cholesterol saturation in gallbladder bile, although after meals the cholesterol level in bile bypassing the gallbladder is unchanged.[91]

Cholescintigraphy and real-time ultrasonography have made possible *in vivo* study of gallbladder emptying.[92] These noninvasive techniques definitely demonstrate gallbladder stasis as a risk factor for cholelithiasis in both studies of patients receiving prolonged parenteral hyperalimentation and in animals with experimentally induced gallbladder stasis.[93–101] Cholelithiasis is associated with impaired gallbladder emptying, thus perpetuating the problem.[102–106]

Two additional situations in females impair emptying and predispose to stone formation: *pregnancy* and *oral contraceptives*. In pregnancy, the gallbladder emptying rate decreases progressively with duration of gestation. Gallbladder volume increases upon fasting, as does residual gallbladder volume after contraction. These changes, indicating stasis, disappear in the postpartum period. Oral contraceptives also cause stasis, in the same ways, albeit less dramatically.[107, 108] These changes in gallbladder function (increased fasting gallbladder volume and a reduced emptying rate) are also found only in the progestational phase of stable menstrual cycles.[109] Thus, it is unclear whether estrogens, progestins, or a combination are principally responsible for these alterations in gallbladder function.

Prolonged parenteral hyperalimentation also causes gallbladder stasis more severe than in other conditions. It causes the formation of an amorphous material termed "biliary sludge" as detected by serial ultrasonography. This term typically refers to a sonographic finding characterized by intraluminal crescentic echoes referred from the dependent portion of the gallbladder.[110] With displacement in the position of the patient from erect to horizontal, the echogenic material can be seen to shift, maintaining its dependent location. Acoustic shadowing, a sonographic feature typical of gallstone disease, is not seen in the presence of biliary sludge.[111]

Microscopically, sludge exhibits both cholesterol monohydrate crystals and bilirubin (presumably insoluble calcium bilirubinate) granules embedded in a matrix of mucus gel. The amount of mucus glycoprotein is strikingly increased compared with bile from patients with gallstones or from normal persons. The origin of the increased mucus in biliary sludge appears to be the gallbladder, the mucosa of which invariably shows evidence of epithelial mucus hypersecretion and early glandular hyperplasia.[112] Serial ultrasonographic studies of patients undergoing total parenteral nutrition (TPN) have revealed that the incidence of sludge increases from 6 per cent during the first three weeks to more than 50 per cent between the fourth and sixth weeks, and reaches 100 per cent after six weeks. Further, gallstones develop in about 50 per cent of sludge-forming patients, but not in patients with no sludge. However, these patients are quite ill and have additional factors, e.g., metabolic, which contribute to stone formation. A majority of patients with sludge due to TPN lose it with restoration of oral feedings. How much TPN-type sludge is formed in patients with a much lesser degree of gallbladder stasis (pregnancy and women taking oral contraceptives) is unknown. If found in these conditions of stasis, hormonal effects will emerge as a common, if not a universal, cause of gallbladder stasis. Certainly, the well-documented higher incidence of cholesterol gallstone disease in premenopausal women than in men lends credence to this view (see p. 1677).

EPIDEMIOLOGY AND NATURAL HISTORY

Epidemiology

The gallstone prevalence rate in England, most of the industrialized countries of Western Europe, and the United States is in the range of 10 to 20 per cent (Fig. 88–7).[113–118] Sweden and Chile previously have been widely held to have the highest prevalence rates for cholesterol gallstones; the figures for the Swedish population are from two autopsy studies in the Malmö area done in the late 1960s.[119, 120] Both were conducted in an area with an autopsy rate of about 90 per cent, but were biased by a strikingly disproportionate number of older persons, thus enhancing the prevalence estimate for an age-correlated disease. Recent prospective population surveys in Sweden, including Malmö, however, indicate a 50 per cent decrease in prevalence since 1970 with a concomitant decrease in the rate of cholecystectomy.[121–123] The reason for this reduction in prevalence, especially among younger patients (age < 40 years) is unclear. It may be peculiar to Sweden, or more likely, it may only reflect a similar, undocumented trend in other Western industrialized countries. Prevalence studies in other Caucasian population groups would be valuable. Two independent 10-year prospective Italian studies of prevalence and natural history of gallstones are under way in two widely different populations: The Grepco Study of civil servants in Rome and the "Sermione Study" surveying the entire population of a rural small-town population on Lake Garda.[124, 125]

Genetic Influences

The prevalence rate in Chile is astonishingly high, about double that of countries with a moderately high prevalence, e.g., Australia, United States, and Japan. Prevalence rates in Afro-Asian countries are very low.[114, 115] The very high prevalence rate from autopsies in Chile, along with anecdotal evidence from neighboring Bolivia, suggests the operation of some as yet undefined ethnic-genetic risk factor in these populations.[126, 127] Because prevalence rates among the Araucanian Indians of Chile are very high and the genetic admixture of indigenous native Americans genetically similar to the Araucanian Indians and the Spanish has been widespread, this genetic factor may explain the high rates in these countries and in adjacent countries of South and Central America.[9, 128, 129]

The extraordinarily high prevalence rates of cholesterol gallstone disease in Native Americans seems to be ubiquitous and not restricted to only one tribe or geographic location. Thus, the earliest reports concerning this linkage provided data on the Navajos and Pimas of the American Southwest.[130, 131] More recent studies have documented a very high prevalence among the Chippewas of northern Minnesota, the Micmacs of Nova Scotia, and Native Americans in Alaska.[132–134] Analogous to the Chilean population, the prevalence of gallbladder disease among Mexican-Americans in Texas is approximately twice that of non-Hispanic Texas Caucasians. This genetic admixture hypothesis is supported by the finding that Mexican-Americans in Texas have a prevalence of gallbladder disease between the rates of Native Americans (e.g., Pimas) and non-Hispanic Caucasians and the strong likelihood that most Mexican-Americans are "mestizos," i.e., a genetic admixture of European Caucasians and Native Americans.[135–141]

The data on prevalence of gallstones derived from autopsies rarely contain information about the composition of stones. Despite this limitation, it is reasonable to believe that the prevalence of pigment gallstones worldwide is small compared to that of cholesterol gallstones. The very high prevalence rates for cholesterol gallstone disease must be due to these genetic influences, especially in smaller isolated population groups and in many family clusters as well as in large ethnic populations and in those with genetic admixtures.[142–144]

Influence of Sex

In addition to the information on worldwide prevalence of gallstone disease in Figure 88–7, prevalence rates for gallstones in females are consistently approximately twice those in males. This phenomenon has been attributed to hormonal factors such as pregnancy and sex hormones, both endogenous and exogenous (oral contraceptives). As noted above, female sex hormones induce gallbladder stasis, and oral contraceptive steroids and pregnancy are associated with hepatic hypersecretion of cholesterol.[12–17, 107–109] Clearly, they are important in pathogenesis of cholelithiasis in women. Yet epidemiologic data on the point are not entirely supportive.[145–147] Thus, an ongoing long-term study has indicated that there is no overall increased risk of gallstones from long-term oral contraceptive use.[148] Both this study and a recent case-control study reconcile some of the disparate findings of previous reports by confirming a previous observation that there is indeed an increased risk of gallstones, but only with short-term (< 5 years) use of oral contraceptives.[148, 149] This risk appears to be due to an acceleration of gallstone disease only in women already predisposed by some metabolic (genetic) defect.[148, 149] The acceleration may affect symptomatic manifestations as well as expression of the disease.[150] With respect to oral contraceptives, the findings of the case-control study also indicate that the risk of associated gallstones is increased only in women up to 29 years of age.[149] With respect to pregnancy, for women under 50 years of age, the relative risk of developing gallstones correlated with the number of pregnancies and was 1.5 to 2.5 times that of the control group.[149] This finding reasonably leads to the deduction that for women who develop gallstones in relation to pregnancy and those in whom stones develop with oral contraceptives the cause is probably the same.

Further support for the endocrine influence in pathogenesis of gallstones in particular women is that the urinary excretion of estrone is significantly higher in women over 50 years of age with gallstones than in control patients over 50, but is not different from female control subjects who have gallstones and are under 50 years old. Neither onset of menopause, nor the mean duration of various indices of ovarian activity (and, therefore, of exposure to endogenous estrogens) differed between the patient groups and their matched control group.

These data suggest the possibility that in postmenopausal women, the increased risk (and indeed the high prevalence) of gallstones is more likely to be due to the intensity of hormonal exposure rather than duration. The pathogenetic mechanism, as noted above, is that oral contraceptives at sufficiently high doses in some women can increase the level of biliary cholesterol secretion, causing a raised level of cholesterol supersaturation and, in addition, partially impair gallbladder contractility.[12, 14, 107, 108] Further, gallstone-promoting effects on bile and gallbladder contractility appear in the last trimester of pregnancy. Taken together, these physiologic effects of hormones are more significant in younger women somehow more susceptible to gallstone formation; certainly, these new observations warrant further investigation of endogenous hormone levels.

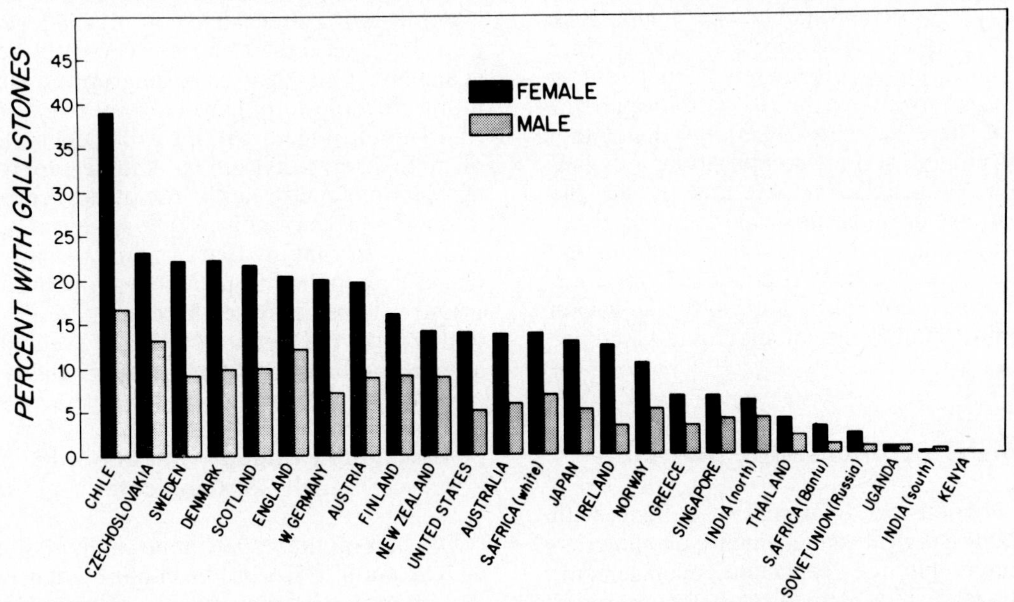

Figure 88–7. Age-standardized, sex-related, worldwide prevalence of gallstones in individuals over 20 years of age at autopsy since 1940. (From data collated by Carey, M. C., and O'Donovan, M. A. Gallstone disease; Current concepts on the epidemiology, pathogenesis, and management. *In* Petersdorf, R. G., et al. [eds]: Harrison's Principles of Internal Medicine–Update V. New York, McGraw-Hill, Inc., 1984, p. 145. Used by permission.)

Natural History of Gallstone Disease

The natural history of gallstone disease has been the subject of much controversy owing to lack of good data. Patients with gallstones may fall into one of several subgroups, based on symptoms, and, perforce, are very likely to have different natural histories. The subgroups may be designated as follows: (1) The totally asymptomatic patient; i.e., in whom the stones are truly "silent." These stones are most commonly discovered by chance in the course of diagnostic studies for other purposes. (2) The patient with nonspecific symptoms, inappropriately attributed to the presence of gallstones, such as dyspepsia, atypical intermittent abdominal right subcostal pain, and fatty food intolerance.[151, 152] (3) The patient with mild but credible symptoms of intermittent biliary pain. (4) The symptomatic patient with unequivocal symptoms due to inflammation and obstruction (see pp. 1691–1695).

For asymptomatic patients (category 1) current data indicate that only about 15 per cent ever have symptoms.[153, 154] In addition, the risk of symptoms diminishes with time and the rare biliary tract complications of this group are usually preceded by warning symptoms.[155] Data for patients in subgroups 2 and 3 are far less adequate than for subgroup 1, in part because the two subgroups, with overlapping and imprecise symptoms, are often difficult to identify adequately. The natural history of patients belonging to subgroup 2 should be identical to that of subgroup 1; however, it is likely that many of these patients have been improperly assigned to subgroup 3. This error adversely influences the already comparatively scant data on the natural history of subgroup 3, making its course appear more benign.[156] Nevertheless, patients in subgroup 3 have a definitely less benign clinical course than patients in subgroup 1.[154, 157, 158] As taken from the best data on natural history available, the cumulative chance for patients in subgroup 3 to move into subgroup 4 is probably approximately 25 per cent at five years, or about five times the risk rate for patients in subgroup 1. There has never been any doubt that the risk of developing serious complications (cholangitis, empyema of gallbladder, etc.) is by far the greatest for patients in subgroup 4 and is cumulatively progressive with time, an observation documented more than two decades ago.[159] The risk rate for complications and progression for patients in this subgroup is probably almost double that of subgroup 3 (see pp. 1693–1695).

TREATMENT OF GALLSTONE DISEASE

Therapeutic options for treatment of patients with gallstones include surgical management, or cholecystectomy; noninterventional, "expectant" management; and interventional, which is medical but nonsurgical management. This latter, most recently developed, therapeutic option now comprises more than one approach and represents the least established of the possibilities (for discussion of surgical management, see pp. 1699–1700).

Each management option ought to be rationally matched to the symptom category of a given patient, based upon what is known of the natural history for that category of gallstone disease. Thus, cholecystectomy is, and probably will remain, the treatment of choice for almost all patients in category 4 and for many in category 3. In contrast, noninterventional or "expectant" management should definitely be the treatment of choice for category 1. A probabilistic quantitative decision analysis study compared survival of patients with asymptomatic (silent) gallstones managed by either prophylactic cholecystectomy or expectant management.[155] The evidence is that prophylactic cholecystectomy slightly decreases survival. Sensitivity analysis spanning a broad range of probability values showed that the differences in survival for the two management strategies for both men and women are small. From this decision analysis approach alone, omitting cost considerations, expectant management should be the treatment of choice for patients of either sex having asymptomatic gallstones. This also applies, despite previous views to the contrary, even if the patient also has diabetes mellitus[160, 161] (see pp. 494–500).

Medical Treatment: The Choices

Other forms of nonsurgical (medical) but interventional therapies are still largely experimental, and various questions remain unanswered. Until very recently, dissolution therapy using bile salts, chenodeoxycholic acid (CDCA), and ursodeoxycholic acid (UDCA) was the only management option. Newer, somewhat more invasive, but nevertheless attractive and interesting alternative nonsurgical forms of therapy have been described and are currently being actively evaluated. One such promising option is rapid dissolution of cholesterol gallstones by direct percutaneous transhepatic puncture of the gallbladder and instillation of methyl tert-butyl ether. Another approach is fragmentation of gallstones by use of extracorporeal acoustic shock waves (lithotripsy), a modification of a device and form of therapy that has only recently been introduced and applied to patients with nephrolithiasis.

One adverse feature characterizing all these modes of therapy is the high probability of eventual recurrence after cessation of the therapeutic modality.[162–166]

Dissolution Therapy with Bile Salts: Selection of Candidates

Dissolution therapy with the cholelitholytic bile acids CDCA and UDCA has been most extensively studied. An intensive investigational effort involving clinical trials has convincingly shown that biliary cholesterol output is significantly reduced in patients thus treated, leading to marked reductions in the level of cholesterol in bile.[167–187] The mechanism of this potent primary therapeutic effect has never been established in humans. There are important metabolic, physical-chemical, and pharmacologic differences between CDCA and UDCA, so that it is entirely possible that the desaturating effect on cholesterol in the bile of treated patients is mediated by differing mechanisms for the two agents.[188–202]

Only mildly symptomatic patients with small, uncalcified stones in a functioning gallbladder are proper subjects for therapy with oral bile salts. The wisdom of this policy is underscored by the lack of justification for either medical or surgical management for asymptomatic patients. The size of the pool of candidates is further severely limited because about 75 per cent of randomly identified, unselected gallstone patients in subgroups 1, 2, and 3 have radiologic features that militate against dissolution therapy, including a nonfunctioning gallbladder, comparatively large stones (> 15 mm diameter), and stone calcification.[203]

Age is important in selection of patients with gallstones for dissolution therapy. Patients 60 years and older would seem more suitable for dissolution therapy; the comparative risks of both treatment failures and recurrence rates are more acceptable than the mortality and complication rates of cholecystectomy in this age group. This small group of remaining patients for whom dissolution therapy appears most suitable is further diminished by three factors that militate against a trial. First, dissolution therapy is too slow, requiring six to nine months in nonobese patients with very small noncalcified stones to more than two years in the obese. Because therapy is continued daily with interval monitoring, patient compliance is difficult to achieve. Second, even among compliant patients the success rate (about 30 per cent) is low when "complete" rather than "partial" dissolution is sought. Third, the recurrence rate after successful dissolution is remarkably high, 50 per cent or greater, upon cessation of therapy. High recurrence rates indicate the need for continuing therapy indefinitely or for instituting another form of preventive ("secondary") therapy; both prospects are not well entertained by patient or doctor.

CDCA Versus UDCA Treatment. The therapeutic regimens for both forms of bile acid dissolution therapy are virtually identical. In optimally selected nonobese patients, an oral cholecystogram is obtained within three months of initiation of treatment. This examination provides useful information not obtainable by ultrasonography; namely, rim calcification of stones, an unfavorable prognostic indicator, and the characteristic floating pattern of cholesterol gallstones, a favorable prognostic omen. The dosage employed for CDCA is about 15 mg/kg per day, whereas the equivalently effective dose for UDCA is about one third less, i.e., about 10 mg/kg per day. Follow-up oral cholecystograms are indicated at six monthly intervals during therapy. In most instances, at least partial stone dissolution will be discernible within six months of therapy, and in some, there will be an apparent complete dissolution of small (i.e., < 5 mm diameter) stones. If there has been no dissolution at six months, therapy is stopped. If no further dissolution has occurred at one year compared with that at six months, further treatment should be abandoned. If continuing partial dissolution is observed up to one year, the therapeutic program is continued for a second year provided that substantial net reduction in size has been observed (say, more than 50 per cent). This caveat will be of particular importance in patients with initially large stones (i.e., > 15 mm diameter) in whom even with continuing partial dissolution, albeit at an extremely slow rate, complete dissolution cannot reasonably be expected even after two years of treatment. In such patients, therapy must also be abandoned. In other patients during the second year, therapy is discontinued if no progressive diminution in stone size has been observed at six months.

During therapy, if oral cholecystography shows no stones, the finding should soon be confirmed by ultrasonography because of its greater sensitivity in detection of small incompletely dissolved fragments. Complete dissolution with either CDCA or UDCA is comparable (i.e., between 20 and 40 per cent), depending upon the stringency of selection criteria of patients. With more stringent patient selection criteria (i.e., small stones, no rim calcification, nonobesity, etc.) efficacy rates are increased.

Toxicity. With CDCA, as opposed to the newer UDCA, there are some special problems of safety and toxicity.[174] At adequate therapeutic dosage levels, i.e., 15 mg/kg per day, these include the following: a high rate of slightly raised liver-specific serum transaminase levels (~ 40 per cent) and mild to marked, usually reversible, histologic hepatitis (~ 3 per cent);[204–206] a mild to moderate incidence of diarrhea (~ 50 per cent) (this can often be managed by drug withdrawal for a few days followed by restoration of therapy at a lower dose); and lastly, a 10 per cent or greater increase in serum LDL-cholesterol which was detected in a large, well-controlled clinical trial.[174] Partially controlled and uncontrolled clinical trials indicate that UDCA does not have these special problems of CDCA and is equally effective. Further, lower dosage levels, i.e., 10 mg/kg per day may be employed. The general shortcomings of dissolution therapy, as outlined above, however, also pertain to UDCA and, in addition (unlike CDCA), some investigators believe that UDCA therapy may actually induce gallstone calcification, possibly by increasing bicarbonate in biliary secretion.[207–209] More recently, however, some investigators have found no greater incidence of stone calcification with UDCA than with CDCA.[210–212]

Combined Bile Salt Therapy. A combination of CDCA and UDCA mitigates the toxic effects of the former and the higher costs of the latter. Further, the efficacy rate of either CDCA or UDCA was achieved by combination therapy.[214–216] Among several entirely new potential candidates for dissolution therapy that differ significantly in mechanism of action from CDCA and UDCA are hyodeoxycholate, ursocholate, and 7-ketolithocholic acid.[217–220] These have not yet, however, been sufficiently tested in humans to permit conclusions regarding safety and efficacy, but the evidence to date, at least regarding efficacy of ursocholate, is unimpressive. Attempts through chemical synthesis to produce more potent and potentially less expensive therapeutic bile acids are being vigorously pursued.[221, 222] Prevention of gallstone disease is conventionally termed primary prevention. As mentioned above, prevention of recurrence is termed secondary prevention. Strong consideration should be given to giving the dissolving agent in low doses or intermittently as the mode for secondary prevention.[223]

Residual Problems of Dissolution Therapies. Despite more than a decade of intense study of dissolution therapy, there persist a number of important unanswered questions. Among these questions are the following: Will some form of lifelong therapy be necessary for a sizeable proportion of responding patients? Will an effective, nontoxic agent be found to prevent stones initially forming in highly susceptible population groups, e.g., Amerindian females? Preliminary evidence has suggested that greatly increasing fiber and reducing refined carbohydrates in the diet is effective in secondary prevention of gallstones after successful dissolution therapy.[213] Could such a program be implemented on a broader-scale basis to reduce recurrence? Finally, what about a cost comparison in the United States of dissolution therapy versus perhaps eventual cholecystectomy? Fees for uncomplicated surgery—surgeons, anesthetists, operating, recovery, and hospital rooms—range from $6000 to $10,000. The estimated complete costs per year of initial dissolution therapy per patient is about $1200. These short-term comparisons appearing to favor dissolution therapy are often more than offset by additional costs of the failure of complete dissolution at one year, of stone recurrence after complete dissolution requiring re-treatment, and possibly eventual need for cholecystectomy because of medical treatment failure or acute complication.

Instillation Therapy (MTBE) and Lithotripsy

Gallstone dissolution by direct instillation of methyl tert-butyl ether (MTBE therapy) and gallstone fragmentation by extracorporeal shock waves are new therapeutic modalities which act rapidly and are apparently effective. Both therapies are best applicable to those who are only mildly symptomatic.

MTBE Therapy. The rationale for use of MTBE therapy is straightforward; it rapidly dissolves cholesterol gallstones upon direct contact *in vivo* as well as *in vitro,* and unlike diethyl ether, it does not volatilize at body temperature because its boiling point is 55.2°C.[224–226]

The procedure for *in vivo* instillation of MTBE into the gallbladder is as follows. After ascertaining that a sufficient area of attachment of the gallbladder to the bed or undersurface of the liver exists by use of a combined oral contrast cholecystogram CT scan, the operator inserts under local anesthesia a 21-gauge transhepatic cholangiographic needle under fluoroscopic guidance into the gallbladder lumen via the liver-gallbladder bed. A wire guide is inserted through the needle; the needle is then removed and replaced by a modified No. 5 French pigtail catheter. Following maximal aspiration of bile from the gallbladder, 5 ml of contrast material is infused which serves both to more sharply outline the stones and to exclude extravasation by catheter cholecystography. Upon aspiration of all contrast material, continuous infusion and aspiration of MTBE are begun. At 15 minute intervals, the syringe is discarded and replaced with another syringe filled with pure MTBE, maintaining a high concentration of unsaturated MTBE in the infusate. Catheter cholecystograms are obtained at hourly intervals as long as necessary to assess stone dissolution. An average duration of treatment for patients is 12 hours. Although published preliminary observations with MTBE includes information on successful treatment in two cases, the study has now been extended to include over 40 patients with similarly favorable results with no untoward complications (references 224 to 226 and Thistle, J. L., personal communication).

Experience with MTBE to date has been confined to treatment of gallbladder stones. Recently reported experience indicates that MTBE therapy for common duct stones through retrograde instillation not only lacks efficacy because of insufficient duration of contact between the solvent and the stone surface but also has undesirable side effects, e.g., effects of MTBE anesthesia, resulting from excessive intestinal absorption.[227, 228]

Limitations of MTBE. MTBE therapy warrants continued careful evaluation before it can be recommended for gallstone patients for the following reasons: First, the technique requires percutaneous transhepatic puncture of the gallbladder, an invasive procedure requiring skill and experience. In addition to local complications of inaccurate insertion, there is risk of bile, blood, or MTBE leaking into the peritoneum, hepatic parenchyma, or blood stream where it could produce tissue necrosis or hemolysis. These complications have not been seen in Thistle's first 40 patients (Thistle, J. L., personal communication). Second, following removal of all the lipid components of the stones after many hours of instillations and aspirations, a small (i.e., about 1 to 3 mm) residue of sonographically detectable, insoluble material (presumably gallstone matrix) resembling biliary sludge remains in about 70 per cent of patients. The material probably is the mucin glycoprotein-bilirubin matrix-like material that provides a lattice structure upon which the cholesterol crystals form a stone.[85] In the majority of these patients, however, follow-up sonographic studies show that this sludge disappears. Although the natural history or pathogenetic significance of this residual sludge is at present unclear, gallstones reappear in some patients who have no residual sludge. Thus, continuing therapy, perhaps UDCA, may also be required in these successfully treated patients for secondary prevention. Third, MTBE is largely excreted in the lungs, and because it has a disagreeable odor, it causes dose-dependent nausea and vomiting. The cost for this form of therapy likely will be lower than either prophylactic cholecystectomy or conventional dissolution therapy.

Lithotripsy. The most recent form of rapid eradication of gallstones is their fragmentation by extracorporeal shockwaves (lithotripsy).[229–233] Earlier favorable European results demonstrated in carefully selected patients with symptomatic upper urinary tract stones that eradication rates of between 60 and 90 per cent could be achieved with minimal complications, depending on stone size, location, composition, and prior percutaneous extraction procedures. Based upon these findings, six American centers participated in premarketing trials in 1984 in which the earlier promising results were quickly confirmed. This report resulted in rapid F.D.A. approval in early 1985 for marketing of the (West German) Dornier devices in America for application to urolithiasis, at a cost of approximately $2 million for each lithotriptor installation. Plans are now in the formulative stage to repeat the previous experience with a new device specifically adapted to gallstone fragmentation with approximately the same installation cost. Premarketing testing of the new device in ten American medical centers is contemplated beginning in late 1987, with the aim of rapid acquisition of sufficient data to secure FDA approval.

In preliminary observations based upon experience with only 14 gallstone patients, investigators from Munich have reported encouraging results in selected patients with gallstones, five of whom had common bile duct stones that were difficult to treat.[229] The procedure for application of extracorporeal shock wave fragmentation therapy is as follows. Only a diminishing minority of patients require either epidural or general anesthesia. The steadily increasing majority are now treated under moderate anesthesia with intravenous administration of diazepam and an opiate. The patient is positioned for ultrasonographic focusing of the acoustic shock waves emitted via a water cushion which covers the discharging electrode and which must be in perfect contact with the patient's body exterior to permit entrance of the shock waves. With proper placement, the shock waves pass (apparently harmlessly) through soft tissues until the stone is encountered, where the large difference in acoustical impedance generates sufficient pressure to shatter the target. Between 600 and 1500 shock waves are delivered over a period of one to two hours, synchronized with the continuously monitored R wave of the patient's electrocardiogram.[229]

Early Results with Lithotripsy. In the initially reported series, two patients experienced three episodes of post-treatment biliary pain, one of whom also experienced a mild bout of pancreatitis. In the remaining four patients, biliary sludge and residual stone fragments disappeared within 1 to 25 weeks with no symptoms. With extension of the series to about 200 patients, only one additional patient has experienced an episode of pancreatitis, including a subset of about 30 patients with stones in the biliary ductular (including intrahepatic ducts) system. Larger (i.e., >30 mm in diameter) stones have been found more resistant to fragmentation. About 30 per cent of patients have experienced one or more post-treatment episodes of biliary pain, most of them mild, related to passage of stone fragments. Many of the patients with biliary ductular stones at the time of treatment were quite ill, and surgery was hazardous because of age and symptoms of biliary tract obstruction, including fever and jaundice. Each had undergone prelithotripsy endoscopic sphincterotomy with no success in removing stones by forceps. In the majority, shock wave lithotripsy resulted in relief of obstruction and acute subsidence of fever, without the complications and the high mortality rate of surgery (Paumgartner, G., personal communication).

Special Problems of Lithotripsy. Special problems relate to use of extracorporeal shock wave treatment of gallstones. First, either epidural or general anesthesia may be required for pain in some patients, carrying risks. Second, should focusing go awry, the shock wave can severely injure gas-filled intestine or lung tissue because of differences in acoustic impedance due to the gas- or air-filled alveoli. Pulmonary or intestinal hemorrhage could conceivably result. Third, not all patients can be accepted as suitable candidates for lithotripsy. Current data indicate, however, that approximately 25 per cent of patients with gallbladder or common duct stones referred for lithotripsy can be accepted as suitable candidates, an almost fourfold increase over the originally published estimate. This probably reflects both a broadening of acceptance criteria as well as the referral of more suitable patients.

Biliary sludge after lithotripsy may differ from "sludge" after MTBE therapy. The sludge found in about 70 per cent of patients following MTBE therapy results from dissolution of lipid (cholesterol), leaving behind the nonlipid matrix. In contrast, acoustic shock wave stone fragmentation physically shatters lipid as well as the nonlipid matrix, leaving fragments of whole stone material.

Although experience must still be considered very preliminary, the newer developments with acoustic shock wave lithotripsy are beginning to make it possible to consider repeat lithotripsy within perhaps as little as two to three months in patients whose residual fragmented stones have not already spontaneously passed.

With more extensive experience and less stringent patient acceptance criteria, acoustic shock wave lithotripsy may well become the treatment of choice for most of the patients for whom medical interventional therapy is preferred. It certainly achieves quicker results than the currently available oral dissolution therapy. Perhaps oral dissolution with the CDCA and UDCA-like drugs will find a role in secondary prevention for those patients whose gallstones have already been acutely treated by MTBE dissolution or acoustic shock wave lithotripsy. Clearly, this aspect of medical therapeutics is rapidly changing, and it is still far too early to forecast the eventual place for all the available medical management approaches either alone or in combination. The needed information is being gathered with extraordinary rapidity, however, and it is entirely conceivable that within the next several years, the places for most of the present medical therapies will have become reasonably well established, providing attractive therapeutic options. Considering both the strong trend to no therapy for the clinically "silent" stone and the present progress in development of medical interventional therapies for those with symptomatic gallstone disease, cholecystectomy may become an operation performed only for serious complications of stones at least in countries where the full panoply of newer medical technologic developments has become available.

PIGMENT STONES

Description and Composition

There are several types of pigment stones, which differ markedly in frequency, composition, and geographic distribution; however, significantly, the pathogenesis is not clearly understood for either.[234, 235] By far the more common type is the pure black pigment stone (see Fig. 88–1*B*). Although relatively infrequent, brown (bile pigment–calcium) pigment stones are next in order of occurrence.[236–238] Brown pigment stones exhibit marked morphologic differences from black pigment stones[239–241] (see Fig. 88–1*C*). They are firmer to the grasp, on average of larger diameter, nongranular, laminated, and have an earthen hue in contrast to the coal-blackness of black pigment stones. Other rarer forms of pigment stones are too rare to discuss.

Black pigment stones show significant composition differences from brown pigment stones, as indicated in Table 88–2. Black pigment stones contain considerably more of a polymerized form of an oxidized bilirubin degradation product, coloring it black.[242–248] This substance is combined with modest amounts of calcium bilirubinate and other calcium salts. Brown pigment stones consist primarily of calcium bilirubinate along with calcium salts of fatty acids derived from bile lecithin, together with small and variable amounts of an oxidatively degraded bilirubin polymer.[249] Study of lipids in both types of stone has suggested that the fatty acid content of stone is largely artifactual and that much more intact lecithin is present in these stones in the fresh state than was formerly believed, particularly in brown pigment stones.[250] Both types of stone contain 10 to 60 per cent by weight of an unmeasured and unidentified residue, most likely consisting primarily of a mucin glycoprotein matrix.[251]

Table 88–2. COMPOSITION OF BLACK AND BROWN PIGMENT GALLSTONES*

Component	Black (%)	Brown (%)
Bile pigment, total	40 (10–90)†	50 (28–79)
Major form	Insoluble polymer	Ca bilirubinate
Calcium	15 (3–40)	5 (3–9)
Calcium salts		
Carbonate	13 (0–65)	None
Phosphate	5 (0–32)	<1
Palmitate + stearate	1 (0–3)	23 (11–67)
Cholesterol (unesterified)	3 (1–13)	10 (2–28)
Unmeasured residue	24 (10–73)	12 (0–30)

*Values are given as a percentage of dry weight of the stone.
†Values are means, with ranges in parentheses.
From Ostrow, J. D. The etiology of pigmented gallstones. Hepatology *4*:215s–222s. © 1984 by The American Association for the Study of Liver Diseases.

Epidemiology

In most American medical centers, the incidence of black and other forms of pigment stones is about 10 per cent of all gallstones, although an exceptionally high incidence (25 per cent) has been reported from a center in Philadelphia.[252] The latter figure approaches the incidence at major medical centers in Japan; however, the types of gallbladder pigment stones found there are about equally divided between the common black pigment stone and an almost uniquely Oriental form of brown (bile pigment–calcium) pigment stone. Brown pigment stones are found more often in rural Japan than in urban Japanese medical centers, and indications are that they are also commonly found at surgery in Taiwan and mainland China. They are exceedingly rare in the United States. Even less common forms of noncholesterol pigment stones composed primarily of calcium salts are found at surgery everywhere.

Clinical Associations

Black pigment stones occur almost invariably in patients who have no readily discernible predisposing condition. Bacterial studies in both America and Japan have indicated that, as a rule, bile from patients with black pigment stones, like those with cholesterol gallstones, is sterile.[253, 254] As shown in Table 88–3, however, there are well-established clinical associations or risk factors for this form of gallstone disease. The most important of these are chronic hemolysis, such as sickle cell disease (30 to 60 per cent incidence), thalassemia, hereditary spherocytosis, and cardiac valve prosthesis. Cirrhosis is another well-known association, possibly related in some patients to chronic or intermittent hemolysis.[255] Age is another established clinical correlate, although its significance is not well understood.[252] In one study, more than 50 per cent of patients age 70 or older undergoing cholecystectomy were found to have black pigment stones.[252]

In contrast to black pigment stones, brown (Oriental) pigment stones have some special correlations with particular situations and unique localized parts of the world. Until about 1960, both the brown pigment stones and biliary bacterial infection were attributed to the biliary parasitism, e.g., ascariasis, especially in

Table 88–3. CLINICAL ASSOCIATIONS OF THE TWO MAJOR TYPES OF PIGMENT GALLSTONES

Characteristics	Black Pigment Stone Type	Brown Pigment Stone Type
Color	Black	Brown to orange
Consistency	Amorphous, powdery	Soft, laminated
Anatomic location	Gallbladder	Gallbladder and bile ducts
Geography	West and Orient	Mostly Orient
Disease association	Hemolysis, cirrhosis	Cholangitis, ova, parasites, sutures
Cultures of bile	Usually sterile	Infected *(E. coli)*
Principal components	Pigment polymer, calcium phosphate, and calcium carbonate	Calcium bilirubinate, calcium soaps of fatty acids, and cholesterol
Etiology	Increased excretion or hydrolysis of conjugated bilirubin	Bacterial hydrolysis of conjugated to unconjugated bilirubin

From Ostrow, J. D. The etiology of pigmented gallstones. Hepatology 215s–222s. © 1984 by The American Association for the Study of Liver Diseases.

rural, Oriental populations. With improved hygiene and living standards, the incidence of biliary parasitism, at least in Japan, has become virtually nil.

Some of the special clinical features associated with brown pigment stones include the following: first, there is a strikingly high coincidence of biliary infection with aerobic *E. coli* as well as with the clostridial and *Bacteroides* forms of anaerobes.[254, 256, 257] Bacterial colonies in the interior of a brown pigment stone are strikingly demonstrated in Figure 88–8.[257a] Moreover, a high incidence of bacterial beta-glucuronidase activity has been reported in association with these biliary bacterial infections, thus lending credence to the original proposal put forward by Maki over 20 years ago regarding brown pigment stone pathogenesis.[240, 258] Second, there is a remarkably high incidence (about 50 per cent) of stones within the common duct and other smaller ducts of brown pigment stones in patients with these gallstones.[254] The high association of brown pigment stone disease with bacterial infections is clearer when intraductal stones cause biliary stasis; however, the basis for infected bile when brown pigment stones are confined solely to the gallbladder is less clear. It has been speculated that even in the absence of coexistent choledocholithiasis, the high incidence of biliary infection may be attributable either to residuals of prior biliary tract parasitism or to idiopathic congenital anomalies, e.g., variants of Caroli's disease with segmental saccular dilatations of the intrahepatic and more distal bile ducts. In any event, either process could cause the biliary duct distortion, stasis, and infection observed in this setting. Patients with brown stones are

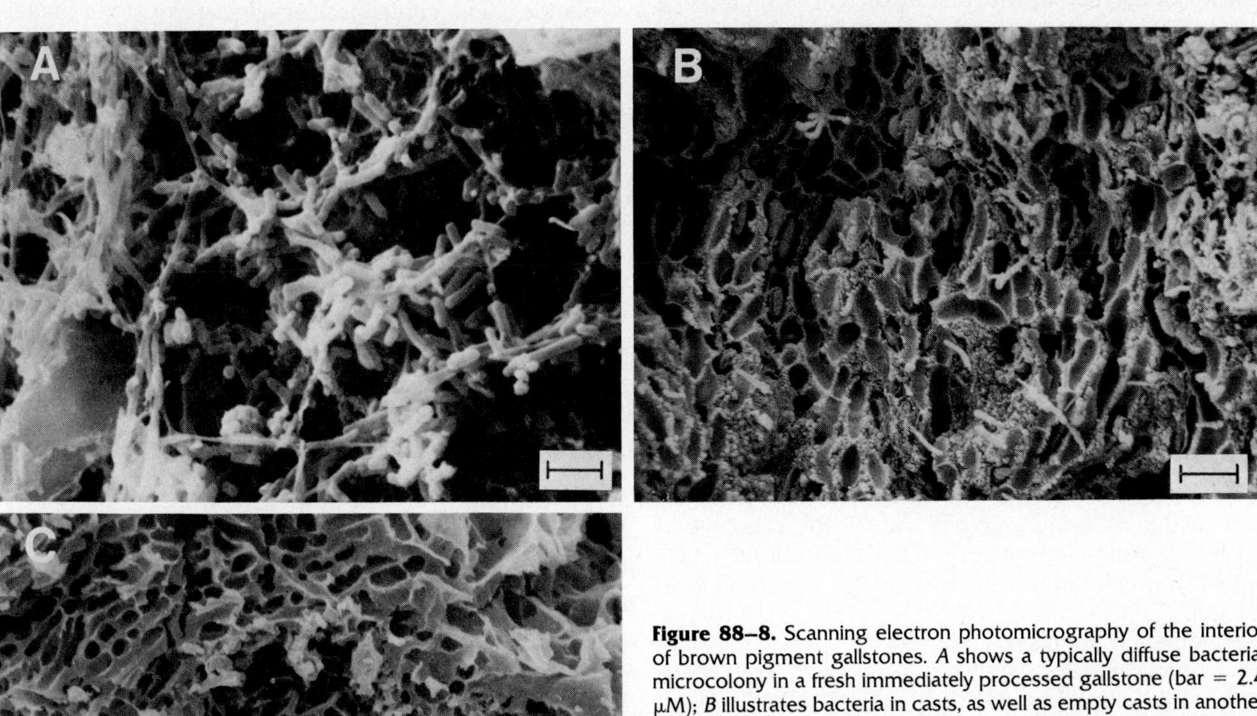

Figure 88–8. Scanning electron photomicrography of the interior of brown pigment gallstones. *A* shows a typically diffuse bacterial microcolony in a fresh immediately processed gallstone (bar = 2.4 μM); *B* illustrates bacteria in casts, as well as empty casts in another similarly processed gallstone (bar = 1.9 μM); *C*, air-dried interior of a brown pigment stone not immediately processed showing bacteria casts but no viable bacteria (bar = 2.3 μM). (From Stewart, L., Smith, A. L., Pelligrini, C. A., et al. Ann. Surg. *206*:242, 1987. Used by permission.)

about 10 years older than patients with the more common black stones.[237] The reason for this distinct age differential between the two patient populations is unknown. Perhaps the presence of these stones primarily in the older age groups in Japan (and elsewhere in the Orient) merely reflects the striking change in incidence of biliary parasitism within the last generation. In any event, by the year 2000, brown pigment stones will probably be as rare in the Orient as they currently are in Western countries.

Pathogenesis

The clinical associations described for brown pigment stones, i.e., stasis and bacterial infection, provide the strongest clues regarding pathogenesis for this form of pigment stone disease. In contrast, biliary bacterial infection clearly has no role in the pathogenesis of the more common black pigment stones.[253–254] Beyond this firm statement, all other considerations of factors potentially applicable to the pathogenesis of black pigment stones are conjectural, resting only upon implication, and lacking in essential corroborating data. The conventional collection of putative pathogenic factors cited as having a role in black pigment stone pathogenesis include the following: an excess (abnormal) amount of insoluble unconjugated bilirubin (UCB), a relative deficiency in the amount of bile salts needed to solubilize the increase in UCB, and other even less substantiated factors including a possible excess of ionized calcium (to form irreversibly insoluble calcium bilirubinate) and a possible excess of gallbladder mucin, which in turn could be related to possibly impaired gallbladder contractility.

One hypothetical view, encompassing some of the potential factors cited, is that like patients with chronic hemolytic anemia (sickle cell disease, thalassemia, valve prosthesis, hereditary spherocytosis, cirrhosis, etc.) in whom as much as a tenfold increase above normal in the secretion of (mainly) conjugated and unconjugated bilirubin can be found in bile collected by T tube, patients with black pigment stones may have at least an intermittent state(s) of supersaturation of bile with insoluble UCB.[234, 235] Because bile salts are an important solubilizer for UCB, even the presence of a relative deficiency of bile salts in the presence of supersaturating amounts of UCB would not only permit UCB precipitation but also slightly increase ionized calcium.[259–261]

Heightened nonbacterial hydrolysis, possibly caused by a glucuronidase secreted by the liver, converting conjugated bilirubin to UCB, is another possible factor in the pathogenesis of black pigment stones, but the data are far from clear.[262, 263] Even more speculative is a role for the presence of excessive gallbladder mucin, known to be an important component of "biliary sludge" (see above). Mucin has the capacity to bind not only to UCB but also to hydrophobic biliary lipids, such as lecithin (which in turn can also bind UCB) and cholesterol.[83]

The probable significance of excess biliary UCB relative to bile salt concentrations in pathogenesis of black pigment stones has recently been underscored by the finding of a strain of mice with an hereditary hemolytic anemia which have a nearly 60 per cent incidence of pigment stones.[264] The stones are comparable in composition to those from patients with hemolytic anemia, with a calcium carbonate content of nearly 70 per cent. Further simulation of the situation in humans includes a large quantity of gallbladder mucin glycoprotein, an increased concentràtion in bile of both total bilirubin and UCB, and a significantly reduced bile salt concentration.[265, 266]

The physical chemistry of these complex interactions has not yet been worked out but what seems clear is that conditions leading to black pigment stone formation entail supersaturation of bile with UCB and concomitant relative deficiency of UCB-solubilizing bile salts, presence of a sufficient calcium concentration to permit calcium bilirubinate precipitation, and possibly in older patients, a relative impairment of gallbladder contractility with mucin accumulation.

Treatment

There exist no medical interventional options, such as dissolution therapy, for pigment stones of the gallbladder. The guidelines for cholesterol stone management apply. If the stones are clinically silent, nonoperative expectant management is appropriate; whereas, if the patient has symptoms, cholecystectomy is the only reasonable therapeutic option. Owing to the frequent coexistence of infection and stasis, treatment of brown pigment stone disease often will require antibiotics and surgical intervention (see pp. 1691–1729). For common duct or other biliary duct stones, the problem must be addressed surgically or by other means of invading the ductal system, e.g., endoscopy, T-tube basket retrieval, or even percutaneous catheter insertion (see pp. 1741–1761).

References

1. Bennion, L. J., and Grundy, S. M. Effects of obesity and caloric intake on biliary lipid metabolism in man. J. Clin. Invest. *56*:996, 1975.
2. Grundy, S. M., Duane, W. C., Adler, R. D., Aron, J. M., and Metzger, A. L. Biliary lipid outputs in young women with cholesterol gallstones. Metabolism *23*:67, 1974.
3. Kesäniemi, Y. A., and Grundy, S. M. Clofibrate, caloric restriction, supersaturation of bile, and cholesterol crystals. Scand. J. Gastroenterol. *18*:897, 1983.
4. Reuben, A., Quareshi, Y., Murphy, G. M., and Dowling, R. H. Effect of obesity and weight reduction on biliary cholesterol saturation and the response to chenodeoxycholic acid. Eur. J. Clin. Invest. *16*:133, 1985.
5. Shaffer, E. A., and Small, D. M. Biliary lipid secretion in cholesterol gallstone disease. The effect of cholecystectomy and obesity. J. Clin. Invest. *59*:828, 1977.
6. Reuben, A., Maton, P. N., Murphy, G. M., and Dowling, R. H. Biliary lipid secretion in obese and non-obese individuals with and without gallstones. Clin. Sci. *69*:71, 1985.

7. Nilsell, K., Angelin, B., Liljeqvist, L., and Einarsson, K. Biliary lipid output and bile acid kinetics in cholesterol gallstone disease. Evidence for an increased hepatic secretion of cholesterol in Swedish patients. Gastroenterology *89*:287, 1985.
8. Leiss, O., and Von Bergmann, K. Comparison of biliary lipid secretion in non-obese cholesterol gallstone patients with normal, young, male volunteers. Klin. Wochenschr. *63*:1163, 1985.
9. Valdivieso, V., Palma, R., Nervi, F., Covarrubias, C., Severin, C., and Antezana, C. Secretion of biliary lipids in young Chilean women with cholesterol gallstones. Gut *20*:997, 1979.
10. Valdivieso, V., Palma, R., Wünkhaus, R., Antezana, C., Severin, C., and Contreras, A. Effect of aging on biliary lipid composition and bile acid metabolism in normal Chilean women. Gastroenterology *74*:871, 1978.
11. Einarsson, K., Nilsell, K., Leijd, B., and Angelin, B. Influence of age on secretion of cholesterol and synthesis of bile acids by the liver. N. Engl. J. Med. *313*:277, 1985.
12. Kern, F., Jr., Everson, G. T., Demark, B., McKinley, C., Showalter, R., Erfling, W., Braverman, D. Z., Szczepanik-Van Leeuwen, P., and Klein, P. D. Biliary lipids, bile acids and gallbladder function in the human female. Effects of pregnancy and the ovulatory cycle. J. Clin. Invest. *68*:1229, 1981.
13. Bennion, L. J., Mott, D. M., and Howard, B. V. Oral contraceptives raise the cholesterol saturation of bile by increasing biliary cholesterol secretion. Metabolism *29*:18, 1980.
14. Kern, F., Jr., Everson, G. T., Demark, B., McKinley, C., Showalter, R., Braverman, D. Z., Szcepanik-Vanleeuwen, P., and Klein, P. D. Biliary lipids, bile acids, and gallbladder function in the human female: Effects of contraceptive steroids. J. Lab. Clin. Med. *99*:798, 1982.
15. Henriksson, P., Einarsson, K., Ericksson, A., Kelter, U., and Angelin, B. Estrogen-induced gallstone formation in males. Relation to changes in serum and biliary lipids during hormonal treatment of prostatic carcinoma. Gastroenterology in press, 1988.
16. Berr, F., Eckel, R. H., and Kern, F., Jr. Contraceptive steroids increase hepatic uptake of chylomicron remnants in healthy young women. J. Lipid Res. *27*:645, 1986.
17. Kern, F., Jr., and Everson, G. T. Contraceptive steroids increase cholesterol in bile: mechanisms of actions. J. Lipid Res. *28*:828, 1987.
18. Vlahcevic, Z. R., Bell, C. C., Jr., Buhac, I., Farrar, J. T., and Swell, L. Diminished bile acid pool size in patients with gallstones. Gastroenterology *59*:165, 1970.
19. Grundy, S. M., Metzger, A. L., and Adler, R. D. Mechanisms of lithogenic bile formation in American Indian women with cholesterol gallstones. J. Clin. Invest. *51*:3026, 1972.
20. Grundy, S. M., and Metzger, A. L. A physiological method for estimation of hepatic secretion of biliary lipids in man. Gastroenterology *62*:1200, 1972.
21. Everson, G. T., Lawson, M. J., McKinley, C., Showalter, R., and Kern, F., Jr. Gallbladder and small intestinal regulation of biliary lipid secretion during intraduodenal infusion of standard stimuli. J. Clin. Invest. *71*:596, 1983.
22. Redinger, R. N. The effect of loss of gallbladder function on biliary lipid composition in subjects with cholesterol gallstones. Gastroenterology *71*:470, 1976.
23. Turley, S. D., Anderson, J. M., and Dietschy, J. M. Rates of sterol synthesis and uptake in the major organs of the rat in vivo. J. Lipid Res. *22*:551, 1981.
24. Long, T. T., III, Jakoi, L., Stevens, R., and Quarfordt, S. The sources of rat biliary cholesterol and bile acid. J. Lipid Res. *19*:872, 1978.
25. Turley, S. D., and Dietschy, J. M. The contribution of newly synthesized cholesterol to biliary cholesterol in the rat. J. Biol. Chem. *256*:2438, 1981.
26. Robins, S. J., and Brunengraber, H. Origin of biliary cholesterol and lecithin in the rat: Contribution of new synthesis and preformed hepatic stores. J. Lipid Res. *23*:604, 1982.
27. Schwartz, C. C., Berman, M., Vlahcevic, Z. R., Halloran, L. C., Gregory, D. H., and Swell, L. Multicompartmental analysis of cholesterol metabolism in man. Characterization of the hepatic bile acid and biliary cholesterol precursor sites. J. Clin. Invest. *61*:408, 1978.
28. Nervi, F. O., and Dietschy, J. M. The mechanism of and the interrelation between bile acid chylomicron-mediated regulation of hepatic cholesterol synthesis in the liver of the rat. J. Clin. Invest. *61*:895, 1978.
29. Turley, S. D., and Dietschy, J. M. Regulation of biliary cholesterol output in the rat: Dissociation from the rate of hepatic cholesterol synthesis, the size of the hepatic cholesteryl pool, and the hepatic uptake of chylomicron cholesterol. J. Lipid Res. *20*:923, 1979.
30. Turley, S. D., Spady, D. K., and Dietschy, J. M. Alteration of the degree of biliary cholesterol saturation in the hamster and rat by manipulation of the pools of preformed and newly synthesized cholesterol. Gastroenterology *84*:253, 1983.
31. Nervi, F. O., Del Pozo, R., Covarrubias, C. F., and Ronco, B. O. The effect of progesterone on the regulatory mechanisms of biliary cholesterol secretion in the rat. Hepatology *3*:360, 1983.
32. Del Pozo, R., Nervi, F. O., Covarrubias, C., and Ronco, B. Reversal of progesterone-induced biliary cholesterol output by dietary cholesterol and ethynylestradiol. Biochim. Biophys. Acta *753*:164, 1983.
33. Nervi, F. O., Bronfman, M., Allalon, W., Depiereux, E., and Del Pozo, R. Regulation of biliary cholesterol secretion in the rat. Role of hepatic cholesterol esterification. J. Clin. Invest. *74*:2226, 1984.
34. Turley, S. D., and Dietschy, J. M. Modulation of the stimulatory effect of pregnenolone-16 α-carbonitrile on biliary cholesterol output in the rat by manipulation of the rate of hepatic cholesterol synthesis. Gastroenterology *87*:284, 1984.
35. Spady, D. K., Bilheimer, D. W., and Dietschy, J. M. Rates of receptor-dependent and independent low density lipoprotein uptake in the hamster. Proc. Natl. Acad. Sci. USA *80*:3499, 1983.
36. Stange, E. F., and Dietschy, J. M. Age-related decreases in tissue sterol acquisition are mediated by changes in cholesterol synthesis and not low density lipoprotein uptake in the rat. J. Lipid Res. *25*:703, 1984.
37. Spady, D. K., Turley, S. D., and Dietschy, J. M. Rates of low density lipoprotein uptake and cholesterol synthesis are regulated independently in the liver. J. Lipid Res. *26*:465, 1985.
38. Spady, D. K., Turley, S. D., and Dietschy, J. M. Receptor-independent low density lipoprotein transport in the rat in vivo. Quantitation, characterization, and metabolic consequences. J. Clin. Invest. *76*:1113, 1985.
39. Spady, D. K., Stange, E. F., Bilhartz, L. E., and Dietschy, J. M. Bile acids regulate hepatic low density lipoprotein receptor activity in the hamster by altering cholesterol flux across the liver. Proc. Natl. Acad. Sci. USA *83*:1916, 1986.
40. Spady, D. K., Meddings, J. B., and Dietschy, J. M. Kinetic constants for receptor-dependent and receptor-independent low density lipoprotein transport in the tissues of the rat and hamster. J. Clin. Invest. *77*:1474, 1986.
41. Carulli, N., Loria, P., Bertolotti, M., Ponz de Leon, M., Menozzi, D., Medici, G., and Piccagli, I. Effects of acute changes of bile acid pool composition on biliary lipid secretion. J. Clin. Invest. *74*:614, 1984.
42. Bilhartz, L. E., and Dietschy, J. M. Bile acid hydrophobicity determines cholesterol recruitment from hepatocytes when cholesterol synthesis and LDL uptake are constant. Gastroenterology in press, 1988.
43. Nervi, F. O., Covarrubias, C. F., Valdivieso, V. D., Ronco, B. O., Solari, A., and Tocornal, J. Hepatic cholesterologenesis in Chileans with cholesterol gallstone disease: Evidence for sex differences in the regulation of hepatic cholesterol metabolism. Gastroenterology *80*:539, 1981.
44. Bilhartz, L. E., and Dietschy, J. M. Lipoprotein metabolism, hepatic cholesterol pools, and cholesterol gallstone formation. *In* Barbara, L., Dowling, R. H., Hofmann, A. F., Roda, E. (eds.): Recent Advances in Bile Acid Research. New York, Raven Press, 1985, pp. 165–171.
45. Admirand, W. H., and Small, D. M. The physico-chemical

basis of cholesterol gallstone formation in man. J. Clin. Invest. *47*:1043, 1968.
46. Holzbach, R. T., Marsh, M., Olszewski, M., and Holan, K. Cholesterol solubility in bile: Evidence that supersaturated bile is frequent in healthy man. J. Clin. Invest. *52*:1467, 1973.
47. Carey, M. C., and Small, D. M. The physical chemistry of cholesterol solubility in bile. J. Clin. Invest. *61*:988, 1978.
48. Sömjen, G. J., and Gilat, T. A non-micellar mode of cholesterol transport in human bile. FEBS Lett. *156*:265, 1983.
49. Mazer, N. A., and Carey, M. C. Quasi-elastic light-scattering studies of aqueous biliary lipid systems. Cholesterol solubilization and precipitation in model bile solutions. Biochemistry *22*:426, 1983.
50. Mazer, N. A., Schurtenberger, P., Carey, M. C., Preisig, R., Weigand, K., and Känzig, W. Quasi-elastic light scattering studies of native hepatic bile from the dog: Comparison with aggregative behavior of model biliary lipid systems. Biochemistry *23*:1994, 1984.
51. Pattinson, N. R. Solubilisation of cholesterol in human bile. FEBS Lett. *181*:339, 1985.
52. Sömjen, G. H., and Gilat, T. Contribution of vesicular and micellar carriers to cholesterol transport in human bile. J. Lipid Res. *26*:699, 1985.
53. Kibe, A., Dudley, M. A., Halpern, Z., Lynn, M. P., Breuer, A. C., and Holzbach, R. T. Factors affecting cholesterol monohydrate crystal nucleation time in model systems of supersaturated bile. J. Lipid Res. *26*:1102, 1985.
54. Halpern, Z., Dudley, M. A., Lynn, M. P., Nader, J. M., Breuer, A. C., and Holzbach, R. T. Vesicle aggregation in model systems of supersaturated bile: Relation to crystal nucleation and lipid composition of the vesicular phase. J. Lipid Res. *27*:295, 1986.
55. Halpern, Z., Dudley, M. A., Kibe, A., Lynn, M. P., Breuer, A. C., and Holzbach, R. T. Rapid vesicle formation and aggregation in abnormal human bile. A time-lapse video-enhanced contrast microscopy study. Gastroenterology *90*:875, 1986.
56. Pattinson, N. R., and Chapman, B. A. Distribution of biliary cholesterol between mixed micelles and nonmicelles in relation to fasting and feeding in humans. Gastroenterology *91*:697, 1986.
57. Ulloa, N., Garrido, J., and Nervi, F. Ultracentrifugal isolation of vesicular carriers of biliary cholesterol in native human and rat bile. Hepatology *7*:235, 1987.
58. Lee, S. P., Park, H. Z., Madani, H., and Kaler, E. W. Partial characterization of a non-micellar system of cholesterol solubilization in bile. Am. J. Physiol. *252*:G374, 1987.
59. Holzbach, R. T. Recent progress in understanding cholesterol crystal nucleation as a precursor to human gallstone formation. Hepatology *6*:1403, 1986.
60. Hofmann, A. F., Molino, G., Milanese, M., and Belforte, G. Description and simulation of a physiological pharmacokinetic model for the metabolism and enterohepatic circulation of bile acids in man. Cholic acid in healthy man. J. Clin. Invest. *71*:1003, 1983.
61. Myant, N. B., and Mitropoulas, K. A. Cholesterol 7α-hydroxylase. J. Lipid Res. *18*:135, 1977.
62. Wagner, C. I., Trotman, W. B., and Soloway, R. D. Kinetic analysis of biliary lipid excretion in man and dog. J. Clin. Invest. *57*:473, 1976.
63. Mok, H. Y. I., von Bergmann, K., and Grundy, S. M. Effects of interruption of enterohepatic circulation on biliary lipid secretion in man. Am. J. Dig. Dis. *23*:1067, 1978.
64. Carey, M. C., and Mazer, N. M. Biliary lipid secretion in health and in cholesterol gallstone disease. Hepatology *4*:315, 1984.
65. Mazer, N. M., and Carey, M. C. Mathematical model of biliary lipid secretion: A quantitative analysis of physiological and biochemical data from man and other species. J. Lipid Res. *25*:932, 1984.
66. Rahman, K., Hammond, T. G., Lowe, P. J., Barnwell, S. G., Clark, B., and Coleman, R. Control of biliary phospholipid secretion. Effect of continuous and discontinuous infusion of taurocholate on biliary phospholipid secretion. Biochem. J. *234*:421, 1986.
67. Holan, K. R., Holzbach, R. T., Hermann, R. E., Cooperman, A. M., and Claffey, W. J. Nucleation time: A key factor in the pathogenesis of cholesterol gallstone disease. Gastroenterology *77*:611, 1979.
68. Sedaghat, A., and Grundy, S. M. Cholesterol crystals and the formation of cholesterol gallstones. N. Engl. J. Med. *302*:1274, 1980.
69. Gollish, S. H., Burnstein, J. M., Ilson, R. G., Petrunka, C. N., and Strasberg, S. M. Nucleation of cholesterol monohydrate crystals from hepatic and gallbladder bile of patients with cholesterol gallstones. Gut *24*:836, 1983.
70. Holzbach, R. T. Metastability behavior of supersaturated bile. Hepatology *4*:155S, 1984.
71. Whiting, M. J., and Watts, J. M. Cholesterol gallstone pathogenesis: A study of potential nucleating agents for cholesterol crystal formation in bile. Clin. Sci. *68*:589, 1985.
72. Holzbach, R. T., Kibe, A., Thiel, E., Howell, J. H., Marsh, M., and Hermann, R. E. Biliary proteins: Unique inhibitors of cholesterol crystal nucleation in human gallbladder bile. J. Clin. Invest. *73*:35, 1984.
73. Whiting, M. J., and Watts, J. M. Supersaturated bile from obese patients without gallstones supports cholesterol crystal growth but not nucleation. Gastroenterology *86*:243, 1984.
74. Burnstein, M. J., Ilson, R. G., Petrunka, C. N., and Strasberg, S. M. Evidence for a potent nucleating factor in the gallbladder bile of patients with cholesterol gallstones. Gastroenterology *85*:801, 1983.
75. Ito, H., and Coe, F. L. Acid peptide and polyribonucleotide crystal growth inhibitors in human urine. Am. J. Physiol. *233*:F455, 1977.
76. Coe, F. L., Margolis, H. C., Deutsch, L. H., and Strauss, A. L. Urinary macromolecular crystal growth inhibitors in calcium nephrolithiasis. Electrolyte Metab. *3*:268, 1980.
77. Nakagawa, Y., Margolis, H. C., Yokayama, S., Kézdy, F. J., Kaiser, E. T., and Coe, F. L. Purification and characterization of a calcium oxalate monohydrate crystal growth inhibitor from human kidney tissue culture medium. J. Biol. Chem. *256*:3936, 1981.
78. Nancollas, G. H. Enamel apatite nucleation and crystal growth. J. Dental Res. *58*:861, 1979.
79. DeVries, A. L. Antifreeze peptides and glycopeptides in cold-water fishes. Annu. Rev. Physiol. *45*:245, 1983.
80. Sutor, D. J., and Percival, J. M. Presence or absence of inhibitors of crystal growth in bile. 1. Effect of bile on the formation of calcium phosphate, a constituent of gallstones. Gut *17*:506, 1976.
81. Lee, S. P., LaMont, J. T., and Carey, M. C. Role of gallbladder mucus hypersecretion in the evolution of cholesterol gallstones. J. Clin. Invest. *67*:1712, 1981.
82. Levy, P. F., Smith, B. F., and LaMont, J. T. Human gallbladder mucin accelerates nucleation of cholesterol in artificial bile. Gastroenterology *87*:270, 1984.
83. Smith, B. F., and LaMont, J. T. Hydrophobic binding properties of bovine gallbladder mucin. J. Biol. Chem. *259*:12170, 1984.
84. Gallinger, S., Taylor, R. D., Harvey, P. R. C., Petrunka, C. N., and Strasberg, S. M. Effect of mucous glycoprotein on nucleation time of human bile. Gastroenterology *89*:648, 1985.
85. Smith, B. F., and LaMont, J. T. Identification of gallbladder mucin-bilirubin complex in human cholesterol gallstone matrix. Effects of reducing agents on in vitro dissolution of matrix and intact gallstones. J. Clin. Invest. *76*:439, 1985.
86. Harvey, P. R. C., Rupar, C. A., Gallinger, S., Petrunka, C. N., and Strasberg, S. M. Quantitative and qualitative comparison of gallbladder mucus glycoprotein from patients with and without gallstones. Gut *27*:374, 1986.
87. Malet, P. F., Williamson, C. E., Trotman, B. W., and Soloway, R. D. Composition of pigmented centers of cholesterol gallstones. Hepatology *6*:477, 1986.
88. Van Berge Henegouwen, G. P., and Hofmann, A. F. Nocturnal gallbladder storage and emptying in gallstone patients and healthy subjects. Gastroenterology *75*:879, 1978.
89. Mok, H. Y. I., Von Bergmann, K., and Grundy, S. M. Kinetics of the enterohepatic circulation during fasting: Biliary lipid secretion and gallbladder storage. Gastroenterology *78*:1023, 1980.

90. Duane, W. C., and Hanson, K. C. Role of gallbladder emptying and small bowel transit in regulation of bile acid pool size in man. J. Lab. Clin. Med. *92*:858, 1978.
91. Jazrawi, R. P., Bridges, C., Joseph, A. E. A., and Northfield, T. C. Effects of artificial depletion of the bile acid pool in man. Gut *27*:771, 1986.
92. Everson, G. T., Braverman, D. Z., Johnson, M. L., and Kern, F., Jr. A critical evaluation of real-time ultrasonography for the study of gallbladder volume and contraction. Gastroenterology *79*:40, 1980.
93. Roslyn, J. J., Pitt, H. A., Mann, L. L., Ament, M. E., and Denbesten, L. Gallbladder disease in patients on long-term parenteral nutrition. Gastroenterology *84*:148, 1983.
94. Messing, B., Bories, C., Kunstlinger, F., and Bernier, J.-J. Does total parenteral nutrition induce gallbladder sludge formation and lithiasis? Gastroenterology *84*:1012, 1983.
95. Pitt, H. A., King, W., III, Mann, L. L., Roslyn, J. J., Berquist, W. E., Ament, M. A., and DenBesten, L. Increased risk of cholelithiasis with prolonged total parenteral nutrition. Am. J. Surg. *145*:106, 1983.
96. Hölzbach, R. T. Gallbladder stasis: Consequence of long-term parenteral hyperalimentation and risk factor for cholelithiasis (editorial). Gastroenterology *84*:1055, 1983.
97. Doty, J. E., Pitt, H. A., Porter-Fink, V., and Denbesten, L. Cholecystokinin prophylaxis of parenteral nutrition-induced gallbladder disease. Ann. Surg. *201*:76, 1985.
98. Cano, N., Cicero, F., Ranieri, F., Martin, J., and DiCostanzo, J. Ultrasonographic study of gallbladder motility during total parenteral nutrition. Gastroenterology *91*:313, 1986.
99. Doty, J. E., Pitt, H. A., Kuchenbecker, S. L., and DenBesten, L. Impaired gallbladder emptying before gallstone formation in the prairie dog. Gastroenterology *85*:168, 1983.
100. Fridhandler, T. M., Davison, J. S., and Shaffer, E. A. Defective gallbladder contractility in the ground squirrel and prairie dog during the early stages of gallstone disease. Gastroenterology *85*:830, 1983.
101. Bernhoft, R. A., Pellegrini, C. A., Broderick, W. C., and Way, L. W. Pigment sludge and stone formation in the acutely ligated dog gallbladder. Gastroenterology *85*:1166, 1983.
102. Fisher, R. S., Stelzer, F., Rock, E., and Malmud, L. S. Abnormal gallbladder emptying in patients with gallstones. Dig. Dis. Sci. *27*:1019, 1982.
103. Spellman, S. J., Shaffer, E. A., and Rosenthall, L. Gallbladder emptying in response to cholecystokinin. Gastroenterology *77*:115, 1979.
104. Forgacs, I. C., Maisey, M. N., Murphy, G. M., and Dowling, R. H. Influence of gallstones and ursodeoxycholic acid therapy on gallbladder emptying. Gastroenterology *87*:299, 1984.
105. Shaffer, E. A., McOrmond, P., and Duggan, H. Quantitative cholescintigraphy: Assessment of gallbladder filling and emptying in a duodenogastric reflux. Gastroenterology *79*:899, 1980.
106. Pomeranz, I. S., and Shaffer, E. A. Abnormal gallbladder emptying in a subgroup of patients with gallstones. Gastroenterology *88*:787, 1985.
107. Braverman, D. Z., Johnson, M. L., and Kern, F., Jr. Effects of pregnancy and contraceptive steroids on gallbladder function. N. Engl. J. Med. *302*:362, 1980.
108. Everson, G. T., McKinley, C., Lawson, M., Johnson, M., and Kern, F., Jr. Gallbladder function in the human female: Effect of the ovulatory cycle, pregnancy, and contraceptive steroids. Gastroenterology *82*:711, 1982.
109. Braun, B., and Dormeyer, H. H. Changes in gallbladder motor function during the female cycle—a risk factor lending to gallstone formation? Klin. Wochenschr. *60*:1357, 1982.
110. Filly, R. A., Allen, B., Minton, M. J., Bernhoft, R., and Way, L. W. In vitro investigation of the origin of echoes within biliary sludge. J. Clin. Ultrasound *8*:193, 1980.
111. Gonzalez, L., and MacIntyre, W. J. Acoustic shadow formation by gallstones. Radiology *135*:217, 1980.
112. Lee, S. P., and Nicolls, J. F. Nature and composition of biliary sludge. Gastroenterology *90*:677, 1986.
113. Friedman, G. D., Kannel, W. B., and Dawber, T. R. The epidemiology of gallstone disease: Observations in the Framingham study. J. Chronic Dis. *19*:273, 1966.
114. Bainton, D., Davies, G. R., Evans, K. T., and Gravelle, I. H. Gallbladder disease: Prevalence in a South Wales industrial town. N. Engl. J. Med. *294*:1147, 1976.
115. Barker, S. J. P., Gardner, M. J., Power, C., and Hutt, M. S. R. Prevalence of gallstone at necropsy in nine British towns: A collaborative study. Br. Med. J. *4*:1392, 1979.
116. Balzer, K., Goebell, H., Breuer, N., Ruping, K. W., and Leder, L. D. Epidemiology of gallstones in a German industrial town (Essen) from 1940–1975. Digestion *33*:189, 1986.
117. Brett, M., and Barker, D. J. P. The world distribution of gallstones. Int. J. Epidemiol. *5*:335, 1976.
118. Lowenfels, A. B. Gallstones and the risk of cancer. Gut *21*:1090, 1980.
119. Záhor, Z., Sternby, N. H., Kagan, A., Uemura, K., Vanecek, R., and Vichert, A. M. Frequency of cholelithiasis in Prague and Malmö: An autopsy study. Scand. J. Gastroenterol. *9*:3, 1974.
120. Lindström, C. G. Frequency of gallstone disease in a well-defined Swedish population. A prospective necropsy study in Malmö. Scand. J. Gastroenterol. *12*:341, 1977.
121. Ahlberg, J., Bergstrand, L. -O., and Sahlin, S. Changes in gallstone morbidity in a community with decreasing frequency of cholecystectomies. A statistical study in the county of Stockholm, Sweden, 1969–1982. Acta Chir. Scand. Suppl. *520*:53, 1984.
122. Janzon, L., Aspelin, P., Eriksson, S., Hildell, J., Trell, E., and Ostberg, H. Ultrasonographic screening for gallstone disease in middle-aged women. Detection rate, symptoms, and biochemical features. Scand. J. Gastroenterol. *20*:706, 1985.
123. Norrby, S., Fagerberg, G., and Sjödahl, R. Decreasing incidence of gallstone disease in a defined Swedish population. Scand. J. Gastroenterol. *21*:158, 1986.
124. Rome Group for the epidemiology and prevention of cholelithiasis (GREPCO). Prevalence of gallstone disease in an Italian adult female population. Am. J. Epidemiol. *119*:796, 1984.
125. Barbara, L., Sama, C., Labate, A. M. M., Taroni, F., Rusticali, A. G., Festi, D., Sapio, C., Roda, E., Banterli, C., Puci, A., Formentini, F., Colasanti, S., and Nardin, F. A population study on the prevalence of gallstone disease: The Sermione Study. Hepatology *7*:913, 1987.
126. Medina, E., Kaempffer, A. M , and de Croizet, V. A. Epidemiologia de las colecistopatias en Chile. II. Factores de importancia en estudios de autopsia. Rev. Med. Chile *100*:1382, 1972.
127. Rios-Dalenz, J., Takabayashi, A., Henson, D. E., Strom, B. L., and Soloway, R. D. Cancer of the gallbladder in Bolivia: Suggestions concerning etiology. Am. J. Gastroenterol. *80*:371, 1985.
128. Marinovic, I., Guerra, C., and Larach, G. Incidencia de litiasis biliar en material de autoposia y analisis de composicion de los calculos. Rev. Med. Chile *100*:1320, 1972.
129. Medina, E., Pascual, J., and Medina, R. Frecuencia de la litiasis biliar en Chile. Rev. Med. Chile *111*:668, 1983.
130. Sampliner, R. E., Bennett, P. H., Commess, L. J., Rose, F. A., and Burch, T. A. Gallbladder disease in Pima Indians: Demonstration of high prevalence and early onset by cholecystography. N. Engl. J. Med. *283*:1358, 1970.
131. Bennion, L. J., Knowler, W. C., Mott, D. M., Spagnola, A. M., and Bennett, P. H. Development of lithogenic bile during puberty in Pima Indians. N. Engl. J. Med. *300*:873, 1979.
132. Williams, C. N., Johnson, J. L., and Weldon, K. L. M. Prevalence of gallstones and gallbladder disease in Canadian Micmac Indian women. Can. Med. Assoc. J. *117*:758, 1977.
133. Thistle, J. L., Eckhart, K. L., Nensel, R. E., Nobrega, F. T., Poehling, G. G., Reimer, M., and Schoenfield, L. J. Prevalence of gallbladder disease among Chippewa Indians. Mayo Clin. Proc. *46*:603, 1971.
134. Boss, L. P., Lanier, A. P., Dohan, P. H., and Bender, T. R. Cancers of the gallbladder and biliary tract in Alaskan natives: 1970–79. J. Natl. Cancer Inst. *69*:1005, 1982.
135. Odom, F. C., Oliver, B. B., Kline, M., and Rogers, W.

Gallbladder disease in patients 20 years of age and under. South. Med. J. *69*:1299, 1976.
136. Morris, D. L., Buechley, R. W., Key, C. R., and Morgan, M. V. Gallbladder disease and gallbladder cancer among American Indians in tricultural New Mexico. Cancer *42*:2472, 1978.
137. Diehl, A. K., Stern, M. P., Ostrower, V. S., and Friedman, P. C. Prevalence of clinical gallbladder disease in Mexican-American, Anglo, and black women. South. Med. J. *73*:438, 1980.
138. Blanco, D., Ross, R. K., Paganini-Hill, A., and Henderson, B. E. Cholecystectomy and colon cancer. Dis. Colon Rectum *27*:290, 1984.
139. Hanis, C. L., Ferrell, R. E., Tulloch, B. R., and Schull, W. J. Gallbladder disease epidemiology in Mexican-Americans in Starr County, Texas. Am. J. Epidemiol. *122*:820, 1985.
140. Diehl, A. K., Rosenthal, M., Hazuda, H. P., Comeaux, P. J., and Stern, M. P. Socioeconomic status and the prevalence of clinical gallbladder disease. J. Chronic Dis. *38*:1019, 1985.
141. Weiss, K. M., Ferrell, R. E., Hanis, C. L., and Styne, P. N. Genetics and epidemiology of gallbladder disease in New World native peoples. Am. J. Hum. Genet. *36*:1259, 1984.
142. Van der Linden, W., and Lindelöf, G. The familial occurrence of gallstone disease. Acta Genet. Statist. *15*:159, 1965.
143. Van der Linden, W., and Simonson, H. Familial occurrence of gallstone disease: Incidence in parents of young patients. Hum. Hered. *23*:123, 1973.
144. Gilat, T., Feldman, C., Halpern, Z., Dan, M., and Bar-Meir, S. An increased familial frequency of gallstones. Gastroenterology *84*:242, 1983.
145. Boston Collaborative Drug Surveillance Programme. Oral contraceptives and venous thromboembolic disease, surgically confirmed gallbladder disease, and breast tumours. Lancet *1*:1399, 1973.
146. Evron, S., Frankel, M., and Diamant, Y. Biliary disease in young women and its association with pregnancy or oral contraceptives. Int. Surg. *67*:488, 1982.
147. Strom, B. L., Tamragouri, R. N., Morse, M. L., Lazar, E. L., West, S. L., Stolley, P. D., and Jones, J. K. Oral contraceptives and other risk factors for gallbladder disease. Clin. Pharmacol. Ther. *39*:335, 1986.
148. Royal College of General Practitioners' oral contraception study. Oral contraceptives and gallbladder disease. Lancet *2*:957, 1982.
149. Scragg, P. K. R., McMichael, A. J., and Seamark, R. F. Oral contraceptives, pregnancy, and endogenous oestrogen in gallstone disease—a case-control study. Br. Med. J. *288*:1795, 1984.
150. Everson, R. B., Byar, D. P., and Bischoff, A. J. Estrogen predisposes to cholecystectomy but not to gallstones. Gastroenterology *82*:4, 1982.
151. Price, W. H. Gallbladder dyspepsia. Br. J. Med. *2*:138, 1963.
152. Koch, J. P., and Donaldson, R. M., Jr. A survey of food intolerances in hospitalized patients. N. Engl. J. Med. *271*:657, 1964.
153. Gracie, W. A., and Ransohoff, D. F. The natural history of silent gallstone: The innocent gallstone is not a myth. N. Engl. J. Med. *307*:798, 1982.
154. McSherry, C. K., Ferstenberg, H., Calhoun, W. F., Lahman, E., and Virshup, M. The natural history of diagnosed gallstone disease in symptomatic and asymptomatic patients. Ann. Surg. *202*:59, 1985.
155. Ransohoff, D. F., Gracie, W. A., Wolfenson, L. B., and Neuhauser, D. Prophylactic cholecystectomy or expectant management for silent gallstones. A decision analysis to assess survival. Ann. Intern. Med. *99*:199, 1983.
156. Thistle, J. L., Cleary, P. A., Lachin, J. M., Tyor, M. P., and Hersh, T. The Steering Committee; and the National Cooperative Gallstone Study Group. The natural history of cholelithiasis: The National Cooperative Gallstone Study. Ann. Intern. Med. *101*:171, 1984.
157. Wenkert, A., and Robertson, B. The natural history of gallstone disease: Eleven-year review of 781 non-operated cases. Gastroenterology *50*:376, 1966.
158. Mok, H. Y. I., Druffel, E. R. M., and Rampone, W. M. Chronology of cholelithiasis. Dating gallstones from atmospheric radiocarbon produced by nuclear bomb explosions. N. Engl. J. Med. *314*:1075, 1986.
159. Lund, J. Surgical indications in cholelithiasis: Prophylactic cholecystectomy elucidated upon the basis of long-term follow-up on 526 non-operated cases. Ann. Surg. *151*:153, 1960.
160. Sandler, R. S., Maule, W. F., and Baltus, M. E. Factors associated with postoperative complications in diabetics after biliary tract surgery. Gastroenterology *91*:157, 1986.
161. Pelligrini, C. A. Asymptomatic gallstones. Does diabetes mellitus make a difference? Gastroenterology *91*:245, 1986.
162. Ruppin, D. C., and Dowling, R. H. Is recurrence inevitable after gallstone dissolution by bile acid treatment? Lancet *1*:183, 1982.
163. Somerville, K. W., Rose, D. H., Bell, G. D., and Knapp, D. R. Gallstone dissolution and recurrence: Are we being mislead? Br. Med. J. *284*:1295, 1982.
164. Shapero, T. F., Rosen, I. E., Wilson, S. R., and Fisher, M. M. Discrepancy between ultrasound and oral cholecystography in the assessment of gallstone dissolution. Hepatology *2*:587, 1982.
165. Gleeson, D., Ruppin, R. C., and the British Gallstone Study Group. Discrepancies between cholecystography and ultrasonography in the detection of recurrent stones. J. Hepatol. *1*:597, 1985.
166. Ruppin, D. C., Murphy, G. M., Dowling, R. H., and The British Gallstone Study Group. Gallstone disease without gallstones—bile acid and bile lipid metabolism after complete gallstone dissolution. Gut *27*:559, 1986.
167. Nakagawa, S., Makino, I., Ishizaki, T., and Dohi, I. Dissolution of cholesterol gallstones by ursodeoxycholic acid. Lancet *2*:367, 1977.
168. Stiehl, A., Czygan, P., Kommerell, B., Weis, H. J., and Holtermüller, K. H. Ursodeoxycholic acid versus chenodeoxycholic acid. Comparison of their effects on bile acid and bile lipid composition in patients with cholesterol gallstones. Gastroenterology *75*:1016, 1978.
169. Makino, I., and Nakagawa, S. Changes in biliary lipid and biliary bile acid composition in patients after administration of ursodeoxycholic acid. J. Lipid Res. *19*:723, 1978.
170. Tokyo Cooperative Gallstone Study Group. Efficacy and indications of ursodeoxycholic acid treatment for dissolving gallstones. A multicenter double-blind trial. Gastroenterology *78*:542, 1980.
171. Stiehl, A., Raedsch, R., Czygan, P., Götz, R., Männer, C. H., Walker, S., and Kommerell, B. Effects of biliary bile acid composition on biliary cholesterol saturation in gallstone patients treated with chenodeoxycholic acid and/or ursodeoxycholic acid. Gastroenterology *79*:1192, 1980.
172. Salen, G., Colalillo, A., Verga, D., Bagan, E., Tint, G. S., and Shefer, S. Effect of high and low doses of ursodeoxycholic acid on gallstone dissolution in humans. Gastroenterology *78*:1412, 1980.
173. Weis, H. J., Holtermüller, K. H., and Gilsdorf, P. Gallstone dissolution with chenodeoxycholic acid: A clinical study. Klin. Wochenschr. *58*:313, 1980.
174. Schoenfield, J. L., Lachin, J. M., The Steering Committee, and the National Cooperative Gallstone Study Group. Chenodiol (chenodoxycholic acid) for dissolution of gallstones: The National Cooperative Gallstone Study: A controlled trial of efficacy and safety. Ann. Intern. Med. *95*:257, 1981.
175. Tint, G. S., Salen, G., Colalillo, A. Ursodeoxycholic acid: A safe and effective agent for dissolving gallstones. Ann. Intern. Med. *97*:351, 1982.
176. Thistle, J. L., LaRusso, N. F., Hofmann, A. F., Turcotte, J., Carlson, G. L., and Ott, B. J. Differing effects of ursodeoxycholic or chenodeoxycholic acid on biliary cholesterol saturation and bile acid metabolism in man. A dose response study. Dig. Dis. Sci. *27*:161, 1982.
177. Bachrach, W. H., and Hofmann, A. F. Ursodeoxycholic acid in the treatment of cholesterol cholelithiasis. Dig. Dis. Sci. *27*:737, 1982.
178. Roda, E., Bazzoli, F., Labate, A. M. M., Mazzella, G., Roda, A., Sama, C., Festi, D., Aldini, R., Taroni, F., and Barbara,

L. Ursodeoxycholic acid vs. chenodeoxycholic acid as cholesterol gallstone-dissolving agents: A comparative randomized study. Hepatology *2*:804, 1982.

179. Meredith, T. J., Williams, G. V., Maton, P. N., Murphy, G. M., Saxton, H. M., and Dowling, R. H. Retrospective comparison of 'Cheno' and 'Urso' in the medical treatment of gallstones. Gut *23*:382, 1982.
180. Maton, P. N., Iser, J. H., Reuben, A., Saxton, H. M., Murphy, G. M., and Dowling, R. H. Outcome of chenodeoxycholic acid (CDCA) treatment in 125 patients with radiolucent stones. Medicine *61*:86, 1982.
181. Neligan, P., Bateson, M. C., Trash, D. B., Ross, P. E., and Bouchier, I. A. D. Ursodeoxycholic acid for the dissolution of radiolucent gallbladder stones. Digestion *28*:225, 1983.
182. Fromm, H., Roat, J. W., Gonzalez, V., Sarva, R. P., and Farivar, S. Comparative efficacy and side effects of ursodeoxycholic and chenodeoxycholic acids in dissolving gallstones. A double-blind controlled study. Gastroenterology *85*:1257, 1983.
183. Maudgal, D. P., Kupfer, R. M., and Northfield, T. C. Factors affecting gallstone dissolution rate during chenic acid therapy. Gut *24*:7, 1983.
184. Stiehl, A., Raedsch, R., Rudolph, G., and Walker, S. Effect of ursodeoxycholic acid on biliary bile acid and bile lipid composition in gallstone patients. Hepatology *4*:107, 1984.
185. Erlinger, S., Go, A. L., Husson, J. M., and Fevery, J. French-Belgian cooperative study of ursodeoxycholic acid in the medical dissolution of gallstones: A double-blind, randomized, dose-response study, and comparison with chenodeoxycholic acid. Hepatology *4*:308, 1984.
186. Fisher, M. M., Roberts, E. A., Rosen, I. E., Shapero, T. F., Sutherland, L. R., Davies, R. S., Bacchus, R., and Lee, S. V. The Sunnybrook Gallstone Study: A double-blind controlled trial of chenodeoxycholic acid for gallstone dissolution. Hepatology *5*:102, 1985.
187. Ros, E., Novarro, S., Fernandez, I., Reixach, M., Ribo, J. M., and Rodes, J. Utility of biliary microscopy for the prediction of the chemical composition of gallstones and the outcome of dissolution therapy with ursodeoxycholic acid. Gastroenterology *91*:703, 1986.
188. Lindblad, L., Lundholm, K., and Scherstén, T. Influence of cholic and chenodeoxycholic acid on biliary cholesterol secretion in man. Eur. J. Clin. Invest. *7*:383, 1977.
189. Anderson, J. M. Chenodeoxycholic acid desaturates bile—but how? Gastroenterology *77*:1146, 1979.
190. Einarsson, K., and Grundy, S. M. Effects of feeding cholic acid and chenodeoxycholic acid on cholesterol absorption and hepatic secretion of biliary lipids in man. J. Lipid Res. *21*:23, 1980.
191. Ahlberg, J., Angelin, B., and Einarsson, K. Hepatic 3-hydroxy-3-methylglutaryl coenzyme A reductase activity and biliary lipid composition in man: Relation to cholesterol gallstone disease and effects of cholic acid and chenodeoxycholic acid treatment. J. Lipid Res. *22*:410, 1981.
192. Sama, C., LaRusso, N. F., Lopez del Pino, V., and Thistle, J. L. Effects of acute bile acid administration on biliary lipid secretion in healthy volunteers. Gastroenterology *82*:515, 1982.
193. Angelin, B., Ewerth, S., and Einarsson, K. Ursodeoxycholic acid treatment in cholesterol gallstone disease: Effects on hepatic 3-hydroxy-3-methylglutaryl coenzyme A reductase activity, biliary lipid composition, and plasma lipid levels. J. Lipid Res. *24*:461, 1983.
194. Nilsell, K., Angelin, B., Leijd, B., and Einarsson, K. Comparative effects of ursodeoxycholic acid and chenodeoxycholic acid on bile acid kinetics and biliary lipid secretion in man. Evidence for different modes of action on bile acid synthesis. Gastroenterology *85*:1248, 1983.
195. Von Bergmann, K., Epple-Gutsfeld, M., and Leiss, O. Differences in the effects of chenodeoxycholic and ursodeoxycholic acid on biliary lipid secretion and bile acid synthesis in patients with gallstones. Gastroenterology *87*:136, 1984.
196. Leiss, O., Von Bergmann, K., Streicher, U., and Strotkoetter, H. Effect of three different dihydroxy bile acids on intestinal cholesterol absorption in normal volunteers. Gastroenterology *87*:144, 1984.
197. Hardison, W. G. M., and Grundy, S. M. Effect of ursodeoxycholic acid and its taurine conjugate on bile acid synthesis and cholesterol absorption. Gastroenterology *87*:130, 1984.
198. Grundy, S. M., Lan, S-P., Lachin, J., The Steering Committee, and The National Cooperative Gallstone Study Group. The effects of chenodiol on biliary lipids and their association with gallstone dissolution in the National Cooperative Gallstone Study (NCGS). J. Clin. Invest. *73*:1156, 1984.
199. Tint, G. S., Salen, G., and Shefer, S. Effect of ursodeoxycholic acid and chenodeoxycholic acid on cholesterol and bile acid metabolism (progress article). Gastroenterology *91*:1007, 1986.
200. Angelin, B., Raviola, C. A., Innerarity, T. L., and Mahley, R. W. Regulation of hepatic lipoprotein receptors in the dog. Rapid regulation of apolipoprotein B, E receptors, but not of apolipoprotein E receptors, by intestinal lipoproteins and bile acids. J. Clin. Invest. *71*:816, 1983.
201. Park, Y. -H., Igimi, H., and Carey, M. C. Dissolution of human cholesterol gallstones in simulated chenodeoxyocholate-rich and ursodeoxycholate-rich biles. An in vitro study of dissolution rates and mechanisms. Gastroenterology *87*:150, 1984.
202. Poupon, R. E., Poupon, R. Y., Duval, M., LeQuernec, L., and Erlinger, S. Chronic administration of chenodeoxycholic acid increases cholesterol saturation in bile in the dog. Eur. J. Clin. Invest. *9*:103, 1979.
203. The Rome Group for the Epidemiology and Prevention of Cholelithiasis (GREPCO). Radiologic appearance of gallstones and its relationship with biliary symptoms and awareness of having gallstones: Observations during epidemiological studies. Dig. Dis. Sci. *32*:349, 1987.
204. Sarva, R. P., Fromm, H., Farivar, S., Sembrat, R. F., Mendelow, H., Shinozuka, H., and Wolfson, S. K. Comparison of the effects between ursodeoxycholic and chenodeoxycholic acids on liver function and structure in the rhesus monkey. Gastroenterology *79*:629, 1980.
205. Fisher, R. L., Anderson, D., Boyer, J. L., Ishak, K., Klatskin, G., Lachin, J. M., and Phillips, M. J., The Steering Committee, and The National Cooperative Gallstone Study Group. A prospective morphologic evaluation of hepatic toxicity of chenodeoxycholic acid in patients with cholelithiasis. The National Cooperative Gallstone Study. Hepatology *2*:187, 1982.
206. Phillips, M. J., Fisher, R. L., Anderson, D. W., Lan, S., Lachin, J. M., and Boyer, J. L., The Steering Committee, and The National Cooperative Gallstone Study Group. Ultrastructural evidence of intrahepatic cholestasis before and after chenodeoxycholic acid (CDCA) therapy in patients with cholelithiasis: The National Cooperative Gallstone Study. Hepatology *3*:209, 1983.
207. Dumont, M., Erlinger, S., and Uchman, S. Hypercholeresis induced by ursodeoxycholic acid and 7-ketolithocholic acid in the rat. Possible role of bicarbonate transport. Gastroenterology *79*:82, 1980.
208. Raedsch, R., Stiehl, A., and Czygan, P. Ursodeoxycholic acid and gallstone calcification. Lancet *2*:1296, 1981.
209. Bateson, M. C., Bouchier, I. A. D., Trash, D. B., Maudgal, D. B., and Northfield, T. C. Calcification of radiolucent stones during treatment with ursodeoxycholic acid. Br. Med. J. *283*:645, 1981.
210. Whiting, M. J., Jarvinen, V., and Watts, J. M. Chemical composition of gallstones resistant to dissolution therapy with chenodeoxycholic acid. Gut *21*:1077, 1980.
211. Whiting, M. J., Bradley, B. M., and Watts, J. M. Chemical and physical properties of gallstones in South Australia: Implications for dissolution treatment. Gut *24*:11, 1983.
212. Freilich, H. S., Malet, P. F., Schwartz, J. S., and Soloway, R. D. Chemical and morphologic characteristics of cholesterol gallstones that failed to dissolve on chenodiol. The National Cooperative Gallstone Study. Gastroenterology *91*:713, 1986.
213. Williams, C. N. Prevention of cholelithiasis: Intervention on risk factors. *In* Capocaccia, L. K., Ricci, G., Angelico, F., Angelico, M., and Attili, A. F. (eds.): Epidemiology and Prevention of Gallstone Disease. Boston, MTP Press Ltd., 1984, pp. 210–222.
214. Podda, M., Zuin, M., Dioguardi, M. G., Festorazzi, S., and

Diguardi, N. A combination of chenodeoxycholic acid and ursodeoxycholic acid is more effective than either alone in reducing biliary cholesterol saturation. Hepatology *2*:334, 1982.
215. Roehrkasse, R., Fromm, H., Malavolta, M., Tunuguntla, A. K., and Ceryak, S. Gallstone dissolution treatment with a combination of chenodeoxycholic and ursodeoxycholic acids. Studies of safety, efficacy and effects on bile lithogenicity, bile acid pool, and serum lipids. Dig. Dis. Sci. *31*:1032, 1986.
216. Podda, M., Zuin, M., De Fazio, C., Dioguardi, M. L., Battezzati, P. M., and Grandinotti, G. Efficacy of combined ursodeoxycholic and chenodeoxycholic acid treatment. Ann. Intern. Med., in press, 1988.
217. Singhal, A. K., Cohen, B. I., Mosbach, E. H., Une, M., Stenger, R. J., McSherry, C. K., May-Donath, P., and Palaia, T. Prevention of cholesterol-induced gallstones by hyodeoxycholic acid in the prairie dog. J. Lipid Res. *25*:539, 1984.
218. McSherry, C. K., Mosbach, E. H., Cohen, B. I., Une, M., Stenger, R. J., and Singhal, A. K. Hyodeoxycholic acid: A new approach to gallstone prevention. Am. J. Surg. *149*:126, 1985.
219. Loria, P., Carulli, N., Medici, G., Menozzi, D., Salvioli, G., Bertolotti, M., and Montanari, M. Effect of ursocholic acid on bile lipid secretion and composition. Gastroenterology *90*:865, 1986.
220. Mazella, G., Bazzoli, F., Villanova, N., Grigola, B., Malavolti, M., Roda, A., Luzza, F., Roda, E., and Barbara, L. 7-ketolithocholic acid administration in man: Effects on biliary lipid composition, serum bile acid pattern and evaluation of the cholelitholytic potential. Ital. J. Gastroenterol. *18*:145, 1985.
221. Gurantz, D., and Hofmann, A. F. Influence of bile acid structure on bile flow and biliary lipid secretion in the hamster. Am. J. Physiol. *247*:G736, 1984.
222. Yoon, Y. V., Hagey, L. R., Hofmann, A. F., Gurantz, D., Michelotti, E. L., and Steinbach, J. H. Effect of side-chain shortening on the physiological properties of bile acids: Hepatic transport and effect on biliary secretion of 23-nor-ursodeoxycholate in rodents. Gastroenterology *90*:837, 1986.
223. Marks, J. W., Lan, S. -P., The Steering Committee, and The National Cooperative Gallstone Study Group. Low dose chenodiol to prevent gallstone recurrence after dissolution therapy. Ann. Intern. Med. *100*:376, 1984.
224. Allen, M. J., Borody, T. J., Bugliosi, T. F., May, G. R., LaRusso, N. F., and Thistle, J. L. Rapid dissolution of gallstones by methyl tert-butyl ether. Preliminary observations. N. Engl. J. Med. *312*:217, 1985.
225. Allen, M. J., Barody, T. J., Bugliosi, T. F., May, G. R., LaRusso, N. F., and Thistle, J. L. Cholelitholysis using methyl tertiary butyl ether. Gastroenterology *88*:122, 1985.
226. Allen, M. J., Barody, T. J., and Thistle, J. L. In vitro dissolution of cholesterol gallstones. A study of factors influencing rate and a comparison of solvents. Gastroenterology *89*:1097, 1985.
227. vanSonnenberg, E., Hofmann, A. F., Neoptolemus, J., Wittich, G. R., Princenthal, R. A., and Wilson, S. A. Gallstone dissolution with methyl-tert-butyl ether via percutaneous cholecystostomy: Success and caveats. Am. J. Roentgenol. *146*:865, 1986.
228. DiPadova, C., DiPadova, F., Montorsi, W., and Tritapepe, R. Methyl tert-butyl ether fails to dissolve retained radiolucent common bile duct stones. Gastroenterology *91*:1296, 1986.
229. Sauerbruch, T., Delius, M., Paumgartner, G., Holl, J., Weiss, O., Weber, W., Hepp, W., and Brendel, W. Fragmentation of gallstones by extracorporeal shock waves. N. Engl. J. Med. *314*:818, 1986.
230. Mulley, A. G., Jr. Shock-wave lithotripsy. Assessing a slam-bang technology (editorial). N. Engl. J. Med. *314*:845, 1986.
231. Riehle, R. A., Jr., Fair, W. R., and Vaughen, E. D., Jr. Extracorporeal shock-wave lithotripsy for upper urinary tract calculi. One year's experience at a single center. JAMA *255*:2043, 1986.
232. Neubrand, M., Sauerbruch, T., Stellaard, F., and Paumgartner, G. In vitro cholesterol gallstone dissolution after fragmentation with shock waves. Digestion *34*:51, 1986.
233. Brendel, W. Shockwaves: A new physical principle in medicine. Eur. Surg. Res. *18*:177, 1986.
234. Trotman, B. W. Insights into pigment stone disease. J. Lab. Clin. Med. *93*:349, 1979.
235. Ostrow, J. D. The etiology of pigment gallstones. Hepatology *4*:215s, 1984.
236. Matsushiro, T., Suzuki, N., Sato, T., and Maki, T. Effects of diet on glucuric acid concentration in bile and the formation of calcium bilirubinate gallstones. Gastroenterology *72*:630, 1977.
237. Nagase, M., Hikasa, Y., Soloway, R. D., Tanimura, H., Setoyama, M., and Kato, H. Gallstones in western Japan. Factors affecting the prevalence of intrahepatic gallstones. Gastroenterology *78*:684, 1980.
238. Hikasa, Y., Takabayashi, A., Sato, T., Takahashi, H., Sekiya, T., Maruyama, K., Kobiashi, N., Tanimura, H., and Soloway, R. D. Mechanism of the formation of bilirubin calcium and black stones. Arch. Jpn. Chir. *55*:3, 1986.
239. Trotman, B. W., and Soloway, R. D. Pigment Gallstone Disease: Summary of the National Institute of Health-International Workshop. Hepatology *2*:879, 1982.
240. Maki, T., Matsushiro, T., and Suzuki, N. Clarification of the nomenclature of pigment stones. Am. J. Surg. *144*:302, 1982.
241. Malet, P. F., Takabayashi, A., Trotman, B. W., Soloway, R. D., and Weston, N. E. Black and brown pigment gallstones differ in microstructure and microcomposition. Hepatology *4*:227, 1984.
242. Suzuki, N., Nakamura, Y., and Sato, T. Infrared absorption spectroscopy of pure pigment gallstones. Tohoku J. Exp. Med. *116*:259, 1975.
243. Wosiewitz, U., and Schroebler, S. On the chemistry of 'black' pigment stones from the gallbladder. Clin. Chim. Acta *89*:1, 1978.
244. Wosiewitz, U., and Schroebler, S. On "polymer pigments" in human pigment gallstones. Naturwissenschaften *65*:162, 1978.
245. Burnett, W., Dwyer, K. R., and Kennard, C. H. L. Black pigment or polybilirubinate gallstones, composition, and formation. Ann. Surg. *193*:331, 1981.
246. Zilm, K. W., Grant, D. M., Englert, E., Jr., and Straight, R. C. The use of ^{13}C-nuclear magnetic resonance for the characterization of cholesterol and bilirubin pigment composition of human gallstones. Biochem. Biophys. Res. Commun. *93*:857, 1980.
247. Black, B. E., Carr, S. H., Ohkubo, H., and Ostrow, J. D. Equilibrium swelling of pigment gallstones: Evidence for network polymer structure. Biopolymers *21*:601, 1982.
248. Ohkubo, H., Ostrow, J. D., Carr, S. H., and Rege, R. H. Polymer networks in pigment and cholesterol gallstones assessed by equilibrium swelling and infrared spectroscopy. Gastroenterology *98*:805, 1984.
249. Masuda, H., and Nakayama, F. Composition of bile pigment in gallstones and bile and their etiological significance. J. Lab. Clin. Med. *93*:353, 1979.
250. Robins, S. J., Fasulo, J. M., and Patton, G. M.: Lipids of pigment gallstones. Biochim. Biophys. Acta *712*:21, 1982.
251. LaMont, J. T., Ventola, A. S., Trotman, B. W., and Soloway, R. D. Mucin glycoprotein content of human pigment gallstones. Hepatology *3*:377, 1983.
252. Trotman, B. W., and Soloway, R. D. Pigment vs. cholesterol cholelithiasis: Clinical and epidemiological aspects. Am. J. Dig. Dis. *20*:735, 1975.
253. Goodhard, G. L., Levison, M. E., Trotman, B. W., and Soloway, R. D. Pigment vs. cholesterol cholelithiasis. Bacteriology of gallbladder stone, bile, and tissue correlated with biliary lipid analysis. Am. J. Dig. Dis. *23*:877, 1978.
254. Tabata, M., and Nakayama, F. Bacteria and gallstones. Etiological significance. Dig. Dis. Sci. *26*:218, 1981.
255. Schull, S. D., Wagner, C. I., Trotman, B. W., and Soloway, R. D. Factors affecting bilirubin excretion in patients with cholesterol or pigment gallstones. Gastroenterology *72*:625, 1977.
256. Soloway, R. D., Trotman, B. W., Maddrey, W. C., and Nakayama, F. Pigment gallstone composition in patients with hemolysis or infection/stasis. Dig. Dis. Sci. *31*:454, 1986.
257. Cetta, F. Bile infection documented as initial event in the

pathogenesis of brown pigment biliary stones. Hepatology *6*:482, 1986.

257a. Stewart, L., Smith, A. L., Pelligrini, C. A., Motson, R. W., and Way, L. W. Pigment gallstones form as a composite of bacterial microcolonies and pigment solids. Ann. Surg. *206*:242, 1987.

258. Maki, T. Pathogenesis of calcium bilirubinate gallstones: Role of E. coli, β-glucuronidase, and coagulation by inorganic ions, polyelectrolytes and agitation. Ann. Surg. *164*:90, 1966.

259. Wosiewitz, U., and Schroebler, S. Solubilization of unconjugated bilirubin by bile salts. Experientia *35*:717, 1979.

260. Moore, E. W., Celic, L., and Ostrow, J. D. Interactions between ionized calcium and sodium taurocholate: Bile salts are important buffers for prevention of calcium-containing gallstones. Gastroenterology *83*:1079, 1982.

261. Rege, R. V., and Moore, E. W. Pathogenesis of calcium-containing gallstones. Canine ductular bile, but not gallbladder bile, is supersaturated with calcium carbonate. J. Clin. Invest. *77*:21, 1986.

262. Boonyapisit, S. T., Trotman, B. W., and Ostrow, J. D. Unconjugated bilirubin and the hydrolysis of conjugated bilirubin in gallbladder bile of patients with cholelithiasis. Gastroenterology *74*:70, 1978.

263. Duvaldestin, P., Mahu, J. -L., Metreau, J. -M., Arondel, J., Preaux, A. -M., and Berthelot, P. Possible role of a defect in hepatic bilirubin glucuronidation in the initiation of cholesterol gallstones. Gut *21*:650, 1980.

264. Trotman, B. W., Bernstein, S. E., Bove, K. E., and Wirt, G. D. Studies on the pathogenesis of pigment gallstones in hemolytic anemia. Description and characteristics of a mouse model. J. Clin. Invest. *65*:1301, 1980.

265. LaMont, J. T., Turner, B. S., Bernstein, S. E., and Trotman, B. W. Gallbladder glycoprotein secretion in mice with hemolytic anemia and pigment gallstones. Hepatology *3*:198, 1983.

266. Trotman, B. W., Bernstein, S. E., Balistreri, W. F., Wirt, G. D., and Martin, R. A. Hemolysis-induced gallstones in mice: Increased unconjugated bilirubin in hepatic bile predisposes to gallstone formation. Gastroenterology *81*:232, 1981.

89 Cholelithiasis; Chronic and Acute Cholecystitis

LAWRENCE W. WAY
MARVIN H. SLEISENGER

Gallstones do not inevitably cause disease. Some remain asymptomatic, some give rise to minor symptoms, and others cause serious complications. This chapter covers the epidemiology and natural history of gallstone disease and the clinical management of gallstone disease of the gallbladder.

EPIDEMIOLOGY OF GALLSTONE DISEASE

Approximately 20 million people in the United States have gallstones, and about 300,000 operations are performed yearly for this disease and its complications. Each year about one third as many individuals are surgically treated for gallstones as newly acquire the disease.

The incidence of gallstone disease is influenced by age, sex, and a variety of cultural, ethnic, and medical factors.[1–9] Cholesterol gallstone disease is two to three times as common in women as in men. The difference begins at puberty, increases until menopause, and then declines. Gender has no influence, however, on the frequency of pigment gallstone disease.

Estimates of the prevalence of gallbladder disease vary, depending on the methods and criteria used to make the diagnosis. Most epidemiologic studies have relied on questionnaires or interviews, basing the diagnosis on a history of cholecystectomy or imaging tests positive for gallstone disease. Studies of this kind have given prevalence rates such as those in Table 89–1 from the article by Diehl and coworkers.[4]

These figures show that racial background has a major influence on the prevalence of gallstones. Blacks are relatively less susceptible; Caucasians have intermediate susceptibility; and American Indians are markedly susceptible. Mexican-Americans, a racially mixed group, have a prevalence between that of American Indians and Caucasians. The relative susceptibility of blacks, Caucasians, and American Indians in the United States is about 1, 1.5, and 3, respectively.

As might be expected, autopsy studies and cholecystographic or ultrasonographic surveys produce prevalence estimates two to three times higher than those derived from patient histories. Representative data from such studies by Godrey,[5] Bateson,[10] Lindstrom,[7] Sampliner,[11] Balzer,[12] and their coworkers are given in Table 89–2. The autopsy study of Balzer et al.[12] demonstrated an increasing prevalence of gallstone disease

Table 89–1. PREVALENCE OF GALLBLADDER DISEASE BASED UPON SYMPTOMS

Age Group	Framingham, Mass.	Pima Indians	Mexican-Americans	Caucasians	Blacks
15–19			0%	0%	0%
20–29			4%	3%	0%
30–39	2%	36%	18%	8%	3%
40–49	6%	40%	25%	25%	12%
50–59	10%	34%	33%	16%	13%

over three 12-year periods from 1940 to 1975, whereas evidence from cholecystographies performed in a defined Swedish population[13] suggested that the prevalence was decreasing between 1972 and 1981.

In most epidemiologic studies, obesity has been found to increase the risk of gallstone disease.[14–17] Bernstein et al.[14] stratified a group of 62,739 American women into five cohorts of different body weight and found a strong progressive correlation between the risk of gallstone disease and increasing levels of obesity. The relative risk of gallstone disease in the most overweight women in the 20- to 29-year-old age group was 6.75 compared with women of the same age of normal weight. The relative risk associated with obesity remained elevated at all age levels examined (i.e., up to age 60), but was greatest in the 20- to 29-year-old cohort.

Layde et al.,[6] using data from a family planning clinic in Oxford, England, found obesity to be the major factor governing variations in the prevalence of gallstone disease in women aged 25 to 39. The relative risk (6.6) for the most overweight group in this study was similar to that in the report by Bernstein et al.[14]

Williams[9] reported that the principal risk factor for gallstones in persons living in a rural Canadian community was obesity. In one study from Australia,[17] the effect of obesity was confined to women under age 50.

Gallstone disease is an ancillary finding in a large percentage of persons who present for surgical therapy of morbid obesity.[18, 19] Thiet et al.[19] calculated the incidence of symptomatic cholelithiasis to be about 70 per cent in a series of 477 morbidly obese patients who had gastric or intestinal bypass operations for obesity. The excess prevalence of gallstone disease in these patients was confined to the women. Because of the technical insensitivity of preoperative ultrasound and cholecystography in the morbidly obese,[20] Thiet et al.[19] and Herbst et al.[21] have found that operative ultrasonography is the most practical and reliable means of diagnosing gallstones in these patients.

The effect of parity has not been conclusively settled. Bernstein et al.,[14] Layde et al.,[6] and a group from Rome[8] found a relationship between increasing parity and gallstone disease, but others have not.[4, 11] Where a positive effect has been found, the contribution of parity appears to be moderate compared with the more striking influence of obesity.

Oral contraceptives do not appear to increase the overall incidence of gallstone disease, but they accelerate the onset, so the disease occurs at a younger age.[22, 23] The influence of some other factors, such as obesity and parity, may also be at least partly explained in this way.

Dietary studies[24, 25] have given conflicting data on the relation of total energy intake to the risk of forming gallstones; the influence of fat intake could not be separated from total caloric intake. Smith and Gee[25] thought there might be a relationship between cholelithiasis and a diet low in protein, fat, and crude fiber intake. Scragg et al.[17] found that sugar intake had an influence, and Capron et al.[26] implicated prolonged fasting as a possible risk factor in some persons.

Along with gallstones and obesity, diabetes mellitus is another common finding in American Indian women. Diabetes has variously been reported to have either a positive effect[4, 26, 27] or no effect[11] on gallstone formation. Bennion and Grundy[28] reported that the cholesterol saturation of bile increased in response to insulin therapy in patients with diabetes. The very high prevalence of gallstones in American Indians cannot be explained as a result of the effects of obesity or diabetes. After taking all other risk factors into account, an inherited predisposition remains as the predominant determinant.

Other factors identified as increasing the incidence of gallstone disease in individual studies include smoking,[6] low socioeconomic status and level of education,[29] low calcium intake,[9] and sedentary life-style.[9] Moderate drinking (i.e., 20 gm of alcohol daily) was found to have a protective effect in one report.[30]

Table 89–2. PREVALENCE OF GALLBLADDER DISEASE BASED UPON DIRECT EVIDENCE

	Pima Indians[11]			Germany[12]		England[5]		Scotland[10]		Sweden[7]	
Age	*Men*	*Women*	**Age**	*Men*	*Women*	*Men*	*Women*	*Men*	*Women*	*Men*	*Women*
15–24	0%	13%	20–29	1%	6%					6%	14%
25–34	4%	73%	30–39	3%	13%	3%	0%			4%	33%
35–44	11%	71%	40–49	7%	22%	0%	13%	4%	0%	13%	15%
45–54	32%	76%	50–59	10%	28%	4%	21%	10%	28%	18%	40%
55–64	66%	62%	60–69	16%	41%	9%	20%	16%	32%	27%	53%
≥65	68%	90%	70–79	22%	46%	17%	21%	23%	34%	36%	63%
			80–89	25%	51%	19%	27%	26%	43%	45%	63%

Cirrhosis of the liver has been noted to be associated with a markedly increased risk of pigment gallstone formation.[31, 32] Diseases known to produce increased rates of hemoglobin turnover (e.g., congenital spherocytosis, sickle cell anemia) have a high incidence of associated pigment gallstone disease, and the explanation for the association in cirrhosis may be related to hypersplenism. The incidence of pigment gallstone disease in cirrhotics with known portal hypertension (40 per cent), for example, was even higher than in cirrhotics without portal hypertension (30 per cent).[31]

NATURAL HISTORY OF GALLSTONE DISEASE

Although estimates vary, of the 70 to 90 per cent of people with gallstones who never come to surgical treatment, about two thirds have mild symptoms or no symptoms at all. Because gallstone disease is so common, the diagnosis is occasionally made in such persons during the course of an evaluation for some other medical problem, and then the question arises as to whether treatment should be recommended. If prophylactic treatment of these cases could be shown to have major health benefits, it would be possible by ultrasound screening to detect the large numbers of subclinical cases of gallstone disease so they could be treated before more severe manifestations develop.

To decide how these mild cases would best be treated, the following information is required: (1) the rate at which symptoms (e.g., colic, dyspepsia) develop in asymptomatic persons; (2) the rate at which complications (e.g., acute cholecystitis, cholangitis, pancreatitis, carcinoma) develop; (3) the likelihood that a complication rather than uncomplicated symptoms will be the initial clinical manifestation; (4) whether the answers to the previous two questions differ in patients with mild symptoms compared with those who have symptoms; (5) the mortality rate of elective cholecystectomy; (6) the mortality rate of complications; and (7) the cost of treatment.

The reports on the natural history of gallstone disease from the 1960s, which were once considered authoritative, have now been superseded by better data. These older articles by Lund[33] and by Wenckert and Robertson[34] traced the natural history of a total of 1307 patients who had not been operated on and reported that 30 per cent of patients experienced attacks of colic, 20 per cent experienced complications, and 50 per cent remained asymptomatic. Concluding that the average patient with gallstone disease had a 50 per cent chance of experiencing significant clinical problems in the next few years, these authors recommended cholecystectomy for all patients, regardless of the severity of their symptoms except when ancillary conditions were present that increased the risks of operation.

The patients who formed the basis of these reports, however, are not as representative of asymptomatic and mildly symptomatic disease as was once assumed. They had all been hospitalized for symptomatic gallstone disease before their course was followed, and many of them (50 to 90 per cent) had nonopacifying gallbladders on oral cholecystography. The latter is a reflection of more advanced disease, seen in less than 30 per cent of asymptomatic persons with gallstones diagnosed by screening examinations.

The natural history of asymptomatic or mildly symptomatic patients is more accurately described in the recent reports from Gracie and Ransohoff,[35] McSherry,[36] and Thistle,[37] and their coworkers.

Gracie and Ransohoff[35] followed 123 asymptomatic patients with gallstones diagnosed by screening oral cholecystograms. The group comprised 110 men and 13 women, whose average age was 54 years (range, 29 to 87 years). The gallbladder opacified on cholecystography in 108 patients (88 per cent) and did not opacify in 15 (12 per cent). Follow-up, which was complete for all patients, ranged from 11 to 24 years. During this time biliary pain developed in 13 per cent (16) of the patients, and complications developed in 2 per cent (three patients). All three complications followed the appearance of episodes of uncomplicated biliary colic. Biliary pain developed in 10 ± 3 per cent of patients within 5 years; 15 ± 4 per cent at 10 years; and 18 ± 4 per cent at both 15 and 20 years. Therefore, among asymptomatic patients, pain developed initially in about 2 per cent per year; at 10 years the rate decreased; and after about 15 years, patients who were still asymptomatic were likely to remain so.

McSherry et al.[36] reported the outcome of expectant management in 691 patients with gallstone disease (65 per cent women, and 35 per cent men) who were followed for an average of 78 ± 62 months. Upon entry into the study, 556 (80 per cent) of the patients had experienced biliary symptoms, and 135 (20 per cent) had been asymptomatic. Symptoms developed in 10 per cent of the asymptomatic patients over an average of five years of follow-up. Only two deaths related to gallstone disease occurred in the entire group of 691 patients, both in patients with chronic symptoms. Therefore, as in the study by Gracie and Ransohoff,[35] asymptomatic patients had about a 2 per cent chance of experiencing colic per year of follow-up. Complications such as acute cholecystitis and pancreatitis were very uncommon, and in 90 per cent of instances they followed rather than preceded the appearance of colic.

Additional information was provided by the National Cooperative Gallstone study, a randomized trial that compared chenodeoxycholate with placebo in the treatment of gallbladder gallstone disease. Data describing the natural history of the disease among the 305 patients in the placebo group were reported by Thistle et al.[37] In order to qualify for entry into the study, the patients initially were required to have opacification of the gallbladder on oral cholecystograms, no calcium in the gallstones seen on plain films, and no symptoms for the three months preceding therapy. During the 24 months of follow-up, biliary colic occurred in 13 per cent of the 305 patients given placebo, and an episode of pain lasting for more than five hours occurred in only 2 per cent. Those who had had an attack of biliary colic in the 12-month period before the study began were more likely than the asymptomatic patients to have an attack during the 24-month follow-up period. Twelve patients (4 per cent), three of whom had gangrenous acute cholecystitis, required cholecystectomy because of biliary symptoms. No deaths occurred as a result of the gallstone disease or its surgical treatment.

Insights into the natural history of gallstone disease can also be gleaned from autopsy studies.[3, 5, 7, 10, 12] They demonstrate, for example, that only 10 to 20 per cent of autopsied persons with gallstone disease have had surgical treatment (i.e., cholecystectomy) before they die, and of those who have not, the gallstones have contributed to death in only a few patients (2 to 5 per cent). The deaths attributable to untreated gallstone disease were almost entirely confined to elderly people and were reasonably well balanced by the few unexpected deaths that followed elective cholecystectomies.

The obvious conclusions from these natural history data are that most persons with gallstones have either no symptoms or symptoms so mild that treatment is not sought. The morbidity rate of asymptomatic gallbladder disease is low and when clinical manifestations appear, they usually consist of colic rather than life-threatening complications. Furthermore, the overall mortality rate of unheralded complications exclusive of carcinoma (i.e., acute cholecystitis, jaundice, or pancreatitis) is below 10 per cent, so even when complications arise, the outcome of treatment is likely to be good.

Nevertheless, the risks of surgical therapy are also low, so careful calculations are required to compare the merits of treatment versus no treatment in asymptomatic or mildly symptomatic patients.

Ransohoff et al.[38] subjected the issue of prophylactic cholecystectomy in asymptomatic persons to decision analysis. The morbidity statistics used in calculating the risks of expectant management were obtained from their earlier article[35] (subsequently supported by the data from McSherry et al.[36]) which had demonstrated about a 2 per cent per year rate of conversion from an asymptomatic to a symptomatic state. The risks of elective and emergency surgery were obtained from 11 representative reports in the literature.

The decision analysis showed that prophylactic cholecystectomy for a 50-year-old man would result in an average loss of 18 days of life expectancy. Choosing cholecystectomy over expectant management for a 30-year-old woman, a 30-year-old man, and a 50-year-old woman, would decrease life expectancy by 1, 4, and 12 days, respectively. Recalculation showed that if operative mortality rates could be reduced to zero, the outcome would now favor surgery, but life expectancy would be enhanced in this theoretical situation by only six to seven days in 30-year-old patients. Taking inflation into account, the costs would be more than sixfold greater with prophylactic surgery than with expectant management.

What all this means is that little is accomplished by aggressive therapy of asymptomatic or mildly symptomatic gallstone disease. Considering the numbers of affected persons, it is obvious that the health care system would be totally overwhelmed by any plan to screen and treat a major proportion of persons who have gallstones, and the costs would amount to billions of dollars. Fortunately, the natural history of the disease proves to be benign in all but a small fraction of cases, so expectant management is not only safe but preferable to surgical treatment in the average case.

On the other hand, even though gallstones pose little threat to the average person, severe, even lethal disease, is occasionally encountered. The next question, therefore, is whether high-risk groups can be identified who do not follow the typical course.

Studies on the epidemiology of gallbladder cancer[39, 40] demonstrate a close association of this tumor with gallstone disease, and it is clear that gallstones constitute a precancerous state. However, the strength of this relationship varies considerably among various ethnic groups,[41, 42] as indicated in Table 89–3.

These figures show that gallbladder cancer, just like gallstone disease, is much more common in American Indians than in other U.S. ethnic groups. The figures in Table 89–3 demonstrate that cancer occurs at an earlier age in American Indians than in other ethnic groups, and it affects a higher proportion of those who have gallstone disease. One other report[40] noted that the frequency of invasive carcinoma or carcinoma in situ found incidentally in gallbladders removed for symptomatic gallstone disease was 0.5 per cent to 1.5 per cent in Caucasians but was as high as 3 per cent to 5 per cent in Mexicans.

Diehl and Beral[43] reported epidemiologic data from various countries which suggested that the incidence of gallbladder cancer was inversely proportional to the cholecystectomy rate the preceding year. Nevertheless, in most patients the threat of gallbladder cancer is too small and remote to have an important influence on the natural history of gallstone disease and to be considered a cogent argument for early therapy of the gallstones. Considering the data in Table 89–3, how-

Table 89–3. INCIDENCE OF GALLBLADDER CANCER IN VARIOUS ETHNIC GROUPS

Race and Sex	Mean Age at Diagnosis	Gallbladder Cancer Incidence (100,000/yr)	Relative Risk	Cancer Risk per 20 Years	Number of Cholecystectomies to Prevent Cancer
Blacks/Women	72.5	3.0	4.5	0.15%	667
Caucasians/Women	73.9	11.5	4.3	0.50%	200
American Indians/Women	64.4	46.4	12.2	1.50%	67

ever, the situation may be different for American Indians, Mexican Americans, and other racially mixed groups that share a similar genetic background. Weiss et al.[41] noted, for example, that the chances of gallbladder cancer developing in American Indian women with gallstone disease is greater than the risk of lung cancer in cigarette smokers. Such data suggest that a more aggressive policy of cholecystectomy may be justified in persons of American Indian ancestry who have gallstone disease in order to prevent this fatal illness.

Amaral and Thompson[18] and Thiet et al.[19] reported that in morbidly obese patients the natural history of gallstone disease seemed to be more aggressive than in others, and for these patients prophylactic cholecystectomy was recommended at the time of gastric bypass if gallstones were present. Calcification in the wall of the gallbladder—an uncommon condition—is associated with gallbladder carcinoma and probably should be handled as if it were a premalignant state.[44, 45] There is also evidence that large gallstones (>2.5 cm) are more likely to precipitate an attack of acute cholecystitis[46] or give rise to gallbladder cancer[47] than are smaller stones. However, there are no good epidemiologic data on the natural history of large stones that would indicate whether these increased risks are great enough to be of clinical importance.

It is commonly assumed that small stones, which can more easily enter the cystic and common ducts, pose a greater potential problem than do larger stones. For example, Houssin et al.[48] recommended cholecystectomy for patients whose gallstones are 3 mm or smaller in diameter because of the risk of pancreatitis. This retrospective study, however, suffers from the same shortcomings as previous surgical assessments of natural history, and if the thesis were valid, support for it might have been expected from the aforementioned observations of Gracie and Ransohoff,[35] Thistle et al.,[37] and McSherry et al.[36]

Asymptomatic patients with stones in the common duct do not appear to have as benign a course as those with stones confined to the gallbladder. There is little written on the natural history of choledocholithiasis, and no prospective studies exist similar to the ones for gallbladder stones. Postmortem surveys indicate, however, that in patients who are found at autopsy to have choledocholithiasis, the ductal stones will have contributed to the patient's death in about half of the cases.[3, 10] Thus, the threat of untreated choledocholithiasis appears to be considerably greater than that of untreated gallbladder stones, and expectant management could not ordinarily be justified for this condition.

Cholelithiasis may occur in children,[49–55] in whom cholecystectomy is probably indicated, regardless of the severity of symptoms. In most children with gallstones a specific etiologic factor can be identified, the most common ones being prolonged total parenteral nutrition, congenital hemolytic disease, or disease of the ileum. Patients without special risk factors resemble their adult counterparts in many ways, because they tend to be female, obese, and older than the others.

Pigment gallstone disease, a result of hemolysis, is seen in about 50 per cent of patients above age 10 with sickle cell disease.[56–58] The abdominal crises of sickle cell disease consist of pain, jaundice, right upper quadrant tenderness, fever, and leukocytosis, a syndrome that may be impossible to distinguish from acute cholecystitis. Because of the similarities between sickle cell crises and acute cholecystitis, coupled with the knowledge that elective—but not emergency—operations are well tolerated in sickle cell disease, prophylactic cholecystectomy is usually recommended for gallstones, even in the absence of symptoms.[58–61]

One commonly accepted notion introduced into the surgical literature 20 to 30 years ago is that associated diabetes mellitus raises the risks of gallstone disease. It is widely believed that complications, such as acute cholecystitis, are more common with this combination, and that when complications occur, they are more likely to be fatal than in the absence of diabetes. More representative statistics fail to support this contention, however.[62–65] The morbidity rate is moderately increased in patients with diabetes, but this can be explained by an increased prevalence in these patients of cardiorespiratory and renal disease. In fact, diabetes seems to be well tolerated in association with a wide variety of surgical conditions, and contrary to previous teaching, it does not by itself seem to increase the morbidity rate for biliary disease or its surgical treatment[62] (see pp. 494–500).

Consequently, if an individual patient is accidentally discovered to have gallstones, the indolent natural history of the disease should be explained. A few patients may wish to proceed with cholecystectomy or therapy with chenodiol (chenodeoxycholic acid). This is acceptable, if only to decrease anxiety, because the risks of either form of treatment are low. In a few patients, special considerations, such as choledocholithiasis, may warrant stronger recommendations for therapy. However, there is no justification for urging treatment in the average patient with gallbladder stones in the hopes of preventing complications in the future. In general, the urgency for treatment in gallbladder disease parallels the severity of symptoms.

BILIARY COLIC AND CHRONIC CHOLECYSTITIS

Biliary colic is the principal complaint in the majority of symptomatic patients with gallstones. Although patients with gallstone disease are usually said to have "chronic cholecystitis," this is not an entirely accurate designation because gallstone formation, not inflammation, is the earliest step in gallbladder disease. Gallstones, as noted previously, are not inevitably symptomatic, and except for patients with advanced disease there is little correlation between the severity and frequency of colic, on the one hand, and the pathologic changes in the gallbladder, on the other.[66, 67] In patients who have never had acute cholecystitis, the histologic changes in the gallbladder wall consist of fibrosis and round cell infiltration with minimal thickening. The mucosa is usually intact. Bacteria can be cultured from gallbladder bile or gallstones in about 10 per cent of patients, but bacterial infection is not thought to contribute to the symptoms or pathologic findings in nonacute gallbladder disease.

Biliary colic, a visceral pain, is the result of transient obstruction of the cystic duct by a stone[68] and, except in patients with acute cholecystitis, is not accompanied by acute inflammation. Therefore, it is possible to have colic with a grossly normal or mildly abnormal gallbladder, or to have no symptoms despite advanced gallbladder scarring.

Clinical Manifestations. About 75 per cent of patients with gallstone disease seek medical attention because of episodic pain (biliary colic). Although the symptoms are not pathognomonic for biliary disease, it is usually possible, when all aspects of the illness are considered, to make a fairly accurate diagnosis from the history. Confirmation of the original impression must then be obtained by demonstrating the presence of gallstones.

In a typical case, the patient experiences episodes of upper abdominal pain, usually in the epigastrium or right upper quadrant, but sometimes in other upper abdominal locations.[69, 70] The pain may be precipitated by eating a meal, but more commonly there is no inciting event, and the pain can even begin at night, although this is uncommon.

Biliary colic is a steady rather than an intermittent pain, as suggested by the word "colic."[69] A typical attack consists of gradually increasing pain over 15 minutes to an hour, which remains at a plateau for an hour or more, and then diminishes slowly. In a third of patients the pain has a sudden onset and, less often, relief is also sudden. Pain lasting more than five to six hours should suggest acute cholecystitis.

In order of decreasing frequency, the pain is felt maximally in the epigastrium, right upper quadrant, left upper quadrant, and various parts of the precordium or lower abdomen.[69, 70] It is incorrect to think that pain located other than in the right upper quadrant is "atypical" of gallstone disease. The pain radiates to other parts of the abdomen or the back, in over one half of patients, often to the scapula, the middle of the back, or the tip of the right shoulder. The attack is associated with vomiting and sweating in most individuals, and vomiting occasionally affords some relief. It is rarely as protracted as in intestinal obstruction, however. As with other kinds of visceral pain, the patient with biliary colic is usually restless and active during an attack.

The interval between attacks may be weeks, months, or years, and the unpredictability of their timing is a hallmark of the disease. As shown in the studies of Thistle et al.[37] the activity of the disease tends to remain about the same over long periods. If the patient has been experiencing frequent attacks, they usually continue with the same frequency.

Dyspepsia is a general term used to refer to a group of ill-defined symptoms associated with gallstone disease and many other abdominal conditions.[71–75] Dyspepsia includes fatty or other kinds of food intolerances; excessive belching or flatus; postprandial abdominal bloating, fullness, and discomfort; inability to finish a normal-sized meal; epigastric burning; regurgitation of bitter fluid (water brash); nausea; and vomiting. One or more of these symptoms are present in about 80 per cent of patients with gallstones who seek medical care. About 25 per cent of patients experience some relief from antacids. About one third of patients have heartburn, some of whom have positive acid infusion (Bernstein) tests.

Prospective studies of middle-aged women have shown that the frequency and severity of dyspeptic complaints are unrelated to the presence of gallstones.[73] This suggests that dyspepsia is randomly distributed in relation to gallstone disease and is not a direct consequence of the stones. On the other hand, most patients with gallstones and dyspepsia obtain some relief following cholecystectomy,[72, 74] which suggests the two are at least to some extent related. Several investigators[70, 71, 73, 74] have noted an inverse correlation between the extent of chronic inflammatory changes in the gallbladder and the magnitude of preoperative dyspepsia. If gallstones are associated with poor function on the oral cholecystogram, dyspepsia is less likely to be cured by cholecystectomy than if the gallbladder functions well.

The physical examination is usually normal, but a few patients have tenderness in the region of the gallbladder during an attack of biliary colic.

Chronic distention of the gallbladder due to *hydrops* may occur with chronic cystic duct obstruction.[76, 77] The gallbladder in this condition contains an uninfected clear mucoid fluid. Patients with hydrops may or may not have symptoms. Hydrops must not be confused with empyema of the gallbladder, which presents as an acute toxic illness.

Diagnosis. About 15 per cent of gallstones contain enough calcium to be seen on plain films of the abdomen, but without additional studies it is not possible to be sure that the stones are actually within the gallbladder.

Ultrasonography and Oral Cholecystography.[78–87] The principal methods of imaging gallstones are ultrasonography and oral cholecystography. The specificity (about 98 per cent) and sensitivity (about 95 per cent) of both tests are very high.

Ultrasound scans may show gallstones (echogenic objects that produce an acoustic shadow) or sludge (echogenic material that layers and does not produce an acoustic shadow).[80] Very small stones may fail to produce shadows and therefore may be either missed or confused with sludge. Rarely, advanced scarring and contraction of the gallbladder around gallstones make it impossible to locate the gallbladder or the stones, a finding that should also raise the possibility of gallbladder cancer. Combining oral cholecystography with ultrasonic scanning may occasionally be useful, for the presence of the dense contrast medium in the gallbladder may cause small stones to float, facilitating their detection by ultrasound.[88]

Sludge, which consists of precipitated calcium bilirubinate, may be seen in association with gallstones or in any condition causing bile stasis.[89, 90] Sludge is common in persons receiving total parenteral nutrition. By itself, sludge is not an indication for cholecystectomy, although it often occurs in conjunction with a surgical lesion such as bile duct obstruction.

Oral cholecystography is an excellent method of diagnosing gallstones, but ultrasonography is just as accurate and requires no preparation of the patient, involves no ionizing radiation, and is simpler to perform. Oral cholecystography, on the other hand, shows whether the gallbladder functions and whether the stones are calcified, information of value if treatment with chenodiol is being contemplated. Because the gallbladder fails to opacify in about 40 per cent of patients in response to the initial dose of contrast agent, ultrasound is much more likely to provide a correct diagnosis during the first examination.

Although ultrasound is the first test ordered in most cases, oral cholecystography must not be considered an outmoded test. If the ultrasound results are negative and gallstone disease still seems to be a possibility, an oral cholecystogram should be obtained. If oral cholecystography is done first, ultrasound may be used if the cholecystogram fails to opacify or if the cholecystogram unexpectedly appears normal.[91–93] It must be remembered that both tests give false negative results in about 5 per cent of cases, and because gallstone disease is so common, difficulties in diagnosis can be expected occasionally by all physicians who see patients with this disease.

About 60 per cent of oral cholecystograms opacify on the initial study.[94] When a single-dose study fails to opacify and there is no reason to suspect problems with intestinal absorption or hepatic excretion of the contrast agent, the patient may be given a second dose, and X-rays are repeated on the following day. This brings about opacification of the gallbladder in about two thirds of the remaining patients. Persistent nonopacification at this point is more than 95 per cent reliable as an indication of gallbladder disease.[94] It is usually easier, however, to study patients with nonopacification by ultrasound rather than proceeding with a double-dose oral cholecystogram.[95] Prolonged opacification of the gallbladder on oral cholecystography is no longer considered to be significant as was once claimed.[96]

If both ultrasound and oral cholecystography are normal and symptoms are highly suggestive, the next test should be either an endoscopic retrograde cholangiogram (with filling of the gallbladder) or examination of duodenal bile for cholesterol crystals or bilirubinate granules.

Endoscopic Retrograde Cholangiopancreatography (ERCP). Venu et al.[97] reported the results of ERCP in 195 patients who were thought clinically to have biliary pain but who had no stones on oral cholecystograms or ultrasound studies of the gallbladder. Thirty-two of these patients had had mild, transient abnormalities of liver function tests that coincided with the attacks of pain. No liver function abnormalities had been detected in the other 163 patients. ERCP demonstrated gallstones in 25 (78 per cent) of the 32 with abnormal test results but in only 4 (25 per cent) of the remainder. The most common ERCP finding in the first group was a layer of very small (3 to 7 mm) stones at the interface between the bile and the contrast medium. The ability of ERCP to partially displace gallbladder bile with contrast medium, which creates an interface where small stones can float, was given the credit for the success of this study.

Duodenal Drainage. Duodenal drainage studies are cumbersome compared with ultrasonography, but they may be useful in diagnosing gallstones when other tests have failed. The test involves duodenal intubation and sampling of gallbladder bile, which is then examined for the presence of cholesterol crystals or calcium bilirubinate granules. This method of diagnosis was first described about 30 years ago, but only recently have the methods been refined, the theory supported with sound evidence, and the reliability validated.[98–100]

The following technique was developed by Strasberg and his colleagues at the University of Toronto.[101] A tube is placed under radiographic control into the duodenum and another tube is placed in the stomach. During the test, gastric secretions are aspirated from the gastric tube and discarded. The duodenal tube is allowed to drain by siphonage, placing the end of the fluid-filled tube below the patient, where it can empty into a collecting receptacle. The patient is given an IV injection of cholecystokinin (CCK) (1.5 U/kg over three minutes) or CCK-octapeptide (0.02 ng/kg over one minute). After the hormone is given, bile issuing from the duodenal tube will be noted to be light yellow (A bile), then dark (B bile), and then light again (C bile). The sequence consists of common duct bile, gallbladder bile, and hepatic bile.

The B bile, which comes from the gallbladder, is used for the examination. A sample is centrifuged at 2000 rpm for 10 minutes, and the pellet is examined by light and polarizing microscopy. Cholesterol crystals have typical plate-like parallelogram shapes, which are birefringent under polarized light. Calcium bilirubinate appears as small red-brown granules in clusters. If gastric acid has not been excluded from the duodenum, a precipitate may appear that resembles calcium bilirubinate granules, so it is important to make sure that the pH of the specimen is above 5.0.

A positive duodenal drainage test consists of 10 or more cholesterol or calcium bilirubinate crystals per slide. Between 1 and 10 crystals is considered suggestive but not diagnostic.

The scientific rationale for using the presence of cholesterol crystals in diagnosing gallstone disease comes from the observations of Sedaghat and Grundy.[100] These workers noted the presence of cholesterol crystals in bile specimens from 25 of 28 patients with cholesterol gallstones but in none of the specimens from 72 patients without cholesterol gallstones, even though the latter group included some patients whose bile was supersaturated with cholesterol. Subsequently, Burnstein[98] and Delchier[99] and their coworkers showed prospectively in a total of 114 patients that the presence of cholesterol crystals or bilirubinate granules in gallbladder bile obtained by duodenal intubation was sensitive and specific for the diagnosis of gallstones in patients with normal cholecystograms and ultrasound studies. Thus, the duodenal drainage test as described above seems to be both useful and reliable, and probably deserves wider use.

Cholecystokinin Cholecystography. There is some evidence that gallbladder disease can be detected if abdominal pain and/or abnormalities in gallbladder motor function occur in response to an intravenous injection of cholecystokinin. Nathan et al.[102] and Davis et al.[103] showed that pain occurs in only 1 per cent of normal subjects when CCK is given during oral cholecystography, so pain during this test could be of significance in the diagnosis of gallbladder disease. This is the theory of the cholecystokinin cholecystogram, which involves using fluoroscopy to observe the response of the opacified gallbladder to an injection of cholecystokinin (or CCK-octapeptide), and correlating abnormalities in gallbladder emptying with the patient's symptoms. Burnstein et al.[98] combined performance of CCK cholecystography with the duodenal drainage test. Cholecystokinin cholecystography can also be performed using ^{99m}Tc-iminodiacetic acid derivatives instead of radiopaque contrast medium to image the gallbladder.

According to Burnstein et al.,[98] the CCK cholecystogram should be considered abnormal if less than 20 per cent (hypocontraction) or more than 80 per cent (hypercontraction) of gallbladder bile is emptied in response to CCK. In their experience, hypercontraction correlated with the presence of abnormal bile (88 per cent specific) on duodenal drainage. Hypocontraction was a less sensitive and specific finding. A "fighting gallbladder," defined as a gallbladder that develops a rounded shape in response to CCK but fails to empty, has also been said to be an important sign.

The diagnostic usefulness of CCK cholecystography is unsettled. Dunn et al.[104] studied the test prospectively in 74 patients with normal cholecystograms who had symptoms of gallbladder disease. In 17 (85 per cent) of 20 patients who had reproduction of their pain in response to CCK, the pain was relieved or lessened by cholecystectomy, but a similar response to cholecystectomy occurred in six (67 per cent) of nine patients with no pain after CCK. There was also a high incidence (14 to 36 per cent) of false positive results in a group of control subjects. These authors concluded that the CCK cholecystogram was of uncertain value, a sentiment shared by Davis et al.[103] Others, however, claim that because a positive test is usually associated with a good clinical result after cholecystectomy, CCK cholecystography can be used clinically as long as it is realized that false negative results may occur.[98, 105–109]

Differential Diagnosis. Because the symptoms of chronic cholecystitis are not highly specific, the patient's history, the findings on physical examination, and the laboratory data must all be carefully evaluated. An upper gastrointestinal series,[110] barium enema, or intravenous pyelogram may be indicated preoperatively in some patients, but ordering an upper gastrointestinal series in the absence of clinical suspicions of gastroduodenal disease, which was routine in the past, has been shown to be unrewarding.[111] The most common diseases to be considered in the differential diagnosis are gastritis, peptic ulcer, reflux esophagitis, pancreatitis, renal disease, lesions of the colon (diverticulitis and carcinoma), radiculitis, and angina pectoris.

An upper gastrointestinal series may show *reflux esophagitis* with or without a hiatus hernia or peptic ulcer disease (see pp. 594–619). Endoscopy of the upper gastrointestinal tract may be indicated in some patients with symptoms of reflux. When available, pH measurements of the lower esophagus may be helpful.

The pain of angina pectoris is of shorter duration than the average episode of biliary colic, but the location of the pain is not as specific for each of these conditions as is sometimes thought. An electrocardiogram should be performed, in some cases during exercise.

The question of whether gallbladder disease may have a direct influence on cardiac disease has been debated for some time. The basis for thinking so has been that arrhythmias or episodes of angina pectoris occasionally subside following cholecystectomy.[112, 113] Experimentally, distention of the bile ducts sometimes induces cardiac arrhythmias, premature ventricular contractions, or angina. However, prospective clinical studies suggest that gallbladder disease only rarely affects the heart, so cholecystectomy should not be performed specifically in the hope of improving cardiac disease.

Patients with *chronic pancreatitis*, many of whom are alcoholics, may have vague upper abdominal complaints similar to those of patients with gallstone disease (see pp. 1842–1872). Even though gallstones may cause acute pancreatitis, gallstone pancreatitis (in contrast with alcoholic pancreatitis) rarely leads to chronic scarring with endocrine and exocrine dysfunction. Special studies (such as glucose tolerance test, endoscopic retrograde pancreatography, or test of exocrine function) may be required if the history or plain films suggest the possibility of pancreatitis. Nevertheless, if a symptomatic patient is discovered to have both chronic pancreatitis and gallstones, cholecystectomy should usually be performed as a first attempt to provide pain relief.

The *irritable bowel syndrome* (IBS), which may produce postprandial abdominal pain, should be considered in the differential diagnosis, especially if there is a distinct relationship of symptoms to bowel movements (see pp. 1402–1418). When both diseases are present, cholecystectomy will usually be indicated because it is usually impossible to exonerate the gallbladder as a cause of the symptoms.

Because colonic function increases after eating (gastrocolic reflex), colonic lesions such as *adenocarcinoma* (see pp. 1519–1547) or *diverticular disease* of the colon (see pp. 1419–1439) may be associated with postprandial discomfort. When the discomfort is on the right side of the abdomen, as it may be with right-sided neoplasms, the syndrome may closely mimic gallstone disease. Awareness of this problem should lead to more thorough study of the colon in appropriate cases.

Renal stones or infection may produce right-sided abdominal pain, but if a urinalysis is obtained routinely and abnormal results are further investigated by intravenous pyelography, renal disease should be overlooked rarely.

Radiculitis from osteoarthritis or peripheral nerve tumors may produce symptoms that resemble those produced by gallstones. Thoracic spine films and, occasionally, myelograms should be obtained in selected patients in whom radicular pain cannot be explained on the basis of the clinical examination.

Treatment. Cholecystectomy is the only definitive treatment and is indicated for most symptomatic patients. The other forms of treatment discussed below are to some extent experimental, impractical, or both. Therapeutic diets (e.g., a low-fat diet), anticholinergic drugs, and antacids are of no value in preventing attacks of colic, although they may provide some relief from dyspeptic symptoms. In fact, gallbladder contraction is just as complete after ingestion of low-fat meals as after a high-fat meal.[114]

Cholecystectomy (Color Figs. 89–1 and 89–2, p. xlv). Cholecystectomy usually relieves preoperative pain if other abdominal disease has been ruled out and if stones are not left behind in the bile duct.[115, 116] It is less possible to be sure that dyspepsia will be eliminated by cholecystectomy, although as indicated earlier, some relief can be expected in most cases. When dyspepsia is the major complaint and pain is not present, the results are unpredictable, so dyspepsia by itself is not an accepted indication for surgery.

In a collected series the overall mortality rate of elective cholecystectomy without common duct exploration or other ancillary procedures was 0.20 per cent (six deaths in 2756 cholecystectomies).[117–120] These reports[117–119] were chosen because they give detailed mortality statistics and the cause of death in each patient. Mortality rates in this range can be expected only when the surgery is performed by fully trained surgeons. In the large experience from the New York Hospital–Cornell Medical Center,[121] the gross mortality rate of cholecystectomy in patients under age 50 was 0.1 per cent and in patients over age 50 it was 0.8 per cent. Cardiovascular complications were the principal cause of death in the latter group.

Many reports on the mortality rates of operations for gallstone disease fail to distinguish between routine operations and cholecystectomies done as an ancillary procedure during laparotomy for some other serious diseases, such as carcinoma of the pancreas.[120–122] In other instances the mortality rate of operations performed for acute cholecystitis is not separated from the rate of those done electively,[123] or the results of simple cholecystectomy are included among those for cholecystectomy plus common duct exploration. These practices inflate the mortality rates attributed to "cholecystectomy" and have sometimes been used inappropriately to estimate the risks of an elective operation in otherwise healthy persons with minimal disease.

Age by itself is not a contraindication to elective cholecystectomy.[124–126] The risks in the elderly are the result of the ancillary diseases that are so often present in this age group. The increased risks in patients with diabetes mellitus are a result of the increased prevalence of renal and cardiovascular disease in patients with this disease.[62–64] Elective cholecystectomy is considerably more hazardous in patients with cirrhosis of the liver than in others, and surgery should be undertaken only if the symptoms are severe or the cirrhosis is mild.[127–129]

Cholecystectomy produces no alterations in digestion and absorption, and, perhaps surprisingly, the concentration of bile acids in intestinal chyme remains in the physiologic range after removal of the gallbladder.[130] There is no need for special diets (e.g., a low-fat diet) or vitamin supplements postoperatively.

In summary, deaths and major complications after cholecystectomy are encountered primarily in the elderly or others who have serious disease in other organ systems.

Dissolution Therapy (see pp. 1678–1680). Chenodeoxycholic acid (CDCA; chenodiol) (12 to 15 mg per kg of body weight per day) will lower the cholesterol saturation of bile enough to bring about gradual dissolution of cholesterol stones in some patients.[131–135] Chenodeoxycholic acid treatment is unsuccessful or otherwise contraindicated in the presence of any of the following: (1) pigment stones; (2) calcified stones; (3) large (>1.5 cm) stones; (4) nonopacifying gallbladder; (5) women who might become pregnant; (6) concomitant liver disease; (7) symptoms too severe to tolerate two years of therapy; (8) obesity (it is difficult to desaturate the bile in obese persons); and (9) lack of signs of dissolution on oral cholecystogram following nine months of treatment. About 85 to 90 per cent of patients now being treated by cholecystectomy would be excluded from consideration for chenodeoxycholic acid therapy for one or more of these reasons.[136]

In the controlled trial of this treatment in the United States, the stones dissolved in 15 per cent of selected patients during two years of continuous therapy.[133] Other studies indicate that more stringent selection criteria and higher doses of the drug would increase the chance of success to 30 to 50 per cent of treated patients.[134]

Ursodeoxycholic acid (UDCA) (10 mg per kg of body weight per day) is preferable to chenodeoxycholic acid (CDCA), because it is just as effective as CDCA but does not produce diarrhea or liver dysfunction.[137–141] A combination of CDCA and UDCA may be more effective than either alone.[142] Ursodeoxycholic acid is not yet available in the United States.

A major weakness of dissolution therapy is the tendency for gallstones to recur in most successfully treated patients after the drug is discontinued;[143, 144] this results from the continued abnormalities in cholesterol saturation.[145] Recurrence may be prevented in some patients by giving a chronic nighttime maintenance dose of the drug,[144, 146, 147] but the safety of this approach is not proved.

At present the indications for dissolution therapy are unclear. More information is needed on its efficacy and on whether the selection of patients can be improved to increase the success rate. Based upon the data available, CDCA or UDCA might be preferable to surgery in appropriately selected patients with serious ancillary disease that increases the risks of surgery. Most such patients would be over 65 years of age. In others, cholecystectomy would be superior.

Lithotripsy (see pp. 1681–1682). Gallstones, like kidney stones, can be fragmented by exposure to extracorporeal shock waves.[148–152] The stones are broken into pieces that range in size from small granules to about 8 mm, which increases the efficacy of dissolution by cheno- or ursodeoxycholic acid.

In the reports by Sauerbruch et al.[148, 151] gallbladder stones were eliminated within 1 to 25 weeks in 75 per cent of 97 patients treated by 430 to 1600 shock wave discharges followed by a combination of UDCA plus CDCA, each given in a daily dose of 7 to 8 mg/kg. Painful episodes experienced by a few patients were thought to coincide with passage of stone fragments through the common duct. The following were considered contraindications to this therapy: stones greater than 25 mm in diameter; more than three stones; calcified stones; nonopacifying gallbladder on oral cholecystogram; concurrent common bile duct stone; and poor general condition of the patient.

Therefore, the ability to fragment gallstones augments the effectiveness of dissolution therapy. This is complex, expensive technology, however, which may have the potential of complications to adjacent organs, and as with CDCA given alone, recurrent stone formation can be expected in most patients. Furthermore, with the present list of exclusions, about 10 per cent of patients with gallstones are candidates for shock wave treatment.

Percutaneous Dissolution. Allen et al.[153] reported dissolving cholesterol gallbladder stones in four patients using methyl tert-butyl ether (MTBE) instilled into a catheter inserted percutaneously into the gallbladder. Using CT scans for guidance, the catheter was passed through the liver and hepatic surface of the gallbladder into the gallbladder lumen. MTBE was chosen as a solvent because it dissolves cholesterol rapidly, and unlike diethyl ether, it remains liquid at body temperature. No serious side effects were described in these four patients, in three of whom the stones were successfully dissolved. A common bile duct stone was also dissolved in one of the patients.

More information will have to be developed concerning the safety and efficacy of this approach before its place in the therapy of gallstone disease can be determined (see pp. 1680–1681).

Incidental Cholelithiasis and Incidental Cholecystectomy. Sometimes patients scheduled for an operation on some other organ are discovered preoperatively or intraoperatively to have gallstones, and a decision must be made concerning whether it is important and safe to remove the gallbladder as an incidental procedure. As mentioned earlier in this chapter, cholecystectomy probably should be performed in morbidly obese patients who have gallstones in conjunction with gastric bypass operations, and this has become fairly standard practice.[18, 19] In other patients, the natural history of untreated gallstones would not be expected to pose risks greater than the minimal ones documented by Gracie and Ransohoff[35] and McSherry et al.;[36] this subject is discussed in detail elsewhere in this chapter.

Cholecystectomy, however, would add few additional risks to most abdominal operations, and there is good evidence that an incidental cholecystectomy is acceptable as long as the incision is adequate and the patient is stable and reasonably healthy.[154–156] Specific discussions have supported incidental cholecystectomy in the elderly[157] and during colectomy,[158] gynecologic operations,[159] and insertion of arterial grafts.[160, 161]

McSherry and Glenn[155] pointed out that it is also safe to treat other abdominal diseases incidentally discovered during planned biliary tract surgery.

CHOLESTEROLOSIS

Cholesterolosis of the gallbladder consists of deposits of cholesterol esters in submucosal macrophages and epithelial cells.[162–165] As viewed from the mucosal surface, the submucosal cholesterol produces a fine yellow reticular pattern on a red background, an appearance similar to a ripe strawberry. The saturation of bile with cholesterol in patients with cholesterolosis is in the range of what is seen in normal subjects, and the pathogenesis of this condition probably differs from that of cholesterol gallstones.[163, 166] Gallstones and cholesterolosis are more often found independent of one another than together.[7] Methyl sterols (cholesterol precursors) are increased in hepatic and gallbladder bile of patients with cholesterolosis, presumably a result of increased hepatic production.[166] It has been postulated that cholesterolosis results from absorption of these free sterols from gallbladder bile by the gallbladder mucosa, followed by accumulation in submucosal macrophages.

In 80 per cent of cases the cholesterol deposits are confined to the mucosa (planar cholesterolosis).[163] In 20 per cent of cases, however, the lesions grow to assume a polypoid configuration, and then the cholesterol polyps may separate from their mucosal attachments and behave like ordinary gallstones. The planar form is usually asymptomatic, but polypoid cholesterolosis may be responsible for biliary colic or biliary pancreatitis. Planar and polypoid cholesterolosis are not distinct conditions but just different degrees of the same process. Because the stones that form from cholesterolosis are usually very small, they may be difficult to detect on oral cholecystograms or ultrasound scans. In some cases the oral cholecystogram may reveal decreased concentration of the contrast medium or one or more small mucosal excrescences (cholesterol polyps) that remain fixed as the patient changes position. Duodenal drainage studies may also be helpful in diagnosis. Symptomatic cases should be treated by cholecystectomy.

GALLSTONE DISEASE, CHOLECYSTECTOMY, AND CANCER

The prevalence of gallstone disease in various cultures has been shown by Lowenfels to correlate with the prevalence of cancer of the uterus, large intestine, and stomach.[167] These findings were interpreted to suggest that common environmental factors, thought most likely to involve dietary habits, influence the rates of all these diseases. In an autopsy study, Lowenfels[168] measured the relationship between the prevalence of gallstone disease and death from colorectal cancer. There was a 13-fold increase in the prevalence of gallstones in women under age 50 with colorectal cancer, but no correlations were found in other groups.

In another case-controlled study,[169] gallstone disease was found to be more prevalent among subjects who died from cancer compared with subjects who died from other causes. When the analysis was restricted to 89 women under age 50 who died from cancer of the breast, reproductive system, or colon, the odds ratio reached its highest value (3.3).

Linos et al.[170] found a relative risk for colon cancer of 1.52 among patients with cholelithiasis. They attributed this result to case-finding bias, however, because the positive correlation was confined to patients whose gallstones were asymptomatic.

Therefore, there is evidence that gallstone disease is more common in societies with a high prevalence of various cancers, but it is not clear that correlations exist between these diseases among individuals in these societies.

There are also theoretical reasons to think that changes in the enterohepatic circulation of bile acids following cholecystectomy might increase the incidence of colon cancer.[171] Cholecystectomy increases cycling of the enterohepatic circulation, which results in greater exposure of bile acids to intestinal bacteria and increased conversion of primary to secondary bile acids. Deoxycholate, the principal secondary bile acid, has been implicated as a possible cofactor in the pathogenesis of several carcinomas. Furthermore, in experimental animals, either cholecystectomy or feeding bile acids increases the frequency of colonic neoplasms in response to exogenous carcinogens.

In recent years, several reports have linked cholecystectomy in humans to an increased risk of colon cancer 10 to 15 years later. Vernick and Kuller[172] performed a case-controlled study of 150 patients with adenocarcinoma of the cecum or ascending colon. Two control groups were used: those with carcinoma of the left colon and neighborhood control subjects. Compared with the control groups, the relative risk for right-sided colon cancer was 1.86 in patients who had had cholecystectomies.

Linos et al.[173] traced the health of 1681 residents of Rochester, Minnesota, who had had cholecystectomies an average of 13 years previously. The relative risk for right-sided colon cancer in the women was found to be 2.1. There was no association in men.

Turunen and Kivilaasko[174] calculated that the relative risk of developing colon cancer after cholecystectomy was 1.59 compared with control subjects and was 3.00 for those with cancer of the right colon. They found no correlation in autopsied subjects between unoperated gallstones and colon cancer.

Dissenting views concerning a cancer-promoting effect of cholecystectomy are as numerous, however. In well-controlled studies Weiss,[175] Adami,[176] Abrams,[177] Spitz,[178] and their coworkers all found no relationship between previous cholecystectomy and cancer of the colon in general, or of the right colon in particular.

Therefore, it is possible that cholecystectomy increases the risk of carcinoma of the right colon, but the data are by no means conclusive, and the effect, if it truly exists, is slight.

ACUTE CHOLECYSTITIS

Acute cholecystitis consists of acute inflammation of the wall of the gallbladder associated with abdominal pain, tenderness, and fever. Somewhat surprisingly, the etiology of this relatively common condition is only vaguely understood, with little empirical evidence to support the most popular theories. Animals other than humans almost never develop acute cholecystitis spontaneously, and the various animal models that have been used to study the disease incompletely reflect the problem in humans.

Etiology and Pathogenesis

Acute cholecystitis can result from stasis, bacterial infection, or ischemia of the gallbladder. All but a few cases are caused by stasis, most often from cystic duct obstruction by a gallstone. Cholelithiasis is present in 90 per cent of cases of acute cholecystitis, the remaining 10 per cent being acalculous. About three quarters of patients with acute cholecystitis have had previous episodes of biliary colic.

Just how obstruction of the cystic duct leads to acute cholecystitis is as yet unclear. The agents postulated to initiate the inflammation include high concentrations of bile salts, cholesterol, or lysolecithin. Experimentally, if one ligates the cystic duct of an animal, the usual result is gradual absorption of the gallbladder contents without the development of inflammation. If the animal is fasted, however, and the gallbladder becomes distended with concentrated bile, cystic duct obstruction sometimes results in acute inflammation. Interpretation of these observations suggests a role for bile salts, when highly concentrated, in causing cholecystitis.[179]

The notion that cholesterol may play a part is supported by experiments on prairie dogs.[180] When the bile in these animals becomes supersaturated with cholesterol as a result of supplemental cholesterol feeding, ligation of the cystic duct results in acute cholecystitis. This happens even before gallstones develop. If the bile is normal, the gallbladder does not become inflamed when the duct is ligated.

Lecithin, a normal constituent of bile, is converted to lysolecithin by phospholipase A, an enzyme present in gallbladder mucosal cells. There is evidence that phospholipase may be released by gallstone-induced mucosal trauma, followed by conversion of lecithin to lysolecithin.[181] Experimentally, lysolecithin instillation into the gallbladder lumen stimulates increased mucosal prostaglandin (PGE_2) production and induces acute cholecystitis,[182] changes that are blocked by administration of the cyclo-oxygenase inhibitor indomethacin.[183] Although normally absent from gallbladder bile, lysolecithin is present in gallbladder contents from patients with acute cholecystitis.[181]

Prostaglandins have been shown to convert fluid absorption by the gallbladder mucosa to secretion and also to stimulate mucus production.[184] Measurements in humans show that pressure within the gallbladder lumen is increased in the presence of acute cholecystitis, probably as a result of fluid secretion by the mucosa.[185] Intravenous indomethacin decreases luminal pressure and decreases the pain of acute cholecystitis.[186]

These data suggest that acute cholecystitis begins when one or more factors (e.g., lysolecithin, cholesterol, bile salts, gallstones) damage the gallbladder mucosa and stimulate increased prostaglandin synthesis. In the presence of an obstructed cystic duct, the resulting fluid secretion causes pressure within the lumen to rise, which produces a vicious cycle of increasing mucosal injury, prostaglandin production, and inflammation.

Although cultures of gallbladder bile are positive for bacteria early in the attack in most patients,[187, 188] bacteria are not thought to contribute to the inception of acute cholecystitis with few exceptions. In other words, the disease is not primarily an infectious process. Nevertheless, in about 20 per cent of cases, conditions in the gallbladder become favorable for bacterial proliferation, and suppurative cholecystitis (empyema) or perforation and abscess formation develop in the absence of treatment.

Acute cholecystitis in the absence of gallstones (*acalculous cholecystitis*)[189–193] is often associated with sudden starvation and immobility, changes that interrupt the usual sequence of gallbladder filling and emptying. Consequently, it is frequently seen in patients hospitalized for another illness, such as cardiovascular disease, acute trauma, burns, or surgery other than on the biliary system. Many of these patients are receiving total parenteral nutrition.[193]

Acute cholecystitis may also result from obstructing adenocarcinoma of the gallbladder or even, in some cases, from obstructing stones or neoplasms of the common bile duct. In Oriental *cholangiohepatitis*, common duct obstruction from primary ductal stones is sometimes complicated by acute acalculous cholecystitis with empyema.[194] For reasons as yet unknown, the use of chlorothiazides is associated with a threefold increase in the risk of acquiring acute cholecystitis.[195]

Rare cases of acute acalculous cholecystitis seem to represent specific bacterial infections. Some cases of salmonella cholecystitis[196] fall into this category, even though salmonella contamination of the gallbladder is more often present without acute inflammation. Cholera has been implicated as the cause of a few cases of acute acalculous cholecystitis, and cytomegalovirus infection of the gallbladder may be responsible for acute cholecystitis in patients with AIDS.[197, 198]

Studies of the vascular supply to acutely inflamed gallbladders show that the small arteries are often occluded.[199] In most cases this is probably a consequence rather than a cause of the illness, although it may contribute to the evolution of gangrenous cholecystitis and perforation. In some situations, arterial ischemia may be an etiologic factor earlier in the disease. This has been postulated to be the case in patients with diabetes mellitus, in whom acute cholecystitis is more likely to involve complications.[200] *Emphysematous cholecystitis* may be primarily an acute ischemic lesion. Acute cholecystitis has also been reported as a complication of polyarteritis nodosa.[201] Finally, torsion of the gallbladder, which can occur if fixation of the gallbladder to the liver is incomplete, produces an acute ischemic cholecystitis.[202, 203]

Pathology

In the initial few days of an attack, the changes in the gallbladder consist principally of hyperemia and edema (Color Fig. 89–3, p. xlv).[204–206] The cystic duct is usually obstructed by a gallstone, and the gallbladder becomes distended with bile, inflammatory exudate, or, rarely, pus. The histologic changes in the mucosa and underlying fibromuscular layers range from mild acute inflammation with edema and cellular infiltration to necrosis and perforation of the gallbladder wall. Early, the bile in the gallbladder is normal in appearance and consistency. Later, bile salts and pigments are absorbed and replaced with thin mucoid material, pus, or blood.

After the initial attack subsides, the mucosal surface heals and the wall becomes scarred. The absorptive capacity of the gallbladder mucosa is usually sufficiently damaged that the gallbladder becomes permanently nonfunctioning by oral cholecystography. If the inflammation subsides but the cystic duct remains obstructed, the lumen may become distended with clear mucoid fluid (hydrops of the gallbladder).[207]

Clinical Manifestations

The typical attack begins with acute abdominal pain and tenderness. The onset is usually similar to previous episodes of self-limited biliary colic, and for this reason the patient may delay seeking medical attention. At first, the pain may be poorly localized or maximally felt in the epigastrium or left upper quadrant before shifting to the right upper quadrant and becoming more severe and associated with tenderness. This pattern reflects the visceral pain of cystic duct obstruction,[208, 209] which evolves into parietal pain as the gallbladder becomes inflamed. It is analogous to the progression that is more often observed in acute appendicitis (see pp. 246–249).

The clinical findings in patients with acute cholecystitis span a wide spectrum.[210–212] The average case consists of moderate pain and localized tenderness with anorexia and vomiting. Usually pain precedes the vomiting, and the vomiting is not so severe as in acute pancreatitis or intestinal obstruction. Rarely, the pain may be more intense in the back or shoulder than in the abdomen. The temperature is usually 99 to 102°F.

During palpation in the right subcostal region, pain and inspiratory arrest occur when the patient takes a deep breath (*Murphy's sign*), a maneuver that brings the inflamed gallbladder into contact with the examiner's hand. In a few patients, the local findings are not very striking and the symptoms consist of a mild ache and anorexia. In other patients, the pain and tenderness are severe, abdominal guarding and localized rebound tenderness are prominent, and fever and other systemic manifestations are more advanced.

In about one third of patients, the gallbladder is palpable, sometimes in its normal location in the midclavicular line but often more lateral. The gallbladder is more often palpable in patients suffering their first attack of acute cholecystitis than in those who have had chronic symptoms for many years. Absence of a palpable gallbladder in the majority of patients is due to chronic scarring, which limits enlargement of the organ; guarding by the patient, which limits the examination; or hepatomegaly, which protects the gallbladder from the examiner's hand.

Jaundice is present in about 20 per cent of patients.[212, 213] It is usually mild (bilirubin <4.0 mg/dl) but occasionally is more severe. Common duct stones are present in only one half of jaundiced patients with acute cholecystitis. The higher the bilirubin, the more likely that stones will be found in the duct. In the other patients, jaundice seems to be due to edema of the ducts or perhaps to direct involvement of the liver by inflammation.

During the acute attack, the leukocyte count averages 12,000 to 15,000 cells per cu mm with a neutrophilic leukocytosis and an increase in band forms. Serum transaminase and alkaline phosphatase values may be mildly elevated even in the absence of intrahepatic infection or common bile duct obstruction.

Sometimes the serum amylase concentration may exceed 1000 U/dl. This usually indicates concomitant acute pancreatitis, but amylase elevations in this range are occasionally seen in acute cholecystitis without any changes in the pancreas. Whenever the amylase level is high, the presence of a common duct stone should be suspected.

Because acute cholecystitis is primarily a chemical inflammation, more than half of cases allowed to run the course of the disease resolve spontaneously without complications. Nevertheless, a substantial portion (e.g., 25 to 35 per cent) become worse. When pain and tenderness become severe, fever exceeds about 102°F, leukocytosis rises above 15,000 cells per μl, and the patient experiences chills, suppurative cholecystitis (empyema)[214, 215] or perforation has developed and requires urgent operation. Advanced gallbladder suppuration may be present, however, even though the local and systemic manifestations are unimpressive.[215]

As a rule, an attack of acute cholecystitis lasts for a week to ten days.[205, 206] However, it is not uncommon to encounter a patient whose acute findings completely resolve within 24 to 48 hours after hospitalization. Less commonly, the disease resolves much more slowly, with localized pain and tenderness persisting for four to six weeks. When operation is performed in these patients, the gallbladder is inflamed, distorted, or shrunken and often has lost full-thickness portions of the wall because of patchy gangrene.

Fever of unknown origin may rarely be due to subacute or chronic cholecystitis in patients without specific symptoms or abnormal physical findings. These patients are often elderly or otherwise debilitated. Sometimes the fever is caused by a slowly resolving perforation. Rarely, it may be secondary to a *subhepatic abscess* following an earlier attack of cholecystitis. Residual *typhoid infection* in the gallbladder may be the cause of mysterious fevers in some areas of the world.

Diagnosis

Because acute cholecystitis is a common disease, the sudden onset of right upper quadrant pain and tenderness should always suggest this diagnosis. The list of conditions that must be considered in the differential diagnosis is long, however, and confirmatory tests are important. Only 40 per cent of patients in whom the diagnosis of acute cholecystitis is seriously considered are ultimately found to have the disease.

Plain films of the abdomen rarely provide specific evidence of acute cholecystitis. They may show gallstones in the 15 per cent of patients whose stones contain enough calcium to render them radiopaque. Emphysematous cholecystitis may be diagnosed when gas in the wall produces a silhouette of the gallbladder. Plain films are probably most important, however, when they provide evidence for some other condition in the differential diagnosis, such as perforated peptic ulcer or intestinal obstruction.

Ultrasonography of the gallbladder should be almost routine.[216–220] In patients with acute cholecystitis, gallstones usually can be demonstrated, and it is also usually possible for the examiner to tell whether tenderness is maximal over the gallbladder or elsewhere. Less reliable clues from ultrasound include a thickened gallbladder wall (> 3 mm), gallbladder distention, or sludge in the lumen. Wall thickening can occur in the presence of any inflammatory process near the gallbladder or with hypoalbuminemia, ascites, or portal hypertension. Marked irregularity of the luminal surface or the presence of intraluminal membranes suggests gangrenous cholecystitis.[220] A pericholecystic fluid collection may be seen with localized gallbladder perforation.

The sensitivity and specificity of an ultrasonographic diagnosis are about 90 and 95 per cent, respectively. False positive diagnoses may occur in patients with chronic cholecystitis, and false negative diagnoses in patients with acalculous cholecystitis. Sonography is useful in patients with jaundice, in whom scintigraphy may be technically unsatisfactory.

Biliary scintigraphy is more sensitive but less specific than sonography (97 and 90 per cent, respectively).[217, 221–228] The imaging agents, ^{99m}Tc-6 labeled derivatives of iminodiacetic acid, are taken up by hepatocytes and excreted in bile in sufficient concentrations to produce a gamma camera image.[229] In normal subjects, scans obtained 15 to 30 minutes after intravenous administration of the radionuclide outline the bile ducts, gallbladder, and proximal intestine. Acute cholecystitis is suggested if the ducts are imaged, but the gallbladder is not. Except for a few cases of acute acalculous cholecystitis, acute cholecystitis is ruled out if the gallbladder fills. An indeterminant study consists of poor imaging of the liver or biliary tree. Although the gallbladder invariably becomes imaged within an hour in normal subjects, gallbladder filling in patients who have nonacute gallstone disease may not occur for one to three hours. Therefore, final scans must be obtained four hours after administration of the radionuclide before a study can be called definitely positive.

False positive scans[230–232] may occur in patients with acute pancreatitis, chronic cholecystitis, alcoholism, neoplasms of the gallbladder and liver, and those who are receiving total parenteral nutrition. False negative scans may be seen in patients with acute acalculous cholecystitis.

Despite the availability of excellent noninvasive tests, it is sometimes impossible to determine with certainty whether acute cholecystitis is the cause of severe right upper quadrant findings. In critically ill patients in whom the diagnosis is in doubt, one may obtain a sample of gallbladder bile by percutaneous transhepatic aspiration performed under ultrasound guidance.[233, 234] The bile is examined for gross appearance and the presence of microorganisms on Gram stain and culture. If the patient is a poor surgical risk, a catheter may be left in the gallbladder as a form of percutaneous cholecystostomy. Complications of this technique are rare.

The findings on CT and magnetic resonance scans are relatively nonspecific, although CT may be of help in diagnosing a pericholecystic abscess.

An oral cholecystogram may be ordered if it is thought that the diagnosis is probably not acute cholecystitis, and if the patient has not been vomiting. Opacification of the gallbladder would largely rule out acute cholecystitis. Nonopacification cannot be interpreted, because it occurs not only with cholecystitis but also with many other acute abdominal illnesses, such as pancreatitis, gastroenteritis, and so forth.

Differential Diagnosis

The principal conditions to consider in the differential diagnosis are acute pancreatitis, appendicitis, pyelonephritis or renal stone, peptic ulcer disease, acute hepatitis, pneumonitis, hepatic abscess or tumor, and gonococcal perihepatitis. Studies of patients admitted to the hospital with acute abdominal pain show that diagnostic errors (among admitting impressions) in patients with acute cholecystitis are more often false negative than false positive.

Acute appendicitis is the disease most often confused with acute cholecystitis, as the initial diagnostic impression is largely based upon localized right abdominal tenderness, which may be lower than expected in cholecystitis or higher than expected in appendicitis. In general, fever, leukocytosis, and tenderness progress more inexorably in appendicitis. Real-time ultrasonography is usually able to identify which of these organs is the one acutely inflamed (see pp. 1382–1389).

Acute pancreatitis may also be difficult to distinguish from acute cholecystitis, because on physical examination the pain and tenderness are in the same area. Many patients with acute pancreatitis are known to have recently been on an alcoholic binge. However, gallstones and cholecystitis are more common in alcoholics than in the general population, and hyperamylasemia, characteristic of acute pancreatitis, is also seen at times in acute cholecystitis even when the pancreas is normal. HIDA scans and ultrasound examination for gallstones will aid in the differentiation of these two conditions (see pp. 1814–1842).

One should also remember that cholelithiasis may cause acute pancreatitis as stones traverse the common bile duct and ampulla of Vater. Moreover, pancreatitis may occur in conjunction with acute cholecystitis or cholangitis.

Renal disease may produce anterior abdominal pain and tenderness typical of cholecystitis. Usually a clue to the presence of urinary disease is found in the urinalysis.

Peptic ulcer disease may also be confused with cholecystitis and should be suspected if there is a past history of ulcers. Perforated peptic ulcer usually produces more striking findings than does cholecystitis and usually is associated with free intra-abdominal air on plain X-ray films. When free air is not seen but peptic ulcer is still suspected, an emergency upper gastrointestinal series with water-soluble contrast medium may demonstrate the perforation. If the clinical findings point more toward acute cholecystitis, an ultrasound examination and HIDA scan should be obtained first (see pp. 925–938).

Pleurisy and *pneumonitis* may cause abdominal pain and tenderness. There usually will be pain on breathing, abnormalities on auscultation of the lungs, and X-ray evidence of pulmonary disease.

Hepatitis, especially alcoholic hepatitis, may be surprisingly similar in presentation to acute cholecystitis. In alcoholic hepatitis, right upper quadrant pain and tenderness may be accompanied by fever and leukocytosis, and the SGOT level is usually only slightly elevated. In some cases, progressive local findings in the right upper quadrant may suggest the development of suppurative cholecystitis and the need for emergency surgery. If alcoholic hepatitis is thought to be a possibility, percutaneous liver biopsy may be indicated.

Gonococcal perihepatitis (Fitz-Hugh–Curtis syndrome) produces right upper quadrant pain, tenderness, and leukocytosis, which often overshadow any pelvic complaints. Nevertheless, adnexal tenderness will be present on physical examination, and a Gram stain of the cervical smear should show gonococci. Laparoscopy has been used successfully to diagnose gonococcal perihepatitis (see pp. 1264–1265).

The symptoms of *pyogenic* or *amebic hepatic abscesses* may at first be thought to be caused by acute cholecystitis. In many cases of hepatic abscess a history of antecedent abdominal sepsis or amebic infection is absent. Often, however, the patient is more septic than expected on the basis of the right upper quadrant findings, pleural fluid is present on chest films, and the liver is enlarged. ^{99m}Tc-colloid liver scan, ultrasound examination, or CT scan will usually delineate the liver abscess (see pp. 1162–1165).

Hepatic tumors, both primary and metastatic, occasionally produce acute symptoms resulting from necrosis or hemorrhage into their substance. The differentiation from acute cholecystitis may be impossible on clinical grounds, even when one knows that the patient's liver contains tumor. A HIDA scan may not image the extrahepatic ducts, and in some cases the severity of the symptoms will justify diagnostic percutaneous transhepatic aspiration of the gallbladder under ultrasonic guidance to obtain a specimen of bile for examination (see pp. 467–487).

Treatment

The patient should be admitted to the hospital for observation and treatment. Dehydration from lack of oral intake and vomiting should be corrected by intravenous fluids and electrolytes to ensure adequate urinary output and normal plasma electrolytes. Oral feeding should be stopped temporarily and nasogastric suction instituted.

Antibiotics should probably be given even in the absence of suppurative complications because bile is known to acquire a resident bacterial population early in the course of acute cholecystitis. On the other hand, antibiotics administered prophylactically do not appear to decrease the incidence of suppuration.[235] The initial regimen should consist of a single agent, such as cefoxitin, 2.0 gm in divided doses four times daily. If sepsis develops, a more aggressive regimen should be prescribed, which would include an aminoglycoside, ampicillin, and a drug effective against anaerobes (e.g., metronidazole, clindamycin).

Three factors should be considered in planning treatment: (1) the severity of the cholecystitis, (2) the general condition of the patient, and (3) the firmness of the diagnosis.

Whenever acute cholecystitis seems on the verge of producing complications, laparotomy must be performed as soon as the patient can be readied. Some of these individuals are seriously ill when they enter the hospital; others become so while being managed on a nonoperative regimen. High doses of antibiotics should be given parenterally and fluid and electrolyte balance restored. This can usually be accomplished within a few hours, and operation is then performed.

Differences of opinion still remain concerning how best to manage an uncomplicated case. Because the disease may resolve spontaneously, there are some who prefer an expectant, nonoperative regimen, and they recommend operation during the acute attack only if the disease becomes more severe. Then interval cholecystectomy is performed six to eight weeks later, after the patient has fully recovered. Others favor cholecystectomy early in the course, provided that the diagnosis has been established and the patient's overall status is suitable for general anesthesia. Because the natural history of the disease is more severe in those over the age of 60, these patients should not be treated expectantly unless there are overriding contraindications to surgery.[236, 237] Everyone agrees, however, that if ancillary problems such as congestive heart failure or pneumonitis are present, further treatment might improve operability, and in this situation the patient should be begun on a nonoperative regimen.

For the average patient, early operation has the following advantages over expectant management, as demonstrated by four randomized clinical trials (Table 89–4):[238–242] (1) By eliminating the possibility of progressive disease, early operation results in a lower mortality; (2) the total morbidity of the illness, includ-

Table 89–4. CONSOLIDATED RESULTS FROM FIVE REPORTS OF FOUR CONTROLLED TRIALS COMPARING EARLY AND INTERVAL CHOLECYSTECTOMY FOR ACUTE CHOLECYSTITIS*

Timing of Cholecystectomy	Number of Patients	Deaths	Duct Injuries	Total Mean Hospital Stay (Days)	Failure of Regimen†
Early	215	0	0	10.9	N/A
Interval	192	5	0	20.1	19%

*References 238–242.
†Failure of regimen means surgery was required for progressive acute disease.

ing days in the hospital and time lost from work, is less with early operation; (3) the operation is technically no easier, and may even be more difficult, if it is delayed; and (4) direct costs of the expectant regimen are several thousand dollars more.[243]

It should be emphasized, however, that early surgery in uncomplicated acute cholecystitis does not imply an emergency operation. Rather, the procedure should be scheduled in the next available opening in the operating schedule during regular working hours with adequate preparations for operative cholangiography.[244]

When surgery is performed, cholecystectomy is possible in 90 per cent of cases. The common bile duct is explored for the same indications as in elective cholecystectomy. If the general condition of the patient is precarious, cholecystostomy may be preferable to cholecystectomy.[245, 246] Cholecystostomy consists of evacuating the gallbladder of gallstones and infected bile and securing a tube (e.g., a large Foley catheter) in the lumen; the tube is then brought out through the abdominal wall and allowed to drain by gravity. If an experienced interventional radiologist is available, a percutaneous cholecystostomy may be performed by inserting a tube through liver and into the gallbladder under ultrasound or CT guidance.[247–249] This is preferable to operation in high-risk patients (see pp. 1751–1758). Cholecystostomy is simpler and less time-consuming than cholecystectomy and resolves sepsis with lower morbidity and mortality rates in the critically ill patient. It is, however, inadequate therapy for common duct obstruction and acute cholangitis.[248, 250] The incidence of cholecystostomy in an institution generally reflects the number of elderly patients who are treated for acute cholecystitis, because it is indicated mainly for those over age 60.

After cholecystostomy, a tube cholangiogram should be performed when the patient has fully recovered from the acute attack. If the patient is under age 65 and in good health, a cholecystectomy should then be performed.[250, 251] Otherwise, the cholecystostomy tube can be removed in about four weeks, and the patient may be followed expectantly so long as there are no residual stones in the gallbladder or bile ducts. If expectant management is indicated, residual stones in the gallbladder can usually be removed percutaneously through the cholecystostomy tube tract, and common duct stones can be eliminated by endoscopic sphincterotomy. Less than one half of patients followed under these circumstances manifest symptoms of gallbladder disease within five years.[252, 253]

ACUTE ACALCULOUS CHOLECYSTITIS

Acute acalculous cholecystitis is important enough to warrant a separate section, for unlike acute cholecystitis in patients with gallstone disease, acalculous cholecystitis progresses rapidly to gangrene and perforation and must not be treated expectantly.[189–192, 254, 255] The condition most often occurs following accidental or surgical trauma or as a complication of another serious illness. An early step in the pathogenesis may involve activation of Factor XII, which in experimental animals results in acute injury to the gallbladder and lungs.[256] Once inflammation begins, it may worsen as a result of prostaglandins released locally in the gallbladder wall.

Men outnumber women by more than 2 to 1, and 80 per cent of patients are over age 50. Sepsis from another condition and diabetes mellitus are common associated findings.

The clinical presentation usually consists of right upper quadrant pain and fever. The diagnosis may be very difficult, however, because in as many as 25 per cent of patients the initial syndrome is fever without pain or local findings.[192] Therefore, when more common problems have been excluded in patients hospitalized for some other condition, unexplained fever should raise the suspicion of acute cholecystitis. Twenty-five per cent of patients have an enlarged, palpable gallbladder. Leukocytosis is usual but not universal.

The diagnosis often can be confirmed by ultrasound scans. Positive findings include thickening of the gallbladder wall to >3 mm (average, 5.5 mm); gallbladder enlargement and tenderness (an ultrasonographic Murphy's sign); and a pericholecystic fluid collection (i.e., an abscess). Biliary scintigraphy is also reasonably accurate.[257, 258] In uncomplicated cases the bile ducts are imaged but not the gallbladder. With gallbladder perforation, an image is obtained of a pericholecystic collection or spillage of bile into the free peritoneal cavity. Despite their proven value, sonography and scintigraphy are not as sensitive in the diagnosis of acalculous cholecystitis as in the diagnosis of calculous cholecystitis.[259] False negative results occur in about 20 per cent of cases, so repeating these tests or performing percutaneous aspiration of the gallbladder or exploratory laparotomy may be indicated in selected cases, depending on the clinical findings.

Gangrene, empyema, or perforation is present by the time of surgery in 75 per cent of cases. In one series, perforation had developed in only 10 per cent of patients who were surgically treated within 48 hours of the onset of symptoms but had developed in 40 per cent of patients treated thereafter.[192]

In most cases, urgent cholecystectomy or cholecystostomy is the appropriate therapy.[189–192] Critically ill patients who are poor surgical risks may be treated by percutaneous, transhepatic cholecystostomy.[260] The catheter is allowed to drain for about three weeks, and then if a tube cholecystogram shows that the biliary tree is patent, the catheter can be removed and the gallbladder left undisturbed.

The disease is fatal in about 10 per cent of patients, most of whom are quite elderly, have serious associated disease, or have experienced complications as a result of a delay in diagnosis and treatment.

EMPHYSEMATOUS CHOLECYSTITIS[261–263]

Emphysematous cholecystitis is a form of acute cholecystitis in which the gallbladder, its wall, and sometimes even the bile ducts or pericholecystic area contain gas. It is a manifestation of infection by gas-producing bacteria and often occurs in the absence of gallstone disease. *Clostridium welchii* has been cultured most often, but *Escherichia coli,* anaerobic streptococci, and other clostridial species have been found in some patients. Clinically, the presentation is typical of acute cholecystitis, except that pain may be more severe and the patient more toxic. The gallbladder may be palpable as a subcostal mass, and it is usually evident, riddled with gas, on abdominal plain films. The findings on ultrasound scan are also characteristic and may be present before gas becomes visible on plain films.[264] About 20 per cent of patients have diabetes mellitus. Men outnumber women by a ratio of 3 to 1. The male preponderance, absence of gallstones, anaerobic infection, and frequency of diabetes mellitus have suggested that ischemia resulting from obstruction of the cystic artery may be the initial event in this illness. The differential diagnosis must consider other causes of gas in the gallbladder, principally cholecystenteric fistula. Lipomatosis of the gallbladder, a rare condition, may give a similar X-ray picture. Initial therapy should consist of high doses of antibiotics in addition to other general supportive measures. Treatment consists of early surgery, preferably cholecystectomy rather than cholecystostomy. True gas gangrene of the abdominal wall (clostridial myositis) is a rare complication of emphysematous cholecystitis. The morbidity and mortality rates of emphysematous cholecystitis are greater than for other forms of acute cholecystitis.

Complications

Perforation of the *gallbladder*, the most serious complication of acute cholecystitis, is seen in about 10 per cent of cases.[265–268] It may occur without a preliminary course of severe symptoms, or it may be the product of progressive disease during expectant management. Acalculous cholecystitis, which evolves into gangrenous cholecystitis in about half of the cases, has become more common, and this variant now makes up 40 per cent of those who develop perforation. Typically, patients with perforation seek medical care later in their illness (about 7.5 days) than do patients without perforation. Even with modern diagnostic tools, perforation is rarely suspected preoperatively.

Three types of perforation occur: localized perforation with abscess formation, free perforation into the peritoneal cavity with generalized peritonitis, and perforation into an adjacent hollow viscus with formation of a cholecystenteric fistula. Surgical intervention is indicated for all three types.

Localized Perforation. *Pericholecystic abscess* is the most common type of perforation resulting from acute cholecystitis. As the inflammatory process evolves, adjacent viscera and omentum become firmly adherent to the gallbladder, so when perforation occurs, the spillage is confined and an abscess results. The relatively slow evolution of acute cholecystitis probably accounts for the high frequency of contained perforations.

Perforations may occur within the first few days of an attack or as late as the second week. High fever, right upper quadrant pain with direct and rebound tenderness, and the presence of a palpable mass all indicate this complication. The features overlap those of uncomplicated cholecystitis, however, and the diagnosis may not be suspected until surgery. Ultrasound and CT scans may demonstrate the abscess adjacent to the gallbladder, but this is unusual.

Surgical treatment is mandatory. In most cases, cholecystectomy can be accomplished, although some unstable patients are better treated by cholecystostomy and drainage of the abscess.

Free Perforation. Generalized bile peritonitis[269–271] is associated with about a 30 per cent mortality rate and fortunately is seen in only 1 to 2 per cent of patients with acute cholecystitis. The perforation usually occurs in the fundus as the result of progressive inflammation and distention. Sometimes the patient experiences transient pain relief following perforation and decompression of the gallbladder into the peritoneal cavity. Then more serious symptoms evolve as purulent peritonitis becomes established. However, most patients present as cases of severe abdominal disease with few clues to implicate the gallbladder, and the diagnosis of free perforation is rarely made preoperatively. Antimicrobial drugs must be given and abdominal exploration performed as an emergency. Cholecystostomy with peritoneal lavage is the surgical treatment in most cases.

Cholecystenteric Fistula. The gallbladder may also perforate into the lumen of an adjacent organ.[272–274] The duodenum is the most common site, and the hepatic flexure of the colon is next. Fistulas to the stomach and jejunum are less common, and instances of perforation into the thoracic cavity and renal pelvis are rare. As the gallbladder contents decompress into the intestine, the attack of acute cholecystitis often subsides. Chronic symptoms may develop later, particularly if gallstones remain in the gallbladder.

Oral cholecystography opacifies neither the gallbladder nor the fistula. In some cases a preoperative diagnosis of chronic cholecystitis is made on the basis of symptoms and a nonopacified gallbladder on cholecystogram, and fistula is unsuspected until discovered at surgery. An ultrasound scan will usually demonstrate the gallstones. Plain films may show air in the biliary tree. If an upper gastrointestinal series is performed, it may demonstrate a cholecystoduodenal fistula. A barium enema may reveal chronic perforation into the colon.

Uncomplicated cholecystenteric fistulas per se rarely produce much morbidity. In fact, deliberate surgical anastomosis of the gallbladder to the intestine is performed commonly to bypass an obstructed common bile duct. Gallstones are usually present in the gallbladder or common duct if the patient has persistent complaints. Cholecystectomy and closure of the affected bowel are curative. Exploration of the common duct will be indicated in many of these patients.

Fistulas from the duodenum or stomach into the gallbladder or bile duct are occasionally seen as complications of peptic ulcer disease. Jaundice or cholangitis may develop, but often the biliary involvement is unsuspected until shown on an upper gastrointestinal series. If the fistula enters the gallbladder, cholecystectomy and an ulcer operation can be performed. The appropriate therapy for a fistula into the duct is an ulcer operation, such as vagotomy and gastroenterostomy, which does not require takedown of the fistula. Technical problems with the bile duct may follow a direct attack on the fistula, whereas healing usually ensues without sequelae if the ulcer can be made to heal.

Prognosis

The overall mortality rate of acute cholecystitis is about 5 per cent, but several factors distinguish patients in whom the death rate is higher. Age is most influential; nearly all who succumb are over 60 years, and those over age 70 have a mortality rate of about 15 per cent. Most deaths are due to *uncontrolled sepsis*, *pneumonitis*, or *cardiovascular complications*. Acute cholecystitis is also more often lethal in patients with diabetes mellitus. The diabetic patient with acute cholecystitis should have cholecystectomy performed as soon as he can be prepared for operation.

Choledocholithiasis, or common duct stones, is not considered a direct complication of acute cholecystitis, but they coexist in about 15 per cent of patients. If acute cholecystitis is accompanied by jaundice and cholangitis, the morbidity rate increases substantially. Pancreatitis is also thought to be more a complication of choledocholithiasis than of acute cholecystitis, but patients simultaneously afflicted by both have a worse prognosis (see pp. 1718–1721).

The stage of the disease in the gallbladder also influences the outcome. Empyema, gangrene, and localized or diffuse peritonitis progressively diminish the chances of recovery, although young persons with these complications do surprisingly well. Because cholecystostomy must be done in the most critically ill patients, clinical reports note mortality rates of about 20 per cent for this procedure.

Carcinoma of the *gallbladder* is found in a small percentage of patients with acute cholecystitis. Although the immediate mortality rate is not excessive, nearly all are dead within one year (see pp. 1734–1740).

GALLSTONE ILEUS

This form of mechanical intestinal obstruction is caused by a gallstone impacted in the intestinal lumen, having entered the bowel through a *cholecystenteric fistula*.[275–282] The stone is nearly always 2.5 cm or greater in diameter. Most of the patients are elderly women, and the diagnosis should always be considered in someone over age 70 with intestinal obstruction. The absence of an external hernia or scars from a previous laparotomy should place gallstone ileus high on the list of possible causes of small bowel obstruction in this age group. Although some patients relate a history compatible with recent acute cholecystitis, the majority do not. It has been suggested that fistula formation in patients with gallstone ileus is most often caused by gradual pressure leading to erosion through the fundus by the large heavy stone, rather than cystic duct obstruction, inflammation, and perforation.

Usually the gallstone enters the bowel through a cholecystoduodenal fistula and travels a varying length aborally before stopping. It may temporarily occlude the lumen in one spot and then dislodge and move farther along. This results in intermittent symptoms and may lead the physician to think that the obstruction is partial and likely to resolve. Then, complete obstruction appears when the stone finally reaches bowel too narrow to allow further progression.

Most gallstone obstructions occur in the ileum because the diameter of the small bowel progressively decreases aborally, and the ileum is the narrowest segment. Less commonly, the stone may enter the colon either after negotiating the entire small intestine or by direct passage through a cholecystocolonic fistula.[281] Gallstone obstruction of the colon is uncommon because of the large size of the colonic lumen. When it does occur, the obstructing stone has usually lodged in a segment narrowed by another disease process, usually chronic sigmoid diverticulitis.

The diagnosis of gallstone ileus may be suspected from clinical data such as coincidental acute cholecystitis, intermittent bowel obstruction, or age of the patient. Abdominal X-rays will show the typical findings of mechanical small bowel obstruction. Air is present in the biliary tree on plain films, but it may be difficult to detect unless carefully sought. Sometimes the stone is radiopaque, but it often goes unrecognized as a gallstone unless gallstone ileus is specifically considered. If gallstone ileus is suspected but the diagnosis is still unclear, an upper gastrointestinal series may resolve the issue by demonstrating a cholecystoduodenal fistula as well as verifying the presence of small bowel obstruction. Duodenal obstruction has been diagnosed when the stone was seen by endoscopy.[283]

The mortality rate of gallstone ileus is high, about 15 to 20 per cent, and can be attributed mainly to delay in surgical treatment. Typically, the patient has been symptomatic for several days before seeking medical care, and further delay is incurred during diagnostic efforts in a puzzling clinical situation. These elderly patients do not tolerate acute illness of this duration, and pneumonitis or cardiovascular complications are frequent.

Gallstone ileus requires an emergency laparotomy. The obstructing stone should be removed through a small enterotomy, which is then closed. The intestine proximal to the obstruction must be carefully examined for the presence of a second stone, which could cause an immediate recurrence postoperatively. Cholecystectomy and closure of the cholecystoduodenal fistula are almost never indicated acutely. Many of these fistulas will close spontaneously because the gallbladder has discharged its only stone.

After recovery from the operation, cholecystectomy is indicated only if chronic symptoms of gallbladder disease are present, but this occurs in less than half the patients. Recurrent gallstone ileus, which has an incidence of 4 per cent, is caused by residual stones.

References

1. Bainton, D., Davies, G. T., Evans, K. T., et al. Gallbladder disease. Prevalence in a South Wales industrial town. N. Engl. J. Med. *294*:1148, 1976.
2. Barker, D. J. P., Gardner, M. J., Power, C., et al. Prevalence of gall stones at necropsy in nine British towns: A collaborative study. Br. Med. J. *2*:1389, 1979.
3. Bateson, M. C., and Bouchier, I. A. D. Prevalence of gall stones in Dundee: necropsy study. Br. Med. J. *4*:4271, 1975.
4. Diehl, A. K., Stern, M. P., Ostrower, V. S., et al. Prevalence of clinical gallbladder disease in Mexican-American, Anglo, and Black women. South. Med. J. *73*:438, 1980.
5. Godrey, P. J., Bates, T., Harrison, M., et al. Gall stones and mortality: A study of all gall stone related deaths in a single health district. Gut *25*:1029, 1984.
6. Layde, P. M., Vessey, M. P., and Yeatles, D. Risk factors for gall-bladder disease: A cohort study of young women attending family planning clinics. J. Epidemiol. Commun. Health *36*:274, 1982.
7. Lindstrom, C. G. Frequency of gallstone disease in a well-defined Swedish population. A prospective necropsy study in Malmo. Scand. J. Gastroenterol. *12*:341, 1977.
8. Rome Group for the Epidemiology and Prevention of Cholelithiasis (GREPO). Prevalence of gallstone disease in an Italian adult female population. Am. J. Epidemiol. *119*:796, 1984.
9. Williams, C. N., and Johnston, J. L. Prevalence of gallstones and risk factors in Caucasian women in a rural Canadian community. Can. Med. Assoc. J. *120*:664, 1980.
10. Bateson, M. C. Gallbladder disease and cholecystectomy rate are independently variable. Lancet *2*:621, 1984.
11. Sampliner, R. E., Bennett, P. H., Comess, L. J., et al. Gallbladder disease in Pima Indians. Demonstration of high prevalence and early onset by cholecystography. N. Engl. J. Med. *283*:1358, 1979.
12. Balzer, K., Goebell, H., Breuer, N., Ruping, K. W., and Leder, L. D. Epidemiology of gallstones in a German industrial town (Essen) from 1940–1975. Digestion *33*:189, 1986.
13. Norby, S., Fagerberg, G., and Sjodahl, R. Decreasing incidence of gallstone disease in a defined Swedish population. Scand. J. Gastroenterol. *21*:158, 1986.
14. Bernstein, R. A., Giefer, E. E., Vieira, J. J., et al. Gallbladder disease. II. Utilization of the life table method in obtaining clinically useful information. A study of 62,739 weight-conscious women. J. Chron. Dis. *30*:529, 1977.
15. Honore, L. H. Cholesterol cholelithiasis in adolescent females. Its connection with obesity, parity, and oral contraceptive use—a retrospective study of 31 cases. Arch. Surg. *115*:62, 1980.
16. Layde, P. M., Vessey, M. P., and Yeates, D. Risk factors for gall-bladder disease: A cohort study of young women attending family planning clinics. J. Epidemiol. Commun. Health *36*:274, 1982.
17. Scragg, R. K. R., McMichael, A. J., and Baghurst, P. A. Diet, alcohol, and relative weight in gall stone disease: A case-control study. Br. Med. J. *288*:1113, 1984.
18. Amaral, J. F., and Thompson, W. R. Gallbladder disease in the morbidly obese. Am. J. Surg. *149*:551, 1985.
19. Thiet, M. D., Mittelstaedt, C. A., Herbst, C. A., Jr., et al. Cholelithiasis in morbid obesity. South. Med. J. *77*:416, 1984.
20. Klingensmith, W. C., III, and Eckhout, G. V. Cholelithiasis in the morbidly obese: Diagnosis by US and oral cholecystography. Radiology *160*:27, 1986.
21. Herbst, C. A., Mittelstaedt, C. A., Staab, E. V., et al. Intraoperative ultrasonography evaluation of the gallbladder in morbidly obese patients. Ann. Surg. *200*:691, 1984.
22. Boston Collaborative Drug Surveillance Programme. Oral contraceptives and venous thromboembolic disease, surgically confirmed gallbladder disease, and breast tumours. Lancet *1*:1399, 1973.
23. Royal College of General Practitioners' Oral Contraception Study. Oral contraceptives and gallbladder disease. Lancet *2*:957, 1982.
24. Sarles, H., Hauton, J., Planche, N. E., et al. Diet, cholesterol gallstones, and composition of the bile. Dig. Dis. *15*:251, 1970.
25. Smith, D. A., and Gee, M. I. A dietary survey to determine the relationship between diet and cholelithiasis. Am. J. Clin. Nutr. *32*:1519, 1979.
26. Capron, J. P., Delamarre, J., and Herve, M. A. Meal frequency and duration of overnight fast: A role in gall-stone formation? Br. Med. J. *283*:1435, 1981.
27. Hanis, C. L., Ferrell, R. E., Tulloch, B. R., et al. Gallbladder disease epidemiology in Mexican Americans in Starr County, Texas. Am. J. Epidemiol. *122*:820, 1985.
28. Bennion, L. J., and Grundy, S. M. Effects of diabetes mellitus on cholesterol metabolism in man. N. Engl. J. Med. *296*:1365, 1977.
29. Diehl, A. K., Rosenthal, M., Hazuda, H. P., et al. Socioeconomic status and the prevalence of clinical gallbladder disease. J. Chron. Dis. *38*:1019, 1985.
30. Thornton, J., Symes, C., and Heaton, K. Moderate alcohol intake reduces bile cholesterol saturation and raises HDL cholesterol. Lancet *2*:819, 1983.
31. Bouchier, I. A. D. Postmortem study of the frequency of gallstones in patients with cirrhosis of the liver. Gut *10*:705, 1969.
32. Nicholas, P., Rinaudo, P. A., and Conn, H. O. Increased incidence of cholelithiasis in Laennec's cirrhosis. A postmortem evaluation of pathogenesis. Gastroenterology *63*:112, 1972.
33. Lund, J. Surgical indications in cholelithiasis: Prophylactic cholecystectomy elucidated on the basis of long-term follow up on 526 nonoperated cases. Ann. Surg. *151*:153, 1960.
34. Wenckert, A., and Robertson, B. The natural course of gallstone disease. Eleven-year review of 781 nonoperated cases. Gastroenterology *50*:376, 1966.
35. Gracie, W. A., and Ransohoff, D. F. The natural history of silent gallstones. The innocent gallstone is not a myth. N. Engl. J. Med. *307*:798, 1982.
36. McSherry, C. K., Ferstenberg, H., Calhoun, W. F., et al. The natural history of diagnosed gallstone disease in symptomatic and asymptomatic patients. Ann. Surg. *202*:59, 1985.
37. Thistle, J. L., Cleary, P. A., Lachin, J. M., et al. The natural history of cholelithiasis: The National Cooperative Gallstone Study. Ann. Intern. Med. *101*:171, 1984.
38. Ransohoff, D. F., Gracie, W. A., Wolfenson, L. B., et al. Prophylactic cholecystectomy or expectant management for silent gallstones. Ann. Intern. Med. *99*:199, 1983.
39. Diehl, A. K. Epidemiology of gallbladder cancer: A synthesis of recent data. JNCI *65*:1209, 1980.
40. Lowenfels, A. B., Lindstrom, C. G., Conway, M. J., et al. Gallstones and risk of gallbladder cancer. JNCI *75*:77, 1985.
41. Weiss, K. M., Ferrell, R. E., Hanis, C. L., et al. Genetics and epidemiology of gallbladder disease in new world native peoples. Am. J. Hum. Genet. *36*:1259, 1984.
42. Strom, B. L., Hibberd, P. L., Soper, K. A., et al. International variations in epidemiology of cancers of the extrahepatic biliary tract. Can. Res. *45*:5165, 1985.
43. Diehl, A. K., and Beral, V. Cholecystectomy and changing mortality from gallbladder cancer. Lancet *2*:187, 1981.
44. Polk, H. C., Jr. Carcinoma and the calcified gallbladder. Gastroenterology *50*:582, 1966.
45. Ashur, H., Siegal, B., Oland, Y., et al. Calcified gallbladder (porcelain gallbladder). Arch. Surg. *113*:594, 1978.
46. Schein, C. J., Hurwitt, E. S., and Rosenblatt, M. A. The

significance of calculus size in determining the indication for elective cholecystectomy. Gastroenterology *29*:377, 1955.
47. Diehl, A. K. Gallstone size and the risk of gallbladder cancer. JAMA *250*:2323, 1983.
48. Houssin, D., Castaing, D., Lemoine, J., et al. Microlithiasis of the gallbladder. Surg. Gynecol. Obstet. *157*:20, 1983.
49. Adye, B., and Ryand, J. A., Jr. Cholecystitis in teenage girls. West. J. Surg. *139*:471, 1983.
50. Henschke, C. I., and Teele, R. L. Cholelithiasis in children: Recent observations. J. Ultrasound Med. *2*:481, 1983.
51. Lau, G. E., Andrassy, R. J., and Mahour, G. H. A 30-year review of the management of gallbladder disease at a children's hospital. Am. Surg. *49*:411, 1983.
52. Pokorny, W. J., Saleem, M., O'Gorman, R. B., et al. Cholelithiasis and cholecystitis in childhood. Am. J. Surg. *148*:742, 1984.
53. Shafer, A. D., Ashley, J. V., Goodwin, C. D., et al. A new look at the multifactoral etiology of gallbladder disease in children. Am. Surg. *49*:314, 1983.
54. Takiff, H., and Fonkalsrud, E. W. Gallbladder disease in childhood. Am. J. Dis. Child. *138*:565, 1984.
55. Lee, S. S., Wasiljew, B. K., and Lee, M. J. Gallstones in women younger than thirty. J. Clin. Gastroenterol. *9*:65, 1987.
56. Lachman, B. S., Lazerson, J., Starshak, R. J., et al. The prevalence of cholelithiasis in sickle cell disease as diagnosed by ultrasound and cholecystography. Pediatrics *64*:601, 1979.
57. Sarnaik, S., Slovis, T. L., Corbett, D. P., et al. Incidence of cholelithiasis in sickle cell anemia using the ultrasonic grayscale technique. J. Pediatr. *96*:1005, 1980.
58. Schubert, T. T. Hepatobiliary system in sickle cell disease. Gastroenterology *90*:2013, 1986.
59. Cameron, J. L., Maddrey, W. C., and Zuidema, G. D. Biliary tract disease in sickle cell anemia: Surgical considerations. Ann. Surg. *174*:702, 1971.
60. Flye, M. W., and Silver, D. Biliary tract disorders and sickle cell disease. Surgery *72*:361, 1972.
61. Stephens, C. G., and Scott, R. B. Cholelithiasis in sickle cell anemia. Surgical or medical management. Arch. Intern. Med. *140*:648, 1980.
62. Walsh, D. B., Eckhauser, F. E., Ramsburgh, S. R., et al. Risk associated with diabetes mellitus in patients undergoing gallbladder surgery. Surgery *91*:254, 1982.
63. Hjoryrup, A., Sorensen, C., Dyremose, E., et al. Influence of diabetes mellitus on operative risk. Br. J. Surg. *72*:783, 1985.
64. Sandler, R. S., Maule, W. F., and Baltus, M. E. Factors associated with postoperative complications in diabetes following biliary tract surgery. Gastroenterology *91*:157, 1986.
65. Ransohoff, D. F., and Gracie, W. A. Assessment of prophylactic cholecystectomy and medical therapy for diabetics with silent gallstones. Gastroenterology *88*:1549, 1985.
66. Edlund, Y., and Zettergren, L. Histopathology of the gallbladder in gallstone disease related to clinical data. Acta Chir. Scand. *116*:450, 1959.
67. Nahrwold, D. L., Rose, R. C., and Ward, S. P. Abnormalities in gallbladder morphology and function in patients with cholelithiasis. Ann. Surg. *184*:415, 1976.
68. Sullivan, F. J., Eaton, S. B., Jr., Ferrucci, J. T., Jr., et al. Cholangiographic manifestations of acute biliary colic. N. Engl. J. Med. *288*:33, 1973.
69. French, E. B., and Robb, W. A. T. Biliary and renal colic. Br. Med. J. *3*:135, 1963.
70. Gunn, A., and Keddie, N. Some clinical observations on patients with gallstones. Lancet *2*:7771, 1972.
71. Johnson, A. G. Cholecystectomy and gallstone dyspepsia. Clinical and physiological study of a symptom complex. Ann. R. Coll. Engl. *56*:69, 1975.
72. Kingston, R. D., and Windsor, W. O. Flatulent dyspepsia in patients with gallstones undergoing cholecystectomy. Br. J. Surg. *62*:231, 1975.
73. Price, W. H. Gall-bladder dyspepsia. Br. Med. J. *2*:138, 1963.
74. Rhind, J. A., and Watson, L. Gall stone dyspepsia. Br. Med. J. *1*:32, 1968.
75. Earlam, R. J., and Thomas, M. The clinical significance of gallstones and their radiological investigation. Br. J. Surg. *65*:164, 1978.
76. Gambill, E. E., Hodgson, J. R., and Priestley, J. T. Painless obstructive cholecystopathy. Arch. Intern. Med. *110*:442, 1962.
77. Gambill, E. E., Hodgson, J. R., and Priestley, J. T. Obstructive cholecystography or primary roentgenographic shadow of the gallbladder. Report on 262 patients. Am. J. Dig. Dis. *10*:939, 1965.
78. Bartum, R. J., Crow, H. C., and Foote, S. R. Ultrasonic and radiographic cholecystography. N. Engl. J. Med. *296*:538, 1977.
79. Boutkan, H., Butzelaar, R. M. J. M., and Davies, G. The diagnosis of gallstones—a prospective comparison of oral cholecystography and real-time ultrasound. Neth. J. Surg. *36*:124, 1984.
80. Cooperberg, P., and Golding, R. H. Advances in ultrasonography of the gallbladder and biliary tract. Radiol. Clin. North Am. *20*:611, 1982.
81. Cooperberg, P., and Burhenne, H. J. Real-time ultrasonography. Diagnostic technique of choice in calculous gallbladder disease. N. Engl. J. Med. *302*:1277, 1980.
82. Detwiler, R. P., Kim, D. S., and Longerbeam, J. K. Ultrasonography and oral cholecystography. A comparison of their use in the diagnosis of gallbladder disease. Arch. Surg. *115*:1096, 1980.
83. Escallon, A., Jr., Rosales, W., and Aldrete, J. S. Reliability of pre- and intraoperative tests for biliary lithiasis. Ann. Surg. *201*:640, 1985.
84. Ferrucci, J. T., Jr., Fordtran, J. S., Cooperberg, P. L., et al. The radiological diagnosis of gallbladder disease. Radiology *141*:49, 1981.
85. Krook, P. M., Allen, F. H., Bush, W. H., Jr., et al. Comparison of real-time cholecystosonography and oral cholecystography. Radiology *135*:145, 1980.
86. Lee, J. K. T., Melson, G. L., Koehler, R. E., et al. Cholecystosonography: Accuracy, pitfalls and unusual findings. Am. J. Surg. *139*:223, 1980.
87. Mogensen, N. B., Madsen, M., Stage, P., et al. Ultrasonography versus roentgenography in suspected instances of cholecystolithiasis. Surg. Gynecol. Obstet. *159*:353, 1984.
88. Lebensart, P. D., Bloom, R. A., Meretyk, S., et al. Oral cholecystosonography: A method for facilitating the diagnosis of cholesterol gallstones. Radiology *153*:255, 1984.
89. Allen, B., Bernhoft, R., Blanckaert, N., et al. Sludge is calcium bilirubinate associated with bile stasis. Am. J. Surg. *141*:51, 1981.
90. Filly, R. A., Allen, B., Minton, M. J., et al. In vitro investigation of the origin of echoes within biliary sludge. J. Clin. Ultrasound *8*:193, 1980.
91. Fiegenschuh, W. H., and Loughry, C. W. The false-normal oral cholecystogram. Surgery *81*:239, 1977.
92. McCluskey, P. L., Prinz, R. A., Guico, R., et al. Use of ultrasound to demonstrate gallstones in symptomatic patients with normal oral cholecystograms. Am. J. Surg. *138*:655, 1979.
93. Somerville, K. W., Rose, D. H., Bell, G. D., et al. Gall-stone dissolution and recurrence: Are we being misled? Br. Med. J. *284*:1295, 1982.
94. Mujahed, Z., Evans, J. A., and Whalen, J. P. The nonopacified gallbladder on oral cholecystography. Radiology *112*:1, 1974.
95. Bartrum, R. J., Jr., Crow, H. C., and Foote, S. R. Ultrasound examination of the gallbladder. An alternative to "double-dose" oral cholecystography. JAMA *236*:1147, 1976.
96. Jacob, C. O., Modan, M., Itzchak, Y., et al. Prolonged opacification of the gallbladder after oral cholecystography: A reevaluation of its clinical significance. Gastroenterology *81*:938, 1981.
97. Venu, R. P., Geenen, J. E., Toouli, J., et al. Endoscopic retrograde cholangiopancreatography. Diagnosis of cholelithiasis in patients with gallbladder x-ray and ultrasound studies. JAMA *249*:758, 1983.
98. Burnstein, M. J., Vassal, K. P., and Strasberg, S. M. Results of combined biliary drainage and cholecystokinin cholecystography in 81 patients with normal oral cholecystograms. Ann. Surg. *196*:627, 1982.
99. Delchier, J. C., Benfredj, P., Preaux, A. M., et al. The usefulness of microscopic bile examination in patients with suspected microlithiasis: A prospective evaluation. Hepatology *6*:118, 1986.

100. Sedaghat, A., and Grundy, S. M. Cholesterol crystals and the formation of cholesterol gallstones. N. Engl. J. Med. *302*:1274, 1980.
101. Strasberg, S. M. Personal communication.
102. Nathan, M. H., Newman, A., and Murray, D. J. Normal findings in oral and cholecystokinin cholecystography. JAMA *240*:2271, 1978.
103. Davis, G. B., Berk, F. N., Scheible, F. W., et al. Cholecystokinin cholecystography, sonography, and scintigraphy: Detection of chronic acalculous cholecystitis. AJR *139*:1117, 1982.
104. Dunn, F. H., Christensen, E. C., Reynold, J., et al. Cholecystokinin cholecystography. Controlled evaluation in the diagnosis and management of patients with possible acalculous gallbladder disease. JAMA *228*:997, 1974.
105. Nora, P. F., Davis, R. P., and Fernandez, M. J. Chronic acalculous gallbladder disease: A clinical enigma. World J. Surg. *8*:106, 1984.
106. Griffen, W. O., Bivins, B. A., Rogers, E. L., et al. Cholecystokinin cholecystography in the diagnosis of gallbladder disease. Ann. Surg. *191*:636, 1980.
107. Proudfoot, R., Mattingly, S. S., Snodgrass, S., et al. Cholecystokinin cholecystography: Is it a useful test? South. Med. J. *78*:1443, 1985.
108. Pickleman, J., Peiss, R. L., Henkin, R., et al. The role of sincalide cholescintigraphy in the evaluation of patients with acalculus gallbladder disease. Arch. Surg. *120*:693, 1985.
109. Rajagopalan, A. E., and Pickleman, J. Biliary colic and functional gallbladder disease. Arch. Surg. *117*:1005, 1982.
110. Choctaw, W. T., Pollack, E. W., and Wolfman, E. F., Jr. Evaluation of associated upper gastrointestinal pathology prior to elective cholecystectomy. Am. J. Surg. *135*:620, 1978.
111. Max, M. H., and Polk, H. C., Jr. Routine preoperative upper gastrointestinal series (UGIS) in patients with biliary tract disease: A plea for more selectivity. Surgery *82*:334, 1977.
112. Friedman, G. D. The relationship between coronary heart disease and gallbladder disease. A critical review. Ann. Intern. Med. *68*:222, 1968.
113. Palmer, E. D. Gallbladder disease and the cardiac status. JAMA *234*:97, 1975.
114. Mogadam, M., Albarelli, J., Ahmed, S. W., et al. Gallbladder dynamics in response to various meals: Is dietary fat restriction necessary in the management of gallstones? Am. J. Gastroenterol. *79*:745, 1984.
115. Bremner, D. N., McCormick, J. S. C., Thomson, J. W. W., et al. A study of cholecystectomy. Surg. Gynecol. Obstet. *138*:752, 1974.
116. Gunn, A. A., and Foubiser, G. Biliary surgery. A 5-year follow-up. R. Coll. Surg. Edinburgh *23*:292, 1978.
117. MacLean, L. D., Goldstein, M., MacDonald, J. E., et al. Results of cholecystectomy in 1000 consecutive patients. Can. J. Surg. *18*:459, 1975.
118. Martin, J. K., Jr., and van Heerden, J. A. Surgery of the liver, biliary tract, and pancreas. Mayo Clin. Proc. *55*:333, 1980.
119. Seltzer, M. H., Steiger, E., and Rosato, F. E. Mortality following cholecystectomy. Surg. Gynecol. Obstet. *130*:64, 1970.
120. Glenn, F., and McSherry, C. K. Etiological factors in fatal complications following operations upon the biliary tract. Ann. Surg. *157*:695, 1963.
121. McSherry, C. K., and Glenn, F. The incidence and causes of death following surgery for nonmalignant biliary tract disease. Ann. Surg. *191*:271, 1980.
122. Weckesser, E. C. Surgery for gallbladder disease in Ohio. A survey of 3,085 operations. Am. J. Surg. *102*:695, 1961.
123. National Halothane Committee. Summary of the National Halothane Study. Possible association between halothane anesthesia and postoperative hepatic necrosis. JAMA *197*:775, 1966.
124. Houghton, P. W. J., Jenkinson, L. R., and Donaldson, L. A. Cholecystectomy in the elderly: A prospective study. Br. J. Surg. *72*:220, 1985.
125. Huber, D. F., Martin, E. W., Jr., and Cooperman, M. Cholecystectomy in elderly patients. Am. J. Surg. *146*:719, 1983.
126. Sullivan, D. M., Hood, T. R., and Griffen, W. O., Jr. Biliary tract surgery in the elderly. Am. J. Surg. *143*:216, 1982.
127. Aranha, G. V., Sontag, S. J., and Greenlee, H. B. Cholecystectomy in cirrhotic patients: A formidable operation. Am. J. Surg. *143*:55, 1982.
128. Bloch, R. S., Allaben, R. D., and Walt, A. J. Cholecystectomy in patients with cirrhosis. A surgical challenge. Arch. Surg. *120*:669, 1985.
129. Castaing, D., Houssin, D., Lemoine, J., et al. Surgical management of gallstone in cirrhotic patients. Am. J. Surg. *146*:310, 1983.
130. Simmons, F., and Bouchier, I. A. D. Intraluminal bile salt concentrations and fat digestion after cholecystectomy. S. Afr. Med. J. *46*:2089, 1972.
131. Tangedahl, T. The present status of agents for dissolving gallstones. Am. J. Gastroenterol. *80*:64, 1985.
132. Kogut, K., Aragoni, T., and Ackerman, N. B. Cholecystectomy in patients with mild cirrhosis. Arch. Surg. *120*:1310, 1985.
133. Schoenfield, L. J., Lachin, J. M., Baum, R. A., et al. Chenodiol (chenodeoxycholic acid) for dissolution of gallstones: The National Cooperative Gallstone Study. Ann. Intern. Med. *95*:257, 1981.
134. Maton, P. N., Iser, J. H., Reuben, A., et al. Outcome of chenodeoxycholic acid (CDCA) treatment in 125 patients with radiolucent gallstones. Factors influencing efficacy, withdrawal, symptoms and side effects and post-dissolution recurrence. Medicine *61*:86, 1982.
135. Fisher, M. M., Roberts, E. A., Rosen, I. E., et al. The Sunnybrook gallstone study: A double-blind controlled trial of chenodeoxycholic acid for gallstone dissolution. Hepatology *5*:102, 1985.
136. Johansson, G. A prospective study of the clinical significance of the treatment of gallstones with chenodeoxycholic acid. Surg. Gynecol. Obstet. *154*:127, 1984.
137. Erlinger, S., Go, A. L., Husson, J. M., et al. Franco-Belgian Cooperative Study of ursodeoxycholic acid in the medical dissolution of gallstones. A double-blind, randomized, dose-response study, and comparison with chenodeoxycholic acid. Hepatology *4*:308, 1984.
138. Roda, E., Bazzoli, F., Morselli, A. M., et al. Ursodeoxycholic acid vs. chenodeoxycholic acid as cholesterol gallstone-dissolving agents: A comparative randomized study. Hepatology *2*:804, 1982.
139. Fromm, H., Roat, J. W., Gonzalez, V., et al. Comparative efficacy and side effects of ursodeoxycholic and chenodeoxycholic acids in dissolving gallstones. A double-blind controlled study. Gastroenterology *85*:1257, 1983.
140. Meredith, T. J., Williams, G. V., Maton, P. N., et al. Retrospective comparison of "cheno" and "urso" in the medical treatment of gallstones. Gut *23*:382, 1982.
141. Stiehl, A., Raedsch, R., Rudolph, G., et al. Effect of ursodeoxycholic acid in biliary bile acid and bile lipid composition in gallstone patients. Hepatology *4*:107, 1984.
142. Podda, M., Zuin, M., Dioguardi, M. L., et al. A combination of chenodeoxycholic acid and ursodeoxycholic acid is more effective than either alone in reducing biliary cholesterol saturation. Hepatology *2*:334, 1982.
143. Ruppin, D. C., and Dowling, R. H. Is recurrence inevitable after gallstone dissolution by bile-acid treatment? Lancet *1*:181, 1982.
144. Gleeson, D., Ruppin, D. C., and the British Gallstone Study Group. Discrepancies between cholecystography and ultrasonography in the detection of recurrent gallstones. J. Hepatol. *1*:597, 1985.
145. Ruppin, D. C., Murphy, G. M., Dowling, R. H., and the British Gallstone Study Group. Gallstone disease without gallstones—bile acid and bile lipid metabolism after complete gallstone dissolution. Gut *27*:559, 1986.
146. Tint, G. S., Salen, G., and Chazen, D. Symptomatic gallstones are likely to reoccur after dissolution with ursodeoxycholic acid (UDCA) but this may be prevented by low-dose UDCA. Gastroenterology *92*:1787, 1987.

147. Villanova, N., Bazzoli, F., Frabboni, R., Mazzela, G., Morselli-Labate, A. M., Barbara, L., and Roda, E. Gallstone recurrence after successful oral bile acid treatment: A follow-up study and evaluation of long term post-dissolution treatment. Gastroenterology *92*:1789, 1987.
148. Sauerbruch, T., Delius, M., Paumgartner, G., et al. Fragmentation of gallstones by extracorporeal shock waves. N. Engl. J. Med. *314*:818, 1986.
149. Mulley, A. G., Jr. Shock-wave lithotripsy. Assessing a slam-bang technology. N. Engl. J. Med. *314*:845, 1986.
150. Neubrand, M., Sauerbruch, T., Stellaard, F., and Paumgartner, G. In vitro cholesterol gallstone dissolution after fragmentation with shock waves. Digestion *34*:51, 1986.
151. Sackmann, M., Delius, M., Sauerbruch, T., Holl, J., Weber, W., Hagelauer, U., Hepp, W., Brendel, W., Paumgartner, G., and Medizintechnik, D. Extracorporeal shock wave lithotripsy of gallbladder stones: Results of 101 treatments. Gastroenterology *92*:1608, 1987.
152. Staritz, M., Floth, A., Rambow, A., Buess, G., Wilpert, D., and Schild, F. Extracorporal shock waves (device of the second generation) for therapy of large common bile duct stones: Success and problems. Gastroenterology *92*:1652, 1987.
153. Allen, M. J., Borody, T. J., Bugliosi, T. F., et al. Rapid dissolution of gallstones by methyl tert-butyl ether. N. Engl. J. Med. *312*:217, 1985.
154. Kovalcik, P. J., Burrell, M. J., and Old, W. L., Jr. Cholecystectomy concomitant with other intra-abdominal operations. Assessment of risk. Arch. Surg. *118*:1059, 1983.
155. McSherry, C. K., and Glenn, F. Biliary tract surgery concomitant with other intra-abdominal operations. Ann. Surg. *193*:169, 1981.
156. Thompson, J. S., Philben, V. J., and Hodgson, P. E. Operative management of incidental cholelithiasis. Am. J. Surg. *148*:821, 1984.
157. Schreiber, H., Macon, W. L., IV, and Pories, W. J. Incidental cholecystectomy during major abdominal surgery in the elderly. Am. J. Surg. *135*:196, 1978.
158. Shennib, H., Fried, G. M., and Hampson, L. G. Does simultaneous cholecystectomy increase the risk of colonic surgery? Am. J. Surg. *151*:266, 1986.
159. Stevens, M. L., Hubert, B. C., and Wenzel, F. J. Combined gynecologic surgical procedures and cholecystectomy. Am. J. Obstet. Gynecol. *149*:350, 1984.
160. Ouriel, K., Ricotta, J. J., Adams, J. T., et al. Management of cholelithiasis in patients with abdominal aortic aneurysm. Ann. Surg. *196*:717, 1983.
161. Tompkins, W. C., Chavez, C. M., Conn, J. H., et al. Combining intra-abdominal arterial grafting with gastrointestinal or biliary tract procedures. Am. J. Surg. *126*:598, 1973.
162. Salmenkivi, K. Cholesterosis of the gall-bladder. A clinical study. Based on 269 cholecystectomies. Acta Chir. Scand. Suppl. *324*:1, 1964.
163. Holzbach, R. T., Marsh, M., and Tang, P. Cholesterolosis: Physical-chemical characteristics of human and diet-induced canine lesions. Exp. Molec. Pathol. *27*:324, 1977.
164. Koga, A., Todo, S., and Nishimura, M. Electron microscopic observations on the cholesterol distributed in the epithelial cells of the gallbladder. Histochemistry *44*:303, 1975.
165. Koga, A. Fine structure of the human gallbladder with cholesterosis with special reference to the mechanism of lipid accumulation. Br. J. Exp. Pathol. *66*:605, 1985.
166. Tilvis, R. S., Aro, J., Strandberg, T. E., et al. Lipid composition of bile and gallbladder mucosa in patients with acalculous cholesterolsis. Gastroenterology *82*:607, 1982.
167. Lowenfels, A. B., Schwaetz, R., and Pitchumoni, C. Cholelithiasis and cancer. Gastroenterology *80*:1218, 1981.
168. Lowenfels, A. B. Gallstones and the risk of cancer. Gut *21*:1090, 1980.
169. Lowenfels, A. B., Domellof, L., Lindstrom, L., et al. Cholelithiasis, cholecystectomy, and cancer: A case-control study in Sweden. Gastroenterology *83*:672, 1982.
170. Linos, D. A., O'Fallon, W. M., Thistle, J. L., et al. Cholelithiasis and carcinoma of the colon. Cancer *50*:1015, 1982.
171. Schottenfeld, D., and Winawer, S. J. Cholecystectomy and colorectal cancer. Gastroenterology *85*:966, 1983.
172. Vernick, L. J., and Kuller, L. H. Cholecystectomy and right-sided colon cancer: An epidemiological study. Lancet *2*:381, 1981.
173. Linos, D. A., Beard, C. M., O'Fallon, W. M., et al. Cholecystectomy and carcinoma of the colon. Lancet *2*:379, 1981.
174. Turunen, M. J., and Kivilaakso, E. O. Increased risk of colorectal cancer after cholecystectomy. Ann. Surg. *194*:639, 1981.
175. Weiss, N. S., Daling, J. R., and Chow, W. H. Cholecystectomy and the incidence of cancer of the large bowel. Cancer *49*:1713, 1982.
176. Adami, H. O., Meirik, O., Gustavsson, S., et al. Colorectal cancer after cholecystectomy: Absence of risk increase within 11–14 years. Gastroenterology *85*:859, 1983.
177. Abrams, J. S., Anton, J. R., and Dreyfuss, D. C. The absence of a relationship between cholecystectomy and the subsequent occurrence of cancer of the proximal colon. Dis. Colon Rectum *26*:141, 1983.
178. Spitz, M. R., Russell, N. C., Guinee, V. F., et al. Questionable relationship between cholecystectomy and colon cancer. J. Surg. Oncol. *30*:6, 1985.
179. Thomas, C. G., Jr., and Womack, N. A. Acute cholecystitis, its pathogenesis and repair. Arch. Surg. *64*:590, 1952.
180. Roslyn, J. J., DenBesten, L., Thompson, J. E., Jr., and Silverman, B. F. Roles of lithogenic bile and cystic duct occlusion in the pathogenesis of acute cholecystitis. Am. J. Surg. *140*:126, 1980.
181. Sjodahl, R. On the development of primary acute cholecystitis. Scand. J. Gastroenterol. *18*:577, 1983.
182. Neiderhiser, D., Thornell, E., Bjorck, S., and Svanvik, J. The effect of lysophosphatidylcholine on gallbladder function in the cat. J. Lab. Clin. Med. *101*:699, 1983.
183. Thornell, E., Jivegard, L., Bukhave, K., Rask-Madsen, J., and Svanvik, J. Prostaglandin E_2 formation by the gallbladder in experimental cholecystitis. Gut *27*:370, 1986.
184. Thornell, E. Mechanisms in the development of acute cholecystitis and biliary pain. A study on the role of prostaglandins and the effects of indomethacin. Scand. J. Gastroenterol. *17*(suppl.):76, 1982.
185. Csendes, A., and Sepulveda, A. Intraluminal gallbladder pressure measurements in patients with chronic or acute cholecystitis. Am. J. Surg. *139*:383, 1980.
186. Jivegard, L., Thornell, E., and Svanvik, J. Pathophysiology of acute obstructive cholecystitis: implications for non-operative management. Br. J. Surg. *74*:1084, 1987.
187. Claesson, B., Holmlund, D., and Matzsch, T. Biliary microflora in acute cholecystitis and the clinical implications. Acta Chir. Scand. *150*:229, 1984.
188. Claesson, B. E. B., Holmlund, D. E. W., and Matzsch, T. W. Microflora of the gallbladder related to duration of acute cholecystitis. Surg. Gynecol. Obstet. *162*:531, 1986.
189. Gately, J. F., and Thomas, E. J. Acute cholecystitis occurring as a complication of other diseases. Arch. Surg. *118*:1137, 1983.
190. Glenn, F., and Becker, C. G. Acute acalculous cholecystitis: An increasing entity. Ann. Surg. *195*:131, 1982.
191. Devine, R. M., Farnell, M. B., and Mucha, P., Jr. Acute cholecystitis as a complication in surgical patients. Arch. Surg. *119*:1389, 1984.
192. Johnson, L. B. The importance of early diagnosis of acute acalculus cholecystitis. Surg. Gynecol. Obstet. *164*:197, 1987.
193. Petersen, S. R., and Sheldon, G. F. Acute acalculous cholecystitis: A complication of hyperalimentation. Am. J. Surg. *138*:814, 1979.
194. Ong, G. G. A study of recurrent pyogenic cholangitis. Arch. Surg. *84*:199, 1962.
195. Rosenberg, L., Shapiro, S., Slone, D., Kaufman, D. W., Miettinen, O. S., and Stolley, P. D. Thiazides and acute cholecystitis. N. Engl. J. Med. *303*:546, 1980.
196. Machemer, W. L., Fuge, W. W., and Mendez, F. L. Typhoid cholecystitis. Surgery *31*:738, 1952.
197. Kavin, H., Jonas, R. B., Chowdhury, L., and Kabins, S. Acalculous cholecystitis and cytomegalovirus infection in the acquired immunodeficiency syndrome. Ann. Intern. Med. *104*:53, 1986.
198. Blumberg, R. S., Kelsey, P., Perrone, T., Dickersin, R.,

Laquaglia, M., and Ferruci, J. Cytomegalovirus and cryptosporidium-associated acalculous gangrenous cholecystitis. Am. J. Med. *76*:1118, 1984.
199. Gordon, K. C. D. Cystic arterial patterns in diseased human gallbladders. Gut *8*:565, 1967.
200. Schein, C. J. Acute cholecystitis in the diabetic. Am. J. Gastroenterol. *51*:511, 1969.
201. Remigio, P., and Zaino, E. Polyarteritis nodosa of the gallbladder. Surgery *67*:427, 1970.
202. Stieber, A. C., and Bauer, J. J. Volvulus of the gallbladder. Am. J. Gastroenterol. *78*:96, 1983.
203. Schlinkert, R. T., Mucha, P., and Farnell, M. B. Torsion of the gallbladder. Mayo Clin. Proc. *59*:490, 1984.
204. Edlund, Y., and Zettergren, L. Histopathology of the gallbladder in gallstone disease related to clinical data. Acta Chir. Scand. *116*:450, 1959.
205. Edlund, Y., Lanner, O., and Olsson, O. Cholecystography and cholegraphy in gallstone disease (with notes on the causation and course of acute cholecystitis). Acta Chir. Scand. *120*:366, 1961.
206. Edlund, Y., and Olsson, O. Acute cholecystitis; its aetiology and course, with special reference to the timing of cholecystectomy. Acta Chir. Scand. *120*:479, 1961.
207. Gambill, E. E., Hodgson, J. R., and Priestly, J. T. Painless obstructive cholecystopathy. Arch. Intern. Med. *110*:442, 1962.
208. French, E. G., and Robb, W. A. T. Biliary and renal colic. Br. Med. J. *2*:135, 1963.
209. Glenn, F. Pain in biliary tract disease. Surg. Gynecol. Obstet. *122*:495, 1966.
210. Gagic, N., Frey, C. F., and Gaines, R. Acute cholecystitis. Surg. Gynecol. Obstet. *140*:868, 1975.
211. Raine, P. A. M., and Gunn, A. A. Acute cholecystitis. Br. J. Surg. *62*:697, 1975.
212. Dumont, A. E. Significance of hyperbilirubinemia in acute cholecystitis. Surg. Gynecol. Obstet. *142*:855, 1976.
213. Edlund, G., Kempi, V., and Van Der Linden, W. Jaundice in acute cholecystitis without common duct stones. Acta Chir. Scand. *149*:597, 1983.
214. Fry, E. E., Cox, R. A., and Harbrecht, P. J. Empyema of the gallbladder: A complication in the natural history of acute cholecystitis. Am. J. Surg. *141*:366, 1981.
215. Thornton, J. R., Heaton, K. W., Espiner, H. J., and Eltringham, W. K. Empyema of the gallbladder—reappraisal of a neglected disease. Gut *24*:1183, 1983.
216. Laing, F. C. Diagnostic evaluation of patients with suspected acute cholecystitis. Radiol. Clin. North Am. *21*:477, 1983.
217. Henriksen, J. H. Acute cholecystitis: Diagnostic impact of ultrasonography and cholescintigraphy. Scand. J. Gastroenterol. *20*:129, 1984.
218. Soiva, M., Haveri, M., Taavitsainen, M., and Suramo, I. The value of routine sonography in clinically suspected acute cholecystitis. Scand. J. Gastroenterol. *21*:70, 1986.
219. Ralls, P. W., Colletti, P. M., Lapin, S. A., Chandrasoma, P., Boswell, W. D., Jr., Ngo, C., Radin, D. R., and Halls, J. M. Real-time sonography in suspected acute cholecystitis. Prospective evaluation of primary and secondary signs. Radiology *155*:767, 1985.
220. Jeffrey, R. B., Laing, F. C., Wong, W., and Callen, P. W. Gangrenous cholecystitis: Diagnosis by ultrasound. Radiology *148*:219, 1983.
221. Samuels, B. I., Freitas, J. E., Bree, R. L., Schwab, R. D., and Heller, S. T. A comparison of radionuclide hepatobiliary imaging and real-time ultrasound for the detection of acute cholecystitis. Radiology *147*:207, 1983.
222. Fink-Bennett, D., Freitas, J. E., Ripley, S. D., and Bree, R. L. The sensitivity of hepatobiliary imaging and real-time ultrasonography in the detection of acute cholecystitis. Arch. Surg. *120*:904, 1985.
223. Gill, P. T., Dillon, E., Leahy, A. L., Reeder, A., and Peel, A. L. G. Ultrasonography, HIDA scintigraphy or both in the diagnosis of acute cholecystitis? Br. J. Surg. *72*:267, 1985.
224. Smith, R., Rosen, J. M., Gallo, L. N., and Alderson, P. O. Pericholecystic hepatic activity in cholescintigraphy. Radiology *156*:797, 1985.
225. Jamieson, N. V., Friend, P. J., and Wraight, E. P. A two year experience with ^{99m}Tc HIDA cholescintigraphy in teaching hospital practice. Surg. Gynecol. Obstet. *163*:29, 1986.
226. Brunkwall, J., Borjesson, B., and Lindberg, B. Cholescintiscan or infusion cholecystography in acute cholecystitis. Acta Chir. Scand. *151*:139, 1985.
227. Mauro, M. A., McCartney, W. H., and Melmed, J. R. Hepatobiliary scanning with ^{99m}Tc PIPIDA in acute cholecystitis. Radiology *142*:193, 1982.
228. Brachman, M. B., Tanasescu, D. E., Ramanna, L., and Waxman, A. D. Acute gangrenous cholecystitis: Radionuclide diagnosis. Radiology *151*:209, 1984.
229. Williams, W., Krishnamurthy, G. T., Brar, H. S., and Bobba, V. R. Scintigraphic variations of normal biliary physiology. J. Nucl. Med. *25*:160, 1984.
230. Serafini, A. N., Al-Sheikh, W., Barkin, J. S., Hourani, M., Sfakiankis, G., Clarke, L. P., and Ashkar, F. S. Biliary scintigraphy in acute pancreatitis. Radiology *144*:591, 1982.
231. Potter, T., McClain, C. J., and Shafer, R. B. Effect of fasting and parenteral alimentation on PIPIDA scintigraphy. Dig. Dis. Sci. *28*:687, 1983.
232. Shuman, W. P., Gibbs, P., Rudd, T. G., and Mack, L. A. PIPIDA scintigraphy for cholecystitis: False positives in alcoholism and total parenteral nutrition. AJR *138*:1, 1982.
233. McGahan, J. P., and Walter, J. P. Diagnostic percutaneous aspiration of the gallbladder. Radiology *155*:619, 1985.
234. Van Sonnenberg, E., Wittich, G. R., Casola, G., Princethal, R. A., Hofmann, A. F., Keightley, A., and Wing, V. W. Diagnostic and therapeutic percutaneous gallbladder procedures. Radiology *160*:23, 1986.
235. Kune, G. A., and Burdon, J. G. W. Are antibiotics necessary in acute cholecystitis? Med. J. Aust. *2*:627, 1975.
236. Glenn, F. Surgical management of acute cholecystitis in patients 65 years of age and older. Ann. Surg. *193*:56, 1981.
237. Morrow, D. J., Thompson, J., and Wilson, S. E. Acute cholecystitis in the elderly. Arch. Surg. *113*:1149, 1978.
238. Jarvinen, H. J., and Hasbacka, J. Early cholecystectomy for acute cholecystitis. A prospective randomized study. Ann. Surg. *191*:501, 1980.
239. Lahtinen, J., Alhava, E. M., and Aukee, S. Acute cholecystitis treated by early and delayed surgery. A controlled clinical trial. Scand. J. Gastroenterol. *13*:673, 1978.
240. McArthur, P., Cuschieri, A., Sells, R. A., and Shields, R. Controlled clinical trial comparing early with interval cholecystectomy for acute cholecystitis. Br. J. Surg. *62*:850, 1975.
241. Van Der Linden, W., and Sunzel, H. Early versus delayed operation for acute cholecystitis. A controlled clinical trial. Am. J. Surg. *120*:7, 1970.
242. Van Der Linden, W., and Edlund, G. Early versus delayed cholecystectomy: The effect of a change in management. Br. J. Surg. *68*:753, 1981.
243. Fowkes, F. G. R., and Gunn, A. A. The management of acute cholecystitis and its hospital cost. Br. J. Surg. *67*:613, 1980.
244. Saltztein, E. C., Peacock, J. B., and Mercer, L. C. Early operation for acute biliary tract stone disease. Surgery *94*:704, 1983.
245. Moore, E. E., Kelly, G. L., Driver, T., and Eiseman, B. Reassessment of simple cholecystostomy. Arch. Surg. *114*:515, 1979.
246. Skillings, J. C., Kumai, C., and Hinshaw, J. R. Cholecystostomy: A place in modern biliary surgery? Am. J. Surg. *139*:865, 1980.
247. Shaver, R. W., Hawkins, I. F., Jr., and Soong, J. Percutaneous cholecystostomy. AJR *138*:1133, 1982.
248. Pearse, D. M., Hawkins, I. F., Jr., Shaver, R., and Vogel, S. Percutaneous cholecystostomy in acute cholecystitis and common duct obstruction. Radiology *152*:365, 1984.
249. Klimberg, S., Hawkins, I., and Vogel, S. B. Percutaneous cholecystostomy for acute cholecystitis in high-risk patients. Am. J. Surg. *153*:125, 1987.
250. Weigelt, J. A., Norcross, J. F., and Aurbakken, C. M. Cholecystectomy after tube chelecystostomy. Am. J. Surg. *146*:723, 1983.
251. Spillers, W. P., and Goldman, L. I. Interval cholecystectomy: An appraisal. South. Med. J. *75*:802, 1982.
252. Gagic, N., and Frey, C. F. The results of cholecystostomy for

the treatment of acute cholecystitis. Surg. Gynecol. Obstet. *140*:255, 1975.
253. Welch, J. P., and Malt, R. A. Outcome of cholecystostomy. Surg. Gynecol. Obstet. *135*:717, 1972.
254. Orlando, R., Gleason, E., and Drezner, A. D. Acute acalculous cholecystitis in the critically ill patient. Am. J. Surg. *145*:472, 1983.
255. Fox, M. S., Wilk, P. J., Weissmann, H. S., Freeman, L. M., and Gliedman, M. L. Acute acalculous cholecystitis. Surg. Gynecol. Obstet. *159*:13, 1984.
256. Becker, C. G., Dubin, T., and Glenn, F. Induction of acute cholecystitis by activation of factor XII. J. Exp. Med. *151*:81, 1980.
257. Ramanna, L., Brachman, M. B., Tanasecu, D. E., Berman, D. S., and Waxman, A. D. Cholescintigraphy in acute acalculous cholecystitis. Am. J. Gastroenterol. *79*:650, 1984.
258. Swayne, L. C. Acute acalculous cholecystitis: Sensitivity in detection using technetium-99m iminodiacetic acid cholescintigraphy. Radiology *160*:33, 1986.
259. Shuman, W. P., Rogers, J. V., Rudd, T. G., Mack, L. A., Plumley, T., and Larson, E. B. Low sensitivity of sonography and cholescintigraphy in acalculous cholecystitis. AJR *142*:531, 1984.
260. Eggermont, A. M., Lameris, J. S., and Jeekel, J. Ultrasound-guided percutaneous transhepatic cholecystostomy for acute acalculous cholecystitis. Arch. Surg. *120*:1354, 1985.
261. May, R. E., and Strong, R. Acute emphysematous cholecystitis. Br. J. Surg. *58*:453, 1971.
262. Rosoff, L., and Meyers, H. Acute emphysematous cholecystitis. Am. J. Surg. *111*:410, 1966.
263. Mentzer, R. M., Jr., Golden, G. T., Chandler, J. G., and Horsley, J. S., III. A comparative appraisal of emphysematous cholecystitis. Am. J. Surg. *129*:10, 1975.
264. Blaquiere, R. M., and Dewbury, K. C. The ultrasound diagnosis of emphysematous cholecystitis. Br. J. Radiol. *55*:114, 1982.
265. Roslyn, J., and Busuttil, R. W. Perforation of the gallbladder: A frequently mismanaged condition. Am. J. Surg. *137*:307, 1979.
266. Williams, N. F., and Scobie, T. K. Perforation of the gallbladder: Analysis of 19 cases. Can. Med. Assoc. J. *115*:1223, 1976.
267. Felice, P. R., Trowbridge, P. E., and Ferrara, J. J. Evolving changes in the pathogenesis and treatment of the perforated gallbladder. A combined hospital study. Am. J. Surg. *149*:466, 1985.
268. Larmi, T. K. I., Kairaluoma, M. I., Junila, J., Laitinen, S., Stahlberg, M., and Fock, H. G. Perforation of the gallbladder. A retrospective comparative study of cases from 1946–1956 and 1969–1980. Acta Chir. Scand. *150*:557, 1984.
269. Abu-Dalu, J., and Urca, I. Acute cholecystitis with perforation into the peritoneal cavity. Arch. Surg. *102*:108, 1971.
270. McCarthy, J. D., and Picazo, J. G. Bile peritonitis. Am. J. Surg. *116*:664, 1968.
271. Ackerman, N. B., Sillin, L. F., and Suresh, K. Consequences of intraperitoneal bile: Bile ascites versus bile peritonitis. Am. J. Surg. *149*:244, 1985.
272. Haff, R. C., Wise, L., and Ballinger, W. F. Biliary-enteric fistulas. Surg. Gynecol. Obstet. *133*:84, 1971.
273. Piedad, O. L. H., and Wells, P. B. Spontaneous internal biliary fistula, obstructive and nonobstructive types. Ann. Surg. *175*:75, 1971.
274. Porter, J. M., Mullen, D. C., and Silver, D. Spontaneous biliary-enteric fistulas. Surgery *68*:597, 1970.
275. Andersson, A., and Zederfeldt, B. Gallstone ileus. Acta Chir. Scand. *135*:713, 1969.
276. Kasahara, Y., Umemura, H., Shiraha, S., Kuyama, T., Sakata, K., and Kubota, H. Gallstone ileus. Review of 112 patients in the Japanese literature. Am. J. Surg. *140*:437, 1980.
277. Heuman, R., Sjodahl, R., and Wetterfors, J. Gallstone ileus: An analysis of 120 patients. World J. Surg. *4*:595, 1980.
278. Svartholm, E., Andren-Sandberg, A., Evander, A., Jarhult, J., and Thulin, A. Diagnosis and treatment of gallstone ileus. Report of 83 cases. Acta Chir. Scand. *148*:435, 1982.
279. Kurtz, R. J., Heimann, T. M., and Kurtz, A. B. Gallstone ileus: A diagnostic problem. Am. J. Surg. *146*:314, 1983.
280. Hesselfeldt, P., and Jess, P. Gallstone ileus. A review of 39 cases with emphasis on surgical treatment. Acta Chir. Scand. *148*:431, 1982.
281. Milsom, J. W., and MacKeigan, J. M. Gallstone obstruction of the colon. Report of two cases and review of management. Dis. Colon Rectum *28*:367, 1985.
282. Deitz, D. M., Standage, B. A., Pinson, C. W., McConnell, D. B., and Krippaehne, W. W. Improving the outcome in gallstone ileus. Am. J. Surg. *151*:572, 1986.
283. Oakland, D. J., and Denn, P. G. Endoscopic diagnosis of gallstone ileus of the duodenum. Dig. Dis. Sci. *31*:98, 1986.

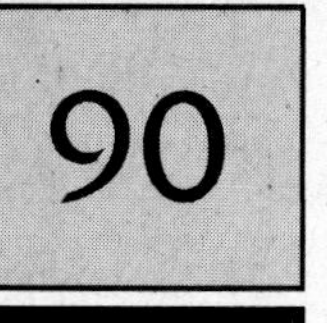

90 Biliary Obstruction, Cholangitis, and Choledocholithiasis

LAWRENCE W. WAY
MARVIN H. SLEISENGER

Gallstones may pass from the gallbladder into the common bile duct, where they remain and give rise to complications by obstructing bile flow. About 15 per cent of patients with cholecystolithiasis (stones in the gallbladder) are found to have concomitant choledocholithiasis; the association increases with the age of the patient. Although the great majority of ductal stones originate in the gallbladder, stones may form in the intrahepatic or common bile ducts in special circumstances. Spontaneous passage of common duct stones into the duodenum has been well documented and may even be common with small stones. However, this event is rarely observed in clinical practice.

The general features of the syndromes produced by the different causes of biliary obstruction overlap considerably. In addition to choledocholithiasis, general aspects of biliary obstruction will be discussed in this chapter.

BILIARY OBSTRUCTION AND THE DIFFERENTIAL DIAGNOSIS OF JAUNDICE

Hyperbilirubinemia may be due to an increase in the unconjugated or conjugated fraction.[1–5] The former characterizes jaundice from hemolysis and Gilbert's syndrome. Conjugated hyperbilirubinemia occurs in hepatocellular dysfunction and bile duct obstruction. When associated with other biochemical evidence of obstruction, such as increased serum levels of alkaline phosphatase, gammaglutamyl transferase, bile salts, cholesterol, and lipoprotein-X, the condition is termed *cholestasis*.[6, 7] It is impossible to differentiate among the various causes of cholestasis from an analysis of the liver function tests alone (see pp. 455–462).

Obstruction of the bile duct may lead to jaundice, cholangitis, pruritus, hepatic abscess formation, and hepatic cirrhosis and its complications.[8] The most common causes of bile duct obstruction are gallstone disease and neoplasms, although there are many others, the most important of which are discussed later in this chapter.

Pathophysiology. Obstruction of the bile duct increases bile pressure upstream from the obstruction[9] and causes the ducts to dilate.[10] Normal pressure in the duct is 10 to 15 cm H_2O and it rises to 25 to 40 cm H_2O with complete obstruction. When the pressure exceeds 15 cm H_2O, bile flow decreases and at 30 cm H_2O it stops.[11–13] When the ducts are obstructed, bile continues to be secreted into the canaliculus. The increased hydrostatic pressure distorts the junctional complexes, increasing their permeability,[6, 7] and stimulates fibrogenesis.[14] During obstruction, bile may reflux into the sinusoids by a transcellular or transjunctional path.

The bilirubin, alkaline phosphatase, 5′-nucleotidase, and leucine aminopeptidase levels begin to increase within one hour of the onset of obstruction.[15] They continue to rise for days to weeks before reaching a plateau. The average peak serum bilirubin concentration with complete obstruction falls in the range of 20 to 30 mg/dl, at which point the daily pigment load is being excreted by the kidneys. Even higher bilirubin levels may occur with concomitant renal dysfunction or hemolysis.

The rise in alkaline phosphatase is more rapid and precedes (i.e., occurs at a lower pressure than) that of bilirubin.[16, 17] Unlike bilirubin, whose increase stems from blocked excretion, the alkaline phosphatase level rises because of increased synthesis of the enzyme by the canalicular epithelium, followed by regurgitation into the sinusoids. This explains why the alkaline phosphatase value may be abnormal and the bilirubin level normal or only mildly elevated with a lesion that only partially blocks the excretory pathway for bilirubin (e.g., hepatic metastasis, Klatskin tumor, or hepatic abscess).[16, 18]

The absolute height of the bilirubin concentration is proportional to the degree of obstruction, but the height of the alkaline phosphatase level bears no relationship to either the degree of obstruction or its cause.[19] The patient becomes jaundiced if the bilirubin level exceeds about 2.5 mg/dl, and dark urine, due to excretion of conjugated bilirubin, may be noted. The rate of appearance of jaundice may vary considerably, depending on the site and degree of obstruction and the presence and functional condition of the gallbladder. If the common duct is obstructed distal to a functioning gallbladder, the gallbladder may dilate, concentrate bile, and delay the appearance of jaundice for a day or two. With obstruction higher in the duct or in the absence of a gallbladder, jaundice develops quickly.

With high-grade obstruction, bilirubin is unable to enter the intestine and the stools may become light ("clay-colored," acholic). However, stool color is not totally dependent on the presence of bile pigment; brown stools are common in the presence of deep jaundice, and, in general, information about stool color is of little diagnostic value. In any event, gallstone obstruction is rarely complete enough to produce clay-colored stools. The latter finding is most often seen in patients with complete or nearly complete obstruction and bilirubin values above 15 mg/dl (i.e., principally in those with neoplastic obstruction).

In the presence of high-grade common duct obstruction the gallbladder may become so dilated that it presents as a mass in the right subcostal region. This finding is most frequent in obstructing malignancies and forms the basis of *Courvoisier's law:* In a jaundiced patient, the presence of a palpable, nontender gallbladder suggests that the biliary obstruction is due to malignancy. An enlarged, palpable gallbladder is unusual in patients with common duct stones, because the obstruction is much less complete and the gallbladder is usually scarred and nondistensible owing to changes from chronic inflammation.

Hepatic enlargement may be detected in patients with biliary obstruction, and mild to moderate tenderness is often present in the right upper quadrant during an attack of cholangitis.

Obstruction usually produces dilatation of the bile ducts, which can be detected by ultrasound or CT scans.[20–25] When obstruction is complicated by infection or cirrhosis, however, dilatation may be restricted by scarring and edema, and the caliber of the ducts may be normal.[26] Furthermore, dilatation is sometimes absent in patients with choledocholithiasis because the obstruction is low-grade and intermittent.[26]

Secondary biliary cirrhosis may result, and the rate at which it develops varies directly with the duration and extent of obstruction.[27] Cirrhosis has been reported as early as three to four months after the onset of high-grade (e.g., neoplastic) obstruction, but the average duration of symptoms in the few patients with choledocholithiasis who progress to cirrhosis is about five years. Once substantial hepatic damage has developed, it may progress slowly to biliary cirrhosis even after the cause has been removed, but this is not invariable, and some patients with secondary cirrhosis have been noted to improve substantially with relief of the obstruction.[28] Hepatic failure may appear as the terminal complication in progressive biliary cirrhosis. Its evolution may be rapid in high-grade obstruction, as with malignancy.

Bleeding esophageal varices caused by portal hypertension is the other major end result of prolonged biliary obstruction and cirrhosis.[29] Varices seem to be more common after prolonged incomplete obstruction, in contrast to complete blockage, which tends to cause hepatic failure.

Diagnosis. The cause of jaundice can be determined in most cases from clinical data and routine laboratory tests,[5, 19, 30–33] including an ultrasound scan.[20, 23, 25] Characteristic syndromes that can be diagnosed readily include acute viral hepatitis in a young person with raised transaminase levels, cirrhosis in a known alcoholic whose deteriorating liver function follows a binge, pancreatic carcinoma in a patient with weight loss and a palpable gallbladder, and so forth. Alcoholic cirrhosis, infectious hepatitis, gallstone disease, and neoplasms are the most common causes. Atypical presentations are fairly frequent, however (see pp. 454–467).

The bilirubin and alkaline phosphatase values in a large group of patients with obstructive jaundice[19] are depicted in Figures 90–1 and 90–2. The alkaline phosphatase value is often elevated when the bilirubin is normal, and in general it is a more sensitive index of obstruction. In patients with choledocholithiasis the bilirubin level rarely exceeds 12 mg/dl and the alkaline phosphatase uncommonly exceeds five times normal.[19]

When jaundice is acute, it is often best to allow the illness to evolve for a few days before scheduling special tests, such as cholangiograms or CT scans. In most cases there is no urgency in establishing a precise diagnosis; delay in therapy for several days holds few risks except in a patient with severe or worsening cholangitis. The only special study that is regularly useful in the early stage is an ultrasound scan of the gallbladder and bile ducts. Ultrasound may demonstrate gallbladder stones or dilatation of the bile ducts, the latter signifying ductal obstruction. A negative study does not prove the absence of stones or obstruction;[34–36] the sensitivity of ultrasound in detecting obstruction is about 85 per cent.[20] Although some workers have been able to demonstrate common duct stones by sonography,[37, 38] this is not the usual experience.[39, 40] CT can also demonstrate dilated bile ducts and estimate the site of blockage.[20] Compared with ultrasound, however, CT is less able to image gallbladder and common duct stones,[41, 42] but is better able to image mass lesions. Consequently, if the clinical find-

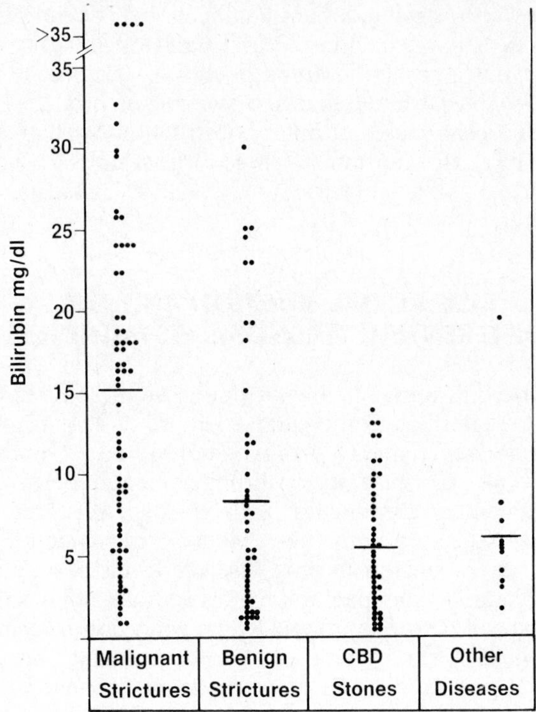

Figure 90–1. Serum bilirubin levels in 178 patients with bile duct obstruction. The mean value ± SD was 15.2 ± 10.8 mg/dl for malignant strictures, 8.3 ± 8.1 mg/dl for benign strictures, and 5.5 ± 3.9 mg/dl for common duct stones. The highest bilirubin value caused by common duct stones was 13.8 mg/dl.

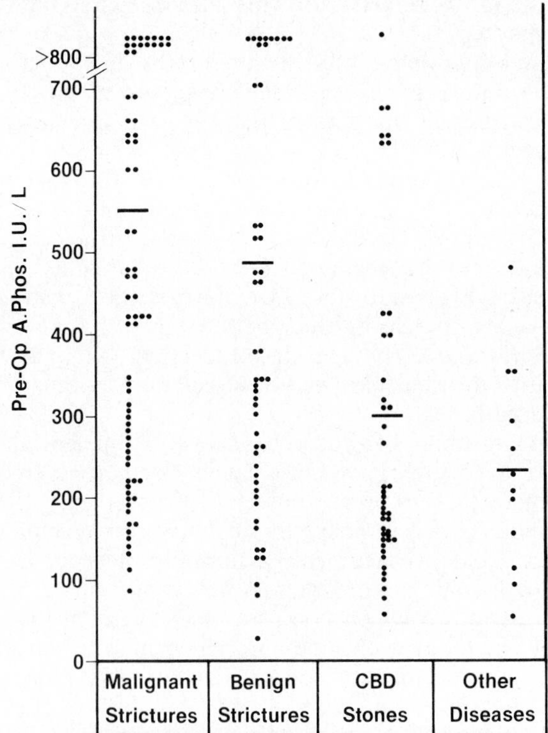

Figure 90–2. Serum alkaline phosphatase values in 178 patients with bile duct obstruction. Normal by this method is less than 71 IU per liter. The alkaline phosphatase exceeded five times normal in 57 per cent of patients with malignant strictures, in 45 per cent of patients with benign strictures, and in 21 per cent of patients with common duct stones.

ings suggest a diagnosis of neoplastic obstruction of the bile duct (e.g., pancreatic tumor), it is most efficient to obtain a CT scan rather than an ultrasound scan as the first specialized test.

If jaundice is intense and dilated bile ducts are not seen on ultrasound or CT scan, the jaundice usually stems from intrahepatic rather than extrahepatic obstructive disease. Liver biopsy is usually indicated in these patients, provided that the coagulation mechanism is intact. Viral hepatitis, alcoholic hepatitis, and primary and secondary hepatic tumors are among the specific conditions that may be diagnosed. A cholestatic picture on liver biopsy does not indicate whether the disease affects primarily the hepatic parenchyma or the ducts.

Although liver scans using Tc-sulfur colloid are often ordered in jaundiced patients, they are of diminishing value. Radionuclide scans are most accurate in detecting mass lesions, but even here there are many false positive and false negative results, and both CT and ultrasound scans are superior tests for obtaining this information.

If the jaundice is mild, transient, and accompanied by fever, and gallstones are present in the gallbladder, the diagnosis is obvious—common duct stones. As mentioned, the bilirubin value in choledocholithiasis usually falls in the range of 2 to 5 mg/dl and rarely surpasses 12 mg/dl.[19, 43, 44] If an ultrasound (or CT) scan shows ductal dilatation, if the bilirubin level is above 10 mg/dl, and if the jaundice has remained steady for several weeks, the most likely diagnosis is neoplastic obstruction,[19, 45] *even if the patient has stones in the gallbladder.*

With the higher levels of jaundice, or when gallstones are not seen on ultrasound, endoscopic retrograde[20, 43–48] or transhepatic cholangiography[49–52] is usually indicated. If the gallbladder is dilated or there are other reasons to suspect that the block is at the lower end of the duct, an ERCP would usually be the procedure of choice. In addition to obtaining an outline of the bile duct and pancreatic duct, an ERCP allows one to detect and biopsy an ampullary carcinoma. When the block is located proximally, as with posttraumatic biliary stricture or proximal carcinoma, a THC is usually indicated as the first test.

The principal weaknesses of ERCP are a moderately high failure rate in attempts to cannulate the duct and poor opacification of the hepatic side of an obstructing lesion. The latter is more common and of greater significance with lesions near the hilum, where the proximal anatomy is of critical importance in planning therapy. The principal weaknesses of THC are the moderately high failure rate in patients with nondilated ducts and the risk of bleeding in patients with an abnormal coagulation mechanism. With either test there is a danger of producing severe septicemia in a patient with active cholangitis.

Efforts should be made to avoid overtesting. For example, in a patient who is thought to have a biliary stricture, a THC should usually be the first test performed, and the addition of an ERCP and CT scan would usually be superfluous. In about 50 per cent of patients, however, both a THC and an ERCP will be needed to obtain all the information desired.

CHOLANGITIS (BACTERIAL CHOLANGITIS)

Cholangitis consists of bacterial infection of bile in the bile duct. Cholangitis is discussed here rather than under a specific disease because it may result from any condition that produces bile duct obstruction. The most common causes are choledocholithiasis, biliary stricture, and neoplasm, but a number of less common causes are discussed at the end of this chapter.

The initial events leading to cholangitis are imperfectly understood. Bile duct obstruction does not always produce cholangitis, but for cholangitis to occur, bile duct obstruction is required. Cholangitis is relatively common in patients with choledocholithiasis, is nearly universal in patients with posttraumatic bile duct stricture, but is seen in only 15 per cent of patients with neoplastic obstruction.[53] Patients with neoplasm average a much higher degree of ductal obstruction than is found in patients with stricture or common duct stones, but the occurrence of cholangitis in neoplastic obstruction is unrelated to the degree of obstruction.[54] The available evidence suggests that cholangitis is most likely to result when obstruction supervenes on a duct that already contains bacteria, which is the case in most patients with choledocholithiasis and stricture but in few with neoplastic obstruction. Iatrogenic contamination or chance factors that seed the duct with organisms are responsible for the infection under other circumstances.

The chills and fever of cholangitis are due to bacteremia from bile duct organisms. In experimental studies, regurgitation into hepatic venous blood of bacteria in bile is directly proportional to the biliary pressure and hence the degree of obstruction.[9, 55, 56] This is the reason that decompression alone (e.g., inserting a T-tube) can reverse the illness so promptly. Intrahepatic abscesses may develop after prolonged or severe cholangitis. Once abscesses become established, neither antibiotics nor surgery are very successful in reversing sepsis, and the patient often succumbs.

The clinical manifestations of cholangitis consist of pain, jaundice, and chills and fever—a syndrome known as *Charcot's triad.* Only 70 per cent of patients exhibit all these features, however, and those with an incomplete triad may be difficult to diagnose.[53, 57, 58] Fever is present in 95 per cent, pain in 90 per cent, but clinically evident jaundice is absent in about 20 per cent of patients.

The physical findings are relatively nonspecific. Abdominal tenderness is present in the majority of patients but is by no means universal, and peritoneal signs (e.g., rebound tenderness) are noted in only 15 per cent. Hypotension and mental confusion each occur in about 15 per cent of patients, often simultaneously.[53]

Leukocytosis is present in 80 per cent of patients. Sometimes a marked shift to the left is the only white blood cell abnormality. Usually the serum bilirubin value exceeds 2.0 mg/dl, but in 20 per cent of patients it is below this value, most often when the blood sample has been drawn shortly after the onset of acute symptoms. The alkaline phosphatase concentration is usually elevated, and the SGOT may also be abnormal.

Blood cultures are usually positive, especially if taken during fever spikes and chills. The organism found in the blood is invariably the same as that in the bile. The bile contains two organisms in about half of the cases. The bacterial species most commonly cultured are *Escherichia coli, Klebsiella, Pseudomonas,* enterococci, and *Proteus.*[53, 57–60] Anaerobic species—for example, *Bacteroides fragilis* or *Clostridium perfringens*—are seen in about 15 per cent of appropriately cultured bile specimens.[61–63] Anaerobes usually accompany aerobes, especially *E. coli.*

The clinical manifestations of cholangitis span a wide spectrum. Many patients experience a transient self-limited illness characterized by a fever spike, chills, dark urine, and abdominal pain. Such a course is typical of those with choledocholithiasis or biliary stricture. In other patients, however, the illness is devastating, consisting of profound toxic sepsis with shock and impaired mental function. This form of the disease is often called suppurative cholangitis,[53, 59, 60, 64–66] but the term is imprecise because the clinical syndrome only loosely correlates with the character of the bile (i.e., whether the bile has the appearance of pus). The most important point, and the major reason for retaining the term "suppurative cholangitis," is to emphasize the existence of a condition characterized by overwhelming sepsis due to biliary obstruction, in which specific signs of biliary disease may be subtle or absent. Often the diagnosis is missed in this setting, the chance of early decisive therapy is lost, and the patient dies. Renal failure is a potential complication in these severely ill patients.[67]

Treatment. Mild to moderate cases of cholangitis usually respond to antibiotic therapy.[53, 57, 58, 68, 69] One should choose drugs effective against the organisms listed above. For mild cases, it is usually sufficient to initiate therapy with a single drug, such as cefoxitin, 2.0 gm intravenously every 6 hours or ampicillin, 1.0 gm intravenously every 4 hours. In severe cases, more intensive therapy (e.g., gentamicin, ampicillin, and clindamycin) is indicated from the start.

Improvement should be expected within 6 to 12 hours, and in most instances the attack will come under control within 48 to 72 hours. If this kind of response is not evident or if the patient is severely toxic at any point, the duct must be decompressed, either surgically,[53, 64, 65] by endoscopic sphincterotomy,[70–72] or by percutaneous transhepatic catheterization.[73–75]

If the illness is due to choledocholithiasis, endoscopic sphincterotomy will usually allow the duct to drain, which will abort the acute attack. Endoscopic sphincterotomy is also effective in some patients with carcinoma of the ampulla of Vater. Laparotomy and surgical decompression of the duct are required in other cases. The patient should never be judged to be too ill for surgery or some other means of decompression, since the effects may be dramatic in the most toxic cases.

CHOLEDOCHOLITHIASIS (COMMON DUCT STONES)

Conclusive evidence concerning the origin of common duct stones is not available, but what is known supports a gallbladder origin for most of them. Nevertheless, stones can form primarily in the duct, but this requires an abnormality that produces bile stasis, such as partial obstruction or marked dilatation. About 15 per cent of patients with gallbladder stones also have stones in the duct. Conversely, of patients with ductal stones, 95 per cent also have gallbladder stones. All gallstones from one patient, whether from the gallbladder or common duct, are of the same kind, either cholesterol or pigment. Chemically and visually, cholesterol stones from the duct are identical with those from the gallbladder.[76, 77] Pigment stones vary somewhat, but in general, the resemblance between gallbladder and ductal stones is close.[76] For example, a patient with an earthy pigment stone in the duct will usually be found to have an earthy stone in the gallbladder. About 40 per cent of common duct stones are pigment stones, considerably higher than the prevalence of pigment stones among gallbladder stones.[76] Most pigment stones probably form as a result of bacterial action, involving deconjugation of bilirubin diglucuronide and agglomeration of the solid pigment with bacteria by bacterial glycocalyx[78] (see pp. 1682–1684). This is why primary common duct stones (e.g., those that form proximal to a biliary stricture) are always pigment stones, and it also explains why sepsis is more common in patients with pigment stones.[76] The available evidence suggests that cholesterol stones in the duct are always secondary stones (i.e., they formed in the gallbladder), while pigment stones can be either primary or secondary. There is evidence, which has been contested,[79] that patients with common duct stones have an associated motor disorder of the sphincter of Oddi characterized by reversal of the normal direction of peristaltic sequences.[80] Whether this is a cause or an effect of the disease is unknown, but it could be a factor contributing to stasis.

In patients who present with choledocholithiasis months or years after cholecystectomy, it may be impossible to determine whether the present stones were overlooked at the earlier operation or have formed since.[81] It is reasonable to conclude from the preceding discussion that cholesterol stones have usually been overlooked, whereas pigment stones could have been overlooked, or if bile flow is sluggish and bacteria have gained a foothold, they could be recurrent.

Clinical Findings. Choledocholithiasis may present in any of the following ways:[43, 82–84] (1) without symptoms; or with (2) biliary colic, (3) jaundice, (4) cholangitis, or (5) pancreatitis. The last four of these may appear in any combination. For example, while pain may be the only symptom in some patients, it may be accompanied by jaundice or cholangitis in others. Pancreatitis may develop without symptoms referable to the biliary system, or it may be accompanied by jaundice or cholangitis.

Not much information is available on the natural history of the asymptomatic state, but it is clear that in many patients common duct stones are asymptomatic for months or years before causing symptoms.[85] Common duct stones probably cause clinical problems more often than asymptomatic gallbladder stones do. There seems to be no justification, however, for screening susceptible populations to detect and treat asymptomatic choledocholithiasis.

The morbidity of choledocholithiasis stems principally from biliary obstruction, which increases biliary pressure and diminishes bile flow. The rate of onset of obstruction, its degree, and the amount of bacterial contamination of the bile are the major factors that determine the resulting syndrome. Thus, acute obstruction usually causes biliary colic and jaundice, whereas obstruction that develops gradually over several months may present at first with pruritus or jaundice alone. If bacteria proliferate, cholangitis may result.

In addition to the primary syndromes, choledocholithiasis may give rise to the following complications: (1) cirrhosis with hepatic failure or portal hypertension or both, and (2) hepatic abscess formation. These complications may also follow biliary obstruction from other lesions, such as biliary stricture and malignant tumors, although cholangitis and abscess formation are considerably less common with malignant obstruction.

Laboratory Findings. The principal laboratory clues to the diagnosis are elevation of the bilirubin or alkaline phosphatase concentration in a patient with abdominal pain, jaundice, infection, or pancreatitis.[19, 43, 44, 82, 84, 86]

The presence of a stone in the duct may be inferred from a history of intermittent mild jaundice and fever and demonstration by ultrasound or oral cholecystography of gallbladder stones. The peak bilirubin value in choledocholithiasis is in the range of 2 to 10 mg/dl in over 90 per cent of jaundiced patients.[19] If the jaundice is steady instead of fluctuating and unassociated with fever, or if the bilirubin level exceeds 10 mg/dl, one should be suspicious of neoplastic obstruction and obtain an ERCP, even though stones are known to be present in the gallbladder.[87] If the patient has had a previous uncomplicated cholecystectomy, an ERCP—and probably an endoscopic sphincterotomy—are indicated.

Differential Diagnosis. Biliary colic may be strongly suspected from the patient's description. Just considering its character, the pain from cystic duct obstruction cannot be distinguished from that of common duct obstruction. If the patient's condition is satisfactory, it is neither practical nor important to determine immediately whether a common duct stone is present. An ultrasound scan will usually demonstrate any stones in the gallbladder. If the ultrasound scan and oral cholecystogram show no stones in the gallbladder, an ERCP should be obtained, because in 5 per cent of patients stones are present only in the duct.

Renal and *intestinal colic* are rarely confused with biliary pain. The pain of renal colic starts in the flank and often radiates downward, especially to the inner surface of the thigh or to the genitalia; dysuria and hematuria are often present.

The pain of intestinal colic is usually generalized and cramping and is often felt most severely below the umbilicus. If it is due to intestinal obstruction, emesis increases, the abdomen distends, and high-pitched borborygmi are heard with the waves of colic.

A *hepatic abscess*, either pyogenic or amebic, may closely simulate cholangitis caused by choledocholithiasis. Patients with solitary abscess experience right upper quadrant pain, which often has an acute onset. Chills and fever are characteristic, but jaundice will be either absent or faint except in advanced cases. Subcostal tenderness is usually present, and the liver may be palpable. An important clue to differentiation in a difficult case may be the detection of pleural fluid on the right side in patients with an abscess. Hepatic ultrasound, scintiscans, and CT scans should be obtained if an abscess is suspected.

The pain of *acute myocardial infarction* and of choledocholithiasis may be similar. In some patients, coronary ischemia causes abdominal distress localized to the right upper quadrant or epigastrium. The electrocardiogram should be helpful. The presence of a pericardial friction rub is distinctive for myocardial infarction. Slight jaundice may follow a myocardial infarction, but it is less common than with biliary calculus, and it usually does not appear until several days after the attack. Although the SGOT may be elevated in both myocardial infarction and choledocholithiasis with cholangitis, it rarely exceeds 100 to 150 units with the former disease except in very severe cases or when shock has supervened; elevation of the SGPT will be noted in the latter, but not in the former, condition.

Jaundice resulting from calculous obstruction of the common bile duct must be differentiated from extrahepatic bile duct obstruction from other causes. This subject was discussed earlier in the chapter.

Acute congestion of the liver, associated with cardiac decompensation, may cause intense right upper quadrant pain and even jaundice. In this condition, however, the temperature is normal, and the white blood cell count is normal or only slightly elevated. The patient has other obvious signs of cardiac decompensation, of which the enlarged tender liver may be only one. Particular findings of constrictive pericarditis, cor pulmonale, or tricuspid valve disease must always be sought.

Treatment. Treatment of cholangitis has been discussed already (see above). In the majority of patients, the attack can be brought under control within a day or two. If not, the duct must be decompressed urgently, either by surgery, endoscopic sphincterotomy, or transhepatic catheterization. In general, surgery will be indicated for patients who are stable and good operative risks, and the other methods will be appropriate for unstable patients or those who are poor risks for other reasons.

If cholangitis resolves under medical therapy, additional diagnostic studies are usually in order. Because cholangitis indicates mechanical obstruction, antibiotic treatment cannot be considered definitive. Percutaneous transhepatic or retrograde cholangiography should be postponed until the cholangitis has resolved.

Once common duct stones have been demonstrated, they should be surgically removed at the earliest convenient date. Preoperative correction of vitamin K deficiency is important.

Many patients with common duct stones come to treatment having suffered nothing more serious than an occasional attack of biliary colic. An ultrasound scan or oral cholecystogram will have demonstrated gallbladder stones, but information on the status of the common duct is not usually available. Under these circumstances, laparotomy and cholecystectomy may be scheduled without a preoperative cholangiogram. If at surgery there is reason to suspect the presence of stones in the common duct, the surgeon will either perform an operative cholangiogram or proceed directly with exploration of the duct after cholecystectomy.[43] Indications for exploring the duct are as follows: a history of (1) cholangitis, (2) jaundice, or (3) pancreatitis; operative evidence of (4) a dilated duct; or (5) palpable stones in the duct. Operative cholangiography is used to decide whether to explore the duct with the first four of these, which are called "relative" indications. Pre-exploratory operative cholangiography is simple, safe, and reliable and is performed liberally during cholecystectomy, even in the absence of clinical findings that suggest choledocholithiasis.

In addition to removing the stones, the surgeon should perform a drainage procedure when the common duct is markedly dilated, when more than about five stones are found, when all the stones cannot be removed, or when there have been one or more previous operations for common duct stones.[81] The term *drainage procedure* refers to any measure that eliminates the narrowing in the duct created by the sphincter. It includes sphincteroplasty, choledochoduodenostomy, and Roux-en-Y choledochojejunostomy. A drainage procedure will allow any residual or recurrent stones to pass into the gut.

Patients found to have choledocholithiasis who have had a cholecystectomy in the past can be treated effectively in most cases by transendoscopic sphincterotomy.[81, 88–94] Contraindications to endoscopic sphincterotomy include very large stones (i.e., >2 cm), bile duct stricture proximal to the ampullary orifice, and termination of the bile duct in a duodenal diverticulum. Endoscopic sphincterotomy may be unable to create adequate drainage when the duct is markedly dilated. In the face of contraindications to endoscopic sphincterotomy or when this technique fails, laparotomy and choledocholithotomy are usually indicated. The indications for a drainage procedure are the same as those listed earlier.

After the common bile duct has been surgically explored and the stones removed, a T-tube is inserted and the duct is closed. The tube provides a vent to decompress biliary pressure, which otherwise could cause a bile leak from the suture line, and it allows cholangiograms to be obtained postoperatively. The T-tube can be removed in the clinician's office 3 weeks after surgery, and the tract between the duct and the abdominal wall closes spontaneously within 24 hours. Before extraction of the T-tube, a cholangiogram should be performed. About 2 per cent of patients undergoing choledochotomy are discovered to have a residual stone on the postoperative cholangiogram.[43, 95–97]

Several methods are available to remove these retained common duct stones. The easiest is to extract the stones with a stone basket passed down the T-tube tract under radiologic[98] or endoscopic control.[99–101] The endoscopic method avoids exposure to radiation and can be done in the office, but it requires a fiberoptic choledochoscope. The radiologic method allows one to keep better track of the stone, but it is slightly more cumbersome and expensive. Using one or both of these techniques, it is possible to remove about 80 per cent of retained stones (although higher success rates are reported by a few individuals with extensive experience).

It may also be possible to dissolve retained stones if they are composed of cholesterol.[102, 103] Both cholic acid[102, 103] and mono-octanoin[103–106] are effective cholesterol solvents, although the latter is somewhat more potent in vitro. Both drugs are nontoxic and may be infused down the T-tube (see pp. 1678–1680). They should not be forced into the duct if it is obstructed, if the patient complains of pain, or if cholangitis appears.[43] Cholestyramine must be administered throughout cholic acid therapy in order to prevent the development of diarrhea. Details of the methods can be found in the literature on this subject.

Retained stones may also be eliminated by transendoscopic sphincterotomy,[107] but this should be reserved for patients in whom extraction from above has failed. Lastly, reoperation[108] or, rarely, expectant management may sometimes be appropriate.

Severe intrahepatic stone formation may present a formidable problem. Sometimes these patients can be managed by repeated stone extractions through a Roux-en-Y choledochojejunostomy placed to allow percutaneous access from the abdominal wall or via endoscopy (e.g., with an anastomosis to the stomach). In some of these patients in whom the disease is confined to a single lobe, hepatic lobectomy may be indicated.[109]

Complications. Spontaneous rupture of the common duct[110] and biliary stricture are rare complications. Acute, recurrent, and chronic pancreatitis are often related to calculous biliary tract disease (see pp. 1814–1872). Patients with obstructive jaundice and cholangitis are especially susceptible to acute renal failure.[67]

Sometimes the renal dysfunction may not improve until the biliary infection is surgically treated. The other complications have already been discussed.

RECURRENT PYOGENIC CHOLANGITIS (ORIENTAL CHOLANGIOHEPATITIS, PRIMARY CHOLANGITIS)

Recurrent pyogenic cholangitis (RPC) is a disease characterized by chronic infection and stone formation in the bile duct. It mainly affects inhabitants of Southeast Asia and is most prevalent in Taiwan and the south of China.[111–120] In Hong Kong it is the most common disease of the biliary tract and is the third most frequent cause of acute abdominal pain requiring surgical intervention. In Western countries, RPC must be considered as a cause of cholangitis in immigrants from Asia. The disease affects males and females equally. Most patients are between the ages of 25 and 80 years, the average being 52 years.

Etiology and Pathology.[111] The most popular etiologic theory postulates portal bacteremia as the initial event. Histologic studies have shown that portal phlebitis is the earliest lesion, antedating changes in the bile ducts. This leads to portal suppuration, which secondarily spreads to the ductal system. *E. coli* can be cultured from the ducts in virtually all cases. This organism produces β-glucuronidase, which deconjugates bilirubin and produces the stone formation. A low-protein diet is thought to contribute by decreasing the glucaro-1:4-lactone in bile, a factor that inhibits β-glucuronidase. The ductal epithelium becomes inflamed at focal points throughout the intra- and extrahepatic biliary tree. Stone formation is facilitated by the inflammation and scarring and may be enhanced by excessive excretion of bilirubin in patients who are also suffering from malaria. Subsequently the stones and debris produce obstruction, which, combined with infection, gives rise to the more serious pathologic and clinical manifestations. Portal vein thrombosis is an occasional complication of the portal inflammation.

The stones and sludge form throughout the biliary ducts, but the gallbladder is involved in only 15 per cent of patients. The material is predominantly calcium bilirubinate (i.e., this is a type of pigment stone disease). Stenosis may develop at any point in the ductal system and may trap stones within more proximal dilated segments.

Secondary changes on liver biopsy are characteristic of obstruction and cholangitis. Portions of the liver may atrophy as a result of long-standing obstruction. If sepsis gets the upper hand, intrahepatic abscess formation may supervene.

About one half of patients with cholangiohepatitis are infested with *Clonorchis sinensis.* This parasitic fluke is acquired by ingesting raw freshwater fish. The parasite migrates from the duodenum into the biliary tree, where it takes up prolonged residence. Whether there truly is an etiologic relationship between RPC and chlonorchiasis is debatable. It is known, for example, that clonorchis infestation is also common in persons from the same area and culture who do not have RPC.

Clinical Manifestations. The patient suffers from recurrent cholangitis and pain in the right upper quadrant or epigastrium. Nausea and vomiting are usually present. Chills, fever, and jaundice may appear, but subclinical elevations of bilirubin are common even in severely toxic patients. RPC must be considered in any patient with right upper quadrant pain who is or was an inhabitant for many years of an indigenous area.

Because the gallbladder may be unscarred, it is often palpable during acute attacks of obstructive cholangitis. Occasionally, pronounced distention of the gallbladder leads to tenderness, empyema, free perforation, and bile peritonitis.

Endoscopic retrograde or transhepatic cholangiography is required to make a definitive diagnosis and plan therapy.[112]

The presence of a palpable gallbladder in this disease enables differentiation from cholangitis caused by cholesterol gallstones. Empyema, carcinoma of the gallbladder, emphysematous cholecystitis, and, occasionally, cholangitis complicating periampullary malignancy may be other causes of a right subcostal tender mass in a patient with acute cholangitis.

Treatment. Endoscopic sphincterotomy is an effective form of therapy for patients with stones confined to the bile ducts who do not have ductal strictures. The success in emptying the ducts of stones and controlling the disease is about 80 per cent (see pp. 1741–1744).

Surgery is indicated for failures of endoscopic sphincterotomy or for advanced disease with complications.[117–120] If the duct does not contain strictures, surgical therapy should consist of choledochotomy and removal of the stones followed by transduodenal sphincteroplasty and cholecystectomy. If the duct is unusually large or sphincterotomy has previously failed, a Roux-en-Y choledochoduojejunostomy is the procedure of choice.[120]

The late results of surgical sphincteroplasty are good (no further symptoms) in 85 per cent of patients.[113] Ten per cent have mild to moderate symptoms, and 5 per cent have a poor result with continued severe cholangitis and its complications. Recurrent symptoms are occasionally the result of narrowing of the sphincteroplasty, which can be corrected by reoperation and conversion to a Roux-en-Y choledochojejunostomy. About 75 per cent of patients treated by Roux-en-Y choledochojejunostomy have a good result.[120] Persistent symptoms are most often caused by recurrent intrahepatic stone formation.

If abscesses have formed in the liver, they may be drained, but the prognosis at this stage is poor. Abscesses more often affect the left lobe of the liver than the right. Hepatic lobectomy is occasionally indicated when one lobe (usually the left) becomes severely scarred and chronically infected and the opposite lobe is relatively spared.

SCLEROSING CHOLANGITIS

Sclerosing cholangitis is an uncommon condition in which the bile ducts are involved by a stenosing inflammatory process of unknown origin.[121–127] Most evidence points toward an immune process to explain the etiology. About 70 per cent of patients manifest the human leukocyte antigen (HLA) B8 or DR3 phenotype, genetic markers associated with various organ specific autoimmune diseases. These antigens are found in about 25 per cent of the general population. Hypergammaglobulinemia is common, especially elevated levels of IgM. More than half of patients with primary sclerosing cholangitis have ulcerative colitis,[128, 129] and of them, two thirds have circulating anticolon antibodies[130] that cross-react with an antigen possessed by most strains of *Escherichia coli* (see p. 1467). Circulating T-8 (suppressor) cells are decreased, and in the liver T-8 cells are concentrated around proliferating bile ductules, while T-4 (helper) cells predominate in inflammatory lesions around portal tracts.[131] The clearance of immune complexes from the circulation is prolonged in primary sclerosing cholangitis,[132] which suggests that macrophages of the reticuloendothelial system are functioning at a subnormal level.

The patient may come to clinical attention for any of the following findings: (1) jaundice, (2) pruritus, (3) portal hypertension, (4) abdominal pain, or (5) an unexplained elevation of the alkaline phosphatase value. Attacks of fever and chills (i.e., bacterial cholangitis) are uncommon in the absence of previous surgery on the biliary system.

The basic lesion is composed of inflammation and fibrosis of the bile ducts; its distinctive radiographic appearance on cholangiography consists of ductal stiffening and irregularity with multiple sites of beading and stenosis. The disease is usually extensive, involving both intrahepatic and extrahepatic ducts, but variants are seen in which the disease is confined to just one of these areas. Endoscopic retrograde cholangiography is the diagnostic procedure of choice.[133]

The changes on liver biopsy are not specific, although they may suggest the correct diagnosis.[134, 136] They consist of periductal fibrosis and inflammation, portal edema and fibrosis, focal proliferation of bile ducts, focal obliteration and loss of bile ducts, deposition of copper, and cholestasis. The most characteristic lesion is the loss in some areas and the proliferation in others of small ducts. It is now apparent that the hepatic changes in patients with ulcerative colitis, previously referred to as pericholangitis, are the same as the early hepatic changes in patients with primary sclerosing cholangitis. Liberal use of ERCP in patients with ulcerative colitis and an elevated alkaline phosphatase concentration (or some other subtle finding of liver disease) has demonstrated that sclerosing cholangitis is more common than was previously recognized, and that it is often subclinical and nonprogressive.[127] In patients with ulcerative colitis, there is no relationship between the severity of the colonic disease and the severity of the sclerosing cholangitis. In fact, in most patients the colitis is mild and it may even be confined to the rectum.

The laboratory findings in most cases are typical of mild cholestasis. Antimitochondrial antibodies usually are absent.

Sclerosing cholangiocarcinoma may occasionally be misdiagnosed as sclerosing cholangitis, but this is not so common as in the past because the diffuse changes demonstrable by ERCP are characteristic in sclerosing cholangitis. However, some patients with sclerosing cholangitis eventually develop biliary carcinoma, and it may be impossible to make the diagnosis without laparotomy and biopsy. The neoplasm may even then go unrecognized. Carcinoma should be suspected clinically whenever the bilirubin value climbs progressively over several months from the usual low range (i.e., around 5 mg/dl) to above 10 mg/dl.

Treatment. Subclinical disease requires no therapy and is unlikely to progress. There is no general agreement on what is the best therapy. Assuming this may be an autoimmune disease, the use of corticosteroids seems logical, but there is no conviction that corticosteroids have a beneficial effect, and they have the potential for aggravating osteoporosis, a common complication of the chronic liver dysfunction. There are no data that support the use of other immunosuppressive agents, such as azathioprine or cyclosporin. At present, these drugs should only be given as part of a randomized trial.

Dominant strictures demonstrated on cholangiograms can sometimes be dilated with balloon catheters passed by a percutaneous transhepatic approach.[137] Treatment by prolonged (e.g., 6 to 12 months) stenting may be more effective, however.[138–141] Stents may be inserted transhepatically, endoscopically, or surgically. Excision of the stricture and Roux-en-Y hepaticojejunostomy is appropriate for the occasional case with a dominant stricture of the lower end of the duct and mild proximal disease, especially with proximal dilatation. Cameron[141] has had good results with resecting the hepatic duct bifurcation (where the disease is usually the most severe) and stenting the lobar ducts after reconstruction by a Roux-en-Y hepaticojejunostomy. Periodic episodes of bacterial cholangitis are fairly common following any of these procedures. Liver transplantation has given good results in patients with progressive advanced disease. Transplantation is more difficult if the patient has had previous surgery of the bile ducts, so the indications for such operations in patients with sclerosing cholangitis must be well thought out.

MISCELLANEOUS UNCOMMON CAUSES OF BILE DUCT OBSTRUCTION

Uncommon causes of bile duct obstruction in adults, clinically manifested by jaundice, colic, cholangitis, or a combination of these, are discussed in this section. Pancreatic and periampullary tumors are discussed on pages 1872 to 1884 and 461 to 462, respectively. Other causes rarely encountered are compression by inflammatory paraductal lymph nodes and duodenal Crohn's disease.

Congenital Choledochal Cysts.[142–145] The principal morphologic variants of congenital cystic disease of the extrahepatic bile duct are (1) fusiform (in adults) or saccular (in children) dilatation of the entire duct (95 per cent), (2) saccular diverticulum projecting from the side of the duct (4 per cent), and (3) saccular dilatation of the very end of the duct at the ampulla (choledochocele) (1 per cent). About 25 per cent of patients also have cystic changes within the intrahepatic ducts (see p. 1650).

In nearly all patients with an extrahepatic cyst, the pancreatic and bile ducts join to form a common channel several centimeters (average, 2.8 cm; range, 1.5 to 4.5 cm) proximal to the connection with the duodenum.[146–148] The length of a common channel in normal subjects ranges from 0.2 to 1.0 cm. It is thought that this is important in the etiology of the cyst because it allows regurgitation of pancreatic juice into the developing bile ducts. The regurgitated pancreatic juice is postulated to weaken the duct wall and damage the mucosa, which allows the duct to dilate. Awareness of the proximal junction is also important to the surgeon, who must avoid injuring the high-lying pancreatic duct when excising the choledochal cyst.

Although it is a congenital disease, about one half of patients with choledochal cysts have their initial clinical manifestations after age 17 years. The patients present with pain, jaundice, cholangitis, and, in some, a right upper quadrant mass consisting of the dilated duct full of stones.[142, 144, 149] A syndrome consisting of abdominal pain and jaundice is most common.

At the time of an attack, the serum bilirubin, alkaline phosphatase, and amylase values are usually elevated. Diagnosis is best accomplished by transhepatic or, preferably, retrograde cholangiography.[145, 150] CT or ultrasound scans may help define the mass and its relationship to other structures. A HIDA scan may give an outline of the cyst.[151] An occasional case is not diagnosed until operation.

Surgical therapy consists of excision of the abnormal duct, if possible, followed by Roux-en-Y jejunal anastomosis to the stump of the hepatic duct.[144, 152–154] A cholecystectomy should also be performed. Anastomosis of the cyst to the intestine (cholecystoduodenostomy or cholecystojejunostomy) is less definitive, but it is simpler and may be required for technical reasons or when the patient's condition is poor. Because the cyst is not lined by normal mucosa, cyst-intestinal anastomoses are prone to gradual stricture formation, so many patients treated by this procedure eventually require reoperation. Congenital choledochal cyst is a premalignant lesion, another reason to prefer resection rather than internal decompression.[142, 155–157]

Caroli's Disease. Caroli's disease consists of multiple congenital saccular dilatations of the intrahepatic bile ducts.[158–161] It is now recognized that cysts of the intrahepatic ducts are common accompaniments of extrahepatic cysts,[162] and the term *Caroli's disease* should probably be reserved for cystic disease confined to the intrahepatic system.

Most patients become symptomatic between the ages of 20 and 50 years owing to intrahepatic stone formation and cholangitis or to complications of portal hypertension. Two forms of Caroli's disease are recognized, one a disease of the ducts only, and the other more common type, which is associated with congenital hepatic fibrosis[161] and medullary sponge kidney. In the former, cholangitis is the mode of presentation. Patients in the latter group often have bleeding from esophageal varices before cholangitis or obstructive jaundice appears. Oral cholecystograms rarely opacify, and direct cholangiography is most often required for diagnosis. The cysts may be imaged by scintiscans (e.g., HIDA scan).[163, 164] Antimicrobial therapy may control attacks of cholangitis, and surgical procedures to facilitate ductal emptying or to extract stones may help in some cases, but the intrahepatic anomaly cannot be definitively corrected. Rarely, the left lobe alone is involved, and lobectomy is curative.[165, 166] In most cases, episodes of cholangitis recur, which may eventually result in lethal sepsis.

Hemobilia.[167–174] Hemobilia presents with the triad of biliary colic, obstructive jaundice, and occult or gross intestinal bleeding. Most cases result from hepatic trauma, in which manifestations of hemobilia present several weeks after the original injury. Hemobilia is also a rare complication of liver biopsy and transhepatic cholangiography. Other causes of hemobilia include biliary or hepatic neoplasms, intraductal rupture of a hepatic artery aneurysm, hepatic abscess, or biliary calculus. Inflammatory hemobilia has been reported mostly from the Orient, where it accompanies biliary parasitism (*Ascaris lumbricoides*) or cholangiohepatitis.

The diagnosis has been made in some cases by detecting biliary extravasation of ^{99m}Tc-labeled red blood cells.[168, 170] It can be verified preoperatively and the site of the leak pinpointed by selective hepatic arteriography. Treatment consists of selective embolization (e.g., with Gelfoam) or hepatic artery ligation for hemobilia secondary to trauma; for the other types, direct surgical management of the lesion is usually necessary. Minor bleeding episodes may resolve completely without operative intervention, but this seems to be uncommon.

Pancreatitis. Inflammatory swelling can produce transient jaundice in acute pancreatitis by obstruction of the distal common duct where it courses through pancreatic tissue.[175] Simultaneous acute pancreatitis and jaundice may also be the manifestations of a common duct stone lodged in the ampulla of Vater (see pp. 1823–1824).

Unremitting obstruction can result from entrapment in pancreatic scarring from chronic pancreatitis.[176–182] Unremitting obstruction is not seen as a complication of pancreatitis due to gallstone disease. The patient may present with elevated serum alkaline phosphatase and bilirubin values and manifestations of (1) pancreatitis (i.e., epigastric pain and tenderness and hyperamylasemia), or (2) bile duct obstruction (i.e., jaundice, pruritus, and/or cholangitis). The most common presenting syndrome consists of episodic relapsing pancreatitis and signs of cholestasis in an alcoholic patient. Only 50 per cent of patients with a significant degree of bile duct obstruction are clinically jaundiced.[178] The diagnosis may go unsuspected in alcoholic patients in whom elevated alkaline phosphatase and bilirubin values may incorrectly be attributed to hepatic parenchymal disease. Still, a disproportionate elevation of the alkaline phosphatase value may occur in alcoholic liver disease in the absence of bile duct obstruction (see pp. 1849 and 1859).[183]

Cholangiograms would routinely be obtained if the patient were thought from clinical findings to have bile duct obstruction, but it is also important to study patients who present with relapsing pancreatitis in whom the alkaline phosphatase and bilirubin values remain elevated as the acute symptoms resolve. If the bilirubin or the alkaline phosphatase remains elevated for a month or two, a fixed bile duct stenosis in need of surgical decompression will almost always be present. Expectant management of such patients is rarely successful, and prolonged nonoperative management runs a risk of secondary biliary cirrhosis developing silently.[176, 184]

The lesion, which appears as a long stricture, is demonstrable by transhepatic or retrograde cholangiography. Pancreatic calcifications are present in about half the cases. Treatment consists of a side-to-side choledochoduodenostomy or a Roux-en-Y choledochojejunostomy. Because the stricture is so long, endoscopic sphincterotomy or surgical sphincteroplasty is unable to provide adequate decompression.

When jaundice develops in a patient with a pancreatic pseudocyst, drainage of the cyst may fail to decompress the bile duct.[185, 186] An ERCP should be performed preoperatively to help decide whether or not an ancillary choledochoduodenostomy is necessary at the time the cyst is surgically treated.

Duodenal Diverticula.[187, 188] Most duodenal diverticula arise within 1 to 2 cm of the hepatobiliary ampulla, and in some patients the common duct empties directly into a diverticulum. Duodenal diverticula may obstruct the common duct by anatomic distortion of its duodenal entry, by diverticulitis, or by an enterolith (of bile acids) in the sac. Even in jaundiced patients, most duodenal diverticula are only incidental findings, but when definite proof implicates them in ductal obstruction, either choledochoduodenostomy or Roux-en-Y choledochojejunostomy is simpler treatment than attempting to excise the diverticulum or surgically to enlarge its entry into the duodenum.

Echinococcosis.[189–192] Echinococcosis, by rupture of a hepatic cyst into the ducts, can give rise to biliary colic, jaundice, and cholangitis. Preoperative ERCP may demonstrate the communication between the cyst and the duct. Treatment involves surgical removal of the obstructing hydatid debris and daughter cysts from the ducts and excision of the parent cyst from the liver. The practice of injecting formalin into the hepatic cysts is no longer used, because in patients with a biliary communication it may injure the bile ducts. Mebendazole or albendazole may be given in conjunction with surgery to help minimize the possibility of peritoneal implantation of the parasite.[193]

Ascariasis. Ascariasis may produce colic, jaundice, cholangitis, and right upper quadrant tenderness by worms that invade the bile duct through the choledochal sphincter from the duodenum.[194, 195] The gallbladder may be dilated and palpable on physical examination. The diagnosis may be suspected from abdominal plain films, which show ascarids in the intestine as clusters of parallel radiolucent lines. The diagnosis can be made from typical findings on CT or ultrasound scans or ERCP.[194–198] Air is sometimes seen in the ducts, presumably having entered through the sphincter with the ascarid. Usually only one worm invades the bile duct, but in extreme cases there may be many more. The worm eventually withdraws into the duodenum or dies but in some cases not until after depositing ova. It may be possible to remove an obstructing worm from the orifice of the duct endoscopically.[199] Complications consist of bile duct stricture, stones, perforation, acute cholecystitis, and liver abscess formation.

Treatment entails antimicrobial drugs and then piperazine after the acute symptoms are controlled. If progressive cholangitis or obstruction occurs despite antimicrobial therapy, common duct exploration and extraction of the parasites may be necessary. Laparotomy is also indicated for complications. After the nonsurgical regimen, follow-up intravenous or direct cholangiograms should be obtained to verify that no worms remain in the duct; if residual worms or their remnants are present, they should be removed surgically or by endoscopic sphincterotomy (see pp. 1173–1174).

Cancer. Metastatic cancer is an occasional cause of bile duct obstruction.[200] The primary tumors most often responsible are adenocarcinoma of the colon, gallbladder, pancreas, small intestine, stomach, breast, and ovary as well as melanoma and lymphoma. Metastatic colonic cancer accounts for about two thirds of cases. Painless jaundice is the most common presentation. Transhepatic cholangiogram or ERCP will demonstrate the block. Surgical decompression into a Roux-en-Y limb of jejunum is indicated if the lesion is not too extensive and a segment of dilated extrahepatic duct is available above the site of obstruction for the anastomosis. If surgical drainage is not feasible, permanent transhepatic intubation will be required. A percutaneous CT-guided aspiration biopsy may provide a specific diagnosis in patients with lymphoma, who usually respond so quickly to radiotherapy that surgical or radiologic intervention is unnecessary.

References

1. Schmid, R. Bilirubin metabolism: State of the art. Gastroenterology *74*:1307, 1978.

2. Billing, B. H. Twenty-five years of progress in bilirubin metabolism (1952–77). Gut *19*:481, 1978.
3. Schiff, L. Jaundice: Five and a half decades in historic perspective. Selected aspects. Gastroenterology *78*:831, 1980.
4. Weiss, J. S., Gautam, A., Lauff, J. J., Sundberg, M. W., Jatlow, P., Boyer, J. L., and Seligson, D. The clinical importance of a protein-bound fraction of serum bilirubin in patients with hyperbilirubinemia. N. Engl. J. Med. *309*:147, 1983.
5. Chopra, S., and Griffin, P. H. Laboratory tests and diagnostic procedures in evaluation of liver disease. Am. J. Med. *79*:221, 1985.
6. Erlinger, S. What is cholestasis in 1985? J. Hepatol. *1*:687, 1985.
7. Phillips, M. J., Poucell, S., and Oda, M. Mechanisms of cholestasis. Lab. Invest. *54*:593, 1986.
8. Malchow-Moller, A., Matzen, P., Bjerregaard, B., Hilden, J., Holst-Christensen, J., Staehr-Johnsen, T., Altman, L., Thomsen, C., and Juhl, E. Causes and characteristics of 500 consecutive cases of jaundice. Scand. J. Gastroenterol. *16*:1, 1981.
9. Williams, R. D., Fish, J. C., and Williams, D. D. The significance of biliary pressure. Arch. Surg. *95*:374, 1967.
10. Schein, C. J., and Beneventano, T. C. Choledochal dynamics in man. Surg. Gynecol. Obstet. *126*:591, 1968.
11. Jonson, G., and Sundman, L. Bile and dry matter output at elevated liver secretion pressure. Acta Chir. Scand. *128*:153, 1964.
12. Strasberg, S. M., Dorn, B. C., Redinger, R. N., Small, D. M., and Egdahl, R. H. Effects of alteration of biliary pressure on bile composition—A method for study: Primate biliary physiology V. Gastroenterology *61*:357, 1971.
13. Strasberg, S. M., Dorn, B. C., Small, D. M., and Egdahl, R. H. The effect of biliary tract pressure on bile flow, bile salt secretion, and bile salt synthesis in the primate. Surgery *70*:140, 1971.
14. Carlson, E., Zukoski, C. F., Campbell, J., and Chvapil, M. Morphologic, biophysical, and biochemical consequences of ligation of the common biliary duct in the dog. Am. J. Pathol. *86*:301, 1977.
15. Corlette, M. B., Mendes-Monteiro, A. C., Bismuth, H., and Morin, J. Transient bile duct obstruction. Arch. Surg. *111*:1017, 1976.
16. Kaplan, M. M. Serum alkaline phosphatase—another piece is added to the puzzle. Hepatology *6*:526, 1986.
17. Komoda, T., Koyama, I., Nagata, A., Sakagishi, Y., Kurata, M., and Kumegawa, M. A possible mechanism of induction and translocation into blood stream of rat alkaline phosphatase activity by bile duct ligation. Arch. Biochem. Biophys. *251*:323, 1986.
18. Braasch, J. W., Whitcomb, F. F., Jr., Watkins, E., Jr., Maguire, R. R., and Khazei, A. M. Segmental obstruction of the bile duct. Surg. Gynecol. Obstet. *134*:915, 1972.
19. Pellegrini, C. A., Thomas, M. J., and Way, L. W. Bilirubin and alkaline phosphatase values before and after surgery for biliary obstruction. Am. J. Surg. *143*:67, 1982.
20. Thomas, M. J., Pellegrini, C. A., and Way, L. W. Usefulness of diagnostic tests for biliary obstruction. Am. J. Surg. *144*:102, 1982.
21. Pedrosa, C. S., Casanova, R., and Rodriguez, R. Computed tomography in obstructive jaundice. Part I: The level of obstruction. Radiology *139*:627, 1981.
22. Pedrosa, C. S., Casanova, R., and Rodriguez, R. Computed tomography in obstructive jaundice. Part II: The cause of obstruction. Radiology *139*:634, 1981.
23. Gibson, R. N., Yeung, E., Thompson, J. N., Carr, D. H., Hemingway, A. P., Bradpiece, H. A., Benjamin, I. S., Blumgart, L. H., and Allison, D. J. Bile duct obstruction: Radiologic evaluation of level, cause, and tumor resectability. Radiology *160*:43, 1986.
24. Baron, R. L., Stanley, R. J., Lee, J. K. T., Koehler, R. E., and Levitt, R. G. Computed tomographic features of biliary obstruction. AJR *140*:1173, 1983.
25. Laing, F. C., Jeffrey, R. B., Jr., Wing, V. W., and Nyberg, D. A. Biliary dilatation: Defining the level and cause by real-time US. Radiology *160*:39, 1986.
26. Schaffer, A. A., Jr., Buschi, A. J., and Brenbridge, N. A. G. Limitations of ultrasonography in evaluating patients with jaundice or cholecystectomy. South. Med. J. *74*:525, 1981.
27. Scobie, B. A., and Summerskill, W. H. J. Hepatic cirrhosis secondary to obstruction of the biliary system. Am. J. Dig. Dis. *10*:134, 1965.
28. Weinbren, K., Hadjis, N. S., and Blumgart, L. H. Structural aspects of the liver in patients with biliary disease and portal hypertension. J. Clin. Pathol. *38*:1013, 1985.
29. Adson, M. A., and Wychulis, A. R. Portal hypertension in secondary biliary cirrhosis. Arch. Surg. *96*:604, 1968.
30. Zimmerman, H. J. The differential diagnosis of jaundice. Med. Clin. North Am. *52*:1417, 1968.
31. Schenker, S., Balint, J., and Schiff, L. Differential diagnosis of jaundice: Report of a prospective study of 61 proved cases. Am. J. Dig. Dis. *7*:449, 1962.
32. Stern, R. B., Knill-Jones, R. P., and Williams, R. Use of computer program for diagnosing jaundice in district hospitals and specialized liver unit. Br. Med. J. *2*:659, 1975.
33. Knill-Jones, R. P., Stern, R. B., Girmes, D. H., Maxwell, J. D., Thompson, R. P. H., and Williams, R. Use of sequential Bayesian model in diagnosis of jaundice by computer. Br. Med. J. *1*:530, 1973.
34. Mueller, P. R., Ferrucci, J. T., Jr., Simeone, J. F., van Sonnenberg, E., Hall, D. A., and Wittenberg, J. Observations on the distensibility of the common bile duct. Radiology *142*:467, 1982.
35. Muhletaler, C. A., Gerlock, A. J., Jr., Fleischer, A. C., and James, A. E., Jr. Diagnosis of obstructive jaundice with nondilated bile ducts. AJR *134*:1149, 1980.
36. Beinart, C., Efremidis, S., Cohen, B., and Mitty, H. A. Obstruction without dilation. Importance in evaluating jaundice. JAMA *245*:353, 1981.
37. Laing, F. C., Jeffrey, R. B., and Wing, V. W. Improved visualization of choledocholithiasis by sonography. AJR *143*:949, 1984.
38. Cronan, J. J. US diagnosis of choledocholithiasis: A reappraisal. Radiology *161*:133, 1986.
39. Gross, B. H., Harter, L. P., Gore, R. M., Callen, P. W., Filly, R. A., Shapiro, H. A., and Goldberg, H. I. Ultrasonic evaluation of common bile duct stones: Prospective comparison with endoscopic retrograde cholangiopancreatography. Radiology *145*:471, 1983.
40. O'Connor, H. J., Hamilton, I., Ellis, W. R., Watters, J., Lintott, D. J., and Axon, A. T. R. Ultrasound detection of choledocholithiasis: Prospective comparison with ERCP in the postcholecystectomy patient. Gastrointest. Radiol. *11*:161, 1986.
41. Baron, R. L. Common bile duct stones: Reassessment of criteria for CT diagnosis. Radiology *162*:419, 1987.
42. Menu, Y., Lorphelin, J. M., Scherrer, A., Grenier, P., and Nahum, H. Sonographic and computed tomographic evaluation of intrahepatic calculi. AJR *145*:579, 1985.
43. Way, L. W., Admirand, W. H., and Dunphy, J. E. Management of choledocholithiasis. Ann. Surg. *176*:347, 1972.
44. Saltzstein, E. C., Peacock, J. B., and Thomas, M. D. Preoperative bilirubin, alkaline phosphatase and amylase levels as predictors of common duct stones. Surg. Gynecol. Obstet. *154*:381, 1982.
45. Matzen, P., Haubek, A., Holst-Christensen, J., Lejerstofte, J., and Juhl, E. Accuracy of direct cholangiography by endoscopic or transhepatic route in jaundice—a prospective study. Gastroenterology *81*:237, 1981.
46. Gregg, J. A., and McDonald, D. G. Endoscopic retrograde cholangiopancreatography and gray-scale abdominal ultrasound in the diagnosis of jaundice. Am. J. Surg. *137*:611, 1979.
47. Silvis, S. E., Rohrmann, C. A., and Vennes, J. A. Diagnostic accuracy of endoscopic retrograde cholangiopancreatography in hepatic, biliary, and pancreatic malignancy. Ann. Intern. Med. *84*:438, 1976.
48. Kullman, E., Broch, K., Tarpila, E., and Liedberg, G. Endoscopic retrograde cholangiopancreatography (ERCP) in patients with jaundice and suspected biliary obstruction. Acta Chir. Scand. *150*:657, 1984.
49. Goldstein, L. I., Sample, W. F., Kadell, B. M., and Weiner, M. Gray-scale ultrasonography and thin-needle cholangiogra-

phy. Evaluation in the jaundiced patient. JAMA *238*:1041, 1977.
50. Kreek, M. J., and Balint, J. A. "Skinny needle" cholangiography—results of a pilot study of a voluntary prospective method for gathering risk data on new procedures. Gastroenterology *78*:598, 1980.
51. Gold, R. P., Casarella, W. J., Stern, G., and Seaman, W. B. Transhepatic cholangiography: The radiological method of choice in suspected obstructive jaundice. Radiology *133*:39, 1979.
52. Gibson, R. N., Yeung, E., Thompson, J. N., Carr, D. H., Hemingway, A. P., Bradpiece, H. A., Benjamin, I. S., Blumgart, L. H., and Allison, D. J. Bile duct obstruction: Radiologic evaluation of level, cause, and tumor resectability. Radiology *160*:43, 1986.
53. Boey, J. H., and Way, L. W. Acute cholangitis. Ann. Surg. *191*:264, 1980.
54. O'Connor, M. J., Schwartz, M. L., McQuarrie, D. G., and Sumner, H. W. Cholangitis due to malignant obstruction of biliary outflow. Ann. Surg. *193*:341, 1981.
55. Huang, T., Bass, J. S., and Williams, R. D. The significance of biliary pressure in cholangitis. Arch. Surg. *93*:629, 1969.
56. Kjellander, J. J., and Rosengren, B. Cholangiovenous reflux. An experimental study. Acta Chir. Scand. *123*:316, 1962.
57. Thompson, J. E., Jr., Tompkins, R. K., and Longmire, W. P., Jr. Factors in management of acute cholangitis. Ann. Surg. *195*:137, 1982.
58. O'Connor, M. J., Schwartz, M. L., McQuarrie, D. G., and Sumner, H. W. Acute bacterial cholangitis. An analysis of clinical manifestation. Arch. Surg. *117*:437, 1982.
59. Kinoshita, H., Hirohashi, K., Igawa, S., Nagata, E., and Sakai, K. Cholangitis. World J. Surg. *8*:963, 1984.
60. Shimada, H., Nakagawara, G., Kobayashi, M., Tsuchiya, S., Kudo, T., and Morita, S. Pathogenesis and clinical features of acute cholangitis accompanied by shock. Jpn. J. Surg. *14*:269, 1984.
61. Bourgault, A. M., England, D. M., Rosenblatt, J. E., Forgacs, P., and Bieger, R. C. Clinical characteristics of anaerobic bactibilia. Arch. Intern. Med. *139*:1346, 1979.
62. Shimada, K., Noro, T., Inamatsu, T., Urayama, K., and Adachi, K. Bacteriology of acute obstructive suppurative cholangitis of the aged. J. Clin. Microbiol. *14*:522, 1981.
63. Finegold, S. M. Anaerobes in biliary tract infection. Arch. Intern. Med. *139*:1338, 1979.
64. Welch, J. P., and Donaldson, G. A. The urgency of diagnosis and surgical treatment of acute suppurative cholangitis. Am. J. Surg. *131*:527, 1976.
65. Weissglas, I. S., and Brown, R. A. Acute suppurative cholangitis secondary to malignant obstruction. Can. J. Surg. *24*:468, 1981.
66. Chock, E., Wolfe, B. M., and Matolo, N. M. Acute suppurative cholangitis. Surg. Clin. North Am. *61*:885, 1981.
67. Bismuth, H., Kuntziger, H., and Corlette, M. B. Cholangitis with acute renal failure: Priorities in therapeutics. Ann. Surg. *181*:881, 1975.
68. Sharia, P. C., and Cameror, J. L. Clinical management of acute cholangitis. Surg. Gynecol. Obstet. *142*:369, 1976.
69. Munro, R., and Sorrell, T. C. Biliary sepsis. Reviewing treatment options. Drugs *31*:449, 1986.
70. Ikeda, S., Tanaka, M., Itoh, H., Kishikawa, H., and Nakayama, F. Emergency decompression of bile duct in acute obstructive suppurative cholangitis by duodenoscopic cannulation: A lifesaving procedure. World J. Surg. *5*:587, 1981.
71. Leese, T., Neoptolemos, J. P., Baker, A. R., and Carr-Locke, D. L. Management of acute cholangitis and the impact of endoscopic sphincterotomy. Br. J. Surg. *73*:988, 1986.
72. Yin, T. P., Frost, R. A., and Goodacre, R. L. The benefit of emergency nasobiliary drain in cholelithiasis with ascending cholangitis, coagulopathy, and thrombocytopenia. Surgery *100*:105, 1986.
73. Nunez, D., Jr., Guerra, J. J., Jr., Al-Sheikh, W. A., Russell, E., and Mendez, G., Jr. Percutaneous biliary drainage in acute suppurative cholangitis. Gastrointest. Radiol. *11*:85, 1986.
74. Pessa, M. E., Hawkins, I. F., and Vogel, S. B. The treatment of acute cholangitis. Percutaneous transhepatic biliary drainage before definitive therapy. Ann. Surg. *205*:389, 1987.
75. Lois, J. F., Gomes, A. S., Grace, P. A., Deutsch, L. S., and Pitt, H. A. Risks of percutaneous transhepatic drainage in patients with cholangitis. AJR *148*:367, 1987.
76. Bernhoft, R. A., Pellegrini, C. A., Motson, R. W., and Way, L. W. Composition and morphologic and clinical features of common duct stones. Am. J. Surg. *148*:77, 1984.
77. Whiting, M. J., and Watts, J. M. Chemical composition of common bile duct stones. Br. J. Surg. *73*:229, 1986.
78. Stewart, L., Smith, A. L., Pellegrini, C. A., Motson, R. W., and Way, L. W. Pigment gallstones form as a composite of bacterial microcolonies and pigment solids. Ann. Surg. *206*:242, 1987.
79. De Masi, E., Corazziari, E., Habib, F. I., Fontana, B., Gatti, V., Fegiz, G. F., and Torsoli, A. Manometric study of the sphincter of Oddi in patients with and without common bile duct stones. Gut *25*:275, 1984.
80. Toouli, J., Geenen, J. E., Hogan, W. J., Dodds, W. J., and Arndorfer, R. C. Sphincter of oddi motor activity: A comparison between patients with common bile duct stones and controls. Gastroenterology *82*:111, 1982.
81. Allen, B., Shapiro, H., and Way, L. W. Management of recurrent and residual common duct stones. Am. J. Surg. *142*:41, 1981.
82. Anciaux, M. L., Pelletier, G., Attali, P., Meduri, B., Liguory, C., and Etienne, J. P. Prospective study of clinical and biochemical features of symptomatic choledocholithiasis. Dig. Dis. Sci. *31*:449, 1986.
83. DenBesten, L., Doty, J. E. Pathogenesis and management of choledocholithiasis. Surg. Clin. North Am. *61*:893, 1981.
84. Hauer-Jensen, M., Karesen, R., Nygaard, K., Solheim, K., Amlie, E., Havig, and Viddal, K. O. Predictive ability of choledocholithiasis indicators. A prospective evaluation. Ann. Surg. *202*:64, 1985.
85. Way, L. W. Retained common duct stones. Surg. Clin. North Am. *53*:1139, 1973.
86. Lacaine, F., Corlette, M. B., and Bismuth, H. Preoperative evaluation of the risk of common bile duct stones. Arch. Surg. *115*:1114, 1980.
87. Gordon, P., Cooperberg, P. L., and Cohen, M. M. Presence of gallstones is a poor indicator of the cause of obstructive jaundice. Surg. Gynecol. Obstet. *151*:635, 1980.
88. Siegel, J. H. Endoscopic papillotomy in the treatment of biliary tract disease. 258 procedures and results. Dig. Dis. Sci. *26*:1057, 1981.
89. Shapiro, H. A. Endoscopic diagnosis and treatment of biliary tract disease. Surg. Clin. North Am. *61*:843, 1981.
90. Silvis, S. E. Current status of endoscopic sphincterotomy. Am. J. Gastroenterol. *79*:731, 1984.
91. Osnes, M., Rosseland, A. R., and Aabakken, L. Endoscopic retrograde cholangiography and endoscopic papillotomy in patients with a previous Billroth-II resection. Gut *27*:1193, 1986.
92. Thompson, M. H. Influence of endoscopic papillotomy on the management of bile duct stones. Br. J. Surg. *73*:779, 1986.
93. Geenen, J. E., Toouli, J., Hogan, W. J., Dodds, W. J., Stewart, E. T., Mavrelis, P., Diedel, D., and Venu, R. Endoscopic sphincterotomy: Follow-up evaluation of effects on the sphincter of Oddi. Gastroenterology *87*:754, 1984.
94. Cotton, P. B. Endoscopic management of bile duct stones (apples and oranges). Gut *25*:587, 1984.
95. Birkett, D. H., and Williams, L. F., Jr. Prevention and management of retained bile duct stones. Surg. Clin. North Am. *61*:939, 1981.
96. Heuman, R., Smeds, S., Hellgren, E., Sjodahl, R., and Wetterfors, J. Evaluation of factors affecting the incidence of retained calculi in the bile ducts. Acta Chir. Scand. *148*:185, 1982.
97. Rogers, A. L., Farha, G. J., Beamer, R. L., and Chang, F. C. Incidence and associated mortality of retained common bile duct stones. Am. J. Surg. *150*:690, 1985.
98. Burhenne, H. J. Percutaneous extraction of retained biliary tract stones: 661 patients. AJR *134*:888, 1980.

99. Birkett, D. H., and Williams, L. F. Choledochoscopic removal of retained stones via a T-tube tract. Am. J. Surg. *139*:531, 1980.
100. Moss, J. P., Whelan, J. G., Jr., Dedman, T. C., III, and Voyles, R. G. Postoperative choledochoscopy through the T-tube tract. Surg. Gynecol. Obstet. *151*:807, 1980.
101. Berci, G., and Hamlin, J. A. A combined fluoroscopic and endoscopic approach for retrieval of retained stones through the T-tube tract. Surg. Gynecol. Obstet. *153*:237, 1981.
102. Way, L. W., and Motson, R. W. Dissolution of retained common duct stones. Adv. Surg. *10*:99, 1976.
103. Neoptolemos, J. P., Hofmann, A. F., and Moossa, A. R. Chemical treatment of stones in the biliary tree. Br. J. Surg. *73*:515, 1986.
104. Tritapepe, R., Di Padova, C., Pozzoli, M., Rovagnati, P., and Montorsi, W. The treatment of retained biliary stones with monooctanoin: Report of 16 patients. Am. J. Gastroenterol. *79*:710, 1984.
105. Butch, R. J., MacCarty, R. L., Mueller, P. R., Ferrucci, J. T., Jr., Simeone, J. F., Teplick, S. K., and Haskin, P. H. Monooctanoin perfusion treatment of intrahepatic calculi. Radiology *153*:375, 1984.
106. Teplick, S. K., and Haskin, P. H. Monooctanoin perfusion for in vivo dissolution of biliary stones. A series of 11 patients. Radiology *153*:379, 1984.
107. O'Doherty, D. P., Neoptolemos, J. P., and Carr-Locke, D. L. Endoscopic sphincterotomy for retained common bile duct stones in patients with T-tube in situ in the early postoperative period. Br. J. Surg. *73*:454, 1986.
108. Broughan, T. A., Sivak, M. V., and Hermann, R. E. The management of retained and recurrent bile duct stones. Surgery *98*:746, 1985.
109. Adson, M. A., and Nagorney, D. M. Hepatic resection for intrahepatic ductal stones. Arch. Surg. *117*:611, 1982.
110. Chu, C. S. Spontaneous perforation of the common hepatic duct: Report of seven cases. Surg. Gastroenterol. *3*:69, 1984.
111. Chou, S. T., and Chan, C. W. Recurrent pyogenic cholangitis: A necropsy study. Pathology *12*:415, 1980.
112. Lam, S. K., Wong, K. P., Chan, P. K. W., Ngan, H., and Ong, G. B. Recurrent pyogenic cholangitis: A study by endoscopic retrograde cholangiography. Gastroenterology *74*:1196, 1978.
113. Choi, T. K., Wong, J., Lam, K. H., Lim, T. K., and Ong, G. B. Late result of sphincteroplasty in the treatment of primary cholangitis. Arch. Surg. *116*:1173, 1981.
114. Nakayama, F., Soloway, R. D., Nakama, T., Miyazaki, K., Ichimiya, H., Sheen, P. C., Ker, C. G., Ong, G. B., Boey, C. J., Foong, W. C., Tan, E. C., Tung, K. H., and Lee, C. N. Hepatolithiasis in East Asia. Retrospective study. Dig. Dis. Sci. *31*:21, 1986.
115. Lam, S. K. A study of endoscopic sphincterotomy in recurrent pyogenic cholangitis. Br. J. Surg. *71*:262, 1984.
116. Kerlan, R. K., Jr., Pogany, A. C., Goldberg, H. I., and Ring, E. J. Radiologic intervention in oriental cholangiohepatitis. AJR *145*:809, 1985.
117. Lau, W. Y., Fan, S. T., Yip, W. C., and Wong, K. K. Surgical management of strictures of the major bile ducts in recurrent pyogenic cholangitis. Br. J. Surg. *74*:1100, 1987.
118. Nakayama, F., and Koga, A. Hepatolithiasis: Present status. World J. Surg. *8*:9, 1984.
119. Koga, A., Miyazaki, K., Ichimiya, H., and Nakayama, F. Choice of treatment for hepatolithiasis based on pathological findings. World J. Surg. *8*:36, 1984.
120. Choi, T. K., Wong, J., and Ong, G. B. Choledochojejunostomy in the treatment of primary cholangitis. Surg. Gynecol. Obstet. *155*:43, 1982.
121. Thompson, H. H., Pitt, H. A., Tompkins, R. K., and Longmire, W. P., Jr. Primary sclerosing cholangitis. A heterogeneous disease. Ann. Surg. *196*:127, 1982.
122. Pitt, H. A., Thompson, H. H., Tompkins, R. K., and Longmire, W. P., Jr. Primary sclerosing cholangitis: Results of an aggressive surgical approach. Ann. Surg. *3*:259, 1982.
123. Chapman, R. W. G., and Jewell, D. P. Primary sclerosing cholangitis—an immunologically mediated disease? West J. Med. *143*:193, 1985.
124. Chapman, R. W. Primary sclerosing cholangitis. J. Hepatol. *1*:179, 1985.
125. Wiesner, R. H., Ludwig, J., LaRusso, N. F., and MacCarty, R. L. Diagnosis and treatment of primary sclerosing cholangitis. Semin. Liv. Dis. *5*:241, 1985.
126. Wiesner, R. H., LaRusso, N. F., Ludwig, J., and Dickson, E. R. Comparison of the clinicopathologic features of primary sclerosing cholangitis and primary biliary cirrhosis. Gastroenterology *88*:108, 1985.
127. Helzberg, J. H., Petersen, J. M., and Boyer, J. L. Improved survival with primary sclerosing cholangitis. A review of clinicopathologic features and comparison of symptomatic and asymptomatic patients. Gastroenterology *92*:1869, 1987.
128. Shepherd, H. A., Selby, W. S., Chapman, R. W. G., Nolan, D., Barbatis, C., McGee, J. O., and Jewell, D. P. Ulcerative colitis and persistent liver dysfunction. Q. J. Med. *208*:503, 1983.
129. Wee, A., and Ludwig, J. Pericholangitis in chronic ulcerative colitis: Primary sclerosing cholangitis of the small bile ducts? Ann. Intern. Med. *102*:581, 1985.
130. Chapman, R. W., Cottone, M., Selby, W. S., Shepherd, H. A., Sherlock, S., and Jewell, D. P. Serum autoantibodies, ulcerative colitis and primary sclerosing cholangitis. Gut *27*:86, 1986.
131. Whiteside, T. L., Lasky, S., Si, L., and Van Thiel, D. H. Immunologic analysis of mononuclear cells in liver tissues and blood of patients with primary sclerosing cholangitis. Hepatology *5*:468, 1985.
132. Minuk, G. Y., Angus, M., Brickman, C. M., Lawley, T. J., Frank, M. M., Hoffnagle, J. H., and Jones, E. A. Abnormal clearance of immune complexes from the circulation of patients with primary sclerosing cholangitis. Gastroenterology *88*:166, 1985.
133. MacCarty, R. L., LaRusso, N. F., Wiesner, R. H., and Ludwig, J. Primary sclerosing cholangitis: Findings on cholangiography and pancreatography. Radiology *149*:39, 1983.
134. Cameron, J. L., Gayler, B. W., Sanfey, H., Milligan, F., Kaufman, S., Maddrey, W. C., and Herlong, H. F. Sclerosing cholangitis. Anatomical distribution of obstructive lesions. Ann. Surg. *200*:54, 1984.
135. Barbatis, C., Grases, P., Shepherd, H. A., Chapman, R. W., Trowell, J., Jewell, D. P. J., and McGee, J. O. Histological features of sclerosing cholangitis in patients with chronic ulcerative colitis. J. Clin. Pathol. *38*:778, 1985.
136. Ludwig, J., MacCarty, R. L., LaRusso, N. F., Krom, R. A. F., and Wiesner, R. H. Intrahepatic cholangiectases and large-duct obliteration in primary sclerosing cholangitis. Hepatology *6*:560, 1986.
137. May, G. R., Bender, C. E., LaRusso, N. F., Wiesner, R. H. Nonoperative dilatation of dominant strictures in primary sclerosing cholangitis. AJR *145*:1061, 1985.
138. Wood, R. A. B., and Cuschieri, A. Is sclerosing cholangitis complicating ulcerative colitis a reversible condition? Lancet *2*:716, 1980.
139. Hamilton, I., Soutar, J. S., Bouchier, I. A. D., and Cuschieri, A. Short-term biliary dilatation and stenting in primary sclerosing cholangitis. J. Clin. Gastroenterol. *9*:70, 1987.
140. Krige, J. E. J., Terblanche, J., Harries-Jones, E. P., and Bornman, P. C. Primary sclerosing cholangitis: Biliary drainage and duct dilatation. Br. J. Surg. *74*:54, 1987.
141. Lillemoe, K. D., Pitt, H. A., and Cameron, J. L. Sclerosing cholangitis. Adv. Surg. *21*:65, 1987.
142. Todani, T., Watanabe, Y., Narusue, M., Tabuchi, K., and Okajima, K. Congenital bile duct cysts. Classification, operative procedures, and review of thirty-seven cases including cancer arising from choledochal cyst. Am. J. Surg. *134*:263, 1977.
143. Yamaguchi, M. Congenital choledochal cyst. Analysis of 1,433 patients in the Japanese literature. Am. J. Surg. *140*:653, 1980.
144. Deziel, D. J., Rossi, R. L., Munson, J. L., Braasch, J. W., and Silverman, M. L. Management of bile duct cysts in adults. Arch. Surg. *121*:410, 1986.
145. Todani, T., Watanabe, Y., Fujii, T., Toki, A., Uemura, S., and Koike, Y. Cylindrical dilatation of the choledochus: A special type of congenital bile duct dilatation. Surgery *98*:964, 1985.

146. Kimura, K., Ohto, M., Ono, T., Tsuchiya, Y., Saisho, H., Kawamura, K., Yogi, Y., Karasawa, E., and Okuda, K. Congenital cystic dilatation of the common bile duct: Relationship to anomalous pancreaticobiliary ductal union. Am. J. Roentgenol. *128*:571, 1977.
147. Matsumoto, Y., Uchida, K., Nakase, A., and Honjo, I. Congenital cystic dilatation of the common bile duct as a cause of primary bile duct stone. Am. J. Surg. *124*:346, 1977.
148. Nagata, E., Sakai, K., Kinoshita, H., and Hirohashi, K. Choledochal cyst: Complications of anomalous connection between the choledochus and pancreatic duct and carcinoma of the biliary tract. World J. Surg. *10*:102, 1986.
149. Okada, A., Oguchi, Y., Kamata, S., Ikeda, Y., Kasashima, Y., and Saito, R. Common channel syndrome—diagnosis with endoscopic retrograde cholangiopancreatography and surgical management. Surgery *93*:634, 1983.
150. Thatcher, B. S., Sivak, M. V., Jr., Hermann, R. E., and Esselstyn, C. B. ERCP in evaluation and diagnosis of choledochal cyst: Report of five cases. Gastrointest. Endosc. *32*:27, 1986.
151. Han, B. K., Babcock, D. S., and Gelfand, M. H. Choledochal cyst with bile duct dilatation: Sonography and ^{99m}Tc IDA cholescintigraphy. AJR *136*:1075, 1981.
152. Powell, C. S., Sawyers, J. L., and Reynolds, V. H. Management of adult choledochal cysts. Ann. Surg. *193*:666, 1981.
153. Todani, T., Watanabe, Y., Mizuguchi, T., Fujii, T., and Toki, A. Hepaticoduodenostomy at the hepatic hilum after excision of choledochal cyst. Am. J. Surg. *142*:584, 1981.
154. Takiff, H., Stone, M., and Fonkalsrud, E. W. Choledochal cysts: Results of primary surgery and need for reoperation in young patients. Am. J. Surg. *150*:141, 1985.
155. Rossi, R. L., Silverman, M. L., Braasch, J. W., Munson, J. L., and ReMine, S. G. Carcinomas arising in cystic conditions of the bile ducts. A clinical and pathologic study. Ann. Surg. *205*:377, 1986.
156. Komi, N., Tamura, T., Tsuge, S., Miyoshi, Y., Udaka, H., and Takehara, H. Relation of patient age to premalignant alterations in choledochal cyst epithelium: Histochemical and immunohistochemical studies. J. Pediatr. Surg. *21*:430, 1986.
157. Komi, N., Tamura, T., Miyoshi, Y., Hino, M., Yada, S., Kawahara, H., Udaka, H., and Takehara, H. Histochemical and immunohistochemical studies on development of biliary carcinoma in forty-seven patients with choledochal cyst—special reference to intestinal metaplasia in the biliary duct. Jpn. J. Surg. *15*:273, 1985.
158. Foulk, W. T. Congenital malformations of the intrahepatic biliary tree in the adult. Gastroenterology *58*:253, 1970.
159. Mercadier, M., Chigot, J. P., Clot, J. P., Langlois, P., and Lansiaux, P. Caroli's disease. World J. Surg. *8*:22, 1984.
160. Dayton, M. T., Longmire, W. P., Jr., and Tompkins, R. K. Caroli's disease: A premalignant condition? Am. J. Surg. *145*:41, 1983.
161. Skummerfield, J. A., Nagafuchi, Y., Sherlock, S., Cadafalch, J., and Scheuer, P. J. Hepatobiliary fibropolycystic diseases. A clinical and histological review of 51 patients. J. Hepatol. *2*:141, 1986.
162. Matsumoto, Y., Uchida, K., Nakase, A., and Honjo, I. Clinicopathologic classification of congenital cystic dilatation of the common bile duct. Am. J. Surg. *134*:569, 1977.
163. Cabrera, J., Quintero, E., Bruguera, M., Alarco, R., Limena, F., Humbert, P., De Las Casas, P., and Rodes, J. Diagnosis of Caroli's disease by technetium-99m DISIDA cholescintigraphy. Report of three cases. Clin. Nucl. Med. *10*:478, 1985.
164. Moreno, A. J., Parker, A. L., Spicer, M. J., and Brown, T. J. Scintigraphic and radiographic findings in Caroli's disease. Am. J. Gastroenterol. *79*:299, 1984.
165. Ramond, M. J., Huguet, C., Danan, G., Rueff, B., and Benhamou, J. P. Partial hepatectomy in the treatment of Caroli's disease. Report of a case and review of the literature. Dig. Dis. Sci. *29*:367, 1984.
166. Nagasue, N. Successful treatment of Caroli's disease by hepatic resection. Report of six patients. Ann. Surg. *200*:718, 1984.
167. Sanblom, P., Saegesser, F., and Mirkovitch, V. Hepatic hemobilia: Hemorrhage from the intrahepatic biliary tract, a review. World J. Surg. *8*:41, 1984.
168. Curet, P., Baumer, R., Roche, A., Grellet, J., and Mercadier, M. Hepatic hemobilia of traumatic or iatrogenic origin: Recent advances in diagnosis and therapy, review of the literature from 1976 to 1981. World J. Surg. *8*:2, 1984.
169. Sandblom, P. Iatrogenic hemobilia. Am. J. Surg. *151*:754, 1986.
170. Jackson, D. E., Jr., Floyd, J. L., and Levesque, P. H. Hemobilia associated with hepatic artery aneurysms: Scintigraphic detection with technetium-99m-labeled red blood cells. J. Nucl. Med. *27*:491, 1986.
171. Kelley, C. J., Hemingway, A. P., McPherson, G. A. D., Allison, D. J., and Blumgart, L. H. Non-surgical management of post-cholecystectomy haemobilia. Br. J. Surg. *70*:502, 1983.
172. Sarr, M. G., Kaufman, S. L., Zuidema, G. D., and Cameron, J. L. Management of hemobilia associated with transhepatic internal biliary drainage catheters. Surgery *95*:603, 1984.
173. Chen, M. F., Chou, F. F., Wang, C. H., and Jang, Y. I. Hematobilia from ruptured hepatic artery aneurysm. Report of two cases. Arch. Surg. *118*:759, 1983.
174. Wilkinson, M., Michell, M., Alexander, G., Ratcliffe, J., Larkworthy, W., and Williams, R. Difficulty in diagnosing hemobilia from a hepatic artery aneurysm: Value of endoscopic retrograde cholangiography. Gastrointest. Radiol. *9*:223, 1984.
175. Bradley, E. L., and Salam, A. A. Hyperbilirubinemia in inflammatory pancreatic disease: Natural history and management. Ann. Surg. *188*:626, 1978.
176. Littenberg, G., Afroudakis, A., and Kaplowitz, N. Common bile duct stenosis from chronic pancreatitis: A clinical and pathologic spectrum. Medicine *58*:385, 1979.
177. Petrozza, J. A., Dutta, S. K., Latham, P. S., Iber, F. L., and Gadacz, T. R. Prevalence and natural history of distal common bile duct stenosis in alcoholic pancreatitis. Dig. Dis. Sci. *29*:890, 1984.
178. Lygidakis, N. J. Biliary stricture as a complication of chronic relapsing pancreatitis. Am. J. Surg. *145*:804, 1983.
179. Newton, B. B., Rittenbury, M. S., and Anderson, M. C. Extrahepatic biliary obstruction associated with pancreatitis. Ann. Surg. *197*:645, 1983.
180. Aranha, G. V., Prinz, R. A., Freeark, R. J., and Greenlee, H. B. The spectrum of biliary tract obstruction from chronic pancreatitis. Arch. Surg. *119*:595, 1984.
181. Sugerman, H. J., Barnhart, G. R., and Newsome, H. H. Selective drainage for pancreatic, biliary, and duodenal obstruction secondary to chronic fibrosing pancreatitis. Ann. Surg. *203*:558, 1983.
182. Petrozza, J. A., and Dutta, S. K. The variable appearance of distal common bile duct stenosis in chronic pancreatitis. J. Clin. Gastroenterol. *7*:447, 1985.
183. Perrillo, R. P., Griffin, R., DeSchryver-Kecshemeti, K., Lander, J. J., and Zuckerman, G. R. Alcoholic liver disease presenting with marked elevation of serum alkaline phosphatase. A combined clinical and pathological study. Am. J. Dig. Dis. *23*:1061, 1978.
184. Afroudakis, A., and Kaplowitz, N. Liver histopathology in chronic common bile duct stenosis due to chronic alcoholic pancreatitis. Hepatology *1*:65, 1981.
185. Skellenger, M. E., Patterson, D., Foley, N. T., and Jordan, P. H., Jr. Cholestasis due to compression of the common bile duct by pancreatic pseudocyst. Am. J. Surg. *145*:343, 1983.
186. Warshaw, A. L., and Rattner, D. W. Facts and fallacies of common bile duct obstruction by pancreatic pseudocysts. Ann. Surg. *192*:33, 1980.
187. McSherry, C. K., and Gleen, F. Biliary tract obstruction and duodenal diverticula. Surg. Gynecol. Obstet. *130*:829, 1970.
188. Scudamore, C. H., Harrison, R. C., and White, T. T. Management of duodenal diverticula. Can. J. Surg. *25*:311, 1982.
189. Lygidakis, N. J. Diagnosis and treatment of intrabiliary rupture of hydatid cyst of the liver. Arch. Surg. *118*:1186, 1983.
190. Dadoukis, J., Gamvros, O., and Aletras, H. Intrabiliary rupture of the hydatid cyst of the liver. World J. Surg. *8*:786, 1984.
191. Ertan, A., Sahin, B., Kandilci, U., Acikalin, T., Cumhur, T., and Danisoglu, V. The mechanism of cholestasis from hepatic hydatid cysts. J. Clin. Gastroenterol. *5*:437, 1983.
192. Ovnat, A., Peiser, J., Avinoah, E., Barki, Y., and Charuzi, I.

Acute cholangitis caused by ruptured hydatid cyst. Surgery 95:497, 1984.
193. Morris, D. L., Dykes, P. W., Marriner, S., Bogan, J., Burrows, F., Sheene-Smith, H., and Clarkson, M. J. Albendazole—objective evidence of response in human hydatid disease. JAMA *253*:2053, 1985.
194. Khuroo, M. S., and Zargar, S. A. Biliary ascariasis. A common cause of biliary and pancreatic disease in an endemic area. Gastroenterology *88*:418, 1985.
195. Davies, M. R. Q., and Rode, H. Biliary ascariasis in children. Progr. Pediatr. Surg. *15*:55, 1982.
196. Radin, D. R., and Vachon, L. A. CT findings in biliary and pancreatic ascariasis. J. Comput. Assist. Tomogr. *10*:508, 1986.
197. Cerri, G. G., Leite, G. J., Simones, J. B., Da Rocha, D. J. C., Albuquerque, F. P., Machado, C. C., and Magalhaes, A. Ultrasonographic evaluation of ascaris in the biliary tract. Radiology *146*:753, 1983.
198. Schulman, A., Loxton, A. J., Heydenrych, J. J., and Abdurahman, K. E. Sonographic diagnosis of biliary ascariasis. AJR *139*:485, 1982.
199. Saul, C., Pias, V. M., Jannke, H. A., and Braga, N. H. M. Endoscopic removal of *Ascaris lumbricoides* from the common bile duct. Am. J. Gastroenterol. *79*:725, 1984.
200. Thomas, J. H., Pierce, G. E., Karlin, C., Hermreck, A. S., and MacArthur, R. I. Extrahepatic biliary obstruction secondary to metastatic cancer. Am. J. Surg. *142*:770, 1981.

91 Postoperative Syndromes

LAWRENCE W. WAY
MARVIN H. SLEISENGER

BILIARY STRICTURE

Benign biliary stricture[1–4] is caused by surgical trauma in about 95 per cent of cases. The remainder are the result of external abdominal trauma, chronic pancreatitis, or rarely, erosion of the duct by a gallstone. Sometimes the operative accident can be attributed to technical problems resulting from advanced disease, but more often the procedure was not especially difficult. Biliary stricture was more frequent in the past, when more cholecystectomies were performed by incompletely trained surgeons. Although this aspect of the problem has not been eliminated, improvement is continuing. Operations in the hilum of the liver require not only technical skill and experience but also a thorough knowledge of the normal anatomy and its variations in order to avoid the pitfalls that result in inadvertent injury to the ducts. However, after all preventive measures have been exhausted, iatrogenic trauma will still be seen occasionally.

The varieties of injury consist of transection, incision, excision of a segment, or occlusion of the duct by a ligature. The surgeon may or may not recognize at the operation that the duct has been damaged. If the injury is seen, it should be repaired and a T-tube inserted through a nearby choledochotomy.

Most injuries go unnoticed by the surgeon, and the first signs of a complication become evident in the postoperative period. If the duct is completely occluded, jaundice will develop rapidly. More often the duct is partially obstructed, and the initial manifestations consist of episodic jaundice or cholangitis. Sometimes there is a rent in the side of the duct, and the earliest sign is excessive or prolonged drainage of bile from the drains after surgery. The drainage predisposes to subhepatic infection, which contributes to stricturing of the duct as it heals. If the gallbladder bed has not been drained, the patient may present with bile ascites.

Clinical Findings. Depending on the severity of the trauma and the amount of infection, symptoms may occur immediately or as late as seven years after the injury. Cholangitis later than two years after cholecystectomy, however, is more likely to be caused by common duct stones than by bile duct stricture.

Cholangitis is the most common manifestation. The typical case consists of episodes of pain, fever, chills, and mild jaundice. Antibiotics are usually successful in controlling the symptoms, but further attacks occur at irregular intervals. The cholangitis may be toxic and refractory to therapy, but milder attacks are much more common. Cholangitis is so typical that biliary stricture may not be seriously considered in a jaundiced afebrile patient who is having little pain. However, this is another mode of presentation.

There may be a history of operative injury during cholecystectomy or a previous operation for stricture repair, in which case the diagnosis is usually obvious. Cholangitis in such patients nearly always signifies recurrent stricture. Another, albeit uncommon, explanation for cholangitis under these circumstances is intrahepatic stone formation with intermittent passage of stones into the gut.

Physical findings are not distinctive. The right upper quadrant may be tender, but it usually is not. Jaundice and dark urine are usually present during an attack of cholangitis. In the rare case of bile ascites, physical examination reveals the typical findings of ascites, usually with nothing to suggest its unique character.

Laboratory Findings. Direct cholangiography is essential for diagnosis. Transhepatic cholangiography (THC) is superior to endoscopic retrograde cholangiography (ERCP) in the average patient because the latter often gives incomplete opacification of the proximal side of the stricture. ERCP may be helpful for patients in whom THC has been unsuccessful or in whom there are special reasons for investigating the duodenal end of the duct. Prophylactic antibiotics should be given before performing either of these studies. In patients with a previous anastomosis between the duct and the duodenum, the stricture can sometimes be outlined by refluxing barium into the biliary tree during an upper gastrointestinal series. No specific information is provided by ultrasound scans or CT scans, although they may demonstrate dilated ducts.

The alkaline phosphatase value is elevated in most cases. The bilirubin may fluctuate in relation to symptoms. Usually it remains below 5 mg/dl.

Blood cultures may be positive during an attack of cholangitis. Bile ascites may be diagnosed by paracentesis.

Differential Diagnosis. *Choledocholithiasis,* the condition that must be differentiated most often, may yield identical clinical and laboratory findings. A history of trauma to the duct would be more indicative of stricture. As mentioned, most patients with stricture manifest cholangitis or jaundice within two years of the cholecystectomy, whereas the symptom-free interval in patients with choledocholithiasis often exceeds two years. The final distinction usually must await the results of the cholangiograms.

Other causes of cholestatic jaundice may have to be ruled out.

Treatment. Strictures of the bile duct should be surgically repaired in all but the few patients who are excessively poor risks for laparotomy.[1–4] Even what appears clinically to be advanced liver disease from chronic bile duct obstruction may respond.[5] Symptomatic treatment with antibiotics should be used to control attacks of cholangitis, but long-term antibiotic treatment is not recommended as a definitive regimen. Although the cholangitis may respond regularly, the liver eventually develops secondary biliary cirrhosis and its complications. Even if the patient has had one or more previous unsuccessful attempts to repair the stricture, there is about a 75 per cent chance that an experienced surgeon can still obtain a definitive repair. Biliary stricture is one lesion that should be referred to a surgeon who specializes in such problems.

The surgical procedure should be selected on the basis of technical considerations presented by the individual patient. The objectives are to re-establish bile flow by anastomosing unscarred duct from the hepatic side of the stricture either to the intestine or to normal duct below the stricture. End-to-end repair may seem to be the simplest approach, but it is technically more difficult, and the results are inferior. There is no physiologic advantage in maintaining bile flow through the lower duct and ampulla. Therefore, the operation usually consists of making an anastomosis directly between the proximal duct and the intestine. In most cases this entails reimplantation of the duct into the duodenum (choledochoduodenostomy) or into a Roux-en-Y segment of jejunum (choledochojejunostomy). The latter procedure is slightly more versatile and is preferred by most surgeons.

If the patient has portal hypertension and esophageal varices, an operative attempt to repair the stricture may be bloody and technically unsuccessful. In such cases, transhepatic dilatation is probably the best initial treatment. If that fails, a prophylactic central splenorenal shunt should be performed and the stricture repaired four to six weeks later.

For patients who are poor risks for surgery, percutaneous transhepatic dilatation with balloon catheters is the most successful treatment.[6–9] Dilatation may also be performed in a retrograde fashion following a previous Roux-en-Y hepaticojejunostomy by percutaneous catheterization of the Roux-en-Y limb. Recurrence is relatively common after dilatation, however, and it has a low success rate in treating the primary stricture (i.e., it is much more likely to be beneficial in patients who have had a previous hepaticojejunostomy). A stenotic hepaticoduodenostomy can be dilated through an endoscope.

Complications. Complications usually result from delay in surgical correction of the stricture or from technical failure. Persistent cholangitis may progress to the formation of multiple intrahepatic abscesses. When this stage has been reached, it may be impossible to reverse the sepsis.

Secondary biliary cirrhosis may develop as a result of prolonged obstruction (i.e., for five years or more).

Prognosis. Surgical correction of the stricture is successful in about 85 per cent of attempts.[1–4] Experience at centers with a special interest in this problem indicates that good results can be obtained even if several previous attempts failed to relieve the obstruction.[10, 11] Therefore, if a stricture is present, the patient should be considered for correction despite a previous history of surgical failure. The death rate from biliary stricture is about 10 to 15 per cent, and the morbidity rate is high. If the stricture is not repaired, episodic cholangitis and secondary liver disease are inevitable.

POSTCHOLECYSTECTOMY SYNDROME

The term *postcholecystectomy syndrome* has become entrenched in the medical literature as a general diagnosis for patients with abdominal pain or other discomfort who have had a cholecystectomy. The term came into use long ago, when the tests available to demonstrate disease of the biliary tree, pancreas, and upper gut were much less sensitive than those currently in use. The problem was also more common then because cholecystectomy was performed more liberally in the absence of gallstones, the presumed cause of symptoms being chronic acalculous cholecystitis.

In most cases the symptoms consist of dyspepsia.[12–16] Since dyspepsia is common in the absence of gallbladder disease, it is not surprising that cholecystectomy often fails to relieve this complaint. Severe pain and other more serious symptoms are seen in a small proportion of individuals.

The notion that loss of the gallbladder may directly contribute to the symptoms has long been known to be incorrect. Removal of the gallbladder produces a variety of changes, but none of them could give rise to pain or dyspepsia. Following cholecystectomy the initial bolus of bile that normally enters the intestine in the first stages of a meal is no longer seen, but the concentration of bile salts in upper intestinal chyme remains in the physiologic range, and digestion and absorption are unimpaired.[17] The bile salt pool recycles faster,[18] which lowers the cholesterol concentration in bile, and, owing to increased exposure to intestinal bacteria, a higher proportion of the pool consists of deoxycholic acid.[19–21] Faster cycling of the pool may also increase the amount of bile salt entering the colon, which may lower the threshold for diarrhea or even cancer.[22]

Therefore, cholecystectomy per se cannot be implicated in the etiology of postcholecystectomy complaints, and "postcholecystectomy syndrome" is a misnomer. Postcholecystectomy "distress" or "symptoms" would be a more precise term. One is left, however, with the task of determining the reason for the patient's symptoms. The causes to consider may be grouped as follows: (1) residual biliary tract disease, (2) nonbiliary digestive disease, (3) nonspecific digestive dysfunction, and (4) psychiatric disorders.

General Considerations

Prospective studies show that about 95 per cent of patients are either cured or substantially relieved of their preoperative symptoms by cholecystectomy.[23] However, severe symptoms are seen in about 5 per cent of patients, and another 30 per cent have some mild discomfort or dyspepsia.[12–16] In one half the cases, postcholecystectomy distress presents within a few weeks of the operation; in the other half, it first appears months or years later. It is three times as common in women as in men.

Postcholecystectomy distress may consist of dyspepsia, mild pain, or severe pain. Patients with severe pain may also be divided into those with and without cholangitis. Mild right upper quadrant pain or dyspepsia or both are the principal complaints in 85 per cent of individuals. Patients with these complaints are rarely found to harbor retained stones or to have a dilated common duct, and an objective abnormality is not often demonstrated on upper gastrointestinal series, endoscopy, or other examinations. More severe symptoms, such as *severe pain, cholangitis,* or *pancreatitis,* occur in about 5 per cent of patients who have had a cholecystectomy. Investigation is much more likely to reveal a distinct, treatable cause in these patients than in those with mild symptoms.

However, the presence of severe pain alone does not entirely correlate with the presence of demonstrable disease. If the pain is continuous and there is no jaundice or other sign of obstruction, the bile duct is usually found to be of normal caliber and without evidence of stones. Evaluation of other systems usually fails to uncover a convincing cause for the complaints. The pain in these patients usually appears soon after operation and persists, in contrast to those with discrete attacks due to common duct stones or stenosis of the papilla. It is in the patients with episodic severe pain or cholangitis or both that diagnostic tests are most likely to demonstrate a significant abnormality.

After cholecystectomy for gallstone disease, postoperative distress is more common if the gallbladder had opacified on oral cholecystography and was histologically uninflamed than when the gallbladder showed signs of acute or chronic inflammation, when it failed to opacify, or when the common duct also contained stones. In other words, the more advanced the pathologic findings, the more likely that cholecystectomy will relieve the preoperative symptoms.

About two thirds of patients whose postcholecystectomy pain resembles the preoperative complaints and almost all of those whose postoperative distress has no resemblance to their preoperative pain are found to have no evidence of residual biliary tract disease. If a specific lesion is found in these patients, it is nearly always in some other organ.

Differential Diagnosis[12–16, 24]

Choledocholithiasis. Choledocholithiasis and pancreatitis are the most common explanations for severe *episodic* pain. If the patient also has cholangitis, it is most often due to common duct stones. Patients with common duct stones are more likely to have had attacks of cholangitis associated with cholelithiasis preoperatively and to have had symptoms over many months or years preoperatively. Physical examination reveals tenderness and guarding with rebound tenderness in the right upper quadrant. During an acute attack the SGOT and SGPT values may be transiently elevated, in which case the condition should not be mistaken for hepatitis (see pp. 1718–1721).

Pancreatitis. Pancreatitis is the basis for the pain in about 10 per cent of patients. It may be associated with retained stones in the common duct, with ampullary stenosis, or with both. The clinical findings in pancreatitis are fairly distinctive. The serum amylase value is usually elevated during an attack. In some cases the syndrome is further complicated by cholangitis. In pancreatitis associated with choledocholithiasis, the bilirubin level rises higher (>3.0 mg/dl) than is usually found in idiopathic or alcoholic pancreatitis, and there is usually an increase in the alkaline phosphatase level. Gallstone pancreatitis is caused by passage of a stone through the ampulla, and the rise in the bilirubin and alkaline phosphatase values is often transient (i.e., it lasts a day or two). Ductal dilatation may be noted on the ultrasound examination (see pp. 1824–1830).

Common Bile Duct Stricture. Stricture of the common bile duct will usually be heralded by cholangitis or jaundice early in the postoperative period. In some instances, the stricture develops more insidiously and symptoms do not appear for weeks or months (see above).

Ampullary Stenosis.[25–28] Also referred to as papillary stenosis, papillitis, or stenosis of the sphincter of Oddi, this condition is a rare cause of abdominal pain and pancreatitis. Ampullary stenosis is usually separated into two varieties, primary and secondary, depending upon whether it is thought to be idiopathic or to be the result of trauma from gallstones. Ampullary stenosis is most often considered in the differential diagnosis of postcholecystectomy complaints, although there is no reason to confine it to this situation.

The term ampullary stenosis actually embraces a broader concept than the words suggest. The central idea is that the terminus of the duct, the region occupied by the sphincter, is obstructing the flow of bile, producing biliary colic and in some cases cholangitis, intermittent jaundice, or pancreatitis. The obstruction could be the result of inflammation and fibrosis (passive obstruction) or spasm of the sphincter (active obstruction). Included in the latter is the hypothetical entity referred to as biliary dyskinesia, a form of motor incoordination of the duct and sphincter.

From the clinical standpoint, ampullary stenosis should be considered in patients who have abdominal pain accompanied by jaundice, cholangitis, and abnormal liver function studies, and whose ducts contain no gallstones when studied by ERCP. Whether the clinical manifestations were caused by a gallstone that passed into the duodenum is often an unanswerable question. Pain without ancillary findings of biliary obstruction is insufficient evidence. The efficacy of manometry in this situation is questionable. The appropriate treatment is sphincterotomy preferably performed through the endoscope,[29–31] but if endoscopic sphincterotomy is unavailable or there are other indications for laparotomy, it should be performed surgically (see pp. 1741–1744).

Cystic Duct Remnant.[32, 33] The cystic duct remnant has been blamed for some cases of postcholecystectomy distress. The postulated mechanisms include a gallstone trapped in the remnant; traction of the remnant distorting the common duct; or cyst, granuloma, or neuroma formation at the cut end.

Evidence to implicate the cystic duct remnant as a cause of postcholecystectomy pain is unconvincing except when there are discrete attacks accompanied by increased bilirubin and alkaline phosphatase levels and radiographic demonstration of residual gallstones in the cystic duct. Although there may be occasional instances in which a neuroma, granuloma, or cyst of the stump could cause pain, there are no reliable diagnostic criteria, and these mechanisms must still be considered hypothetical.

Diagnosis

Patients with postcholecystectomy complaints should have the usual liver function tests (e.g., serum alkaline phosphatase, bilirubin, SGOT) and amylase determinations. The presence of common duct stones or papillary stenosis does not correlate closely with the laboratory findings. For example, an anatomic abnormality may be found despite a normal alkaline phosphatase level; conversely, only two thirds of patients with an elevated alkaline phosphatase value have a demonstrable anatomic cause for their symptoms. The same inexact correlation has been noted between the findings on ERCP and elevations of the SGOT. Still, if the alkaline phosphatase, bilirubin, SGOT, and amylase values are all normal, the likelihood of finding a significant lesion on ERCP is low.

Sonography, ERCP, and transhepatic cholangiography are indicated in many cases. When ultrasonography shows a dilated common duct, ERCP will usually demonstrate a lesion. A normal sonogram, however, does not rule out biliary disease.

Endoscopic retrograde cholangiopancreatography is the test of choice because it allows investigation of the stomach, duodenum, biliary tree, and pancreatic duct, the location of most of the lesions responsible for postcholecystectomy pain.[34–36] As a general rule, ERCP should be performed in any patient with severe upper abdominal symptoms following cholecystectomy. An abnormality is nearly always found in patients with jaundice, cholangitis, or pancreatitis and in more than half of those with severe pain and dyspepsia. If the common duct cannot be successfully cannulated, a transhepatic cholangiogram should be performed. In the absence of jaundice, pancreatitis is the most common finding, but common duct stones are found in almost 10 per cent of such patients. Occasionally, a peptic ulcer that was missed on an earlier upper gastrointestinal series is discovered. In the presence of jaundice, common duct stones is the most common explanation, but benign and malignant strictures are also seen. Other conditions that may be diagnosed include biliary stricture, biliary carcinoma, ampullary stenosis, chronic pancreatitis, pancreas divisum, sclerosing cholangitis, incomplete cholecystectomy, pancreatic cyst, and pancreatic carcinoma.

Psychiatric Aspects

Patients with postcholecystectomy distress but without objective evidence for an anatomic abnormality of the biliary tree or for other intra-abdominal disease (reflux esophagitis, peptic ulcer, irritable colon, and so forth) often have psychiatric problems. Many have long histories of abdominal pain and a nonfunctioning or poorly functioning gallbladder or a gallbladder with stones but without inflammation. Cholecystectomy is often performed in such individuals in the vain hope of providing relief. Most of these patients are women. Psychiatric problems often underlie the complaints in patients with other plausible causes of postcholecystectomy distress (reflux esophagitis, and so forth) that do not respond to conventional therapy. One large study cited a 43 per cent incidence of psychiatric disturbances in patients who still had symptoms after cholecystectomy.[13]

Treatment

Treatment should be determined by the specific diagnosis. Patients who have considerable morbidity but no discernible organic disease may be benefited by psychiatric therapy.

References

1. Way, L. W., Bernhoft, R. A., and Thomas, M. J. Biliary stricture. Surg. Clin. North Am. *61*:963, 1981.
2. Way, L. W. Biliary stricture. *In* Way, L. W., and Pellegrini, C. A. (eds.): Surgery of the Gallbladder and Bile Ducts. Philadelphia, W. B. Saunders, 1987, Chap. 27.
3. Blumgart, L. H., and Thompson, J. N. The management of benign strictures of the bile ducts. Curr. Probl. Surg. *24*:1, 1987.
4. Genest, J. F., Nanos, E., Grundfest-Broniatowsik, S., Bogt, D., and Hermann, R. E. Benign biliary strictures: An analytic review (1970 to 1984). Surgery *99*:409, 1986.
5. Weinbren, K., Hadjis, N. S., and Blumgart, L. H. Structural aspects of the liver in patients with biliary disease and portal hypertension. J. Clin. Pathol. *38*:1013, 1985.
6. Mueller, P. R., vanSonnenberg, E., Ferrucci, J. T., Jr., Weyman, P. J., Butch, R. J., Malt, R. A., and Burhenne, H. J. Biliary stricture dilatation: Multicenter review of clinical management in 73 patients. Radiology *160*:17, 1986.
7. Russell, E., Yrizarry, J. M., Huber, J. S., Nunez, D., Jr., Hutson, D. G., Schiff, E., Reddy, K. R., Jeffers, L. J., and Williams, A. Percutaneous transjejunal biliary dilatation: Alternate management for benign strictures. Radiology *159*:290, 1986.
8. Vogel, S. B., Howard, R. J., Caridi, J., and Hawkins, I. F., Jr. Evaluation of percutaneous transhepatic balloon dilatation of benign biliary strictures in high-risk patients. Am. J. Surg. *149*:73, 1985.
9. Hutson, D. G., Russell, E., Schiff, E., Levi, J. J., Jeffers, L., and Zeppa, R. Balloon dilatation of biliary strictures through a choledochojejuno-cutaneous fistula. Ann. Surg. *199*:637, 1984.
10. Pellegrini, A. A., Thomas, M. J., and Way, L. W. Recurrent biliary stricture. Patterns of recurrence and outcome of surgical therapy. Am. J. Surg. *147*:175, 1984.
11. Pitt, H. A., Miyamoto, T., Parapatis, S. K., Tompkins, R. K., and Longmire, W. P. Factors influencing outcome in patients with postoperative biliary strictures. Am. J. Surg. *144*:14, 1982.
12. Bodvall, B. The postcholecystectomy syndromes. Clin. Gastroenterol. *2*:103, 1973.
13. Christiansen, J., and Schmidt, A. The postcholecystectomy syndrome. Acta Chir. Scand. *137*:789, 1971.
14. Ros, E., and Zambon, D. Postcholecystectomy symptoms. A prospective study of gall stone patients before and two years after surgery. Gut *28*:1500, 1987.
15. Schofield, G. E., and Macleod, R. G. Sequelae of cholecystectomy. Br. J. Surg. *53*:1042, 1966.
16. Duncan, A. W., Tibballs, J., and Sugherland, S. K. Investigation of postcholecystectomy problems. Med. J. Aust. *1*:214, 1982.
17. Simmons, F., and Bouchier, I. A. Intraluminal bile salt concentrations and fat digestion after cholecystectomy. S. Afr. Med. J. *46*:1089, 1972.
18. Roda, E., Aldini, R., Mazzella, G., Roda, A., Sama, C., Festi, D., and Barbara, L. Enterohepatic circulation of bile acids after cholecystectomy. Gut *19*:640, 1978.
19. Redinger, R. N. The effect of loss of gallbladder function on biliary, lipid composition in subjects with cholesterol gallstones. Gastroenterology *71*:470, 1976.
20. Shaffer, E. A., and Small, D. M. Biliary lipid secretion in cholesterol gallstone disease. The effect of cholecystectomy and obesity. J. Clin. Invest. *59*:828, 1977.
21. Palmer, R. H. The gallbladder and bile composition. Am. J. Dig. Dis. *21*:795, 1976.
22. Vernick, L. J., and Kuller, L. H. Cholecystectomy and right-sided colon cancer: An epidemiological study. Lancet *2*:381, 1981.
23. Gunn, A. A., and Foubister, G. Biliary surgery. A 5-year followup. Ann. R. Coll. Surg. Edinburgh *23*:292, 1978.
24. Glenn, F., and McSherry, C. K. Secondary abdominal operations for symptoms following biliary tract surgery. Surg. Gynecol. Obstet. *121*:979, 1965.
25. Cattell, R. B., Colcock, B. P., and Pollack, J. L. Stenosis of the sphincter of Oddi. N. Engl. J. Med. *256*:429, 1957.
26. Acosta, J. M., and Nardi, G. L. Papillitis. Inflammatory disease of the ampulla of vater. Arch. Surg. *92*:354, 1966.
27. Shingleton, W. W., and Gamburg, D. Stenosis of the sphincter of Oddi. Am. J. Surg. *119*:34, 1970.
28. Gregg, J. A., Clark, G., Barr, C., McCartney, A., Milano, A., and Volcjak, C. Postcholecystectomy syndrome and its association with ampullary stenosis. Am. J. Surg. *139*:374, 1980.
29. Shapiro, H. A. Endoscopic diagnosis and treatment of biliary tract disease. Surg. Clin. North Am. *61*:834, 1981.
30. Viceconte, G., Viceconte, G. W., Pietropaolo, V., and Montori, A. Endoscopic sphincterotomy: Indications and results. Br. J. Surg. *68*:376, 1981.
31. Siegel, J. H. Endoscopic papillotomy in the treatment of biliary tract disease. Dig. Dis. Sci. *26*:1057, 1981.
32. Larmi, T. I. I., Mokka, R., Kemppainen, P., and Seppala, A. A critical analysis of the cystic duct remnant. Surg. Gynecol. Obstet. *141*:48, 1975.
33. Hopkins, S. F., Bivins, B. A., and Griffen, W. O., Jr. The problem of the cystic duct remnant. Surg. Gynecol. Obstet. *148*:531, 1975.
34. Cooperman, M., Ferrara, J. J., Carey, L. C., Thomas, F. B., Martin, E. W., Jr., and Fromkes, J. J. Endoscopic retrograde cholangiopancreatography. Arch. Surg. *116*:606, 1981.
35. Blumgart, L. H., Carachi, R., Imrie, C. W., Benjamin, I. S., and Duncan, J. G. Diagnosis and management of postcholecystectomy symptoms: The place of endoscopy and retrograde choledochopancreatography. Br. J. Surg. *64*:809, 1977.
36. Ruddell, W. S. J., Ashton, M. G., Lintott, D. J., and Axon, A. T. R. Endoscopic retrograde cholangiography and pancreatography in investigation of post-cholecystectomy patients. Lancet *1*:444, 1980.

92 Neoplasms of the Gallbladder and Bile Ducts

LAWRENCE W. WAY
DAVID F. ALTMAN

CARCINOMA OF THE GALLBLADDER[1–10]

Etiology and Incidence

Primary carcinoma of the gallbladder is the most common malignant tumor of the biliary tract and in the United States is the fifth most frequent digestive tract malignancy. There are over 6000 new cases each year in the United States, and over 95 per cent of affected patients succumb to their disease. Gallstones are present in 80 per cent of individuals with gallbladder cancer, an association that accounts for the prevalence of women and certain racial and ethnic groups.[11, 12] Cancer of the gallbladder is two to six times more common in native Americans or persons of a mixed racial background that includes native American ancestry.[13] The risk of gallbladder cancer, for example, reaches 4 to 5 per cent in female native Americans by age 85, which is just about the same as the risk of lung cancer in a lifelong heavy smoker of the same age.[13] The risk in these peoples is high enough that cholecystectomy should be considered more pressing for minimally symptomatic gallstone disease than it is in Caucasians. Gallstones are probably etiologic; in patients with gallstone disease, atypical mucosal hyperplasia and carcinoma in situ develop in the gallbladder with increasing frequency with age.[14] Furthermore, large gallstones (i.e., >2 cm) appear to carry a greater risk than do small ones.[15] Environmental factors, chemical carcinogens, and parasitic disease of the biliary passages may play a role as well, and certain occupational groups may be at increased risk, especially workers in the rubber and automotive industries.[11] The incidence of gallbladder cancer increases steadily with age, the average patient being 69 years old. There is evidence that the incidence is decreasing in countries where cholecystectomy is performed liberally for symptomatic gallstone disease.[16]

Evidence from Japan[17, 18] indicates that many patients with gallbladder cancer have an anomalous union between the pancreatic duct and bile duct, the junction occurring outside the duodenal wall, 1.5 cm or more upstream from the papilla of Vater. This condition, which has also been implicated in the pathogenesis of congenital choledochal cyst, is thought to produce harmful effects by allowing reflux of pancreatic juice into the biliary tree. In one study[18] consisting of 96 patients with gallbladder cancer and 65 patients with anomalous union, the anomaly was present in 17 per cent of patients with cancer, and cancer was present in 25 per cent of patients with the anomaly.

Pathology

Adenocarcinoma accounts for more than 80 per cent of gallbladder malignancies, with squamous cell carcinomas, adenocanthomas, and others making up the remainder.[19–21] Dysplasia may be a histologic precursor of carcinoma in some cases.[22, 23] The tumors grow rapidly, and, by the time symptoms appear, spread beyond the gallbladder is common. Spread is most commonly via the lymphatics, generally first involving the cystic duct nodes and the pericholedochal nodes along the right side of the common bile duct.[24, 25] The system used to stage gallbladder cancer is described in Table 92–1.[24] Most long-term survivors following cholecystectomy have stage I or II disease. Unfortunately, 75 per cent of patients have stage IV or V disease by the time they present for medical care. Venous metastases may occur, principally via the cholecystic veins into the quadrate lobe of the liver. Papillary adenocarcinomas may spread directly via the cystic and common bile ducts into the liver. Metastases deep in the substance of the liver and distant spread represent a late stage of the disease.

Clinical and Radiologic Findings

Although there may be evidence of widespread intra-abdominal tumor, more frequently the patients present with jaundice or manifestations of chronic or acute cholecystitis.[1–10] A palpable right upper quadrant mass in an elderly patient with cholecystitis should strongly suggest the diagnosis of gallbladder carcinoma. If a mass can be felt, the lesion is virtually always incurable. Substantial weight loss may be an additional clue to the diagnosis. Tumors obstructing the biliary tree produce jaundice and occasionally cholangitis or even

Table 92–1. STAGING OF GALLBLADDER CARCINOMA

Stage	Extent of Involvement
I	Intramucosal
II	Submucosa and muscularis
III	Serosa
IV	Serosa plus regional lymph nodes
V	Extension into liver or distant metastases

hepatic abscess formation. Local abscesses may also occur adjacent to the gallbladder.

Oral cholecystograms usually do not opacify. Ultrasound scans may show gallstone disease, a mass, or in early cases a polypoid intraluminal tumor.[26, 27] The findings on CT scan[10, 26] may include the following: a mass filling or replacing the gallbladder; irregularity of the gallbladder wall; a soft tissue mass in the gallbladder lumen; a nonenhancing soft tissue mass in the hilum of the liver; low attenuation areas in the liver adjacent to the gallbladder (i.e., segments IV and V) and absence of a normal gallbladder outline; or dilatation of the intrahepatic bile ducts due to obstruction of the common hepatic duct near the bifurcation. Angiography is not particularly useful, but it may demonstrate stricturing or occlusion of the portal vein or encasement of the hepatic artery.

Because the findings are so often subtle or nonspecific, the correct diagnosis is made preoperatively in less than 10 per cent of cases.

Treatment

As the tumor is generally unsuspected preoperatively, most patients with gallbladder cancer undergo laparotomy for cholecystitis, jaundice, or cholangitis. In most patients, distant metastases or, more often, local invasion rules out any attempt at a curative resection.[1–10, 24] Tumors that obstruct the bile duct by direct extension are nearly always unresectable. These cases are best treated by a bile duct stent placed by a percutaneous transhepatic or endoscopic approach. In the 25 per cent of cases in which the tumor is confined to the gallbladder or spread is limited to adjacent areas, where it can be removed, there may be a chance for cure.[1] Cholecystectomy alone is sufficient for carcinoma in situ (stage I disease), which is usually an incidental finding.[7, 28] For invasive disease confined to the gallbladder, cholecystectomy, resection of a 3- to 5-cm wedge of liver constituting the gallbladder bed, and resection of the cystic duct and pericholedochal lymph nodes is the procedure of choice.[1, 7] This operation is indicated even in patients with invasive tumors confined to the mucosal or submucosal layers of the gallbladder, because their five-year survival rate is only 65 per cent with cholecystectomy alone.[29] In 25 per cent of patients the diagnosis is first made by the pathologist when examining a gallbladder removed for symptomatic gallstone disease. Although there is no proof that survival is prolonged, reoperation is recommended in these cases to resect the gallbladder bed and the nearby lymph nodes that tend to be involved early. More extensive operations, such as right hepatic lobectomy, appear only to add greater surgical risk. Adjunctive radiation and chemotherapy may also add to survival, but experience is limited.[2, 8, 30, 31]

A trial of chemotherapy that compared 5-FU, 5-FU plus streptozotocin, and 5-FU plus methyl-CCNU for advanced carcinoma of the gallbladder showed about a 10 per cent response rate with each regimen.[32] The efficacies of the regimens were similar, but toxicity of the two combinations was substantially greater than that of 5-FU alone.

Prognosis

For the majority of patients who have widespread disease at the time of diagnosis, there is no effective treatment; the operative mortality rate of 15 per cent reflects this hopeless situation. Median survival after diagnosis is six months. Only 5 per cent of patients survive for five years; in almost all these individuals, the tumor is discovered incidentally.[2, 8, 28, 29, 33] Furthermore, the survivors are almost entirely from among those whose tumors were confined to the mucosa and submucosa without invasion of the muscular layers or metastases to lymph nodes. Although early cholecystectomy would provide effective prophylaxis, only in native Americans is carcinoma frequent enough as a complication of gallstone disease for it to weigh heavily in favor of this approach.[13]

CANCER OF THE EXTRAHEPATIC BILE DUCTS

For unknown reasons, the incidence of primary neoplasms of the extrahepatic bile ducts, especially those at the bifurcation of the common hepatic duct, is increasing. The etiology of bile duct cancer is unclear.[34] Gallstones, which are present in 85 per cent of patients with gallbladder cancer, are found in only 30 per cent of those with bile duct neoplasms. A few other diseases are associated with biliary cancer, but they are absent in the majority of cases. Biliary cancer, for example, is more common in patients with ulcerative colitis.[35, 36] However, the risk of developing the biliary lesion is unrelated to the severity of the colitis. Congenital choledochal cysts, including those in Caroli's disease, are predisposed to malignant transformation.[37] The greater incidence of biliary carcinoma in the Orient is at least partly a result of the effects of *Clonorchis sinensis* infestation.[34] Workers in aircraft, automotive, chemical, rubber, and wood-finishing industries have a higher than average incidence of carcinoma of the extrahepatic bile ducts.[40]

The average age of affected persons is about 60 years; the range extends from 25 to 85 years. The frequency with which the tumors are found at various levels of the duct is as follows:[41–49] upper one third, 50 per cent; middle one third, 20 per cent; lower one third, 20 per cent; and diffuse, 10 per cent. A few arise from the cystic duct.[50]

Pathologically, most malignant bile duct tumors are adenocarcinomas.[41–49] The histologic appearance may be well differentiated, poorly differentiated, or anaplastic. The gross morphologic appearance may be infiltrating, nodular, scirrhous, or papillary. The last of these, which has a relatively good prognosis, is the least common. Multicentricity has been reported but does not seem to be common. The scirrhous variety constricts the duct in a manner resembling sclerosing cholangitis, and on microscopic section it may be difficult to identify the neoplastic cells amidst the fibrous stroma. These scirrhous lesions have occasionally been incorrectly diagnosed as benign; they may require multiple biopsies before an adequate specimen is obtained.

Because of the strategic location of the tumors, jaundice develops while they are still small, but local invasion of the portal vein, hepatic artery, or liver parenchyma is often present by the time of diagnosis. Metastases are initially present in only 20 per cent of patients, and even late in the course of the disease the morbidity more often results from effects of expansion of the primary lesion than from metastases.

Tumors at the very terminus of the common bile duct are difficult to distinguish from *carcinoma* of the *ampulla of Vater*. This latter cancer originates in tissue of the ampulla, is slow growing, and frequently exhibits only mild or no symptoms. Jaundice is common, is usually mild or only slowly progressive, and may even fluctuate. Weight loss is not marked, and stools may be guaiac positive for occult bleeding. On physical exam the gallbladder may be palpable. Rarely, the patient has intermittent fever, as in choledocholithiasis. As with patients who have other biliary tract cancer, the incidence of gallstones also is high in these patients.

Laboratory studies reveal elevated bilirubin (3.0 to 10.0 mg/dl) and alkaline phosphatase (two or more times normal) with good liver function. Ultrasound and CT examinations usually show dilated common bile duct and often dilation of proximal ducts as well. CT may show the tumor itself; however, investigations with contrast usually reveal only dilatation and a discrete terminal narrowing of the duct. Diagnosis is often confirmed by visualization of the tumor at endoscopy with biopsy. The importance of accurate diagnosis of this periampullary type of malignancy is the success of radical surgery (Whipple procedure), which carries a 50 per cent, 5-year cure rate, in marked contrast to cancer of the pancreas (see p. 1879). (Local excision is another option for elderly or poor risk patients. If the head of the pancreas is uninvolved, cure rate may be as high as 30 per cent.) Poor risk patients may be treated with endoscopic sphincterotomy, which provides good palliation (see pp. 1741–1744).

Clinical Manifestations[41–49]

Obstructive jaundice is usually the first clinical manifestation, although in 15 per cent of patients it is preceded by pruritus. Weight loss occurs in most patients. Cholangitis and biliary colic are uncommon, and the bile is usually sterile. The patient may experience a deep-seated dull pain, or there may be no pain. The stools may be clay-colored. Obstruction, however, may be minimal with tumors at the junction of the right and left hepatic ducts, in which alkaline phosphatase is disproportionately elevated (Klatskin cancer of the bifurcation).

The liver becomes enlarged and firm; the spleen is not enlarged unless obstruction has been present long enough to produce biliary cirrhosis. A palpable gallbladder is present if the obstruction is confined to the common bile duct and the cystic duct is uninvolved. If the cystic duct is obstructed, the gallbladder usually collapses and contains only a small volume of clear, thin fluid. Alternatively, obstruction of the cystic duct occasionally produces a distended hydrops of the gallbladder. Gallbladder distention is absent when the tumor arises from or involves the common hepatic duct.

Diagnosis[41–49, 51–59]

Primary bile duct tumors should be considered in the differential diagnosis of any case of obstructive jaundice. Malignant obstruction generally produces higher bilirubin levels (mean value, 18 mg/dl) than does choledocholithiasis (mean value, 5 mg/dl). In the early stages the intensity of the jaundice may fluctuate. The alkaline phosphatase values are nearly always elevated. The serum albumin level is below 3.5 gm/dl in half the patients. The SGOT is often elevated but rarely exceeds 200 U/dl.

Ultrasound and CT scans show dilated intra- and extrahepatic bile ducts down to the site of the lesion. Dilatation is rarely absent in neoplastic obstruction, and it is rarely missed on the scan. In advanced disease, a mass may be identified in the hilum or metastases may be seen. Cholangiography, either transhepatic or retrograde endoscopic, should be performed to demonstrate the site and extent of the block. If the cholangiogram shows a focal, high-grade obstruction and marked dilatation of the proximal ducts, the pattern is almost pathognomonic for malignancy.

It is important to remember that the demonstration of gallbladder stones by ultrasound is not reliable evidence that obstructive jaundice is caused by gallstones.[54] In fact, if the bilirubin value exceeds 10 mg/dl, the cause is most likely to be neoplastic obstruction.[51] A useful rule is to perform direct cholangiography in any patient whose bilirubin value is this high, unless a diagnosis of neoplastic obstruction is obvious from ultrasound and CT scans and treatment can be initiated without additional preoperative tests (as in some cases of pancreatic cancer).

In general, transhepatic cholangiography (THC) is more apt to be helpful than endoscopic cholangiography (ERCP), particularly for proximal lesions. The reason is that the block is so complete that the endoscopist is often unable to obtain complete opacification of the ducts on the hepatic side of the lesion, an area that must be well seen in order to plan therapy. On the other hand, for periampullary lesions, ERCP often provides information (e.g., about the pancreatic duct and the ampulla) not available from THC. For these reasons, a reasonable strategy is to perform THC if the gallbladder is not palpable and ERCP if the gallbladder is palpable, if the bilirubin level is below 10 mg/dl, or if there are contraindications (e.g., abnormal clotting) to THC. Then, if the first cholangiogram does not provide all the information desired, another one should be performed by the alternate technique.

Angiography is recommended preoperatively by some surgeons to help determine the resectability of the lesion and the anatomy of the hilar vessels.[57] Encasement of the hepatic artery or obstruction of the main portal vein suggests that the tumor is unresectable. On the other hand, occasionally a vessel appears to be involved, whereas exploration reveals it to be distorted but not invaded, and furthermore, it is sometimes possible to resect portions of involved vessels. Consequently, we no longer perform angiography in most patients.

Cytologic examination of bile obtained during THC reveals typical malignant cells in 25 to 50 per cent of cases.[59, 60] Direct percutaneous aspiration biopsy of the lesion is rarely feasible for biliary tumors because they are so small. Most often the histologic diagnosis is made by frozen section at the time of surgery. Nevertheless, the diagnosis is usually fairly certain preoperatively from the cholangiographic findings.

Differential Diagnosis

Other causes of obstructive jaundice must be considered in the differential diagnosis. Choledocholithiasis rarely yields bilirubin levels above 12 mg/dl, the usual range for neoplastic obstruction, and the levels in choledocholithiasis usually fluctuate. Calculous obstruction often produces colic and cholangitis, uncommon manifestations of neoplasms. Other types of neoplastic obstruction, such as gallbladder cancer, pancreatic cancer, metastatic carcinoma in hilar lymph nodes, and hilar lymphoma, may give similar findings. Extrinsic lesions may produce bowing of the duct, whereas intrinsic lesions appear to pinch off the lumen. However, obstruction due to hilar metastases sometimes gives a cholangiographic picture identical to that of a primary biliary tumor.[61]

The presence of a subcostal mass palpable on physical examination would suggest gallbladder or pancreatic cancer, or metastases from some remote site, rather than biliary cancer. Lesions of the distal bile duct may be difficult to differentiate from other periampullary tumors (e.g., pancreas or ampulla of Vater), and some middle-third lesions thought to originate in the duct are eventually shown to have arisen from the gallbladder and secondarily invaded the duct. There are rare cases of benign focal stenosis of the bifurcation that closely resemble a neoplasm.

Patients without a palpable gallbladder often present a difficult diagnostic problem. The gradual onset of jaundice or pruritus with little pain and no fever may suggest intrahepatic cholestasis. Occasionally these patients have been followed for months with a presumptive diagnosis of primary biliary cirrhosis or toxic (drug) hepatitis with cholestasis. An ultrasound scan is usually all that is necessary to suggest the correct diagnosis. Liver biopsy is usually inadequate to differentiate intrahepatic from extrahepatic cholestasis. As a general rule, one should assume that persistent cholestatic jaundice has an obstructive cause until cholangiography has proved otherwise.

Primary biliary cirrhosis occurs mainly in women between the ages of 40 and 60 years. Antimitochondrial antibodies can be demonstrated in about 90 per cent of patients with primary biliary cirrhosis, and the serum IgM value is elevated. In the early stages of primary biliary cirrhosis, the changes on liver biopsy are specific.

Treatment and Prognosis

Resection of the tumor is the best treatment. If resection is impossible, the obstructed duct should be decompressed by inserting tube stents or by anastomosing proximal dilated ducts to the gut.

Because renal failure sometimes develops postoperatively in severely jaundiced patients[62, 63] and experimental studies demonstrate that high bilirubin levels may impair renal function,[64–66] it became common practice several years ago to decompress the bile duct with a percutaneous transhepatic catheter for a week or so preoperatively.[67, 68] This allows the bilirubin level to decrease substantially, but every so often it is followed by complications (e.g., bleeding, cholangitis, and so forth).[69, 70] Meanwhile, in centers that specialize in complex biliary surgery, the incidence of complications and death after bile duct resections in deeply jaundiced patients has been dropping,[46, 71, 72] probably from improvements in many areas of surgical care. Subsequently, three controlled trials[71, 73, 74] all failed to show superior results with preoperative decompression, and at present there seems to be no definite indication for this technique.

Tumors at the bifurcation of the common hepatic duct (Klatskin tumors) are difficult to manage.[44–48, 75–80] Resection is preferred, and although technically demanding, it can be accomplished in about one half of patients. In many cases the tumor involves one of the two lobar ducts (usually the left) more extensively than the other (types IIIA and IIIB, Fig. 92–1), and the best operation consists of hepatic lobectomy in addition to resection of the bifurcation of the hepatic duct. It may sometimes be necessary to remove a short segment of focally involved portal vein. The length and quality of survival after resection is about twice that which is achieved with percutaneous or surgically placed stents. After the tumor is removed, bile drainage is re-established by constructing a Roux-en-Y hepaticojejunostomy to the liver hilum. Transhepatic tubes placed during surgery are usually left in place for a year or more to prevent recurrent tumor from blocking the ducts.

Unresectability is usually the result of spread of tumor into the adjacent hilar vessels. In these patients, the best treatment consists of an endoprosthesis (stent) placed percutaneously or endoscopically.[84–88] Today permanent external biliary catheters are rarely used for palliation. The stents range from 10 to 15 F in diameter, and the larger ones remain patent longer (see p. 1746).

The various configurations of hilar carcinoma are illustrated in Figure 92–1. For tubes to be effective in relieving jaundice, they must drain at least one entire lobe. Unfortunately, tumors with a type III or type IV configuration are most often unresectable, and they are not well drained by catheters either (Fig. 92–2). For example, a catheter in any duct of the right lobe in the presence of a type IIIA lesion will decompress only one segment; therefore, jaundice persists, often accompanied by refractory cholangitis in the undrained ducts. Treatment of a type IIIA lesion must entail drainage of the left duct and possibly one of the right ducts. The general rule is to obtain decompression of at least one lobe to correct the jaundice, but to anticipate the possibility that other large undrained ducts may be the site of continuing cholangitis. Then, additional catheters may be inserted into them as necessary.

Another surgical procedure occasionally used for palliation consists of anastomosing a dilated intrahepatic duct (usually the left duct) to a Roux-en-Y limb of jejunum.[81–83]

Tumors of the middle third of the bile duct may be resected or, if unresectable, either stented or bypassed internally into the gut. Tumors of the lower third require a pancreaticoduodenectomy (Whipple procedure) for removal.

Most experts favor the use of radiotherapy postoperatively either as definitive treatment for an unresectable primary tumor or as adjuvant therapy in the case of a resectable tumor. Treatment usually consists of 4500 to 5000 rads delivered by external supervoltage

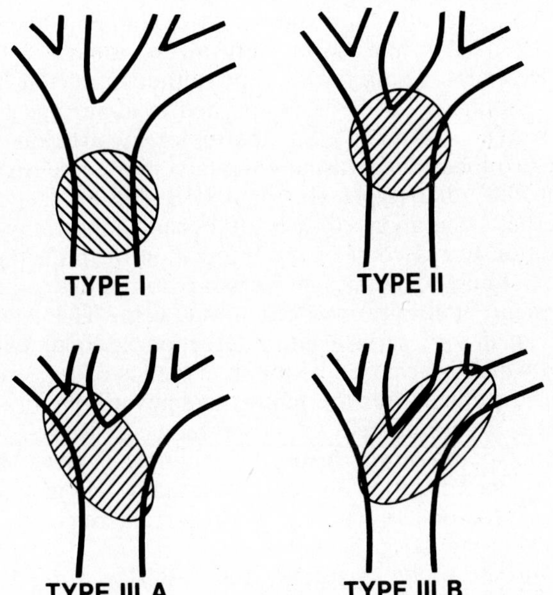

Figure 92–1. Various patterns of blockage produced by hilar bile duct carcinomas. Type IV (not illustrated) is a combination of types IIIA and IIIB. Resection of the right or left hepatic lobe would be required in the treatment of type IIIA or IIIB, respectively. The plan for obtaining decompression using percutaneous or surgically placed stents must differ for the different patterns of obstruction.

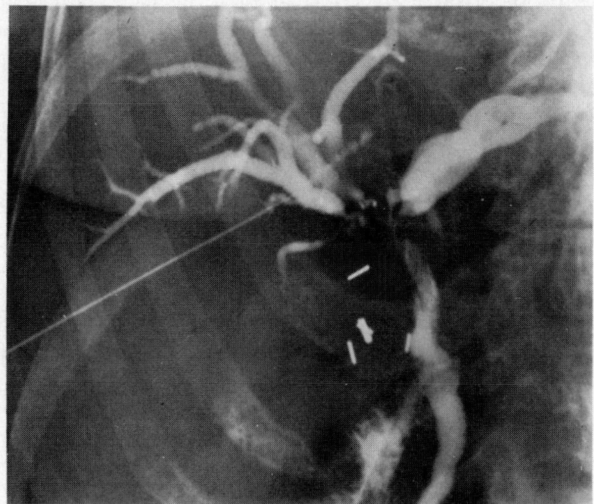

Figure 92–2. An example of the type IV pattern of bile duct obstruction due to an adenocarcinoma of the hepatic duct. In this kind of lesion, it is difficult with transhepatic tubes to obtain drainage that is adequate to return the bilirubin level to normal and avoid repeated attacks of cholangitis.

techniques.[89–91] To provide a target for postoperative treatment, the surgeon should place a few metal clips at the borders of the tumor during laparotomy. A new method involves passing a wire containing iridium-192 through a transhepatic catheter so that the radiation source is positioned within the tumor.[91, 92] The catheter is left in place for 48 hours and is then removed. X-rays emitted by iridium-192 penetrate only a few centimeters into the adjacent tissues, which allows a maximum dose to be delivered to the tumor with relative protection of the liver, intestine, and kidney. The results with iridium have so far been disappointing.[92] Radiotherapy is occasionally complicated by duodenitis or a radiation ulcer of the hepatic artery or portal vein.

Average survival following resection of all gross tumor is 20 months; after incomplete tumor removal, it is eight months; and after other procedures, it is three months. Most five-year survivors have had lesions of the middle or lower third of the duct. The five-year survival rate after a Whipple procedure for a lower-third lesion without distant spread is about 30 per cent.

References

1. Adson, M. A., and Farnell, M. B. Hepatobiliary cancer—Surgical considerations. Mayo Clin. Proc. *56*:686, 1981.
2. Roberts, J. W., and Daugherty, S. F. Primary carcinoma of the gallbladder. Surg. Clin. North Am. *66*:743, 1986.
3. Donaldson, L. A., and Busuttil, A. A clinicopathological review of 68 carcinomas of the gallbladder. Br. J. Surg. *26*:62, 1975.
4. Klamer, T. W., and Max, M. H. Carcinoma of the gallbladder. Surg. Gynecol. Obstet. *156*:641, 1983.
5. Hamrick, R. E., Jr., Liner, F. J., Hastings, P. R., and Cohn, I., Jr. Primary carcinoma of the gallbladder. Ann. Surg. *195*:270, 1982.
6. Koo, J., Wong, J., Cheng, F. C. Y., and Ong, G. B. Carcinoma of the gallbladder. Br. J. Surg. *68*:161, 1981.
7. Piehler, J. M., and Crichlow, R. W. Primary carcinoma of the gallbladder. Surg. Gynecol. Obstet. *147*:929, 1978.
8. Morrow, C. E., Sutherland, D. E. R., Florack, G., Eisenberg,

M. M., and Grage, T. B. Primary gallbladder carcinoma: significance of subserosal lesions and results of aggressive surgical treatment and adjuvant chemotherapy. Surgery *94*:709, 1983.

9. Shukla, V. K., Khandelwal, C., Roy, S. K., and Vaidya, M. P. Primary carcinoma of the gallbladder: a review of a 16-year period at the University Hospital. J. Surg. Oncol. *28*:32, 1985.
10. Collier, N. A., Carr, D., Hemingway, A., and Blumgart, L. H. Preoperative diagnosis and its effect on the treatment of carcinoma of the gallbladder. Surg. Gynecol. Obstet. *159*:465, 1984.
11. Diehl, A. K. Epidemiology of gallbladder cancer: a synthesis of recent data. J. Natl. Cancer Inst. *65*:1209, 1980.
12. Lowenfels, A. B. Gallstones and the risk of cancer. Gut *21*:1090, 1980.
13. Weiss, K. M. Phenotype amplification, as illustrated by cancer of the gallbladder in new world peoples. *In* Chakraborty, R., and Szathmary, E. J. (eds.). Diseases of Complex Etiology in Small Populations: Ethnic Differences and Research Approaches. New York, Alan R. Liss, 1985, pp. 179–198.
14. Albores-Saavedra, J., Alcantra-vasquez, A., Cruz-Ortiz, H., and Herrera-Goepfert, R. The precursor lesions of invasive gallbladder carcinoma. Hyperplasia, atypical hyperplasia and carcinoma in situ. Cancer *45*:919, 1980.
15. Diehl, A. K. Gallstone size and the risk of gallbladder cancer. JAMA *250*:2323, 1983.
16. Diehl, A. K., and Beral, V. Cholecystectomy and changing mortality from gallbladder cancer. Lancet *2*:187, 1981.
17. Nagata, E., Sakai, K., Kinoshita, H., and Kobayashi, Y. The relation between carcinoma of the gallbladder and an anomalous connection between the choledochus and the pancreatic duct. Ann. Surg. *202*:182, 1985.
18. Kimura, K., Ohto, M., Saisho, H., Unozawa, T., Tsuchiya, Y., Morita, M., Ebara, M., Matsutani, S., and Okuda, K. Association of gallbladder carcinoma and anomalous pancreaticobiliary ductal union. Gastroenterology *89*:1258, 1985.
19. Brandt-Rauf, P. W., Pincus, M., and Adelson, S. Cancer of the gallbladder: a review of forty-three cases. Hum. Pathol. *13*:48, 1982.
20. Sons, H. U., Borchard, F., and Joel, B. S. Carcinoma of the gallbladder: autopsy findings in 287 cases and review of the literature. J. Surg. Oncol. *28*:199, 1985.
21. Laitio, M. Histogenesis of epithelial neoplasms of human gallbladder. II. Classification of carcinoma on the basis of morphological features. Pathol. Res. Pract. *178*:57, 1983.
22. Ojeda, V. J., Shilkin, K. B., and Walters, M. N. I. Premalignant epithelial lesions of the gallbladder: a prospective study of 120 cholecystectomy specimens. Pathology *17*:451, 1985.
23. Laitio, M. Histogenesis of epithelial neoplasms of human gallbladder. I. Dysplasia. Pathol. Res. Pract. *178*:51, 1983.
24. Nevin, J. E., Moran, T. J., Kay, S., and King, R. Carcinoma of the gallbladder. Staging, treatment, and prognosis. Cancer *37*:141, 1976.
25. Fahim, R. B., McDonald, J. R., Richards, J. C., and Ferris, D. O. Carcinoma of the gallbladder: A study of its modes of spread. Ann. Surg. *156*:114, 1962.
26. Weiner, S. N., Koenigsberg, M., Morehouse, H., and Hoffman, J. Sonography and computed tomography in the diagnosis of carcinoma of the gallbladder. AJR *142*:735, 1984.
27. Koga, A., Yamauchi, S., Izumi, Y., and Hamanaka, N. Ultrasonographic detection of early and curable carcinoma of the gallbladder. Br. J. Surg. *72*:728, 1985.
28. Albores-Saavedra, J., Manrique, J. de J. Angeles-Angeles, A., and Henson, D. E. Carcinoma in situ of the gallbladder. A clinicopathologic study of 18 cases. Am. J. Surg. Pathol. *8*:323, 1984.
29. Bergdahl, L. Gallbladder carcinoma first diagnosed at microscopic examination of gallbladders removed for presumed benign disease. Ann. Surg. *191*:19, 1980.
30. Whetstone, M. R., Saltzstein, E. C., and Mercer, L. C. Demographic characteristics of gallbladder cancer in an area endemic for biliary calculi. Am. J. Surg. *152*:728, 1986.
31. Kopelson, G., and Gunderson, L. L. Primary and adjuvant radiation therapy in gallbladder and extrahepatic biliary tract carcinoma. J. Clin. Gastroenterol. *5*:43, 1983.
32. Falkson, G., Macintyre, J. M., and Moertel, C. G. Eastern cooperative oncology group experience with chemotherapy for inoperable gallbladder and bile duct cancer. Cancer *54*:965, 1984.
33. Appleman, R. M., Morlock, C. G., Dahlin, D. C., and Adson, M. A. Long term survival in carcinoma of the gallbladder. Surg. Gynecol. Obstet. *117*:459, 1963.
34. Bismuth, H., and Malt, R. A. Carcinoma of the biliary tract. N. Engl. J. Med. *301*:704, 1979.
35. Wee, A., Ludwig, J., Coffey, R. J., Jr., LaRusso, N. F., and Wiesner, R. H. Hepatobiliary carcinoma associated with primary sclerosing cholangitis and chronic ulcerative colitis. Hum. Pathol. *16*:719, 1985.
36. Mir-Madjlessi, S. H., Farmer, R. G., and Sivak, M. V., Jr. Bile duct carcinoma in patients with ulcerative colitis. Relationship to sclerosing cholangitis: report of six cases and review of the literature. Dig. Dis. Sci. *32*:145, 1987.
37. Rossi, R. L., Silverman, M. L., Braasch, J. W., Munson, J. L., and ReMine, S. G. Carcinomas arising in cystic conditions of the bile ducts. A clinical and pathologic study. Ann. Surg. *205*:377, 1986.
38. Nakanuma, Y., Terada, T., Tanaka, Y., and Ohta, G. Are hepatolithiasis and cholangiocarcinoma aetiologically related? A morphological study of 12 cases of hepatolithiasis associated with cholangiocarcinoma. Virchows Arch. Pathol. Anat. *406*:45, 1985.
39. Koga, A., Ichimiya, H., Yamaguchi, K., Miyazaki, K., and Nakayama, F. Hepatolithiasis associated with cholangiocarcinoma. Possible etiologic significance. Cancer *55*:2826, 1985.
40. Krain, L. S. Gallbladder and extrahepatic bile duct carcinoma. Analysis of 1,808 cases. Geriatrics *27*:111, 1972.
41. Tompkins, R. K., Thomas, D., Wile, A., and Longmire, W. P., Jr. Prognostic factors in bile duct carcinoma. Analysis of 96 cases. Ann. Surg. *194*:447, 1981.
42. Alexander, F., Rossi, R. L., O'Bryan, M., Khettry, U., Braasch, J. W., and Watkins, E., Jr. Biliary carcinoma. A review of 109 cases. Am. J. Surg. *147*:503, 1984.
43. Anderson, J. B., Cooper, M. J., and Williamson, R. C. N. Adenocarcinoma of the extrahepatic biliary tree. Ann. R. Col. Surg. Engl. *67*:139, 1985.
44. Gibby, D. G., Hanks, J. B., Wanebo, H. J., Kaiser, D. L., Tegtmeyer, C. J., Chandler, J. G., and Jones, R. S. Bile duct carcinoma. Diagnosis and treatment. Ann. Surg. *202*:139, 1985.
45. Tsunoda, T., Tsuchiya, R., Harada, N., Noda, T., and Yamamoto, K. Surgical treatment for carcinoma of the extrahepatic bile duct. Jpn. J. Surg. *15*:123, 1985.
46. Langer, J. C., Langer, B., Taylor, B. R., Zeldin, R., and Cummings, B. Carcinoma of the extrahepatic bile ducts: results of an aggressive surgical approach. Surgery *98*:752, 1985.
47. Roberts, J. W. Carcinoma of the extrahepatic bile ducts. Surg. Clin. North Am. *66*:751, 1986.
48. Blumgart, L. H., and Thompson, J. N. The management of malignant strictures of the bile duct. Curr. Probl. Surg. *24*:69, 1987.
49. Bruggen, J. T., McPhee, M. S., Bhatia, P. S., and Richter, J. M. Primary adenocarcinoma of the bile ducts. Clinical characteristics and natural history. Dig. Dis. Sci. *31*:840, 1986.
50. Manabe, T., and Sugie, T. Primary carcinoma of the cystic duct. Arch. Surg. *113*:1202, 1978.
51. Pellegrini, C. A., Thomas, M. J., and Way, L. W. Bilirubin and alkaline phosphatase values before and after surgery for biliary obstruction. Am. J. Surg. *143*:67, 1982.
52. Thomas, M. J., Pellegrini, C. A., and Way, L. W. Usefulness of diagnostic tests for biliary obstruction. Am. J. Surg. *144*:102, 1982.
53. Okuda, K., Ohto, M., and Tsuchiya, Y. The role of ultrasound, percutaneous transhepatic cholangiography, computed tomographic scanning and magnetic resonance imaging in the preoperative assessment of bile duct cancer. World J. Surg. *12*:18, 1988.
54. Gordon, P., Cooperberg, P. L., and Cohen, M. M. Presence of gallstones is a poor indicator of the cause of obstructive jaundice. Surg. Gynecol. Obstet. *151*:635, 1980.
55. Nichols, D. A., MacCarty, R. L., and Gaffey, T. A. Cholangiographic evaluation of bile duct carcinoma. AJR *141*:1291, 1983.
56. Beazley, R. M., Hadjis, N., Benjamin, I. S., and Blumgart, L.

H. Clinicopathological aspects of high bile duct cancer. Experience with resection and bypass surgical treatments. Ann. Surg. *199*:623, 1984.
57. Voyles, C. R., Bowley, N. J., Allison, D. J., Benjamin, I. S., and Blumgart, L. H. Carcinoma of the proximal extrahepatic biliary tree radiologic assessment and therapeutic alternatives. Ann. Surg. *197*:188, 1983.
58. Dooms, G. C., Kerlan, R. K., Jr., Hricak, H., Wall, S. D., and Margulis, A. R. Cholangiocarcinoma: Imaging by MR. Radiology *159*:89, 1986.
59. Cohan, R. H., Illescas, F. F., Newman, G. E., Braun, S. D., and Dunnick, N. R. Biliary cytodiagnosis. Bile sampling for cytology. Invest. Radiol. *20*:177, 1985.
60. Harrell, G. S., Anderson, M. F., and Berry, P. F. Cytologic bile examination in the diagnosis of biliary duct neoplastic strictures. Am. J. Roentgenol. *137*:1123, 1981.
61. Warshaw, A. L., and Welch, J. P. Extrahepatic biliary obstruction by metastatic colon carcinoma. Ann. Surg. *188*:593, 1978.
62. Allison, M. E. M., Prentice, C. R. M., Kennedy, A. C., and Blumgart, L. H. Renal function and other factors in obstructive jaundice. Br. J. Surg. *66*:392, 1979.
63. Dawson, J. L. The incidence of postoperative renal failure in obstructive jaundice. Br. J. Surg. *52*:663, 1965.
64. Koyama, K., Ito, K., Fukaya, H., Okabe, K., and Sato, T. Experimental and clinical studies on renal disturbance in obstructive jaundice. Jpn. J. Surg. *11*:440, 1981.
65. Masumoto, T., and Masuoka, S. Kidney function in the severely jaundiced dog. Am. J. Surg. *140*:426, 1980.
66. Ozawa, K., Yamada, T., Tanaka, J., Ukikusa, M., and Tobe, T. The mechanism of suppression of renal function in patients and rabbits with jaundice. Surg. Gynecol. Obstet. *149*:54, 1979.
67. Denning, D. A., Ellison, E. C., and Carey, L. C. Preoperative percutaneous transhepatic biliary decompression lowered operative morbidity in patients with obstructive jaundice. Am. J. Surg. *141*:61, 1981.
68. Gobien, R. P., Stanley, J. H., Soucek, C. D., Anderson, M. C., Vujic, I., and Gobien, B. S. Routine preoperative biliary drainage: effect on management of obstructive jaundice. Radiology *152*:343, 1984.
69. Stambuk, E. C., Pitt, H. A., Pais, O. S., Mann, L. L., Lois, J. F., and Gomes, A. S. Percutaneous transhepatic drainage. Risks and benefits. Arch. Surg. *118*:1388, 1983.
70. Nilsson, U., Evander, A., Ihse, I., Lunderquist, A., and Mocibob, A. Percutaneous transhepatic cholangiography and drainage. Risks and complications. Acta Radiol. *24*:433, 1983.
71. Pitt, H. A., Gomes, A. S., Lois, J. F., Mann, L. L., Deutsch, L. S., and Longmire, W. P., Jr. Does preoperative percutaneous biliary drainage reduce operative risk or increase hospital cost? Ann. Surg. *201*:545, 1985.
72. Pellegrini, C. A., Allegra, P., Bongard, F. S., and Way, L. W. Risk of biliary surgery in patients with hyperbilirubinemia. Am. J. Surg. *154*:111, 1987.
73. Hatfield, A. R. W., Terblanche, J., Fataar, S., Kernoff, L., Tobias, R., Girdwood, A. H., Harries-Jones, R., and Marks, I. N. Preoperative external biliary drainage in obstructive jaundice. Lancet 2:896, 1982.
74. McPherson, G. A. D., Benjamin, I. S., Hodgson, H. J. F., Bowley, N. B., Allison, D. J., and Blumgart, L. H. Preoperative percutaneous transhepatic biliary drainage: The results of a controlled trial. Br. J. Surg. *71*:371, 1984.
75. Iwasaki, Y., Okamura, T., Ozaki, A., Todoroki, T., Takase, Y., Ohara, K., Nishimura, A., and Otsu, H. Surgical treatment for carcinoma at the confluence of the major hepatic ducts. Surg. Gynecol. Obstet. *162*:457, 1986.
76. Mizumoto, R., Kawarada, Y., and Suzuki, H. Surgical treatment of hilar carcinoma of the bile duct. Surg. Gynecol. Obstet. *162*:153, 1986.
77. Bismuth, H., Castaing, D., and Traynor, O. Resection or palliation: priority of surgery in the treatment of hilar cancer. World J. Surg. *12*:39, 1988.
78. Pinson, C. W., and Rossi, R. L. Extended right hepatic lobectomy, left hepatic lobectomy, and skeletonization resection for proximal bile duct cancer. World J. Surg. *12*:52, 1988.
79. Sakaguchi, S., and Nakamura, S. Surgery of the portal vein in resection of cancer of the hepatic hilus. Surgery *99*:344, 1986.
80. Cameron, J. L., Broe, P., and Zuidema, G. D. Proximal bile duct tumors. Surgical management with silastic transhepatic biliary stents. Ann. Surg. *196*:412, 1982.
81. Cahow, C. E. Intrahepatic cholangiojejunostomy: A new simplified approach. Am. J. Surg. *137*:443, 1979.
82. Dudley, S. E., Edis, A. J., and Adson, M. A. Biliary decompression in hilar obstruction. Round ligament approach. Arch. Surg. *114*:519, 1979.
83. Cameron, J. L., Gayler, B. W., and Harrington, D. P. Modification of the Longmire procedure. Ann. Surg. *187*:379, 1978.
84. Mueller, P. R., Ferrucci, J. T., Teplick, S. K., Van Sonnenberg, E., Haskin, P. H., Butch, R. J., and Panicoalaou, N. Biliary stent endoprosthesis: analysis of complications in 113 patients. Radiology *156*:637, 1985.
85. Lammer, J., Neumayer, K., and Steiner, H. Biliary endoprostheses in tumors at the hepatic duct bifurcation. Europ. J. Radiol. *6*:275, 1986.
86. Siegel, J. H. Improved biliary decompression with large caliber endoscopic prostheses. Gastrointest. Endosc. *30*:21, 1984.
87. Yamakawa, T., Esguerra, R. D., Kaneko, H., and Fukuma, E. Percutaneous transhepatic endoprosthesis in malignant obstruction of the bile duct. World J. Surg. *12*:78, 1988.
88. Siegel, J. H., and Daniel, S. J. Endoscopic and fluoroscopic transpapillary placement of a large caliber biliary endoprosthesis. Am. J. Gastroenterol. *79*:461, 1984.
89. Fields, J., and Bahman, E. Carcinoma of the extrahepatic biliary system—results of primary and adjuvant radiotherapy. Int. J. Radiat. Oncol. Biol. Phys. *13*:331, 1987.
90. Buskirk, S. J., Gunderson, L. L., Adson, M. A., Martinez, A., May, G. R., McIlrath, D. C., Nagorney, D. M., Edmundson, G. K., Bender, C. E., and Martin, J. K., Jr. Analysis of failure following curative irradiation of gallbladder and extrahepatic bile duct carcinoma. Int. J. Radiat. Oncol. Biol. Phys. *10*:2013, 1984.
91. Johnson, D. W., Safai, C., and Goffinet, D. R. Malignant obstructive jaundice: treatment with external-beam and intracavitary radiotherapy. Int. J. Radiat. Oncol. Biol. Phys. *11*:411, 1985.
92. Molt, P., Hopfan, S., Watson, R. C., Botet, J. F., and Brennan, M. F. Intraluminal radiation therapy in the management of malignant biliary obstruction. Cancer *57*:536, 1986.

93

Endoscopic/Radiologic Treatment of Biliary Tract Diseases

HOWARD A. SHAPIRO
TIMOTHY P. MARONEY
ERNEST J. RING

DIRECT CHOLANGIOGRAPHY

Direct cholangiography has proved to be the most reliable method of evaluating biliary tract disease.[1–4] Although important for screening, the noninvasive imaging techniques, ultrasonography and computed tomography, are far less accurate in portraying ductal anatomy and demonstrating specific disease.[5–8] Often, the choice between performing endoscopic retrograde cholangiopancreatography (ERCP) or percutaneous transhepatic cholangiography (PTC) has depended on whether the biliary tree is dilated. In major medical centers where operators are becoming increasingly experienced, the success rate of both methods approximates 90 to 95 per cent with an acceptably low complication rate of 3 to 5 per cent. In smaller centers the choice between ERCP and PTC is usually based on local expertise. When operators have equivalent expertise with PTC and ERCP, the decision should rest on the potential therapeutic maneuvers of each technique.[9, 10]

It is not surprising that technical advances have extended these diagnostic modalities into important therapeutic tools for the management of biliary tract disease. The relatively simple drainage function of the biliary tree and the mechanical nature of the disease processes which affect it lend themselves to innovative therapies. Moreover, the poor prognosis for most malignancies causing ductal obstructions and the high morbidity and mortality rates associated with surgical bypass procedures in patients with extensive tumor have encouraged the development of nonoperative methods of palliation.

Three potential access routes exist through which biliary interventions can be performed: endoscopic retrograde catheterization, surgical drainage tracts, and direct percutaneous puncture. Endoscopy provides excellent visibility to permit a variety of interventions in the periampullary area including sphincterotomy. Fluoroscopy provides an overview of ductal anatomy to guide manipulations within the duct for placement of stents through obstructing lesions, removal of ductal stones, and positioning of balloon dilating catheters into benign strictures.

In this chapter we focus on the current status of biliary interventions from these approaches including the indications, therapeutic potential, and limitations of each technique as well as experience with combined approaches that further extend the range of nonoperative treatment of biliary tract disease.

ENDOSCOPIC SPHINCTEROTOMY

Approximately 600,000 cholecystectomies are performed each year in the United States. Although it is unusual for a surgeon to overlook or leave stones within the common bile duct during a biliary tract operation, about 30,000 patients each year will have retained, residual, or recurrent common duct stones i.e., *choledocholithiasis*, at some time after cholecystectomy[11–13] (see pp. 1718–1721).

Indications

Transendoscopic incision of the papilla of Vater and extraction of common duct stones first became possible with the development of the side-viewing duodenoscope and diathermy sphincterotomes. In 1974, studies from Japan and Germany first reported experience with this operation,[14, 15] and in the ensuing three years worldwide interest grew regarding the application of this technique as an alternative to operative choledochotomy and stone extraction.[16–18] Large series of patients have been reported demonstrating that endoscopic sphincterotomy is clearly the procedure of choice for the management of common duct stones after cholecystectomy.[19–21]

In patients with retained common duct stones and a suitable T-tube in place, percutaneous extraction of the stone through the T-tube tract is preferred and endoscopic sphincterotomy should be performed only if the safer percutaneous approach fails.[22]

In patients at high surgical risk who have an intact gallbladder and choledocholithiasis, combined endoscopic sphincterotomy and stone extraction is excellent treatment. Prompt resolution of symptoms also follows when the same treatment is applied to cases of acute gallstone pancreatitis.[23] Similarly, acute cholangitis resolves most dramatically following endoscopic sphincterotomy. In frail or elderly patients with intact gallbladders, endoscopic sphincterotomy will clear the common duct, and cholecystectomy can be performed at a later time if cholecystitis ensues. Recent large European series report a 6 to 10 per cent incidence of subsequent cholecystitis during a one- to six-year follow-up.[24, 25] For patients with intact gallbladders at standard risk for surgery, the question of whether endoscopic sphincterotomy is indicated remains unanswered, but current judgment in the United States favors surgery.

Stenosis of the *papilla of Vater* is difficult to diagnose.[26–28] The most notable symptom is recurrent epigastric or right upper quadrant abdominal pain similar to that of biliary or pancreatic origin. There is biochemical evidence of intermittent or constant cholestasis (elevated levels of serum bilirubin or alkaline phosphatase) or pancreatitis (elevated serum amylase), and it is a condition common to patients after cholecystectomy. On sonography and ERCP, the common bile duct is often dilated and has delayed (longer than 45 minutes) drainage of contrast material. The value of sphincter of Oddi manometry in confirming pressure elevations and predicting a good clinical result from endoscopic sphincterotomy is argued persuasively by the Milwaukee group.[28, 29] Other investigators, however, have found no predictive value from endoscopic manometry[30] (see p. 1732). The clinical application of this tool remains unresolved. With our present knowledge, sphincterotomy should be performed for papillary stenosis only in patients with prolonged symptoms and severe disability who have been unresponsive to symptomatic therapy.[31] The greatest danger of endoscopic sphincterotomy in papillary stenosis is indiscriminate use which might subject patients to risks higher than those of endoscopic sphincterotomy for choledocholithiasis and with less chance of lasting benefits.

The *sump syndrome* is an infrequent complication of side-to-side choledochoduodenostomy. Foreign debris may accumulate in the bypassed segment of the common duct and act as a nidus for recurrent cholangitis. Endoscopic sphincterotomy permits clearance of debris or biliary stones from the distal common duct and is highly successful in resolving the pain and recurrent cholangitis typical of this syndrome.[32, 33]

In patients with *tumors* of the *papilla of Vater*, jaundice and pruritus are palliated after endoscopic sphincterotomy.[34] However, this procedure should only be performed in patients at significant surgical risk because definitive surgery has a high cure rate in otherwise healthy patients. Endoscopic sphincterotomy can also be used as a temporizing measure when attempting to convert a poor-risk patient into a surgical candidate. Endoscopic placement of biliary endoprostheses in these patients provides an alternative measure of palliation[35] (see p. 1879).

Contraindications

Significant coagulation defects are detected by always obtaining a screening prothrombin time, partial thromboploastin time, and platelet count and can generally be corrected by administration of the appropriate coagulation factors. A long stricture of the distal common duct would increase the risk of retroduodenal perforation or pancreatic damage. In patients with large common duct stones; i.e., greater than 2 cm to 2.5 cm in diameter or in those with smaller stones but a short intraduodenal segment of the common bile duct, operative choledochotomy is preferable to endoscopic sphincterotomy. However, in poor-risk patients with large stones, several nonoperative options exist if sphincterotomy is performed. Some surprisingly large stones pass spontaneously. A long biliary retention catheter (nasobiliary drain) can be placed in the proximal common duct following sphincterotomy with the other end routed out the nose and left in place for days to weeks.[36, 37] This allows performance of frequent cholangiograms to see if the stones have passed and also functions to decompress the biliary tree if retained stones impact the distal bile duct. Infusion of a gallstone-dissolving agent such as mono-octanoin through a nasobiliary drain is sometimes effective in reducing the stone size and facilitating passage through the sphincterotomy opening.[38] One or several double-pigtail catheters can be placed in the bile duct, preventing the stone from impacting distally. One patient in our series is doing well five years after placement of a biliary stent and is without evidence of recurrent jaundice or cholangitis. A new mechanical lithotripsy device that has become available[39] is composed of a basket with high tensile strength wires for mechanical cutting and a coil spring sheath for firm traction on the stone. Still in preliminary development, the device is unfortunately quite difficult to maneuver; future versions may prove even more promising. Electric spark pulsing lithotripsy, extracorporeal ultrasonic lithotripsy, and YAG laser are also in the early stages of experimental development.

Peri-Vaterian duodenal diverticuli, impacted gallstones, and prior *subtotal gastrectomy* with Billroth II anastomosis are *not* contraindications for endoscopic sphincterotomy. Although failure may be caused by technical difficulties encountered in identifying the papilla or properly seating the sphincterotomy, neither should preclude attempting the procedure.

Technique

Prior to performance of endoscopic sphincterotomy, informed consent must be obtained after careful explanation to the patient and family of alternative treatments, procedural details, and the relative risks and benefits. In case of complications expert surgical backup is essential. Antibiotics are used prophylactically in patients with common duct obstruction or recent cholangitis, but are usually discontinued shortly after successful relief of obstruction.

The initial diagnostic ERCP is crucial to determining the feasibility or advisability of sphincterotomy. Findings that influence advisability include the size and number of intraductal calculi, the presence of biliary stricture, the length of the intraduodenal segment of the bile duct, the presence and location of peri-Vaterian diverticuli, and the presence or absence of associated diseases whose management might require surgery.

Following the diagnostic ERCP, the sphincterotome is passed deeply and selectively into the common bile duct (Fig. 93–1). The Erlangen model is most frequently used in the United States and consists of an electrosurgical wire enclosed in a Teflon catheter, an adjusting handle, and a sideport for injecting contrast material. The exposed distal 2 cm to 4 cm of wire is the electrosurgical cutting edge. The adjusting handle attached to the diathermy unit is used to flex the cutting wire. After fluoroscopy demonstrates proper placement of the sphincterotome within the bile duct, the sphincterotome is withdrawn so that approximately one half to two thirds of the wire is visible in the duodenum outside the papillary orifice. The length of the intramural segment of the common duct is usually visible as a bulge superior to the papillary orifice. The wire is oriented in a twelve o'clock position in relation to the papilla by gentle flexion of the cutting wire and manipulation of the directional tip of the duodenoscope. Short bursts of a blended diathermy current are then applied so that a measured cut of sufficient length can be made through the sphincter muscle to allow passage of all stones. In order to determine the necessary size of the orifice, a balloon-tipped catheter can be inflated within the bile duct and pulled into the duodenal lumen.

To prevent reimpaction and subsequent cholangitis, removal of stones is optimally performed at the time of sphincterotomy. A balloon-tipped catheter, the safest and most preferred stone extractor, is inflated after deep passage into the proximal bile duct and, under fluoroscopic guidance, is then pulled down the bile duct, sweeping the stone before it (Fig. 93–2). With extensively dilated bile ducts or large stones, this technique may fail. Insertion of a Dormia basket under fluoroscopic guidance may then be required to attempt extraction by engagement of the stone within the basket (Fig. 93–3). If this technique also proves unsuccessful, a nasobiliary drain is usually left in the bile duct, and time is allowed for spontaneous passage of the stone (Fig. 93–4). If this maneuver is not successful, alternative therapies include a repeat attempt at stone extraction, lithotriptic stone crushing, mono-octanoin infusion, palliative endoscopic biliary stent placement, or surgery. In the uncomplicated patient, however, the average duration of hospitalization is 48 hours.

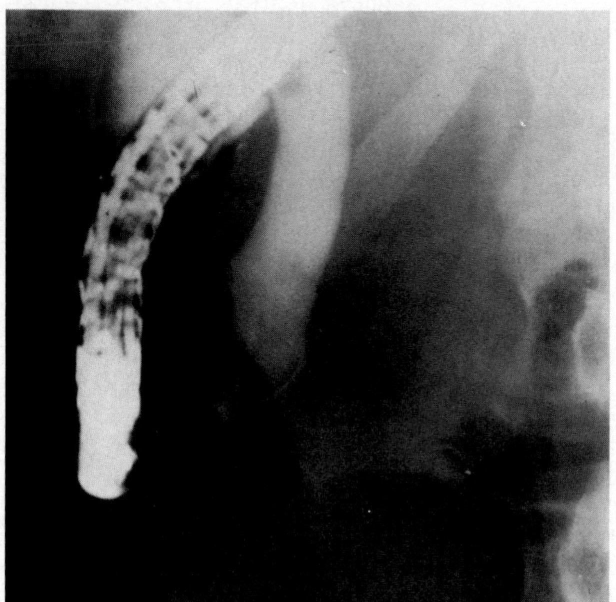

Figure 93–1. The sphincterotome is properly seated in the distal bile duct and bowel. The papilla of Vater is tented into the doudenal lumen and is seen in profile. A small stone is seen in the bile duct.

Results

By 1984, the tenth anniversary of endoscopic sphincterotomy, more than 50,000 had been performed worldwide.[21] The unqualified acceptance of this new technique is based upon a worldwide success rate for endoscopic sphincterotomy and stone extraction of 80 to 90 per cent.[20, 21] Failures are most often secondary to either large stones or disordered anatomy (papilla within a diverticulum, Billroth II gastrectomy). Experience favors success; the results are not so good during the learning phase. The best results may not be from the centers with the largest experience because these institutions treat the most difficult patients (usually referred), and further, the initial attempts at sphincterotomy are often made by trainees.

Complication rates are acceptably low universally. They range from 6 to 10 per cent with a need for urgent surgery in 1 to 2 per cent of cases, and an overall mortality rate of 0.4 to 1.4 per cent.[20, 21] Bleeding is the most frequent complication and is directly the cause of one half of the deaths. It is generally treated conservatively because surgical procedures to arrest bleeding are difficult to perform. Arteriographic embolization may be a reasonable alternative, if the vessel can be located. Pancreatitis is difficult to differentiate from a contained perforation in the pancreas. Both are treated conservatively and rarely require surgical drainage. Free retroduodenal perforation is also best managed conservatively unless a retroperitoneal abscess develops. This can be drained percutaneously under ultrasound guidance as an alternative to surgery. Cholangitis should become diminishingly rare as better technique is used to prevent stone impaction, such as the routine use of nasobiliary drains in failed stone extractions.

Common duct stones in patients with intact gallbladders represent a special situation. In several European series between 6 and 10 per cent will require cholecystectomy for biliary pain or cholecystitis in a six-year follow-up period after endoscopic removal of common duct stones.[21, 25] Preliminary data from the United States support these figures.[40] Most patients do not have complications from the remaining gallbladder stones; hence, an elective cholecystectomy is generally not indicated.

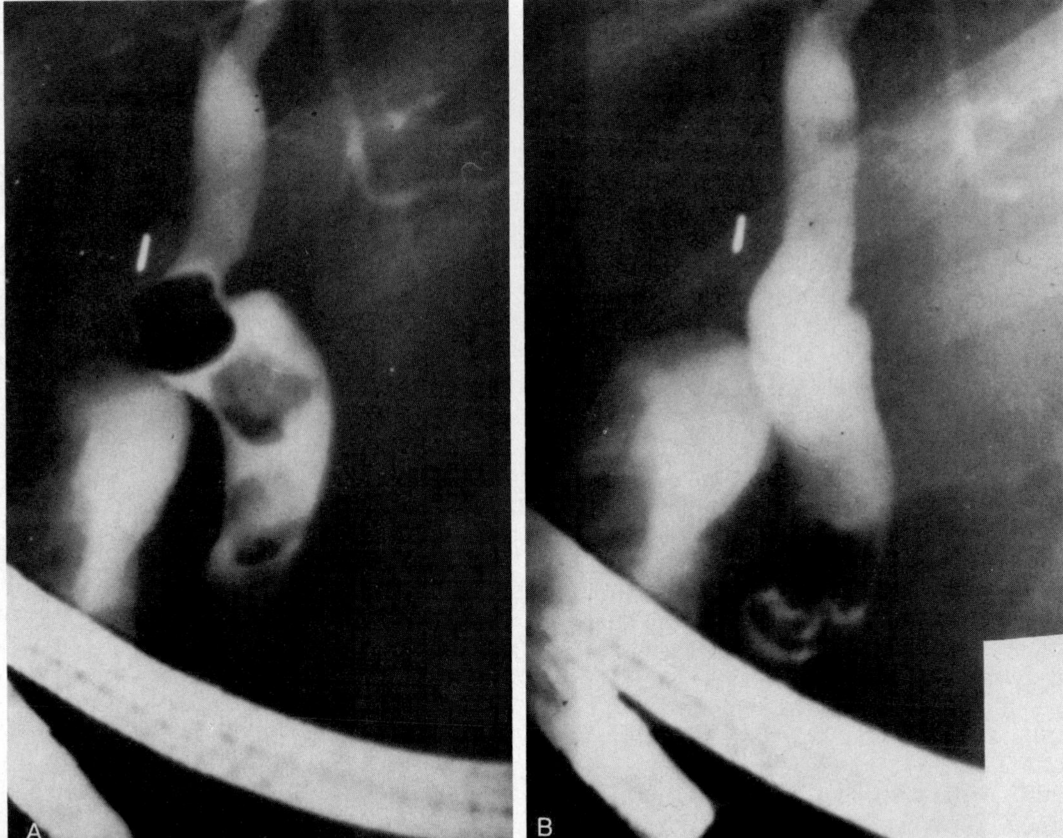

Figure 93–2. *A*, A balloon catheter is inflated in the bile duct proximal to several common duct stones. *B*, The balloon catheter has been pulled into the distal bile duct, sweeping the stones before it and extruding them into the duodenal lumen.

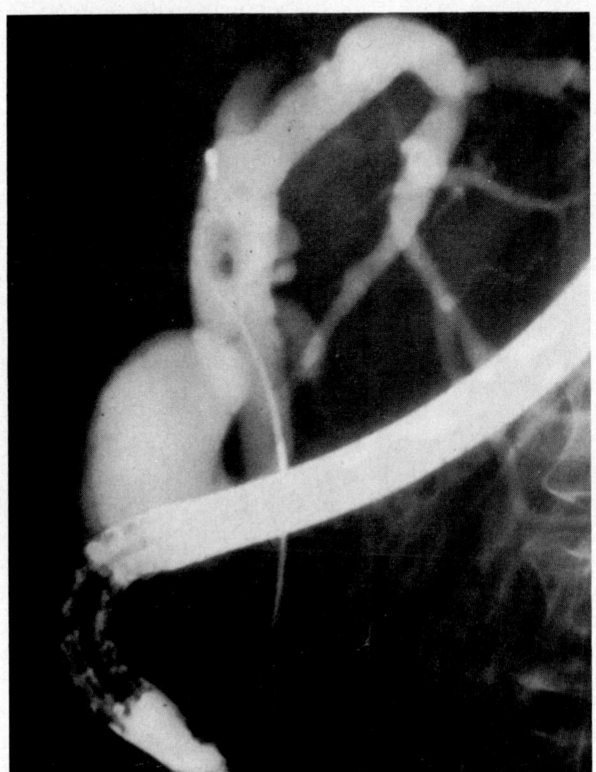

Figure 93–3. A stone is entrapped in a Dormia basket in the common bile duct prior to extraction.

Late complications are difficult to assess because they can be answered only in the long term. In several studies, however, 5 to 10 per cent will develop either new stones, or distal duct stenosis, or both in one to seven years after sphincterotomy.[21, 25, 41] These complications also can generally be treated endoscopically.

These results compare quite favorably with surgical series that report a 3 to 4.5 per cent mortality rate and a delayed complication rate of up to 10 per cent following choledochotomy.[42, 43] Cost analyses have been done comparing surgery and endoscopic sphincterotomy, with the latter being far less expensive. The occasional failure of endoscopic sphincterotomy does not preclude surgery.

ENDOSCOPIC METHODS FOR RELIEF OF BENIGN AND MALIGNANT BILIARY STRICTURES

Shortly after endoscopic sphincterotomy became standard acceptable treatment for extraction of common duct stones in high-risk patients, techniques for endoscopic decompression of the intractably obstructed biliary tree were developed. These approaches were a direct outgrowth of the technical refinements of those groups with large experiences and include endoscopic drainage of obstructed bile ducts, dilation of both

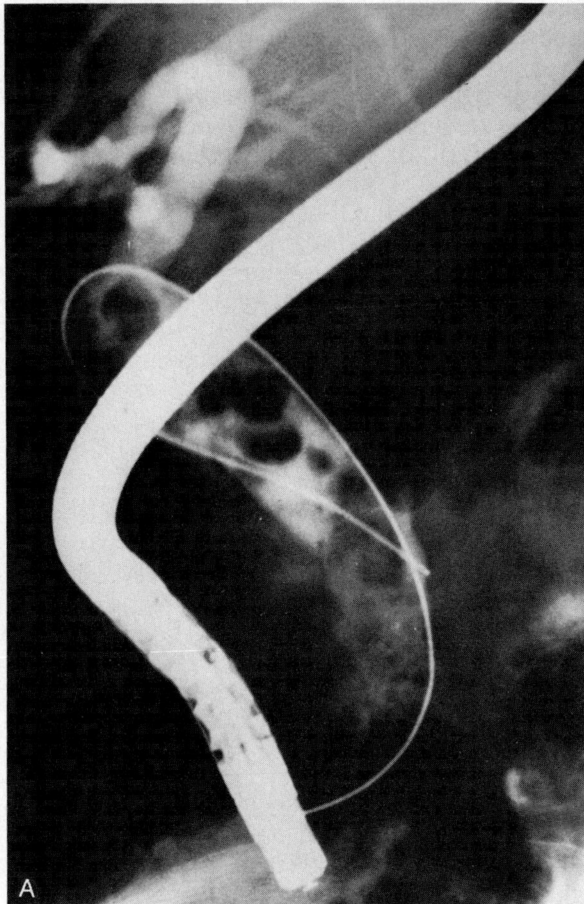

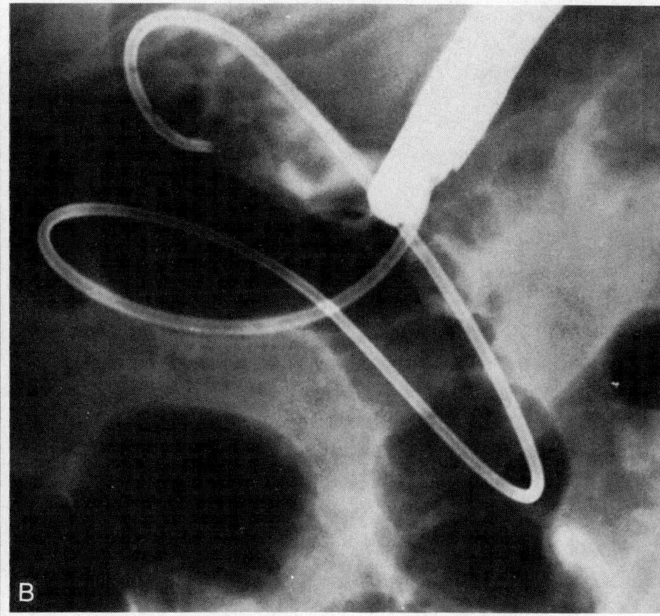

Figure 93–4. *A*, There are multiple stones within the bile duct. A nasobiliary drain has been placed in a looped position. *B*, The duodenoscope is being removed, leaving the transbiliary drain within the bile duct.

benign and malignant strictures, and the placement of endoscopic stents to traverse biliary strictures and promote biliary drainage. All are now being done in many medical centers throughout the world. These techniques reflect developments in angioradiologic procedures encompassing the use of flexible guidewires and exchange catheters, balloons, and stents which can be introduced once the guidewire has traversed the stricture.

Nasobiliary Drainage

The technique of nasobiliary drainage is well established and frequently useful in patients with stones or biliary strictures[36, 37] (Fig. 93–4). Through a transendoscopic catheter placed selectively into the common bile duct, a guidewire is passed through the strictured area or past the retained stone so the tip of the guidewire is high in the common hepatic duct. The diagnostic catheter is then withdrawn over the guidewire using fluoroscopy to monitor proper position of the guidewire. A suitable drainage tube is then advanced through the endoscope over the guidewire to its tip. The guidewire is withdrawn, and the endoscope is carefully removed, leaving the biliary drain in place. The proximal end of the tube is rerouted through the nose with the help of temporary nasopharyngeal intubation. The tube is then taped to the patient's cheek and attached to drainage by a three-way stopcock so that the system can be aspirated, closed, or flushed, as required. Nasobiliary catheters are not difficult to place, provide drainage when needed to prevent septic complications, and provide continuous radiologic access to the biliary tree. They can also provide access for the administration of biliary solvents such as monooctanoin.[38]

Balloon Dilatation

Angiographic dilating balloon catheters have been modified for use in the biliary tree and are available in 4, 6, and 8 mm diameters.[44–46] The catheter is passed over a previously placed guidewire. A limited endoscopic sphincterotomy facilitates this maneuver. Radiographic confirmation of its exact position is aided by using dilute contrast medium for inflating the balloon. This technique generally has been applied to benign biliary strictures but also has been reported useful in the management of malignant strictures, dominant strictures in sclerosing cholangitis, and stenotic biliary enteric anastomoses. Most investigators are impressed by the ease with which it is done and the X-ray appearance of immediate improvement, but intermediate and long-term results are discouraging. The major use of dilating balloons may be in the temporary dilation of a stricture which will then allow the long-term placement of a biliary endoprosthesis.[46]

Biliary Prostheses

The prognosis of most patients with incurable malignant disease of the biliary tract is so dismal that nonoperative positioning of a prosthesis is the best palliative treatment for relief of jaundice, pruritus, and biliary sepsis[35, 47, 48] (see pp. 1724 and 1737–1738). The recent development of large-channel endoscopes and an impressive array of 7- to 15-French plastic endoprostheses of varying lengths has allowed endoscopists to provide long-term palliation of biliary tract obstruction.

Once diagnostic ERCP has been obtained outlining the disordered anatomy, a limited endoscopic sphincterotomy may be done to facilitate access to the common bile duct. A guidewire with a flexible atraumatic tip is then placed through the stricture with a stiffening outer Teflon catheter. When the stricture is traversed, an endoprosthesis of proper length is pushed over the guidewire and catheter with a pusher tube so that it rests with the proximal end above the stricture and the lower end lying free in the duodenal lumen.

The ideal prosthesis has yet to be designed. Initial experience showed that prostheses obstruct quickly, and has led to the current use of larger prostheses of 10- and 12-French diameters, extending the average prosthesis life to six or seven months. A straight prosthesis is easier to insert than a pigtail catheter and lasts a longer time before becoming clogged.

The endoscopic placement of a biliary stent can usually be performed in 30 to 60 minutes, but difficult cases may take longer. The procedure is well tolerated and most patients need only be hospitalized for two or three days. Relief of pruritus and jaundice and a return of sense of well-being is gratifyingly rapid. Failure to improve suggests poor prosthesis position, early blockage due to blood clot, poor liver function due to obstruction, or extensive involvement of the liver with tumor. The best way to differentiate these factors is to repeat the diagnostic ERCP. Prostheses generally are not checked routinely following hospital discharge, but patients are instructed to return at first sign of sepsis or jaundice. This usually indicates stent blockage and need for stent replacement. This is easily accomplished after the original stent is grasped with a snare or basket and removed through the mouth.

Results

Large Stones

Until the perfect lithotripter or stone dissolving agent is discovered there will still be an occasional patient with a large common duct stone that defies endoscopic management. In these patients surgery is advisable, but in the poor-risk patient it is usually possible to place one or two 7-French pigtail catheters in the bile duct in such a position as to keep the stones from impacting in the distal bile duct (Fig. 93–5). These catheters can be left in place for long periods of time because, even if they become clogged, bile will drain adequately around the catheter(s) through the patient's sphincterotomy.

Benign Strictures

Postoperative biliary strictures occur in 0.20 to 0.25 per cent of patients following cholecystectomy and may present early with jaundice, fever, or biliary fistula, or

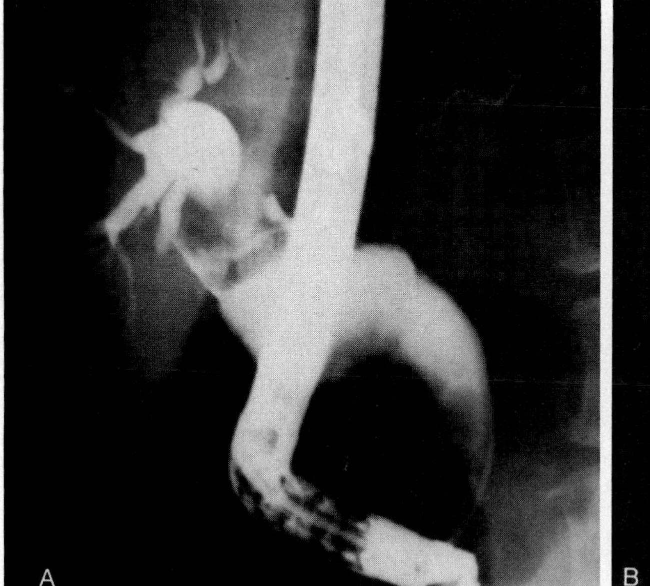

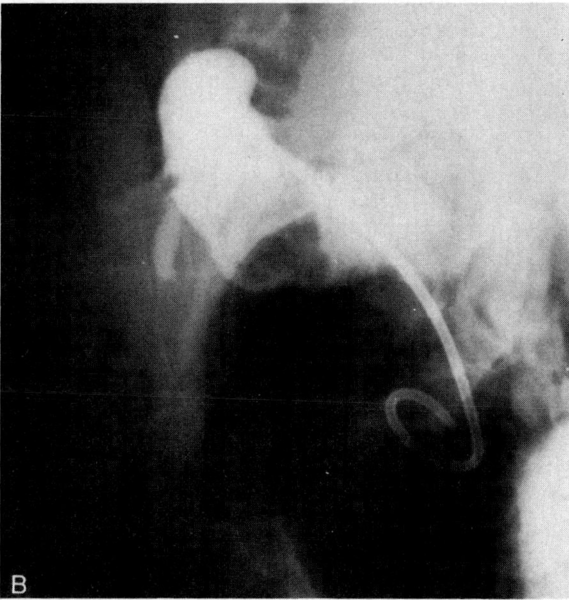

Figure 93–5. *A*, A large square stone is present within the proximal bile duct. Attempts at extraction and dissolution have been unsuccessful. *B*, The stone has been encircled with the proximal limb of a 7-French pigtail stent. The distal end lies free in the duodenal lumen.

late with jaundice or cholangitis (see pp. 1729–1730). Surgical treatment aimed at restoring continuity of bile flow is associated with a mortality rate of 4 to 13 per cent and a morbidity rate as high as 25 per cent. Recurrent strictures are common, necessitating repeat operations in 25 to 35 per cent of patients. It is doubtful also that balloon dilatation alone, either transhepatic or endoscopic, leads to better than transient success.[46] Recent experience with endoscopically placed biliary endoprostheses is promising. In 29 consecutive patients with benign postoperative strictures successful endoscopic stent placement and subsequent improvement were achieved in 27 patients.[46] They suggest prophylactic replacement of the stents at three-month intervals, and removal, if all is well, at six months. Although other operators with less extensive experience are also enthusiastic, long-term results are not yet available.

Sclerosing Cholangitis

Primary sclerosing cholangitis (see p. 1722) is a chronic fibrosing inflammatory condition of extra- and intrahepatic bile ducts of unknown etiology.[49] It is related to inflammatory bowel disease in the majority of cases (see pp. 1467 and 1722). Medical treatment with corticosteroids, immunosuppressive agents, or penicillamine has been disappointing. Surgical relief is aimed at the bypass of a dominant stricture should there be one. Percutaneous transhepatic or endoscopic dilatation of these strictures may afford temporary but seldom long-term relief. Endoscopic placement of biliary stents is sometimes attended by excellent palliation, but the number of patients so treated is presently too small to yield statistically relevant data. One group has undertaken a pilot study of nasobiliary steroid installation and topical lavage in eight patients with encouraging results.[50] Validation of this trial is needed before there is general application of the technique.

Periampullary Tumors

See page 1879.

The treatment of choice is surgical in carcinoma of the papilla of Vater, with an approximately 50 per cent five-year cure rate. In poor-risk patients extended endoscopic sphincterotomy alone provides excellent palliation.[34] Because of a slightly increased risk of hemorrhage during sphincterotomy, most centers now prefer the placement of short, large-bore biliary endoprostheses.[35] This is effective; if in the long-term sepsis or jaundice returns, the stent can be pulled and replaced.

Distal Duct Obstruction

Distal common bile duct obstruction may be due to cholangiocarcinoma, but the usual cause is encircling and invading pancreatic cancer. If the lesion is considered incurable, i.e., not amenable to possible cure by a Whipple procedure, endoscopic placement of a biliary stent will provide good palliation in most patients with jaundice[35, 47, 48] (Fig. 93–6). Success rates in experienced hands are 80 to 90 per cent. An extensive experience indicates a 30-day mortality rate of 10 per cent, but two thirds of these deaths are not directly due to complications from the procedure. A lower 30-day mortality rate after surgery may simply reflect selection bias—fitter patients are selected for surgery with the hope of curative resection, and higher risk patients are referred for stenting. An alternative approach is percutaneous transhepatic biliary stenting; however, the morbidity and mortality rates with it are higher than with endoscopic prosthesis placement. Thus, in patients with unresectable distal bile duct tumors, endoscopic stenting is preferable with transhepatic stenting reserved for patients in whom stents have failed.

Mid-Duct Obstruction

Mid–bile duct obstruction must be considered malignant in the absence of prior biliary surgery. It may be due to cholangiocarcinoma, gallbladder carcinoma with a contiguous spread, or peripancreatic or hilar lymph node enlargement secondary to lymphoma or metastatic tumor (see pp. 1735–1738). Endoscopic stenting can be accomplished with the same high success rate as with distal bile duct tumors.[35, 48] Prognostic factors should influence the decision, for the large stents have a limited patency of approximately six months. Gallbladder carcinoma carries a poor prognosis regardless of the form of treatment and is thus ideal for stenting. Cholangiocarcinoma generally has a more favorable prognosis, making surgical resection, if technically feasible, the treatment of choice. Nodal compression of the mid-duct can be palliated with stents. The time gained may allow other treatment modalities (chemotherapy, X-ray therapy) to shrink the tumor and stunt its growth. The selection of the proper treatment in these patients is more varied than in patients with cancer of the pancreas.

Bifurcation Tumors

The treatment of cancer at the bifurcation of the right and left hepatic ducts (Klatskin tumor) with endoscopic biliary stents is more difficult.[35, 48] Ideally, palliation of these tumors requires placement of two endoprostheses, one in each interhepatic duct. This maneuver is successful only in a minority of cases and reaches only 30 per cent with the best operators. Incomplete drainage of the biliary tree leads inevitably to infection of the proximal undrained segment of the tract. Reasons for failure include tortuous, irregular, and narrow strictures, or a stenotic area that starts at the acute angle to the main biliary axis. Technical failures can usually be solved by transhepatic biliary drainage and stent placement.

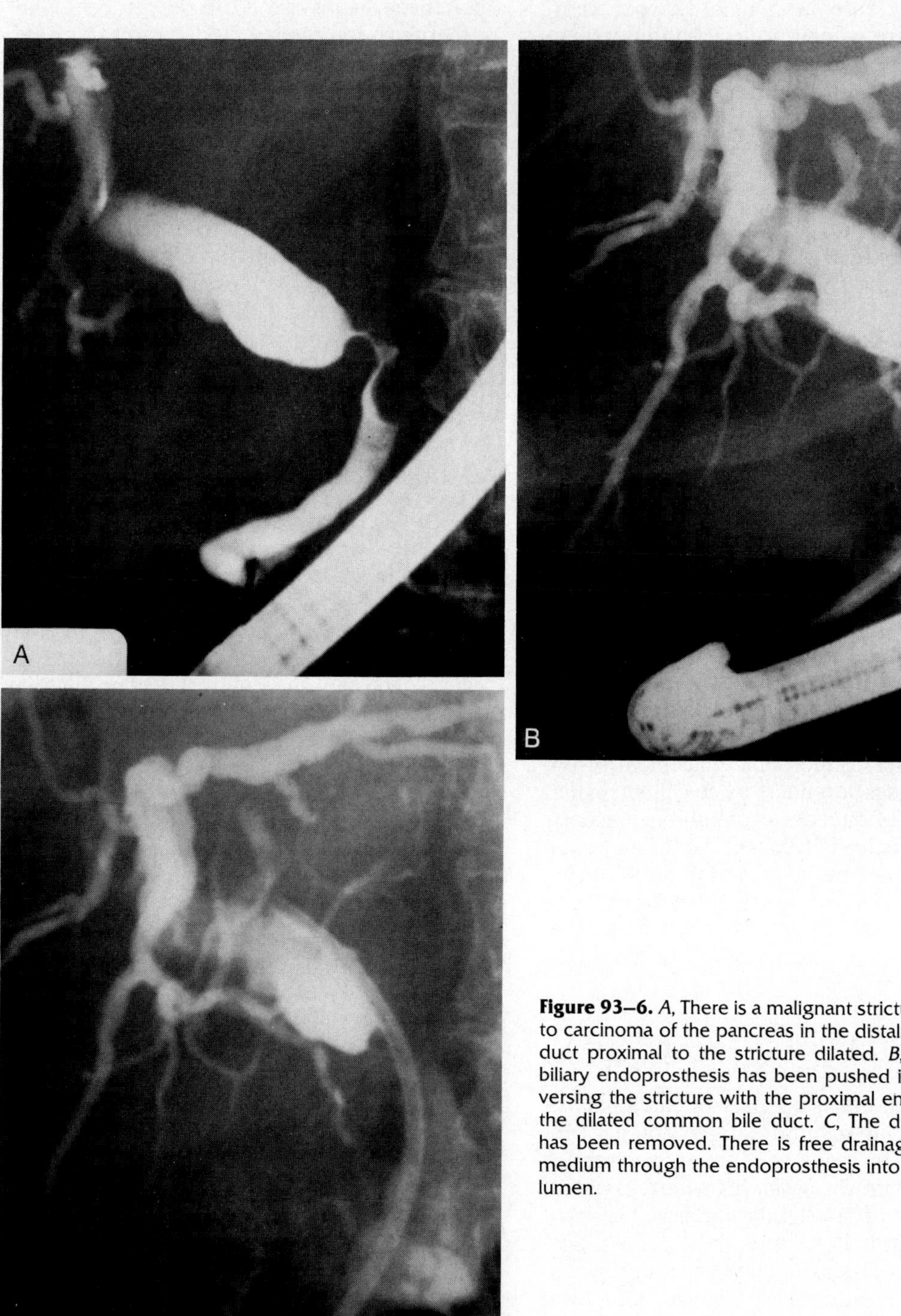

Figure 93–6. *A*, There is a malignant stricture secondary to carcinoma of the pancreas in the distal bile duct. The duct proximal to the stricture dilated. *B*, A 10-French biliary endoprosthesis has been pushed into place traversing the stricture with the proximal end lying within the dilated common bile duct. *C*, The duodenoscope has been removed. There is free drainage of contrast medium through the endoprosthesis into the duodenal lumen.

Complications

The most important early complications of endoscopic stent placement are sepsis (2 per cent), bleeding (1 per cent), and bile duct perforation (less than 1 per cent).[35, 47, 48] The septic complications result from early stent clogging with a coagulum or incomplete biliary drainage. All patients undergoing prosthesis placement should receive prophylactic antibiotics in an attempt to prevent biliary sepsis.

The major late complication is clogging of the endoprosthesis. The 10-French stent has a half-life of six to seven months.[35, 47, 48] Many patients will die sooner as a result of their underlying malignancy, but in those who survive, endoprosthesis blockage will eventually cause chills, fever, and deteriorating liver function. The endoprosthesis should then be removed with a snare or Dormia basket. Replacement is usually accomplished easily and is followed by a subsidence of jaundice and cholangitis.

PROCEDURES PERFORMED THROUGH SURGICALLY CREATED TRACTS

Removal of retained calculi was the initial radiologically guided intervention performed in the bile ducts. During the late 1960s and early 1970s, various instruments, including Fogarty catheters, angiographic catheters, baskets, and forceps were passed under fluoroscopic guidance through the mature T-tube tract to remove retained stones within the biliary tree.[51] Widespread acceptance of the technique awaited the series of 220 cases reported by Mazzariello in 1973.[52] Further technical modifications popularized steerable catheters to position retrieval basket systems more precisely.[22, 53] With the advent of ultrasonic electrohydraulic lithotripsy[54] and stone dissolution technique in the early 1980s,[55–57] even very large retained calculi can be fragmented and removed so that the success of this approach now exceeds 95 per cent.

Another important indication for intervention is the possibility of a retained common duct calculus in a patient who has had biliary tract surgery. At the time of surgery a 14-French, or larger, T-tube is brought out through a lateral, subcostal stab wound. The lateral T-tube entry site facilitates fluoroscopic manipulations and reduces the radiation exposure to the radiologist's hands. Before attempting stone extraction, the T-tube tract is allowed to mature for four to six weeks. The mature tract enables instrumentation within the biliary tree and minimizes the risk of losing continuity with the ductal system.

For the majority of patients, the stone extraction procedure can be performed on an outpatient basis. However, in elderly or debilitated individuals, brief hospitalization for postprocedural observation may be warranted. Prophylaxis with a broad-spectrum antibiotic such as cefoxitin, 1.0 gm every six hours IV, is initiated 24 hours prior to the procedure and continued for two to three days. On the day of the examination, the patient is placed on a clear liquid diet. Although the procedure usually is not painful, selected patients may benefit from administration of a mild sedative.

The patient is placed supine on a tilting fluoroscopic table, and the T-tube is removed by gentle traction. The skin surrounding the tube entry site is cleansed with antiseptic solution and sterilely draped.

To avoid creation of false passages, the tract is catheterized with a soft, red rubber catheter or a blunt-tipped, steerable catheter (Meditech, Watertown, MA). If a red rubber catheter is placed through the tract first, it is exchanged for a Dormia basket sheath over a guidewire. When the steerable catheter is used, it is directed to a point adjacent to the stone. The basket sheath is then passed through the catheter beyond the stone.

The diameter of the retrieval basket should be selected to match the segment of duct in which the stone is located. The basket is advanced to the tip of the sheath and positioned so the midportion of the basket is adjacent to the stone. The sheath is then withdrawn while the basket is held in place, allowing the basket (Fig. 93–7) to open in the appropriate position. The basket is rotated, entrapping the stone within the wire mesh. The sheath is gently advanced, locking the calculus within the basket, and the stone is removed through the tract. Conventional baskets are

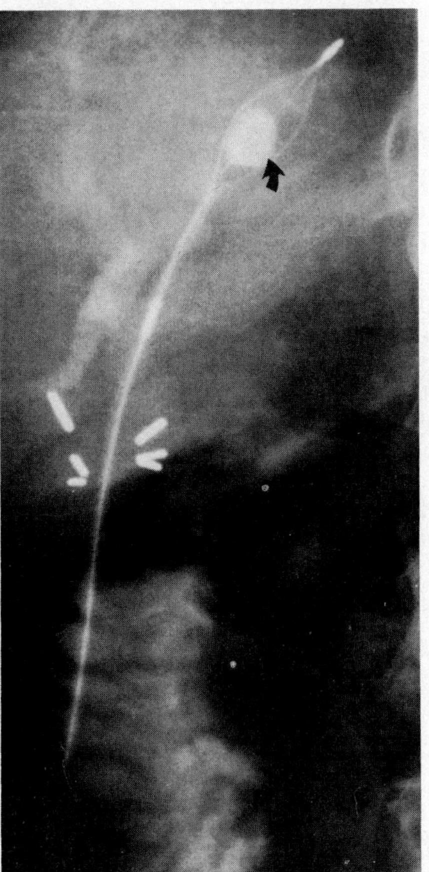

Figure 93–7. An opaque intrahepatic stone *(arrow)* is trapped within a Dormia basket placed through a T-tube tract.

constructed with four wires arranged in a helical configuration. Baskets made with three or six wires may be helpful to trap stones when there is a marked discrepancy between stone size and ductal diameter.

Occasionally, resistance is encountered in extracting the stone through the choledochotomy site. However, if continuous traction is applied under moderate tension, the vast majority of stones can be extracted through 14-French, or larger, surgical tracts, despite the fact that the stone is larger than the tract itself. Damage to the ductal system is exceedingly rare.

Following the removal of all stones, the cholangiogram is repeated to ensure that no additional stones are present. Unfortunately, owing to the introduction of small amounts of air and the formation of blood clots, the postextraction cholangiogram may be difficult to interpret. It is therefore advisable to reinsert a drainage tube through the tract and perform a follow-up cholangiogram in 24 to 48 hours. Only when the cholangiogram is unequivocally normal should the drainage tube be removed, allowing the tract to heal.

Indications

Any patient with a retained common duct stone and an indwelling T-tube is a candidate for the procedure. As an alternative, it is possible to remove retained stones from an endoscopic retrograde approach in conjunction with endoscopic sphincterotomy. If postoperative cholangiographic findings suggest that a sphincterotomy is necessary, the endoscopic approach is warranted.

Contraindications

There are no absolute contraindications to stone removal through a mature T-tube tract. Even very large stones can be removed with this technique, although in selected cases electrohydraulic or ultrasonic lithotripsy may be required to fragment enormous calculi (see pp. 1681–1682).

Stones lodged in cystic duct remnants or in diverticular outpouchings of the extrahepatic bile duct may be impossible to retrieve. When a stone is demonstrated to be in one of these locations, the removal procedure should be deferred. Often, after approximately one week of normal activity, the stone will migrate into a position more conducive to removal.

Results

The overall success rate of stone removal through a T-tube tract approaches 95 per cent.[22, 52] It is important to note that patients with multiple stones will often require more than one procedure to remove all the calculi.

Complications

The complication rate of the procedure is reported to be less than 5 per cent.[58] Only one patient has been reported to have died from the procedure.[59] Low-grade fever is not uncommon, but clinical sepsis is quite unusual.

T-Tube Replacement

History

For many years, T-tubes have been used to provide bile drainage after biliary tract operation. Usually the tube remains in place for only a few weeks and causes few clinical problems. However, when a T-tube is intended to act as a long-term stent for a malignant obstruction or complicated stricture, the tube will eventually dislodge, displace, or become obstructed with sludge. Progressive tumor growth can extend beyond the ends of the tube and cause recurrent jaundice. Prior to the 1970s, replacement or repositioning of an indwelling T-tube required a surgical procedure. During the early 1970s, techniques were developed to disimpact T-tubes occluded by debris, but malpositioned tubes continued to require surgical replacement. In 1977, Crummy and Turnipseed described a technique whereby T-tubes could be replaced percutaneously under fluoroscopic observation.[60]

Technique

The indwelling T-tube is removed by gentle traction over a guidewire. The removed T-tube serves as a model for the limb length of the new tube. Limb length adjustments can be made easily on the basis of the cholangiogram.

Owing to the friction between the rubber of the tube and the stainless steel of the guidewire, replacement is greatly facilitated by coating the T-tube generously with sterile water-soluble lubricant. The proximal limb of the T-tube is threaded over the guidewire, and the wire end is directed through the long external limb. The T-tube is advanced over the wire with the distal limb trailing alongside the external limb. The tube is advanced until the tip of the trailing limb springs freely into the bile duct. The long external limb is retracted, seating the internal limbs into appropriate position.

Obviously, the T-tube may also be inserted with the distal limb leading, if the biliary anatomy is more suitable for this approach.

Complications

As with any manipulation of the biliary tract, sepsis may be precipitated if excessive amounts of contrast medium are injected in the presence of infected bile. Therefore, when manipulations of this type are performed, pretreatment with a broad-spectrum antibiotic is warranted.

In addition, if the T-tube tract has not matured, access to the biliary tree may be lost during the procedure. Although this is an infrequent occurrence, reoperation may be necessary when biliary obstruction is present.

PROCEDURES PERFORMED THROUGH A DIRECT PERCUTANEOUS APPROACH

Percutaneous Transhepatic Cholangiography and Biliary Drainage

History

Percutaneous transhepatic cholangiography (PTC) was first attempted in Southeast Asia during the late 1930s.[61] However, the technique was rarely used in the United States and Europe until the 1960s.[62, 63] Even with technical modifications, at that time most centers considered PTC excessively dangerous unless the procedure was followed immediately by surgical decompression. In the early 1970s, it was shown that when PTC was performed with a fine needle (22- or 23-gauge), there were few risks even in the presence of complete ductal obstruction. Opacification of the biliary tree with the fine needle technique approaches 100 per cent when the ducts are dilated, and is over 80 per cent in most series even when the ducts are of normal caliber.[64] The ease in performance of this technique encouraged its rapid dissemination.

Percutaneous Biliary Drainage

Before the advent of the thin needle technique, attempts were made to enhance the safety of PTC by leaving a small catheter within the biliary tree and allowing temporary decompression of the bile ducts. This avoided the risks of bile leakage after the procedure. However, stable catheter position was difficult to achieve, and complications were frequent. In the mid-1970s, the feasibility of manipulating modified angiographic catheters through the biliary system and across obstructing lesions was demonstrated.[65] Transhepatic catheters could be securely anchored distal to the obstruction, and the sideholes arranged on either side of the obstruction, to permit internal drainage of bile into the duodenum (Fig. 93–8). This procedure gained considerable popularity in the late 1970s as technical refinements were made and large series of patients were reported.[66, 67]

Technique

The patient is given broad-spectrum antibiotic, cefoxitin, 1.0 gm every six hours IV, on the day prior to the procedure; if clinical evidence of cholangitis is present, the dose is 2.0 gm every six hours and an aminoglycoside, 1.5 mg/kg every eight hours IV. A combination sedative hypnotic and narcotic analgesic is administered immediately prior to the procedure. Additional analgesic medication may be administered intravenously during the procedure as needed, but general anesthesia is usually unnecessary.

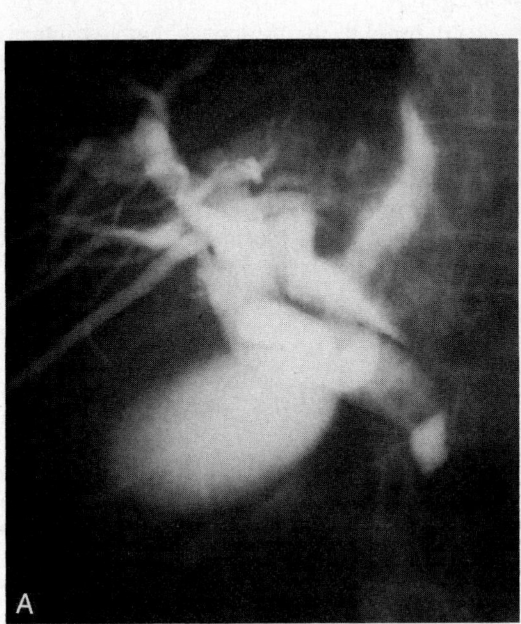

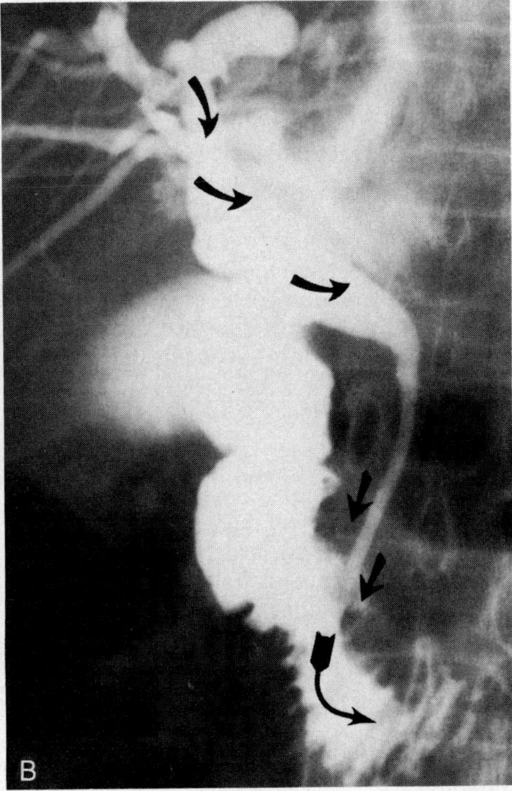

Figure 93–8. A 62-year-old woman with a carcinoma of the pancreas obstructing the distal bile duct. *A*, A percutaneous transhepatic cholangiogram demonstrates obstruction of the pancreatic segment of the duct. *B*, After insertion of an 8.3-French biliary drainage catheter through the obstruction. Antegrade drainage can be established through inflow sideholes above the obstruction and outflow sideholes below the obstruction. Arrows indicate the direction of bile flow.

The skin over the right upper quadrant and right lateral abdomen is cleansed with an antiseptic solution, and sterilely draped. The diaphragmatic border is identified fluoroscopically, and an entry point for a percutaneous transhepatic cholangiogram is selected in the midaxillary line, usually immediately above the tenth or eleventh rib.

A complete transhepatic cholangiogram is performed with a thin-walled, 22-gauge needle passed in a slightly cephalad direction through the liver parenchyma to a point just to the right of the vertebral body. Contrast material is injected through the needle as it is slowly withdrawn through the parenchyma. When the tip of the needle communicates with the ductal system, the contrast will begin to outline the biliary tree. If no contact is made with a duct, the needle is withdrawn to a point within the liver capsule and another pass is made more anterior or posterior to the original needle tract. Caution should be used to avoid overdistention of the biliary system with contrast medium, as this may precipitate septicemia. The transhepatic cholangiogram is reviewed to determine the feasibility of percutaneous drainage.

When percutaneous drainage is deemed appropriate, an entry site is selected in the midaxillary line that provides an almost horizontal approach to a right hepatic duct. After the administration of local anesthesia, a 16-gauge sheathed needle is advanced into the duct, and the stylet is removed. Bile returns freely through the sheath when its tip is within a bile duct. The sheath is then directed through the biliary ductal system and site of obstruction using specially designed steerable guidewires. When the sheath has been advanced into the duodenum, an extremely stiff guidewire is inserted. The sheath is removed, and a drainage catheter is inserted over the guidewire. The multiple sideholes of the drainage catheter are positioned both above and below the site of obstruction. This allows bile to flow in an antegrade direction into the duodenum when the tube is capped externally. The drainage tube is secured in place, and the patient is returned to the ward. Close observation for evidence of intraperitoneal hemorrhage or the development of sepsis is maintained for four to six hours following the procedure.

Indications

Patients considered for percutanteous transhepatic biliary drainage can be divided into two groups: patients requiring only temporary drainage and those requiring permanent intubation. The former group includes some benign causes of biliary obstruction as well as selected patients with malignant obstruction prior to a curative or palliative surgical procedure. The latter group includes patients with advanced tumors for which percutaneous drainage is performed exclusively for palliation.

Indications for Temporary Biliary Drainage

Malignant Obstruction

The utility of temporary transhepatic biliary drainage as a preoperative measure in jaundiced patients with malignant biliary obstruction prior to surgical intervention has been controversial. Several major series have found no benefit with regard to perioperative morbidity and mortality rates in patients undergoing preoperative transhepatic biliary drainage.[68, 69] Another controlled trial of 50 patients was reported that concluded that preoperative percutaneous biliary drainage (PTBD) reduced perioperative morbidity and mortality rates. In this series, major disease occurred in 52 per cent who were operated upon without prior drainage, compared with only 8 per cent in patients in which PTBD was performed prior to surgery.[70] At the present time, however, there is very little other support for the routine use of PTBD prior to surgical resection.

Benign Strictures

Although benign strictures may result from trauma and pancreatitis, most are attributable to prior biliary tract surgery. Of these patients, 80 per cent usually present with symptoms of cholangitis or jaundice within two years of previous surgery. The surgical outcome is successful in approximately 70 per cent of the cases[71] (see pp. 1729–1730).

Portal hypertension, liver disease, infection, and elevated serum bilirubin are major influences on the success of surgical repair.[72] Preoperative transhepatic drainage relieves the obstruction, thus reducing the serum bilirubin and decreasing the risk of biliary infection. Placement of the catheter through the stricture may aid in identification of the extrahepatic bile duct at surgery.

Traditional therapy of benign strictures has been surgical repair; however, recent reports of percutaneous stricture dilatation have been encouraging. A recent multicenter review with a 36-month follow-up had patency rates of 67 per cent in anastomotic strictures, 76 per cent in iatrogenic strictures, and 42 per cent in sclerosing cholangitis.[73] The use of long-term internal-external stenting following stricture dilatation is somewhat controversial.[70, 73]

Cholangitis

Emergent surgical decompression in patients with acute obstructive cholangitis carries a mortality rate ranging from 50 to 75 per cent[74–76] (see pp. 1714–1726). If drainage can be established percutaneously, medical management of the sepsis may be possible in most cases, with the considerable help of multiple antibiotics (see p. 1718). In addition, after the sepsis is controlled, tube cholangiography will demonstrate the precise location of the obstruction. An elective surgical procedure may be performed subsequently to remove or bypass the obstructing lesion when the patient's condition has improved. Using this approach, a 17 per cent mortality rate has been reported in a series of 28 patients with acute obstructive cholangitis.[77]

As an alternative, patients suspected of having obstructive biliary sepsis on the basis of common bile duct calculi may be drained by the endoscopically guided retrograde technique. Endoscopic sphincterotomy can provide definitive therapy in this group of patients, thus avoiding the necessity of an additional procedure.

Indications for Long-Term Drainage

The utility of long-term biliary drainage in malignant disease is controversial. In patients with malignant disease, endoprosthesis placement, either percutaneously or via endoscopy, will provide sufficient palliation. Patients with complex, benign biliary disease such as sclerosing cholangitis or Oriental cholangiohepatitis will require repeated manipulations and should not have an endoprosthesis placed.

Sclerosing cholangitis[78] is a progressive disease that ultimately leads to hepatic failure. Diagnosis is usually made with thin needle cholangiography or ERCP. Management is by a combined surgical or biologic approach. A surgical drainage is performed and a conduit is created so that intermittent biliary toilet can be performed under fluoroscopic guidance. Traditionally, one or more tubes are placed in the biliary tree, allowing repeated access.

Surgeons can now perform a Roux-en-Y hepaticojejunostomy and place a portion of the jejunal loop under the abdominal wall and mark the loop with metal clips. Simple access can then be achieved for biliary interventions by directly puncturing the extraperitoneal portion of the jejunal loop (Fig. 93–9). The catheter can be removed and the tract closes quickly[79] (see p. 1722).

Not all Roux-en-Y hepaticojejunostomies are constructed in this fashion, but percutaneous procedures, including diagnostic cholangiograms, stricture dilatation, and stone removal, are still possible. The location of the specific loop is identified by CT or at fluoroscopy by the presence of catheters or other devices which have been previously placed. Postoperative adhesions around the loop help to fix it and facilitate the puncture by preventing buckling away from the needle. The risk of percutaneous catheterization of Roux-en-Y jejunal loops is minimal, and the mechanical advantages of manipulation in the biliary tree from this subhepatic approach are considerable.

Clinical Contraindications to Percutaneous Transhepatic Biliary Drainage

Severe Bleeding Diathesis

Because PTBD can require several hepatic punctures, patients with bleeding diathesis deserve special consideration. Moderate or marked prolongation of the prothrombin time or partial thromboplastin time as well as a platelet count under 50,000 should be considered contraindications. In such patients administration of vitamin K, fresh frozen plasma, or platelet transfusions is warranted to improve the coagulation status prior to the procedure.

Ascites

The presence of moderate or massive ascites creates several problems for transhepatic drainage. First, the procedure is technically more difficult because guidewires and catheters tend to buckle within the peritoneal cavity, making the application of coaxial force much more difficult. Second, the risk of hemorrhage related to the procedure is greater in the presence of ascites. Finally, even after a successful drainage has been performed, ascitic fluid tends to leak around the catheter entry site. In some cases, relief of the biliary obstruction will be followed by a decrease or disappearance of the ascites. However, in other cases, persistent leakage will continue to burden the patient. Therefore, only patients with ascites who have compelling reasons for it and in whom other therapies have failed should be drained percutaneously.

Intraductal Tumor

Rarely, a neoplastic lesion will establish itself and grow diffusely throughout the ductal system. This occurs rarely with cholangiocarcinoma but also may be observed with intraductal papillomas, rare sarcomas, and some metastases. When the ducts are filled with tumor, biliary drainage by any route is ineffective and percutaneous drainage should not be attempted.

Results

A number of published series have documented the effectiveness of percutaneous biliary drainage in lowering the serum bilirubin level and relieving symptoms of obstructive jaundice.[80–83] The success of the procedure as defined by the establishment of effective bile drainage in most of these series is above 90 per cent. Although statistics vary with regard to the rate of successful negotiation of the obstructing lesion and placement of the catheter into the duodenum, the experienced operator achieves it in more than 95 per cent of cases.

Clinically, in the vast majority of patients with pruritus, the itching disappears within 24 to 48 hours following drainage. In patients being decompressed for sepsis, improvement with defervescence is generally noted in 28 to 24 hours.[80]

Serum bilirubin diminishes at an average rate of 1.4 mg/dl per day.[83] Although patients without underlying liver disease eventually will return to a normal level of serum bilirubin, those with diffuse metastatic disease to the liver or underlying hepatic dysfunction may not respond well. In patients with malignant obstruction, serum bilirubin declines 10 mg/dl or more in 76 per

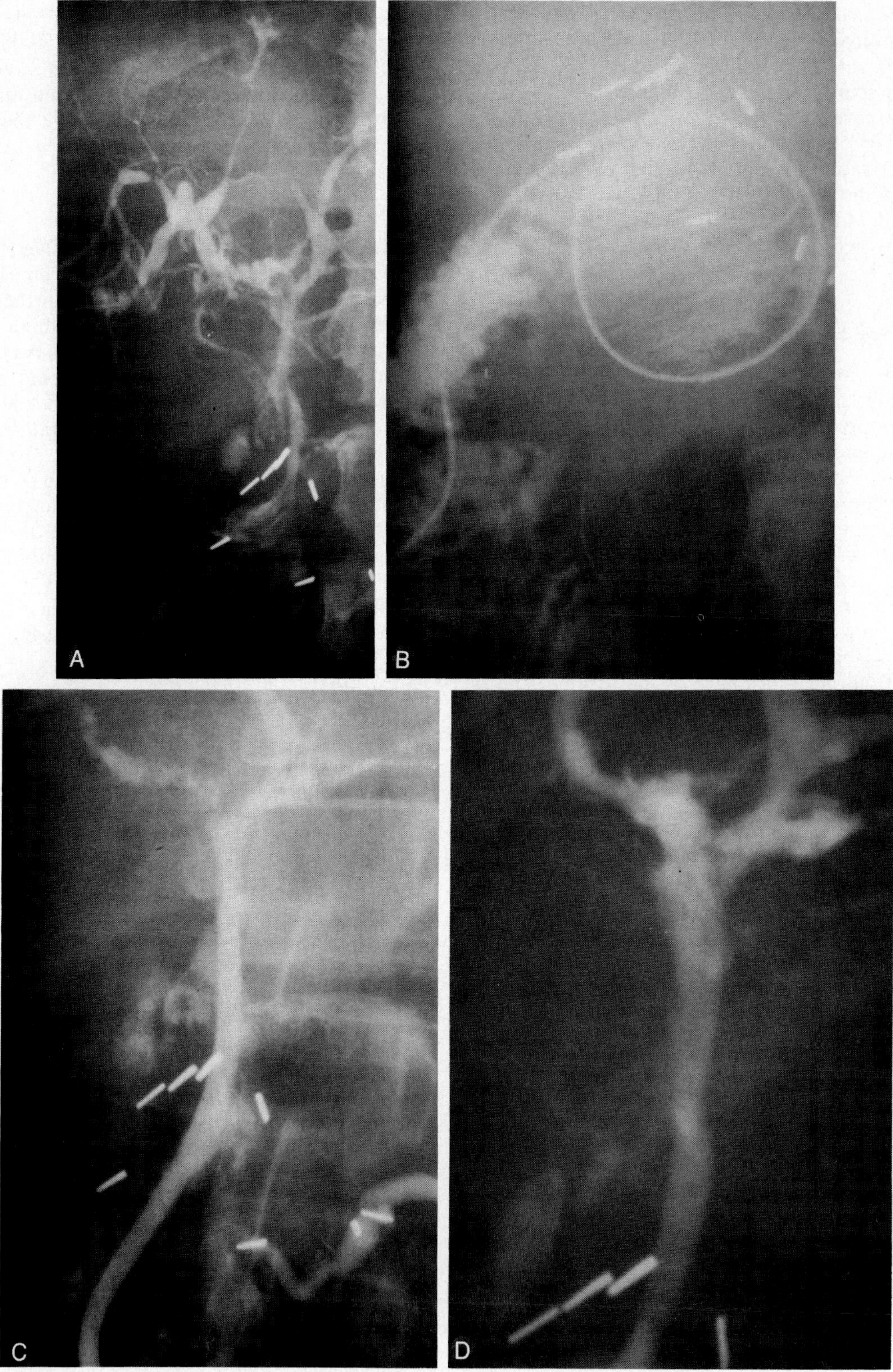

Figure 93–9. Percutaneous puncture of a Roux-en-Y jejunostomy for interventions in sclerosing cholangitis. *A,* A transhepatic cholangiogram performed on a 42-year-old woman with sclerosing cholangitis and a previous choledochojejunostomy anastomosis. Multiple strictures are identified as well as a stone at the confluence of the right and left hepatic duct. *B,* The Roux-en-Y had been constructed so that a segment was extraperitoneal and marked with metallic clips. The jejunal loop is easily punctured with a 22-gauge needle, and a guidewire is passed into the loop. *C,* The stone was crushed into multiple small fragments and a drainage tube was left in the common hepatic duct. *D,* Four days later the debris had cleared. A final cholangiogram demonstrated considerable improvement in the appearance of the bile ducts. The tube was removed and the percutaneous tract closed within 24 hours.

cent of patients and declines 5 mg/dl to 10 mg/dl in 10 per cent.[81]

Complications

The most frequent serious complication of transhepatic biliary drainage is sepsis, reported in slightly over 10 per cent of patients.[84, 85] However, septic shock is unusual and is seen in less than 2 per cent of cases. As noted above, cefoxitin alone or with gentamicin or tobramycin is given for cholangitis (see p. 1718).

Although a minimal degree of bleeding is encountered in the majority of patients, serious hemorrhage is distinctly rare, complicating in less than 2 per cent of cases.[85] Bleeding can be divided into two types: biliary and intraperitoneal.

Bleeding into the biliary tract is not uncommon. It occurs when a sidehole on the biliary drainage catheter is malpositioned proximally into the hepatic parenchyma. This is easily corrected by advancing the drainage catheter to a point where all the sideholes are within the ductal system.

Death from severe bleeding is rare. In one series of 200 patients, two patients died from uncontrollable hemorrhage.[84] Death has also been reported from inadvertent transpleural puncture complicated by pneumothorax and bilious pleural effusion.[86]

Other complications are observed, but are surprisingly infrequent, being noted in less than 1 per cent of patients. These complications include bile leakage into the peritoneal cavity, hepatic or perihepatic abscess, and pancreatitis.

In patients in whom internal drainage cannot be established, fluid and electrolyte loss may become a problem. This is most often observed in the first two or three days following biliary drainage in which a postdrainage biliuresis may develop.

Late complications are common but easily managed in most cases. They include local skin infections and granulomas at the catheter entry site. Catheter occlusion is generally prevented by routine flushing with 3 to 5 ml of sterile saline on a daily basis. Routine catheter exchanges should also be performed every two to three months to prevent build-up of biliary sludge and debris within the catheter lumen.

Sporadic reports of carcinomatous extension along the transhepatic catheter tracts have appeared, but this complication is exceedingly rare. Skin implantation as well as peritoneal seeding has been documented.[87, 88]

Insertion of Completely Indwelling Biliary Stents

History

The development of percutaneous biliary drainage in the mid-1970s stimulated interest in the feasibility of inserting completely indwelling biliary stents by the transhepatic route. In 1978, Pereiras developed a practical endoprosthesis that he inserted successfully in a small group of patients.[89] Subsequently, other prostheses were developed that were easier to insert and evaluated in larger groups of patients.[90–92] Currently, transhepatic insertion of biliary stents has become a common procedure and is performed in most major medical centers throughout the United States and Europe.

Technique

Prior to the insertion of a completely indwelling biliary stent, a standard percutaneous transhepatic drainage is performed. In most cases, the transhepatic tube is left in place for one to two weeks prior to insertion of the endoprosthesis. The procedure is usually performed on an outpatient basis. As with all catheterizations involving the bile ducts, broad-spectrum antibiotic coverage is recommended prior to the procedure, and the patient is placed on a clear liquid diet. The patient is placed supine on the fluoroscopic table, and a cholangiogram is performed through the transhepatic drainage catheter. A stiff guidewire is inserted through the tube into the duodenum, and the drainage catheter is removed. Using coaxial Teflon dilators, the tract is enlarged to 12- or 16-French.

An appropriate length endoprosthesis is selected and advanced through the tract into the appropriate position with a pushing catheter. Once in position, the guidewire is removed and a cholangiogram is performed. In most cases, a temporary transhepatic drainage catheter is left indwelling for the first 24 hours to evacuate any debris that may have formed during the procedure. This catheter is then removed, and the transhepatic tract heals in two or three days.

Several types of biliary stents have been designed to ensure against migration of the endoprosthesis. One type of stent is a 12- to 16-French Teflon tube with eccentric flaps at its proximal end to anchor the catheter[90] (Fig. 93–10). These flaps collapse as the stent is advanced through the transhepatic tract. When the flaps reach the ductal system, they spring open, anchoring the endoprosthesis in proper position. This catheter is used for patients with obstructions above the pancreas. Teflon is a rigid material and may theoretically damage the ampulla or duodenum.

Patients who have pancreatic malignancy require an endoprosthesis with sideholes in the duodenum. A soft endoprosthesis (Carey-Coons) with a distal gentle L curve that rests in the duodenum is used.

Indications

There are several advantages to completely indwelling biliary stents. The large endhole efficiently conducts bile into the duodenum. There is no associated discomfort, and the patient does not need to perform any type of routine tube maintenance. Most important, the quality of life is dramatically improved by not having the nuisance of maintaining an external segment of a drainage tube.

For these reasons, completely indwelling stents are indicated for all patients with malignant biliary obstruc-

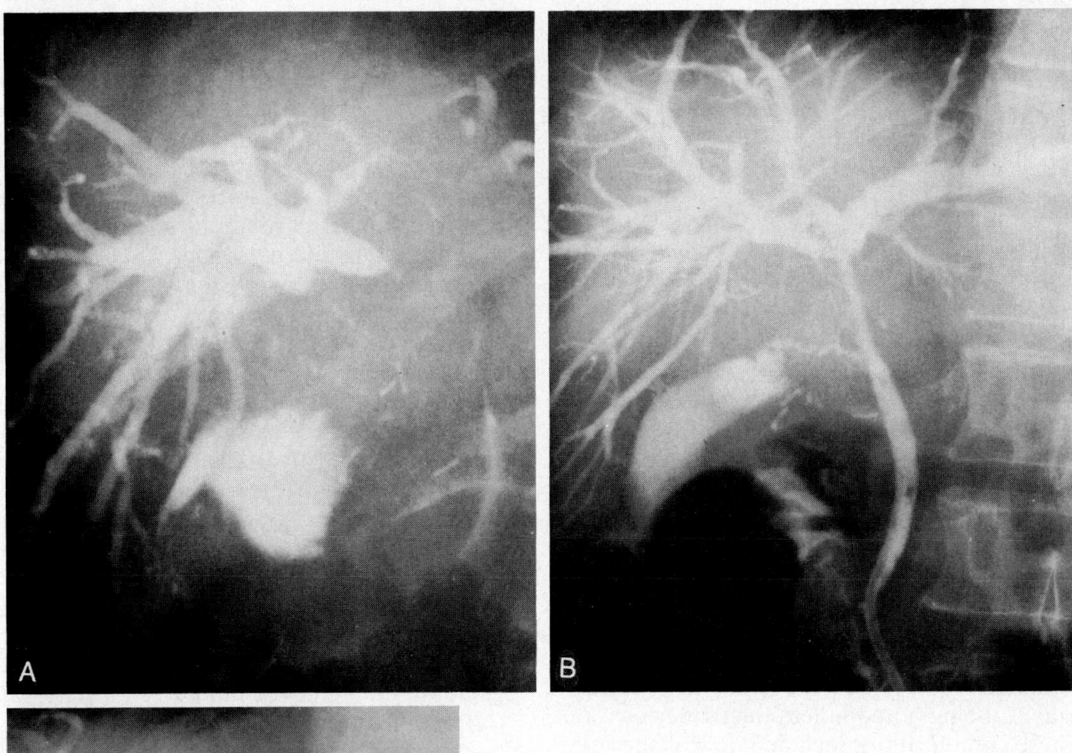

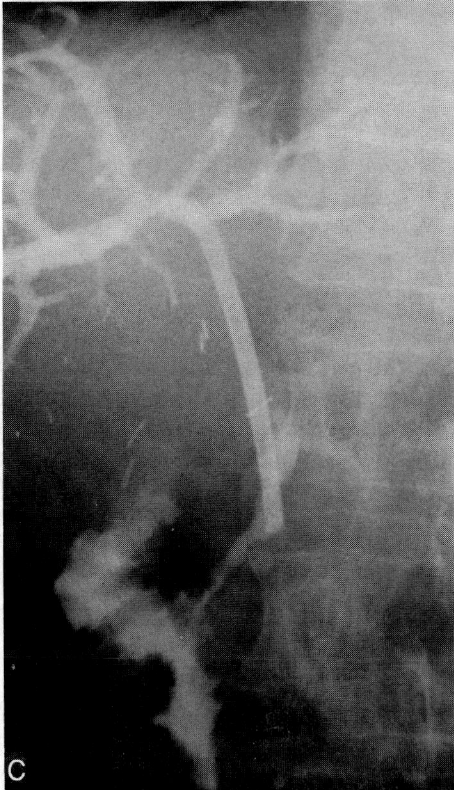

Figure 93–10. A 53-year-old man with malignant obstruction at the porta hepatis. *A*, A thin needle cholangiogram demonstrates complete obstruction of the bile duct. *B*, An 8.3-French catheter was manipulated across the obstruction into the distal duct and duodenum. *C*, One week later the 8.3-French catheter was substituted for a 12-French Teflon endoprosthesis. External segment of catheter was removed. Patient survived for two and a half years without recurrent jaundice.

tion where endoprosthesis placement is technically feasible. This includes patients with obstructing lesions of the extrahepatic bile duct as well as those patients with obstruction of the main right and left hepatic ducts. In the latter case, two stents may be necessary to achieve drainage of the isolated left and right systems.

Results

Transhepatic insertion of biliary stents is a successful procedure in the vast majority of patients. In one series of 162 patients the initial bilirubin level was 15.7 mg/dl and ten days later it was 4.9 mg/dl.[92] Excellent stent patency was noted, for only 6 per cent of the patients presented with occluded stents. Those patients who survived the initial 30 days had a mean survival of 26 weeks (overall survival was 20 weeks). Three patients had functioning endoprostheses two years after placement.

Complications

The complications of endoprosthesis placement include all the hazards previously mentioned for percutaneous transhepatic biliary drainage. In addition, there are two unique complications of this procedure: *stent migration* and *occlusion*. In a series of 102 stent placements,[93] 6 per cent of the stents migrated requiring replacement. These stents are removed endoscopically to avoid complications in the bowel. If possible, the stent is replaced endoscopically; if not, the entire procedure must be repeated. Occlusion of indwelling stents by biliary sludge and debris is also infrequent—6 per cent of cases.[92] Occlusion necessitates removal of the stent and insertion of a new one. Finally, because endoprostheses are placed for malignant disease, inevitable progression of cancer, although rare (3 per cent), may occlude the stent, requiring repositioning or replacement.[93] However, most patients die of complications associated with advanced malignancy rather than recurrent obstructive jaundice.

Percutaneous Cholecystostomy

History

Percutaneous puncture of the gallbladder is not a new procedure. It was originally performed in the early 1920s for diagnostic purposes.[94] However, because of the well-established surgical techniques for gallbladder decompression and fear of intraperitoneal spillage of infected bile, percutaneous catheter decompression has not been attempted until recently. In 1979, a case report appeared establishing feasibility of this procedure.[95]

Technique

The patient is prepared with a clear liquid diet and broad-spectrum antibiotic coverage (see p. 1751). In 1988, this procedure will be very commonly performed.[96, 97]

Ultrasonic guidance is required to localize the optimal position for puncture. The optimal entry site is anterior, where the margin of the liver is insinuated between the anterior abdominal wall and gallbladder. Puncturing through the hepatic parenchyma is recommended. This route allows entry into the gallbladder wall where it is attached to the undersurface of the liver, minimizing the possibility of peritoneal spillage of infected bile.

After the entry site is selected, generous amounts of local anesthesia are administered. The puncture is made with an 18-gauge, sheathed needle, and the stylet is removed. When bile freely returns, a guidewire is advanced through the sheath and is coiled within the gallbladder. The sheath is removed, and a 10- or 12-French drainage tube is inserted over the guidewire. The drainage tube is then secured in place.

Indications

The indications for percutaneous cholecystostomy are identical to the indications for surgical cholecystostomy. This includes elderly and debilitated patients with acute cholecystitis who are poor candidates for immediate cholecystectomy.

After percutaneous cholecystostomy, three management alternatives are available. If the patient's medical condition improves substantially, an elective cholecystectomy may be performed. As an alternative, the percutaneous tract may be dilated and stones removed under fluoroscopic guidance. Finally, in some patients, permanent tube drainage of the gallbladder may be warranted.

Results

The procedure is not technically difficult and is successful in most patients. In a recently published series of 24 patients who underwent 20 diagnostic and 13 therapeutic procedures, eleven had percutaneous cholecystostomy, eight to relieve hydrops and cholecystitis and three for gallstone dissolution and extraction.[96] Other authors have had similar results.[97]

Complications

Bile leakage was not a problem in either of the above series.[96, 97] No clinical evidence of this complication has been reported when the catheter has been securely placed in the gallbladder. A case of fatal bile peritonitis has been reported to occur when the drainage catheter was dislodged. This may be avoided by using a transhepatic tract, a Cope loop in the gallbladder, and secure fixation of the tube.

Sepsis, which is present in virtually all patients who are candidates for percutaneous cholecystostomy, may be transiently aggravated by the procedure. As with cholangitis associated with these procedures, broad-spectrum antibiotics, cefoxitin and either tobramycin or gentamicin, should be given (see p. 1755). This may be minimized by small injections of contrast material used only to confirm catheter placement. Maintaining patency of the catheter averts subsequent sepsis in all instances.[96, 97]

COMBINED TRANSHEPATIC AND ENDOSCOPIC INTERVENTIONS

This chapter has described the progress that has been made in developing nonoperative therapy for biliary tract diseases over the past few years. Both endoscopic and transhepatic biliary interventions are advocated for a variety of clinical problems. In some centers, the overlap in these modalities has led to competition between interventional radiologists and gastroenterologists and conflicting recommendations as to the best method for any given problem. We have been impressed that a cooperative approach can take advantage of the strengths of each technique and extend the range of nonoperative therapies.[98] The following are our indications for each approach and the settings in which we combine the two methods to permit treatment that would not be feasible using only a single approach.

Transhepatic Interventions

The principal advantage of the transhepatic approach to biliary intervention is the controlled manipulations that can be achieved within the ductal system. The short length of the transparenchymal tract and the high degree of maneuverability of transhepatic catheters and guidewires enable therapy of specific intrahepatic ductal disease and consistently allow catheterization through even very complicated biliary strictures, across the ampulla to the duodenum. When necessary, considerable leverage can be achieved through the transhepatic tract so that sufficient force can be applied to introduce very large devices. Transhepatic catheterization is not limited by previous surgical bypass procedures (in either the gastrointestinal tract or the biliary tree). Modifications of transhepatic techniques through subhepatic approaches (via surgically created drainage tracts or Roux-en-Y hepatojejunostomies) facilitate management of very complicated biliary problems such as sclerosing cholangitis and pyogenic cholangiohepatitis.

The major disadvantage of the transhepatic approach is the morbidity associated with the capsular puncture and transparenchymal tract. The liver capsule is extremely sensitive so that transhepatic manipulations can be very painful. Ascites makes catheter insertion more difficult, and once the catheter is in place, the ascitic fluid leaks around the percutaneous entry site. Most important, when a transhepatic procedure is unsuccessful and drainage cannot be achieved, the consequences of failure are usually devastating—bile leakage, peritonitis, and uncontrolled sepsis.[99] The only major consequence of an unsuccessful endoscopic intervention is failure of access to the ampulla or to the duct above an obstruction, and morbid consequences are thus much less than with an unsuccessful transhepatic procedure.

Endoscopic access to the ampulla has three compelling advantages over the transhepatic approach which we believe make it the initial procedure of choice for most biliary interventions. First, the direct visualization of the periampullary area allows controlled sphincterotomy and biopsy or even fulguration of periampullary lesions. Second, interventions can be performed relatively painlessly and require only a brief period of recuperation. Third, endoscopic procedures can be readily repeated so that endoscopically placed stents can be replaced at intervals if they should become obstructed with biliary sludge. Transhepatic stents are either of the internal-external type, which require frequent maintenance, or endoprostheses that can be replaced only by repeating the entire procedure should they become obstructed.

Combined Endoscopic and Transhepatic Approach

Whenever endoscopic catheterization is not possible a combined procedure is employed that takes advantage of the maneuverability of the transhepatic catheter to gain access to the duodenum and engage the endoscopically placed catheter.[100–105] The endoscopic catheter is then brought securely into the biliary tree to perform the intervention. In this way, a major intervention can be performed with as small a transhepatic catheter as possible to minimize pain and reduce the risk of complications.

Technique

The patient is placed supine on a fluoroscopic table. A percutaneous transhepatic biliary drainage is performed in the standard fashion from a right intercostal approach. A 5-French angiographic catheter is advanced over a torque control guidewire through the ampulla, well into the duodenum. A second guidewire is passed to act as a safety wire so that, if necessary, repeated access to the duodenum can be easily achieved. The sheath of a Dormia basket is then passed over one of the guidewires. The guidewire is removed and a four wire basket is introduced through the sheath, but not out the tip. The catheter entry site is then covered with a sterile dressing and the patient is placed in the prone oblique position.

The endoscope is introduced and advanced until the ampulla and basket-catheter are visible to the endoscopist. The basket is opened and repositioned so that it can be seen endoscopically projecting from the ampulla. The tip of the papillotome or endoscopic guidewire is advanced into the basket. The basket is closed and withdrawn, pulling the papillotome into the common duct or the guidewire through the obstructing lesion. For sphincterotomy, the basket is opened and the sphincterotome is released; for insertion of an endoprosthesis, the guidewire is held in the basket until the endoprosthesis has been positioned.

Following completion of the endoscopic procedure, the patient is returned to the supine position. A pigtail drainage catheter is placed over one of the guidewires and attached to a closed drainage system. The following day, a cholangiogram is performed through the transhepatic catheter, and it is removed if there is no residual debris and there is free flow into the duodenum. Occasionally, we have used the transhepatic access to introduce a basket and crush residual ductal stones.

Results

We have successfully performed combined procedures in 32 patients. This includes 27 patients who have had failed attempts at selective cannulation of the bile ducts, four patients in whom endoscopic catheters could not be advanced through obstructing lesions, and one patient with a Billroth II anastomosis. There was one major bleeding complication which required selective hepatic arterial embolization. Two other patients had minor bleeding requiring no therapy, and two patients developed transient sepsis.

References

1. Cotton, P. B. Progress report, ERCP. Gut *18*:316, 1977.
2. Silvis, S. E., Rohrmann, C. A., and Vennes, J. A. Diagnostic accuracy of endoscopic retrograde cholangiopancreatography in hepatic, biliary, and pancreatic malignancy. Ann. Intern. Med. *84*:438, 1976.
3. Okuda, K., Tanikawa, K., Imura, T., et al. Nonsurgical percutaneous transhepatic cholangiography—diagnostic significance in medical problems of the liver. Am. J. Dig. Dis. *19*:21, 1974.
4. Gold, R. P., Casavella, W. J., Stern, G., et al. Transhepatic cholangiography: the radiological method of choice in suspected obstructive jaundice. Radiology *133*:39, 1979.
5. Vallon, A. G., Lees, W. R., and Cotton, P. B. Grey-scale ultrasonography in cholestatic jaundice. Gut *20*:51, 1979.
6. Goldberg, H. I., Filly, R. A., Korobkin, M., et al. Capability of CT body scanning and ultrasonography to demonstrate the status of the biliary ductal system in patients with jaundice. Radiology *129*:731, 1978.
7. Matzen, P., Malchow-Moller, A., Brun, B., et al. Ultrasonography, computed tomography and cholescintigraphy in suspected obstructive jaundice—a prospective comparative study. Gastroenterology *81*:1492, 1983.
8. Matzen, P., Gaubek, A., Holst-Christensen, J., et al. Accuracy of direct cholangiography by endoscopic or transhepatic route in jaundice—a prospective study. Gastroenterology *81*:237, 1981.
9. Scharschmidt, B. F., Goldberg, H. I., and Schmid, R. Medical intelligence—approach to the patient with cholestatic jaundice. N. Engl. J. Med. *308*:1515, 1983.
10. Vennes, J. A., and Bond, J. H. Approach to the jaundiced patient. Gastroenterology *84*:1615, 1983.
11. Girard, R. M., and Legros, G. Retained and recurrent bile duct stones—surgical or nonsurgical removal? Ann. Surg. *193*:150, 1981.
12. Den Besten, L., and Doty, J. E. Pathogenesis and management of choledocholithiasis. Surg. Clin. North Am. *61*:893, 1981.
13. Allen, B., Shapiro, H. A., and Way, L. W. Management of recurrent and residual common duct stones. Am. J. Surg. *142*:41, 1981.
14. Koch, H., Classen, M., Schaffner, O., et al. Endoscopic papillotomy. Experimental studies and initial clinical experience. Scand. J. Gastroenterol. *10*:441, 1975.
15. Kawai, K., Akasaka, Y., Murakami, K., et al. Endoscopic sphincterotomy of the ampulla of Vater. Gastrointest. Endosc. *20*:148, 1974.
16. Cotton, P. B., Chapman, M., Whiteside, C. G., et al. Duodenoscopic papillotomy and gallstone removal. Br. J. Surg. *63*:709, 1976.
17. Osnes, M., and Kahrs, T. Endoscopic choledochoduodenostomy for choledocholithiasis through choledochoduodenal fistula. Endoscopy *9*:162, 1977.
18. Safrany, L. Duodenoscopic sphincterotomy and gallstone removal. Gastroenterology *72*:338, 1977.
19. Cotton, P. B., and Vallon, A. G. British experience with duodenoscopic sphincterotomy for removal of bile duct stones. Br. J. Surg. *68*:373, 1981.
20. Geenan, J. E., Vennes, J. A., and Silvis, S. E. Resume of a seminar on endoscopic retrograde sphincterotomy (ERS). Gastrointest. Endosc. *27*:31, 1981.
21. Cotton, P. B. Endoscopic management of bile duct stones (apples and oranges). Gut *25*:587, 1984.
22. Burhenne, H. G. Percutaneous extraction of retained biliary stones: 661 patients. AJR *134*:889, 1980.
23. Slater, N. D., London, N., Neoptolemos, J. P., et al. Prospective randomized study of ERCP and endoscopic sphincterotomy in acute pancreatitis. Gut *26*:A541, 1985.
24. Lesse, T., Neoptolemos, J. P., Baker, A. R., et al. Management of acute cholangitis and the impact of endoscopic sphincterotomy. Gut *26*:A553, 1985.
25. Escourrou, J., Cordova, J. A., Lazorthes, F., et al. Early and late complications after endoscopic sphincterotomy for biliary lithiasis with and without gallbladder "in situ." Gut *25*:598, 1984.
26. Siegel, J. H. Endoscopic management of choledocholithiasis and papillary stenosis. Surg. Gynecol. Obstet. *148*:747, 1979.
27. Classen, M. Endoscopic approach to papillary stenosis (PS). Endoscopy *13*:154, 1981.
28. Bar-Meir, S., Geenan, J. E., Hogan, W. J., et al. Biliary and pancreatic duct pressures measured by ERCP manometry in patients with suspected papillary stenosis. Dig. Dis. Sci. *24*:209, 1979.
29. Geenan, J. E., Hogan, W. J., Toouli, J., et al. A prospective and randomized study of the efficacy of endoscopic sphincterotomy in patients with presumptive sphincter of Oddi disfunction. Gastroenterology *86*:1086, 1984.
30. Roberts-Thomson, I. C., and Toouli, J. Is endoscopic sphincterotomy for disabling biliary-type pain after cholecystectomy effective? Gastrointest. Endosc. *31*:370, 1985.
31. Silvis, S. E. What is the post-cholecystectomy pain syndrome? Gastrointest. Endosc. *31*:401, 1985.
32. Tanaka, M., Ideda, S., and Yoshimoto, H. Endoscopic sphincterotomy for the treatment of biliary sump syndrome. Surgery *93*:264, 1983.
33. Barkin, J., Silvis, S. E., and Greenwald, R. Endoscopic therapy of sump syndrome. Dig. Dis. Sci. *26*:77, 1980.
34. Sufrany, L. Palliative endoscopic therapy of ampullary cancer. Gastrointest. Endosc. *26*:77, 1980.
35. Huibregtse, K., and Tytgat, G. N. Palliative treatment of obstructive jaundice by transpapillary introduction of a large bore bile duct endoprosthesis. Gut *23*:371, 1982.
36. Cotton, P. B., Burney, P. G., and Mason, R. P. Transnasal bile duct catheterization after endoscopic sphincterotomy: method for biliary drainage, perfusion, and sequential cholangiography. Gut *20*:285, 1979.
37. Wurbs, D., Phillip, J., and Classen, M. Experience with longstanding nasobiliary tube in biliary disease. Endoscopy *12*:219, 1980.
38. Palmer, K. R., and Hofmann, A. F. Intraductal mono-octanoin for the direct dissolution of bile duct stones: experience in 343 patients. Gut *27*:196, 1986.
39. Riemann, J. F., Senberth, K., and Demling, L. Mechanical lithotripsy of common bile duct stones. Gastrointest. Endosc. *31*:207, 1985.
40. Silvis, S. E., and Vennes, J. A. Endoscopic retrograde sphinc-

humans because of rapid autolysis after death and because of the scarcity of normal surgical biopsy specimens. The state of preservation of the specimen, functional status, and fixative used are all critical. For most histologic purposes, Zenker-formol fixation and hematoxylin and eosin staining are suitable.

Acinar cells are tall pyramidal or columnar epithelial cells with their broad bases on a basal lamina and their apices converging on a central lumen (Fig. 94–6). In the resting state, numerous refractive eosinophilic zymogen granules fill the apical portion of the cell. These granules also give a weak periodic acid–Schiff reaction for proteoglycans,[12] but they are nonetheless thought to be serous rather than seromucous in nature. The basal portion of the cells contains one or two centrally located, spherical nuclei and extremely basophilic cytoplasm (i.e., it stains dark purple with hematoxylin). This intense staining reaction is due to the large amounts of ribonucleoprotein present in the ribosomes of the granular endoplasmic reticulum (ergastoplasm of light microscopic sections). Nucleic acids in the nucleus or basal cytoplasm may be specifically stained by the Feulgen reaction or methylgreen-pyronin staining.[12] The Golgi complex lies between the nucleus and zymogen granules and can be seen as a clear, nonstaining region (Fig. 94–6).

The acinar cells undergo cyclic changes in morphology in response to feeding and digestion.[13–15] After a large meal, the zymogen granule content of the cells is depleted. This apparently occurs by a decrease in both the size and the number of granules.[13] After depletion of the granules, which is more rapid and more complete after injection of a gastrointestinal hormone or a cholinergic drug, the Golgi apparatus may be observed at the apex of the cell and appear more extensive than in the resting state. The reduction in size and number of granules occurs with a substantial increase in pancreatic enzyme secretion.

The subcellular structure of the acinar cells can be visualized at the electron microscopic level (Fig. 94–7). The acinar cell has several short, slender microvilli about 0.2 μm in length, which extend into the lumen of the acinus. The lumen frequently contains flocculent electron-dense material, which presumably is the secreted digestive enzymes. Thin filaments form the axis of the microvilli and also form a network beneath the apical plasmalemma.[16] These microfilaments apparently play a structural role, as their disruption causes expansion of the acinar lumen and loss of microvilli.[16] Adjacent cells are joined at the apical surface by electron-dense intercellular junctions. Tight junctions form a belt-like band around the apical end of the cell and are produced by the apposition of the external membrane leaflets of neighboring cells.[17] These junctions prevent the reflux of secreted substances from the duct into the intercellular space. Gap junctions are

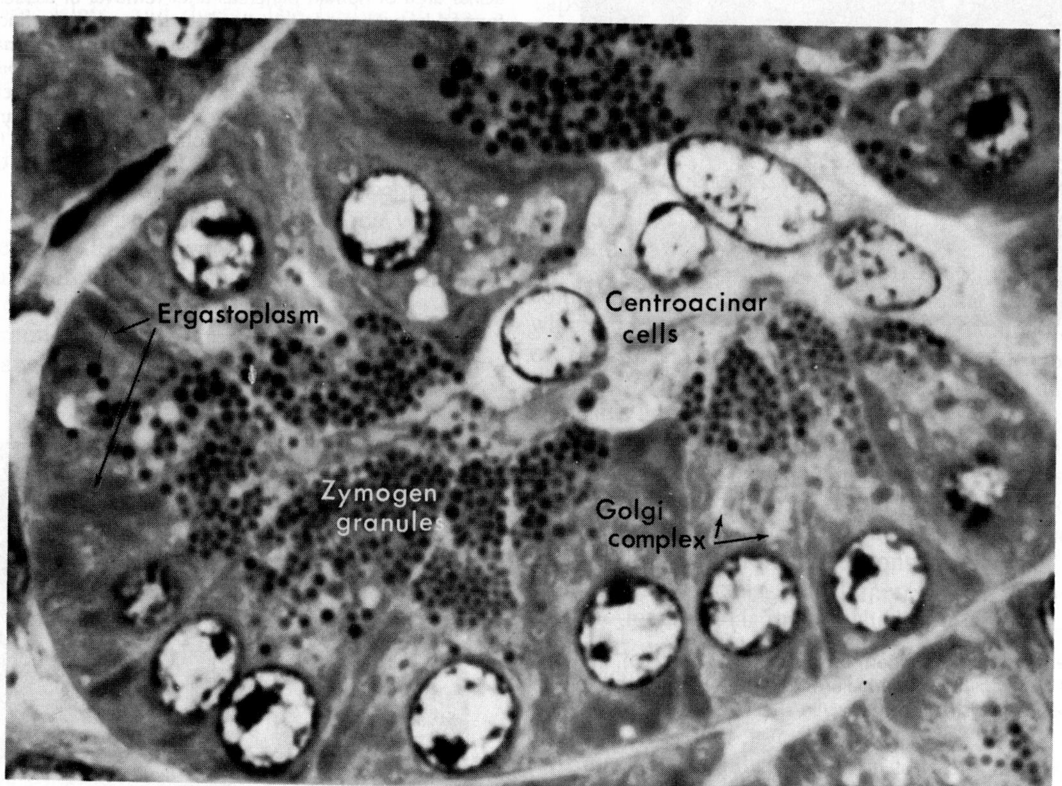

Figure 94–6. Photomicrograph of a human acinus, showing acinar and centroacinar cells. The acinar cell ergastoplasm, Golgi complex, and zymogen granules are easily identifiable. Formalin, osmium fixation. Epon-embedded section. Toluidine blue stain, × 3200. (From Bloom, W., and Fawcett, D. W. A Textbook of Histology, 11th ed. Philadelphia, W. B. Saunders Company, 1986. Courtesy of Susumu Ito, M.D.)

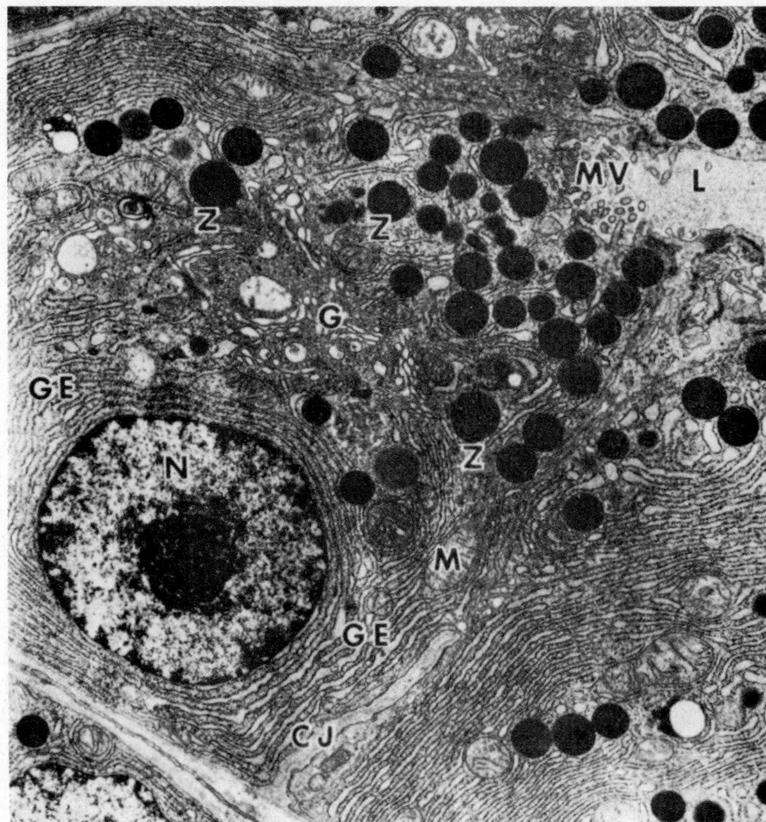

Figure 94–7. Electron micrograph of a human acinar cell. N, Nucleus; GE, granular endoplasmic reticulum; G, Golgi complex; Z, zymogen granules; MV, microvilli; L, lumen of acinus; M, mitochondria; CJ, intercellular space. × 15,000. (Courtesy of Susumu Ito, M.D.)

distributed on the lateral cellular membranes and are formed by the apposition of larger, disk-shaped membrane plaques. They allow communication between cells. Below the junctions, the lateral cell borders are relatively straight and have a few, small interdigitations.

The nucleus is usually spherical, about 6 μm in diameter,[18] with one or more nucleoli in the interior and patches of dense heterochromatin along the inner nuclear membrane. Numerous conspicuous nuclear pores are located at regions where the lightly stained euchromatin makes contact with the nuclear membrane. These pores presumably are the sites where messenger and transfer RNAs are transported out of the nucleus into the cytoplasm. Binucleate cells are also seen occasionally.

Mitochondria are elongate, cylindrical structures that may appear oval in cross section and may contain well-developed cristae and many matrix granules. They occur throughout the cytoplasm, among the granular endoplasmic reticulum or zymogen granules, and adjacent to the basolateral cell border. The cytoplasmic matrix, although inconspicuous to the eye, occupies about 45 per cent of the cell volume.[19] Much of its content (ions, small molecules) is washed out of the cell during routine fixation procedures.

Granular endoplasmic reticulum (Fig. 94–7) occupies about 20 per cent of the cell volume[19, 20] and fills most of the basal region of the acinar cells, although small amounts also occur in the apical region adjacent to and among the zymogen granules. It is composed of numerous parallel cisternal membranes covered with closely spaced attached ribosomes, giving the structures a granular appearance. Free ribosomes or polysomes also occur in the cytoplasmic matrix. On the basis of studies with experimental animals, the ribosomes of the granular endoplasmic reticulum have been found to be the site of protein synthesis.[21, 22]

The Golgi complex (Fig. 94–7) is located between the nucleus and the mass of zymogen granules present in the resting gland and consists of flattened membranous saccules as well as small vesicles or vacuoles containing flocculent electron-dense material. On occasion lysosomes are also observed in the Golgi region.

The Golgi complex is believed to play an important role in the transport of secretory proteins and the formation of zymogen granules. However, the mechanisms by which these processes occur are still unresolved. Around the Golgi complex, numerous small vesicles about 50 nm in diameter are commonly found.[23] On the basis of autoradiographic studies, it has been proposed that these vesicles bud from portions of the granular endoplasmic reticulum and carry secretory proteins to condensing vacuoles or the Golgi complex.[21, 22] It has also been proposed that proteins are transported through specialized connections between the endoplasmic reticulum and condensing vacuoles called GERL (Golgi-endoplasmic reticulum-lysosomes), membrane lamellae rich in hydrolase activity and located adjacent to the Golgi complex.[24, 25] Conclusive evidence for either of these pathways has yet to be presented, and it has been questioned whether proteins are transported through vesicular compartments at all.[26, 27]

The secretory granules of the pancreas are usually divided into two types: electron-lucent condensing vacuoles and electron-dense zymogen granules. The condensing vacuoles are usually seen in the vicinity of the Golgi complex and, on the basis of autoradiographic data,[21, 22] are believed to be precursors of the zymogen granules. They are membrane-bound vesicles slightly larger than zymogen granules and much less numerous, occupying only about 2 per cent of the cytoplasm.[20]

Zymogen granules (Fig. 94–7) are also spherical, membrane-bound vesicles, slightly under 1 μm in diameter,[13, 28, 29] and filled with electron-dense material, which apparently represents the digestive enzymes. The membrane of the granule is difficult to distinguish owing to the electron density of the granule content.

Studies on the chemical composition of the granules have shown that they contain about 12 to 15 different digestive enzymes, which make up about 90 per cent of the granule protein.[30–33] Each granule apparently contains the entire complement of secreted enzymes (i.e., those for breakdown of carbohydrates, proteins, lipids, and nucleic acids), as labeled antibodies to several different enzymes have been located over single zymogen granules from different cells.[34, 35] Individual zymogen granules, however, can differ markedly in the concentration of specific digestive enzymes contained within the granules.[36] The digestive enzymes within the granules apparently are not in solution or suspension but in a solid state array, which exhibits specific binding between the enzymes themselves and between the enzymes and the granule membrane.[37–40] Isolated zymogen granules are stable at slightly acid pH; however, at alkaline pH, they release their enzymes into solution.[38, 40, 41] This behavior may account for the solubilization of digestive enzymes within the alkaline duct lumen.

The size, size distribution, number, and volume fraction of zymogen granules varies with physiologic state.[13, 14] In the fasted adult, granules occupy about 15 to 20 per cent of the cell volume and, with secretion, the volume fraction decreases dramatically. After stimulation with a cholinergic drug or a gastrointestinal hormone such as cholecystokinin, the cells can be virtually depleted of zymogen granules.[42] The remaining granules are smaller, about one fifth the diameter of full-sized granules in adults. After feeding, the depletion of granules is not so extensive as after stimulation, and a large portion of the decrease in volume results from a decrease in granule size.[13]

The most widely accepted mechanism for the secretion of digestive enzymes involves the process of exocytosis, or the fusion of the granule membrane with the apical cell membrane and subsequent release of granule content into the duct lumen.[43] Because this process has never been shown to account completely for the secretion of digestive enzymes, this hypothesis has been challenged and an alternative route for secretion proposed, on the basis of evidence for the permeability of the granule and apical cell membranes.[26, 27]

Along the basal surface of the acinar cells but not extending between adjacent cells is a thin basal lamina below which occur collagen fibers and a rich capillary network. Efferent nerve fibers, derived from the sympathetic and parasympathetic systems, penetrate the basal lamina and terminate adjacent to the acinar cells.

The centroacinar cells (Fig. 94–8) and duct cells have electron-lucent cytoplasm containing few cytoplasmic organelles or specializations. They typically contain free ribosomes and small, round mitochondria. They contain virtually no granular endoplasmic reticulum and therefore are not active in protein synthesis for secretion. Farther down the ducts, the cells contain more mitochondria, but they are never associated with invaginations of the basolateral surface, as occurs in the transporting ductal epithelium of the salivary glands. Both centroacinar and duct cells apparently secrete bicarbonate and water. Carbonic anhydrase, the enzyme responsible for formation of bicarbonate, has been demonstrated in the epithelium.[12]

The islets of Langerhans number about one million in the human pancreas and consist of anastomosing cords of polygonal endocrine cells (Fig. 94–3). Each islet is about 0.2 mm in diameter, much larger than an acinus, and is separated from the surrounding exocrine tissue by fine connective tissue fibers, which are continuous with those of the exocrine gland. Occasionally, a close association is observed between the islets and the pancreatic ducts.

Each islet is surrounded and penetrated by a rich network of capillaries lined by a fenestrated endothelium. The capillaries are arranged in a portal system that conveys blood from the islets to acinar cells (Fig. 94–9).[44–48] This insulo-acinar portal system consists of afferent arterioles that enter the islet, form a capillary glomerulus, and leave the islet as efferent capillaries passing into the exocrine tissue. A parallel arterial system supplies blood directly to the exocrine pancreas (Fig. 94–9), and yet the portal system permits the local action of islet hormones, especially insulin, on the exocrine pancreas.[46–48] Acinar cells surrounding islets of Langerhans, termed peri-insular acini, are morphologically and biochemically different from acini situated further away (tele-insular acini).[49, 50] Peri-insular acini have larger cells, nuclei, and zymogen granule regions[49] and different ratios of specific digestive enzymes.[50]

Although one cell type secretes several different digestive enzymes in the exocrine pancreas, each cell type in the endocrine pancreas appears to secrete a single hormone. Four major types of cells are found: B cells, A cells, D cells and PP cells.[51, 52] B cells are the most numerous, constituting 50 to 80 per cent of pancreatic islet volume, and secrete insulin.[51] A cells occupy about 5 to 20 per cent of the cell mass and secrete glucagon. These two hormones are important in carbohydrate metabolism. PP cells account for 10 to 35 per cent of islet volume and secrete pancreatic

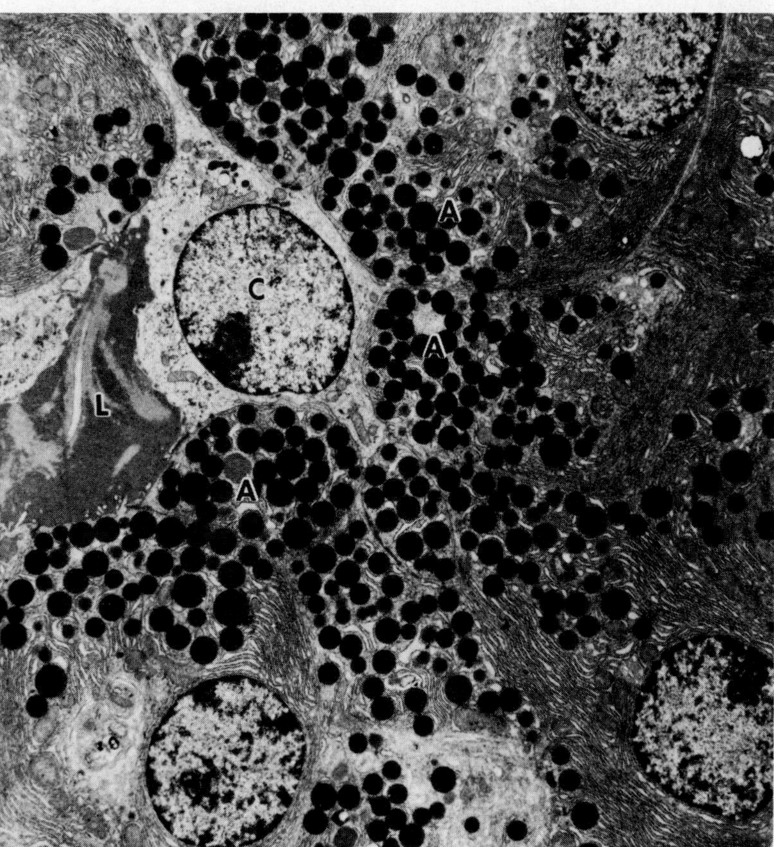

Figure 94–8. Electron micrography of a centroacinar cell (C) and several acinar cells (A). Note the electron-lucid cytoplasm, scattered mitochondria, and lack of other membranous organelles in the centroacinar cell. L is the lumen of the acinus. × 9000. (Courtesy of Susumu Ito, M.D.)

polypeptide. D cells are the least abundant, constituting about 5 per cent of the islets, and secrete somatostatin. Other rare cell types occur in the islet.[53]

The different cell types have traditionally been distinguished at the light microscopic level by specific histochemical stains such as Mallory-azan, which stains the cytoplasm of A cells brilliant red, B cells brownish-orange, and D cells blue.[8, 53, 54] At the ultrastructural level, the different cell types can be distinguished by the structure of the secretion granules, which are about one third the diameter of the zymogen granules of the pancreas. The granules differ slightly in size (from 250 to 300 nm), in the presence or absence of an electron-lucent space within the granule membrane, and in the electron density of the granule core.[54, 55]

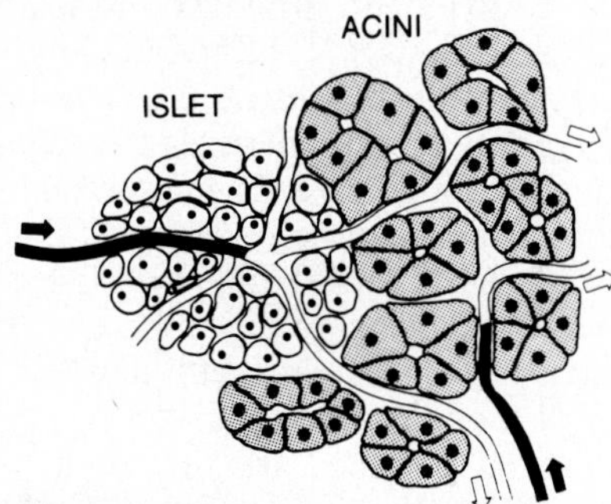

Figure 94–9. Schematic diagram of the insulo-acinar portal system illustrating the dual blood supply to the exocrine pancreas. (From Goldfine, I. D., and Williams, J. A. Int. Rev. Cytol. *85*:1, 1983. Used by permission.)

The cells have also been differentiated by specific immunofluorescence techniques using antisera directed against insulin, glucagon, somatostatin, and pancreatic polypeptide.[51, 52, 56–58] In experimental animals, insulin-secreting B cells tend to be centrally located, whereas the other cell types tend to have a peripheral location.[52, 53] In humans, the islets are subdivided into units, each of which exhibits a central aggregation of B cells surrounded by varying numbers of peripherally located cells secreting the other endocrine hormones.[52] The islets display a heterogeneous cellular composition depending on their anatomic position in the pancreas.[52, 56–58] Immunohistochemical studies sampling different portions of the pancreas indicate a regional partition of glucagon and pancreatic polypeptide. Islets derived from the ventral pancreatic bud are rich in pancreatic polypeptide–secreting cells, whereas islets derived from the dorsal pancreatic bud are rich in glucagon-secreting cells.[52, 56–58]

EMBRYOLOGY

The pancreas first appears in embryos of approximately 4 mm size in the fourth week of gestation.[59, 60] Two outpouchings from the endodermal lining of the

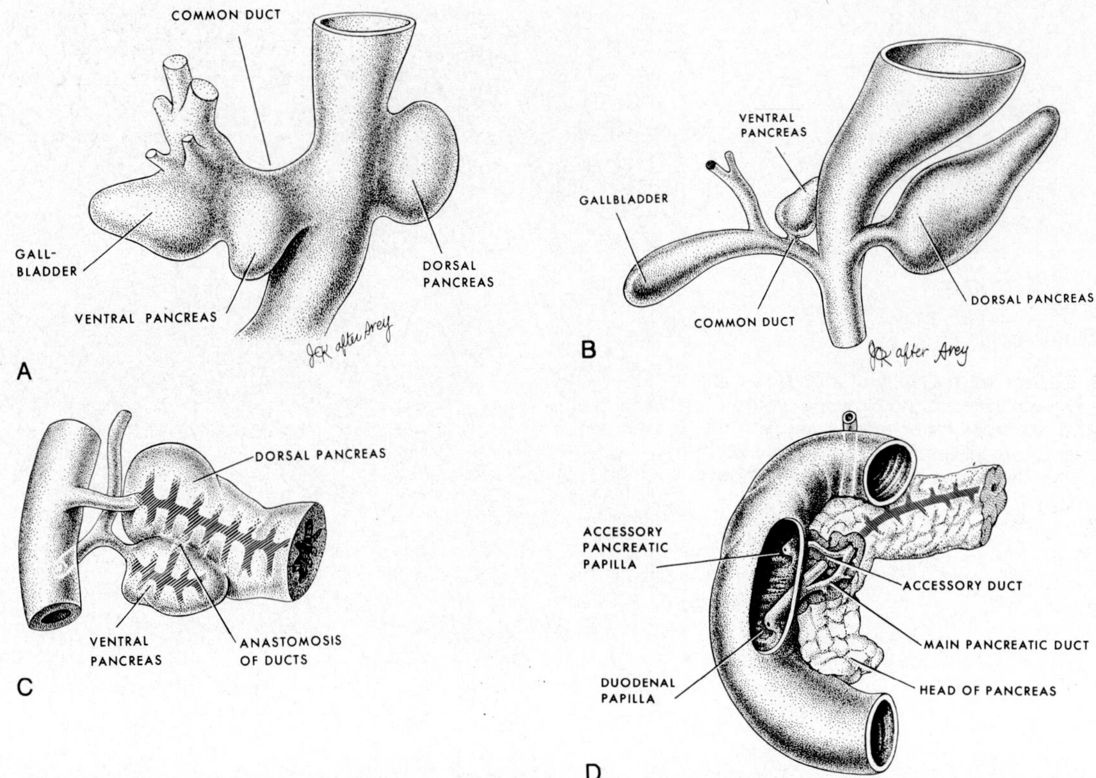

Figure 94–10. Stages in the embryologic development of the pancreas. *A*, At approximately four weeks of gestation, dorsal and ventral buds are formed. *B*, At six weeks, the ventral pancreas extends toward the dorsal pancreas. *C*, By about seven weeks, fusion of dorsal and ventral pancreas has occurred, and ductular anastomosis is beginning. *D*, At birth, the pancreas is a single organ, and ductular anastomosis is complete. (Modified after Arey.)

duodenum develop at this time: the ventral pancreas and the dorsal pancreas (Fig. 94–10*A*). The dorsal anlage grows more rapidly, and by the sixth week it is an elongated nodular structure extending into the dorsal mesentery, within which its growth continues (Fig. 94–10*B*). The ventral pancreas remains smaller and is carried away from the duodenum by its connection with the common bile duct. The two primordia are brought into apposition by the uneven growth of the duodenum and fuse by the seventh week (Fig. 94–10*C*). The tail, body, and part of the head of the pancreas are formed by the dorsal component, the remainder of the head and the uncinate process derive from the ventral pancreas. These primitive relationships are still distinguishable in the adult pancreas.[60]

Both of the primitive pancreata contain an axial duct. The dorsal duct arises directly from the duodenal wall and the ventral duct arises from the common bile duct. On fusion of the ventral and dorsal components, the ventral duct anastomoses with the dorsal one, forming the main pancreatic duct (Fig. 94–10*D*). The proximal end of the dorsal duct becomes the accessory duct in the adult and is patent in 70 per cent of specimens.[61] The common outlet of the bile duct and pancreatic duct observed in most adults is the result of the common origin of the bile duct and the ventral pancreas.

The pancreatic acini appear in the third month as derivatives of the side ducts and termini of the primitive ducts. The acini remain connected to the larger pancreatic ducts by small secretory ductules. The primitive pancreas is composed of relatively undifferentiated epithelial cells, similar in morphology to duct cells. Mesenchymal tissue in which the gland grows provides the thin connective tissue capsule and divides the gland into lobes and lobules.

Distinct differences in morphology, enzyme content, and secretory capacity exist between the embryonic and the adult pancreas.[62–71] Early in development, the pancreas has no zymogen granules and little granular endoplasmic reticulum,[62–66] although low levels of digestive enzymes can be detected in the cells at this time.[67, 68] In humans, the pancreas is composed of undifferentiated epithelial cells at 9 weeks of gestation.[62] During subsequent cell differentiation, the specific activity of the digestive enzymes increases some thousandfold,[67, 68] and the granules increase in size and come to occupy most of the cytoplasm of the cells, including the basolateral regions.[63–66] At 12 weeks in humans, zymogen granules are first seen by electron microscopy. The cells also contain a Golgi complex and granular endoplasmic reticulum in relatively small amounts. By 20 weeks, larger zymogen granules typical of the adult are seen.[62] Each digestive enzyme has a characteristic rate of accumulation and increases in concentration at different times.[67, 68] At birth, the granules in experimental animals are the largest normally found in the pancreas, being about six times the volume of the granules in adults.[72, 73] At about this time, the capacity for stimulated secretion is attained.[69–71] Differentiation of the pancreas continues beyond birth with regard to both the size of the zymogen granules and the amount of granular endoplasmic reticulum,[72–74] as well as the enzyme content of the tissue.[75, 76]

The endocrine pancreas differentiates on roughly the same time course as the exocrine portion,[77, 78] and the appearance of islet hormones also precedes the appearance of secretion granules in the cells. In humans, endocrine cells are first observed singly or in small clusters along the basolateral portion of undifferentiated acinar cells (9 to 10 weeks), but by 12 to 16 weeks distinct islets in various stages of complexity can be observed. The development of islets in the PP-rich regions lags slightly behind that of the glucagon-rich regions.[79] Insulin cells increase continuously with age, whereas glucagon cells increase during fetal life and then decrease in infants and adults. Somatostatin cells are elevated in fetal and infant stages, whereas pancreatic polypeptide cells are the least abundant cells during these stages.[79]

RELATION TO OTHER ORGANS

The pancreas is strategically situated close to a number of important structures in the posterior abdomen (Fig. 94–11). Beginning at the head of the gland and progressing toward the tail, the pancreas has the following relationships with adjacent structures. The posterior surfaces of the head and body are devoid of peritoneum. The inferior vena cava runs behind the head of the pancreas. This surface also overlies the terminal parts of the right renal veins and the right crus of the diaphragm. The common bile duct is situated either in a groove in the upper lateral surface or in the substance of the gland. The posterior surface of the neck overlies the superior mesenteric vein and the origin of the superior portal vein. The body is in contact with the aorta and the origin of the superior mesenteric artery, the left crus of the diaphragm, the left adrenal gland, and the left kidney and its vasculature. The splenic vein courses between the pancreas and the preceding structures (Fig. 94–11). The kidney is separated from the pancreas by the perirenal fat and fascia. The tail of the pancreas is located within the two layers of the splenorenal ligament along with the splenic vessels.

The anterior surface of the head is separated from the transverse colon only by areolar tissue. The caudal surface of the gland is covered with peritoneum, which is continuous with the transverse mesocolon and lies close to a coil of the jejunum. The uncinate process of the head is anterior to the aorta and is traversed by the superior mesenteric vessels, which pass between

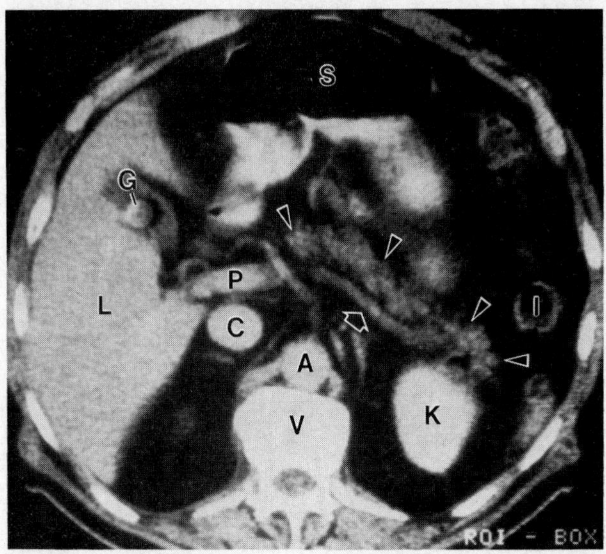

Figure 94–11. Normal anatomic relationship of the pancreas to other intra-abdominal structures as shown by computed tomographic (CT) scanning. The borders of the pancreas are indicated by arrowheads. The splenic vein is indicated by an arrow. A, Aorta; C, vena cava; G, incidental gallstone; I, small intestine; K, left kidney; L, liver; P, portal vein; S, stomach; V, vertebra. (Courtesy of M. P. Federle, M.D.)

the pancreas and the duodenum. The anterior surface of the neck is covered with peritoneum and abuts on the pylorus, separated by a part of the lesser sac of the peritoneum. The anterior surface of the body is separated from the stomach by the lesser sac. The inferior surface of the body is also peritonealized and is close to the duodenojejunal junction and the splenic flexure of the colon. The superior border of the body is in contact with the posterior aspect of the lesser omentum. The splenic artery has its tortuous course along this border. The superior mesenteric arteries and veins pass under the body at its junction with the uncinate process.

The pancreatic duct (duct of Wirsung) begins near the tail and is formed from anastomosing ductules draining the lobules of the gland. It courses from the left to right and is enlarged by additional ducts of various sizes until it reaches the neck, where it turns caudal and posterior, and where it usually joins the common bile duct (Fig. 94–12*A*). The short common segment is the ampulla of the bile duct, which terminates in the duodenal papilla. An accessory pancreatic duct (duct of Santorini) is frequently present; it may terminate in the main pancreatic duct or separately in the accessory pancreatic papilla. The accessory duct is patent in 70 per cent of autopsy specimens.[61] In 10 per cent the main duct drains into the accessory papilla and has no connection with the common bile duct.[61]

CONGENITAL ANOMALIES

Pancreatic *agenesis* occurs only rarely, either in association with other anomalies or as an apparently isolated anomaly.[80] Persons affected with this condition

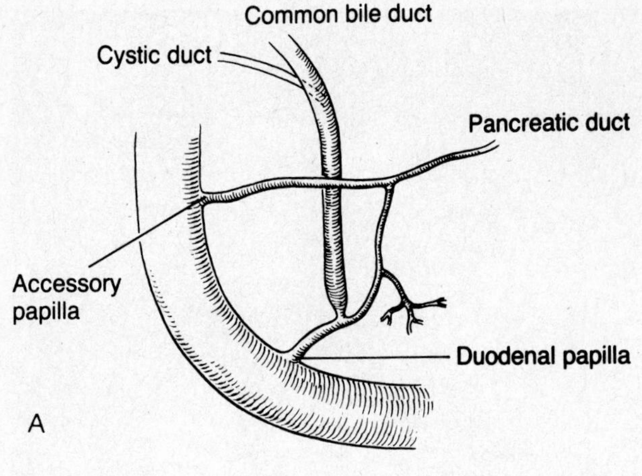

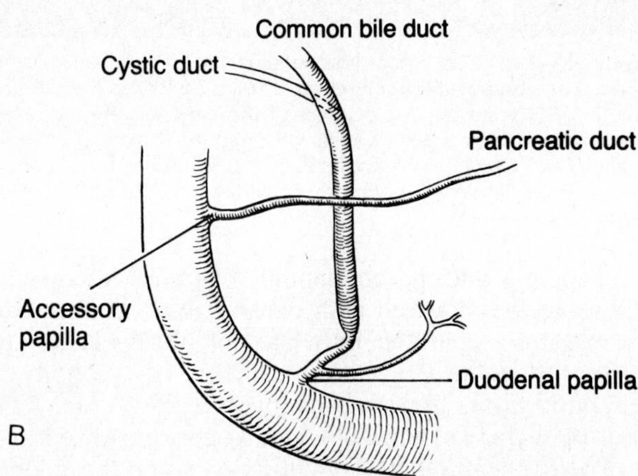

Figure 94–12. Anatomic arrangement of the pancreatic duct system. *A*, The most common arrangement. Most of the pancreatic secretion empties into the duodenum along with bile through the duodenal papilla. The proximal portion of the embryologic dorsal duct remains patent in about 70 per cent of adults and empties through the accessory papilla. *B*, Pancreas divisum. The embryologic dorsal and ventral ducts fail to fuse. Most of the pancreatic secretion empties through the small accessory papilla. Only pancreatic secretion from the uncinate process and part of the head of the pancreas (which are derived from the embryologic ventral pancreas) drain through the duodenal papilla.

generally have died soon after birth. In addition, agenesis can also occur of either the dorsal or the ventral pancreas, although more commonly it involves the dorsal segment.[81] In this situation, normal pancreatic tissue may still be formed. Hypoplasia has also been recognized. Although the larger ducts and islets are normal, there is a reduction in the number of smaller ducts and a lack of differentiation in the terminal duct system.[82]

Accessory pancreata and *ectopic pancreatic tissue* are common and occur at diverse areas in the gastrointestinal tract. The frequency of ectopic pancreatic tissue has been reported from autopsy material to range from 0.55 to 13.7 per cent.[83] The most common sites are the stomach, duodenum, and proximal jejunum. Foci of pancreatic tissue are also found in Meckel's diverticula, ileum, common bile duct, gallbladder, hilus of spleen, and umbilicus, as well as in perigastric and periduodenal locations.

During early embryologic development, part of the ventral pancreas may encircle the duodenum, forming an *annular pancreas*. This entity is the most common anomaly obstructing the duodenum in infancy and, in such cases, usually involves growth of pancreatic tissue into the wall of the duodenum. In one large series of patients, the annulus was almost always proximal to the ampulla of Vater, involving the second portion of the duodenum in 85 per cent of cases.[84] Annular pancreas may be associated with other congenital anomalies, including atresia of the duodenum, and with Down's syndrome (trisomy 21).[85] It may also be present without producing symptoms or may be only an incidental finding at surgery or autopsy. In some cases, symptoms may appear for the first time in the adult. Because pancreatic tissue often extends into the duodenal wall and because the annular tissue may contain a large pancreatic duct or the common bile duct, symptomatic cases are best treated by surgical bypass rather than division of the pancreatic tissue.[84]

Pancreas divisum results from failure of the ducts of the embryologic dorsal and ventral pancreata to fuse (Fig. 94–12). This leads to a situation in which most of the pancreatic exocrine secretion drains through the relatively small duct of Santorini and the accessory papilla. Whether pancreas divisum represents an anatomic variant of no pathologic significance or a congenital anomaly responsible for recurrent acute pancreatitis or chronic abdominal pain in some patients is a matter of considerable ongoing controversy. Pancreas divisum has been observed in about 5 to 10 per cent of autopsy series[61, 86–90] and in about 2 to 7 per cent of patients undergoing endoscopic retrograde pancreatography.[91–94] An association of pancreas divisum with recurrent idiopathic acute pancreatitis has been suggested in some clinical series[91–94] but was not observed in others.[95–97] It has been proposed that both pancreas divisum and a relatively stenotic accessory papilla must be present for clinically evident pancreatic disease to occur. Although dilatation of the duct of Santorini is not frequently seen on pancreatography in the setting of recurrent acute pancreatitis and pancreas divisum, as would be expected if the accessory papilla were acting as a site of obstruction, histopathologic studies of surgically resected specimens have shown involvement with pancreatitis of the segment of the pancreas derived from the embryologic dorsal pancreas (drained through the accessory papilla) and sparing of regions derived from the ventral pancreas, which drain through the ampulla of Vater and duodenal papilla.[97]

Because of the uncertainty concerning the importance of pancreas divisum as an etiologic factor in recurrent acute pancreatitis or abdominal pain, patients with this finding should in general be managed conservatively, without operative or endoscopic intervention. A variety of approaches have been employed to treat patients with frequent episodes of recurrent acute pancreatitis or disabling pain without other apparent cause. These have included surgical sphincteroplasty of either the accessory papilla alone[93, 98–100] or of both the accessory and duodenal papillas;[101, 102] pancreaticoduodenectomy;[103] endoscopic sphincterotomy of the accessory papilla;[97, 104] and endoscopic placement of stents through the accessory papilla.[97] The results of these various therapeutic interventions are mixed but suggest some benefit, at least short-term, of procedures that include surgical accessory sphincteroplasty in patients with idiopathic recurrent acute pancreatitis and pancreas divisum. There appears to be little beneficial effect of operative or endoscopic interventions in patients with pancreas divisum and chronic unexplained abdominal pain who do not have definable episodes of recurrent acute pancreatitis.[97] The clinical significance of the relatively frequent finding of pancreas divisum still remains to be clarified, as does the most appropriate therapeutic management, if it is found to be a significant factor in the production of pancreatic disease in some individuals.

References

1. Clarke, E. S. History of gastroenterology. *In* Paulson, M. (ed.). Gastroenterologic Medicine. Philadelphia, Lea & Febiger, 1969.
2. Garrison, F. H. An Introduction to the History of Medicine. 4th edition. Philadelphia, W. B. Saunders Company, 1929.
3. Major, R. H. A History of Medicine. Springfield, Illinois, Charles C Thomas, 1954.
4. Heidenhain, R. Beiträge Zur Kenntnis Des Pankreas. Pflügers Arch. *10*:557, 1875.
5. Basmajian, J. V. Grant's Method of Anatomy. 10th edition. Baltimore, Williams & Wilkins Co., 1980.
6. Clemente, C. D. (ed.). Gray's Anatomy of the Human Body. 30th ed. Philadelphia, Lea & Febiger, 1985.
7. Munger, B. L. The ultrastructure of the exocrine pancreas. *In* Carey, L. C. (ed.). The Pancreas. St. Louis, C. V. Mosby Co., 1973, p. 17.
8. Bloom, W., and Fawcett, D. W. A Textbook of Histology. 11th edition. Philadelphia, W. B. Saunders Company, 1986.
9. Tompkins, R. K., and Traverso, L. W. The exocrine cells. *In* Keynes, W. M., and Keith, R. G. (eds.). The Pancreas. New York, Appleton-Century-Crofts, 1981, p. 23.
10. Rhodin, J. A. G. Histology; A Test and Atlas. New York, Oxford University Press, 1974.
11. Bockman, D. E., Boydston, W. R., and Parsa, I. Architecture of human pancreas: implications for early changes in pancreatic disease. Gastroenterology *85*:55, 1983.
12. Becker, V. Histochemistry of the exocrine pancreas. *In* de Reuck, A. V. S., and Cameron, M. P. (eds.). The Exocrine Pancreas. Boston, Little, Brown and Co., 1961, p. 56.
13. Ermak, T. H., and Rothman, S. S. Zymogen granules of pancreas decrease in size in response to feeding. Cell Tissue Res. *214*:51, 1981.
14. Ermak, T. H. The size secretory cycle of the pancreatic zymogen granule. *In* Rothman, S. S., and Ho, J. J. L. (eds.). Nonvesicular Transport. New York, John Wiley, 1984, p. 325.
15. Uchiyama, Y., and Saito, K. A morphometric study of 24-hour variations in subcellular structures of the rat pancreatic acinar cell. Cell Tissue Res. *226*:609, 1982.
16. Bauduin, H., Stock, C., Vincent, D., and Grenier, J. F. Microfilamentous system and secretion of enzyme in the exocrine pancreas. Effect of cytochalasin B. J. Cell Biol. *66*:165, 1975.
17. Metz, J., Forssman, W. G., and Ito, S. Exocrine pancreas under experimental conditions. III. Membrane and cell junctions in isolated acinar cells. Cell Tissue Res. *177*:459, 1977.
18. Nevalainen, T. J. Effects of pilocarpine stimulation on rat pancreatic acinar cells. An electron microscopic study with morphometric analysis. Acta Pathol. Microbiol. Scand. Suppl. *210*:1, 1970.
19. Bolender, R. P. Stereological analysis of the guinea pig pancreas. I. Analytical model and quantitative description of nonstimulated pancreatic acinar cells. J. Cell Biol. *61*:269, 1974.
20. Amsterdam, A., and Jamieson, J. D. Studies on dispersed pancreatic exocrine cells. I. Dissociation technique and morphologic characteristics of separated cells. J. Cell Biol. *63*:1037, 1974.
21. Palade, G. E. Intracellular aspects of the process of protein synthesis. Science *189*:347, 1975.
22. Jamieson, J. D., and Palade, G. E. Production of secretory proteins in animal cells. *In* Brinkley, B. R., and Porter, K. R. (eds.). International Cell Biology 1976–1977. New York, Rockefeller University Press, 1977.
23. Jamieson, J. D., and Palade, G. E. Intracellular transport of secretory proteins in the pancreatic exocrine cell. I. Role of the peripheral elements of the Golgi complex. J. Cell Biol. *34*:577, 1967.
24. Novikoff, A. B., Mori, M., Quintana, N., and Yam, A. Studies of the secretory process in the mammalian exocrine pancreas: I. The condensing vacuoles. J. Cell Biol. *75*:148, 1977.
25. Hand, A. R., and Oliver, C. Cytochemical studies of GERL and its role in secretory granule formation in exocrine cells. Histochem. J. *9*:375, 1977.
26. Rothman, S. S. Protein transport by the pancreas. Science *190*:747, 1975.
27. Rothman, S. S. The passage of proteins through membranes—old assumptions and new perspectives. Am. J. Physiol. *238*:G391, 1980.
28. Liebow, C., and Rothman, S. S. Distribution of zymogen granule size. Am. J. Physiol. *225*:258, 1973.
29. Nadelhaft, I. Measurement of the size distribution of zymogen granules from rat pancreas. Biophys. J. *13*:1014, 1973.
30. Greene, L. J., Hirs, C. H. W., and Palade, G. E. On the protein composition of bovine pancreatic zymogen granules. J. Biol. Chem. *238*:2054, 1963.
31. Keller, P. J., and Cohen, E. Enzymic composition of some cell fractions of bovine pancreas. J. Biol. Chem. *236*:1407, 1961.
32. Tartakoff, A., Greene, L. J., and Palade, G. E. Studies on the guinea pig pancreas. Fractionation and partial characterization of exocrine proteins. J. Biol. Chem. *249*:7420, 1974.
33. Scheele, G., Bartelt, D., and Bieger, W. Characterization of human exocrine proteins by two-dimensional isoelectric focusing/sodium dodecyl sulfate gel electrophoresis. Gastroenterology *80*:461, 1981.
34. Kraehenbuhl, J. P., Racine, L., and Jamieson, J. D. Immunocytochemical localization of secretory proteins in bovine pancreatic exocrine cells. J. Cell Biol. *72*:406, 1977.
35. Geuze, J. J., Slot, J. W., and Tokuyasu, K. T. Immunocytochemical localization of amylase and chymotrypsinogen in the exocrine pancreatic cell with special attention to the Golgi complex. J. Cell Biol. *82*:697, 1979.
36. Mroz, E. A., and Lechene, C. Pancreatic zymogen granules differ markedly in protein composition. Science *232*:871, 1986.
37. Burwen, S. J., and Rothman, S. S. Zymogen granules: osmotic properties, interaction with ions, and some structural implications. Am. J. Physiol. *222*:1177, 1972.
38. Rothman, S. S. The behavior of isolated zymogen granules: pH-dependent release and reassociation of protein. Biochim. Biophys. Acta *241*:567, 1971.
39. Rothman, S. S. Association of bovine alpha-chymotrypsinogen and trypsinogen with rat zymogen granules. Am. J. Physiol. *222*:1299, 1972.
40. Ermak, T. H., and Rothman, S. S. Internal organization of the zymogen granule: formation of reticular structures in vitro. J. Ultrastruct. Res. *64*:98, 1978.
41. Hokin, L. E. Isolation of the zymogen granules of dog pancreas and a study of their properties. Biochim. Biophys. Acta *18*:379, 1955.
42. Jamieson, J. D., and Palade, G. E. Synthesis, intracellular transport, and discharge of secretory proteins in stimulated pancreatic exocrine cells. J. Cell Biol. *50*:135, 1971.
43. Palade, G. E. Functional changes in the structure of cell components. *In* Hayashi, T. (ed.). Subcellular Particles. New York, Ronald Press Co., 1959, p. 64.

44. Fujita, T. Insulo-acinar portal system in the horse pancreas. Arch. Histol. Jpn. *35*:161, 1973.
45. Fujita, T., and Murakami, T. Microcirculation of monkey pancreas with special reference to the insulo-acinar portal system. A scanning electron microscope study of vascular casts. Arch. Histol. Jpn. *35*:255, 1973.
46. Bonner-Weir, S., and Orci, L. New perspectives on the microvasculature of the islets of Langerhans in the rat. Diabetes *31*:883, 1982.
47. Williams, J. A., and Goldfine, I. D. The insulin-pancreatic acinar axis. Diabetes *34*:980, 1985.
48. Lifson, N., Kramlinger, K. G., Mayrand, R. R., and Lender, E. J. Blood flow to the rabbit pancreas with special reference to the islets of Langerhans. Gastroenterology *79*:466, 1980.
49. Kramer, M. F., and Tan, H. T. The peri-insular acini of the pancreas of the rat. Z. Zellforsch. *86*:163, 1968.
50. Malaisse-Lagae, F., Ravazzola, M., Robberecht, P., Vandermeers, A., Malaisse, W. J., and Orci, L. Exocrine pancreas: evidence for topographic partition of secretory function. Science *190*:795, 1975.
51. Stefan, Y., Orci, L., Malaisse-Lagae, F., Perrelet, A., Patel, Y., and Unger, R. H. Quantitation of endocrine cell content in the pancreas of nondiabetic and diabetic humans. Diabetes *31*:694, 1982.
52. Orci, L. Macro- and micro-domains in the endocrine pancreas. Diabetes *31*:538, 1982.
53. Boquist, L. The endocrine cells. *In* Keynes, W. M., and Keith, R. G. (eds.). The Pancreas. New York, Appleton-Century-Crofts, 1981, p. 31.
54. Munger, B. L. Morphological characterization of islet cell diversity. *In* Cooperstein, S. J., and Watkins, D. (eds.). The Islets of Langerhans; Biochemistry, Physiology, and Pathology. New York, Academic Press, Inc. 1981, p. 3.
55. Greider, M. H., Howell, S. L., and Lacy, P. E. Isolation and properties of secretory granules from rat islets of Langerhans. II. Ultrastructure of the beta granule. J. Cell. Biol. *41*:162, 1969.
56. Malaisse-Lagae, F., Stefan, Y., Cox, J., Perrelet, A., and Orci, L. Identification of a lobe in the adult human pancreas rich in pancreatic polypeptide. Diabetologia *17*:361, 1979.
57. Gersell, D. J., Gingerich, R. L., and Greider, M. H. Regional distribution and concentration of pancreatic polypeptide in the human and canine pancreas. Diabetes *28*:11, 1979.
58. Rahier, J., Wallon, J., Gepts, W., and Haot, J. Localization of pancreatic polypeptide cells in a limited lobe of the human neonate pancreas: remnant of the ventral primordium? Cell Tissue Res. *200*:359, 1979.
59. Arey, L. B. Developmental Anatomy. A Textbook and Laboratory Manual of Embryology. 7th edition. Philadelphia, W. B. Saunders Company, 1974.
60. Patten, B. M. Human Embryology. 3rd edition. New York, The Blakiston Division, McGraw-Hill Book Co., 1968.
61. Kleitsch, W. P. Anatomy of the pancreas. A study with special reference to the duct system. Arch. Surg. *71*:795, 1955.
62. Laitio, M., Lev, R., and Orlic, D. The developing human fetal pancreas: an ultrastructural and histochemical study with special reference to exocrine cells. J. Anat. *117*:619, 1974.
63. Parsa, I., Marsh, W. H., and Fitzgerald, P. J. Pancreas acinar cell differentiation. I. Morphologic and enzymatic comparisons of embryonic rat pancreas and pancreatic anlage grown in organ culture. Am. J. Pathol. *57*:457, 1969.
64. Pictet, R. L., Clark, W. R., Williams, R. H., and Rutter, W. J. An ultrastructural analysis of the developing embryonic pancreas. Dev. Biol. *29*:436, 1972.
65. Ermak, T. H., and Rothman, S. S. Increase in zymogen granule volume accounts for increase in volume density during prenatal development of pancreas. Anat. Rec. *207*:487, 1983.
66. Uchiyama, Y., and Watanabe, M. A morphometric study of developing pancreatic acinar cells of rats during prenatal life. Cell Tissue Res. *237*:117, 1984.
67. Rutter, W. J., Kemp, J. D., Bradshaw, W. S., Clark, W. R., Ronzio, R. A., and Sanders, T. G. Regulation of specific protein synthesis in cytodifferentiation. J. Cell. Physiol. *72*(Suppl. 1):1, 1968.
68. Sanders, T. G., and Rutter, W. J. The developmental regulation of amylolytic and proteolytic enzymes in the embryonic rat pancreas. J. Biol. Chem. *249*:3500, 1974.
69. Doyle, C. M., and Jamieson, J. D. Development of secretagogue response in rat pancreatic acinar cells. Dev. Biol. *65*:11, 1978.
70. Larose, L., and Morisset, J. Acinar cell responsiveness to urecholine in the rat pancreas during fetal and postnatal growth. Gastroenterology *73*:530, 1977.
71. Werlin, S. L., and Grand, R. J. Development of secretory mechanisms in rat pancreas. Am. J. Physiol. *236*:E446, 1979.
72. Ermak, T. H., and Rothman, S. S. Large decrease in zymogen granule size in the postnatal rat pancreas. J. Ultrastruct. Res. *70*:242, 1980.
73. Uchiyama, Y., and Watanabe, M. Morphometric and fine structural studies of rat pancreatic acinar cells during early postnatal life. Cell Tissue Res. *237*:123, 1984.
74. Sesso, A., Carneiro, J., Cruz, A. R., and De Arruda Leite, J. B. Biochemical, cytochemical and electron microscopic observations of the enhancement of the pancreatic acinar cell secretory activity in the rat during early postnatal growth. Arch. Histol. Jpn. *35*:343, 1973.
75. Deschodt-Lanckman, M., Robberecht, P., Camus, J., Baya, C., and Christophe, J. Hormonal and dietary adaptation of rat pancreatic hydrolases before and after weaning. Am. J. Physiol. *226*:39, 1974.
76. Robberecht, P., Deschodt-Lanckman, M., Camus, J., Bruylands, J., and Christophe, J. Rat pancreatic hydrolases from birth to weaning and dietary adaptation after weaning. Am. J. Anat. *221*:376, 1971.
77. Like, A. A., and Orci, L. Embryogenesis of the human pancreatic islets: A light and electron microscopic study. Diabetes *21*:511, 1972.
78. Baxter-Grillo, D., Blazquez, E., Grillo, T. A. I., Sodoyez, J., Sodoyez-Goffaux, F. and Foa, P. P. Functional development of the pancreatic islets. *In* Cooperstein, S. J., and Watkins, D. (eds.). The Islets of Langerhans. New York, Academic Press, Inc., 1981, p. 35.
79. Stefan, Y., Grasso, S., Perrelet, A., and Orci, L. A quantitative immunofluorescent study of the endocrine cell populations in the developing human pancreas. Diabetes *32*:293, 1983.
80. Warkany, J., Passarge, E., and Smith, L. B. Congenital malformations in autosomal trisomy syndromes. J. Dis. Child. *112*:502, 1966.
81. Seifert, G. Die Pathologie Des Kindlichen Pankreas. Leipzig, Georg Thieme, 1956.
82. Bodian, M. Fibrocystic Disease of the Pancreas. New York, Grune and Stratton, 1953.
83. Dolan, R. V., ReMine, W. H., and Dockerty, M. B. The fate of heterotopic pancreatic tissue. Arch. Surg. *109*:762, 1974.
84. Ravitch, M. M. The pancreas in infants and children. Surg. Clin. North Am. *55*:377, 1975.
85. Silverberg, M., and Davidson, M. Pediatric gastroenterology. A review. Gastroenterology *58*:229, 1970.
86. Millbourn, E. Calibre and appearance of pancreatic ducts and relevant clinical problems. Acta Chir. Scand. *118*:286, 1959.
87. Birastingl, M. A study of pancreatography. Br. J. Surg. *47*:728, 1959.
88. Berman, L. G., Prior, J. T., Abraham, S. M., and Ziegler, D. D. A study of the pancreatic duct system in man by the use of vinyl acetate casts of postmortem preparations. Surg. Gynecol. Obstet. *110*:391, 1966.
89. Dawson, W., and Langman, V. An anatomical-radiological study of the pancreatic duct pattern in man. Anat. Rec. *139*:59, 1961.
90. Smanio, T. Proposed nomenclature and classification of the human pancreatic ducts and duodenal papillae. Study based on 200 postmortems. Int. Surg. *52*:125, 1969.
91. Cotton, P. B. Congenital anomaly of pancreas divisum as cause of obstructive pain and pancreatitis. Gut *21*:105, 1980.
92. Tulassy, Z., and Papp, J. New clinical aspects of pancreas divisum. Gastrointest. Endoscopy *26*:143, 1980.
93. Richter, J. M., Schapiro, R. H., Mulley, A. G., and Warshaw, A. L. Association of pancreas divisum and pancreatitis, and its

treatment by sphincteroplasty of the accessory ampulla. Gastroenterology *81*:1104, 1981.
94. Sahel, J., Cros, R., Bourry, J., and Sarles, H. Clinicopathological conditions associated with pancreas divisum. Digestion *23*:1, 1982.
95. Delhaye, M., Engelholm, L., and Cremer, M. Pancreas divisum: congenital anatomic variant or anomaly? Contribution of endoscopic retrograde dorsal pancreatography. Gastroenterology *89*:951, 1985.
96. Rosch, W., Koch, H., Schaffner, O., and Demling, L. The clincal significance of pancreas divisum. Gastrointest. Endosc. *22*:206, 1976.
97. Mitchell, J., Lintott, D. J., Ruddell, W. S. J., Losowsky, M. S., and Axon, A. T. R. Clinical relevance of an unfused pancreatic duct system. Gut *20*:1066, 1979.
98. Cooperman, M., Ferrara, J. J., Fromkes, J. J., and Carey, L. C. Surgical management of pancreas divisum. Am. J. Surg. *143*:107, 1982.
99. Warshaw, A. L., Richter, J. M., and Schapiro, R. H. The cause and treatment of pancreatitis associated with pancreas divisum. Ann. Surg. *198*:443, 1983.
100. Russell, R. C. G., Wong, N. W., and Cotton, P. B. Accessory sphincterotomy (endoscopic and surgical) in patients with pancreas divisum. Br. J. Surg. *71*:954, 1984.
101. Gregg, J. A., Monaco, A. P., and McDermott, W. V. Pancreas divisum. Results of surgical intervention. Am. J. Surg. *145*:488, 1983.
102. Madura, J., Fiore, A. C., O'Connor, K. W., Lehman, G. A., and McCammon, R. L. Pancreas divisum. Detection and management. Am. Surg. *51*:353, 1985.
103. Blair, A. J., Russell, R. C. G., and Cotton, P. B. Resection for pancreatitis in patients with pancreas divisum. Ann. Surg. *200*:590, 1984.
104. Sahel, J., Boustiere, C., Sarles, J. C., Chevilotte, G., and Sarles, H. Traitement du "pancreas divisum." Resultats preliminaires. Gastroenterol. Clin. Biol. *7*:293, 1983.

95

Pancreatic Physiology

JAMES H. MEYER

Although it is a small organ (less than 110 gm), the pancreas has been the focus of considerable investigation and controversy among physicians and physiologists. The physician understands the pancreas as (1) an endocrine gland essential for life (secretion of insulin and glucagon from the islets of Langerhans); (2) an exocrine gland providing the intestinal lumen with sodium bicarbonate and digestive enzymes that greatly facilitate intestinal assimilation of foodstuffs; and (3) the seat of a painful, debilitating, poorly understood, and even lethal, disease—pancreatitis. The pancreas has provided physiologists with models for classic studies of a variety of secretory phenomena, including (1) the first demonstration of hormone action; (2) later, a dramatic bioassay model for the elucidation of hormone-hormone interactions and the study of hormone receptors; and (3) a model for the study of protein synthesis and export. Despite this prominence in the history of biologic science, the pancreas continues to astonish scientists and physicians with its complexities. Speculations on the role of newly discovered endocrine functions (secretion of pancreatic peptide and somatostatin) are as yet unsubstantiated; the control of normal exocrine function eludes exact definitions; and pancreatitis remains an obscure disease. This chapter will briefly describe the exocrine pancreas as it is currently understood.

ANATOMY

The head of the gland (about 30 per cent of the pancreas) is cradled by the concave medial border of the first, second, and third portions of the duodenum. The remainder consists of the body and tail, which extend retroperitoneally in a transverse and slightly cephalad direction to the hilus of the spleen. The exocrine gland is drained by two ductular systems. The major duct (duct of Wirsung) traverses the gland centrally from the tail through the body and head; it enters the duodenum at the ampulla of Vater, usually alongside the common bile duct (which passes through the posterior head of the pancreas). Both ducts are encased by the sphincter of Oddi. In 30 to 40 per cent of persons, the duct of Wirsung and the common bile duct form a common channel before terminating. The minor (accessory) duct (duct of Santorini) usually joins the main, central ductular system in the body of the gland but runs a separate course through the head of the pancreas, entering the duodenum a few centimeters more cephalad than the main duct in about 70 per cent of persons. Throughout their course, both ducts receive tributaries from the pancreatic lobules.

The exocrine pancreas consists of clusters of *acini* (from the Greek, meaning grapes) that form lobules separated by areolar tissue. The individual acinus is a sphere composed of pyramidal acinar cells arrayed with their broad bases around the circumference and their pointed apices in the central lumen. Each acinus is drained by a ductule. The ductular epithelium extends into the lumen of the acinus, forming the so-called centroacinar cells. The ductules drain into intralobular ("intercalated") ducts; these join interlobular ducts, which finally enter the duct of Wirsung. Interspersed in the loose connective tissue between lobules are the islets of Langerhans, containing the cells of the endocrine pancreas.

COMPOSITION AND FORMATION OF PANCREATIC JUICE

Water and Electrolyte Secretion

Pancreatic juice is isotonic with extracellular fluid at all rates of secretion, indicating that water enters the juice passively along osmotic gradients established by the active secretion of electrolytes or other solutes. The principal anions in pancreatic juice are Cl^- and HCO_3^-. The principal cations, Na^+ and K^+, are secreted at fixed concentrations similar to those in extracellular fluid. Pancreatic juice also contains Ca^{2+} (1 to 2 mEq/L) and traces of Mg^{2+}, Zn^{2+}, HPO_4^{2-}, and So_4^{2-}.

The concentrations of the two principal anions vary reciprocally and together total about 150 mEq/L. At high flow rates, HCO_3^- concentrations are high and Cl^- concentrations are low; at low flow rates, this ratio is reversed. At maximum flow rates, the concentration of HCO_3^- approaches 150 mEq/L and the pH of the juice is about 8.3, corresponding to that of a solution of 150 mM HCO_3^- at a pCO_2 of 40 mm Hg (Fig. 95–1).

The relationships between concentrations of HCO_3^- and Cl^- in pancreatic juice are entirely analogous to the relationship between H^+ and Na^+ in gastric juice (see pp. 713–734) and correspondingly analogous theories have been postulated to explain the anion content of pancreatic juice.[1] One theory, the two-component hypothesis, states that one cell type (i.e., the acinar cell) secretes Cl^- and another cell type (i.e., the centroacinar or ductular cell) secretes HCO_3^-. The Cl^- and HCO_3^- content of the juice would depend on admixture of the secretions from the two cell types. Another theory, the unicellular hypothesis, proposes that all cells secrete both Cl^- and HCO_3^- but that relative rates of secretion of Cl^- and HCO_3^- vary. A third theory (exchange diffusion hypothesis) holds that the principal anion secreted is HCO_3^-, but that as the juice traverses the ductal system, HCO_3^- is exchanged for Cl^-; a low flow rate would increase the time for this exchange, producing juice low in HCO_3^-, whereas a high flow rate would preclude a large exchange of Cl^- for secreted HCO_3^-.

Two independent lines of evidence support the two-component hypothesis that the ductular cells add bicarbonate to chloride-rich juice from the acini. The first comes from analyses of juice from micropunctures of the cat pancreas during high rates of volume and bicarbonate secretion.[2] Juice collected from the intralobular ducts (close to the acini) is richer in chloride (112 mEq/L) than bicarbonate (52 mEq/L). There is a progressive decline in chloride and a rise in bicarbonate secretion on sampling from larger and larger interlobular ducts, until the fluid in the main duct consists primarily of bicarbonate (118 mEq/L) and little chloride (46 mEq/L). Under these same conditions, the extralobular ducts are adding volume to their contents. The simplest explanation of these findings is that most of the water and bicarbonate is contributed by the ducts, which add juice containing 140 mEq/L of bicarbonate to fluid rich in chloride from the acini. The second line of evidence is provided by studies in rats in which 98 per cent of acinar cells are replaced by adipose cells after 100 days of a diet deficient in copper and supplemented with D-penicillamine.[3] These animals are almost completely incapable of secreting amylase in response to exogenous cholecystokinin, confirming a functional loss of acinar cells. Microscopic examination shows that their ductular cells are preserved, and they are capable of responding to secretin by increasing bicarbonate secretion fivefold over basal rates. The preservation of bicarbonate secretion in the

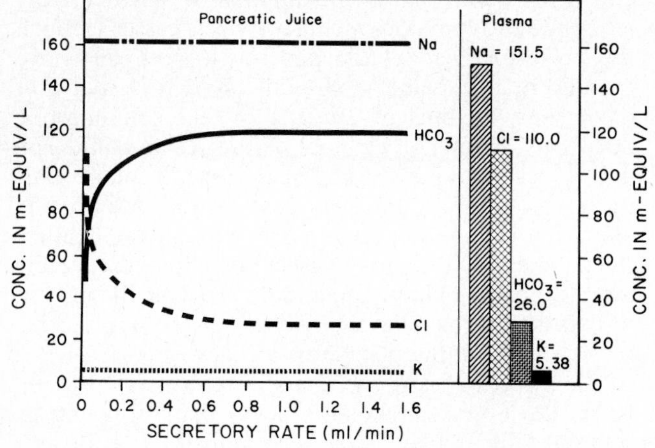

Figure 95–1. Relationship of pancreatic secretion and concentration of electrolytes. (Adapted from Bro-Rasmussen, F., Kilman, S. A., and Thaysen, J. H. Acta Physiol. Scand. *37*:97, 1956. Used by permission.)

almost complete absence of acinar cells supports the idea that the ducts are the major secretors of bicarbonate.

Because, at high flow rates, the concentration of bicarbonate in pancreatic juice greatly exceeds that in extracellular fluid, it would appear that HCO_3^- is secreted actively. Indeed, the electropotential difference across the ductular mucosa during stimulated secretion is 5 to 9 mV, lumen negative, an electric potential gradient indicating active ductular transport of HCO_3^-. Nevertheless, recent work suggests that the primary active process is transport of H^+ from lumen to cell cytoplasm, in exchange for Na^+ moving from cytoplasm to lumen (a slight excess in movement of H^+ out of the lumen relative to rate of entry of Na^+ into the juice could account for the aforementioned electronegativity on the lumen side). This active transport of H^+ lowers the H^+ concentration in the lumen but raises the H^+ concentration in the cell. Cellular CO_2 then diffuses into the lumen, dissociating into H^+ + HCO_3^- in the relatively alkaline luminal juice. Continued transport of H^+ out of the lumen thus leads to the formation of juice containing Na^+ and HCO_3^-.[4]

Enzyme Proteins: Content, Formation, and Secretion

More than 90 per cent of the protein in pancreatic juice consists of enzymes or proenzymes; the rest is composed of trypsin inhibitors, plasma proteins, and small amounts of mucoproteins. Pancreatic proteases account for the majority of enzymic proteins. They are secreted as enzymatically inactive proenzymes that are activated in the lumen of the proximal intestine. Secreted by mucosa of the proximal bowel, the peptidase enterokinase converts the proenzyme trypsinogen to active trypsin by splitting a small peptide fragment off trypsinogen. Once formed, trypsin activates all other pancreatic proteases, as well as pancreatic phospholipase (lecithinase). Lipase, amylase, and ribonuclease are secreted by the acinar cell in the active form. Pancreatic juice also contains a small (molecular weight 9000) peptide cofactor called co-lipase, which combines stoichiometrically with lipase. Co-lipase prevents inhibition of lipase activity by bile salts and, in the presence of bile salts, lowers the pH optimum of lipase from 8.5 to 6.5, the normal luminal pH in the proximal intestine.[5]

All of these enzymes are synthesized in the acinar cells at very rapid rates; time required from synthesis to secretion into the acinar lumen is of the order of 50 minutes. The most widely accepted analysis[6] of this process envisions six steps from synthesis to secretion: (1) The protein enzymes are formed at the ribosomes attached to the cytoplasmic surface of the cisternae of the rough endoplasmic reticulum. (2) The newly formed enzyme then is segregated from the rest of the cell by moving across the cisternal membrane into the adjacent cisternal space. This first step of segregation is an irreversible process, possibly the result of a change in molecular configuration of the newly formed protein on entering the cisternal space, rendering it impermeable to the cisternal membrane. Once in the cisternal space, enzymes remain membrane-bound within the acinar cell. (3) The enzymic protein is moved through the cell by way of the rough endoplasmic reticulum and Golgi complex to condensing vacuoles in the apical region of the cell. Energy (ATP) is required for this intracellular transport. (4) Once in the condensing vacuoles, the enzymic proteins are concentrated in these membrane-bound vacuoles. The concentrated vacuoles are visible as zymogen granules. (5) Here, in the zymogen granules, they remain stored until called forth during periods of stimulation. (6) The final step is discharge. Extrusion (exocytosis) results after the membrane of the zymogen granule fuses with the apical cell membrane, followed by elimination of membrane layers at the point of fusion and ultimate rupture of the membrane, with disgorgement of zymogen contents into the acinar lumen. The fusion of membranes in this final step is a highly organized process, initiated by depolarization of the plasma membrane and involving specific reception between the apical plasma membrane and the zymogen membrane. Although this formulation is widely accepted, details of the various steps have not been described,[6,7] and some observations indicate alternative pathways. For example, during high rates of enzyme secretion zymogen granules may be depleted; but enzyme secretion continues unabated (from smaller vacuoles). Likewise, there is some evidence of movement of enzymic proteins between cytosol and membrane-bound compartments of the cells.[7]

In short-term experiments in humans[8] or animals,[9] the relative concentrations of various pancreatic enzymes remain constant; that is, under a variety of stimuli, over a range of secretory rates, and throughout the periods of observation, the various enzymes are secreted in parallel with one another (so-called "parallel secretion"). Moreover, analyses of enzyme contents in subfractions of the acinar cells (zymogen granules, condensing vacuoles, Golgi), have revealed the same ratios of one enzyme to another as in secreted juice. Such observations have supported the view that the mix of enzymic proteins in secreted juice is fixed at the time of synthesis. Nevertheless, some workers claim to have observed significant deviations from parallel secretion; perhaps the most dramatic example was the threefold increase in pancreatic secretion of chymotrypsinogen while lipase output remained unchanged after an intravenous injection of the peptide "chymodenin" in the anesthetized rabbit.[10] The deviation from parallel secretion occurred too quickly after chymodenin injection to be accounted for by a change in the ratio of enzymic proteins synthesized at the ribosomes. Two other explanations have been put forward: (1) that the composition of enzymic proteins in the zymogen granule (and hence the secreted juice) is not immutable but can be changed by various stimuli through equilibration with traces of individual enzymes in the cytosol; or (2) that there are subpopulations of acinar cells having different proportions of enzymes in zymogen storage; deviations from parallel secretion thus represent selective discharge of one of these subpopulations with a different zymogen content. Recent studies in humans of the turnover of ^{75}Se-methionine–labeled pancreatic enzymes indicate that there are subpopulations of acinar cells that discharge their enzyme contents differentially under varying conditions of stimulation.[11]

The rat pancreas exemplifies regional differences among lobules of acini. As in other mammals, the ventral and dorsal portions of the rat pancreas have different embryologic origins, but the diffuse spread of rat pancreas in mesentery allows easy separation of dorsal from ventral secretion. At maturity, the composition and number of islets differ in the ventral and dorsal portions so that more pancreatic polypeptide is stored and presumably secreted in the ventral pancreas and more insulin is stored and secreted in the dorsal portion. The amylase content per gram of tissue is about 30 per cent higher in the dorsal pancreas, and both basal and stimulated amylase output from the isolated dorsal pancreas were two to three times that from the ventral portion of the gland.[12] Insulin stimulates an increased production of amylase by stimulating an increase in messenger RNA for amylase.[13] Furthermore, pancreatic islets communicate with acini via a portal system,[14] so that high levels of insulin may stimulate amylase production from the dorsal pancreas. The differences in amylase content and output between ventral and dorsal portions of the rat pancreas may thus reflect regional differences in islet-acinar interactions. That this idea is true is supported by the observations that regional differences disappeared when acinar cells were dispersed, and thus removed from the influence of islet hormones, and that making rats diabetic lowered amylase secretion from the *ex vivo* dorsal, but not ventral, pancreas.

Although short-term deviations from parallel secretion are disputed among groups of scientists, there seems to be little question that there can be long-term adaptations, at least in the rat.[15] Thus, prolonged feeding of diets high in carbohydrate raises the amylase content and proportion of amylase in the rat pancreas, whereas isocaloric diets high in complete protein or fat elevate trypsinogen and lipase content relative to that of amylase. Moreover, the size of the rat pancreas can be modified experimentally by manipulating hormonal or stimulatory mechanisms. For example, administration of exogenous cholecystokinin (CCK) to rats sharply increases DNA synthesis and content in the pancreas. Secretin by itself is a weak stimulus of pancreatic cell proliferation, but exogenous secretin potentiates the effect of CCK, much in the same way these two hormones interact on pancreatic bicarbonate secretion. (Penta)gastrin probably has weak trophic effects on rat pancreas.

Dietary adaptation and trophic stimuli have been demonstrated convincingly only in rat pancreas. Whether these phenomena pertain to humans as well is unknown. Some studies suggest a high correlation between gastric capacity to secrete acid and pancreatic capacity to secrete bicarbonate;[16, 17] trophic influences in humans (for example, the release of secretin by luminal acid) might account for this relationship. In humans, protein malnutrition produces a fall in pancreatic secretory capacity which can be reversed by resumption of protein intake;[18] with more prolonged protein malnutrition there is atrophy of acinar cells and acinar endoplasmic reticulum, loss of lobular architecture, and finally fibrosis.[19] As human starvation progresses, lipase disappears from duodenal juice before trypsin, which in turn disappears before amylase.[19]

STIMULATION OF PANCREATIC SECRETION (Table 95–1)

Hormonal Regulation

The gut hormone *secretin* is a potent stimulant of pancreatic secretion from either the *in vivo* or the isolated perfused pancreas. Its main effects are on water and bicarbonate secretion, producing a copious outflow of juice high in bicarbonate concentration.

Secretin has two effects on protein or enzyme secretion. The juice stimulated initially contains relatively high concentrations of protein (enzyme), so the output of protein also rises sharply. However, as high rates of secretin-stimulated secretion continue, protein concentration in the juice falls until a steady, low concentration is reached. The initial surge of protein output after secretin injection is thought to represent the washing out of protein-rich basal fluid, which had collected in the ductular system. As protein output after sustained stimulation with secretin is somewhat greater than rates of basal secretion, secretin is a weak stimulus of protein secretion.

The other classic gut hormone, *cholecystokinin* (CCK), stimulates the pancreas *in vivo* or *in vitro* to secrete a juice that is relatively low in volume and bicarbonate concentration but very high in protein (enzyme) concentration. Gastrin, which shares the C-terminal structure of CCK, stimulates a juice similar in character to that stimulated by CCK, but in humans gastrin is considerably less potent than CCK.[20]

Given together, secretin and cholecystokinin augment each other's actions. In animals, these two hormones exhibit marked interactions affecting pancreatic volume and bicarbonate secretion. For example, simultaneous administration of a dose of each, which given alone would evoke 25 per cent of the maximal response to secretin, produces a bicarbonate output that is much more than 50 per cent of the maximum to secretin. Also, the highest observed bicarbonate response to combinations of the two hormones greatly exceeds the maximum response to either hormone alone or the sum of the two maximal responses.[21] This type of strong interaction is called potentiation. These two hormones also interact on protein (enzyme) secretion, but the interaction is less dramatic than on bicarbonate. Secretin combined with submaximal doses

Table 95–1. PATHWAYS STIMULATING PANCREATIC EXOCRINE SECRETION

Bicarbonate Secretion			Enzyme Secretion		
Site	*Mode*	*Stimulus*	*Site*	*Mode*	*Stimulus*
?	Vagus (VIP)	?	Brain	Vagus	Sight, smell, or taste of food
Small gut	Secretin	Acid, oleate	Brain	Vagus	Hypoglycemia
Small gut	Potentiation (secretin + CCK, gastrin, or vagal drive)	Acid + fatty acids, amino acids, peptides	Stomach	Vagus	Distention (body and antrum)
			Stomach	Gastrin	Distention, food bathing antrum
			Small gut	Vagus	Oleate, L-tryptophan
			Small gut	Hormone (?CCK)	Fatty acids, neutral amino acids, small peptides, polypeptides (after peptic digestion of protein)

of CCK raises protein secretion to levels above those after CCK alone, but maximal responses to CCK alone are not clearly exceeded by adding secretin. Carefully designed studies on interactions between secretin and CCK on pancreatic secretion in humans have not been undertaken. In general, humans seem to respond to combinations of these two agents like experimental animals; that is, combinations of secretin and CCK produce volume, bicarbonate, and enzyme outputs which exceed rates of secretion expected from the sum of responses to similar doses of each agent alone.[22]

Both secretin and cholecystokinin exert their full effects on the pancreas within minutes after their entry into the bloodstream. Similarly, both hormones are inactivated rapidly in the body, and pancreatic secretion stimulated by them ceases within minutes after they stop entering the blood.[23]

Vasoactive intestinal peptide (VIP) is structurally similar to secretin[24] and exhibits secretin-like effects on pancreatic secretion; it stimulates a large volume of bicarbonate-rich juice, low in protein, and can potentiate the action of CCK on bicarbonate output.[25] It is a weaker agonist than secretin and when given together with secretin may competitively inhibit the effects of secretin.[25] *Glucagon* also shares portions of its peptide structure with secretin and VIP,[24] and it is claimed to be an inhibitor of pancreatic volume secretion in animals and man.[26, 27]

In vitro incubates of fragments of pancreatic tissue or of suspensions of acini or acinar cells have been used increasingly to study hormone receptors and cellular mechanisms of hormone actions.[28] Such studies have revealed a multitude of receptors on the acinar cell for peptide hormones or neurotransmitters. Secretin and cholecystokinin have separate receptors. VIP shares affinity with secretin for the secretin receptors; gastrin and the C terminal octapeptide of cholecystokinin interact with the CCK receptors, which have affinity for the common sequence of amino acids near the C termini of these peptides. The cholinergic neurotransmitter carbachol has an acinar cell receptor. There are also separate receptors each for bombesin and substance P, both of which are probable neuropeptide transmitters in mammalian tissues.

Human or canine pancreatic enzyme secretion never reaches maximum after meals. Typically,[29, 30] output approaches maximum in the first hour but then falls to less than 50 per cent of the sustained, maximal output that can be stimulated by exogenous CCK. It is unclear whether this decline is the result of stimulus decay with time or of active inhibition by neural or hormonal signals to limit pancreatic output, or both. As pancreatic secretion in response to intravenous secretin plus CCK in humans can be inhibited by instillation of 50 per cent glucose into the duodenum, or in animals by perfusion of the distal ileum with fat,[31] there is good experimental evidence for inhibitory mechanisms. Several hormones could mediate such inhibition. Of these, the best studied is pancreatic polypeptide (PP), found in the pancreatic islets. This hormone does not have receptors on acinar cells but appears to inhibit secretion by acting on intrapancreatic nerves. When given in amounts that reproduce postprandial blood levels of endogenous hormone, exogenous intravenous PP inhibits pancreatic secretion. A structurally related peptide, peptide YY (PYY), is located in the mucosal endocrine cells along the intestine, predominantly in the ileum. When PYY is given in sufficient amounts to achieve postprandial blood concentrations, inhibition of pancreatic output varies among species. In humans PYY does not inhibit, leaving the role of this hormone as an inhibitor of postcibal secretion open to question. Other candidates for hormonal inhibition are somatostatin or glucagon, but evidence supporting their roles as inhibitors of postcibal pancreatic secretion is even less convincing than that for PYY. Of course, neural mechanisms, acting alone or together with inhibiting hormones, could also give rise to postcibal inhibition (see pp. 78–107).

Neural Regulation

In anesthetized animals, pancreatic secretion can be evoked by electrical stimulation of the peripheral ends of the transected vagus nerve. In all species tested, electrical stimulation of the vagus excites the secretion of amylase or protein. Similarly, pancreatic enzyme secretion can be stimulated by cholinergic drugs. Both modes of stimulation can be blocked with atropine. The various observations indicate vagal pathways with cholinergic mediation.

In the pig, electrical stimulation of the vagus also evokes moderate outputs of bicarbonate. This effect is not blocked by atropine but is blocked by ganglionic blockers, such as hexamethonium. Fahrenkrug and coworkers[32] reported a rise in concentrations of VIP in pancreatic venous blood, which paralleled the rise in bicarbonate secretion on electrical stimulation of the vagus. Because studies with immunofluorescent antibodies have indicated there are VIP-containing nerves in the pancreas, the sum of observations suggests that bicarbonate secretion in the pig can be excited via vagal pathways with VIP (peptidergic) mediation.

In humans, insulin-induced hypoglycemia (a presumed vagal excitant) augments pancreatic protein outputs secreted in response to secretin. In both humans and experimental animals, vagal transection reduces pancreatic responses to perfused intestinal stimulants.[33, 34] Likewise, postcibal trypsin secretion is reduced by truncal vagotomy.[29, 35]

Stimulus-Secretion Coupling

Despite the multitude of acinar cell receptors and agonists, studies on stimulation of amylase secretion have revealed only two pathways that couple stimuli with secretion.[28, 36] Secretin and VIP stimulate intracellular adenylcyclase and, thus, the formation of cyclic adenosine monophosphate (cAMP). All other agents, including CCK and acetylcholine, trigger the activation of phospholipase C and therefore the hydrolysis of membrane phosphatidyl-inositol to inositol triphosphate and diacylglycerol. Each pathway then continues through the activation of various protein kinases: cAMP directly activates a protein kinase; the formation of inositol phosphate signals the release of membrane calcium and build-up of intracellular calcium, which, through action of calmodulin, activates another protein kinase and phosphatase; and the release of diacylglycerol from membrane phosphatidyl-inositol also activates yet another phospholipid-dependent protein kinase (Fig. 95–2). Through the interaction between the cAMP pathway and the phosphatidyl-inositol pathway, the combined actions of secretin plus CCK or of secretin plus acetylcholine are potentiated. For example, when acinar cells are exposed to agents that excite each pathway, such as secretin plus CCK, the amount of amylase secreted is higher than the sum of responses to each agent alone. Agonists of phosphatidyl-inositol pathway also trigger the build-up of intracellular cyclic guanosine monophosphate (cGMP), but as accumulation of intracellular cGMP does not stimulate amylase release from cells permeated by 8Br-cyclic GMP, the action of cGMP is unknown.

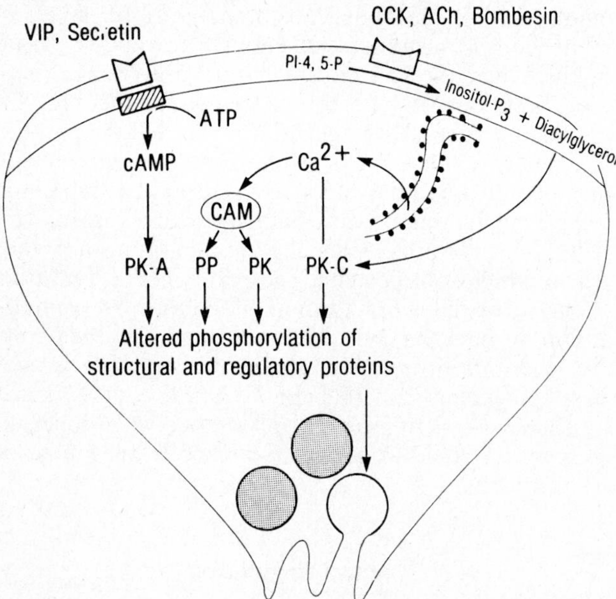

Figure 95–2. A schematic diagram of stimulus-secretion coupling of pancreatic acinar cell protein secretion. VIP, Vasoactive intestinal peptide; CCK, cholecystokinin; ACh, acetylcholine; cAMP, cyclic AMP; PK-A, cyclic-AMP-activated protein kinase; CAM, calmodulin; PP, protein phosphatase; PK, protein kinase; PK-C, phospholipid-dependent protein kinase; PI-4,5-P, phosphatidylinositol-4,5-bisphosphate; inositol-P_3, inositol-1,4,5-trisphosphate. (From Hartman, S. R., and Williams, J. A. *In* Johnson, J. R., et al. [eds.]: Physiology of the Gastrointestinal Tract. 2nd edition. Vol. 2. New York, Raven Press, 1987, p. 1129. Used by permission.)

Phases of Pancreatic Secretion

The exact mechanisms controlling pancreatic exocrine secretion remain obscure. Technical problems make the elucidation of these mechanisms much more difficult than comparable studies of gastric secretion. The surgical preparation of innervated or denervated chronic pancreatic fistulas is far more difficult than the preparation of gastric fistulas or Heidenhain (vagally denervated) pouches for physiologic studies. Moreover, sufficiently sensitive and reliable radioimmunoassays for serum secretin or cholecystokinin have been far more difficult to develop than useful immunoassay systems for gastrin; consequently, the role of these hormones in regulating postcibal secretion is unsettled. Nevertheless, as amply illustrated by the foregoing, both *in vitro* and *in vivo* studies indicate major effects of hormones and neurotransmitters on pancreatic secretion. It is probable, therefore, that some mix of neural-hormonal interaction controls pancreatic output during normal alimentation. Until the details of such interactions are forthcoming, it is only possible to describe what happened under one or another controlled experimental circumstance and speculate on relevance to normal alimentation. This information can be conveniently catalogued according to phases of pancreatic secretion.

Basal Secretion. Basal rates of secretion in normal humans are low and difficult to measure accurately. Basal secretion of bicarbonate is about 2 per cent, and of enzymes about 15 per cent, of maximal. The stimuli of basal secretion are not known. Some basal secretion apparently is intrinsic to the pancreas, because the isolated perfused pancreases (free of endogenous hormonal and neural stimuli) exhibit a basal secretion. As atropine sharply reduces basal output, it is likely that intrapancreatic nerves stimulate basal secretion through the release of acetylcholine. Like gastric, biliary, and duodenal secretion, basal pancreatic output fluctuates in cycles with the migrating myoelectric complex (MMC) (see pp. 675–713 and 1090–1091), so that output crests during phase III of the MMC. Coordination with the MMC must have a large neural component, because either atropine or ganglionic blockade[37] abolishes cyclic secretion.

Cephalic Stimulation. The sight and smell of appetizing food stimulates a modest output of volume from the pancreas of humans, producing a juice high in enzyme concentration but low in bicarbonate concentration.[38, 39] Sham feeding in humans stimulates enzyme secretion at about 50 per cent of maximum;[40] this response is largely abolished by atropine, an observation that indicates that the response is neurally mediated. Sham feeding also evokes the secretion of bicarbonate, but as bicarbonate secretion under sham feeding is almost entirely eliminated by cimetidine, the response is indirectly mediated through the stimulation of gastric acid and the entry of acid into the duodenum. In dogs, cephalic stimulation of the pancreas (produced by sham feeding) is mediated largely by vagal release of antral gastrin, because pancreatic response can be almost abolished by prevention of gastrin release.[41] Because parallel experiments cannot be easily performed in humans, it is uncertain whether cephalic stimulation is mediated directly by neural impulses to the pancreas or indirectly by neurally mediated release of gastrin, but radioimmunoassays for gastrin in subjects who underwent sham feeding suggest that too little gastrin was released to account for the observed output of pancreatic enzymes at 50 per cent of maximal rates.[40]

Gastric Phase. In humans, as in dogs, balloon distention of the body of the stomach evokes the output of modest volumes of pancreatic juice high in enzyme concentration but low in bicarbonate.[42] In dogs, this response is considerably reduced or abolished by vagal transection, indicating that it is at least in part neurally mediated.

In the dog, distention of the gastric antrum also evokes pancreatic secretion of an enzyme-rich juice, low in volume. As the effect of antral distention is blocked by atropine or by truncal vagotomy but not by antral acidification (which prevents the release of gastrin), an antropancreatic reflex has been postulated.[43] The importance of gastric distention is indicated by recent observations in humans with 500-ml meals of glucose versus glucose plus amino acids.[44] Both meals emptied from the stomach at identical rates. Trypsin output was high and was about the same after either meal, even though amino acids, but not glucose, released large amounts of CCK. With either meal, trypsin secretion continued at a high rate until less than 10 per cent of the meal remained in the stomach. The observations indicate that the glucose meal was as potent as the glucose plus amino acid meal because both meals distended the stomach equally and for a similar duration.

Gastrin may also be a stimulus as it is released by food in the stomach. Nevertheless, gastrin is a considerably weaker stimulus of pancreatic enzyme secretion than is CCK,[20] and gastrin release probably begins only minutes before food enters the small intestine and releases the more potent CCK. Through its modifications of chyme, the stomach contributes to the subsequent intestinal phase of stimulation. On entry into the duodenum, gastric acid evokes bicarbonate and volume secretion from the pancreas. Peptic digestion cleaves proteins into polypeptides, which are potent intestinal stimuli of pancreatic enzyme secretion.[45] Similarly, the intragastric breakdown of triglycerides may release products that stimulate the pancreas on arrival in the duodenum. In addition to chemical digestion, gastric grinding of food into tiny particles greatly speeds subsequent digestion in the small intestine to release stimulating products.

Intestinal Phase. The delivery of food into the proximal intestine of humans evokes outputs of pancreatic enzymes that are about 70 per cent of maximal.[29, 30] Volume and bicarbonate secretion cannot be measured accurately during and after feeding, but parallel experiments in animals have shown that food entering the gut from the stomach evokes a moderate output of pancreatic volume and bicarbonate.

Volume and bicarbonate outputs increase as the pH of the meal decreases and acid load increases.[46, 47] Furthermore, neutralizing duodenal content by instilling sodium bicarbonate halves the postcibal output of bicarbonate and volume.[48, 49] The P_{CO_2} in the postcibal duodenum approaches 800 mm Hg at the site of entry of the pancreatic duct,[50] indicating a large amount of neutralization of incoming acid by bicarbonate. These various observations strongly implicate the role of acid contents in the intestine as stimuli of pancreatic volume and bicarbonate outputs. Instillation of acid into the proximal bowel is a known stimulus of pancreatic bicarbonate secretion.[51] As the juice evoked is most similar to that stimulated by exogenous intravenous secretin, the presumption has been that acid contents in the duodenum release endogenous secretin and so stimulate bicarbonate output. Recently, radioimmunoassays have confirmed release of endogenous secretin during intestinal perfusion with acid.[52]

Nevertheless, under feeding conditions, the pH of duodenal contents never falls so low as during these acid perfusion experiments, and postcibal rises in serum secretin concentrations are hardly detectable.[52–55] Because of the possibility, or indeed the probability, of strong neural-hormonal or hormone-hormone interactions on bicarbonate secretion during feeding conditions (see earlier discussion), the release of tiny quantities of endogenous secretin could suffice to evoke modest secretion of bicarbonate. Such small quantities of secretin probably can be released by acidic contents in the pH range of 3 to 5,[51] yet may not be easily distinguished by existing immunoassay systems from basal circulating concentrations of secretin. Because titratable acid (that is, bound plus free H^+), rather than free H^+ ions alone, drives bicarbonate output, duodenal pH poorly reflects how much buffered H^+

enters the duodenum to stimulate pancreatic secretion. Also, postcibal pHs recorded in the duodenum fluctuate widely. As food-bound H^+ ions dissociate slowly from food particles,[56] fluctuations of duodenal pH toward neutrality may represent a transitory disequilibration between incoming acid and incoming pancreatic bicarbonate at the recording site. For both reasons, the intensity of acid drive is underestimated by measurement of duodenal pH.

A variety of different food products in the gut evoke pancreatic secretion, which varies in relative contents of bicarbonate and volume.[57] As indicated in the preceding paragraph, intestinally perfused acid stimulates secretion of a juice high in bicarbonate and low in protein, a juice with a ratio of HCO_3^- to protein only slightly lower than that stimulated by pure secretin. On the other hand, some amino acids, peptides, and protein digests stimulate a juice low in volume and bicarbonate but high in protein concentration, a juice similar to that evoked by exogenous CCK or by neural stimulation. Fatty acids in the intestinal lumen stimulate a modest output of volume. The bicarbonate-protein ratios in pancreatic juice evoked by fatty acid vary with (1) the concentration of the fatty acid and (2) the chain length of the fatty acid.[57] It has been assumed that these variations in response to fatty acids might reflect variations in the proportions of gut hormones released—for example, the ratio of secretin to CCK.

Faichney and coworkers have confirmed that intraluminal oleate releases endogenous secretin.[58] Nevertheless, other recent studies also indicate the importance of enteropancreatic neural pathways that mediate responses to intraluminal nutrients. Studying secretory responses of a denervated, autotransplanted portion of the canine pancreas, Solomon and Grossman[59] found enzyme secretion from the denervated pancreas in response to intestinal oleate or tryptophan was unaffected by systemic atropine or truncal vagotomy; however, both atropine and vagotomy reduced responses of the innervated pancreas to these luminal stimuli by about 50 per cent. The findings were consistent with the idea that about 50 per cent of the secretory response of the innervated gland was mediated by cholinergic, vagal reflexes sensitive to atropine or vagal transection: As the denervated gland no longer had these reflexes, its responses were unaffected. An independent line of evidence for enteropancreatic reflexes was provided by Singer and colleagues,[60] who studied latency for the increase in amylase secretion after bolus injection of oleate or tryptophan into the proximal segment of the bowel of dogs with pancreatic fistulas. The lag between injection and increase in amylase secretion was only 0.3 minute after intestinal oleate or tryptophan, much shorter than the 0.5-minute lag between bolus injection of CCK into the portal vein and increase in amylase secretion. Atropine or truncal vagotomy markedly prolonged latency after intestinal instillation of oleate or tryptophan but had no effect on latency after intraportal CCK. These studies confirm the idea that pancreatic enzyme secretion in response to intestinal stimuli is also in part mediated by hormonal mechanisms, as a portion of these responses remained after pancreatic denervation.

Whatever the detailed mechanisms of stimulation, the potency of intestinal contents appears to arise from the cumulation of effects along the proximal segment of the small intestine. Thus, confining acid or amino acids or peptide digests to short segments of intestine evokes much less of a pancreatic response than that produced when longer lengths of small bowel are similarly exposed to these products.[61–63]

Such observations indicate receptors mediating pancreatic responses to intestinal stimuli are arrayed along much of the intestine, but the response that can be triggered from any localized segment is small. Because products of fat and protein digestion are released postcibally along most of the small intestine, a cumulative stimulus of considerable magnitude can be generated by these products as long as chyme continues to traverse the small bowel. On the other hand, acid is generated at one point (the stomach) along the alimentary tract and is quickly dissipated in the duodenum. Thus, the length of gut exposed to acids is short, and correspondingly the intensity of stimulation from acid (i.e., the amount of endogenous secretin released) may be small.

Postabsorptive Phase. Little is known of the effects of absorbed digestive products on pancreatic secretion. Hyperglycemia, induced by an intravenous infusion of glucose, inhibits trypsin output in response to a liquid meal of protein plus fat.[64] Likewise, intravenous infusions of amino acids inhibit pancreatic enzyme secretion in response to intestinally perfused amino acids.[65] Postulated but unsubstantiated mechanisms for these observed inhibitions are (1) the suppression of central nervous impulses by hyperglycemia, (2) the release of glucagon by amino acids, or (3) the release of somatostatin by both.[66]

DIGESTIVE FUNCTIONS OF PANCREATIC SECRETION

Pancreatic Bicarbonate Secretion

The stomach increases its output of acid and pepsin promptly after eating. Initially, much of the hydrogen ion secreted into the meal contents in the stomach is bound as undissociated hydrogen ion by food protein or peptides; however, with the continued secretion of hydrogen ion and with the gastric emptying of food buffers, the pH shifts downward, ultimately dropping as low as pH 2. The peak load of titratable acid (free hydrogen ion plus bound or undissociated hydrogen ion) delivered from stomach to duodenum after a meal is about 20 to 30 mEq/hour, roughly equal to the maximal capacity of the stomach to secrete acid and of the secretin-stimulated pancreas to secrete bicarbonate.[16] Both free and bound (undissociated) hydrogen ion must be neutralized or dissipated to raise the pH of the duodenal contents to optimum for enzymatic digestion of the chyme (about pH 6). At any one moment, hydrogen ion accounts for the pH of the contents, but bound hydrogen ion is in equilibrium with free hydrogen ion and will dissociate from the proteins or peptides as free hydrogen ion is neutralized or absorbed, thus resisting a change in pH. As a result, the pH in the small intestinal lumen will not rise until most or all of the titratable acid has been dissipated.

Despite the high load of titratable acid that enters the duodenum, the pH of chyme is quickly raised from 2 at the pylorus to above 4 beyond the duodenal bulb.[67] Bringing the pH to above 5 ensures solubility of bile salts and high activity of pancreatic enzymes. If the pH in the duodenum is allowed to drop below 4, pancreatic enzymes are irreversibly inactivated (see pp. 263–282). To accomplish this rapid neutralization, a large amount of bicarbonate must be added within this short segment of duodenum. Some neutralization is achieved by the duodenal mucosa, which may both absorb hydrogen ion and secrete bicarbonate. Nevertheless, the capacity of the proximal duodenum to dissipate hydrogen ion is modest. Because bile contains only small amounts of bicarbonate, most (probably about two thirds) titratable acid entering the duodenum is dissipated as the result of neutralization by pancreatic bicarbonate. In turn, the pancreas adjusts its rate of bicarbonate secretion in response to the rate of entry of titratable acid into the duodenum.[51, 61]

Patients with pancreatic insufficiency cannot secrete normal amounts of bicarbonate and therefore do not neutralize duodenal infusions of hydrochloric acid nearly as well as normal subjects.[68] In view of this observation, it is somewhat surprising that postcibal duodenal pH in these patients differs only a little from that in normal subjects.[69, 70] At least two mechanisms other than pancreatic secretion of bicarbonate control duodenal pH: (1) Gastric emptying is increasingly inhibited as the amount of titratable acid entering the duodenum increases.[71] As a result, the entry of acid is slowed toward amounts that can be neutralized by extrapancreatic mechanisms. (2) Acid entering the intestine also inhibits gastric secretion of acid,[72] further reducing the load of acid that must be neutralized (see pp. 713–734).

Pancreatic Enzymes[73]

Amylase. Pancreatic amylase is an alpha-1,4-glycosidase. It splits straight-chain glucose polysaccharides (amyloses in starch), which have only 1,4 linkages, into maltose and maltotriose. Branched-chain glucose polysaccharides (amylopectins in starch) have 1,6 glycosidic linkages at the branching points, which cannot be cleaved by pancreatic amylase, so the end products are maltose, maltotriose, and dextrins containing the 1,6 glycosidic bonds. These products are then further cleaved into glucose by brush border enzymes in the gut mucosa.

Lipase. Pancreatic lipase splits fatty acids from alpha positions of triglyceride, forming two molecules of fatty acid and one molecule of beta monoglyceride. As lipase is a water-soluble enzyme and triglyceride is water-insoluble, lipase can act on triglyceride only at the interface between the fat (triglyceride) and water phases. Emulsification of triglyceride, in which the fat phase is broken into many small droplets dispersed evenly throughout the water phase, greatly increases this surface (interfacial) area and correspondingly accelerates the rate at which lipase can hydrolyze triglyceride. The products of lipolysis (fatty acids and monoglyceride) inhibit further action of the lipase. Thus, lipolysis is also speeded by the process of micelle formation with bile salts, which solubilizes these hydrolytic products and moves them away from the interface between lipase and triglyceride. The pancreas secretes two other lipases: phospholipase A_2, which cleaves lecithin into lysolecithin, and cholesterol esterase, which hydrolyzes cholesterol esters but also has very broad specificity and can hydrolyze many kinds of lipids.

Protease. The pancreas secretes a variety of proteases. Trypsin, chymotrypsin, and elastase are endopeptidases; that is, they cleave peptide bonds in the middle of protein or polypeptide chains. Each enzyme has particular specificities for peptide bonds adjacent to certain amino acids. Carboxypeptidases are exopeptidases; that is, they split peptide bonds adjacent to the amino acid residues at the carboxyl terminus of the peptide chain.

The final hydrolytic products formed in the lumen by these proteases are oligopeptides (peptides of fewer than four amino acids) and free amino acids, particularly neutral amino acids and dibasic amino acids. Amino acids are transported directly by the gut mucosa. The oligopeptides either are split further by peptidases in the brush border of the mucosa or are directly transported by the mucosa with subsequent intracellular digestion to amino acids.

Alternative Pathways of Digestion

From the foregoing, it might be assumed that pancreatic enzymes perform essential digestive functions without which people would die from failure to absorb food. On the contrary, both humans and animals may survive total or near total pancreatic insufficiency without replacement of enzymes. After exclusion of pancreatic juice from the intestinal lumen of pigs,[74] nearly 40 per cent of ingested protein and fat was absorbed despite the absence of detectable pancreatic enzymes postcibally in the jejunum. Likewise, in humans,[75] 20 to 40 per cent of dietary fat and protein may be absorbed when postcibal secretion of enzymes from a diseased gland is less than 1 per cent of normal. Despite survival under these circumstances, health is impaired: Body weight and muscle mass are lost, and the patient is frequently incapacitated by diarrhea associated with the profound steatorrhea. Nevertheless, the fact that up to 40 per cent of dietary fat and protein may be assimilated in the absence of pancreatic enzymes suggests alternative, less efficient pathways of digestion.

The salivary glands secrete an alpha-1,4-amylase with similar specificity to that of pancreatic amylase. Some starch digestion can therefore take place in the absence of the pancreas. Humans secrete a pharyngeal lipase[76] and possibly another lipase from the stomach;[77] in addition, the gut mucosa contains some nonspecific esterases that might serve as inefficient lipases. Peptic digestion in the stomach cleaves much of ingested protein into polypeptides; peptidases in the brush borders of gut mucosal cells probably have some inefficient capacity to split some of these peptides into amino acids.[78] All of these potential alternative pathways for digestion in the absence of pancreatic juice are poorly defined.

The pancreas normally secretes more enzymes than are required for complete digestion. Even with liquid test meals, which are transported through the gastrointestinal tract more rapidly than solid food, digestion and absorption are nearly completed in the proximal two thirds of the gut. These findings indicate that pancreatic enzymes are secreted at rates more than sufficient to accomplish digestion in the length of gut available. It has been estimated that postcibal enzyme secretion must fall below 10 per cent of normal before maldigestion or malabsorption occurs.[75]

TESTS OF PANCREATIC EXOCRINE FUNCTION (Table 95–2)

A variety of tests have been utilized to diagnose abnormally low pancreatic secretion and thus disease of the pancreas.[79] Two questions often have clinical relevance: (1) Is the pancreas so diseased that the patient is experiencing malabsorption on that basis? (2) Is the pancreas abnormal (from cancer or chronic pancreatitis)? In the patient with pancreatogenous malabsorption, nearly all capacity to secrete has been lost, so results of tests that measure secretory capacity will be markedly abnormal. On the other hand, in the absence of malabsorption pancreatic disease may produce only minor reductions in secretory capacity, which are difficult to distinguish from normal. The problem is compounded by the wide variation in normal secretory responses to one or another stimulus of secretion.[80] In this situation of mild impairment, tests demonstrating anatomic disease (CT scan, ultrasonography, endoscopic pancreatography) may be more sensitive than secretory testing.

Two types of secretory tests are commonly used. In the first, the fasting subject undergoes duodenal intubation. Increases in volume, bicarbonate, and amylase secretion are measured in duodenal aspirates after pancreatic secretion is stimulated with intravenous exogenous hormones. The most widely employed test uses a maximal or near-maximal dose of intravenously administered secretin as the stimulus. Some investigators use combinations of secretin and cholecystokinin; however, as CCK may cause abdominal cramps, diarrhea, and hypotension, the dose used is submaximal for pancreatic enzyme secretion. Obviously, the duodenal aspirates will consist of pancreatic and duodenal juices, as well as bile. In addition, not all of the secreted juice will be aspirated. Some clinicians try to correct for the last problem by using a dilution indicator. No matter what method is employed, the results are only approximate. From this description, it is quite understandable how minor reductions in secretory capacity may escape detection. Nevertheless, patients with pancreatogenous malabsorption almost always have a bicarbonate concentration below 80 mEq/L in aspirated duodenal juice after stimulation with intravenous secretin.

Another commonly used test is the Lundh test. In this method the patient undergoes duodenal intubation, but the gland is stimulated with a liquid test meal containing fat, protein, and sugar. What is measured is the average trypsin concentration in duodenal aspirates obtained over several hours after the patient drinks the test meal. In the normal patient, trypsin output doubles or triples over basal rates of secretion with distention of the stomach and emptying of the test meal into the duodenum. As the meal empties slowly, trypsin concentration remains the same or even rises over basal values despite the flow of meal and secretions through the duodenum. In patients with pancreatogenous malabsorption, there is virtually no rise in trypsin secretion after the meal, so postcibal trypsin concentrations fall below 10 per cent of normal values in most cases. Quite obviously the test result depends on the relationship between pancreatic secretion and gastric emptying of the meal, so that the test may be less reliable in patients who have had ulcer surgery (in whom the test meal empties precipitously).[81]

A number of oral tolerance tests have been utilized for the diagnosis of pancreatogenous malabsorption (pancreatic insufficiency). These tests depend on the detection of a metabolite in the breath, blood, or urine of an ingested test substance that is absorbed by the intestine only after luminal hydrolysis by pancreatic

Table 95–2. RANGE OF NORMAL RESPONSES TO SECRETORY TESTS OF THE PANCREAS

1. *Secretin test**
   - Volume (ml/80 min): 117–392
   - HCO_3^- concentration (mEq/L): 88–137
   - HCO_3^- output (mEq/80 min): 16–33
   - Amylase output (units/80 min): 439–1921
2. *Secretin + CCK**
   - Volume (ml/80 min): 111–503
   - HCO_3^- concentration (mEq/L): 88–144
   - HCO_3^- output (mEq/80 min): 10–86
   - Amylase output (units/80 min): 441–4038
3. *Lundh test†*
   - Mean tryptic activity (IU/L):61

*Modified from Dreiling, D. A., Janowitz, H. D., and Perrier, C. V. Pancreatic Inflammatory Disease. A Physiologic Approach. New York, Hoeber Medical Division, Harper & Row, Publishers, 1964.

†Value from Mottaleb et al.[81]

enzymes. Most of these indirect tests assume uniform rates of gastric emptying, intestinal absorption (after luminal hydrolysis), metabolism, and secretion. Hence, these indirect tests of pancreatic function are generally less reliable than the secretin or Lundh tests.[80]

References

1. Makhlouf, G. M., and Blum, A. L. An assessment of models for pancreatic secretion. Gastroenterology *59*:896, 1970.
2. Lightwood, R., and Reber, H. A. Micropuncture study of pancreatic secretion in the cat. Gastroenterology *72*:61, 1977.
3. Fölsch, U. R., and Creutzfeldt, W. Pancreatic duct cells in rats: secretory studies in response to secretin, cholecystokinin-pancreozymin and gastrin in vivo. Gastroenterology *73*:1053, 1977.
4. Swanson, C. H., and Solomon, A. K. Micropuncture analysis of the cellular mechanisms of electrolyte secretion by the in vitro rabbit pancreas. J. Gen. Physiol. *65*:22, 1975.
5. Borgström, B., and Erlanson, C. Pancreatic lipase and colipase. Interactions and effects of bile salts and other detergents. Eur. J. Biochem. *37*:60, 1973.
6. Palade, G. Intracellular aspects of the process of protein synthesis. Science *189*:347, 1975.
7. Rothman, S. S. Protein transport by the pancreas. Science *190*:747, 1975.
8. Wormsley, K. G., and Goldberg, D. M. Progress report: the interrelationships of the pancreatic enzymes. Gut *13*:398, 1972.
9. Steer, M. I., and Glazer, G. Parallel secretion of digestive enzymes by the in vitro rabbit pancreas. Am. J. Physiol. *231*:1860, 1976.
10. Adelson, J. W., and Rothman, S. S. Chymodenin, a duodenal peptide: specific stimulation of chymotrypsinogen secretion. Am. J. Physiol. *229*:1680, 1975.
11. Robberecht, P., Cremer, M., and Christophe, J. Discharge of newly synthesized proteins in pure juice collected from the human pancreas. Indication of more than one pool of intracellular digestive enzymes. Gastroenterology *72*:417, 1977.
12. Bruzzone, R., Trimble, E. R., Gjinovci, A., and Renold, A. E. Differences in pancreatic enzyme release from ventral and dorsal areas of the rat pancreas. Am. J. Physiol. *251*:G56, 1986.
13. Korc, M., Owerbach, D., Quinto, C., and Rutter, W. J. Pancreatic islet–acinar cell interaction: amylase messenger RNA levels are determined by insulin. Science *213*:351, 1981.
14. Bonner-Weir, S., and Orci, L. New perspectives on the microvasculature of the islets of Langerhans in the rat. Diabetes *31*:883, 1982.
15. Solomon, T. E. Regulation of exocrine pancreatic cell proliferation and enzyme synthesis. *In* Johnson, L. R., Christensen, J., Grossman, M. I., Jacobsen, E. D., and Schulz, S. G. (eds.). Physiology of the Gastrointestinal Tract. Vol. 2. New York, Raven Press, 1981, p. 873.
16. Petersen, H. The relationship between the gastric and pancreatic secretion in man. Scand. J. Gastroenterol. *4*:345, 1969.
17. Petersen, H. Relationship between gastric and pancreatic secretion in patients with duodenal ulcer. Scand. J. Gastroenterol. *5*:321, 1970.
18. Kumar, R., Banks, P. A., George, P. K., and Tanden, B. Early recovery of exocrine pancreatic function in adult protein-calorie malnutrition. Gastroenterology *68*:1593, 1975.
19. Pitchumoni, C. S. Pancreas in primary malnutrition disorders. Am. J. Clin. Nutr. *26*:374, 1973.
20. Valenzuela, J. W., Walsh, J. H., and Isenberg, J. I. Effect of gastrin on pancreatic enzyme secretion and gallbladder emptying in man. Gastroenterology *71*:409, 1976.
21. Meyer, J. H., Spingola, L. J., and Grossman, M. I. Endogenous cholecystokinin potentiates exogenous secretin on pancreas of dog. Am. J. Physiol. *221*:742, 1971.
22. Wormsley, K. G. Response to secretin and pancreozymin in man. Scand. J. Gastroenterol. *6*:342, 1971.
23. Robberecht, P., Cremer, M., Vandermeers, A., Vandermeers-Piret, M. C., Cotton, P., De Neef, P., and Christophe, J. Pancreatic secretions of total protein and of three hydrolases collected in healthy subjects via duodenoscopic cannulation. Effects of secretin, pancreozymin, and caerulein. Gastroenterology *69*:374, 1975.
24. Bodanski, M. Gastrointestinal hormones: families of oligoelectrolytes. *In* Chey, W. Y., and Brooks, F. P. (eds.). Endocrinology of the Gut. Thorofare, N.J., Charles B. Slack, 1974, p. 3.
25. Konturek, S. J., Thor, P., Dembinski, A., and Krol, R. Vasoactive intestinal peptide: comparison with secretin for potency: spectrum of physiological action. *In* Thompson, J. C. (ed.). Symposium on Gastrointestinal Hormones. Austin, University of Texas Press, 1975, p. 611.
26. Dyck, W. P., Rudick, H., Hoexter, B., and Janowitz, H. D. Influence of glucagon on pancreatic exocrine secretion. Gastroenterology *56*:531, 1969.
27. Dyck, W. P., Texter, E. C., Lasater, J. M., and Hightower, N. C. Influence of glucagon on pancreatic secretion in man. Gastroenterology *58*:532, 1970.
28. Gardiner, J. D., and Jensen, R. T. Secretagogue receptors on pancreatic acinar cells. *In* Johnson, J. R., Christensen, J., Jackson, M. J., Jacobson, E. D., and Walsh, J. H. (eds.). Physiology of the Gastrointestinal Tract. 2nd edition, Vol. 2. New York, Raven Press, 1987, p. 1109.
29. MacGregor, I. L., Parent, J. A., and Meyer, J. H. Gastric emptying of liquid meals and pancreatic and biliary secretion after subtotal gastrectomy or truncal vagotomy and pyloroplasty in man. Gastroenterology *72*:195, 1977.
30. Beglinger, C., Fried, M., Whitehouse, I., Jansen, J. B., Lamers, C. B., and Gyr, K. Pancreatic enzyme response to a liquid meal and to hormonal stimulation. Correlation with plasma secretin and cholecystokinin levels. J. Clin. Invest. *75*:1471, 1985.
31. Solomon, T. E. Control of exocrine pancreatic secretion. *In* Johnson, J. R., Christensen, J., Jackson, M. J., Jacobson, E. D., and Walsh, J. H. (eds.). Physiology of the Gastrointestinal Tract. 2nd edition. Vol. 2. New York, Raven Press, 1987, p. 1173.
32. Fahrenkrug, J., Schaffalitzky de Muckadell, O. B., Holst, J., and Lindkaer Jensen, S. Vasoactive intestinal polypeptide in vagally mediated pancreatic secretion of fluid and HCO_3. Am. J. Physiol. *237*:E535, 1979.
33. Debas, H. T., Konturek, S. J., and Grossman, M. I. Effect of extragastric and truncal vagotomy on pancreatic secretion in the dog. Am. J. Physiol. *228*:1172, 1975.
34. Malagelada, J. R., Go, V. L. W., and Summerskill, W. H. J. Altered pancreatic and biliary function after vagotomy and pyloroplasty. Gastroenterology *66*:22, 1974.
35. Mayer, E. A., Thomson, J. B., Jehn, D., Reedy, T., Elashoff, J., Deveny, C., and Meyer, J. H. Gastric emptying and sieving of solid food and pancreatic and biliary secretions after solid meals in patients with nonresective ulcer surgery. Gastroenterology *87*:1264, 1984.
36. Hootman, S. R., and Williams, J. A. Stimulus-secretion coupling in the pancreatic acinus. *In* Johnson, J. R., Christensen, J., Jackson, M. J., Jacobson, E. D., and Walsh, J. H. (eds.). Physiology of the Gastrointestinal Tract. 2nd edition. Vol. 2. New York, Raven Press, 1987, p. 1129.
37. Magee, D. F., and Naruse, S. Neural control of periodic secretion of the pancreas and stomach in fasting dogs. J. Physiol. *344*:153, 1983.
38. Sarles, H. R., Dani, G., Prezelin, E., Souville, C., and Figarella, C. Cephalic phase of pancreatic secretion in man. Gut *9*:214, 1968.
39. Novis, D. H., Bank, S., and Marks, I. M. The cephalic phase of pancreatic secretion in man. Scand. J. Gastroenterol. *6*:417, 1971.
40. Anagnosstides, A., Chadwick, V. S., Selden, A. C., and Maton, P. N. Sham feeding and pancreatic secretion. Evidence for direct vagal stimulation of enzyme output. Gastroenterology *87*:109, 1984.
41. Preshaw, R. M., Cooke, A. R., and Grossman, M. I. Sham feeding and pancreatic secretion in the dog. Gastroenterology *50*:171, 1966.
42. White, T. T., McAlexander, R. A., and Magee, D. F. The effect of gastric distension on duodenal aspirates in man. Gastroenterology *44*:48, 1963.
43. Debas, H. T., and Yamagishi, T. Evidence of pyloropancreatic reflex for pancreatic exocrine secretion. Am. J. Physiol. *234*:E468, 1978.

44. Fried, M., Meyer, J. H., Jehn, D., Reedy, T., and Elashoff, J. Gastric phase of pancreatic secretion in humans. (Abstract). Dig. Dis. Sci. *31*:1130, 1986.
45. Meyer, J. H., and Kelly, K. A. Canine pancreatic responses to intestinally perfused proteins and protein digests. Am. J. Physiol. *231*:682, 1976.
46. Grossman, M. I., and Konturek, S. J. Gastric acid does drive pancreatic bicarbonate secretion. Scand. J. Gastroenterol. *9*:299, 1974.
47. Moore, E. W., Verine, H. J., and Grossman, M. I. Pancreatic bicarbonate response to a meal. Acta Hepatogastroenterol. *26*:30, 1979.
48. Annis, D., and Hallenbeck, G. A. Effect of excluding pancreatic juice from duodenum on secretory response of pancreas to a meal. Proc. Soc. Exp. Biol. Med. *77*:383, 1951.
49. Cooke, A. R., Nahrwold, D. L., and Grossman, M. I. Diversion of pancreatic juice on gastric and pancreatic response to a meal stimulus. Am. J. Physiol. *213*:637, 1967.
50. Rune, S. J., and Henriksen, F. W. Carbon dioxide tensions in the proximal part of the canine gastrointestinal tract. Gastroenterology *56*:758, 1970.
51. Meyer, J. H., Way, L. W., and Grossman, M. I. Pancreatic bicarbonate response to various acids in duodenum of dog. Am. J. Physiol. *219*:964, 1970.
52. Lee, K. Y., Tai, H. H., and Chey, W. Y. Plasma secretin and gastrin responses to a meal and duodenal acidification in dogs. Am. J. Physiol. *230*:784, 1976.
53. Schaffalitzky de Muckadell, O. B., and Fahrenkrug, J. Secretion pattern of secretin in man: regulation by gastric acid. Gut *19*:812, 1978.
54. Schafmayer, A., Teichmann, R. K., Rayford, P. L., and Thompson, J. C. Physiological release of secretin measured in peripheral and portal venous blood of dogs. Digestion *17*:509, 1978.
55. Kim, M. S., Lee, K. Y., and Chey, W. Y. Plasma secretin concentrations in fasting and postprandial states in dog. Am. J. Physiol. *236*:E539, 1979.
56. Meyer, J. H., and Fink, A. S. Pancreatic bicarbonate response to food-bound hydrogen ion along the gut. Gastroenterology *87*:586, 1984.
57. Meyer, J. H. Release of secretin and cholecystokinin. *In* Thompson, J. C. (ed.). Symposium on Gastrointestinal Hormones. Austin, University of Texas Press, 1975, p. 475.
58. Faichney, A., Chey, W. Y., Kim, Y. C., Lee, K. Y., Kim, M. S., and Chang, T. M. Effect of sodium oleate on plasma secretin concentrations and pancreatic secretion in dog. Gastroenterology *81*:458, 1981.
59. Solomon, T. E., and Grossman, M. I. Effect of atropine and vagotomy on response of transplanted pancreas. Am. J. Physiol. *236*:E186, 1979.
60. Singer, M. V., Solomon, T. E., Wood, J., and Grossman, M. I. Latency of pancreatic enzyme response to intraduodenal stimulants. Am. J. Physiol. *238*:G23, 1980.
61. Meyer, J. H., Way, L. W., and Grossman, M. I. Pancreatic response to acidification of various length of intestine in dog. Am. J. Physiol. *219*:971, 1970.
62. Meyer, J. H., Kelly, K. A., Spingola, L. J., and Jones, R. S. Canine gut receptor system mediating pancreatic responses to luminal L-amino acids. Am. J. Physiol. *231*:669, 1976.
63. Fink, A. S., Luxemburg, M., and Meyer, J. H. Regionally perfused fatty acids augment acid-induced canine pancreatic secretion. Am. J. Physiol. *245*:G78, 1983.
64. MacGregor, I. L., Deveney, C., Way, L. W., and Meyer, J. H. The effect of acute hyperglycemia on meal stimulated gastric, biliary, and pancreatic secretion and serum gastrin. Gastroenterology *70*:197, 1976.
65. DiMagno, E. P., Go, V. L. W., and Summerskill, W. H. J. Intraluminal and postabsorptive effects of amino acids on pancreatic enzyme secretion. J. Lab. Clin. Med. *82*:241, 1973.
66. Wilson, R. M., Boden, G., Shore, L. S., and Essa-Kaumer, N. Effect of somatostatin on meal-stimulated pancreatic exocrine secretion in dogs. Diabetes *26*:7, 1976.
67. Rhodes, J., and Prestwich, C. J. Acidity at different sites in proximal duodenum of normal subjects and patients with duodenal ulcers. Gut *7*:509, 1966.
68. Dutta, S. K., Russell, R. M., and Iber, F. I. Impaired acid neutralization in the duodenum in pancreatric insufficiency. Dig. Dis. Sci. *24*:775, 1979.
69. Ovesen, L., Bendtsen, F., Tage-Jensen, U., Pedersen, N. T., Gram, B. R., and Rune, S. J. Intraluminal pH in the stomach, duodenum, and proximal jejunum in normal subjects and patients with pancreatic insufficiency. Gastroenterology *90*:958, 1986.
70. Youngberg, C. A., Berardi, R. R., Howatt, W. F., Hyneck, M. L., Amidon, G. L., Meyer, J. H., and Dressman, J. B. Comparison of gastrointestinal pH in cystic fibrosis and healthy subjects. Dig. Dis. Sci. (in press).
71. Williams, N. S., Elashoff, J., and Meyer, J. H. Abnormalities of gastric emptying of liquids in duodenal ulcer disease. Dig. Dis. Sci. *31*:943, 1986.
72. Debas, H. T. Peripheral regulation of gastric acid secretion. *In* Johnson, J. R., Christensen, J., Jackson, M. J., Jacobson, E. D., and Walsh, J. H. (eds.). Physiology of the Gastrointestinal Tract. 2nd edition. Vol. 2. New York, Raven Press, 1987, p. 931.
73. Beck, I. The role of pancreatic enzymes in digestion. Am. J. Clin. Nutr. *26*:311, 1973.
74. Imondi, A. R., Stradley, P., and Wolgemuth, R. Enzyme replacement therapy in the pancreatic duct ligated swine. Proc. Soc. Exp. Biol. Med. *141*:367, 1972.
75. DiMagno, E. P., Go, V. L. W., and Summerskill, W. H. J. Relations between pancreatic enzyme outputs and malabsorption in severe pancreatic insufficiency. N. Engl. J. Med. *288*:813, 1973.
76. Hamosh, M., Klaeveman, H. L., Wolf, R. O., and Scow, R. O. Pharyngeal lipase and digestion of dietary triglyceride in man. J. Clin. Invest. *55*:908, 1975.
77. Cohen, M., Morgan, R. G. H., and Hoffman, A. F. Lipolytic activity of human gastric and duodenal juice against medium and long chain triglycerides. Gastroenterology *60*:1, 1971.
78. Kurtis, K. J., Gaines, H. D., and Kim, Y. S. Protein digestion and absorption in rats with pancreatic duct occlusion. Gastroenterology *74*:1271, 1978.
79. Goff, J. S. Pancreatic exocrine function testing. West. J. Med. *135*:368, 1981.
80. Meyer, J. H. Tests of pancreatic function (editorial). West. J. Med. *135*:401, 1981.
81. Mottaleb, A., Kapp, F., Noguera, E., Kellock, T. D., Wiggins, H. S., and Waller, S. L. The Lundh test in the diagnosis of pancreatic disease: a review of five year's experience. Gut *14*:835, 1973.

96

Pancreatic Disorders in Childhood

JEFFREY A. BILLER
RICHARD J. GRAND

HEREDITARY DISEASES

Although cystic fibrosis is the most common of the hereditary disorders affecting the pancreas, other congenital and familial diseases may present difficult diagnostic challenges (Table 96–1). In this section are reviewed those disorders of the exocrine pancreas that present in the infant as well as in the older child.

CYSTIC FIBROSIS

Epidemiology

Cystic fibrosis is the most common lethal genetic defect of Caucasian populations.[1] The disease was once limited to infants and children, but because the immediate prognosis has changed drastically over the last three decades, the majority of patients now survive into adolescence, and nearly 80 per cent live beyond their twentieth birthday.[2–4] In most patients the diagnosis is made in the first several years of life; however, in 2 per cent of cases the diagnosis is first established after 18 years of age. The disorder is a genetic syndrome of apparent exocrine dysfunction, characterized by ductal obstructive lesions throughout multiple organ systems and disturbances of mucus and electrolyte secretion.[3, 5, 6] Although reported in various racial groups, cystic fibrosis is more common in Caucasians. It is inherited in an autosomal recessive fashion and is estimated to occur in 1 in 2000 live Caucasian births, with a gene frequency of 4 to 5 per cent.[5] The specific genetic defect appears to reside on chromosome 7, and prenatal diagnosis is becoming a reality.[7] The diagnosis still rests on demonstration of elevated concentrations of sodium and chloride in sweat.[8] Cystic fibrosis is a major cause of malabsorption in infants and children in the United States and is responsible for a large proportion of the chronic pulmonary disease encountered during childhood. Indeed, chronic obstructive pulmonary disease is eventually present in all cases and accounts for much of the morbidity and almost all of the mortality associated with cystic fibrosis beyond the neonatal period. Gastrointestinal symptoms are less consistent, but steatorrhea occurs in 85 to 90 per cent of patients with cystic fibrosis.[9]

Table 96–1. HEREDITARY DISEASE OF THE EXOCRINE PANCREAS

A. Exocrine Pancreatic Insufficiency
   1. Cystic fibrosis
   2. Shwachman's syndrome
   3. Isolated enzyme deficiency
      a. Lipase
      b. Co-lipase
      c. Trypsin
      d. Enterokinase
B. Pancreatitis
   1. Hereditary
   2. Metabolic
      a. Hyperlipidemias
      b. Hyperparathyroidism
      c. Alpha$_1$-antitrypsin deficiency
C. Miscellaneous

Etiology

Cystic fibrosis has been classified as an inborn error of metabolism. The exact nature of the primary defect is unknown, and no single biochemical aberration has been detected that accounts for the varied manifestations of the disease.

Conflicting pathogenetic hypotheses, including autonomic dysfunction, defects in glycoprotein biochemistry (perhaps reflected in altered membrane structure or permeability), structural aberrations in mucosubstances, or abnormalities in a variety of regulatory factors (hormones, antibodies, neurohumoral transmitters, and kallikreins) have been suggested.[5] None of these reconciles the unique sweat gland defect with the abnormal characteristics of mucus secretion or the abnormalities in the male genital tract. Environmental and exogenous influences, such as climate, diet, and familial patterns of response to infection, as well as intrauterine insults and vitamin deficiencies, have all been discarded as causative factors in the disease. At present, cystic fibrosis cannot be reproduced in animals.

Pathogenesis

Although early observations appeared promising concerning the pathogenesis of some of the manifestations of cystic fibrosis,[6] most have not proved helpful in understanding the basic abnormality of the disease. Early research centered on the glycoproteins and mucosubstances in patients with cystic fibrosis. Although increased numbers of mucus-secreting cells with increased amounts of intracellular glycoprotein had been found in the secretory cells, histochemical techniques have failed to reveal any unique characteristics differentiating mucus in patients with cystic fibrosis from those with other conditions associated with mucus hypersecretion. The importance of the relative concentrations of fucose and sialic acid in salivary and respiratory glycoproteins in patients with cystic fibrosis compared with those of controls remains debated.[10] Interest had centered on humoral factors accounting for ciliary dyskinesia in various tissues.[11] Perfusion of such materials into the parotid duct of rats or into human sweat glands can lead to abnormal sodium reabsorption. The clinical significance, however, of these various factors remains unclear. Other studies investigating host defenses have revealed that the IgG respiratory opsonins in patients with cystic fibrosis are fragmented and may inhibit the killing of the *Pseudomonas* organism by macrophages.[12] Further studies are being conducted to expand on this observation.

The most promising area of research at this time involves that centered on electrolyte secretion and chloride channel regulation. Abnormal electrolyte secretion in the exocrine glands, present from birth, is the most characteristic and constant finding in cystic fibrosis.[5] Elevation of the sodium and chloride concentrations in the sweat is most common, although the potassium concentration is also elevated but less consistently. All patients with clinical manifestations of the disease show this sweat abnormality.

Electrophysiologic studies on sweat gland ducts[13] and airway epithelia[14] have documented decreased chloride ion transport in patients with cystic fibrosis. The presence of selective channels for chloride ion in the apical membrane of tracheal epithelial cells has been described by several groups in both normal subjects and patients with cystic fibrosis.[15–17] In contrast to that found in tracheal epithelial cells of normal patients, chloride ion channel activity was not elicited by epinephrine or cyclic adenosine monophosphate (cAMP) in these cells of patients with cystic fibrosis. Further studies suggest that, in affected tissues of cystic fibrosis patients, alteration in a common intracellular mediator or inhibitor protein distal to the site of generation of cAMP is more likely to be the underlying abnormality rather than one of the chloride ion channel itself.[18]

Diagnosis

The diagnosis of cystic fibrosis begins with a suspicion of the disease. Greater than 95 per cent of children with pancreatic insufficiency, most of those with meconium ileus, 30 per cent with meconium peritonitis, and 15 per cent with small bowel atresia will have cystic fibrosis. Other indications for evaluation include unexplained chronic pulmonary disease, chronic hepatobiliary disease, hypoproteinemia and edema, and failure to thrive. Siblings of an affected family member should also be screened.

The diagnosis rests primarily on the finding of abnormal sweat electrolytes. The sodium and chloride concentrations in sweat are elevated in 98 to 99 per cent of patients with cystic fibrosis, as determined by quantitative pilocarpine iontophoresis.[8] The test, although simple, is a demanding one to perform well, and considerable variation in reliability exists among testing centers. In addition, as noted in Table 96–2, many conditions other than cystic fibrosis are associated with elevated sweat concentrations of electrolytes. In many of these situations the abnormalities in electrolytes in sweat are transient. False negative sweat test results have been recognized in infants with cystic fibrosis with edema as well as when the amount of sweat obtained is insufficient (less than 100 mg).[19] Steroid medications, diuretics, and high- or low-sodium diets may also affect results. These observations demand, therefore, that sweat electrolyte determination be conducted with great care at centers performing the test frequently, using a standardized method.[8] Other, simpler methods for sweat electrolyte determination exist, although reproducibility is lower, and standard deviations for the Orion and Medtherm methods can be expected to be as large as ±52 and ±35 mEq/L, respectively. Positive or questionable results should be confirmed at least once, preferably at a major Cystic Fibrosis Center. Results must then be correlated with clinical findings, family history, and pulmonary and gastrointestinal findings.

It can be stated with a confidence level of 99 per cent that most patients with cystic fibrosis will have sweat chloride and sodium concentrations above 77 mEq/L and 74 mEq/L, respectively (Fig. 96–1). Also, in patients with cystic fibrosis, the concentration of chloride is slightly greater than that of sodium, the reverse of normal subjects. Large discrepancies be-

Table 96–2. CONDITIONS REPORTED WITH ELEVATED SWEAT ELECTROLYTE CONCENTRATION

Cystic fibrosis
Ectodermal dysplasia
Glycogen storage disease, type I
Adrenal insufficiency
Familial hypoparathyroidism
Malnutrition
Fucosidosis
Nephrosis with edema
Pitressin-resistant diabetes insipidus
Mucopolysaccharidosis
Hypothyroidism
Mauriac syndrome
Familial cholestasis syndrome
Environmental deprivation syndrome
Acute respiratory disorders (croup, epiglottitis, viral pneumonia)
Chronic respiratory disorders (bronchopulmonary dysplasia, $alpha_1$-antitrypsin deficiency)

Adapted from Christoffel, K., Lloyd-Still, J., Brown, G., and Shwachman, H. J. Pediatr. *107*:231, 1985.

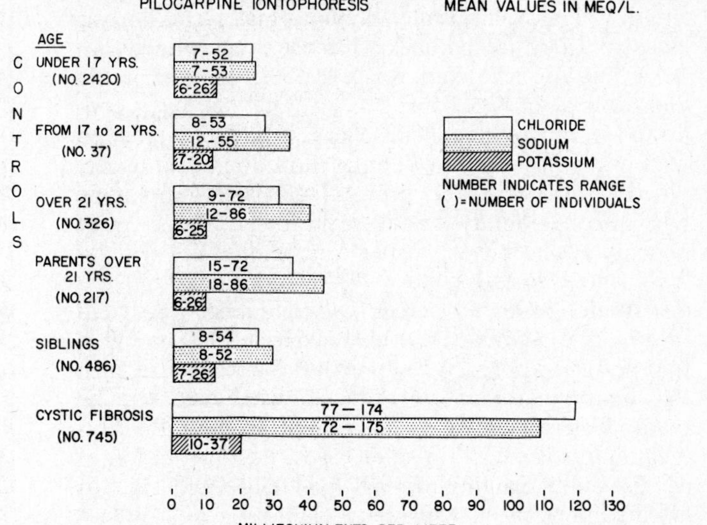

Figure 96–1. Sweat test results: pilocarpine iontophoresis.

tween sodium and chloride determinations suggest technical problems and an unreliable result. Borderline values (i.e., between 47 and 74 mEq/L for sodium and between 47 and 77 mEq/L for chloride) remain a difficult problem, requiring careful clinical correlations with family history, pulmonary findings, and analysis of pancreatic secretion after stimulation with CCK and secretin (see p. 1786). Indications for sweat testing are shown in Table 96–3. Investigators have demonstrated an increased bioelectric potential difference across nasal epithelium and sweat glands in patients with cystic fibrosis.[14, 20] This observation may prove important, especially in the evaluation of patients with suspected cystic fibrosis who have borderline sweat electrolyte concentrations.

Neonatal Screening. Most infants with cystic fibrosis have been found to have elevated levels of immunoreactive trypsinogen in their serum or in dried blood spots obtained within the first year of life.[21, 22] This test has therefore been advocated as a screen for cystic fibrosis in newborn infants.[23, 24] Concerns have been raised, however, regarding large numbers of false positive results on initial screening. Although serum lipase activity is also elevated in infants with cystic fibrosis, the test does not improve accuracy of serum trypsinogen as a screening test for cystic fibrosis.[25] It remains unclear whether early diagnosis before onset of clinical symptoms will significantly reduce morbidity of these patients.[26–28] For this reason, in the United States neonatal screening for cystic fibrosis using serum trypsinogen levels is not being performed routinely, although investigation continues. With advancing age, there is a progressive decline in the serum level of trypsinogen.[25] Cystic fibrosis patients over five years of age with pancreatic insufficiency have low or undetectable levels, whereas those with intact pancreatic exocrine function have significantly higher levels. This test may therefore serve to identify pancreatic insufficiency in the older patient with cystic fibrosis.[29–31]

Table 96–3. INDICATIONS FOR THE SWEAT TEST (QUANTITATIVE PILOCARPINE IONTOPHORESIS)

Siblings of patients with cystic fibrosis
Chronic pulmonary symptoms
Cough
Recurrent respiratory infection
Bronchitis
Bronchiectasis
Lobar atelectasis
Failure to thrive (stunting of growth)
Rectal prolapse
Nasal polyposis
Intestinal obstruction of newborn
Jaundice in early infancy
Cirrhosis in childhood or adolescence
Portal hypertension
Adult males with aspermia
Heat stroke
Hypoproteinemia
Hypoprothrombinemia

Prenatal Diagnosis. Although early attempts at prenatal diagnosis of cystic fibrosis had failed, several newer techniques appear very promising. During the second trimester of pregnancy, low levels of intestinal alkaline phosphatase have been found in the amniotic fluid from pregnant women subsequently giving birth to a child with cystic fibrosis.[32–34] This technique employs a monoclonal antibody specific for this microvillus enzyme. It appears to have a high sensitivity (greater than 90 per cent), especially at 17 to 18 weeks' gestation, with very few false positive and false negative results when used for screening of families in which there is already an affected child. Its usefulness in those families without an affected child remains unclear.

The recent use of DNA probes has allowed determination of linkage between a restriction fragment length polymorphism and the abnormal cystic fibrosis locus. With this technique, it has been determined that the cystic fibrosis locus resides in the middle of the long arm of chromosome 7.[7, 35–36] This has been confirmed in studies involving over 200 families affected with cystic fibrosis representing more than 1200 genotyped individuals. The prenatal diagnosis employing DNA probes tightly linked to the cystic fibrosis gene appears applicable in 80 per cent of families with at least one affected child.[37, 38] As more markers are determined, a higher percentage of families may yield informative results using this technique. The implications of this approach for prenatal diagnosis are such that genotypic diagnosis of the affected fetus can be made at 11 to 12 weeks' gestation. In addition, this technique will allow, in some cases, documentation of carrier status among siblings and close relatives of affected persons.

Clinical Picture

The clinical manifestations of cystic fibrosis are shown in Table 96–4. The general appearance of the cystic fibrosis patient may vary considerably from that of a severely malnourished, stunted person to one who appears healthy. The disease should be suspected in any child having chronic or recurrent symptoms involving the upper or lower respiratory tract. Well over 90 per cent of patients show respiratory tract involvement during childhood, and the majority of patients have evidence of pulmonary disease during infancy. The gastrointestinal symptoms are primarily malabsorption and maldigestion caused by exocrine pancreatic insufficiency (see pp. 263–282). Bulky and frequent stools may be a minor complaint. In small infants, diarrhea and failure to gain weight are often noted. The stools are usually described as large, gray-colored, poorly formed, oily, and foul-smelling. The odor is often so pungent that a child not yet diagnosed as having the disease may be suspected to have it on this account. The stool changes are more noticeable as the infant's diet is increased with a variety of foods. A simple diagnostic clue is the detection of excess neutral fat or of decreased stool trypsin or chymotrypsin concentrations (see p. 1794). The development of a protuberant abdomen is common in untreated patients, as is rectal prolapse.

By the age of three years, approximately 20 per cent of untreated children have a history of rectal prolapse, a symptom easily avoided by medical therapy. The prolapse may indeed be the initial complaint in some patients. Although this entity is also seen in patients with other intestinal disorders, such as celiac disease (celiac sprue), infectious enteritis, kwashiorkor, and severe functional chronic constipation, its occurrence in infancy in the United States is highly suggestive of cystic fibrosis. The cause of this abnormality is related to poor nutrition, frequent voluminous bowel movements, and increased intra-abdominal pressure associated with chronic cough. Prolapse rarely or never requires surgery for correction. Proper dietary management with restriction of fat intake and pancreatic supplementation usually leads to rapid improvement and prevents recurrences.

Table 96–4. CLINICAL MANIFESTATIONS OF CYSTIC FIBROSIS

Viscid secretions: small duct obstruction
- Respiratory
  - Upper
    - Sinusitis
    - Mucous membrane hypertrophy; nasal polyposis
  - Lower
    - Atelectasis
    - Emphysema
    - Infections
      - Bronchitis
      - Bronchopneumonia, bronchiectasis, lung abscess
      - Respiratory failure; right heart failure; death
- Gastrointestinal
  - Gastroesophageal reflux
  - Peptic ulcer disease
  - Meconium ileus
  - Volvulus
  - Peritonitis
  - Ileal atresia
  - Distal intestinal obstruction syndrome
    - Fecal masses
    - Obstruction
- Pancreas
  - Nutritional failure due to pancreatic insufficiency
  - Diabetes
  - Calcification
  - Maldigestion
  - Vitamin deficiencies
  - Loss of bile salts
  - Steatorrhea and azotorrhea
- Hepatobiliary
  - Mucus hypersecretion
  - Atrophic gallbladder
  - Focal biliary cirrhosis
  - Cirrhosis
  - Portal hypertension
  - Esophageal varices
  - Hypersplenism
- Reproductive system
  - Females: increased viscosity of vaginal mucus and decreased fertility
  - Males: failure of wolffian duct development; sterility; absent ductus deferens, epididymis, and seminal vesicles
- Skeletal
  - Retardation of bone age
  - Demineralization
  - Hypertrophic pulmonary osteoarthropathy
- Eye
  - Venous engorgement
  - Retinal hemorrhage
- Other
  - Salt depletion through excessive loss of salt through skin
  - Heat stroke
  - Hypertrophy of apocrine glands

The diagnosis of cystic fibrosis should also be suspected in infants with hypoproteinemic edema. Another condition that may lead to the diagnosis of cystic fibrosis is vitamin K deficiency in infancy, in which the initial manifestation may be hemorrhage into the skin or elsewhere. All patients suspected of having celiac disease should have sweat tests (see Table 96–3). The concurrence of these two diseases is indeed rare. However, a number of patients with cystic fibrosis have been misdiagnosed as having celiac disease and may respond very satisfactorily to dietary therapy at first. It may be discovered a number of months or years later, when pulmonary lesions appear, that the original diagnosis was incorrect.[9]

Infrequently the child presents with signs and symptoms of cirrhosis of the liver and portal hypertension, often with associated hypersplenism. All children with unexplained cirrhosis of the liver should be investigated for cystic fibrosis, and a diagnostic sweat test should be performed. The pulmonary changes may be minimal when the patient is first seen.

During warm weather and during febrile episodes, some patients will suffer from heat exhaustion. All such persons should have sweat tests. The loss of water and electrolytes through excessive sweating may result in hypovolemia and shock.

The clinical symptoms of cystic fibrosis most often are present in the first few months; however, they may be delayed for years with considerable variability in severity. Some infants have severe manifestations, have a rapidly deteriorating course, and succumb in the first year of life. However, the majority of patients have a milder course and, with early recognition and constant medical supervision and therapy, may reach adulthood. Still others, a smaller group, have their first symptoms after four or five years of age. In approximately 15 to 20 per cent of patients, the pulmonary disease predominates in the clinical picture at the time the diagnosis of cystic fibrosis is made, and there are no signs or symptoms of pancreatic involvement. On the other hand, the gastrointestinal manifestations may antedate chronic pulmonary disease for months or years. By far the largest number of infants and children with this disease have both pulmonary and pancreatic involvement. The frequency of gastrointestinal manifestations of cystic fibrosis is shown in Table 96–5.

Table 96–5. FREQUENCY OF GASTROINTESTINAL MANIFESTATIONS IN CYSTIC FIBROSIS

Organ or Other Structure	Complication	Percentage of Patients
Pancreas	Total achylia	85–90
	Partial or normal function	10–15
	Pancreatitis	
	Abnormal glucose tolerance	20–30
	Diabetes	1–2
Intestine	Meconium ileus	10–15
	Rectal prolapse	20
	Distal intestinal obstruction syndrome ("meconium ileus equivalent")	
	Intussusception	10–20
	Pneumatosis intestinalis	1–5
	? Mucosal function impairment	
Liver	Fatty liver	15–30
	Focal biliary cirrhosis	25
	Portal hypertension	2–5
Biliary tract	Gallbladder abnormal, nonfunctional, or small	45
	Gallstones	
	Cholecystitis	4–12
Esophagus	Gastroesophageal reflux	
	Esophagitis	

Pancreas in Cystic Fibrosis

Eighty-five to 90 per cent of patients with cystic fibrosis present with evidence of exocrine pancreatic dysfunction, and although initial pancreatic involvement may be minimal, it may be progressive. It is thought that in patients who lack pancreatic involvement early in the course of their disease, progression may be less common.

Pathology. When the patient is severely affected, the pancreas is shrunken, with marked fibrosis, fatty replacement, and cysts.[39] The extent of involvement is variable, however. Infants and children with cystic fibrosis have been reported in whom the pancreas was histologically normal at autopsy. Stenosis of large pancreatic ducts is seen occasionally, but, in general, the pancreatic lesions are caused by obstruction of small ducts by secretions and cellular debris. Histologically, hyperplasia and eventual necrosis of ductular and centroacinar cells, together with inspissated secretions, block pancreatic ductules and subsequently encroach upon acini, causing flattening and atrophy of lining epithelium (Fig. 96–2). Cystic spaces fill with calcium-rich, eosinophilic concretions. A mild inflammatory reaction may be present around obstructed acini, and progressive fibrosis gradually separates and replaces the pancreatic lobules. The islets of Langerhans are spared in most cases until late in the process and are concentrated in the shrinking pancreas. Nesidioblastosis (neoformation of islets) has been described

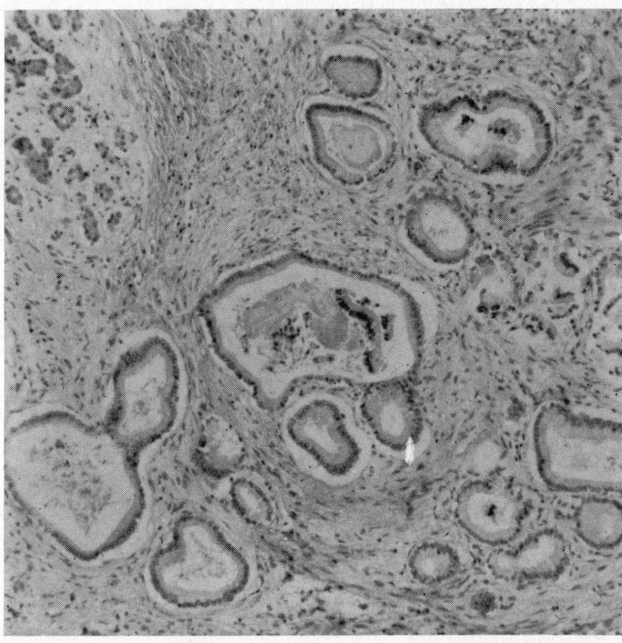

Figure 96–2. Pancreas from patient with cystic fibrosis, showing characteristic histologic changes. Hematoxylin and eosin stain, × 150.

in cystic fibrosis. Calcification, although rare, may be apparent on radiographs.

Functional Abnormalities

Exocrine Dysfunction. Fat and protein maldigestion and fecal loss are the primary manifestations of pancreatic involvement in cystic fibrosis, although there may be considerable variation in severity from one patient to another. Early studies demonstrated evidence of residual lipolysis even in the absence of pancreatic lipase, the amount of steatorrhea being roughly proportional to dietary intake of fat. Gastric lipolysis was suggested as a possible explanation, and Roulet and coworkers have shown increased gastric lipolysis in patients with cystic fibrosis compared with normal subjects.[40] Steatorrhea and azotorrhea generally are greater with pancreatic insufficiency than with mucosal malabsorption but are not observed in exocrine pancreatic insufficiency until the secretion of lipase and trypsin falls below 5 to 10 per cent of normal.[41] In cystic fibrosis, the vast majority of patients satisfy this criterion.

Recurrent, acute pancreatitis may complicate the course of cystic fibrosis in those patients who do not have complete loss of pancreatic enzymatic activity. The diagnosis of cystic fibrosis commonly is delayed in these individuals, as they lack classic gastrointestinal symptoms, and pancreatitis may be the presenting complaint. In these patients, pancreatic insufficiency may develop later.

Duodenal aspirates from patients with cystic fibrosis and complete pancreatic achylia are of small volume, are viscous, and contain low concentrations of pancreatic enzymes and bicarbonate. Cholecystokinin (CCK) and secretin fail to stimulate flow of enzyme secretion. Those patients without absorptive defects may have normal or even elevated concentrations of pancreatic enzymes, but pancreatic secretions remain scanty and viscid and contain low concentrations of bicarbonate even after stimulation.[42–44]

Tests of Pancreatic Exocrine Function. Numerous indirect tests of exocrine pancreatic function have been used in patients with cystic fibrosis, but none gives the quantitative information available from a CCK-secretin test, as discussed on pages 1780 to 1786. A new test using an artificial substrate bentiromide BT-PABA (*N*-benzoyl-L-tyrosyl-*p*-amino-benzoic acid) has been described.[45, 46] Ingested BT-PABA is hydrolyzed in the proximal small intestine by chymotrypsin, with subsequent release of para-aminobenzoic acid (PABA), which can be measured either in the serum or in the urine. Because the PABA is absorbed across intestinal mucosa, subsequently conjugated in the liver, and excreted by the kidneys, falsely abnormal test results may be found in patients with bowel, liver, or renal disease. This problem may be avoided by the separate administration of PABA alone and subsequently BT-PABA in order to calculate a PABA excretion index.[47] Pancreatic dysfunction is not reliably detected when pancreatic enzyme output is greater than 5 per cent of normal or when steatorrhea is absent.[48] Serum levels of PABA obtained 90 minutes after ingestion of BT-PABA appear more specific in teenagers and adults than urinary levels.[49, 50] Early studies in infants and children with cystic fibrosis have suggested that this test may help identify patients with pancreatic insufficiency.[45] However, low urinary excretion of PABA in some patients without cystic fibrosis may limit its usefulness.[46] Recent studies in adults with cystic fibrosis have documented that the BT-PABA test does differentiate those patients with pancreatic exocrine insufficiency from those with exocrine sufficiency.[49]

Another test that reflects altered pancreatic acinar integrity is the serum cationic trypsinogen and trypsin levels measured by radioimmunoassay.[51] Low level of serum trypsin-like immunoreactivity has been shown to be a reliable test in adults with pancreatic insufficiency as well as in older children with cystic fibrosis when steatorrhea is present.[52]

Fecal excretion of trypsin and chymotrypsin have been used as a measure of pancreatic function in infants with cystic fibrosis. Because stool trypsin is more susceptible to inactivation by colonic bacteria, stool chymotrypsin is more reliable.[53] Both tests are relatively insensitive, however, and are of value only in cases of severe pancreatic insufficiency.[54]

Endocrine Dysfunction. Glucose intolerance has been found in approximately 30 per cent of patients with cystic fibrosis and clinically significant diabetes mellitus in 1 to 2 per cent (the normal pediatric population has an incidence of diabetes mellitus of 1:2500). In patients over 25 years of age, diabetes mellitus was found in 13 per cent.[55] The carbohydrate intolerance in these patients is accompanied by insulinopenia, an increase in the number of insulin receptors on peripheral blood monocytes, and a decrease in the affinity of these receptors for insulin.[56]

Data concerning other exocrine abnormalities and responses of gastrointestinal hormones in cystic fibrosis are conflicting.[9]

Treatment

Pancreatic Extracts. Pancreatic enzyme replacement is standard practice in patients with cystic fibrosis, although fat absorption may not return completely to normal. Numerous pancreatic preparations are available commercially, but enzyme activities vary considerably from one product to another, and low levels of lipase remain a problem.[57] Cotazym, Viokase, and Pancrease are the products used most frequently in the United States and all are roughly equivalent in their clinical effectiveness. The goal of pancreatic enzyme replacement is to deliver adequate concentrations of digestive enzymes into the duodenum, but DiMagno and coworkers found that only about 22 per cent of the ingested trypsin activity and 8 per cent of the lipase activity reached the ligament of Treitz and provided less than 2 per cent of the normal enzyme activity.[58] Even massive doses commonly fail to normalize digestion and eliminate steatorrhea and azotorrhea, and increasing the dose of enzyme predisposes to uricosuria.[59] Lipase is inactivated below pH 4.5 and trypsin below pH 3.5, so that increased gastric acid secretion in cystic fibrosis accompanied by low pancreatic bicarbonate secretion interferes with the efficacy of pancreatic enzyme replacement. Enteric-coated preparations, although protected from acid, need an alkaline solution in which to dissolve and therefore may be ineffective in patients with cystic fibrosis and exocrine pancreatic insufficiency.

Sodium bicarbonate has been administered with pancreatic extracts and improves fat absorption in some patients;[60] generally, however, the effects are modest, and large doses of bicarbonate are difficult to administer to children and may constitute a considerable sodium load. Cimetidine has been shown to improve the effectiveness of pancreatic enzyme replacement,[61–63] but long-term administration to children is not practical. Nevertheless, this treatment may allow relatively normal fat absorption. Initial therapy should consist of pancreatic extract totalling from 3000 to 15,000 units of lipase activity, given just before each meal and with snacks. The exact dose prescribed depends on the individual's age, the degree of pancreatic insufficiency, the amount of fat ingested, and the commercial preparation chosen. The response to the administered dose—that is, the change in coefficient of fat absorption, bowel symptoms, and growth—determines adequacy.

Pancreatic enzyme replacement is not without potential complications. Perioral and perianal irritation are common in infants. Attention has been focused on the high purine content of pancreatic extracts, and hypouricosuria has been reported in patients taking large doses of enzyme preparations.[59] Powdered preparations of pancreatic extracts have caused immediate hypersensitivity reactions in parents who administer the product to their children, although there are no reports of allergic reactions in patients with cystic fibrosis.[64, 65]

Intestine in Cystic Fibrosis

Pathology. The mucosal glands of the small intestine may contain variable quantities of inspissated secretions within the lumen but rarely have increased numbers of goblet cells. Brunner's glands may show dilatation, flattening of epithelial lining cells, and stringy secretions within their lumens. Meconium ileus is often associated with severe alterations in the intestinal glands of the small bowel.[66] Even in patients without meconium ileus, however, these findings are common and appear unrelated to the severity of gastrointestinal symptoms or changes in other organs. The small intestinal mucosa in older patients with the distal intestinal obstruction syndrome often shows markedly increased mucus.[67] Normal small intestinal villous and microvillous architecture is the rule in cystic fibrosis.[68, 69] Electron microscopy generally is normal except for an adherent film of mucus on the luminal surface.[68]

Rectal biopsy specimens from patients with cystic fibrosis often show widely dilated crypts packed with mucus.[70–73] Often, the mucus appears laminated or may extrude from a gaping crypt. Bulging goblet cells seem to crowd out the intervening columnar epithelium. Variable cellular infiltration may be present in the lamina propria. Histochemical studies of mucus have not demonstrated any significant qualitative difference between cystic fibrosis patients and control subjects, although mucus in cystic fibrosis generally is more abundant, stains more intensely, and contains more weak acid groups and protein.

Characteristic changes of cystic fibrosis are seen in the appendix.[74] Increased numbers of goblet cells distended with mucus line dilated crypts. Eosinophilic casts of these crypts are extruded into the lumen of the appendix. The diagnosis of cystic fibrosis may be suspected on the basis of the histologic appearance of the appendix.[75] Although chronic changes in the appendix are common at autopsy, the incidence of acute appendicitis is apparently not increased in cystic fibrosis, only four cases being found in one study over 22 years in 250 children with cystic fibrosis.[76]

Radiology of the Intestine. Typical radiographic features of the intestine are often seen in cystic fibrosis (Fig. 96–3). In approximately 80 per cent of patients, thickened duodenal folds, nodular filling defects, mucosal smudging, dilatations, and redundancy are seen.[77] The findings are not age-related. Duodenal biopsies do not adequately explain the radiographic appearance. Radiographically, similar changes occur in the small bowel, including thickening and distortion of jejunal folds and variable dilatation of loops from the jejunum to the rectum.[78] Pneumatosis coli is considered a benign condition secondary to chronic pulmonary disease and fecal impaction.[79]

Functional Abnormalities. Small bowel mucosal dysfunction in cystic fibrosis has been suggested by studies that demonstrate absorptive defects that apparently are unexplained by exocrine pancreatic insufficiency or that persist after adequate pancreatic replacement therapy. Decreased activity of certain cytoplasmic peptide

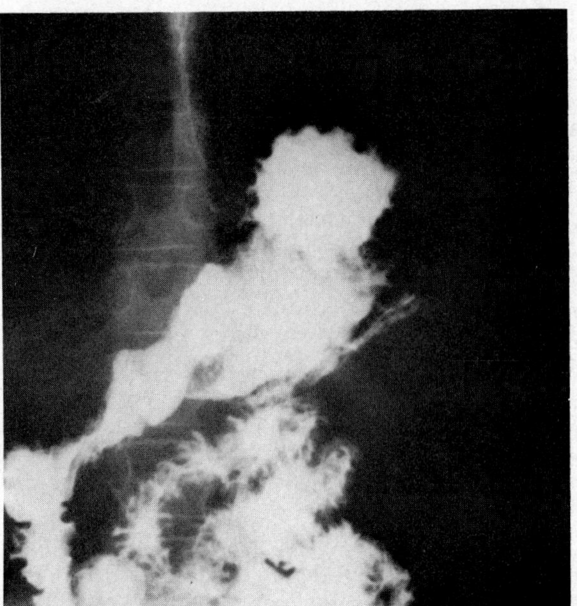

Figure 96–3. X-ray: Upper gastrointestinal barium series in a patient with cystic fibrosis showing thickened folds, nodular filling defects, and variable dilatation of the loops.

hydrolases in intestinal mucosa and reduced uptake of phenylalanine, cycloleucine, and glycine occur in patients with cystic fibrosis compared with control subjects.[80, 81]

Intestinal lactase activity has been a controversial topic until recently. Older reports suggested an association between cystic fibrosis and low lactase levels in jejunal biopsy samples.[82] However, with further study, it has become clear that lactase deficiency in cystic fibrosis is not related to the disease entity but merely reflects a normal ethnic and age-related phenomenon.[83, 84] Interestingly, young children with cystic fibrosis often have elevated lactase values when compared with age-matched controls.[84] This finding may be a response to pancreatic insufficiency, as suggested by Alpers and Tedesco.[85] Xylose absorption is normal in patients with cystic fibrosis.[86]

Meconium Ileus. Meconium ileus is the presenting symptom in 10 to 15 per cent of infants with cystic fibrosis.[87–90] A striking decrease in the content of water and the presence of undegraded serum proteins, intestinal disaccharidases, and some lysosomal enzymes are also found. Sodium, potassium, magnesium, copper, zinc, and manganese concentrations are reduced and calcium greatly increased in concentration in meconium from infants with meconium ileus. Pancreatic insufficiency developing in utero could be the factor predisposing to meconium ileus. However, pancreatic involvement often appears to be mild in infants with meconium ileus, whereas the presence or absence of meconium ileus may be directly related to the severity of involvement of the intestinal glands.[66] Infants dying with meconium ileus often have a completely normal pancreas.[91] Meconium ileus rarely occurs in infants without cystic fibrosis but has been reported in infants with stenosis of the pancreatic duct or partial pancreatic aplasia and in infants with otherwise normal gastrointestinal tracts as a familial occurrence or as an isolated incident.

Pathology. Uncomplicated meconium ileus characteristically demonstrates a narrow distal ileum with beaded appearance owing to waxy gray pellets of inspissated meconium, beyond which the colon is unused. Proximally, the ileal wall is hypertrophied; it then becomes greatly distended with extremely sticky, dark green to black meconium. As many as half the cases of meconium ileus are complicated by volvulus, atresia, or meconium peritonitis. Extravasation of meconium into the fetal peritoneal cavity causes an intense inflammatory reaction that shows variable resolution at birth (depending on when the perforation occurred); it may present clinically merely as intra-abdominal calcifications, a meconium pseudocyst, generalized adhesive meconium peritonitis, or meconium ascites. Fetal volvulus and vascular compromise may cause atresia.

Radiology. Characteristic radiologic findings may be present in meconium ileus[87, 92] (Fig. 96–4). Unevenly distended loops of bowel with absent or scarce air-fluid levels may be seen and presumably reflect the viscid nature of the intestinal secretions. Small bubbles of gas trapped in the sticky meconium may be scattered throughout the distal segment of the small bowel. Barium enema study demonstrates a microcolon and may outline the obstructing meconium mass in the distal ileum. Abdominal calcification reflects meconium peritonitis (Fig. 96–5), and a meconium pseudocyst may displace loops of bowel.

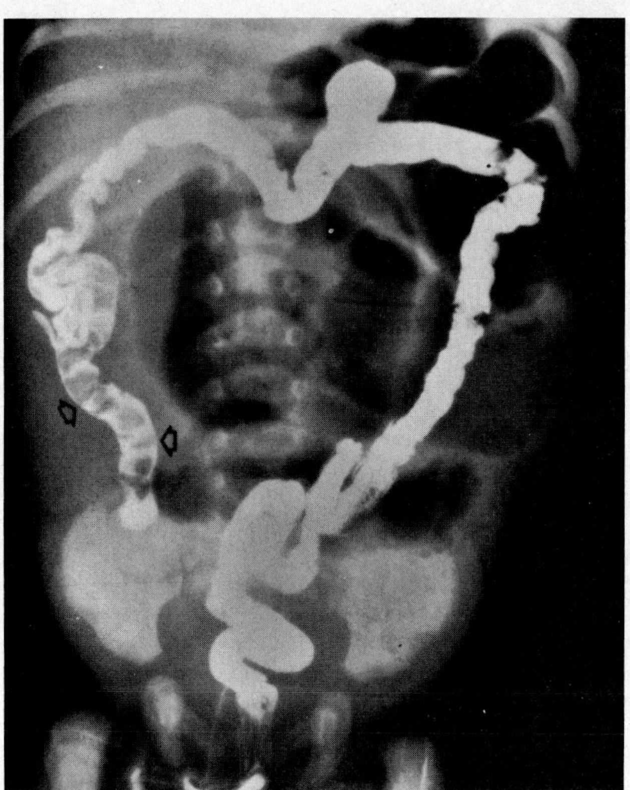

Figure 96–4. Barium enema in an infant with meconium ileus demonstrating a microcolon as well as meconium in the distal ileum *(arrows).* Distended small bowel loops are also noted.

Clinical Features. Meconium ileus classically presents with signs of intestinal obstruction within 48 hours of birth in an infant who is otherwise well; infants with complicated meconium ileus present earlier and appear much sicker. Polyhydramnios is common. A family history of cystic fibrosis is helpful. There seems to be an increased frequency of meconium ileus in some families with cystic fibrosis. In simple meconium ileus, no meconium is passed, and there is progressive abdominal distention and, eventually, bilious vomiting. Dilated, firm, rubbery loops of bowel are visible and palpable through the abdominal wall, particularly in the right lower quadrant, and rectal examination is tight, productive of only a small mucus plug or a small amount of sticky meconium.

Sweat tests should be done in all infants with jejunal and ileal atresia, volvulus, or meconium ileus; the results are likely to be positive in 30 per cent of patients with meconium peritonitis and in 15 to 20 per cent of those with atresia of the small intestine.[87] Although occasionally infants with meconium plug syndrome have cystic fibrosis, it must be stressed that meconium

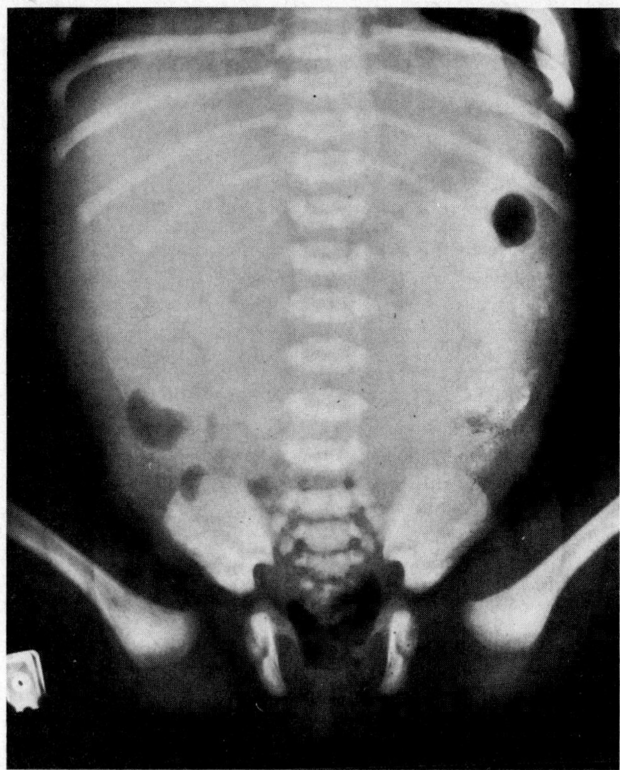

Figure 96–5. Abdominal radiograph in an infant with meconium peritonitis. Calcification is noted in left flank.

plug syndrome and meconium ileus must be carefully differentiated.

Treatment. Meconium ileus was considered invariably fatal until 1948, when the first patients were treated successfully by surgery. More recent reports document an operative mortality rate of about 30 per cent and a long-term survival rate of greater than 50 per cent.[87] Various irrigating solutions have been used during the operation and postoperatively to dissolve and dislodge the abnormal meconium. *N*-Acetylcysteine (Mucomyst), which reduces the viscosity of mucoprotein solutions by cleaving disulfide bonds in the mucoprotein molecule, and polysorbate 80 (Tween 80), a mild industrial detergent and preservative, are now generally recognized as safe and effective. Nonoperative relief of obstruction with Gastrografin enemas[87] has virtually eliminated prolonged hospitalization and early respiratory complications for many infants with uncomplicated meconium ileus. Gastrografin is a radiopaque, aqueous solution that contains a small amount of Tween 80 and has an osmolality of 1900 mOsm. Presumably the detergent action of Tween 80 helps the fluid pass around and into other inspissated meconium, whereas the hypertonicity and mild mucosal irritation draw fluid into the bowel to soften and loosen the meconium. Hypaque enemas have also been employed successfully. Enemas using water-soluble, hypertonic solutions, however, may cause dangerous fluid and electrolyte shifts, especially in small, sick infants. Colonic perforation from enemas has been reported in meconium ileus. Gastrografin enemas are not appropriate therapy for complicated meconium ileus.

A diagnostic barium enema examination should precede therapeutic Gastrografin enemas.[87] Infants with cystic fibrosis and meconium ileus who survive beyond six months of age have the same prognosis as any patient with cystic fibrosis and do not have more severe disease, although they are at somewhat greater risk for episodes of distal intestinal obstruction later in life.

Distal Intestinal Obstruction Syndrome. Intestinal impaction and obstruction remain common and troublesome features in cystic fibrosis beyond the neonatal period. The term "meconium ileus equivalent" is a misnomer; the authors prefer the term "distal intestinal obstruction syndrome."

Pathogenesis. Mechanisms other than inspissated intestinal secretions and pancreatic achylia are probably operative and include undigested food residues, possible disturbances of motility, dilatation of the bowel leading to fecal stasis, and dehydration. Intussusception and, less frequently, volvulus may complicate the distal intestinal obstruction syndrome.[93, 94]

The frequency of the distal intestinal obstruction syndrome is estimated to be as high as 10 per cent among patients with cystic fibrosis. It may even be the presenting symptom of the disease.

Clinical Features. A spectrum of clinical conditions result from partial or complete obstruction of the bowel by abnormal intestinal contents, including (1) abdominal pain from constipation or fecal impaction, (2) palpable cecal masses that may eventually pass spontaneously, and (3) complete obstruction of the bowel by firm, putty-like fecal material in the terminal ileum or right colon or both.[67, 95, 96]

Abdominal pain, usually recurrent and cramping in nature, is the most common symptom of the distal intestinal obstruction syndrome. This may be the only symptom or may persist for years before obstructive symptoms occur. Insufficient doses or cessation of pancreatic enzyme replacement, recent or concomitant respiratory infection, and dietary changes have been incriminated as precipitating factors.[76] Frequently, symptoms appear without warning in patients receiving presumably adequate medical management. The distal intestinal obstruction syndrome should be suspected in any patient with cystic fibrosis who has abdominal pain, a palpable right lower quadrant abdominal mass, or bowel obstruction. The soft, indentable, nontender nature of the palpable fecal mass on examination of the abdomen may be a diagnostic aid. The plain radiograph of the abdomen characteristically shows the proximal segment of the colon and distal portion of the small bowel packed with bubbly-appearing fecal material. The fecal bolus can be identified on barium enema examination but may have to be differentiated from a cecal neoplasm or appendiceal abscess.[97]

Treatment. Uncomplicated distal intestinal obstruction syndrome, once a surgical problem, now usually responds to medical management. Those patients with inadequately controlled steatorrhea may be at higher risk for development of this problem.[95] Vigorous medical therapy includes regular oral doses of pancreatic enzymes and stool softeners, oral or rectal administration of *N*-acetylcysteine, and Gastrografin enemas.

Maintenance treatment with oral doses of *N*-acetylcysteine has been employed successfully to prevent recurrent episodes of the syndrome. Recently, treatment of this disorder using balanced intestinal lavage solutions has been shown to be helpful.[98]

Complications

Intussusception. Intussusception, most often ileocolic in location, is a complication of the distal intestinal obstruction syndrome reported in approximately 1 per cent of patients with cystic fibrosis followed over 17 years.[93] Presumably, a tenacious fecal bolus adherent to the intestinal mucosa acts as the lead point of the intussusception. Most of the patients present acutely with intermittent, severe cramping abdominal pain, although some experience pain for several months before the diagnosis is recognized. Only 25 per cent of the patients note blood in their stools. Efforts should be made to reduce intussusceptions by barium enema. Intussusception has been reported as the presenting symptom of cystic fibrosis, and cystic fibrosis is a major cause of intussusception beyond infancy.

Rectal Prolapse. Rectal prolapse is common in cystic fibrosis, with a frequency of 22 per cent in a series of 386 patients with cystic fibrosis, including 16 cases in which prolapse was the presenting symptom.[99] It is usually recurrent, and patients diagnosed early in life are much less likely to experience rectal prolapse except when stools are voluminous. Additional factors thought to be responsible for the high rate of rectal prolapse in cystic fibrosis include frequent bowel movements, varying degrees of malnutrition, and increased intra-abdominal pressure. Medical management is almost always successful, and a low-fat diet and adequate replacement of pancreatic enzymes usually result in rapid improvement.[55]

Liver in Cystic Fibrosis

The frequency of hepatic abnormalities in cystic fibrosis varies from 20 to 50 per cent of cases studied, although only about 5 per cent of patients with the disease develop cirrhosis, and approximately 2 per cent progress to clinically apparent or important liver disease. A familial tendency to develop cirrhosis has been seen in some patients.

Pathology. Hepatic changes may be present at any age and may be progressive.[100] Excessive biliary mucus associated with mild periportal inflammation and early fibrosis is common in infants under one year of age. Focal biliary fibrosis, characterized by inspissated granular eosinophilic material in ductules, bile duct proliferation, chronic inflammatory infiltrates, and variable fibrosis, is uncommon in infants but present in more than 20 per cent of surviving children and adolescents (Fig. 96–6). In time, focal lesions coalesce in some patients and progress to multilobular biliary cirrhosis. Bile-plugged ducts may be present, but bile stasis within lobules is conspicuously rare beyond the neonatal period, even in advanced liver disease caused by cystic fibrosis.[100–102]

Cholestasis is not uncommon in neonates and young infants; it may be prolonged and associated with excessive biliary mucus and mild periportal changes. Approximately one half of the reported cases were associated with meconium ileus.[103]

Fatty liver, often independent of nutritional status, remains one of the most common hepatic abnormalities encountered in cystic fibrosis. Unexplained hemosiderin deposits in hepatocytes, as well as Kupffer cells, may be prominent in infants and persist beyond four to six months of age.

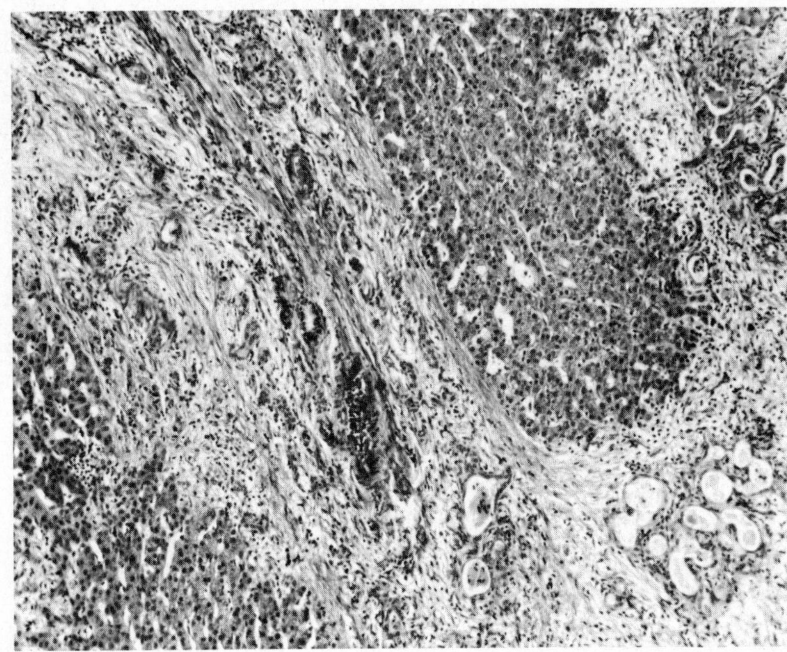

Figure 96–6. Liver from a patient with cystic fibrosis, showing focal biliary fibrosis. Masson stain, × 250.

Radiology. As in other liver disorders, assessment of hepatic disease may be achieved by use of a variety of studies. The abdominal flat film or ultrasonography may suggest hepatomegaly, whereas upper gastrointestinal barium series may indicate the presence of esophageal varices. With progressive involvement, ultrasonographic examination may reveal fibrosis or a dilated portal vein indicative of portal hypertension. Enlarged hepatic veins may be seen as a consequence of congestive heart failure or because of poor outflow secondary to constriction of the inferior vena cava by an enlarged liver at or above the entrances of the hepatic veins. Endoscopic retrograde cholangiopancreatography (ERCP) may reveal irregular filling defects throughout the biliary tree with cystic dilatations of the intrahepatic bile ducts and intrahepatic cholelithiasis.[104] In addition, irregularities of the smaller proximal ducts have been noted, presumably owing to focal biliary cirrhosis.

Functional Abnormalities. Tests of hepatic function in cystic fibrosis may be normal even in cases of overt cirrhosis.[101, 105] An elevated serum alkaline phosphatase value is the most common chemical abnormality indicative of hepatic involvement, although the high values commonly seen in normal infants and children (mainly due to the bone isoenzyme) may conceal increased levels of the hepatic isoenzyme.[106] Serum enzyme levels reflecting hepatocellular injury may be moderately elevated and fluctuate over the course of the illness. Prothrombin time usually is normal but may become prolonged as a consequence of reduced dietary intake or suppression of colonic flora by antibiotics, independent of changes in other liver function tests. Hypoalbuminemia is often found as liver disease progresses.[107]

Bile acid metabolism is disturbed in patients with cystic fibrosis and exocrine pancreatic insufficiency.[108–111] Fecal losses are high and may approach those of patients with ileal resections. Pancreatic enzyme replacement reduces fecal bile acid excretion and corrects steatorrhea and azotorrhea. The fractional turnover rate of the bile acid pool is increased and the total bile acid pool size is diminished in the absence of pancreatic enzymes,[111] whereas the biliary lipid composition and saturation index approach those of patients with cholelithiasis.[109] Treatment with pancreatic supplements returns abnormal values toward normal.

Clinical Features. Symptoms of liver disease in patients with cystic fibrosis are rare and often subtle, although occasionally they can be the presenting complaint. Clinical findings in neonates and young infants may include obstructive jaundice.[103, 112] Hepatomegaly caused by fatty metamorphosis commonly is present in infants and children with the disease. Hepatosplenomegaly, esophageal varices, and, occasionally, ascites can be the first clinical indications of hepatic involvement in cystic fibrosis. Hepatocellular failure has been reported but is distinctly uncommon.

Treatment. The treatment of symptomatic liver disease in cystic fibrosis is identical to that in any other condition associated with hepatic failure. Portosystemic shunts have been performed effectively in patients with cystic fibrosis and portal hypertension.[105, 113] Although some groups have suggested that cystic fibrosis patients with portal hypertension are a special group in whom prophylactic shunt surgery is reasonable,[113] the authors' more recent experience suggests that the same indications should be applied in cystic fibrosis as in any other disorder when deciding on shunt surgery, and prophylactic shunting is not recommended. Liver transplantation may be appropriate treatment for liver failure when pulmonary function is not impaired.[114]

Gallbladder and Biliary System in Cystic Fibrosis

The gallbladder and cystic duct are abnormal in approximately one third of patients with cystic fibrosis, independent of age, clinical course, or hepatic pathology.[104, 109–111]

Pathology. "Microgallbladders" commonly are reported, characteristically containing thick, colorless white bile. Mucus is present within the epithelial lining cells, and numerous mucus-filled cysts may be present immediately beneath the mucosa. The cystic duct may be atrophic or occluded with mucus, but obstruction of the hepatic or common ducts by mucus plugs does not occur.

Radiology. Oral cholecystograms often identify nonfunctioning gallbladders, of which a significant fraction fail to opacify after intravenous cholangiography. Functional and anatomic abnormalities, however, are not usually associated with symptoms.[104]

Clinical Features. Gallstones and their clinical complications have been reported in patients with cystic fibrosis, and intrahepatic cholelithiasis has been seen.

Treatment. Cholecystectomy is indicated in cystic fibrosis whenever clinical disease demands it. Indications are those frequently applied to gallstone disease of other causes (see pp. 1691–1714).

Respiratory Tract in Cystic Fibrosis

Pathology. Most deaths are due to respiratory failure attributed to the severe, extensive chronic pulmonary infection. Autopsy usually reveals the trachea and bronchi to be filled with tenacious mucopurulent material from which *Pseudomonas aeruginosa* or *Staphylococcus aureus* may be cultured. The thorax is rounded, and the lungs are voluminous. Pleural adhesions, emphysematous blebs, hemorrhage, areas of consolidation, abscesses of varying sizes, and massive lung destruction are often noted. Histologically, there are areas of bronchopneumonia, emphysema, and atelectasis, with widespread thick, dilated bronchi. The bronchiectasis generally involves all lobes; often the upper lobes show greater changes than the lower lobes. The hilar lymph nodes are enlarged.

The initial lesion in the lung is bronchial obstruction. Infection supervenes, and a chronic inflammatory process occurs, in which *Staphylococcus aureus* predominates. When the bronchi become colonized with *Pseudomonas,* the mucoid strain often predominates and

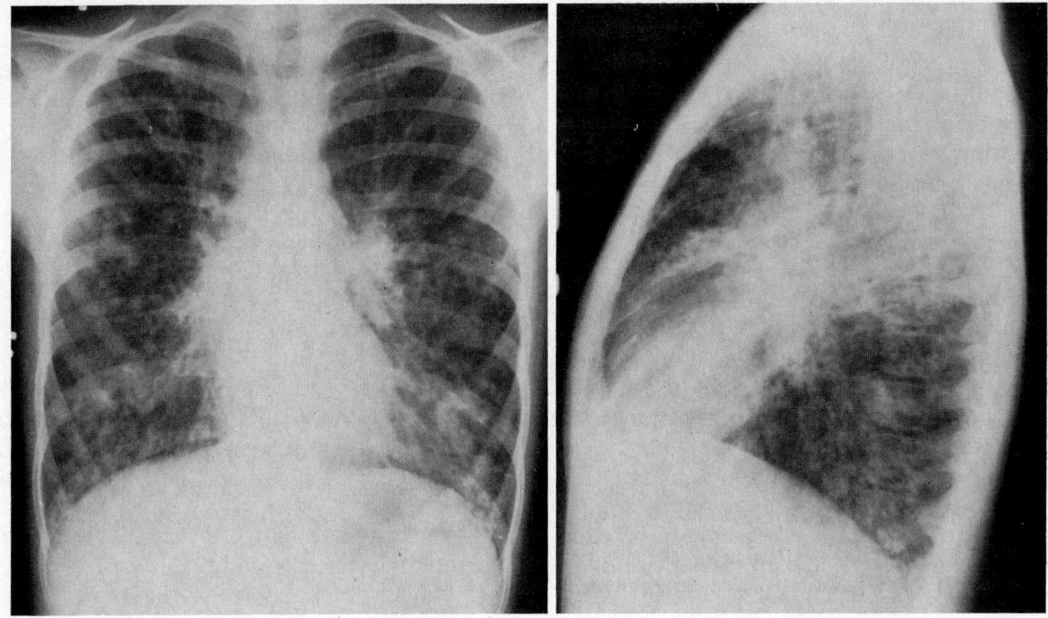

Figure 96–7. Chest X-rays of a patient with severe pulmonary involvement.

adds further metabolic debris. It has been impossible to eradicate *Pseudomonas* completely once it has become established within the bronchi.

The upper respiratory tract is usually affected. Chronic sinus infection is present in the majority of patients. The mucus-secreting cells may be hyperactive. Nasal polyposis is of frequent occurrence and is present in approximately 10 per cent of patients over ten years of age. It may be noted as early as two years. Often polyps are bilateral and cause nasal obstruction. They may be multiple, requiring surgical removal, and frequently recur.

Clinical Manifestations. One of the earliest symptoms is cough. At first it may attract little attention, but it soon becomes chronic and more frequent, results in vomiting, and may even become paroxysmal, suggesting pertussis. Symptoms may be present at two or three months of age. By two years of age, over 75 per cent of children with cystic fibrosis have had the aforementioned symptoms. The x-ray of the chest may reveal evidence of irregular aeration and scattered areas of segmental or lobar atelectasis. The lungs are hyperinflated, and the diaphragm may be depressed. The peribronchial markings become pronounced. A characteristic X-ray with advanced disease is shown in Figure 96–7.

The earliest functional changes may be reflected in a lowered Po_2 and a prolongation of the expiratory flow rate (FEV). The physical findings may often be minimal despite the presence of widespread pulmonary lesions noted by X-ray. Digital clubbing and cyanosis are often present. Some of the serious complications include pneumothorax, hemoptysis, and cor pulmonale. The cause of death is usually respiratory failure accompanied by a fall in Po_2 and a rise in Pco_2. Detailed discussions of pulmonary features of cystic fibrosis are found in recent textbooks.[3, 6]

Genital Abnormalities in Male Patients

The most striking changes in the male genital tract occur in the wolffian duct derivatives, namely, the epididymis, the ductus deferens, and the seminal vesicles. The epididymis is poorly developed, and the body and tail are rudimentary or absent. Upon dissection, the efferent ductules of the head are found to end blindly. The rete testes are intact. The ductus deferens in most cases cannot be identified. Sometimes a solid smooth muscle cord of varying thickness is found in place of the ductus deferens. Multiple sections of spermatic cords rarely show histologic patency at more than one level. Seminal vesicles cannot be identified positively. In addition to these defects, there is a striking increase in abnormalities associated with testicular descent, such as inguinal hernia, hydrocele, and undescended testes. Approximately 97 per cent of males are sterile as a result of these changes. These abnormalities are unique; they have not been noted in any other genetic disease. The defects may be found in male infants shortly after birth and may be useful in supporting the diagnosis of cystic fibrosis in atypical cases.

Treatment of Cystic Fibrosis

Therapy in cystic fibrosis is designed essentially for both prophylaxis and clinical symptoms, because the basic nature of the disorder is unknown. It is also individualized because of the wide range of clinical manifestations and the varying degrees of involvement of affected organs. As the disease is lifelong, therapy must be continuous and comprehensive. For children, particularly infants, in whom the diagnosis is strongly suspected but not confirmed, treatment should not wait until clear-cut clinical evidence appears. Such delay could result in premature development of advanced or irreversible changes and early death.

Pulmonary System

The main considerations are twofold: the relief or prevention of bronchial obstruction, and the treatment of the pulmonary infection.[115]

Obstruction. A variety of measures are employed to remove viscid secretions, which include postural drainage, bronchodilators, and expectorant drugs. Bronchodilators given by aerosol are used in patients with bronchospastic and moderately severe disease. A recent study has suggested improved pulmonary function in those patients treated with alternate-day corticosteroids.[116] Currently, a multihospital cooperative study is under way evaluating the use of alternate-day corticosteroids and home prophylactic oral antibiotics in managing pulmonary complications.

Pulmonary resection has been carried out in carefully selected patients with long-standing areas of persistent atelectasis and underlying abscess formation or bronchiectasis, and in whom the remainder of the lungs is reasonably free of serious disease. Patients with cor pulmonale are treated effectively with digitalis and, if necessary, restriction of salt and fluid, diuretics, and spironolactone.

Infection. Therapy is directed toward those organisms most often implicated in acute and chronic pulmonary infections in these patients (*Staphylococcus aureus, Pseudomonas aeruginosa,* and *Klebsiella pneumoniae*). Sputum cultures may be helpful in following bacterial colonization. With the changing resistance patterns of these bacteria, it is suggested that antibiotics be chosen according to the sensitivities of these organisms. Home parenteral antibiotic treatment is possible for those patients requiring prolonged intravenous therapy. The efficacy of inhaled aerosolized antibiotics remains controversial and currently is not recommended.

Nutritional Management

See also pages 1971 to 2028.

In the routine clinical setting, the nutritional management of patients with cystic fibrosis is based on an assessment of requirements, taking into consideration age, height, weight and anthropometrics, severity of lung disease, anorexia, pancreatic insufficiency, other intraluminal phase abnormalities, and mucosal dysfunction. Ideally, a normal diet for age should be encouraged, with adequate pancreatic replacement therapy provided (and bicarbonate or cimetidine if indicated) to achieve as normal a fat balance as possible.[117, 118] Rigid restrictions of fat intake may lead to reduced energy intake. Medium-chain triglycerides and glucose polymers (Polycose) may be used to improve caloric intake. The long-term impact of such improved nutritional status on growth and development, pulmonary disease, and survival remains controversial. Several studies have suggested that improved nutrition may either improve or at least slow progression of the pulmonary disease.[119–121] The relationship between improved nutrition (via oral, nasogastric, gastrostomy, jejunostomy, or intravenous routes) and pulmonary function will be examined further in future studies. Increased intake of a multivitamin preparation is customary (usually two "high-potency" tablets a day). Vitamin E (in aqueous form) is provided at a dose of 5 units/kg body weight/day. Additional fat-soluble vitamin or mineral supplements are recommended when necessary; infants usually receive daily vitamin K.

Although a great deal has been written regarding defined-formula diets as supplements or replacement for food in patients with cystic fibrosis, there is no evidence that these are better than a balanced diet providing appropriate protein, energy, and essential nutrients.

Prognosis

Currently, between 80 and 90 per cent of patients with cystic fibrosis survive beyond 20 years. Male patients tend to live longer than females by about four years. Most significant morbidity and mortality are related to the chronic obstructive pulmonary disease. The relative influence of nutritional support, pancreatic enzyme replacement, and aggressive treatment of pulmonary disease on improving the quality and duration of life remains uncertain, although the last-mentioned is most likely predominant. It has been reported that patients with intact pancreatic function have better pulmonary status than those with pancreatic insufficiency. This suggests either a heterogeneous form of the disease or better survival with better nutrition.

SHWACHMAN'S SYNDROME

The combination of exocrine pancreatic insufficiency, hematologic abnormalities, and normal sweat electrolytes typifies this syndrome, which has been expanded greatly in the last 25 years to include abnormalities in most organ systems. It is said to be the second most frequently recognized cause of pancreatic insufficiency in children.[122, 123]

Etiology

Analysis of sibship segregation ratios and familial incidence support an autosomal recessive mode of inheritance.[123–124] However, the factors leading to multisystem disease are unidentified. It has been suggested that an abnormality in microtubular or microfilament function may be at fault. Such malfunction may produce diminished neutrophil chemotaxis, poor enzyme secretion, and intracellular inclusions, all of which occur in the disease.[124] Abnormalities of the cytoskeleton of neutrophils as reflected by an abnormal distribution of concanavalin A receptors has been demonstrated in patients with Shwachman's syndrome.[125, 126] Other theories invoke fetal injury, as pancreatic exocrine tissue and the myeloid population of the bone marrow both develop at approximately the fifth month of gestation. However, this would not explain the familial incidence. At present, these and other pathogenetic mechanisms remain speculative.

Pathology

The pancreas at laparotomy varies in size from normal to small and usually has a fatty appearance. The main pancreatic ducts are normal. At microscopic examination, the "lipomatous" appearance is confirmed by the predominance of fat cells, with scattered normal islets and minimal remaining acinar tissue. This lipomatous change can also be suspected from ultrasonography and CT scan.[127] The inflammatory reaction is scant, and mild to moderate fibrosis may present around ductules. These changes may be late and may result from progressive degeneration and fatty metamorphosis.[124]

Clinical Features

The clinical manifestations of Shwachman's syndrome are given in Table 96–6. The sexes are affected equally, and children almost always become ill with symptoms of malabsorption by four to six months of age.[123, 124, 128] There may be other early problems, including failure to thrive and feeding problems. Growth soon becomes suboptimal, with only a rare patient exceeding the third percentile for height; this deficit worsens with age. Infections are also an early problem and are severe in at least 85 per cent, occasionally leading to death. Most patients are diagnosed in the first two years of life, although occasionally recognition of symptoms is delayed.[129]

Table 96–6. SHWACHMAN'S SYNDROME

Genetics:	Autosomal recessive	
Clinical Features:	General:	Failure to thrive
	Digestive:	Pancreatic exocrine insufficiency Normal results on sweat test
	Hematologic:	Neutropenia Thrombocytopenia Anemia
	Skeletal:	Metaphyseal chondrodysplasia, especially of the femur
	Immune:	Increased propensity to infection
	Liver:	Elevated aminotransferase Liver biopsy periportal fibrosis Fatty change Cirrhosis (rare)
	Cardiac:	Endocardial fibrosis Myocardial infarction
	Miscellaneous:	Ichthyosis Testicular fibrosis Developmental delay
Treatment:		Pancreatic enzyme replacement Caloric supplementation Vigorous treatment of infections

Digestive Symptoms. Diarrhea is almost always present, with onset in infancy. The fecal fat content is excessive, as judged either by Sudan staining or by quantitative analysis. Although methods by which pancreatic secretion has been analyzed vary considerably, low to absent activities of lipase, amylase, and trypsin are usual. Other parameters of pancreatic function, including volume and bicarbonate content, are also reported to be slightly low.[128, 130] The serum amylase activity may be low, and pancreatic isoamylase may be absent from the serum of patients with the syndrome. The response of these patients to pancreatic replacement therapy is said to be good, although this has been quantified infrequently.[128, 131] Growth failure, however, does not abate with this therapy although weight gain is noted. In addition, many older patients seem able to discontinue this therapy with little change in clinical status despite pancreatic achylia. Endocrine pancreatic function is only rarely abnormal. The concentrations of sweat electrolytes are normal.

Hematologic Manifestations. Neutropenia (less than 1500 neutrophils/μL) is seen at some time in at least 95 per cent of patients. This is often, although not necessarily, intermittent, with fluctuation occurring over periods as brief as one to two days. Patients are usually able to muster a normal or elevated count in response to infection. Regardless of the underlying mechanism of neutropenia, clinical sequelae are frequent in that severe infections (pneumonia, meningitis, sepsis) occur in up to 85 per cent of patients, and in the past, 15 to 25 per cent have died as a result.[124] The cyclic nature of this neutropenia demands that serial blood counts be performed for diagnostic purposes and that close attention be paid to infectious complications.

Thrombocytopenia (less than 100,000 platelets/μL) is seen in 60 to 70 per cent of patients and is also usually a cyclic phenomenon.[124] Purpura with counts of less than 60,000/μL have been seen, but severe bleeding is unusual. Increased plasma acid phosphatase levels have suggested to some researchers that this thrombocytopenia is the result of inadequate production.

Anemia (hemoglobin less than 10 gm/dl) has been the least common hematologic abnormality in most series, with a maximum frequency of about 50 per cent. The anemia tends to be mild and usually resistant to iron, folic acid, and vitamin B_{12} therapy. Elevated fetal hemoglobin (HbF) levels have been confirmed in 45 per cent of patients, usually with a reciprocal drop in hemoglobin A_2. The presence of HbF at high levels has suggested a predisposition to malignant disease. Indeed, various malignancies have been reported in patients with Shwachman's syndrome, including leukemia.[124]

Bone marrow biopsy in patients with Shwachman's syndrome reveals variable but often decreased cellularity, with normal, increased, or decreased granulocytic elements. A maturation arrest in the granulocyte series may be seen, and occasionally, marrow replacement by fibrosis and fat may be severe. Normal marrow aspirates have been documented in neutropenic patients.[123, 124] Occasionally a reduction in the number of megakaryocytes is noted.

Finally, a decrease in serum immunoglobulins (especially IgA) has been noted in a few patients and their relatives. The relationship of this finding to infectious sequelae is not clear.

Skeletal Abnormalities. Although originally not part of the clinical description, bone lesions have been repeatedly documented[123, 124, 128, 131] in 10 to 15 per cent of patients. Metaphyseal chondrodysplasia of the femur, tibia, and ribs is the most common bone lesion (Fig. 96–8). The pattern in Shwachman's syndrome seems unique, in that involvement is predominantly at the femoral neck and usually is evident there if present at any other location. The lesion is commonly symmetric and may be progressive, occasionally leading to coxa vara deformities and pseudofractures. Diagnosis before the age of one year is unusual.

Serum calcium, phosphorus, and alkaline phosphatase levels usually are normal, and bone lesions do not seem related to malnutrition, particularly because the lesions are not diffuse. Bone age has been reported to be near normal.

Liver Dysfunction. Abnormalities in liver structure and function are not uncommon. In a large series, hepatomegaly was found in about two thirds of patients less than five years of age but far less frequently in older children.[124] Similarly, the serum aminotransferase levels are elevated in 50 to 75 per cent, again most significantly in young children and tending to fall with age. The serum bilirubin value is usually normal, with minimal elevation of alkaline phosphatase levels. Chronic liver disease has been documented; biopsy reveals nonspecific changes of periportal fibrosis, mononuclear infiltrates, fatty change, and, rarely, cirrhosis.[130, 132]

Other Manifestations. Many other conditions have been reported infrequently in association with Shwachman's syndrome. Among these are cardiac lesions, including endocardial fibrosis with development of myocardial infarction[133, 134] and right-sided hypertrophy secondary to chronic lung disease,[124, 135] ichthyosis, testicular fibrosis, pubertal delay, renal tubular malfunction, developmental and intellectual delay, incoordination of osseous maturation, and abnormal results of pulmonary function tests. Small intestinal biopsy has shown mild villous blunting with normal disaccharidase levels.[123]

Diagnosis

The diagnosis should be suspected in any child with exocrine pancreatic insufficiency and is established by careful documentation of normal sweat electrolyte concentrations and serial hematologic studies revealing neutropenia, thrombocytopenia, or anemia. The presence of metaphyseal chondrodysplasia at the hips is a supportive, but not essential, finding. In young children, the disease may present with nonspecific extraintestinal symptoms, but diarrhea soon develops in most.

Prognosis

The mortality rate has been reported to be between 15 and 25 per cent, usually because of severe infection, although hemorrhage from thrombocytopenia plus the development of neoplasia may contribute. Full stature may not be obtained despite vigorous therapy, particularly if hip disease is severe.

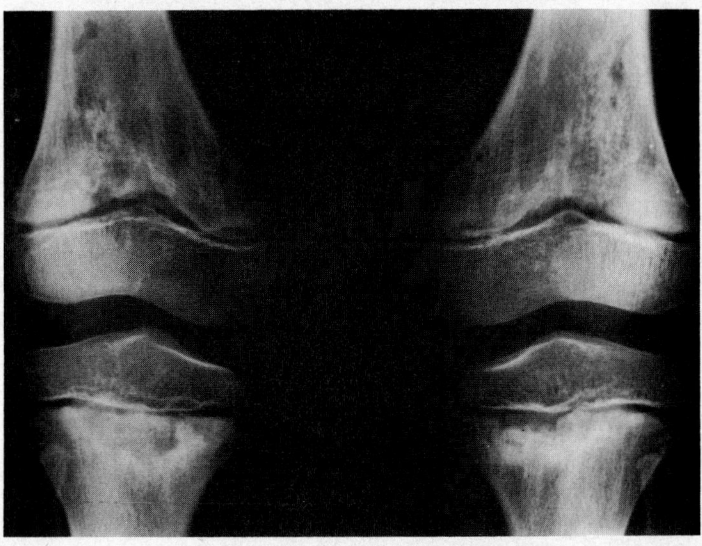

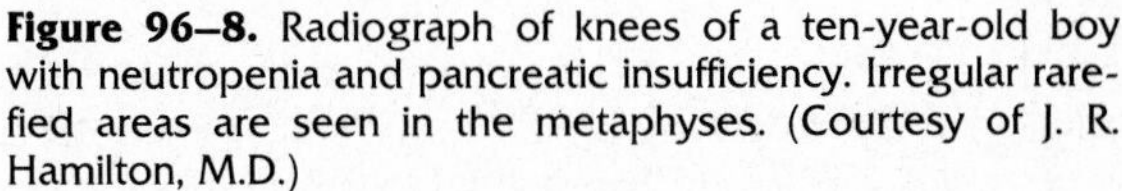

Figure 96–8. Radiograph of knees of a ten-year-old boy with neutropenia and pancreatic insufficiency. Irregular rarefied areas are seen in the metaphyses. (Courtesy of J. R. Hamilton, M.D.)

Treatment

Optimal pancreatic enzyme replacement should be initiated, with an expectation of diminished steatorrhea and improved weight gain but not necessarily enhanced growth. Fat-soluble vitamins, medium-chain triglycerides, and other calorie supplements may be needed, as discussed for cystic fibrosis.

During periods of granulocytopenia, febrile episodes should be evaluated and treated with particular vigor. Episodes of bleeding or severe anemia may require transfusion. Hip disease should be monitored, with intervention if progression occurs.

ISOLATED ENZYME DEFECTS OF THE PANCREAS

Lipase Deficiency

Congenital deficiency of pancreatic lipase is a rare disorder accompanied by variable preservation of other enzymes.[135–138] The cause of the enyzme deficiency is unknown. Persons of both sexes are affected. The more common causes of pancreatic disease have not been found. The earliest and most characteristic manifestation of this disease seems to be the passage of stool with a usual amount of readily separable oil, which is often responsible for soiling. Failure to thrive is noted only occasionally, and systemic manifestations are absent.

The concentration of pancreatic lipase activity within duodenal content is low to absent. Both trypsin and amylase activities have been somewhat diminished in some patients; however, other parameters of exocrine function, including co-lipase, phospholipase A_2, and HCO_3^- concentration and volume, are usually normal. Any residual lipase activity has been suggested to be due to lingual or gastric lipase activity. Bile salt metabolism in this disease has not been investigated extensively.

In addition to its functional absence, no immunologically active lipase could be detected.[138] This suggested either the complete absence of pancreatic lipase or the occurrence of a major structural change affecting both immunogenicity and function.

The biochemical response to exogenous pancreatic enzyme therapy is suboptimal, and limitation in dietary fat usually is necessary to avoid oily stools and incontinence. However, extensive data regarding therapy do not exist.

Co-lipase deficiency has been described in brothers born in a consanguineous marriage.[139] These patients presented with loose stools and steatorrhea; growth and development were normal. Co-lipase activity was markedly reduced, with otherwise normal pancreatic enzyme secretion. Fat absorption improved dramatically with the intraduodenal instillation of purified co-lipase. Co-lipase is probably secreted in the less active form proco-lipase, which requires cleavage of the N terminal pentapeptide by trypsin to form an active co-lipase.[140] Very low levels of trypsin could therefore impair co-lipase activity. In studies of patients with pancreatic insufficiency associated with cystic fibrosis and Shwachman's syndrome, steatorrhea occurred only when lipase and co-lipase secretion were diminished to less than 2 per cent or less than 1 per cent of mean normal values, respectively.[141]

Trypsin Deficiency

Townes reported two unrelated children who presented in infancy with severe growth failure, hypoproteinemia, and edema.[142, 143] Evaluation of unstimulated duodenal fluid revealed absent trypsin and chymotrypsin and carboxypeptidase activity that reverted to normal with the addition of exogenous trypsin. Lipase and amylase levels returned rapidly to normal, and growth failure and edema were corrected with the introduction of predigested protein to the diet, therefore suggesting a nutritional basis. The relationship between this disorder and enterokinase deficiency has not been fully delineated.

Enterokinase Deficiency

Although few reports of congenital absence of enterokinase have appeared since the original description in 1969,[144] a familial nature was suggested by its documentation in siblings.[145] These patients presented with malabsorption, hypoproteinemia, and severe growth retardation. Evaluation included normal amylase and lipase activities and very low trypsin activity in the duodenum, with normal concentrations of sweat electrolytes. Luminal trypsinogen could be activated by the addition of exogenous enterokinase. Small intestinal morphology and disaccharidase levels were normal.

The steatorrhea associated with enterokinase deficiency may be related to a deficiency of phospholipase, the activation of which requires trypsin, which in turn is activated by enterokinase. Patients with cystic fibrosis and Shwachman's syndrome have increased intraluminal and normal mucosal enterokinase activities.[145] However, in untreated celiac sprue, normal mucosal and normal intraluminal enterokinase activities have been reported.[146]

HEREDITARY PANCREATITIS

Hereditary pancreatitis is the second most commonly identified inherited disease of the pancreas. This entity, first reported in 1952,[147] has been found in more than 200 patients.[147–152]

Etiology

The disease has repeatedly been confirmed to be inherited in an autosomal dominant manner. Estimates of penetrance have varied, however, from 40 to 80 per cent, depending on the rigor of the diagnostic criteria applied and the characteristics of the families studied. Despite knowledge of inheritance, the pathophysiology leading to chronic pancreatitis remains obscure. An anatomic defect or the presence of a structurally abnormal, nonenzymatic protein may be the underlying abnormality.[153] In this regard, abnormalities of the pancreatic ducts have been seen frequently, but it is unclear whether they are primary or secondary to chronic pancreatitis.[149–151] Surgical procedures to relieve these abnormalities have achieved varied success; it may be, however, that these anomalies were corrected too late to affect the course of the disease.[152–155]

Pathology

Pathologic observations are usually from surgical or autopsy specimens and thus consistent with long-standing pancreatitis. On gross examination, the pancreas is found to be shrunken and indurated, and calculi are often present within the pancreatic ducts. By light microscopy, extensive interstitial fibrosis, near-total loss of acinar tissue, and relative preservation of normal-appearing islets are seen, not unlike the features in cystic fibrosis.

Clinical Features

Consistent with an autosomal dominant inheritance, males and females are affected with equal frequency and severity. Onset of symptoms occurs under age 20 years in approximately 80 per cent of patients, with a mean of approximately 10 to 12 years[153, 155, 156] and a range of from 11 months to very old age. There is evidence for a second peak age at 17 years, possibly secondary to the introduction of alcohol into the diet. Pain usually heralds the presence of the disease, sometimes precipitated by fasting, ingestion of a fatty meal, alcohol, or stress. Its character is comparable with that of pancreatic pain of any cause, and it is often accompanied by nausea and vomiting. Episodes occur with variable frequency, separated by months to years. It has been stated that episodes usually are not severe and, in fact, often become less severe with age.[155] This is by no means universal, as many patients require extensive abdominal surgery before pain is relieved.[152, 154, 155] Hemorrhagic pancreatitis may supervene.[153] Between episodes, patients are well unless pancreatic insufficiency has developed.

The physical examination and laboratory test results during an exacerbation are typical of acute pancreatitis. Abdominal X-ray may reveal large, rounded calcifications in the pancreas even in early childhood, suggesting hereditary pancreatitis (cystic fibrosis is rarely associated with such marked calcification). Calcification occurs during the course of hereditary pancreatitis in approximately 50 per cent of patients. If pancreatitic insufficiency has developed, findings related to diabetes mellitus or malabsorption may be present.

One of the most significant associations of hereditary pancreatitis has been the development of intra-abdominal carcinoma. Among 54 deceased patients with definite or suspected hereditary pancreatitis in 21 kindreds, there were eight cases of pancreatic carcinoma and five other abdominal tumors (15 per cent and 9 per cent, respectively, of those deceased).[156] Family members without apparent pancreatitis have developed pancreatic adenocarcinomas, and large kindreds have been reported without known carcinomas.[155] Suspicion of the presence of neoplasm should be aroused when changes in the patients' course occur, such as alteration in the usual pain pattern, weight loss, icterus, thrombotic phenomena, or lassitude.

Complications

Early studies documented an aminoaciduria in two families among both affected and nonaffected members.[157] The major amino acids secreted were cystine and lysine, with lesser amounts of arginine, consistent with "incompletely recessive form of cystinuria." The aminoaciduria and pancreatitis were not necessarily linked etiologically or pathogenetically, their association perhaps representing the chance inheritance of unrelated abnormalities. It appears, therefore, that the associated aminoaciduria noted in less than 50 per cent of families represents either the simultaneous occurrence of two diseases or a nonspecific defect in renal tubular function that may accompany acute pancreatitis of any cause.[153, 158]

Diabetes mellitus is said to occur in 10 to 25 per cent of patients with hereditary pancreatitis, although abnormalities in the glucose tolerance test are seen in up to 40 per cent.[155, 156] Steatorrhea and malabsorption have been reported in 5 to 45 per cent of patients.[155, 156] Systematic testing of pancreatic secretion after stimulation has been performed rarely, but limited studies of patients with definite pancreatitis as well as some normal family members reveal compromise of both ductular and acinar function, consistent with chronic pancreatitis.[156]

Pseudocysts complicate hereditary pancreatitis with variable frequency, ranging from 5 to 10 per cent;[155, 159] Portal vein and splenic vein thrombosis are infrequent.[160]

Diagnosis

The diagnosis of hereditary pancreatitis should be suspected if multiple family members develop pancreatitis at an early age in the absence of known etiologic factors, such as alcohol or gallstones. The presence of large, rounded calcifications in the region of the pancreatic duct on abdominal X-ray tends to support the diagnosis, but this and other investigations are of little help other than to rule out known causes of pancreatitis and to detect complications of the disease. The sweat sodium and chloride concentrations, serum calcium and phosphorus levels, alpha$_1$-antitrypsin level and typing, serum triglyceride concentrations, and abdominal ultrasonography findings should be normal during quiescence. The usefulness of invasive studies of the pancreatic ducts is uncertain. Although abnormalities such as intraductal stones, pseudocysts, and dilatations or narrowing may be found, their relationship to the pathogenesis of disease remains uncertain. Therefore, ERCP should be employed early for staging and later for preoperative assessment.[149]

Treatment

Supportive care, such as nasogastric suction; maintenance of proper fluid, electrolyte, and nutrient balance; and anticipation of complications are necessary during acute flare-up. Prevention of exacerbation has been claimed for dietary manipulation, including the avoidance of fatty foods and the administration of pancreatic extracts even if steatorrhea is not present. These are empirical observations only, and the benefit of these measures is unclear. Patients should abstain from alcohol ingestion. Diabetes mellitus and documented exocrine insufficiency should be treated as usual. As stated earlier, the results of surgical intervention are variable. Incapacitating refractory pain or well-defined duct obstruction warrant surgical consideration. Chronic jejunostomy feeding may be helpful.

METABOLIC PANCREATITIS

Hyperlipidemia

Incidence figures for associated pancreatitis in familial hyperlipidemia are approximately 30 per cent for type I, 15 per cent for type IV, and 30 to 40 per cent for type V.[160] The pancreatitis is usually acute and recurrent, although pancreatic insufficiency has been reported with both type I and type V.[161, 162]

The mechanism whereby high serum triglyceride levels lead to pancreatic injury is unknown, although the most popular and well-substantiated theory involves breakdown of excessive triglyceride within the pancreas and release of noxious free fatty acids.[163]

The finding of an elevated triglyceride value in the serum of a patient with pancreatitis should raise suspicion of an underlying error in lipid metabolism. The serum of such a patient should be retested serially under appropriate conditions after resolution of the acute episode.

Hyperparathyroidism

The relationship between hyperparathyroidism and acute and chronic pancreatitis is less clear. In one series, the authors calculated a frequency of 7 per cent among all cases of hyperparathyroidism.[164] Later reports, however, suggested a frequency of approximately 15 per cent of all patients with surgically confirmed hyperparathyroidism[165–167] (see pp. 490–491).

MISCELLANEOUS ANOMALIES

ALPHA$_1$-ANTITRYPSIN DEFICIENCY

An association between alpha$_1$-antitrypsin deficiency and pancreatitis has been reported, but its significance remains unclear.[168]

CONGENITAL ANOMALIES OF THE PANCREAS AND ADJACENT STRUCTURES

Several developmental anomalies of the pancreas or of neighboring structures lead to pancreatic disease (see Table 96–7). Pancreas divisum, annular pancreas, and ectopic pancreas are thought to be attributable to errors in the migration and fusion of the dorsal and ventral pancreatic anlagen. In other, more sporadically reported conditions, maldevelopment of adjacent bowel has been implicated in the induction of pancreatic disease.

Annular Pancreas

Symptomatic annular pancreas has been reported as often in adults as in children.[169, 170] Children usually present in the neonatal period with inability to swallow or with vomiting, whereas abdominal pain is a more frequent symptom in adults. Jaundice and hematemesis are less frequent findings. Plain abdominal X-ray may reveal a "double bubble" sign (Fig. 96–9); contrast studies classically show a smooth, circumferential filling defect in the second portion of the duodenum with proximal dilatation. Stasis and duodenal ulceration may occur. Surgical repair is oriented toward bypass of the obstruction using a gastroenterostomy or duodenojejunostomy rather than resection of the anulus itself, as coexistent atresia is usually encountered. Associated anomalies include trisomy 21, malrotation,

Table 96–7. PANCREATIC DISEASE INDUCED BY ANOMALIES OF THE PANCREAS OR ADJACENT STRUCTURES

A. Pancreas
   1. Annular pancreas
   2. Ectopic pancreas
   3. Pancreas divisum
B. Adjacent Structures
   1. Intraduodenal duplication
   2. Malrotation
   3. Duodenal diverticulum
   4. Choledochal cyst
   5. Anomalous insertion of common bile duct

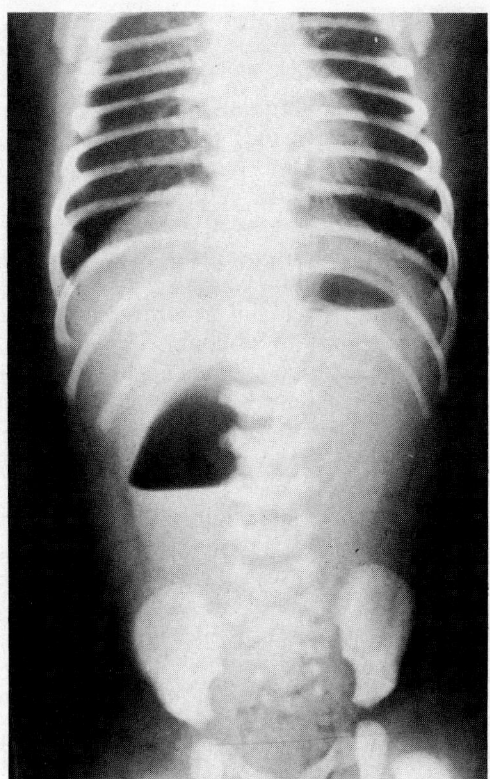

Figure 96–9. Duodenal stenosis in a newborn with annular pancreas. Plain film without contrast material. Note "double bubble" sign and no air in the remaining intestine. (Courtesy of Prof. M. Bettex, Department of Pediatric Surgery, University of Berne.)

cardiac defects, and tracheoesophageal fistula. Separation of this condition into two subtypes depending on the presence of intramural pancreatic tissue has been proposed to explain the predominance of obstructive or ulcerative symptoms.[170]

Ectopic Pancreas

Ectopic pancreatic tissue is usually appreciated as an incidental finding at autopsy (0.5 to 14 per cent) or upper abdominal surgery (0.2 per cent)[171–174] and is found most often in the stomach, duodenum, or jejunum as an isolated anomaly. Radiographically, a smooth, dome-shaped mass less than 4 cm in diameter is seen; a central umbilication is characteristic. In the stomach, the tissue is usually located on the greater curve within 5 cm of the pylorus. At endoscopy, a corresponding submucosal nodule is seen. Whether this lesion can truly be associated with clinical symptoms remains uncertain. The clinical importance lies in preoperative differentiation from other, more clearly significant lesions, particularly neoplasia. True symptoms probably result only when the location and size of the tissue lead to obstruction or when rare complications, such as ulceration, pancreatitis, pseudocyst, or neoplastic degeneration, arise within the ectopic tissue.

Pancreas Divisum

Pancreas divisum, found at autopsy in 4 to 11 per cent of patients and at ERCP in about 5 per cent, is said to be the most common congenital lesion of the pancreas.[175, 176] The condition arises when ventral and dorsal pancreatic buds fail to fuse. The body and tail of the pancreas drain via the accessory duct (Santorini) and papilla; the head drains as usual via the main papilla of Vater and duct of Wirsung. The ERCP findings are shown in Figure 96–10. It has been argued that poor drainage of the bulk of the pancreas predisposes to recurrent pancreatitis, particularly in younger patients. For more detailed discussion of the association of pancreas divisum and pancreatitis, see page 1822.

DEVELOPMENTAL ANOMALIES

Developmental anomalies adjacent to the pancreas have been reported infrequently in association with pancreatic disease. These include duodenal duplication, choledochal cyst, duodenal diverticulum, and anomalous insertion of the common bile duct.[177–182] The pathogenesis of pancreatitis in these disorders has been postulated to include duct obstruction and poor drainage of the gland.

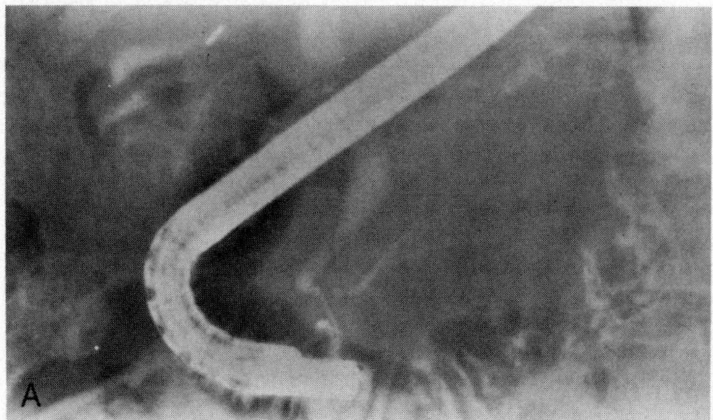

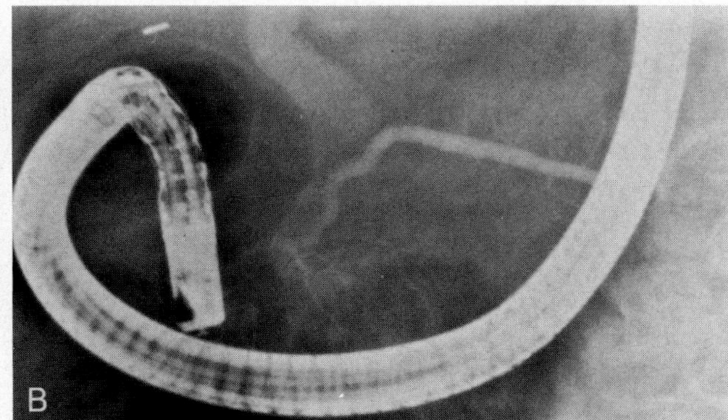

Figure 96–10. Endoscopic retrograde cholangiopancreatogram (ERCP) in a patient with pancreas divisum. *A*, Injection into the ampulla of Vater fills the duct of Wirsung supplying the head of the pancreas but does not opacify the duct to the body or tail of the pancreas. In addition, extrahepatic bile ducts are filled. *B*, Injection into the accessory duct (Santorini) opacifies the duct draining the body and the tail of the pancreas.

ACQUIRED PANCREATITIS

Acquired pancreatic disease (pancreatitis) is not commonly reported in children. In addition, diagnostic criteria and the rigor with which they have been applied vary considerably.[183–186]

ETIOLOGY

The causes of acquired pancreatitis in children are listed in Table 96–8. Trauma, usually blunt and associated with injuries to other abdominal viscera, is responsible for pancreatitis in 13 to 33 per cent of children.[182, 183, 187] Onset of symptoms is usually soon after injury,[188] although injury apparently may precede the presentation of pancreatitis by several weeks. In such an instance, a precise relationship is unclear. Perhaps more importantly, the possibility of injury to the pancreas is often not considered in a severely injured or battered child.[187]

Drugs are said to be one of the most frequent causes of pancreatitis in children, although affected children have usually been treated for significant underlying disease that is perhaps equally likely to cause pancreatitis.[189] As discussed in the literature, few drugs have been clearly incriminated, but among those used with frequency in children are valproic acid and azathioprine.[189–194] Other drugs associated with pancreatitis include prednisone, L-asparaginase, thiazides, and tetracycline.[195–197] The relationship between corticosteroid use and pancreatitis remains controversial.[195] The development of persistent abdominal pain in a child receiving any medication should suggest the possibility of drug-induced pancreatitis. This is confirmed only by documentation of pancreatic disease, improvement on drug withdrawal, and return of disease when the drug is reintroduced.

Table 96–8. REPORTED CAUSES OF ACQUIRED PANCREATITIS IN CHILDREN

A. Trauma
   Child abuse
B. Drug-induced
   1. Azathioprine
   2. Valproic acid
   3. L-Asparaginase
   4. Thiazides
   5. Tetracycline
   6. Sulfonamides
   7. Furosemide
   8. Estrogen
C. Infection
   1. Mumps virus
   2. Enterovirus
   3. Epstein-Barr virus
   4. Hepatitis A virus
   5. Coxsackie B virus
   6. Influenza A virus
   7. Measles virus
   8. Leptospirosis
   9. Mycoplasmosis
   10. Typhoid fever
   11. Ascariasis
   12. Malaria
   13. Rubella
D. Biliary Tract Disease
E. Metabolic
   1. Protein-calorie malnutrition
   2. Hypercalcemia
   3. Reye's syndrome
   4. Hypertriglyceridemia
   5. Cystic fibrosis
F. Miscellaneous
   1. Henoch-Schönlein purpura
   2. Systemic lupus erythematosus
   3. Perforated duodenal ulcer
   4. Kawasaki's disease
   5. Congenital partial lipodystrophy
   6. Juvenile tropical pancreatitis

Infection is a relatively frequent cause of childhood pancreatitis; a partial list of putative agents appears in Table 96–8. Enteroviruses, particularly coxsackievirus and echovirus, have been documented by stool isolation and concomitant serum titer rise in up to 8 per cent of adults with "idiopathic" pancreatitis. As in aseptic meningitis, only about one half of virus isolations are associated with an antibody rise.[198–200] Pancreatitis has been reported in Epstein-Barr virus infection in children, appearing, interestingly, after an initial clinical improvement.[201, 202] Interstitial pancreatitis has been described in the congenital rubella syndrome.[203] Pancreatitis in children is often attributed to mumps virus on the basis of abdominal pain and an elevated serum amylase value, with parotitis or waxing mumps antibody titers, or both.[182, 183, 204] Confirmation via isoamylase determinations and abdominal ultrasonography is lacking, however, and the frequency of this entity may be overestimated. Bacterial pancreatitis has been described,[205] although this patient had other reasons to develop pancreatitis, including antecedent hypotension. *Mycoplasma pneumoniae* infection followed one to two weeks later by clinically apparent pancreatitis has been seen in an estimated 8 per cent of patients with that disease. Complement fixation titers and serum IgM values were elevated, and other causes of pancreatitis were absent.[206] Typhoid fever often presents with abdominal pain; pancreatitis has been suggested as one possible cause.[207] Although it is uncommon in the United States, ascariasis is the most frequent cause of pancreatitis in children in regions such as South Africa and India.[208–210] Worms can be found within the pancreatic duct and are usually vomited as the initial diagnostic clue. Malaria has also been reported to cause pancreatitis.[211]

Biliary tract disease and specifically gallstone pancreatitis is less common in children than in adults[182] and is probably a reflection of the relative infrequency of cholelithiasis in most populations below puberty. However, as almost 10 per cent of children with pancreatitis in some series had cystic duct stones or common bile duct disease, this diagnosis should certainly be considered regardless of age.[182] Little is known of the natural history of this disease in children (see pp. 1640–1655).

Acquired metabolic derangements have been associated with the development of pancreatic disease in children. Perhaps the most common of these is seen in children with protein-calorie malnutrition. In severely malnourished children, pancreatic enzyme secretion is often compromised, while volume and bicarbonate secretion are preserved.[212, 213] Recovery of function is said to follow more promptly after kwashiorkor than after marasmus, but in either case the pancreatic disease may contribute to malabsorption during convalescence. Vigorous early refeeding of malnourished children has been associated with the development of clinically significant pancreatitis.[214, 215] Hypercalcemia during parenteral nutrition leading to pancreatitis was first described in a child; similar reports have followed.[216–218] Other causes of pancreatitis were not apparent in these patients, although it has been suggested that the calcium content of the solutions infused may not have been the only factor involved in the development of hypercalcemia and disease.[217] Histologic changes have been known to occur in the pancreas during Reye's syndrome.[219, 220] Usually this complication has been signaled by hypotension and rapid clinical deterioration during the treatment of advanced illness. Whether the pancreatitis is a cause of or a sequel to the clinical deterioration is not clear.

Several other conditions have been associated infrequently with the development of pancreatitis in children. Both children and adults with Henoch-Schönlein purpura and pancreatitis have been reported,[221, 222] suggesting another cause of abdominal pain in this syndrome. Other systemic diseases, such as systemic lupus erythematosus, have been reported in association with pancreatitis.[183] Pancreatitis in children has also been described with perforated duodenal ulcer and diabetic ketoacidosis.[182] Recently two cases of clinically significant pancreatitis have been documented in association with Kawasaki disease.[223] Patients with partial lipodystrophy have been described with pancreatitis, which was accompanied by eosinophilia and renal disease.[224] Tropical juvenile pancreatitis is characterized by abdominal pain, malabsorption, diabetes mellitus, and pancreatic calcifications and is seen only in countries within 15 degrees of the equator. Although a nutritional cause has been proposed, this has not been confirmed.[225–226]

CLINICAL FEATURES

Children with pancreatitis usually present with pain of less than two months' duration, although longer illnesses occur. Age at onset is commonly greater than ten years, although the disease is reported in infancy.[182–185] The pain is usually supraumbilical, is made worse by eating, and is often accompanied by nausea, and vomiting; occasionally jaundice occurs as well. A transient fever is also often present. Laboratory diagnosis centers on an elevated serum amylase value. Normal values increase with age,[182] explained perhaps by the delayed appearance of pancreatic isoamylase, which usually is not present in infants under three months old and often is not detected until 11 months; even then it is not present at adult levels until the age of 10 years. Salivary isoamylase appears and matures much sooner. The serum amylase concentration, however, may be normal despite other evidence of pancreatitis.[186] An elevated amylase–creatinine clearance ratio may be helpful in those cases in which the diagnosis is unclear, although false positive results occur in states of diabetic ketoacidosis and burns.[227] Other laboratory abnormalities include hypocalcemia in 27 per cent, hyperbilirubinemia in 22 per cent, and hyperglycemia in 15 per cent. A "sentinel loop" is seen on abdominal X-ray in 29 per cent[182] (see pp. 1823–1830).

COMPLICATIONS OF PANCREATITIS

Most often, pancreatitis is not severe in children, although hemorrhagic pancreatitis occurs in up to 13 per cent, with a mortality rate of 86 per cent, versus 18 per cent for those with less severe disease.[182] This complication is usually suggested by severe abdominal pain, peritoneal signs, protracted vomiting, and circulatory compromise.

Pancreatic pseudocysts, as diagnosed by ultrasonography, have been reported in 15 per cent of children with pancreatitis, although the frequency is probably higher.[228] The majority of these are secondary to trauma,[188, 229, 230] and child abuse should be remembered, especially in a preschool child. Symptoms of abdominal cysts include pain in two thirds of patients, emesis in one half, and fever in one fourth; a mass is palpable in two thirds; and an elevated amylase value will be found in almost 90 per cent of cases.[229] An extra-abdominal location is reported in children.[231] Management is dictated by the location, presence or absence of infection, and, perhaps, age of the cyst.

The frequency of pancreatic abscess during childhood is unknown, but the diagnosis should be considered whenever fever and clinical disease are present for a prolonged time. Disseminated fat necrosis occurs infrequently in association with pancreatitis in children. Symptoms include subcutaneous nodules, polyarthritis, fever, eosinophilia, soft tissue swelling, and bone pain.[232] Children may display multiple osteolytic lesions occurring three to six weeks after clinical pancreatitis. These are most easily appreciated in the hands and feet and tend to heal over a period of months. It is important to differentiate these lesions from hematogenous osteomyelitis, disseminated neoplasia, or sickle cell disease.[232] The indications for performing an ERCP to evaluate pancreatic disease in childhood are similar to those in adults. In the setting of recurrent pancreatitis, an ERCP is helpful in planning medical and surgical management.[233]

TREATMENT

The treatment of acute pancreatitis in children and adolescents is similar to that in adults and is discussed on pages 1832 to 1839.

References

1. Steinberg, A., and Brown, D. On the incidence of cystic fibrosis of the pancreas. Am. J. Hum. Genet. *12*:416, 1960.
2. Corey, M. Longitudinal studies in cystic fibrosis. *In* Sturges, J. M. (ed.). Perspectives in Cystic Fibrosis. Toronto, Canadian Cystic Fibrosis Foundation, 1980, p. 246.
3. Taussig, L. (ed.). Cystic Fibrosis. New York, Thieme-Stratton, 1984.
4. Davis, P. Cystic fibrosis in adults. *In* Lloyd-Still, J. (ed.). Textbook of Cystic Fibrosis. Boston, John Wright PSG, 1983, p. 351.
5. Talamo, R. C., Rosenstein, B. J., and Berninger, R. W. Cystic fibrosis. *In* Stanbury, J., Wyngaarden, J., and Fredrickson, D. (eds.). The Metabolic Basis of Inherited Disease. New York, McGraw-Hill, 1982, p. 1889.
6. Lloyd-Still, J. (ed.). Textbook of Cystic Fibrosis. Boston, John Wright PSG, 1983.
7. Wainwright, B., Scambler, P., Schmidtke, J., Watson, E., Law, H. -Y., Farrall, M., Cooke, H., Eiberg, H., and Williamson, R. Localization of cystic fibrosis locus to the human chromosome 7cen-q22. Nature *318*:384, 1985.
8. Shwachman, H., and Mahmoodian, A. Pilocarpine iontophoresis sweat testing: results of seven years' experience. Med. Probl. Pediatr. *10*:158, 1967.
9. Park, R. W., and Grand, R. J. Gastrointestinal manifestations of cystic fibrosis: a review. Gastroenterology *81*:1143, 1981.
10. Boat, T., and Cheng, P. Glycoproteins. *In* Lloyd-Still, J. (ed.). Textbook of Cystic Fibrosis. Boston, John Wright PSG, 1983, p. 53.
11. Davis, P. Cystic fibrosis factors. *In* Lloyd-Still, J. (ed.). Textbook of Cystic Fibrosis. Boston, John Wright PSG, 1983, p. 71.
12. Fick, R., Naegel, G., Squier, S., Wood, R., Gee, J., and Reynolds, H. Proteins of the cystic fibrosis respiratory tract. J. Clin. Invest. *74*:236, 1984.
13. Quinton, P. Chloride impermeability in cystic fibrosis. Nature *301*:421, 1983.
14. Knowles, M., Gatzy, J., and Boucher, R. Increased bioelectric potential difference across respiratory epithelia in cystic fibrosis. N. Engl. J. Med. *305*:1489, 1981.
15. Welsh, M., and Liedtke, C. Chloride and potassium channels in cystic fibrosis airway epithelia. Nature *322*:467, 1986.
16. Welsh, M. An apical membrane chloride channel in human tracheal epithelium. Science *232*:1648, 1986.
17. Frizzell, R., Rechkemmer, G., and Shoemaker, R. Altered regulation of airway epithelial cell chloride channels in cystic fibrosis. Science *233*:558, 1986.
18. McPherson, M., Dormer, R., Goodchild, M., and Dodge, J. Biochemical basis of cystic fibrosis. Nature *323*:400, 1986.
19. Christoffel, K., Lloyd-Still, J., Brown, G., and Shwachman, H. Environmental deprivation and transient elevation of sweat electrolytes. J. Pediatr. *107*:231, 1985.
20. Quinton, P., and Bijman, J. Higher bioelectric potentials due to decreased chloride absorption in sweat glands of patients with cystic fibrosis. N. Engl. J. Med. *308*:1185, 1983.
21. Crossley, J. R., Elliot, R. B., and Smith, P. A. Dried blood spot screening for cystic fibrosis in the newborn. Lancet *1*:472, 1979.
22. Heeley, A. F., Heeley, M. E., King, D. N., Kuzemko, J. A., and Walsh, M. P. Screening for cystic fibrosis by dried blood spot trypsin assay. Arch. Dis. Child. *57*:18, 1982.
23. Wilcken, B., Brown, A. R. D., Urwin, R., and Brown, D. A. Cystic fibrosis screened by dried blood spot trypsin assay. Results in 75,000 newborn infants. J. Pediatr. *102*:1383, 1983.
24. Cassio, A., Bernardi, F., Piazzi, S., Capelli, M., Frejaville, E., Villa, M. P., Martelli, E., Balsamo, A., Salardi, S., Merighi, R., and Cacciari, E. Neonatal screening for CF by dried blood spot trypsin assay. Acta Pediatr. Scand. *73*:554, 1984.
25. Cleghorn, G., Benjamin, L., Corey, M., Forstner, G., Dati, F., and Durie, P. Age-related alterations in immunoreactive pancreatic lipase and cationic trypsinogen in young children with cystic fibrosis. J. Pediatr. *107*:377, 1985.
26. Phelan, P. D. Screening for cystic fibrosis. *In* Meadow, S. R. (ed.). Recent Advances in Pediatrics. Vol. 7. Edinburgh, Churchill Livingstone, 1983, pp. 103–120.
27. Orenstein, D. M., Boat, T. F., Stern, R. C., Tucker, A. S., Charnock, E. L., Matthews, L. W., and Doershuk, C. F. The effect of early diagnosis and treatment in cystic fibrosis. A seven year study of 16 sibling pairs. Am. J. Dis. Child. *131*:973, 1977.
28. Wilcken, B., and Chalmers, G. Reduced morbidity in patients with cystic fibrosis detected by neonatal screening. Lancet *2*:1319, 1985.
29. Ad Hoc Committee Task Force on Neonatal Screening, Cystic Fibrosis Foundation: Neonatal screening for cystic fibrosis. Position paper. Pediatrics *72*:741, 1983.
30. Durie, P., Gaskin, K., Corey, M., Kopelman, H., Weizman, Z., and Forstner, G. Pancreatic function testing in cystic fibrosis. J. Pediatr. Gastroenterol. *3*(Suppl. 1):S89, 1984.
31. Durie, P., Forstner, G., Gaskin, K., Moore, D., Cleghorn, G., Wong, S., and Corey, M. Age related alterations of immunoreactive pancreatic cationic trypsinogen in sera from cystic fibrosis patients with and without pancreatic insufficiency. Pediatr. Res. *20*:209, 1986.
32. Brock, D., Bedgood, D., Barron, L., and Hayward, C. Prospective prenatal diagnosis of cystic fibrosis. Lancet *1*:1175, 1985.
33. Muller, F., Berg, S., Frot, J. F., Bove, J., and Bove, A. Alkaline phosphatase isoenzyme assays for prenatal diagnosis of cystic fibrosis. Lancet *1*:8376, 1984.
34. Muller, F., Berg, S., Frot, J. C., Bove, J., and Bove, A. Prenatal diagnosis of cystic fibrosis. I. Prospective study of 51 pregnancies. Prenat. Diagn. *5*:97, 1985.
35. White, R., Woodward, S., Leppert, M., O'Connell, P., Hoff, M., Herbst, J., Lalouel, J. M., Dean, M., and Woude, G. A closely linked genetic marker for cystic fibrosis. Nature *318*:382, 1985.
36. Eiberg, H., Mohr, J., Schmiegelow, K., Nielsen, L., and Williamson, R. Linkage relationships of paraoxonase (PON) with other markers. Indication of PON-cystic fibrosis synteny. Clin. Genet. *28*:265, 1985.
37. Farrall, M., Law, H. Y., Rodeck, C., Warren, R., Stainer, P., Super, M., Lissens, W., Scambler, P., Watson, E., et al. First-trimester prenatal diagnosis of cystic fibrosis with linked DNA probes. Lancet *1*:1402, 1986.
38. Tsui, L. C., Buchwald, M., Barker, D., et al. Cystic fibrosis locus defined by a genetically linked polymorphic DNA marker. Science *230*:1054, 1985.
39. Oppenheimer, E., and Esterly, J. Pathology of cystic fibrosis, review of the literature and comparison with 146 autopsied cases. Perspect. Pediatr. Pathol. *2*:241, 1975.
40. Roulet, M., Weber, A., and Roy, C. Increased gastric lipolytic activity in cystic fibrosis. *In* Sturgess, J. M. (ed.). Perspectives in Cystic Fibrosis. Toronto, Canadian Cystic Fibrosis Foundation, 1980, p. 172.
41. DiMagno, E., Go, V., and Summerskill, W. Relations between pancreatic enzyme outputs and malabsorption in severe pancreatic insufficiency. N. Engl. J. Med. *288*:813, 1973.
42. Hadorn, B., Johansen, P., and Anderson, C. Pancreozymin secretin test of exocrine pancreatic function in cystic fibrosis and the significance of the results for the pathogenesis of the disease. Can. Med. Assoc. J. *98*:377, 1968.
43. Hadorn, B., Zoppi, G., Shmerling, D., Prader, A., McIntyre, I., and Anderson, C. Quantitative assessment of exocrine pancreatic function in infants and children. J. Pediatr. *73*:39, 1968.
44. Zoppi, G., Shmerling, H., Gaburro, D., and Prader, A. The electrolytes and protein contents and outputs in duodenal juice after pancreozymin and secretin stimulation in normal children and in patients with cystic fibrosis. Acta Paediatr. Scand. *59*:692, 1970.

45. Nousia-Arvanitakis, S., Arvanitakis, C., and Greenberger, N. Diagnosis of exocrine pancreatic insufficiency in cystic fibrosis by the synthetic peptide N-benzoyl-L-tyrosyl-p-aminobenzoic acid. J. Pediatr. *92*:734, 1978.
46. Sacher, M., Kobsa, A., and Shmerling, D. PABA screening test for exocrine pancreatic function in infants and children. Arch. Dis. Child. *53*:639, 1978.
47. Mitchell, C. J., Humphrey, C. S., Bullen, A. W., Kelleher, J., and Losowsky, M. S. Improved diagnostic accuracy of a modified oral pancreatic function test. Scand. J. Gastroenterol. *14*:737, 1979.
48. Hubbard, V., Wolf, R., Lester, L., and Egge, A. Diagnostic and therapeutic application of Bentiromide. Screening test for exocrine pancreatic insufficiency in patients with cystic fibrosis. Comparison with other tests of exocrine pancreatic disease. Dig. Dis. Sci. *29*:881, 1984.
49. Weizman, Z., Forstner, G., Gaskin, K., Kopelman, H., Wong, S., and Durie, P. Bentiromide test for assessing pancreatic dysfunction using analysis of PABA-aminobenzoic acid in plasma and urine. Studies in cystic fibrosis and Shwachman's syndrome. Gastroenterology *89*:596, 1985.
50. Delchier, J. L., and Soule, J. C. BT-PABA test with plasma PABA measurements: evaluation of sensitivity and specificity. Gut *24*:318, 1983.
51. Brodrick, J., Geokas, M. M., and Largman, C. Molecular forms of immunoreactive pancreatic cationic trypsin in a pancreatitis patient sera. Am. J. Physiol. *237*:E474, 1979.
52. Jacobson, D., Curington, C., Connery, K., and Toskes, P. Trypsin-like immunoreactivity as a test for pancreatic insufficiency. N. Engl. J. Med. *310*:1307, 1984.
53. Barbero, G., Sibinga, M., and Marino, J. Stool trypsin and chymotrypsin. Value in the diagnosis of pancreatic insufficiency in cystic fibrosis. Am. J. Dis. Child. *112*:536, 1966.
54. Haverback, B., Dyce, B., and Gutentag, P. Trypsin and chymotrypsin in stool. A diagnostic test for pancreatic exocrine insufficiency. Gastroenterol. *34*:588, 1963.
55. Shwachman, H. Cystic fibrosis. Curr. Probl. Pediatr. *8*:1, 1978.
56. Lippe, B., Kaplan, S., Neufeld, N., Smith, A., and Scott, M. Insulin receptors in cystic fibrosis: increased receptor number and altered affinity. Pediatrics *65*:1018, 1980.
57. Graham, D. Enzyme replacement therapy of exocrine pancreatic insufficiency in man, relation between in vitro enzyme activities and in vivo potency in commercial pancreatic extracts. N. Engl. J. Med. *296*:1314, 1977.
58. DiMagno, E., Malagelada, J., Go, V., and Moertel, C. Fate of orally ingested enzymes in pancreatic insufficiency. N. Engl. J. Med. *296*:1318, 1977.
59. Stapelton, F., Kennedy, J., Nousia-Arvanitakis, S., and Linshaw, M. Hyperuricosuria due to high-dose pancreatic extract therapy in cystic fibrosis. N. Engl. J. Med. *295*:246, 1976.
60. Kattwinkel, J., Agus, S., Taussig, L., di Sant'Agnese, P., and Laster, L. The use of L-arginine and sodium bicarbonate in the treatment of malabsorption due to cystic fibrosis. Pediatrics *50*:134, 1972.
61. Cox, K., Isenberg, J., Osher, A., and Dooley, R. The effect of cimetidine on maldigestion in cystic fibrosis. J. Pediatr. *94*:488, 1979.
62. Hubbard, V., Dunn, G., and Laster, L. Effectiveness of cimetidine as an adjunct to supplemental pancreatic enzymes in patients with cystic fibrosis. Am. J. Clin. Nutr. *33*:2281, 1980.
63. Durie, P., Bell, L., Linton, W., Corey, M. L., and Forstner, G. G. Effect of cimetidine and sodium bicarbonate on pancreatic replacement therapy in cystic fibrosis. Gut *21*:778, 1980.
64. Bergner, A., and Bergner, R. Pulmonary hypersensitivity associated with pancreatin powder exposure. Pediatrics *55*:814, 1975.
65. Twarog, F., Weinstein, S., Khaw, K., Strieder, D., and Colten, H. Hypersensitivity to pancreatic extracts in parents of patients with cystic fibrosis. J. Allergy Clin. Immunol. *59*:35, 1977.
66. Thomaidis, T., and Arey, J. The intestinal lesions in cystic fibrosis of the pancreas. J. Pediatr. *63*:444, 1963.
67. Matseshe, J., Go, V., and DiMagno, E. Meconium ileus equivalent complicating cystic fibrosis in postneonatal children and young adults. Gastroenterology *72*:732, 1977.
68. Freye, H., Kurtz, S., Spock, A., and Capp, M. Light and electron microscopic examination of the small bowel of children with cystic fibrosis. J. Pediatr. *64*:575, 1964.
69. Rubin, C., and Dobbins, W. Peroral biopsy of the small intestine. A review of its diagnostic usefulness. Gastroenterology *49*:676, 1965.
70. Martin, L., Landing, B., and Nakai, H. Rectal biopsy as an aid in the diagnosis of diseases of infants and children. J. Pediatr. *62*:197, 1963.
71. Parkins, R., Ruben, C., Eidelman, S., and Dobbins, W. The diagnosis of cystic fibrosis by rectal suction biopsy. Lancet *2*:851, 1963.
72. Jabro, I., and Gibbs, G. Rectal mucosal biopsies as a diagnostic aid in cystic fibrosis. Lancet *86*:385, 1966.
73. Johansen, P., and Kay, R. Histochemistry of rectal mucus in cystic fibrosis of the pancreas. J. Pathol. *99*:299, 1969.
74. Andersen, D. Pathology of cystic fibrosis. Ann. N.Y. Acad. Sci. *93*:500, 1962.
75. Shwachman, H., and Holsclaw, D. Examination of the appendix at laparotomy as a diagnostic clue in cystic fibrosis. N. Engl. J. Med. *286*:1300, 1972.
76. Jaffe, B., Graham, W., and Goldman, L. Postinfancy intestinal obstruction in children with cystic fibrosis. Arch. Surg. *92*:337, 1966.
77. Taussig, L., Saldino, R., and di Sant'Agnese, P. Radiographic abnormalities of the duodenum and small bowel in cystic fibrosis of the pancreas (mucoviscidosis). Radiology *106*:369, 1973.
78. Grossman, H., Berdon, W., and Baker, D. Gastrointestinal findings in cystic fibrosis. AJR *97*:227, 1966.
79. Wood, R., Herman, C., Johnson, K., and di Sant'Agnese, P. Pneumatosis coli in cystic fibrosis: clinical radiological and pathological features. Am. J. Dis. Child. *129*:246, 1975.
80. Morin, C., Roy, C., Lasalle, R., and Bonin, A. Small bowel mucosal dysfunction in patients with cystic fibrosis. J. Pediatr. *88*:213, 1976.
81. Milla, P., Rassam, U., Kilby, A., Ersser, R., and Harries, J. T. Small intestinal absorption of amino acids and dipeptide in pancreatic insufficiency. *In* Sturgess, J. M. (ed.). Perspectives in Cystic Fibrosis. Toronto, Canadian Cystic Fibrosis Foundation. 1980, p. 177.
82. Antonowicz, I., Reddy, V., Khaw, K., and Shwachman, H. Lactase deficiency in patients with cystic fibrosis. Pediatrics *42*:492, 1968.
83. Lebenthal, E., Antonowicz, I., and Shwachman, H. Correlation of lactase activity, lactose tolerance and mild consumption in different age groups. Am. J. Clin. Nutr. *28*:595, 1975.
84. Antonowicz, I., Lebenthal, E., and Shwachman, H. Disaccharidase activities in small intestinal mucosa in patients with cystic fibrosis. J. Pediatr. *92*:214, 1978.
85. Alpers, D., and Tedesco, F. The possible role of pancreatic proteases in the turnover of intestinal brush border proteins. Biochim. Biophys. Acta *401*:28, 1975.
86. Buts, J. P., Morin, C. L., Roy, C. C., Weber, A., and Bonin, A. One-hour blood xylose test: a reliable index of small bowel function. J. Pediatr. *92*:729, 1978.
87. Noblett, H. Meconium ileus. *In* Ravitch, M., Welch, K., Benson, C., Aberdeen, E., and Randolph, J. (eds.). Pediatric Surgery. Chicago, Year Book Medical Publishers, 1979, p. 943.
88. Holsclaw, D., Eckstein, H., and Nixon, H. Meconium ileus, a 20 year review of 109 cases. Am. J. Dis. Child. *109*:101, 1965.
89. Donnison, A., Shwachman, H., and Gross, R. A review of 164 children with meconium ileus seen at the Children's Hospital Medical Center, Boston. Pediatrics *37*:833, 1966.
90. McPartlin, J., Dickson, J., and Swain, V. Meconium ileus, immediate and long term survival. Arch. Dis. Child. *47*:207, 1972.
91. Oppenheimer, E., and Esterly, J. Cystic fibrosis of the pancreas, morphologic findings in infants with and without pancreatic lesions. Arch. Pathol. *96*:149, 1973.
92. Weiner, E. S. Meconium peritonitis. *In* Welch, K. J., Randolph, J. G., Ravitch, M., O'Neill, J. A., Jr., and Rowe, M. I. (eds.). Pediatric Surgery. Chicago, Year Book Medical Publishers, 1986, p. 929.

93. Holsclaw, D., Rocmans, C., and Shwachman, H. Intussusception in patients with cystic fibrosis. Pediatrics *48*:51, 1971.
94. Mullins, F., Talamo, R., and di Sant'Agnese, P. Late intestinal complications of cystic fibrosis. JAMA *192*:741, 1965.
95. Rubinstein, S., Moss, R., and Lewiston, N. Constipation and meconium ileus equivalent in patients with cystic fibrosis. Pediatrics *78*:473, 1986.
96. Hubbard, V. Gastrointestinal complications in cystic fibrosis. Semin. Resp. Med. *6*:299, 1985.
97. Berk, R., and Lee, F. The late gastrointestinal manifestations of cystic fibrosis of the pancreas. Radiology *106*:377, 1973.
98. Cleghorn, G., Forstner, G., Stringer, D., and Durie, P. Treatment of distal intestinal obstruction syndrome in cystic fibrosis with a balanced intestinal lavage solution. Lancet *1*:8, 1986.
99. Kulczycki, L., and Shwachman, H. Studies in cystic fibrosis of the pancreas: occurrences of rectal prolapse. N. Engl. J. Med. *259*:409, 1958.
100. Oppenheimer, E., and Esterly, J. Hepatic changes in young infants with cystic fibrosis: possible relation to focal biliary cirrhosis. J. Pediatr. *86*:683, 1975.
101. di Sant'Agnese, P., and Blanc, W. A distinctive type of biliary cirrhosis of the liver associated with cystic fibrosis of the pancreas. Pediatrics *18*:387, 1956.
102. Craig, M., Haddad, H., and Shwachman, H. The pathological changes in the liver in cystic fibrosis of the pancreas. Am. J. Dis. Child. *93*:357, 1957.
103. Valman, H., France, N., and Wallis, P. Prolonged neonatal jaundice in cystic fibrosis. Arch. Dis. Child. *46*:805, 1971.
104. Bass, S., Cannon, J., and Ho, C. Biliary tree in cystic fibrosis. Gastroenterology *84*:1592, 1983.
105. Stern, R., Stevens, D., Boat, T., Doershuk, C., Izant, R., and Matthews, L. Symptomatic hepatic disease in cystic fibrosis: incidence, course and outcome of portal systemic shunting. Gastroenterology *70*:645, 1976.
106. Kattwinkel, J., Taussig, L., Statland, B., and Verter, J. The effects of age on alkaline phosphatase and other serologic liver function tests in normal subjects and patients with cystic fibrosis. J. Pediatr. *82*:234, 1973.
107. Feigelson, J., Pecau, Y., Cathelineau, L., and Navarro, J. Additional data on hepatic function tests in cystic fibrosis. Acta Paediatr. Scand. *64*:337, 1975.
108. Weber, A., Roy, C., Chartrand, L., Lepage, G., Dufour, O., Morin, C., and Lasalle, R. Relationship between bile acid malabsorption and pancreatic insufficiency in cystic fibrosis. Gut *17*:295, 1976.
109. Roy, C., Weber, A., Morin, C., Combes, J., Nussle, D., Megevand, A., and Lasalle, R. Abnormal biliary lipid composition in cystic fibrosis, effect of pancreatic enzymes. N. Engl. J. Med. *297*:1301, 1977.
110. Weber, A., Roy, C., Morin, C., and LaSalle, R. Malabsorption of bile acids in children with cystic fibrosis. N. Engl. J. Med. *289*:1001, 1973.
111. Watkins, J., Tercyak, A., Szczepanik, P., and Klein, P. Bile salt kinetics in cystic fibrosis: influence of pancreatic enzyme replacement. Gastroenterology *73*:1023, 1977.
112. Perkins, W., Klein, G., and Beckerman, R. Cystic fibrosis mistaken for idiopathic biliary atresia. Clin. Pediatr. *24*:107, 1985.
113. Schuster, S., Shwachman, H., Toyama, W., Rubino, A., and Khaw, K. The management of portal hypertension in cystic fibrosis. J. Pediatr. Surg. *12*:201, 1977.
114. Cox, K. L., Ward, R. E., Farguide, T. L., Cannon, R. A., Sanders, K. D., and Kurland, G. Orthotopic liver transplantation in patients with cystic fibrosis. Pediatrics *80*:571, 1987.
115. Mischler, E. Treatment of pulmonary disease in cystic fibrosis. Semin. Resp. Med. *6*:271, 1985.
116. Auerbach, H., Kirkpatrick, J., Williams, M., and Colten, H. Alternate day prednisone reduces morbidity and improves pulmonary function in cystic fibrosis. Lancet *2*:686, 1985.
117. Chase, H. P., Long, M., and Lavin, M. Cystic fibrosis and malnutrition. J. Pediatr. *95*:337, 1979.
118. Hubbard, V. Nutritional considerations in cystic fibrosis. Semin. Resp. Med. *6*:308, 1985.
119. Boland, M., MacDonald, N., Stoski, D., Soucy, P., and Patrick, J. Chronic jejunostomy feeding with a non-elemental formula in undernourished patients with cystic fibrosis. Lancet *1*:232, 1986.
120. Shepherd, R. W., Holt, T. L., Thomas, B. J., Kay, L., Isles, A., Francis, P. J., and Ward, L. C. Nutritional rehabilitation in cystic fibrosis: Controlled studies of effects on nutritional growth retardation, body protein turnover and the course of pulmonary disease. J. Pediatr. *109*:788, 1986.
121. Levy, L. D., Durie, P. R., Pencharz, P. B., and Corey, M. L. Effects of long term nutritional rehabilitation on body composition and clinical status in malnourished children and adolescents with cystic fibrosis. J. Pediatr. *107*:225, 1985.
122. Stafford, R. J., and Grand, R. J. Hereditary disease of the exocrine pancreas. Clin. Gastroenterol. *11*:141, 1982.
123. Shwachman, H., Diamond, L. K., Oski, F. A., and Khaw, K. T. The syndrome of pancreatic insufficiency and bone marrow dysfunction. J. Pediatr. *65*:645, 1964.
124. Aggett, P. J., Cavanagh, N. P. C., Matthew, D. J., Pincott, J. R., Sutcliff, J., and Harries, J. T. Shwachman's syndrome. Arch. Dis. Child. *55*:331, 1980.
125. Rothbaum, R., Williams, D., and Daugherty, C. Unusual surface distribution of Concanavalin A reflects a cytoskeletal defect in neutrophils in Shwachman's syndrome. Lancet *2*:800, 1982.
126. Oliver, J., and Berlin, R. Surface and cytoskeletal events regulating leukocyte membrane topography. Semin. Hematol. *20*:282, 1983.
127. Robberecht, E., Nachtegaele, P., VanRattinghe, R., Afschrift, M., and Kunnen, M. Pancreatic lipomatosis in Shwachman-Diamond syndrome. Pediatr. Radiol. *15*:348, 1985.
128. Shmerling, D. H., Prader, A., Hitzig, W. H., Giedion, A., Hadorn, B., and Kuhni, M. The syndrome of exocrine pancreatic insufficiency, neutropenia, metaphyseal dysostosis and dwarfism. Helv. Paediatr. Acta *24*:547, 1969.
129. Hislop, W., Hayes, P., and Boyd, E. Late presentation of Shwachman's syndrome. Acta Paediatr. Scand. *71*:677, 1982.
130. Havlikova, D., Vychytil, O., and Jelinek, J. The syndrome of congenital pancreatic insufficiency, chronic respiratory disease and chronic liver damage. Acta Paediatr. Scand. *56*:676, 1967.
131. Stanley, R., and Sutcliff, J. Metaphyseal chondrodysplasia with dwarfism, pancreatic insufficiency and neutropenia. Pediatr. Radiol. *1*:119, 1973.
132. Liebman, W. M., Rosental, E., Hirschberger, M., and Thaler, M. M. Shwachman-Diamond syndrome and chronic liver disease. Clin. Pediatr. *18*:695, 1979.
133. Perez, N., Calvo, C., Malo, P., Ruiz, A., and Ruza, F. Myocardial infarction in newborn children and infants not secondary to an abnormal coronary. An. Esp. Pediatr. *19*:255, 1983.
134. Savilahti, E., and Rapola, J. Frequent myocardial lesions in Shwachman's syndrome. Acta Paediatr. Scand. *73*:642, 1984.
135. Graham, A. R., Walson, P. D., Paplanus, S. H., and Payne, C. M. Testicular fibrosis and cardiomegaly in Shwachman's syndrome. Arch. Pathol. Lab. Med. *104*:242, 1980.
136. Muller, D. P. R., McCollum, J. P. K., Trompeter, R. S., and Harries, J. T. Studies on the mechanism of fat absorption in congenital isolated lipase deficiency. Gut *16*:838, 1975.
137. Figarella, C., DeCaro, A., Leupold, D., and Poley, J. Congenital pancreatic lipase deficiency. J. Pediatr. *96*:412, 1980.
138. Figarella, C., Negri, G. A., and Sarles, H. Presence of colipase in congenital pancreatic lipase deficiency. Biochim. Biophys. Acta *280*:205, 1972.
139. Hildebrand, H., Borgstrom, B., Bekassy, A., Erlanson-Albertsson, C., and Helin, I. Isolated co-lipase deficiency in two brothers. Gut *23*:243, 1981.
140. Borgstrom, B., Wieloch, T., and Erlanson-Albertsson, C. Evidence for a pancreatic pro-colipase and its activation by trypsin. FEBS Lett. *108*:407, 1979.
141. Gaskin, K., Durie, P., Lee, L., Hill, R., and Forstner, G. Colipase and lipase secretion in childhood-onset pancreatic insufficiency. Gastroenterology *86*:1, 1984.
142. Townes, P. L. Trypsinogen deficiency disease. J. Pediatr. *66*:275, 1965.
143. Townes, P. L., Bryson, M. F., and Miller, G. Further observations on trypsinogen deficiency disease: report of a second case. J. Pediatr. *71*:220, 1967.

144. Hadorn, B., Tarlow, M. J., Lloyd, J. K., and Wolff, O. H. Intestinal enterokinase deficiency. Lancet *1*:812, 1969.
145. Lebenthal, E., Antonowicz, I., and Shwachman, H. Enterokinase and trypsin activities in pancreatic insufficiency and diseases of the small intestine. Gastroenterology *70*:508, 1976.
146. Lebenthal, E., Antonowicz, I., and Shwachman, H. The interrelationship of enterokinase and trypsin activities in intractable diarrhea of infancy, celiac disease, and intravenous alimentation. Pediatrics *56*:585, 1975.
147. Comfort, M. W., and Steinberg, A. G. Pedigree of a family with hereditary chronic relapsing pancreatitis. Gastroenterology *21*:54, 1952.
148. Erbe, R. W. Current concepts in genetics. N. Engl. J. Med. *294*:480, 1976.
149. Perrault, J., Gross, J. B., and King, J. E. Endoscopic retrograde cholangiopancreatography in familial pancreatitis. Gastroenterology *71*:138, 1976.
150. Rohrmann, C., Surawicz, C., Hutchinson, D., Silverstein, F., White, T., and Marchioro, T. The diagnosis of hereditary pancreatitis by pancreatography. Gastrointestinal Endoscopy *27*:168, 1981.
151. Vantini, I., Piubello, W., Ederle, A., Adamo, S., Cavallini, G., and Scuro, L. Hereditary pancreatitis: morphological pictures (ERCP) in the youngest member of a family. Acta Hepatogastroenterol. *26*:253–256, 1979.
152. Appel, M. F. Hereditary pancreatitis. Arch. Surg. *108*:63, 1974.
153. Riccardi, V. M., Shih, V. E., Holmes, L. B., and Nardi, G. L. Hereditary pancreatitis. Arch. Intern. Med. *135*:822, 1975.
154. Sato, T., and Saitoh, Y. Familial chronic pancreatitis associated with pancreatic lithiasis. Am. J. Surg. *127*:511, 1974.
155. Lilja, P., Evander, A., and Ihse, I. Hereditary pancreatitis—a report on two kindreds. Acta Chir. Scand. *144*:35, 1978.
156. Kattwinkel, J., Lapey, A., di Sant'Agnese, P. A., Edwards, W. A., and Hufty, M. P. Hereditary pancreatitis: three new kindreds and a critical review of the literature. Pediatrics *51*:55, 1973.
157. Gross, J. B., Gambill, E. E., and Ulrich, J. A. Hereditary pancreatitis. Am. J. Med. *33*:358, 1961.
158. Lapey, A., Kattwinkel, J., di Sant'Agnese, P., and Laster, L. Steatorrhea and azotorrhea and their relations to growth and nutrition in adolescents and young adults with cystic fibrosis. J. Pediatr. *84*:328, 1974.
159. Fried, A., and Selke, A. Pseudocyst formation in the hereditary pancreatitis. J. Pediatr. *93*:950, 1978.
160. McElroy, R., and Christiansen, P. A. Hereditary pancreatitis in a kinship associated with portal vein thrombosis. Am. J. Med. *52*:228, 1972.
161. Krauss, R. M., and Levy, A. G. Subclinical chronic pancreatitis in Type 1 hyperlipoproteinemia. Am. J. Med. *62*:144, 1977.
162. Salen, S., Kessler, J. I., and Janowitz, H. D. The development of pancreatic secretory insufficiency in a patient with recurrent pancreatitis and type V hyperlipoproteinemia. Mt. Sinai J. Med. *37*:103, 1970.
163. Saharia, P., Margolis, S., Zuidema, G. D., and Cameron, J. L. Acute pancreatitis with hyperlipemia: studies with an isolated canine pancreas. Surgery *82*:60, 1977.
164. Mixer, C. G., Jr., Keynes, W. M., and Cope, O. Further experience with pancreatitis as a diagnostic clue to hyperparathyroidism. N. Engl. J. Med. *266*:265, 1962.
165. Bess, M. A., Edis, A. J., and van Heerden, J. A. Hyperparathyroidism and pancreatitis. JAMA *243*:246, 1980.
166. Romanus, R., Heimann, P., Nilsson, O., and Hansson, G. Surgical treatment of hyperparathyroidism. Prog. Surg. *12*:22, 1973.
167. Werner, S., Hjern, B., and Sjoberg, H. E. Primary hyperparathyroidism: analysis of findings in a series of 129 patients. Acta Chir. Scand. *140*:618, 1974.
168. Mihas, A. A., and Hirschowitz, B. I. Alpha 1-antitrypsin and chronic pancreatitis. Lancet *2*:1032, 1976.
169. Kiernan, P. D., ReMine, S. G., Kiernan, P. C., and ReMine, W. H. Annular pancreas: Mayo Clinic experience from 1957–1976 with review of the literature. Arch. Surg. *115*:46, 1980.
170. Johnston, D. W. B. Annular pancreas: a new classification and clinical observation. Can. J. Surg. *21*:241, 1978.
171. Thoeni, R. F., and Gedgaudas, R. K. Ectopic pancreas: usual and unusual features. Gastrointest. Radiol. *5*:37, 1980.
172. Dolan, R. V., ReMine, W. H., and Dockerty, M. B. The fate of heterotopic pancreatic tissue. Arch. Surg. *109*:762, 1974.
173. Strobel, C. T., Smith, L. E., Fonkalsrud, E. W., and Isenberg, J. N. Ectopic pancreatic tissue in the gastric antrum. J. Pediatr. *92*:586, 1978.
174. Green, P. H. R., Barratt, P. J., Percy, J. P., Cumberland, V. H., and Middleton, W. R. J. Acute pancreatitis occurring in gastric aberrant pancreatic tissue. Dig. Dis. *22*:734, 1977.
175. Cotton, P. B. Congenital anomaly of pancreas divisum as cause of obstructive pain and pancreatitis. Gut *21*:105, 1980.
176. Richter, J. M., Schapiro, R. H., Mulley, A. G., and Warshaw, A. L. Association of pancreas divisum and pancreatitis and its treatment by sphincteroplasty of the accessory ampulla. Gastroenterology *81*:1104, 1981.
177. Williams, W. H., and Hendren, W. H. Intrapancreatic duodenal duplication causing pancreatitis in a child. Surgery *60*:708, 1971.
178. Dine, M. S., and Martin, L. W. Malrotation with gastric volvulus, midgut volvulus, and pancreatitis. Am. J. Dis. Child. *131*:1345, 1977.
179. Agrawall, R. M., and Brodmerkel, G. J. Choledochal cyst presenting as pancreatitis. Am. J. Gastroenterol. *71*:408, 1979.
180. Leinkram, C., Roberts-Thomson, I. C., and Kune, G. A. Juxtapapillary duodenal diverticula: association with gallstones and pancreatitis. Med. J. Aust. *8*:209, 1980.
181. Griffin, M., Carey, W. D., Hermann, R., and Buonocore, E. Recurrent acute pancreatitis and intussusception complicating an intraluminal duodenal diverticulum. Gastroentrology *81*:345, 1981.
182. Jordan, S. C., and Ament, M. E. Pancreatitis in children and adolescents. J. Pediatr. *91*:211, 1977.
183. Buntain, W. L., Wood, J. B., and Woolley, M. M. Pancreatitis in childhood. J. Pediatr. Surg. *13*:143, 1978.
184. Sibert, J. R. Pancreatitis in childhood. Postgrad. Med. J. *55*:171, 1979.
185. Rubin, S. Z., and Ein, S. H. The unusual presentation of pancreatitis in infancy. J. Pediatr. Surg. *14*:146, 1979.
186. Samuels, B. I., Culbert, S. J., Okamura, J., and Sullivan, M. P. Early detection of chemotherapy-related pancreatic enlargement in children using abdominal sonography. Cancer *38*:1515, 1976.
187. Pena, S. D. J., and Medovy, H. Child abuse traumatic pseudocyst of the pancreas. J. Pediatr. *83*:1026, 1973.
188. Pokorny, W. J., Raffensperger, J. G., and Harberg, F. J. Pancreatic pseudocysts in children. Surg. Gynecol. Obstet. *151*:182, 1980.
189. Mallory, A., and Kern, F. Drug-induced pancreatitis: a critical review. Gastroenterology *78*:813, 1980.
190. Parker, P. H., Helinek, G. L., Ghishan, F. K., and Greene, H. L. Recurrent pancreatitis induced by valproic acid. Gastroenterology *80*:826, 1981.
191. Allen, R. J., and Coulter, D. L. Valproic acid induced pancreatitis in children. Pediatrics *65*:1194, 1980.
192. Batalden, P. B., VanDyne, B. J., and Cloyd, J. Pancreatitis associated with valproic acid therapy. Pediatrics *64*:520, 1979.
193. Sturdevant, R. A. L., Singleton, J. W., Deren, J. J., Law, D. H., and McCleary, J. L. Azathioprine-related pancreatitis in patients with Crohn's disease. Gastroenterology *77*:883, 1979.
194. Isenberg, J. N. Pancreatitis, amylase clearance and azathioprine. J. Pediatr. *93*:1043, 1978.
195. Steinberg, W. M., and Lewis, J. H. Steroid-induced pancreatitis: does it really exist? Gastroenterology *81*:799, 1981.
196. Land, V. J., Sutow, W. W., Fernback, D. J., Lane, D. M., and Williams, T. E. Toxicity of L-asparaginase in children with advanced leukemia. Cancer *30*:339, 1972.
197. Elmore, M. F., and Rogge, J. S. Tetracycline-induced pancreatitis. Gastroenterology *81*:1134, 1981.
198. Arnesjo, B., Eden, T., Ihse, I., Nordenfelt, E., and Ursing, B. Enteroviral infections in acute pancreatitis—a possible etiologic connection. Scand. J. Gastroenterol. *11*:645, 649, 1976.
199. Ursing, B. Acute pancreatitis in Coxsackie B infections. Br. Med. J. *3*:524, 1973.
200. Capner, P., Lendrum, R., Jeffries, D. J., and Walker, G. Viral antibody studies in pancreatic disease. Gut *16*:866, 1975.

201. Lifschitz, C., and LaSala, S. Pancreatitis, cholecystitis, and choledocholithiasis associated with infectious mononucleosis. Clin. Pediatr. *20*:131, 1981.
202. Werbitt, W., and Mohsenifar, Z. Mononucleosis pancreatitis. South. Med. J. *71*:1094, 1980.
203. Bunnell, C. E., and Monif, G. R. G. Interstitial pancreatitis in the congenital rubella syndrome. J. Pediatr. *80*:465, 1972.
204. Naficy, K., Nategh, R., and Ghadimi, H. Mumps pancreatitis without parotitis. Br. Med. J. *1*:529, 1973.
205. Bell, M. J., Ternberg, J. L., and Feigin, R. D. Surgical complications of leptospirosis in children. J. Pediatr. Surg. *13*:325, 1978.
206. Mardh, P., and Ursing, B. The occurrence of acute pancreatitis in *Mycoplasma pneumoniae* infection. Scand. J. Infect. Dis. *6*:167, 1974.
207. Russell, I. J., Forgacs, P., and Geraci, J. E. Pancreatitis complicating typhoid fever. JAMA *235*:753, 1976.
208. Gilbert, M. G., and Carbonnell, M. L. Pancreatitis in childhood associated with ascariasis. Pediatrics *33*:589, 1964.
209. Marks, I. N., Bank, S., and Louw, J. H. Chronic pancreatitis in the Western Cape. Digestion *9*:447, 1973.
210. Das, S. Pancreatitis in children associated with round-worms. Indian Pediatr. *14*:81, 1977.
211. Johnson, R. C., DeFord, J. W., and Carlton, P. K. Case report: pancreatitis complicating falciparum malaria. Postgrad. Med. *6*:181, 1977.
212. Danus, O., Urbena, A. M., Valenzuela, I., and Solimano, G. The effect on pancreatic exocrine function in marasmic infants. J. Pediatr. *77*:334, 1970.
213. Barbezat, G. O., and Hansen, J. D. L. The exocrine pancreas and protein-calorie malnutrition. Pediatrics *42*:77, 1968.
214. Gryboski, J., Hillemeier, C., Kocoshis, S., Anyan, W., and Seashore, J. S. Refeeding pancreatitis in malnourished children. J. Pediatr. *97*:441, 1980.
215. Keane, F. B. V., Fennell, J. S., and Tomkin, G. H. Acute pancreatitis, acute gastric dilatation and duodenal ileus following refeeding in anorexia nervosa. Irish J. Med. Sci. *147*:191, 1978.
216. Ulstrom, R. A., and Brown, D. M. Hypercalcemia as a complication of parenteral alimentation. J. Pediatr. *81*:419, 1972.
217. Izsak, E. M., Shike, M., Roulet, M., and Jeejeebhoy, K. N. Pancreatitis in association with hypercalcemia in patients receiving total parenteral nutrition. Gastroenterology *79*:555, 1980.
218. Manson, R. R. Acute pancreatitis secondary to iatrogenic hypercalcemia. Arch. Surg. *108*:213, 1974.
219. Chaves-Carballo, E., Menezes, A. H., Bell, W. E., and Henriquez, E. M. Acute pancreatitis in Reye's syndrome: a fatal complication during intensive supportive care. South. Med. J. *73*:152, 1980.
220. Ellis, G. H., Mirkin, L. D., and Mills, M. C. Pancreatitis and Reye's syndrome. Am. J. Dis. Child. *133*:1014, 1979.
221. Puppala, A. R., Cheng, J. C., and Steinheber, F. U. Pancreatitis—a rare complication of Schönlein-Henoch purpura. Am. J. Gastroenterol. *60*:101, 1978.
222. Garner, J. A. Acute pancreatitis as a complication of anaphylactoid (Henoch-Schoenlein) purpura. Arch. Dis. Child. *52*:971, 1977.
223. Stoler, J., Biller, J., and Grand, R. Pancreatitis in Kawasaki disease. Am. J. Dis. Child. *141*:306, 1987.
224. Smith, P. M., Morgans, M. E., Clark, C. G., Lennard Jones, J. E., Gunnlaugsson, O., and Jonasson, T. A. Lipodystrophy, pancreatitis and eosinophilia. Gut *16*:230, 1975.
225. Nwokolo, C., and Oli, J. Pathogenesis of juvenile tropical pancreatitis syndrome. Lancet *1*:456, 1980.
226. Pitchumoni, C. S. Juvenile tropical pancreatitis. Lancet *2*:1028, 1980.
227. Levitt, M., and Cooperland, S. Increased renal clearance of amylase in pancreatitis. N. Engl. J. Med. *292*:364, 1975.
228. Cox, K. L., Ament, M. E., Sample, W. F., Sarti, D. A., O'Donnell, M., and Byrne, W. J. The ultrasonic and biochemical diagnosis of pancreatitis in children. J. Pediatr. *96*:407, 1980.
229. Cooney, D. R., and Grosfeld, J. L. Operative management of pancreatic pseudocysts in infants and children. A review of 75 cases. Ann. Surg. *182*:590, 1975.
230. Wool, G., and Goldring, D. Pseudocyst of the pancreas. J. Pediatr. *70*:586, 1967.
231. Mallard, R. E., Stilwell, C. A., O'Neill, J. A., and Karzon, D. T. Mediastinal pancreatic pseudocyst in infancy. J. Pediatr. *91*:445, 1977.
232. Shackelford, P. G. Osseous lesions and pancreatitis. J. Dis. Child. *131*:731, 1977.
233. Blustein, P., Gaskin, K., Filler, R., Ho, C. S., and Cannon, J. Endoscopic retrograde cholangiopancreatography in pancreatitis in children and adolescents. Pediatrics *68*:387, 1981.

Acute Pancreatitis

KONRAD H. SOERGEL

DEFINITION

Acute pancreatitis typically presents with abdominal pain and is usually associated with elevation of pancreatic enzymes in the blood. There are two definitive diagnostic criteria: (1) elevation of plasma levels of two pancreatic enzymes greater than five times the upper limit of normal (greater than 10 SD above the laboratory mean), and (2) evidence of acute pancreatitis from ultrasonographic, computed tomographic, surgical, or autopsy findings. The disease may be manifested as an initial or recurrent attack and its course may be mild, severe, or complicated. The complete description of an attack of acute pancreatitis includes degree of severity (mild, severe), occurrence of local (e.g., abscess, pseudocyst) and systemic complications, initial or recurrent episode, and the underlying cause, if known. After the attack, exo- and endocrine pancreatic function may remain impaired for variable periods of time. Morphologically, the pancreas usually recovers completely, although pseudocysts and limited scarring may persist. Histologic criteria, so useful in the categorization of many other diseases, play little role in the clinical decision process because pancreatic tissue rarely becomes available for histologic study during the evolution of pancreatitis.

Acute pancreatitis very rarely progresses to chronic pancreatitis, which is characterized by continuing inflammation leading to irreversible structural changes and by permanent impairment of exocrine and endocrine pancreatic function. In the individual acutely ill patient, the clinical distinction between acute and chronic pancreatitis cannot always be made. Particularly during the early stages of chronic alcoholic pancreatitis, exacerbations closely resemble attacks of acute pancreatitis and should be treated as such.

The definitions given here are based on two recent attempts at the classification of pancreatitis,[1, 2] which effectively replace the earlier "Marseilles" classification of 1963.[3] The earlier terms "relapsing acute pancreatitis" and "chronic relapsing pancreatitis" have been discarded.

PATHOLOGY

The retroperitoneal location of the pancreas is the key to understanding the involvement of adjacent organs in the course of acute pancreatitis. The absence of a well-developed pancreatic capsule allows the inflammatory process to spread freely and to affect any of the following organs: duodenum, terminal common bile duct, splenic artery and vein, spleen, mesocolon, greater omentum, small bowel mesentery, the celiac and superior mesenteric ganglia, the lesser omental sac, posterior mediastinum, the pararenal spaces, and the diaphragm.

The morphologic appearance of acute pancreatitis represents a spectrum of severity but gives no clue to its cause. Early stages are characterized by confluent peripancreatic fat necrosis extending along interstitial septa into the gland and containing small numbers of polymorphonuclear leukocytes. The still-intact parenchyma shows interstitial edema. Only the acinar cells abutting on the fat necrosis are involved; they appear flattened with loss of luminal microvilli, depletion and fusion of zymogen granules, and cisternal dilatation of the endoplasmic reticulum and Golgi complex. Autophagic vacuoles appear, which contain various cell elements, including zymogen granules.[4] These changes are consistent with initial release of active enzymes across the basolateral wall of peripherally located acinar cells, and they are similar to the evolutionary changes of cerulein-induced pancreatitis in the rat.[5] This stage is called *acute edematous pancreatitis.* The disease may progress to coagulation necrosis of glandular elements and the surrounding fatty tissue, termed *necrotizing pancreatitis.* The factors determining this progression are unknown, but disruption or thrombotic occlusion of blood vessels, possibly mediated by pancreatic elastase, may be important. Necrosis usually does not affect the gland uniformly: Red, friable areas of frank necrosis with grayish zones of ischemic necrosis, and white areas indicating fat necrosis with deposition of calcium soaps alternate with regions of preserved architecture to give the pancreas a mottled appearance. The connective tissue elements remain reasonably well preserved. Such a mass of inflamed pancreas containing patchy areas of necrosis is designated a phlegmon.

Frank hemorrhage from rupture of blood vessels within or around the gland[6] may lead to collections of blood within the pancreas or the surrounding retroperitoneal spaces. This stage is described as *hemorrhagic pancreatitis.* Extravasated blood dissecting along tissue planes may result in a bluish discoloration surrounded by diffuse induration in the costovertebral angle (Turner's sign) or the periumbilical area (Cullen's sign).

Tissue debris, pancreatic juice, blood, and fat droplets from disrupted adipose cells may accumulate within confluent areas of necrosis, forming so-called pseudocysts. These arise within or adjacent to the pancreas and may extend into the transverse mesocolon, into the hilus of the spleen, or along the lateral retroperitoneal space. Similarly, accumulations of activated pancreatic enzymes and polymorphonuclear leukocytes may inflame the peritoneal surfaces, leading to fluid accumulation in the lesser omental sac. This process may extend to the peritoneal cavity (pancreatic ascites) or through the diaphragmatic lymphatics to cause a sterile pleural effusion and pneumonitis.[7] Pseudocysts may resolve spontaneously as the pancreatic inflammation subsides. They will persist if a pancreatic duct has ruptured during the course of pancreatitis, leading to continued secretion of pancreatic juice into a closed space.[8] Pancreatic and peripancreatic abscesses result from secondary infection of necrotic tissue and fluid collections by enteric bacteria. The route of this bacterial spread is unknown. Areas of fat necrosis are common in the retroperitoneal area. Grossly, they appear opaque and yellowish, acquiring a white stippled appearance with the precipitation of calcium salts of free fatty acids liberated by the action of pancreatic lipase. Eventually, inflammatory cells and macrophages surround the area of necrotic adipose cells; small cysts may develop and a foreign body type of giant cells may appear.

Distant lesions occasionally arise during the course of acute and chronic pancreatitis: subcutaneous or intramedullary osseous fat necrosis; aseptic epiphyseal necrosis;[9] or polyserositis involving articular synovium, pleura, or pericardium. Arthritis, thought to be caused by fat necrosis adjacent to the synovium, is accompanied by clear to cloudy synovial fluid with a high white cell count.[10] Pathogenetically, tissue injury by circulating pancreatic lipase is implicated by experimental evidence.[11] Distant fat necrosis is recognized clinically in less than 1 per cent of cases, whereas autopsy studies reveal a frequency of 10 per cent.[12]

PATHOGENESIS

Acute pancreatitis is a process of autodigestion caused by the premature activation of zymogens to active proteolytic enzymes within the pancreas. In accord with the generally accepted classifications,[1, 2] chronic pancreatitis is best considered a different disease rather than a late stage of the acute variety (see pp. 1842–1872). The events that trigger the sequence of enzymatic reactions that initiate acute pancreatitis remain unknown. There is good reason to believe that more than one etiologic mechanism is responsible. However, the search for the cause of acute pancreatitis has been frustrated by the fact that none of the various experimental animal models that have been devised mimics the situations in which the human disease occurs. In the clinical setting, acute pancreatitis clearly is associated with several other conditions, but the sequence that would explain a cause-and-effect relationship has, so far, eluded medical investigators. With these reservations in mind, current pathogenetic hypotheses will be discussed first, followed by a description of the pathophysiologic events of pancreatic autodigestion.

Pathogenetic Hypotheses

Obstruction-Secretion

A popular opinion holds that acute pancreatitis results from obstruction to the outflow of pancreatic juice. Indeed, an 18-year-old boy developed severe pancreatitis after a fast and a subsequent large meal.[13] He was later cured of recurrences by division of a fibrotic sphincter of Oddi. Similarly, about 40 per cent of patients with acute pancreatitis at a hospital in mainland China presented with a history of dietary surfeit following a brief period of food deprivation.[13a] Permanent decompression of a choledochocele has prevented further pancreatitis attacks in several patients, presumably by removing intermittent pancreatic outflow obstruction.[14] However, there is evidence against obstruction as the major cause of acute pancreatitis. For example, duct dilatation is not a feature of this disease. Ligation of the pancreatic duct or its occlusion by tumor[15] generally does not cause acute pancreatitis. Furthermore, although an association between acute pancreatitis and duodenal periampullary diverticula appears established,[16] it is not clear how such diverticula might interfere with pancreatic juice flow. Finally, the experience with indiscriminate surgical sphincterotomy and sphincteroplasty in patients with relapsing acute pancreatitis has been disappointing when no attempt was made to preselect those few who have demonstrable sphincter of Oddi dysfunction.

Reflux of Duodenal Contents

Reflux of duodenal contents was proposed because retrograde injection of activated pancreatic enzymes mixed with bile into the pancreatic duct system produces pancreatitis in experimental animals. More recently it has been shown that prograde perfusion under physiologic pressure from the pancreatic tail produces pancreatitis as well, provided that the perfusate contains active pancreatic enzymes and that pancreatic duct permeability has been increased by the addition of bile salts or by preadministration of various drugs, including ethanol.[17] The hypothesis is supported by the occurrence of acute pancreatitis in dogs after creation of a closed duodenal loop and by the occasional association of duodenal obstruction and pancreatitis in patients.[18] Arguments against this hypothesis are the pressure gradient of about 12 mm Hg between pancreatic duct and duodenum,[19] the finding of normal sphincter of Oddi and pancreatic duct resting pressures in the majority of patients with acute recurrent pancreatitis, and the absence of ill effects after sphincteroplasty, which allows intermittent free reflux into the duct of Wirsung. Thus, duodenal regurgitation may be a factor in some patients with pancreatitis, but no evidence exists to support this assumption in the majority of cases.

Bile Reflux

The bile reflux, or common channel, hypothesis is limited mainly to pancreatitis associated with cholelithiasis. It was formulated by Opie at the beginning of this century[20] when he described a gallstone impacted in the ampulla of Vater of a patient with fatal pancreatitis and reasoned that this enabled bile to reflux into the pancreatitic duct. Although stone impaction in the ampulla is found in fewer than 5 per cent of patients who die of pancreatitis, transitory impaction may occur in 92 per cent of patients with acute pancreatitis who are jaundiced as a result of choledocholithiasis.[21] This postulated mechanism can cause bile reflux only if two conditions are met: (1) that the simultaneous obstruction of both ducts leads to a reversal of the normal pressure gradient from pancreatic to common bile duct, and (2) that a common channel exists that is long enough to permit confluence of bile and pancreatic juice proximal to a common bile duct stone impacted in the ampulla of Vater. Such a channel, however, is present in only 18 per cent of the population.[22] Finally, pure bile flowing through the pancreatic duct at near physiologic pressures does not cause pancreatitis in experimental animals.[23] In summary, there is a strong association between the passage of gallstones from common bile duct into the duodenum and some cases of acute pancreatitis; transient pancreatic duct obstruction, rather than bile reflux, is likely to be the precipitating factor in these patients.

Intracellular Protease Activation

Two models of experimental pancreatitis receive much current interest: (1) feeding a choline-deficient, ethionine-supplemented (CDE) diet, which causes severe pancreatitis in female mice, and (2) injection of supramaximal doses of cerulein, an analogue of cholecystokinin, which causes mild pancreatitis in rats and the necrotizing form in mice. To understand the pathogenesis of these two types of experimental pancreatitis, it should be recalled that lysosomal and digestive enzymes are synthesized together in the rough-surfaced endoplasmic reticulum and are then transported intracellularly in condensing vacuoles. These enzymes are then segregated into lysosomes and zymogen granules, respectively. In CDE-induced pancreatitis, these two intracellular structures fuse by a process termed crinophagy. In the cerulein-induced disease the condensing vacuoles never segregate. Eventually, these zymogen-containing vacuoles are extruded across the basolateral cell wall of the acinar cell, leading to delivery of digestive and lysosomal enzymes to the interstitial and peripancreatic fatty tissue.[5, 23a] Thus, both disease models have in common the intracellular admixture of digestive proenzymes and lysosomal hydrolases, including cathepsin B. Cathepsin B can activate trypsinogen, and trypsin will then activate the other protease precursors. Furthermore, the intrinsic pancreatic trypsin inhibitor protein is inactive at the acidic pH known to exist in lysosomes.[24]

The observation that two different methods of producing experimental pancreatitis exhibit the same intracellular mechanism for protease activation as well as the clinical morphologic observations already mentioned[4] suggests that clinical acute pancreatitis is initiated by similar mechanisms of intracellular trypsin activation.

Miscellaneous Hypotheses

The effect of ethanol on the pancreas is discussed on pages 1844 to 1845 because ethanol-associated pancreatitis is considered chronic.[1, 2] Embolic occlusion of small pancreatic blood vessels produces pancreatitis in experimental animals. Clinical pancreatitis associated with visceral vasculitis tends to be segmental in nature but is exceedingly rare. Viral infection may play a role in juvenile-onset diabetes mellitus but very rarely in acute pancreatitis. The association with hypertriglyceridemia is discussed later.

Pathogenetic Role of Pancreatic Enzymes: Autodigestion Hypothesis

Regardless of the manner by which pancreatic enzymes are activated, this activation is the central step in the pathogenesis of acute pancreatitis. Experimentally, activated trypsin and chymotrypsin by themselves do not cause the coagulation necrosis and mild inflammatory response of the pancreas that are characteristic of early human pancreatitis. Trypsinogen undergoes slow spontaneous autoactivation at slightly alkaline pH. The trypsin so formed is then rapidly inactivated by a specific trypsin inhibitor present in pancreatic tissue and secretions.[25] The immeasurably small amounts of trypsin needed for activation of other proenzymes may exist under certain conditions, enough to trigger the cascade of autodigestion known as acute pancreatitis. Purified phospholipase A_2 causes severe pancreatic parenchymal and adipose tissue necrosis in the presence of low concentrations of bile acids. This effect is mediated by the cytotoxic properties of lysolecithin and lysocephalin, substances that are produced by partial hydrolysis of cell membrane phospholipids. Fatty acids, including arachidonic acid, are the other products of phospholipid hydrolysis. Liberated arachidonic acid is converted by the cyclo-oxygenase and lipoxygenase pathways into various bioactive substances, including prostaglandin (prostacyclin) I_2 and thromboxanes, which are vasoactive and affect blood coagulation. Elastase, also activated by trypsin, mainly dissolves the elastic fibers of blood vessels, and its action is strongly implicated in human necrotizing pancreatitis associated with hemorrhage.[26] Furthermore, trypsin activates the classical and alternative complement pathways with local production of cytotoxic substances. Lastly, blood coagulation is altered by the activation of thrombolytic (e.g., plasmin) and thrombotic (e.g., thrombin) factors.[27]

In summary, once trypsin activation has been triggered, the balance between activated proteases and protease inhibitors determines the subsequent course of acute pancreatitis. The major protease inhibitors are the locally produced pancreatic trypsin inhibitor and circulating alpha-macroglobulin, alpha$_1$-antitrypsin and the C_1-esterase inhibitor.[28] Much of the histologic appearance of acute human pancreatitis is explained by the effects of phospholipase A_2 and elastase. Any reflux of bile into the pancreatic duct would intensify this deleterious sequence by enhancing the cytotoxic effects of phospholipase A_2, by activating lipase, and by the detergent effect of bile acids on cell membranes. This working hypothesis is illustrated in Figure 97–1, but it provides no answer to the central question: What event allows trypsin activity to become high enough for activation of several locally and systemically deleterious biochemical cascades?

PATHOPHYSIOLOGY

Several substances are released from the acutely injured pancreas that are responsible for the signs and symptoms of pancreatitis. The following discussions center on these substances and on the changes in homeostasis that characterize acute pancreatitis.

Kallikrein-Kinins and Shock

Some of the local and systemic features of acute pancreatitis can be attributed to the actions of two low-molecular-weight vasoactive peptides, bradykinin and kallidin. These kinins are cleaved from kininogens, alpha$_2$-globulins present in plasma and lymph, by kallikrein. The latter enzyme is present as inactive kalli-

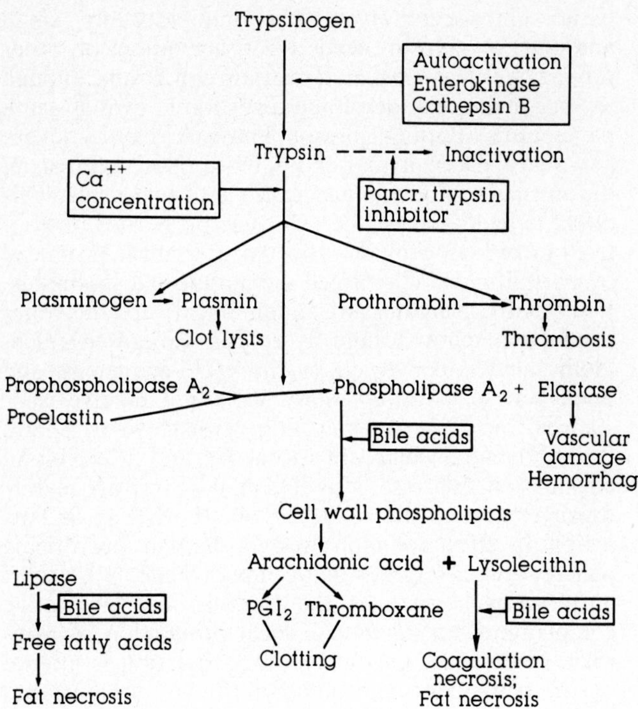

Figure 97–1. Working hypothesis for pathophysiology of pancreatic autodigestion.

kreininogen in pancreas, salivary glands, and plasma, and it is activated to kallikrein by plasmin, by kallikrein itself, and by trypsin. The generation of kinins is, in turn, inhibited by circulating alpha$_1$-antitrypsin, alpha$_2$-macroglobulin, and, experimentally, by aprotinin, a protein found in bovine lung and parotid gland. The kinins, once liberated, are rapidly inactivated by a variety of local pancreatic and systemic factors[27] (Fig. 97–2). They have a broad spectrum of biologic activity, which includes vasodilation and increase in vascular permeability (both promoting shock), pain, and leukocyte accumulation. Although elevated concentrations of these vasoactive peptides have been demonstrated in pancreatic and in systemic venous blood in patients with acute pancreatitis, their precise pathophysiologic role is difficult to define for lack of reproducible assay methods.

Serum Calcium: Hypocalcemia

Transient hypocalcemia develops in about one third of patients during acute pancreatitis, although the appearance of clinical or subclinical tetany is extremely rare.[29] The frequency and degree of hypocalcemia parallel the clinical severity of the disease. In many cases the fall in serum calcium concentration is merely a reflection of decreased binding to serum proteins because of rapidly developing hypoalbuminemia. In patients with severe pancreatitis, however, the hypocalcemia may be accompanied by a decrease in ionized serum calcium.[30, 31] Although calcium sequestration in areas of fat necrosis explains the initial fall in serum calcium concentration,[32] the adequacy of normal homeostatic mechanisms that restore serum calcium to normal is a matter of debate. Thus, one report states that the serum immunoreactive parathyroid hormone (iPTH) concentration fails to rise in response to the hypocalcemia, signifying a relative iPTH deficiency,[31] whereas appropriate rises in iPTH were found in patients studied by other groups.[29, 30] End-organ resistance to the calcium-mobilizing effect of PTH on bone is unlikely.[31] Another potential cause of hypocalcemia is the calcium-lowering effect of pancreatic glucagon,

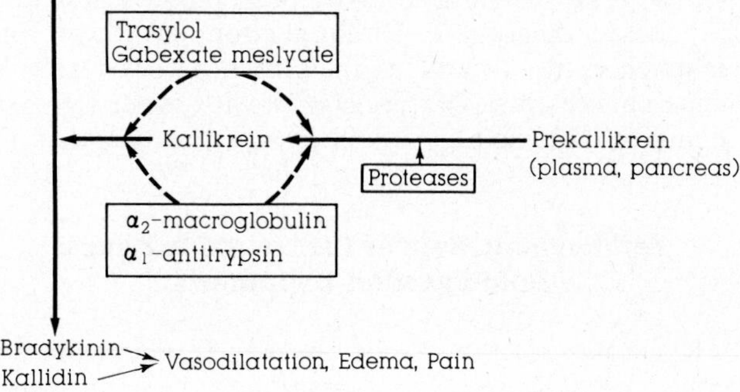

Figure 97–2. Activation and role of vasoactive polypeptides in acute pancreatitis. Kallikrein activation and the generation of bradykinin and kallidin are proteolytic reactions. Both reactions are accelerated when the binding sites of protease inhibitors are occupied by the excess trypsin and other activated proteases liberated during acute pancreatitis. These reactions can be inhibited by exogenous protease inhibitors, such as trasylol and gabexate mesylate. Neither compound has yet been shown to be effective in the treatment of acute pancreatitis, however. Interrupted lines indicate inhibiting effects.

which is probably mediated by glucagon-induced release of thyrocalcitonin. However, the glucagon levels required for this action are higher than the degree of hyperglucagonemia found during pancreatitis; furthermore, serum thyrocalcitonin levels are not measurably elevated in patients with severe pancreatitis.[30]

Insulin and Glucagon: Hyperglycemia

Damage to the islets of Langerhans during acute pancreatitis is reflected by mild, transient hyperglycemia in 15 to 25 per cent of patients. This is associated with an excess of glucagon and inappropriately low plasma insulin levels. The lipolytic effects of inadequate circulating insulin and elevated cortisol and glucagon levels combine to produce a rise in plasma nonesterified free fatty acid concentration.[33] Hypoglucagonemia and increasingly severe insulin deficiency appear as irreversible pancreatic damage develops during the course of chronic pancreatitis.[34]

Impaired Pulmonary Function

A majority of patients with moderately severe or severe pancreatitis develop arterial hypoxia. The arterial PO_2 falls to 50 to 70 mm Hg between the first and sixth days without parenchymal changes on chest radiographs. The major abnormality responsible for the hypoxia is intrapulmonary right-to-left shunting, possibly caused by pulmonary intravascular microthrombi formed as a result of subclinical disseminated intravascular coagulation.[35]

Diffuse pulmonary infiltrates and severe progressive hypoxemia with tachypnea appear in 5 to 10 per cent of patients three or more days after the onset of acute pancreatitis. The frequency of this type of adult respiratory distress syndrome (ARDS) rises with the increasing clinical severity of the attack and with coexisting hyperlipidemia. The pulmonary edema is due to a reversible disruption of the alveolar-capillary membrane with loss of the normal size selectivity for diffusion of plasma proteins.[36] Hyaline membranes and fibrinogen deposits lining the alveolar surface frequently are present. The pulmonary capillary hydrostatic forces, however, remain unaltered, as determined by hemodynamic studies. The protein content of the edema fluid approaches that of serum. The initiating factors may be circulating phospholipase A[37] and high concentrations of free fatty acids, as both have been shown to damage the pulmonary surfactant layer and to produce pulmonary edema in experimental animals.

Altered Renal Function

Renal impairment, ranging from mild dysfunction to anuria, is a recognized complication of acute pancreatitis. It is the consequence of hypovolemia with a rising hematocrit and declining plasma protein levels, reflecing the generalized increase in capillary permeability.[37a] Associated factors are a selective increase in renal vascular resistance with reduction in renal blood flow and oxygen uptake[38] and decreased renal tubular reabsorption of low-molecular-weight serum proteins.[39] Therapy with vasodilator drugs provides no benefit.[38]

Miscellaneous Problems: Circulatory Shock and DIC

Patients with increasingly severe acute pancreatitis develop a hyperdynamic circulatory state characterized by decreased peripheral vascular resistance and an increase in the shunt fraction of the pulmonary circulation—both contributing to a rise of the cardiac index and a decrease in the arteriovenous oxygen gradient.[40] Eventually, circulatory shock may supervene, which is not accounted for by the reduction of intravascular volume. Myocardial contractility is preserved, in contrast to some forms of experimental pancreatitis, in which the appearance of a myocardial depressant factor (MDF) was demonstrated. Disseminated intravascular coagulation (DIC), with development of microthrombi and consumption of clotting factors as well as complement components, is another complication occasionally documented in life-threatening pancreatitis. This chain of events may be initiated by release of active pancreatic proteases into the circulation.[41] Mild forms of DIC, detectable only by serial laboratory studies, may contribute to the early hypoxia and the renal functional impairment just described.

CONDITIONS ASSOCIATED WITH ACUTE PANCREATITIS

Some conditions that are definitely associated with acute pancreatitis are listed in Table 97–1. Their prompt identification in individual patients is important for two reasons: In some instances the condition can be dealt with immediately, which may favorably influence the course of the current attack; in others the elimination of the underlying cause will prevent further attacks of this life-threatening disease.

Table 97–1. CONDITIONS ASSOCIATED WITH ACUTE PANCREATITIS

Cholelithiasis Ethanol abuse Idiopathic	90% of all cases
Abdominal operations	
Hyperlipemia	
Injection into pancreatic duct	
Trauma	
Hypercalcemia	
Pregnancy	
Peptic ulcer	
Outflow obstruction	
Pancreas divisum	
Organ transplantation	
End-stage renal failure	
Hereditary (Familial pancreatitis)	
Scorpion bite	
Miscellaneous:	hypoperfusion, viral infections, *Mycoplasma pneumoniae* infection, intraductal parasites

Gallstones

Gallstones are present in about 50 per cent of patients with acute pancreatitis admitted to private hospitals and in 30 per cent of patients admitted to public hospitals. The difference is attributable to the higher prevalence of another associated condition, alcoholism, among patients in city, county, and Veterans Administration hospitals.[42] The frequency of gallstone-associated pancreatitis parallels that of cholelithiasis: The peak occurrence is at 50 to 70 years of age; women outnumber men by 2:1. With a gallstone prevalence of 20 to 35 per cent in the general population aged 50 to 70 years,[43] the possibility of a chance association between these two diseases has to be considered. However, the following observations argue strongly for a causal relationship. First, the risk of attacks of recurrent pancreatitis is about 50 per cent unless all gallstones are removed.[42] Secondly, if the stools of patients with pancreatitis and gallstones are strained for ten days after the onset of an attack of pancreatitis, gallstones are detected in 92 per cent, compared with 12 per cent of patients with gallstones but no pancreatitis, and with 0 per cent in attacks of alcoholic pancreatitis in patients with or without coexisting gallstones.[21] This observation clearly links the passage of small gallstones into the duodenum with acute pancreatitis. Thirdly, the relative risk of developing acute pancreatitis is 25 to 30 times higher in patients carrying gallstones compared with the expected rate in the general population. Cholecystectomy, performed before or after pancreatitis has occurred, eliminates the excess risk of developing first or recurrent attacks of acute pancreatitis.[44] The association between gallstones and pancreatitis has been firmly established in populations in which cholesterol gallstones predominate. Whether bile pigment stones, prevalent in cirrhosis, in hemolytic anemia, and in Far Eastern populations, present a similar risk has been less well documented (see pp. 1682–1684).

The mortality of gallstone-associated pancreatitis is about 12 per cent during the first attack and tends to be lower during subsequent attacks.[45] Chronic pancreatitis with pancreatic insufficiency develops rarely, if ever, even after multiple episodes of pancreatitis associated with gallstones.[42]

Alcohol Abuse

An association between excessive alcohol consumption and pancreatitis is well documented. Up to 66 per cent of first episodes of pancreatitis belong in this category. The mortality rate is less than that of the gallstone-associated or the idiopathic variety,[45] partly because of the younger age of these patients, most of whom are 30 to 45 years old. Men outnumber women by about 3:1. Although most alcoholic patients with pancreatitis acquire irreversible functional and structural damage of the organ and, therefore, chronic pancreatitis,[1, 2] they may also develop all the complications of acute pancreatitis during the initial attacks of this disease. When alcoholism and gallstones coexist, the pancreatitis nearly always follows the pattern of alcoholism-related pancreatitis, and removal of the gallstones will not prevent further attacks.[42]

Idiopathic Pancreatitis

In 8 to 25 per cent of patients with acute pancreatitis, none of the conditions known to be associated with pancreatitis have been identified. This figure is considerably lower when careful endoscopic retrograde cholangiopancreatography (ERCP) and sphincter of Oddi manometry have been performed after the first or second attack of "idiopathic" pancreatitis (see pp. 1837–1839). The male-to-female ratio, age incidence, and mortality rate are similar to those of gallstone-associated pancreatitis. Some patients with radiologically undetectable gallstones are mistakenly included in this idiopathic group.[46]

Medications

Several drugs, particularly antimetabolites and sulfonamide derivatives, are known to cause acute pancreatitis on occasion.[47, 48] These are listed in Table 97–2. The association may be an indirect one: The proximate cause of pancreatitis with sulfonamide adminis-

Table 97–2. DRUG- AND POISON-INDUCED PANCREATITIS

		Comments
Definite	Ethyl alcohol	Dose-related; mild to severe
	Methyl alcohol	Dose-related; mild to severe[49]
	Organophosphorus insecticides	Dose-related; cholinergic stimulation[50]
	6-Mercaptopurine	Mild pancreatitis; not dose-related[51]
	(Hydro)chlorothiazide	Mild to severe; related to duration of therapy
	Furosemide	Very rare
	Sulfonamides	Including salicylazosulfapyridine, sulfamethoxazole; rare
	Tetracyclines	Associated with acute fatty degeneration of liver and renal failure; mainly ante and post partum; very rare
	Estrogens	Associated with hyperlipemia (type IV or V pattern)
	Intravenous lipid infusion	Dose-related[52]
	Valproic acid	Anticonvulsant; may be fatal
	L-Asparaginase	Incidence 7%; high mortality rate
		Patients on multiple drugs
Probable	Chlorthalidone	Several case reports
	Ethacrynic acid	Several case reports
	Phenformin	Several case reports
	Nonsteroidal anti-inflammatory agents	Several case reports
	Nitrofurantoin	Single well-documented case
	Methyldopa	Single well-documented case
	Corticosteroids	Higher incidence at autopsy than recognized clinically; mild to severe
	Iatrogenic hypercalcemia	Mild

tration may be coexistent allergic vasculitis, and the pancreatitis observed during estrogen therapy is attributable to hormone-induced hyperlipemia.

Additional drugs have been implicated in only a few patients with sufficient proof for a causal role in pancreatitis: Amphetamine abuse by intravenous injection, propoxyphene improperly administered intravenously, diaxozide, histamine, azathioprine, the metabolic precursor of 6-mercaptopurine, rifampicin, cimetidine, acetaminophen, and opiates.

Abdominal Operations

Postoperative pancreatitis has a high mortality rate, 25 to 50 per cent.[53] Operations on and near the pancreas are involved in the majority of cases. The frequency after gastrectomy and after biliary tract surgery is between 0.2 and 0.8 per cent. Prompt recognition is difficult because abdominal pain, ileus, and elevations of serum amylase levels may be nonspecific sequelae of abdominal operations.

Hyperlipemia

Lipemic serum is frequently found in patients hospitalized for an attack of acute pancreatitis. The evidence points toward the sequence of lipemia preceding pancreatitis rather than lipemia representing a manifestation of pancreatic inflammation. Hyperlipemia and pancreatitis combine in several distinct settings: (1) Patients with Fredrickson type I, IV, or V hyperlipoproteinemia frequently develop attacks of abdominal pain, some of which are due to pancreatitis that usually progresses to chronic pancreatitis.[54] (2) Ten to 20 per cent of alcoholic patients with an acute episode of pancreatitis have lipemic serum. Serum triglyceride levels are greatly elevated, and the cholesterol concentration is normal or slightly raised (type V pattern). Minor elevations in fasting serum triglycerides persist during pain-free intervals in about 80 per cent of those patients. The observation that over 90 per cent respond to a high fat intake with excessive hypertriglyceridemia and that 60 per cent of these patients develop pancreatitis during this type of fat challenge[55, 56] is of considerable clinical significance. (3) Most patients who develop pancreatitis during estrogen therapy exhibit type IV or V hyperlipemia. The serum lipoprotein pattern in such patients may be unremarkable after the attack, but there is an abnormal serum triglyceride response to oral carbohydrate loads.[57]

The mechanism by which elevated circulating triglycerides trigger attacks of pancreatitis is unknown, but local lipolysis with liberation of cytotoxic free fatty acids is one possibility. Two features of lipemia-associated pancreatitis are of special clinical importance: First, attacks frequently are not accompanied by measurable increases in serum amylase values. Secondly, recurrences can be prevented by treatment aimed at avoiding peak elevations in serum triglycerides. Depending on the type of the underlying disorder, this involves weight reduction, low fat intake (Fredrickson type I and V), carbohydrate restriction (type IV), and clofibrate or nicotinic acid therapy (type V).[58]

Injections into Pancreatic Duct

Retrograde injections of the pancreatic ducts during endoscopic retrograde pancreatography (ERP) are followed by transient elevations in serum lipase and amylase in the majority of cases and by mild clinical pancreatitis in 1 per cent. The rise in total serum amylase concentration is attributable mainly to the isoamylase of pancreatic origin.[59] The frequency of clinical pancreatitis after this procedure rises with overdistention of the duct system ("acinar staining") by contrast material, and it is low in the hands of experienced operators. Bacterial infection of partially obstructed pancreatic ducts and of pseudocysts may follow ERP.[60] Neither complication is prevented by prophylactic administration of antibiotics,[61] glucagon, or aprotinin, and the treatment consists of urgent surgical operation under broad-spectrum antibiotic coverage. Low-pressure reflux of duodenal contents or radiologic contrast material into the pancreatic duct after sphincterotomy and during T-tube cholangiography is well tolerated.

Trauma

Physical trauma to the pancreas is the most common cause of pancreatitis in children and teenagers. With penetrating injuries, the prognosis is determined by the severity of damage to adjacent organs and blood vessels. Blunt trauma (compression by bicycle handle bars, steering wheels) may result in disruption of pancreatic ducts and in pancreatic contusion with resultant pseudocyst or fistula formation. The diagnosis of pancreatic injuries usually is made during thorough surgical exploration of the abdomen. Serum amylase elevations provide an unreliable guide in situations in which small intestinal trauma may coexist.[62]

Hypercalcemia

The frequency of pancreatitis in patients with hyperparathyroidism has been reported to vary between 1.5 per cent and 19 per cent.[63] The pancreatitis is acute and severe in one third and chronic in the remainder. The association between hypercalcemia and pancreatitis may be transiently obscured by the calcium-lowering effect of acute pancreatitis discussed earlier. Experimental and clinical evidence argue against a primary role of parathyroid hormone and of pancreatic intraductal formation of calcific concretions in initiating the pancreatitis. An alternative theory, activation of trypsinogen in the presence of increased calcium concentration, although lacking experimental verification, is supported by occasional reports of acute pancreatitis during iatrogenic hypercalcemia induced by calcium infusion or vitamin D poisoning.[64] Limited studies suggest a high frequency of pancreatic exocrine dysfunction in patients with hyperparathyroidism without clinical evidence of pancreatitis (see pp. 490–491).

Pregnancy

More than 150 cases of acute pancreatitis during pregnancy have been reported. Most of the episodes occur during the third trimester and the post-partum period. Coexisting cholelithiasis is present in about 90 per cent of patients. The prognosis is good, and the disease does not recur after surgical correction of the underlying cause carried out post partum (see p. 500).

Peptic Ulcer

Penetration of a duodenal ulcer into the pancreas causes local injury to the gland with pain and hyperamylasemia, but this usually does not progress to overt clinical pancreatitis.

Outflow Obstruction

Several reports claim an association between mechanical resistance to pancreatic secretion and acute pancreatitis. These conditions include annular pancreas, periampullary duodenal diverticula,[16] duodenal Crohn's disease, and afferent loop obstruction after gastrojejunostomy.[65] The possible causative role of pancreas divisum and that of sphincter of Oddi abnormalities and choledochocele are discussed later (next section and pp. 1837–1839). Primary and metastatic neoplasms obstructing portions of the pancreatic duct system account for 1 to 2 per cent of acute pancreatitis attacks.[53] Experimental evidence suggests that the pressure generated by stimulation of pancreatic secretion against obstruction at the level of the ampulla of Vater or the duodenal lumen must mechanically disrupt acinar cells before pancreatitis supervenes.

Pancreas Divisum

Pancreas divisum (PD) represents the absence of fusion between the ventral and dorsal pancreatic ducts during embryologic development. As a result, the ventral duct (Wirsung) drains only the posterior-inferior portion of the pancreatic head through the major papilla, whereas the rest of the pancreas drains separately via the dorsal duct (Santorini) through the accessory (minor) papilla. This congenital abnormality is found in 5 to 10 per cent of the population, and in an additional 2 per cent the ventral duct is absent altogether.[66] Patients undergoing ERCP examination in search of the cause of recurrent acute pancreatitis occasionally are discovered to have pancreas divisum, raising the question of a cause-and-effect relationship. This issue remains unsettled. Those who support such a relationship claim an increased occurrence of PD in patients with idiopathic pancreatitis and postulate functional outflow obstruction through the small orifice of the minor papilla as the proximate cause.[67] Other authors found the frequency of PD to be the same among patients with and without pancreatitis.[68] The clinician caring for a patient with recurrent acute pancreatitis and PD demonstrated by endoscopic pancreatography (ERP), therefore, faces a difficult choice; that is, to decide whether to recommend surgical or endoscopic decompression of the dorsal pancreatic duct in the light of conflicting epidemiologic evidence and uncontrolled observations regarding the benefits derived from such a decompression procedure. This is discussed further on page 1839.

Organ Transplantation

Acute pancreatitis follows renal and cardiac transplantation in 2 to 9 per cent of patients. About half of these attacks occur more than six months postoperatively and the mortality rate varies between 20 and 70 per cent. In some patients the condition progresses to chronic calcific pancreatitis.[69, 70] Various factors may contribute to post-transplant pancreatitis: secondary hyperparathyroidism, hyperlipemia, viral infections, vasculitis and—most important—immunosuppressive therapy with corticosteroids, L-asparaginase, or azathioprine. Thus, the appearance of this complication presents the clinician with the difficult choice between continued immunosuppression to prevent transplant rejection and reduction of this therapy to improve the prognosis of the pancreatitis.

End-stage Renal Failure

Patients with end-stage renal disease develop acute pancreatitis at rates of 0.03 per patient year when treated by peritoneal dialysis, and of 0.01 per patient year when treated by hemodialysis. The mortality is high at 21 per cent. About one half of these patients have mild to moderate type IV hyperlipemia.[71]

Hereditary Pancreatitis

The clinical onset of hereditary pancreatitis usually occurs during childhood (see pp. 1804–1806). Although the disease may begin with an acute attack, the course is dominated by the symptoms and signs of chronic calcific pancreatitis (see pp. 1846–1848). An increased frequency of pancreatic adenocarcinoma in affected families has been reported.[72]

Scorpion Bite

In the West Indies, bites by the scorpion *Tityus trinitatis* of the Buthidae family are followed by mild pancreatitis in at least half of the cases. Excessive salivation, sweating, dyspnea, and cardiac arrhythmias are the most prominent symptoms.[73] The mechanism of action is increased acetylcholine release by postganglionic cholinergic neurons,[74] which suggests that therapy with anticholinergic agents may be beneficial. Immunity does not develop.

Miscellaneous Causes

In isolated instances, acute pancreatitis is precipitated by decreased blood supply, as during severe systemic hypotension, after cardiopulmonary bypass,[75] with cholesterol embolization, and with angiitis. Among viral diseases, mumps is very rarely complicated by clinically significant pancreatitis.[76] The role of Coxsackie virus and cytomegalovirus infections remains speculative. Pancreatic duct obstruction by the fluke of *Clonorchis sinesis* and by *Ascaris* worms is another rare cause of pancreatitis. Finally, mild acute pancreatitis frequently accompanies Reye's syndrome and fulminant viral hepatitis but causes few, if any, symptoms in these settings.

INCIDENCE

It is difficult to compare the incidence of acute pancreatitis in different geographic areas and at different times because uniform diagnostic criteria and efforts at case finding have not been applied. During the 1960s, the incidence was about 10 per 100,000 population per year, and the mortality rate was 1.0 per 100,000 per year in Rochester, Minnesota. The median age of patients was 53 years, the male-to-female ratio was nearly equal, and the incidence rose steadily from the third to the seventh decade.[77] In England during the late 1970s, the yearly incidence of first attacks of acute pancreatitis was 9 per 100,000, and the mortality rate was 1.6 per 100,000 per year.[53] In 1979–1980, the incidence in Copenhagen was higher, at 28.1 per 100,000 population aged 20 years or older; in contrast to other studies, these figures were obtained by a prospective search for patients with acute pancreatitis.[78] The mortality rate of initial attacks is 1.6 times higher than that of recurrences, and it is equal or slightly higher when associated with gallstones than with alcoholism.[53]

CLINICAL PRESENTATION

Symptoms and Physical Findings

Steady, dull, or boring pain in the epigastrium or left upper abdominal quadrant is the hallmark of acute pancreatitis. It is poorly localized and reaches peak intensity within 15 minutes to one hour, in contrast to the more abrupt onset of pain with perforation of a viscus. The pain radiates to the midline of lower thoracic vertebral region in about 50 per cent of patients, and it is usually worse in the supine position. With standard medical management, the pain disappears within three to seven days. Painless acute pancreatitis occurs in fewer than 2 per cent of patients, but has a grave prognosis because the presenting symptom frequently is shock or coma.[79]

Localized epigastric tenderness to deep palpation is intense; signs of peritoneal irritation, such as abdominal wall rigidity and rebound tenderness, are absent on initial presentation, consistent with the retroperitoneal location of the pancreas. The combination of severe abdominal pain and a "soft" abdomen (as with early, severe mesenteric ischemia) is a valuable clue for the early diagnosis of acute pancreatitis. Bowel sounds are diminished but not absent. Mild abdominal distention develops in most patients during the first two days. Complete paralytic ileus signifies extension of the disease process into the small intestinal and colonic mesentery or chemical peritonitis caused by pancreatic ascites. Nausea and vomiting ensue in 80 per cent of patients and may be aggravated by opiate analgesic medications. Vomiting is rarely protracted and is effectively eliminated by nasogastric suction. The body temperature is elevated to 100° to 101° F in most patients, probably as a result of the entry of products of tissue injury into the circulation. A septic fever curve suggests the development of a complicating bacterial infection in the form of pancreatic abscess, pneumonitis, cholecystitis, or cholangitis (see pp. 238–250 and 1714–1729).

Hypotension or circulatory shock is noted in 30 to 40 per cent of patients. Several factors contribute to this circulatory instability: Hypovolemia caused by plasma exudation into the retroperitoneal space, fluid accumulation in an atonic intestine, vomiting, and hemorrhage. Additional causes include peripheral vasodilatation as well as increased vascular permeability caused by excessive circulating kinins. Bluish-brown discoloration of the flanks (Grey Turner's sign) or the periumbilical area (Cullen's sign) owing to dissection of peripancreatic bleeding into subcutaneous tissue are uncommon findings and develop only after several days. Hypocalcemic tetany is exceedingly rare (less than 1 per cent) and indicates a poor prognosis. Subcutaneous fat necrosis is detected occasionally on physical examination. These lesions occur late in the course of the disease and appear mainly over the extremities; they resemble erythema nodosum or nonsuppurative panniculitis. Patients with severe pancreatitis may present in coma or shock or with a toxic psychosis. More frequent is the development of delirum tremens in the alcoholic patient, complicating medical management considerably.

Effects on Contiguous Organs

Mild hyperbilirubinemia is observed in 40 per cent of all patients. Extrinsic compression of the terminal common bile duct by the inflamed pancreas is the cause of cholestasis in half these cases. In this instance, the hyperbilirubinemia rarely exceeds 2.5 mg/dl. When pancreatitis is associated with persisting impaction of a common bile duct stone, however, bilirubin concentration usually is higher than 2.5 mg/dl, and signs and symptoms of cholangitis are usually present, with temperatures of 101° to 103° F. In extreme instances, gram-negative bacteremia supervenes. The medial portion of the duodenum (C loop) and the greater curvature aspect of the gastric antrum frequently become involved by direct extension of the inflammation. This is readily recognized by barium contrast studies but rarely is severe enough to cause mechanical obstruction of antrum or duodenum. However, the spreading inflammation may reach the mucosa and cause acute antral gastritis and duodenitis with erosions or small superficial ulcerations. This results in minor mucosal bleeding in 10 to 20 per cent of patients, generally not severe enough to require blood transfusions. Spasm and edema of intestinal segments result from spread of the inflammation into the mesentery. Segmental obstruction or intestinal paralysis may develop, manifesting as the "cut-off sign" in the transverse colon or the "sentinel loop" of distended small bowel on radiographs of the abdomen. These findings are rare and nonspecific and do not affect clinical management, except for the 10 per cent of patients whose condition progresses to fully developed paralytic ileus.

Pulmonary manifestations caused by the spread of inflammatory exudate through diaphragmatic lymphatics are observed during 20 per cent of the attacks. Several of these manifestations may develop in the same patient. Thus, during 45 pancreatitis episodes in which such changes were identified on chest radiographs, the diaphragm was elevated in 20 (left, 9; right, 6; bilateral, 5) and pleural effusion was present in 15 (left, 8; right, 1; bilateral, 6). In addition, infiltration of the lower pulmonary lobes occurred in 16 episodes, basilar disk atelectasis in 14, and minor pleural reactions in 19.[80] Pleural effusions are exudative and frequently hemorrhagic and have a high amylase and lipase content. Irritation of the diaphragm may result in hiccups and referred shoulder pain. Pleuritic pain with pleural effusions and pulmonary infiltrates is one cause of impaired ventilation during acute pancreatitis.

Table 97–3. MANIFESTATIONS OF ACUTE PANCREATITIS

Local:	Mild: Edema, inflammation, fat necrosis
	Severe: Phlegmon, necrosis, hemorrhage; pseudocyst, abscess
Extension:	Retroperitoneum, perirenal spaces, mesocolon, major and minor omentum, mediastinum I
	Adjacent viscera: ileus, obstruction, perforation
	Exudative effusion: Lesser sac, peritoneum, pleural cavity
Systemic:	Hypovolemia
	Peripheral vasodilatation
	Pulmonary edema—adult respiratory distress syndrome
	Renal dysfunction, including acute tubular necrosis
	Coagulopathy—disseminated intravascular coagulation
	Hypocalcemia
	Hyperglycemia
	Distant fat necrosis (skin, bones, joints)

DIAGNOSIS

General Approach

When confronted with a patient suspected of having acute pancreatitis, several questions should be asked. (1) *What is the correct diagnosis?* The urgency lies in excluding other acute conditions that require different, usually surgical, management. Examples are perforated peptic ulcer, acute cholangitis, and mesenteric infarction (see pp. 1830–1832). (2) *What is the prognosis?* Although mild attacks usually subside within less than one week and require little active therapeutic intervention, a severe clinical course should be recognized early to institute major supportive measures without delay. (3) *Are complications developing?* Table 97–3 lists the possible local complications of acute pancreatitis, the manifestations of contiguous extension of the inflammatory process, and the systemic complications that may develop. It serves as a general guide for the continuing evaluation of the patient with established acute pancreatitis. When complications are suspected, appropriate diagnostic studies need to be selected to confirm this impression, followed by therapy directed specifically toward the complication. (4) *Can an associated condition be identified?* For example, is choledocholithiasis present? Correction of this problem may be required to treat the current attack of pancreatitis. In general, recurrences can be prevented if a cause is identified and promptly corrected.

Acute pancreatitis should be suspected in any patient with upper abdominal pain, shock, or elevated levels of serum pancreatic enzymes. Because there is no clinical or laboratory finding completely specific for this disease, the final diagnosis rests as much on findings consistent with pancreatitis as it does on the exclusion of other diseases that could account for the patient's condition. A past history of similar attacks diagnosed as pancreatitis or biliary colic and a history of alcoholism provide valuable clues, as does the finding of lipemic serum on admission. Two common mistakes are to base the decision for or against pancreatitis on the serum amylase level alone and to use this value as a prognostic indicator.

Early recognition of severe pancreatitis, which requires intensive clinical monitoring and more aggressive therapy, is faciliated by the use of standard assessment criteria. Those listed in Table 97–4 *A*,[81] apply to patients suffering predominantly from alcohol-associated acute pancreatitis. A complicated course, defined by the need for intensive care for longer than one week or for emergency laparotomy, is likely to ensue only when more than two of these criteria are met; the mortality rate rises steeply in the presence of four or more of the signs listed. Further analysis of risk factors by the same group of investigators showed that patients with poor prognosis had experienced fewer or no preceding attacks and that they had lower serum amylase levels on admission than patients with a favorable clinical course.[82]

The criteria in Table 97–4*B*, are based on an older patient population in which biliary tract disease was the most common precipitating factor. One advantage over the list of criteria in Table 97–4*A*, is that the

Table 97–4. FINDINGS CORRELATED WITH SEVERE OR COMPLICATED COURSE AND INCREASING MORTALITY RISK

A. Acute, Ethanol-Associated Pancreatitis[81]	
At admission:	(1) Age over 55 years
	(2) White blood cell count > 16,000 cells/cu mm
	(3) Blood glucose > 200 mg/dl (no history of prior hyperglycemia)
	(4) Serum LDH > 350 IU/L (normal, up to 225 IU/L
	(5) AST (SGOT) > 250 Sigma Frankel units/L (normal, up to 40 units/L)
During initial 48 hours:	(6) Hematocrit drop > 10 percentage points
	(7) BUN rise > 5 mg/dl
	(8) Arterial Po_2 < 60 mm Hg
	(9) Base deficit > 4 mEq/L
	(10) Serum calcium < 8.0 mg/dl
	(11) Estimated fluid sequestration > 6 L
B. Acute Pancreatitis Not Related to Ethanol Intake[83]	
Any time during first 48 hours after hospitalization:	(1) White blood cell count > 15,000 cells/cu mm
	(2) Blood glucose >180 mg/dl (no history of prior hyperglycemia)
	(3) BUN >45 mg/dl (after adequate hydration)
	(4) Arterial Po_2 < 60 mm Hg
	(5) Serum calcium < 8.0 mg/dl
	(6) Serum albumin < 3.2 gm/dl
	(7) Serum LDH > 600 units/L (normal, up to 250 units/L)
	(8) AST (SGOT) or ALT (SGPT) > 200 units/L (normal, up to 40 units/L)

LDH, Lactic dehydrogenase; IU, international units; AST, aspartate aminotransferase; BUN, blood urea nitrogen; ALT, alanine aminotransferase.

patient can be classified before the start of the third hospital day. A severe course can be predicted with a high degree of accuracy when three or more of these criteria are fulfilled.[83]

Laboratory Studies

Serum Amylase

Determination of total serum amylase activity remains the laboratory test used most frequently for the diagnosis of acute pancreatitis. Although methods for measuring additional pancreatic enzymes exist, these are not yet widely available, take longer to perform, and generally are not offered on a 24-hour basis.[84] The serum amylase level rises 2 to 12 hours after onset of symptoms and remains elevated for three to five days in most cases. The serum levels of other pancreatic enzymes, such as lipase and the pancreatic amylase isoenzyme, tend to stay increased about ten days longer.[85] In 5 to 10 per cent of cases, however, hyperamylasemia lasts for longer than ten days without persisting symptoms or the development of complications. The magnitude of serum amylase elevation provides no clue to the prognosis of the pancreatitis attack. In fact, serum amylase remains normal in 10 per cent of cases of lethal pancreatitis.[86] On the other hand, serum amylase level may be elevated in many other conditions. Total output and concentration of urinary amylase provide no additional useful information with the following exception: In the presence of marked hyperlipemia (serum triglyceride levels greater than 2000 mg/dl) and acute pancreatitis, measured serum amylase (and lipase) activity frequently is normal whereas urinary amylase concentration is markedly elevated.[87] Elevation of urinary amylase in the face of normal serum amylase may very rarely be found in factitious pancreatitis, in which the patient feigns abdominal pain and expectorates into the urine. In such a case, the high level in urine is due to salivary amylase.

Total serum amylase content can be separated into pancreatic (P) and salivary (S) isoenzymes. The assay method in widest use employs a wheat protein that selectively inhibits the activity of the S isoenzyme.[84] About 40 per cent of normal serum amylase activity is derived from the pancreas—that is, the normal P/S ratio is about 0.7. Determination of the amylase isoenzyme activity is clinically useful only when total amylase activity is increased. An increased P/S ratio is present in all types of pancreatic diseases and with gastric and small intestinal perforation.

The renal clearance of serum amylase in relation to the creatinine clearance rises early during the course of acute pancreatitis. The mechanism has been identified as decreased renal tubular reabsorption of this small enzyme protein (55,000 molecular weight) from the glomerular filtrate.[88] The amylase-creatinine clearance ratio (ACR), expressed as a percentage, is obtained as follows:

$$\text{ACR} = \frac{\text{A (urine)} \times \text{Cr (serum)}}{\text{A (serum)} \times \text{Cr (urine)}} \times 100$$

where A and Cr represent amylase and creatinine concentration, respectively. The normal range is 1 to 4 per cent, but this varies with the laboratory methods employed. Although the ACR is increased in acute pancreatitis, the clinical diagnostic value of this determination is limited mainly to the detection of macroamylasemia.

Macroamylasemia is a rare condition in which most of the elevated circulating amylase activity is in the form of macromolecular aggregates of amylase or of amylase complexed with immunoglobulin A. These aggregates do not undergo glomerular filtration; hence, the ACR is abnormally low (less than 0.2 per cent). The majority of these patients show no evidence of salivary gland or pancreatic disease.[89]

Table 97–5 lists the large number of conditions other than acute pancreatitis in which total serum amylase activity may be elevated. Group A can be distinguished from acute pancreatitis only by clinical and radiologic observations. This applies also to group B, except that the rise in serum amylase activity tends to be less than twice the upper limit of normal. Groups C and D can be differentiated from acute pancreatitis by the additional determination of the amylase isoenzyme ratio and the ACR value, respectively.

Measurement of amylase in pleural fluid can help greatly in diagnosis of acute pancreatitis, particularly when associated with an inflammatory pseudocyst. The level is usually three or more times the simultaneously determined serum values and often as high as ten times greater (see p. 1856).

Other Serum Pancreatic Enzymes

Serum lipase activity is elevated in about 87 per cent of patients with acute pancreatitis but tends to remain normal in instances in which total serum amylase is falsely elevated (see Table 97–5).[84, 96] Thus, this test is less sensitive but more specific than the total serum amylase level for acute pancreatitis. Elevations of serum lipase persist longer than those of amylase during the healing phase of acute pancreatitis.[84]

Serum immunoreactive trypsinogen/trypsin (IRT) concentrations can be measured routinely by radioimmunoassay. The finding of elevated serum IRT is about as specific and as sensitive for diagnosing acute pancreatitis as is hyperamylasemia.[84, 90, 96]

The relative merits of serum total amylase, amylase isoenzyme, lipase, and IRT determinations in the diagnosis of acute pancreatitis have been summarized.[84, 90, 96] Ideally, any two of these tests should be available in the clinical laboratory 24 hours a day.

Table 97–5. CONDITIONS OTHER THAN ACUTE PANCREATITIS OCCASIONALLY ASSOCIATED WITH HYPERAMYLASEMIA

Group A	Chronic pancreatitis
	Pancreatic pseudocyst
	Carcinoma of pancreas
	Perforation of stomach, duodenum, jejunum
	Mesenteric infarction
	Opiate administration
	After ERCP
Group B	Common bile duct obstruction
	Acute cholecystitis
	Burn injury
Group C	Salivary adenitis
	Postoperative state
	Renal insufficiency[90]
	Metabolic, including diabetic, acidosis[91]
	Admission to intensive care unit[92]
	Acute alcoholism[93]
	Acute and chronic hepatocellular disease[90]
	Anorexia nervosa, bulimia[94]
	Ovarian neoplasm
	Salpingitis; ruptured ectopic pregnancy
	Incidental finding[95]
	Upper gastrointestinal endoscopy[94a]
Group D	Macroamylasemia[88]

Group A: Entry of pancreatic enzymes into blood stream directly from pancreas or via peritoneal surfaces. Indistinguishable from acute pancreatitis by measurements of serum pancreatic enzyme levels.

Group B: Generally minor total serum amylase elevation. Coexisting mild pancreatitis difficult to rule out without surgical exploration, US, or CT scanning.

Group C: Minor total serum amylase elevation, mainly owing to elevation of salivary isoenzyme. Serum lipase and immunoreactive trypsin (IRT) levels generally normal.

Group D: No symptoms of current pancreatic disease; low amylase-creatinine clearance ratio.[88]

Liver Function Tests

The serum aspartate aminotransferase (AST; SGOT) level is elevated up to 15 times above the upper limit of normal in about 50 per cent of patients. Alcoholic liver disease, common bile duct obstruction, and acute pancreatitis all may cause raised AST values. By contrast, the presence of elevated alanine aminotransferase (ALT; SGPT) and alkaline phosphatase values should raise the suspicion of associated biliary tract disease. Minor increases in serum bilirubin concentrations are common and can be caused by alcoholic liver disease or extrinsic compression of the intrapancreatic portion of the common bile duct. With cholestasis due to coexisting choledocholithiasis, the degree of hyperbilirubinemia is variable; however, this condition should be suspected when the serum bilirubin level exceeds 2.5 mg/dl and continues to rise.[97]

The following laboratory results obtained on admission are of value in predicting whether a pancreatitis attack is associated with gallstones: (1) alkaline phosphatase level greater than twice the upper limit of normal, (2) ALT (SGPT) level greater than 2.2 times the upper limit of normal, and (3) serum bilirubin level greater than 2.5 mg/dl. When "negative" is defined as all three criteria being negative, and "positive" as any one of the three being positive, these three laboratory tests predict associated gallstones with a sensitivity of 73 per cent and exclude this association with a specificity of 94 per cent.[98] As noted earlier, persisting choledocholithiasis underlying acute pancreatitis not only causes bilirubin elevations well above 2.5 mg/dl but may also cause acute cholangitis.

Methemalbumin

Brown discoloration of the serum by methemalbumin has been observed in some patients with necrotizing pancreatitis. This phenomenon is due to breakdown of hemoglobin in and around the pancreas, followed by entry of hematin into the plasma, where it combines with albumin. The serum haptoglobin concentration remains normal, in contrast to the methemalbuminemia caused by acute hemolysis. The value of this determination is limited, however, because it may be positive with any hemorrhagic or necrotizing intra-abdominal event.[99]

Other Determinations

Transient, mild hyperglycemia is common, particularly during initial attacks of acute pancreatitis, when excess glucagon is released from alpha cells of the islets of Langerhans.[32, 34] Sustained fasting hyperglycemia of greater than 200 mg/dl reflects widespread pancreatic necrosis and is a poor prognostic sign.

Previously normoglycemic patients do not develop diabetic ketoacidosis during acute pancreatitis.

Hypocalcemia can be detected in up to 30 per cent of patient when daily measurements are obtained. It appears two to three days after onset of the disease, rarely requires treatment, and may persist for several weeks after recovery. Calcium levels below 8.0 mg/dl signify a poor prognosis. Acute pancreatitis arising in a patient with hypercalcemia due to hyperparathyroidism may result in a normal serum calcium concentration (see pp. 490–491). Associated hypercalcemia, therefore, can be ruled out only several weeks after recovery. The hematocrit frequently is elevated on admission owing to hemoconcentration as a manifestation of extensive fluid sequestration. A continuing or dramatic fall in hematocrit value after correction of the volume deficit requires prompt diagnostic efforts to identify a bleeding site. Acute hemolysis is an exceedingly rare complication of acute pancreatitis.

Leukocytosis of 10,000 to 25,000 cells/cu mm is present in 80 per cent of patients. Moderate hypoproteinemia and hypoalbuminemia are common after restoration of the intravascular fluid volume. A progressive fall in arterial PO_2 several days after onset of symptoms accompanies the development of ARDS, the pulmonary edema caused by increased permeability of the alveolar-capillary membrane.

The hyperlipemia associated with some causes of pancreatitis has been discussed earlier. The serum usually is lactescent, with the serum triglyceride level exceeding 1700 to 2000 mg/dl; serum cholesterol level is normal or only moderately elevated. The lactescence clears slowly over a period of five to seven days.

A preliminary report suggests that marked elevation of the serum C-reactive protein concentration on the first hospital day predicts progression to severe, necrotizing pancreatitis with an accuracy of 95 per cent.[100] It remains to be seen whether this simple laboratory value can eventually replace the prognostic criteria listed in Table 97–4.

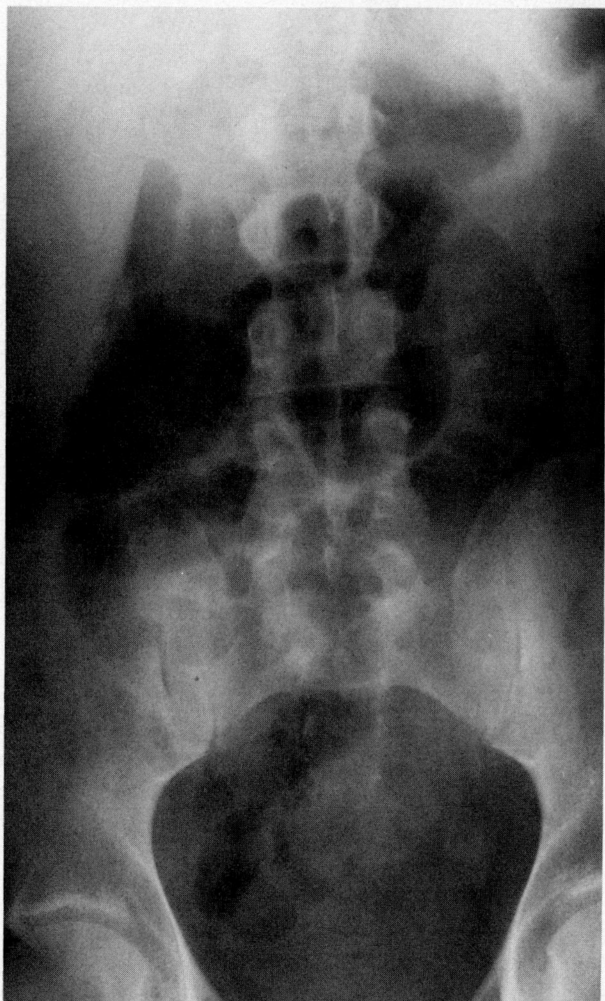

Figure 97–3. Sentinel loop. Recumbent abdominal radiograph demonstrating several loops of proximal small bowel distended by gas: focal small bowel ileus in acute pancreatitis. (Courtesy of Edward T. Stewart, M.D.)

Radiologic Features

Radiographic studies, including ultrasonography (US), computed tomography (CT), and selective angiography, play an important role in the management of acute pancreatitis. They are particularly helpful for establishing the presence of pancreatic disease, for detecting local complications and involvement of contiguous organs, and for demonstrating associated conditions, particularly cholelithiasis and choledocholithiasis.

Plain Abdominal Radiographs

Plain films of the abdomen should be obtained in every patient admitted with known or suspected acute pancreatitis. They may show a sentinel loop (a distended small intestinal loop near the pancreas) (Fig. 97–3), paralytic ileus involving the entire small intestine, the colon cut-off sign (spasm in the transverse colon or at the splenic flexure with absent colonic gas beyond this point), loss of the preperitoneal fat line, indistinct organ contours (psoas muscle, kidneys), and the diffuse haziness indicating ascites. Although these findings are neither specific for nor frequent in acute pancreatitis, they do point to the presence of an acute intra-abdominal or retroperitoneal process. Specific abnormalities are the diffuse pancreatic calcification diagnostic of advanced chronic pancreatitis and the extraluminal gas bubbles seen in about 10 per cent of patients with pancreatic abscess formation (Fig. 97–4).[101] A major use of this examination lies in ruling out the presence of free intraperitoneal air caused by gastric and intestinal perforation and the thickening and "thumb-printing" of the intestinal wall accompanying mesenteric infarction.

Chest Radiographs

The diaphragmatic involvement and pulmonary complications of acute pancreatitis are easily recognized[80] but entirely nonspecific. It should be recalled that these

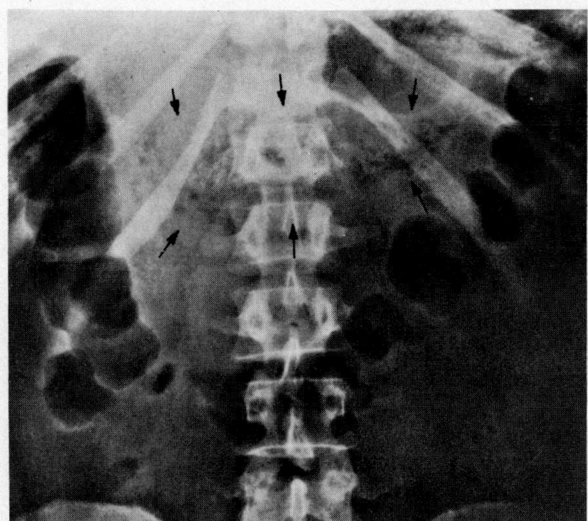

Figure 97–4. Pancreatic abscess: extraluminal gas collections (soap bubble sign) *(arrows)*. The transverse colon is displaced caudad. (From Woodard S., Kelvin, F. M., Rice, R. P., and Thompson, W. M. AJR *136*:871. © 1981, American Roentgen Ray Society.)

changes are not confined to the left side but may be bilateral or entirely right-sided. Interstitial fluffy infiltrates in a distribution characteristic of pulmonary edema but without associated cardiomegaly are the hallmark of the respiratory failure syndrome arising during severe pancreatitis. A pleural effusion visible on a chest radiograph in a patient with suspected acute pancreatitis or in one with an established diagnosis indicates marked activity. Such fluid contains a very high concentration of amylase, many times the serum level; hence, this measurement can significantly help in diagnosis of acute pancreatitis or of inflammatory pseudocyst (see pp. 1825, 1856, and 1867).

Contrast Studies

Contrast studies of the upper gastrointestinal and biliary tracts during acute pancreatitis rarely provide important information and have largely been replaced by abdominal ultrasonography and computed tomography and by endoscopy. The upper gastrointestinal series frequently exhibits evidence of pancreatic enlargement and peripancreatic inflammation. The duodenal C-loop may be widened and the mucosal folds swollen or effaced (Fig. 97–5). An enlarged papilla of Vater may appear as a hemispheric or lobulated filling defect. The stomach may be displaced anteriorly or medially by retroperitoneal swelling or a developing pseudocyst or abscess. Finally, delayed gastric emptying from extrinsic compression of the antrum or the pylorus may be observed. Oral cholecystograms and intravenous cholangiograms rarely, if ever, allow visualization of the biliary tract during the acute stage of pancreatitis; they are poor choices for determining associated biliary tract disease and should not be ordered in the acutely ill patient (see pp. 1691–1714 for discussion of newer techniques for visualizing the biliary tract in inflammatory states).

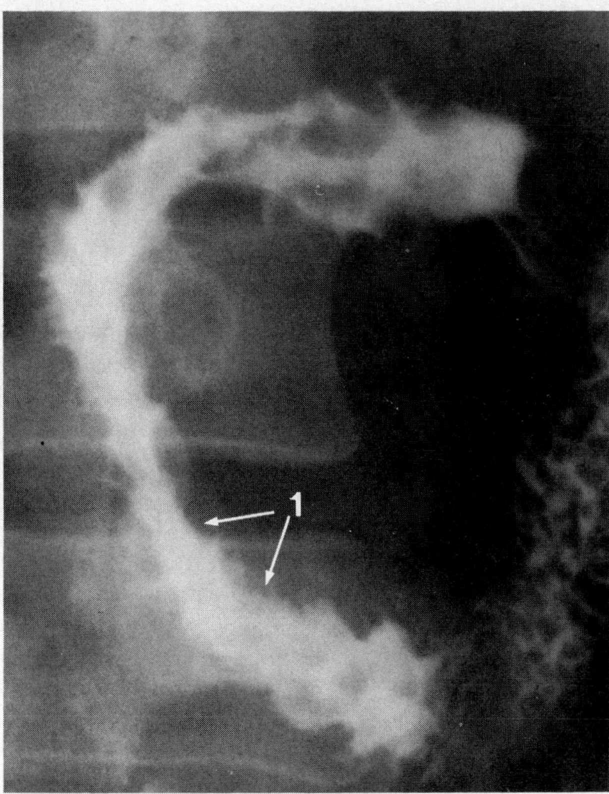

Figure 97–5. Duodenal involvement: Oblique film from an upper gastrointestinal series. Resolving acute pancreatitis; same patient as in Figure 97–3 but one week later. There is marked edematous thickening of the duodenal folds. Note the mass effect along the medial aspect of the C-loop (1) caused by enlargement of head of pancreas. (Courtesy of Edward T. Stewart, M.D.)

Ultrasonography and Computed Tomography

US and CT are employed mainly for the following three purposes: (1) to determine the presence of pancreatic disease, (2) to assess the severity of pancreatitis and the development of local complications, and (3) to evaluate the biliary tract for the presence of stones and dilatation. Following are considerations regarding the relative merits of these two noninvasive imaging methods: Arguments for the use of US are that it is less expensive, can be performed at the bedside, and it does not involve the use of peroral and intravenous contrast media. Furthermore, US yields unsurpassed sensitivity (98 per cent) and specificity (93.5 per cent) for the diagnosis of cholelithiasis,[102] and it provides equal or better information on dilatation of intra- and extrahepatic bile ducts than does CT imaging. The major disadvantage to the use of abdominal US is the high rate of technically unsatisfactory examinations, usually owing to bowel gas overlying the area of interest; this rate is between 14 per cent[103] and 38 per cent[104] in acute pancreatitis, compared to a 1 per cent technical failure rate with abdominal CT.[103]

CT is considered the imaging method of choice for any pancreatic disease, especially in patients with suspected complications of acute pancreatitis. When intravenous contrast medium is given during the CT

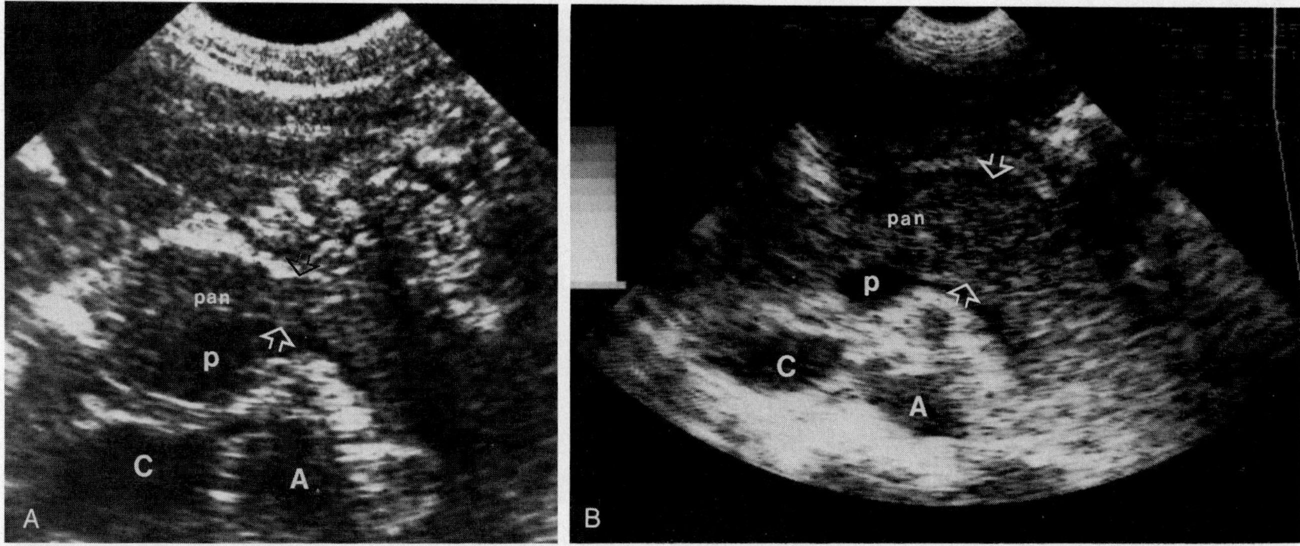

Figure 97–6. Axial ultrasonograms at the level of the pancreatic head. *A*, Normal; *B*, mild acute pancreatitis: Diffuse pancreatic enlargement. A, aorta; C, inferior vena cava; P, portal vein; PAN, pancreas; *arrows*, width of pancreas. (Courtesy of Edward T. Stewart, M.D.)

examination, areas of high attenuation suggest fresh hemorrhage and the patency of the portal and splenic vessels can be assessed; pancreatic areas of low contrast may reflect necrosis of the organ.[105] However, allergy to contrast medium or compromised renal function precludes the use of intravenous contrast material. The sensitivity and specificity of CT for identifying changes consistent with acute pancreatitis are 92 and 90 per cent, respectively; the corresponding figures for US are 78 and 89 per cent.[103] Similarly, 74 per cent of surgically confirmed pancreatic abscesses were identified by CT, but only 38 per cent by US.[106] Unfortunately, neither method can determine whether pseudocysts and areas of pancreatic phlegmon or peripancreatic necrosis are infected, nor are they reliable for detecting common bile duct stones impacted in the ampulla of Vater.

US and CT show a morphologically normal pancreas in approximately 10 per cent and 28 per cent, respectively, of patients with acute, uncomplicated pancreatitis.[103] Either examination occasionally documents pancreatitis in situations in which the clinical diagnosis has remained unclear. The abnormalities produced by mild pancreatitis on US and CT studies are shown in Figure 97–6, *A* and *B*, and Figure 97–7, *A* and *B*, respectively. The appearance of severe pancreatitis on CT scans, progressing from phlegmon and retroperitoneal edema (Fig. 97–8) to pancreatic pseudocyst and ascites formation (Fig. 97–9) and, finally, to a pancreatic abscess (Fig. 97–10), is illustrated in these figures, which emphasize the value of CT examinations in the evaluation of complicated acute pancreatitis.

The current development of nuclear magnetic resonance facilities promises an alternative method of

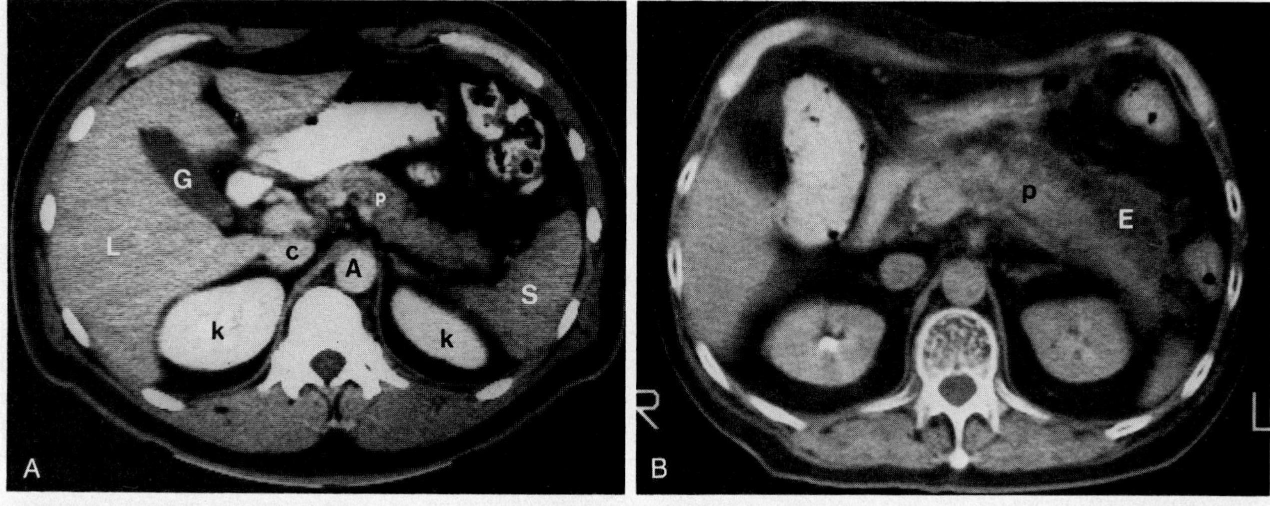

Figure 97–7. Computerized tomographic (CT) scans after intravenous contrast administration at the level of the pancreatic body and tail. *A*, Normal pancreas and its relation to intra-abdominal and retroperitoneal organs. The presence of fat allows good discrimination of anatomic structures. *B*, Acute pancreatitis with thickening of the organ and peripancreatic edema (E). A, aorta; C, inferior vena cava; K, kidney; G, gallbladder; L, liver; S, spleen; E, edema; p, pancreas. (Courtesy of Edward T. Stewart, M.D.)

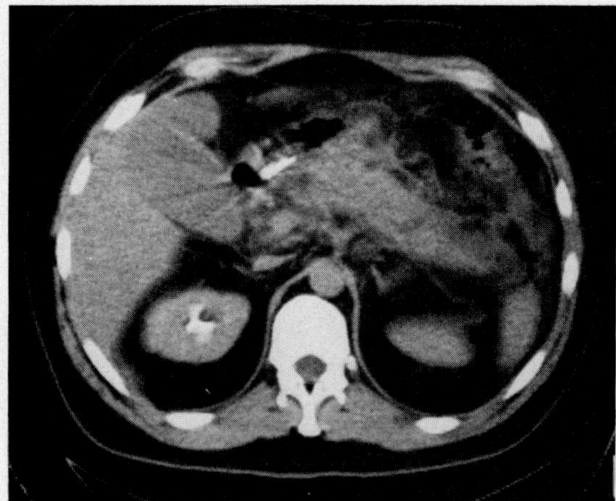

Figure 97–8. CT scan of developing pancreatic phlegmon. Striking peripancreatic eema can no longer be differentiated from the pancreas. Inflammatory edema extends to anterior pararenal spaces, especially on the left, and into the base of mesentery anteriorly. There are no discrete fluid collections. (Courtesy of Edward T. Stewart, M.D.)

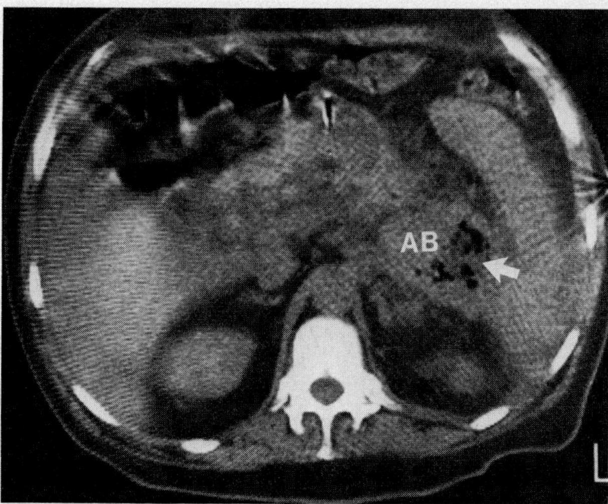

Figure 97–10. CT scan of pancreatic abscess. Patient with severe pancreatitis, 16 days after onset of symptoms. An abscess (AB) is seen in the tail of the pancreas near the hilus of the spleen; characteristic gas bubbles are found within the abscess *(arrow)*. (Courtesy of Edward T. Stewart, M.D.)

pancreatic imaging, the usefulness of which has yet to be defined[107] (Fig. 97–11).

Angiography

The major indication for selective mesenteric arteriography in acute pancreatitis is the rare occurrence of hemosuccus pancreaticus, that is, bleeding through the pancreatic duct. The bleeding is acute and may be massive. Through the endoscope, blood may be seen to emanate from the papilla of Vater. Emergency mesenteric arteriography during active severe bleeding will distinguish hemosuccus pancreaticus from hemobilia, will identify the arterial or venous source of the bleeding, and will determine whether the blood first appears in a pancreatic pseudocyst or abscess before entering the pancreatic duct system (Fig. 97–12). Finally, arteriography offers the option of arterial embolization as a temporizing or permanent means of hemostasis[108] (see pp. 401–402).

DIFFERENTIAL DIAGNOSIS

The problem of differentiating acute pancreatitis from other conditions faces the clinician in a variety of distinct settings: (1) In a patient with acute epigastric pain and elevated serum amylase, other causes of hyperamylasemia need to be ruled out; (2) when acute epigastric pain is accompanied by normal serum amylase, pancreatitis remains a diagnostic possibility, especially when the onset of pain occurred several days before medical attention was sought, and when the

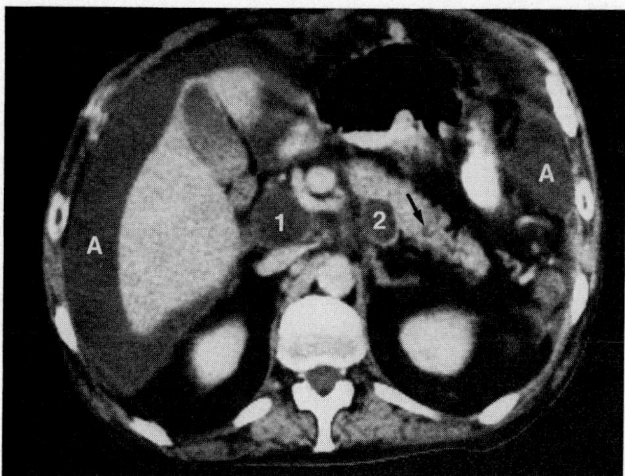

Figure 97–9. CT scan of complicated acute pancreatitis. There is generalized pancreatic ascites (A). Two fluid collections[1,2] are seen posterior to the pancreas; these represent acute pseudocysts without evident wall formation. Note that the appearance of the pancreatic tail approaches normal except for mild dilatation of the main pancreatic duct *(arrow)*. (Courtesy of Edward T. Stewart, M.D.)

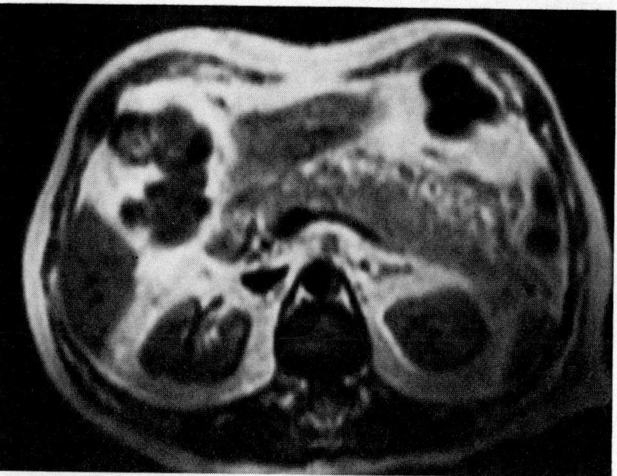

Figure 97–11. Magnetic resonance scan of mild acute pancreatitis. The inflammatory process appears similar to that on CT scan of the same patient (see Fig. 97–7*B*). Notice high signal intensity from areas of fatty tissue, lower intensity, from pancreas and prepancreatic edema, and low intensity from flowing blood, in contrast to the findings on CT scanning. (Courtesy of Edward T. Stewart, M.D.)

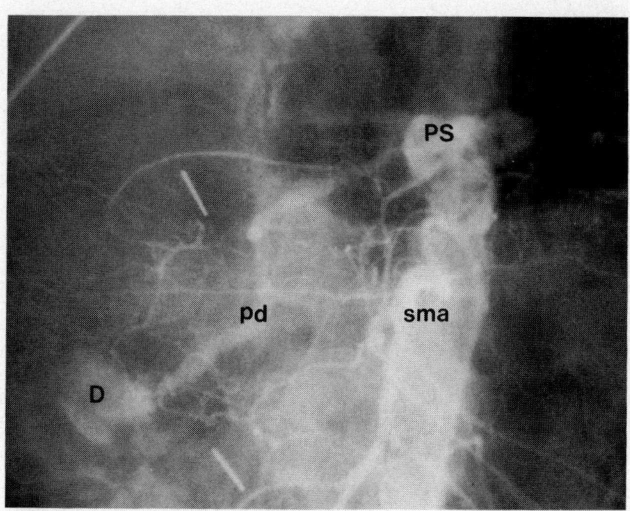

Figure 97–12. Selective arterogram of patient with hemosuccus pancreaticus. Patient with resolving acute pancreatitis developed sudden massive bleeding through the papilla of Vater. Contrast injection into the superior mesenteric artery (sma) was followed by collection of contrast in a small pancreatic pseudocyst (PS) in communication with the pancreatic duct (pd), from where contrast is seen entering the duodenum (D). Blood flow is from the sma through collateral vessels, including inferior and superior pancreaticoduodenal arteries, to the splenic artery, which developed a pseudoaneurysm that ruptured into a small pseudocyst. (Courtesy of Elliott Lipchik, M.D.)

patient appears severely ill when first seen; in this situation, US or CT scan may show positive evidence of pancreatitis; (3) in a patient presenting in shock or coma of unknown cause but without abdominal pain, a serum amylase determination should always be obtained to help rule out painless, often fatal, pancreatitis.

Perforated Peptic Ulcer

Perforated peptic ulcers may mimic pancreatitis. Serum pancreatic enzyme concentrations frequently rise owing to spillage of upper gastrointestinal contents into the peritoneal cavity, from where pancreatic enzymes gain access to the circulation. The amylase-creatinine clearance ratio (ACR) usually is not elevated. With free perforation of a peptic ulcer, the patient has a more abrupt onset of pain and shows more evidence of peritoneal irritation than with acute pancreatitis. The radiologic detection of free intraperitoneal air is diagnostic of a perforated viscus, but this sign gradually disappears as the interval from the onset of pain to plain radiographs of the abdomen lengthens. A swallow of water-soluble contrast material (Gastrografin) may demonstrate extravasation, but endoscopy is not part of the initial diagnostic approach.

Acute Cholecystitis

Acute cholecystitis may be accompanied by mild hyperamylasemia. Here, again, the clinical examination is most important: The pain tends to be maximal in the right upper abdominal quadrant, it frequently radiates to the right infrascapular area, and a tender, distended gallbladder may be palpable. ^{99m}Tc-HIDA or ^{99m}Tc-PIPIBA scanning provides additional diagnostic information (see p. 1704). In acute cholecystitis, the radioisotope scan is abnormal (visualization of the common bile duct but not the gallbladder 60 minutes after intravenous injection) in greater than 95 per cent of cases, although the specificity of the test (normal examination in patients without the disease) is only about 85 per cent. Thus, cholescintigraphy excludes acute cholecystitis more reliably than it establishes this diagnosis.[109] Acute cholecystitis may actually coexist with acute, generally mild pancreatitis. When the cholecystitis requires emergency surgery, laparotomy should not be delayed because of the known or suspected presence of acute pancreatitis.

Simultaneous Occurrence of Acute Bile Duct Disease and Pancreatitis

Biliary colic owing to choledocholithiasis presents with midepigastric or right upper quadrant pain and tenderness, mild hyperamylasemia, and nausea. Serum bilirubin, AST (SGOT), and alkaline phosphatase levels tend to be elevated to a greater extent than with acute pancreatitis.[97] The diagnosis can often be confirmed by US. The coexistence of acute pancreatitis with a gallstone impacted in the ampulla of Vater presents difficult diagnostic and therapeutic challenges. Pain localization and laboratory studies provide no completely reliable clues, although steadily rising serum bilirubin, alkaline phosphatase, and ALT (SGPT) levels should alert the clinician to this possibility.[97, 98] The stone itself may be too small to be detected by present-day US and CT equipment. The demonstration of dilated extrahepatic bile ducts and of obstruction to flow of a radiolabeled scanning agent from choledochus into the duodenum[109] does not distinguish between extrinsic compression of the common bile duct and stone impaction. When jaundice and clinical condition continue to worsen, the choledochus should be cleared of all stones without delay to reestablish biliary, as well as pancreatic, drainage. This aim can be achieved by surgical common bile duct exploration, usually with added cholecystectomy and duodenotomy. The currently preferred way of dealing with this situation less traumatically is to undertake an ERCP procedure with endoscopic sphincterotomy. Any choledochal stones that fail to pass into the duodenum after the sphincterotomy are then removed by endoscopically introduced baskets or balloons. This approach, under antibiotic cover with a third-generation cephalosporin plus gentamycin, is highly successful in the hands of experienced endoscopists.[98, 110] An elective cholecystectomy should follow as soon as the patient has recovered. Not surprisingly, the majority of these patients have multiple gallstones of a diameter smaller than that of the cystic bile duct.[111]

Ascending bacterial cholangitis in a patient with acute pancreatitis presents with the same clinical features as those just described for gallstone impaction in the ampulla of Vater, with the added signs of bacteremia, usually gram-negative. Hyperbilirubinemia and common bile duct dilatation may be absent or mild because the stone(s) may be impacted only intermittently. Most patients give a history of symptomatic cholelithiasis and, frequently, cholecystectomy. Spiking fevers (101° to 104° F), chills, tachycardia, and hypotension, with a shift to immature forms in the white blood cell differential count, are the hallmarks of this condition. Antibiotic treatment (a cephalosporin [cefoxitin, 1.0 to 2.0 gm every six hours intravenously], or ampicillin, 1.0 gm, with clindamycin, 600 mg intravenously every six hours, plus gentamycin or tobramycin, 2 mg/kg intravenously, then maintenance doses as calculated from plasma drug levels) should be started before the results of blood cultures become known. Definitive treatment consists of immediate decompression of the biliary tree. This can be accomplished surgically or endoscopically as described in the preceding paragraph. As a temporary measure, external catheter drainage of dilated bile ducts by the percutaneous transhepatic route may be instituted (see pp. 1751–1752).

Mesenteric Vascular Occlusion

The early symptoms and signs are quite nonspecific. Abdominal pain tends to be diffuse and steady. Tenderness, abdominal guarding, and blood in the stool appear only after some delay. This condition must be considered in elderly atherosclerotic patients who have hours of unremitting abdominal pain and become severely ill (see pp. 1903–1916).

Uncertain Diagnosis

The clinician occasionally is confronted with an acutely ill patient in whom clinical examination, serum pancreatic enzyme levels, plain abdominal radiographs, abdominal CT, and examination of the biliary system by US or radionuclide scanning have not resulted in a firm diagnosis nor in exclusion of acute pancreatitis (see pp. 238–250). At this point, urgent surgical consultation must be obtained. Unless the clinical condition improves rapidly, a laparotomy should be performed, generally within 48 hours of admission. Should only uncomplicated pancreatitis be found, the abdomen is closed, and the prognosis is not adversely affected by this surgical diagnostic procedure. If any condition masquerading as acute pancreatitis, such as intestinal strangulation-obstruction, mesenteric infarction, or perforation of a viscus, is present, it must be corrected surgically, even in the presence of coexisting pancreatitis.

THERAPY

No specific therapy is available that interrupts the process of autodigestion that is central to acute pancreatitis. The overall mortality rate per attack is about 9 per cent, and this is largely accounted for by those 15 to 20 per cent of patients who develop a severe or complicated course. In essence, the mortality rate can be decreased by standard medical therapy of systemic complications as they arise, by timely therapy of local complications (such as endoscopic or surgical removal of impacted common duct stones), and, ultimately, by the prevention of recurrent episodes through correction of associated conditions (e.g., removal of common duct stones or cholescystectomy for cholelithiasis (see pp. 1691–1714 and 1741–1761).

Mild Pancreatitis

Overall Aims

An empirical goal of medical therapy is to stop pancreatic autodigestion by reducing pancreatic enzyme synthesis and secretion (i.e., putting the pancreas at rest) or by inactivating pancreatic hydrolases. There is no evidence that any treatment method tested so far is of specific clinical benefit (Table 97–6). This is explained, in part, by the fact that pancreatic execrine secretion during experimental, as well as clinical, acute pancreatitis already is greatly reduced. A second aim is the prevention of potentially disastrous infectious complications, such as pancreatic abscess, ascending cholangitis, and bacterial pneumonia. However, there is no evidence that prophylactic treatment with antibiotics is effective in this regard.[118] The mainstays of the management of mild pancreatitis are good general supportive care and an alert watch for the development of severe disease and localized complications (see Tables 97–3 and 97–4).

General Supportive Care

Supportive care of acute pancreatitis consists of analgesia, restoration and maintenance of intravascular volume, and frequent monitoring of physical findings and vital signs. The patient should receive sufficient

Table 97–6. TREATMENT OF ACUTE PANCREATITIS: RANDOMIZED STUDIES

Treatment	Type of Pancreatitis	Effect	Reference
Nasogastric suction	Mild	None	112
Cimetidine	All	None	113
Anticholinergic drugs	Mild	None	114
Aprotinin	All	None	115, 116
Glucagon	All	None	115
Calcitonin	All	None	112, 117
Antibiotic agents	Mild	None	118
Indomethacin	All	Less pain	119
$CaNa_2$ EDTA*	All	None	120
Peritoneal lavage	All	None	116, 121
Parenteral alimentation	All	None	122
Somatostatin	All	None	123
Fresh frozen plasma	All	None	123a

*A phospholipase A_2 inhibitor.

analgesic medication to relieve pain. The frequently observed transient rise in serum amylase and lipase levels after opiate administration is not deleterious to the patient, and narcotics should not be withheld or curtailed for this reason. Meperidine hydrochloride (Demerol) in doses of 75 to 125 mg intramuscularly may be given every three to four hours. This drug induces less spasm of the sphincter of Oddi than does morphine. Thirty per cent or more of the circulating plasma volume may be sequestered as peripancreatic exudate. Additional sources of fluid loss are vomiting and nasogastric aspiration. The fluid deficit must be assessed at regular intervals by charting pulse rate, postural changes in blood pressure, urine output, skin turgor, hematocrit, and plasma urea nitrogen level. The choice of replacement solution is less important than rapidity and adequacy of volume restoration. When the estimated volume deficit exceeds 3 to 4 L, one unit of human serum albumin (12.5 gm) may be given per liter infused. Continuous hemodynamic and arterial blood gas monitoring are not indicated in mild pancreatitis. Chest radiographs and plain films of the abdomen (upright and supine) should be obtained on admission and repeated as the clinical situation dictates.

Reducing Secretions

To achieve the empiric goal of minimizing pancreatic secretions, the patient should be given nothing by mouth. The decision whether to institute continuous gastric suction with a double-lumen sump tube rests on general indications, not on the presence of pancreatitis.[112] Thus, nasogastric suction is indicated in the presence of vomiting, severe nausea, and developing or complete paralytic ileus. Hourly antacids (e.g., 30 to 45 ml of a potent aluminum-magnesium hydroxide preparation, with clamping of the tube, if in place, for 15 minutes), or 300 mg of cimetidine or 50 mg of ranitidine hydrochloride, or 20 mg of famotidine intravenously twice daily, is advisable when the gastric aspirate reveals evidence of upper gastrointestinal bleeding. Once the pain has subsided, small feedings of a diet high in carbohydrate but low in protein and fat are begun. Regular food may be taken several days later, but large meals are best avoided. Pain recurs on refeeding in 10 to 20 per cent of patients and is an indication for resumption of no oral intake. Repeat disappearance of pain and decrease in serum amylase or lipase levels, or both, serve as approximate guides for the timing of resumption of oral intake. With prolonged hyperamylasemia, a developing pancreatic pseudocyst should be suspected, but this laboratory finding otherwise has no adverse clinical consequences, particularly when it is accounted for by elevation of the salivary isoenzyme. Usually an enlarging inflammatory pseudocyst will be associated with continuing or recurrent postprandial pain (see p. 1835).

Attempts at reducing pancreatic secretion by dietary manipulations have met with little success. Thus, there is no evidence that pancreatic juice flow is lower with feeding elemental diets than with regular food, and pancreatic enzyme output in humans is stimulated as much by intrajejunal as by gastric feedings.[124] Intravenously administered glucose and fat do not affect basal gastric and pancreatic secretion, whereas intravenous infusion of an amino acid mixture stimulates gastric acid and pancreatic chymotrypsin and trypsin outputs.[125] Total parenteral nutrition should be considered only in patients with complicated or prolonged pancreatitis.[122]

Additional drugs and hormones, evaluated because of their pancreatic antisecetory or enzyme-inhibitory potential, are listed in Table 97–6. Controlled clinical studies have not shown any benefit from H_2 blockers, anticholinergics, glucagon, calcitonin, somatostatin, prostaglandin synthetase inhibitors, inhibitors of trypsin and phospholipase A_2, and infusions of fresh frozen plasma on the course or outcome of acute pancreatitis.

Summary

Following is a suggested outline for the management of mild acute pancreatitis:

On Admission. Chest and supine abdominal radiographs; nothing by mouth; frequent charting of vital signs, intake, output, and daily weight; intravascular volume restitution to maintain urine output above 40 ml/hour. Pain medication. Omit medications listed on Table 97–2. Laboratory tests: Perform the test listed in Table 97–4, plus determination of serum creatinine and triglyceride levels.

Later. Continue charting intake and output; daily determinations of hematocrit, white blood cells, blood urea nitrogen, creatinine, serum electrolytes, and glucose. As pain subsides: Repeat serum amylase and lipase determinations; cautious refeeding; discontinue daily laboratory tests.

Near Discharge. Serum amylase and lipase determinations; abdominal ultrasonography (gallstones?); schedule studies to determine possible associated conditions (see pp. 1819–1820).

Necrotizing and Prolonged Pancreatitis

Definition

Mild pancreatitis is conventionally separated from severe and fulminant disease by the terms "edematous" and "hemorrhagic," respectively. Use of these terms is not advised, however, because the actual appearance of the pancreas usually is not known. Furthermore, the spread of peripancreatic necrosis and the appearance of infection, not hemorrhage, determine the severity of an attack. Prolonged pancreatitis means an extended hospital course caused by severe necrotizing pancreatitis itself, by localized complications, or by both. Patients with mild disease whose course is lengthy because of recurrences of pain and hyperamylasemia on refeeding have been discussed above.

Criteria of Severity and General Approach

The criteria listed in Table 97–4 provide a reliable guide for evaluating patients who on admission to hospital cannot easily be categorized by brief clinical assessment alone. Alcoholic patients who meet three or more criteria of Table 97–4, *A*, nonalcoholics fulfilling three or more criteria of Table 97–4, *B*, and all patients with hypotension or oliguria persisting after initial rehydration efforts should be admitted to an intensive care unit and should be managed jointly with an experienced surgeon. The proximate causes of early death with acute pancreatitis are cardiovascular collapse, probably mediated by circulating vasoactive substances; the type of adult respiratory distress syndrome (ARDS) typical of necrotizing pancreatitis; acute intra-abdominal hemorrhage; acute renal failure; and complicating acute cholangitis. Septic complications, pneumonitis, and—particularly—pancreatic abscess tend to occur after the first week of illness and account for late mortality. The progression of the intra-abdominal and retroperitoneal disease process should be defined by repeat CT scans. The patient with necrotizing pancreatitis requires close monitoring of central venous pressure, urine output, body weight, and temperature. Serial laboratory determinations should include arterial blood gases, serum bilirubin and calcium, blood glucose, and hematocrit. Urgent laparotomy is indicated when the diagnosis remains in doubt, and when acute cholecystitis progresses despite antiobiotic treatment. Common duct stones impacted in the ampulla of Vater should be removed by surgical or endoscopic means regardless of coexisting cholangitis. The choice of the procedure depends on the patient's overall condition and on the expertise available locally. These problems have been discussed on pages 1691 to 1729 and 1741 to 1761.

Management of Life-threatening Complications

Patients who are still hypotensive after adequate volume replacement require placement of a Swan-Ganz catheter and a trial of intravenously administered pressor substances, such as dopamine or isoproterenol hydrochloride (Isuprel). With persistent hypotension and clinical deterioration during the early course of acute pancreatitis, the issue arises whether removal of the pancreatic exudate or of the necrotic pancreas will benefit the patient. To this end, peritoneal lavage,[121] peritoneal dialysis,[126] sump drainage of the necrotic pancreas,[127] and partial to total pancreatectomy[128, 129] have been evaluated in largely uncontrolled clinical studies. Although no consensus exists regarding the merits of any one of these procedures, the preponderance of the evidence argues against their value in decreasing mortality rate or the frequency of subsequent pancreatic abscess formation.[130, 131] As a general rule, surgical intervention should be reserved for those situations in which secondary infection in or around the pancreas is known to be present, or, at least, strongly suspected. In summary, proper management of necrotizing pancreatitis is predicated on the capability of making difficult decisions promptly and of providing a high level of medical, radiologic, and surgical skills.

Additional supportive measures include intravenous calcium to combat severe hypocalcemia, correction of magnesium deficiency, found especially in malnourished alcoholic patients, and administration of small doses of regular insulin when marked hyperglycemia occurs.

Respiratory insufficiency (ARDS), manifested by pulmonary edema and hypoxemia, develops mainly in patients with associated hyperlipemia, marked hypocalcemia, and massive requirements for intravenous colloid. Chest radiographs show interstitial fluffy infiltrates; heart size and central venous pressure are normal. These patients require endotracheal intubation and controlled ventilation with application of positive end-expiratory pressure (PEEP). With early recognition and skilled treatment, the immediate prognosis of this complication is quite good.[37]

Renal insufficiency is a serious complication of severe pancreatitis, associated with a mortality rate of up to 50 per cent. Acute tubular necrosis may develop with prolonged hypovolemia and shock. Oliguria (urine volume less than 400 ml/day) ensues, but anuria is rare. Urinalysis reveals hematin casts, red cells, and protein; the urine osmolarity is approximately isotonic to plasma, and urine sodium concentration exceeds 30 mEq/L. Plasma blood urea nitrogen and creatinine concentrations rise steadily. Treatment is the same as for acute tubular necrosis arising in any setting: Volume and electrolyte intake are restricted; nitrogen should be administered mainly as intravenous essential amino acids, and hyperkalemia and metabolic acidosis need to be corrected. Hemodialysis or continued peritoneal dialysis may become necessary. A very similar type of acute renal failure may develop in the absence of hypotension.[132] The prognosis is good, and the pathogenesis probably involves selective renal vasoconstriction, which has been documented in acute pancreatitis.[38] Bilateral renal vein thrombosis and renal cortical necrosis are very rare but grave complications of necrotizing pancreatitis.

Nutritional Aspects

Caloric and amino nitrogen maintenance need to be provided when a complicated and prolonged course of the pancreatitis precludes feeding for more than 10 to 14 days. Nutritional deficits develop rapidly in the presence of fever and widespread tissue necrosis and with surgical operations. In patients undergoing laparotomy, a feeding jejunostomy should be constructed. In nonoperated patients, total parenteral nutrition should be instituted before nutritional and nitrogen depletion become advanced (see pp. 2007–2027). Either method of supplying calories and nitrogen should be viewed as supportive and not as primary therapy.[122]

Localized Complications

The widespread use of US and CT scanning revealed that intra- and peripancreatic fluid collections arise frequently during acute pancreatitis. These begin as areas of liquefaction necrosis containing tissue debris and pancreatic juice and may mature to well-defined pseudocysts surrounded by a capsule of granulation and fibrous tissue. Either type may become infected secondarily.

Pseudocysts

Pseudocysts, that is, fluid collections within or adjacent to the pancreas (Fig. 97–9), the lesser omental sac, the pararenal spaces, the mediastinum, or surrounding the spleen or liver, complicate the course of severe pancreatitis in up to 50 per cent of patients.[7] About 30 per cent of these present as a palpable mass. At least one half of these acute pseudocysts resolve spontaneously during the succeeding six weeks.[133] The treatment consists of an uneasy watch for signs of bacterial infection, bleeding into the cyst, and rapid expansion. Enlarging and infected acute pseudocysts require surgical intervention. In skilled hands, repeat percutaneous aspiration or catheter drainage under US or CT guidance has been reported to be safe and effective.[134]

Pseudocysts persisting for longer than six weeks are considered chronic and should then undergo a surgical drainage procedure, preferably internal.[135] Massive pancreatic ascites, a chemical peritonitis caused by pancreatic juice within the peritoneal cavity, is a rare occurrence. Both of these complications are more common with chronic pancreatitis and are discussed on pages 1855 to 1859.

Pancreatic Phlegmon

A pancreatic phlegmon is a mass of inflamed pancreas often containing patchy areas of necrosis (Fig. 97–8). This inflammatory process usually subsides within two weeks. Blood vessels in contact with the phlegmon may thrombose, causing infarction of the transverse colon or of the spleen, with eventual development of gastric fundic varices caused by splenic vein thrombosis. The management consists of close observations for the appearance of infection, thrombosis, or localized hemorrhage.[136]

Secondary Bacterial Infection; Pancreatic Abscess

Bacterial infection of devitalized tissue within and around the pancreas is the major life-threatening complication of acute pancreatitis, occurring in 3 to 7 per cent of patients.[106, 129] The infection may arise in an acute pseudocyst or in areas of peripancreatic and pancreatic necrosis, and it may present as diffuse bacterial inflammation or a discrete abscess. The occurrence of secondary bacterial infection is strongly correlated with the initial severity of the pancreatitis attack (see Table 97–4), and it usually is recognized two to four weeks after the onset of symptoms. The timely diagnosis of this complication remains a clinical challenge: (1) Fever greater than 101° F occurs in 85 per cent, increasing pain in 80 per cent, a palpable mass in 33 per cent, and leukocytosis greater than 10,000 cells/cu mm in nearly 100 per cent. Tachycardia, chills, and hypotension are common; the serum amylase level frequently does not rise again after the initial decline.[137] However, all of these features are frequently observed in necrotizing pancreatitis without infection.[129] (2) Typical radiographic (Fig. 97–4) and CT findings (Fig. 97–10) occasionally are present, but neither imaging method is capable of ruling out the presence of infection.[106, 129] (3) Blood cultures are neither consistently positive nor specific for the site of infection. Direct demonstration of bacteria on a gram-stain of a percutaneous aspirate obtained under sonographic or CT guidance represents the fastest, most reliable method for establishing or excluding the presence of bacterial infection.[131, 138]

Cultures of these aspirates show enteric microorganisms; frequently only a single species can be identified. Combining the results of two reported series, *Escherichia coli* is present in 51 per cent of cases; *Enterococcus* in 19 per cent; *Proteus, Klebsiella,* and *Pseudomonas* species in 10 per cent each; *Staphylococcus* in 18 per cent; *Streptococcus faecalis* in 7 per cent; and *Bacteroides* species in 6 per cent of cases.[106, 129]

The treatment consists of wide surgical debridement followed by percutaneous catheter drainage and lavage of the infected area. Attempts at percutaneous drainage guided by US or CT have been made, but the standard surgical approach is preferred.[106, 131] Antibiotic coverage should be instituted before the results of bacterial culture and microbial sensitivity are known. A combination of piperacillin, 3 gm every four hours, and gentamycin, 1.5 mg/kg body weight every eight hour intravenously, is recommended. The abscesses frequently are multiloculated. The need for reoperation arises in at least 25 per cent of patients owing to further abscess formation, acute bleeding into infected spaces, and involvement of adjacent organs. Local bacterial infection supervenes in a patient population with a high frequency of ARDS, renal failure, and hypotension. Thus, the mortality rate of this complication remains at 25 to 35 per cent.[106, 129]

Bleeding

Gastrointestinal bleeding during acute pancreatitis results from several mechanisms. First, diffuse mucosal bleeding from duodenal and antral erosions may be caused by inflammation spreading from the head of the pancreas. The rate of bleeding is usually slow, and surgical intervention is rarely necessary. Second, limited intra- and peripancreatic hemorrhage occurs in the course of severe pancreatitis with a frequency of approximately 6 per cent. Third, acute pseudocysts and abscesses may show either oozing of blood into the cavity or brisk bleeding arising from erosion of the splenic or gastroduodenal arteries. At times, the blood gains access to a pancreatic duct and can then be seen by the endoscopist to gush from the main pancreatic duct into the duodenum (hemosuccus pancreaticus; see Fig. 97–12). Finally, bleeding may signal the fistulization of an abscess or pseudocyst into colon, duodenum, stomach, or, very rarely, the esophagus or common bile duct. Massive bleeding in this setting constitutes an emergency that requires close and prompt collaboration between surgeon, radiologist, and gastroenterologist. The results of emergency upper gastrointestinal endoscopy and of selective mesenteric arteriography usually enable the surgeon to identify and treat the bleeding site successfully.

Involvement of Adjacent Organs

Spreading peripancreatic necrosis and infection may involve the duodenum, small bowel, and transverse colon (see Table 97–3). It may cause transient obstruction owing to edema, or it may progress to necrosis and perforation with fistula formation. Fibrotic obstruction may develop as a late consequence.[139] The spleen may become involved by direct extension or, secondarily, by splenic vein thrombosis, leading to splenic abscess, infarction or hemorrhage, or the formation of gastric fundic varices. Extension of peripancreatitic inflammation into the pleural space or mediastinum, (including, later, inflammatory pseudocysts) and extrinsic compression of the distal common bile duct were mentioned earlier in this chapter.

PREVENTION OF RECURRENCE

Once the patient has recovered from a first attack of acute pancreatitis, the chances of a recurrence in the next one to two years are between 25 and 60 per cent.[140] A systematic search for an associated and correctable condition must, therefore, be undertaken promptly so that repeated attacks may be prevented. A second important question to answer is whether the attack was a manifestation of chronic pancreatitis according to current definitions.[1, 2] In this regard, evidence of persistent structural or functional impairment of the gland signifies chronic disease. This may be manifested as persistent pain, as pancreatic calcifications seen on plain abdominal radiographs, by the appearance of diabetes mellitus during or shortly after the attack, or by clinical signs of malabsorption confirmed by quantitative stool fat analysis. A more detailed search for evidence of chronic pancreatitis by pancreatic function testing (see pp. 1786–1787 and 1845–1848), US, or CT scanning is not routinely indicated. Diagnostic ERCP may show unexpected evidence of chronic pancreatitis (Fig. 97–13); the indications for this procedure are stated on page 1837. When pancreatitis is associated with alcoholism (see pp. 1844–1845), hyperparathyroidism, or hyperlipemia, or when it is familial, it may safely be assumed to be of the chronic variety.

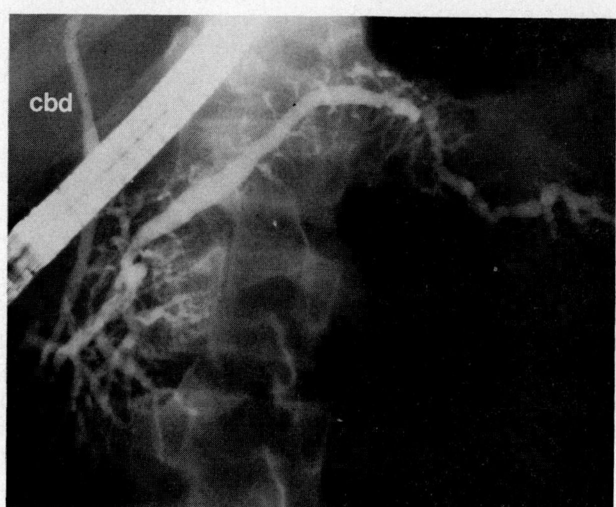

Figure 97–13. ERCP showing chronic pancreatitis. This nonalcoholic patient, who was investigated for four attacks of idiopathic recurrent pancreatitis, currently is asymptomatic. Mild ectasia and irregularity of main pancreatic duct and its lateral branches without obstruction to flow are seen. Common bile duct (cbd) is normal, as are manometry findings of the sphincter of Oddi. This case illustrates rare progression of acute to chronic pancreatitis. (Courtesy of Edward T. Stewart, M.D.)

During and shortly after recovery from the attack, serum calcium, triglyceride, and cholesterol levels should be measured. If calcium concentration is elevated, hyperparathyroidism should be suspected, particularly when the serum phosphate level is low and the alkaline phosphatase level is elevated. If triglyceride concentrations are elevated, with or without increased serum cholesterol level, a formal definition of the hyperlipemia should be established so that proper therapy can be instituted (see pp. 511 and 1821). The evidence for and against the possibility of medication-induced pancreatitis (Table 97–2) should be reviewed, although a challenge trial to confirm this cause is rarely justifiable on clinical and ethical grounds.

The Importance of Gallstones

The search for biliary tract calculi should begin before the patient is discharged from the hospital, because a second attack of pancreatitis will occur within a few weeks in about one third of patients who continue to harbor gallstones.[141] Real-time ultrasonography has replaced oral cholecystography as the method of choice for finding gallbladder stones, and it has replaced intravenous cholangiography for the diagnosis of choledocholithiasis and bile duct dilatation.[102] The recommended approach consists of US while the attack is subsiding. When gallstones are demonstrated, elective cholecystectomy with careful examination of the choledochus is performed during the same hospitalization without added surgical mortality or morbidity as compared with operating during a later, elective hospital admission.

"Idiopathic" Cases

Until recently, the conventional search for conditions associated with acute pancreatitis was considered to be complete at this stage, and the patient was assumed to have idiopathic pancreatitis when no associated condition had been identified. Current evidence indicates, however, that diagnostic ERCP examination, performed a few weeks after the first or second attack of acute pancreatitis, frequently reveals additional remediable causes of pancreatitis.

ERCP Examination

The results of diagnostic ERCP performed in several hundred patients considered to have idiopathic pancreatitis have been reported.[142, 143] Surgically remediable abnormalities were detected in 35 to 40 per cent of patients, excluding the diagnoses of sphincter spasm and fibrosis, which are discussed below. The list of conditions includes US-negative choledocholithiasis and cholelithiasis; obstruction of the pancreatic duct by calculi, strictures, small pseudocysts, annular pancreas, or carcinoma; and tumors of the papilla of Vater. Follow-up observations revealed that in most patients recurrences of pancreatitis were eliminated by operative correction of these lesions. Two additional identified abnormalities require special comment: choledochocele and pancreas divisum.

A choledochocele may be found in a few patients with recurrent acute pancreatitis. This structure represents a prolapse of the intramural segment of the common bile duct or the common channel into the duodenum and leads to intermittent obstruction to the flow of pancreatic juice or bile, or both (Color Fig. 97–14 [p. xlv], and Fig. 97–15). Its recognition requires special endoscopic and radiologic expertise. Endoscopic sphincterotomy or transduodenal surgical unroofing of this structure alleviates further pancreatitis attacks.[14]

A certain number of patients will be found to have pancreas divisum (see p. 1822); the clinical implications of this congenital abnormality remain controversial. However, there exist some reports of cessation of pancreatitis attacks after surgical[144] or endoscopic[145] decompression of the dorsal pancreatic duct. On the basis of limited clinical experience, the author's group currently recommends endoscopic dilation of the minor papilla, followed by placement of a stent catheter extending from dorsal duct to duodenal lumen in patients with recurrent acute pancreatitis, pancreas divisum, and no other identifiable causes.[145]

Spincter of Oddi Dysfunction

The sphincter of Oddi, including those circular muscle bundles that surround only the terminal portion of

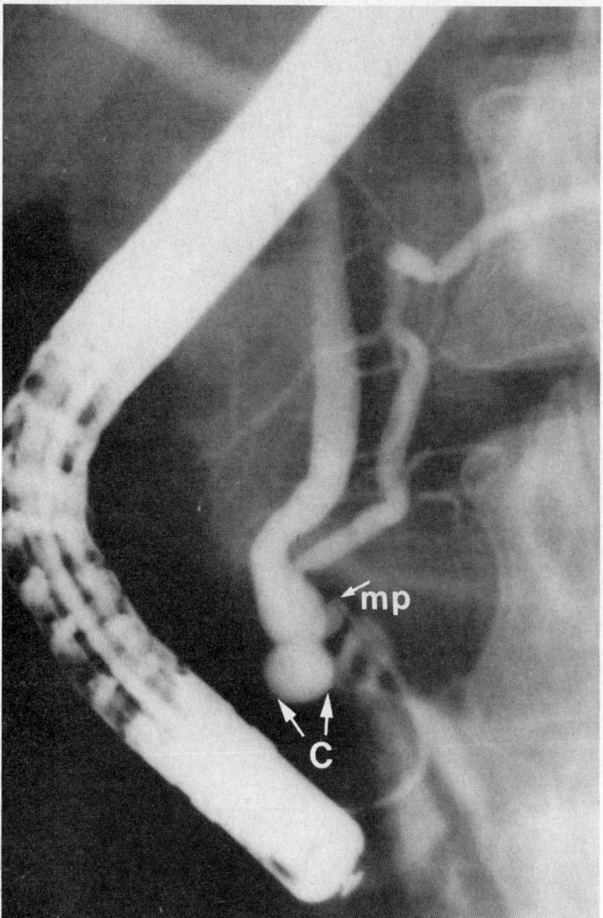

Figure 97–15. ERCP demonstration of choledochocele. The patient had recurrent attacks of acute pancreatitis. The cannula is seen entering the major papilla (mp). The choledochocele (C) within the duodenal wall is well demonstrated (same patient as in Fig. 97–14). There is a long common channel: pancreatic and common bile ducts join proximal to the choledochocele. No further pancreatitis attacks occurred after endoscopic incision of the choledochocele through the duodenal mucosa. (Courtesy of Joseph E. Gennen, M.D. and R. Venu, M.D.)

the main pancreatic duct, may cause increased resistance to pancreatic juice flow and, hence, pancreatitis. The causes of this type of sphincter dysfunction are (1) fixed stenosis owing to fibrosis or inflammation and (2) functional sphincter abnormalities, termed dyskinesia. The preoperative diagnosis of abnormal sphincter function rested on uncertain grounds until recently for the following reasons: (1) sphincter stenosis caused by preceding intraoperative trauma or by inflammation cannot reliably be assessed by examination of endoscopic biopsy samples.[146] (2) Pharmacologic testing with morphine sulfate, 10 mg, plus neostigmine sulfate, 1 mg, intramuscularly (Nardi test) results in elevation of serum amylase, lipase, and AST (SGOT) levels in many normal subjects. Thus, the Nardi test lacks specificity as well as sensitivity for the diagnosis of stenosis or hypercontractility (spasm) of the sphincter. (3) The inability of an experienced endoscopist to cannulate the papilla of Vater is an unreliable criterion

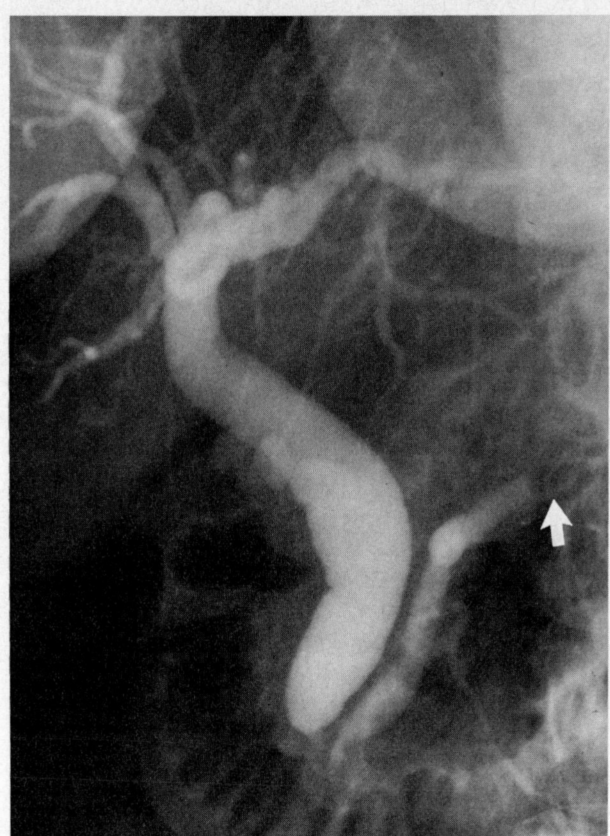

Figure 97–16. ERCP in papillary stenosis. Patient with three attacks of recurrent pancreatitis. The endoscope has been withdrawn, but a portion of the pancreatic duct is still filled; an air bubble is present in the duct at the junction of the pancreatic head and body *(arrow)*. Prior cholecystectomy had been performed. Mild dilatation of the common bile and of the pancreatic duct are seen; there was delayed drainage of contrast material from both duct systems. These findings are consistent with, but not diagnostic of, sphincter of Oddi dysfunction. (Courtesy of Edward T. Stewart, M.D.)

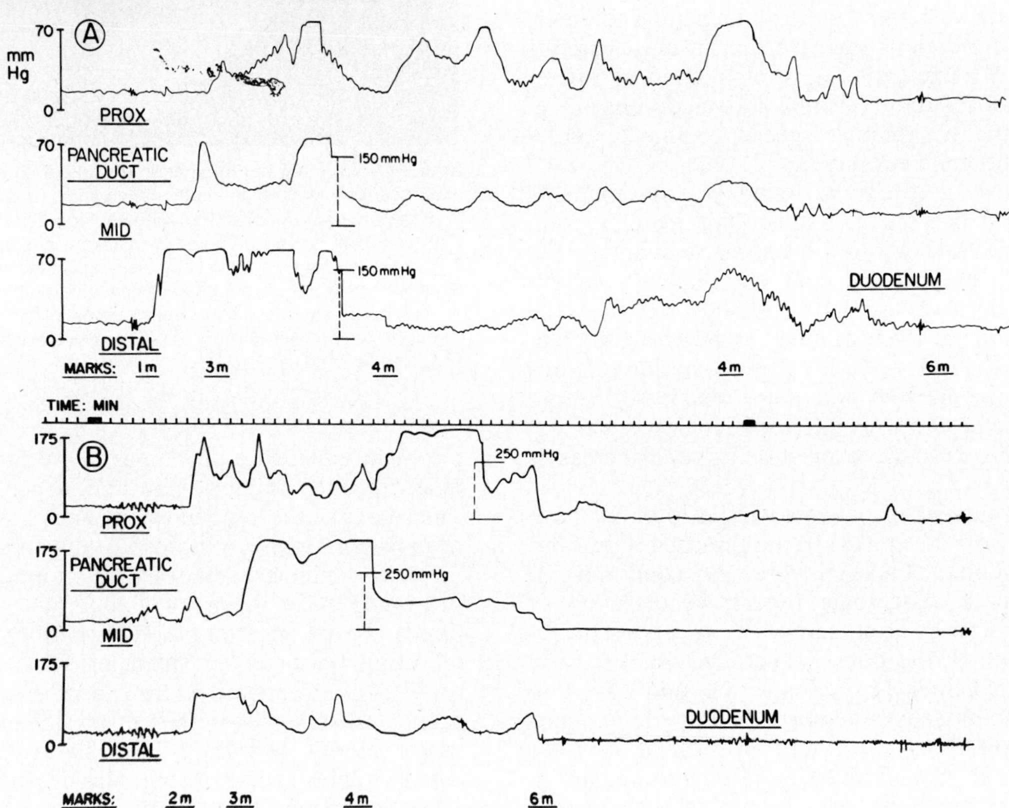

Figure 97–17. Manometric recordings of the sphincter of Oddi with triple-lumen catheter withdrawn from the pancreatic duct. *A*, Normal. *B*, Patient with recurrent acute pancreatitis, later cured by surgical sphincterotomy with septectomy. Three side-hole recording ports are spaced 2 mm apart in a 120-degree radial orientation. The lowest tracing (distal) is from the port closest to the duodenum. Ring marks on catheter are 2 mm apart. Mark 6m coincides with distal port. 4m: Endoscopist sees four rings; hence, the distal port is 4 mm inside the papilla. Pressures are in mm Hg above the duodenal lumen. Pancreatic duct: *A*, 8 mm Hg; *B*, 10 mm Hg: Normal. Sphincter: *A*, 25 mm Hg; *B*, 100 mm Hg. Patient has elevated sphincter of Oddi pressure indicative of dyskinesia. Note rhythmic pressure peaks in sphincter zone, best seen in the proximal traces.

for this diagnosis.[142] (4) "Delayed drainage" of contrast material and mild dilatation of the pancreatic duct system observed during ERCP (Fig. 97–16) lack precise definition because the volume injected, the intraductal pressures achieved, the counteracting pancreatic secretory pressure, and the effect of opiate analgesics on sphincter contraction cannot be quantitated during the standard diagnostic ERCP examination.

Sphincter of Oddi manometry, performed during ERCP, is becoming the standard tool for evaluating sphincter dysfunction.[19] This investigation is technically demanding and only a few centers currently are equipped to perform this study reliably. It is indicated when prior injection of contrast material into the pancreatic and bile duct systems revealed no organic lesion as the likely cause of acute pancreatitis. Briefly, the patient is sedated only with a benzodiazepine, and a three-lumen, water-perfused catheter is introduced through the papilla of Vater into the pancreatic duct. Under close endoscopic observation, the recording catheter is withdrawn into the duodenum in 2-mm steps. Pressures are recorded from the pancreatic duct and from the sphincter zone and are expressed in millimeters of mercury above duodenal lumen resting pressure. A normal tracing shows a pancreatic duct pressure of about 10 mm Hg; the sphincter baseline pressure is 15 to 25 mm Hg and exhibits superimposed phasic (3 to 5 cycles/minute) pressure peaks with an amplitude of 50 to 200 mm Hg (Fig. 97–17*A*).[147] The majority of these phasic waves show antegrade propagation through the sphincter zone.[148] Pharmacologic testing during sphincter manometry includes (1) intravenous injection of cholecystokinin octapeptide (CCK-OP), which causes phasic wave activity to disappear, and (2) inhalation of the smooth muscle relaxant amyl nitrite, which eliminates sphincter pressures unless an organic stenosis is present. Abnormal sphincter function has been identified in about 20 per cent of patients with "idiopathic" recurrent pancreatitis who had normal findings on diagnostic ERCP examination.[148, 149] The most common abnormality is an elevation of the sphincter resting pressure above 30 mm Hg (Fig. 97–17*B*). Surgical sphincteroplasty combined with septectomy[150] or endoscopic sphincterotomy of the pancreatic—not common bile duct—sphincter has eliminated further attacks of pancreatitis in a number of patients with sphincter of Oddi dysfunction as defined by manometry. Wider application and better standardization of sphincter of Oddi manometry in the diagnostic evaluation of pancreatic and biliary tract disorders is expected in the coming years.[149]

References

1. Sarner, M., and Cotton, P. B. Classification of pancreatitis. Gut 5:756, 1984.
2. Singer, M. V., Gyr, K., and Sarles, H. Editorial. Revised classification of pancreatitis. Gastroenterology *89*:683, 1985.
3. Sarles, H. Clinical classification. Bibl. Gastroenterol. 7:7, 1965.
4. Klöppel, G., Dreyer, T., Willemer, S., Kern, H. F., and Adler, G. Human acute pancreatitis: its pathogenesis in the light of immunocystochemical and ultrastructural findings in acinar cells. Virchows Arch. (Pathol. Anat.) *409*:791, 1986.
5. Adler, G., Rohr, G., and Kern, H. F. Alteration of membrane fusion as a cause of acute pancreatitis in the rat. Dig. Dis. Sci. *27*:993, 1982.
6. Isikoff, M. B., Hill, M. C., Silverstein, W., and Barkin, J. The clinical significance of acute pancreatitis hemorrhage. AJR *136*:679, 1981.
7. Siegelman, S. S., Copeland, B. E., Saba, G. P., Cameron, J. L., Sanders, R. C., and Zerhouni, E. A. CT of fluid collections associated with pancreatitis. AJR *134*:1121, 1980.
8. Karlan, M., McPherson, R. C., and Watman, R. N. Experimental production of pseudocysts of the pancreas of the dog. Surg. Gynecol. Obstet. *107*:221, 1958.
9. Gerle, R. D., Walker, C. A., Achord, J. L., and Weens, H. S. Osseous changes in chronic pancreatitis. Radiology *85*:330, 1965.
10. Gibson, T. J., Schumacher, H. R., Pascual, E., and Brighton, C. Arthropathy, skin and bone lesions in pancreatic disease. J. Rheumatol. *2*:7, 1975.
11. Lee, P. C., and Howard, J. M. Fat necrosis. Surg. Gynecol. Obstet. *148*:785, 1979.
12. Scarpelli, D. G. Fat necrosis of bone marrow in acute pancreatitis. Am. J. Pathol. *32*:1077, 1956.
13. McDermott, W. V., Jr., Bartlett, M. K., and Culver, P. J. Acute pancreatitis after prolonged fast and subsequent surfeit. N. Engl. J. Med. *254*:379, 1956.

13a. Ming-Chai, C.: Diet-induced pancreatitis in China. J. Clin. Gastroenterol *8*:611, 1987.

14. Venu, R. P., Geenen, J. E., Hogan, W. J., Dodds, W. J., Wilson, S. W., Stewart, E. T., and Soergel, K. H. Role of endoscopic retrograde cholangiopancreatography in the diagnosis and treatment of choledochocele. Gastroenterology *87*:1144, 1984.
15. Nakamura, K., Sarles, M., and Payan, H. Three-dimensional reconstruction of the pancreatic ducts in chronic pancreatitis. Gastroenterology *62*:942, 1972.
16. Lotveit, T., Aune, S., Johnsrud, N. K., and Osnes, M. The clinical significance of juxta-papillary duodenal diverticula. Scand. J. Gastroenterol. *10*(Suppl. *34*):22, 1975.
17. Farmer, R. C., Maslin, S. C., and Reber, H. A. Acute pancreatitis—role of duct permeability. Surg. Forum *34*:224, 1983.
18. Creutzfeldt, W., and Schmidt, H. Aetiology and pathogenesis of pancreatitis. Scand. J. Gastroenterol. *5*(Suppl. 6):47, 1970.
19. Geenen, J. E., Hogan, W. J., Dodds, W. J., Stewart, E. T., and Arndorfer, R. C. Intraluminal pressure recording from the human sphincter of Oddi. Gastroenterology *78*:317, 1980.
20. Opie, E. L. The etiology of acute hemorrhagic pancreatitis. Bull. Johns Hopkins Hosp. *12*:182, 1901.
21. Acosta, J. M., Rossi, R., and Ledesma, C. L. The usefulness of stool screening for diagnosing cholelithiasis in acute pancreatitis. A description of the technique. Am. J. Dig. Dis. *22*:168, 1977.
22. DiMagno, E. P., Shorter, R. G., and Taylor, W. F. Relationships between pancreaticobiliary ductal anatomy and pancreatic ductal parenchymal histology. Cancer *49*:361, 1982.
23. Anderson, M. C., Mehn, W. H., and Methad, H. L. An evaluation of the common channel as a factor in pancreatic or biliary disease. Ann. Surg. *151*:379, 1960.

23a. Scheele, G., Adler, G., and Kern, H.: Exocytosis occurs at the lateral plasma membrane of the pancreatic acinar cell during supramaximal secretagogue stimulation. Gastroenterology *92*:345, 1987.

24. Steer, M. L., Meldolesi, J., and Figarella, C. Pancreatitis: the role of lysosomes. Dig. Dis. Sci. *29*:934, 1984.
25. Pubols, M. H., Bartelt, D. C., and Greene, L. J. Trypsin inhibitor from human pancreas and pancreatic juice. J. Biol. Chem. *249*:2235, 1974.
26. Geokas, M. C., Rinderknecht, H., Swanson, V., and Haverback, B. J. The role of elastase in acute hemorrhagic pancreatitis in man. Lab. Invest. *19*:235, 1968.
27. Lasson, Å. Acute pancreatitis in man. A clinical and biochemical study of pathophysiology and treatment. Scand. J. Gastroenterol. *19*(Suppl. 99):1, 1984.
28. Borgström, A., and Lasson, Å. Trypsin-alpha$_1$-protease inhibitor complexes in serum and clinical course of acute pancreatitis. Scand. J. Gastroenterol. *19*:1119, 1984.

29. Allam, B. F., and Imrie, C. W. Serum ionized calcium in acute pancreatitis. Br. J. Surg. *64*:665, 1977.
30. Weir, G. C., Lesser, P. B., Drop, L. J., Fischer, J. E., and Warshaw, A. L. The hypocalcemia of acute pancreatitis. Ann. Intern. Med. *83*:185, 1975.
31. Robertson, G. M., Jr., Moore, E. W., Switz, D. M., Sizemore, G. W., and Estep, E. L. Inadequate parathyroid response in acute pancreatitis. N. Engl. J. Med. *294*:512, 1976.
32. Stewart, A. F., Longo, W., Kreutter, D., Jacob, R., and Burtis, W. J. Hypocalcemia associated with calcium-soap formation in a patient with a pancreatic fistula. N. Engl. J. Med. *315*:496, 1986.
33. Drew, S. I., Joffe, B., Vinik, A., Seftel, H., and Singer, F. The first 24 hours of acute pancreatitis. Changes in biochemical and endocrine homeostasis in patients with pancreatitis compared with those in control subjects undergoing stress for reasons other than pancreatitis. Am. J. Med. *64*:795, 1978.
34. Donowitz, M., Hendler, R., Spiro, H. M., Binder, H. J., and Felig, P. Glucagon secretion in acute and chronic pancreatitis. Ann. Intern. Med. *83*:778, 1975.
35. Murphy, D., Pack, A. I., and Imrie, C. W. The mechanism of arterial hypoxia occurring in acute pancreatitis. Q. J. Med. *49*:151, 1980.
36. Holter, J. F., Weiland, J. E., Pacht, E. R., Gadek, J. E., and Davis, W. B. Protein permeability in the adult respiratory distress syndrome: loss of size selectivity of the alveolar epithelium. J. Clin. Invest. *78*:1513, 1986.
37. Warshaw, A. L., Lesser, P. B., Rie, M., and Cullen, D. J. The pathogenesis of pulmonary edema in acute pancreatitis. Ann. Surg. *182*:505, 1975.
37a. Levy, M., Geller, R., and Hymovitch, S.: Renal failure in dogs with experimental acute pancreatitis: role of hypovolemia. Am. J. Physiol. *251*:F969, 1986.
38. Werner, M. H., Hayes, D. F., Lucas, C. E., and Rosenberg, I. K. Renal vasoconstriction in association with acute pancreatitis. Am. J. Surg. *127*:185, 1974.
39. Meier, P. B., and Levitt, M. D. Urine protein excretion in acute pancreatitis. J. Lab. Clin. Med. *108*:628, 1986.
40. Beger, H. G., Bittner, R., Büchler, M., Hess, W., and Schmitz, J. E. Hemodynamic data pattern in patients with acute pancreatitis. Gastroenterology *90*:74, 1986.
41. Goldstein, I. M., Cala, D., Radin, A., Kaplan, H. B., Horn, J., and Ranson, J. Evidence of complement catabolism in acute pancreatitis. Am. J. Med. Sci. *275*:257, 1978.
42. Howard, M. J.: Gallstone pancreatitis. *In* Howard, J. M., Jordan, G. L., Jr., and Reber, H. A. (eds.): Surgical Diseases of the Pancreas. Philadelphia, Lea & Febiger, 1987, p. 269.
43. Zahor, Z., Sternby, N. H., Kagan, A., Uemura, K., Vanecek, R., and Vichert, A. M. Frequency of cholelithiasis in Prague and Malmo. Scand. J. Gastroenterol. *9*:3, 1974.
44. Moreau, J. A., Zinsmeister, A. R., Melton, J. L., and DiMagno, E. P. Gallstone pancreatitis and the effect of cholecystectomy: a population-based cohort study. Mayo Clin. Proc., June, 1988 (in press).
45. Medical Research Council Multicentre Trial of Glucagon and Aprotinin. Death from acute pancreatitis. Lancet *2*:632, 1977.
46. Block, M. A., and Priest, R. J. Acute pancreatitis related to grossly minute stones in radiographically normal gallbladder. Am. J. Dig. Dis. *12*:934, 1967.
47. Mallory, A., and Kern, F., Jr. Drug-induced pancreatitis: a critical review. Gastroenterology *78*:813, 1980.
48. Dobrilla, G., Felder, M., and Chilovi, F. Medication-induced acute pancreatitis. Schweiz. Med. Wschr. *115*:850, 1985.
49. Bennett, I. L., Jr., Cary, F. H., Mitchell, G. L., Jr., and Cooper, M. N. Acute methyl alcohol poisoning: a review based on experience in an outbreak of 323 cases. Medicine *32*:431, 1953.
50. Dressel, T. D., Goodale, R. L., Arneson, M. A., and Borner, J. W. Pancreatitis as a complication of anticholinesterase insecticide intoxication. Ann. Surg. *189*:199, 1978.
51. Haber, C. J., Meltzer, S. J., Present, D. H., and Korelitz, B. I. Nature and course of pancreatitis caused by 6-mercaptopurine in the treatment of inflammatory bowel disease. Gastroenterology *91*:982, 1986.
52. Lashner, B. A., Kirsner, J. B., and Hanauer, S. B. Acute pancreatitis associated with high-concentration lipid emulsion during total parenteral nutrition therapy for Crohn's disease. Gastroenterology *90*:1039, 1986.
53. Corfield, A. P., Cooper, M. J., and Williamson, R. C. N. Acute pancreatitis: a lethal disease of increasing incidence. Gut *26*:724, 1985.
54. Herfort, K., Sobra, J., Fric, P., and Heyrovsky, A. Familial hyperlipoproteinemia and exocrine pancreas. Scand. J. Gastroenterol. *6*:139, 1971.
55. Cameron, J. L., Capuzzi, D. M., Zuidema, G. D., and Margolis, S. Acute pancreatitis with hyperlipemia. Evidence for a persistent defect in lipid metabolism. Am. J. Med. *56*:482, 1974.
56. Cameron, J. L., Zuidema, G. D., and Margolis, S. A pathogenesis of alcoholic pancreatitis. Surgery *77*:754, 1975.
57. Editorial. Pancreatitis from oral contraceptives. Br. Med. J. *3*:688, 1973.
58. Levy, R. I., Morgenroth, J., and Rifkind, B. M. Treatment of hyperlipidemia. N. Engl. J. Med. *20*:1295, 1974.
59. Fjøsne, U., Waldum, H. L., Romslo, I., Kleveland, P. M., Johnsen, H., and Engebretsen, L. F. Amylase, pancreatic isoamylase and lipase in serum before and after endoscopic pancreatography. Acta Med. Scand. *219*:301, 1986.
60. Bilbao, M. K., Dotter, C. T., Lee, T. G., and Katon, R. M. Complications of endoscopic retrograde cholangiopancreatography (ERCP). Gastroenterology *70*:314, 1976.
61. Brandes, J.-W., Scheffer, B., Lorenz-Meyer, H., Korst, H. A., and Littmann, K.-P. ERCP: complications and prophylaxis. A controlled study. Endoscopy *13*:27, 1981.
62. Northrup, W. F., III, and Simmons, R. L. Pancreatic trauma. A review. Surgery *71*:27, 1972.
63. Bess, M. A., Edis, A. J., and van Heerden, J. A. Hyperparathyroidism and pancreatitis. Chance or a causal association? JAMA *243*:246, 1980.
64. Hochgelernt, E. L., and David, D. S. Acute pancreatitis secondary to calcium infusion in a dialysis patient. Arch. Surg. *108*:218, 1974.
65. Banks, P. A. Pancreatitis. New York, Plenum Medical Book Company, 1979.
66. Sigfusson, B. F., Wehlin, L., and Lindström, C. G. Variants of pancreatic duct system of importance in endoscopic retrograde cholangiopancreatography. Acta Radiol. Diagn. *24*:113, 1983.
67. Cotton, P. B. Pancreas divisum—curiosity or culprit? (Editorial.) Gastroenterology *89*:1431, 1985.
68. Delhaye, M., Engelholm, L., and Cremer, M. Pancreas divisum: congenital anatomic variant or anomaly? Contribution of endoscopic retrograde dorsal pancreatography. Gastroenterology *89*:951, 1985.
69. Corrodi, P., Knoblauch, M., Binswanger, U., Scholzel, E., and Largiader, F. Pancreatitis after renal transplantation. Gut *16*:285, 1975.
70. Aziz, S., Bergdahl, L., Baldwin, J. C., Weiss, L. M., Jamieson, S. W., Oyer, P. E., Stinson, E. B., and Shumway, N. E. Pancreatitis after cardiac and cardiopulmonary transplantation. Surgery *97*:653, 1985.
71. Rutsky, E. A., Robards, M., Van Dyke, J. A., and Bostand, S. G. Acute pancreatitis in patients with end-stage renal disease without transplantation. Arch. Intern. Med. *146*:1741, 1986.
72. Horstkotte, H., Freise, J., Gebel, M., Burdelski, M., Rumpf, K. D., and Schmidt, F. W. Hereditäre chronisch-calcifizierende Pankreatitis. Dtsch. Med. Wschr. *110*:753, 1985.
73. Bartholomew, C. Acute scorpion pancreatitis in Trinidad. Br. Med. J. *1*:666, 1970.
74. Gallagher, S., Sankaran, H., and Williams, J. A. Mechanisms of scorpion toxin-induced enzyme secretion in rat pancreas. Gastroenterology *80*:970, 1981.
75. Haas, G. S., Warshaw, A. L., Daggett, W. M., and Aretz, H. T. Acute pancreatitis after cardiopulmonary bypass. Am. J. Surg. *149*:508, 1985.
76. Feldstein, J. D., Johnson, F. R., Kallick, C. A., and Doolas, A. Acute hemorrhagic pancreatitis due to mumps. Ann. Surg. *180*:85, 1974.
77. O'Sullivan, J. N., Nobrega, F. T., Morlock, C. G., Brown, A.

L., Jr., and Bartholomew, L. G. Acute and chronic pancreatitis in Rochester, Minnesota, 1940–1969. Gastroenterology *62*:373, 1972.

78. The Copenhagen Pancreatitis Study Group. An interim report from a prospective epidemiological multicenter study. Scand. J. Gastroenterol. *16*:305, 1981.
79. Toffler, A. H., and Spiro, H. M. Shock or coma as the predominant manifestation of painless acute pancreatitis. Ann. Intern. Med. *57*:655, 1962.
80. Roseman, D. M., Kowlessar, O. D., and Sleisenger, M. H. Pulmonary manifestations of pancreatitis. N. Engl. J. Med. *263*:294, 1960.
81. Ranson, J. H. C., Rifkind, K. M., and Turner, J. W. Prognostic signs and nonoperative peritoneal lavage in acute pancreatitis. Surg. Gynecol. Obstet. *143*:209, 1976.
82. Ranson, J. H. C., and Pasternack, B. S. Statistical methods for quantifying the severity of clinical acute pancreatitis. J. Surg. Res. *22*:79, 1977.
83. Osborne, D. H., Imrie, C. W., and Carter, D. C. Biliary surgery in the same admission for gallstone-associated pancreatitis. Br. J. Surg. *68*:758, 1981.
84. Eckfeldt, J. H., Kolars, J. C., Elson, M. K., Shafer, R. B., and Levitt, M. D. Serum tests for pancreatitis in patients with abdominal pain. Arch. Pathol. Lab. Med. *109*:316, 1985.
85. Kolars, J. C., Ellis, C. J., and Levitt, M. D. Comparison of serum amylase pancreatic isoamylase and lipase in patients with hyperamylasemia. Dig. Dis. Sci. *29*:289, 1984.
86. Peterson, L. M., and Brooks, J. R. Lethal pancreatitis: a diagnostic dilemma. Am. J. Surg. *137*:491, 1979.
87. Dickson, A. P., O'Neill, J., and Imrie, C. W. Hyperlipidaemia, alcohol abuse and acute pancreatitis. Br. J. Surg. *71*:685, 1984.
88. Johnson, S. G., Ellis, C. J., and Levitt, M. D. Mechanism of increased renal clearance of amylase/creatinine in acute pancreatitis. N. Engl. J. Med. *295*:1214, 1976.
89. Levitt, M. D., Duane, W. C., and Cooperband, S. R. Study of macroamylase complexes. J. Lab. Clin. Med. *80*:414, 1972.
90. Tietz, N. W., Huang, W. Y., Rauh, D. F., and Shuey, D. F. Laboratory tests in the differential diagnosis of hyperamylasemia. Clin. Chem. *32*:301, 1986.
91. Eckfeldt, J. H., Leatherman, J. W., and Levitt, M. D. High prevalence of hyperamylasemia in patients with acidemia. Ann. Intern. Med. *104*:362, 1986.
92. Kameya, S., Hayakawa, T., Kameya, A., and Watanabe, T. Hyperamylasemia in patients at an intensive care unit. J. Clin. Gastroenterol. *8*:438, 1986.
93. Bloch, R. S., Weaver, D. W., Bouwman, D. L., and Berger, G. Alcohol-induced salivary hyperamylasemia. J. Surg. Res. *36*:389, 1984.
94. McClain, C. J., Humphries, L., Adams, L., Eckfeldt, J., and Levitt, M. Hyperamylasemia in patients with eating disorders. Gastroenterology *90*:1541, 1986.

94a. Pellethier, G., Nee, N., Brivet, M., Etienne, J-P., and Lemonnier, A.: Upper gastrointestinal endoscopy. An unrecognized cause of hyperamylasemia. Dig. Dis. Sci. *32*:254, 1987.

95. Levitt, M. D. Clinical use of amylase clearance and isoamylase measurements. Mayo Clin. Proc. *54*:428, 1979.
96. Steinberg, W. M., Goldstein, S. S., Davis, N. D., Shamma'a, J., and Anderson, K. Diagnostic assays in acute pancreatitis. A study of sensitivity and specificity. Ann. Intern. Med. *102*:576, 1985.
97. Lesser, P. B., and Warshaw, A. L. Differentiation of pancreatitis from common bile duct obstruction with hyperamylasemia. Gastroenterology *68*:636, 1975.
98. Goodman, A. J., Neoptolemos, J. P., Carr-Locke, D. L., Finlay, D. B. L., and Fossard, D. P. Detection of gallstones after acute pancreatitis. Gut *26*:125, 1985.
99. Bank, S., Barbezat, G. O., Marks, I. N., and Silber, W. Methaemalbuminaemia in acute abdominal emergencies. Br. Med. J. *2*:86, 1968.
100. Büchler, M., Malfertheiner, P., Uhl, W., and Beger, H. G. A new staging system in patients with acute pancreatitis (Abstract). Gastroenterology *90*:1361, 1986.
101. Woodard, S., Kelvin, F. M., Rice, R. P., and Thompson, W. M. Pancreatic abscess: importance of conventional radiology. AJR *136*:871, 1981.
102. Cooperberg, P. L., and Burhenne, H. J. Real-time ultrasonography. Diagnostic technique of choice in calculus gallbladder disease. N. Engl. J. Med. *302*:1277, 1980.
103. Van Dyke, J. A., Stanley, R. J., and Berland, L. L. Diagnosis and treatment. Pancreatic imaging. Ann. Intern. Med. *102*:212, 1985.
104. Silverstein, W., Isikoff, M. B., Hill, M. C., and Barkin, J. Diagnostic imaging of acute pancreatitis: prospective study using CT and sonography. AJR *137*:497, 1981.
105. Block, S., Maier, W., Bittner, R., Büchler, M., Malfertheiner, P., and Beger, H. G. Identification of pancreas necrosis in severe acute pancreatitis: imaging procedures versus clinical staging. Gut *27*:1035, 1986.
106. Warshaw, A. L., and Gongliang, J. Improved survival in 45 patients with pancreatic abscess. Ann. Surg. *202*:408, 1985.
107. Stark, D. D., Moss, A. A., Goldberg, H. I., Davis, P. L., and Federle, M. P. Magnetic resonance and CT of the normal and diseased pancreas. A comparative study. Radiology *150*:153, 1984.
108. Steckman, M. L., Dooley, M. C., Jaques, P. F., and Powell, D. W. Major gastrointestinal hemorrhage from peripancreatic blood vessels in pancreatitis. Treatment by embolotherapy. Dig. Dis. Sci. *29*:486, 1984.
109. Freitas, J. E., and Gulati, R. M. Rapid evaluation of acute abdominal pain by hepatobiliary scanning. JAMA *244*:1585, 1980.
110. Safrany, L., and Cotton, P. B. A preliminary report: urgent duodenoscopic sphincterotomy for acute gallstone pancreatitis. Surgery *89*:424, 1981.
111. Armstrong, C. P., Taylor, T. V., Jeacock, J., and Lucas, S. The biliary tract in patients with acute gallstone pancreatitis. Br. J. Surg. *72*:551, 1985.
112. Sarr, M. G., Sanfey, H., and Cameron, J. L. Prospective randomized trial of nasogastric suction in patients with acute pancreatitis. Surgery *100*:500, 1986.
113. Regan, P. T., Malagelada, J. R., Go, V. L. W., Wolf, A. M., and DiMagno, E. P. A prospective study of the antisecretory and therapeutic effects of cimetidine and glucagon in human pancreatitis. Mayo Clin. Proc. *56*:449, 1981.
114. Soergel, K. H. Medical treatment of acute pancreatitis. What is the evidence? Gastroenterology *74*:620, 1978.
115. Medical Research Council Multicentre Trial. Morbidity of acute pancreatitis: the effect of aprotinin and glucagon. Gut *21*:334, 1980.
116. Balldin, G., Borgström, A., Genell, S., and Ohlsson, K. The effect of peritoneal lavage and aprotinin in the treatment of severe acute pancreatitis. Res. Exp. Med. *183*:203, 1983.
117. Goebell, H., Amman, R., Herfath, C., Horn, J., Hotz, J., Knoblauch, M., Schmid, M., Jaeger, M., Akovbiantz, A., Linder, E., Abt, K., Nuesch, E., and Barth, E. A double-blind trial of synthetic salmon calcitonin in the treatment of acute pancreatitis. Scand. J. Gastroenterol. *14*:881, 1979.
118. Howes, R., Zuidema, G. D., and Cameron, J. L. Evaluation of prophylactic antibiotics in acute pancreatitis. J. Surg. Res. *18*:197, 1975.
119. Ebbehøj, N., Friis, J., Srendsen, L. B., Bülow, S., and Madsen, P. Indomethacin treatment of acute pancreatitis. A controlled double-blind trial. Scand. J. Gastroenterol. *20*:798, 1985.
120. Tykkä, H. T., Vaittinen, E. J., Mahlberg, K. L., Railo, J. E., Pantzar, P. J., Sarna, S., and Tallberg, T. A randomized double-blind study using $CaNa_2$ EDTA, a phospholipase A_2 inhibitor, in the management of human acute pancreatitis. Scand. J. Gastroenterol. *20*:5, 1985.
121. Mayer, A. D., McMahoy, M. J., Corfield, A. P., Cooper, M. J., Williamson, R. C. N., Dickson, A. P., Shearer, M. G., and Imrie, C. W. Controlled clinical trial of peritoneal lavage for the treatment of severe acute pancreatitis. N. Engl. J. Med. *312*:399, 1985.
122. Goodgame, J. T., and Fischer, J. E. Parenteral nutrition in the treatment of acute pancreatitis. Effects on complications and mortality. Ann. Surg. *186*:651, 1977.
123. Leuschner, U., Ueberla, K., and Usadel, K.-H.: Somatostatin in der Therapie der akuten Pankreatitis. Z. Gastroenterologie, Verh. Bd. *22*:138, 1987.

123a. Leese, T., Holliday, M., Heath, D., Hunt, D., Scott, J.,

Withers, D., Brett, M. C. A., and Hall, A. W.: Preliminary results of a multicentre prospective trial of fresh frozen plasma in the treatment of acute pancreatitis. (Abstract.) Gut *27*:A 1279, 1986.

124. DiMagno, E. P., and Go, V. L. W. Intraluminal postabsorptive effects of amino acids on pancreatic enzyme secretion. J. Lab. Clin. Med. *82*:241, 1973.
125. Niederau, C., Sonnenberg, A., and Erckenbrecht, J. Effects of intravenous infusion of amino acids, fat or glucose on unstimulated pancreatic secretion in healthy humans. Dig. Dis. Sci. *30*:445, 1985.
126. Stone, H. H., and Fabian, T C. Peritoneal dialysis in the treatment of acute alcoholic pancreatitis. Surg. Gynecol. Obstet. *150*:878, 1980.
127. Waterman, N. G., Walsky, R., Kasdan, M. L., and Abrams, B. L. The treatment of acute hemorrhagic pancreatitis by sump drainage. Surg. Gynecol. Obstet. *126*:963, 1968.
128. Nordback, I. H., and Auvinen, O. A. Long-term results after pancreas resection for acute necrotizing pancreatitis. Br. J. Surg. *72*:687, 1985.
129. Beger, H. G., Bittner, R., Block, S., and Buchler, M. Bacterial contamination of pancreatic necrosis. A prospective clinical study. Gastroenterology *91*:433, 1986.
130. Pellegrini, C. A. The treatment of acute pancreatitis: a continuing challenge. (Editorial.) N. Engl. J. Med. *312*:436, 1985.
131. Reber, H. A. Surgical intervention in necrotizing pancreatitis. (Editorial.) Gastroenterology *91*:479, 1986.
132. Goldstein, D. A., Llach, F., and Massry, S. G. Acute renal failure in patients with acute pancreatitis. Arch. Intern. Med. *136*:1363, 1976.
133. Bradley, L. E., III, Gonzalez, A. C., and Clements, J. L., Jr. Acute pancreatitis pseudocysts. Incidence and implications. Ann. Surg. *184*:734, 1976.
134. MacErlean, D. P., Bryan, P. J., and Murphy, J. J. Pancreatic pseudocyst: management by ultrasonically guided aspiration. Gastrointest. Radiol. *5*:255, 1980.
135. Warshaw, A. L., and Rattner, D. W. Timing of surgical drainage for pancreatic pseudocyst. Clinical and chemical criteria. Ann. Surg. *202*:720, 1985.
136. Sostre, C. F., Flournoy, J. G., Bova, J. G., Goldstein, H. M., and Schenker, S. Pancreatic phlegmon. Clinical features and course. Dig. Dis. Sci. *30*:918, 1985.
137. Cramer, S. J., Tan, E. G. C., Warren, K. W., and Braasch, J. W. Pancreatic abscess. A critical analysis of 113 cases. Am. J. Surg. *129*:426, 1975.
138. Gerzof, S. G., Banks, P. A., Robbins, A. H., Johnson, W. C., Speckler, S. J., Wetzner, S. M., Snider, J. M., Langevin, R. E., and Jay, M. E.: Early diagnosis of pancreatic infection by computed tomography–guided aspiration. Gastroenterology *93*:1315, 1987.
139. Bradley, E. L., III Enteropathies. *In* Bradley, E. L., III (ed.). Complications of Pancreatitis. Medical and Surgical Management. Philadelphia, W. B. Saunders Company, 1982, p. 265.
140. Trapnell, J. E., and Ducan, E. H. L. Patterns of incidence in acute pancreatitis. Br. Med. J. *2*:179, 1975.
141. Ranson, J. H. C. The timing of biliary surgery in acute pancreatitis. Ann. Surg. *189*:654, 1979.
142. Cotton, P. B., and Beales, J. S. M. Endoscopic pancreatography in management of relapsing acute pancreatitis. Br. Med. J. *1*:608, 1974.
143. Feller, E. R. Endoscopic retrograde cholangiopancreatography in the diagnosis of unexplained pancreatitis. Arch. Intern. Med. *144*:1797, 1984.
144. Warshaw, A. L., Richter, J. M., and Schapiro, R. H. The cause and treatment of pancreatitis associated with pancreatic divisum. Ann. Surg. *198*:443, 1983.
145. Satterfield, S. T., Geenen, J. E., Hogan, W. J., Venu, R. P., Dodds, W. J., Johnson, G. K., and McKinney, J. Clinical experience in 82 patients with pancreas divisum: preliminary results of manometry and endoscopic therapy (Abstract). Gastroenterology *88*:1572, 1985.
146. Stolte, M. Some aspects of the anatomy and pathology of the papilla of Vater. *In* Classen, M., Geenen, J. E., and Kawai, K. (eds.). The Papilla of Vater and Its Diseases. New York, Gerhard Witzstrock, 1979.
147. Bar-Meir, S., Geenen, J. E., Hogan, W. J., Dodds, W. J., Stewart, E. T., and Arndorfer, R. C. Biliary and pancreatic duct pressures measured by ERCP manometry in patients with suspected papillary stenosis. Dig. Dis. Sci. *24*:209, 1979.
148. Toouli, J., Roberts-Thomson, I. C., Dent, J., and Lee, J. Sphincter of Oddi motility disorders in patients with idiopathic recurrent pancreatitis. Br. J. Surg. *72*:859, 1985.
149. Venu, R. P., Geenen, J. E., Hogan, W. J., Stewart, E. T., Dodds, W. J., and Johnson, G. K. Idiopathic recurrent pancreatitis (IRP): diagnostic role of ERCP and sphincter of Oddi manometry. Gastrointest. Endosc. *31*:141, 1985.
150. Moody, F. G., Berenson, M. M., and McCloskey, D. Transampullary septectomy for postcholecystectomy pain. Ann. Surg. *186*:415, 1977.

98

Chronic Pancreatitis

JAMES H. GRENDELL
JOHN P. CELLO

As the problem of chronic alcoholism has grown in the Western world, so has the frequency of chronic, irreversible damage to the pancreas. A multiplicity of causes may lead to chronic pancreatitis; however, chronic alcohol abuse appears to be the etiologic basis in more than 90 per cent of adult patients. Although recognition of the disease may be delayed in the minority of patients who are relatively pain-free, the vast majority have a clinical course that is readily recognizable; that is, one of progressive damage to the gland marked by episodes of pain with or without incontrovertible evidence of acute inflammation. Owing to the degree of disability and discomfort, which may extend over a period of years, caring for patients with chronic pancreatitis is often difficult.

Because chronic pancreatitis results in permanent destruction of pancreatic tissue, exocrine or endocrine pancreatic insufficiency, or both, often follows. However, owing to the tremendous reserve of pancreatic function, insufficiency may be subclinical and pancreatic function tests may be necessary to demonstrate it. Regardless of the degree of insufficiency, most patients with chronic pancreatitis generally have continuous or intermittent abdominal pain. It is this symptom more than any other that brings an individual to the physician for relief. Unrelenting pain is also the principal indication for surgical intervention. About five per cent of patients with chronic pancreatitis have no pain yet may require treatment for malabsorption or diabetes.

DEFINITION

Several recent international meetings have attempted to refine the definition of chronic pancreatitis.[1–3] The revised Marseilles classification defines chronic pancreatitis clinically as a disease characterized by recurrent or persisting abdominal pain with evidence in some patients of pancreatic exocrine or endocrine insufficiency in the absence of pain. On the basis of morphology, chronic pancreatitis is characterized by irregular sclerosis of the gland with inflammation and destruction of exocrine tissue in a pattern that may be focal, segmental, or diffuse. In addition, stricturing and dilatation of the pancreatic ducts may be present, as well as intraductal protein plugs and calculi (stones). Endocrine pancreatic tissue (islets of Langerhans) tends to be more slowly destroyed than exocrine (acinar) tissue. Although these morphologic changes appear to be progressive and irreversible, the revised Marseilles classification recognizes a particular subset of chronic pancreatitis, termed obstructive chronic pancreatitis, in which pancreatic function and morphologic changes may improve after relief of obstruction of the main pancreatic duct.[4]

States of pancreatic insufficiency as a consequence of surgical pancreatectomy, hereditary isolated pancreatic enzyme deficiencies, cystic fibrosis, and the syndrome of congenital pancreatic insufficiency combined with neutropenia (see pp. 1765–1777 and 1789–1814), although manifested by impaired pancreatic function, are considered separate diagnostic entities. Pancreatic fibrosis and atrophy without evident inflammation are considered under the heading of chronic pancreatitis primarily because it may be impossible to document the morphologic evolution of pancreatic disease in clinical practice.

Symptomatic episodes during the course of chronic pancreatitis, particularly that associated with alcohol, may be clinically indistinguishable from acute pancreatitis. Thus, patients with chronic pancreatitis may suffer fatal pancreatic necrosis, hemorrhage, acute pseudocysts, and pancreatic abscess. Except for pseudocysts, these acute complications are considered on pages 1814 to 1842.

PATHOLOGY

The pathologic changes of chronic pancreatitis explain many, but not all, of its clinical features, particularly those of endocrine and exocrine insufficiency. The histopathologic changes consist mainly of irregularly distributed fibrosis, reduced number and size of acini and islets of Langerhans, and variable obstruction of pancreatic ducts of all sizes. Proliferating fibroblasts, collagen fibers, and interspersed collections of lymphocytes and plasma cells surround single or small groups of pancreatic acini (intralobular fibrosis). The duct system may show fibrotic strictures, squamous metaplasia of the epithelial lining, and minute disruption surrounded by areas of necrotic debris or cystic spaces. Three-dimensional reconstruction of the pancreatic ducts in chronic pancreatitis associated with alcoholism[5] suggests the following sequence of events: protein precipitation in lobular and interlobular ducts as the initial manifestation, leading to formation of plugs that calcify by surface accretion; the development of foci of acinar ectasia, acinar atrophy, chronic inflammation, and fibrosis in areas of ductal obstruction; and the appearance of concentric, lamellar protein precipitates in the major pancreatic ducts, which subsequently also calcify. The presence of these concretions, together with stricture formation owing to periductal fibrosis, eventually leads to the duct ectasia recognized during pancreatography. By contrast, extrinsic obstruction of the main pancreatic duct at or near the duodenal papilla by a tumor leads to more uniform and less pronounced dilatation of the ductal system with sparing of the minor branches; protein plugs are rarely formed, and the foci of parenchymal destruction are more evenly distributed throughout the gland.[5] The calcified plugs or calculi contain mainly calcium carbonate, whereas the less frequent focal calcifications of parenchymal and intervening adipose tissue consist of hydroxyapatite, a mixture of calcium phosphate and calcium carbonate.[6] The chronic inflammatory and fibrotic process may extend to adjacent organs, causing constriction of the proximal duodenum, antrum, common bile duct, or transverse colon.

Although the role of repeated bouts of acute inflammation and necrosis in the development of chronic pancreatitis has not been investigated extensively, it is generally believed that chronic pancreatitis is primarily the result of an insidious sclerosing process, analogous to the pathogenesis of hepatic cirrhosis. In one autopsy series,[7] histologic features suggestive of chronic pancreatitis were found in 52 of 394 consecutive autopsies on adults, whereas chronic pancreatitis had been diagnosed clinically in only two of these persons. This suggests that chronic inflammation and fibrosis of the pancreas commonly are occult processes.

Rare reports exist of primary atrophy and lipomatosis of the pancreas in adults presenting with pancreatogenous steatorrhea or diabetes mellitus, or both.[8] This condition probably represents an end stage of painless chronic pancreatitis rather than a separate disease entity, particularly because some of these patients are alcohol abusers.[9]

HISTORY AND INCIDENCE

The first comprehensive description of chronic pancreatitis was published by Comfort and his associates at the Mayo Clinic in 1946;[10] in this report they emphasized its association with long-standing heavy alcohol intake and the chronic relapsing nature of the disease. The dominant role of alcohol intake in the pathogenesis and prevalence of chronic pancreatitis was documented in a series of epidemiologic studies conducted by Sarles' group in Marseilles, France.[11]

Few reliable studies have been performed concerning the incidence of chronic pancreatitis. During 1978 and 1979, the incidence of hospitalization for chronic pancreatitis in Copenhagen, Denmark, was 4.0 per 100,000 inhabitants aged 20 years old or older.[12] The male-to-female ratio was 3:1, and the overall median age at onset was 49 years. An earlier study estimating the annual incidence of chronic pancreatitis in Rochester, Minnesota, between 1960 and 1969[13] found a similar value of 3.5 per 100,000 population.

ETIOLOGY AND PATHOGENESIS

The cause and pathogenesis of the disease are both unknown. Associative factors, some of which are probably casual, are well recognized, however. Why or how these factors damage the pancreas either acutely or chronically remains largely unknown.

Ethanol

The epidemiologic evidence supporting ethanol abuse as the major cause of chronic pancreatitis is convincing, although obviously it is impossible to establish the point by controlled studies in human subjects. At autopsy the morphologic changes of chronic pancreatitis are present in 45 per cent of alcoholics who had no symptoms of pancreatic disease during life; this rate is 40 to 50 times higher than in nondrinkers.[14] These findings correlate well with a report that 54 per cent of asymptomatic alcoholics exhibit abnormal pancreatic exocrine function after secretin-pancreozymin stimulation.[15] The daily intake of ethanol by patients with chronic pancreatitis was 141 gm, compared with 83 gm in a matched control population in France;[16] the corresponding figures in Sweden were 82 gm/day and 18 gm/day, respectively. There does not appear to be a "threshold" value of ethanol consumption in terms of the risk of developing chronic pancreatitis. The risk for total abstainers from ethanol is significantly lower than the risk for individuals consuming a low quantity (1 to 20 gm/day).[17]

There is no evidence that either protein or calorie malnutrition plays a role in the development of chronic pancreatitis owing to alcohol use. In fact, the authors of one study have proposed that a high intake of protein and fat are factors in the development of chronic pancreatitis.[17] However, a subsequent study did not confirm such an association.[18] The form in which ethanol is ingested (hard liquor, wine, beer) does not appear to influence the risk of developing chronic pancreatitis.[17, 18]

Most alcoholic patients already have sustained permanent structural and functional damage to the pancreas by the time of their first attack of symptoms related to pancreatic disease; hence alcoholic pancreatitis, even when acutely symptomatic, is a chronic disease.[19] Usually the initial symptoms appear in patients who have been drinking excessively for 10 to 20 years and are in their late 30s or 40s. However, the variability is considerable, and some patients may have their first attack of pancreatitis before age 25. Coexisting alcoholic liver disease is not as rare as had previously been believed. In two prospective studies of patients with chronic pancreatitis,[20, 21] 40 to 50 per cent had alcoholic liver disease (cirrhosis, alcoholic hepatitis, or fatty liver).

Although a number of ingenious experimental studies have been performed in animals, they have failed to resolve the question of how alcohol causes chronic pancreatitis in humans. In one study, more than 50 per cent of a group of rats fed 20 per cent ethanol for 20 to 30 months developed chronic pancreatitis that was morphologically similar to human disease,[22] including the precipitation of protein plugs early in the development of the disease. In those rats in which it was measured, the protein concentration of pancreatic juice was higher in ethanol-treated animals than in controls.[22] Dogs on a diet rich in fat and protein who received 2 gm/kg of body weight per day of ethanol for two years likewise had pancreatic lesions comparable to the stages of human pancreatitis, with protein precipitates (some of which were calcified) obstructing the pancreatic ducts, pericanalicular fibrosis, and atrophy of the acinar cells.[23] Although chronic ethanol ingestion can produce lesions in experimental animals similar to those seen in clinical chronic pancreatitis, the mechanism of injury in the experimental models remains unclear.

Until relatively recently, studies to investigate the pathogenesis of alcohol-related chronic pancreatitis in humans have been limited by the inability both to obtain pure pancreatic juice and to visualize directly the pancreatic ducts early in the course of the disease. Advances in endoscopic equipment and techniques now permit retrograde cannulation of the pancreatic duct for the collection of pure pancreatic juice and the injection of contrast media for pancreatography. After administration of secretin and cholecystokinin (CCK), the protein concentration in pancreatic juice is higher both in patients with alcohol-related chronic pancreatitis and in those with a history of heavy alcohol use without pancreatitis than in control patients.[24] In addition, pancreatic bicarbonate concentration was decreased in individuals with either alcohol-related chronic pancreatitis or a history of heavy alcohol use.[24]

Another group of investigators has demonstrated a significantly elevated protein concentration in pancreatic juice in alcoholics without pancreatic insufficiency compared with controls.[25] They found that this was caused by a selective increase in the concentration of trypsinogen, which resulted in a marked increase in the ratio of trypsinogen to trypsin inhibitor in pancreatic juice. An additional patient with a history of chronic alcoholism was studied during and after an episode of acutely symptomatic pancreatitis. The pancreatic juice from that patient showed an increased concentration of protein and an elevated ratio of trypsinogen relative to trypsin inhibitor. In addition there was evidence for intraductal activation of proteozytic enzymes. After clinical recovery and ten weeks' abstention from alcohol, both protein and trypsinogen concentrations in pure pancreatic juice had returned to almost normal.[26]

Because of the frequent finding of intraductal plugs and calculi in alcohol-related chronic pancreatitis, considerable interest has been aroused by the discovery of a small (molecular weight about 13,500) protein in pancreatic juice and in pancreatic calculi that is capable of inhibiting the formation of insoluble calcium salts in a supersaturated milieu.[27] This protein, named pancreatic stone protein, has been reported to be decreased in the pancreatic juice of patients with alcohol-related chronic pancreatitis and to be totally absent in the pancreatic juice of a woman with chronic pancreatitis and large intraductal calculi who did not use alcohol.[28] The role of pancreatic stone protein in the pathogenesis of chronic pancreatitis remains to be established more clearly by further clinical studies. The secretion of citrate is also reduced in patients with alcohol-related chronic pancreatitis and in heavy alcohol users without pancreatitis.[29] Because citrate chelates calcium, a reduction in citrate level in pancreatic juice may predispose individuals to the development of intraductal plugs and calculi.

In addition to the hypothesis that the intraductal precipitation of plugs occurs early in the course of chronic pancreatitis owing to an increase in overall protein concentration in pancreatic juice coupled with a decrease in the concentration of pancreatic stone protein,[30] other proposals have been that precipitation is linked to an increase in the viscosity of pancreatic juice caused by an increase in mucosubstance[31] or to a series of partial enzyme activations.[32]

Further information on the evolution of alcohol-related chronic pancreatitis has come from serial endoscopic retrograde pancreatography.[33] This work suggests that the branch ducts are deformed early in the course of the disease, before the lumen of the main duct becomes increasingly damaged. Very significantly, these ductal abnormalities, once initiated, often progress despite reduction in, or abstinence from, drinking. In contrast, no remarkable ductal changes were seen in patients with nonalcoholic chronic pancreatitis.[33]

A variety of histologic changes in the pancreas have been described in patients with alcohol-related chronic pancreatitis or with a history of heavy alcohol use without pancreatitis and also in experimental animals chronically ingesting ethanol.[34] These include dedifferentiation of acinar cells into ductular-type cells; accumulation of lipid droplets within, and mucous metaplasia of, pancreatic parenchymal cells; and loss of the epithelial basal lamina barrier. The significance of these cellular alterations is not known.

In summary, although chronic heavy alcohol ingestion appears to produce changes in the composition of pancreatic juice, the pathogenetic sequence of events leading from excessive alcohol use to chronic pancreatitis remains largely unknown. Nor can the continued progression of the disease in some patients after alcohol intake has stopped[33] be explained. The general hypothesis that "alcohol does no more than promote duct obstruction through precipitation of pancreatic secretory proteins,"[11] however, still can account for many of the experimental and clinical observations.

Gallstone Disease

All evidence suggests that repeated acute attacks of gallstone-associated pancreatitis rarely, if ever, progress to any form of chronic pancreatitis. The possible pathogenetic mechanisms for these attacks are discussed on page 1820. However, chronic pancreatitis may coexist with cholelithiasis, and most series of chronic pancreatitis in alcoholic patients report the same prevalence of gallstones as in the general population of the same age and sex. When both alcoholism and gallstones are present in patients with chronic pancreatitis, the pattern and course of the disease usually resemble those of alcohol-related pancreatitis.[35] Cholecystectomy usually does *not* alter the course of the disease. The higher frequency of cholelithiasis in cirrhosis is due to pigment (calcium bilirubinate) stones. Although these types of stones may be associated with acute pancreatitis, they are not responsible for alcohol-related chronic pancreatitis.

Other Causes of Chronic Pancreatitis

A variety of chronic pancreatitis is seen in certain tropical areas, including Southern India, Indonesia, and several Central and South African countries.[36] It is a disease of young adults with a fairly equal distribution between the sexes. Although many patients give a history of abdominal pain beginning as teenagers, patients are usually diagnosed on the basis of diabetes mellitus or intrapancreatic calcifications discovered on radiographs of the abdomen. Steatorrhea is uncommon because of the low fat intake in the diet; however, pancreatic secretory studies show decreases in the volume of secretion and in the concentrations of bicarbonate and digestive enzymes, with greater reductions in the concentrations of trypsin and lipase than of amylase. The cause of this form of chronic pancreatitis remains unknown. There is no evidence of a relationship to alcohol consumption. Malnutrition appears to play a major contributory role, although chronic pancreatitis is not found in other areas where protein and caloric intake are similar to those regions in which chronic pancreatitis is prevalent.[37] However, nutritional repletion may lead to a return to normal of pancreatic exocrine secretory function,[38] presumably if instituted before the development of extensive atrophy and fibrosis of the gland. Other dietary factors have been proposed to play a role in tropical chronic pancreatitis, including the consumption of cassava[39] and sorghum.[40] The importance of these factors, if any, remains to be clarified.

Although *hyperparathyroidism* (and other hypercalcemic states) and hyperlipidemia have been proposed to produce chronic pancreatitis resulting from recurrent acute attacks, this relationship has not been clearly established (see pp. 491 and 511).

Pancreatic *trauma* can produce acute pancreatitis. Subsequent healing may not be complete, with severe parenchymal injury or disruption of pancreatic ducts. Ductal strictures and compression by pseudocysts may also contribute to the development of chronic inflammation and fibrosis. Unlike alcohol-related chronic pancreatitis, abnormalities in trauma-related pancreatitis may be focal, leaving the remainder of the gland entirely normal.

Hereditary pancreatitis is discussed on pages 1804 to 1806. Intraductal calcifications are common.

Pancreas divisum (discussed on p. 1822) is a congenital anomaly occurring because embryologic dorsal and ventral pancreatic ducts fail to fuse into a single structure. When this occurs, most of the pancreatic juice must drain through the accessory papilla. Clinically, pancreas divisum has been most closely associated with episodes resembling recurrent acute pancreatitis. However, surgical specimens from some patients with pancreas divisum have shown histologic changes consistent with chronic pancreatitis in the portions of the pancreas derived from the embryologic dorsal pancreas, which drains through the small accessory papilla.[41]

The number of patients placed in the "idiopathic" category depends to a great extent on the type of patient population and on the diligence with which known associated factors (such as chronic alcohol use) have been excluded. The literature suggests a frequency ranging between 5[42] and 50[12] per cent, with figures at the low end of this range reported from populations in which high alcohol intake is common.

CLINICAL COURSE AND COMPLICATIONS

Course

The principal and most dramatic clinical events in the course of chronic pancreatitis in about 50 per cent of patients are episodes of acute pancreatitis as described on pages 1814 to 1842. In this situation, however, acute inflammation is superimposed on an irreversibly damaged organ. In about 35 per cent of patients, these acute exacerbations are absent and the disease is heralded by the insidious onset of pain that is continuous or intermittent and varying in intensity. Newly appearing symptoms of diabetes mellitus or of malabsorption, jaundice, and upper gastrointestinal bleeding lead to the diagnosis in the remaining 15 per cent.[43, 44] Pain is absent or a minor component of the clinical history in 10 to 15 per cent of patients with alcohol-related chronic pancreatitis and as many as 23 per cent of patients with nonalcoholic chronic pancreatitis.[44, 45] The erroneous notion that chronic pancreatitis need not be considered in patients presenting with malabsorption or obstructive jaundice who are pain-free may cause unnecessary delay in reaching the correct diagnosis.

The "typical" patient develops an initial attack of pancreatitis at age 35 to 40 years and recovers, but continues to drink, setting the stage for recurring exacerbations. The second attack often occurs one to two years later. Finally, patients have more frequent but less severe attacks that evolve into a clinical picture dominated by continuous or intermittent pain. Weight loss, diabetes, and steatorrhea may develop, and intrapancreatic calcifications may appear on abdominal X-rays. The mortality rate is approximately 3 to 4 per cent a year, but fewer than half of the deaths are a direct result of pancreatic disease. Additional causes of death include acute gastrointestinal bleeding, hypoglycemia, cancer, and complications of alcoholism, such as cirrhosis, tuberculosis, other infections, and trauma. With the possible exception of hereditary pancreatitis (see p. 1805), the frequency of pancreatic carcinoma does not appear to be increased substantially in patients with chronic pancreatitis.[46] There is an added risk of carcinoma of the lungs, mouth, and larynx, probably accounted for by the habit of heavy smoking, in which alcoholics often indulge.[47]

The Pain of Chronic Pancreatitis

The pathway of pancreatic pain fibers passes to the celiac plexus and then to the right and left paravertebral sympathetic ganglia (T6 to T11) via the right and left splanchnic nerves (see pp. 239–242). The events that trigger the pain of chronic pancreatitis are poorly understood. Pancreatic pseudocysts may be the source of pain in a minority of patients. Histologic examination of surgical specimens could not correlate severity of pain and either degree of perineural inflammation or fibrosis. However, the degree of perineural eosinophilic infiltration did correlate with severity of pain.[48] Studies evaluating the importance of increased pancreatic ductal pressure or the degree of duct obstruction in the production of pain in chronic pancreatitis have yielded mixed results.[49–52]

It is well known that the great majority of patients with chronic pancreatitis are afflicted with pain, either intermittently or chronically. It is the predominant symptom of this illness, the one that most determines the effect of chronic pancreatitis on a patient's lifestyle, career, and family relationships. The pain, often accompanied by nausea and vomiting, is boring, dull, or sharp and is steady rather than colicky. It is generally perceived in the epigastrium, in the right or left subcostal areas, and, occasionally, in the periumbilical region or lower abdomen. Pain radiates directly through to the back in about 65 per cent of patients and to the left shoulder in about 5 per cent. Attacks of pain usually last from several days to several weeks, are gradual in onset, and are not accompanied by signs suggesting an inflammatory process. Patients often find that pain can be lessened by leaning forward from a sitting position or by the analgesic effect of ethanol. The pain may be aggravated by eating or by lying supine and sometimes begins some hours after imbibing ("pain in the afternoon after the night before"). About 20 per cent of patients require frequent doses of narcotics for pain relief.[12] Up to 8 per cent of alcoholic patients from a low socioeconomic background become addicted;[19] the percentage of addiction is lower in patients who are better integrated into society. Indeed, the combination of continuing or intermittently severe pain and alcoholism often destroys careers and marriages. When addiction to narcotics supervenes, patients' problems are greatly aggravated.

It is not clear whether abstinence from alcohol decreases the frequency or severity of pain from alcohol-related chronic pancreatitis. Substantial relief of pain may be enjoyed by 75 per cent of patients after cessation of drinking.[53] However, in another group of patients no such relationship could be demonstrated between alcohol avoidance and pain.[54, 55] In most patients the pain of chronic pancreatitis appears to "burn out" over long periods of time. Data on the average duration of pain per year for patients with chronic pancreatitis as related to the total number of years these patients have experienced pain from this disorder are given in Table 98–1.[16] During the first four years, more than 80 per cent of patients had pain at some point each year. However, by five years after the onset of this symptom, one third of the patients were pain-free, and an additional 40 per cent had painful symptoms for a total of less than one month each year. These findings are supported by a recent report of a longitudinal study over 20 years of 245 patients with chronic pancreatitis, which also demonstrated that patients tended to experience relief of pain over time (85 per cent of patients at a median time of 4½ years) and that this pain relief was correlated with the development of pancreatic calcifications and exocrine or endocrine insufficiency.[56] Knowledge of the unpredictable course of the pain of chronic pancreatitis, with spontaneous and permanent relief of pain in a substantial number of patients, is important in assessing the results of operations and other therapeutic interventions designed to relieve this symptom.

Table 98–1. PERCENTAGE OF PATIENTS WITH ALCOHOLIC CHRONIC PANCREATITIS EXPERIENCING PAIN, IN RELATION TO THE TIME FROM ONSET OF PAIN

Pain Duration per Year	Years from Pain Onset			
	0–4	5–9	10–14	15–19
None	17	33	35	32
0–29 days	42	38	41	45
2–4 months	28	16	13	9
5–12 months	12	11	9	13

Modified from Gastard, J., Jouband, F., Farbos, T., et al.: Digestion 9:416, 1973.

Weight Loss and Malabsorption

Patients with chronic pancreatitis initially tend to be overweight.[16] Accordingly, weight loss is common during the course of the disease. Malabsorption is one of several important causes for it. Many patients limit their food intake because of the pain caused by eating or because of anorexia resulting from the use of narcotics or of ethanol. The glycosuria of untreated diabetes, iatrogenic food deprivation during hospitalizations, and insufficient funds for food after the purchase of spirits may also contribute to malnutrition. During pain-free periods, however, patients with chronic pancreatitis frequently have good to excellent appetites and, by eating more, often limit the weight loss from malabsorption.

Secretion of pancreatic digestive enzymes decreases early in the course of chronic pancreatitis, but fat and protein are not malabsorbed until at least 90 per cent of the secretory capacity is lost.[57] Because lipase secretion decreases more rapidly than secretion of proteolytic enzymes,[58] the development of steatorrhea often precedes that of azotorrhea (protein malabsorption) and is usually more severe. Steatorrhea and azotorrhea are found in up to 70 per cent of patients eight or more years after the onset of symptoms at a time when pancreatic calcifications are frequently seen on radiographs. If a patient attempts to compensate for malabsorption by overeating, increased fat intake leads not only to more fat absorption but also to more abdominal discomfort associated with more voluminous diarrhea. By contrast, increased protein intake causes additional nitrogen absorption with no increase in symptoms.[59] Given equal degrees of steatorrhea, the stool volume in patients with chronic pancreatitis is smaller than in patients with primary intestinal disease.[60] This is probably attributable in part to concomitant impairment in absorption of fluid in patients with primary intestinal disease and in part to a lower ratio of free to esterified dietary fatty acids entering the colon in pancreatic insufficiency (a digestive disorder) than in intestinal disease affecting absorption.[61] Because some free fatty acids inhibit absorption of sodium and water by the colon, their effect is proportionately diminished in chronic pancreatitis, despite some hydrolysis of dietary triglycerides by bacterial lipases in the colon.[62] The use of fecal fat concentration has been proposed as a means of discriminating between pancreatitic and nonpancreatic causes of steatorrhea, with values higher than 9.5 per cent in patients with fecal fat outputs of 21 gm or more suggestive of pancreatic insufficiency.[60] However, the use of antidiarrheal drugs, by increasing water absorption in the intestine, may result in elevated fecal fat concentrations in patients with steatorrhea resulting from primary disease in the small intestine (see pp. 263–282).

Although carbohydrate malabsorption has not been investigated extensively in pancreatic insufficiency, symptomatic carbohydrate malabsorption with abdominal cramping and bloating or watery diarrhea appears to be uncommon in chronic pancreatitis, probably for two reasons: (1) salivary amylase secretion remains unimpaired, and (2) pancreatic amylase secretion must be reduced by greater than 97 per cent before the rate of intraluminal starch digestion is slowed.[63] Because pancreatic proteases are involved in the degradation or release of intestinal brush border hydrolases, one of the consequences of reduced protease activity is an increase in the jejunal mucosal content of sucrase, maltase, and lactase activity in patients with pancreatic insufficiency.[64]

In view of the intact absorptive capacity and enterohepatic circulation of bile salts, the malabsorption of chronic pancreatitis is rarely associated with vitamin, iron, or calcium deficiency. The contrast with the clinical presentation of untreated celiac sprue is well illustrated in Table 98–2[65] (see also pp. 263–282 and 1134–1152).

About 40 per cent of patients with pancreatic insufficiency demonstrate malabsorption of cobalamin (vitamin B_{12}), although overt cobalamin deficiency rarely develops.[66] In this setting, cobalamin malabsorption appears to be attributable to reduced degradation by pancreatic proteases of cobalamin–R protein complexes, resulting in decreased availability of cobalamin to bind to intrinsic factor in the small intestine[67, 68] (see also p. 265).

Table 98–2. MANIFESTATIONS OF MALABSORPTION WITH CHRONIC PANCREATITIS AND WITH CELIAC SPRUE

	Pancreatic Insufficiency (Per Cent)	Celiac Sprue (Per Cent)
Gross oil separates from stool	57	0
Edema or ascites	12	50
Weakness	7	5
Tetany	0	40
Glossitis, stomatitis	0	66
Bleeding due to vitamin K deficiency	0	23
Bone pain	0	19
Stool fat (gm/day)	48	25
Anemia	0	21
Serum total protein (6.0 gm/dl)	14	71

Modified from Evans, W. B., and Wollaeger, E. E. Am. J. Dig. Dis. *11*:594, 1966.

Diabetes Mellitus

Insulin release in response to a glucose load is impaired early in the course of chronic pancreatitis, at a time when the rise in plasma glucose may still be normal. This may be due to a concomitant decrease in glucagon release. Eventually overt diabetes develops in 30 per cent of patients before, and in 70 per cent after, they develop pancreatic calcifications.[69]

Diabetic ketoacidosis and nephropathy are unusual in diabetes mellitus resulting from chronic pancreatitis. Neuropathy may be seen more frequently, possibly owing to the additional effects of chronic alcoholism and malnutrition. The prevalence of retinopathy has been reported to be similar in patients with diabetes secondary to chronic pancreatitis as in patients with idiopathic diabetes mellitus if corrected for the duration of diabetes.[70] Patients with chronic pancreatitis and diabetes may be at increased risk of hypoglycemia because of the combination of glucagon deficiency, irregular eating habits, malnutrition, and the effects of alcohol.

DIAGNOSIS

The diagnosis of chronic pancreatitis is not difficult in the alcoholic patient with documented attacks of pancreatitis, nor is it in the patient with pancreatic calcifications on radiographs. Diagnostic efforts in these patients should be limited to situations in which the detection of complications such as pseudocysts, malabsorption, or diabetes mellitus has important therapeutic implications. Diagnostic challenges are provided by patients with painless disease and by those in whom it is difficult to differentiate between recurrences of acute pancreatitis (e.g., attributable to gallstone disease) and chronic pancreatitis. Patients with recurrences of acute pancreatitis have few to many discrete attacks of pancreatitis without evidence of irreversible damage to the gland. On the other hand, patients with chronic pancreatitis may have recurrent acute exacerbations similar to attacks of acute pancreatitis. Unfortunately, there are no reliable clinical criteria for diagnosing early or mild chronic pancreatitis, nor, in fact, for differentiating it from pancreatic carcinoma. At present direct tests of pancreatic exocrine function and pancreatic imaging studies provide the most sensitive indicators of chronic pancreatic disease (see Table 95–2).

Physical Findings in Chronic Pancreatitis

Patients with advanced disease and untreated malabsorption are underweight and have varying degrees of malnutrition. Aside from occasional epigastric tenderness and evidence of some weight loss, physical findings are of little diagnostic help. Occasionally, distant subcutaneous fat necrosis, pancreatic ascites, or jaundice is evident. A palpable epigastric mass may be a pancreatic pseudocyst. Unlike in malabsorption owing to small intestinal disease, signs of fat-soluble vitamin deficiencies in skin and in skeletal or neuromuscular systems usually are absent.

Laboratory Studies

Routine Blood Tests and Urinalysis. Results of routine blood tests, including the complete blood count, are usually normal unless the patient has diabetes and glycosuria. Levels of blood electrolytes and minerals (e.g., calcium, magnesium) are also usually normal. If the patient has become diabetic, the fasting blood glucose level will be elevated and carbohydrate tolerance will be abnormal. Prothrombin time and partial thromboplastin times, unless the patient also has significant liver disease, are normal.

Serum and Urinary Measurements of Pancreatic Enzymes. Serum amylase and lipase concentrations frequently are normal during attacks of pain. This may be explained by several factors: the acute inflammation may be mild and thus acinar cell destruction may be minimal; the entry of extracellular hydrolases into blood and lymph may be restricted by periacinar and periductal fibrosis; and the acinar cell mass may decrease as the disease progresses (smoldering inflammation in a "burned-out" gland). Although increased levels of these enzymes are occasionally sustained in the presence of pseudocysts or pancreatic ascites, chronic elevations of the serum amylase concentration in patients who are asymptomatic or who have nonspecific symptoms are usually *not* attributable to the presence of pancreatic disease.[71] Determination of amylase isoenzyme levels in such patients (including, in one series, patients with alcoholism[72]) has demonstrated that the increase in serum amylase concentration is usually the result of an excess of the salivary (S) type of isoenzyme.[72, 73]

Some patients with chronic pancreatitis and pancreatic insufficiency have been found to have decreased circulating levels of the pancreatic (P) isoenzyme of amylase[74] as well as of other pancreatic enzymes, such as trypsin[75] and lipase.[76] Conversely, elevated serum concentrations of the pancreatic enzymes elastase,[77] DNase,[78] and RNase[78] have also been reported in patients with chronic pancreatitis. The use of these relatively simple blood tests have been proposed for the laboratory confirmation of the diagnosis of chronic pancreatitis. However, these serum enzyme assays so far have not demonstrated a sufficient degree of sensitivity or specificity, especially in early or mild chronic pancreatitis, to be useful in this regard.[78]

The amylase-creatinine clearance ratio (see p. 1825) is usually normal in chronic pancreatitis. The trypsin-creatinine clearance ratio has been reported to be elevated in both patients with chronic pancreatitis and those with cancer of the pancreas.[79, 80] Its clinical value remains to be established.

Serum Bilirubin and Alkaline Phosphatase Concentrations. Serum bilirubin or alkaline phosphatase concentrations, or both, may be elevated owing to concomitant liver disease. However, a rise in the alkaline phosphatase level greater than five times the upper limit of normal (even without hyperbilirubinemia) that persists for more than four weeks is a strong indication of common bile duct stenosis caused by fibrosis of pancreatic tissue surrounding the distal common bile duct.[81] This type of obstructive jaundice affects 5 to 10 per cent of patients with chronic pancreatitis. The serum bilirubin value is usually only mildly to moderately elevated (3 to 10 mg/dl). Further evidence for obstruction can be obtained by sonography or computed tomography (CT), whereas confirmation requires direct cholangiography (see pp. 1716 and 1741).

Lactoferrin Levels in Pancreatic Juice. Lactoferrin is an iron-binding protein found in a variety of human secretions (e.g., salivary, lacrimal) and also in neutrophils and pancreatic acinar cells. The concentration of lactoferrin in pure pancreatic juice obtained by endoscopic retrograde cannulation has been reported to be increased in patients with chronic pancreatitis but not in those with acute pancreatitis, pancreatic cancer, or other disease.[82–84]

After stimulation of patients with secretin and cerulein (a cholecystokinin analogue), the ratio of lactoferrin to lipase in duodenal juice collected by intubation is increased in chronic pancreatitis. This ratio is quite sensitive and specific in distinguishing patients with chronic pancreatitis from normal subjects and patients with other pancreatic or digestive diseases, including pancreatic cancer, gallstone-related acute pancreatitis, and pancreas divisum.[85, 86] In addition, the lactoferrin-to-lipase ratio is elevated in patients with chronic pancreatitis with chronic pain and reduced bicarbonate secretion after secretin stimulation but with normal fat absorption, absence of pancreatic calcification on abdominal X-rays, and normal pancreatic duct anatomy on ERCP.[85, 86]

These initial studies are very promising in suggesting that the measurement of the lactoferrin-to-lipase ratio in dudoenal juice may be quite sensitive and specific in the diagnosis of early or mild chronic pancreatitis. However, its adaptability to routine clinical use remains to be established.

Tests of Pancreatic Exocrine Function. Accurate assessment of pancreatic exocrine function by a test of stimulation is useful in the diagnosis of the relatively few patients whose chronic pancreatitis is not already obvious clinically. Examples are the differential diagnosis between recurrences of acute pancreatitis and steatorrhea of unknown cause. Chronic pancreatitis cannot be ruled out by the finding of a normal duct system by ERCP, especially in nonalcoholic patients. In some patients, chronic pancreatitis can be diagnosed with certainty only by demonstrating diminished function during adequate stimulation of the gland. No pancreatic function test can reliably distinguish between cancer and chronic pancreatitis.[87]

Exogenous Stimulation: Secretin and Secretin plus Cholecystokinin or Cerulein. Aspiration and analysis of duodenal contents after injection of pure synthetic or natural secretin remains the most reliable, commonly used test of pancreatic exocrine function. Secretin is injected intravenously or subcutaneously to stimulate pancreatic water and bicarbonate secretion, and duodenal juice is aspirated continuously. The volume of secretion and the concentration and output of bicarbonate are determined. The injection of cholecystokinin (CCK) or cerulein along with secretin has been used with measurement in duodenal juice of digestive enzymes (e.g., amylase, trypsin, lipase) in addition to the volume of secretion and bicarbonate. Whether this modification of the basic secretin stimulation test enhances diagnostic accuracy has not been established.[88] The sensitivity of the secretin stimulation test (with or without CCK or cerulein) appears to be in the range of 80 to 90 per cent.[88] The secretin stimulation test is expensive and technically demanding, requiring trained personnel and fluoroscopic placement of the duodenal tube (see p. 1786 and Table 95–2). The use of a nonabsorbable marker has been advocated to correct for incomplete aspiration of duodenal juice.[88] The response to secretin stimulation as measured in pure pancreatic juice collected after endoscopic retrograde cannulation of the pancreatic duct has been evaluated in normal subjects and in patients with chronic pancreatitis.[89] This approach has not been shown to be superior to duodenal intubation.

Endogenous Stimulation: Perfusion and Feedings. Pancreatic secretion in response to endogenous hormones released by perfusion of the duodenum with amino or fatty acids can be measured quantitatively using a multilumen tube.[90] This test is too complex, however, for routine clinical use. In the Lundh test meal, the mean concentration of digestive enzymes in the proximal jejunum is determined for two hours after ingestion of a standard test meal. This procedure is relatively simple to perform but not as sensitive as the secretin test in detecting impaired pancreatic function.[88] Measurement of chymotrypsin in random stool samples from patients on their regular diet represents an attempt to assess pancreatic digestive enzyme secretion without the need for intestinal intubation. Although measurement of fecal chymotrypsin is a reliable test for advanced chronic pancreatitis, most cases of mild or early disease are missed.[88]

Indirect or "Tubeless Tests" of Secretory Function. Two tests have been developed to evaluate pancreatic secretory function without the need for duodenal intubation.[91] In the *bentiromide* (NBT-PABA) *test,* a synthetic peptide (*N*-benzoyl-L-tyrosyl-*p*-aminobenzoic acid) is given orally and cleaved in the small intestine by pancreatic chymotrypsin, releasing para-aminobenzoic acid (PABA). The free PABA is absorbed by the intestine, conjugated by the liver, and excreted in urine. Concentrations in urine or serum of arylamines (PABA and its metabolites) are measured and reflect pancreatic exocrine secretory activity. The *pancreolauryl* (fluorescein dilaurate) *test* operates on similar principles. Fluorescein dilaurate is hydrolyzed by pancreatic arylesterases to water-soluble fluorescein, which is absorbed by the small intestine, conjugated by the liver, and excreted into urine. The concentration of fluorescein in the urine or blood reflects pancreatic exocrine secretory activity.

These tests are noninvasive and relatively inexpensive and have a sensitivity of about 80 per cent for the diagnosis of severe chronic pancreatitis when compared to the secretin stimulation test.[88] However, in early or mild chronic pancreatitis, the sensitivity is less than 50 per cent.[88] Falsely abnormal results occur in renal insufficiency, intestinal and liver diseases, and diabetes mellitus.[88] Modifications of both tests have been proposed to correct for some of these factors and improve the specificity.[88]

Other Tests of Pancreatic Function. A variety of other laboratory tests have been proposed for use in the diagnosis of chronic pancreatitis. These include the dual-labeled Schilling test[92] and measurement after stimulation of exocrine pancreatic secretion of human pancreatic polypeptide (decreased compared to normal),[93] of the rate of synthesis of pancreatic digestive enzymes using a radiolabeled amino acid (increased compared to normal),[94] and of plasma amino acid levels (decreased total amino acid levels; altered kinetics of serine, valine, leucine, and histidine).[95] The clinical value of all of these approaches remains to be determined.

Malabsorption in Chronic Pancreatitis: Clinical Insufficiency. The diagnosis of malabsorption owing to pancreatic exocrine insufficiency depends primarily on the direct measurement of increased fecal fat excretion. Neither weight loss nor the finding of reduced pancreatic enzyme output constitutes acceptable evidence of insufficiency because of the enormous reserve of the gland: approximately 90 per cent of function must be lost before malabsorption supervenes. Only the quantity of fat lost in the stool definitively establishes steatorrhea and helps gauge response to therapy. A three-day stool collection is usually obtained but one- or two-day collections may be sufficient in patients with frequent bowel movements. Patients should be consuming 70 to 100 gm of fat/day. The normal fecal fat excretion of 5 to 7 gm/day (depending on daily fat intake) is exceeded in pancreatic insufficiency, usually by a large margin. Indeed, some of the highest values for stool fat excretion are found in patients with chronic pancreatitis and pancreatic insufficiency (Table 98–2). Because of the unpopularity with both patients and laboratory personnel of fecal fat determination on 72-hour stool collections, other approaches are being evaluated to quantify degrees of fat malabsorption. These include a two-stage triolein breath test[96] and NMR spectrometry of lyophilized samples of three consecutive stools.[97] Neither of these techniques is currently available routinely.

Azotorrhea (greater than 2.5 gm/day of fecal nitrogen) usually accompanies steatorrhea, but the stool nitrogen determination is cumbersome and adds little information useful to the clinician (see pp. 263–282). Recent studies using H_2 breath tests have demonstrated carbohydrate malabsorption in pancreatic insufficiency.[98, 99] However, the clinical value of this type of information remains to be demonstrated.

Radiologic Diagnosis

In about 30 per cent of patients with chronic pancreatitis, plain radiographs of the abdomen reveal diffuse or focal pancreatic calcification (Fig. 98–1). When calcification is present, the diagnosis of chronic pancreatitis is almost certain, even if there is no clinical evidence of pancreatic disease. Progressive displacement of calcium on serial films may provide a clue to the presence of an enlarging tumor or pseudocyst in a patient with underlying chronic pancreatitis. Approximately 5 per cent of patients with chronic pancreatitis have radiographically demonstrated osseous abnormalities, such as medullary infarcts or aseptic necrosis of the femoral or humeral heads. These may result from necrosis of medullary fat during episodes of acute pancreatitis, when intraperitoneal fat is also necrosed. The long bones of the hands and feet are affected most often.

Barium Contrast Studies

Barium contrast radiographic studies are insensitive and nonspecific for chronic pancreatitis. Occasionally, however, the findings on these radiographic techniques may suggest the diagnosis of pancreatic disease and lead to more exacting diagnostic procedures. Extrinsic displacement of the greater curvature of the stomach or the medial aspect of the duodenum is seen in 10 to 15 per cent of patients, but these abnormalities are not diagnostic of chronic pancreatitis. Effacement of the normal mucosal pattern along the medial descending duodenum is the most frequent finding on air-contrast barium upper gastrointestinal series. Enlargement of the papilla of Vater, spiculation of the mucosa, and "thumbprinting" in the duodenal bulb are other nonspecific changes and suggest an acute inflammatory component to the chronic pancreatitis. Pancreatic cancer, acute pancreatitis, or hemorrhage, however, may produce similar radiographic abnormalities. The barium contrast examination may likewise be helpful in the diagnosis of pancreatic pseudocyst (Figs. 98–2 and 98–3). Depending on its size and location, the pseudocyst may also displace the stomach anteriorly or otherwise distort normal anatomy. Cysts in the head of the pancreas may compress the medial aspect of the duodenum. Barium enema radiographs may likewise show extrinsic narrowing and displacement of the midtransverse colon. Rarely, a pseudocyst will fill during a barium enema study. Sonography and, in particular, CT and magnetic resonance imaging scanning are far more accurate methods of detecting localized or generalized enlargements or abnormalities of shape and contour of the pancreas than are conventional radiographic techniques, including the use of barium contrast studies (see pp. 1796 and 1828).

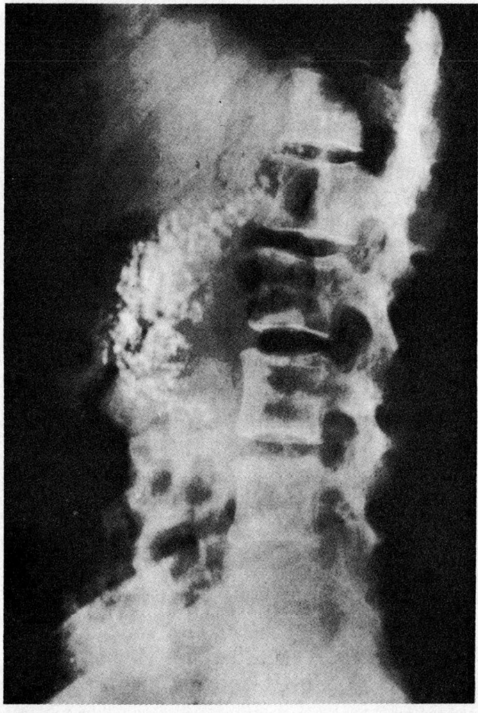

Figure 98–1. Lateral plain radiograph of abdomen, demonstrating diffuse pancreatic calcification seen in chronic pancreatitis. (Courtesy of O. D. Kowlessar, M.D.)

Noninvasive Cholangiography

With chronic pancreatitis, no specific abnormalities of the gallbladder are found on oral cholecystography. Although used with decreasing frequency, intravenous cholangiography (IVC) may demonstrate a smoothly tapered narrowing of the distal common bile duct in chronic pancreatitis, provided that the serum bilirubin concentration is less than 2 to 3 mg/dl. More recently, biliary tract scintigraphy has also been shown to demonstrate these same distortions of the terminal portion of the common bile duct. The precise anatomic details are rarely evident by noninvasive cholangiography and when substantial liver function test abnormalities are present, direct cholangiography is essential (Fig. 98–4).

ERCP and Transhepatic Cholangiography

Endoscopic retrograde cholangiopancreatography (ERCP) often is extremely helpful in the diagnosis and management of patients with pancreatic disease. The average normal diameters of the pancreatic duct are 4 mm, 3 mm, and 2 mm in the head, body, and tail, respectively (Fig. 98–5). With early chronic pancreatitis and in some patients with advanced disease, ductal changes may be minimal. In many patients with ad-

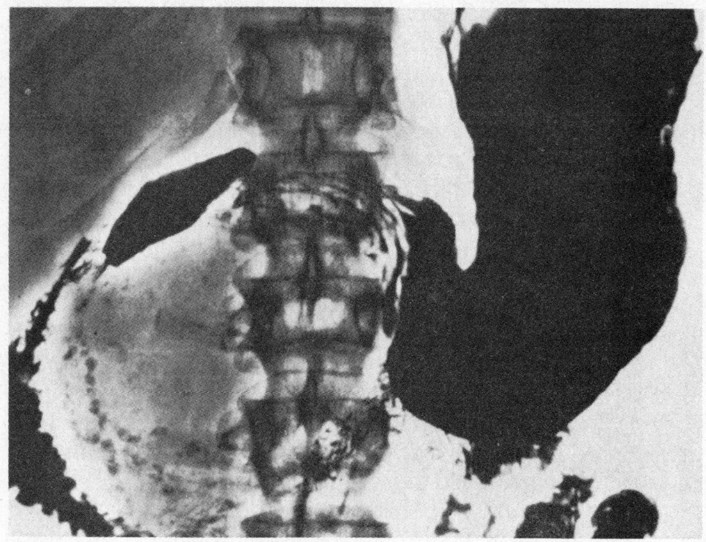

Figure 98–2. Upper gastrointestinal series, demonstrating a pseudocyst in the head of the pancreas causing peripheral displacement of pancreatic calcification and upward and medial deviation of the gastric antrum. Note the flattened mucosal folds of the antrum. This same radiographic feature may be seen, however, in pancreatic cancer.

vanced disease, however, the main pancreatic duct may be dilated to 1 cm or more with intermittent points of obstruction (Fig. 98–6) producing a "chain of lakes" appearance. Strictures, cysts, and ductal calculi may likewise be seen on pancreatography in patients with chronic pancreatitis. In most instances, the pancreatogram does distinguish pancreatic cancer from chronic pancreatitis. Contiguous, irregular, nodular, or "rattailed" obstruction of both common bile duct and pancreatic duct (see Fig. 99–5, p. 1878), the so-called "double duct sign," is strongly suggestive of pancreatic cancer, especially when the remainder of the pancreatic duct is normal. These changes may occasionally be encountered, however, in patients with chronic pancreatitis.[100] As opposed to the single focus of pancreatic duct stricturing in pancreatic cancer, pancreatography in patients with chronic pancreatitis demonstrates multiple pancreatic ductal stenoses or a single, smooth, tapering stenosis together with intraductal calculi and irregular branching ducts. Repeat pancreatography in patients with chronic alcoholic pancreatitis may demonstrate progressive ductal disease in spite of abstinence from alcohol.[33]

Endoscopic manometric studies of the sphincter of Oddi and the pancreatic duct in patients with chronic pancreatitis have revealed conflicting results, probably in part related to varying equipment and techniques.[101–103] When compared with those of controls, papillary

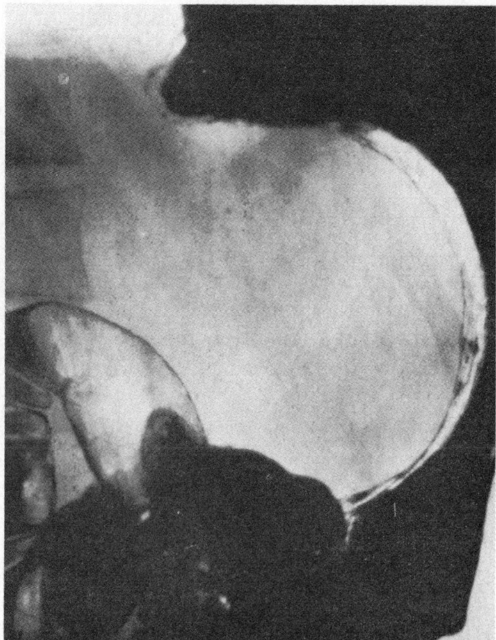

Figure 98–3. Barium in the stomach is displaced forward by a retrogastric pseudocyst in the body of the pancreas, which smoothes but does not invade the gastric wall draped over it. Note that the vertebral-gastric distance exceeds the normal limit of approximately one anteroposterior width of a vertebral body.

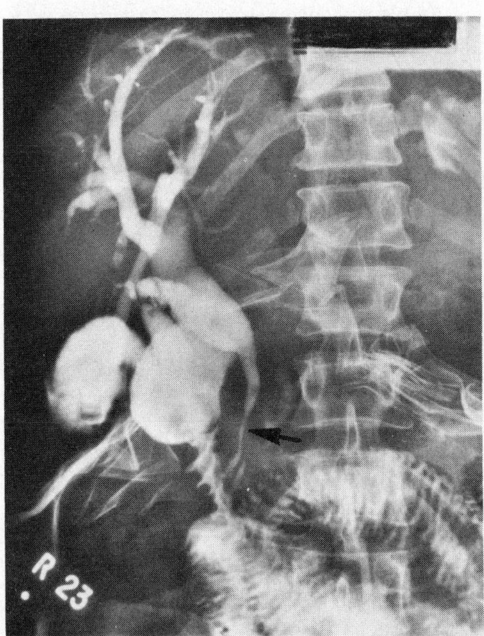

Figure 98–4. Operative cholangiogram in a patient with chronic pancreatitis. The patient had obstructive jaundice caused by compression of the intrapancreatic portion of the common bile duct *(arrow)*.

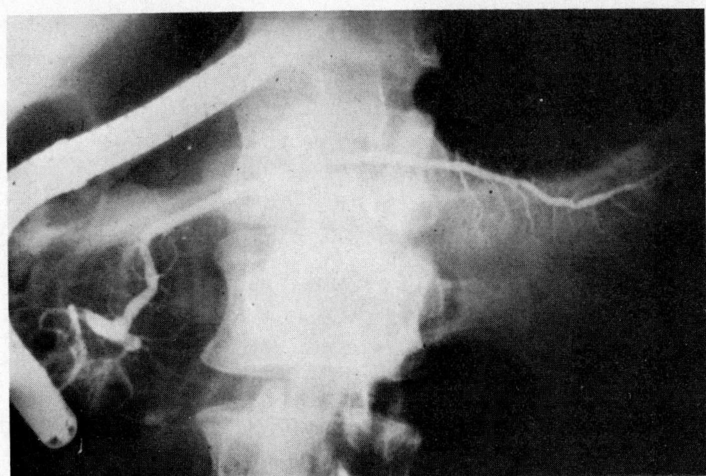

Figure 98–5. Normal retrograde pancreatogram obtained by endoscopic cannulation of the pancreatic duct. The main duct is opacified, along with primary and some secondary branches.

sphincter zone peak and basal pressures are normal in most patients with chronic pancreatitis.[102, 103] With perfusion catheter techniques, pancreatic duct pressures were not significantly different from those of control patients in two clinical studies.[101] However, using a 4-French size microtransducer catheter, Okazaki and associates noted pancreatic ductal pressures in 20 patients with chronic pancreatitis (mean pressure, 54.5 ± 29.9 mm Hg) significantly greater than control patients (mean pancreatic duct pressure, 16.2 ± 8.7 mm Hg).[101] Furthermore, patients with moderate-change chronic pancreatitis had higher pancreatic duct pressures than those with minimal-change pancreatitis, whereas the patients with advanced changes of chronic pancreatitis were noted to have duct pressures lower than those in patients with less severe pancreatitis.[101] Further studies will be needed before routine pancreatic duct and sphincter of Oddi pressure measurements can be accepted as being either necessary or useful for patients with chronic pancreatitis.

ERCP permits the preoperative identification of potentially surgically correctable lesions (strictures, cysts) and provides useful information to the surgeon (see p. 1863). It may also be an important means of excluding chronic pancreatitis in the alcoholic patient demanding more narcotics for relief of chronic abdominal pain. Complications of ERCP include cholangitis (in about 5 per cent of patients with pre-existing obstructive jaundice) and pancreatitis (in less than 3 per cent).[104] An occasional fatality from severe pancreatitis induced by ERCP has been reported; thus, this procedure should not be undertaken unless there is a clear-cut diagnostic or therapeutic indication.

In all patients with the suspicion of chronic pancreatitis, contrast material must be injected carefully during ERCP while the pancreatic duct is viewed under fluoroscopy (with the image screen close by the endoscopist and fluoroscopist) to avoid rupture of smaller pancreatic ducts (so-called "acinarization") or overdistention of pseudocysts.

For those patients undergoing ERCP in preparation for a planned surgical procedure (e.g., pseudocyst drainage or pancreatic duct–enterostomy), the authors recommend performing the ERCP within 12 to 24 hours before the intended surgery to ensure adequate drainage of ERCP-injected ducts and pseudocysts.

Good-quality radiographs of the intra- and extrahepatic bile ducts but not pancreatic ducts may also be

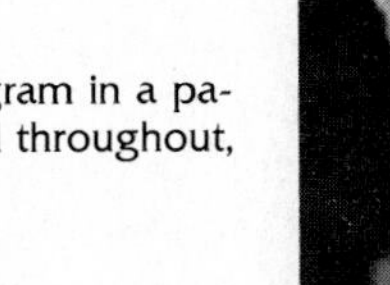

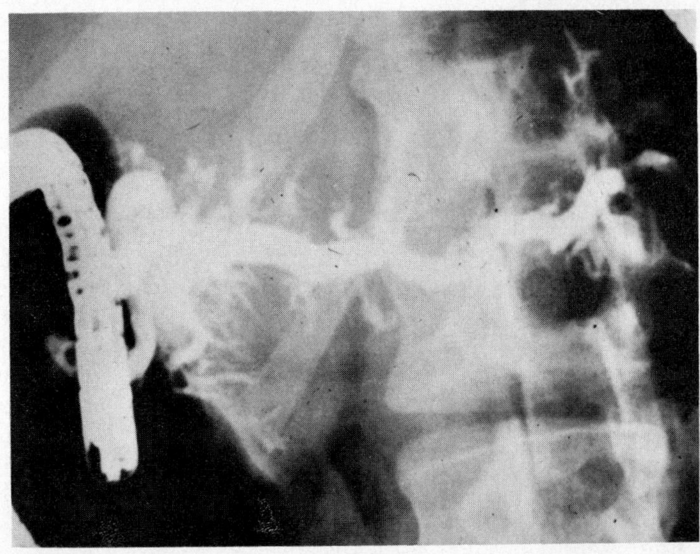

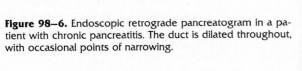

Figure 98–6. Endoscopic retrograde pancreatogram in a patient with chronic pancreatitis. The duct is dilated throughout, with occasional points of narrowing.

obtained when contrast material is injected directly percutaneously through the liver (transhepatic cholangiography) or at operation (operative cholangiography). Chronic pancreatitis characteristically produces angulation of the distal common bile duct with a smooth, tapering narrowing of its intrapancreatic portion (Fig. 98–4).

Ultrasonography and Computed Tomography (CT)

With uncomplicated chronic pancreatitis, ultrasonographic (Fig. 98–7) and CT (Fig. 98–8) examinations of the pancreas are usually unremarkable except for irregularity of the contour of the gland, dilatation of the pancreatic duct, or the possible presence of calcification.[105] In a comparison of these methods, the CT scan was found to be superior for detecting pseudocysts and delineating their anatomic relationships.[106] Because of its lower costs, however, ultrasonography should usually be the first of these two noninvasive imaging techniques to be employed. In the presence of overlying gas-filled loops of bowel, common in patients with an acute inflammatory process in the pancreas, the ultrasonographic examination will not be adequate in visualizing the entire pancreas, and CT scanning should be employed.[107] With both techniques, an enlarged pancreatic duct can be determined with great accuracy. This finding plus evidence of small pseudocysts and pancreatic calcification makes the diagnosis of chronic pancreatitis certain. When surgical decompression of pseudocysts is planned, a CT scan just prior to surgery is essential to characterize the pseudocysts. Intraoperative ultrasonography may likewise be helpful in localizing difficult-to-find smaller fluid collections.

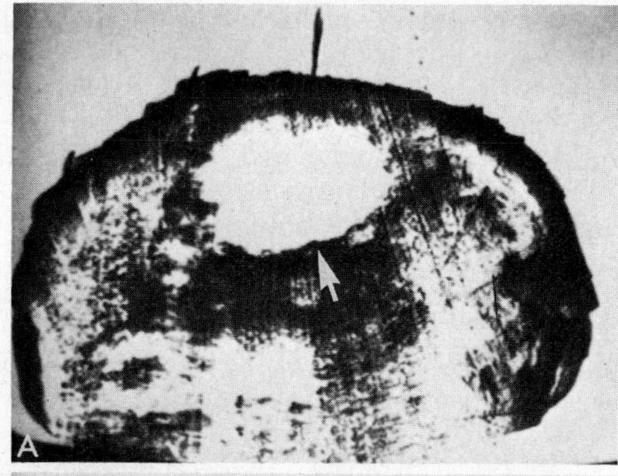

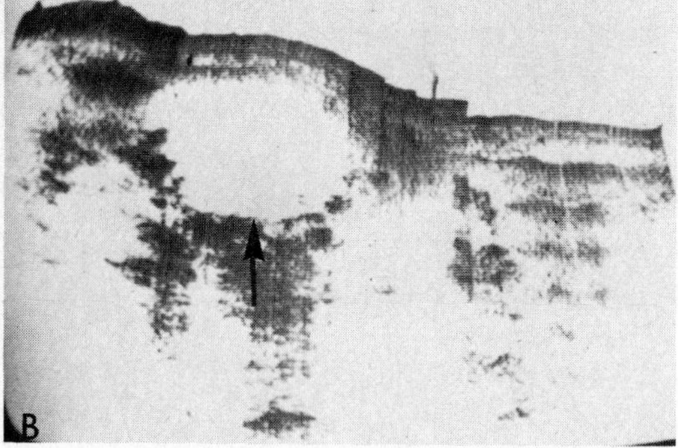

Figure 98–7. Abdominal ultrasonographic scans in a patient with chronic pancreatitis and pancreatic pseudocyst *(arrows)*. *A*, Transverse section. *B*, Longitudinal section; the patient's head is to the left. The pseudocyst presented through the transverse colon as a bulging mass behind and below the stomach. Its fluid nature was suggested by the absence of echoes on the ultrasonogram and was confirmed by surgical drainage.

Angiography

Pancreatic angiography is not used routinely to diagnose chronic pancreatitis. In patients with advanced disease, it may show that the intrapancreatic arteries have alternating dilated and narrow segments or arterial aneurysms, or both, and the veins may be narrowed or occluded. This technique is particularly helpful in revealing obstruction of the splenic vein in patients with gastric and, in some cases, esophageal varices, an infrequent but important complication of acute and chronic pancreatitis. All of these angiographic abnormalities, however, may also be seen with pancreatic cancer (see pp. 1872–1884). Thus, angiography is rarely helpful in distinguishing chronic pancreatitis from pancreatic cancer.

Differential Diagnosis of Chronic Pancreatitis

In most patients, the diagnosis of chronic pancreatitis is straightforward. A history of alcoholism combined with recurrent episodes of abdominal pain, the presence of clinical diabetes mellitus or elevated fasting blood glucose level, pancreatic calcifications, weight loss, and some evidence of malabsorption are found in some combination in most patients. Occasionally the presentation is less clear, and the distinction of *chronic pancreatitis* from pancreatic cancer may be difficult, particularly when there is little or no antecedent history of alcoholism or pancreatitis, when jaundice results from compression of the intrapancreatic portion of the common bile duct, when pain is of relatively recent onset, and when weight loss is significant. Although chronic pancreatitis usually produces characteristic features on ultrasonography, CT, and ERCP, distinction between the two diseases may be difficult.[87] Cytologic examination of ultrasonographically or CT-guided aspiration specimens may show evidence of malignancy in 80 per cent of patients with cancer, but negative findings on cytologic study do not absolutely rule out cancer.[86] In such patients, operation with transduodenal or wedge pancreatic biopsy may be necessary to make the diagnosis.

Chronic pancreatitis cannot be cured. Medical treatment is directed toward alleviating the symptoms, particularly pain and weight loss. Properly timed surgical interventions aim at the correction of complications such as severe pain, pancreatic ascites, large pseudocysts, and compression or involvement of adjacent organs or structures (common bile duct or

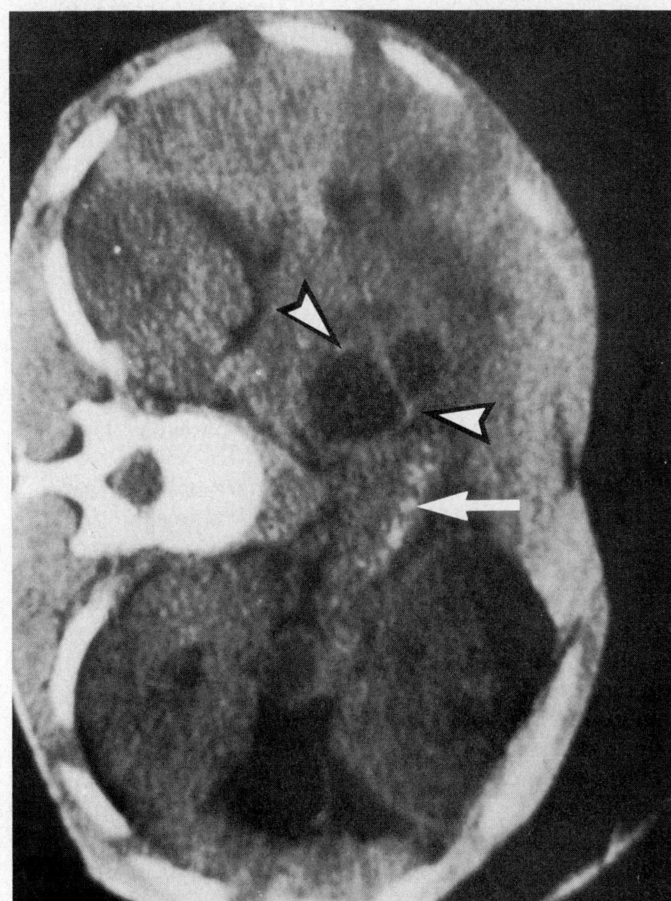

Figure 98–8. Computed tomography in patient with pancreatic pseudocyst. Three low-density fluid collections are visible in the head of the pancreas *(arrowheads),* and an additional cyst is seen in the tail of the gland. *Arrow* points to calcifications in the body of the pancreas, a typical finding on computed tomography in chronic pancreatitis.

splenic vein). Correction of the condition causing the pancreatitis should be attempted, although progression of the disease may not be arrested despite abstinence from alcohol. On occasion, patients with *mesenteric vascular disease* can present with a clinical picture similar to that encountered in patients with chronic pancreatitis (see pp. 1903–1916). Angiographic studies will usually be needed to clarify the nature of the vascular disease in these patients who will invariably have normal findings on ultrasonographic, CT, or ERCP studies of the pancreas.

It would be well to remember that some patients with *celiac sprue* have a subnormal response of the pancreas to endogenous stimulation, ostensibly because of mucosal inflammation of the duodenum, resulting in deficient release of secretin and CCK. As with malabsorption attributable to other diseases that severely affect the upper small intestine and cause steatorrhea, the correct diagnosis often rests on findings on the peroral jejunal biopsy and the absence of other evidence of pancreatic disease (see pp. 263–282 and 1134–1152).

COMPLICATIONS

Although most patients with chronic pancreatitis are affected by varying degrees of pain, malnutrition, and often by the consequences of continuing alcohol and narcotic abuse, a substantial minority develop rather more clinically dramatic complications. These include inflammatory pseudocyst, abscess of the pancreas, obstruction of the common bile duct, splenic vein thrombosis, and, possibly, peptic ulcer.

Pseudocysts

Pancreatic pseudocysts are encapsulated collections of fluid with high concentrations of pancreatic enzymes. They arise from the pancreas, usually communicate with the pancreatic duct, and are usually within or adjacent to the pancreas in the lesser peritoneal sac. Occasionally, pseudocysts dissect retroperitoneally and may be found outside the peritoneal cavity (e.g., mediastinum or pelvis). They may also dissect through the mesentery and be found virtually anywhere in the abdomen. Unlike true cysts, these cysts do not have an epithelial lining of their walls, hence the term "pseudocysts."

Discussion of pseudocysts of the pancreas is included here because the majority of these cysts appear during the course of chronic pancreatitis, at times as a consequence of an attack of acute inflammation; in most instances, however, they appear insidiously and cannot be clearly related to such acute attacks. Thus, two different mechanisms are responsible for the development of pancreatic pseudocysts, and their recognition is important for proper therapy (see pp. 1866–1867). In the first mechanism, the cyst forms after an episode of acute pancreatitis, no matter whether it is an initial episode or one of many. The cyst is composed initially of exudate from within or on the surface of the inflamed gland, and if the ductal system has been disrupted, pancreatic juices are walled off by a barrier formed by adjacent serosal, mesenteric, and peritoneal surfaces. Although the contained fluid may be partially reabsorbed, movement of material out of the sac is increasingly impeded by progressive thickening and fibrosis of the cyst surface. At a certain point, the surface becomes a cyst wall, and the patient has an inflammatory pseudocyst.

The second and more common pathogenetic mechanism for pseudocyst formation is part of the evolution of the chronic pancreatic disease and is unrelated to a bout of clinically recognizable acute pancreatitis. It results from obstruction and dilation of small ducts and acinar spaces, caused by occluded larger ducts in chronic pancreatitis. With atrophy of the epithelial cells, a retention cyst is formed that may grow beyond the confines of the pancreas. This accumulation also results in a thick cyst wall.

Clinically palpable pseudocysts develop in only about 2 per cent of patients with acute pancreatitis and, when present, are single in 85 per cent of cases. Many more patients with acute pancreatitis will be found to have small fluid collections when studied by the newer imaging techniques. In one series of 36 patients with severe acute pancreatitis, noninfected pancreatic or extrapancreatic fluid collections were noted in 10 patients on routine CT scans.[108] Among 923 patients admitted for pancreatic disease, pseudocysts were identified sonographically in 93.[109] According to the original Marseilles classification, the diagnoses were categorized as acute pancreatitis, 7; relapsing acute pancreatitis, 24; chronic relapsing pancreatitis, 46; and chronic pancreatitis, 16. Pseudocysts are clinically apparent in 5 to 10 per cent of all instances because of their size or location. Pseudocysts may also develop after the disruption of the ductal system owing to trauma (usually deceleration injuries to the epigastrium) or surgical injury (e.g., after subtotal gastrectomy or splenectomy, operations in which the gland is vulnerable to injury). In these patients, symptoms attributable to the pseudocyst may not be evident until several weeks after the traumatic injury or operation.

Clinical Findings. When a patient with acute pancreatitis either fails to recover after a week of treatment or, after improving for a time, again has symptoms, a pseudocyst should be suspected. It must be distinguished from a tender epigastric mass that may be palpable early in the episode of acute inflammation. This collection, termed a phlegmon, is formed by the inflamed and edematous pancreas and surrounding tissues; it usually recedes as the pancreatitis improves, in contrast to a pseudocyst, which may persist and enlarge (see p. 1835).

When a pseudocyst develops insidiously, the patient is usually seen because of the symptoms of the cyst per se. Regardless of the way in which it develops, the most frequent symptom is pain. Pain is usually located in the upper abdomen, with radiation to the back. Other important symptoms are low-grade fever, usually no more than 100° to 101° F daily, and weight loss primarily as a result of greatly reduced food intake because of anorexia and the pain that follows eating. Nausea and vomiting are also common.

A tender, palpable abdominal mass or fullness is present in only about one half of patients. Jaundice and, more rarely, cholangitis may reflect compression of the common bile duct by the enlarging pseudocyst. Although this latter complication is infrequent, it is important because it increases the risk of serious infection. Occasionally, the cyst may cause gastric outlet obstruction by duodenal compression.

Pseudocysts may occasionally inflame the overlying diaphragm (usually the left) and exude fluid into the pleural spaces and, rarely, even into the mediastinum. Patients with this complication will complain of pleuritic or chest pain and sometimes have dyspnea. If infection is present, the patient will be febrile with high, spiking fever. Chest radiographs and CT scans will usually show the subdiaphragmatic pseudocyst and pleural fluid. Strangely, a rare patient may be free of pain, in which case the diagnosis of underlying pancreatic inflammation is suspected based on a high diaphragm and/or pleural effusion.

Laboratory Findings. An elevated serum amylase concentration and mild leukocytosis (10,000 to 15,000 cells/cu mm) are present in about one half of the patients. Persistence of an elevated serum amylase concentration for more than five to seven days in a patient with acutely symptomatic pancreatitis who is otherwise improving clinically should suggest the presence of a pseudocyst. The amylase-creatinine clearance ratio may be normal if acute pancreatic inflammation has subsided; this test is not helpful in diagnosing pancreatic pseudocysts. If extrahepatic biliary obstruction is present, the serum bilirubin and alkaline phosphatase concentrations are usually elevated.

Abdominal ultrasonographic examination is a reliable way to diagnose pseudocysts and should be used in most cases to screen for their presence (Fig. 98–7).[109] On occasion, adjacent ileus may interfere with good-resolution ultrasonography. CT scans also provide useful diagnostic information (Fig. 98–8). With these two techniques, the size of the cyst can be determined accurately. Serial studies may reveal changes in size and configuration. Occasionally, acute pseudocysts will disappear as the fluid is reabsorbed. Fluid-filled cysts can be distinguished reliably from a pancreatic phlegmon. The distinction from pancreatic abscess may be less clear, however. Because ultrasonography and CT scanning can detect lesions as small as a few centimeters in diameter, small asymptomatic pseudocysts are now being diagnosed whereas previously most went undetected. As far as is known, such cysts (less than 5 cm) do not require therapy and most will resolve spontaneously.

In most cases, the upper gastrointestinal series will

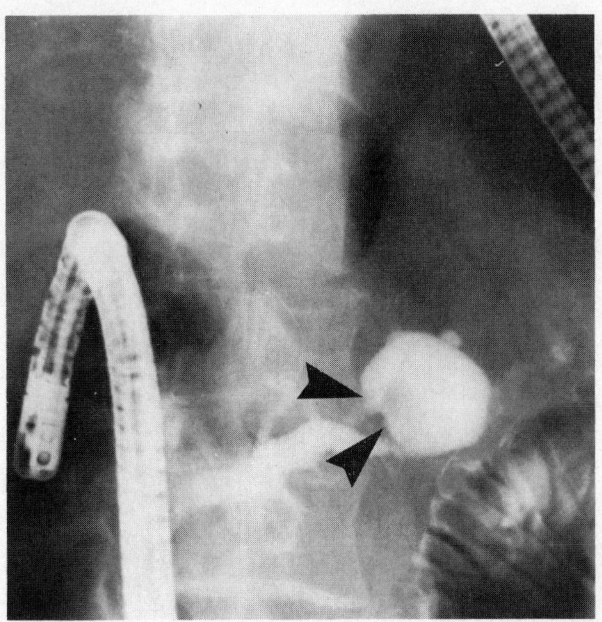

Figure 98–9. ERCP in a patient with a pancreatic pseudocyst. The contrast material first fills a dilated irregular pancreatic duct, then a 3 to 4 cm rounded collection *(arrows)* arising from the midbody of the duct. The contrast injection is made directly under fluoroscopic guidance and is stopped when the pseudocyst fills.

reveal a lesser sac mass that distorts the stomach or duodenum. However, a pseudocyst cannot be distinguished reliably from a phlegmon, pancreatic cancer, or pancreatic abscess by conventional barium radiographic studies.

Although endoscopic retrograde cholangiopancreatography (ERCP) will usually cause filling of the cyst, demonstrating its location and showing multiple cysts in 10 to 15 per cent of cases, the role of ERCP lies in the demonstration of the anatomy of the pancreatic duct and the pseudocyst itself immediately prior to scheduled surgical intervention.[110] When it is performed, the patient should receive prophylactic antibiotics before endoscopic cannulation of the pancreatic duct, because there is some danger of introducing infection during the study (see p. 1858 for antibiotics used for infection). The duct must be filled cautiously, with careful fluoroscopic monitoring (Fig. 98–9). To minimize the frequency of complicating infections, surgical treatment of the cyst is usually done within 12 to 24 hours of ERCP.

Thoracentesis of pleural fluid caused by a subdiaphragmatic inflammatory pseudocyst will reveal fluid with a high protein level, a high white cell count, and an amylase concentration three to ten times the level that is measured simultaneously in serum. If grossly infected, the fluid may contain frank pus or be very cloudy and have a white cell count of 10,000/mm^3 or higher.

Differential Diagnosis. Pancreatic pseudocyst must be distinguished from pancreatic abscess, which usually produces clinical toxicity with higher fever (103° to 104° F) and marked leukocytosis (greater than 15,000 cells/cu mm) (see p. 1835).

Neoplastic cysts, such as cystadenoma or cystadenocarcinoma, account for about 10 per cent of pancreatic masses that are cystic. Although ultrasonographic examination may suggest neoplasm (neoplastic cysts are usually multiloculated and have thicker irregular walls), preoperative distinction between pseudocysts and cystic tumors is not always possible. Sonography and CT scanning techniques are steadily improving, however, and both examinations are enhanced when combined with directed percutaneous aspiration cytology of the cyst fluid and wall. The diagnosis is established at operation from histologic study of tissue from the cyst wall (see pp. 1878–1879).

Natural History and Complications of Pseudocysts. The natural history of any individual pseudocyst is difficult to predict. A sizable percentage of acute cystic fluid collections of the pancreas resolve with conservative management. In one series of 54 patients followed by serial clinical and sonographic evaluations, of the 24 for whom the presumed duration of the pseudocyst was less than six weeks, spontaneous resolution occurred in ten (40 per cent).[109] Only 1 of 13 pseudocysts present between 7 and 12 weeks resolved spontaneously, whereas none of the 17 present for longer than 13 weeks resolved. In the patient groups with pseudocysts of less than one to six, 7 to 12, and 13 weeks' duration, the complication rates were 21 per cent, 46 per cent, and 65 per cent, respectively. Thus, pseudocysts present for more than six weeks are unlikely to resolve spontaneously and more likely to result in complications. Infection, rupture, and hemorrhage complicate the course of a sizable number of patients with pseudocysts, but because the larger pseudocysts of most patients are treated surgically within several months of diagnosis, the true frequency of these complications is unknown.[111] In a patient with a known or suspected pseudocyst, however, the pseudocyst must always be considered the likely source of unexplained sepsis, abdominal pain, or marked hemorrhage until proved otherwise.

Infection. Although infection of a pseudocyst is rare, the clinical picture is usually striking, as this complication usually produces high fever, severe pain, shaking chills, and leukocytosis. It may be startling because its expression is often sudden in patients who are otherwise doing well. The source of the organism is presumed to be the adjacent stomach, small intestine, and large bowel, as cultures yield a variety of enteric organisms. Except for the obvious introduction of organisms by the injection of contrast agents during ERCP, the mechanism of infection by bowel organisms of the stagnant cyst fluid is unknown. Diagnosis of infection should be suspected in the presence of fever, often spiking to 103° to 104° F or more, upper abdominal tenderness, and marked leukocytosis (>15,000 cells/cu mm). Blood cultures may be positive. On occasion, plain radiography of the abdomen or CT scans may show pancreatic gas (Fig. 98–10). However, the absence of gas in the pseudocyst *does not exclude* an infection. In patients in whom the suspicion of an infected pseudocyst is raised, CT- or ultrasonographi-

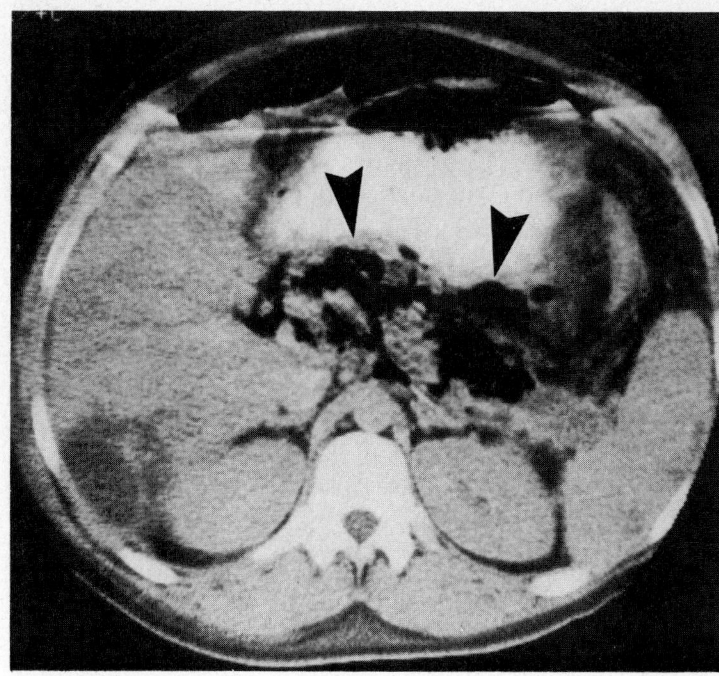

Figure 98–10. Computed tomography in a patient with an infected acute pseudocyst. Multiple low-density gas-filled cystic spaces are noted throughout the pancreas *(arrows)*. Free peritoneal air was introduced during peritoneal dialysis and is to be seen anterior to the stomach.

cally guided fine needle aspiration for Gram stain and aerobic and anaerobic bacterial cultures must be undertaken.[112]

As soon as the diagnosis is suspected, the patient must be started on broad-coverage antibiotics intravenously: ampicillin (1 gm intravenously every four hours); clindamycin (600 mg intravenously every six hours); and an aminoglycoside, such as gentamicin or tobramycin (3 to 5 mg/kg/day in three divided doses). Other antibiotic combinations, such as the newer cephalosporins and metronidazole, are also acceptable, although extensive series have not established the most appropriate antibiotic coverage. Surgical drainage must be performed promptly; otherwise the patient is at risk for serious intra-abdominal spread of infection or gram-negative septicemia, or both. Because anastomoses do not heal in the presence of infection, external drainage frequently is necessary for infected pseudocysts. If the pseudocyst is intimately adherent to the posterior wall of the stomach, internal drainage into the stomach (cystogastrostomy) may be possible.

The role of percutaneous transabdominal catheter drainage of infected pseudocysts is being actively studied in several centers. The catheter is placed under CT or ultrasonographic guidance. Large catheters (at least No. 8 French) must be used. Complex infected pseudocysts with internal septations or a large amount of necrotic solid material, or both, may not drain well using the percutaneous techniques. At present, this method of infected cyst drainage remains promising and worthy of controlled clinical trials.[113, 114]

Rupture. Sudden perforation of a pseudocyst into the free peritoneal cavity produces a severe chemical peritonitis with boardlike abdominal rigidity and intense pain.[115] Rapid enlargement of the pseudocyst, verifiable by sonography, sometimes precedes perforation and is an indication for operation. The treatment for perforation is emergency operation with irrigation of the peritoneal cavity and the drainage of the cyst. Even with prompt treatment, perforation is often fatal.

Rarely, the pseudocyst will erode into an adjacent viscus (the stomach or colon most frequently) and drain spontaneously into the gastrointestinal tract rather than freely into the peritoneal space. The palpable mass disappears, and ultrasonography confirms its collapse. With perforation into the colon, vague abdominal pain and a self-limited bloody diarrhea may be the only findings. Perforation into the stomach may produce even fewer symptoms. Unless bleeding or infection requires operation, a patient whose cyst spontaneously decompresses into the stomach and not into the colon does not require further treatment.

Hemorrhage. Hemorrhage from pancreatic pseudocyst results from erosion of small vessels lining the cyst wall (thus hemorrhaging into the cyst), from erosion of the cyst into nearby major vessels (e.g., splenic or gastroduodenal arteries, forming pseudoaneurysms, thus bleeding into the peritoneum or cyst, or both), or from cyst perforation into an adjacent viscus.[116] When a cyst bleeds into the stomach or duodenum directly, the patient usually has massive hematemesis and shock. With intracystic bleeding, rapid enlargement of the cyst may be confirmed on physical examination and by sonography; however, severe pain and shock may be the only clues. Some bleeding into the pancreatic duct (hemosuccus pancreaticus) may occur.[117, 118] In patients with vigorous hemorrhage into the pancreatic duct, endoscopy may visualize blood flowing from the duodenal papilla; however, in most instances endoscopy will fail to visualize a source of hemorrhage. In patients with known pseudocysts who develop significant hemorrhage without clear-cut findings on endoscopy, mesenteric arteriography is essential. In many instances, interventional techniques such as selective arterial embolization with metal coils will control the hemorrhage without the need for surgical ligation.

If the cyst bleeds into the peritoneal cavity, hemorrhagic shock may develop rapidly with no early clues for either site or cause of bleeding. Unfortunately, the patient's condition usually deteriorates so rapidly that angiography may be impractical, but it should be attempted. Emergency operation, although technically quite difficult, may ultimately be necessary to identify and stop the hemorrhage. The mortality rate of this complication is high even with prompt therapy.

Pancreatic Ascites

Pancreatic ascites is the result of a persistent leak of pancreatic juice from a pseudocyst or, less frequently, directly from a disrupted pancreatic duct.[111, 119] It is an uncommon condition and constitutes less than 5 per cent of the causes of ascites (see pp. 428–454).

Clinical Findings. Pancreatic ascites is painless and usually massive, as pancreatic secretions may exceed 1 L/per day. It usually develops insidiously in a chronic alcoholic patient and most often is misdiagnosed as cirrhotic ascites. In most patients, there is no previous history of pancreatic disease. Occasionally it is a complication of severe acute pancreatitis, in which case the pancreatic origin of the problem is more obvious. In children, trauma is responsible for most cases. Whereas sudden rupture of a pseudocyst presents as a major abdominal catastrophe with a high mortality rate, swelling of the abdomen with pancreatic ascites runs a much more benign and chronic course. Indeed, many patients have pancreatic ascites for weeks or months before diagnosis. Marked recent weight loss is the major clinical manifestation, aside from an enlargement of the abdomen. When the leak is confined by adjacent structures, the pancreatic juice does not empty into the free peritoneal cavity and may be loculated at some distance from the pancreas. Thus, even mediastinal and pleural pancreatic effusions may be found occasionally; the fluid in these loci has the same composition as the fluid in the abdomen. The physician should be especially alert to the diagnosis of pancreatic ascites in the alcoholic patient with ascites whose liver function is not significantly impaired and in whom the liver is not significantly enlarged.

Laboratory Findings. Definitive diagnosis of pancreatic ascites is based on chemical analysis of the ascitic fluid (straw-colored or blood-tinged), which shows a high amylase concentration (greater than 1000 IU/L)—much higher than the serum amylase concentration, which may indeed be normal. A high protein concentration (greater than 3.0 gm/dl) of the ascitic fluid is also characteristic. Rarely, the albumin concentration of the fluid is low because of severe hypoproteinemia, usually associated with evidence of liver disease or severe malnutrition.

Initial management of this problem is medical; however, inasmuch as the majority of these patients require it, surgical treatment of pancreatic ascites is discussed on page 1867.

Common Bile Duct Obstruction

The intrapancreatic portion of the common bile duct is obstructed in 5 to 10 per cent of persons with chronic pancreatitis but requires treatment in only a fraction of these patients.[88, 120] This complication should always be suspected in patients with chronic pancreatitis who have persistent hyperbilirubinemia or marked elevation of the serum alkaline phosphatase value (greater than five times normal limits), or both. The diagnosis of extrahepatic bile duct obstruction can also be suggested by liver biopsy findings, 80 per cent of the patients in one series showing pathologic changes of the liver consistent with common duct obstruction.[121] The diagnosis may be further supported by ultrasonography and CT scanning (noting dilated bile ducts) and made definitively by retrograde or percutaneous cholangiography (Fig. 98–11). Intervention to relieve the obstruction is warranted, however, only in those whose liver function results or histologic findings show progressive damage attributable to chronic stasis. The gastric outlet as well as the common duct occasionally is obstructed, usually as the result of duodenal or antral compression by a large inflammatory pseudocyst or pancreatic phlegmon. The clinical pictures of cholangitis and

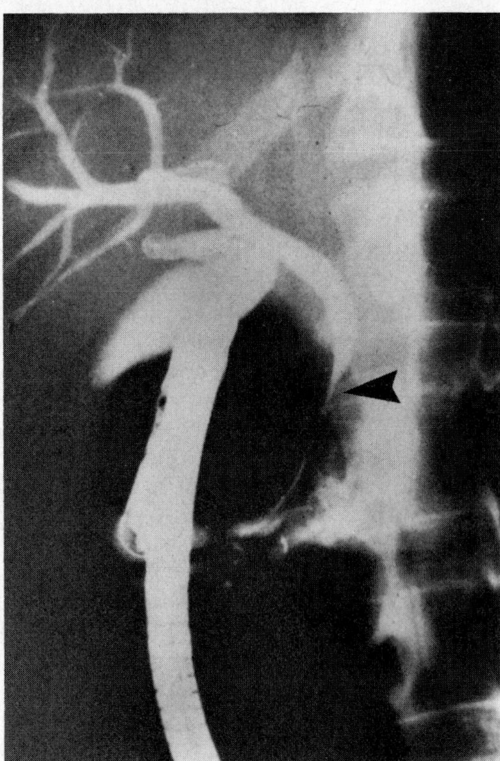

Figure 98–11. ERCP in patient with chronic pancreatitis with obstructive jaundice. A symmetric, smoothly tapered common bile duct stricture is injected with contrast material *(arrow)*. Only a small portion of the pancreatic duct is filled.

gastric outlet obstruction are presented in detail on pages 1717 and 932, respectively.

Portal and Splenic Vein Thrombosis

Rarely, extrahepatic portal hypertension may result from the compression of the portal or splenic veins, or both, by a fibrotic pancreas or a pseudocyst. Splenic vein thrombosis with concomitant splenomegaly may also be a complication resulting from the contiguity of the inflamed pancreas and the splenic vein. Thrombosis of the splenic vein causes intrasplenic venous hypertension leading to collateral circulation through gastric fundic varices, upper gastrointestinal bleeding, and evidence of hypersplenism. The physician must be especially alert to the possibility of splenic vein thrombosis as the cause of gastric varices and bleeding in alcoholic patients with pancreatic disease. As in the instance of the misdiagnosis of pancreatic ascites for hepatic ascites in the alcoholic patient, so bleeding varices may be attributed to intrahepatic portal hypertension rather than splenic vein thrombosis. Clinically, the differential diagnosis may be difficult because the spleen is enlarged in both situations (although a rapidly enlarging spleen makes splenic vein thrombosis more likely), because the patient may have concomitant liver disease, and because splenic vein thrombosis is also a complication of portal hypertension. Splenic vein thrombosis must be strongly suspected, however, in the alcoholic patient with probable or known pancreatitis—acute or chronic—with gastric variceal bleeding. The diagnosis may be suggested by ultrasonography but is made by selective splenic artery angiography or splenoportography with careful study of the anatomy of the splenic vein and search for prominent perisplenic vessels that may be collaterals associated with gastric varices.

Peptic Ulcer Disease

The prevalence of peptic ulcer disease in chronic pancreatitis is about 20 per cent.[12, 19] This figure may be an underestimate because the available information is not based on a systematic endoscopic search for gastroduodenal ulceration. Thus, its accuracy is not established. Although decreased availability of bicarbonate in pancreatic juice for gastric acid neutralization may be responsible for the development of duodenal ulcers, gastric acid secretion is decreased in patients with chronic pancreatitis who also have a high frequency of achlorhydria.[122] The relationship, if any, of chronic pancreatitis to duodenal ulcer thus remains obscure.

TREATMENT

Treatment of uncomplicated chronic pancreatitis is usually nonsurgical, with care directed to preventing further intake of alcohol (if this is the cause of the disease), relief of acute and chronic pain, nutritional support, and oral replacement of missing digestive enzymes. Surgical intervention may be necessary in certain situations.

Acute Exacerbations of Chronic Pancreatitis

When patients have attacks that are clinically indistinguishable from those of acute pancreatitis during the course of their chronic illness, they should be treated as described on pages 1832 to 1836. Often these attacks are brief and mild, requiring only a few days of hospitalization with a treatment program consisting primarily of rest and restriction of food and fluid by mouth. Of course, such patients may have more severe episodes, including symptoms due to inflammatory pseudocysts. In these instances, more comprehensive evaluation and management are indicated (see pp. 1855–1859).

Chronic Pain

Pain is the chief symptom for which most patients with chronic pancreatitis seek relief. Abstention from alcohol and from consumption of large meals is helpful in some instances. Unremitting pain causes decreased food intake and weight loss. The physician should first prescribe non-narcotic analgesics, such as acetaminophen, aspirin, or other nonsteroidal anti-inflammatory drugs. However, narcotics are frequently required and should not be withheld because pain relief, not the risk of inducing opiate addiction, is the immediate concern of patient and physician.

Destruction of the celiac plexus by alcohol injection under radiographic guidance was reported to reduce pain for greater than six months in about one half of patients so treated in one study,[123] but produced no measurable benefit at six months in two other studies.[124, 125] Because of the questionable benefits of this procedure and potential complications, it is not to be recommended for the treatment of intractable pain in chronic pancreatitis, although it may palliate pain in some patients with pancreatic cancer.[124] In a prospective, randomized investigation, neither electroacupuncture nor transcutaneous electric nerve stimulation resulted in an improvement in patients' sense of well-being or a reduction in use of analgesics.[126]

Considerable interest has recently been generated by reports that administration of pancreatic digestive enzyme supplements may produce an improvement in chronic pain in patients with chronic pancreatitis.[127, 128] The proposed mechanism of action is by intraduodenal feedback inhibition of cholecystokinin-stimulated pancreatic secretion by proteases present in the enzyme supplements. Evidence for the existence of such feedback regulation has been observed in humans;[129] in addition, several,[130, 131] but not all,[132] studies have demonstrated elevated plasma cholecystokinin levels in patients with chronic pancreatitis.

The two studies suggesting a benefit from enzyme

supplement therapy for pain indicate that women with idiopathic chronic pancreatitis[127, 128] and patients with normal fecal fat excretion[128] are most likely to respond. A subsequent study[133] failed to show a significant reduction in pain in patients receiving enzyme supplements.

The efficacy of digestive enzyme supplementation in treating the pain of chronic pancreatitis is difficult to evaluate owing to frequent spontaneous remissions of this symptom, either temporary or permanent, in this group of patients. However, pending the results of future prospective, randomized clinical trials, it is reasonable to institute a therapeutic trial with an enzyme supplement (e.g., Viokase or Ilozyme, eight tablets four times a day) for one to two months in patients being considered for surgical procedures to alleviate the pain of chronic pancreatitis. If suppression of pancreatic stimulation by cholecystokinin does prove to be of benefit in reducing the pain of chronic pancreatitis, it is possible that treatment with potent cholecystokinin-receptor antagonists currently being developed[134] may prove to be a more direct means of accomplishing this goal. Surgery as treatment of pain is discussed on pages 1863 to 1866.

Malabsorption

The clinical expression of chronic pancreatitis that has led to pancreatic insufficiency is malabsorption (see also pp. 263–282), which results from impaired digestion in the lumen of the small intestine. Malabsorption requires specific medical treatment only after steatorrhea has been documented quantitatively and after weight loss has persisted despite efforts to correct factors that limit food intake, such as pain, high doses of opiates, and irregular eating habits. The treatment is based on digestive enzyme substitution with orally administered extracts of pancreas. The results are commonly expressed as the reduction in the degree of steatorrhea because the secretion of lipase tends to decrease more rapidly than secretion of proteolytic enzymes in chronic pancreatitis. Hence, steatorrhea is often an earlier and more severe problem.

Pancreatic Enzyme Supplementation. Success with enzyme supplementation is not always easily achieved. It requires some understanding of the factors determining the enzyme activities that will occur intraluminally after digestion.[135, 136] Four important points need to be considered.

1. The commercially available enzyme preparations are of relatively low potency. Thus, if *no* inactivation of contained lipase occurred, eight or more tablets or capsules of such preparations as pancreatin (Viokase) or pancreatolipase (Cotazym) with meals would be necessary to abolish steatorrhea. This amount is roughly equivalent to 5 to 10 per cent of total lipase secretion after maximal stimulation of the pancreas that usually reaches the duodenum.[57, 137]

2. Once ingested, lipase is rapidly inactivated at a pH below 4.0, whereas trypsin inactivation proceeds more slowly and is mediated by pepsin at a pH of less than 3.5.[138]

3. The duodenal pH in patients with chronic pancreatitis is lower than in control subjects late in the postprandial period[139] and is frequently less than 5.0—a pH at which bile acids precipitate. This reduced availability of conjugated bile acids for fat solubilization and micelle formation is an additional cause of impaired fat absorption.[140]

4. Because enzyme supplements are expensive and must be taken with every meal and snack to be maximally effective, compliance is often poor, especially among alcoholics.

Clinical studies have shown that eight pancreatin tablets taken with a meal results in the delivery to the duodenum of only 8 per cent of the lipase activity contained in the tablets, amounting to less than 1 per cent of normal output of meal-stimulated lipase. The corresponding values for trypsin are 22 per cent and 1.4 per cent, respectively. However, even these small increments in duodenal digestive enzyme content are sufficient to reduce stool fat by about 60 per cent and stool nitrogen output by about 75 per cent.[139] Other studies have also indicated that the efficacy of enzyme substitution therapy decreases in parallel with the mean postprandial pH in the stomach or duodenum.

These observations have led to efforts to improve the efficacy of therapy in patients who do not have an adequate response to pancreatic enzyme supplementation by avoiding the acid pH that inactivates the oral enzyme preparations. Two different approaches have been tried: the use of antacids or cimetidine to raise the gastric and intestinal pH and the use of pancreatic enzymes in microencapsulated enteric pH-coated forms.

The use of antacids has yielded mixed results. Whereas coadministration of enzyme tablets with either sodium bicarbonate or aluminum hydroxide resulted in a greater reduction of steatorrhea than did enzyme tablets alone, the use of calcium carbonate or magnesium-aluminum hydroxide actually tended to worsen steatorrhea.[141, 142] Sodium hydroxide was effective only if given prior to, or at the beginning of, a meal rather than after a meal.[141] The worsening of steatorrhea with the use of calcium carbonate or magnesium-aluminum hydroxide appears to result mainly from the formation of poorly soluble calcium or magnesium soaps and to the intraluminal precipitation of glycine-conjugated bile salts.[143, 144]

The use of cimetidine (300 mg 30 minutes before meals) as an adjunct to pancreatic enzyme supplementation has produced modest to major reductions in steatorrhea in most studies;[142, 145–148] no effect was seen in another study, however.[141] It appears that cimetidine is more likely to be beneficial in patients with hyperchlorhydria than in patients with relatively low rates of gastric acid secretion and when given in conjunction with large amounts of pancreatic enzymes (approximately 30,000 IU of lipase per meal).[136] In addition to reducing inactivation of pancreatic enzymes by maintaining gastric and duodenal pH greater than 4.0, cimetidine may also be effective in reducing steatorrhea by decreasing the total volume of fluid in the duodenum (by reducing gastric secretion), thus resulting in less dilution of ingested pancreatic enzymes.[142]

In a different approach to the prevention of pH-dependent inactivation of enzyme, a lipase-enriched pancreatic extract is enclosed by a pH-dependent polymer to produce granules 1.5 to 2.5 mm in diameter (Pancrease brand of pancrelipase). When swallowed encased in a capsule, the granules are released in the stomach; their protective coating, however, dissolves only when the pH is 6.0 or higher. Thus, the enzymes are designed to go into solution only in the distal duodenum or jejunum. Unlike some earlier enteric-coated "delayed-release" preparations, Pancrease is effective in reducing steatorrhea owing to pancreatic insufficiency.[149] However, it has not been shown to be more effective than conventional enzyme preparations,[142, 149, 150] which generally are less expensive. The failure of this type of enteric-coated preparation to be more effective than potent conventional forms may be due to incomplete release of enzymes in the proximal intestine of patients with chronic pancreatitis (who may have an intraluminal pH for extended periods of time that is less than the 6.0 required for dissolution of the enzyme-containing granules), delayed emptying of the granules from the stomach,[150] or inactivation of granules in the stomach if the intragastric pH first rises above 6.0 (releasing the enzymes from the granules) and subsequently falls to less than 4.0 during the digestion of a meal. It has been proposed that patients with hyperchlorhydria (often present in children with cystic fibrosis) may benefit most from this enteric-coated preparation.[136]

Despite the potential complexity of enzyme replacement therapy in chronic pancreatitis, most patients will respond to a restricted-fat diet (60 to 80 gm/day) and treatment with conventional enzyme preparations (six to eight tablets or capsules of Viokase, Cotazym, or Ilozyme taken throughout each meal) with stabilization or gain of weight and a reduction in diarrhea, abdominal cramps, and bloating. The efficacy of therapy can be assessed objectively by comparing the 24-hour stool fat excretion during enzyme supplementation to that measured prior to enzyme therapy. If this approach is unsuccessful, the dose of the original preparation should be increased. If the exocrine insufficiency remains substantially unimproved, the use of the enteric-coated preparation (Pancrease, three to four capsules/meal) or addition of cimetidine (300 mg 30 minutes before each meal) should be tried. Continued failure should lead the physician to consider other potential causes of malabsorption (e.g., intestinal parasites, celiac sprue) instead of, or in addition to, pancreatic insufficiency.

Pancreatic extracts contain 8 to 10 per cent by weight of nucleic acids. When given in therapeutic doses, this increased dietary purine content results in an additional uric acid load of up to 500 mg/day. This explains why considerable hyperuricosuria and occasional hyperuricemia have been reported in children with cystic fibrosis receiving large amounts of supplemental pancreatic enzymes.[151] Renal urate stone formation, however, has not been observed. This issue has not been investigated in adult patients with chronic pancreatitis.

Nutritional Support. Although many patients with chronic pancreatitis and malnutrition (in part attributable to malabsorption) are able to maintain weight and strength because of good appetite and high caloric intake, some require measures to improve and maintain good nutrition. For those who are chronically debilitated or whose nutrition may be jeopardized by an acute complication of their chronic disease, modern measures for supplementing protein and calories should be employed. Total parenteral nutrition (TPN) or enteral feeding may be needed for weeks to months (details for these regimens as well as for more conventional modes of supplementation are found on pp. 1994–2027). As patients improve, frequent feedings high in protein, supplemented by fat to make the diet palatable, and the addition of a pancreatic enzyme preparation will usually suffice to maintain weight and strength. In some patients, however, this approach will not be adequate, and greater emphasis must be placed on fat intake, particularly the use of medium-chain triglycerides.

Medium-Chain Triglycerides (MCT). In patients with weight loss refractory to diet and enzyme substitution therapy, supplementation with MCT is a theorectically attractive step. MCT is prepared from coconut oil and consists of approximately 75 per cent trioctanoate (C_8) and 25 per cent tridecanoate (C_{10}). MCT differs from dietary long-chain triglycerides (LCT) in the following ways: It is partly water-soluble; hydrolysis by gastric and pancreatic lipase proceeds much faster than for LCT; and some MCT is absorbed intact. Absorbed medium-chain fatty acids enter the portal vein rather than intestinal lymph, and more MCT than LCT is metabolized to CO_2 and ketone bodies.[152] MCT may be used to replace part of the dietary LCT and to increase total fat intake as high as tolerated. About 25 per cent of patients, however, develop nausea and increased diarrhea when consuming 40 gm/day or more of MCT. The coefficient of fat absorption rises invariably when MCT is added to the diet, but, curiously, weight gain is achieved with regularity only in children with cystic fibrosis and rarely in adults with advanced chronic pancreatitis.[152] MCT is available in formula diet (Portagen), but many patients prefer to use pure MCT oil for food preparation.[153]

Management of Diabetes Mellitus. The principal steps in the management of diabetes mellitus associated with chronic pancreatitis consist of correction of irregular food intake and malnutrition, reduction of alcohol intake, treatment of malabsorption, and reversal of the poor attitudes of patients concerning this disease. Oral hypoglycemic agents may improve glucose tolerance and are worth a trial if the patient has significant glycosuria.[154] Eventually many patients require insulin, which, however, must be administered with extreme caution. Although the daily insulin requirement is usually between 20 and 40 units, single doses of 10 to 15 units may reduce very high blood glucose levels to dangerously low values. This tendency to hypoglycemia is unpredictable and may be attributable in part to the deficiency of glucagon secretion in chronic pancreatitis.[155] In one series of 18 patients with chronic pancreatitis requiring insulin treatment, six patients developed severe hypoglycemic episodes, which were fatal in three patients over a nine-year period. The safe course is to give sufficient insulin to prevent large urinary glucose losses rather than attempt to achieve normal blood glucose concentrations. This approach carries little risk because the patient with pancreatic diabetes appears less prone to develop either ketoacidosis or the severe microvascular disease so common in hereditary diabetes. Because of the frequency and dangers of hypoglycemia, the patient with pancreatitis who is taking insulin must be thoroughly instructed in its prevention and symptoms as well as modes of self-treatment.

Hyperoxaluria. An additional risk of untreated steatorrhea is increased renal oxalate excretion (see pp. 263–282 and 1106–1112). With a high concentration of long-chain fatty acids in the colon, intraluminal calcium is bound by the formation of insoluble calcium soaps. Consequently, less calcium is available for the precipitation of unabsorbed dietary oxalate as calcium oxalate; the oxalate remains in solution and diffuses passively across the colonic mucosa and is then excreted in the urine. The result is that a patient with steatorrhea of any cause may exhibit hyperoxaluria (greater than 40 to 50 mg/day of urinary oxalate) provided that the colon is intact. The hyperoxaluria can be corrected by four different approaches: a low dietary oxalate intake, a diet low in long-chain triglycerides, pancreatic enzyme substitution therapy, and an increased intake of either calcium (2 to 3 gm/day) or aluminum in the form of antacids (3.5 gm/day of aluminum). With severe steatorrhea (greater than 30 gm/day of fecal fat), any two of these four methods should be employed.[157, 158] The risk of renal oxalate stone formation in patients with pancreatic insufficiency is not known but probably is quite low. In this setting, the detection and specific treatment of hyperoxaluria may therefore be reserved for those few patients who develop nephrolithiasis.

SURGERY FOR PAIN

Surgical procedures for the management of pain in chronic pancreatitis should be limited to those patients who meet certain specific criteria: (1) constant disabling pain that interferes with life-style *or* several relapses of substantial pain per year *or* several months of loss of work per year because of pain, *and* (2) failure to respond to a conservative medical program, including pain medications and a trial of exocrine pancreatic enzyme replacement.[159–162] Exocrine insufficiency alone must not be the sole indication for surgery in patients with chronic pancreatitis. The decision to operate on these individuals is difficult because the pain of this disease often remits spontaneously after several years' duration. Patients should be advised, therefore, to postpone an operation in hope of a permanent remission or substantial improvement of symptoms. Additional deterrents to surgery are the high likelihood of long-term postoperative morbidity in the alcoholic or the narcotic addict; the psychologic, physical, and economic toll of the commonly used surgical procedures; and the unpredictability of a successful result even under the best of circumstances.

Choice of operation is best made with the knowledge of the anatomy of the pancreatic duct system, which should be obtained preoperatively by ERCP and CT scanning. Because dilated ducts imply obstruction, drainage operations (Fig. 98–12) are more likely to succeed when ducts are dilated. Subtotal pancreatectomy may be indicated when the ducts are small (less than 8 mm diameter), when disease is confined to a segment of the gland and the remainder is relatively normal, and when a previous drainage procedure has been unsuccessful. Results of operative procedures generally are better in patients who abstain from alcohol postoperatively (if alcohol was the primary etiologic agent in the development of pancreatitis).[162–165]

Drainage Operations

Longitudinal Pancreaticojejunostomy (Puestow-Gillesby Procedure). At present, this is the most widely performed and accepted drainage operation; it is usually done in patients with pain and an irregular, widely dilated pancreatic duct (8 mm or more diameter) with alternating segments of narrowing and dilatation ("chain of lakes" appearance) (Fig. 98–12*C*). The entire main duct is opened longitudinally, and any stones are extracted. A defunctionalized jejunal segment (Roux-en-Y loop) is opened longitudinally and sewn over the open duct so that pancreatic juice can empty into the lumen over the length of the gland.

Surgical mortality rate for this drainage procedure generally is less than 4 per cent.[162] In general, nearly 80 per cent of patients undergoing longitudinal pancreaticojejunostomy can be expected to have substantial pain relief at six months, whereas at five years, 50 per cent of alcohol abusers and 60 per cent of nonalcoholics have continued pain relief.[162] In one study of the long-term results of pancreaticojejunostomy in chronic pancreatitis patients, 60 per cent reported complete or excellent pain relief, whereas 12 per cent noted good relief for an overall good to excellent result in 72 per cent of patients followed for a mean of over eight years.[166] For those who fail to respond, a postoperative ERCP is indicated to look for undrained segments of the pancreatic duct or for nonopacification of the Roux-en-Y loop.[167] Redrainage rather than resection may provide good to excellent pain relief in as many as 70 per cent of patients.[167]

Caudal Pancreaticojejunostomy (Du Val Procedure) (Fig. 98–12*B*). Rarely, a single point of ductal obstruction may be present in the middle of the pancreas with

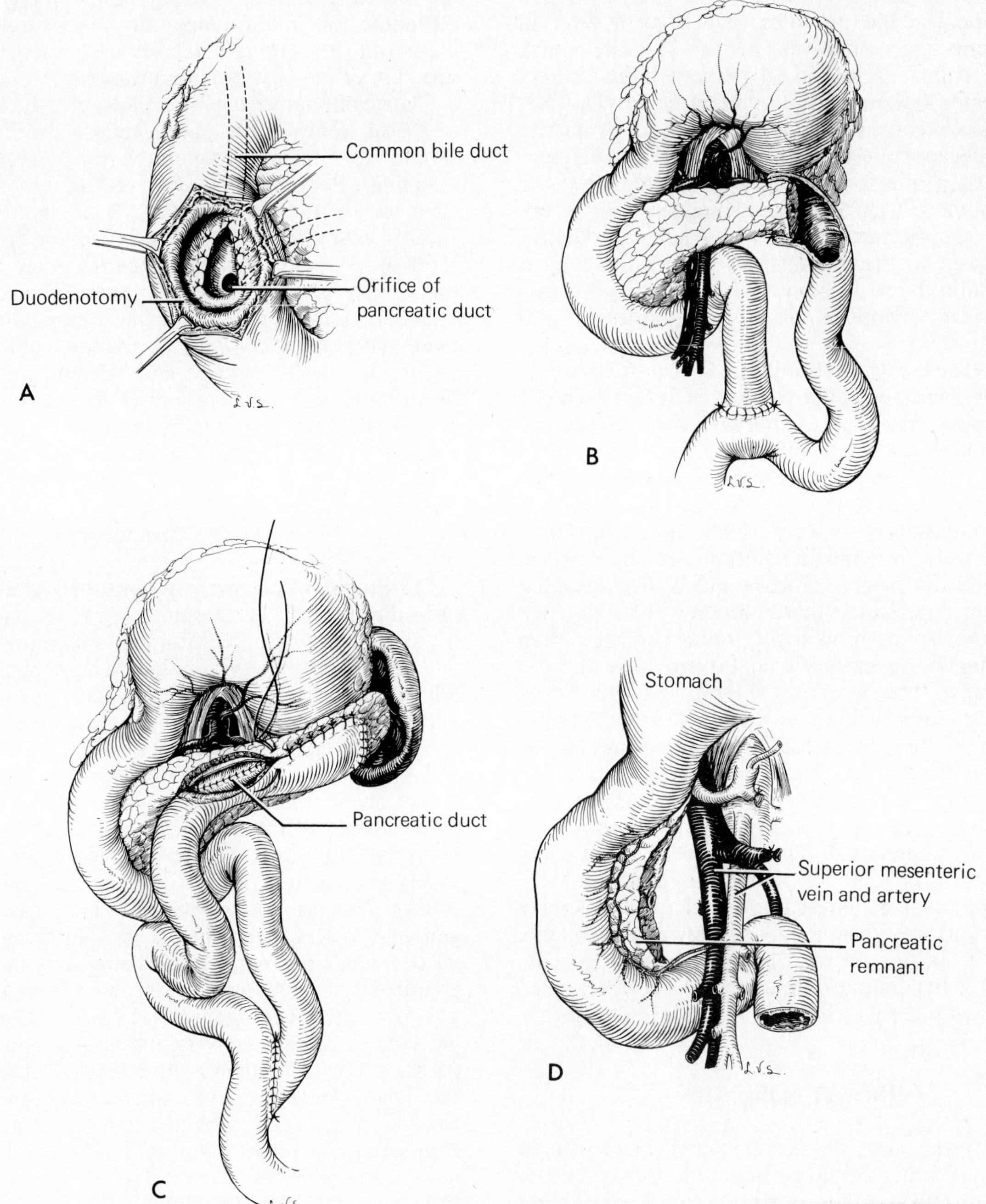

Figure 98–12. *A*, Sphincteroplasty. *B*, Caudal pancreaticojejunostomy (Du Val procedure). *C*, Longitudinal pancreaticojejunostomy (Puestow procedure). *D*, Ninety-five per cent pancreatectomy. (From Dunphy, J. E., and Way, L. W. [eds.]. Current Surgical Diagnosis and Treatment. 2nd edition. Los Altos, Calif., Lange Medical Publications, 1975. Used by permission.)

distal duct dilatation. Retrograde drainage into a defunctionalized segment of jejunum placed end-to-end with the tail of the pancreas may be effective in relieving pain. In this setting, however, removal of the distal part of the pancreas containing the obstructed duct segment may often be preferable, so that caudal pancreaticojejunostomy is infrequently used today.

Sphincteroplasty (Fig. 98–12*A*). Although this surgical procedure was once employed in the treatment of chronic pancreatitis, it is useful only when an isolated obstruction is present at the sphincter of Oddi. For those patients with pancreas divisum *and* chronic pancreatitis *and* a dilated pancreatic ductal system, limited experience and some success have been reported employing sphincteroplasties of the major and minor papillae[164] (see pp. 1814–1842).

Endoscopic Therapy

An increase in pressure within the pancreatic duct behind a pancreatic stone or stricture has been postulated to be associated with the acute symptomatic relapses and the pain of chronic pancreatitis. Although considerable controversy still remains concerning pancreatic ductal pressures in chronic pancreatitis, the favorable response to surgical decompression has stimulated preliminary studies of endoscopic management. For those patients with chronic pancreatitis who have ampullary stenosis or retained common bile duct stones, a standard common bile duct endoscopic sphincterotomy should be considered. Pancreatic duct sphincterotomy, whether alone or in combination with basket extraction of pancreatic duct stones and pancreatic duct endoprosthesis, has been the subject of a few studies.[169, 170] Among 10 patients treated by pancreatic endoscopic sphincterotomy, Fuji and colleagues noted symptomatic improvement in nine patients,[170] whereas Schneider and Lux reported symptomatic relief in all three patients treated with pancreatic endoscopic papillotomy and stone removal.[169] Given the potential risks and the lack of larger series with long-term follow-up, pancreatic sphincterotomy and endoprosthesis placement should be performed only in the context of controlled clinical trials (see pp. 1741–1746).

Resection

In the absence of a dilated pancreatic duct on ERCP or intraoperative pancreatography or when previous decompressive procedures have failed, pancreatic resection has been performed in the hope of relieving intractable pain.[171–177] Preoperative ERCP may be very helpful in determining the extent of resection.[171] If the abnormal findings are confined exclusively to the distal part of the body or tail of the gland, as is often the case with traumatic pancreatitis caused by duct rupture or stricture, a limited (40 to 80 per cent) resection can be performed with the likelihood that the patient's pain will be relieved. In general, when the duct is occluded completely at only one point, whatever the cause of the pancreatitis, resection of the pancreas distal to that point often is the best procedure.

However, chronic pancreatitis caused by alcoholism usually involves the gland diffusely, and for this reason a 40 to 80 per cent pancreatic resection often is ineffective in relieving pain.[163, 173] In this situation, subtotal pancreatectomy (95 per cent) has been performed, leaving a small remnant of the head of the gland attached to the duodenum (Fig. 98–12).[163, 175, 176] This operation is also used after failure of a drainage procedure. Pancreaticoduodenectomy (Whipple's procedure) has been done when severe pancreatitis is confined to the head of the gland.[163, 175, 176] In rare cases, total pancreatectomy has been performed when severe pain has persisted after lesser resections.[163, 176, 177]

Pancreatic resections, like drainage procedures, have been reported to relieve pain completely or substantially for short periods of follow-up in 75 to 80 per cent of patients.[173–175, 177] However, retrospective comparisons indicate that drainage procedures are as effective[162] or more effective[172] than resection in relieving chronic pain. In addition, resection of more than 50 per cent of the pancreas in patients with chronic pancreatitis carries a substantial risk of pancreatic insufficiency and diabetes mellitus. With 95 per cent resection, about 75 per cent of patients will have diabetes mellitus requiring insulin, and all will require exocrine enzyme replacement therapy.[176] These factors must be considered when contemplating 95 per cent or total pancreatectomy or pancreaticoduodenectomy in active alcoholic patients known to lack compliance and emotional stability. The vast majority of these patients will require multiple subsequent hospitalizations for unstable diabetes mellitus or malnutrition, or both.[162]

Islet Cell and Segmental Pancreatic Autotransplantation

In an attempt to prevent diabetes mellitus by preserving pancreatic endocrine function after subtotal or total pancreatectomy, islet cell autotransplantation by infusion of islet cell preparations into the portal system has been employed.[178, 179] This approach has met with limited success because of the difficulty in obtaining adequate numbers of islet cells from a fibrotic, calcified pancreas. For this reason, vascularized, denervated, and neoprene-injected duct segments of pancreas have been autotransplanted in a small number of patients after pancreatic resection.[180–183] These appear to have been successful in maintaining normal glucose homeostasis. The use of a closed-loop insulin infusion system (artificial pancreas) is another potential approach to this problem.

Celiac Ganglionectomy (Splanchnicectomy)

This procedure interrupts efferent fibers from the pancreas and has been used to treat chronic pancreatic pain. However, the results are short-lived (less than 10 per cent relief over five years), and this approach has not found general acceptance.[162, 175]

SURGICAL MANAGEMENT OF PSEUDOCYSTS

Because ultrasonography has demonstrated that perhaps as many as 20 per cent or more of acute pseudocysts will resolve spontaneously, it is reasonable to follow the patient who has no complications with serial ultrasonographic examinations. This has the advantage of not only allowing time for spontaneous resolution but also, in the case of acute pseudocysts, permitting the wall of the pseudocyst to "mature" so that it is sufficiently firm to hold the sutures for internal drainage. If complications such as abscess formation, rupture into the abdominal cavity, hemorrhage into the pseudocyst, or biliary or gastric outlet obstruction occur during the period of observation, emergency surgical intervention will be required.

The appropriate length of time that acute pseudocysts can be observed safely in the hope of spontaneous resolution prior to nonemergency surgery has not been firmly established. In one series,[109] 90 per cent of pseudocysts that resolved spontaneously did so within six weeks of discovery, whereas 70 per cent of complications of pseudocysts appeared after seven weeks. About six weeks is generally required for the cyst wall to mature. However, if a pseudocyst is asymptomatic, small (less than 5 cm), and continuing to decrease in size after six weeks (as assessed sonographically), further close observation alone is indicated.

Chronic pseudocysts behave quite differently from acute pseudocysts.[184, 185] Over 90 per cent of chronic pseudocysts can be drained internally, whereas the vast majority of acute pseudocysts (of less than six weeks' age clinically) requiring drainage because of complication need external drainage. Moreover, nearly all patients with pseudocysts of indeterminate age (no recent bout of clinically acute pancreatitis) can undergo internal drainage.[185] The presence in the serum of an "old" amylase, an electrophoretically more mobile pancreatic (P) isoamylase, has been shown to correlate with the ability to perform internal drainage.[185] All 14 patients with serum "old" amylase could undergo internal drainage, whereas only 1 of 5 patients without "old" amylase could be drained internally.[185]

Pseudocysts developing in patients with chronic pancreatitis behave differently from those of acute pancreatitis and do not carry the same risk of serious complication. Most often, these patients come to surgical treatment because of the belief that the pseudocyst(s) may be responsible for intractable chronic pain or because of symptoms caused by compression of an important neighboring structure, such as the duodenum or common bile duct. However, in patients with chronic pain, when surgical drainage of a pseudocyst is done alone, without either a drainage procedure of the pancreatic duct or pancreatic resection, there is often little improvement in pain after the operation.[106, 163]

Excision, internal drainage, and external drainage are the three surgical procedures used in treatment of pseudocysts. In addition, there have been several reports of successful percutaneous drainage of pseudocysts by aspiration or catheter drainage guided by ultrasonography or computed tomography.[186–189] However, more experience will be required to determine if this approach is a feasible alternative to surgery.

Excision

Excision of the pseudocyst is the most definitive treatment but cannot be done frequently. It may be feasible for cysts of the pancreatic tail when the rest of the pancreas is normal (e.g., some traumatic pseudocysts).

Internal Drainage[190, 191]

If excision is impractical, internal drainage is the preferred method of treatment for most patients. An anastomosis is created between the pseudocyst and the stomach (cystogastrostomy), duodenum (cystoduodenostomy), or small bowel (cystojejunostomy), according to the location of the pseudocyst. The cyst fluid drains into the gastrointestinal tract, and the cyst cavity rapidly becomes obliterated. Even after cystogastrostomy, the patient can be allowed to eat an unrestricted diet within one week of surgery, and radiographs taken at this time usually show only a small residual cyst cavity.

External Drainage[190, 192]

External drainage is used for critically ill patients, those with infected pseudocysts, or those in whom the wall is not mature enough to hold sutures. A large catheter is sewn into the cyst lumen, and the other end is brought out through the abdominal wall. Postoperatively, the cyst collapses as the fluid drains externally, and with time the cyst becomes obliterated. Marsupialization, a technique rarely used today, consists of suturing the ends of the cyst wall to an opening in the peritoneum, through which the cyst fluid drains. Pancreatic fistulas, which may persist for months or years, develop in 30 per cent of patients treated by external drainage (see p. 395). These fistulas usually close in about five months without further surgery.

Operations for pancreatic pseudocysts generally are safe and effectively treat the immediate problem. The recurrence rate for pancreatic pseudocysts after surgery is about 10 per cent; recurrence is more frequent after external drainage.[191, 193] New cysts occasionally develop as manifestations of the underlying chronic pancreatitis, a disease process unaltered by cyst drainage. Major hemorrhage from the pseudocyst is a rare but serious complication of the drainage procedure.

MANAGEMENT OF PANCREATIC ASCITES AND PANCREATIC PLEURAL EFFUSION[114, 194, 195]

If the patient has lost more than 10 per cent of normal body weight, initial management should consist of total parenteral nutrition (TPN). In addition to correcting malnutrition, TPN obviates oral intake, thus removing a stimulus of pancreatic secretion (see pp. 1777–1788). Diuretics are ineffective in decreasing the amount of ascites. Although repeated paracentesis may keep the patient comfortable, complete removal of the recurring ascites is unnecessary and will not hasten resolution of this problem. The use of anticholinergic agents or of acetazolamide to reduce pancreatic secretion has been proposed but is of uncertain clinical value.

In a substantial number of patients, the leak of pancreatic fluid will spontaneously close, and ascites will begin to resolve during nutritional therapy.[188] When the amount of ascites has not decreased significantly after two to three weeks of medical management, an operation should be performed. Preoperative ERCP to identify the site of the leak (disruption of a duct or pseudocyst) will substantially improve the likelihood of successful surgery and reduce the frequency of recurrence.[195] If the site of the leak is the distal part of the pancreas, distal resection (with or without a drainage procedure, depending upon the state of the remainder of the duct system) may suffice. If the lesion is more proximal, it should be drained into the intestinal lumen via a Roux-en-Y jejunal anastomosis to the pseudocyst or the pancreatic duct, whichever is the source of the leak. Occasionally distal resection or internal drainage may be difficult to perform, and external drainage with a tube may be necessary. Eighty per cent of patients are relieved of their ascites, and the mortality rate for the operation is low if the patient's fluid, electrolyte, and nutritional deficiencies are corrected before surgery.

Intractable pancreatic pleural effusions may be drained via a large chest tube. Once again, adequate visualization of the ductal anatomy by ERCP is mandatory. In addition to adequate chest tube drainage, total parenteral nutrition and elimination of oral intake is indicated. The physician should not, however, expect medical conservative therapy to be successful in more than 50 per cent of patients; thus, continuation of this therapy is not justified for more than a few weeks.[162] The surgical approach for patients with pancreatic pleural effusions due to inflammatory pseudocysts is similar to that in patients with pancreatic ascites, i.e., drainage by Roux-en-Y jejunal anastomosis to the source of the leak, or, rarely, distal resection.

MISCELLANEOUS SURGICAL PROBLEMS: OBSTRUCTION OF COMMON BILE DUCT OR STOMACH AND SPLENIC VEIN THROMBOSIS

Common bile duct obstruction may occur in patients with chronic pancreatitis owing to constriction of the duct by fibrosis in the head of the pancreas or by compression as a result of a pseudocyst.[120, 121, 196, 197] A biliary-enteric drainage procedure (choledochoduodenostomy or cholecystojejunostomy) as well as drainage of pseudocysts in the head of the pancreas (if present) should be performed in patients with evidence of persistent stenosis of the intrapancreatic portion of the common bile duct. This will prevent the development of secondary biliary cirrhosis, which can occur in this setting even in the absence of clinical symptoms or signs of biliary obstruction.[121] Similarly, gastric outlet obstruction may occur owing to compression by a pseudocyst or the inflammatory process around the pancreas. Gastrojejunostomy will relieve this obstruction if there is no immediate remedy for the complication of chronic pancreatitis causing the blockage.

Extrahepatic portal hypertension from splenic vein thrombosis can be associated with gastric varices that may bleed. Splenectomy is curative because, unlike the case of portal hypertension from cirrhosis, the venous hypertension is restricted to those tributaries that drain into the splenic vein. Splenic vein thrombosis must be suspected in patients with acute and chronic pancreatitis, particularly alcoholics, who have upper gastrointestinal bleeding, gastric varices, but no significant liver disease or portal hypertension. The problem can be managed successfully with simple splenectomy. The physician must be sure preoperatively, however, via angiography, that the splenic vein indeed is occluded, that the varices represent perisplenic venous collaterals, and that the portal vein is patent.

References

1. Frey, C. F. Classification of pancreatitis: state of the art 1986. Pancreas *1*:62, 1986.
2. Sarles, H. Revised classification of pancreatitis—Marseille 1984. Dig. Dis. Sci. *30*:573, 1985.
3. Singer, M. V., Gyr, K., and Sarles, H. Revised classification of pancreatitis. Gastroenterology *89*:683, 1985.
4. Payan, H., Sarles, H., Demirdjian, M., Gauthier, A. P., Cros, R. C., and Durbel, J. P. Study of the histological features of chronic pancreatitis by correspondence analysis. Identification of chronic calcifying pancreatitis as an entity. Biomedicine *18*:663, 1972.
5. Nakamura, K., Sarles, H., and Payan, H. Three-dimensional reconstruction of the pancreatic ducts in chronic pancreatitis. Gastroenterology *62*:942, 1972.
6. LaGergren, C. Calcium carbonate precipitation in the pancreas, gallstones and urinary calculi. Acta Chir. Scand. *124*:320, 1962.
7. Olsen, T. S. The incidence and clinical relevance of chronic inflammation in the pancreas in autopsy material. Acta Pathol. Microbiol. Scand. (Sect. A) *86*:361, 1978.
8. Bartholomew, L. G., Baggenstoss, A. H., Morlock, C. G.,

and Comfort, M. W. Primary atrophy and lipomatosis of the pancreas. Gastroenterology *36*:563, 1959.
9. Patel, S., Bellon, E. M., Haala, J., and Park, C. H. Fat replacement of the exocrine pancreas. Am. J. Radiol. *135*:843, 1980.
10. Comfort, M. W., Gambill, E. E., and Baggenstoss, A. H. Chronic relapsing pancreatitis. In a study of twenty-nine cases without associated disease of the biliary or gastrointestinal tract. Gastroenterology *6*:239, 376, 1946.
11. Sarles, H. Alcoholism and pancreatitis. Scand. J. Gastroenterol. *6*:193, 1971.
12. The Copenhagen Pancreatitis Study Group. An interim report from a prospective epidemiological multicenter study. Scand. J. Gastroenterol. *16*:305, 1981.
13. O'Sullivan, J. N., Nobrega, F. T., Morlock, C. G., Brown, A. L., and Bartholomew, L. G. Acute and chronic pancreatitis in Rochester, Minnesota, 1940 to 1969. Gastroenterology *62*:373, 1972.
14. Clark, E. Pancreatitis in acute and chronic alcoholism. Am. J. Dig. Dis. *9*:428, 1942.
15. Goebell, H., Bode, C., Bastian, R., and Strohmeyer, G. Clinical asymptomatic functional disorders of the exocrine pancreas in chronic alcoholics. Dtsch. Med. Wochenschr. *95*:808, 1970.
16. Gastard, J., Jobaud, F., Farbos, T., Loussovarn, J., Marion, J., Pannier, M., Renaudet, F., Valdazo, R., and Gosselin, M. Etiology and course of primary chronic pancreatitis in Western France. Digestion *9*:416, 1973.
17. Durbel, J. P., and Sarles, H. Multicenter survey of the etiology of pancreatic disease. Relationship between the relative risk of developing chronic pancreatitis and alcohol, protein, and lipid consumption. Digestion *18*:337, 1978.
18. Wilson, J. S., Bernstein, L., McDonald, D., Tait, A., McNeil, D., and Pinola, R. C. Diet and drinking habits in relation to the development of alcoholic pancreatitis. Gut *26*:882, 1985.
19. Strum, W. B., and Spiro, H. M. Chronic pancreatitis. Ann. Intern. Med. *74*:264, 1971.
20. Dutta, S. K., Mobrahan, S., and Iber, F. L. Associated liver disease in alcoholic pancreatitis. Am. J. Dig. Dis. *23*:618, 1978.
21. Angelini, G., Merigo, F., Degani, G., Camplani, N., Bovo, P., Passini, A. F., Cavallini, G., Brocco, G., and Scuro, L. A. Association of chronic alcoholic liver disease and pancreatic disease: a prospective study. Am. J. Gastroenterol. *80*:998, 1985.
22. Sarles, H., Lebrevil, G., Tasso, F., Figarella, C., Clemente, F., Devaux, M. A., Fagonde, B., and Payan, H. A comparison of alcoholic pancreatitis in rat and man. Gut *12*:377, 1971.
23. Sarles, H., Sahel, J., Lebrevil, G., and Tiscornia, O. Pancreatite alcoolique chronique experimentalle du chien. Etude anatomo-pathologique. Forum de Recherches de Saerbrooke, 16–17 June. Biol. Gastroenterol. *9*:25, 1975.
24. Sahel, J., and Sarles, H. Modifications of pure human pancreatic juice induced by chronic alcohol consumption. Dig. Dis. Sci. *24*:897, 1979.
25. Renner, I. G., Rinderknecht, H., Valenzuela, J. E., and Douglas, A. P. Studies of pure pancreatic secretions in chronic alcoholic subjects without pancreatic insufficiency. Scand. J. Gastroenterol. *15*:281, 1980.
26. Renner, I. G., Rinderknecht, H., and Douglas, A. P. Profiles of pure pancreatic secretions in patients with acute pancreatitis: the possible role of proteolytic enzymes in pathogenesis. Gastroenterology *75*:1090, 1978.
27. Multigner, L., Sarles, H., Lombardo, D., and DeCaro, A. Pancreatic stone protein. I. Implications in stone formation during the course of chronic calcifying pancreatitis. Gastroenterology *89*:381, 1985.
28. Sarles, H., DeCaro, A., Multigner, L., and Martin, E. Giant pancreatic stones in teetotal women due to absence of the "stone protein"? Lancet *2*:714, 1982.
29. Boustiene, C., Sarles, H., Lohse, J., Durbec, J. P., and Sahel, J. Citrate and calcium secretion in the pure human pancreatic juice of alcoholic and nonalcoholic men and of chronic pancreatitis patients. Digestion *32*:1, 1985.
30. Sarles, H. Etiopathogenesis and definition of chronic pancreatitis. Dig. Dis. Sci. *31* (Suppl. 9):915, 1986.
31. Wakabayashi, A., and Takeda, Y. The behavior of mucopolysaccharide in the pancreatic juice in chronic pancreatitis. Am. J. Dig. Dis. *21*:607, 1976.
32. Allan, J., and White, T. T. An alternate mechanism for the formation of protein plugs in chronic calcifying pancreatitis. Digestion *11*:428, 1974.
33. Nagata, A., Homma, T., Tamai, K., Ueno, K., Shimakura, K., Oguchi, H., Furuta, S., and Oda, M. A study of chronic pancreatitis by serial endoscopic pancreatography. Gastroenterology *81*:884, 1981.
34. Bockman, D. E., Singh, M., Laugier, R., and Sarles, H. Alcohol and the integrity of the pancreas. Scand. J. Gastroenterol. *20* (Suppl. 112):106, 1985.
35. Howard, J. M., and Jordan, G. L., Jr. Surgical Diseases of the Pancreas. Philadelphia, J. B. Lippincott Company, 1960, p. 170.
36. Pitchumoni, C. S. "Tropical" or "nutritional" pancreatitis—an update. *In* Gyr, K. E., Singer, M. V., and Sarles, H. (eds.). Pancreatitis Concepts and Classification. Amsterdam, Elsevier, 1984, p. 359.
37. Vakil, B. J. Chronische Pankreatitis in Indien. Leber Magen Darm *6*:276, 1976.
38. Barbezat, G. O., and Hansen, J. D. L. The exocrine pancreas and protein-calorie malnutrition. Pediatrics *42*:77, 1968.
39. Pitchumoni, C. S., and Thomas, E. Chronic cassava toxicity: possible relationship to chronic pancreatic disease in malnourished populations. Lancet *2*:1397, 1973.
40. Kakrani, A. L., Parajpe, S. M., and Kakrani, V. A. Pancreatic fibrosis—calcification with diabetes in South Maharashtra, India. Trop. Geogr. Med. *37*:276, 1985.
41. Cotton, P. B. Pancreas divisum—curiosity or culprit? (Editorial). Gastroenterology *89*:1431, 1985.
42. Mott, C. B., Guanita, D. R., Machado, M. C. C., and Bettadrello, A. Epidemiology and etiology of chronic pancreatitis in São Paulo (Brazil): a prospective study of 200 cases. *In* Gyr, K. G., Singer, M. V., and Sarles, H. (eds.). Pancreatitis, Concepts and Classification. Amsterdam, Elsevier, 1984, p. 355.
43. Ammann, R. W., Hammer, B., and Fumagalli, I. Chronic pancreatitis in Zurich, 1963–1972. Clinical findings and follow up studies of 102 cases. Digestion *9*:404, 1973.
44. Marks, I. N., Banks, S., and Louw, J. H. Chronic pancreatitis in the Western Cape. Digestion *9*:447, 1973.
45. Kalthoff, L., Layer, P., Claiw, J. E., and Di Magno, E. P. The course of alcoholic and nonalcoholic chronic pancreatitis. Dig. Dis. Sci. *29*:553, 1984.
46. Wyndner, E. L., Mabuchi, K., Maruchi, N., and Fortner, J. G. Epidemiology of cancer of the pancreas. J. Natl. Cancer Inst. *50*:645, 1973.
47. Ammann, R. W., Knoblauch, M., Moehr, P., Deyhle, P., Larginader, R., Akovbiantz, A., Schueler, A., and Schneider, J. High incidence of extrapancreatic carcinoma in chronic pancreatitis. Scand. J. Gastroenterol. *15*:395, 1980.
48. Keith, R. G., Keshvjee, S. H., and Kerenyi, N. R. Neuropathology of chronic pancreatitis in humans. Can. J. Surg. *28*:207, 1985.
49. Bradley, E. L., III. Pancreatic duct pressure in chronic pancreatitis. Am. J. Surg. *144*:313, 1982.
50. Keith, R. A. Effect of a low fat elemental diet on pancreatic secretion during pancreatitis. Surg. Gynecol. Obstet. *151*:337, 1980.
51. Girdwood, A. H., Hatfield, A. R. W., Bornman, P. C., Denyer, M. E., Fottler, I. N. Structure and function in noncalcific pancreatitis. Dig. Dis. Sci. *29*:721, 1984.
52. Jensen, A. R., Matzen, P., Mollhow-Moller, A., and Christoffersen, I. Pattern of pain, duct morphology, and pancreatic function in chronic pancreatitis—a comparative study. Scand. J. Gastroenterol. *19*:334, 1984.
53. Trapnell, J. E. Chronic relapsing pancreatitis: a review of 64 cases. Br. J. Surg. *66*:471, 1979.
54. Bornman, P. C., Marks, I. N., Girdwood, A. H., Clain, J. E., Narunsky, L., Clain, D. J., and Wright, J. P. Is pancreatic duct obstruction or stricture a major cause of pain in calcific pancreatitis? Br. J. Surg. *67*:425, 1980.
55. Marks, I. N., Girdwood, A. H., Banks, S., and Louw, J. H.

The prognosis of alcohol-induced chronic pancreatitis. S. Afr. Med. J. *57*:640, 1980.
56. Ammann, R. W., Akovbiantz, A., Largiader, F., Schueler, G. Course and outcome of chronic pancreatitis. Longitudinal study of a mixed medical surgical series of 245 patients. Gastroenterology *86*:820, 1984.
57. DiMagno, E. P., Go, V. L. W., and Summerskill, W. H. J. Relations between pancreatic enzyme outputs and malabsorption in severe pancreatic insufficiency. N. Engl. J. Med. *288*:813, 1973.
58. DiMagno, E. P., Malagelada, J. R., and Go, V. L. W. Relationship between alcoholism and pancreatic insufficiency. N.Y. Acad. Sci. *252*:200, 1975.
59. Wollaeger, E. E., Comfort, M. M., Glagett, O. T., and Osterberg, A. E. Efficiency of gastrointestinal tract after resection of head of pancreas. JAMA *137*:348, 1948.
60. Bo-Linn, G. W., and Fordtran, J. S. Fecal fat concentration in patients with steatorrhea. Gastroenterology *87*:319, 1984.
61. Kim, Y. A., and Spritz, H. Hydroxy acid excretion in steatorrhea of pancreatic and non pancreatic origin. N. Engl. J. Med. *279*:1424, 1968.
62. Ammon, H. V., and Phillips, S. F. Inhibition of colonic water and electrolyte absorption by fatty acids in man. Gastroenterology *65*:744, 1973.
63. Fogel, R. M., and Gray, G. M. Starch hydrolysis in man: an intraluminal process not requiring membrane digestion. J. Appl. Physiol. *35*:263, 1973.
64. Arvanitakis, C., and Olsen, W. A. Intestinal mucosal disaccharidases in chronic pancreatitis. Am. J. Dig. Dis. *19*:417, 1974.
65. Evans, W. B., and Wollaeger, E. E. Incidence and severity of nutritional deficiency states in chronic exocrine pancreatic insufficiency: comparison with nontropical sprue. Am. J. Dig. Dis. *11*:594, 1966.
66. Toskes, P. P., Hansell, J., Cerda, J., and Deren, J. J. Vitamin B_{12} malabsorption in chronic pancreatic insufficiency. Studies suggesting the presence of a pancreatic "intrinsic factor." N. Engl. J. Med. *284*:627, 1971.
67. Allen, R. H., Seetharam, B., Podell, E., and Alpers, D. H. Effect of proteolytic enzymes on the binding of cobalamin to R protein and intrinsic factor. J. Clin. Invest. *61*:47, 1978.
68. Gueant, J. L., Djalali, M., Aouadj, R., Gaucher, P., Monin, B., and Nicholas, J. P. In vitro and in vivo evidences that the malabsorption of cobalamin is related to its binding on haptocorrin (R binder) in chronic pancreatitis. Am. J. Clin. Nutr. *44*:265, 1986.
69. Stasiewicz, J., Adler, M., and Delcourt, A. Pancreatic and gastrointestinal hormones in chronic pancreatitis. Hepatogastroenterology *27*:152, 1980.
70. Covet, C., Genton, P., Pointel, J. P., Gross, P., Saudax, E., DeBry, G., and Drovin, P. The prevalence of retinopathy is similar in diabetes mellitus secondary to chronic pancreatitis with or without pancreatectomy and in idiopathic diabetes mellitus. Diabetes Care *8*:323, 1985.
71. Levitt, M. D. Clinical use of amylase clearance and isoamylase measurements. Mayo Clin. Proc. *54*:428, 1979.
72. Dutta, S. F., Douglass, W., Smalls, U. A., Nipper, H. C., and Levitt, M. D. Prevalence and nature of hyperamylasemia in acute alcoholism. Dig. Dis. Sci. *26*:136, 1981.
73. Kameya, S., Hayakawa, T., Kameya, A., and Watanabe, T. Clinical value of routine isoamylase analysis of hyperamylasemia. Am. J. Gastroenterol. *81*:358, 1986.
74. Skude, G., and Eriksson, S. Serum isoamylases in chronic pancreatitis. Scand. J. Gastroenterol. *11*:525, 1976.
75. Koop, H., Lankisch, P. G., Stoeckmann, F., and Arnold, R. Trypsin radioimmunoassay in the diagnosis of chronic pancreatitis. Digestion *20*:151, 1980.
76. Lesi, C., Melzi-Deril, G. U., Pavesi, F., Scandellani, A., Faccenda, F., Grazia-Lasertano, M., Savoia, M., Zoni, L., and Peppi, M. Clinical significance of serum pancreatic enzymes in the quiescent phase of chronic pancreatitis. Clin. Biochem. *18*:235, 1985.
77. Del Favero, G., Fabris, C., Plebani, M., Panucci, A., Piccoli, A., Perobelli, L., Burlina, A., and Naccarato, R. Serum elastase in chronic pancreatic disease. Klin. Wochenschr. *63*:603, 1985.
78. Basso, D., Fabris, C., Meani, A., Del Favero, G., Panucci, A., Vianezlo, D., Piccoli, A., and Naccarato, R. Serum deoxyribonuclease and ribonuclease in pancreatic cancer and chronic pancreatitis. Tumori *71*:529, 1985.
79. Lake-Bakaar, G., McKavanagh, S., and Summerfield, J. A. Urinary immunoreactive trypsin excretion: a non-invasive screening test for pancreatic cancer. Lancet *2*:878, 1979.
80. Del Favero, G., Fabris, C., Bonvicini, P., Piccoli, A., Baccaglini, V., Pedrazzoli, S., Burlina, A., and Naccarato, R. Trypsin/creatinine clearance ratio and serum immunoreactive trypsin in digestive and pancreatic diseases. Ric. Clin. Lab. *15*:343, 1985.
81. Littenberg, G., Afroudakis, A., and Kaplowitz, N. Common bile duct stenosis from chronic pancreatitis. Medicine *58*:385, 1979.
82. Fedail, S. S., Harvey, R. F., Salmon, P. R., and Read, P. E. Radioimmunoassay of lactoferrin in pancreatic juice as a test for pancreatic diseases. Lancet *1*:181, 1978.
83. Fedail, S. S., Harvey, R. F., Salmon, P. R., Brown, P., and Read, A. E. Trypsin and pure lactoferrin levels in pure pancreatic juice in patients with pancreatic disease. Gut *20*:893, 1979.
84. Multigner, L., Figarella, C., Sahel, J., and Sarles, H. Lactoferrin and albumin in human pancreatic juice. A valuable test of diagnosis of pancreatic diseases. Dig. Dis. Sci. *25*:173, 1980.
85. Multigner, L., Figarella, C., and Sarles, H. Diagnosis of chronic pancreatitis by measurement of lactoferrin in duodenal juice. Gut *22*:350, 1981.
86. Gaia, E., Figarella, C., Piantino, P., Rucca, G., Iuliano, R., Calcamuggi, G., and Emanuelli, G. Duodenal lactoferrin in patients with chronic pancreatitis and gastrointestinal diseases. Digestion *32*:229, 1985.
87. Reber, H., Tweedie, J. H., and Austin, J. L. Pancreatic secretions as clue to the presence of cancer. Cancer *47*:1646, 1981.
88. Niederau, C., and Grendell, J. H. Diagnosis of chronic pancreatitis. Gastroenterology *88*:1973, 1985.
89. Denyer, M. E., and Cotton, P. B. Pure pancreatic juice studies in normal subjects and patients with chronic pancreatitis. Gut *20*:89, 1979.
90. Go, V. L. W., Hofmann, A. F., and Summerskill, W. H. J. Pancrozymin bioassay in man based on pancreatic enzyme secretion: potency of specific amino acids and other digestive products. J. Clin. Invest. *49*:1558, 1970.
91. Lankisch, P. G., Brauneis, J., Otto, J., and Göke, B. Pancreolauryl and NBT-PABA tests. Are serum tests more practicable alternatives to urine tests in the diagnosis of exocrine pancreatic insufficiency? Gastroenterology *90*:350, 1986.
92. Brugge, W. R., Goff, J. S., Allen, N. C., Podell, E. R., and Allen, R. H. Development of a dual label Schilling test for pancreatic exocrine function based on the differential absorption of cobalamin bound to intrinsic factor and R protein. Gastroenterology *78*:937, 1980.
93. Koch, M. B., Go, V. L. W., and DiMagno, E. P. Can pancreatic polypeptide detect diseases of the exocrine pancreas? Mayo Clin. Proc. *60*:259, 1985.
94. Hamilton, I., Boyd, E. J., Penston, J. G., Soutar, J. S., and Bouchier, I. A. Pancreatic function and enzyme synthesis rates in mild chronic pancreatitis. Scand. J. Gastroenterol. *21*:542, 1986.
95. Domschke, S., Heptner, G., Kolb, S., Sailer, D., Schneider, M. U., and Domschke, W. Decrease in plasma amino acid level after secretin and pancreozymin as an indicator of exocrine pancreatic function. Gastroenterology *90*:1031, 1986.
96. Goff, J. S. Two-stage triolein breath test differentiates pancreatic insufficiency from other causes of malabsorption. Gastroenterology *83*:44, 1982.
97. Schneider, M. U., Demling, L., Domschke, S., Heptner, G., Merkel, I., Domschke, W. NMR spectrometric stool fat analysis—a new technique for quantifying steatorrhea and establishing the indication for enzyme replacement in chronic pancreatitis. Hepatogastroenterology *32*:210, 1985.
98. Mackie, R. D., Levine, A. S., and Levitt, M. D. Malabsorption of starch in pancreatic insufficiency. (Abstract). Gastroenterology *80*:1220, 1981.
99. Jain, N. K., Patel, V. P., Agarwal, N., Khawaja, F. I.,

Geevarghese, P. J., and Pitchumoni, C. S. A comparative study of bentiromide test (BT) vs rice flour breath hydrogen test (RFBHT) in the detection of exocrine pancreatic insufficiency (EPI). (Abstract.) Gastroenterology *88*:1429, 1985.
100. Ralls, P. W., Halls, J., Renner, I., and Juttner, H. Endoscopic retrograde cholangiopancreatography (ERCP) in pancreatic disease. Radiology *134*:347, 1980.
101. Okazaki, K., Yamamoto, Y., Ito, K. Endoscopic measurement of papillary sphincter zone and pancreatic main ductal pressure in patients with chronic pancreatitis. Gastroenterology *91*:409, 1986.
102. Rolny, P., Arleback, A., Jarnerot, G., and Anderson, T. Endoscopic manometry of the sphincter of Oddi and pancreatic duct in chronic pancreatitis. Scand. J. Gastroenterol. *21*:415, 1986.
103. Novis, B. H., Bornman, P. C., Girdwood, A. W., Marks, I. N. Endoscopic manometry of the pancreatic duct and sphincter zone in patients with chronic pancreatitis. Dig. Dis. Sci. *30*:225, 1985.
104. Zimmar, D. S., Falkenstein, D. B., Riccobono, C., and Aaron, B. Complications of endoscopic retrograde cholangiopancreatography. Analysis of 300 consecutive cases. Gastroenterology *69*:303, 1975.
105. Ferrucci, J. T., Wittenberg, J., Black, E. B., Kirkpatrick, R. H., and Hall, D. A. Computed body tomography in chronic pancreatitis. Radiology *130*:175, 1979.
106. Foley, D. W., Stewart, E. T., Lawson, T. L., Geenen, J., LoGindice, J., Maher, L., and Unger, G. F. Computed tomography, ultrasonography, and endoscopic retrograde cholangiopancreatography in the diagnosis of pancreatic disease: a comparative study. Gastrointest. Radiol. *5*:29, 1980.
107. Silverstein, W., Isikoff, M. B., Hill, M. C., and Barkin, J. Diagnostic imaging of acute pancreatitis: prospective study using CT scan and sonography. Am. J. Radiol. *137*:497, 1981.
108. Jeffrey, R. B., Federle, M. P., Cello, J. P., and Crass, R. A. Early computed tomographic scanning in acute severe pancreatitis. Surg. Gynecol. Obstet. *154*:170, 1982.
109. Bradley, E. L., Clements, J. L., and Gonzales, A. C. The natural history of pancreatic pseudocysts: a unified concept of management. Am. J. Surg. *137*:135, 1979.
110. Sugawa, C., and Walt, A. J. Endoscopic retrograde pancreatography in the surgery of pancreatic pseudocysts. Surgery *86*:639, 1979.
111. Sankaran, S., and Walt, A. J. The natural and unnatural history of pancreatic pseudocysts. Br. J. Surg. *62*:37, 1975.
112. Federle, M. P., Jeffrey, R. B., Crass, R. A., and Van Dalsem, V. Computed tomography of pancreatic abscesses. AJR *136*:879, 1981.
113. MacErlean, D. P., Bryan, P. J., and Murphy, J. J. Pancreatic pseudocyst: management by ultrasonically guided aspiration. Gastrointest. Radiol. *5*:255, 1980.
114. Barkin, J. S., Smith, F. R., Perieras, R., Isikoff, M., Levi, J., Livingstone, A., Hill, M., and Rogers, A. I. Therapeutic percutaneous aspiration of pancreatic pseudocysts. Dig. Dis. Sci. *26*:585, 1981.
115. Hanna, W. A. Rupture of pancreatic cysts: report of a case and review of the literature. Br. J. Surg. *47*:495, 1980.
116. Frey, C. F. Pancreatic pseudocyst: operative strategy. Ann. Surg. *188*:652, 1978.
117. Lam, A. Y., and Bricker, R. S. Pancreatic pseudocyst with hemorrhage into the gastrointestinal tract through the duct of Wirsung. Am. J. Surg. *129*:694, 1975.
118. Starling, J. R., and Crummy, A. B. Hemosuccus pancreaticus secondary to ruptured splenic artery aneurysm. Dig. Dis. Sci. *24*:726, 1979.
119. Sankaran, S., and Walt, A. J. Pancreatic ascites: recognition and management. Arch. Surg. *111*:430, 1976.
120. Snape, W. J., Long, W. B., Trotman, B. W., Marin, G. A., and Czaja, A. J. Marked alkaline phosphatase elevation with partial common bile duct obstruction due to calcified pancreatitis. Gastroenterology *70*:70, 1976.
121. Afroudakis, A., and Kaplowitz, N. Liver histopathology in chronic common bile duct stenosis due to chronic alcoholic pancreatitis. Hepatology *1*:65, 1981.
122. Banks, S., Marks, I. N., and Groll, A. Gastric acid secretion in pancreatic disease. Gastroenterology *51*:639, 1966.
123. Bell, S., Cole, R., and Robert-Thomson, I. C. Coeliac plexus block for control of pain in chronic pancreatitis. Br. Med. J. *281*:1604, 1980.
124. Leung, J. W. C., Bowen-Wright, M., Aveling, W., Shorvon, P. J., and Cotton, P. B. Coeliac plexus block for pain in pancreatic cancer and chronic pancreatitis. Br. J. Surg. *70*:730, 1983.
125. Madsen, P., and Hansen, E. Coeliac plexus block versus pancreaticogastrostomy for pain in chronic pancreatitis. A controlled randomized trial. Scand. J. Gastroenterol. *20*:1217, 1985.
126. Ballegaard, S., Christophersen, S. J., Pawids, S. G., Hesse, J., and Olsen, N. V. Acupuncture and transcutaneous electric nerve stimulation in the treatment of pain associated with chronic pancreatitis. A randomized study. Scand. J. Gastroenterol. *20*:1249, 1985.
127. Isaksson, G., and Ihse, I. Pain reduction by an oral pancreatic enzyme preparation in chronic pancreatitis. Dig. Dis. Sci. *28*:97, 1983.
128. Slaff, J., Jacobson, D., Tillman, C. R., Curington, C., and Toskes, P. Protease-specific suppression of pancreatic exocrine secretion. Gastroenterology *87*:44, 1984.
129. Owyang, C., May, D., and Louie, D. S. Trypsin suppression of pancreatic enzyme secretion. Differential effect on cholecystokinin release and the enteropancreatic reflex. Gastroenterology *91*:637, 1986.
130. Schafmayer, A., Becker, H. D., Werner, M., Folsch, V. R., and Creutzfeldt, W. Plasma cholecystokinin levels in patients with chronic pancreatitis. Digestion *32*:136, 1985.
131. Slaff, J. I., Wolfe, M. M., and Toskes, P. R. Elevated fasting cholecystokinin lévels in pancreatic exocrine impairment: evidence to support feedback regulation. J. Lab. Clin. Med. *105*:282, 1985.
132. Funakoshi, A., Nakano, I., Shinozaki, H., Ibayashi, H., Tateishi, K., and Hamaoka, T. Low plasma cholecystokinin response after ingestion of a test meal in patients with chronic pancreatitis. Am. J. Gastroenterol. *80*:937, 1985.
133. Halgreen, H., Thorsgaard Pedersen, N., and Worning, H. Symptomatic effect of pancreatic enzyme therapy in patients with chronic pancreatitis. Scand. J. Gastroenterol. *21*:104, 1986.
134. Niederau, C., Niederau, M., Williams, J. A., and Grendell, J. H. New proglumide-analogue CCK receptor antagonists: very potent and selective for peripheral tissues. Am. J. Physiol. *251*:G856, 1986.
135. Di Magno, E. P. Medical treatment of pancreatic insufficiency. Mayo Clin. Proc. *54*:435, 1979.
136. Di Magno, E. P. Controversies in the treatment of exocrine pancreatic insufficiency. Dig. Dis. Sci. *27*:481, 1982.
137. Graham, D. Y. Enzyme replacement of pancreatic insufficiency in man. Relation between in vitro enzyme activities and in vivo potency in commercial pancreatic extracts. N. Eng. J. Med. *296*:1314, 1977.
138. Heizler, W. D., Cleveland, C. R., and Iben, F. L. Gastric inactivation of pancreatic supplements. Bull. Johns Hopkins Hosp. *116*:261, 1965.
139. Di Magno, E. P., Malagelada, J. R., Go, V. L. W., and Moertel, C. G. Fate of orally ingested enzymes in pancreatic insufficiency. Comparison of two dosage schedules. N. Engl. J. Med. *296*:1318, 1977.
140. Regan, P. T., Malagelada, J. R., Di Magno, E. P., and Go, V. L. W. Reduced intraluminal bile acid concentrations and fat malabsorption in pancreatic insufficiency: correction by treatment. Gastroenterology *77*:285, 1979.
141. Graham, D. Y. Pancreatic enzyme replacement. The effect of antacid or cimetidine. Dig. Dis. Sci. *27*:485, 1982.
142. Regan, P. T., Malagelada, J. R., Di Magno, E. P., Glanzman, S. L., and Go, V. L. W. Comparative effects of antacids, cimetidine, and enteric coating on the therapeutic response to oral enzymes in severe pancreatic insufficiency. N. Engl. J. Med. *297*:854, 1977.
143. Hofmann, A. F., and Small, D. M. Detergent properties of

bile salts: correlation with physiological function. Annu. Rev. Med. *18*:333, 1967.

144. Graham, D. Y., and Sackman, J. W. Mechanism of increase in steatorrhea with calcium and magnesium in exocrine pancreatic insufficiency: an animal model. Gastroenterology *83*:6388, 1982.
145. Cox, F. L., Isenberg, J. W., Asher, A. P., and Douley, R. R. The effect of cimetidine on maldigestion in cystic fibrosis. J. Pediatr. *99*:448, 1979.
146. Durie, P., Bell, L., Linton, W., Corey, M. L., and Forstner, G. G. Effect of cimetidine and sodium bicarbonate on pancreatic replacement therapy in cystic fibrosis. Gut *21*:778, 1980.
147. Boyle, B. J., Long, W. B., Balisteri, W. F., Widzer, S. J., and Huant, N. Effect of cimetidine and pancreatic enzymes on serum and fecal bile acids and fat absorption in cystic fibrosis. Gastroenterology *78*:950, 1980.
148. Gow, R., Francis, P., Bradbear, R., and Shepherd, R. Comparative studies of varying regimens to improve steatorrhea and creatorrhea in cystic fibrosis: effectiveness of an enteric-coated preparation with and without antacids and cimetidine. Lancet *2*:1071, 1981.
149. Graham, D. Y. An enteric-coated pancreatic enzyme preparation that works. Dig. Dis. Sci. *24*:906, 1979.
150. Dutta, S. K., Rubin, J., and Harvey, J. Comparative evaluation of the therapeutic efficacy of a pH sensitive enteric coated pancreatic enzyme preparation with conventional pancreatic enzyme therapy in the treatment of exocrine pancreatic insufficiency. Gastroenterology *84*:476, 1983.
151. Stapleton, F. B., Kennedy, J., Nousia-Arvanitakis, S., and Linshaw, M. A. Hyperuricosuria due to high-dose pancreatic extract therapy in cystic fibrosis. N. Engl. J. Med. *295*:246, 1976.
152. Greenberger, N. J., and Skillman, T. G. Medium-chain triglycerides. Physiologic considerations and clinical implications. N. Engl. J. Med. *280*:1045, 1969.
153. Schizas, A. A., Cremen, J. A., Larson, E., and O'Brien, R. Medium-chain triglycerides—use in food preparation. J. Am. Diet. Assoc. *51*:228, 1967.
154. Joffe, B. I., Jackson, W. P. H., Bank, S., and Vinik, A. I. Effect of oral hypoglycaemic agents on glucose tolerance in pancreatic diabetes. Gut *13*:285, 1972.
155. Donowitz, M., Hendler, R., Spiro, H. M., Binder, H. J., and Felig, P. Glucagon secretion in acute and chronic pancreatitis. Ann. Intern. Med. *83*:778, 1975.
156. Linde, J., Nillson, H., and Barany, F. R. Diabetes and hypoglycemia in chronic pancreatitis. Scand. J. Gastroenterol. *12*:369, 1977.
157. Earnest, D. L., Johnson, G., Williams, H. E., and Admirand, W. H. Hyperoxaluria in patients with ileal resection: an abnormality in dietary calcium in regulating intestinal oxalate absorption. Gastroenterology *66*:1114, 1974.
158. Stauffer, J. Q. Hyperoxaluria and intestinal disease. The role of steatorrhea and dietary calcium in regulating intestinal oxalate absorption. Am. J. Dig. Dis. *22*:921, 1977.
159. Priestley, J. T., Remine, W. H., Barber, K. W., Jr., and Gambill, E. E. Chronic relapsing pancreatitis: treatment by surgical drainage of the pancreas. Ann. Surg. *161*:838, 1965.
160. Arnesjo, B., Ihse, I., Kugelberg, C., and Tyler, U. Pancreaticojejunostomy in chronic pancreatitis. An appraisal of 29 cases. Acta Chir. Scand. *141*:139, 1975.
161. Warshaw, A. L., Popp, J. W., Jr., and Schapiro, R. H. Long-term patency, pancreatic function, and pain relief after lateral pancreatico-jejunostomy for chronic pancreatitis. Gastroenterology *79*:289, 1980.
162. Rossi, R. L., Heiss, F. W., Braasch, J. W. Surgical management of chronic pancreatitis. Surg. Clin. North Am. *65*:79, 1985.
163. Traverso, L. W., Tompkins, R. K., Urrea, P. T., and Longmire, W. P. Surgical treatment of chronic pancreatitis. Twenty-two years' experience. Ann. Surg. *290*:312, 1979.
164. Ammann, R. W., Largiader, F., and Akovbiantz, A. Pain relief by surgery in chronic pancreatitis? Relationship between pain relief, pancreatic dysfunction, and alcohol withdrawal. Scand. J. Gastroenterol. *14*:209, 1979.
165. Prinz, R. A., and Greenlee, H. R. Pancreatic duct drainage in 100 patients with chronic pancreatitis. Ann. Surg. *194*:313, 1981.
166. Holmberg, J. T., Isaksson, G., and Ihse, I. Long-term results of pancreaticojejunostomy in chronic pancreatitis. Surg. Gynecol. Obstet. *160*:339, 1985.
167. Prinz, R. A., Aranha, G. V., and Greenlee, H. B. Redrainage of the pancreatic duct in chronic pancreatitis. Am. J. Surg. *151*:150, 1986.
168. Warshaw, A. L., Richter, J. M., and Schapiro, R. H. The cause and treatment of pancreatitis associated with pancreas divisum. Ann. Surg. *198*:443, 1983.
169. Schneider, M. U., and Lux, G. Floating pancreatic duct concrements in chronic pancreatitis—pain relief by endoscopic removal. Endoscopy *17*:8, 1985.
170. Fuji, T., Amano, H., Harima, K., Aibe, T., Asagami, F., Kinukawa, K., Ariyama, S., and Takemoto, T. Pancreatic sphincterotomy and pancreatic endoprosthesis. Endoscopy *17*:69, 1985.
171. Cooperman, A. M., Sivak, M. V., Sullivan, B. H., Jr., and Hermann, R. E. Endoscopic pancreatography. Its value in preoperative and postoperative assessment of pancreatic disease. Am. J. Surg. *129*:38, 1975.
172. Proctor, H. J., Mendes, O. C., Thomas, C. G., Jr., and Herbst, C. A. Surgery for chronic pancreatitis: drainage versus resection. Ann. Surg. *189*:664, 1979.
173. White, T. T., and Hart, M. J. Pancreaticojejunostomy versus resection in the treatment of chronic pancreatitis. Am. J. Surg. *138*:129, 1979.
174. Taylor, R. H., and Bagley, F. H. Ductal drainage or resection for chronic pancreatitis. Am. J. Surg. *141*:28, 1981.
175. White, T. T., and Slavotinek, A. H. Results of surgical treatment of chronic pancreatitis. Report of 142 cases. Ann. Surg. *189*:217, 1979.
176. Frey, C. F., Child, C. G., and Fry, W. Pancreatectomy for chronic pancreatitis. Ann. Surg. *184*:403, 1976.
177. Braasch, J. W., Vito, L., and Nugent, F. W. Total pancreatectomy for end-stage chronic pancreatitis. Ann. Surg. *188*:317, 1978.
178. Najarian, J. S., Sutherland, D. E. R., Baumgartner, D., Burke, B., Rynasiewicz, J. J., Matas, A. J., and Goetz, F. C. Total or near total pancreatectomy and islet autotransplantation for treatment of chronic pancreatitis. Ann. Surg. *192*:526, 1980.
179. Hinshaw, D. B., Jolley, W. B., Hinshaw, D. B., Kaiser, J. E., and Hinshaw, K. Islet autotransplantation after pancreatectomy for chronic pancreatitis with a new method of islet preparation. Am. J. Surg. *142*:118, 1981.
180. Rossi, R. L., Braasch, J. W., O'Bryan, E. M., and Watkins, E. Segmental pancreatic autotransplantation for chronic pancreatitis—a preliminary report. Gastroenterology *84*:621, 1983.
181. Rossi, R. L., Heiss, F. W., Watkins, E., Soeldner, J. S., Shea, J. A., Silverman, M. L., Braasch, J. W., Nugent, F. W., and Bolton, J. Segmental pancreatic autotransplantation with pancreatic ductal occlusion after near total or total pancreatic resection for chronic pancreatitis—results at 5- to 54-month follow-up evaluation. Ann. Surg. *203*:626, 1986.
182. Hogle, H. H., and Roemtsma, K. Pancreatic autotransplantation following resection. Surgery *83*:359, 1978.
183. Tosatti, E., Valente, U., Campisi, C., Barabino, C., and Pozzati, A. Segmental pancreas autotransplantation in man following total or near total pancreatectomy for serious recurrent chronic pancreatitis. Transplant. Proc. *12*(Suppl. 2):15, 1980.
184. Crass, R. A., and Way, L. W. Acute and chronic pancreatic pseudocysts are different. Am. J. Surg. *142*:660, 1981.
185. Warshaw, A. L., Rattner, D. W. Timing of surgical drainage for pancreatic pseudocyst—clinical and chemical criteria. Ann. Surg. *202*:720, 1985.
186. Gronvall, J., Gronvall, S., and Hegebus, V. Ultrasound-guided drainage of fluid-containing masses using angiographic catheterization techniques. Am. J. Radiol. *129*:997, 1977.
187. Hancke, S., and Pederson, J. F. Percutaneous puncture of pancreatic cysts guided by ultrasound. Surg. Gynecol. Obstet. *142*:551, 1976.

188. Cooperman, A. M. Chronic pancreatitis. Surg. Clin. North Am. *61*:71, 1981.
189. Karlson, K. B., Martin, E. C., Fankuchen, E. I., Mattern, R. F., Schultz, R. W., and Casarella, W. J. Percutaneous drainage of pancreatic pseudocysts and abscesses. Radiology *142*:619, 1982.
190. Martin, E. W., Catalano, P., Copperman, M., Hecht, C., and Carey, L. C. Surgical decision-making in the treatment of pancreatic pseudocysts: internal versus external drainage. Am. J. Surg. *138*:821, 1979.
191. Ravelo, H. R., and Aldrete, J. S. Analysis and forty-five patients with pseudocysts of the pancreas treated surgically. Surg. Gynecol. Obstet. *148*:735, 1979.
192. Elechi, E. N., Callender, C. O., Leffall, L. D., and Kurtz, L. H. The treatment of pancreatic pseudocysts by external drainage. Surg. Gynecol. Obstet. *148*:707, 1979.
193. Shatney, C. H., and Lillehei, R. C. Surgical treatment of pancreatic pseudocysts. Ann. Surg. *189*:386, 1979.
194. Cameron, J. L. Chronic pancreatic ascites and pancreatic pleural effusions. Gastroenterology *74*:134, 1978.
195. Sankaran, S., Sugawa, C., and Walt, A. J. Value of endoscopic retrograde pancreatography in pancreatic ascites. Surg. Gynecol. Obstet. *148*:185, 1979.
196. Schulte, W. J., LoPorta, A. J., Condin, R. E., Unger, G. F., Geenen, J. E., and DeCosses, J. J. Chronic pancreatitis: a cause of biliary stricture. Surgery *82*:303, 1977.
197. Gregg, J. A., Carr-Locke, D. L., and Gallagher, M. M. Importance of common bile duct stricture associated with chronic pancreatitis. Diagnosis by endoscopic retrograde cholangiopancreatography. Am. J. Surg. *141*:199, 1981.

Carcinoma of the Pancreas

JOHN P. CELLO

Carcinoma of the pancreas is an insidiously developing, relentlessly progressive, and nearly universally fatal malignancy. Histologically, over 90 per cent of carcinomas of the pancreas are moderately well differentiated mucinous adenocarcinomas of pancreatic ductal origin, derived from the cuboidal epithelium of the pancreatic duct.[1] Approximately 5 per cent of adenocarcinomas of the pancreas are of islet cell origin, and these tumors often are manifested early by the secretion of hormones. Islet cell tumors of the pancreas are discussed on pages 1888 to 1890 and will not be reviewed in this chapter. Occasionally, even rarer forms of pancreatic malignancies may be encountered, such as acinar cell, giant cell, and epidermoid carcinomas, adenoacanthomas, sarcomas, and cystadenocarcinomas.

INCIDENCE AND EPIDEMIOLOGY

Carcinoma of the pancreas is responsible for over 24,000 new cases of cancer and 20,000 cancer-related deaths annually in the United States. The frequency in Western society is nearly 10 per 100,000 total population, with up to 100 cases per 100,000 population over age 75 years.[2] This malignancy currently ranks as the fourth most common cause of cancer death in men (after lung, colon, and prostate) and the fifth leading cause of cancer death in women (after breast, lung, colon, and ovary-uterus).[3] Carcinoma of the pancreas is more frequent in men than in women (2:1 in most patient series). Pancreatic carcinoma affects all age groups (although rarely before age 25 years), but the mean age of onset is in the seventh and eighth decades of life. Blacks in the United States, native Polynesians in Hawaii, Maoris in New Zealand, and urban dwellers throughout the world appear to have an increased rate of pancreatic cancer.[2] A strong positive association between latitude and pancreatic cancer and a strong negative association with the average ambient temperature has also been noted, even after controlling for per capita consumption of foods related to cancer mortality internationally.[3]

A few other etiologic factors have been suggested to explain the recent increase in frequency of carcinoma of the pancreas: cigarette smoking, dietary agents, environmental agents, diabetes mellitus, and chronic pancreatitis. Men smoking more than one and one-half packs of cigarettes per day have a threefold enhanced risk of pancreatic cancer, whereas women who smoke more than one pack per day have double the risk for pancreatic cancer than for nonsmokers.[4] As with so many other malignancies, a search for dietary factors associated with pancreatic cancer has yielded several possible factors, particularly increased consumption of fat, protein, and highly refined flour breads. Coffee consumption, once linked to pancreatic cancer in earlier studies, has more recently been shown to have no association with pancreatic cancer.[4–6] Various environmental agents have likewise been suggested to be associated with a high frequency of pancreatic cancer. In one study of a large pancreatic cancer cluster in the southern United States, oil refining and paper manufacturing were noted to be associated with higher risks for this malignancy.[7] Chronic pancreatic diseases have not been identified as important risk factors for carcinoma of the pancreas, although juvenile-onset diabetes may be associated with an increased risk of pancreatic cancer. No substantial evidence links either acute or chronic pancreatitis or increased alcohol consumption with pancreatic cancer. On occasion, however, patients with pancreatic cancer present with signs and symptoms of pancreatitis. In nonalcoholic patients with pancreatitis, particularly elderly persons, pancreatic cancer should be considered as a possible etiologic factor.

PATHOPHYSIOLOGY AND CLINICAL MANIFESTATIONS

Adenocarcinoma of the pancreas is characterized pathologically by a dense fibrotic, scirrhous, or desmoplastic reaction producing a compact hard mass of tissue in the retroperitoneum (Fig. 99–1). As the pancreas lacks a mesentery, lies adjacent to the common bile duct and other vital porta hepatis structures, and is surrounded by duodenum, stomach, and colon, the most common clinical manifestations are those related to the encroachment on these adjacent structures. For the vast majority of patients, there are few characteristic signs or symptoms early in the course of the disease that suggest the diagnosis of pancreatic cancer. A substantial number of patients will complain of a vague, dull, midepigastric abdominal pain, occasionally going through to the back. For patients with pancreatic cancer, this usually implies direct invasion of adjacent retroperitoneal organs or splanchnic nerves. An insidious weight loss with anorexia, occasionally associated with a curious aversion for meats, accompanied by a metallic taste in the mouth, diarrhea, weakness, and vomiting may also be seen in a large percentage of patients with carcinoma of the pancreas.[8] Vomiting may signal gastric or duodenal invasion with outlet obstruction or extensive peritoneal metastases. Jaundice is noted in over 50 per cent of patients with carcinoma of the pancreas, the vast majority of whom unfortunately have large, bulky tumor masses encasing the distal part of the common bile duct.

On occasion, however, a small focal mass in the head of the pancreas in the immediate periampullary area will obstruct the distal part of the common bile duct and produce jaundice at a relatively early stage in the disease. For patients with carcinoma of the pancreas arising in the body or tail of the gland, jaundice is an extremely late manifestation of the disease, usually associated with a large tumor mass or with hepatic metastasis. About one fourth of patients with pancreatic malignancy will be noted to have a large, hard, palpable abdominal mass at the time of presentation.[8] Moreover, the jaundice and weight loss in some patients with pancreatic cancer may be accompanied by a palpable, distended, nontender gallbladder, termed Courvoisier's sign, which may also be seen in patients with other tumors obstructing the distal portion of the bile duct, such as carcinoma of the ampulla of Vater, duodenal carcinoma and cholangiocarcinoma.

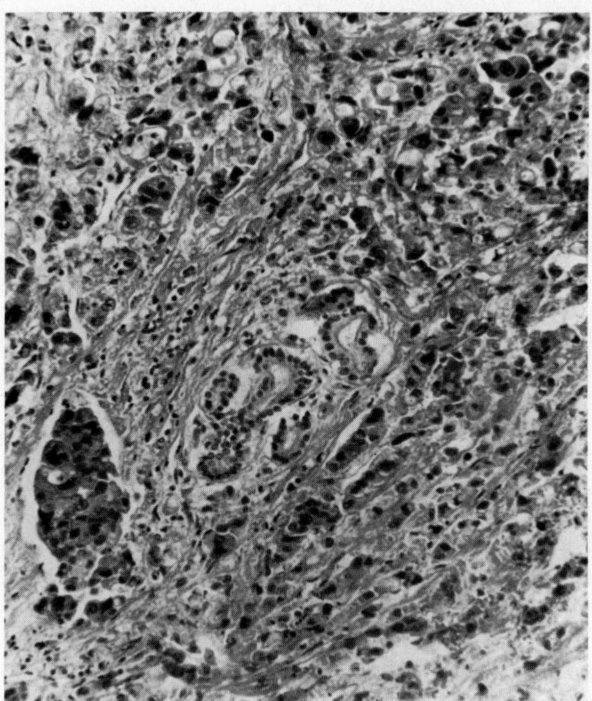

Figure 99–1. Adenocarcinoma of the pancreas, light microscopy. Nests and cords of malignant cells are separated by strands of dense fibrous tissue. In some areas, the malignant cells form structures resembling ductules.

On even rarer occasions (less than 5 per cent of patients), severe back pain, migratory thrombophlebitis, intense pruritus, acute pancreatitis, psychiatric disturbance (particularly depression), or new onset of brittle diabetes mellitus may be an early manifestation of carcinoma of the pancreas.[6] Hematemesis and melena may occasionally be noted late in the course of disease in patients with duodenal or gastric involvement as the tumor erodes into these richly vascularized adjacent structures.

Given the distinct lack of characteristic historical and physical features in patients with pancreatic malignancy, the appearance of the aforementioned signs or symptoms in a reliable, observant, previously healthy patient should lead to at least the suspicion of underlying pancreatic malignancy and appropriate diagnostic tests.

DIAGNOSIS

An Overview of the Challenge

The insidious development of pancreatic cancer without characteristic clinical features and its dismal five-year survival rate of under 2 per cent have given rise to the search for newer, more sensitive, and more specific diagnostic tests to detect the early stages. Many of these diagnostic tests were reported initially with great enthusiasm and were alleged to be accurate in the early diagnosis of potentially resectable pancreatic malignancy. Much more experience is required, however, including extensive controlled clinical trials, before any new diagnostic procedure can be labeled a true breakthrough in the early diagnosis of carcinoma of the pancreas.

In evaluating the plethora of newer diagnostic tests, the physician must keep in mind several points. First, any ideal diagnostic tool for evaluating pancreatic malignancy must have a high sensitivity for detecting small pancreatic mass lesions, that is, tumors less than 2 to 3 cm in diameter. The emphasis must be on detecting such small lesions, which are possibly resectable for cure. Mass lesions of the pancreas larger than 3 to 4 cm in diameter almost invariably will involve adjacent great vessels or will have spread beyond the confines of the pancreatic bed. These are unlikely to be resectable for cure, rendering fruitless even the highest degree of accuracy of their detection. Second, a truly superior diagnostic tool for pancreatic cancer must be available for use at an extremely low threshold of clinical suspicion. Because so many of the presenting complaints of patients subsequently found to have pancreatic cancer, such as weight loss, anorexia, and abdominal pain, are common to many abdominal diseases and disorders and thus are nonspecific, any proposed screening test should be low risk, low cost, noninvasive or minimally invasive, and available for use on an outpatient basis. Third, in view of the necessity of resecting cancer of the pancreas early, a sensitive diagnostic test for it must also be specific (i.e., when the disease is absent, the test result must be negative). A negative result from a highly specific diagnostic test—that is, one with a low false positive rate—logically directs the physician's focus away from a particular diagnosis. Unfortunately, tests that are very sensitive are usually not very specific, as those with low false negative rates (sensitive tests) usually have a significant rate of false positive results. Thus, a new diagnostic technique for diagnosing carcinoma of the pancreas with a 1 to 5 per cent false positive rate might result in subjecting a large number of patients without cancer to further unnecessary, possibly invasive diagnostic procedures and even exploratory laparotomy. No single diagnostic test currently available for pancreatic malignancy fulfills the requirements for both great sensitivity and high specificity that would facilitate the early diagnosis of resectable and curable lesions.

Laboratory Tests

Most patients with pancreatic cancer will be found to have an anemia from nutritional deficiency, indolent blood loss into the bowel, or the anemia of "chronic disease"; however, early in the disease the hematocrit value often is normal. An elevated erythrocyte sedimentation rate is common, as is the presence of occult blood in the stool. Rarely, the obstructive jaundice caused by an extensive mass in the head of the pancreas together with the blood loss into the duodenum from an eroding pancreatic tumor may produce a characteristic silver-colored stool.

Available serologic and biochemical tests cannot definitively make or exclude the diagnosis of carcinoma of the pancreas. On rare occasions, patients with pancreatic malignancy will have an elevated serum amylase value.[8] In some patients, this may be due to the uncommon development of acute pancreatitis in association with pancreatic malignancy; in others, the elevated amylase level will be an S-type isoamylase. This isoamylase variant is neither sensitive nor specific for pancreatic cancer and may be seen in a variety of tumors, such as bronchogenic cancers of the lung. Alkaline phosphatase elevation is also commonly noted in patients with pancreatic malignancy from either bile duct obstruction or multiple large bulky hepatic metastases.[8] For those with bile duct obstruction, the serum alkaline phosphatase level not infrequently is greater than five times the upper limits of normal, a situation unusual for gall-stone disease. In patients with bile duct obstruction, relentlessly progressive hyperbilirubinemia is observed, with the direct-reacting component predominant. Once again, the serum bilirubin levels often are greater than 15 mg/dl, levels uncommon for benign bile duct obstruction, particularly choledocholithiasis. A variable number of patients will be found to have mildly to moderately elevated lactic dehydrogenase (LDH), aspartate aminotransferase (AST, SGOT), and glucose values and a depressed serum albumin level (Table 99–1).[8, 9]

No tumor markers can be considered helpful in detecting the patient with pancreatic cancer. Elevated carcinoembryonic antigen (CEA) has been noted in some series in over 70 per cent of patients with subsequently confirmed pancreatic malignancy.[10–12] In other studies, CEA was elevated in little more than one half the patients with pancreatic malignancy, the majority of whom had tumors that were already nonresectable for cure.[10] Concentrations of other tumor markers, such as alpha-fetoprotein (AFP) and onco-

Table 99–1. LABORATORY TESTS IN CARCINOMA OF THE PANCREAS

Test	Per Cent Abnormal
Alkaline phosphatase	82
5′-Nucleotidase	71
Aspartate aminotransferase (SGOT)	64
Lactic dehydrogenase (LDH)	69
Bilirubin	55
Serum albumin	60
Serum protein	17
Amylase	17

Adapted from Fitzgerald, P. J., Fortner, J. G., Watson, R. C., et al. Cancer *41*:868, 1978.

fetal antigen, reportedly have been elevated in small numbers of patients with pancreatic malignancy. Small numbers of patients with carcinoma of the pancreas have also been reported to have increased parathyroid hormone, calcitonin, glucagon, insulin, pancreas cancer–associated antigen (PCAA), pancreatic RNase, C-peptide, and even gastrin levels.[10, 13, 14] Human chorionic gonadotropin (HCG) has been reported to be increased in from 33 to 50 per cent of patients with carcinoma of the pancreas. Fewer than 20 per cent of patients with pancreatic cancer have been shown to have increased levels of HCG-beta, and none had raised serum levels of HCG-alpha.[11] A serum mucin antigen has been detected in patients with gastrointestinal and pancreatic cancer employing a monoclonal antibody 19–9 produced by a hybridoma.[15, 16] Results of this test (also called CA 19–9 antibody) have been positive in up to 90 per cent of patients with pancreatic cancer. Further studies are necessary to document the future clinical impact of this new serologic test system.

Galactosyltransferase isoenzyme II (GT-II) has been suggested as a serologic marker for pancreatic malignancy, and in one survey it was more sensitive and specific than other "tumor" markers. Sixty-seven per cent of patients with pancreatic cancer had detectable serum levels of GT-II, compared with only 1.7 per cent of patients with benign disease.[12] However, GT-II was likewise noted in 71 per cent of patients with other gastrointestinal tract cancers and in 21 per cent of patients with other malignancies (Table 99–2).

An elevated trypsin-creatinine clearance has likewise been demonstrated in patients with carcinoma of the pancreas but not in normal control subjects or in patients with chronic pancreatitis.[17] The elevated trypsin-creatinine clearance can also be demonstrated in patients with acute pancreatitis. Future studies of these and other biochemical and serologic tests for pancreatic malignancy will need extensive evaluation in large prospective trials. For the present, none of these tests should be relied on to make or exclude the diagnosis of pancreatic cancer.

IMAGING TECHNIQUES IN DETECTING PANCREATIC CANCER

Noninvasive Techniques

The upper gastrointestinal series may demonstrate widening of the duodenal loop and a mass indentation along the medial aspect of the second portion of the duodenum in patients with carcinoma of the head of the pancreas (Fig. 99–2). Anterior displacement of the stomach or displacement of the ligament of Treitz from the greater curvature of the stomach, or both, may be noted in patients with large tumors involving the body or tail of the pancreas. The upper gastrointestinal series must, however, be considered a poor screening test in establishing the early diagnosis of resectable pancreatic malignancy, especially in patients with carcinoma of the body or tail of the pancreas. Selenium-75-selenomethionine pancreatic nuclear scanning cannot be recommended as a routine, sensitive, and specific test for pancreatic cancer.[18] Newer radioisotope scans of the pancreas with better radiospecificity for the pancreas and higher resolution for focal defects may improve this unacceptably poor yield for the selenomethionine scan.

Newer abdominal imaging techniques of ultrasonography, computed tomography (CT scans) and magnetic resonance imaging (MRI scanning) have markedly enhanced the ability to visualize the pancreas noninvasively.[19–24] Pancreatic malignancy is characteristically noted on scanning as an asymmetrically or uniformly enlarged pancreatic mass. Loss of tissue fat planes between the pancreas and other retroperitoneal structures is also suggestive of carcinoma of the pancreas (see Fig. 99–6). In addition to the mass enlargement of the pancreas, marked dilatation of the extrahepatic and intrahepatic bile ducts will be readily apparent in most patients with malignant bile duct obstruction. A dilated pancreatic duct may also be noted in patients with carcinoma of the head of the pancreas. Metastases to the liver and retroperitoneum may likewise be

Table 99–2. PERCENTAGE OF POSITIVE FINDINGS SUGGESTIVE OF PANCREATIC CANCER

Diagnostic Test*	Pancreatic Cancer (61)	Other Gastrointestinal/ Unknown Primary (28)	Nongastrointestinal Cancer (14)	Benign Disease (167)
Ultrasonography (n = 236)	64	19	0	1
Computed tomography (n = 74)	79	0	25	4
ERCP (n = 79)	93	0	0	0
Angiography (n = 12)	100	—	—	0
Alpha-fetoprotein (n = 270)	3	6	7	1
Ferritin (n = 270)	50	45	64	22
RNase (n = 270)	30	39	8	14
Carcinoembryonic antigen (CEA) >4 ng/dl (n = 270)	34	38	7	2
GT-II (n = 270)	67	71	21	2

Adapted from Podolsky, D. K., McPhee, M. S., Alpert, E., et al. N. Engl. J. Med. *304*:1313, 1981.
*ERCP, Endoscopic retrograde cholangiopancreatography; GT-II, galactosyltransferase isoenzyme II.

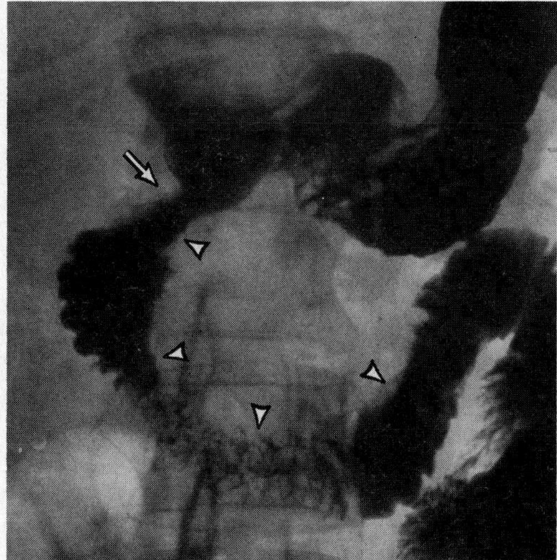

Figure 99–2. An upper gastrointestinal barium study, demonstrating displacement and infiltration of the medial aspect of the duodenal loop by pancreatic adenocarcinoma *(arrowheads)* and compression of the lateral aspect of the upper duodenum by an enlarged gallbladder *(arrow).*

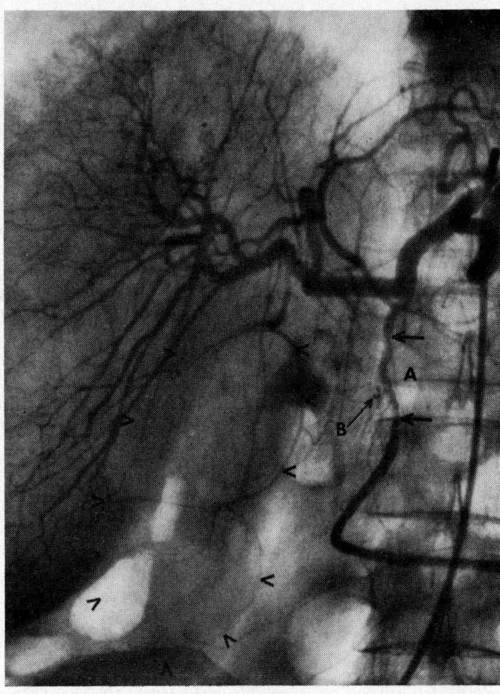

Figure 99–3. Angiogram of pancreatic adenocarcinoma, showing tumor encasement of gastroduodenal artery (A, between arrows), increased and abnormal vascularity in the head of the pancreas (B), and enlarged gallbladder manifest by elongation and displacement of cystic artery branches (outlined by open arrows).

detected by either ultrasonography, CT, or MRI scanning. The sensitivity and specificity of both ultrasonography and CT in pancreatic cancer exceed 90 per cent.[23] The larger mass lesions will almost certainly be demonstrated by either ultrasonography or CT. However, the lower limits of resolution for both these methods are in the range of 1 to 2 cm; thus, small foci of potentially resectable malignancy in the pancreas, especially those not altering the contour of the gland or obstructing ductal structures, may easily be overlooked by both of these techniques. In patients with suspected pancreatic cancer, ultrasonography with its lower cost, greater availability, absence of radiation, and rapidity of scanning is an ideal diagnostic screening procedure. When the ultrasonographic examination does not show the pancreas or records atypical findings, CT should be considered the next procedure for diagnosis because it is accurate and noninvasive. The role of MRI scanning in evaluating patients with suspected pancreatic cancer has not yet been established but appears promising. When a pancreatic mass is not demonstrable by either ultrasonography or CT techniques, in the face of dilation of common bile and pancreatic ducts, the suspicion of a small periampullary tumor is sufficient to warrant an endoscopic retrograde cholangiopancreatography (ERCP) examination (see p. 1877).

Invasive Techniques

Many invasive diagnostic procedures are available for investigating tumors of the pancreas. Angiography will usually demonstrate displacement of the pancreatic arcades or tumor encasement of the celiac, splenic, gastroduodenal, or superior mesenteric arteries (Fig. 99–3).[25] Moreover, the venous phase of the angiogram may demonstrate occlusion of the splenic vein. Most pancreatic adenocarcinomas are "hypovascular" and do not enhance with selective angiography. Small islet cell carcinomas, on the other hand, may be detected by selective angiography. Given the advancements in noninvasive imaging, such as ultrasonography, CT, and MRI scanning, routine angiograms play little role in diagnosing pancreatic cancer.

Secretin or cholecystokinin (CCK) stimulation of the pancreas with collection of pancreatic juice by a duodenal sump tube is a relatively insensitive and nonspecific test for the diagnosis of pancreatic malignancy. Low bicarbonate output, primarily owing to decreased secretion of pancreatic juice, is neither sensitive nor specific enough to serve as an acceptable screening test for patients with the suspicion of pancreatic malignancy.[26] Collections of pure pancreatic juice at the time of directed endoscopic cannulation of the pancreatic duct may enhance the diagnostic sensitivity and specificity of the secretin-CCK stimulation test of the pancreas. The distinction of patients with pancreatic cancer from those with chronic pancreatitis is not easily made by this pancreatic function test alone.

Transhepatic cholangiography (THC) in patients with pancreatic malignancy obstructing the common bile duct usually demonstrates a long, irregularly strictured, and tapered segment of the distal part of the common bile duct as it passes through the pancreatic malignancy (Fig. 99–4). Because the THC, unlike ERCP, does not demonstrate the pancreatic duct, difficulty may be encountered in differentiating a ma-

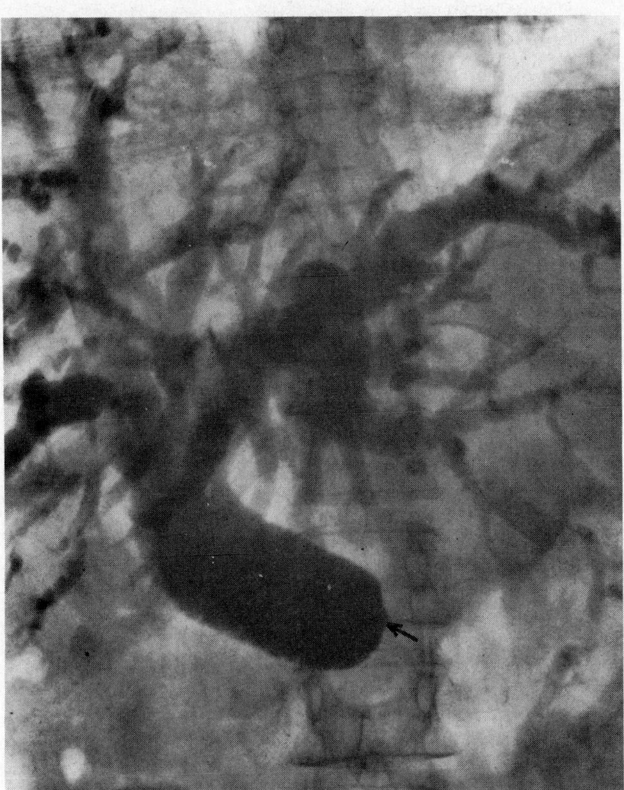

Figure 99–4. Percutaneous cholangiogram, showing massively dilated and completely obstructed common bile duct by pancreatic adenocarcinoma *(arrow)*. Note degree of intrahepatic bile duct dilatation.

lignant stricture of the distal portion of the common bile duct from a scarred bile duct associated with chronic pancreatitis (see pp. 1851–1854). Transhepatic cholangiography when combined with cytologic study of aspirates obtained percutaneously by a fine needle inserted into the area of the pancreas under suspicion, may reveal that cancer is causing the obstruction. Moreover, transhepatic insertion of a bile duct stent may assist in the nonoperative decompression of the bile duct, relieving the patient of jaundice and pruritus. This procedure is of distinct benefit to many patients with nonresectable pancreatic cancer obstructing the common bile duct (see pp. 1751–1757).

ERCP provides the only nonsurgical means of visualizing the entire pancreatic duct (Fig. 99–5). As the vast majority of pancreatic cancers are ductal adenocarcinomas, even small mass lesions generally will produce occlusion or stenosis of the main pancreatic duct or its branches. Sensitivities in excess of 90 per cent have been reported in most series of patients with carcinoma of the pancreas.[12, 21, 25, 27–30] Several changes may be noted in the pancreatograms of patients with pancreatic cancer. These include a solitary irregular pancreatic ductal stenosis with or without prestenotic ectasia of the main duct, abrupt or gradual occlusion of the main duct, displacement of Wirsung's duct, changes in the side branches in the vicinity of the tumor (such as cystic destruction, fragmentation, and displacement of ductules), and pooling of the contrast agent in irregular pockets of necrotic tumor mass.[30] In addition to pancreatic duct changes, stenosis of the common bile duct with an irregular stricture may be noted in the cholangiographic phase of the ERCP (Fig. 99–5). Some of these same ductal changes may be encountered in patients with chronic pancreatitis.[27, 30] The best criteria for the diagnosis of carcinoma of the pancreas by ERCP appear to be a single, irregular, abrupt focal stricture of the pancreatic duct and the absence of other changes characteristic of chronic pancreatitis in the remainder of the ductal system. Multiple stenoses or a single smooth stenosis of the pancreatic duct is, on the other hand, more commonly due to chronic pancreatitis. An additional diagnostic benefit of ERCP is its concomitant endoscopic examination of the duodenum in patients with suspected pancreatic malignancy. Although the majority of patients with pancreatic cancer will undergo a successful pancreatogram, the procedure is impossible to perform in some. In many of these patients, endoscopic examination of the medial wall of the descending duodenum may demonstrate an irregular tumor invading and eroding the bowel, making cannulation of the pancreatic duct impossible. However, biopsy of the mass will confirm the endoscopic impression of carcinoma.[28] In some patients, tumor invading the ampulla or pancreatic duct close to the papillary orifice but not extending into the duodenal lumen will prevent contrast material from filling the ducts. In some of these patients, pure pancreatic juice or directed brushings of ductal occlusions may be collected endoscopically for cytologic study, which in some centers has often been found to demonstrate malignant cells. In this way, cytologic examination enhances the diagnostic accuracy of the ERCP procedure in patients with pancreatic cancer.

ERCP and CT are complementary, not competitive, in the diagnosis of pancreatic malignancy.[18] In one series of patients with suspected pancreatic cancer, the overall diagnostic accuracy of the ERCP in those patients who were successfully cannulated was nearly 90 per cent, about the same accuracy as that for CT scanning. The combined accuracy of ERCP and CT in patients with pancreatic malignancy was 100 per cent in this limited series. Therefore, a definite abnormality on either CT scan or ERCP that is strongly suggestive of pancreatic cancer should prompt further evaluation, as there is a strong likelihood that a pancreatic malignancy is present. Even with the combined use of these two sophisticated diagnostic techniques, the physician is cautioned against accepting negative results as an absolute guarantee that pancreatic cancer is not present. Small focal mass lesions under 1 cm, especially those deep in the body or tail, neither deforming the gland contour nor obstructing the pancreatic duct, could still be missed by both techniques. These are early, theoretically curable lesions.

Histologic demonstration of malignancy by intraoperative transduodenal biopsy or intraoperative wedge biopsy of the pancreas had previously been

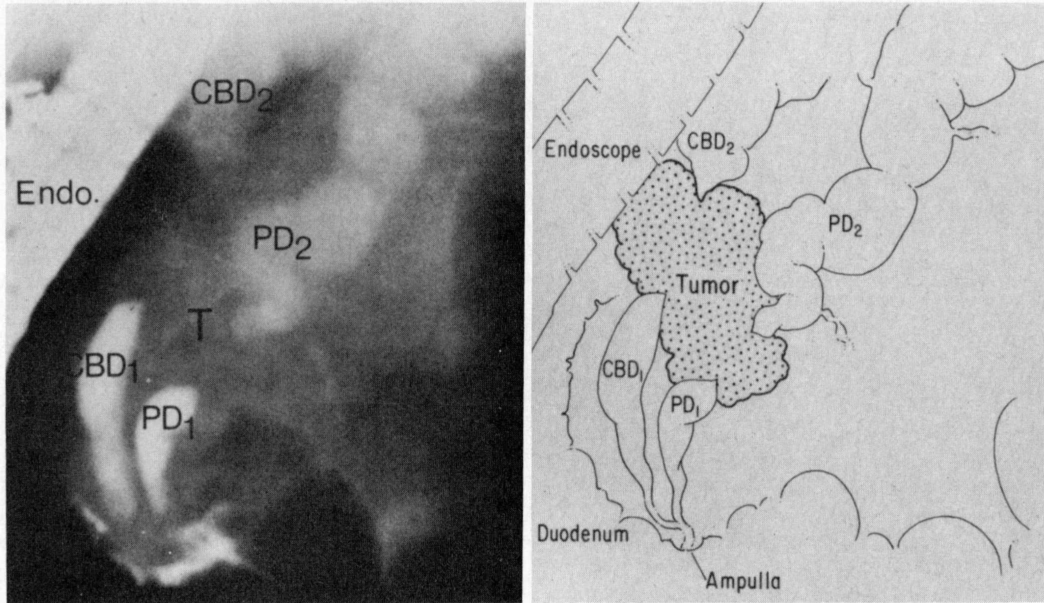

Figure 99–5. An endoscopic retrograde cholangiopancreatogram showing a 4-cm pancreatic carcinoma (T) obstructing both the common bile duct (CBD) and the main pancreatic duct (PD) ("double-duct sign"). Injection of contrast medium into the ampulla opacifies the normal proximal pancreatic duct (PD_1) and distal common bile duct (CBD_1); the obstructed distal pancreatic duct (PD_2) and proximal common bile duct (CBD_2) are markedly dilated.

considered to be the only definitive means of obtaining tissue for diagnosis. This technique is safe as well as highly sensitive and specific.[31] As mentioned, on occasion the endoscopic biopsy of a mass eroding the medial wall of the duodenum may reveal carcinoma of the pancreas.[28] In addition, cytologic study of pure pancreatic juice or of fluid collected by duodenal aspiration at the time of exogenous stimulation of the pancreas (secretin test, CCK-pancreozymin stimulation) may demonstrate malignant cells in approximately 25 per cent of patients with pancreatic cancer.

Fine needle aspiration biopsy of the pancreas has rapidly become one of the principal procedures available for pancreatic cancer diagnosis (Fig. 99–6).[31–35] Using either ultrasonographic or CT guidance, the operator passes a No. 22 gauge needle directly into the mass lesion. In most series, 80 to 90 per cent sensitivity and 100 per cent specificity in the presence of pancreatic cancer have been demonstrated.[33–35] Of great importance is the absence of false positive biopsy results in patients with chronic inflammatory disease of the pancreas. The absence of malignant cells in an aspirated biopsy or cytologic examination of the pancreas, however, does not definitively exclude pancreatic cancer. Several attempts at aspiration may be necessary to secure an adequate number of cells for cytologic examination. The presence of a cytologist in the examining room to prepare the cytology slides immediately and fix them in alcohol quickly will enhance the accuracy of this technique. Although complications are notably infrequent after this technique, there has been one report of seeding of malignant cells along the needle tract after aspiration of the pancreas with a fine needle.[36] The accuracy of this technique, of course, depends greatly on the skill of the operator as well as on the experience of the cytologist in reading specimens obtained from deep needle aspiration.

Schematic Approach to Diagnosis

In view of the large number of invasive and noninvasive techniques for imaging the pancreas, a schematic approach to the diagnosis of pancreatic cancer is helpful (Fig. 99–7). The patient suspected of harboring this disease should first have ultrasonography, which is easily done on an outpatient basis and is inexpensive. If the ultrasonographic examination is deemed inadequate in visualizing the pancreas completely, it should

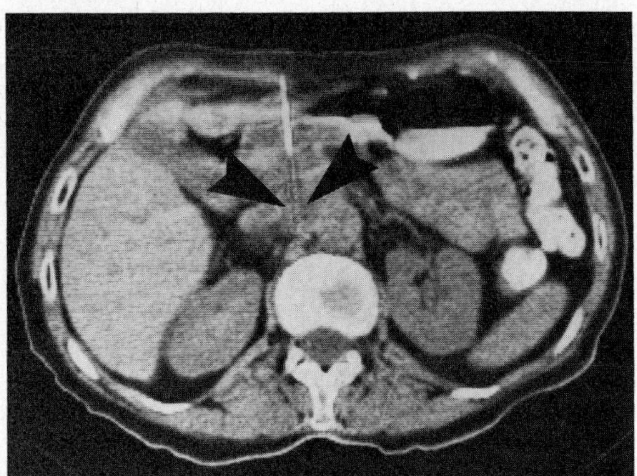

Figure 99–6. Computed tomography-directed aspiration cytology of the pancreas. A fine needle has been placed deeply within a mass in the region of the head of the pancreas *(black arrows).* Multiple passes are necessary to ensure adequate numbers of cells for cytologic examination. (Courtesy of R. Brooke Jeffrey, M.D.)

be followed immediately by an outpatient CT study. In patients with large, readily identifiable pancreatic masses, cytologic examination of an aspirate by guided needle using ultrasonographic or CT assistance may then be performed. In patients with cytologic confirmation of malignancy, appropriate therapy should be instituted without delay. Those patients with negative results on guided aspiration cytologic studies should undergo ERCP to support the suspicion of chronic pancreatitis. In patients with small focal mass lesions, diffuse enlargement of the pancreas with calcification, or equivocal findings on noninvasive imaging studies, ERCP should be performed. This examination may also be done on an outpatient basis. Normal ultrasonographic and CT scans of the pancreas, on the other hand, with persistence of symptoms should lead to additional diagnostic tests to evaluate other potential causes of abdominal complaints. Only if other features suggest pancreatic disease (intermittent serum amylase elevations, new onset of midepigastric pain with back radiation) should ERCP be performed in patients with completely normal findings on ultrasonography and CT.

Carcinoma of the ampulla of Vater must be differentiated from pancreatic carcinoma in patients with obstructive jaundice. Most patients with ampullary cancer present early in the stage of the disease with jaundice and moderate pruritus. Laboratory evaluation for these patients demonstrates increased levels of serum alkaline phosphatase and bilirubin (usually less than 10 mg/dl). In addition, some anemia and guaiac-positive stools may be noted owing to the bleeding of ampullary cancer into the duodenal lumen. The diagnosis of carcinoma of the ampulla of Vater is usually suggested by computed tomography and/or ultrasonography demonstrating dilation of the extrahepatic bile duct and pancreatic duct down to the level of the duodenum *without* a detectable mass. Endoscopic visualization of the medial wall of the duodenum is mandatory in these patients prior to surgery. Visualization of the papilla, endoscopic biopsy, and confirmatory cholangiopancreatography should be performed prior to surgical exploration. For patients judged not to be good candidates for pancreaticoduodenectomy, a surgical ampullectomy, or an endoscopic papillotomy with or without stent placement should be considered.

TREATMENT OF CANCER OF THE PANCREAS

Surgery

In general, only one fourth of patients with pancreatic cancer have lesions that are surgically resectable, and only one tenth have potentially curable disease at the time of clinical presentation.[37–40] In a survey of nearly 1300 patients referred to the Mayo Clinic during a 24-year period, only 162 (13 per cent) were able to undergo a resection for cure.[40] Among 101 patients with cancer of the pancreas referred to the Surgical Service at the Peter Bent Brigham Hospital, 21 patients could not undergo exploratory surgery because of gross metastases and poor physical status.[41] Of the remaining 80 patients in the Brigham study, 25 underwent intraoperative biopsy alone, 35 underwent a palliative by-

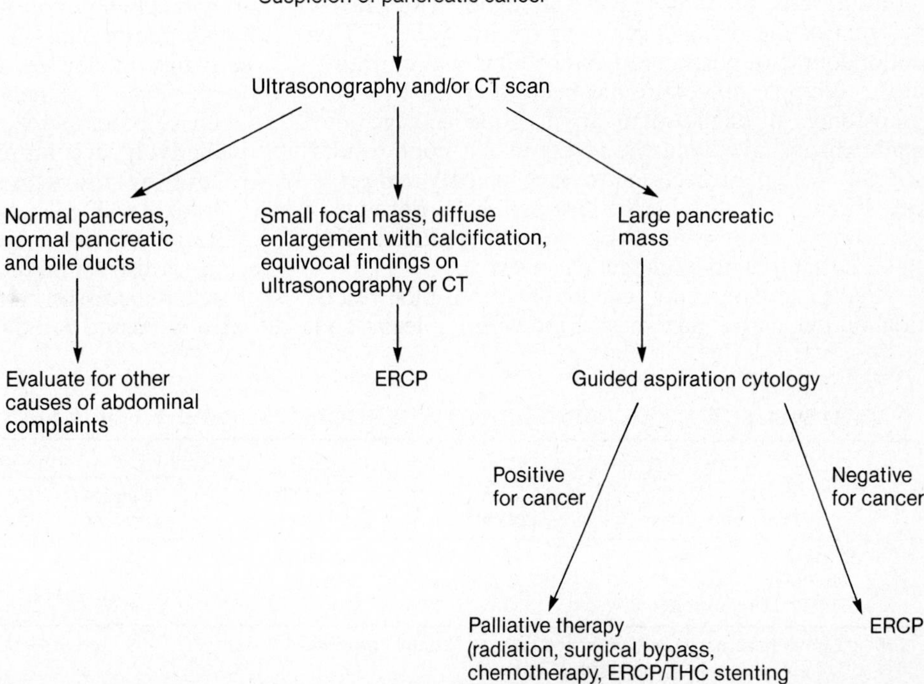

Figure 99–7. Scheme for diagnosis of pancreatic cancer. ERCP, endoscopic retrograde cholangiopancreatography; THC, transhepatic cholangiography.

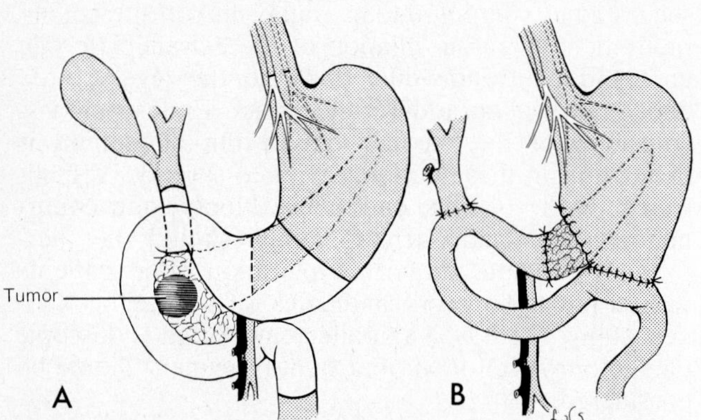

Figure 99–8. *A*, An en bloc resection of the distal stomach, duodenum, common duct, and head of the pancreas containing the pancreatic neoplasm is performed (areas removed are not shaded). In addition, a cholecystectomy and truncal vagotomy are also done. *B*, Gastrointestinal continuity is restored by performing a pancreaticojejunostomy, a choledochojejunostomy, and a gastrojejunostomy. The cholecystectomy prevents the development of gallstones which might occur because of stasis of bile in the gallbladder. The vagotomy minimizes the chance for peptic ulceration in the jeunum near the gastrojejunostomy (marginal ulcer). (From Reber, H. A., and Way, L. W.: The pancreas. *In* Dunphy, J. E., and Way, L. W. [eds.]. Current Surgical Diagnosis and Treatment. 3rd edition. Los Altos, Calif., Lange Medical Publications, 1977. Used by permission.)

pass, and only 20 underwent an attempted curative resection.

The Whipple resection remains the surgical procedure of choice for patients with small resectable carcinomas of the head of the pancreas (Fig. 99–8). In this situation it is not attended by the appreciable mortality rate that is seen when the resection is performed in patients with large bulky tumors of the pancreatic head. Of nearly 500 patients undergoing a Whipple resection for large carcinomas, an operative mortality rate of 21 per cent was noted, with only 4 per cent of the patients surviving for five years.[42] The major source of postoperative morbidity and mortality in the Whipple procedure has been the pancreaticojejunostomy, through which anastomotic leakage and hemorrhage have occurred. Despite the poor results overall, Whipple resection provides the only real prospect of cure and may be the best palliative procedure, particularly among good-risk younger patients with small periampullary pancreatic cancer.

Total pancreatectomy, combining an en bloc resection of the entire pancreas, duodenum, spleen, and greater omentum with subtotal gastrectomy and a careful lymphadenectomy, has been reported to have several distinct advantages over the Whipple procedure for patients with carcinoma of the pancreas.[41, 43–45] The total pancreatectomy avoids the need for a difficult pancreaticojejunal anastomosis. In many patients with carcinoma of the head of the pancreas, the entire gland is expendable, as the remainder of the gland is fibrotic and will not function normally postoperatively. Moreover, in many patients with carcinoma of the head of the pancreas, microscopic or macroscopic tumor foci can be found in the pancreas far from the main lesion and well beyond the usual margin of pancreatic resection. A mean survival of 40 months has been reported in some centers, compared with a 13-month mean survival for patients undergoing the Whipple procedure (Table 99–3).[41] Even in experienced hands, however, the total pancreatectomy carries an operative mortality rate in excess of 15 per cent.[40, 41]

The view that total pancreatectomy is superior to Whipple resection has been challenged in one series of 162 patients from the Mayo Clinic.[45] The overall surgical mortality rate for each operation was 16 per cent, and there was no difference in mean five-year survival between Whipple procedure and total pancreatectomy patients. Total pancreatectomy among persons in this survey, however, revealed multiple foci of cancer in 30 per cent of patients, many of which were far removed from the main tumor mass.

For symptomatic patients (i.e., those with considerable pruritus, fever, or jaundice) who have large, bulky tumor masses that are clearly nonresectable, some consideration should be given to a palliative procedure to decompress the dilated biliary tree. The mean survival time after palliative biliary surgical bypass is only 6 months. A cholecystojejunostomy can be performed rapidly and safely and usually drains as well as a choledochojejunostomy. For patients with large, bulky tumor masses of the pancreatic head eroding into the duodenum, a gastrojejunostomy should also be performed. Percutaneous transhepatic stenting may likewise be employed, by experienced radiologists, to palliatively decompress the dilated biliary tree and relieve the obstructive jaundice and pruritus.

In skilled hands, endoscopic biliary stenting is possible in the vast majority of patients with pancreatic cancer obstructing the distal portion of the bile duct.[46, 47] After successful cannulation of the bile duct, a guide wire is passed proximal to the obstruction. Over the

Table 99–3. SURVIVAL IN PATIENTS UNDERGOING SURGERY FOR CARCINOMA OF THE PANCREAS

Procedure	Number of Patients	Surgical Mortality (%)	Survival (Mean, in Months)		
			Stages I and II	*Stage III*	*All Stages*
Bypass	35	14	5.8	5.4	5.6
Whipple	11	21	12.7	6.0	7.6
Total pancreatectomy	16	13	40.0*	6.0	23.0†

*P<.03, total pancreatectomy versus bypass and Whipple procedure.
†P<.03, total pancreatectomy versus bypass.
Adapted from Brooks, J. R., and Culebras, J. M. Am. J. Surg. *131*:516, 1976.

guide wire the stent is passed through the obstruction. Occasionally a papillotomy is necessary to facilitate passage of the larger No. 10 French stents. Unlike many percutaneous transhepatic stenting and drainage procedures, no external catheter remains in place after endoscopic stenting, and catheter exchange can be accomplished readily in the event of stent blockage. Additional studies will be needed to compare the costs, risks, and quality of life among patients with surgical, transhepatic, and endoscopic drainage techniques (see pp. 1741–1761).

Chemotherapy

Single-agent chemotherapy offers little, if any, palliation and no significant improvement in survival for patients with nonresectable pancreatic malignancy, especially those with widespread hepatic metastases. 5-Fluorouracil (5-FU) administered in doses of 400 to 500 mg/sq m/day for five days produces a partial response rate of only 10 to 15 per cent of patients.[48] Median survival time after the administration of 5-FU is less than 20 weeks. When used as single agents, methotrexate, actinomycin D, doxorubicin, carmustine (BCNU), and semustine (methyl-CCNU) cannot be demonstrated to produce significant activity in the palliation of pancreatic cancer.[49] Most chemotherapeutic regimens used in treating patients with nonresectable pancreatic cancer have relied on combinations of 5-FU and other agents.[50–55] Fluorouracil, doxorubicin (Adriamycin), and mitomycin (Mitomycin C)—the so called FAM regimen—was reported in preliminary studies to produce "response rates" in the range of 9 per cent to 40 per cent of patients treated. This efficacy has been refuted, however, by a large study comparing fluorouracil alone, fluorouracil and doxorubicin, and FAM among 144 patients with pancreatic cancer.[56] The median survival time (22 weeks for the entire group of 144 patients), the median interval to progression of tumor (nine weeks for the entire group), and the objective response rates (only 21 per cent for the entire group) were not significantly better for the combination chemotherapeutic regimens than for fluorouracil alone. Toxic reactions, specifically thrombocytopenia, anorexia, nausea, and vomiting were, however, more frequent with the doxorubicin-containing program. In addition to overall lack of efficacy, the FAM regimen was estimated to cost $500 for eight weeks, compared to $30 for fluorouracil alone.

Other combination chemotherapeutic regimens have produced variable response rates. Five of 23 (22 per cent) patients in one study with advanced pancreatic cancer achieved a partial remission with 5-FU, doxorubicin, mitomycin, and semustine (FAMMc).[57] In another series, streptozotocin, mitomycin, and 5-FU (SMF) produced 34 per cent response rates among patients with pancreatic cancer.[58] Median survival time was only 21 weeks, however, and was not significantly better than with that achieved by mitomycin and fluorouracil alone. In general, studies to date have not provided convincing evidence that combination chemotherapy either prolongs survival or enhances the quality of life among patients with advanced pancreatic cancer. As such, although chemotherapy holds the promise of future advances in the therapy of pancreatic cancer, extensive controlled studies are required before the routine use of chemotherapy outside of rigorous controlled clinical trials can be recommended for patients with advanced pancreatic cancer.

Radiation Therapy

Therapy with 4000 to 6000 rad from cobalt or linear accelerator sources to a reduced field consisting of only pancreas and tumor enhances median survival time compared with results in control groups.[59, 60] Prior to the availability of megavoltage radiation, this type of treatment was not commonly employed in pancreatic cancer because of the high radioresistance of pancreatic cancer, the relative inaccessibility of the gland in the retroperitoneum, and the radiosensitivity of adjacent structures, such as small bowel, spinal cord, liver, and

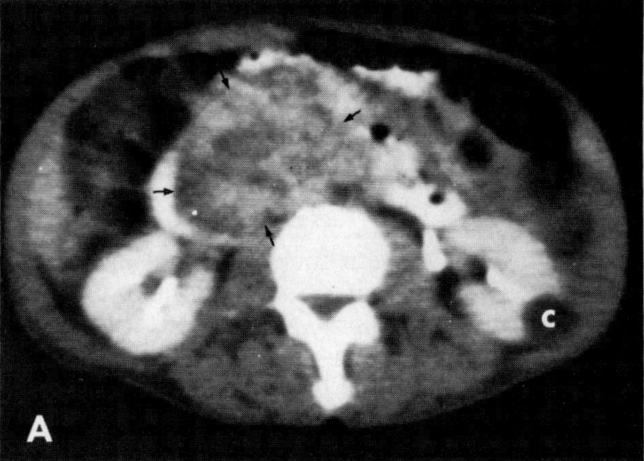

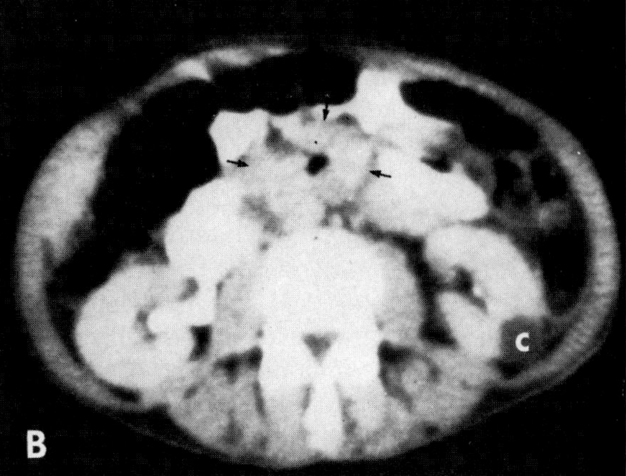

Figure 99–9. Computed tomography in carcinoma of the pancreas before *(A)* and after *(B)* heavy charged particle Bragg peak radiation therapy. Substantial decrease in tumor volume is evident. (Courtesy of Jeanne M. Quivey, M.D.)

kidneys. Megavoltage external beam radiation therapy, however, achieves the delivery of high-dose, small-volume radiation therapy with high minimum tumor doses to much smaller target areas over shorter periods of time. The combined use of radiation therapy and 5-FU appears promising. Combinations of 4000 to 6000 rad from cobalt or linear accelerator sources to a reduced field and administration of 5-FU produce a median survival time significantly better than that achieved by 6000 rad of radiation therapy alone.[61]

In a limited number of patients, high linear energy transfer (LET) particle (neutron or heavy ion) radiation therapy has been demonstrated to produce substantial decrease in tumor bulk.[62, 63] Computed tomography may serve as a valuable means of estimating quantitative tumor response in patients treated by radiation therapy alone or by combinations of radiation therapy and chemotherapy (Fig. 99–9). In a study of 77 patients with locally advanced, nonresectable pancreatic adenocarcinoma, intensive neutron beam irradiation of the primary site (15 to 25 Gy or 1500 to 2500 rad) achieved symptomatic palliation in the majority of patients.[63] The median survival time was only 6 months in these patients, however, which does not differ from previous reports of patients treated with standard radiation therapy. Two of 19 autopsied patients who had been treated with particle radiation therapy were free of tumor, whereas the entire group demonstrated massive tumor fibrosis, focal necrosis, and collagen hyalinization. Substantial morbidity was noted, particularly gastrointestinal ulceration, among patients treated with high dosages (24 Gy [2400 rad] or more). Future studies of this technique are necessary, particularly those comparing particle with standard radiation therapy.

PANCREATIC CYSTADENOMA, CYSTADENOCARCINOMA, AND ADENOACANTHOMA

Pancreatic malignancy other than adenocarcinoma is uncommon. In one series of 205 patients with pancreatic cancer, malignancies other than adenocarcinoma constituted only 5 per cent of pancreatic cancers.[1] The most frequent of these atypical malignancies is the cystadenocarcinoma, accounting for 1 per cent of primary pancreatic malignancy. The cystadenocarcinomas often arise within cystadenomas of the pancreas. The latter tumors, composing about 10 per cent of the cystic lesions of the pancreas, occur predominantly in middle-aged women.[64–66] In one series, 82 per cent of patients with cystadenomas of the pancreas were women, with a mean age of onset of 55 years.[64] The symptoms of cystadenomas and cystadenocarcinomas are predominantly pain (56 per cent), weight loss (40 per cent), nausea and vomiting (25 per cent), and belching and gaseousness (25 per cent). Jaundice and upper gastrointestinal tract hemorrhage are uncommon manifestations of cystadenocarcinomas of the pancreas. Infrequently, a patient with this tumor will have attacks of acute pancreatitis with elevated serum amylase values. Sonograms or CT scans of such patients may reveal a mass that can be confirmed by ERCP. A common presentation of cystadenoma with focal cystadenocarcinoma of the pancreas is a well-nourished patient with a large, protruding abdominal mass.

The most common physical finding in patients with cystadenomas and cystadenocarcinomas of the pancreas is a palpable mass in the epigastrium.[64] Not surprisingly, noninvasive imaging by CT or ultrasonography will demonstrate a large cystic mass lesion. About 10 per cent of the cystadenomas and cystadenocarcinomas have foci of calcification. A disproportionate number of cystadenomas and cystadenocarcinomas arise in the body and tail of the pancreas, in comparison with other, more common pancreatic tumors, which are located in the head of the gland. Differentiation of these cystic neoplasms from benign pancreatic pseudocysts is sometimes difficult, although the absence of a history of trauma, alcoholism, clinical pancreatitis, or biliary tract disease makes cystic neoplasia more likely.[65]

Diagnosis of these tumors is made most commonly by laparotomy with resection and pathologic confirmation. Cystic masses as large as 30 cm in diameter have been reported in patients with cystadenomas and cystadenocarcinomas of the pancreas. Therapy consists primarily of surgical resection. Because long-term survival in patients undergoing Whipple procedure or distal pancreatectomy for cystadenocarcinoma of the pancreas is considerably better than for those with adenocarcinoma of the pancreas, these patients should be considered for resection even if large, bulky tumors are demonstrated.

On occasion, adenocarcinoma of the pancreas may be found to have squamous components. These tumors, adenoacanthomas, represent about 2 per cent of malignant neoplasms of the pancreas.[1] Generally, adenoacanthoma behaves like adenocarcinoma. The sex ratio, age incidence, distribution of cancer in the pancreas, sites of metastases, and survival statistics are similar for adenoacanthoma and adenocarcinoma of the pancreas.[67] It is important to recognize, however, that the pancreas may be the site of origin of metastatic squamous cell carcinoma or of a mixed tumor of squamous cell carcinoma and adenocarcinoma.

CONCLUSION

Carcinoma of the pancreas is currently a major cause of death in Western society. It remains a substantial therapeutic problem, primarily because of its insidious onset and the advanced stage of disease at the time of clinical manifestations. Although techniques in diagnosis and methods of treatment have advanced considerably over the past decades, carcinoma of the pancreas remains a disease with a dismal outlook.

References

1. Kissane, J. M. Carcinoma of the exocrine pancreas: pathologic aspects. J. Surg. Oncol. *7*:167, 1975.
2. MacMahon, B. Risk factors for cancer of the pancreas. Cancer *50*:2676, 1982.
3. Kato, I., Tajima, K., Kuroishi, T., and Tominaga, S. Latitude and pancreatic cancer. Jpn. J. Clin. Oncol. *15*:403, 1985.
4. Wynder, E. L., Hall, N. E., and Polansky, M. Epidemiology of coffee and pancreatic cancer. Cancer Res. *43*:3900, 1983.
5. MacMahon, B., Yen, S., Trichopoulos, D., Warren, K., and Nardi, G. Coffee and cancer of the pancreas. N. Engl. J. Med. *304*:630, 1981.
6. Gold, E. B., Gordis, L., Diener, M. D., Seltser, R., Boitnott, J. K., Bynum, T. E., and Hutcheon, D. F. Diet and other risk factors for cancer of the pancreas. Cancer *55*:460, 1985.
7. Pickle, L. W., and Gottlieb, M. S. Pancreatic cancer mortality in Louisiana. Am. J. Public Health *70*:256, 1980.
8. Weingarten, L., Gelb, A. M., and Fischer, M. G. Dilemma of pancreatic ductal carcinoma. Am. J. Gastroenterol. *71*:473, 1979.
9. Fitzgerald, P. J., Fortner, J. G., Watson, R. C., Schwartz, M. K., Sherlock, P., Benua, R. S., Cubilla, A. L., Schottenfeld, D., Miller, D., Winower, S. J., Lightdale, C. J., Leidner, S., and Nesselbaum, J. S. The value of diagnostic aids in detecting pancreas cancer. Cancer *41*:868, 1978.
10. Mackie, C. R., Moosa, A. R., Go, V. L. W., Noble, G., Sizemore, G., Cooper, M. J., Wood, R. A. B., Hall, A. W., Waldmann, T., Gelder, F., and Rubenstein, A. H. Prospective evaluation of some candidate tumor markers in the diagnosis of pancreatic cancer. Dig. Dis. Sci. *25*:161, 1980.
11. Bender, R. A., Weintraub, B. D., and Rosen, S. W. Prospective evaluation of two tumor-associated proteins in pancreatic adenocarcinoma. Cancer *43*:591, 1979.
12. Podolsky, D. K., McPhee, M. S., Alpert, E., Warshaw, A. L., and Isselbacher, K. J. Galactosyltransferase isoenzyme II in the detection of pancreatic cancer: comparison with radiologic, endoscopic, and serologic tests. N. Engl. J. Med. *304*:1313, 1981.
13. Weickmann, J. L., Olson, E. M., and Glitz, D. G. Immunological assay of pancreatic ribonuclease in serum as an indicator of pancreatic cancer. Cancer Res. *44*:1682, 1984.
14. Kurihara, M., Ogawa, M., Ohta, T., Kurokawa, E., Kitahara, T., Murata, A., Matsuda, K., Kosaki, G., Watanabe, T., and Wada, H. Radioimmunoassay for human pancreatic ribonuclease and measurement of serum immunoreactive pancreatic ribonuclease in patients with malignant tumors. Cancer Res. *44*:2240, 1984.
15. Magnani, J. L., Steplewski, Z., Koprowski, H., and Ginsburg, V. Identification of the gastrointestinal and pancreatic cancer-associated antigen detected by monoclonal antibody 19–9 in the sera of patients as a mucin. Cancer Res. *43*:5489, 1983.
16. Brockhaus, M., Wysocka, M., Magnani, J. L., Steplewski, Z., Kaprowski, H., and Ginsburg, V. Normal salivary mucin contains the gastrointestinal cancer-associated antigen detected by monoclonal antibody 19–9 in the serum mucin of patients. Vox Sang. *48*:34, 1985.
17. Lake-Bakaar, G., McKavanagh, S., and Summerfield, J. A. Urinary immunoreactive trypsin excretion: a noninvasive screening test for pancreatic cancer. Lancet *2*:878, 1979.
18. Hall, T. J., Cooper, M., Hughes, R. G., Levin, B., Skinner, D. B., and Moossa, A. R. Pancreatic cancer screening—analysis of the problem and the role of radionuclide imaging. Am. J. Surg. *134*:544, 1977.
19. Cotton, P. B., Denyer, M. E., Kreel, L., Husband, J., Meire, H. B., and Lees, W. Comparative clinical impact of endoscopic pancreatography, grey-scale ultrasonography, and computed tomography (EMI scanning) in pancreatic disease: preliminary report. Gut *19*:679, 1978.
20. Foley, W. D., Stewart, E. T., Lawson, T. L., Grenan, J., Loguidice, J., Maher, L., and Unger, G. F. Computed tomography, ultrasonography, and endoscopic retrograde cholangiopancreatography in the diagnosis of pancreatic disease: a comparative study. Gastrointest. Radiol. *5*:29, 1980.
21. Moss, A. A., Federle, M., Shapiro, H. A., Ohto, M., Goldberg, H., Korobkin, M., and Clemett, A. The combined use of computed tomography and endoscopic retrograde cholangiopancreatography in the assessment of suspected pancreatic neoplasm: a blind clinical evaluation. Radiology *134*:159, 1980.
22. Simeone, J. F., Wittenberg, J., and Ferrucci, J. T. Modern concepts of imaging of the pancreas. Invest. Radiol. *15*:6, 1980.
23. Van Dyke, J. A., Stanley, R. J., and Berland, L. L. Pancreatic imaging. Ann. Intern. Med. *102*:212, 1985.
24. Stark, D. D., Moss, A. A., Goldberg, H. I., Davis, P., and Federle, M. P. Magnetic resonance and CT of the normal and diseased pancreas: a comparative study. Radiology *150*:153, 1984.
25. Suzuki, T., Imamura, M., Tamura, K., Sumiyoshi, A., Sakanashi, S., Nishimura, I., and Tobe, T. Correlative evaluation of angiography and pancreatoductography in relation to surgery for cancer of the pancreas. Surgery *85*:644, 1979.
26. Rolny, P., Lukes, P. J., Gamklow, R., Jagenburg, R., and Nelson, A. A comparative evaluation of endoscopic retrograde pancreatography and secretin CCK test in the diagnosis of pancreatic disease. Scand. J. Gastroenterol. *13*:777, 1978.
27. Ralls, P. W., Halls, J., Renner, I., and Juttner, H. Endoscopic retrograde cholangiopancreatography (ERCP) in pancreatic disease. Radiology *134*:347, 1980.
28. Reuben, A., and Cotton, P. B. Endoscopic retrograde cholangiopancreatography in carcinoma of the pancreas. Surg. Gynecol. Obstet. *148*:179, 1979.
29. Lawson, T. L., Irani, S. K., and Stock, M. Detection of pancreatic pathology by ultrasound and endoscopic retrograde cholangiopancreatography. Gastrointest. Radiol. *3*:335, 1978.
30. Anacker, H., Weiss, H. D., and Kramann, B. Endoscopic retrograde pancreaticocholangiography in chronic diseases of the pancreas and in papillary stenoses. Gastrointest. Radiol. *3*:325, 1978.
31. Tweedle, D. E. F. Peroperative transduodenal biopsy of the pancreas. Gut *20*:992, 1979.
32. Dekker, A. Fine-needle aspiration biopsy in ampullary and pancreatic carcinoma. Arch. Surg. *114*:592, 1979.
33. Itoh, K., Yamanaka, T., Kasahara, K., Koiki, M., Nakamura, A., Hayaski, A., Kimura, K., Morioka, Y., and Kawai, T. Definitive diagnosis of pancreatic carcinoma with percutaneous fine needle aspiration biopsy under ultrasonic guidance. Am. J. Gastroenterol. *71*:469, 1979.
34. Yamanaka, T., and Kimura, K. Differential diagnosis of pancreatic mass lesion with percutaneous fine-needle aspiration biopsy under ultrasonic guidance. Dig. Dis. Sci. *24*:694, 1979.
35. Taylor, K. J. W., and Brand, M. H. Ultrasonic biopsy guidance in the management of patients with pancreatic cancer. J. Clin. Gastroenterol. *1*:267, 1979.
36. Ferrucci, J. T., Wittenberg, J., Margolis, M. N., and Carey, R. W. Malignant seeding of the tract after thin-needle aspiration biopsy. Radiology *130*:345, 1979.
37. Moossa, A. R. Pancreatic cancer: approach to diagnosis, selection for surgery and choice of operation. Cancer *50*:2689, 1982.
38. Andrew-Sandberg, A., and Ihse, I. Factors influencing survival after total pancreatectomy in patients with pancreatic cancer. Ann. Surg. *198*:605, 1983.
39. Appelquist, P., Viren, M., Minkkinen, J., Kajanti, M., Kostianinen, S., and Rissanen, P. Operative finding, treatment, and prognosis of carcinoma of the pancreas: an analysis of 267 cases. J. Surg. Oncol. *23*:143, 1983.
40. Edis, A. J., Kiernan, P. D., and Taylor, W. F. Attempted curative resection of ductal carcinoma of the pancreas. Mayo Clin. Proc. *55*:531, 1980.
41. Brooks, J. R., and Culebras, J. M. Cancer of the pancreas-palliative operation, Whipple procedure, or total pancreatectomy? Am. J. Surg. *131*:516, 1976.
42. Shapiro, T. M. Adenocarcinoma of the pancreas: a statistical analysis of biliary bypass vs Whipple resection in good risk patients. Ann. Surg. *182*:715, 1975.
43. Ruilova, L. A., and Hershey, C. D. Experience with 21 pancreaticoduodenectomies. Arch. Surg. *111*:27, 1976.
44. Pliam, M. D., and ReMine, W. H. Further evaluation of total pancreatectomy. Arch. Surg. *110*:506, 1975.

45. Ihse, I., Lilja, B., Arnesjo, B., and Bengmark, S. Total pancreatectomy for cancer—an appraisal of 65 cases. Ann. Surg. *186*:675, 1977.
46. Siegel, J. H. Improved biliary decompression with large caliber endoscopic prostheses. Gastrointest. Endoscopy *30*:21, 1984.
47. Marks, W. M., Freeny, P. C., Ball, T. J., and Gannan, R. M. Endoscopic retrograde biliary drainage. Radiology *152*:357, 1984.
48. Moertel, C. G., Engstrom, P., Lavin, P. T., Gelber, R. D., and Carbone, P. P. Chemotherapy of gastric and pancreatic carcinoma. Surgery *85*:509, 1979.
49. Schein, P. S., Lavin, P. T., Moertel, C. G., Frytak, S., Hahn, R. G., O'Connell, M. J., Reitemeier, R. J., Rubin, J., Schutt, A. J., Weiland, L. H., Kalser, M., Barkin, J., Lessner, H., Mann-Kaplan, R., Redlhammer, D., Silverman, M., Troner, M., Douglass, H., Milliron, S., Lokich, J., Brooks, J., Chaffe, J., Like, A., Zamcheck, N., Ramming, K., Bakman, J., Spiro, H., Livstone, E., and Knowlton, A. Randomized phase II clinical trial of adriamycin, methotrexate, and actinomycin-D in advanced measurable pancreatic carcinoma. Cancer *42*:19, 1978.
50. Moertel, C. G., Douglas, H. O., Hanley, J., and Carbone, P. P. Treatment of advanced adenocarcinoma of the pancreas with combinations of streptozotocin plus 5-fluorouracil and streptozotocin plus cyclophosphamide. Cancer *40*:605, 1977.
51. Wiggans, R. G., Wooley, P. V., MacDonald, J. S., Smythe, T., Veno, W., and Schein, P. S. Phase II trial of streptozotocin, mitomycin-C and 5-fluorouracil (SMF) in the treatment of advanced pancreatic cancer. Cancer *41*:387, 1978.
52. Stephens, R. L., Hoogstraten, B., and Clark, G. Pancreatic cancer treated with carmustine, fluorouracil, and spironolactone. Arch. Intern. Med. *138*:115, 1978.
53. Mallinson, C. N., Rake, M. O., Cocking, J. B., Fox, C. A., Cwynarski, M. T., Diffey, B. L., Jackson, G. A., Hanley, J., and Wass, V. J. Chemotherapy in pancreatic cancer: results of a controlled, prospective, randomized, multicentre trial. Br. Med. J. *281*:1589, 1980.
54. Bruckner, H. W., Storch, J. A., Brown, J. C., Goldberg, J., and Chamberlin, K. Phase II trial of combination chemotherapy for pancreatic cancer with 5-fluorouracil, mitomycin C, and hexamethylmelamine. Oncology *40*:165, 1983.
55. Smith, F. P., Stablein, D., Korsmeyer, S., Neefe, J., Chun, B. K., Woolley, P. V., and Schein, P. S. Combination chemotherapy for locally advanced pancreatic cancer: equivalence to external beam irradiation and implication for future management. J. Clin. Oncol. *1*:413, 1983.
56. Cullinan, S. A., Moertel, C. G., Fleming, T. R., Rubin, J. R., Krook, J. E., Everson, L. K., Windschitl, H. E., Twito, D. I., Marschke, R. F., Foley, J. F., Pfeifle, D. M., and Barlow, J. F. A comparison of three chemotherapeutic regimens in the treatment of advanced pancreatic and gastric carcinoma. JAMA *253*:2061, 1985.
57. Karlin, D. A., Stroehlein, J. R., Bennetts, R. W., Jones, R. D., Heifetz, L. J., and Mahal, P. S. Phase I-II study of the combination of 5-FU, doxorubicin, mitomycin, and semustine (FAMMe) in the treatment of adenocarcinoma of the stomach, gastroesophageal junction, and pancreas. Cancer Treat. Rep. *66*:1613, 1982.
58. Bukowski, R. M., Balcerzak, S. P., O'Bryan, R. M., Bonnet, J. D., and Chen, T. T. Randomized trial of 5-fluorouracil and mitomycin C with or without streptozotocin for advanced pancreatic cancer. A Southwest Oncology Group Study. Cancer *52*:1577, 1983.
59. Dobelbower, R. R., Borgett, B. B., Suntharalingam, N., and Strubler, K. A. Pancreatic carcinoma treated with high-dose, small-volume irradiation. Cancer *41*:1087, 1978.
60. Komaki, R., Wilson, J. F., Cox, J. D., and Kline, R. W. Carcinoma of the pancreas: results of irradiation for unresectable lesions. J. Radiat. Oncol. Biol. Phys. *6*:209, 1980.
61. Gastrointestinal Tumor Study Group. A multi-institutional comparative trial of radiation therapy alone and in combination with 5-fluorouracil for locally unresectable pancreatic cancer. Ann. Surg. *189*:205, 1979.
62. Quivey, J. M., Castro, J. R., Chen, G. T. Y., Moss, A., and Marks, W. M. Computerized tomography in the quantitative assessment of tumor response. Br. J. Cancer *41*(Suppl. 4):30, 1980.
63. Cohen, L., Woodruff, K. H., Hendrickson, F. R., Kurup, P. D., Mansell, J., Awschalom, M., Rosenberg, I., and Ten Haken, R. K. Response of pancreatic cancer to local irradiation with high-energy neutrons. Cancer *56*:1235, 1985.
64. Hodgkinson, D. J., ReMine, W. H., and Weiland, L. H. Pancreatic cystadenoma—a clinicopathologic study of 45 cases. Arch. Surg. *113*:512, 1978.
65. Corrente, R. F. Cystadenocarcinoma of the pancreas. Am. J. Surg. *139*:265, 1980.
66. Golematis, B., Georgakakis, A., Bastounis, E., Bramis, J., and Dreiling, D. A. Papillary cystadenocarcinoma of the pancreas. Am. J. Gastroenterol. *67*:600, 1977.
67. Weitzner, S. Adenoacanthoma of the pancreas—report of four cases and literature review. Am. Surg. *44*:206, 1978.

Secretory Tumors of the Pancreas

JOHN DELVALLE
TADATAKA YAMADA

The discovery of insulin by Banting and Best[1] in 1922 permitted the first documentation five years later of a hormone-producing tumor, an insulinoma, in a patient with severe hypoglycemia resulting from a metastatic islet cell carcinoma.[2] Since then, numerous clinical syndromes attributable to the hypersecretion of one or more peptides by neoplastic lesions in the pancreas have been described. Indeed, in recent years, hormone secretion has been a frequently encountered characteristic of many non-neuroendocrine tumors as well. The consequences of these accidents of nature have provided valuable insight into some of the functions of gastroenteropancreatic peptides. Moreover, the molecular structures of many human peptide hormones and the cDNAs encoding them have been obtained from pancreatic endocrine tumors. With the advent of radioimmunoassay techniques first described by Yalow and Berson[3] in 1959, the list of peptides associated with tumors of the pancreas has grown rapidly, even to include peptide-containing neoplasms that are associated with no clinical symptoms. The prevalence of endocrine neoplasms in unselected autopsy studies approximates 0.5 to 1.5 per cent,[4] yet the reported frequency of symptomatic endocrine tumors is less than 1 per 100,000.[5] The high frequency of endocrine neoplasms that remain undetected may be attributed to subthreshold presentation of signs and symptoms, low hormone secretion rates, altered peptide structure resulting in diminished biologic activity, and production of peptides with no clearly recognizable functions.

Although pancreatic tumors associated with excessive hormone production are frequently called islet cell tumors, the bulk of evidence points to a non-islet ductular origin.[6] The tumors are thought to arise from pluripotent stem cells in the duct epithelium. Under normal conditions in the fetus these stem cells, called *nesidioblasts*, give rise to islets by budding,[7] but under pathologic conditions they may differentiate into neoplasms producing ectopic hormones. This hypothesis is supported by the observations of Heitz and coworkers[8] that endocrine cells could be found in close contact with ductules at sites distant from the primary location of pancreatic endocrine tumors. Such a derivation may explain the presence in these tumors of several hormones that are not present in normal adult islet cells.

A basic assumption in most theories on the evolution of hormone-producing pancreatic neoplasms is that the cells producing hormones are embryologically related. Pearse[9] coined the acronym APUD (*A*mine *P*recursor *U*ptake and *D*ecarboxylation) to describe a family of cells that possessed a number of cytochemical and ultrastructural properties in common. APUD cells were identified by their fluorescence on ultraviolet illumination after fixation with formaldehyde vapor following accumulation of injected monoamines.[10] Such techniques have identified most of the gastroenteropancreatic peptide-containing cells as APUD cells; hence tumors secreting these peptides have been referred to as *apudomas*.

Polak and coworkers[11] have shown that calcitonin-producing C cells of the thyroid gland, known to be APUD cells, are derived from the neural crest. The authors used the technique of Le Douarin,[12] in which the neural tube and crest of quail embryos were grafted to chick embryos. Because the nuclei of quail cells could be distinguished readily from those of chick cells, the origin of C cells in the adult chick could be traced to the quail embryo neural crest. These experiments, in addition to the common property of APUD cells and nerves to accumulate amines and the observations that APUD cells contain enzymes previously thought to be present only in nerves (neuronal specific enolase[13] and tyrosine hydroxylase[14]) provide the basis of support for the theory proposed by Pearse[15] that all gastroenteropancreatic peptide-containing cells originate from the neural crest and not from the endoderm. Thus, the APUD cells have been proposed as a third division of the nervous system, with effector activities slower in onset and of longer duration than the effectors of the central and peripheral systems.[16]

Recently, however, some skepticism has arisen regarding the neural crest origin of all APUD cells.[17, 18] Le Douarin and Teillet,[19] using the aforementioned technique, were unable to find quail cells in gut epithelium of chickens that received quail neural crest heterografts. Likewise, Lamers and colleagues[20] were unable to find neural crest derivatives in the gastrointestinal epithelium of fish embryo injected with ^{3}H-labeled neural crest cells. Consistent with these observations were those of Pictet and coworkers,[21] who examined the effect of peeling the entire ectodermal sheet from nine-day rat embryos prior to the four-somite stage. At this time the neural crest is yet unformed; thus, removing the ectodermal sheet removed the source of all neural crest cells. After culturing of the remaining embryo for 11 more days to allow the pancreas to develop, the embryos were examined. Immunoassayable insulin and histologically identifiable B cells were found in normal proportions, suggesting that B cells do not arise from the neural crest but from an endodermal precursor. In other experiments, Andrew and coworkers[22] demonstrated the endodermal origin of gut endocrine cells by demonstrating their development in co-cultures of quail endoderm with chick mesoderm that had been stripped of ectoderm. In light of such evidence, Pearse[23] has revised his original theory by suggesting that APUD cells are derived from epiblastic elements preprogrammed to develop into neuroendocrine cells. None of these studies, however, precludes the possibility that cells of ectodermal origin migrate to endoderm prior to the earliest stage of the embryo studied. Anderson and Axel examined the developmental fate of a bipotential neuroendocrine precursor in the adrenal medulla.[24] They demonstrated that a given progenitor cell will differentiate into a neuron if exposed to neural growth factor and into an adrenomedullary endocrine cell if exposed to corticosteroids. Thus, the microenvironment appears to play a critical role in the final phenotypic expression of a specific progenitor cell. Definitive examination of Pearse's APUD theory may require an analogous experiment in which gut endocrine cell development is studied after progenitor cells of either ectodermal or endodermal origins are exposed to factors found within the gastrointestinal microenvironment.

MULTIPLE ENDOCRINE NEOPLASIA, TYPE I

Multiple endocrine neoplasias (MEN) are syndrome complexes associated with tumors or hyperplasia identified in two or more endocrine organs. These disorders are divided into three categories according to their patterns of organ involvement: type I (Wermer's syndrome), associated with lesions of the pancreas, parathyroid, pituitary, adrenal cortex, and thyroid; type II (Sipple's syndrome), associated with lesions of the adrenal medulla, parathyroid, and thyroid; and type III (multiple mucosal neuroma syndrome), associated with lesions of the adrenal medulla, thyroid, parathyroid, mucosal tissues, and bones (see pp. 491–494). As the subject of this chapter is secretory tumors of the pancreas, only type I (MEN I) is considered in detail here.

Despite numerous earlier reports of multiple endocrine tumors in patients,[25–27] it was not until 1954, when Wermer[28] first reported a family in which the father and four of his nine children were found to have tumors in two or more endocrine organs, that MEN I became recognized as a syndrome complex. As suggested in Wermer's initial report, subsequent studies have confirmed that MEN I is inherited as an autosomal dominant trait with a high degree of penetrance. Anderson[29] reported that 76 of 145 offspring over age 20 years of patients with MEN I also had evidence of the syndrome. The occasional patients with MEN I who do not have an affected parent despite thorough search for evidence of the disease are thought to have had new mutations. Although detailed epidemiologic information is unavailable, MEN I is estimated to occur at a rate of 0.02 to 0.2 per 1000 population.[30] It is rare in childhood and usually does not present after the age of 60 years. The penetrance of the gene is probably complete if the entire lifespans of the afflicted individuals are considered.[31]

The clinical features of MEN I are variable and depend on the endocrine organs involved (Table 100–1). In one of the largest series reported, Ballard and associates[32] found that 87 per cent of 85 patients with MEN I had involvement of the parathyroids, 81 per cent had disorders of the endocrine pancreas, and 65 per cent had lesions in the pituitary. Although only one third of the patients exhibited clinically evident involvement of these three organs simultaneously, autopsy studies[33] indicate a much higher frequency at time of death. A minority of patients also had evidence of disease in the adrenal cortex (38 per cent) and thyroid gland (19 per cent). Occasionally patients had carcinoid tumors (see pp. 1560–1570). Although multiple organs are diseased in MEN I, patients seldom present with clinical signs of more than one endocrinopathy. Furthermore, patients may have tumors that are "nonfunctioning," in that they do not secrete quantities of peptide sufficient to produce symptoms. In addition, overproduction and hypersecretion of some hormones, such as prolactin in men or in children of both sexes or pancreatic polypeptide (PP), may produce no symptoms or clinically recognizable signs of illness.

The clinical manifestations of parathyroid involvement in MEN I, including hypercalcemia, subperiosteal bone resorption, bone cysts, nephrolithiasis, and renal failure, are no different from those encountered in primary hyperparathyroidism of other causes, although patients with MEN I tend to be diagnosed at a somewhat younger age.[34] Roughly one in six patients with primary hyperparathyroidism is found to have MEN I.[35] Chief cell hyperplasia is the most common pathologic finding, although this diagnosis is difficult to differentiate from adenoma. Perhaps more characteristic is that multicentric lesions are found in MEN I in 50 per cent of patients,[29, 32] although solitary lesions are the rule in other causes of primary hyperparathy-

Table 100–1. CLINICAL FEATURES OF MEN I ACCORDING TO SITE OF LESION AND HORMONE SECRETED

Lesion	Hormones	Clinical Symptoms
Pituitary tumor or hyperplasia, or both	GH →	Acromegaly
	ACTH →	Cushing's disease
	Prolactin →	Asymptomatic Amenorrhea Galactorrhea
	Nonfunctioning →	Hypopituitarism Visual field defect Asymptomatic
Parathyroid tumor or hyperplasia, or both	PTH →	Hypercalcemia Urolithiasis Osteitis fibrosa cystica
Pancreatic endocrine tumor or hyperplasia, or both	Gastrin →	Zollinger-Ellison syndrome
	Insulin →	Hypoglycemia
	VIP →	WDHA syndrome
	Glucagon →	Diabetes mellitus Skin lesion
	Calcitonin →	Asymptomatic
	Pancreatic polypeptide →	Asymptomatic?

From Yamaguchi, K., Kameya, T., and Abe, K. Clin Endocrinol. Metab. 9:261, 1980. Used by permission.

GH, Growth hormone; ACTH, adrenocorticotropic hormone; PTH, parathyroid hormone; VIP, vasoactive intestinal peptide; WDHA, watery diarrhea–hypokalemia-achlorhydria syndrome.

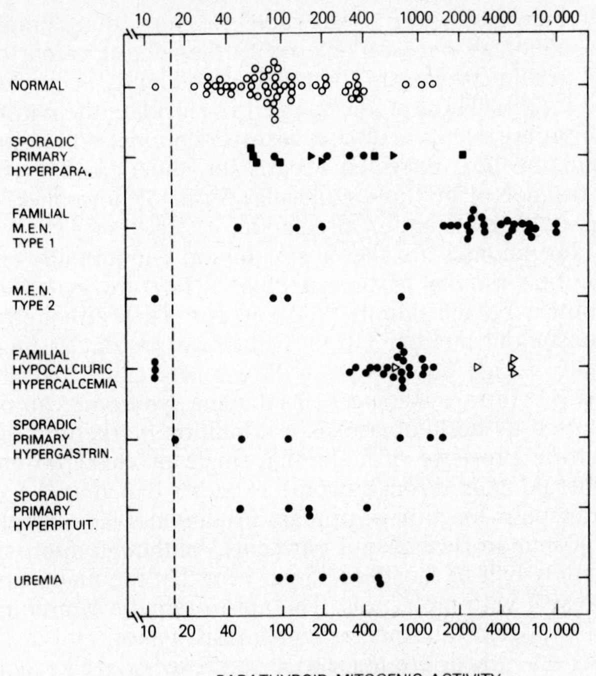

Figure 100–1. Effect of plasma on ^{3}H-thymidine incorporation by bovine parathyroid cells, according to diagnosis. The group with sporadic primary hyperparathyroidism is subdivided according to histologic diagnosis, as follows: parathyroid adenoma (●), parathyroid hyperplasia (■), and parathyroid cancer (▲). △ denotes five members of the same kindred with familial hypocalciuric hypercalcemia. Mean activity in the group with MEN type I was greater than that for ech other group ($P < 0.05$). The broken line indicates the lower limit of detectability. (From Brandi, M. L., Aurbach, G. D., Fitzpatrick, L. A., et al. Reprinted by permission of The New England Journal of Medicine *314*:1287, 1986.)

roidism.[36] Brandi and associates[37] have detected parathyroid mitogenic activity in plasma of patients with MEN I (Fig. 100–1); thus, the high frequency of parathyroid involvement may have a humoral basis. Such studies provide more general support for the role of a circulating oncogenic factor in the pathogenesis of multiple endocrine neoplasia.[38] It is important to remember that hypercalcemia without hyperparathyroidism may be encountered in MEN I in patients with gastrinoma[39] (see pp. 909–925) or watery diarrhea–hypokalemia-achlorhydria syndrome (WDHA, see p. 1890). As in sporadic hyperparathyroidism, the indications for parathyroidectomy in patients with MEN I include evidence of bone disease, urolithiasis, altered mental status, and a persistently elevated serum calcium level to values exceeding 11.5 mg/dl.[40] The surgical procedure of choice is subtotal parathyroidectomy, although some investigators have reported success with total parathyroidectomy following autotransplantation of resected parathyroid tissue into the forearm musculature.[41]

The most common pituitary lesion in MEN I is a "nonfunctioning" chromophobe adenoma,[32] which can present as blindness secondary to optic nerve compression or as hypopituitarism. Hyperprolactinemia has been reported in as many as 94 per cent of patients with pituitary tumors[42]; thus, serum prolactin may prove to be the most sensitive test for diagnosing pituitary involvement in MEN I. In children of both sexes and in men, prolactin-producing tumors would, of course, appear as "nonfunctioning" tumors. Growth hormone–secreting tumors may account for as many as 25 per cent of pituitary tumors in patients with MEN I, some of whom may manifest frank acromegaly.[32] Cushing's syndrome secondary to overproduction of adrenocorticotropin is much less common. Patients with growth hormone and adrenocorticotropin-secreting pituitary tumors should undergo a transsphenoidal hypophysectomy, followed by postoperative radiation therapy if complete tumor resection is not feasible. Some physicians treat their patients with prolactin-secreting microadenomas with transphenoidal hypophysectomy or bromocriptine therapy, but others advocate simple observation with no definitive treatment.[40]

The clinical features of pancreatic involvement in MEN I, discussed later in this chapter and on pages 909 to 925, result in the major morbidity and mortality associated with MEN I syndrome (Table 100–2). Roughly one fourth of all patients with gastrinoma[43] and 4 per cent of patients with insulinoma[44] have MEN I, which has also been reported in association with WDHA syndrome[45] and glucagonoma.[46] Elevated pancreatic polypeptide (PP)[47] and calcitonin levels[44] have also been observed in patients with MEN I. In contrast to isolated peptide-secreting tumors, pancreatic tumors associated with MEN I are nearly always multicentric.[32] Interestingly, the hormone composition of each of the pancreatic tumors in a single patient with MEN I may be quite different.[45, 48] In addition, any single tumor may have more than one secretory product. Generally, only one of the hormones is secreted predominantly into the plasma, and this hormone determines the clinical features.

Once a secretory endocrine tumor is diagnosed, patients should be evaluated carefully for the presence of other endocrinopathies. A thorough medical and family history should be obtained. Routine diagnostic studies should include skull and bone X-rays and evaluation of visual fields and of fasting blood glucose, serum calcium, and serum prolactin levels; evaluation for pancreatic secretory tumors should also be done as described later. The most important aspects of managing patients with MEN I are genetic counseling and

Table 100–2. CAUSES OF DEATH RELATED TO MEN I

Cause of Death	Patients
Ulcer complications (perforation, bleeding)	12
Following laparotomy for (sub) total gastrectomy or pancreatectomy, or both	7
Sequel of other operations	3
Metastatic tumors, cachexia	4
Hyperparathyroid crisis	4
Pituitary tumor	3
Infections	2
Hypoglycemic coma	1

Adapted from Eberle, F., and Grun, R. Ergbnisse der Inneren Medizin und Kinderheil Kunde *46*:75, 1981. Used by permission.

Table 100–3. PREVALENCE OF ABNORMAL LABORATORY TESTS IN KNOWN CARRIERS OF THE MEN I GENE

Test	Subjects Tested (n)	Abnormally High Result (%)
Calcium	18	50
Albumin-corrected calcium	18	95
Parathyroid hormone	17	65
Prolactin (females)	21	29
Prolactin (males)	14	7
Gastrin	34	38
Pancreatic polypeptide	34	12
Glucagon	34	18
Glicentin	34	15
Insulin	33	3
Motilin	16	16
Somatostatin	16	0
Growth hormone	34	3

From Marx, S. J., Vinik, A. I., Santen, R. J., et al. Medicine *65*:226, 1986. Used by permission.

careful screening of family members, all of whom should be followed regularly if they are not affected. The disease should become manifest by 20 years of age.[29] Marx and coworkers[49] performed extensive laboratory studies on a large kindred (221 members) of MEN I patients with the hope of identifying a potential genetic basis for the disorder. Among presumed carriers of the MEN I gene, the most frequently encountered abnormal serum values were albumin-adjusted calcium, parathyroid hormone, gastrin, and prolactin (in women) (Table 100–3). Primary hyperparathyroidism was the most common clinical expression of the MEN I gene, and penetrance for this trait increased from almost zero before the age of 15 years to nearly 100 per cent after 40 years.

Treatment of MEN I is complicated by the fact that the tumors are usually multicentric; thus, removal of all tumors from any single organ is difficult. However, dangerous clinical problems, such as progressive visual field defects from pituitary tumors or hypercalcemia from parathyroid lesions, should be treated by surgical resection if possible. Treatment of pancreatic tumors is described later in this chapter.

INSULINOMA

As noted at the beginning of this chapter, insulinoma was the first syndrome attributable to the hypersecretion of a substance produced by neoplastic cells. In 1927, Wilder and colleagues[2] reported a patient with severe hypoglycemia on whom Mayo operated and found a pancreatic islet cell tumor with liver metastasis. Whipple[50] in 1935 described the typical triad of symptoms associated with this syndrome: (1) symptoms of insulin shock with fasting, (2) fasting blood sugar of less than half normal, and (3) relief of symptoms with infusion of glucose. The use of radioimmunoassay techniques developed by Yalow and Berson[3] for measurement of insulin provided confirmation of hyperinsulinemia in patients with the syndrome. In 1967, Steiner and Oyer[51] were able to show that human insulinomas were capable of synthesizing a precursor of insulin (proinsulin) that was subsequently converted to insulin. These studies helped to elucidate the nature of prohormones and their post-translational processing and, further, provided a basis for understanding the existence of multiple molecular forms of hormones in tissue extracts and in circulation.

Insulinomas are the most common symptomatic endocrine tumors of the pancreas. They are generally solitary benign tumors (70 to 80 per cent), although a substantial number (10 per cent) can present as multiple benign adenomas or diffuse islet cell hyperplasia.[52–55] In rare instances, insulinoma syndrome can be caused by nesidioblastosis, a condition marked by the diffuse presence of additional single or clustered endocrine cells throughout the exocrine pancreas.[56] Extrahepatic location of primary insulinomas is relatively uncommon (less than 1 per cent),[57] although approximately half of the 10 to 15 per cent that are malignant present with metastasis. The most dramatic symptoms of hypoglycemia such as diaphoresis, pallor, and tachycardia, which are associated with excessive catecholamine release, frequently are *not* observed in patients with insulinoma because their blood glucose levels decrease gradually with prolonged fasting. Instead, their symptoms are often subtle and hidden by the tendency of the patients to compensate for their hypoglycemia by overeating. Neuropsychiatric manifestations of hypoglycemia ranging from mild personality changes to confusion, seizures, and coma may lead to difficulty in the diagnosis of insulinoma. Minor symptoms, such as hunger, fatigue, nausea and vomiting, lightheadedness, paresthesias, peripheral neuropathy,[58] and blurred vision, may be the only ones encountered. The worst symptoms are more likely to be observed in the morning after an overnight fast.

Diminished plasma glucose concentrations, defined as less than 55 mg/dl in men and less than 35 mg/dl in women,[59] are encountered in 80 per cent of patients with insulinoma after 24 hours of fasting and in more than 95 per cent after a 48-hour fast followed by exercise.[60] The diagnostic accuracy of fasting hypoglycemia is improved if plasma insulin values obtained concomitantly are inappropriately elevated above 15 mU/L.[61] Patients with the disorder generally have ratios of plasma insulin (in mU/L) to serum glucose (in mg/dl) that are greater than 0.4.[62]

The development of radioimmunoassays for proinsulin and C-peptide, the short peptide that is cleaved during the conversion of proinsulin to insulin, has greatly facilitated the diagnosis of insulinomas. A plasma proinsulin value of greater than 40 fmol/ml was considered to be virtually diagnostic of insulinoma in the past; however, more recent studies indicate that 10 to 25 per cent of patients with this disorder have normal proinsulin levels,[63] and, on the other hand, there may be overlap with the high levels found in obese patients without insulinomas.[64] An important and distinctive feature of the elevated proinsulin levels in insulinoma patients is that it cannot be suppressed by infusion of exogenous insulin.[64] The mechanism for the autonomous high proinsulin secretion is unknown, but Creutzfeldt and associates[65] have proposed that decreased peptide storage capacity is a characteristic defect in insulinoma cells. This hypothesis is supported by observations that insulinoma cells do not stain as well as normal beta cells by immunochemistry.[66] Indeed, the regularity of immunostaining may divide insulinomas into two classes: those with clearly stainable granulated cells that have modest proinsulin levels and serum insulin elevations that can be suppressed with somatostatin and diazoxide, and those with poor immunostaining that have very high proinsulin levels and insulin secretion that cannot be suppressed.[66] Measurement of serum C-peptide concentrations is useful in diagnosing insulinoma in patients who do not manifest fasting hypoglycemia. Artificial lowering of blood glucose level by injection of commercial pork insulin in these patients will fail to suppress endogenous insulin release. However, since pork insulin cross reacts with human insulin in radioimmunoassay, measurements of endogenous insulin release cannot be made easily. Measurement of C-peptide, which is produced in equimolar concentrations with insulin during cleavage of proinsulin, will provide a more accurate gauge of B cell function.[67] Alternatively, fish insulin, which is biologically active but which does not cross react with human insulin, has been infused to suppress endogenous insulin.[68] A serum endogenous insulin value of greater than 4 mU/L or a C-peptide concentration of greater than 60 pg/ml in the presence of insulin-induced hypoglycemia supports the diagnosis of insulinoma. In the past, other agents such as tolbutamide[69] or glucagon[70] were used to provoke tumor insulin release, but they were only moderately successful, and tests using these agents have become obsolete. More recently, promising results have been obtained using the euglycemic hyperinsulinemia clamp technique in diagnosing endogenous hyperinsulinism without exposing patients to the risk of hypoglycemia.[64, 71–73]

Most clinical disorders that can mimic the syndrome of insulinoma, such as liver disease, adrenal insufficiency, nonpancreatic tumors, hypopituitarism, and alcoholic hypoglycemia, are easily differentiated from insulinoma because they are not associated with inappropriate hyperinsulinism. Elevation of proinsulin or C-peptide concentrations will help to distinguish insulinoma patients from those taking insulin surreptitiously. The most difficult diagnostic challenge is to identify patients who are abusing oral sulfonylureas. In these patients, the drugs themselves must be identified in the plasma[74] for the diagnosis to be certain.

Diagnosis and Treatment

Because surgical resection is the treatment of choice in insulinoma, and because the vast majority of tumors are solitary benign lesions, accurate diagnosis is crucial. Numerous tests and procedures have been advocated as aids in location of the tumors. Noninvasive techniques, such as computed tomography and ultrasonography, would be preferred, but, unfortunately, most insulinomas are less than 1 cm in diameter and thus are difficult to detect by these techniques.[75] Other diagnostic methods, such as nuclear magnetic resonance, intra-arterial dynamic computed tomography[76] and intraoperative ultrasonography,[77, 78] have been applied, but further experience is necessary to establish their sensitivity and specificity. Arteriography has been useful in identifying some insulinomas,[79] but the procedure has been associated with a high frequency of false positive and false negative results.[80] Fortunately, more than 90 per cent of insulinomas can be palpated by the surgeon at laparotomy; thus, most other localization procedures may be superfluous.[80] However, there is no substitute for knowing the precise location of a tumor at the time of surgery. One test that has proved to be useful in this regard is selective portal and splenic vein catheterization for mapping the sources of elevated insulin levels in plasma.[81, 82] Although reported success rates in tumor localization have varied, perhaps reflecting differences in technical experience, selective angiography is clearly indicated in patients undergoing reoperation after their tumors were found not to be palpable on initial exploration.

A generalized approach to treating patients with a confirmed diagnosis of insulinoma is provided in Figure 100–2. Patients should be given a trial of therapy with diazoxide, a drug known to inhibit insulin release, in doses of 100 to 600 mg/day.[83] If symptoms can be controlled satisfactorily, the patient may undergo laparotomy without further testing, as the likelihood of identifying and excising a resectable lesion is high. If no lesion can be identified, the patient can be managed safely with diazoxide until a second operation is undertaken after samples of portal vein blood, obtained selectively by a transhepatic approach, demonstrate an elevated insulin value that corresponds to a segment of the pancreas. If the patient's symptoms of hypoglycemia cannot be managed with diazoxide, a great effort should be made to ensure that the first operation is definitive by measuring insulin levels in selective portal vein samples to locate the tumor before laparotomy. If no tumor can be identified by laparotomy, a blind distal pancreatectomy should be attempted. Serum glucose levels should be monitored during this operation as the pancreas is resected in segments, starting with the tail, to minimize the loss of pancreatic tissue.[84]

Numerous therapeutic options can be considered in managing patients with unresectable lesions. Diazoxide, a nondiuretic benzothiadiazine that inhibits the release of secretory granules from normal B cells and insulinoma tissues, can control insulin secretion in some patients.[85] Other treatment methods, such as phenytoin,[86] diltiazam,[86] verapamil,[87] and mithramycin,[88] have been reported to be effective. Propranolol has been used to treat some patients with insulinoma;[89] however, the risks of masking the symptoms of hypoglycemia in these patients must be considered. The

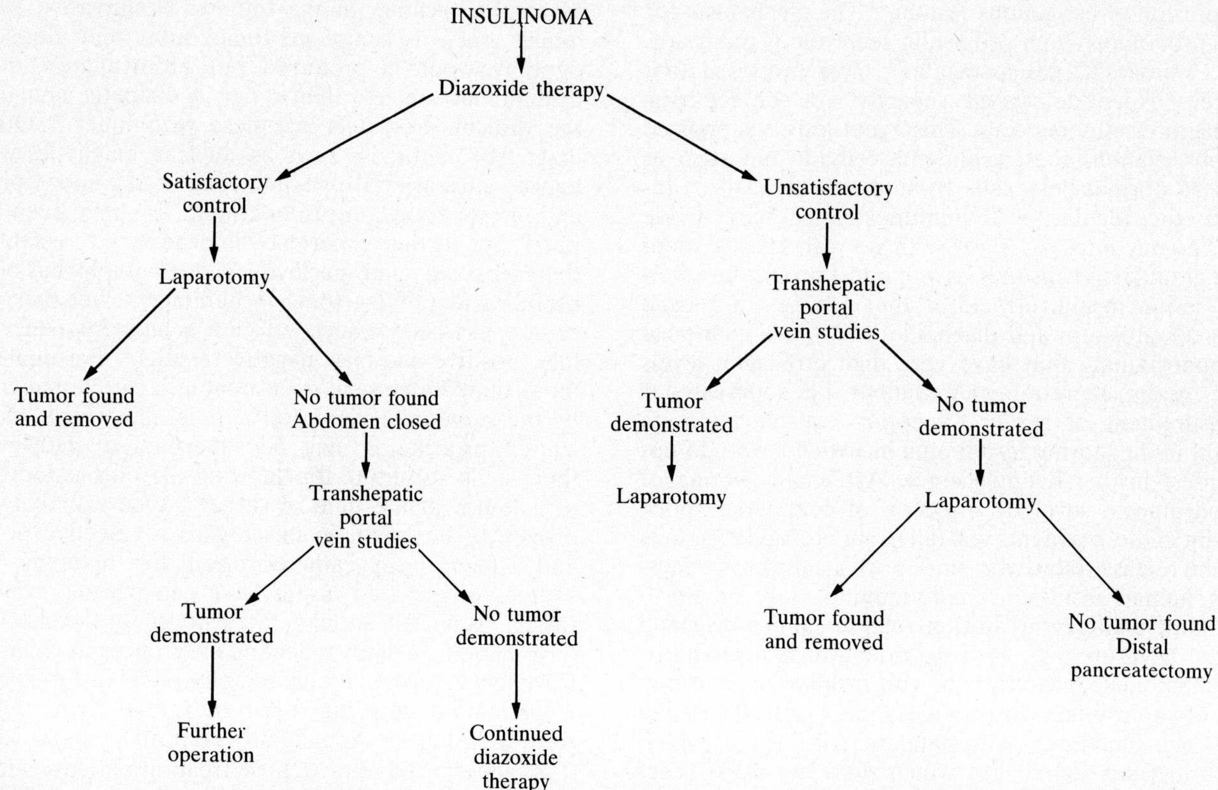

Figure 100–2. Scheme for management of patients with insulinoma. (From Le Quesne, L. P., Nabarro, J. D. N., Kurtz, A., and Zweig, S. Br. J. Surg. *66*:373, 1979. Used by permission.)

usefulness of somatostatin and its long-acting analogues in the treatment of symptomatic pancreatic endocrine neoplasms is discussed on page 1892. Streptozotocin has produced short-lived remissions in about one half of patients with malignant insulinomas. Improved response rates (63 per cent complete or partial remission) were obtained with the combination of streptozotocin and 5-fluorouracil.[90] Successful therapy of refractory metastatic endocrine neoplasms with human leukocyte interferon[91] has been reported, but further studies will be required to assess the potential benefit of this treatment regimen.

WATERY DIARRHEA–HYPOKALEMIA-ACHLORHYDRIA (WDHA) SYNDROME

In 1958, Verner and Morrison[92] described two patients with a syndrome of profuse watery diarrhea, severe hypokalemia, dehydration, and shock in whom non-B cell pancreatic islet adenomas were found at autopsy. Subsequently, achlorhydria was associated with this syndrome by Murray and coworkers,[93] hence the derivation of the name WDHA syndrome. The disease has been termed pancreatic cholera by Mellinkoff in recognition of the pancreatic origin of the tumor and the major clinical features of this disease.[94] This term was later deemed inappropriate when patients were identified in whom the syndrome resulted from neural crest tumors arising outside the pancreas. The association of vasoactive intestinal peptide (VIP)[95] with WDHA suggested the term "VIPoma;" however, some controversy has arisen regarding the pathogenetic role of VIP in WDHA syndrome.

Clinically, the hallmark of the disease is profuse watery diarrhea in association with symptoms of hypokalemia and dehydration.[96] The diarrhea may be constant or intermittent but generally worsens with time. The stool has the appearance of weak tea, and the volume ranges from 1 to more than 6 L/day. The diarrhea is secretory (see pp. 290–316) and thus persists despite cessation of oral intake of all liquids or solids. Twice the sum of the stool K^+ plus Na^+ concentrations should account for nearly all the osmolarity of the stool water. Net secretion of water, Na^+, and Cl^- from the intestine has been documented in these patients.[97] Generally, patients have been said not to manifest abdominal cramping or steatorrhea, although a series reported by Bloom and colleagues[98, 99] indicates that both problems are more frequent than had previously been reported. As many as 20 per cent of patients exhibit flushing in association with their diarrhea. Severe hypovolemia and electrolyte depletion from diarrhea can produce lethargy, muscle weakness, cramping, nausea, and vomiting. Transient renal tubular dysfunction, manifested by a defect in concentrating ability, may result from hypovolemia, but prolonged hypercalcemia may lead to progressive renal failure.

Hypercalcemia has been observed in as many as 76 per cent of patients with WDHA syndrome.[95] In a few patients this finding may be explained by primary hyperparathyroidism in association with MEN I, but the cause in most patients is undetermined. It is possible that a secretory product of the tumor may produce hypercalcemia directly. VIP[100] and prostaglandin E_2,[101] both implicated in the pathophysiology of WDHA syndrome, have been shown to increase serum calcium levels when infused into animals. In addition, calcitonin has been shown to be released from the pancreas of two patients with WDHA syndrome with metastatic VIPoma.[102] Hyperglycemia and impaired glucose tolerance are observed in nearly one half of the patients with WDHA syndrome,[95] and this has been attributed either to the inhibitory effect of prolonged hypokalemia on islet B cells or to a direct hyperglycemic effect of a tumor product, such as VIP. Basal achlorhydria is observed in two thirds of patients with WDHA syndrome, but the rest have low or normal acid secretion. Most patients with basal achlorhydria will exhibit a small secretory response to pentagastrin or histamine.

The observation that excision of the pancreatic tumor (if possible) results in disappearance of symptoms suggested that a diarrheogenic secretion of the tumor is the cause of WDHA syndrome. Among the other substances that have been implicated in patients with the syndrome are secretin,[103] gastrin inhibitory polypeptide (GIP),[104] PP,[105] and prostaglandins.[106] However, only VIP levels have been found to be elevated in virtually all patients with WDHA syndrome associated with neoplasm of the pancreatic islets or other tissues of presumed neural crest origin (Fig. 100–3).[107, 108] In addition, VIP is capable of producing most of the symptoms associated with WDHA syndrome, including the characteristic secretory diarrhea.[109] Nevertheless, the etiologic role of VIP has been questioned because elevated plasma VIP levels have been reported in some patients without watery diarrhea.[110] Furthermore, there appears to be a subpopulation of patients with all the clinical manifestations of WDHA syndrome but without any evidence of tumor. These patients have sometimes been referred to as having "pseudo–Verner-Morrison" or "pseudo-WDHA" syndrome. In the experience of one group, plasma VIP of greater than 60 pmol/L is absolutely diagnostic of VIP-producing tumor as the cause of symptoms in a patient with WDHA syndrome.[98] At present, plasma VIP assay is the only diagnostic test that is highly specific for the disease. A high plasma VIP level should rule out most other causes of secretory diarrhea. Bloom and coworkers[111] have found that diarrhea in a VIPoma patient was associated with co-secretion of a second active peptide, peptide histidine isoleucine (PHI). PHI was first isolated from pig intestine[112] and was found to have tissue distribution similar to that of VIP. Studies indicating that peptide histidine methionine (PHM), the human form of PHI (see pp. 78–107), is co-localized and co-secreted with VIP and, in fact, is a product of the same RNA transcript, suggest its potential usefulness as a marker for VIPomas.[113] Because PHM has a longer plasma half-life than VIP, its circulating concentrations are higher than those of VIP given the same rate of secretion. In a review of 42 patients with VIPoma, Bloom and coworkers[111] found that all had elevated PHI concentrations.

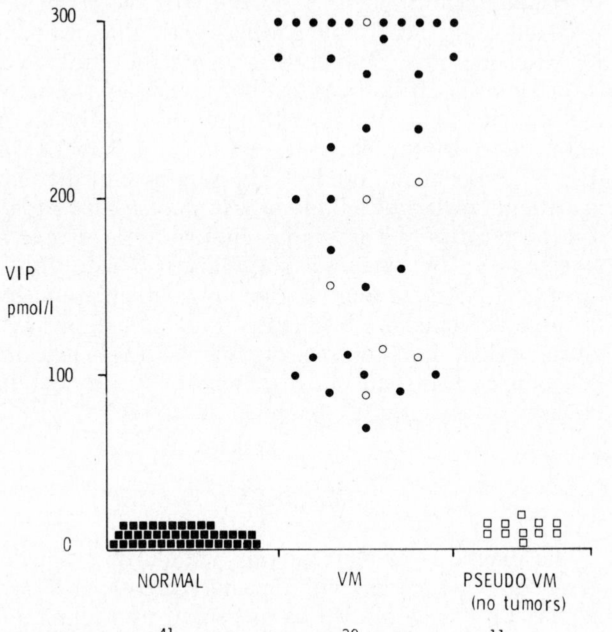

Figure 100–3. Plasma VIP concentrations in normal subjects, patients with WDHA syndrome (VM) with pancreatic tumors (●) and ganglioneuroblastomas (○), and patients with watery diarrhea syndrome in whom no evidence of tumor was discovered. (From Bloom, S. R. Am. J. Dig. Dis. *23*:373, 1978. Used by permission.)

In Verner and Morrison's[114] review of 55 cases of WDHA syndrome, 37 per cent of patients were found to have malignant lesions, 43 per cent had benign lesions that were potentially resectable, and 20 per cent had diffuse hyperplasia of the pancreatic islets. More recent reports,[115] however, suggest a higher rate of malignancy (50 to 60 per cent) in WDHA syndrome. In Long and colleagues' series[98] of 60 patients, 17 per cent had ganglioneuromas and the rest had pancreatic lesions. All children under ten years of age with WDHA syndrome had ganglioneuromas, and they constituted 70 per cent of all patients with ganglioneuromas.

Treatment

Once the diagnosis of tumor-associated WDHA syndrome is made and the patient's dehydration and electrolyte abnormalities are corrected, some effort at definitive therapy must be attempted. Because steroids have been shown to diminish diarrhea markedly in some patients, a trial of therapy with prednisone at a dose of 40 mg/day is indicated. Patients who fail to respond should undergo immediate surgery, and if a tumor is found, it should be resected. Patients who respond to steroid therapy may be managed conservatively until they have improved clinically and diagnostic studies are unable to rule out a surgically resectable secretory tumor. An operation should then be performed to make the diagnosis. If no discrete pancreatic tumor is observed at surgery, a thorough abdominal exploration should be performed. In the event that no lesions, benign or malignant, are found, a 75 per cent pancreatectomy has been advocated,[110] as some patients with diffuse islet cell hyperplasia have been shown to respond to this resection. For inoperable malignant lesions, the combination of streptozotocin and 5-fluorouracil has proved to be effective with response rates in the range of 66 per cent.[90] Dimethyltriazeno-imidazole-carboxamide (DTIC)[116] and human leukocyte interferon[91, 117] show promise in therapy of metastatic disease. In some patients for whom no definitive therapy is possible, symptomatic relief has been reported with a variety of agents, including corticosteroids, indomethacin,[118] and trifluoperazine.[119] Long-acting somatostatin analogues have been effective in controlling diarrhea in some patients with WDHA syndrome,[120, 121] and even in shrinking of a metastatic tumor in the liver.[122] Symptoms of WDHA eventually recur despite continued treatment with somatostatin analogue,[123] perhaps reflecting further growth of the tumor. One interesting complication of successful therapy in patients with WDHA is the occurrence of gastric acid hypersecretion, lending support to the theory that the agent responsible for the syndrome is a potent inhibitor of acid secretion. Thus, a prophylactic regimen of antisecretory therapy may be indicated in the postoperative management of these patients.[62]

GLUCAGONOMA

The first report of a patient with skin rash, diabetes mellitus, and anemia in association with a tumor arising from glucagon-producing cells of the pancreatic islets (a glucagonoma) was presented by Becker and coworkers as early as 1942.[124] Subsequently, in 1963 Unger and coworkers[125] described four patients with high concentrations of immunoreactive glucagon in their pancreatic tumors. McGavran and Unger[126] reported a patient with diabetes, skin rash, anemia, elevated serum glucagon level, and an alpha cell tumor of the pancreas in 1966. However, it was not until 1974 that Mallinson and coworkers[127] described the glucagonoma syndrome in a series of nine patients with elevated plasma glucagon levels and glucagon-producing tumors of the pancreas. Since then, the diagnosis of glucagonoma has been made with increasing frequency. It occurs in adult patients of all age groups, ranging from 20 to 73 years.[128] Although initially it was thought to occur more frequently among women, the disease appears to be just as common in men.

The most characteristic clinical finding in glucagonoma is a form of eczematous dermatitis referred to as migratory necrolytic erythema (Fig. 100–4).[129] The skin lesion has a characteristic evolution, progressing over 7 to 14 days from erythematous macules to larger fluid-filled bullae, followed by central necrosis, by scaly eczematoid lesions with erythematous margins, and finally by central clearing and scaling. A bronze discoloration may persist after clearing. Not uncommonly, the lesions may become superinfected with bacteria or fungi. The lesions occur most prominently in areas associated with friction, such as the groin, perineum, breasts, and buttocks, as well as on the face and distal extremities. On biopsy,[130] the appearance of the lesions can vary from superficial epidermal necrosis to suppurative folliculitis. The patients also present with atrophic glossitis and stomatitis. The mechanism by which these cutaneous manifestations develop is unclear, but it does not appear to be related to the levels of plasma glucagon. The resemblance of the lesions to those seen with zinc deficiency has prompted trials of therapy with zinc, with some remarkable responses.[131] Deficiencies of amino acids and essential fatty acids observed in patients with glucagonoma, presumably resulting from the metabolic actions of the hormone, have been implicated in the pathogenesis of the skin rash.[129] Norton and associates[132] have reported that parenteral administration of amino acids without added zinc or fatty acids results in a rapid clearance of the skin lesions. However, resolution of skin rash has been reported to occur after simple hydration with glucose, saline,[133] and somatostatin[134]; thus, further investigation is required to confirm the cause of migratory necrolytic erythema.

In addition to the skin lesions, glucagonoma is associated with a number of other characteristic clinical features. The patients all tend to exhibit substantial weight loss, even when the tumor is small and nonmalignant, because of the general catabolic activity of glucagon. The same mechanism is thought to be responsible for normocytic normochromic anemia, which is observed in nearly all patients with glucagonoma. Diabetes mellitus or demonstrable glucose intolerance is observed in virtually all patients as well. In general, the diabetes is mild and easily controlled with diet or small doses of insulin, but occasionally diabetic ketoacidosis is encountered.[133] The presence of diabetes in patients with glucagonoma has interested investigators because of the potential etiologic role of excess glucagon in the glucose intolerance of adult-onset diabetics. As mentioned earlier, hypolipemia and hypoaminoacidemia are frequently noted in patients with glucagonoma. In a minority of patients, psychiatric and neurologic disturbances, diarrhea, and thromboembolic phenomena have also been observed.[127, 131, 135]

Diagnosis

The diagnosis of glucagonoma should be suspected in any diabetic patient with the characteristic skin rash. A plasma glucagon level as measured by radioimmunoassay should exceed 500 pg/ml.[136] Although normal plasma glucagon level should be less than 150 pg/ml, occasional patients with diabetes mellitus, renal failure, cirrhosis, acute injury, bacteremia, or Cushing's syndrome will have levels between 150 and 500 pg/ml. Intravenous glucose administration decreases plasma

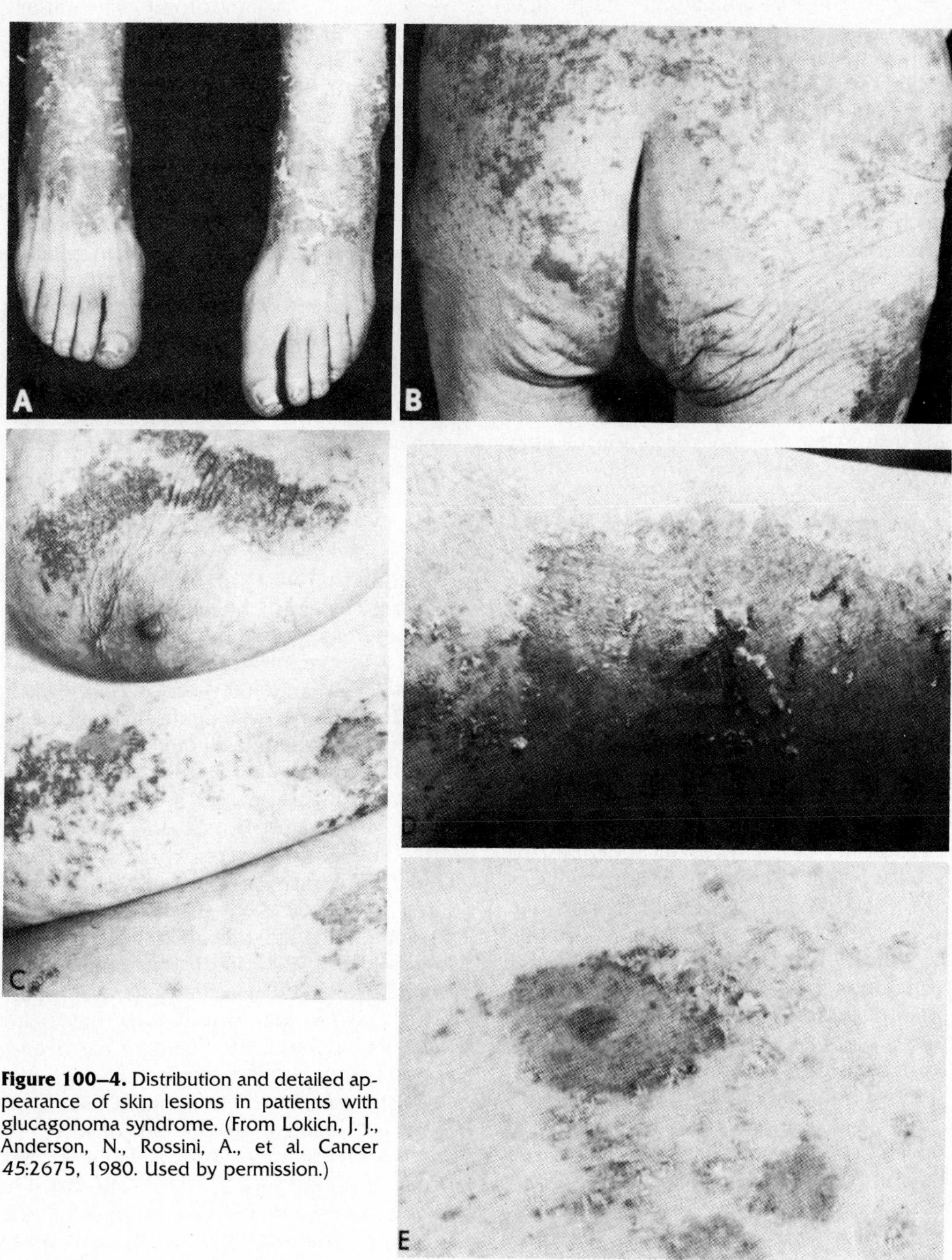

Figure 100–4. Distribution and detailed appearance of skin lesions in patients with glucagonoma syndrome. (From Lokich, J. J., Anderson, N., Rossini, A., et al. Cancer *45*:2675, 1980. Used by permission.)

glucagon concentration in patients with glucagonoma but, paradoxically, oral carbohydrates cause an increase.[136] This may result from a massive release of enteroglucagon, which may cross react somewhat with the antibody used in the glucagon radioimmunoassay. Alternatively, it may simply be a manifestation of the abnormal regulation of the neoplastic cells. The molecular forms of glucagon that circulate in the plasma of patients with glucagonoma are somewhat different from those in normal subjects. Four molecular forms with glucagon-like immunoreactivity have been detected by gel filtration of normal plasma: big glucagon (MW 30,000), proglucagon (MW 9,000), glucagon (MW 35,000), and a 2,000-MW form termed glucagon-like immunoreactivity.[136, 137] In patients with glucagonoma, elevations are mostly found in the proglucagon and glucagon fractions.[137–139] The release of both glucagon and proglucagon from glucagonomas[140] appears to be stimulated by arginine, tolbutamide, calcium, and calcitonin; these forms were suppressed by somatostatin. Despite the relative abundance of the large molecular forms of glucagon in the circulation, chromatographic profiles of plasma glucagon-like immunoreactivity are insufficient for differentiation of normal subjects from patients with glucagonoma.[141] Bordi and coworkers[142] have described glicentin-like immunoreactivity by histochemistry in a glucagonoma. Glicentin is the 69–amino acid peptide from gut tissues that contains glucagon sandwiched between carboxyl- and amino-terminal extensions. Elevations in glicentin would not be detected in plasma unless specifically sought for, as the peptide does not cross react with most antibodies used for assay of pancreatic glucagon.

Course and Treatment

As with other pancreatic islet cell tumor syndromes, glucagonomas are slowly progressive, but the majority of patients have malignant lesions with metastasis. Higgins and coworkers[128] reported in their review that only 20 of 47 patients had tumors confined to the pancreas at the time of diagnosis, and three of those patients subsequently manifested hepatic metastasis. Most of the primary tumors (30 of 47) were found in the body and tail of the pancreas, a few (4 of 47) were found in the head, and the rest were too extensive to discern their site of origin. In contrast to insulinomas, the vast majority of glucagonomas are greater than 3 cm in size at the time of diagnosis and therefore can be localized by noninvasive means, such as ultrasonography or computed tomography. The diagnosis of glucagonoma at an earlier stage in its development may be difficult because the associated symptoms are somewhat more insidious than those of insulinoma.

Bordi and coworkers[142] have described a group of patients without the glucagonoma syndrome but with benign alpha cell tumors of the pancreas. The tumors in these patients were usually multiple and small, ranging from 0.5 mm to 1 cm in size. As might be expected, the ultrastructure of the cells contained within these tumors resembled normal human alpha cells more closely than they did the usual glucagonoma cells. Boden and Owen[143] reported a patient with glucagonoma in whom hyperglucagonemia occurred in family members in an autosomal dominant pattern. No obvious tumor could be detected in the hyperglucagonemic family members, although none of them underwent exploratory laparotomy. The patients reported in these two studies may represent variants of the initial stage of the glucagonoma syndrome.

Resection of a glucagonoma localized to the pancreas can be curative; thus, surgery is the treatment of choice. Unfortunately, some of these patients manifest evidence of metastasis at a later date. Kaplan and Michelassi[62] and Montenegro and colleagues[144] have reported that even in the face of metastatic glucagonoma, surgical debulking by distal pancreatectomy can result in substantial clinical improvement. Chemotherapy with streptozotocin or streptozotocin plus 5-fluorouracil results in objective regression of tumor and symptomatic improvement in most patients with glucagonoma,[136, 145] although the long-term outlook is unclear. Another drug that has been useful in treating some patients is DTIC.[133, 146, 147]

SOMATOSTATINOMA

Within four years after the discovery of somatostatin by Brazeau and colleagues,[148] patients with tumors of the pancreas containing somatostatin-like immunoreactivity were reported in Europe[149] and in the United States.[150] In both of these patients, the diagnosis of somatostatinoma was made incidentally at the time of surgery for gallstones. The similarity between the immunoreactive somatostatin found in the blood and tumor tissue extracts of these patients and the peptide originally isolated from ovine hypothalamus was confirmed by Larsson and coworkers[149] in chromatographic studies indicating the co-elution of the two on gel filtration. Bioassay of the tumor extract revealed that it contained a substance that, like somatostatin, could inhibit the release of insulin and glucagon from the isolated perfused porcine pancreas. Since these initial case reports, somatostatinoma has been recognized more widely, and the diagnosis has been made preoperatively in a number of patients. As with all the other secretory tumors of the pancreas, some of the patients have had excess production of other hormones in addition to somatostatin, specifically adrenocorticotropic hormone (ACTH)[151, 152] and calcitonin.[153, 154]

The highly variable clinical presentation of patients with these tumors has led to some controversy over the existence of a distinct "somatostatinoma syndrome."[155] However, the triad of symptoms most frequently encountered in somatostatinoma are gallstones, diabetes, and diarrhea with steatorrhea.[154] The manifestations of the disease are a reflection of the pharmacologic actions of somatostatin and provide important insight into the physiologic actions of the peptide (Table 100–4). Because somatostatin inhibits

Table 100–4. PREDICTED AND OBSERVED EFFECTS OF SOMATOSTATIN EXCESS ON DIGESTIVE ORGANS

Target Organ	Pharmacologic Action	Predicted Findings *Laboratory*	Predicted Findings *Clinical*	Observed Findings *Laboratory*	Observed Findings *Clinical*
Stomach	↓ Hydrochloride response to pentagastrin, histamine, and meal		"Dyspepsia," postprandial fullness	Basal acid output 0.04 mEq/hr Peak acid output 2.84 mEq/hr (after pentagastrin)	"Dyspepsia," postprandial fullness
	↓ Pepsin response to meal	Same*		Not tested	
				100% of ^{99m}Tc-labeled meal remaining in stomach at 60 min (normal: 50%)	
Intestine	↓ Gastric emptying ↓ Absorption of sugars, amino acids, and fat	Same*	"Indigestion"	Delayed postprandial rise in plasma nutrients; low sugar and amino acid absorption on intestinal perfusion studies	"Indigestion"
	Motility changes	Increased frequency of interdigestive migrating complexes		Interdigestive migrating complexes at mean interval of 38 min (normal: 120 min)	
Gallbladder	↓ Contractility	Same*	Gallstones	X-ray evidence of gallstones	Gallstones (cholecystectomy in 1974)
Exocrine pancreas	↓ Volume, bicarbonate, and enzyme response to stimuli	Same*	Maldigestion, steatorrhea	↓ Volume, bicarbonate, and enzyme response (secretin test and Lundh meal)	Maldigestion, steatorrhea responsive to replacement therapy
Salivary glands	Not tested	Somatostatin effect has not been studied	Dry mouth	Not studied	Dry mouth
Splanchnic blood flow	Reduced	Same*	?	Not tested	?

*Same as pharmacologic action.
From Krejs, G. J., Orci, L., Conlon, J. M., et al. Reprinted by permission of the New England Journal of Medicine. *301*:285, 1979.

both insulin and glucagon, only a mild diabetic syndrome is encountered in most patients with somatostatinoma. Severe hypoglycemia or ketosis is unusual, although both complications have been reported.[156, 157] Inhibition of cholecystokinin-induced gallbladder contraction may result in bile stasis with subsequent stone formation. The combination of impaired gallbladder contraction, delayed intestinal absorption of nutrients, and diminished pancreatic enzyme secretion results in diarrhea with steatorrhea. Delayed gastric emptying may produce dyspepsia and abdominal fullness. Inhibition of acid secretion results in basal achlorhydria, although no inhibition of basal gastrin is observed. This suggests that the gastric parietal cell is more sensitive to the inhibitory actions of somatostatin than is the G cell. Plasma growth hormone level is diminished, and insulin requirements are low even in the presence of overt diabetes.

Diagnosis

In the past, diagnosis of somatostatinoma has been made most frequently at surgery for another problem, such as cholecystitis. Early diagnosis required a high index of suspicion on the part of the examining physician and a knowledge of the classic triad of symptoms. Plasma immunoreactive somatostatin levels have been difficult to obtain in the past, but, when measured, they are usually elevated to more than ten times normal. In some instances, tumor release of somatostatin must be enhanced with tolbutamide to elicit elevations in plasma concentrations.[158] Gel filtration of plasma from patients with somatostatinoma has revealed at least one, and as many as three, larger molecular forms of somatostatin-like immunoreactivity, in addition to the one that corresponds to somatostatin tetradecapeptide.[149, 152–154, 157, 159] The presence of the larger molecular forms is not diagnostic, however, as these forms may also be present in the plasma of normal subjects. Patel and coworkers[160] found concentrations of the amino-terminal dodecapeptide of somatostatin-28 to be greater than those of somatostatin-14 both in the plasma and in the tumor extracts of patients with somatostatinoma. A few tests of endocrine function may support the diagnosis of somatostatinoma. Diminished plasma growth hormone and glucagon levels have been reported. Suppressed insulin response to glucose may also be observed.

Treatment

The relatively mild and nonspecific clinical symptoms associated with somatostatinoma may lead to delays in diagnosis and, therefore, of treatment. Indeed, Bloom and Polak[99] reported a patient who had evidence of a somatostatinoma for as long as 15 years before he died and postmortem examination revealed the diagnosis. Perhaps for this reason, most of the patients are diagnosed with late-stage malignant lesions. The primary tumors are distributed in both the head and the tail of the pancreas, with metastatic lesions occurring in the liver. Primary tumors in the duodenum[161, 162] and metastatic lesions in the bone, skin,[157] and cystic duct[163] have also been reported. In one patient with a benign lesion, surgical resection with a Whipple's procedure resulted in a long-term cure.[150] However, Whipple's procedure in patients with malignant somatostatinoma has proved to be fatal in two of the three reported cases in which it has been attempted.[154] Treatment with streptozotocin or 5-fluorouracil, or both, has been reported to be successful in a number of patients, although no controlled studies have been undertaken.

MISCELLANEOUS HORMONES

In addition to the neoplastic syndromes associated with the hormones described, tumors of the pancreas have been associated with a number of other hormones, including ACTH, calcitonin, PP, alpha-endorphin, beta-melanocyte stimulating hormone, motilin, secretin, growth hormone releasing factor (GRF), neurotensin, and growth hormone. It is common to find more than one type of hormone associated with endocrine tumors of the pancreas. Although symptoms generally are associated with overproduction of only one of the hormones, a series of patients with combined syndromes has recently been described. Asa and coworkers[164] described a patient who initially presented with Zollinger-Ellison syndrome and metastatic pancreatic islet cell tumor, then subsequently developed signs and symptoms of Cushing's syndrome. Immunoreactive gastrin, ACTH, beta-endorphin, somatostatin, and calcitonin were all found in the tumor tissue. Other reported multihormonal clinical presentations of pancreatic endocrine neoplasms include VIP and insulin,[165] VIP and gastrin,[166] glucagon and gastrin,[167] and GRF and gastrin.[168] One patient presented with a tumor producing both somatostatin and GRF, two hormones with opposing effects on growth hormone release.[169] The patient manifested diabetes, steatorrhea, hypochlorydria, anemia, and cholelithiasis, all consistent with a somatostatinoma picture, but, in addition, there was evidence of acromegaly. Although, as in this case, GRF in pancreatic endocrine neoplasms can be biologically active, some patients with GRF in their tumors show no evidence of acromegaly.[170] Absence of a growth hormone response to exogenously administered GRF points to the ectopic production of GRF in these patients.[171]

Of the many gut peptides, PP deserves special mention. After Floyd and coworkers'[47] initial report that patients with insulinomas had elevated PP levels, Polak and colleagues[172] suggested that PP could serve as a general marker for hormone-secreting tumors of the pancreas. However, subsequent studies have indicated that PP elevations are not particularly useful tools for this purpose.[173] PP may be present in pancreatic tumors as one of many hormones, or as a single hormone, that is overproduced.[174] Until recently, no specific symptoms have been associated with elevated serum PP levels. However, Strodel and coworkers[175] have found that of eight patients with tumors that appeared to secrete only PP, all had a variety of symptoms, including upper abdominal pain, gastrointestinal hemorrhage, weight loss, jaundice, and diarrhea. The possibility that these symptoms result from the effects of an unmeasured hormone cannot be excluded.

Another potentially useful marker for hormone-secreting tumors is chromogranin A, a substance found in secretory granules of most neuroendocrine cells.[176, 177] O'Connor and Duftos[178] reported that chromogranin A levels were significantly elevated in plasma of patients with endocrine tumors with a sensitivity of 81 per cent and a specificity of 100 per cent. The observation that the recently isolated peptide pancreastatin[179] may be a product of the chromogranin A gene[180, 181] suggests another possible marker that may be of use in diagnosing hormone-secreting tumors.

References

1. Banting, F. G., and Best, C. H. The internal secretion of the pancreas. J. Lab. Clin. Med. 7:251, 1922.
2. Wilder, R. M., Allan, F. N., Power, M. H., and Robertson, H. E. Carcinoma of the islands of the pancreas. Hyperinsulinism and hyperglycemia. JAMA *89*:348, 1927.
3. Yalow, R. S., and Berson, S. A. Assay of plasma insulin in human subjects by immunologic methods. Nature *184*:1648, 1959.
4. Grimelius, L., Hultquist, G. T., and Stenkiuist, B. Cytological differentiation of asymptomatic pancreatic islet cell tumors in autopsy material. Virchows Arch. [Pathol. Anat.] *365*:275, 1975.
5. Schein, P. S., DeLellis, R. A., Kahn, C. R., Gorden, P., and Kraft, A. R. Islet cell tumors. Current concepts and management. Ann. Intern. Med. *79*:239, 1973.
6. Larsson, L. I. Endocrine pancreatic tumors. Hum. Pathol. 9:401, 1978.
7. Pictet, R. L., and Rutter, W. J. Development of the embryonic pancreas. *In* Steiner, D., and Freinkel, N. (eds.). Handbook of Physiology. Vol. 1, Sect. 7. Baltimore, Williams & Wilkins Company, 1972, p. 25.
8. Heitz, P. U., Kasper, M., Polak, J. M., and Kloppel, G. Pancreatic endocrine tumors: immunocytochemical analysis of 125 tumors. Hum. Pathol. *13*:263, 1982.
9. Pearse, A. G. E. Common cytochemical and ultrastructural characteristics of cells producing polypeptide hormones (the APUD series) and their relevance to thyroid and ultimobranchial C cells and calcitonin. Proc. R. Soc. Lond. *107*:71, 1968.
10. Falck, B. Observations on the possibilities of the cellular localization of monoamines by a fluorescence method. Acta Physiol. Scand. *56*(Suppl. 197):1, 1962.
11. Polak, J. M., Pearse, A. G. E., Le Lievre, C., Fontaine, C., and Le Douarin, N. M. Immunocytochemical confirmation of the neural crest origin of avian calcitonin-producing cells. Histochemistry *40*:209, 1973.
12. Le Douarin, N. Particularities du noyau interphasique chez la Caille japonaise *(Coturnix coturnix japonica)*. Utilisation de ces particularities comme "marque biologique" dans les recherches sur les interactions tissulaires et les migrations cellulaires au cours de l'ontogenese. Bull. Biol. Fr. Belg. *103*:435, 1969.

13. Schmechel, D., Marangos, P. J., and Brightman, M. Neurone-specific enolase is a molecular marker for peripheral and central neuro-endocrine cells. Nature *276*:834, 1978.
14. Teitelman, G., Joh, T. H., and Reis, J. Transformation of catecholaminergic precursors in glucagon (A) cells in mouse embryonic pancreas. Proc. Natl. Acad. Sci. USA *78*:5225, 1981.
15. Pearse, A. G. E. The cytochemistry and ultrastructure of polypeptide hormone producing cells of the APUD series and the embryologic, physiologic and pathologic implications of the concept. J. Histochem. Cytochem. *17*:303, 1969.
16. Pearse, A. G. E. Peptides in brain and intestine. Nature *262*:92, 1976.
17. Andrews, A. Gut and pancreatic amine precursor uptake and decarboxylation cells are not neural crest derivatives. Gastroenterol. *84*:429, 1983.
18. Stevens, R. E., and Moore, G. E. Inadequacy of APUD concept in explaining production of peptide hormones by tumors. Lancet *1*:118, 1983.
19. Le Douarin, N. M., and Teillet, M.-A. The migration of neural crest cells to the wall of the digestive tract in avian embryo. J. Embryol. Exp. Morphol. *30*:31, 1973.
20. Lamers, C. H. J., Rombout, J. W. H. M., and Timmermans, L. P. M. An experimental study on neural crest migration in *Barbus conchonius* (Cyprinidae, Teleostei), with special reference to the origin of the enteroendocrine cells. J. Embryol. Exp. Morphol. *62*:309, 1981.
21. Pictet, R. L., Rall, L. B., Phelps, P., and Rutter, W. J. The neural crest and the origin of the insulin-producing and other gastrointestinal hormone-producing cells. Science *191*:191, 1976.
22. Andrew, A., Kramer, B., and Rawdon, B. B. The embryonic origin of endocrine cells of the gastrointestinal tract. Gen. Comp. Endocrinol. *47*:249, 1982.
23. Pearse, A. G. E. Islet cell precursors are neurons. Nature *295*:96, 1982.
24. Anderson, D. J., and Axel, R. A bipotential neuroendocrine precursor where choice of cell fate is determined by NGF and glucocorticoids. Cell *47*:1079, 1986.
25. Erdheim, J. Zur normalen und pathologisenen Histologic der glandula Thyreoidea, Parathyroidea und Hypophysis. Beitr. Pathol. *33*:158, 1903.
26. Cushing, H., and Davidoff, L. M. The Pathological Findings in Four Autopsied Cases of Acromegaly with a Discussion of Their Significance (Monograph 22). New York, Rockefeller Institute for Medical Research, 1927.
27. Underdahl, L. O., Woolner, L. B., and Black, B. M. Multiple endocrine adenomas: report of 8 cases in which the parathyroids, pituitary and pancreatic islets are involved. J. Clin. Endocrinol. Metab. *13*:20, 1953.
28. Wermer, P. Genetic aspects of adenomatosis of endocrine glands. Am. J. Med. *16*:363, 1954.
29. Anderson, D. E. Genetic varieties of neoplasia. *In* Anderson, D. E. Genetic Concepts and Neoplasia. Baltimore, Williams & Wilkins Company, 1970, p. 85.
30. Eberle, F., Grun, R. Multiple endocrine neoplasia type I (MEN I). Ergeb. Inn. Med. Kinderheilkd. *46*:76, 1981.
31. Schimke, R. N. Genetic aspects of multiple endocrine neoplasia. Annu. Rev. Med. *35*:25, 1984.
32. Ballard, H. S., Frame, B., and Hartsock, R. J. Familial multiple endocrine adenoma–peptic ulcer complex. Medicine *43*:418, 1964.
33. Majewski, J. T., and Wilson, S. D. The MEA-I syndrome: an all or none phenomenon? Surgery *86*:475, 1979.
34. Lamers, C. B. H. W., and Froeling, P. G. A. M. Clinical significance of hyper-parathyroidism in familial multiple endocrine adenomatosis type I (MEA I). Am. J. Med. *66*:422, 1979.
35. Mallette, L. E., Bilezikian, J. P., Heath, D. A., and Aurbach, G. D. Primary hyperparathyroidism; clinical and biochemical features. Medicine *53*:127, 1974.
36. Hellstrom, J., and Ivemark, B. I. Primary hyperparathyroidism; clinical and structural findings in 138 cases. Acta Chir. Scand. (Suppl.)*294*:1, 1962.
37. Brandi, M. L., Aurbach, G. D., Fitzpatrick, L. A., Quarto, R., Spiegel, A. M., Bliziotes, M. M., Norton, J. A., Doppman, J. L., and Marx, S. J. Parathyroid mitogenic activity in plasma from patients with familial multiple endocrine neoplasia type I. N. Engl. J. Med. *314*:1287, 1986.
38. Schmike, R. N. Multiple endocrine neoplasia. Search for an oncogenic trigger. N. Engl. J. Med. *314*:1315, 1986.
39. Cryer, P. E., and Kissane, J. Fasting hypoglycemia, hypercalcemia and hyperprolactinemia. Am. J. Med. *57*:611, 1974.
40. Leshin, M. Multiple endocrine neoplasia. *In* Wilson, J. D., and Foster, D. W. (eds.). Williams Textbook of Endocrinology. Philadelphia, W. B. Saunders Co., 1985, p. 1274.
41. Wells, S. A., Jr., Ellis, G. J., and Gunnells, J. C. Parathyroid auto transplantation in primary parathyroid hyperplasia. N. Engl. J. Med. *295*:57, 1976.
42. Frantz, A. G. Prolactin. *In* Degroot, L. J., Chahill, G. F., Jr., Odell, W. D., Martini, L., Potts, J. T., Jr., Steinberger, D. H., and Winegrad, A. I. (eds.). Endocrinology. New York, Grune & Stratton, 1979, p. 153.
43. Wilson, S. D. Ulcerogenic tumors of the pancreas: the Zollinger-Ellison syndrome. *In* Casey, L. C. (ed.). The Pancreas. St. Louis, C. V. Mosby Company, 1973, p. 295.
44. Stefanini, P., Carboni, M., and Patrassi, N. Surgical treatment and prognosis of insulinoma. Clin. Gastroenterol. *3*:697, 1974.
45. Yamaguchi, K., Kameya, T., and Abe, K. Multiple endocrine neoplasia type I. Clin. Endocrinol. Metab. *9*:261, 1980.
46. Holst, J. J. Gut endocrine tumour syndromes. Clin. Endocrinol. Metab. *8*:413, 1979.
47. Floyd, J. C., Jr., Fajans, S. S., Pek, S., and Chance, R. E. A newly recognized pancreatic polypeptide; plasma levels in health and disease. Recent Prog. Horm. Res. *33*:519, 1977.
48. Yamaguchi, K., Abe, K., Miyakawa, S., Ohnami, S., Adachi, I., Oka, Y., Ueda, M., Kameya, T., and Yanaihara, N. Multiple hormone production in endocrine tumors of the pancreas. *In* Miyoshi, A. (ed.). Gut Peptides. Tokyo, Kodansha, 1979, p. 343.
49. Marx, S. J., Vinik, A. I., Santen, R. J., Floyd, J. C., Mills, J. L., Green, J. Multiple endocrine neoplasia type I: assessment of laboratory tests to screen for the gene in a large kindred. Medicine *66*:226, 1986.
50. Whipple, A. O. The surgical therapy of hyperinsulinism. J. Int. Chir. *3*:237, 1938.
51. Steiner, D. F., and Oyer, P. E. The biosynthesis of insulin and a probable precursor of insulin by a human islet cell adenoma. Proc. Natl. Acad. Sci. USA *57*:473, 1967.
52. Howard, J. M., Moss, N. H., and Rhoads, J. E. Collective review: hyperinsulinism and islet cell tumors of the pancreas with 398 recorded tumors. Surg. Gynecol. Obstet. *90*:417, 1950.
53. Scholz, D. A., Re Mine, W. H., and Priestly, J. T. Hyperinsulinism: review of 95 cases of functioning islet cell tumors. Mayo Clin. Proc. *35*:545, 1960.
54. Stefanini, P., Carboni, M., Patrassi, N., and Baroli, A. Beta-islet cell tumors of the pancreas: results of a study of 1,067 cases. Surgery *4*:597, 1974.
55. Service, F. J., Dale, A. J. D., Elveback, L. R., and Liang, N. S. Insulinoma: clinical and diagnostic features of 60 consecutive cases. Mayo Clin. Proc. *51*:417, 1976.
56. Bani, D., Sacch, T., and Biliotti, G. Nesidioblastosis and intermediate cells in the pancreas of patients with hyperinsulinemic hypoglycemia. Virchows Arch. [Cell Pathol.] *48*:19, 1985.
57. Elfvirg, G., and Hastbacka, J. Pancreatic heterotopia and its clinical importance. Acta Chir. Scand. *130*:593, 1965.
58. Jaspan, J. B., Wollman, R. L., Berstein, L., and Rubenstein, A. H. Hypoglycemic peripheral neuropathy in association with insulinoma: implication of glucopenia rather than hyperinsulinism. Medicine *61*:33, 1982.
59 Merimee, T. J., and Tyson, J. E. Stabilization of plasma glucose during fasting. N. Engl. J. Med. *291*:1275, 1974.
60. Marks, V. The investigation of hypoglycaemia. Br. J. Hosp. Med. *11*:731, 1974.
61. Turner, R. C., Oakley, N. W., and Nabarro, J. D. N. Control of basal insulin secretion with special reference to the diagnosis of insulinomas. Br. Med. J. *2*:132, 1971.
62. Kaplan, E. L., and Michelassi, F. Endocrine tumors of the pancreas and their clinical syndromes. Surg. Annu. *18*:181, 1986.

63. Service, F. J. Clinical presentation and laboratory evaluation of hypoglycemic disorders in adults. *In* Service, F. J. (ed.). Hypoglycemic Disorders: Pathogenesis and Treatment. Boston, G. K. Hall, 1983, p. 73.
64. Koivisto, V. A., Yki-Jarvinen, H., Hartling, S. G., and DelKoren, R. The effects of exogenous hyperinsulinemia on proinsulin secretion in normal man, obese subjects and patients with insulinoma. J. Clin. Endocrinol. Metab. *63*:1117, 1986.
65. Creutzfeldt, W. A. R., Creutzfeldt, C., Deuticke, U., Frerichs, H., and Track, N. S. Biochemical and morphological investigations of 30 insulinomas. Diabetologia *9*:217, 1973.
66. Berger, M., Bordi, C., Cuppers, H. J., Berchtold, P., Gries, A. F., Munterfering, H., Sailer, R., Zimmerman, H., and Orci, L. Functional and morphological characterization of human insulinomas. Diabetes *32*:921, 1983.
67. Rubenstein, A. H., Block, M. B., Starr, J., and Steiner, D. F. Proinsulin and C-peptide in blood. Diabetes *21*(Suppl. 2):661, 1972.
68. Turner, R. C., and Harris, E. Diagnosis of insulinomas by suppression tests. Lancet *2*:188, 1974.
69. Fajans, S. S., Schneider, J. M., Schteingart, D. E., and Conn, J. W. The diagnostic value of sodium tolbutamide in hypoglycaemic states. J. Clin. Endocrinol. Metab. *21*:371, 1961.
70. Marks, V., and Samols, E. Glucagon test for insulinoma: a chemical study in 25 cases. J. Clin. Pathol. *21*:346, 1968.
71. Pontiroli, A. E., Secchi, A., Dabandi, M., Alberetto, N., Bosi, E., Fautaguzzi, S., and Dozza, G. Study of hypoglycemic patients by the glucose clamp technique using the artificial pancreas. J. Clin. Endocrinol. Metab. *57*:1297, 1983.
72. Reynolds, J. H., Kanunsby, N. I., Schade, D. S., and Eaton, R. P. Use of computerized glucose clamp technique to diagnose an insulinoma. Ann. Intern. Med. *101*:648, 1984.
73. Yhi-Jaroinen, H., Peldonen, R., and Koivisto, V. A. Failure to suppress C-peptide secretion by euglycemic hyperinsulinemia: a new diagnostic test for insulinoma? Clin. Endocrinol. *23*:461, 1985.
74. Sved, S., McGilveray, I. J., and Beadoin, N. Assay of sulfonylureas in human plasma by high-performance liquid chromatography. J. Pharm. Sci. *65*:1356, 1976.
75. Le Quesne, L. P., Nabarro, J. D. N., Kurtz, A., and Zweig, A. The management of insulin tumours of the pancreas. Br. J. Surg. *66*:373, 1979.
76. Fink, I. J., Krudy, A. G., Shawker, T. H., Norton, J. A., Gorden, P., and Doppman, J. L. Demonstration of an angiographically hypovascular insulinoma with intraarterial dynamic CT. AJR *144*:555, 1985.
77. Rueckert, K. F., Klotter, H. J., and Kummerle, F. Intraoperative ultrasonic localization of endocrine tumors of the pancreas. Surgery *96*:1045, 1984.
78. Gorman, B., Charboneau, J. W., James, E. M., Reading, C. C., Galiber, A. K., Grant, C. S., VanHeerden, J. A., Telander, R. L., and Service, F. J. Benign pancreatic insulinoma: preoperative and intraoperative sonographic localization. AJR *147*:929, 1986.
79. Gray, R. K., Rosch, J., and Grollman, J. H. Arteriography in the diagnosis of islet-cell tumours. Radiology *97*:39, 1970.
80. Daggert, P. R., Goodburn, A. E., Kurtz, A. B., Le Quesne, L. P., Nabarro, J. D. N., and Raphael, M. J. Is preoperative localization of insulinomas necessary? Lancet *1*:483, 1981.
81. Roche, A., Raisonnier, A., and Gillon-Savouret, M. L. Pancreatic venous sampling and arteriography in localizing insulinomas and gastrinomas: procedure and results in 55 cases. Radiology *145*:621, 1982.
82. Glaser, B., Valtysson, G., Fajans, S. S., Vinik, A. J., Cho, K., and Thompson, N. Gastrointestinal/pancreatic hormone concentrations in the portal venous system of nine patients with organic hyperinsulinism. Metabolism *30*:1001, 1981.
83. Marks, V., and Samols, E. Diazoxide therapy of intractable hypoglycaemia. Ann. N.Y. Acad. Sci. *150*:442, 1968.
84. Stringel, G., Dalpe-Scott, M., Perelman, A. H., and Heick, H. M. C. The occult insulinoma operative localization by quick insulin radioimmunoassay. J. Pediatr. Surg. *20*:734, 1985.
85. Goode, P. N., Farndon, J. R., Anderson, J., Johnston, I. D. A., and Ahscalmorte, J. Diazoxide in the management of patients with insulinoma. World J. Surg. *10*:586, 1986.
86. Imanaka, S., Matsada, S., Ito, K., Matsuoka, T., and Okada, Y. Medical treatment for inoperable insulinoma: clinical usefulness of diphenylhydantoin and diltiazem. Jpn. J. Clin. Oncol. *16*:66, 1986.
87. Ulbrecht, J. S., Schneltz, R., Aarons, J. H., and Green, D. A. Insulinoma in a 94 year old woman: long term therapy with verapamil. Diabetes Care *9*:186, 1986.
88. Kiang, D. T., Frenning, D. H., and Bauer, G. E. Mithramycin for hypoglycemia in malignant insulinoma. N. Engl. J. Med. *299*:134, 1978.
89. Scandarelli, C., Zaccaria, M., DePalo, C., Sicolo, N., Erle, G., and Federspil, G. The effects of propranolol on hypoglycaemia: observations in 5 insulinoma patients. Diabetologia *15*:297, 1978.
90. Moertel, C. G., Hanley, J. A., and Johnson, L. A. Streptozotocin alone compared with streptozotocin plus fluorouracil in the treatment of advanced islet-cell carcinoma. N. Engl. J. Med. *303*:1189, 1980.
91. Eriksson, B., Alm, G., Lundquist, G., Wilander, E., Oberg, K., Karlsson, A., Andersson, T., and Wide, L. Treatment of malignant endocrine pancreatic tumours with human leukocyte interferon. Lancet *2*:1307, 1986.
92. Verner, J. V., and Morrison, A. B. Islet cell tumor and a syndrome of refractory watery diarrhea and hypokalemia. Am. J. Med. *25*:374, 1958.
93. Murray, J. S., Paton, R. R., and Pope, C. E., II. Pancreatic tumor associated with flushing and diarrhea. Report of a case. N. Engl. J. Med. *264*:436, 1961.
94. Matsumoto, K. K., Peter, J. B., Schultze, R. G., Hakim, A. A., and Frauck, P. T. Watery diarrhea and hypokalemia associated with pancreatic islet-cell adenoma. Gastroenterology *50*:231, 1966.
95. Bloom, S. R., Polak, J. M., and Pearse, A. G. E. Vasoactive intestinal peptide and watery diarrhea syndrome. Lancet *2*:14, 1973.
96. Kraft, A. R., Tompkins, R. K., and Zollinger, R. M. Recognition and management of the diarrheal syndrome caused by nonbeta islet cell tumors of the pancreas. Am. J. Surg. *119*:163, 1970.
97. Krejs, G. J., Walsh, J. H., Morawski, S. G., and Fordtran, J. S. Intractable diarrhea. Intestinal perfusion studies and plasma VIP concentrations in patients with pancreatic cholera syndrome and surreptitious ingestion of laxatives and diuretics. Am. J. Dig. Dis. *22*:280, 1977.
98. Long, R. G., Mitchell, S. J., Bryant, M. G., Polak, J. M., and Bloom, S. R. Clinicopathological study of pancreatic and neural VIPomas. Gut *20*:A934, 1979.
99. Bloom, S. R., and Polak, J. M. Glucagonomas, VIPomas, and somatostatinomas. Clin. Endocrinol. Metab. *9*:285, 1980.
100. Makhlouf, G. M., Said, S. I., and Yau, W. M. Interplay of vasoactive intestinal polypeptide (VIP) and synthetic VIP fragments with secretin and octapeptide of cholecystokinin (Octa-CCK) on pancreatic and biliary secretion. Gastroenterology *66*:737, 1974.
101. Franklin, R. B., and Tachjian, A. H. Intravenous infusion of prostaglandin E_2 raises plasma calcium concentration in the rat. Endocrinology *97*:240, 1975.
102. Oberg, K., Lööf, L., Boström, H., Grimelius, L., Fahrenkrug, J., and Lundqvist, G. Hypersecretion of calcitonin in patients with Verner-Morrison syndrome. Scand. J. Gastroenterol. *16*:135, 1981.
103. Schmitt, M. G., Jr., Soergel, K. H., Hensley, G. T., and Chey, W. Y. Watery diarrhea associated with pancreatic islet cell carcinoma. Gastroenterology *69*:206, 1975.
104. Elias, E., Bloom, S. R., Welbourn, R. B., Kuzio, M., Polak, J. M., Pearse, A. G. E., Booth, C. C., and Brown, J. C. Pancreatic cholera due to production of gastric inhibitory polypeptide. Lancet *2*:791, 1972.
105. Tomita, T., Kimmel, J. R., Friesen, S. R., and Mantz, F. A., Jr. Pancreatic polypeptide cell hyperplasia with and without watery diarrhea syndrome. J. Surg. Oncol. *14*:11, 1980.
106. Jaffe, B. M., and Condon, S. Prostaglandins E and F in endocrine diarrheogenic syndromes. Ann. Surg. *184*:516, 1976.
107. Bloom, S. R. Vasoactive intestinal peptide, the major mediator of the WDHA (pancreatic cholera) syndrome: value of meas-

urement in diagnosis and treatment. Am. J. Dig. Dis. *23*:373, 1978.

108. Said, S. I., and Faloona, G. R. Elevated plasma and tissue levels of vasoactive intestinal polypeptide in the watery diarrhea syndrome due to pancreatic, bronchogenic and other tumors. N. Engl. J. Med. *293*:155, 1975.
109. Kane, M. G., O'Dorisio, T. M., and Krejs, G. J. Production of secretory diarrhea by intravenous infusion of vasoactive intestinal polypeptide. N. Engl. J. Med. *309*:1482, 1983.
110. Gardner, J. D., and McCarthy, D. M. VIP and watery diarrhoea I-arguments against VIP being the cause of watery diarrhoea syndrome. *In* Bloom, S. R. (ed.). Gut Hormones. London, Churchill Livingstone, 1978, p. 570.
111. Bloom, S. R., Delamarter, J., Kawashima, E., Chistofides, N. D., Buell, G., and Polak, J. M. Diarrhoea in VIPoma patients associated with cosecretion of a second active peptide (peptide histidine isoleucine) explained by single coding gene. Lancet *2*:1163, 1983.
112. Tatemoto, K., and Mutt, V. Isolation and characterization of the intestinal peptide porcine PHI (PHI-27), a new member of the glucagon-secretin family. Proc. Natl. Acad. Sci. USA *78*:6603, 1981.
113. Fahrenkrug, J., and Pedersen, J. H. Secretion of peptide histidine methonine (PHM) and vasoactive intestinal peptide (VIP) in patients with VIP producing tumors. Peptides *7*:717, 1986.
114. Verner, J. V., and Morrison, A. B. Endocrine pancreatic islet disease with diarrhea; report of a case due to diffuse hyperplasia of nonbeta islet tissue with a review of 54 additional cases. Arch. Intern. Med. *133*:492, 1974.
115. Capella, C., Polak, J. M., Buffa, R., Tapia, F. J., Heitz, P., Usellini, L., Bloom, S. R., and Solicia, E. Morphologic patterns and diagnostic criteria of VIP producing endocrine tumors. Cancer *52*:1860, 1983.
116. Kessinger, A., Foley, J. F., and Lemon, H. M. Therapy of malignant APUD cell tumors. Effectiveness of DTIC. Cancer *51*:790, 1983.
117. Oberg, K., Lindstrom, H., Alm, G., and Lindquist, G. Successful treatment of therapy resistant pancreatic cholera with human leukocyte interferon. Lancet *1*:725, 1985.
118. Jaffe, B. M., Kopen, D. F., DeSchryver-Kecskemeti, K., Gengerich, R. L., and Greider, M. Indomethacin-responsive pancreatic cholera. N. Engl. J. Med. *297*:817, 1977.
119. Donowitz, M., Elta, G., Bloom, S. R., and Nathanson, L. Trifluoroperazine reversal of secretory diarrhea in pancreatic cholera. Ann. Intern. Med. *93*:284, 1980.
120. Santangelo, W. C., O'Dorisio, T. M., Kim, J. G., Severiro, G., and Krejs, G. J. Pancreatic cholera syndrome: effect of a synthetic somatostatin analog on intestinal water and ion transport. Ann. Intern. Med. *103*:363, 1985.
121. Wood, S. M., Kraezzlin, M. E., Adrian, T. E., and Bloom, S. R. Treatment of patients with pancreatic endocrine tumors using a new long acting somatostatin analogue symptomatic and peptide response. Gut *26*:438, 1985.
122. Kraezlin, M. E., Ching, J. L. C., Wood, S. M., Carr, D. H., and Bloom, S. R. Long-term treatment of a VIPoma with somatostatin analogue resulting in remission of symptoms and possible shrinkage of metastasis. Gastroenterology *88*:185, 1985.
123. Koel, A., Kraenzlin, M., Gyr, K., Meier, V., Bloom, S. R., Heitz, P., and Stalder, H. Escape of the response to a long acting somatostatin analogue (SMS-201-995) in patients with VIPoma. Gastroenterology *92*:527, 1987.
124. Becker, S. W., Kahn, P., and Rothman, S. Cutaneous manifestations of internal malignant tumors. Arch. Dermatol. *45*(Suppl.):1069, 1942.
125. Unger, R. H., Eisentraut, A. M., and Lochner, J. D. V. Glucagon producing tumors of the islets of Langerhans. J. Clin. Invest. *42*:987, 1963.
126. McGavran, M. H., and Unger, R. H. A glucagon secreting alpha cell carcinoma of the pancreas. N. Engl. J. Med. *274*:1408, 1966.
127. Mallinson, C. N., Bloom, S. R., Warin, A. P., Salmon, P. R., and Cox, B. A glucagonoma syndrome. Lancet *2*:1, 1974.
128. Higgins, G. A., Recant, L., and Fischman, A. B. The glucagonoma syndrome: surgically curable diabetes. Am. J. Surg. *137*:142, 1979.
129. Kahan, R. S., Perez-Figaredo, R. A., and Neumanis, A. Necrolytic migratory erythema: distinctive dermatosis of the glucagonoma syndrome. Arch. Dermatol. *113*:792, 1977.
130. Kheir, S. M., Onuna, E. F., Grizzle, W. E., Herrera, G. A., and Lee, I. Histologic variation in the skin lesions of the glucagonoma syndrome. Am. J. Surg. Pathol. *10*:445, 1986.
131. Tasman-Jones, C., and Kay, R. G. Zinc deficiency and skin lesions. N. Engl. J. Med. *293*:830, 1975.
132. Norton, J. A., Kahn, C. R., Scheibinger, R., Gorschboth, C., and Brennan, M. F. Amino acid deficiency and the skin rash associated with glucagonoma. Ann. Intern. Med. *91*:213, 1979.
133. Marynick, S. P., Fagadau, W. R., and Duncan, L. A. Malignant glucagonoma syndrome: response to chemotherapy. Ann. Intern. Med. *93*:453, 1980.
134. Elsborg, L., and Glenthoj, A. Effect of somatostatin in necrolytic migratory erythema of glucagonoma. Acta Med. Scand. *218*:245, 1985.
135. Khandekar, J. D., Oyer, D., Miller, H. J., and Vick, N. A. Neurologic involvement in glucagonoma syndrome: response to combination chemotherapy with 5-fluorouracil and streptozotocin. Cancer *44*:2014, 1979.
136. Leichter, S. B. Clinical and metabolic aspects of glucagonoma. Medicine *59*:100, 1980.
137. Valverde, I., Lemon, H. M., Kessinger, A., and Unger, R. H. Distribution of plasma glucagon immunoreactivity in a patient with suspected glucagonoma. J. Clin. Endocrinol. Metab. *42*:804, 1976.
138. Recant, L., Perrino, P. V., Bhathena, S. J., Danforth, D. H., and Lavine, R. L. Plasma immunoreactive glucagon fractions in four cases of glucagonoma: increases "large glucagon-immunoreactivity." Diabetologia *12*:319, 1976.
139. Villar, H. V., Johnson, D. G., Lynch, P. J., Pond, G. D., and Smith, P. H. Pattern of immunoreactive glucagon in portal, arterial and peripheral plasma before and after removal of glucagonoma. Am. J. Surg. *141*:148, 1981.
140. Hendriks, T. H., Jansen, J. B. J. M., and Tongeren, J. H. M. The glucagonoma syndrome: stimulus induced plasma responses of circulating glucagon components IRG^{9000} and IRG^{3500}. Acta Endocrinol. *105*:226, 1984.
141. Holst, J. J. Molecular heterogeneity of glucagon in normal subjects and in patients with glucagon producing tumors. Diabetologia *24*:359, 1983.
142. Bordi, C., Ravazzola, M., Baetens, D., Gorden, P., Unger, R. H., and Orci, L. A study of glucagonomas by light and electron microscopy and immunofluorescence. Diabetes *28*:925, 1979.
143. Boden, G., and Owen, O. E. Familial hyperglucagonemia—an autosomal dominant disorder. N. Engl. J. Med. *296*:534, 1977.
144. Montenegro, F., Lawrence, G. D., Macon, W., and Pass, C. Metastatic glucagonoma: improvement after surgical debulking. Am. J. Surg. *139*:424, 1980.
145. Lokich, J., Anderson, N., Rossini, A., Hadley, W., Federman, M., and Legg, M. Pancreatic alpha cell tumors: case report and review of the literature. Cancer *45*:2675, 1980.
146. Kessinger, A., Lemon, H. M., and Foley, J. F. The glucagonoma syndrome and its management. J. Surg. Oncol. *9*:419, 1977.
147. Strauss, G. M., Weitzman, S. A., and Aoki, T. T. Dimethyltriazeno-imidazole carboxamide therapy of malignant glucagonoma. Ann. Intern. Med. *90*:57, 1979.
148. Brazeau, P., Vale, W., Burgus, R., Ling, N., Butcher, M., Rivier, J., and Guillemin, R. Hypothalamic polypeptide that inhibits the secretion of immunoreactive pituitary growth hormone. Science *178*:77, 1973.
149. Larsson, L.-I., Hirsch, M. A., Holst, J. J., Ingemansson, S., Kuhl, C., Lindkaer Jensen, S., Lundqvist, G., Rehfeld, J. F., and Schwart, T. W. Pancreatic somatostatinoma: clinical features and physiological implications. Lancet *1*:666, 1977.
150. Ganda, O. P., Weir, G. C., Sveldner, J. S., Legg, M. A., Chick, W. L., Patel, Y. C., Ebeid, A. M., Gabbay, K. M.,

and Reichlin, S. R. "Somatostatinoma": a somatostatin-containing tumor of the endocrine pancreas. N. Engl. J. Med. *296*:963, 1977.
151. Kovacs, K., Horvath, E., Ezrin, C., Sepp, H., and Elkan, I. Immunoreactive somatostatin in pancreatic islet-cell carcinoma accompanied by ectopic A.C.T.H. syndrome. Lancet *1*:1365, 1977.
152. Penman, E., Lowry, P. J., Wass, J. A. H., Marks, V., Dawson, A. M., Besser, G. M., and Rees, L. H. Molecular forms of somatostatin in normal subjects and in patients with pancreatic somatostatinoma. Clin. Endocrinol. *12*:611, 1980.
153. Galmiche, J. P., Chayvialle, J. A., Dubois, P. M., David, L., Deseos, F., Paulin, C., Ducastelle, T., Colin, R., and Geffroy, Y. Calcitonin-producing pancreatic somatostatinoma. Gastroenterology *78*:1577, 1980.
154. Krejs, G. J., Orci, L., Conlon, J. M., Ravazzola, M., Davis, G. R., Raskin, P., Collins, S. M., McCarthy, D. M., Baetens, D., Rubenstein, A., Aldor, T. A. M., and Unger, R. H. Somatostatinoma syndrome: biochemical, morphologic, and clinical features. N. Engl. J. Med. *301*:285, 1979.
155. Stacpoole, P. W., Kasselberg, A. G., Berelowitz, M., and Chey, W. Y. Somatostatinoma syndrome: does a clinical entity exist? Acta Endocrinol. *102*:80, 1983.
156. Wright, J., Abolfathi, A., Penman, E., and Marks, V. Pancreatic somatostatinoma presenting with hypoglycemia. Clin. Endocrinol. *12*:613, 1980.
157. Axelrod, L., Bush, M. A., Hirsch, H. J., and Loo, S. W. H. Malignant somatostatinoma: clinical features and metabolic studies. J. Clin. Endocrinol. Metab. *52*:886, 1981.
158. Pipeleers, D., Somers, G., Gepts, W., De Nuttie, N., and De Vroede, M. Plasma pancreatic hormone levels in a case of somatostatinoma: diagnostic and therapeutic implications. J. Clin. Endocrinol. Metab. *49*:572, 1979.
159. Conlon, J. M., McCarthy, D., Krejs, G., and Unger, R. H. Characterization of somatostatin-like components in the tumors and plasma of a patient with a somatostatinoma. J. Clin. Endocrinol. Metab. *52*:66, 1981.
160. Patel, Y. L., Ganda, O. M. P., and Benoit, R. Pancreatic somatostatinoma: abundance of somatostatin-28 (1-12)-like immunoreactivity in tumor and plasma. J. Clin. Endocrinol. Metab. *57*:1048, 1983.
161. Kaneko, H., Yanaihara, N., Ito, S., Kusumoto, Y., Fujita, T., Ishikawa, S., Sumida, T., and Sekiya, M. Somatostatinoma in the duodenum. Cancer *44*:2273, 1979.
162. Dayal, Y., Doos, W. G., O'Brien, M. J., Nennemacher, G., De Lellis, R. A., and Wolfe, H. J. Psammomatous somatostatinomas of the duodenum. Am. J. Surg. Pathol. *7*:653, 1983.
163. Zachary, M., Goodman, D., Saavedra, J. A., and Lundblad, A. M. Somatostatinoma of the cystic duct. Cancer *53*:498, 1984.
164. Asa, S. L., Kovaes, K., Killinger, D. W., Marcon, N., and Platts, M. Pancreatic islet cell carcinoma producing gastrin, ACTH, alpha endorphin, somatostatin and calcitonin. Am. J. Gastroenterol. *74*:30, 1980.
165. Long, R. G, Bryant, M. G., Yuille, P. M., Polak, J. M., and Bloom, S. R. Mixed pancreatic apudoma with symptoms of excess vasoactive intestinal polypeptide and insulin: improvement of diarrhea with metoclopramide. Gut *22*:505, 1981.
166. Barragry, T. P., Wick, M. R., and Delaney, J. P. Pancreatic islet cell carcinoma with gastrin and vasoactive intestinal polypeptide production. Arch. Surg. *120*:1178, 1985.
167. Ferrara, J. J., Fucii, J. C., and Benson, J. B. Metastatic pancreatic islet cell carcinoma causing manifestations of glucagon and gastrin hypersecretion. Conn. Med. *49*:777, 1985.
168. Wilson, D. M., Ceda, G. P., Bostwick, D. G., Webber, R. J., Minkoff, J. R., Pont, A., Hintz, R. L., Bensch, K. G., Kraemer, F. B., Rosenfeld, R. G., and Hoffman, A. R. Acromegaly and Zollinger-Ellison syndrome secondary to an islet cell tumor: characterization and quantification of plasma and tumor human growth hormone releasing factor. J. Clin. Endocrinol. Metab. *59*:1002, 1984.
169. Chadenas, D., Pinsard, D., Messiere, D., Trouillas, J., Zafrani, E. S., Pradayrol, L., Sassolas, G., Li, Y., Girod, G., and Aumaitre, J. Tumeur pancreatique endocrine secretant de la somatostatine et de la somatocrinine. La Presse Med. *14*:2129, 1985.
170. Dayal, Y., Hong, D., Tallberg, K., Reichlin, S., De Lellis, R. A., and Wolfe, H. J. Immunocytochemical demonstration of growth hormone releasing factor in gastrointestinal and pancreatic endocrine tumors. Am. J. Clin. Pathol. *85*:13, 1986.
171. Schulte, H. M., Benher, G., Weindeck, R., Olbrich, T., and Reinwein, D. Failure to respond to growth hormone releasing hormone (GHRH) in acromegaly due to a GHRH secreting pancreatic tumor: dynamics of multiple endocrine testing. J. Clin. Endocrinol Metab. *61*:585, 1985.
172. Polak, J. M., Bloom, S. R., Adrain, T. E., Heitz, P., Bryant, M. G., and Pearse, A. G. E. Pancreatic polypeptide in insulinomas, gastrinomas, vipomas, and glucagonomas. Lancet *1*:328, 1976.
173. Taylor, I. L., Walsh, J. H., Rotter, J., and Passaro, E., Jr. Is pancreatic polypeptide a marker for Zollinger-Ellison syndrome? Lancet *1*:845, 1978.
174. Schwartz, T. W. Pancreatic-polypeptide (PP) endocrine tumors of the pancreas. Scand. J. Gastroenterol. *14*(Suppl. 53):93, 1979.
175. Strodel, W. E., Vinik, A. I., Lloyd, R. V., Glaser, B., Eckhauser, F. E., Fiddian Green, R. G., Turcotte, J. G., and Thompson, N. W. Pancreatic polypeptide-producing tumors. Silent lesions of the pancreas? Arch. Surg. *119*:508, 1984.
176. Wilson, B. S., and Lloyd, R. V. Detection of chromogranin in neuroendocrine cells with a monoclonal antibody. Am. J. Pathol. *115*:458, 1984.
177. Lloyd, R. V., Mervak, T., Schmidt, K., Warner, T. F. C. S., and Wilson, B. S. Immunohistochemical detection of chromogranin and neuron specific enolase in pancreatic endocrine neoplasms. Am. J. Surg. Pathol. *8*:607, 1984.
178. O'Connor, D. T., and Deftos, L. J. Secretion of chromogranin by peptide producing endocrine neoplasms. N. Engl. J. Med. *314*:1145, 1986.
179. Tatemoto, K., Etendic, S., Mutt, V., Makk, G., Feistner, G. J., and Barchas, J. D. Pancreastatin, a novel pancreatic peptide that inhibits insulin secretion. Nature *324*:476, 1986.
180. Iacangelo, A., Affolter, H. U., Eiden, L. E., Herbert, E., and Grimes, M. Bovine chromogranin A sequence and distribution of its messenger RNA in endocrine tissues. Nature *323*:82, 1986.
181. Eiden, L. E. Is chromogranin a prohormone? Nature *325*:301, 1987.

VIII

DISEASES OF THE INTRA-ABDOMINAL VASCULATURE AND SUPPORTIVE STRUCTURES

101

Vascular Diseases of the Bowel

JAMES H. GRENDELL
ROBERT K. OCKNER

Recent advances in angiography and vascular surgery and in the management of nutrition and fluid balance after intestinal resection have permitted a more aggressive approach to the diagnosis and treatment of vascular syndromes of the gastrointestinal tract.[1–3] The prognosis of a number of these conditions remains grave, but in certain situations early diagnosis and appropriate management may significantly improve the outlook. A sound clinical approach to these disorders is necessarily based upon an understanding of the basic concepts of anatomy and physiology of the mesenteric circulation. In this chapter, the anatomy, physiology, and pathophysiology of the mesenteric circulation will be reviewed, followed by discussions of chronic and acute intestinal ischemic syndromes and of other vascular disorders affecting the bowel.

BLOOD SUPPLY OF THE GUT AND THE PATHOPHYSIOLOGY OF ISCHEMIC DISEASE

Anatomy of the Mesenteric Circulation

The intra-abdominal portions of the digestive tract are nourished almost entirely by three major unpaired arterial trunks arising from the ventral aspect of the abdominal aorta: the *celiac axis,* the *superior mesenteric artery,* and the *inferior mesenteric artery*. The anatomy of these vessels, including their anatomic interrelationships and potential for collateral formation, determines the consequences of acute or chronic vascular occlusion.

Celiac Axis. This large vessel usually originates at a level between the twelfth thoracic and the first lumbar vertebrae, passes next to the median arcuate ligament of the diaphragm, and almost immediately gives rise to three major branches: the splenic, left gastric, and hepatic arteries (Fig. 101–1). All three branches contribute to the blood supply of the stomach. The splenic artery supplies the greater curvature via the short gastric and left gastroepiploic branches. The left gastric artery supplies primarily the lesser curvature of the stomach and may anastomose with the right gastric branch of the hepatic artery. The hepatic artery also gives rise to the gastroduodenal artery; this vessel, in turn, divides into the right gastroepiploic and superior pancreaticoduodenal arteries. Because of this rich network about both the greater and the lesser curvatures of the stomach, ischemic infarction of this organ in the absence of more generalized mesenteric ischemia is most unusual, but it has been reported.[4, 5]

Of particular importance are those vessels derived from the hepatic artery that supply the pancreas and duodenum. As noted, the gastroduodenal artery gives rise to the superior pancreaticoduodenal arteries (anterior and posterior). These, in turn, form anastomotic connections about the duodenum in the region of the

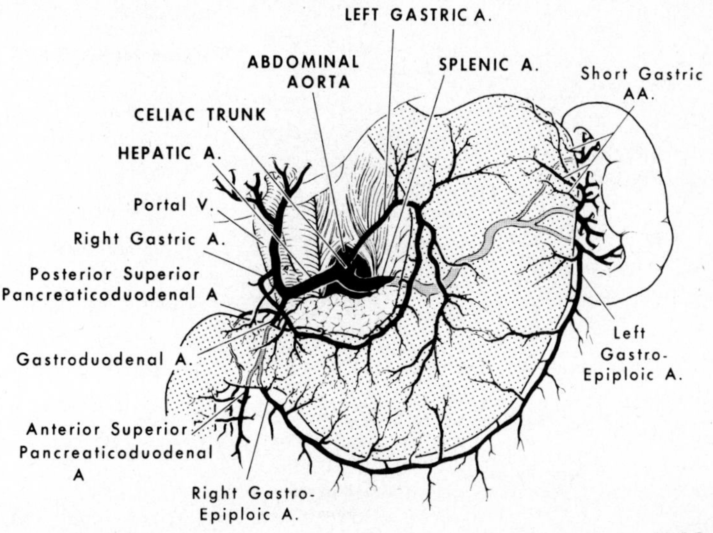

Figure 101–1. Blood supply to the stomach and duodenum. Each of the three major branches of the celiac axis supplying the stomach and the anastomotic connections to the superior mesenteric artery near the duodenum are illustrated.

head of the pancreas with branches of the inferior pancreaticoduodenal arteries, which are derived from the superior mesenteric artery. These interconnections, designated the pancreaticoduodenal arcades, constitute anastomotic routes of major importance between the celiac and the superior mesenteric arteries (Figs. 101–1 and 101–2).

Superior Mesenteric Artery. This vessel (Fig. 101–2) originates behind the pancreas at the level of the first lumbar vertebra, just caudal to the celiac axis. It emerges from behind the lower border of the body of the pancreas and passes anterior to the uncinate process of the pancreas and third portion of the duodenum. Distal to the origin of the inferior pancreaticoduodenal artery, the superior mesenteric artery gives rise to three major branches—the middle colic, right colic, and ileocolic arteries—and also to a series of smaller intestinal branches that nourish the jejunum and ileum. The intestinal branches form a series of three or four arcades before entering the wall of the intestine as the arteriae rectae. Although there is considerable potential for collateral flow within the primary and secondary arcades, the arteriae rectae appear to represent end-arteries, and few, if any, important anastomotic connections are present within the bowel wall itself. Accordingly, selective occlusion of these more distal vessels, as may occur in vasculitis, may lead to segmental infarction. The ileocolic artery forms anastomoses in the vicinity of the cecum with the continuation of the main trunk of the superior mesenteric artery and supplies the terminal ileum, cecum, and proximal ascending colon. The right colic artery (which may arise from either the superior mesenteric or the middle colic artery) is responsible primarily for supplying the ascending colon and hepatic flexure, whereas the middle colic artery supplies the proximal portion of the transverse colon. Anastomotic connections of major clinical importance exist between the middle colic artery and branches of the inferior mesenteric artery, as noted below.

Inferior Mesenteric Artery. This vessel, smaller in caliber than the celiac and superior mesenteric arteries, originates at the left of the third lumbar vertebra and carries blood to the distal transverse colon, the descending and sigmoid colon, and the proximal portions of the rectum (Fig. 101–2). The left colic branch supplies the distal transverse and descending colon and may, in addition, connect directly with the middle colic artery through the *arc of Riolan*, or "meandering mesenteric" artery (Fig. 101–3).[6, 7] The inferior mesenteric artery also gives rise to two or three sigmoidal arteries and finally terminates as the superior rectal artery. In addition to the arc of Riolan, the adjacent branches of the sigmoidal, left colic, middle colic, right colic, and ileocolic arteries form an arterial channel that parallels the large intestine along its mesenteric aspect. This channel, the *marginal artery of Drummond,* gives rise to arteriae rectae that enter the wall of the colon itself. In some individuals, this channel is of adequate caliber to function as a route for collateral supply in the event that one of the larger vessels from which it is derived is occluded. In many, however, the marginal artery is not an important collateral channel, and the arc of Riolan (meandering mesenteric artery) serves as the major connection between superior and inferior mesenteric arterial systems.[2]

The distal portions of the rectum are supplied primarily by the middle rectal and inferior rectal arteries, derived from the hypogastric (internal iliac) arteries.

General Anatomic Considerations. From this brief review of the mesenteric vascular anatomy, it is evident that the blood supply to the intra-abdominal portion of the gastrointestinal tract is richly endowed with several anastomotic interconnections that help protect against the consequences of occlusive vascular disease. In the presence of chronic progressive occlusive disease, these anastomotic interconnections, including the pancreaticoduodenal arcades, the arc of Riolan, and the marginal artery of Drummond, are usually capable of developing sufficiently to permit collateral flow. In

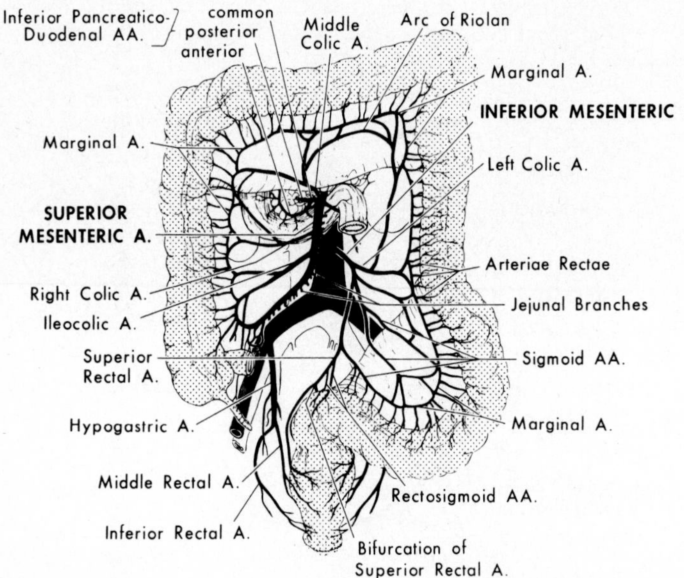

Figure 101–2. Blood supply to the small and large intestines. Anastomotic connections to the celiac axis in the region of the duodenum are shown, as are those between the superior and inferior mesenteric arteries. Illustrated here are those branches of the left and middle colic arteries which in a number of patients connect directly (and apart from the marginal artery) to form the arc of Riolan, or "meandering mesenteric" artery.

fact, it is possible for all the intra-abdominal viscera to be adequately supplied by only one of the three major mesenteric vessels.[8]

Conversely, the collateral supply may be only marginally adequate in certain areas. For example, occlusion of the arteriae rectae and intramural arteries may lead to segmental ischemia of the small or large intestine. Also potentially vulnerable are the "watershed" areas in the distal transverse colon and splenic flexure and at the junction of the superior and middle portions of the rectum, where branches of the inferior mesenteric artery anastomose with branches of the superior mesenteric and hypogastric arteries, respectively. This may, in part, account for the fact that segmental infarction in ischemic colitis occurs most commonly in the region of the splenic flexure and rectosigmoid, although the basis for this predilection is not entirely clear.[9]

Venous Circulation. In general, veins parallel arteries in the smaller branches and for portions of the main mesenteric trunks. However, rather than entering the vena cava, the superior mesenteric and splenic veins join to form the portal vein, which enters the liver after receiving additional blood from the gastric circulation via the coronary vein. The inferior mesenteric vein usually drains into the splenic vein. Connections between the splanchnic and systemic venous beds become enlarged and serve as collateral channels in the presence of portal venous hypertension or inferior vena cava occlusion. These collaterals, most prominent at the gastroesophageal junction, the hemorrhoidal plexus, the residual umbilical circulation, and a variety of sites at which abdominal viscera are in contact with retroperitoneal structures, become clinically significant as sites of bleeding (see pp. 397–427) or in the pathogenesis of portal-systemic encephalopathy.

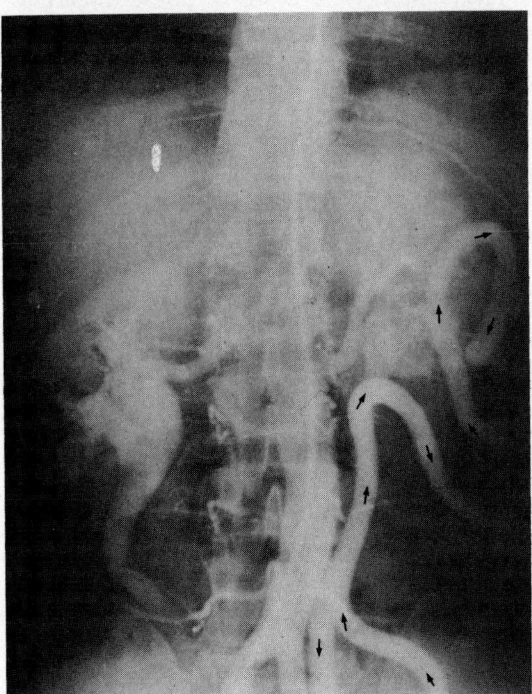

Figure 101–3. Arteriographic demonstration of the meandering mesenteric artery. In this patient with extensive mesenteric arterial disease, the inferior mesenteric artery and the meandering mesenteric artery *(arrows)* play a major role in the blood supply to the entire intra-abdominal gastrointestinal tract via anastomotic connections with the superior mesenteric artery. (From Sacks, R. P., Sheft, D. J., and Freeman, J. H. The demonstration of the mesenteric collateral circulation in young patients. AJR *102*:401–406. © by The American Roentgen Ray Society, 1968.)

Regulation of Blood Flow

The flow of blood to the abdominal viscera is modulated by a variety of mechanisms that can be considered either intrinsic (local response to alterations in pressure or to an increase in tissue metabolites) or extrinsic (autonomic nervous system). In addition, a variety of circulating vasoactive substances, both endogenous and exogenous, may significantly affect intra-abdominal blood flow. Methodologic advances in recent years have led to an improvement in our understanding of the regulation of mesenteric blood flow and the intestinal microcirculation.[2, 9–12] The intestinal microcirculation has at least two functionally and anatomically distinct control points—the arteriole, which as the major site of resistance is the most important local determinant of overall mesenteric flow, and the precapillary sphincter, which determines capillary perfusion.

Intrinsic or local modulation of blood flow occurs in response to changes in arteriolar transmural pressure or to alterations in tissue oxygenation in order to maintain adequate blood flow and oxygen delivery. In addition, vasodilatation occurs following brief periods of arterial occlusion (reactive hyperemia)[13, 14] and during digestion of a meal (functional hyperemia).[15–17] Intrinsic modulation appears to involve changes in both arteriolar resistance and precapillary sphincter activity. A controversy exists as to whether the predominant stimulus for intrinsic regulation is an alteration in arteriolar transluminal pressure (myogenic hypothesis)[18–20] or an increase in vasodilator metabolites entering the circulation as the result of a fall in tissue oxygen tension (metabolic hypothesis).[12, 21, 22]

Extrinsic neurologic regulation of mesenteric and intestinal blood flow is mediated by sympathetic postganglionic fibers originating from the splanchnic nerves, which cause constriction of arteries and arterioles and a reduction in intestinal blood flow. However, continued stimulation of these nerves leads to a partial or, in some cases, complete recovery of flow (autoregulatory escape).[10] The mechanisms involved in this escape have not been determined.[23–25] Currently available evidence does not support a physiologically significant role for direct parasympathetic regulation of mesenteric blood flow.[26] Other possible neurologic regulatory pathways (e.g., purinergic, dopaminergic) have been suggested but have not been extensively studied.[2, 10]

The possibility that the arteriole and precapillary sphincter may respond selectively to various agents is suggested by canine studies, which showed that whereas vasopressin and epinephrine caused similar decreases in intestinal blood flow (i.e., increased arteriolar resistance), vasopressin diminished intestinal oxygen consumption but epinephrine did not. Norepinephrine is similar in these respects to vasopressin. One possible explanation is that epinephrine constricts arteriolar smooth muscle but not that of the precapillary sphincter. Alternatively, epinephrine may alter tissue metabolism, lowering intracellular oxygen tension and thereby increasing the capillary-to-cell oxygen gradient.[27] In primates, epinephrine acts as a vasodilator at low doses and a vasoconstrictor at higher doses.[28] Beta-receptor blockade abolishes the vasodilator effect, whereas alpha-receptor blockade potentiates it. This suggests that, at low concentrations, epinephrine produces vasodilatation by stimulating beta-receptors, whereas alpha-receptor-mediated vasoconstriction predominates at higher concentrations.[28–31]

In addition to intrinsic and neurologic regulation of mesenteric blood flow, circulating endogenous and exogenous agents may exert an effect. The observation that nutrients present in the intestinal lumen result in increased intestinal blood flow and oxygen consumption suggests a possible regulatory role for gastrointestinal hormones.[17] Administration of both cholecystokinin and gastrin has been shown to increase intestinal blood flow, as has infusion of other peptides isolated from the intestine for which physiologic roles have yet to be proved.[2, 10] Whether any of these peptides are important regulators of the mesenteric circulation remains to be determined. Regulatory roles for histamine, serotonin, and the prostaglandins have also been suggested, although conclusive data have not yet been obtained to establish a physiologic role for any of these.[10] A vasoconstrictor role has been demonstrated for the digitalis glycosides.[32–34]

Some studies of the microcirculation in the intestinal mucosa have suggested the presence of a *countercurrent exchange* or multiplier in the intestinal villus resulting from blood flow in the central villus arteriole parallel but opposite in direction to that in the subepithelial villus venules.[35, 36] It has been postulated that this relationship would lead to a gradient in oxygen tension between arteriole and venule, most prominent at the base of the villus. Diffusion along this gradient would tend to result in a progressive decrease in oxygen tension as blood in the central arteriole flows toward the villus tip.[37, 38] Important species differences exist, however; and the significance of this proposed countercurrent mechanism in the development of intestinal ischemia and necrosis remains unproved.

Most of the physiologic studies of the regulation of the mesenteric circulation have been done in experimental animals. Thus, the applicability of many of the findings to humans has not been established.

Pathophysiologic Considerations

The ability of the visceral circulation to provide an adequate supply of oxygen and nutrients to meet tissue needs is dependent on both the anatomic and the physiologic determinants described previously. In disease, additional temporal factors are important in determining the extent, severity, and possible reversibility of ischemic processes or events.

Temporal Factors. If occlusion of a large vessel is gradual, adequate collateral circulation may develop so that ischemia may be minimized or prevented even if the large vessel becomes completely blocked. Thus, chronic arterial occlusive disease ordinarily does not cause symptoms or signs of ischemia unless two or more major vessels are affected, because of the large number of collateral channels that interconnect the major arterial trunks. In the absence of additional acute superimposed factors (e.g., hypotension, hypoxia, embolization of an atherosclerotic plaque), it would be unusual for a patient with chronic atherosclerotic disease limited to a single vessel to develop symptoms of intestinal ischemia. A possible exception to this generalization is the suggested association of chronic occlusive disease of the celiac axis alone with recurrent abdominal pain in the absence of other mesenteric arterial disease (see p. 1907 for a discussion of this association).

In contrast, occlusion of a vessel over a period of time too brief to allow for development of adequate collateral circulation may result in ischemic necrosis. A classic example of this is embolization to the superior mesenteric artery in a young person with mitral stenosis but normal mesenteric arteries. Undue delay in recognition and treatment of this event may result in intestinal infarction, even though only one major vessel is occluded and adequate potential collateral channels are present.

Anatomic Factors. Disease processes (such as certain forms of vasculitis) that affect smaller vessels, particularly the arteriae rectae or the intramural arteries and arterioles, may cause segmental infarction of either small or large bowel, because anastomotic connections between these vessels are limited. Arterial emboli to the viscera most commonly lodge in the superior mesenteric artery, probably because of its oblique take-off from the aorta. The celiac axis, although comparable in caliber, originates at nearly a right angle to the aorta, whereas the inferior mesenteric artery, although oblique in its take-off, is relatively small in caliber. As a result, these latter vessels are less frequent sites of arterial embolization.

Similarly, anatomic factors are important in the development of ischemia following thrombosis of the mesenteric veins. Thrombosis of the superior mesenteric vein may not result in intestinal ischemia because of the large capability for collateral flow through the mesenteric venous arcades and vasa recta. However, involvement of these smaller veins in the thrombotic process typically will lead to intestinal infarction.

Physiologic Factors. An extreme example of the importance of physiologic factors in determining the oxygen supply to the intestine is represented by the syndrome of *nonocclusive intestinal infarction.* In this disorder, widespread ischemic necrosis of the intestine may occur in hypoxic patients or those with reduced cardiac output (e.g., as the result of an acute myocardial infarction or congestive heart failure) or hypotension, despite the absence of mesenteric vascular occlusion. A variety of mechanisms have been proposed. It has been suggested that the putative countercurrent exchange in the intestinal villus[35, 36] would result in a marked reduction in oxygen tension in the villus tip with slowing of flow in the mesenteric arteriole, a hypothesis that remains unproved.[38, 39] Other experimental studies have led to the proposal that ischemia renders the brush border glycoproteins and proteins susceptible to the destructive effects of intraluminal pancreatic enzymes, such as elastase. Disruption of the brush border then exposes the underlying mucosa to the effects of intraluminal proteolytic enzymes and subsequent invasion by bacteria.[40] Support for this concept comes from experiments that show a marked reduction in mucosal necrosis in experimental mesenteric low-flow states following diversion of pancreatic enzymes from the bowel or intraluminal instillation of aprotinin, a trypsin inhibitor.[41] Other recent animal studies have suggested that superoxide anion formation during reperfusion following ischemia plays an important role in ischemic nonocclusive injury to the small intestine and that pretreatment with superoxide dismutase or allopurinol significantly reduces ischemic tissue necrosis.[42, 43]

In the final analysis, adequate oxygenation of the abdominal viscera depends upon many factors, including patency of the major arterial trunks, arteriolar resistance, adequacy of perfusion pressure, arterial oxygen saturation, and the oxygen requirement of the tissues themselves. Any or all of these factors may change gradually or abruptly, depending upon the clinical circumstances, and may result in visceral ischemia.

HISTOPATHOLOGIC AND FUNCTIONAL SEQUELAE OF VISCERAL ISCHEMIA

Ultrastructural changes are evident in the absorptive cells within five minutes after occlusion of the superior mesenteric artery.[44–47] The epithelium then becomes detached from the basement membrane, especially at the villus tips, and subepithelial blebs form. Within 30 to 60 minutes the upper portions of the villi are denuded of epithelium, whereas crypt cells are more resistant. The mucosa undergoes necrosis and ulceration, and a variable inflammatory cell infiltrate appears, presumably in response to both tissue necrosis and secondary bacterial invasion. Among the phenomena that characterize acute ischemic necrosis is an increase in capillary permeability,[48] followed by loss of capillary integrity as reflected by submucosal edema and hemorrhage. The muscular layers of the bowel are more resistant than is the epithelium to oxygen deprivation; only with more prolonged or severe ischemia do they undergo necrosis.

Viewed in the context of these events, certain of the clinical phenomena associated with bowel ischemia are readily understandable. For example, submucosal edema and hemorrhage are the basis for the so-called thumbprint pattern seen radiographically in patients with acute ischemic disease (see Fig. 101–7). Later, the exudation of protein-rich fluid (and ultimately bleeding) into the lumen of the bowel reflects extensive loss of vascular and epithelial integrity. Finally, the development of peritonitis suggests that even the relatively resistant muscular layers have become necrotic and that perforation has occurred or is imminent. In those ischemic episodes that are self-limited (i.e., those that do not perforate or require immediate resection), the resolution of the acute inflammatory reaction is accompanied by granulation tissue, fibrosis, and finally, the scar and stricture that often characterize this process.[2]

GENERAL DIAGNOSTIC CONSIDERATIONS

Clinical diagnosis of visceral ischemic syndromes may be extremely difficult. The patient's symptoms are usually nonspecific. Routine radiographic procedures (plain films and barium contrast studies) are often not helpful. Furthermore, even the angiographic demonstration of stenosis, narrowing, or occlusion of a major vessel, or the presence of a meandering mesenteric artery, does not establish ischemia as the cause of the patient's symptoms, because such anatomic abnormalities are frequently noted in asymptomatic individuals. Indeed, as shown by angiography, vessel caliber may correlate poorly with clinical symptoms in the individual patient.[49–51] Conversely, the demonstration of patent vessels by arteriography does not exclude ischemic disease, both because of the critical dependence of mesenteric blood flow on circulatory, hormonal, and metabolic factors and because of the possibility that an occlusive process may be localized to smaller, less well visualized, intramural vessels. Accordingly, diagnosis of the visceral ischemic syndromes requires not only a high index of suspicion but a careful and continuing evaluation of all available clinical, laboratory, and radiographic information.

CHRONIC INTESTINAL ISCHEMIC SYNDROMES

Most patients with clinically significant occlusive disease of the mesenteric vasculature present with one of the acute syndromes to be described in the following section. "Chronic" (actually, recurrent acute) ischemia is uncommon. It is represented by two conditions that differ greatly in virtually every respect but between them illustrate most of the priniciples and problems with which the clinician must deal in approaching the patient with suspected mesenteric vascular disease.

Intestinal Angina

Occlusive vascular disease, usually atherosclerotic and affecting at least two of the three major splanchnic vessels, rarely may be associated with a syndrome of intermittent dull or cramping midabdominal pain, or intestinal angina.[51–53] The pain characteristically appears from 15 to 30 minutes after a meal and lasts for up to a few hours. It is during this period that nutrients are undergoing digestion and absorption in the small intestine, and adequate vascular perfusion is required to permit increased intestinal blood flow and oxygen consumption. Because the superior mesenteric artery and other vascular channels that might provide effective collateral supply are partially or completely occluded, however, there is relative ischemia, and the patient experiences pain that may be analogous to that of angina pectoris.

Clinical Picture. Patients with this syndrome are usually in the older age group, although it may rarely affect children.[54] They quickly discover the relationship between eating and the initiation or aggravation of their pain. As a result, they develop a fear of eating and tend to decrease both the size of individual meals ("small meal syndrome") and total food intake. Consequently, marked weight loss is the rule, and this may be aggravated to some degree by mild to moderate steatorrhea. Other digestive symptoms such as diarrhea, constipation, nausea, vomiting, and abdominal bloating may be reported but are less constant. In one report, gastric ulceration was attributed to chronic mesenteric ischemia,[55] and in another, rectal ischemia was implicated as the cause of fecal incontinence.[56] The duration of the symptoms from onset to diagnosis may vary considerably, depending upon the severity of the symptoms and the awareness of the physician. Retrospectively, however, it is clear that many patients who present with frank infarction of the intestine have had antecedent symptoms suggestive of abdominal angina for periods of weeks to months.[2] Accordingly, this syndrome is significant not only because of the disability and discomfort that it causes but also because it may be a harbinger of imminent catastrophe.

Physical examination in these patients, in addition to showing evidence of marked weight loss, will usually disclose findings of advanced atherosclerotic disease. An abdominal bruit may be detectable, but neither its presence not its absence carries major diagnostic weight, because many patients with advanced mesenteric vascular disease have no bruits, and totally insignificant abdominal bruits are well described in normal individuals.[57, 58] Possibly, phonoangiographic documentation of a diastolic phase may discriminate significant bruits.[59]

Laboratory findings are generally nonspecific. In a number of patients, however, steatorrhea has been well documented (see pp. 263–282). As a rule, it is mild to moderate, up to about 20 gm of fecal fat per day;[60] in the case of atherosclerotic mesenteric insufficiency, it is almost always associated with pain.[61] In some patients, steatorrhea may contribute to malnutrition, the cause of which is not well understood. Although it presumably reflects reduced mesenteric blood flow,[62] the correlation between intestinal function and angiographic findings is poor.[51] Specific alterations in mucosal morphologic appearance have been described in such patients,[60] but steatorrhea may persist after revascularization, even though bowel morphologic appearance is normal.[63] Possibly, ischemic injury to autonomic nerves or stricture formation may alter intestinal motility and lead to bacterial overgrowth. In most patients, diminished food intake is the major factor, and malabsorption is ordinarily not an important clinical problem.

Diagnosis and Treatment. The presentation of an older patient with recurrent severe abdominal pain and progressive weight loss may suggest a diagnosis of intra-abdominal malignancy. However, on careful questioning it is usually possible to elicit the fact that fear of eating rather than lack of appetite accounts for decreased food intake. Advanced atherosclerotic vascular disease is often present. A systolic abdominal bruit may be heard, but as noted, this clinical sign (or its absence) is usually of no help. Barium contrast studies do not usually disclose abnormalities sufficient to account for the clinical picture. If the diagnosis of abdominal angina is suspected, other possible causes of pain are excluded, and if the patient's condition is such that corrective surgery would be undertaken were the diagnosis to be established, then angiographic study of the splanchnic circulation is indicated. A positive study will disclose significant (> 50 per cent) narrowing in at least two of the three major arteries and often evidence for collateral flow (Fig. 101–4). Because blood flow rather than vessel caliber determines the adequacy of tissue oxygenation, it is understandable why many patients with apparently severe mesenteric vascular disease (as judged by angiography) have no clinical evidence of vascular insufficiency.[50] For this reason, one cannot look to angiography as a means of positively establishing the diagnosis of abdominal angina. Rather, the presumptive diagnosis must be made on the basis of compatible symptoms and the exclusion of other conditions; the angiogram may either substantiate the diagnosis or, by revealing normal splanchnic vasculature, exclude it. Thus, if there is serious doubt that the clinical history and findings are consistent with abdominal angina, then angiography will be most helpful if it is negative and rules out the diagnosis. Conceivably, the diagnostic accuracy of angiography eventually may be improved by combining it with other methods that more directly reflect blood flow, such as radioxenon washout.[64]

The decision to undertake reconstructive vascular surgery for abdominal angina should be made only when other significant and potentially contributory abdominal disease has been excluded and when angiography shows significant narrowing near the ostia (i.e., in a surgically accessible area), usually of at least two major vessels. Even with these preconditions, however, errors in diagnosis must be anticipated. At surgery, a gradient of more than 33 mm Hg across a

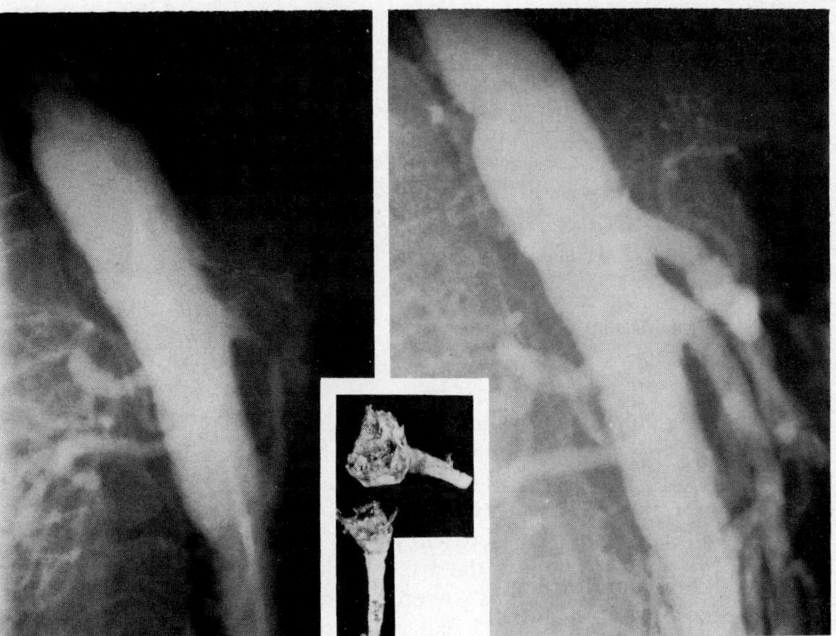

Figure 101–4. Diffuse atherosclerosis of splanchnic vessels in a patient with abdominal angina. Lateral aortogram, before and after endarterectomy, demonstrating the virtually complete occlusion of both the celiac and the superior mesenteric arteries at their take-off. The inset shows the atherosclerotic plaques that were removed at surgery. (Courtesy of William Ehrenfeld, M. D., Department of Surgery, University of California, San Francisco.)

stenotic area will confirm the hemodynamic significance of the block.[65, 66] Bypass, endarterectomy, and reimplantation procedures have all been effective.[65–73] Stoney and coworkers[66, 70, 71] emphasize the importance of antegrade graft placement and report favorable experience with a thoracoretroperitoneal approach to transaortic endarterectomy. The general experience with such corrective surgery has been that results are favorable, in regard to relief of pain and correction of malabsorption. Accumulating experience with percutaneous transluminal angioplasty offers the possibility that nonsurgical approaches may also prove useful in selected patients.[74–77]

Celiac Compression Syndrome

In a number of individuals, recurrent abdominal pain has been associated with narrowing of the celiac axis alone.[78–85] This disorder, the so-called *celiac compression syndrome*, would seem to be an exception to the general rule that at least two major visceral arteries must be narrowed before symptoms occur. Its validity is questionable.

Most patients have been women, younger than those expected to have significant atherosclerotic disease, who describe epigastric pain of variable frequency and duration. The pain may or may not be related to meals, is infrequently associated with nausea and vomiting, and is accompanied by an epigastric bruit which does not radiate to the lower abdomen. Other gastrointestinal disease has not been demonstrable in most cases. Angiographically, the celiac axis is narrowed near its origin, with poststenotic dilatation; other vessels are normal. At surgery, the celiac axis may have a high take-off and be compressed by the median arcuate ligament of the diaphragm or by neurofibrous tissue of the celiac ganglion. In some cases, stenosis is ascribed to intimal fibrosis.

Some important problems remain to be clarified before this syndrome can be placed in proper clinical and pathophysiologic perspective. One problem is that the cause of the pain remains obscure, because it is clear that in most patients the pancreaticoduodenal arcades are adequate collateral routes for supply of blood to the distribution of the celiac axis. Possibly, it is the diversion of blood from areas normally supplied by the superior mesenteric artery that accounts for the pain.[82] It has also been suggested that the celiac ganglion itself may be the source of the pain.[80–81] Because the surgical approach to the vessel essentially requires removal of the celiac ganglion, it is entirely possible that any symptomatic relief that may be obtained results from this part of the procedure, rather than from the correction of vascular compression or stenosis.

A second unresolved and possibly related problem is that significant stenosis of the celiac axis may be found incidentally at autopsy[50, 86] or on abdominal angiography,[79, 87–90] indicating that this lesion may be asymptomatic in many or most individuals.

If celiac compression syndrome is indeed a valid entity, it awaits far more convincing clinical and pathophysiologic definition than is currently available. At present, it is not possible to predict which patients may benefit from surgery,[91] nor is it clear which phase of the surgical procedure is responsible for symptomatic relief when it is obtained. It may be that surgery will be effective in selected cases, but the present state of affairs is clearly unsatisfactory.[92–94]

ACUTE INTESTINAL ISCHEMIC SYNDROMES

Most patients with ischemic bowel disease present with an acute episode. Because of the various anatomic, temporal, physiologic, and etiologic factors that may be operating, these acute syndromes are quite heterogeneous and may present very difficult challenges to the clinician in the evaluation and management of the patient. Among these, several more or less well characterized entities have been defined, and they are described in the following pages. In addition, the material dealing with acute mesenteric arterial occlusion includes a discussion of the assessment and management of patients with bowel infarction from any cause.

Acute Mesenteric Arterial Occlusion

When intestinal blood flow falls below a critical level, ischemic necrosis of the supplied areas of bowel will result.[2] Commonly, this is due to advanced atherosclerotic disease affecting at least two of the major visceral branches of the aorta. In atherosclerosis, it is usually the most proximal segment of the artery, near its takeoff from the aorta, that is most severely involved, but the process may involve more distal portions of the arteries or their branches. Other conditions may also cause mesenteric artery occlusion, including embolism (see below), dissecting aortic aneurysm, and fibromuscular hyperplasia; there is also an association with the use of oral contraceptive agents.[95–99] Oral contraceptives have also been associated with mesenteric venous thrombosis and with segmental ischemic colitis (see below). Systemic diseases associated with vasculitis may involve the mesenteric arterial tree at any of the several points from the major arterial trunks to the intramural arterioles. Vasculitis, as it affects the bowel, is considered separately on pages 1916 to 1918.

Clinical Presentation of Infarction. Acute infarction of the small intestine is dominated clinically by severe abdominal pain that initially may be colicky in nature and periumbilical in location. Early in the clinical presentation, the patient's complaint of pain often appears out of proportion to physical findings or laboratory studies. In this phase of the disease, bowel sounds may be not only intermittently heard but may also even be hyperactive. As ischemia progresses over a period of four to eight hours, pain becomes constant and poorly localized. The only other clinical clue is some elevation of white blood cell count, not always universal, however. At this time examination may reveal nontenderness or slight midabdominal tenderness; although clear signs of infarction with necrosis usually are not yet evident, bowel sounds may noticeably diminish, and the abdomen may be slightly distended. Eight or more hours later in the course, manifestations reflecting progressing infarction and necrosis appear. The abdomen is distended (variably), is tender to palpation midabdominally, and usually rebound tenderness may be elicitable. The patient may pass blood per rectum or via nasogastric tube. Systemic signs appear and are usually striking; these signs include tachycardia, hypotension, fever, hemoconcentration, and marked leukocytosis (often in excess of 30,000 cells with a left shift). Ultimately, in 12 to 24 hours, ischemic necrosis becomes transmural, and unequivocal signs of peritonitis appear. At this point, the patient has signs of intestinal ileus and peritonitis and usually has passed blood per rectum, and the diagnosis of bowel infarction is almost inescapable. Unfortunately, it is also at this point that prognosis (with or without surgery) is extremely poor. Accordingly, the chances for the patient's survival will be maximized if the diagnosis of bowel ischemia is considered and established early in the course. This goal can be achieved only if the suspicion of its possibility is high.

Diagnosis. The history and physical examination are often of little help in arriving at a diagnosis. Significant clues may include the history or physical findings of occlusive vascular disease elsewhere in the body, recurrent postprandial abdominal pain suggestive of abdominal angina (in some series as many as 50 per cent of patients presenting with acute thrombotic infarction have given such a history[65]), recent episodes of significant hypotension or anoxia, and evidence of arterial embolization (see below). Laboratory studies are often nonspecific. In addition to the hemoconcentration and leukocytosis noted above, the serum amylase value may be elevated. It has been suggested, based on small numbers of patients and experimental animal studies, that elevations in serum and peritoneal fluid phosphate concentration may be sensitive indicators of intestinal infarction.[100–103] In addition, elevations in serum of intestinal alkaline phosphatase[104] and of N-acetylhexosaminidase, a lysosomal enzyme found in the mucosa of the small intestine,[105] have been proposed as early indicators of intestinal necrosis. The clinical value of these determinations in making an earlier diagnosis of intestinal ischemia and improving patient outcome remains to be proved.

Metabolic acidosis also is often noted, especially late in the course.[106] Blood may be present in nasogastric aspirate or vomitus or in the stool, and there may be clinical and radiographic evidence of ileus, including distended loops of bowel with air-fluid levels (Fig. 101–5). Other radiographic changes, such as the appearance of gas in the bowel wall or in the portal vein (Fig. 101–6), are less frequently seen and usually appear late in the course, but may be helpful when present. Abdominal sonography[107] and, in particular, computed tomography[108] are useful in some patients in suggesting the diagnosis of acute intestinal ischemia or bowel infarction and in differentiating these entities from other conditions which may mimic them, such as acute pancreatitis or a perforated viscus. The sensitivity and specificity of these newer imaging techniques remain to be defined. Experimental animal studies suggest that phosphorus nuclear magnetic resonance spectroscopy may be a sensitive noninvasive diagnostic tool in intestinal ischemia.[109] However, this technique is not currently clinically applicable. A decision regarding angiography in patients with suspected bowel infarction must be individualized.[110, 111] In the patient in whom signs of peritonitis are present, suggesting that perforation may already have occurred, the information to be gained from studies may not justify the necessary

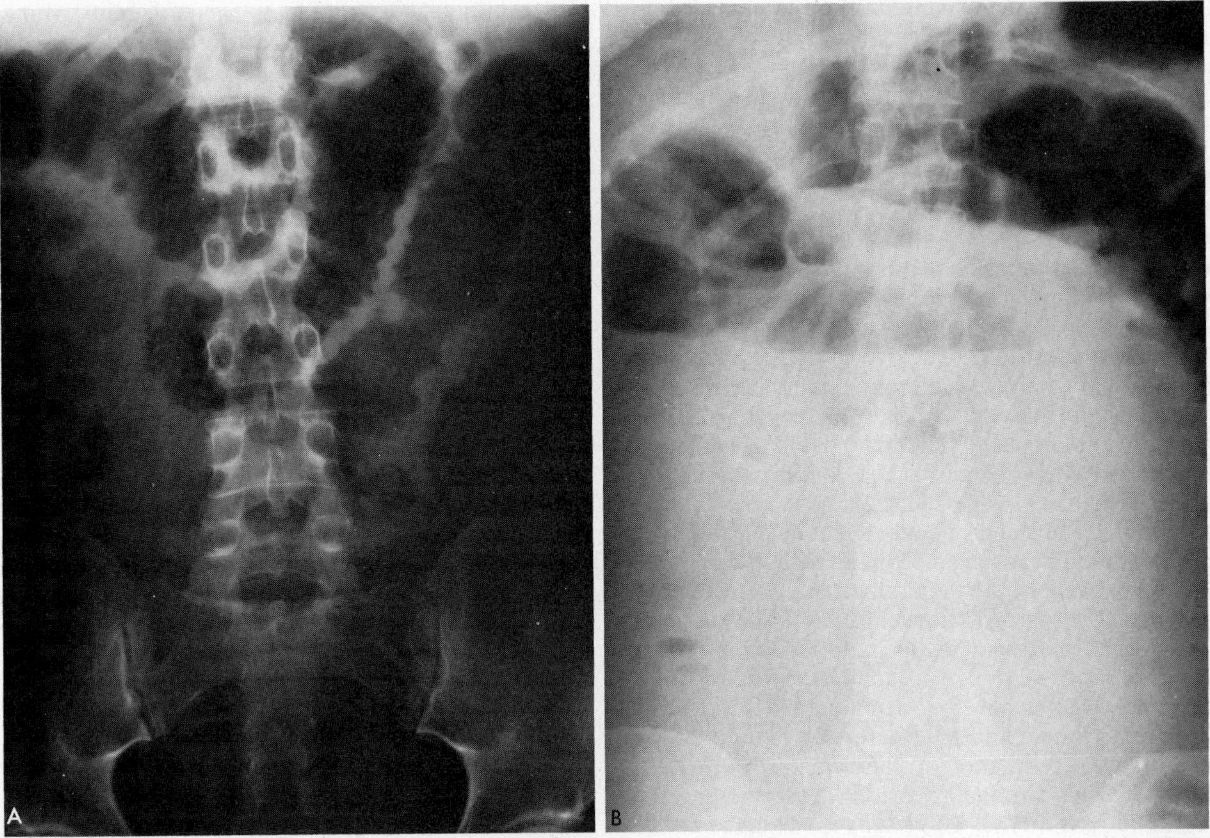

Figure 101–5. Abdominal X-rays in a patient with acute infarction of the small intestine. The supine film *(A)* shows dilatation of loops of small bowel with irregular thickening of the bowel wall. The upright view *(B)* shows small bowel dilatation and multiple air-fluid levels. These radiographic findings should suggest the diagnosis of bowel infarction but may be seen with intestinal obstruction of various causes.

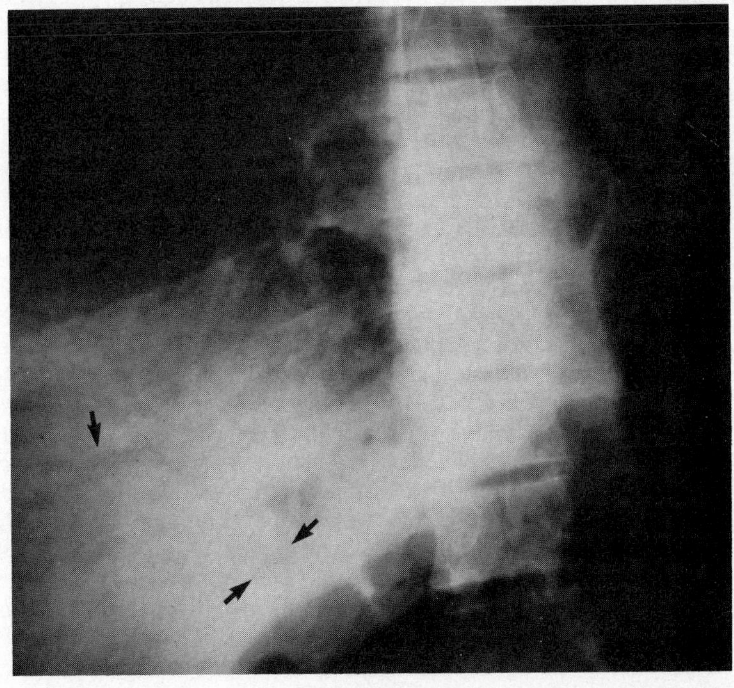

Figure 101–6. In this plain film of the right upper quadrant, gas may be seen in the portal vein and its intrahepatic radicles *(arrows.)* This phenomenon does not occur until an advanced stage of acute bowel infarction is reached, and represents extensive loss of epithelial and vascular integrity with invasion of gas-forming organisms. (Courtesy of Henry I. Goldberg, M.D.)

delay in surgical management. If the patient is seen early, however, angiography may help define the nature and extent of the occlusive process or, in the absence of major vessel occlusion, suggest the diagnosis of nonocclusive infarction (see below).

The keys to correct diagnosis and possible salvage, in addition to suspicion, are alertness to the disparity between pain and physical findings in the early hours of the event, and the recognition that diminution of pain and bowel sounds and the appearance of early ileum with abdominal tenderness are evidence of beginning infarction. Evidence—local and systemic (bleeding, lactic acidosis, unequivocal ileus, or signs of peritonitis)—of completed infarction with necrosis and perforation help the clinician only to realize that the opportunity for effective treatment has been missed. Ideally, surgery must be performed within six hours of the onset of pain.

Treatment. The management of patients with progressing bowel infarction can be divided into two major categories: supportive and operative. Supportive management includes nasogastric suction, appropriate fluid and electrolyte replacement (including albumin, fresh frozen plasma, or blood), and administration of antibiotics after cultures have been obtained.

Fluid replacement must be carefully monitored in order to avoid precipitation of acute congestive cardiac failure. Although cardiac glycosides cause mesenteric vasoconstriction and thus potentially may reduce intestinal perfusion even further, these agents should not be withheld if they are otherwise indicated. In the management of shock not correctable by appropriate volume replacement, those sympathomimetic amines (e.g., norepinephrine) which adversely affect intestinal perfusion and may precipitate renal failure by reducing blood flow to the kidneys should be avoided. Dopamine, in low doses, may be used if a pressor agent is necessary. Because congestive heart failure or uncorrectable shock or both worsen the already poor prognosis of bowel infarction, the primary objective of initial management should be to prepare the patient for possible surgery before these complications arise.

In the treatment of patients judged to be sufficiently stable to tolerate angiography, the use of vasodilators infused through a catheter placed at angiography has been advocated to treat the severe vasospasm frequently observed in the setting of intestinal ischemia.[2, 112] Papaverine (30 to 90 mg per hour) has been the agent most commonly employed.[2, 112] Tolazoline has also been used in this setting.[2] In experimental studies of intestinal ischemia in rats, intravenous infusions of glucagon, methylprednisolone, or prostacyclin have also been shown to be beneficial.[113] Although appealing on a theorectical basis, the efficacy of vasodilator therapy in this situation has yet to be established conclusively in good prospective clinical trials.

At surgery, revascularization of viable bowel or resection of necrotic bowel is the primary objective. Revascularization of yet viable intestine or of viable intestine remaining after resection of infarcted segments is via bypass graft, embolectomy, or endarterectomy in selected cases. In those patients who have had resection, revascularization procedures can be undertaken only if their condition is sufficiently stable to permit the additional surgery.[111, 114] A major problem faced by the surgeon at the time of operation is to define the limits of viable bowel in order to limit resection to completely irreversibly diseased intestine, thus minimizing postoperative malabsorption due to the short bowel syndrome (see pp. 1106–1112). In addition to the visual assessment of intestinal coloration and peristalsis and the palpation of mesenteric pulses, other recent intraoperative techniques to assess viability have included electromyography,[115] Doppler ultrasonography,[116] the injection of radioactive microspheres,[117] and intraoperative fluorescein angiography.[118] Because of the difficulty in determining intestinal viability at surgery, it is often necessary for the surgeon to perform a "second-look" operation 12 to 36 hours after the initial exploration to identify and resect any additional bowel that in the interim proved to be nonviable.[119]

Mesenteric Arterial Embolization

When arterial *emboli* interfere with the blood supply to the abdominal viscera, they most commonly lodge in the superior mesenteric artery.[2] As noted earlier, the caliber of this vessel and the obliquity of its takeoff from the abdominal aorta account for this predisposition. Emboli to the celiac axis, and particularly to the inferior mesenteric artery, are less common. The vast majority of mesenteric emboli occur in patients who have valvular or atherosclerotic heart disease with mural thrombi in the heart. Emboli may also arise from vegetations of *bacterial endocarditis, valvular prostheses,* or *atrial myxomas* or from *atherosclerotic plaques* in the thoracic or upper abdominal aorta, either spontaneously or during angiography.[120] Patients may give a history of previous embolic episodes, or there may be evidence of simultaneous peripheral embolization (brain or extremities). Typically, the event is signaled by a very abrupt onset of severe midabdominal cramping pain, accompanied by vomiting or diarrhea. Bleeding and evidence of intestinal obstruction are absent initially, and although the subjective impression of severe illness is obvious to both patient and physician, objective findings are deceptively sparse because the abdomen is soft and bowel sounds are active. If the process is not recognized and treated properly, mesenteric embolus will lead to bowel infarction and the clinical manifestations described on page 1910.

On the other hand, the characteristic clinical setting in which this event occurs (a patient with atrial fibrillation or other known heart disease) and its abrupt, almost unmistakable onset offer a greater opportunity for early diagnosis and operative treatment. For these reasons as well as the fact that the patients are on the average younger, the prognosis is generally more favorable than with nonembolic causes of bowel infarction.[119, 122]

As soon as the diagnosis is apparent and the patient's condition suitable, laparotomy with embolectomy should be carried out. Preoperative angiography, if performed, will confirm the presence of an occluded vessel. The use of intra-arterial infusion of vasodilators for this disorder has been advocated.[112, 123] Often the absence of collateral flow will indicate the acute nature of the process. Fortunately, the majority of emboli lodge within the proximal few centimeters of the superior mesenteric artery and are accessible at the time of surgery. As is the case with thrombotic infarction, it may not be possible for the surgeon to determine reliably the extent of viable bowel, and a "second-look" operation may be necessary. However, early operation after superior mesenteric embolization may permit complete recovery of the intestine with no resection being required.[119] Such patients generally fare quite well, although a transient but self-limited malabsorption syndrome may persist for several months.

Nonocclusive Intestinal Infarction

In many patients with intestinal infarction, occlusion of the mesenteric arteries cannot be demonstrated. This syndrome of nonocclusive intestinal infarction has been recognized with increasing frequency and in some series is the most common cause of visceral ischemia.[1, 2] Usually, these patients tend to be younger than patients with mesenteric vascular obstruction; they exhibit severe congestive cardiac failure, shock, or anoxia; or they may have sustained a recent myocardial infarction. Occasionally, however, a precipitating event is not identifiable.[1, 2, 111, 124–128] In the presence of inadequate cardiac output and generally poor tissue perfusion, blood flow distribution favors the brain and other vital organs, and mesenteric flow falls disproportionately. The use of α-adrenergic vasoconstrictors in such patients with shock adds to the effect of an already increased secretion of endogenous catecholamines and further reduces mesenteric flow. As perfusion pressure falls in the splanchnic bed to below a critical level (closing pressure), tension in the arteriolar walls may lead to collapse of vessels. Many patients with this syndrome have been receiving digitalis glycosides as well; although these agents cause mesenteric vasoconstriction, their role in the pathogenesis of nonocclusive infarction remains uncertain. Some patients with this disorder may have evidence of occlusive disease in the smaller splanchnic vessels, and these lesions may contribute to the ischemia.[129]

Of the various layers of the intestinal wall, the mucosa has the greatest requirement for blood flow because of its high degree of metabolic activity. Thus, it is most sensitive to anoxia. In some patients, only this portion of the bowel will undergo hemorrhagic necrosis. In others, infarction is transmural, resulting in a clinical picture indistinguishable from mesenteric artery thrombosis. At surgery or autopsy, areas of infarction are often found to be patchy and irregular in distribution and do not necessarily conform to the area supplied by a major vessel.

The diagnosis of nonocclusive intestinal infarction should be suspected in patients with recent myocardial infarction, congestive cardiac failure, shock, or anoxia who develop signs of intestinal infarction, with or without bleeding. Early angiography in this setting has been proposed.[111, 124, 130–133] Demonstrated absence of major vessel occlusion excludes thrombotic or embolic infarction, and it has been suggested that a pattern of angiographic findings is relatively specific for the syndrome. These include (1) narrowed and irregular branches of the superior mesenteric artery, (2) spasm of the arcades, and (3) impaired filling of the intramural vessels.[127] These angiographic findings are present in perhaps 50 per cent of such patients.[134]

Angiography in this syndrome may be useful for two major reasons. First, by excluding occlusive arterial disease, it may provide additional time for resuscitation and stabilization of the patient prior to surgery. Second, there may be a role for intra-arterial vasodilators in the nonoperative or preoperative management of these patients,[111, 124, 133–136] as mesenteric vasoconstriction may persist even after the hemodynamic factors that precipitated the event have been corrected. Despite the physiologic and clinical attractiveness of this approach, it is based on limited clinical experience. Although a number of potential vasodilators have been considered (including histamine, phenoxybenzamine, isoproterenol, papaverine, dopamine, methylprednisolone, gut peptides, and PGE_1), the therapeutic efficacy of such an approach remains to be established. Furthermore, there is a significant error in angiographic diagnosis.[134] In view of these considerations and the very poor prognosis associated with the syndrome, there is ample clinical, scientific, and ethical justification for a controlled prospective evaluation of these new therapeutic approaches in centers with adequate angiographic and surgical capability.

As with thrombotic infarction, supportive management is directed at maintaining blood pressure, oxygenation, and cardiac output; treating infection, if present; and replacing fluid and electrolytes. A major dilemma arises in weighing the decision to operate on a patient with cardiac failure and signs suggestive of bowel infarction. It is clear that, unoperated, this circumstance carries an exceedingly high mortality rate. Conversely, the surgical procedure itself may prove fatal in patients with decompensated heart disease. Generalizations are impossible in such matters, but the presumptive diagnosis of intestinal infarction accompanied by peritonitis should be regarded as an indication for surgical exploration as soon as the patient's condition permits so that necrotic bowel may be resected. If there is no evidence of peritonitis, then angiography, in addition to the usual resuscitative measures, may facilitate the evaluation and management of these patients.

Colonic Ischemia

As with the small intestine, the response of the colon to vascular insufficiency depends on several factors, including the location and extent of occlusive disease and possible associated systemic disorders.[137] Thus, ischemia of the colon may accompany nonthrombotic infarction of the small intestine in patients with cardiac failure or may result from interruption of the colonic blood supply during an abdominal aortic aneurysmectomy or abdominoperineal resection. Following aortoiliac reconstruction, the incidence of colonic ischemia reportedly approximates 0.5 to 2.0 per cent,[138–141] although it seems likely that in many patients with mild or transient symptoms, the syndrome may go unrecognized.[138] In support of this concept, an incidence of 6.8 per cent was reported among patients undergoing routine colonoscopy an average of 2.8 days after abdominal aortic reconstruction.[142] Colonic ischemia usually appears within the first few postoperative days but may be seen as late as two weeks.[138] To reduce the incidence of this potentially lethal complication, it has been suggested that preoperative angiography and intraoperative evaluation of the inferior mesenteric and other visceral arteries (e.g., by Doppler ultrasound) be performed.[143] Ischemic colitis attributed to loss of the inferior mesenteric artery or of an important collateral is not as common after abdominoperineal resection of the rectum.[144, 145] In many cases, symptoms develop in the early postoperative period, but in some, ischemia may not present until several years have elapsed. For this reason, the validity of the relationship has been questioned.[144, 145]

Colonic ischemia may result from localized occlusive disease in the inferior mesenteric artery or in its critical collateral channels.[124, 137] Less commonly, the syndrome is associated with hypercoagulable states, amyloid, vasculitis,[146, 147] ruptured aortic aneurysm,[148] obstructing colorectal cancer,[149, 150] bilateral nephrectomy or renal transplanation,[151] or the use of ergots,[158] vasopressin,[159] or oral contraceptive agents.[96, 99, 152–157] Oral contraceptive–associated ischemic colitis is typically segmental in its distribution. It should be noted, however, that a cause-and-effect relationship has not been conclusively established and that similar colonic lesions of uncertain cause have been observed in young persons not using these agents.[160] These same reservations apply to small bowel infarction and mesenteric venous thrombosis associated with oral contraceptives.

It has become evident that the syndrome of ischemic colitis may be quite variable in its extent, severity, and prognosis. Extensive infarction, gangrene, or perforation may result from occlusive disease, nonocclusive ischemia, or surgical interruption of the blood supply affecting all or a portion of the colon. This severe form of colonic ischemia appears to be infrequent, however. More common are the less catastrophic variants that seem to be associated with localized or segmental ischemia. Particularly vulnerable are those areas of the colon that lie on the "watershed" between two adjacent arterial supplies—i.e., the splenic flexure (superior and inferior mesenteric arteries) and the rectosigmoid area (inferior mesenteric and internal iliac arteries).[161–163] As noted, however, the vascular basis for this predilection is not established.[9] Moreover, in small vessel disease any portion of the colon may be affected.

Most patients with ischemic colitis are over 50 years of age and have evidence of vascular disease, usually atherosclerotic. They characteristically present with abrupt onset of lower abdominal cramping pain, rectal bleeding, and variable vomiting and fever. Physical and laboratory findings of left-sided peritonitis may suggest the diagnosis of acute diverticulitis. Some patients give a history of similar symptoms several weeks to months prior to presentation. This clinical course is also typical of younger individuals with segmental ischemic colitis, including those using oral contraceptive agents.

Initial management consists of general supportive measures and broad-spectrum antibiotics.[137, 161, 164, 165] Rarely, the severity of the clinical picture may suggest local or generalized peritonitis; in these cases, because of the possibility of a perforated or infarcted viscus, surgical exploration may be indicated early in the course. In some of these patients, ischemic bowel will require resection and a temporary colostomy with subsequent reanastomosis when the patient's condition improves. In most patients, however, although the process appears acute in onset, clinical signs do not suggest the presence of peritonitis; such patients must be closely observed. Many will stabilize, and pain, distention, and fever will subside without surgical intervention. Subsequent barium enema examination will often show the characteristic picture of intramural hemorrhage and edema, including "thumbprinting," tubular narrowing, "sawtooth" irregularity, and sacculations (Figs. 101–7 and 101–8*A*). In many patients, the clinical process may subside completely with disappearance of symptoms and return of X-rays to normal.[161, 164] In others, however, a residual stricture will remain (Fig. 101–8), and resection may be required.[2]

As noted, ischemic disease may also affect the rectosigmoid area.[137, 162] These patients, also in the older age group, present with abdominal pain, rectal bleeding, and a change in bowel habits. Unlike those with more proximal involvement, however, signs of peritonitis are unusual. Sigmoidoscopic findings are variable and include a picture suggestive of nonspecific proctitis, multiple discrete ulcers, polypoid or nodular lesions that occasionally are blue-black (reflecting underlying hemorrhage), or an adherent pseudomembrane.[162] Rectal biopsy may show ischemic necrosis; in most patients, however, the histologic picture is nonspecific, with variable ulceration, crypt abscesses, submucosal inflammation and fibrosis, and thrombosis in small vessels.[137, 162] Radiographic changes, if present, are similar to those noted previously, i.e., thumbprinting early and, perhaps, smooth narrowing after recovery.[162]

The differentiation of ischemic colitis from nonspecific ulcerative colitis or proctitis, infections of the colon, Crohn's disease of the colon, or other forms of colitis may be difficult or impossible on the basis of

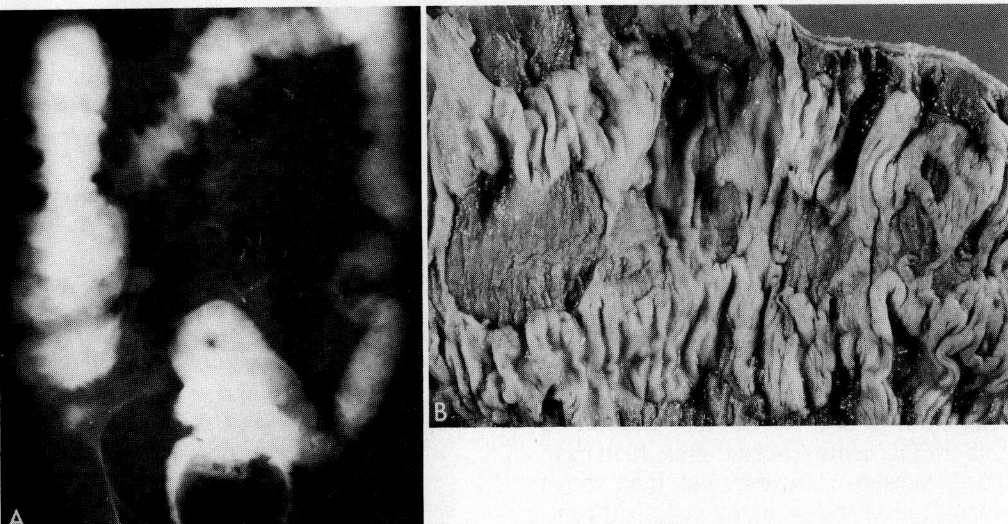

Figure 101–7. *A,* Barium enema, showing large nodular impressions (thumbprinting) in ascending and transverse colon of a patient with ischemic colitis, with ulcerations in the descending colon *(B).* (Courtesy of Henry I. Goldberg, M.D.)

clinical evidence alone. It may occur in younger patients, not all of whom have an apparent predisposing cause.[166] Furthermore, ischemic colitis has even been reported to cause a picture of "toxic dilatation."[167, 168] Histologic examination may also fail to differentiate these various diseases. However, it is important to consider the diagnosis of ischemic colitis in patients in the older age group who present with what appears to be an initial episode of acute ulcerative colitis.[169, 170] Angiography may rarely be helpful in establishing the presence of vascular disease, but occlusions that are localized to smaller vessels may not be detectable. Moreover, as noted, the presence of mesenteric vascular disease does not by itself establish the diagnosis of ischemic bowel disease. For these reasons, angiography is of very limited value in the evaluation of patients with suspected ischemic colitis.[171, 172]

Mesenteric Venous Thrombosis

Acute thrombosis in the mesenteric venous system occurs less frequently than arterial occlusion, account-

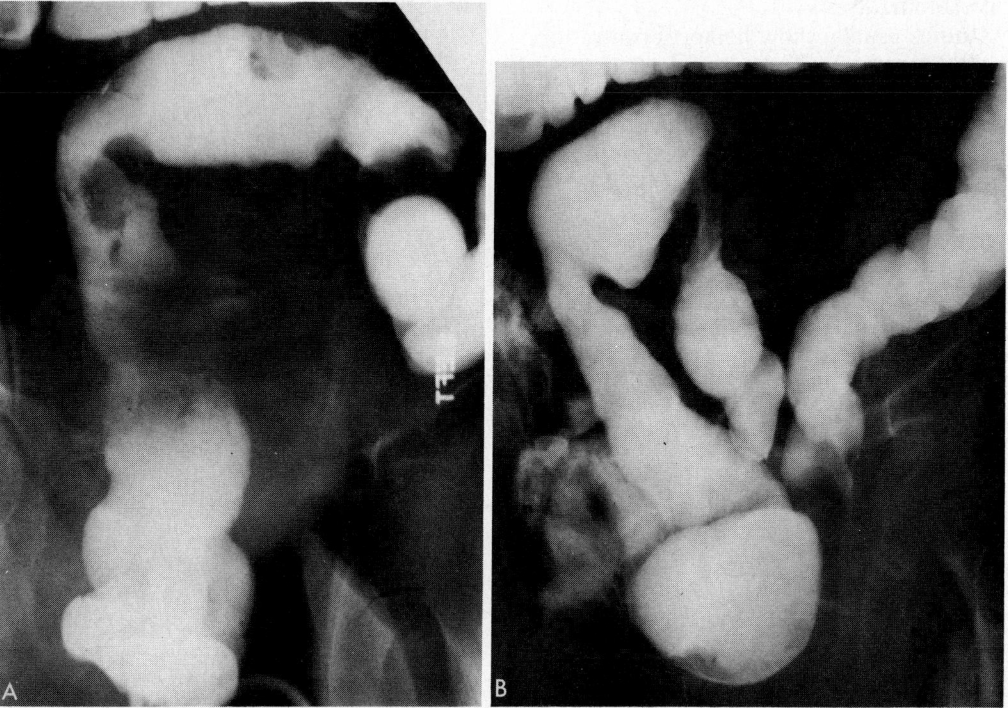

Figure 101–8. Ischemic colitis secondary to amyloid disease. *A,* Large impressions in the sigmoid colon reflect intramural hemorrhage. Sigmoidoscopy showed blue nodular masses. *B,* Follow-up study, three weeks later, shows healing with two strictures present in sigmoid colon. (Courtesy of Henry I. Goldberg, M.D.)

ing for approximately 5 to 15 per cent of patients with intestinal ischemia in recent reports. Within this group, the thrombotic process involves the superior mesenteric vein in about 95 per cent of patients.[172]

Mesenteric venous thrombosis is associated with a variety of conditions. These include disorders predisposing to stasis in the mesenteric venous bed (portal hypertension, congestive heart failure), abdominal neoplasms, intra-abdominal inflammation (peritonitis, abscess, inflammatory bowel disease), abdominal surgery or trauma, and a variety of presumed hypercoagulable states (including antithrombin III deficiency, polycythemia vera, and migratory thrombophlebitis).[173] It has also been reported to occur in association with the use of oral contraceptives.[173, 174] In addition, a substantial number of patients reported since 1950 have had no evident predisposing cause and have been regarded as having primary mesenteric venous thrombosis.[175–177] It is possible that many of the patients included in this latter group could be demonstrated to have a coagulation inhibitor deficiency or some other change in their thrombostatic system if subjected to extensive coagulation studies.

Clinically, the disease may present as an acute abdominal catastrophe, similar to that observed in infarction secondary to acute arterial insufficiency. In many cases, however, the process may be more gradual, with development of progressive abdominal discomfort over a period of weeks. Nausea and vomiting are present in about one half of patients, whereas changes in bowel habits, hematemesis, and melena or hematochezia are less frequent. Physical findings are nonspecific, and patients usually appear sicker and in more pain than would be expected from other aspects of the physical examination.

Laboratory studies usually show hemoconcentration and a moderate leukocytosis. The presence of a small amount of bloody peritoneal fluid is typical and may be an important clue to the diagnosis in patients with a subacute clinical course. X-ray studies are often abnormal, demonstrating dilatation of the small intestine with thickening and irregularity of the bowel wall.[178, 179] Both computed tomography (Fig. 101–9)[180] and abdominal sonography[107] have been reported as offering an early, noninvasive means of establishing the diagnosis in some patients. Selective superior mesenteric angiography shows intense spasm of the arteries to the involved segment of bowel and absence of venous drainage.[178, 181]

The diagnosis is confirmed at surgery by the persistence of arterial pulsations coupled with extrusion of thrombus from cut venous surfaces. Histologic examination of resected bowel demonstrates thrombosed veins accompanied by totally patent arteries (Fig. 101–10). Treatment, as with other forms of bowel infarction, is supportive and operative. Infarcted bowel is resected along with its mesentery. Reconstructive venous surgery is not generally practical, although in a few selected cases, thrombectomy alone without intestinal resection apparently has been successful.[173] Because about 25 per cent of patients may experience a

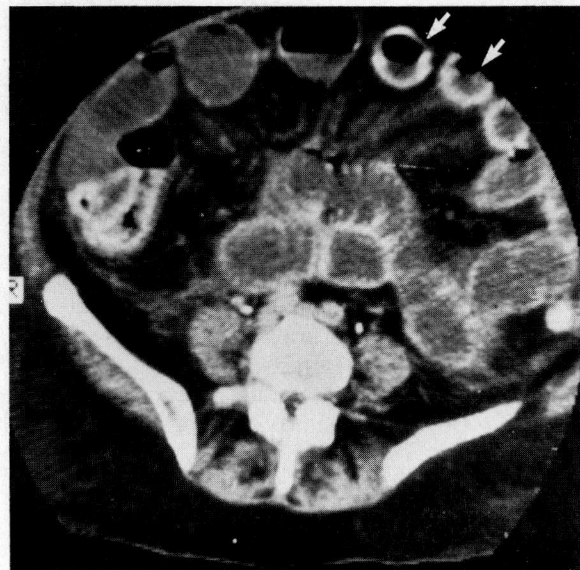

Figure 101–9. Computed tomography (CT) following intravenous injection of a contrast medium in a patient with mesenteric venous thrombosis. The small bowel loops *(arrows)* show air-fluid levels and marked enhancement of the bowel wall due to stasis resulting from the venous thrombosis. (Courtesy of Peter Humphreys, M.D., and Robert Berk, M.D.)

recurrence within the first several weeks postoperatively, anticoagulation is recommended except in individuals who have underlying disease processes that would make this hazardous (e.g., in patients with cirrhosis and portal hypertension, severe trauma, polycythemia vera, neoplasms).[173, 176, 182] In addition, patients should undergo prompt surgical re-exploration in a search for recurrent thrombosis if there is unexplained clinical deterioration following initial surgery.

In general, the overall prognosis of mesenteric venous occlusion is more favorable than that of arterial disease. The mortality rate, reported earlier to be from 50 to 80 per cent,[176] may now be as low as 20 per cent,[2] although it remains higher in some series.[175]

OTHER DISORDERS AFFECTING THE SPLANCHNIC CIRCULATION

Vasculitis

Occlusive disease of the visceral arteries may complicate a variety of systemic conditions associated with vasculitis. This large and diverse group of disorders has been classified on the basis of the nature of the vascular lesion and the vessels involved.[183–185] Depending on the particular disease, the inflammatory occlusive process may involve the larger main arterial trunks, the smaller vasa recta, or the intramural vessels. When larger vessels are involved, as in polyarteritis nodosa or the vasculitis associated with rheumatoid arthritis,[186] the patient is somewhat more likely to present with symptoms and signs of an acute abdomen than is the case in small vessel disease,[187] but there are

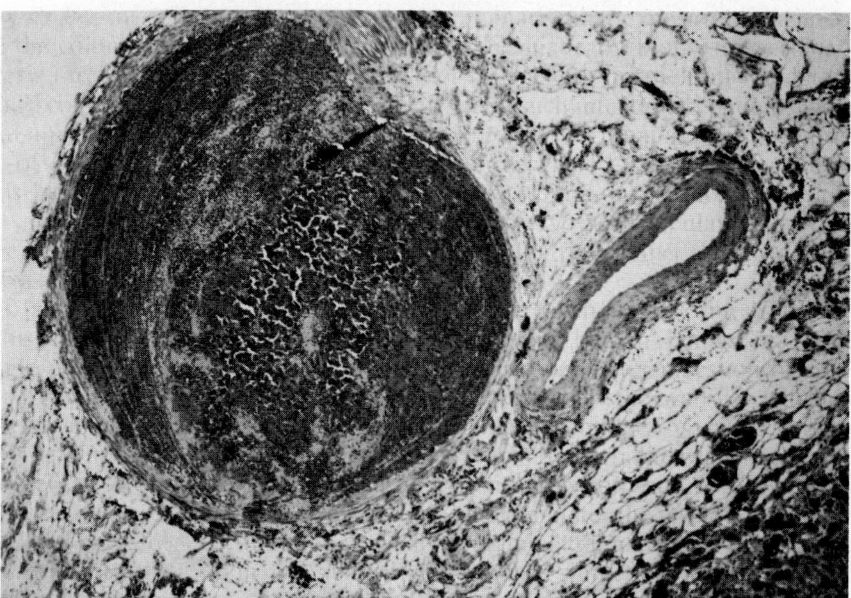

Figure 101–10. Photomicrograph of a section taken from an operative specimen of small intestine in a patient with mesenteric venous thrombosis. This shows a completely thrombosed mesenteric vein adjoining a totally patent artery. (× 20.) (Courtesy of Edward Smuckler, M.D.)

exceptions. Although the abdominal findings may be indistinguishable from those of atherosclerotic or embolic infarction, mesenteric and intestinal vasculitis is usually associated with other evidence of systemic disease; for example, renal involvement, eosinophilia, and hypertension in polyarteritis, or rheumatoid nodules and a very high serum titer of rheumatoid factor in rheumatoid vasculitis.[185, 188] Involvement of medium-sized arteries by vasculitis may also lead to the formation of aneurysms, the demonstration of which is strongly suggestive of polyarteritis nodosa,[184, 185] and the rupture of which may be a cause of gastrointestinal or intra-abdominal hemorrhage.

Vasculitis may affect primarily the vasa recta and intramural arteries and arterioles in virtually all the disorders associated with systemic vasculitis, including lupus erythematosus,[189–192] dermatomyositis, polyarteritis, Henoch-Schönlein purpura ("anaphylactoid purpura"),[193, 194] rheumatoid vasculitis,[185, 187, 188, 190] Wegener's granulomatosis,[185] and Churg-Strauss syndrome[185] (see pp. 505–508). Patients present with abdominal pain, fever, gastrointestinal bleeding (usually, but not invariably occult), diarrhea, or variable evidence of intestinal obstruction; they may develop signs of frank perforation or infarction. Barium contrast studies may show a segment of variable length which is marked by ulceration or a spiculated or thumbprint appearance, reflecting submucosal hemorrhage and edema (Fig. 101–12). This picture may not be distinguishable radiographically from that of regional enteritis. Similar to other forms of ischemic injury, the resulting ischemic necrosis may lead to ulceration, to stricture formation, or less commonly, to perforation.

In *polyarteritis nodosa*, abdominal pain and other gastrointestinal symptoms have been reported in up to 65 per cent of cases.[185, 187, 188] Moreover, about 50 per cent of autopsied cases show vasculitis involving the intestinal tract and liver. Although clinically significant liver disease is uncommon as a result of this process, hepatic artery thrombosis caused by polyarteritis has accounted for approximately half of the reported cases of spontaneous infarction of the liver. Clinically apparent ischemic disease of the bowel is more frequent, and may range from massive infarction to segmental ischemia with ulceration, hemorrhage,[195] or perforation.[184, 185, 187, 190, 196] The finding that up to 50 per cent of cases of polyarteritis nodosa are associated with evidence of hepatitis B virus infection is well established,[184, 197–199] and bowel involvement also occurs in this setting.[200]

Lupus erythematosus causes gastrointestinal involvement in 10 to 60 per cent of cases,[184, 191, 201] usually manifest clinically as abdominal pain. Most frequently, such symptoms reflect an arteritis of smaller vessels; and massive bowel infarction is uncommon. However, segmental lesions leading to necrosis and perforation of small bowel or colon have been reported.[146, 191] Venulitis involving the submucosa and muscularis has also been reported, in association with apparent protein-losing enteropathy.[192] In addition, abdominal pain in lupus may be due to serositis or to acute pancreatitis. Furthermore, there is an uncommon but well-documented association of either classic ulcerative colitis or Crohn's disease with lupus erythematosus,[202] and vasculitic changes may be seen in resected specimens in more than 20 per cent of cases of Crohn's disease.[203] Accordingly, gastrointestinal symptoms in patients with lupus may be particularly difficult to evaluate.

Dermatomyositis is noteworthy because of the increased incidence of associated gastrointestinal malignancies in this disorder. Vasculitis may occur, however, and be associated with ischemic bowel ulceration and hemorrhage.

Henoch-Schönlein or anaphylactoid purpura is a disorder of unknown cause associated with small vessels.[183, 187, 188, 193, 194] Classically, it is associated with the clinical triad of palpable purpura, arthritis, and abdominal pain. It affects all ages, and in adults appears to have a mean age at onset of 43 years.[194, 204, 205] The gastrointestinal tract is involved in more than 50 per cent of patients, manifested most commonly by abdominal pain and gastrointestinal bleeding (either upper or lower) and reflecting localized or segmental ischemia and ulceration (Fig. 101–11). Intussusception, gross infarction, and perforation are rare, but all these problems have been reported.[204, 205] In most patients the disease is self-limited, but it has been suggested that the outlook is less favorable in adults, possibly because the syndrome in the older age group is etiologically more diverse.[183, 184, 206] As in the case of lupus erythematosus, distinction of the vasculitis of anaphylactoid purpura from inflammatory bowel disease may be difficult. Corticosteroid therapy has been advocated for protracted or recurrent disease.[183, 184, 207] It is advisable to remember that many of these patients also have evidence of an active glomerulitis.

A number of less common vascular disorders have been associated with ischemic lesions of the bowel. One rare syndrome of progressive occlusive vascular disease (*Köhlmeier-Degos disease*) affects small and medium-sized arteries.[208] It was described initially by Köhlmeier[209] and Degos et al.[210] and involves chiefly the skin ("malignant atrophic papulosis") and intestine. It primarily affects young men, and terminates in intestinal infarction and perforation. This disease is recognized by its characteristic cutaneous lesions.[211] Takayasu's ("pulseless") disease may also affect mesenteric arteries.[212–214] It has been suggested that its reported occurrence in association with Crohn's disease[215] reflects an extraintestinal manifestation of the underlying bowel disease. Giant cell arteritis of the temporal arteritis type has also been reported in association with Crohn's disease.[216] Vasculitis affecting the intramural vessels also occurs in patients using enteric-coated potassium chloride tablets,[217, 218] in Kawasaki disease,[219] in essential mixed cryoglobulinemia[220–221] in C2 deficiency vasculitis,[222] and in radiation injury to the bowel (see pp. 1369–1382). In two reports the association of vasculitis with inflammatory or hyperplastic colonic polyps has been noted.[223, 224] Recently, a new familial syndrome has been described in which hyaline changes of small vessels in the intestine and kidney are associated with various systemic abnormalities and signs of ischemic enteritis.[225]

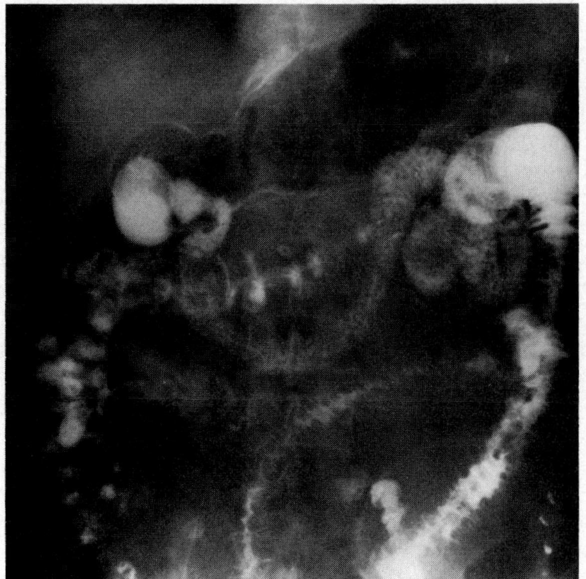

Figure 101–11. Small bowel X-ray series in a patient with anaphylactoid (Henoch-Schönlein) purpura, showing diffuse involvement of the distal jejunum and ileum with thumbprinting and spiculation.

Diagnosis and Management. Usually, the diagnosis of vasculitis of the bowel will be suggested more by the systemic and laboratory features of the disease than by the abdominal findings, which are nonspecific. In contrast to most patients with chronic atherosclerotic mesenteric insufficiency, patients with vasculitis may have steatorrhea in the absence of pain;[226] the mechanism for this has not been established. A radiographic picture of mucosal ulceration or edema (thumbprinting, spiculation) may not be distinguishable from Crohn's disease in either appearance or location (Fig. 101–12). The diagnostic problem is compounded by reports that inflammatory bowel disease may be associated with cutaneous or systemic vasculitis.[203, 207, 215, 216, 227, 228] Although abdominal angiography has been employed to advantage in these disorders,[229] it is principally of value in demonstrating aneurysms at the bifurcations of medium-sized arteries, thereby suggesting the diagnosis of polyarteritis nodosa. Its accuracy in this setting is approximately 75 per cent.[184] Colonoscopic biopsy may be useful in selected cases[230] but often is unrewarding.[185]

As with other types of mesenteric vascular processes, the acute management decisions revolve to a large extent around the question of surgical exploration for possible infarction or perforation. If clinical signs of an acute abdomen are present, surgical exploration may be indicated. The clinical assessment is made more difficult by the fact that many patients with systemic vasculitis are already receiving corticosteroids, and these agents may mask important signs of a serious intra-abdominal process. Continuing clinical, laboratory, and radiographic reassessment is mandatory in such patients, with the expectation that emergency exploration may be required at any time.

Intramural Intestinal Hemorrhage

Bleeding into the wall of the small intestine may occur in a wide variety of clinical situations, including blunt or penetrating abdominal trauma, pancreatic disease, ischemic bowel infarction, vasculitis, uremia, spontaneous or anticoagulant-induced bleeding diatheses, or in unusual association with a variety of conditions such as hiccoughs and duplication of the jejunum.[231–237] Such bleeding may be localized, with formation of a hematoma, or may be more diffuse.

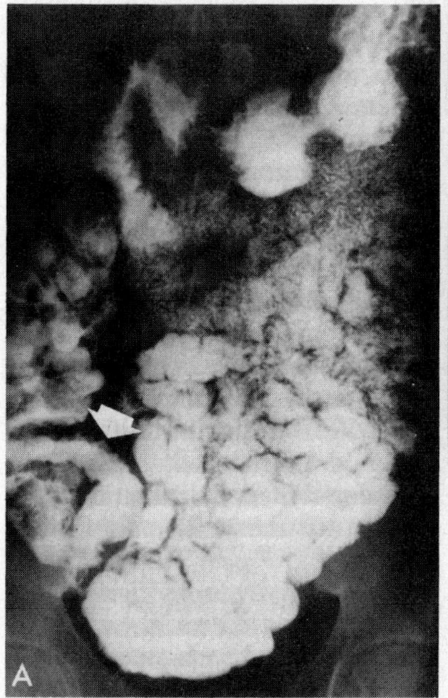

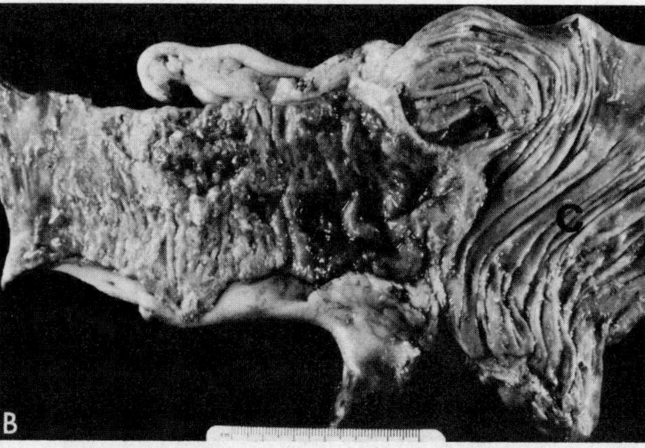

Figure 101–12. Vasculitis affecting the terminal ileum. *A,* The terminal ileum is ulcerated, and separation of bowel loops reflects a thickened mesentery. This patient presented with abdominal pain and diarrhea and was treated with corticosteroids for a diagnosis of regional enteritis. Several months later, significant lower gastrointestinal bleeding occurred, requiring surgery. The terminal ileum was found to be involved by a diffuse vasculitis, affecting the intramural arteries and arterioles. *B,* This is the resected specimen from the case described in *A;* it shows the extensive ischemic ulceration, hemorrhage, and necrosis caused by the vasculitis, involving terminal ileum but not cecum (C). (Courtesy of Henry I. Goldberg, M.D.)

In those cases associated with trauma, the intramural hemorrhage occurs almost always in the duodenum or proximal jejunum, presumably because the bowel at this location is fixed in position and may be compressed against the spine.[231, 232] Clinically, patients may present in one of two ways. A few develop severe abdominal pain, tenderness, absent bowel sounds, and leukocytosis immediately after the traumatic episode. These may be diagnosed erroneously as having a perforated viscus because trauma may perforate the bowel immediately or as a result of necrosis following a latent period.[233] A larger group of patients may not seek medical attention until several days after the traumatic episode, which in some circumstances may have been so slight as to have been disregarded. These patients exhibit the signs and symptoms of partial or complete small bowel obstruction, with pain, vomiting, and occasionally, a palpable mass caused by the presence of the hematoma.

Spontaneous intramural hemorrhage may also develop, either abruptly or over a period of several days, with cramping abdominal pain and variable tenderness, mass, or signs of intestinal obstruction. Hematemesis or melena and fever may be present.[234, 235]

The diagnosis of intramural hemorrhage may be suggested by its characteristic, but nonspecific, radiographic features.[232, 238] On plain film it may be possible to delineate a segment of bowel, separated from adjacent loops, with a narrowed lumen and thickened walls. Barium contrast studies show "cat's paw" or "thumbprint" defects, or a typical "coil spring" or "stacked coins" appearance (Fig. 101–13). The occurrence of this lesion (also seen in bowel infarction) in a patient with heart disease who is being treated with antiocoagulants may raise the diagnostic dilemma of whether one is dealing with hemorrhage or ischemia. In those cases associated with trauma and a large localized hematoma, a mass may be evident.

The treatment of patients with intramural hemorrhage varies with the clinical situation. If the patient is completely obstructed, or if there is strong evidence for peritonitis, the patient should be explored, particularly if seen early after trauma. In most other cases, however, it is possible to manage the patient conservatively, with nasogastric suction, fluid replacement, and correction of a bleeding diathesis.[231, 234–237] Necrosis of the bowel wall is unusual in these patients. Usually, pain and other evidence of obstruction will subside within a few days to a few weeks. The characteristic X-ray findings, likewise, are gone in seven to ten days.

Abdominal Aortic Aneurysm

Abdominal aortic aneurysms are usually atherosclerotic in origin but may occasionally be due to syphilis, trauma, polyarteritis nodosa, or infection (mycotic aneurysm). Atherosclerotic aneurysms nearly always affect the aorta below the origin of the renal arteries and may extend distally to involve the common iliac arteries as well. The aneurysm may be fusiform or saccular in shape; although the true significance of this distinction is uncertain, the latter may be more prone to rupture, an event which is uncommon (fewer than 10 per cent of cases) overall, but which clearly is more likely with those larger than 6.0 cm in diameter.[239]

Most patients with abdominal aortic aneurysms are asymptomatic, but in those who come to elective

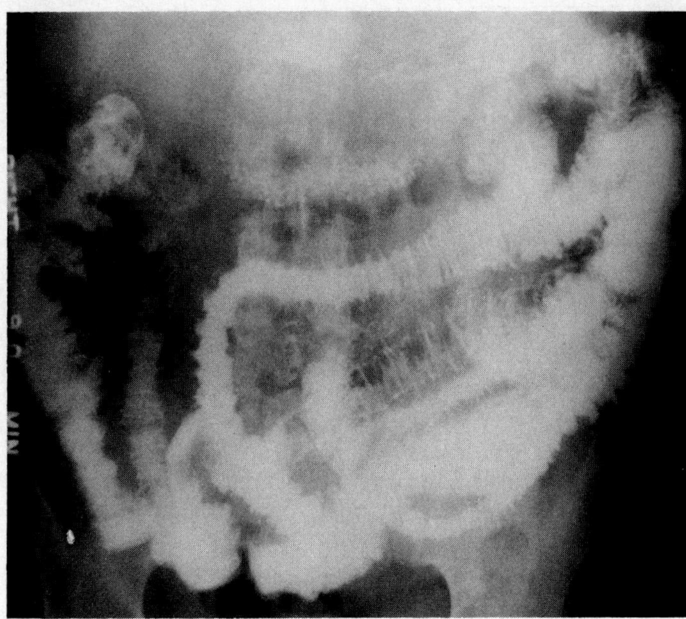

Figure 101–13. Intramural intestinal hemorrhage. This small bowel examination shows separation of loops and thickened mucosal folds, reflecting mucosal, intramural, and intramesenteric hemorrhage, occurring spontaneously in a patient on anticoagulant therapy. (Courtesy of Henry I. Goldberg, M.D.)

surgery there may be abdominal pain, back pain, or leg ischemia.[240–242] On physical examination, a pulsatile mass is often detectable, usually in the epigastrium (the bifurcation of the aorta corresponds roughly to the location of the umbilicus). The pulsations are expansile; differentiation of an aneurysm from an overlying abdominal mass with transmitted pulsations may be facilitated by demonstrating that the pulsations not only are felt directly over the mass but also displace the examining fingers laterally. A bruit may be present, but is usually of no help in diagnosis.

In the uncomplicated aneurysm, laboratory studies are not helpful. Radiographic examination, however, will often show the presence of a soft tissue mass in the region of the abdominal aorta, usually with peripheral calcification. Depending upon the size of the aneurysm, erosion of the lower dorsal and upper lumbar vertebrae or displacement of surrounding viscera, including bowel, kidneys, and ureters, may be evident. Because conventional radiology may not be sufficient to establish the presence or size of an aneurysm, other techniques have gained in popularity. Ultrasound is simple, safe, and highly accurate in the diagnosis and sizing of aneurysms.[243–245] Occasionally, however, sonographic images may be obscured by bowel gas, and this procedure appears to be less sensitive than computed tomography in determining the extent of the process.[245–249]

The major complication is "leakage" or rupture. This event is associated with pain in the abdomen, flank, or back, which may present for several weeks preceding overt rupture. Occasionally, the pain may be worse in the recumbent position and may be relieved by sitting up or by leaning forward, thus suggesting a diagnosis of pancreatic disease. In one series, only 14 per cent of patients referred for treatment of rupture had been known previously to have an aneurysm.[250]

Abdominal aortic aneurysms may rupture in one or more of several directions. Most commonly, bleeding is into the retroperitoneal tissues surrounding the aorta. The predilection for this site probably is due to erosion of the expanding vessel wall by the vertebral column. Abdominal X-rays in this circumstance may show areas of lucency resulting from dissection of blood through the retroperitoneal fat, suggesting the appearance of gas.[251] Less frequently, the aneurysm may bleed into the free peritoneal cavity; in this event, shock supervenes rapidly and the outlook is extremely grave, even when appropriate therapeutic measures (transfusion and surgery) are immediately at hand. An additional site of rupture is into the small intestine, most commonly the third portion of the duodenum, presumably because in this area the intestine is fixed retroperitoneally in close proximity to the aorta itself. Such patients usually present with massive gastrointestinal bleeding, but occasionally bleeding may occur intermittently over a period of weeks.[250–252] Rarely abdominal aneurysms may rupture into the inferior vena cava.

Management. Depending on size and other factors, management of an abdominal aortic aneurysm may include resection or bypass of the involved portions.[253] In elective cases, preoperative angiography has been recommended for demonstrating other significant vascular disease, including stenosis or occlusion of the celiac or superior mesenteric arteries.[240, 254–256] Because these vessels will be important in providing collateral flow to the colon if the inferior mesenteric artery is sacrificed, postoperative bowel ischemia may be avoided by appropriate vascular reconstruction or bypass at the time of aneurysmectomy. As noted in the section dealing with colonic ischemia, it may also be possible to preserve the inferior mesenteric artery.[140] Other authors suggest that aortography should be reserved for those patients with evidence of atherosclerotic or peripheral ischemia, or uncontrolled hypertension or other evidence of renal artery involvement.[257]

The patient with an asymptomatic abdominal aneurysm which has not ruptured may present a major therapeutic dilemma. Factors to be taken into consideration include the propensity of the aneurysm to rupture and the condition of the patient as affected by age and the presence of associated diseases, such as hypertension and coronary artery disease. The operative mortality rate for an elective aneurysmectomy has ranged in the past from 0.8 to 18 per cent, but has decreased significantly in recent years to consistently below 5 per cent in major centers.[240, 258–261] Moreover, the mortality rate increases to 34 to 85 per cent when the procedure is done as an emergency.[241, 242, 250, 253, 262–269] Thus, it is desirable to avoid the need for emergency treatment of ruptured aneurysm by performing an elective aneurysmectomy, but without subjecting patients whose aneurysm may not be a threat, or who are very poor operative risks, to unnecessary surgery.

Opinions on elective surgery vary. Most would agree that aneurysms larger than 6 cm, or demonstrably symptomatic or enlarging aneurysms of any size, should be electively resected in good risk patients.[270] Indeed, a number of centers are finding that the elective operative mortality rate approximates 5 per cent even in high-risk groups.[271–273] Some patients in this latter category may be successfully managed by an alternative surgical procedure in which the aneurysm is reinforced by the introduction into it of 100 to 300 feet of stainless steel wire.[274] The patient with an asymptomatic and nonexpanding aneurysm between 4 and 6 cm in diameter should also be regarded as a candidate for elective aneurysmectomy if the operative risk is acceptable, for the incidence of rupture in this size range approximates 25 per cent.[240] However, the recommended minimum size for elective resection of relatively stable and asymptomatic aneurysms varies from 4.5 cm to 6.0 cm.[271, 272] All would agree, however, that aneurysms that are not treated surgically should be followed ultrasonographically at 3- to 6-month intervals, with the expectation that the size of these aneurysms will increase by an average of 0.40 to 0.48 cm per year.[275, 276] Thus, all would eventually reach a size which would dictate elective resection, if the patient were to live long enough. Asymptomatic aneurysms smaller than 4 cm in diameter have a less than 10 per cent incidence of rupture and are not generally felt to require surgery.[250, 262, 264] However, because these smaller aneurysms do occasionally rupture,[240, 260, 265, 266] they should be followed carefully by periodic ultrasonography;[276] an increase in size or the development of symptoms is an indication for resection.

Paraprosthetic Enteric and Aortoenteric Fistula. An uncommon but potentially catastrophic complication of aortic aneurysmectomy and other procedures in which vascular prostheses are placed in the retroperitoneum or abdomen is the formation of a fistula between the graft and the adjacent bowel, usually the third portion of the duodenum.[277–286] Its incidence is between 0.6 and 2.3 per cent;[264, 287, 288] it may present as early as 21 days postoperatively, but in most cases it is delayed beyond two years and has been reported 14 years later.[277] The complication is thought to result from local conditions at the time of, or subsequent to, the placement of the graft. These include infection, damage to the duodenum or to its blood supply during the dissection, and subsequent erosion of the duodenal wall by the graft.[289] Newer surgical techniques, including the use of nonabsorbable sutures and antibiotics, strict hemostasis, and covering of suture lines with retroperitoneal tissue and peritoneum, may reduce the incidence.

Clinically, patients present with upper or lower gastrointestinal bleeding which may be massive and rapidly fatal if untreated. In a significant number of these patients, however, bleeding may be intermittent, as clot alternately forms and is dislodged from the eroded bowel or fistulous opening. Indeed, often these patients will have a "herald bleed" to be followed by a massive outpouring of blood in hours or a few days. Thus, the pattern of bleeding may superficially resemble that from a number of more common lesions. Upper gastrointestinal endoscopy, to exclude other lesions, and computed tomography, if the patient's condition permits, are helpful in preoperative diagnosis.[290] It is well to remember, also, that the grafts may be infected and a low-grade fever may be present in some patients.

Superior Mesenteric Artery Syndrome

A syndrome of postprandial epigastric pain, distention, and vomiting occasionally may be caused by compression of the third portion of the duodenum between the superior mesenteric artery anteriorly and the fixed retroperitoneal structures posteriorly.[291–293] It is called superior mesenteric artery syndrome and appears to affect most commonly those individuals who are of the "asthenic habitus" who have lost substantial weight. In children, it is seen in those who are growing rapidly, especially in the absence of corresponding gain in weight, or who are fixed in a position of hyperextension by a cast after spinal injury or surgery.[294–297] When possible, assumption of the knee-chest or prone position may afford relief of symptoms, presumably because of an increase in the anatomic angle in which the duodenum lies. Barium contrast studies which show a distended proximal duodenum may suggest the diagnosis,[298] and lateral aortograms have shown a narrowed angle between the aorta and superior mesenteric artery.[299, 300] Generalized disorders of bowel motility, such as scleroderma, must be considered in the differential diagnosis,[300] and the clinical presentation may suggest a diagnosis of anorexia nervosa.[301] Recommended treatment for this syndrome includes the use of small feedings or elemental diets, with the patient lying prone or on the left side after eating. Successful use of parenteral nutrition has been described in several reports.[292, 302, 303] If medical management fails and surgery appears necessary, duodenal mobilization or duodenal-jejunal bypass is reportedly effective in relieving symptoms.[282, 284, 304] Despite these encouraging reports, however, it is important to recognize that apparent compression of the duodenum by the superior mesenteric artery does not reliably indicate that it is causing clinically significant obstruction. For this reason diagnosis of the syndrome must be made only after other possible causes of duodenal stasis have been excluded.

Vascular Malformations of the Gastrointestinal Tract

See also pages 1363 to 1368.

Hemangiomas. Hemangiomas with direct, rapid arteriovenous shunting of blood, are found in the small intestine or colon[305] and are an infrequent cause of gastrointestinal bleeding.[306] These lesions are usually not identified on barium contrast studies and, if in the small intestine, are not readily accessible by endoscopy. Abdominal angiography appears to be a reliable means of establishing the diagnosis.[306] Surgical removal of the involved segment of bowel is the usual treatment.

Vascular Ectasia. Vascular ectasias (also referred to as angiodysplasia) can occur in the gastrointestinal tract in association with diseases involving the skin such as hereditary hemorrhagic telangiectasia (Osler-Weber-Rendu syndrome), blue rubber bleb nevus syndrome, and the CREST syndrome (calcinosis, Reynaud's phenomenon, esophageal hypomotility, sclerodactyly, and telangiectasia).[307] In addition, vascular ectasias may be found as a primary process in the colon or, less commonly, in the stomach or small intestine.[308–310] Vascular ectasias may be responsible both for acute bleeding from either the upper or, more commonly, lower gastrointestinal tract and for chronic gastrointestinal blood loss and anemia.

An association of vascular ectasias with aortic stenosis has been reported but not fully established.[309, 311] In addition, in one series vascular ectasias were reported to be the most common cause of upper gastrointestinal bleeding in patients with chronic renal failure.[312]

Vascular ectasias are composed of ectatic, tortuous submucosal veins and groups of ectatic mucosal vessels lying just under the surface epithelium or, in some cases, on the luminal surface unprotected by any gastrointestinal epithelium.[308] The etiology of these lesions remains uncertain. One theory suggests that in the colon they develop as a result of chronic low-grade or recurring obstruction of submucosal veins as they penetrate the muscularis propria (Fig. 101–14).[308] Another theory proposes that these lesions develop as a result of chronic mucosal ischemia.[313] Others have proposed that vascular ectasia are true congenital arteriovenous malformations.[307] Patients with bleeding from primary gastrointestinal vascular ectasias tend to be over 60 years of age.[308] Vascular ectasias are frequently multiple and are most common in the colon (about 80 per cent).[308]

Vascular ectasias are generally not seen on barium contrast studies of the gastrointestinal tract. Although larger vascular ectasias may be visualized by selective mesenteric angiography, many of the lesions are small and best demonstrated by endoscopy.

Because as many as 25 per cent of individuals over the age of 60 without a history of gastrointestinal bleeding may have vascular ectasias of the colon,[314] asymptomatic individuals should not be treated if vascular ectasias are incidentally discovered at endoscopy. For those patients who have chronic or recurrent gastrointestinal blood loss without other apparent cause, surgery has frequently been recommended if vascular ectasias could be identified and localized (e.g., right colectomy for lesions in the cecum or ascending colon).[308] However, this approach is often unsatisfactory with recurrent bleeding in 15 to 37 per cent of patients[311] either because of the presence of lesions in other parts of the gastrointestinal tract which were not identified at the initial evaluation or because new lesions may subsequently develop. For this reason nonoperative endoscopic approaches are now commonly being employed to obliterate vascular ectasias. Reductions in bleeding episodes and transfusion requirements have been reported following endoscopic treatment with the argon laser, heater probe, or multipolar electrical coagulation (BICAP).[310, 315–317] In addition, use of coagulation biopsy has been described as effective in one study.[318] Following argon laser therapy, patients who had vascular ectasias in the upper gastrointestinal tract were more likely to rebleed than patients with lesions confined to the colon.[310] This may be due to the presence in the former group of additional vascular ectasias in the small intestine beyond the reach of the endoscope (see pp. 416–417).

Varices Resulting from Portal Hypertension

See also pages 405 to 409.

As a consequence of portal hypertension, splanchnic venous blood may be diverted away from the portal vein and liver to the systemic venous system by means of collateral anastomotic channels. Because of their propensity to cause significant upper gastrointestinal bleeding, those venous channels near the esophagogastric junction are the most clinically significant. Esophageal and gastric varices represent massively dilated submucosal veins conveying splanchnic venous blood from the high-pressure portal system to the low-pressure azygous and hemiazygous thoracic veins.

Although variceal hemorrhage most commonly occurs in the distal esophagus or proximal stomach, varices in the colon or small intestine, especially in patients who form vascular adhesions following laparotomy, may cause vigorous variceal hemorrhage.

In the patient with active or recent upper gastrointestinal bleeding, the diagnosis of variceal hemorrhage is best made by upper gastrointestinal endoscopy following adequate resuscitation with intravenous fluids and blood and airway protection, if indicated. Care

VASCULAR ECTASIAS OF THE COLON

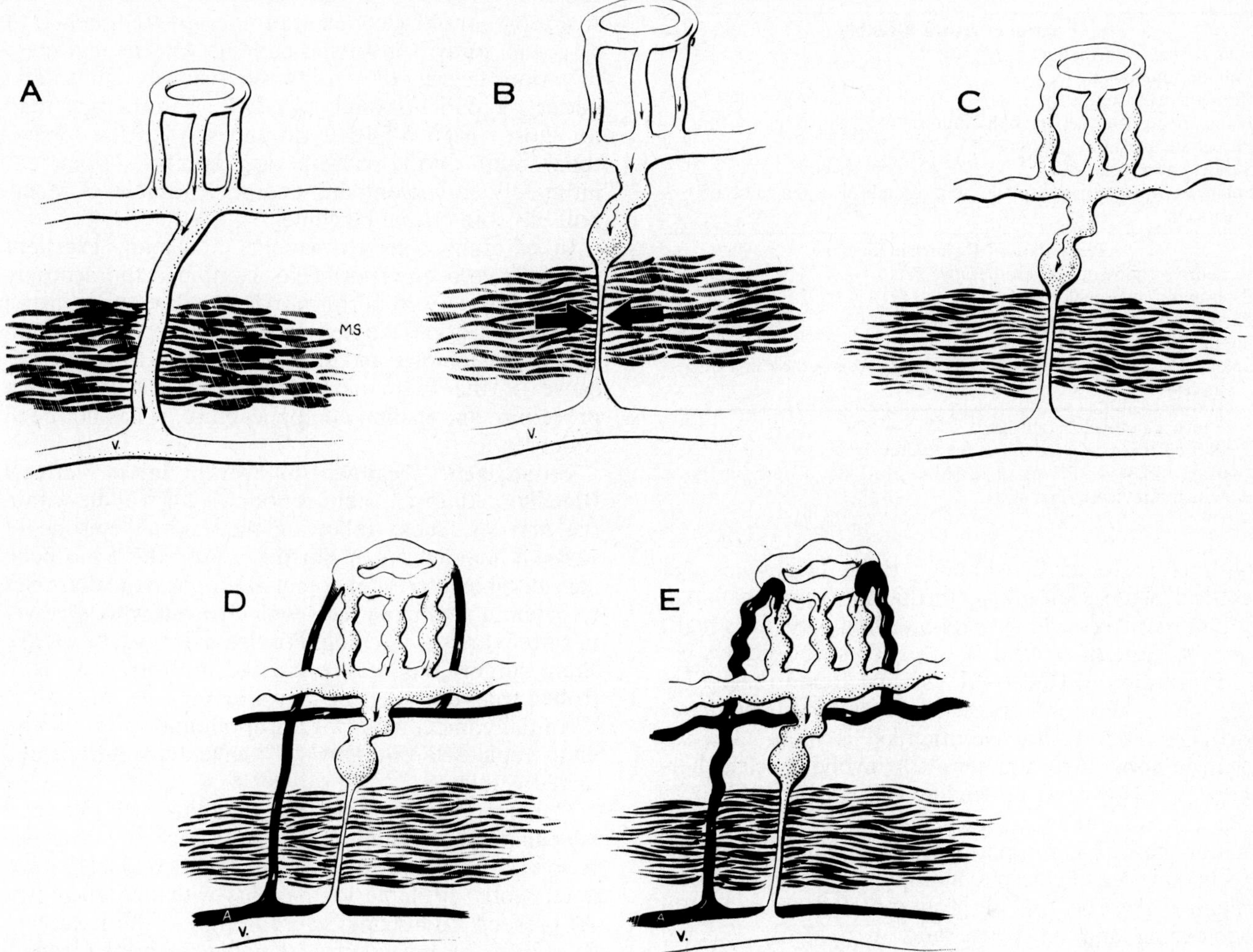

Figure 101–14. Proposed pathophysiology for the development of vascular ectasias. *A,* Normal submucosal vein draining blood from the mucosal capillary ring (top) and venules and passing through the muscularis propria of the bowel wall. *B,* Partial obstruction *(arrows)* due to contraction of muscle or increase in intraluminal pressure. *C,* Continued or repeated obstruction resulting in dilatation and tortuosity of submucosal vein. *D,* Dilatation and tortuosity extending to involve veins and venules draining into submucosal vein. *E,* Dilatation of capillary ring with loss of precapillary sphincter resulting in creation of a small arteriovenous communication through the vascular ectasia. (Reprinted with permission from: On the nature and etiology of vascular ectasias of the colon, by Boley, S. J., Sammartano, R. D., Biase, A., and Sprayregen, S. Gastroenterology *72*[4 Pt. 1]:650–660. Copyright 1977 by The American Gastroenterological Association.)

should be taken not to be overly vigorous in rehydrating patients, because this may elevate central venous pressure, worsen portal hypertension and ascites, if present,[317] and probably exacerbate variceal hemorrhage.

Control of Active Variceal Hemorrhage (Table 101–1). For control of active variceal hemorrhage, endoscopic sclerotherapy is now the procedure of choice with control of bleeding in about 90 per cent of patients.[319, 320] Balloon tamponade therapy can control bleeding in 78 per cent of patients[321] but was less effective than endoscopic selenotherapy in controlled trials,[322, 323] In addition, unlike endoscopic sclerotherapy, balloon tamponade does nothing to alter the rate of rebleeding following acute therapy. Studies evaluating the efficacy of vasopressin have yielded mixed results concerning efficacy and indicate the potential for toxicity.[319] The addition of sublingual or intravenous nitroglycerin in patients receiving intravenous vasopressin has been proposed to ameliorate adverse effects of vasopressin and enhance the reduction in portal pressure.[324] However, this approach has not been shown to improve survival in controlled trials. Control of active variceal hemorrhage has been reported by means of percutaneous transhepatic obliteration of varices. However, this technique has not been widely used because of the technical difficulty of the procedure and high morbidity and rebleeding rates.[325, 326]

Emergency portal-systemic shunt surgery can control active variceal hemorrhage in about 95 per cent of patients but with an operative mortality rate of about 50 per cent.[327] Other operative approaches have included ligation of varices and esophageal transection

Table 101–1. THERAPEUTIC APPROACHES TO THE CONTROL OF VARICEAL HEMORRHAGE

Control of Active Bleeding
Endoscopic sclerotherapy
Balloon tamponade
Intravenous vasopressin*
Percutaneous transhepatic obliteration†
Portasystemic shunt surgery
Surgical devascularization†
Splenectomy (if isolated splenic vein thrombosis is the cause of varices)
Prevention of Recurrent Bleeding
Repetitive endoscopic sclerotherapy
Propranolol hydrochloride*
Portasystemic shunt surgery
Surgical devascularization†
Splenectomy (if isolated splenic vein thrombosis is the cause of varices)

*Efficacy not well established.

†Not currently in wide use in the United States.

From Cello, J. P., et al. JAMA *256*:1481. Copyright 1986, American Medical Association.

with reanastomosis. Although these techniques can control acute variceal hemorrhage in most patients, the mortality rate in actively bleeding patients is high, as is the rate of rebleeding in patients who survive.[328]

Prevention of Recurrent Variceal Hemorrhage (Table 101–1). For prevention of recurrent variceal hemorrhage, endoscopic sclerotherapy is more effective than nonoperative regimens not involving sclerotherapy.[329–333] However, rebleeding still occurs in 13 to 75 per cent of patients, and a number of patients ultimately have required portal-systemic shunt surgery for recurrent bleeding despite multiple sclerotherapy treatments.[329–335] The use of propranolol decreased both rebleeding and mortality rates in a highly selected group of patients with good liver function in France.[336] However, other studies in unselected patients with either good[337] or poor[338] liver function failed to show a benefit.

Although portal-systemic shunt therapy has been shown to be very effective in preventing rebleeding from varices, it does not improve survival compared to nonshunted control patients and results in substantial morbidity from hepatic encephalopathy.[339–342] The selective distal splenorenal shunt was devised to reduce the incidence of postshunt encephalopathy and, perhaps, improve survival by maintenance of portal blood flow to the liver. Some,[343–345] but not all,[346–348] prospective studies indicate a reduction in encephalopathy following distal splenorenal shunt compared to nonselective portal-systemic shunt operations, but no improvement in survival has been observed. In addition difficult-to-control ascites has been a frequent problem following distal splenorenal shunt surgery.[349]

Endoscopic sclerotherapy has been compared with shunt surgery in two prospective controlled trials. In a study of Child's C patients,[335] neither survival nor cost of care was significantly different in patients initially randomized to sclerotherapy compared to those assigned to shunt surgery. Nearly half of the patients randomized to sclerotherapy who survived the index hospitalization ultimately required shunt surgery because of recurrent variceal bleeding despite an intensive program of follow-up sclerotherapy treatments. In a second study[334] involving patients with liver disease of various degrees of severity, survival was significantly better for patients randomized to sclerotherapy than for those assigned initially to undergo a distal splenorenal shunt. Of the sclerotherapy patients, 31 per cent ultimately underwent shunt surgery because of recurrent gastrointestinal bleeding.

In carefully selected patients in Japan, excellent results have been reported for combined thoracotomy and laparotomy to perform extensive esophagogastric devascularization coupled with esophageal transection and reanastomosis and splenectomy.[350] However, because of the tremendous technical difficulty of the procedure and its limited applicability, it has not been widely used.

Prophylactic Treatment to Prevent Initial Variceal Bleeding. Almost 40 per cent of patients will die within the first six weeks following their initial episode of variceal hemorrhage.[351] For this reason there has been considerable interest in potential prophylactic therapies to be employed in patients with cirrhosis who have yet to suffer variceal bleeding. Prophylactic portal-systemic shunt surgery has been evaluated in prospective controlled trials and was not shown to improve survival.[352, 353] Initial clinical trials with propranolol[354, 355] and with endoscopic sclerotherapy[356–360] have thus far yielded mixed results.

Current Approach to the Patient with Variceal Bleeding. The continued high mortality rate resulting from variceal hemorrhage is proof that no ideal therapy is currently available for patients with this diagnosis. At present, endoscopic sclerotherapy is the treatment of choice for the control of active variceal bleeding with employment of balloon tamponade and intravenous vasopressin if sclerotherapy is unsuccessful. Emergency shunt surgery should be reserved only for those patients whose bleeding cannot be controlled by these other means.

For prevention of rebleeding, an attempt should be made to obliterate varices by repeated endoscopic sclerotherapy, although some advocate shunt surgery for Child's A patients. Patients who have three episodes of rebleeding despite this approach should be considered for shunt surgery.

The role of pharmacologic therapy with propranolol or other agents to prevent rebleeding and the efficacy of pharmacologic therapy or endoscopic sclerotherapy as prophylactic treatments remains to be established in well-controlled, randomized clinical trials.

References

1. Boley, S. J., Brandt, L. U., and Vieth, F. V. Ischemic disorders of the intestines. Curr. Probl. Surg. *15*:1, 1978.
2. Marston, A. Vascular Disease of the Gastrointestinal Tract. Pathophysiology, Recognition and Management. Baltimore, Williams & Wilkins, 1986.
3. Clark, R. D., and Gallant, T. E. Acute mesenteric ischemia: Angiographic spectrum. Am. J. Roentgenol. *142*:555, 1984.

4. Cohen, E. B. Infarction of the stomach: Report of three cases of fatal gastric infarction and one case of partial infarction. Am. J. Med. *11*:645, 1951.
5. Kerstein, J. D., Goldberg, B., Panter, B., Tilson, M. D., and Spiro, H. Gastric infarction. Gastroenterology *67*:1238, 1974.
6. Moskowitz, M., Zimmerman, H., and Felson, B. The meandering mesenteric artery of the colon. Am. J. Roentgenol. *92*:1088, 1964.
7. Gonzales, L. L., and Jaffe, M. S. Mesenteric arterial insufficiency following abdominal aortic resection. Arch. Surg. *93*:10, 1966.
8. Reiner, L. Mesenteric arterial insufficiency and abdominal angina. Arch. Intern. Med. *114*:765, 1964.
9. Binns, J. C., and Isaacson, P. Age-related changes in the colonic blood supply: their relevance to ischaemic colitis. Gut *19*:384, 1978.
10. Granger, D. N., Richardson, P. D. I., Kvietys, P. R., and Mortillaro, N. A. Intestinal blood flow. Gastroenterology *78*:837, 1980.
11. Shepherd, A. P. Local control of intestinal oxygenation and blood flow. Annu. Rev. Physiol. *44*:13, 1982.
12. Lanciault, G., and Jacobson, E. D. The gastrointestinal circulation. Gastroenterology *71*:851, 1976.
13. Selkurt, E. E., Rothe, C. F., and Richardson, D. Characteristics of reactive hyperemia in canine intestine. Circ. Res. *15*:532, 1964.
14. Mortillaro, N. A., and Granger, H. J. Reactive hyperemia and oxygen extraction in the feline small intestine. Circ. Res. *41*:859, 1977.
15. Vatner, S. F., Franklin, D., and Van Citter, R. L. Mesenteric vasoactivity associated with eating and digestion in the conscious dog. Am. J. Physiol. *219*:170, 1970.
16. Vatner, S. F., Patrick, T. A., Higgins, C. B., and Franklin, D. Regional circulatory adjustments to eating and digestion in conscious unrestrained primates. J. Appl. Physiol. *36*:525, 1974.
17. Norryd, C., Dencker, H., Lundenquist, A., Olm, T., and Tylen, V. Superior mesenteric blood flow during digestion in man. Acta Chir. Scand. *141*:197, 1975.
18. Folkow, B. Description of the myogenic hypothesis. Circ. Res. *15*(suppl. 1):279, 1964.
19. Johnson, P. C. Origin, localization and homeostatic significance of autoregulation in the intestine. Circ. Res. *15*(suppl. 1):225, 1964.
20. Johnson, P. C. Review of previous studies and current theories of autoregulation. Circ. Res. *15*(suppl. 1):2, 1964.
21. Shepherd, A. P., and Granger, H. J. Autoregulatory escape in the gut: a systems analysis. Gastroenterology *65*:77, 1973.
22. Banks, R. O., Gallavan, R. H., Jr., Zinner, M. J., Bulkley, G. B., Harper, S. L., Granger, D. N., and Jacobson, E. D. Vasoactive agents in control of the mesenteric circulation. Fed. Proc. *44*:2743, 1985.
23. Richardson, D. R. Interaction of systemic and local vascular regulation of the intestinal circulation during systemic infusion of norepinephrine. Cardiovasc. Res. *8*:496, 1974.
24. Guth, P. H., Ross, G., and Smith, E. Changes in intestinal vascular diameter during norepinephrine vasoconstrictor escape. Am. J. Physiol. *230*:1466, 1976.
25. Lautt, W. W., and Graham, S. C. Effect of nerve stimulation of precapillary sphincters, oxygen extraction and hemodynamics in the intestine of the cat. Circ. Res. *41*:32, 1977.
26. Kewenter, J. The vagal control of jejunal and ileal motility and blood flow. Acta Physiol. Scand. *65*(supp. 251):1, 1965.
27. Shepherd, A. P., Pawlik, W., Mailman, D., Burks, T. F., and Jacobson, E. D. Effects of vasoconstrictors on intestinal vascular resistance and oxygen extraction. Am. J. Physiol. *230*:298, 1976.
28. Kern, J. C., Reynolds, D. G., and Swan, K. G. Adrenergic stimulation and blockade in mesenteric circulation of the baboon. Am. J. Physiol. *234*:E457, 1978.
29. Green, M. D. Discussion of intestinal vascular responses to naturally occurring vasoactive substances. Gastroenterology *52*:451, 1967.
30. Swan, K. G., and Reynolds, D. G. Effects of intra-arterial catecholamine infusions on blood flow in the canine gut. Gastroenterology *61*:863, 1971.
31. Pawlik, W., Shepherd, A. P., and Jacobsen, E. D. Effects of vasoactive agents on intestinal oxygen consumption and blood flow in dogs. J. Clin. Invest. *56*:484, 1975.
32. Pawlik, W., and Jacobson, E. D. Effects of digoxin on the mesenteric circulation. Cardiovasc. Res. Cent. Bull. *12*:80, 1974.
33. Ferrer, M. I., Bradley, S. E., Wheeler, H. O., Enson, Y., Preisig, R., and Harvey, R. M. The effect of digoxin in the splanchnic circulation in ventricular failure. Circ. Res. *32*:524, 1965.
34. Bynum, T. E., Hanley, H., and Cole, J. S. Effect of digitalis glycosides on splanchnic blood flow in man. Clin. Res. *22*:509, 1974.
35. Lundgren, O. The circulation of the small bowel mucosa. Gut *15*:1005, 1974.
36. Jodal, M., and Lundgren, O. Countercurrent mechanisms in the mammalian gastrointestinal tract. Gastroenterology *91*:225, 1986.
37. Kampp, M., Lundgren, O., and Nilsson, N. J. Extravascular shunting of oxygen in the small intestine of the cat. Acta Physiol. Scand. *72*:396, 1968.
38. Bond, J. H., Levitt, D. G., and Levitt, M. D. Use of inert gases and carbon monoxide to study the possible influence of countercurrent exchange on passive absorption from the small bowel. J. Clin. Invest. *54*:1259, 1974.
39. Mickflikier, A. B., Bond, J. H., Sircar, B., and Levitt, M. D. Intestinal villus blood flow measured with carbon monoxide and microspheres. Am. J. Physiol. *230*:916, 1976.
40. Bounos, G., Menard, D., and DeMedicis, E. Role of pancreatic proteases in the pathogenesis of ischemic enteropathy. Gastroenterology *73*:102, 1970.
41. Bounos, G. Acute necrosis of the intestinal mucosa. Gastroenterology *82*:1457, 1982.
42. Granger, D. N., Rutili, G., and McCord, J. Superoxide radicals in feline intestinal ischemia. Gastroenterology *81*:22, 1981.
43. Parks, D. A., Bulkley, G. B., Granger, D. N., Hamilton, S. R., and McCord, J. M. Ischemic injury in the cat small intestine: role of superoxide radicals. Gastroenterology *82*:9, 1982.
44. Brown, R. A., Chiv, C., Scott, H. J., and Gurd, F. N. Ultrastructural changes in the canine mucosal cell after mesenteric arterial occlusion. Arch. Surg. *101*:290, 1970.
45. Whitehead, R. The pathology of ischemia of the intestines. Pathol. Annu. *11*:1, 1976.
46. Yamamoto, M., Plessow, B., Koch, H. K., and Oehlert, W. Electron microscopic studies on the small intestinal mucosa of rats after mechanical intestinal obstruction and ischemia. Virchows Arch. B. Cell. Pathol. *32*:157, 1980.
47. Robinson, J. W. L., Mirmovitch, V., Winistorfer, B., and Saegesser, F. Response of the intestinal mucosa to ischemia. Gut *22*:512, 1981.
48. Granger, D. N., Sennett, M., McEleanney, P., and Taylor, A. E. Effect of local arterial hypotension on cat intestinal capillary permeability. Gastroenterology *79*:474, 1980.
49. Dick, A. P., Gruff, R., and Gregg, D. An arteriographic study of mesenteric arterial disease. Gut *8*:206, 1967.
50. Croft, R. J., Menon, G. P., and Marston, A. Does "intestinal" angina exist? A critical study of obstructed visceral arteries. Br. J. Surg. *68*:316, 1967.
51. Marston, A., Clarke, J. M. F., Garcia Garcia, J., and Miller, A. L. Intestinal function and intestinal blood supply: a 20 year surgical study. Gut *26*:656, 1985.
52. Mikkelson, W. P. Intestinal angina: its surgical significance. Am. J. Surg. *94*:262, 1957.
53. Gillespie, I. E. Intestinal ischemia. Gut *26*:653, 1985.
54. Meacham, P. W., and Dean, R. H. Chronic mesenteric ischemia in childhood and adolescence. J. Vasc. Surg. *2*:878, 1985.
55. Cherry, R. D., Jabbari, M., Goresky, C. A., Herba, M., Reich, D., and Blundell, P. E. Chronic mesenteric vascular insufficiency with gastric ulceration. Gastroenterology *91*:1548, 1986.
56. Devroede, G., Vobecky, S., Masse, S., Arhan, P., Zleger, C., Dugay, C., and Hemond, M. Ischemic fecal incontinence and rectal angina. Gastroenterology *83*:970, 1982.

57. Watson, W. C., Williams, P. B., and Duffy, G. Epigastric bruits in patients with and without celiac axis compression. Ann. Intern. Med. *79*:211, 1973.
58. Babb, R. R. Auscultation of the abdomen with reference to vascular sounds. Am. J. Dig. Dis. *18*:1085, 1973.
59. Sarr, M. G., Dickinson, E. R., and Newcomer, A. D. Diastolic bruit in chronic intestinal ischemia. Recognition by abdominal phonoangiography. Dig. Dis. Sci. *25*:761, 1980.
60. Watt, J. K., Watson, W. C., and Haase, S. Chronic intestinal ischemia. Br. Med. J. *2*:199, 1967.
61. Ingelfinger, F. J. Chronic vascular insufficiency of the gastrointestinal tract: abdominal angina. Gastroenterology *45*:789, 1963.
62. Bynum, T. E., and Jacobson, E. D. Blood flow and gastrointestinal function. Gastroenterology *60*:325, 1971.
63. Dardik, H., Seidenberg, B., Parker, J., and Hurwitt, E. Intestinal angina with malabsorption treated by elective revascularization. JAMA *194*:1206, 1967.
64. Williams, R. A., and Wilson, S. E. Radioxenon washout for the diagnosis of low-flow mesenteric ischemia. J. Surg. Res. *28*:217, 1980.
65. Williams, L. F., Jr. Vascular insufficiency of the intestine. Gastroenterology *61*:757, 1971.
66. Stoney, R. J., Ehrenfeld, W. K., and Wylie, E. J. Revascularization methods in chronic visceral ischemia caused by atherosclerosis. Ann. Surg. *186*:468, 1977.
67. Crawford, E. S., Morris, G. C., Myhre, H. O., and Roehm, J. O. F. Celiac axis, superior mesenteric artery occlusion: surgical consideration. Surgery *82*:856, 1977.
68. Hertzer, N. R., Beven, E. G., and Humphries, A. W. Chronic intestinal ischemia. Surg. Gynecol. Obstet. *145*:321, 1977.
69. Connolly, J. E., and Kwaan, J. H. M. Prophylactic revascularization of the gut. Ann. Surg. *190*:514, 1979.
70. Stoney, R. J., and Olcott, C., IV. Visceral artery syndromes and reconstructions. Surg. Clin. North Am. *59*:637, 1979.
71. Rapp, J. H., Reilly, L. M., Qvarfordt, P. G., Goldstone, J., Ehrenfeld, W. K., and Stoney, R. J. Durability of endarterectomy and antegrade grafts in the treatment of chronic visceral ischemia. J. Vasc. Surg. *3*:799, 1986.
72. Connelly, T. L., Perdue, G. D., Smith, R. B., III, Ansley, V. D., and McKinnon, W. M. Elective mesenteric revascularization. Am. Surg. *47*:19, 1981.
73. Stanton, P. E., Hollier, P. A., Seidel, T. W., Rosenthal, D., Clark, M., and Lammis, P. A. Chronic intestinal ischemia: diagnosis and therapy. J. Vasc. Surg. *4*:388, 1986.
74. Furrer, J., Gruntzig, A., Kugelmeier, J., and Goebel, N. Treatment of abdominal angina with percutaneous dilatation of an arterial mesenteric superior stenosis. Cardiovasc. Intervent. Radiol. *3*:43, 1980.
75. Uflacker, R., Goldany, M. A., and Constant, S. Resolution of mesenteric angina with percutaneous transluminal angioplasty of a superior mesenteric artery stenosis using a balloon catheter. Gastrointest. Radiol. *5*:367, 1980.
76. Golden, D. A., Ring, E. J., McLean, G. K., and Freiman, D. B. Percutaneous transluminal angioplasty in the treatment of abdominal angina. Am. J. Roentgenol. *139*:247, 1982.
77. Roberts, L., Wertman, D. A., Mills, S. R., Moore, A. V., and Heaston, D. K. Transluminal angioplasty of the superior mesenteric artery: an alternative to surgical revascularization. Am. J. Roentgenol. *141*:1039, 1983.
78. Dunbar, J. D., Molnar, W., Beman, F. M., and Marable, S. A. Compression of the celiac trunk and abdominal aorta. Am. J. Roentgenol. *95*:731, 1965.
79. Stoney, R. J., and Wylie, E. J. Recognition and management of visceral ischemic syndromes. Ann. Surg. *164*:714, 1966.
80. Snyder, M. A., Mahoney, E. B., and Rob, C. G. Symptomatic celiac artery stenosis due to constriction by the neurofibrous tissue of the celiac ganglion. Surgery *61*:372, 1967.
81. Marable, S. A., Kaplan, M. F., Beman, F. M., and Molnar, W. Celiac compression syndrome. Am. J. Surg. *115*:97, 1968.
82. Edwards, A. J., Hamilton, J. D., Nichol, W. D., Taylor, G. W., and Dawson, A. M. Experience with coeliac axis compression syndrome. Am. J. Surg. *115*:97, 1968.
83. Watson, W. C., and Sadikali, F. Celiac axis compression. Experience with 20 patients and a critical appraisal of the syndrome. Ann. Intern. Med. *86*:278, 1977.
84. Lord, R. S. A., and Tracy, G. D. Celiac artery compression. Br. J. Surg. *67*:590, 1980.
85. Lord, R. S., Stoney, R. J., and Wylie, E. J. Coeliac-axis compression. Lancet *2*:795, 1968.
86. Derrick, J. R., Pollard, H. S., and Moore, R. M. The pattern of arteriosclerotic narrowing of the celiac and superior mesenteric arteries. Ann. Surg. *149*:684, 1959.
87. Charrette, E. P., Iyengar, R. K., Lynn, R. B., Paloschi, G. B., and West, R. O. Abdominal pain associated with celiac artery compression. Surg. Gynecol. Obstet. *132*:1009, 1971.
88. Levin, D. C., and Baltaxe, H. A. High incidence of celiac axis narrowing in asymptomatic individuals. Am. J. Roentgenol. *116*:426, 1972.
89. Szilagyi, D. E., Rian, R. L., Elliott, J. P., and Smith, R. F. The celiac artery compression syndrome: does it exist? Surgery *72*:849, 1972.
90. Colapinto, R. F., McCoughlin, M. J., and Weisbrod, G. L. The routine lateral aortogram and the celiac axis syndrome. Radiology *103*:557, 1972.
91. Evans, W. E. Long term evaluation of the celiac band syndrome. Surgery *76*:867, 1974.
92. Sleisenger, M. H. The celiac artery syndrome—again? Ann. Intern. Med. *86*:355, 1977.
93. Editorial. Coeliac axis compression—a non-syndrome. S. Afr. Med. J. *52*:907, 1977.
94. Brandt, L. J., and Boley, S. J. Celiac axis compression syndrome. A critical review. Am. J. Dig. Dis. *23*:633, 1978.
95. Brennen, M. F., Clarke, A. M., and Macbeth, W. A. A. G. Infarction of the midgut associated with oral contraceptives. N. Engl. J. Med. *279*:1213, 1968.
96. Morowitz, D. A., and Epstein, B. H. Spectrum of bowel disease associated with use of oral contraceptives. Med. Ann. D. C. *42*:6, 1973.
97. Nothmann, B. J., Chittinand, S., and Schuster, M. M. Reversible mesenteric vascular occlusion associated with oral contraceptives. Am. J. Dig. Dis. *18*:361, 1973.
98. Martel, A. J., Lillie, H. J., Jr., and Sawaicki, J. E. Hemorrhage and stenosis of the jejunum following course of progestational agent. Am. J. Gastroenterol. *57*:261, 1972.
99. Schneiderman, D. J., and Cello, J. P. Intestinal ischemia and infarction associated with oral contraceptives. West. J. Med. *145*:350, 1986.
100. Jamieson, W. G., Lozon, A. P., Durand, D., and Wall, W. Changes in serum phosphate levels associated with intestinal infarction and necrosis. Surg. Gynecol. Obstet. *140*:19, 1975.
101. Sawyer, B. A., Jamieson, W. G., and Durand, D. The significance of elevated peritoneal fluid phosphate level in intestinal infarction. Surg. Gynecol. Obstet. *146*:43, 1978.
102. Jamieson, W. G., Marchuk, S., Rowson, J., and Durand, J. The early diagnosis of massive acute intestinal ischemia. Br. J. Surg. *69*:552(suppl.), 1982.
103. Ferretis, C. B., Koborozos, B. A., Vyssoulis, G. P., Manouras, A. J., Apostolidis, N. S., and Golematis, B. C. Serum phosphate levels in acute bowel ischemia. An aid to early diagnosis. Am. Surg. *51*:242, 1985.
104. Barnett, S. M., Davidson, E. D., and Bradley, E. L., III. Intestinal alkaline phosphatase and base deficit in mesenteric occlusion. J. Surg. Res. *20*:243, 1976.
105. Polson, H., Mowat, C., and Himal, H. S. Experimental and clinical studies of mesenteric infarction. Surg. Gynecol. Obstet. *153*:360, 1981.
106. Cooke, M., and Sande, M. A. Diagnosis and outcome of bowel infarction on an acute medical service. Am. J. Med. *75*:984, 1983.
107. Phillips, G., and Dimitrieva, Z. Sonographic diagnosis of thrombosis of the superior mesenteric vein and small bowel infarction. J. Ultrasound Med. *4*:565, 1985.
108. Federle, M. P., Chun, G., Jeffrey, R. B., and Rayor, R. Computed tomographic findings in bowel infarction. Am. J. Radiol. *142*:91, 1984.

109. Blum, H., Summers, J. J., Schnall, M. D., Barlow, C., Leigh, J. S., Jr., Chance, B., and Buzby, G. P. Acute intestinal ischemia studies by phosphorus nuclear magnetic resonance spectroscopy. Ann. Surg. *204*:83, 1986.
110. Koehler, R. E., and Kressel, H. Y. Arteriographic examination in suspected small bowel ischemia. Am. J. Dig. Dis. *23*:853, 1978.
111. Boley, S. J., Sprayregan, S., Siegelman, S., and Veith, F. J. Initial results from an aggressive roentgenological and surgical approach to acute mesenteric ischemia. Surgery *82*:848, 1977.
112. Borden, C. B., and Boley, S. J. Acute mesenteric ischemia: treat aggressively for best results. J. Critical Illness *1*:52, 1986.
113. Kazmers, A., Zwolak, R., Appelman, H. D., Whitehouse, W. M., Jr., Wu, S. -C. H., Zelenock, G. B., Cronewett, J. L., Lindenauer, S. M., and Stanley, J. C. Pharmacologic interventions in acute mesenteric ischemia: improved survival with intravenous glucagon, methylprednisolone, and prostacyclin. J. Vasc. Surg. *1*:472, 1984.
114. Bergan, J. J., Dean, R. H., Conn, D. J., Jr., and Yao, J. S. T. Revascularization in treatment of mesenteric ischemia. Ann. Surg. *182*:430, 1975.
115. Katz, S., Wahab, A., Murray, W., and Williams, L. F. New parameters of viability in ischemic bowel disease. Am. J. Surg. *127*:136, 1974.
116. Coopermen, M., Martin, E. W., and Carey, L. C. Evaluation of ischemic intestine by Doppler ultrasound. Am. J. Surg. *139*:83, 1980.
117. Zianns, C. K., Skinner, D. B., Rhodes, B. A., and James, A. E. Prediction of the viability of revascularized intestine with radioactive microspheres. Surg. Gynecol. Obstet. *138*:576, 1974.
118. Bulkley, G. B., Zuidema, G. D., Hamilton, S. R., O'Mara, C. S., Klacsman, P. G., and Horn, S. Intraoperative determination of small intestinal viability following ischemic injury. Ann. Surg. *193*:628, 1981.
119. Ottinger, L. W. The surgical management of acute occlusion of the superior mesenteric artery. Ann. Surg. *188*:721, 1978.
120. Lande, A., and Meyers, M. A. Iatrogenic embolization of the superior mesenteric artery: Arteriographic observations and clinical implications. Am. J. Roentgenol. *126*:822, 1976.
121. Rogers, D. M., Thompson, J. E., Garrett, W. V., Talkington, C. M., and Patman, R. D. Mesenteric vascular problems. A 26-year experience. Ann. Surg. *195*:554, 1982.
122. Krausz, M. M., and Manny, J. Acute superior mesenteric arterial occlusion: a plea for early diagnosis. Surgery *83*:482, 1978.
123. Boley, S. J., Feinstein, F. R., Sammartano, R., Brandt, L. J., and Sprayregen, S. New concepts in the management of emboli of the superior mesenteric artery. Surg. Gynecol. Obstet. *153*:561, 1981.
124. Williams, L. F., Jr. Vascular insufficiency of the bowels. DM August 1970.
125. Williams, L. F., Jr., Anastasia, L. F., Hasiotis, C. A., Bosniak, M. A., and Bynne, J. J. Nonocclusive mesenteric infarction. Am. J. Surg. *114*:376, 1967.
126. Jordan, P. H., Jr., Boulafendis, D., and Guinn, G. A. Factors other than major vascular occlusion that contribute to intestinal infarction. Ann. Surg. *171*:189, 1970.
127. Watt-Boolsen, S. Non-occlusive intestinal infarction. Acta Chir. Scand. *143*:365, 1977.
128. Haglund, J., and Lundgren, O. Non-occlusive acute intestinal vascular failure. Br. J. Surg. *66*:155, 1979.
129. Arosemena, E., and Edwards, J. E. Lesions of the small mesenteric arteries underlying intestinal infarction. Geriatrics *22*:122, 1967.
130. Ottinger, L. W. Nonocclusive mesenteric infarction. Surg. Clin. North Am. *54*:689, 1974.
131. Habboushe, F., Wallace, H. W., Nusbaum, M., Baum, S., Dratch, P., and Blakemore, W. Nonocclusive mesenteric vascular insufficiency. Ann. Surg. *180*:819, 1974.
132. Siegelman, S. S., Sprayregen, S. S., and Boley, S. J. Angiographic diagnosis of mesenteric arterial vasoconstriction. Radiology *112*:533, 1974.
133. Athanasoulis, C. A., Wittenberg, J., Bernstein, R., and Williams, L. W. Vasodilatory drugs in the management of nonocclusive bowel ischemia. Gastroenterology *68*:146, 1975.
134. Wittenberg, J., Athanasoulis, C. A., Shapiro, J. H., and Williams, L. F., Jr. A radiologic approach to the patient with acute extensive bowel ischemia. Radiology *106*:13, 1973.
135. Davis, L. J., Anderson, J., Wallace, S., and Jacobson, E. D. Experimental use of prostaglandan E1 in nonocclusive mesenteric ischemia. Am. J. Roentgenol. *125*:99, 1975.
136. Boley, S. J., and Brandt, L. J. Selective mesenteric vasodilators—a future role in acute mesenteric ischemia? (Editorial.) Gastroenterology *91*:247, 1986.
137. Fagin, R. R., and Kirsner, J. B. Ischemic diseases of the colon. Adv. Intern. Med. *17*:343, 1971.
138. Ottinger, L. W., Darling, R. C., Nathan, M. J., and Linton, R. R. Left colon ischemia complicating aorto-iliac reconstruction. Causes, diagnosis, management and prevention. Arch. Surg. *105*:841, 1972.
139. Papadopoulos, C. D., Mancini, H. W., and Martin Marino, A. W., Jr. Ischemic necrosis of the colon following aortic aneurysmectomy. Collective review and case reports. J. Cardiovasc. Surg. *15*:494, 1974.
140. Johnson, W. C., and Nabseth, D. C. Visceral infarction following aortic surgery. Ann. Surg. *180*:312, 1974.
141. Launer, D. P., Miscall, B. G., and Beil, A. R., Jr. Colorectal infarction following resection of abdominal aortic aneurysms. Dis. Colon Rectum *21*:613, 1978.
142. Hagihara, P. F., Ernst, C. B., and Griffen, W. O., Jr. Incidence of ischemic colitis following abdominal aortic reconstruction. Surg. Gynecol. Obstet. *149*:571, 1979.
143. Hobson, R. W., Wright, C. B., Rich, N. M., and Collins, G. J., Jr. Assessment of colonic ischemia during aortic surgery by Doppler ultrasound. J. Surg. Res. *20*:231, 1976.
144. Thomas, M. L., and Wellwood, J. M. Ischemic colitis and abdomino-perineal excision of the rectum. Gut *14*:64, 1973.
145. Henberg, J. W., O'Sullivan, P., and Williams, L., Jr. Ischemic colitis after abdominoperineal resection. Gastroenterology *69*:1321, 1975.
146. Kistin, M. G., Kaplan, M. M., and Harrington, J. T. Diffuse ischemic colitis associated with systemic lupus erythematosus—response to subtotal colectomy. Gastroenterology *75*:1147, 1978.
147. Ferrari, B. T., Ray, J. E., Robertson, H. D., Bonau, R. A., and Gathright, J. B., Jr. Colonic manifestations of collagen vascular disease. Dis. Colon Rectum *23*:473, 1980.
148. Bandyk, D. F., Florence, M. G., and Johansen, K. H. Colon ischemia accompanying ruptured aortic aneurysm. J. Surg. Res. *30*:297, 1981.
149. Seagesser, F., and Sandblom, P. Ischemic lesions of the distended colon. A complication of obstructive colorectal cancer. Am. J. Surg. *129*:309, 1975.
150. Whitehouse, G. H., and Walt, J. Ischemic colitis associated with carcinoma of the colon. Gastrointest. Radiol. *2*:31, 1977.
151. Margolis, D. M., Etheredge, E. E., and Garza-Garza, R. Ischemic bowel disease following bilateral nephrectomy or renal transplant. Surgery *82*:667, 1971.
152. Kilpatrick, Z. M., Silverman, J. F., Betancourt, E., Farman, J., and Lawson, J. P. Vascular occlusion of the colon and oral contraceptives: possible relation. N. Engl. J. Med. *278*:438, 1968.
153. Hurwitz, R. L., Martin, A. J., Grossman, B. E., and Waddell, W. R. Oral contraceptives and gastrointestinal disorders. Ann. Surg. *172*:892, 1970.
154. Cotton, P. B., and Thomas, M. L. Ischaemic colitis and the contraceptive pill. Br. Med. J. *3*:27, 1971.
155. Egger, G., and Mangold, R. Ischemic colitis and oral contraceptives: Case report and brief review of the literature. Acta Hepatogastroenterol. *21*:221, 1974.
156. Cello, J. P., and Thoeni, R. F. Ischemic disease of the colon and oral contraceptives. West. J. Med. *126*:378, 1977.
157. Ghahremani, G. G., Myers, M. A., Farmer, J., and Port, R. B. Ischemic disease of the small bowel and colon associated with oral contraceptives. Gastrointest. Radiol. *2*:221, 1977.

158. Stillman, A. E., Weinberg, M., Mast, W. C., and Palpant, S. Ischemic bowel disease attributable to ergot. Gastroenterology *72*:1336, 1977.
159. Lambert, M., dePeyer, R., and Mullen, A. F. Reversible ischemic colitis after intravenous vasopressin therapy. JAMA *247*:666, 1982.
160. Clark, A. W., Lloyd-Mostyn, R. H., and Sadler, M. R. deC. "Ischemic" colitis in young adults. Br. Med. J. *4*:70, 1972.
161. Marston, A., Pheils, M. T., Thomas, M. L., and Morson, B. C. Ischemic colitis. Gut *7*:1, 1966.
162. Kilpatrick, Z. M., Farman, J., Yesner, R., and Spiro, H. M. Ischemic proctitis. JAMA *205*:74, 1968.
163. O'Connell, T. X., Kadell, B., and Tompkins, R. K. Ischemia of the colon. Surg. Gynecol. Obstet. *142*:337, 1976.
164. de Dombal, F. T., Fletcher, D. M., and Harris, R. S. Early diagnosis of ischemic colitis. Gut *10*:131, 1969.
165. Byrne, J. J., Wittenberg, J., Grimes, E. T., and Williams, L. F. Ischemic diseases of the bowel. II. Ischemic colitis. Dis. Colon Rectum *13*:283, 1970.
166. Barcewicz, P. A., and Welch, J. P. Ischemic colitis in young adult patients. Dis. Colon Rectum *23*:109, 1980.
167. Miller, W. T., Scott, J., Rosato, E. F., Rosato, F. A., and Crow, H. Ischemic colitis with gangrene. Radiology *94*:291, 1970.
168. Robertson, R. H., McDowell, H. A., Jr., Vanden, H. P., and Groakke, J. F. Toxic megacolon due to ischemic enterocolitis associated with retroperitoneal fibrosis. Gastroenterology *78*:585, 1980.
169. Eisenberg, R. L., Montgomery, C. K., and Margulis, A. R. Colitis in the elderly: Ischemic colitis mimicking ulcerative and granulomatous colitis. Am. J. Roentgenol. *33*:1113, 1979.
170. Brandt, L. J., Goldberg, L., Boley, S. J., Mitsudo, S., and Berman, A. Ulcerating colitis in the elderly. (Abstract.) Gastroenterology *76*:1106, 1979.
171. Wescott, J. L. Angiographic demonstration of arterial occlusion in ischemic colitis. Gastroenterology *63*:486, 1972.
172. Wittenberg, J., Athanasoulis, C. A., Williams, L. F., Jr., Paredes, S., O'Sullivan, P., and Brown, B. Ischemic colitis. Radiology and pathophysiology. Am. J. Roentgenol. *123*:287, 1975.
173. Grendell, J. H., and Ockner, R. K. Mesenteric venous thrombosis. Gastroenterology *82*:358, 1982.
174. Nesbit, R. R., Jr., and Dewesse, J. A. Mesenteric venous thrombosis and oral contraceptives. South. Med. J. *70*:360, 1977.
175. Matthews, J. E., and White, R. R. Primary mesenteric venous occlusive disease. Am. J. Surg. *122*:579, 1971.
176. Naitove, A., and Weismann, R. Primary mesenteric venous thrombosis. Ann. Surg. *161*:516, 1965.
177. Anane-Sefah, J. C., Blair, E., and Reckler, S. Primary mesenteric venous occlusive disease. Surg. Gynecol. Obstet. *141*:740, 1975.
178. Clemett, A. R., and Chang, J. The radiologic diagnosis of spontaneous mesenteric venous thrombosis. Am. J. Gastroenterol. *63*:209, 1975.
179. Wang, C. C., and Reeves, J. D. Mesenteric vascular disease. Am. J. Roentgenol. *83*:895, 1960.
180. Rosen, A., Korobkin, M., Silverman, P. M., Dunnick, N. R., and Kelvin, F. M. Mesenteric vein thrombosis: CT identification. Am. J. Radiol. *143*:83, 1984.
181. Barth, K. H., Scott, W. W., Jr., Harrington, D. P., and Siegelman, S. S. Abnormalities in the sequence of filling and emptying of mesenteric arteries and veins. A guide to ischemic disease of the bowel. Gastrointest. Radiol. *3*:85, 1978.
182. Jona, J., Cummins, G. M., Jr., Head, H. B., and Govostis, M. C. Recurrent primary mesenteric venous thrombosis. JAMA *227*:1033, 1974.
183. Gilham, J. R., and Smiley, J. D. Cutaneous nectrotizing vasculitis and related disorders. Ann. Allerg. *37*:328, 1976.
184. Fauci, A. S., Haynes, B. F., and Katz, P. The spectrum of vasculitis. Clinical, pathologic, immunologic, and therapeutic considerations. Ann. Intern. Med. *89*:660, 1978.
185. Camilleri, M., Pusey, C. D., Chadwick, V. S., and Rees, A. J. Gastrointestinal manifestations of systemic vasculitis. Q. J. Med. *52*:141, 1983.
186. Schmid, F. R., Cooper, N. S., Ziff, M., and McEwen, C. Arteritis in rheumatoid arthritis. Am. J. Med. *30*:56, 1961.
187. Lopez, L. R., Schocket, A. L., Stanford, R. E., Claman, H. N., and Kohler, P. F. Gastrointestinal involvement in leukocytoclastic vasculitis and polyarteritis nodosa. J. Rheumatol. *7*:677, 1980.
188. Scott, D. G. I., Bacon, P. A., and Tribe, C. R. Systemic rheumatoid vasculitis: A clinical and laboratory study of 50 cases. Medicine *60*:288, 1981.
189. Pollack, V., Grove, W., Kark, R., Muehrcke, R. C., Priani, C. L., and Steck, I. E. Systemic lupus erythematosus simulating acute surgical conditions of the abdomen. N. Engl. J. Med. *259*:258, 1958.
190. Finkbiner, R. B., and Decker, J. P. Ulceration and perforation of the intestine due to necrotizing arteriolitis. N. Engl. J. Med. *268*:14, 1963.
191. Zizic, T. M., Schulman, L. E., and Stevens, M. B. Colonic perforations in systemic lupus erythematosus. Medicine *54*:411, 1975.
192. Weiser, M. M., Andries, G. A., Brentjens, J. R., Evans, J. T., and Reichlen, M. Systemic lupus erythematosus and intestinal venulitis. Gastroenterology *81*:570, 1981.
193. Blazer, S., Aton, U., Berant, M., and Korman, S. H. Henoch-Schönlein syndrome—paucity of renal disease. Review of 71 children. Isr. J. Med. Sci. *17*:41, 1981.
194. Rogh, D. A., Wilz, D. R., and Theil, G. B. Schönlein-Henoch syndrome in adults. Q. J. Med. *53*:145, 1985.
195. Cabal, E., and Holtz, S. Polyarteritis as a cause of intestinal hemorrhage. Gastroenterology *61*:99, 1971.
196. Miller, D. R., and O'Farrell, T. P. Perforation of the small intestine secondary to necrotizing vasculitis. Ann. Surg. *162*:81, 1965.
197. Sergent, J. S., Lockshin, M. D., Christian, C. L., and Gocke, D. V. Vasculitis with hepatitis B antigenemia: long term observations. Medicine *55*:1, 1976.
198. Duffy, J., Lidsky, M. D., and Sharp, J. T. Polyarthritis, polyarteritis, and hepatitis B. Medicine *56*:255, 1972.
199. Boyer, T. D., Jong, M. J., Rakela, J., and Reynolds, T. B. Immunologic studies and clinical follow-up of HB Ag-positive polyarteritis nodosa. Am. J. Dig. Dis. *22*:497, 1977.
200. Anuras, S., McMahon, B. J., Chow, K. C., and Summers, R. W. Severe abdominal vasculitis with hepatitis B antigenemia. Am. J. Surg. *140*:692, 1980.
201. Mendeloff, A. I., and Shulman, L. E. Gastrointestinal responses in connective tissue diseases. *In* Gamble, J. R., and Wilber, D. L., (eds.): Current Concepts of Clinical Gastroenterology. Boston, Little, Brown and Co., 1965, pp. 107–123.
202. Kurlander, D. J., and Kirsner, J. B. The association of chronic "non-specific" inflammatory bowel disease with lupus erythematosus. Ann. Intern. Med. *60*:799, 1964.
203. Geller, S. A., and Cohen, A. Arterial inflammatory cell infiltration in Crohn's disease. Arch. Pathol. Lab. Med. *107*:473, 1983.
204. Rodriguez-Erdmann, F., and Levitan, R. Gastrointestinal and roentgenological manifestations of Henoch-Schönlein purpura. Gastroenterology *54*:260, 1968.
205. Cream, J. J., Gumpel, J. M., and Peachey, R. D. G. Schönlein-Henoch purpura in the adult. A study of 77 adults with anaphylactoid or Schönlein-Henoch purpura. Q. J. Med. *39*:461, 1970.
206. Editorial. Schönlein-Henoch purpura in adults. Lancet *1*:437, 1971.
207. McDermott, V., and McCarthy, C. F. A case of ulcerative colitis presenting as vasculitic purpura. Dig. Dis. Sci. *30*:495, 1985.
208. Strole, W. E., Jr., Clark, W. H., and Isselbacher, K. J. Progressive arterial occlusive disease (Kohlmeier-Degos). N. Engl. J. Med. *276*:195, 1967.
209. Kohlmeier, W. Multiple Hautnekrosen bei Thromboangitis obliterans. Arch. Dermatol. Syph. *181*:783, 1941.
210. Degos, R., Delort, J., and Tricot, R. Dermatite papulosquameuse atrophiante. Bull. Soc. Franc. Dermatol. Syph. *49*:148, 281, 1942.
211. Pallesen, R. M., and Rasmussen, N. R. Malignant atrophic Papulosis-Degos syndrome. Acta Chir. Scand. *145*:279, 1979.

212. Kirshbaum, J. D. Abdominal aortitis with stenosis (Takayasu's disease) and occlusive superior mesenteric arteritis associated with renal artery stenosis and hypertension. Am. Heart J. *80*:811, 1970.
213. Lupi-Herrera, E., Sanchez-Torres, G., Marcushamer, J., Mispireta, J., Horowitz, S., and Vela, J. E. Takayasu's arteritis. Clinical study of 107 cases. Am. Heart J. *93*:94, 1977.
214. Sheldammer, J. H., Volkman, D. J., Partillo, J. E., Lawley, T. M., Johnston, M. R., and Fauci, A. S. Takayasu's arteritis and its therapy. Ann. Intern. Med. *103*:121, 1985.
215. Owyang, C., Miller, L. J., Lie, J. T., and Fleming, C. R. Takayasu's arteritis in Crohn's disease. Gastroenterology *76*:825, 1979.
216. Teja, K., Crum, C. P., and Friedman, C. Giant cell arteritis and Crohn's disease. An unreported association. Gastroenterology *78*:796, 1980.
217. Allen, A. C., Boley, S. J., Schultz, L., and Schwartz, S. Potassium-induced lesions of the small bowel. II. Pathology and pathogenesis. JAMA *193*:1001, 1965.
218. Schwartz, S., Boley, S., Schultz, L., and Allen, A. A survey of vascular diseases of the small intestine. Semin. Roentgenol. *1*:178, 1966.
219. Mercer, S., and Carpenter, B. Surgical complications of Kawasaki disease. J. Pediatr. Surg. *16*:444, 1981.
220. Reza, M. J., Roth, B. E., Pops, M. A., and Goldberg, L. S. Intestinal vasculitis in essential mixed cryoglobulinemia. Ann. Intern. Med. *81*:632, 1974.
221. Scully, R. E., Mark, E. J., and McNeely, B. V. Case records of the Massachusetts General Hospital. N. Engl. J. Med. *311*:904, 1984.
222. Matsuura, H., Murai, M., Hashimoto, T., Matsumoto, T., and Fukui, O. C2 deficiency vasculitis: complications of entercolitis, cutaneous ulcers, and neuropsychiatric disorder. Am. J. Gastroenterol. *78*:1, 1983.
223. Parsa, C. Cronkhite-Canada syndrome associated with systemic vasculitis: an autopsy study. Hum. Pathol. *13*:758, 1982.
224. Tulman, A. B., Bludford, S., Lee, E., and Brady, P. G. Giant hyperplastic polyps associated with vasculitis of colon. J. Florida Med. Assn. *69*:380, 1982.
225. Rambaud, J. -C., Galian, A., Touchard, G., Morel-Maroger, L., Mikol, J., Van Effenterre, G., Leclerc, J. -P., Le Charpenter, Y., Haut, J., Matuchansky, C., and Zittouh, R. Digestive tract and renal small vessel hyalinosis, idiopathic nonarteriosclerotic intracerebral calcifications, retinal ischemic syndrome, and phenotypic abnormalities. A new familial syndrome. Gastroenterology *90*:930, 1986.
226. Carron, D. B., and Douglas, A. P. Steatorrhea in vascular insufficiency of the small intestine. Q. J. Med. *34*:331, 1965.
227. Solley, G. O., Winkelmann, R. K., and Rovelstad, R. A. Correlation between regional entercolitis and cutaneous polyarteritis nodosa. Two case reports and review of the literature. Gastroenterology *69*:235, 1975.
228. Yassinger, S., Adelman, R., Cantor, D., Halsted, C. H., and Bolt, R. J. Association of inflammatory bowel disease and large vascular lesions. Gastroenterology *71*:844, 1976.
229. Philips, J. C., and Howland, W. J. Mesenteric arteritis in systemic lupus erythematosus. JAMA *206*:1569, 1968.
230. Korn, J. E., and Weaver, G. D. Vasculitis of the colon diagnosed by colonoscopy. Gastrointest. Endosc. *25*:136, 1979.
231. Judd, D. R., Taybi, H., and King, H. Intramural hematoma of the small bowel. Arch. Surg. *89*:527, 1964.
232. Wiot, J. F. Intramural small intestinal hemorrhage—a differential diagnosis. Semin. Roentgenol. *1*:219, 1966.
233. Johansson, L., Norrby, K., Nystrom, P.-O., and Lennquist, S. Intestinal intramural hemorrhage after abdominal missile trauma—clinical classification and prognosis. Acta Clin. Scand. *150*:54, 1984.
234. Killian, S. T., and Heitzman, E. J. Intramural hemorrhage of small intestine due to anticoagulants. JAMA *200*:591, 1967.
235. Birns, M. T., Katon, R. M., and Keller, F. Intramural hematoma of the small intestine presenting as major upper gastrointestinal hemorrhage. Case report and review of the literature. Gastroenterology *77*:1094, 1979.
235a. Kolodny, M., Mushlin, A. I., Baker, W. G., Jr., Sleisenger, M. H., and Nachman, R. L. Intramural small intestinal hematoma. Arch. Intern Med. *121*:438, 1968.
236. Babb, R. R., Spittell, J. A., Jr., and Bartholomew, L. G. Gastroenterologic complications of antiocoagulant therapy. Mayo Clin. Proc. *43*:738, 1968.
237. Leatherman, L. L. Intestinal obstruction caused by anticoagulants. Am. Heart J. *76*:534, 1968.
238. Khilnani, M. T., Marshak, R. H., Eliasoph, J., and Wolf, B. S. Intramural intestinal hemorrhage. Am. J. Roentgenol. *92*:1061, 1964.
239. Scully, R. E. (ed.). Case records of the Massachusetts General Hospital. N. Engl. J. Med. *295*:1309, 1976.
240. Darling, R. C., and Brewster, D. C. Elective treatment of abdominal aortic aneurysms. World J. Surg. *4*:661, 1980.
241. Volpetti, G., Barker, C. F., Berkowitz, H., and Roberts, B. A twenty-two year review of elective resection of abdominal aortic aneurysms. Surg. Gynecol. Obstet. *142*:321, 1976.
242. Fielding, J. W. L., Black, J., Ashton, F., Scaney, G., and Campbell, D. J. Diagnosis and management of 528 abdominal aneurysms. Br. Med. J. *283*:355, 1981.
243. Freimanis, A. K. Echographic diagnosis of lesions of the abdominal aorta and lymph nodes. Radiol. Clin. North Am. *13*:557, 1975.
244. Gordon, D. H., Martin, E. C., Schneider, M., Staiano, S. J., and Noyes, M. B. The complementary role of sonography and arteriography in the evaluation of the atheromatous abdominal aorta. Cardiovasc. Radiol. *1*:165, 1978.
245. Eriksson, I., Hemmingsson, A., and Lindgren, P. G. Diagnosis of abdominal aortic aneurysm by aortography, computer tomography, and ultrasound. Acta Radiol. Diagn. *21*(2A):209, 1980.
246. Gomes, M. N., Schellinger, D., and Hufnagel, C. A. Abdominal aortic aneurysms: Diagnostic review and new technique. Ann. Thorac. Surg. *27*:479, 1979.
247. Dixon, A. K., Springall, R. G., Kellsey-Fry, I., and Taylor, G. W. Computed tomography (CT) of abdominal aortic aneurysms: determination of longitudinal extent. Br. J. Surg. *68*:47, 1981.
248. Pond, G. D., and Hillman, B. Evaluation of aneurysms by computed tomography. Surgery *89*:216, 1981.
249. Wolk, L. A., Pasdar, H., McKeown, J. J., Jr., Leibowitz, H., and Scott, M. Computerized tomography in the diagnosis of abdominal aortic aneurysms. Surg. Gynecol. Obstet. *153*:229, 1981.
250. Ottinger, L. W. Ruptured arteriosclerotic aneurysms of the abdominal aorta. JAMA *233*:147, 1975.
251. Nichols, G. B., and Schilling, P. J. Pseudoretroperitoneal gas in rupture of aneurysm of abdominal aorta. Am. J. Roentgenol. *125*:134, 1975.
252. Rosato, F. E., Barker, C., and Roberts, B. Aortico-intestinal fistula. J. Thor. Cardiovasc. Surg. *53*:511, 1967.
253. DeBakey, M. D., Crawford, E. S., Cooley, D. A., Morris, G. C., Royster, T. S., and Abbot, W. P. Aneurysm of abdominal aorta. Analysis of results of graft replacement therapy one to eleven years after operation. Ann. Surg. *160*:622, 1964.
254. Connolly, J. E., and Stemmler, E. A. Intestinal gangrene as the result of mesenteric arterial steal. Am. J. Surg. *126*:197, 1973.
255. Brewter, D. C., Retana, A., Waltman, A. C., and Darling, R. C. Angiography in the management of aneurysms of the abdominal aorta. N. Engl. J. Med. *292*:822, 1975.
256. Alexander, R. H., Evans, M. T., and Blikken, W. C. Angiography in patients with abdominal aortic aneurysms. South. Med. J. *74*:669, 1981.
257. Nuno, I. N., Collins, G. M., Bardin, J. M., and Bernstein, E. F. Should aortography be used routinely in the elective management of abdominal aortic aneurysm? Am. J. Surg. *144*:53, 1982.
258. Crawford, E. S., Palamara, A. E., Salem, S. A., and Roehm, J. O. F., Jr. Aortic aneurysm: Current status of surgical treatment. Surg. Clin. North Am. *59*:597, 1979.
259. Crawford, E. S., Salem, S. A., Babb, J. W., III, Glaeser, D. H., Vaccaro, P. S., and Silvers, A. Infrarenal abdominal aortic aneurysm. Factors influencing survival after operation performed over a 25-year period. Ann. Surg. *193*:699, 1981.

260. Wittemore, A. D., Clowes, A. W., Hechtiman, H. L. B., and Mannick, J. A. Aortic aneurysm repair. Reduced operative mortality associated with maintenance of optimal cardiac performance. Ann. Surg. *192*:414, 1980.
261. McCube, C. J., Coleman, W. S., and Brewster, D. C. The advantage of early operation for abdominal aortic aneurysm. Arch. Surg. *116*:1025, 1981.
262. Fomon, J. J., Kurzweg, F. T., and Broadaway, R. Aneurysms of the aorta: a review. Ann. Surg. *165*:557, 1967.
263. Bernstein, E. F., Fisher, J. C., and Varco, R. L. Is excision the optimum treatment for all abdominal aortic aneurysms? Surgery *61*:83, 1967.
264. Smith, G. Clinical aspects of aneurysms and their management. Practitioner *206*:338, 1971.
265. Szilagyi, D. E., Smith, R. F., DeRusso, F. J., Elliott, J. P., and Sherrin, F. W. Contribution of abdominal aortic aneurysmectomy to prolongation of life. Ann. Surg. *164*:678, 1966.
266. Falkenberg, M., Gabel, H., Gothman, B., Holm, J., Norback, B., and Schersten, T. Abdominal aortic aneurysm. An interhospital study of 171 surgically treated patients. Scand. J. Thor. Cardiovasc. Surg. *9*:271, 1975.
267. Moore, H. D. Abdominal aortic aneurysms. J. Cardiovasc. Surg. *17*:47, 1976.
268. Sink, J. D., Myers, R. T., and James, P. M., Jr. Ruptured abdominal aortic aneurysms. Review of 33 cases treated surgically and discussion of prognostic indications. Am. Surgeon *42*:538, 1976.
269. Stenstrom, J. D., Ford, H. S., MacKay, M. I., Hosie, R. T., and Donald, J. C. Ruptured abdominal aortic aneurysm. Am. Surgeon *42*:538, 1976.
270. Cooley, D. A., and Carmichael, M. J. Abdominal aortic aneurysm. Circulation *70*(suppl. 1):I-5, 1984.
271. Bernstein, E. F., and Chan, E. L. Abdominal aortic aneurysm in high-risk patients. Outcome of selective management based on size and expansion rate. Ann. Surg. *200*:255, 1984.
272. Sterpelti, A. V., Schultz, R. D., Feldhaus, R. J., Peetz, D. J., Jr., Fasciano, A. J., and McGill, J. R. Abdominal aortic aneurysm in elderly patients. Selective management based on clinical status and aneurysmal expansion rate. Am. J. Surg. *150*:772, 1985.
273. Hollier, L. H. Surgical management of abdominal aortic aneurysm in the high-risk patient. Surg. Clin. North Am. *66*:269, 1986.
274. Hicks, G. L., Jr., and Rob, C. Abdominal aortic aneurysm wiring: an alternative method. Am. J. Surg. *131*:664, 1976.
275. Fortner, G., and Johanssen, K. Abdominal aortic aneurysm. West. J. Med. *140*:50, 1984.
276. Bernstein, E. F., Dilley, R. B., Goldberger, L. E., Gosink, B. B., and Leopold, G. R. Growth rates of small aortic aneurysms. Surgery *80*:765, 1976.
277. Elliott, J. P., Jr., Smith, R. F., and Szilagyi, D. E. Aortoenteric and paraprosthetic-enteric fistulas. Arch. Surg. *108*:479, 1974.
278. Keeffe, E. B., Krippaehne, W. W., Rosch, J., and Melnyk, C. S. Aortoduodenal fistula: complication of renal artery bypass graft. Gastroenterology *67*:1240, 1974.
279. Skibba, R. M., Greenberger, N. J., and Hardin, C. A. Paraprosthetic-enteric fistula. Dig. Dis. *20*:1081, 1975.
280. Howard, R. V., Leonard, J. J., and Howard, B. D. Renal artery cholecystoduodenal fistula. Arch. Surg. *113*:888, 1978.
281. Campbell, H. C., and Earnst, C. B. Aortoenteric fistual following renal revascularization. Am. Surg. *44*:155, 1978.
282. Kleinman, L. H., Towne, J. B., and Bernhard, V. M. A diagnostic and therapeutic approach to aortoenteric fistulas: clinical experience with twenty patients. Surgery *86*:868, 1979.
283. Wexler, R. M., Falchuk, K. R., Horst, D. A., Bothe, A., Jr., McDermott, W. V., Jr., and Trey, C. Duodenal erosion of mesocaval graft: an unusual complication of mesocaval shunt interposition surgery. Gastroenterology *79*:729, 1980.
284. Kiernan, P. D., Pairoleru, P. C., Hubert, J. P., and Wallace, R. B. Aortic graft-enteric fistula. Mayo Clin. Proc. *55*:731, 1980.
285. Perdue, G. D., Smith, R. B., III, Anseley, J. D., and Constantino, M. J. Impending aortoenteric hemorrhage. The effect of early recognition of improved outcome. Ann. Surg. *192*:237, 1980.
286. O'Mara, C. S., Williams, G. M., and Ernst, C. B. Secondary aortoenteric fistula. A 20 year experience. Am. J. Surg. *142*:203, 1981.
287. O'Hara, P. J., Hertzer, N. R., Beven, E. G., and Krajewski, L. P. Surgical management of infected abdominal grafts: review of a 25-year experience. J. Vasc. Surg. *3*:725, 1986.
288. Tierney, J. M., Jr. Aortoenteric fistula—Medical Staff Conference. University of California, San Francisco. West. J. Med. *134*:242, 1981.
289. Ikenomopoulos, D. C., Spanos, P. K., and Lazariders, D. P. Pathogenesis of aortoenteric fistula. An experimental study. Int. Angiol. *5*:33, 1986.
290. Mark, A. S., Moss, A. A., McCarthy, S., and McCowin, M. CT of aortoenteric fistulas. Invest. Radiol. *20*:272, 1985.
291. Akin, J. T., Skandalakis, J. E., and Gray, S. W. The anatomic basis of vascular compression of the duodenum. Surg. Clin. North Am. *54*:1361, 1974.
292. Hines, J. R., Gore, R. M., and Ballantyne, G. H. Superior mesenteric artery syndrome. Diagnostic criteria and therapeutic approaches. Am. J. Surg. *148*:630, 1984.
293. Cohen, L. B., Field, S. P., and Sacher, D. B. The superior mesenteric artery syndrome. The disease that isn't, or is it? J. Clin. Gastroenterol. 7:113, 1985.
294. Burrington, J. D., and Wayne, E. R. Obstruction of the duodenum by the superior mesenteric artery—does it exist in children? J. Pediatr. Surg. *9*:733, 1974.
295. Burrington, J. D. Superior mesenteric artery syndrome in children. Am. J. Dis. Child. *130*:1367, 1976.
296. Shandling, B. The so-called superior mesenteric artery syndrome. Am. J. Dis. Child. *130*:1371, 1976.
297. Editorial. Gellis, S. S. Am. J. Dis. Child. *130*:1373, 1976.
298. Lukes, P. J., Rolny, P., Nilson, A. E., Gamklow, R., Danle, N., and Botevall, A. Diagnostic value of hypotonic duodenography in superior mesenteric artery syndrome. Acta Chir. Scand. *144*:39, 1978.
299. Gustafson, L., Falk, A., Lukes, P. J., and Gamblow, R. Diagnosis and treatment of superior mesenteric artery syndrome. Br. J. Surg. *71*:499, 1984.
300. Gundos, B. Duodenal compression defect and the "superior mesenteric artery syndrome." Radiology *123*:575, 1977.
301. Froese, A. P., Szmuilowicz, J., and Baily, J. D. The superior-mesenteric-artery syndrome. Cause or complication of anorexia nervosa. Can. Psych. Assn. J. *23*:325, 1978.
302. Walker, C., and Kahanowitz, N. Recurrent superior mesenteric artery syndrome complicating staged reconstructive spinal surgery. Alternative methods of conservative treatment. J. Pediatr. Orthop. *3*:77, 1983.
303. Munns, S. W., Morrissy, R. T., Golladay, E. S., and McKenzie, C. N. Hyperalimentation for superior mesenteric-artery (Cast) syndrome following corrections of spinal deformity. J. Bone Joint Surg. *66A*:1175, 1984.
304. Appel, M. F., Bentilif, P. S., and Dickson, J. H. Arteriomesenteric duodenal compression syndrome: comparison of methods of treatment. South. Med. J. *69*:340, 1976.
305. Kaijser, R. Hemangiomas of the gastrointestinal tract. Arch. Klin. Chir. *187*:351, 1936.
306. Sutton, D., Murfitt, J., and Howarth, F. Gastrointestinal bleeding from large angiomas. Clin. Radiol. *32*:629, 1981.
307. Richardson, J. D., Max, M. H., Flint, L. M., Schweisinger, W., Howard, M., and Aust, J. B. Bleeding vascular malformations of the intestine. Surgery *840*:430, 1978.
308. Boley, S. J., and Brandt, L. J. Colonic ectasias and lower intestinal bleeding. Hosp. Prac. *17*:137, 1982.
309. Weaver, G. A., Alpern, H. D., Davis, J. S., Ramsey, W. H., and Reichelderfer, M. Gastrointestinal angiodysplasia associated with aortic valve disease: part of a spectrum of angiodysplasia of the gut. Gastroenterology *77*:1, 1979.
310. Cello, J. P., and Grendell, J. H. Endoscopic laser treatment for gastrointestinal vascular ectasias. Ann. Intern. Med. *104*:352, 1986.
311. Meyer, C. T., Troncale, F. J., Galloway, S., and Sheahan, D.

G. Arteriovenous malformations of the bowel: an analysis of 22 cases and a review of the literature. Medicine *60*:36, 1981.

312. Zuckerman, G. R., Cornette, G. L., Clouse, R. E., and Harter, H. R. Upper gastrointestinal bleeding in patients with renal failure. Ann. Intern. Med. *102*:588, 1985.
313. Baum, S., Athanasoulis, C., Waltman, A., Galdabini, J., Schapiro, R., Warshaw, A., and Ottinger, L. Angiodysplasia of the right colon. A cause of gastrointestinal bleeding. Am. J. Radiol. *129*:789, 1977.
314. Boley, S. J., Sammartano, R. D., Biase, A., and Sprayregen, S. On the nature and etiology of vascular ectasias of the colon. Gastroenterology *72*:650, 1977.
315. Bowers, J. H., and Dixon, J. A. Argon laser photo-coagulation of vascular malformations in the GI tract: short term results. Gastrointest. Endosc. *28*:126, 1982 (abstract).
316. Jensen, D. M., Machicado, G. A., Tapia, J. I., and Beilin, B. B. Endoscopic treatment of hemangiomata with argon laser in patients with gastrointestinal bleeding. (Abstract.) Gastroenterology *82*:1093, 1982.
317. Jensen, D. M., and Machicado, G. A. Bleeding colonic angioma: endoscopic coagulation and follow-up. (Abstract.) Gastroenterology *88*:1433, 1985.
318. Howard, O. M., Buchanan, J. D., and Hunt, R. H. Angiodysplasia of the colon. Experience of 26 cases. Lancet *2*:16, 1982.
319. Cello, J. P., Crass, R. A., Grendell, J. H., and Trunkey, D. D. Management of the patient with hemorrhaging esophageal varices. JAMA *256*:1480, 1986.
320. Johnston, G. W., and Rodgers, H. W. A review of 15 years' experience in the use of sclerotherapy in the control of acute hemorrhage from oesophageal varices. Br. J. Surg. *60*:797, 1973.
321. Chojkier, M., and Conn, H. O. Esophageal tamponade in the treatment of bleeding varices. A decadal process report. Dig. Dis. Sci. *25*:267, 1980.
322. Barsoum, M. S., Bolous, F. I., El-Rooby, A. A., Rizk-Allah, M. A., and Ibrahim, A. S. Tamponade and injection sclerotherapy in the management of bleeding oesophageal varices. Br. J. Surg. *69*:76, 1982.
323. Paquet, K.-J., and Feussner, H. Endoscopic sclerosis and esophageal balloon tamponade in acute hemorrhage from esophagogastric varices: a prospective controlled randomized trial. Hepatology *5*:580, 1985.
324. Conn, H. O. Vasopressin and nitroglycerin in the treatment of bleeding varices: the bottom line. Hepatology *6*:523, 1986.
325. Smith-Laing, G., Scott, J., Long, R. G., Dick, R., and Sherlock, S. Role of percutaneous transhepatic obliteration of varices in the management of hemorrhage from gastroesophageal varices. Gastroenterology *80*:1031, 1981.
326. Sos, T. A. Transhepatic portal venous embolization of varices: Pros and cons. Radiology *148*:569, 1983.
327. Orloff, M. J., Charters, A. C., III, Chandler, J. G., Condon, J. K., Grambort, D. E., Modaffeni, T. R., Levin, S. E., Brown, N. B., Sviokla, S. C., and Knox, D. G. Portacaval shunt as emergency procedure in unselected patients with alcoholic cirrhosis. Surg. Gynecol. Obstet. *141*:59, 1975.
328. Keagy, B. A., Schwartz, J. A., and Johnson, G., Jr. Should ablative operations be used for bleeding esophageal varices? Ann. Surg. *203*:563, 1986.
329. MacDougall, B. R. D., Westaby, D., Theodossi, A., Dawson, J. L., and Williams, R. Increased long term survival in variceal hemorrhage using injection sclerotherapy. Lancet *1*:124, 1982.
330. Yassin, Y. M., and Sherif, S. M. Randomized controlled trial of injection sclerotherapy for bleeding oesophageal varices—an interim report. Br. J. Surg. *70*:20, 1983.
331. Terblanche, J., Bornman, P. C., and Kirsch, R. E. Sclerotherapy for bleeding esophageal varices. Ann. Rev. Med. *35*:83, 1984.
332. The Copenhagen Esophageal Varices Sclerotherapy Project. Sclerotherapy after first variceal hemorrhage in cirrhosis. A randomized multicenter study. N. Engl. J. Med. *311*:1594, 1984.
333. Korula, J., Balart, L. A., Radvan, G., Zweiban, B. E., Larson, A. W., Kao, H. W., and Yamada, S. A prospective, randomized controlled trial of chronic esophageal variceal sclerotherapy. Hepatology *5*:584, 1985.
334. Warren, W. D., Henderson, J. M., Millikan, W. J., Galambos, J. T., Brooks, W. S., Riepe, S. P., Salam, A. A., and Kutner, M. H. Distal splenorenal shunt versus endoscopic sclerotherapy for long-term management of variceal bleeding. Preliminary report of a prospective randomized trial. Ann. Surg. *203*:454, 1986.
335. Cello, J. P., Grendell, J. H., Crass, R. A., Weber, T. E., and Trunkey, D. D. Endoscopic sclerotherapy versus portacaval shunt in patients with severe cirrhosis and acute variceal hemorrhage: long-term follow-up. N. Engl. J. Med. *316*:11, 1987.
336. Lebrec, D., Poynard, T., Bernau, J., Bercoff, E., Novel, O., Capron, J.-P., Poupon, R., Bouvry, M., Rueff, B., and Benhamou, J.-P. A randomized controlled study of propranolol for prevention of recurrent gastrointestinal bleeding in patients with cirrhosis: a final report. Hepatology *4*:355, 1984.
337. Burroughs, A. K., Jenkins, W. J., Sherlock, S., Dunk, A., Walt, R. P., Osuafor, T. O. K., Mackie, S., and Dick, R. Controlled trial of propranolol for the prevention of recurrent variceal hemorrhage in patient with cirrhosis. N. Engl. J. Med. *309*:1539, 1983.
338. Villeneuve, J.-P., Pomier-Layrargues, G., Infante-Rivard, C., Willems, B., Huet, P.-M., Marleau, D., and Viallet, A. Propranolol for the prevention of recurrent variceal hemorrhage: a controlled trial. Hepatology *6*:1239, 1986.
339. Jackson, F. C., Perrin, E. B., Felix, R., and Smith, A. G. A clinical investigation of the portacaval shunt: V. Survival analysis of the therapeutic operation. Ann. Surg. *174*:672, 1971.
340. Resnick, R. H., Iber, F. L., Isihara, A. M., Charlmers, T. C., and Zimmerman, H. A controlled study of the therapeutic portacaval shunt. Gastroenterology *67*:843, 1974.
341. Rueff, B., Degos, F., Degos, J. D., Maillard, J. N., Prandi, D., Sicot, J., Sicot, C., Fauvert, R., and Benhamou, J. P. A controlled study of therapeutic portacaval shunt in alcoholic cirrhosis. Lancet *1*:655, 1976.
342. Reynolds, T. B., Donovan, A. J., Mikkelsen, W. P., Redeker, A. G., Turrill, F. L., and Weiner, J. M. Results of a 12 year randomized trial of portacaval shunt in patients with alcoholic liver disease and bleeding varices. Gastroenterology *80*:1005, 1981.
343. Millikan, W. J., Jr., Warren, W. D., Henderson, J. M., Smith, R. B., III, Salam, A. A., Galambos, J. T., Kutner, M. H., and Keen, J. H. The Emory prospective randomized trial: selective versus nonselective shunt to control variceal bleeding. Ten-year follow-up. Ann. Surg. *201*:712, 1985.
344. Langer, B., Taylor, B. R., Mackenzie, D. R., Gilas, T., Stone, R. M., and Blendis, L. Further report of a prospective randomized trial comparing distal splenorenal shunt with end-to-side portacaval shunt. An analysis of encephalopathy, survival, and quality of life. Gastroenterology *88*:424, 1985.
345. Reichle, F. A., Fahmy, W. F., and Golsorkhi, M. Prospective comparative clinical trial with distal splenorenal and mesocaval shunts. Am. J. Surg. *137*:13, 1979.
346. Fischer, J. E., Bower, R. H., Atamian, S., and Welling, R. Comparison of distal and proximal splenorenal shunts. A randomized prospective trial. Ann. Surg. *194*:531, 1981.
347. Conn, H. O., Resnick, R. H., Grace, N. D., Atterbury, C. E., Horst, D., Groszmann, R. J., Gazmuri, P., Gusberg, R. J., Thayer, B., Berk, D., Wright, S. C., Vollman, R., Tilson, D. M., McDermott, W. V., Cohen, J. A., Kerstein, M., Toole, A. L., Maselli, J. P., Razvi, S., Ishihara, A., Stern, H., Trey, C., O'Hara, E. T., Widrich, W., Aisenberg, H., Stansel, H. C., and Zinny, M. Distal splenorenal shunt vs. portal-systemic shunt: current status of a controlled trial. Hepatology *1*:151, 1981.
348. Harley, H. A. J., Morgan, T., Redeker, A. G., Reynolds, T. B., Villamil, F., Weiner, J. M., and Yellin, A. Results of a randomized trial of end-to-side portacaval shunt and distal splenorenal shunt in alcoholic liver disease and variceal bleeding. Gastroenterology *91*:802, 1986.
349. Warren, W. D., Millikan, W. J., Jr., Henderson, J. M., Wright, L., Kutner, M., Smith, R. B., Fulenwider, J. T., Salem, A.

A., Galambos, J. T. Ten years portal hypertensive surgery at Emory: results and new perspectives. Ann. Surg. *195*:530, 1982.
350. Sugiura, M., and Futagawa, S. Further evaluation of the Sugiura procedure in the treatment of esophageal varices. Arch. Surg. *112*:1317, 1977.
351. Graham, D. Y., and Smith, J. L. The course of patients after variceal hemorrhage. Gastroenterology *80*:800, 1981.
352. Resnick, R. H., Schimmel, E. M., O'Hara, E. T., and the Boston Inter-Hospital Liver Group. A controlled study of the prophylactic portacaval shunt—a final report. Ann. Intern. Med. *70*:675, 1969.
353. Jackson, F. C., Perrin, E. B., Smith, A. G., Dagradi, A. E., and Nadal, H. M. A clinical evaluation of the portacaval shunt. II. Survival analysis of the prophylactic operation. Am. J. Surg. *115*:22, 1968.
354. Pascal, J. P. A Multicenter Study Group—CHR PURPAN. Prophylactic treatment of variceal bleeding in cirrhotic patients with propanolol: a multicentric randomized study. (Abstract.) Hepatology *4*:1092, 1984.
355. Pagliaro, L., Pasta, L., D'Amico, G., Filippazo, M. G., Tine, Morabito, A., Ferrari, A., Marenco, G., DePretis, G., and The Italian Multicentric Project for Propranolol in the Prevention of Bleeding. A randomized clinical trial of propranolol for the prevention of initial bleeding in cirrhosis with portal hypertension (letter). N. Engl. J. Med. *314*:244, 1986.
356. Witzel, L., Wolbeargs, E., and Merki, H. Prophylactic endoscopic sclerotherapy of oesophageal varices. a prospective controlled trial. Lancet *1*:773, 1985.
357. Paquet, K. J., and Koussoris, P. Is there an indication for prophylactic endoscopic paravericeal injection sclerotherapy in patients with liver cirrhosis and portal hypertension? Endoscopy *18*:32, 1986.
358. Koch, H., Henning, H., Grimm, H., and Soehendra, N. Prophylactic sclerosing of esophageal varices—results of a prospective controlled study. Endoscopy *18*:40, 1986.
359. Burroughs, A. K., D'Heygere, F., and McIntyre, N. Pitfalls in studies of prophylactic therapy for variceal bleeding in cirrhotics. Hepatology *6*:1407, 1986.
360. Gregory, P., Hartigan, P., Amodeo, D., Baum, R., Camara, D., Colcher, H., Fye, C., Gebhard, R., Goff, J., Kruss, D., McPhee, M., Meier, P., Rankin, R., Reichelderfer, R., Sanouski, R., Shields, D., Silvis, S., Wesner, R., Winship, D., and Young, H. Prophylactic sclerotherapy for esophageal varices in alcoholic liver disease: Results of a VA cooperative randomized trial. (Abstract.) Gastroenterology *92*:1414, 1987.

102 Diseases of the Peritoneum, Mesentery, and Diaphragm

MICHAEL D. BENDER

ANATOMY AND PHYSIOLOGY OF THE PERITONEUM

Gross Anatomy

The peritoneum is the mesothelial lining of the peritoneal cavity and its contained viscera; its total surface area is thought to approximate the surface area of skin (1 to 2 m^2). It forms a closed sac, except at the fimbriated ostia of the fallopian tubes, and is divided into visceral and parietal portions. The visceral peritoneum encloses the intraperitoneal organs and forms the mesenteries by which they are suspended. The parietal peritoneum lines the anterior, lateral, and posterior abdominal walls, the undersurface of the diaphragm, and the pelvic floor. Those abdominal viscera that are retroperitoneal, including the duodenum, the ascending and descending colon, and portions of the pancreas, kidneys, and adrenals are covered anteriorly by the parietal peritoneum. Diseases involving these structures, particularly the peritoneum, often cause ascites (see pp. 428–454).

The peritoneal cavity is subdivided by peritoneal reflections and mesenteric attachments into several compartments and recesses. These are clinically important because they determine the location and spread of pathologic processes, such as abscesses and intraperitoneal metastases.[1, 1a] The omentum develops from dorsal mesogastrium that subsequently fuses with the transverse colon and mesocolon. It is formed by a double layer of fused peritoneum, enclosing lymphatic vessels and blood vessels. The omentum plays an important role in peritoneal defense mechanisms by closing perforations, containing infection, and providing blood supply.[2]

Blood Supply. The greater part of the peritoneal surface (mainly visceral) and mesentery is supplied by the splanchnic blood vessels and drained via the splanchnic venous system and portal vein. A smaller area (mainly parietal) is supplied by the branches of the lower intercostal, subcostal, lumbar, and iliac arteries and is drained by veins that enter the inferior vena cava via the lumbar and iliac veins. The microvascular anatomy of the peritoneum has been studied by scanning electron microscopy. It consists of a capillary plexus of long straight vessels arranged in two layers at right angles to each other. This arrangement of two layers of closely packed, long, straight vessels must account in large part for the efficiency of the peritoneal membrane as an exchange interface[3] (see pp. 1903–1906).

Innervation. The innervation of the parietal peritoneum also differs from that of the visceral peritoneum. The parietal peritoneum is innervated by twigs from the same spinal nerves that supply the abdominal wall. As a result, irritation of the parietal peritoneum gives rise to afferent stimuli that are transmitted via the intercostal nerves and are perceived as somatic pain. In contrast, there are no pain receptors in the visceral peritoneum, and afferent stimuli are conducted in the general distribution of the visceral sympathetic nervous system. These differences in innervation account for the sharp quality and more precise localization of pain and the other physical signs, such as muscle spasm, that result from irritation of the parietal peritoneum, on the one hand, and the poorly characterized and localized nature of visceral pain on the other (see pp. 239–243).

The diaphragmatic peritoneum has dual innervation. The central portion is supplied by the phrenic nerve (C3–C5), whereas the peripheral portion is innervated by branches of the intercostal nerves. Thus, depending on the location of the pathologic process, irritation of the diaphragmatic peritoneum may cause pain to be referred to either the shoulder (phrenic distribution) or the thoracic or abdominal wall (intercostal distribution) (see pp. 239–243).

Microscopic Anatomy

The mesothelium consists of a single layer of cells resting on a thin basement membrane supported by connective tissue stroma. The cells are flat in their resting state, and cuboidal in their active state. The cell surface has a well-developed microvillous border, which increases the cell surface and produces glycoproteins which prevent friction of the peritoneal surfaces. Mesothelial cell junctions show overlapping and interdigitation, which may aid structural integrity and transport processes. The most common junctions are tight junctions, but gap junctions are also present.[4–6] Whether these tight junctions provide a complete or partial seal around the cell is particularly important in intracellular fluid transport.

Physiology

On the basis of anatomic structure, two different pathways for solute transport are possible: via intracellular vesicles (pinocytosis) or extracellular junctions (pores). Radiolabeled solute studies suggest that transport is accomplished by passive diffusion through cellular junctions.[7] On the other hand, evidence of an active process in mesothelial transport is provided by demonstrations that (1) higher concentrations of enzymes are associated with transport (ATPase and 5′-nucleotidase) within mesothelium; (2) mesothelial transport is sensitive to temperature, oxygen tension, pH, and metabolic inhibitors; and (3) tracers are present in the vesicles of mesothelial cells.[4–6] However, changes in blood flow and capillary permeability make these studies difficult to interpret, and tracer studies have been equivocal or conflicting.

By electron microscopy, a close approximation of the peritoneal cavity and subperitoneal capillaries is demonstrable; molecules less than 30 Å in diameter and with a molecular weight of less than 2000 daltons tend to enter the capillaries and portal vein, whereas larger molecules are absorbed by lymphatics.[8]

The peritoneal lymphatics, especially the diaphragmatic lymphatics, play a major role in removing both particulate matter and solutions from the peritoneal cavity. Early experimental work provides evidence that particles injected into the peritoneum pass between mesothelial cells and into lymphatics on the diaphragmatic surface. Electron microscopic studies of diaphragmatic peritoneum have demonstrated the presence of an anatomic arrangement that facilitates absorption from the peritoneal cavity. In areas where peritoneal mesothelial cells contact the terminal lymphatics (lacunae), gaps are present between mesothelial cells, the submesothelial connective tissue is scant or absent, and the lymphatic endothelium lacks a basement membrane. As a result, particles and large molecules may move through the intercellular gaps between mesothelial and endothelial cells into the terminal lymphatics.[9] This process is further aided by respiratory movements. During inspiration, filamentous processes of the lacunar cells overlap and gaps close, intraperitoneal pressure is increased, and the lacunae are emptied through the combined effects of local compression and increased intra-abdominal and reduced intrapleural pressure. During expiration, the gaps are opened and free communication is re-established.[10]

The importance of these diaphragmatic lymphatics has been demonstrated in animal studies in which obliteration of the diaphragmatic peritoneum by abrasion significantly delays the absorption of serum from the peritoneal cavity and increases the propensity of portal hypertension to produce ascites.[11] The resulting decrease in resorptive capacity is accompanied by a disproportionate reduction in permeability to larger molecules, so that the normally slower resorption rate of protein-containing solutions, as compared with saline solutions, is exaggerated after abrasion.[12]

Studies of the clearance of peritoneal fluid from the abdominal cavity in animals demonstrate a rapid initial reabsorption phase followed by a constant clearance rate. Studies in humans in which intraperitoneal saline and labeled albumin are used confirm that equilibration of saline between serum and peritoneal fluid occurs within two hours, after which fluid is absorbed at a relatively constant rate of 33 ml per hour. The rate of absorption during the initial two hours depends upon the transperitoneal osmotic gradient.[13, 14] Thus, transperitoneal fluid exchange is rapid, but this process mainly participates in equilibration of hyposmotic and hyperosmotic solutions. Removal of isosmotic solutions is slower, occurs via diaphragmatic lymphatic drainage, and depends upon intraperitoneal pressure.[15, 16]

The importance of transperitoneal fluid exchange can be appreciated in peritoneal dialysis, in which hyperosmolar solutions can cause a net flow of water into the peritoneal cavity of up to 500 ml per hour. Also, in peritonitis, transperitoneal capillary fluid movement caused by increased vascular permeability can be rapid and massive and may lead to hypotension and shock.

Normally, only small amounts of fluid are present in the peritoneal cavity. Most males have no measurable fluid, but females have from 1 to 20 ml, depending upon the phase of the menstrual cycle. This fluid probably is of ovarian origin and is formed as the result of increased capillary permeability of ovarian vessels, caused by estrogens and prostaglandins.[17]

The defensive role of the peritoneum against microorganisms is not yet well defined. Peritoneal fluid has been shown to have antimicrobial activity against gram-negative organisms and *Candida*; lysozyme, complement, and other identified factors play a role.[18, 19] Inhibitors of neutrophil chemotaxis may also be present, which prevents the development of unprovoked inflammatory reactions.[20] Peritoneal fluid also contains cells, including macrophages, lymphocytes, and small numbers of polymorphonuclear leukocytes.[21, 22] In mice, normal peritoneal lymphocytes were shown to be endocytically active and become phagocytic in culture.[23] Activated peritoneal T lymphocytes and local antibody production have also been demonstrated experimentally.[24] This may take place in specialized areas, such as omental stomata, where lymphocytes have ready access to the peritoneal cavity.[25, 25a]

Peritoneal Response to Injury

The peritoneal mesothelium is easily damaged and, judging from experimentally induced defects in the peritoneum, heals readily. This does not occur by ingrowth of mesothelium from the edges; rather, the entire surface becomes covered by mesothelium and heals within eight days. The origin of new mesothelial cells is due to differentiation of subperitoneal fibroblasts and to free-floating macrophages or mesothelial cells that repopulate the peritoneal surface.[4, 26, 27]

Mesothelial damage may lead to formation of adhesions. Serosal injury causes peritoneal mast cells to release histamine or other factors that promote increased vascular permeability and release of fibrinogen into the peritoneal cavity. With the release of thromboplastin from the injured cells, fibrinogen is converted to fibrin. Fibrinous adhesions may be removed from the peritoneal cavity by fibrinolysis. Although regenerating mesothelial cells demonstrate increased fibrinolytic activity, this activity is depressed in the injured cell.[4, 27–29] This temporary supression of fibrinolysis may provide time for fibroblasts to convert fibrinous to fibrous adhesions. Normally, however, peritoneal injuries or defects heal without formation of fibrous adhesions unless other factors such as infections, ischemia, or foreign bodies are associated or superimposed.[30]

DIAGNOSIS OF PERITONEAL DISEASE

History and Physical Examination

The cardinal symptoms of peritoneal disease are abdominal pain and ascites; more variable in their occurrence are fever, distention, nausea, vomiting, and altered bowel habits. Direct tenderness, rebound tenderness, and involuntary spasm of the anterior abdominal musculature are the major signs of irritation of the parietal peritoneum. These signs and symptoms may be minimal or absent in the elderly or debilitated patient and will vary, depending upon the location, cause, and acuteness of the underlying process (see below).

Radiology

Conventional X-Ray. Plain films of the abdomen may reveal peritoneal calcifications, but these calcifications are unusual and have been reported mainly in association with neoplasms, such as pseudomyxoma peritonei and ovarian carcinoma, and less commonly in association with renal, pancreatic, and gastrointestinal neoplasms.[31, 32] Ascites may also be diagnosed on abdominal plain films (see p. 428). Barium contrast studies may indirectly reflect involvement of visceral peritoneum by changes similar to those seen with transmural involvement of the bowel wall by other processes. Bizarre angular patterns of intestinal loops, rigidity of the bowel with diminished peristalsis, or altered mucosal patterns with filling defects or flattened folds are suggestive of primary disease of the bowel with secondary peritoneal involvement. Peritoneography with intraperitoneal Renografin has been used by some to allow definition of the peritoneum and its reflections and recesses, serosal surfaces, and mesenteric attachments.[1, 33] However, this technique is not widely used, and most clinicians use CT scanning to get similar information.

Ultrasonography. Ultrasonography is an excellent method to demonstrate ascites. In addition, peritoneal masses and nodules may be delineated, but this requires special attention to scanning technique and gain settings.[34] The sensitivity of ultrasound in detecting peritoneal implants is not fully described. In their early stage, implants characteristically appear as small nodules, occasionally as protrusions from the peritoneal surface, and are most readily detected if ascites is present. These nodules may grow, fuse, and form sheet-like masses that can be recognized by ultrasonography.

Computed Tomography. Computed tomography (CT) also identifies ascites and may demonstrate peritoneal implants.[35] The lateral margin of the liver appears to be especially well suited for the latter, because imaging in this area is relatively unhampered by small bowel loops and may be facilitated by adjacent ascitic fluid. Lesions have also been demonstrated in other areas of the peritoneum, but most identified implants are over 1 cm in diameter. The overall sensitivity of CT scanning in recognizing peritoneal implants is discussed below (see pp. 1943–1944). Attempts have been made to increase sensitivity by prior installation of contrast medium, but the value of this manuever has not been determined.[36]

Gallium-67 Scanning. Peritoneal inflammatory cells may take up radioactive gallium, and a diffuse pattern of uptake has been demonstrated in a variety of disorders, including tuberculous peritonitis, secondary bacterial peritonitis, and starch granulomatous peritonitis.[37] This finding obviously is not specific, but it may be a useful clue to peritoneal disease in difficult cases.

Paracentesis

All patients with ascites and suspected peritoneal disease should undergo paracentesis to permit analysis of the ascitic fluid. The technique of paracentesis and interpretation of fluid analysis are discussed on pages 430 to 431.

Peritoneal Biopsy

Percutaneous peritoneal biopsy may yield a tissue diagnosis of the cause of peritoneal disease, but its use is limited to patients with ascites (see p. 431).

Peritoneoscopy

Peritoneoscopy is an excellent diagnostic tool for visualization and directed biopsy of observed lesions of the peritoneum (see pp. 431–432). It is widely applicable, because it can be performed in patients without ascites and in those who may be poor candidates for general anesthesia.

DISEASES OF THE PERITONEUM

(Table 102–1)

Table 102–1. DISEASES OF THE PERITONEUM

- I. Infections
  - A. Bacterial peritonitis
    - 1. Acute bacterial peritonitis
    - 2. Primary (spontaneous) bacterial peritonitis
  - B. Tuberculous peritonitis
  - C. Fungal peritonitis
    - 1. *Candida albicans*
    - 2. *Histoplasma*
    - 3. *Coccidioides*
    - 4. *Cryptococcus*
  - D. Parasitic peritonitis
    - 1. *Schistosoma*
    - 2. *Enterobius*
    - 3. *Ascaris*
    - 4. *Strongyloides*
    - 5. *Entamoeba histolytica*
- II. Neoplasms
  - A. Mesothelial hyperplasia and benign neoplasms
    - 1. Mesothelial hyperplasia and metaplasia
    - 2. Benign adenomatoid mesothelioma
    - 3. Benign cystic mesothelioma
    - 4. Benign papillary mesothelioma
  - B. Primary malignant mesothelioma
  - C. Secondary carcinomatosis
  - D. Pseudomyxoma peritonei
- III. Granulomatous peritonitis
  - A. Exogenous
  - B. Endogenous
  - C. Iatrogenic
- IV. Familial paroxysmal polyserositis
- V. Vasculitis
  - A. SLE and other collagen-vascular diseases
  - B. Allergic vasculitis (Henoch-Schönlein purpura)
  - C. Köhlmeier-Degos disease
- VI. Sclerosing peritonitis
  - A. Toxic
  - B. Indwelling foreign bodies
  - C. Idiopathic
- VII. Miscellaneous peritoneal diseases
  - A. Eosinophilic peritonitis
  - B. Whipple's disease
  - C. Gynecologic lesions
    - 1. Endometriosis and deciduosis
    - 2. Teratoma (gliosis)
    - 3. Leiomyomatosis
    - 4. Dermoid cyst
    - 5. Melanosis
  - D. Splenosis
  - E. Peritoneal lymphangiectasis
  - F. Peritoneal cysts
  - G. Peritoneal encapsulation

Infections of the Peritoneum

Acute Bacterial Peritonitis

Bacterial peritonitis most commonly results from perforation of an abdominal viscus (e.g., perforated ulcer or diverticulum, ruptured appendix, or following abdominal trauma).[38] The peritoneum has several defense mechanisms that are available in response to bacterial contamination.[29] First, bacteria may be cleared from the peritoneum via the diaphragmatic lymphatics. Second, opsonins, polymorphonuclear leukocytes, and macrophages enter the peritoneal cavity where phagocytosis and destruction of bacteria can occur. Finally, the peritoneum and omentum can contain localized infections and close small visceral perforations, in part by the exudation of fibrin-containing fluid.

Clinical Features. The etiology and details of differential diagnosis are discussed on pages 238 to 250. Regardless of etiology, abdominal pain, nausea, vomiting, tachycardia, tachypnea, and fever are usually present. The severity of these symptoms is related to the extent of contamination;[39] in generalized peritonitis, shock is also present and may be profound, whereas symptoms and signs may be minimal if infection is localized. Indeed, an important cause of unexplained fever is a clinically inapparent intra-abdominal abscess. In severe cases, there may be exquisite diffuse tenderness and rigidity of the abdomen; bowel sounds are usually diminished or absent, and distention may be present.

Laboratory findings are nonspecific. Leukocytosis is usually present and may be marked; hemoconcentration may result from loss of fluid into the peritoneal space. Electrolyte concentrations vary, but metabolic acidosis and respiratory alkalosis are often seen. Plain abdominal films show distention of small and large intestine and air-fluid levels. On upright films, air may be seen beneath the diaphragm if a viscus is perforated. In debilitated, obtunded, or elderly patients, peritoneal lavage may help establish the presence of peritonitis. One liter of fluid is instilled through a peritoneal dialysis catheter; a positive lavage fluid contains more than 500 white blood cells per milliliter of fluid or more than 50,000 red blood cells per milliliter, or a Gram stain reveals bacteria.[40] Recent studies document this to be a reliable, safe procedure which may be quite helpful in these selected patients.[40, 41]

The principal systemic complications of peritonitis are septicemia, shock, ileus, and widespread organ failure, including respiratory, renal, hepatic, and cardiac failure.[39, 42, 43] Local complications include wound infection, intraperitoneal abscesses, anastomotic breakdown, and fistula formation. These latter complications are discussed on pages 381 to 397.

Treatment. Patients with milder forms of peritonitis, especially those in whom the process is well localized or in whom the risks of surgery are judged unacceptable, may be managed nonoperatively. Measures employed should include nasogastric suction, antibiotics, analgesics, appropriate administration of fluids (this may need to be aggressive), and monitoring of volume, acid base, and electrolyte status as well as cardiopulmonary and renal function. There has been increasing experience with percutaneous drainage of localized abscesses, and this procedure appears quite promising in selected circumstances (see pp. 388–389).

In patients with advanced peritonitis in whom surgery is indicated, a period of preoperative preparation is often necessary to restore fluid balance and stabilize circulatory and pulmonary function.[42, 43] Nasogastric suction reduces distention and may help improve pulmonary function, and adequate volumes of electrolyte and colloid solutions are administered to correct hypovolemia. Complete blood counts, serum electrolytes, creatinine concentrations, and levels of arterial pH, pO_2, and pCO_2 should be monitored. Depending upon the severity of the illness, urinary, central venous, or pulmonary artery catheters may be placed. Analgesics are administered as needed to control pain, and oxygen may be administered to deal with hypoxemia due to abdominal distention or increased metabolic demand. Respiratory-assist devices or endotracheal intubation may be required.

Antibiotic therapy is essential in treatment and should be initiated early. This will control bacteremia, reduce suppurative complications, and prevent local spread of infection. Bacteriologic findings will vary, depending upon the site of intestinal perforation, the disease process responsible, and the time elapsed after initiation. In advanced peritonitis, however, a single organism is rarely found, and in most cases there is a polymicrobial flora consisting of one or two aerobic and two or three anaerobic species. Approximately 30 per cent of patients have septicemia, usually with *Escherichia coli* and *Bacteroides fragilis.*[29]

Most systemically administered antibiotics reach adequate therapeutic concentrations in intraperitoneal fluid. A frequently used regimen combines an aminoglycoside for aerobes with clindamycin or metronidazole for anaerobes. Cephalosporins are popular for their low toxicity and broad-spectrum coverage, especially the third-generation compounds such as cefoxitin and ceftazidime, which provide broad aerobic and anaerobic coverage.[29, 44–46] However, the role of these newer drugs as single agents, particularly in severe infections, remains to be determined. Ampicillin may be added to ensure coverage of enterococci, although this is not necessary routinely. It should be used only in patients at high risk of enterococcal infections, such as those with persistent or recurrent infection, shock, or immunosuppression.[45, 47]

The nutritional requirements of patients with severe peritonitis are enormous, and resting metabolic rate may increase up to 40 per cent above normal. Thus total parenteral nutrition, providing 3000 to 4000 calories per day via a central venous catheter, is often necessary to avoid major catabolic losses (see pp. 2019–2023).

The appropriate operative procedure in peritonitis is determined by the primary cause, but the basic objectives are to stop the continuing bacterial contamination, reduce the numbers of bacteria, remove foreign material, and provide drainage of purulent collections. The role and value of adjunctive treatments have been difficult to define; management of residual sepsis within the peritoneal cavity is the controversial issue. The traditional method relies on natural defenses of the peritoneal cavity to localize and resolve residual infection. A more aggressive approach has been used in diffuse, poorly localized peritonitis and is designed to remove residual necrotic debris and bacteria using continuous peritoneal lavage, intraperitoneal antibiotic or antiseptic agents, and radical peritoneal debridement.[29, 44, 48–50] Although some experimental models and clinical studies suggest that these procedures may be effective, others have not confirmed these results.[45, 51] These procedures may have value in certain subgroups or high-risk patients, but their overall place in the treatment of peritonitis remains to be defined.

Prognosis. Despite the use of antibiotics, modern anesthesia, and intensive support systems, the mortality rate of generalized peritonitis remains at 50 per cent. The factors adversely affecting prognosis include older age, fecal peritonitis, shock, and organ failure (pulmonary, renal, hepatic).[29, 39, 52]

Bacterial Peritonitis in Chronic Peritoneal Dialysis

In the last decade, peritoneal dialysis has been reintroduced as a long-term treatment option for end-stage renal disease. This increased use is the result of the development of permanent indwelling peritoneal catheters, automated dialysate delivery systems, and the view that peritoneal dialysis may be a physiologically preferred mode of therapy. The reported incidence of peritonitis is variable, ranging from 0.1 to 10 per cent of dialyses, affecting 20 to 85 per cent of patients, and with a frequency of 0.4 to 1.8 episodes per patient year.[53–56] A recent multicenter registry report put the frequency at 1.7 episodes per patient year.[55] This incidence may be reduced to under 1 per cent of dialyses when measures are taken to assure strict asepsis. Chronic ambulatory peritoneal dialysis may have up to twice the incidence of peritonitis as intermittent dialysis, possibly reflecting more prolonged contact with the dialysate or difficulty with patient adherence to sterile routine.[57] Adherence to strict aseptic technique, specially trained personnel, use of air-tight and water-tight catheter dressings, careful screening of potential infection sources, and shortened dialysis times all contribute to a reduction in the incidence of peritonitis.[53]

Although peritonitis is explained by contamination of the abdominal cavity through the catheter, clinically apparent infection may develop due to host factors. In chronic dialysis, actively phagocytic cells and opsonins are removed and diluted, and this may compromise host defenses.[58, 59]

Peritonitis in this setting usually produces a mild clinical syndrome of fever, abdominal pain, and cloudy dialysate drainage. Over one half of the episodes are caused by gram-positive organisms, mainly *Staphylococcus epidermidis, Staphylococcus aureus*, and *Streptococcus* species. Gram-negative organisms are responsible for 15 per cent of infections and tend to occur in later episodes, possibly owing to a change in body flora. Anaerobic organisms are rarely implicated, but unusual organisms such as *Mycobacteria, Candida, Aspergillus*, and *Nocardia* are occasionally seen (see below).[60–62] In addition, 15 to 30 per cent of clinical episodes of peritonitis are aseptic, presumably owing to a chemical constituent in the dialysate, possibly endotoxin.[60, 63, 64]

Eosinophilic peritonitis may occur in 6 to 20 per cent of patients within a few weeks of initiation of dialysis. It presents concern clinically because of cloudy dialysate, but it is usually asymptomatic, cultures are negative, and it requires no treatment.[63, 65]

Elevation of the dialysate polymorphonuclear leukocyte count may precede the clinical symptoms of peritonitis by up to one week. Cell counts in peritonitis are greater than 300 cells per milliliter with greater than 75 per cent neutrophils.[60, 66] Gram stains of peritoneal dialysate are positive in only about 10 per cent of samples. Following successful therapy, the elevated neutrophil count returns to normal in four to five days.

Outpatient treatment is often initiated with broad-spectrum intraperitoneal antibiotics, such as cephalosporin, occasionally supplemented by an oral agent.[67–68a] Increased frequency of exchanges may also be helpful for 24 to 48 hours, with continuation of intraperitoneal antibiotics for two weeks. The treatment of fungal peritonitis is discussed on page 1939. If peritonitis fails to resolve, the dialysis catheter should be removed. If multiple enteric organisms are cultured, if infection persists despite antibiotics and catheter removal, or if the clinical condition is deteriorating, exploratory laparotomy should be considered to rule out another cause of peritonitis.[69, 70]

Patients generally respond well to this approach, and in all cases antibiotic regimens and removal of the catheter as required lead to resolution of peritonitis.[60] Although there are no deaths in many series, as the numbers of patients have increased, mortality rates of 1 to 4 per cent have been reported.[67] Approximately 4 per cent of the patients on maintenance dialysis may develop peritoneal sclerosis (see p. 1949).

Primary (Spontaneous) Bacterial Peritonitis

Primary or spontaneous peritonitis is an acute or subacute bacterial infection of the peritoneum that develops without the usual underlying etiologic factors, such as perforated viscus, abscess, or penetrating abdominal wound. It is most common in children; primary peritonitis accounts for 2 per cent of all pediatric abdominal emergencies and 13 per cent of cases of diffuse peritoneal sepsis in children. In the past, spontaneous peritonitis was mainly a disease of children with nephrotic syndrome; at the present time, two thirds of children with gram-positive peritonitis are nephrotics, and 2 to 5 per cent of nephrotic children still develop gram-positive peritonitis.[71, 72] In recent years, only a small number of children with primary peritonitis have underlying nephrotic syndrome; an upper respiratory or urinary tract infection may precede the onset of peritonitis, but cultures from these areas often do not correlate with peritoneal cultures.[73–76]

The clinical signs and symptoms are similar to those of secondary peritonitis. As mentioned above, gram-positive organisms (*Pneumococcus, Staphylococcus, Streptococcus*) are common in primary peritonitis. Since the start of the antibiotic era, however, a shift has taken place from a preponderance of gram-positive organisms (50 to 80 per cent of pneumococci) to gram-negative organisms (15 to 20 per cent pneumococci[77]), although in some series pneumococci remain the predominant organisms.[71, 75] Anaerobic organisms are rare.

Primary peritonitis in children probably reflects hematogenous spread, because in two thirds of cases the peritoneal bacteria can be cultured elsewhere; i.e., extra-abdominal pathogens.[74, 78] In nephrotics, serum immunoglobulin levels and ascitic fluid immunoglobulins, complement, and bactericidal activity are all diminished, but the immunologic status of non-nephrotics is unknown.[71, 72, 79]

Because the condition mimics peritonitis caused by an acute surgical emergency, laparotomy is almost always undertaken unless the patient is known to have the nephrotic syndrome. If that is so, or the diagnosis is otherwise suspected, abdominal paracentesis and lavage may confirm the diagnosis. If gram-positive organisms are found, the patient may be treated with antibiotics; otherwise, exploratory laparotomy is warranted to rule out a ruptured viscus.[72–75] With the advent of the antibiotic era, the mortality rate has decreased from 40 to 50 per cent to 5 to 10 per cent.

The most common setting for primary, spontaneous peritonitis in adults is cirrhosis with ascites, complicating the course of the illness in up to 10 per cent of cirrhotic patients with portal hypertension and overt ascites. (Because ascites is almost invariably present, this particular form of peritonitis is discussed on pages 433 to 443.) Spontaneous peritonitis is rare in patients with systemic lupus erythematosus, neoplasms, or other reasons for immunosuppression, and is uncommon in transplant patients.[78, 80–84] The rarity in this setting is probably due to the normal levels of complement, opsonic, and antibacterial activity in the ascitic fluid, all of which have also been demonstrated in patients with malignant ascites.[83] Mortality and morbidity rates are higher in these sicker adults with primary peritonitis than in children.

The diagnosis of spontaneous peritonitis should be considered in (1) patients with existing ascites who develop fever or changing abdominal signs or symptoms, (2) patients with a focus for bacteremia, such as indwelling catheters, cellulitis, or urinary, biliary, or pulmonary infection; and (3) patients with decreased immunologic competence. In these circumstances, paracentesis may disclose the presence of gram-positive organisms and justify antibiotics as the sole therapy. Surgery for this group is indicated only if there is an intra-abdominal abscess or perforated viscus.

Tuberculous Peritonitis

Although peritonitis is an unusual form of tuberculosis, it is one of the most important diseases of the peritoneum. It has been reported to represent 0.5 per cent of new cases of tuberculosis and 4 to 10 per cent of cases of extrapulmonary tuberculosis;[85] in developing countries it has been reported in 1.5 per cent of new cases.[86, 87] Its insidious nature and the clinical circumstances in which it occurs often cause it to be mistaken for neoplastic disease or ascites caused by cirrhosis.

Pathogenesis. Most cases of tuberculous peritonitis are not due to contiguous extension of active disease in or adjacent to the peritoneal cavity. Rather, they appear to reflect reactivation of latent tuberculous foci in the peritoneum, established at the time of earlier hematogenous spread from a primary focus, usually in the lung.[86, 88] Thus, many patients with tuberculous peritonitis do not have currently active pulmonary, intestinal, or genital tuberculosis. On the other hand, hematogenous spread from pulmonary or generalized miliary tuberculosis can cause concurrent tuberculous peritonitis, and autopsy series in patients with late generalized tuberculosis suggest that reactivated tuberculous lymph nodes are a source of tuberculous peritonitis.[89] A number of cases have been described in which tuberculous peritonitis developed within a few weeks of laparotomy, but a causal relationship between the surgery and reactivation of peritoneal foci has not been definitely established.[90]

Epidemiology. In the United States, the disease is most commonly encountered in the municipal hospital setting with its large population of cirrhotics and poorly nourished debilitated patients.[85, 91, 92] There is no age or sex predilection, but from 80 to 90 per cent of patients in reported series are black. This distribution may reflect socioeconomic rather than genetic factors.

Tuberculosis is common in patients with acquired immunodeficiency syndrome (AIDS) and is often extrapulmonary or disseminated.[93] Although tuberculous peritonitis has been reported rarely in this setting, it may become more common[94] (see pp. 1233–1257).

Clinical Features. The clinical features of tuberculous peritonitis vary with the population studied.[95] Generally, the onset is insidious, and over 70 per cent of the patients have had symptoms for four months or longer. The most common complaints are constitutional, with fever, anorexia, weakness, malaise, and weight loss occurring in 80 per cent. Abdominal pain is reported in only 50 per cent, and this is usually described as a vague, dull, diffuse discomfort. The incidence and intensity of vomiting, constipation, and diarrhea are variable. The major objective finding is ascites, which is clinically evident in 75 per cent of the patients. Abdominal tenderness, usually diffuse, is present in 65 per cent; despite classic descriptions, the so-called doughy abdomen is rare. Hepatomegaly may be found in 25 per cent, and a mass caused by loculated fluid or an inflamed omentum or mesentery may be palpated in 20 per cent. Lymphadenopathy may be present. It is evident from the clinical description that the signs and symptoms of tuberculous peritonitis are nonspecific and variable. Therefore, tuberculous peritonitis must be suspected in any patient with ascites, fever, unexplained constitutional symptoms, or diffuse abdominal pain or tenderness. This is especially true of the patient being treated for disease in which other reasons for peritonitis might allow tuberculous peritonitis to be overlooked, such as cirrhosis, chronic peritoneal dialysis, or peritoneal carcinomatosis.[85, 96, 97]

Laboratory Findings. Routine blood studies are rarely helpful; there is a normal white blood cell count in 70 to 90 per cent and anemia is only variably present. The tuberculin skin test is negative in about 20 per cent of reported cases, although many of these are in patients with extraperitoneal and miliary disease. If tuberculosis is confined to the peritoneum, the first strength purified protein derivative test may be positive in virtually 100 per cent.[88] A negative test may become positive during treatment, suggesting that the patient may have been anergic initially.[92]

Other studies may prove useful, especially if the disease is more generalized. Pulmonary infiltrates are seen in about one half of the patients, and 40 per cent have pleural effusions. Barium studies of the intestine, pyelograms, or salpingograms are rarely helpful, although bizarre angular or rigid small bowel loops and altered mucosal patterns may suggest mesenteric involvement. Occasionally, tuberculous enteritis may coexist and be demonstrable by barium contrast studies of the intestine.[98] There are no computed tomographic findings that are pathognomonic of peritoneal tuberculosis, but it is suggested by mesenteric adenopathy, low-density centers within the enlarged nodes, mesenteric and omental thickening, peritoneal enhancement, and high-density loculated ascites (see Fig. 102–2*B*).[99] Percutaneous liver biopsy or lymph node biopsy may show granulomas, but this finding is not necessarily diagnostic of active intra-abdominal tuberculosis. Fewer than one half of patients with tuberculous peritonitis will have evidence of disease elsewhere in the body.

Examination of the peritoneal fluid is the most important initial diagnostic test (see p. 430). Protein exceeds 2.5 gm/100 ml in 85 to 100 per cent of patients. Most patients have over 250 leukocytes per milliliter; 90 to 100 per cent have more than 80 per cent mononuclear cells on differential count. Acid-fast stains of the peritoneal fluid will demonstrate the organisms in only about 5 per cent of patients. Cultures of the fluid are also disappointing, for they are positive in only about 40 per cent of patients. However, the yield may be improved to 80 per cent by concentrating up to 1 liter of fluid by centrifugation and by guinea pig inoculation.[87, 91] Tuberculous peritonitis is almost always caused by *Mycobacterium tuberculosis*, but rare cases due to atypical mycobacteria (*Mycobacterium avium-intracellulare, M. fortuitum, M. gordonae*) have been reported.[100, 101] Peritoneal biopsy for granulomas is positive in 30 to 50 per cent of patients with the Vim-Silverman needle, and the use of the Cope needle has been reported to increase the yield substantially.[88] The biopsy specimen should be cultured, but data on the sensitivity of this procedure are limited.

The diagnosis is often suggested at peritoneoscopy by the appearance of the peritoneum, which will show scattered or confluent miliary nodules of uniform size, with adhesions between bowel loops, liver capsule, and abdominal walls.[102, 103] Direct biopsy through the peritoneoscope may improve the chance for diagnosis over that of needle biopsy by 20 to 30 per cent.[87] Because the diagnosis is easily made at laparotomy, this diagnostic approach is preferred by some.[92, 104–107] Although in 80 to 85 per cent of patients the diagnosis may be established by fluid analysis, peritoneal biopsy, and peritoneoscopy, in approximately 15 to 20 per cent laparotomy may be needed. Laparotomy is generally well tolerated in these patients in the absence of serious contraindications.

Prognosis and Treatment. Prior to the availability of chemotherapy, the mortality rate of tuberculous peritonitis was as high as 60 per cent. However, the disease is now curable with antituberculous agents. Therapy with isoniazid and a second agent, usually rifampin, is adequate if the incidence of isoniazid-resistant strains is low in the local population. Three or four drugs should be used if isoniazid-resistant strains are common or if they develop. In the past, 18 to 24 months of therapy was recommended, but nine months of therapy has been found to be successful; this is due to the presence of small bacterial populations in extrapulmonary lesions.[108–110]

Fungal and Parasitic Infection

Peritoneal inflammation caused by fungi and parasites is very uncommon. *Candida albicans* has been reported to cause massive ascites by direct peritoneal involvement, but it is usually in patients with a pathologic or artificial route for contamination of the peritoneal cavity. Because *Candida* organisms enter the peritoneal cavity via contamination, their presence may be a clue to occult gastrointestinal perforation.[111] The usual precipitating factors are perforated peptic ulcers, traumatic intestinal perforations, gastrointestinal surgery, and peritoneal dialysis. *Candida* peritonitis usually remains localized to the abdominal cavity; although the infection disseminates in 10 to 15 per cent, the risk is significant only in patients taking corticosteroids or antibiotics.[112]

Fungal peritonitis is becoming increasingly frequent in patients on peritoneal dialysis, and in a recent series occurred in 4 per cent of patients on intermittent dialysis and 18 per cent of patients on chronic ambulatory peritoneal dialysis.[113, 114] This incidence is related to the presence of a foreign body, high glucose solutions, use of corticosteroids and antibiotics, and the relatively poor phagocytosis of *Candida* by peritoneal macrophages.[115] *Candida* species remain the major pathogen in this setting, but other rare saprophytic organisms such as *Fusarium, Drechslera, Torulopsis, Rhodotorula, Trichosporon, Aspergillus*, or *Mucor* have been reported.[113, 116, 117]

The incidence of *Candida* peritonitis is 1 per cent in renal transplant patients and is related to intestinal perforation or other intraperitoneal disease.[84] Its contribution to peritonitis in other patients with polymicrobial enteric flora is poorly understood. Recently it has been suggested that *Candida* may worsen existing sepsis and may disseminate (even causing acute endocarditis), suggesting that early and vigorous treatment is indicated in patients in whom the organism is cultured.[118] This view has been disputed in a subsequent report.[118a]

The treatment of *Candida* peritonitis consists of drainage and administration of systemic or intraperitoneal anticandidal agents. Fifty per cent of patients with a perforated viscus may be adequately treated with surgical repair and drainage. If these measures are insufficient, antifungal agents should be added. In cases associated with dialysis, the catheter often has to be removed to effect cure.[113, 116] Often intraperitoneal instillation of amphotericin B is the treatment of choice for fungal peritonitis. That the intravenous route appears to establish adequate intraperitoneal concentrations of amphotericin B is important, averting painful intraperitoneal installation. Average total doses of amphotericin B are 250 to 500 mg intravenously and 1600 mg intraperitoneally, and cure is usually established in 2 to 3 weeks.[112] Intraperitoneal miconazole, oral ketoconazole, and 5′-fluorocytosine have also been used in small numbers of patients.[113, 117]

If *Candida* peritonitis is untreated, the mortality rate approaches 100 per cent. When treated with abdominal drainage, surgical repair, and antifungal therapy, however, most patients survive.[112]

Peritoneal involvement by *Histoplasma capsulatum* is very rare, being present in only 1 of 530 patients with active histoplasmosis in a sanitorium population, and in 2 to 4 per cent with disseminated histoplasmosis.[119] *Coccidioides immitis* causes granulomatous peritonitis in 1 to 2 per cent of cases of disseminated coccidioidomycosis. It also may appear without evidence of generalized dissemination, probably secondary to hematogenous spread from a subclinical pulmonary focus. Coccidioidin skin tests are negative, and the diagnosis can be confirmed microscopically by finding spherules of *C. immitis* in wet mounts of ascitic fluid or in histologic sections of peritoneal biopsies. Coccidioidal peritonitis is usually self-limited, and amphotericin B treatment is indicated only in patients with acute peritonitis, disseminated infection, or rising or persistently high complement fixation titers.[120, 121] *Cryptococcus neoformans* rarely involves the peritoneum alone, but cryptoccocal peritonitis and ascites may appear in patients who are immunosuppressed.[122, 123]

Parasitic infestation seldom leads to clinical peritoneal disease; its major importance lies in its ability to mimic peritoneal carcinomatosis or tuberculosis at laparotomy. Cases of granulomatous peritonitis caused by *Schistosoma mansoni*, without other extraintestinal involvement, have been reported. Schistosomal peritonitis is rarely symptomatic and may be due to the escape of eggs from intestinal veins.[124] *Enterobius vermicularis* has been reported to give rise to a granulomatous peritonitis in women, apparently after migration through the upper genital tract.[125] Although most patients are asymptomatic, they may present with lower abdominal pain. *Ascaris lumbricoides* also causes granulomatous peritonitis; the peritoneal nodules reveal evidence of both typical *Ascaris* ova and degenerating fragments of the adult worm.[126]

Two parasites, *Strongyloides stercoralis* and *Entamoeba histolytica*, cause more fulminant peritonitis and ascites after penetrating the intestinal wall.[127, 128] Patients with these diseases are severely ill, with ascites, pain, distention, and diarrhea; peritoneal signs are often mild. Because the peritonitis of these parasites is often not associated with frank intestinal perforation, specific antimicrobial treatment should be started and its effect assessed before surgical intervention is considered. Either infection may disseminate, especially in immunocompromised patients.

Neoplasms of the Peritoneum

Mesothelial Hyperplasia and Benign Mesothelial Neoplasms

In recent years, a spectrum of clinical syndromes and pathologic appearances has been firmly associated with mesothelial hyperplasia and metaplasia. In the presence of inflammation or in the course of undergoing regeneration, mesothelial cells may take on atypical hyperplastic appearances or undergo squamous metaplasia, particularly in localized areas such as hernia sacs.[4, 129] Although these changes are often merely reactive, they may well be preneoplastic or neoplastic and may have papillary or cystic appearances.[130] Three well-characterized types of mesothelial tumors in addition to malignant mesotheliomas discussed below have been delineated: (1) benign adenomatoid mesotheliomas, (2) benign cystic mesotheliomas, and (3) benign papillary mesotheliomas. They are more common in women, probably because the mesothelium covering the ovary and peritoneum in women has a metaplastic or neoplastic potential to produce epithelial elements resembling those found in various parts of the primary müllerian system.[131, 132]

Benign adenomatoid mesotheliomas are benign, gland-like neoplasms usually located in or near the genital tract or on the peritoneum. They usually are incidental findings and do not recur. They consist of irregularly arranged cords, tubules, or gland-like structures with benign histologic features in a fibrous stroma and are important mainly because they may simulate a malignant tumor.[133]

Benign cystic mesotheliomas, on the other hand, usually present with abdominal pain or as a mass in women of childbearing age. The diagnosis may be suspected on CT and ultrasound by the presence of multiseptated thin-walled cystic masses in the lower abdomen and pelvis.[134] The lesion consists of cysts containing watery secretions and lined by a single layer of mesothelial cells with typical microvilli on electron microscopy. The prognosis is excellent with no mortality rate; however, it recurs in 25 to 50 per cent. Surgical resection is the only treatment, with no known role for radiation or chemotherapy.[135–137]

Benign papillary mesotheliomas may also present with abdominal pain, or the lesion may be an incidental finding at surgery. They also cause exudative ascites and effusions in other mesothelium-lined cavities (pericardial or pleural).[138] The lesion may be solitary or disseminated over the peritoneum. It consists of a single layer of mesothelial cells covering a papillary stroma, with absence of infiltrative growth or neoplastic cytologic changes. The prognosis is excellent, and adjunctive therapy is not indicated. Because this lesion is mistaken for ovarian carcinoma in up to 7 per cent of women, it must be recognized as a benign lesion to ensure that inappropriate treatment for cancer is not initiated.[139–142]

Although the etiology of all the above lesions is unclear, they may be induced in women by retrograde spread from the genital canal of agents that can induce mesothelial hyperplasia or dysplasia.[140] These benign hyperplastic and neoplastic lesions do not appear to progress to malignant mesothelioma; however, it is difficult to establish that chronic inflammatory lesions can progress through dysplasia to mesothelioma, for early mesothelial dysplasia is nearly impossible to identify.[143]

Lastly, benign *fibrous mesotheliomas* are solitary tumors of the pleura. However, they are very rare in the peritoneum and may not be mesothelial in origin.[4, 144, 145]

Primary Malignant Mesotheliomas

Primary mesotheliomas are tumors rising from the epithelial and mesenchymal elements of the mesothelium. Approximately 25 per cent of mesotheliomas involve the peritoneum, 65 per cent are pleural, and 10 per cent are pericardial.[146] Mesotheliomas have been considered very rare, but since the 1950s many reports indicate a marked increase in the frequency of their diagnosis.[147, 148]

Epidemiology. Asbestos is the only substance that has been shown to have epidemiologically meaningful association with mesothelioma, and the apparent increased incidence can be related to expansion of the asbestos industry.[146–150] Asbestos is a generic term for a variety of hydrated silicate minerals defined by the attribute of breaking down into fibers when crushed or processed. Their chemical and physical properties make them useful as electrical and thermal insulators and permit them to be woven or otherwise fabricated into a variety of textiles, friction materials, and other products. There are two main types: amphibole and serpentine. The amphiboles used in industry are crocidolite, amosite, and anthrophyllite. The serpentine crysotile is the most common type in nature.[147, 151–153]

The percentage of mesothelioma patients exposed to asbestos has varied from 20 to 90 per cent and is determined by the occupational pattern of the region studied. An average of 50 per cent of patients of several large series had occupational exposure.[148–150, 154] This occupational exposure usually involves insulators, asbestos producers, heating trade workers, shipyard workers, and construction workers, with insulators having the highest relative risk.[148] The factors that influence the incidence of mesothelioma are the type of asbestos fiber used, the duration of exposure, and the concentration of asbestos to which the workers are exposed.

Most evidence suggests that crocidolite is the most potent inducer of mesothelioma, followed by amosite and then crysotile.[147, 150, 151] The duration of exposure is usually prolonged but may be very short, as many patients report only a few months of incidental exposure.[150] Asbestos exposure may be high in certain occupations, but mesothelioma is not always associated with occupational exposure; 20 per cent of all patients give a "bystander" history of para-occupational exposure, such as exposure in the home, contact with a worker or his clothing, or residence near a mine, factory, or shipyard using asbestos.[147, 150, 151] The effect of even lower concentrations of asbestos is still uncertain, since a threshold below which asbestos is safe or above which it is dangerous has not been demonstrated.[149] Asbestos fibers have been demonstrated in ambient air, water supplies, and food, and asbestos bodies may be found in the lungs of almost everybody when suitable techniques are used.[155–157] However, long-term high-level ingestion of various types of asbestos in animal models has failed to produce any carcinogenic effect.[153, 158] The balance of evidence so far does not point to a risk of ingested asbestos in the general population, but further data on the risk of low concentrations are still needed.[153, 158, 159]

The mean time interval between exposure to asbestos and development of mesothelioma is 35 to 40 years, and peak mesothelioma rates may occur after 45 years.[160] The latency period may be shorter for peritoneal than for pleural mesotheliomas.[161] Thus, increased numbers of mesothelioma cases may be anticipated, and it is estimated that about 5 per cent of asbestos workers may develop mesothelioma.

Some epidemiologic studies have suggested that occupational asbestos exposure is associated with a higher incidence of tumors of the esophagus, stomach, and colon, but the data are still inconclusive.[162, 163]

Pathogenesis. In addition to historical evidence of asbestos exposure, 50 per cent of patients with mesotheliomas may have pathologic evidence of pulmonary asbestosis, including pulmonary fibrosis, pleural hyaline plaques, and asbestos bodies in the lungs. It has also been demonstrated that one third of patients with peritoneal mesotheliomas have asbestos fibers in peritoneal tissue if proper techniques are used to demonstrate them.[164] Asbestos fibers are found significantly more frequently and in greater numbers in patients with mesothelioma than in normal individuals. Further, direct injection of asbestos into the pleural and peritoneal cavities of animals has produced mesotheliomas.[153]

No chemical factor has been established as significant in relation to asbestos pathogenicity; rather, emphasis has been placed on the size and shape of the asbestos fibers.[147, 152, 153, 165]

In vitro studies of the effect of asbestos on cells have demonstrated cytotoxicity and proliferative activity of mesothelial cells and fibroblasts, but the cellular action of asbestos is not yet understood.[147, 165] Asbestos is a weak mutagenic agent, so it probably acts as a promoter rather than an initiator of carcinogenesis.[153, 158] The pathogenesis of peritoneal mesothelioma is unclear. Patients with heavy asbestos exposure of large amount and long duration are more likely to present with a peritoneal lesion.[147, 165, 166] In heavily exposed populations, the peritoneum accounts for 50 per cent of all cases; in moderately exposed, 20 per cent; and in minimally exposed, 10 per cent.[154] Peritoneal exposure is presumably due to transport of asbestos fibers from the lungs to the abdomen via lymphatic transport.[147, 165] Asbestos is also transported across the gut mucosa after ingestion, although as mentioned above, feeding experiments have failed to produce peritoneal mesotheliomas.[158]

Because at least 30 per cent of the patients with mesothelioma have no history of asbestos exposure, other factors eventually may be uncovered.[150, 167] As mentioned, the role of environmental pollution is still unclear. In experimental studies, other synthetic fibers that approximate the physical characteristics of asbestos have been shown to produce mesotheliomas. Recently, another fibrous material, zeolite, has been implicated in an area where asbestos is absent.[167, 168] Finally, isolated cases of mesothelioma have been reported following Thorotrast exposure or radiotherapy.[167, 169] Although familial clustering has been reported and a genetic predisposition has been suggested, in most cases this is due to nonoccupational exposure.[170–172] HLA antigen studies have not demonstrated that any particular subtype exhibits increased susceptibility to asbestos.[173]

Clinical Features and Diagnosis. Mesotheliomas, especially peritoneal ones, are more common in males, possibly reflecting occupational factors.[146, 174] The highest prevalence is in the sixth decade, but the condition has been recorded in children.[175] Twenty per cent of mesotheliomas in children are peritoneal, presumably unrelated to asbestos exposure. Patients without asbestos exposure may present earlier and lack male predominance.[176]

Patients presenting with peritoneal primary tumors ordinarily complain first of abdominal pain, an abdominal mass, or increased abdominal girth along with anorexia, nausea, vomiting, constipation, and weight loss.[146, 174, 177] Fever of unknown origin may be the only complaint.[178] Physical examination is often normal early in the disease; later, ascites and abdominal masses become detectable. Signs of asbestos are evident on chest X-rays in 50 per cent, and early pleural mesothelioma may also be apparent with chest pain, dyspnea, or cough.[146, 177]

Usually blood counts and chemistries are not helpful, although the sedimentation rate may be elevated. Rarely, findings associated with ectopic hormone production are noted, such as hypoglycemia or marked electrolyte abnormalities.[178] Barium contrast films also reveal nonspecific findings: fixation, angulation, or narrowing of bowel loops with extrinsic defects on intra-abdominal organs.[179] Ultrasound and CT scans demonstrate sheet-like masses involving the omentum, mesentery, and peritoneum; although the sheet-like nature is not specific, it may suggest the diagnosis.[180–182] Ascites is usually present, but the amount of ascites may be disproportionately small in relation to the degree of tumor dissemination. The diagnosis of mesothelioma, as opposed to peritoneal carcinomatosis, may be suspected on radiologic grounds if the amount of ascites is disproportionately small to the tumor load, if the mesentery is thickened, or if pleural plaques are seen.[181, 183]

Paracentesis yields an exudate that may be hemorrhagic. Fluid hyaluronic acid levels above 120 μg/ml are suggestive of mesothelioma, but because the majority of patients have intermediate levels that may also be seen in metastatic carcinoma, this test may not be diagnostic. A recent modification of technique using a liquid chromatographic method may be more diagnostic.[184] Peritoneal cytologic studies and biopsy may suggest the diagnosis. However, the overlap of morphologic features with other tumors and the tremendous microscopic variability are such that only experienced workers in this area are able to diagnose definitively the disorder on the basis of biopsy and cytologic findings.[147, 149, 185] Unfortunately, this overlap also makes the more easily obtained CT-guided fine needle aspiration biopsies less definitive for diagnosis.[181] Peritoneoscopy reveals extensive studding of all peritoneal surfaces with nodules and plaques, which may be strongly suggestive of mesothelioma.[186] Laparotomy is usually necessary to provide adequate biopsy samples for definitive diagnosis and to rule out a primary neoplasm.[149, 177, 178]

Pathology. On gross examination, primary mesotheliomas of the peritoneum may be extremely difficult to differentiate from secondary carcinomatosis. They usually involve both the visceral and the parietal peritoneum extensively, although they also form discrete plaques and nodules; less than 2 per cent are localized.[174] Superficial capsular invasion of viscera and local lymph node involvement are common. Although visceral metastases are found in up to 50 per cent of patients, they usually are clinically silent.[174, 177]

The histologic characteristics are quite variable. Individual cells are rarely pleomorphic or mitotic. Epithelial elements predominate in 70 per cent, with tubular, papillary, sheet-like, cleft-like, or solid nest-like patterns. Sometimes mesenchymal elements predominate, with a prominent fibromatous component and spindle-shaped cells, but these are rare in peritoneal mesotheliomas. Many mesotheliomas have both epithelial and mesenchymal elements present in a single tumor, and this finding will make the diagnosis of mesothelioma more certain. A negative periodic acid–Schiff stain for mucin and positive stain for hyaluronic acid with colloidal iron or alcian blue are further suggestive, but not diagnostic, of mesothelioma.[147, 149, 174, 177]

Newer pathologic techniques may help in diagnosis. Electron microscopy reveals abundant long microvilli and intermediate filaments, findings that support the diagnosis of mesothelioma.[187–189] Immunopathologic diagnosis has been attempted, using antimesothelial cell serum to stain mesothelial cells, but this technique has not yet been adequately evaluated.[190] Immunochemical staining with monoclonal antibodies promises an advance in cytologic diagnosis. Mesothelioma cells fail to react with anticarcinoembryonic antigen, but give positive staining with certain antiepithelial antibodies (epithelial membrane antigen and Ca antigen) and certain intermediate-sized filaments of the intracellular matrix (cytokeratin and vimentin). Differential staining can thus separate mesotheliomas from carcinomas.[191–193] Electrophoretic analysis of tissue glycosaminoglycans may improve the diagnostic yield.[194] A combination of several or all of the aforementioned techniques usually allows a diagnosis of mesothelioma.

Prognosis and Treatment. The prognosis of mesothelioma is poor, and most patients survive only one year after diagnosis.[146] Peritoneal disease results in cachexia or small bowel obstruction, and death generally results from these complications rather than from metastatic disease. Clotting abnormalities with disseminated intravascular coagulation, thrombosis, phlebitis, or pulmonary emboli may complicate the course.[178] In some series, peritoneal disease and spindle or sarcomatous histologic patterns indicate a worse prognosis than pleural involvement and an epithelial pattern.[177] Other favorable prognostic variables may include limited disease, indolent disease with long symptom duration before diagnosis, and female sex.[195, 196]

Optimal therapeutic regimens for peritoneal mesothelioma remain to be defined. There has been little role for surgery, except for cytoreductive surgery, which may be considered in selective cases (see below). There is little evidence that radiotherapy alone is effective in peritoneal mesothelioma,[197] although radiotherapy has produced some long-term disease-free survivors.[198] Local treatments such as standard low-volume intraperitoneal chemotherapy or radioactive gold have rarely been successful, the latter because of its limited tissue penetration. In recent years, doxorubicin has proved to be an active drug, and a number of studies have demonstrated up to 50 per cent response, with increased survival.[195, 196, 199, 200] However, poor responses to this drug in some large series have encouraged new approaches to treatment.[201] Intracavitary cisplatin has shown promise in early trials.[202] Combined modality therapy has always seemed attractive,[196, 199, 202a] and in a recent report on the treatment of early stage 1 disease, cytoreductive surgery, radiation, and intracavitary doxorubicin and cisplatin have shown good results in a small number of cases.[203]

Secondary Carcinomatosis

Incidence and Etiology. Peritoneal involvement by spread from a primary neoplasm is one of the most common causes of peritoneal disease. Pathologic study of unselected open peritoneal biopsy specimens in a large general hospital shows that 65 per cent are neoplastic. Over 75 per cent of these are metastatic adenocarcinomas; other tumors such as sarcomas, carcinoids, teratomas, lipomas, or nervous tissue tumors are rare.[204] The primary site varies with the population studied, but intra-abdominal primary sites are most common. In one recent series, tumors of the ovary and pancreas were most common, followed by tumors of the colon, lymphatics, stomach, and uterus.[205] Extra-abdominal tumors such as lung and breast may also spread to the peritoneum.

Malignancies of lymphoid or myeloid tissue can also infiltrate the peritoneum. Up to one third of patients with leukemia may have peritoneal fluid, but fewer than 5 per cent have more than 1 liter of ascites.[206] Malignant lymphoma invades the serosa in about 20 per cent of patients, is most often associated with bowel wall invasion, and may cause ascites. Peritoneal disease has been found in up to one third of patients with non-Hodgkin's lymphomas but in a much lower number with Hodgkin's disease.[207] In a recent study of gastrointestinal lymphomas, 10 per cent had documented peritoneal disease.[208] Multiple myeloma has rarely been reported to cause peritoneal infiltration with ascites.[209] Ascites occurs in about 10 per cent of patients with myeloid metaplasia. Ectopic peritoneal implantation of myeloid tissue may also cause ascites, either due to multicentric extramedullary hematopoietic foci or due to implants from occult splenic rupture.[210]

Pathophysiology. Alterations in diaphragmatic lymphatic absorption and peritoneal capillary permeability both play a role in ascites formation associated with peritoneal carcinomatosis.[211, 211a] The physiologic importance of the diaphragmatic lymphatics has been discussed (see p. 1933). Radiologic, scintigraphic, and histopathologic techniques demonstrate obstruction of channels that connect the peritoneal cavity to the subdiaphragmatic lymphatic plexus, thereby preventing adequate drainage from the peritoneal cavity.[212, 213] Dye-injection studies of peritoneal capillaries and the success of sclerosing agents in ameliorating ascites together suggest that altered capillary permeability underlies ascites formation in peritoneal carcinomatosis. Chemical mediators that increase capillary permeability may be liberated by neoplasms, and pharmacologically active substances such as prostaglandins and kinin-like vasoactive polypeptides have been isolated from peritoneal neoplasms.[214]

Immunology. The immunologic consequences of malignant ascites have been extensively studied experimentally, but their clinical implications are as yet unclear. In malignant ascites there is an increased percentage of T lymphocytes, some of which may show cytotoxic activity.[215] On the other hand, malignant ascites may be associated with a general impairment of immune responsiveness.[216, 217]

Clinical Features and Diagnosis. Patients with peritoneal carcinomatosis present with ascites, diffuse abdominal pain, and weight loss, and less frequently with nausea and vomiting. Ascites is the major complaint in about one half of patients.[205] Barium contrast studies may show nodular indentations of the intestine or angulated, fixed, or displaced intestinal loops, especially if attention is paid to the areas of intraperitoneal seeding. These areas include the pouch of Douglas at the rectosigmoid, the right lower quadrant at the small bowel mesentery, the left lower quadrant along the superior border of the sigmoid mesocolon and the colon, and the right paracolic gutter lateral to the cecum and ascending colon.[1, 218]

Ultrasound or CT scan may help confirm the presence of ascites and associated mass lesions, but CT scans have a 30 to 40 per cent false negative rate in diagnosing neoplastic peritoneal lesions.[219, 220] In a recent study, CT scan detected 10 per cent of tumor nodules to be 1 cm or less, 37 per cent of nodules greater than 1 cm, and 42 per cent greater than 2 cm.[221] Thus, although CT scan may be very helpful, it cannot rule out peritoneal spread of tumor.

Paracentesis yields fluid that is usually, but not always, an exudate and often has significant numbers of red blood cells or is grossly hemorrhagic (see pp. 430–431).

The diagnosis is made most directly by cytologic examination, peritoneal biopsy, or peritoneoscopy (see pp. 431–432).

Cytologic findings are positive in the ascitic fluid in 50 to 80 per cent of cases and may also be obtained from peritoneal washings at laparotomy.[191, 222] Both false negative studies and the difficulty in differentiating malignant cells from atypical mesothelial cells are sources of error and confusion. Newer techniques have been employed to decrease the false negative rate and differentiate atypical mesothelial cells. These include electron microscopy, transmission and scanning electron microscopy, tissue culture, cytogenetic analysis, and immunochemical analysis.[189, 223] Only immunochemical analysis seems likely to become routinely useful. With the introduction of immunologic markers and monoclonal antibodies, it is possible to determine the presence or absence of a variety of tumor or tissue markers on specific cells in ascites fluids and in tissues.[191] Antibodies have been raised to carcinoembryonic antigen; cancer-associated antigen (CA1); epithelial-membrane antigen (EMA) and human milk fat globulin (HMFG), both of which are glycoprotein determinants in a variety of carcinomas; and keratin and vimentin (filaments of the intracellular matrix). These antibodies may increase the diagnostic accuracy of cytologically negative or suspicious samples, identify reactive mesothelial cells, or differentiate different types of malignant cells.[191, 193, 224, 225] The specificity and reliability of these methods are currently being clarified and refined. Early reports suggest that identifying abnormal DNA content with flow cytometry may be a valuable technique.[225a]

It is important to remember that many peritoneal diseases may present with a clinical picture mimicking that of peritoneal carcinomatosis. Tuberculous peritonitis and spontaneous bacterial peritonitis associated with cirrhosis must be ruled out, especially because they are treatable. Meigs' syndrome, myxedema, hypoalbuminemic ascites, and Budd-Chiari syndrome may be confused with peritoneal carcinomatosis in certain clinical settings.

Prognosis and Treatment. Once the neoplasm has spread to the peritoneum, the prognosis is poor. Once ascites forms, the mean survival time is less than 20 weeks, with a few long-term survivors and apparent cures noted in patients with ovarian cancers.[205] Six-month survival rate is 12 per cent, one-year survival rate is 4 per cent, and two-year survival, 1 per cent.[226] Because the pathogenesis of malignant ascites is different from that of cirrhosis, simple measures such as salt restriction and diuretics are only occasionally helpful.[227] This may be particularly true in a subgroup of patients with sodium retention and hyperreninemia, which may be due to a reduction in effective circulating blood volume from transfer of fluid into the peritoneal cavity, with secondary activation of the renin-angiotensin system. A therapeutic trial of spironolactone, especially if urinary sodium is low, is often worth while.[228] There are no trials comparing different classes of diuretics in the setting of malignant ascites.

Paracentesis is useful, and removal of large volumes of fluid may be well tolerated without hemodynamic problems.[229] Although repeated paracentesis may reduce body protein stores, increased tumor mass, impaired liver function, and poor alimentation may be more important causes of protein malnutrition.[230]

A variety of agents have been instilled into the peritoneal cavity in an attempt to decrease tumor growth or accumulation of ascites. Cytotoxic agents, radioisotopes, and sclerosing agents have been used with variable temporary success, but no definitive study is available to compare their efficacy. In earlier reports, they were used mainly in advanced disease, and the agents were probably acting as sclerosing agents.

Sclerosing agents include quinacrine (400 mg for three to five days) and tetracycline (500 mg). Cytotoxic agents that produce sclerosis have included nitrogen mustard (0.4 mg/kg), 5-flourouracil (2 to 3 gm), thiotepa, doxorubicin (30 mg), and bleomycin (60 to 120 ml). All these agents have reported response rates of 20 to 70 per cent and variable toxicity, including abdominal pain, nausea, fever, ileus, or bone marrow suppression.[227, 231–234] Tetracycline and bleomycin have been widely used in recent years. Drainage of as much fluid as possible before instilling the drug is important to assure the best possible result.

The cytotoxic action of chemotherapeutic agents is being re-examined. In contrast to the methods of intracavitary treatment aimed at palliation of malignant ascites, by which drugs are administered in high concentrations and small volume, in recent trials of intracavitary therapy a large volume (2 liters) of drug has been used. This is administered through a semipermanent Tenckhoff-type catheter (with or without a subcutaneous port) to allow for uniform drug distribution and to facilitate repetitive treatments. This new approach is based on pharmacologic modeling, suggesting that the administration of certain chemotherapeutic agents directly into the peritoneal cavity could result in significantly higher exposure of the peritoneum to the drug. Experimental evaluation has confirmed the modeling predictions for several antineoplastic drugs including cisplatin, doxorubicin, 5-fluorouracil, methotrexate, mitomycin C, and cytarabin. The peritoneal cavity has been exposed to 1 to 3 logs higher concentration than in plasma. This approach holds the promise of increasing the efficacy of treatment while decreasing the systemic toxicity.[235–237]

Clinical trials have been carried out, mainly in ovarian carcinoma, mesothelioma, and colon cancer, to evaluate the role of intracavitary therapy using different agents, singly and in combination. Cisplatin appears to have potentially important efficacy and has not produced the local toxic effects associated with methotrexate, bleomycin, 5-fluorouracil, and doxorubicin.[235–237] Additional practical problems associated with the peritoneal catheters include catheter obstruction, perforation, ileus, peritonitis, sepsis, bleeding, and adhesion.[238, 239]

Intraperitoneal chemotherapy is still experimental. For patients with extensive peritoneal disease it may be palliative. Because it will probably not improve overall survival, it may not be worth the morbidity and cost. Nonetheless, patients with minimal or microscopic peritoneal disease are the best candidates for this therapy.[239a] Optimal drugs and dosages remain to be established, and the eventual role of intracavitary administration of chemotherapeutic drugs remains to be defined by controlled clinical trials.

Installation of radioactive isotopes such as ^{32}P palliates 40 to 60 per cent of patients.[240] Isotopes are preferred by some over chemotherapeutic or sclerosing agents because of the lower incidence of nausea, vomiting, and bone marrow depression. The radiation effect is due to beta emission and is limited to the peritoneal surface and the tissue 8 mm below it. The major morbidity is due to nonuniform abdominal distribution with focal aggregation of radiocolloid, causing abdominal pain and possible tissue damage.[241] Because of the limited energy deposition of ^{32}P, it is most useful in early peritoneal involvement, where tumor bulk is low and nodules measure less than a few millimeters.[242] The mechanism of radiocolloid activity is probably both inhibition of tumor cell growth and fibrosis of the peritoneal membrane and lymphatics.

There is only limited study and clinical information regarding the role of immunotherapy in the treatment of peritoneal carcinomatosis. Possible therapeutic approaches include administration of (1) nonspecific systemically active agents (*C. parvum*, streptococcal preparation OK432, and BCG), (2) specific tumor antigens, (3) monoclonal antibodies as carriers or agents or as local macrophage activators, (4) autologous leukocytes to act as killer cells or lymphokine releasers, and (5) specific leukokine immunomodulators or antitumor substances, such as interleukin-2 or interferons.[243] Encouraging results from small series have been reported for peritoneal tumors with the use of streptococcal preparation OK432 in gastric and colon carcinoma, and *C. parvum* and interferon in ovarian carcinoma.[244–246] As in other areas of oncology, the role of adjuvant or therapeutic immunotherapy is exciting but remains to be defined.

Surgery is rarely indicated in these patients. However, intestinal obstruction is frequent and is often unresponsive to the usual conservative measures. In this situation surgery is necessary for palliation. It relieves obstructive symptoms in 60 to 80 per cent of patients, with a 15 per cent operative mortality rate and a 20 to 30 per cent incidence of recurrent obstruction.[247]

Peritoneovenous shunting has become more widely used as a method of palliation for malignant ascites, with a reported palliation rate of 75 per cent.[248] Complications similar to those noted in cirrhotics, such as infection, coagulopathy, heart failure, thromboemboli, and shunt occlusion, attend it in approximately 25 per cent, a much lower rate than in cirrhosis.[249] Coagulopathy is rare (2 per cent), especially if ascitic fluid is discarded and replaced with saline.[248, 250, 251] Tumor emboli may be found in up to 15 per cent of patients but are clinically silent and do not affect their otherwise limited survival.[250] Neither the LeVeen nor the Denver shunt is better, and both types have the problem of occlusion. Relative contraindications to shunt placement include the presence of loculated, viscous, or hemorrhagic ascites, because early shunt occlusion is the rule in such settings.[252]

The management of malignant ascites is summarized in Figure 102–1.

Pseudomyxoma Peritonei

Etiology. Pseudomyxoma peritonei is a rare condition in which the peritoneal cavity becomes distended with a pale, translucent, semisolid material that has been shown biochemically and histochemically to be a mucin. There are two major causes of this "mucinous ascites": mucinous cystadenomas and cystadenocarcinomas of the ovary and appendix. Approximately 45 per cent have an ovarian origin, 29 per cent an appendiceal origin, and 26 per cent an indeterminate origin.[253] Only 1 to 2 per cent of patients with ovarian tumors develop pseudomyxoma peritonei.[254] Other less common antecedent lesions include ovarian teratomas, ovarian fibromas, uterine carcinomas, mucinous adenocarcinomas of the bowel, adenocarcinoma in urachal cysts, mucoid omphalomesenteric cysts of the navel, carcinoma of the bile duct, and colloid carcinoma of the pancreas.[255]

Clinical and Pathologic Features. Pseudomyxoma presents primarily with increasing abdominal girth, usually with a disparity between the amount of ascites and the clinical state of the patient. The diagnosis may be suspected if characteristic curvilinear calcifications are seen on abdominal radiographs.[256] Ultrasonography and CT scans are not specific, but may suggest the diagnosis by demonstrating peritoneal and omental sheets, highly echogenic masses due to numerous tiny mucinous cysts, ascites with numerous echoes or septations, and multiple semisolid masses indenting the bowel or scalloping the margin of the liver, due to pressure from adjacent implants. Unlike the ordinary ascites in which bowel floats freely to the anterior abdominal wall and shifts with position, in pseudomyxoma the gelatinous mass is fixed in position. Lastly, an underlying appendiceal or ovarian mass may be present.[257, 258]

At laparotomy, the peritoneal cavity is filled with a mucinous material lying freely as a homogeneous mass or multiple cystic masses, whereas in other places it may be firmly attached to the peritoneum, where nests

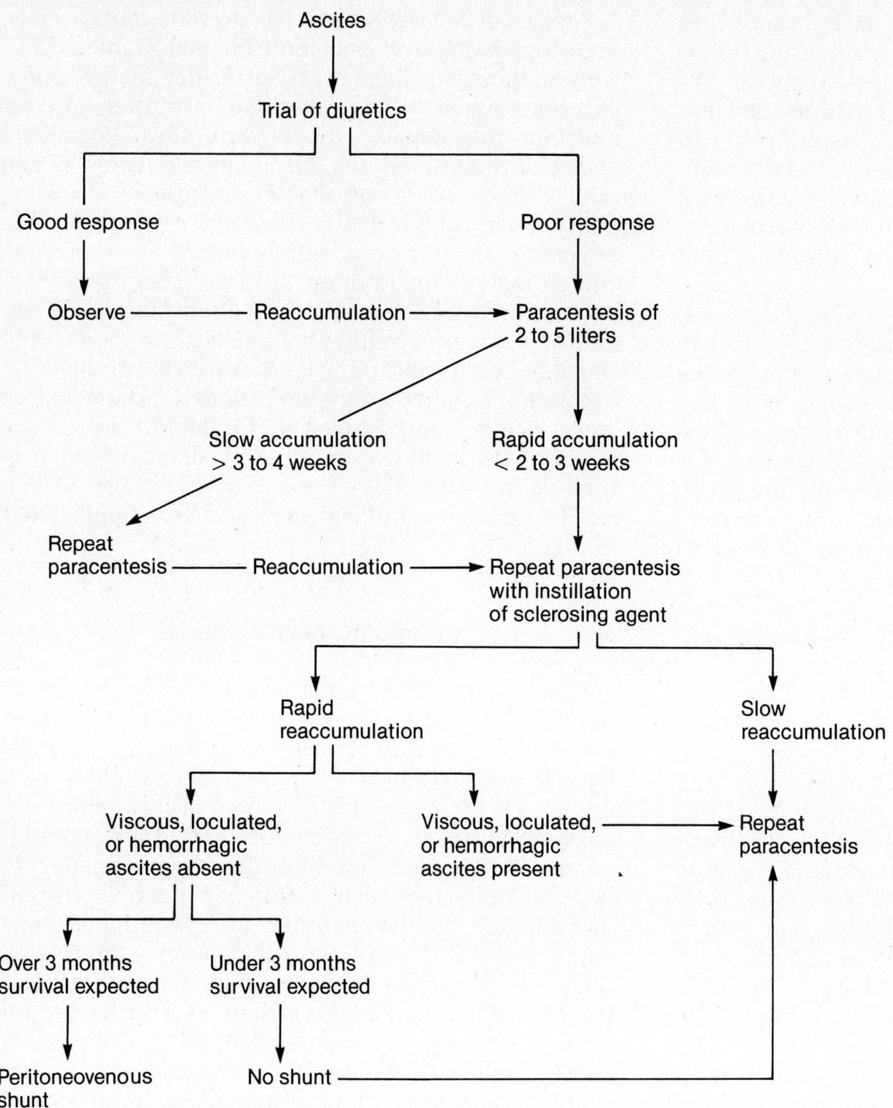

Figure 102–1. Management of malignant ascites. (Adapted from Souter et al.[252])

of the columnar epithelial cells characteristic of the syndrome are located. This epithelium may be quite sparse in relation to the amount of mucin present.

The major point of controversy concerns the malignant nature of the epithelial cells. Although some investigators believe that pseudomyxoma can be caused by rupture of a single mucocele with benign epithelium,[259] others have reported that careful examination of serial sections of the appendix has shown cellular atypia, indicating that these are highly differentiated carcinomas of low biologic malignancy.[260, 261] These two views are reconciled in further studies that correlate clinical and pathologic data.[262] About 20 per cent of benign cystadenomas have periappendiceal mucus, but the process is usually localized, is not associated with free epithelial cells, and has a benign, self-limited course. True pseudomyxoma is almost invariably associated with cystadenocarcinomas, which show stromal invasion by neoplastic glands and epithelial cells in the mucinous implants. Both morbidity, from mucinous accumulation, and mortality rates are much greater in these cases.[263] Similarly, some have claimed that 90 to 95 per cent of mucinous cystadenomas of the ovary are benign, but others have found evidence of low-grade malignancy in a large percentage of those tumors previously thought to be benign. The electron microscopic finding of intracytoplasmic vesicles or canaliculi, often found in carcinomas, supports this concept.[255] Pseudomyxoma develops in many tumors of grade 1 malignancy but is very rare in benign cystadenomas. Rupture of the cyst can also be demonstrated in patients who develop pseudomyxoma. Pseudomyxoma may simultaneously affect the ovary and appendix, and bilateral ovarian tumors may occur.[264]

Prognosis and Treatment. Because the tumor is either benign or of low-grade malignancy, it rarely metastasizes and the course of the disease is often long. The survival rate is 54 per cent at five years, and 18 per cent at 10 years.[253] Death is usually the result of intestinal obstruction and fistula formation.[265] A more aggressive combined surgical and chemotherapeutic approach involves removal of both ovaries, appendix, peritoneal nodules, and omentum; evacuation of mucin; and installation of an alkylating agent.[266] Various other pharmacologic agents have been tried without success, including trypsin, hyaluronidase, and acetylcysteine.[267] The role of single systemic and combination drug regimens is still unclear, although melphalan has been used most often.[253, 268] Abdominal radiation may offer another modality that can improve survival.

Granulomatous Peritonitis

The peritoneum responds to a wide variety of stimuli with a granulomatous inflammatory reaction. The etiology may be exogenous, endogenous, or iatrogenic.

Exogenous Causes

A variety of infectious agents may cause granulomatous peritonitis, including mycobacteria (discussed above), parasites such as *Ascaris, Enterobius*, and *Schistosoma*, as well as fungi such as *Coccidioides immitis*.[120–126] Ingested organic material entering the peritoneal cavity via an intestinal perforation may also cause granulomatous peritonitis.[269] After intestinal perforation, food starch may also enter the peritoneal cavity and cause granulomatous reaction.[270] (Iatrogenic glove starch reaction is discussed below.)

Endogenous Causes

Granulomatous peritonitis is a response to keratin due to ruptured cystic teratomas or squamous metaplasia in adenocarcinomas.[271] In pregnant women, reflux of maternal vernix caseosa (containing fetal epidermal elements) due to premature rupture of the fetal membranes and meconium spillage at the time of cesarean section may cause an acute granulomatous peritonitis and should be considered in women with abdominal pain in pregnancy and following cesarean section.[272, 273] Rarely, adenocarcinoma may produce a granulomatous peritonitits, possibly due to a response to extracellular mucin.[274]

Very rarely sarcoidosis affects the peritoneum, causing granulomatous peritonitis and ascites.[275] The diagnosis can be made only by exclusion, with negative mycobacterial and fungal cultures, positive Kveim tests, and perhaps lack of response to antituberculous therapy. Despite the presence of noncaseating granulomas and response to steroids, it may be reasonable to treat all such patients in whom the diagnosis is uncertain for tuberculosis.

Crohn's disease rarely presents with "miliary" serosal nodules composed of noncaseating granulomas and minimal (but definite) abnormalities of the bowel wall. The major importance of this rare manifestation of Crohn's disease is its confusion with tuberculous peritonitis at laparotomy. The early age of the patients reported and the subsequent disappearance of the miliary lesions suggest that this represents a transient early stage of classic Crohn's disease.[276]

Iatrogenic Causes

A number of foreign bodies may cause a granulomatous peritoneal reaction by contamination of the peritoneal cavity at the time of surgery. The most common cause is starch from surgical gloves, although talc, cotton fibers, and wood fibers originating from disposable surgical gowns and drapes have also been implicated.[277–280]

The syndrome of *starch granulomatous peritonitis* follows about 0.15 per cent of surgical abdominal operations.[281] This syndrome appears two to nine weeks postoperatively but has been seen after four months. Signs and symptoms are consistent with intestinal obstruction or peritonitis (i.e., pain, tenderness, fever, nausea, vomiting and abdominal distention). The small bowel obstructs in 25 per cent of patients, suggesting postoperative complications such as adhesions or abscesses; however, these patients often do not look severely ill. The diagnosis can be made by demonstration of starch granules in fluid obtained by paracentesis, sparing poor-risk patients a second operation.[282] If surgery is necessary because of obstruction, biopsy of adhesions causing the recurrent intestinal obstruction may demonstrate granulomas, granules, or fibers. This confirmation is important because corticosteroids or indomethacin decreases morbidity and speeds improvement in some patients.[281, 283] The prognosis is good, with no progression to chronic disease; however, occasionally the serosal nodules persist or adhesions cause obstruction up to 18 months later.[284, 285]

The peritoneal cavity in starch peritonitis contains miliary peritoneal nodules, adhesions, and ascites. This appearance may be confused with carcinomatosis, especially in patients who have previously undergone surgery for cancer. Pathologically, the lesions consist of granulomas with epithelioid cells, giant cells, and an intense mononuclear infiltrate. Starch granules are easily identified by the characteristic Maltese cross appearance under polarized light microscopy. Lint granulomas reveal a polarized light appearance of coiled linear and trilaminar fibers, and may be demonstrated with special stains (GMS, serius red, and cyaninerythrosin).[279] Rarely, granulomas may be present with caseous necrosis, which can lead to an erroneous diagnosis of tuberculosis.[286] Starch granules are also present in these patients and help make the diagnosis.

The pathogenesis of the granulomatous reaction to starch is unclear, although the time interval, the characteristic histologic appearance, and the response to corticosteroids are consistent with a cell-mediated immune response to starch antigen(s).[287, 288] Lymphocytes sensitized to cornstarch have been demonstrated in patients with starch peritonitis, but more data are needed to support this concept.

Barium peritonitis may occur as a complication of a barium contrast X-ray examination, usually barium enema. It results from the escape of barium sulfate into the peritoneal cavity, via either a pre-existing perforation in diseased bowel or a traumatic perforation during the procedure. In addition to the fact that normal intestinal contents, including bacteria, may cause peritonitis under these conditions, barium sulfate itself is deleterious. In animals, sterile preparations of barium sulfate elicit an early inflammatory response and exudation of fluid. With time, the barium becomes dispersed in small nodules, associated with phagocytes and foreign body giant cells, and accompanied by fibrosis and adhesions. Perforation due to a barium enema has a 50 to 70 per cent mortality rate if surgery is not performed early. At surgery, the perforation is closed and the peritoneum is extensively lavaged to remove as much barium sulfate as possible. Aggressive volume replacement may be necessary perioperatively. Adhesions follow not infrequently and may lead eventually to bowel obstruction.[289–291]

Familial Paroxysmal Polyserositis (Familial Mediterranean Fever)

Etiology and Pathogenesis. Familial paroxysmal polyserositis (FPP), or familial Mediterranean fever (FMF), is a disease characterized by recurrent episodes of acute, self-limited serositis, especially peritonitis. It is an inherited disease, transmitted as an autosomal recessive trait, and occurs predominately in Mediterranean peoples. An FPP-like illness with autosomal dominant inheritance and somewhat atypical clinical features has been reported recently.[291a] Sephardic Jews account for 50 per cent of cases; Armenians, 22 per cent; Arabs, 11 per cent; Turks, 7 per cent; Ashkenazi Jews, 5 per cent; other ethnic groups, 5 per cent.[292] The genetic basis for the disease is securely established and has been thought to be expressed through a metabolic abnormality. However, extensive studies of possible allergic, metabolic, or endocrine factors have been negative. Nonspecific changes in circulating complement components, immune complexes, immunoregulatory abnormalities, cyclic nucleotides, and leukocyte function are part of the disease, but are not yet clearly tied to pathogenesis.[293–296] Recently, the peritoneal fluid of patients was found to be deficient in an inhibitor of inflammation.[297] This factor normally inhibits neutrophil chemotaxis by antagonizing the complement-derived factor (C5a), which may normally be released into the peritoneum in small amounts. These studies remain to be confirmed and extended.

Clinical Features. The onset of the disease is usually within the first two decades of life, but 20 per cent of patients may have their first episode after the age of 20, and 4 per cent after the age of 30.[292] Approximately 60 per cent of patients are males.

The disease usually appears suddenly with an attack of serositis; it takes the form of peritonitis in 55 per cent, arthritis in about 25 per cent, and pleuritis in about 5 per cent.[298] During the course of FPP, 95 per cent of the patients eventually develop peritonitis, which is the sole manifestation in 30 per cent.[292, 299] The search for a precipitating event has been unsuccessful, although stress, heavy activity, and cold exposure have been implicated.

The attack consists of a sudden onset of fever, usually 101 to 103°F, with localized or diffuse abdominal pain. Almost invariably, there is exquisite direct abdominal tenderness, with marked rebound in two thirds of patients. Involuntary spasm and guarding may be striking in one fourth of patients and may be generalized, with a board-like abdomen. Leukocytosis is present in almost 90 per cent, and plain film of the abdomen shows air-fluid levels. After 6 to 12 hours, these signs and symptoms recede, and the patient usually recovers within 24 to 48 hours. These attacks occur at irregular and unpredictable intervals, and between attacks the patient is entirely well. Except for the usual rapid resolution and the recurrent nature of the disease, it presents all the characteristics of an acute surgical abdomen. Occasionally, any of the symptoms of FPP may be mild.

Although peritonitis is the major manifestation during the course of FPP, 50 per cent of patients develop pleuritis, 60 per cent develop arthritis (usually monoarticular and rarely protracted), and 30 per cent develop an erysipelas-like erythema on the lower extremities.[292] Pericarditis has also been noted. Arthritis can be prolonged, and sacroileitis has also been observed.[300] The only fatal complication, amyloid nephropathy, develops in about 25 per cent of patients.[298] Other investigators have found lower incidences of the joint, skin, and renal manifestations, and there is a striking absence of amyloidosis in some ethnic groups.[292, 301–303] Turks and Sephardic Jews have the highest frequency of amyloidosis, but it is extremely uncommon in Arabs and Armenians.

The diagnosis of FPP is based on a knowledge of ethnic background, family history, its characteristic clinical features, and of course, appropriate exclusion of other diseases. Infusion of 10 mg of metaraminol may provoke a typical attack of serositis in these patients but not in control subjects.[304] The usefulness of this test, however, remains to be confirmed.

Pathology. At peritoneoscopy or laparotomy during an acute attack, the peritoneum is lusterless and hyperemic, with occasional scattered areas of fibrin-like material; the peritoneal cavity contains some serous fluid. Peritoneal biopsy shows acute inflammation with polymorphonuclear infiltration, vascular dilatation, and edema. Between attacks, the peritoneum almost always returns to normal. Rarely, organization of the exudate has led to the formation of adhesions.[298, 305]

Prognosis and Treatment. The prognosis of FPP is excellent, and many patients have been followed for years with good general health despite hundreds of attacks. Attacks may increase in frequency with age, but occasionally there are remissions or periods in which the disease is quite intractable. The development of amyloid nephropathy heralds a poor prognosis, with subsequent renal failure and death in 90 per cent of affected patients under the age of 40 years.

In the past, no treatment was of much value in FPP. Controlled studies indicate that colchicine, in doses of 0.6 mg two to three times per day, decreases both the severity and frequency of attacks.[306, 307] Longer-term studies report continued suppression of attacks with little evidence of adverse effects such as sterility, teratogenicity, or chromosome damage.[308, 309] Continuous treatment with colchicine appears to prevent amyloidosis. It reduces the cumulative rate of proteinuria from 49 to 1.7 per cent after nine years, and the prevalence of nephropathy is reduced by two thirds. Colchicine can prevent deterioration of renal function only if minimal proteinuria is present, but probably has little effect on the nephrotic and uremic stages of the disease. Since amyloidogenesis is suppressed, daily lifelong administration (especially in susceptible ethnic groups) is recommended.[310]

In patients with infrequent attacks, colchicine may be taken intermittently at the first premonition of an episode and will abort or ameliorate a significant number of them.[311] Some patients do not respond to chronic or intermittent colchicine and may have inadequate absorption or altered disposition of the drug, and thus higher doses may be necessary.[312] The reasons for the efficacy of colchicine are still unclear, although it does inhibit leukocyte function *in vitro* through interference with microtubular function and neutrophil degranulation and may modulate immunoregulatory cells.[309, 313]

Treatment of patients with amyloid nephropathy includes colchicine, hemodialysis, and renal transplantation, although in the latter circumstance recurrence in the graft has been reported.[303] Anticoagulants may be necessary to treat the hypercoagulable state and renal vein thrombosis that may develop with nephrotic syndrome in these patients.[314]

Vasculitis

See also pages 1916 to 1918.

The systemic vasculitides (e.g., systemic lupus erythematosus, or SLE, and polyarteritis nodosa) may involve the vessels of the gut wall, but the peritoneum is usually affected only after the gut wall is diseased. About 20 per cent of patients with SLE, polyarteritis, scleroderma, and dermatomyositis develop acute abdominal problems (i.e., ulceration, hemorrhage, perforation, obstruction, or infarction); isolated peritonitis not associated with these complications is found in fewer than 1 per cent.[315] Peritoneal permeability is altered in patients with systemic vasculitis, for peritoneal clearances of solutes such as creatinine and urate are decreased.[316]

Peritonitis resulting from arteritis of subserosal arteries most commonly occurs in SLE and manifests the usual signs and symptoms of acute peritonitis and ascites. Acute lupus peritonitis is responsive to steroids, but clearly laparotomy may be needed to rule out a surgically correctable lesion. Indications that the acute episode may be caused by SLE per se include the presence of other clinical and laboratory signs of SLE, changing abdominal findings, or the presence of antinuclear antibodies, LE cells, and decreased complement in the peritoneal fluid.[317] Painless ascites may be a manifestation of SLE.[318–320] Peritoneal nodules or erythema is seen at the time of peritoneoscopy or laparotomy, although the peritoneum may appear normal. Biopsy may show lymphocytic infiltration, perivascular cuffing, or hematoxylin bodies, and immunofluorescent microscopy of the biopsies shows an immune complex vasculitis with immunoglobulin M and complement deposition in the tissues.[318, 319] There are many other causes of ascites that may also need to be ruled out in this setting, including tuberculosis, nephrotic syndrome, or constrictive pericarditis, but if extensive evaluation fails to suggest another cause, a therapeutic trial of high-dose corticosteroids is reasonable.

Allergic vasculitis caused by Henoch-Schönlein purpura rarely causes exudative ascites, and it resolves with steroid therapy.[321] Köhlmeier-Degos disease (malignant atrophic papulosis) is a rare form of systemic vasculitis affecting small and medium-sized arteries and mainly involving the skin and gut.[322] The disease usually begins with the onset of atrophic skin lesions, which after a variable period of weeks to years is followed by abdominal pain, weight loss, diarrhea, and, rarely, neurologic symptoms. Hyaline degeneration and endothelial proliferation in the small intestinal arteries cause vascular thromboses and infarcts, and approximately 50 per cent of patients die of peritonitis due to infarction and perforation of the bowel within two years after onset.

Toxemia of pregnancy has rarely been associated with ascites, presumably secondary to a generalized "capillary leak" syndrome that may rarely include the small subperitoneal vessels.[323]

Sclerosing Peritonitis

Sclerosing peritonitis is a clinical syndrome associated with abdominal pain, intestinal obstruction, and thickening of the peritoneum with massive adhesions. It probably represents a form of peritoneal reactivity to a variety of stimuli. Several causes have been reported: (1) toxins such as practolol and silica, (2) foreign bodies attributable to peritoneovenous shunts, chronic ambulatory peritoneal dialysis with indwelling catheters, and ventriculoperitoneal shunts, and (3) idiopathic causes.

The first toxic form of sclerosing peritonitis described was that due to the beta-adrenergic blocking drug practolol, which is no longer available.[324] Most patients had been on the drug for two years or longer and presented with an oculocutaneous syndrome of rash and dry eyes. Other symptoms included abdominal pain, vomiting, weight loss, and abdominal mass. Patients present with a radiologic picture of intestinal obstruction. At laparotomy they have massive peritoneal adhesions with thickening and contraction of the visceral and parietal peritoneum, affecting the entire small intestine. Histologically, there is nonspecific focal inflammation, granulation tissue, fibrinous exudation, and a peculiar laminated fibrosis; panniculitis and vasculitis are absent. The cause is unknown, but it has been suggested that practolol may block the normal inhibitory effect of catecholamines on lysosomal release. So far, beta blockers other than practolol have not been conclusively implicated in sclerosing peritonitis.[325] One case has been reported of a drug abuser with sclerosing peritonitis, in whom birefringent material was found to contain silica, possibly localizing in the peritoneum by hematogenous spread or inadvertent abdominal drug injections.[326]

Indwelling foreign bodies are becoming increasingly recognized as causes of sclerosing peritonitis. The incidence in chronic peritoneal dialysis is 1.5 to 6 per cent, and may be as high as 18 per cent in those with fungal peritonitis.[114] Although it may appear soon after initiation of dialysis, it usually is manifested after one to two years. There may be a spectrum of peritoneal structural changes from peritoneal thickening and destruction of the mesothelium to a thick, firm tissue which encases the small intestine in a "cocoon" similar to that in practolol peritonitis. The peritoneum may even develop calcifications.[326a] A variety of etiologies has been considered, including recurrent infections, peritonitis, dialysis solutions and their additives or contaminants, or the catheter itself.[327–329] The pathogenesis is unknown, but could involve the stimulation of peritoneal macrophages to produce interleukin-1, a stimulant of fibroblast formation.[330] Sclerosing peritonitis has also been described in 2 per cent of patients with peritoneovenous shunts, in 6 per cent of patients with intraperitoneal chemotherapy, and after ventriculoperitoneal shunt.[239, 331–334]

Idiopathic sclerosing peritonitis ("abdominal cocoon") presents in adolescent females with a clinical picture of small intestinal obstruction due to a dense white membrane surrounding the small intestine. It is felt to be a sequel to peritonitis, but an organism has not been isolated.[335, 336] A case secondary to spontaneous bacterial peritonitis has recently been reported.[336a]

Miscellaneous Peritoneal Diseases

Eosinophilic Gastroenteritis

Eosinophilic gastroenteritis usually presents with peripheral eosinophilia and symptoms caused by mucosal or submucosal involvement (i.e., malabsorption and obstruction). Patients, however, have predominantly subserosal disease causing eosinophilic ascites.[337] Paracentesis yields fluid containing many eosinophils, often well over 50 per cent of total leukocytes. At laparotomy, a thickened, edematous serosa infiltrated with eosinophils, lymphocytes, and plasma cells may be found. The response to steroids is often dramatic, with complete clearing of the ascites (see also pp. 1123–1131).

Other causes of eosinophilic ascites are quite rare. It may be part of the hypereosinophilic syndrome, in which eosinophilic infiltration is present in multiple organs in addition to the intestine and peritoneum. Isolated cases of eosinophilic ascites have been associated with chronic peritoneal dialysis (see p. 1937), vasculitis, lymphoma, metastatic malignancy, ruptured hydatid cyst, and spontaneous bacterial peritonitis.[338, 339]

Whipple's Disease

The broad spectrum of Whipple's disease is discussed separately (see pp. 1297–1306). Significantly, a few patients present primarily with peritoneal manifestations. A picture very similar to tuberculous peritonitis has been described, with ascites, low-grade fever, weight loss, and multiple peritoneal nodules on peritoneoscopy.[340] Histologically, the nodules are composed of chronic inflammatory cells with periodic acid–Schiff positive material in macrophages, similar to the findings in small intestinal mucosa and other tissues. Long-term antibiotic treatment with antimicrobial agents (penicillin, tetracycline) leads to resolution of peritoneal disease and disappearance of ascites.

Whipple's disease may cause ascites in ways other than by direct peritoneal involvement. Indeed, 5 to 10 per cent of patients have ascites, caused by protein-losing enteropathy with hypoalbuminemia, lymphatic obstruction by involved mesenteric nodes, or rupture of dilated serosal lymphatics. Chylous ascites also may be caused by direct involvement of lymphatics (see pp. 445–446).

Gynecologic Lesions

Because the female genital tract opens into the peritoneal cavity, endometrial and decidual tissue occasionally may implant on the peritoneum and cause symptoms. Endometriosis may involve the bowel wall and cause ascites, but symptomatic cases limited to peritoneum are rare (see pp. 1592–1595). Surgical treatment is usually indicated, but hormonal control with danazol has led to resolution of the hemorrhagic ascites.[341] Postpartum abdominal pain with peritoneal signs has been reported, caused by diffuse peritoneal decidual reaction involving the omentum.[342]

Certain gynecologic neoplasms present with diffuse peritoneal implants that may be interpreted erroneously as an end-stage malignant process. Ovarian teratomas can seed the peritoneum with 1 to 3 mm gray implants, presumably from defects in the capsule of the tumor. These implants consist of glial tissue and in most cases are histologically and biologically benign. In long-term follow-up these implants remain asymptomatic, do not progress, and need no definitive treatment.[343] Genital leiomyomas are rarely accompanied by multiple leiomyomatous nodules in the peritoneum, mesentery, and omentum. This leiomyomatosis peritonealis disseminata is a non-neoplastic, multicentric proliferation of smooth muscle in the subperitoneal connective tissue. This condition usually affects women in their reproductive years, often in association with pregnancy or oral contraceptives. It probably represents an abnormal response of the subperitoneal connective tissue to hormonal stimulation and not intraperitoneal seeding.[344] The spectrum may be wider, however, because it has also been reported in women with normal or low hormone levels, including postmenopausal women.[345] In all reported cases, the tumor has been clinically benign, but rarely may be malignant.[346] (Neoplasms arising from the mesothelium—benign adenomatoid, cystic, and papillary mesotheliomas—are discussed above on p. 1940.)

Unusual peritoneal reactions are associated with other gynecologic lesions. The oily contents of a ruptured dermoid cyst of the ovary evokes a marked granulomatous reaction with the formation of dense adhesions, peritoneal cysts, and nodules. The diagnosis is suggested by the finding of oily, cheesy material in the peritoneum or ascitic fluid, or the presence of hair in the peritoneal nodules.[347] It may be suspected on CT scan by finding a fatty tumor with solid components and calcified rims.[348] Benign ovarian cysts occasionally have melanin-containing tissue in their wall. Leakage or rupture of these cysts produces black streaking of the peritoneum and mesentery. This peritoneal melanosis, therefore, does not necessarily imply the presence of malignant melanoma.[349] Malakoplakia of the pelvic peritoneum has been reported recently; it is unknown how frequently it involves the peritoneum, but it must be very rare.[350] (Malakoplakia is discussed further on pp. 1612–1614.)

Infectious agents may enter the peritoneal cavity through the female genital tract and cause peritonitis. Gonococci and *Chlamydia trachomatis* may pass from the fallopian tubes into the paracolic gutters and then to the subphrenic space, causing perihepatitis (Fitz-Hugh–Curtis syndrome) in up to 15 to 30 per cent of women with pelvic inflammatory disease[351, 352] (see pp. 1264–1265). It is very rare in men, and its spread is probably via hematogenous or lymphatic routes.[353] Pelvic symptoms may be minimal, but right upper quadrant pain and tenderness, fever, and a hepatic friction rub may be present. Laparoscopy or surgery reveals the typical "violin string" adhesions between the parietal peritoneum and the anterior surface of the liver. Recent reports suggest that a more extensive peritonitis may rarely occur, presenting with diffuse abdominal symptoms and ascites.[354–356] Ascites could be due to increased capillary permeability secondary to extensive inflammatory changes, or to decreased fluid resorption due to obstruction of the lymphatics at the right hemidiaphragm.

Occasionally, foreign bodies may enter the peritoneum via the genital tract. Douche powders containing starch have been reported to cause granulomatous pelvic peritonitis.[357]

Splenosis

Splenosis is essentially the autotransplantation of splenic tissue to unusual sites after splenic trauma. Splenic pulp is seeded, and implants appear as multiple reddish blue nodules on the peritoneum, omentum, and mesentery. The lesions are usually encapsulated and sessile, although they may be pedunculated, and vary in size from several millimeters to 2 to 3 cm. Large lesions have been demonstrated by radioisotope imaging techniques.

Splenosis is of little clinical significance, and it is usually an incidental finding at autopsy or abdominal surgery many years after splenectomy for traumatic rupture. Rarely, however, it may cause intestinal obstruction or pain secondary to twisting of the pedicle of an implant, and has been reported to cause splenic rupture.[358, 359] The major significance of splenosis is that it simulates a mass lesion or neoplasm. Although metastatic carcinoma, endometriosis, or hemangiomatosis must be considered in the differential diagnosis, the history of splenic trauma, the gross appearance, and the histologic appearance will readily distinguish splenosis.

Splenosis may frequently follow splenic trauma and this splenic tissue may be functional, accounting for the low incidence of bacterial sepsis following splenectomy for trauma.[360] Splenic function in this situation is suggested by the absence of Howell-Jolly bodies in blood smears. That splenosis can be functional is illustrated by a case of idiopathic thrombocytopenic purpura occurring in a splenectomized patient with splenosis.[361]

Peritoneal Lymphangiectasis

Peritoneal lymphangiectasis is a rare condition in which there is a communication between distended peritoneal lymphatics and the vascular system, leading to bloody ascites, hemorrhage, and death in severe cases.[362] Patients may be asymptomatic or may present with abdominal pain or an abdominal mass caused by distended lymphatics. At laparotomy, pedunculated and nonpedunculated blood-filled cysts are found. It is not clear whether this condition is congenital or acquired.

Peritoneal Cysts

A small number of patients have been reported in whom loose peritoneal cysts have been found associated with nonspecific abdominal pain. These probably represent benign cystic mesothelioma (discussed on p. 1940).

Iatrogenic peritoneal pseudocysts may follow ventriculoperitoneal shunts for hydrocephalus.[363] These complicate 0.7 per cent of shunted cases owing to shunt malfunction, and cause abdominal distention, pain, nausea, vomiting, and a localized mass. The wall of the pseudocysts is formed by inflammatory reaction around the catheter tip secondary to low-grade infection and localized peritonitis. The cysts are filled with cerebrospinal fluid, and cerebrospinal fluid ascites may complicate cyst leakage.[364] Abdominal symptoms can arise years after the shunting and may long precede the appearance of neurologic symptoms. The diagnosis of CSF pseudocysts has been simplified by CT scan and ultrasonography, which demonstrate the mass with the ventriculoperitoneal shunt tubing in or adjacent to it.[365]

Chronic pelvic inflammatory disease may lead to the formation of large tubal pseudocysts.[366, 367] The disease may present with abdominal pain, fever, distention, abdominal masses, and exudative ascites and may be difficult to distinguish from ovarian, omental, mesenteric, or peritoneal cysts, from abscesses, or from malignancy.

Peritoneal Encapsulation

Peritoneal encapsulation is a rare developmental anomaly in which the entire small bowel is enclosed in a peritoneal sac, without other evidence of abnormality or malrotation. It has been suggested that the abnormal peritoneal sac is derived from the peritoneum of the normal umbilical hernia, the neck of which becomes adherent to the duodenum. The peritoneum of the umbilical hernia is then drawn into the abdominal cavity with the intestines when they are suddenly retracted in the twelfth gestational week. The condition is generally asymptomatic, is usually found incidentally at surgery, and need not be treated because complications do not arise.[336, 368]

DISEASES OF THE MESENTERY AND OMENTUM

General Clinical Features

Patients with mesenteric disease usually present with nonspecific symptoms, such as abdominal pain, abdominal distention, or intestinal obstruction. The most frequent physical finding is a mass, which may be mobile. Associated lymphatic obstruction may cause steatorrhea, chylous ascites, or protein-losing enteropathy, with hypoalbuminemia and edema.

Although there are no specific laboratory findings, mesenteric disease may be suspected if calcifications, displacement of bowel loops, or pressure deformities are observed radiographically. Omental tumors are suggested by the pattern of gastrocolic separation (i.e., superior or posterior displacement of the stomach with inferior and anterior displacement of the transverse colon by an extrinsic mass[369]). Angiographic diagnosis of mesenteric and omental lesions is disappointing, as small masses are poorly visualized and angiographic findings suggestive of malignancy can be mimicked by inflammatory changes in benign tumors.[370]

Ultrasonography and computed tomography are less invasive and more useful in detecting or confirming the presence and nature of mesenteric and omental disease, with CT generally giving clearer and more complete images (Fig. 102–2). Although certain CT patterns may be correlated with specific diseases, this is by no means invariable, and benign inflammatory diseases can cause similar patterns.[371–373] Therefore, definitive diagnosis of mass lesions of the mesentery and omentum usually depends upon direct inspection or biopsy, either by CT-guided percutaneous biopsy, or at the time of peritoneoscopy or laparotomy.

Diffuse mesenteric disease may be suggested by CT density changes of mesenteric tissue. Mesenteric edema is suggested by increased density of mesenteric fat and poor definition of mesenteric vessels.[374] Excessive mesenteric fat (mesenteric lipomatosis) may present as abdominal distention and simulate ascites or malignancy. The diagnosis is made on CT by the very low attenuation coefficient of fat, and will obviate the necessity for further studies or surgery.[375–377] Lipomatous neoplasms are suspected if there is inhomogeneity, poor margination or infiltration, higher attenuation numbers, or contrast enhancement.[378]

Mesenteric Inflammatory Disease

Mesenteric inflammatory disease comprises a spectrum ranging from inflammatory to fibrotic lesions of the mesentery, called mesenteric panniculitis and retractile mesenteritis, respectively. Other terms applied to these conditions have included primary liposclerosis, lipogranuloma, isolated lipodystrophy, and mesenteric Weber-Christian disease.

Etiology and Pathogenesis. The etiology may include trauma, infection, or ischemia. Mesenteric panniculitis has been reported as part of generalized Weber-Christian disease involving multiple organs, but this entity is probably unrelated to isolated mesenteric inflammatory disease.

It has been postulated that the underlying pathogenetic defect involves excessive growth of morphologically normal fat tissue, with subsequent degeneration, fat necrosis, and xanthogranulomatous inflammation. It is suggested that after the degeneration of hyperplastic mesenteric adipose tissue, lipid material, perhaps abnormal, is released from degenerating fat cells. This evokes granulomatous infiltration, with eventual progression to fibrotic scarring. Mesenteric inflammatory disease also may be a nonspecific response to any form of injury.[379]

Clinical Features. Mesenteric panniculitis is mainly a disease of late adulthood, with a median age of 60 years. The male-to-female ratio is 1.8 to 1. It presents as recurrent episodes of crampy abdominal pain, either localized or generalized, with weight loss, nausea, vomiting, and low-grade fever in about 60 per cent of patients. Rarely, it may present with signs of an acute abdomen. The other 40 per cent are discovered only by the incidental finding of a mass at examination or laparotomy.[380, 381] A mass is palpable in 60 per cent, with local tenderness but usually without peritoneal signs. Leukocytosis may be present. Radiologic evaluation may reveal displacement of intestinal segments, extrinsic pressure deformity, separation of jejunal-ileal loops with kinking or angulation, and rugal distortions of the mesenteric border of compressed loops. Angiography demonstrates nonspecific stretching of the vasa recta, and areas of irregularity may suggest vascular encasement. CT scanning reveals a low-density mass, which is usually not homogeneous and contains areas of fat density interspersed with areas of water or soft-tissue density, depending upon the amount of edema, inflammation, or fibrosis.[382]

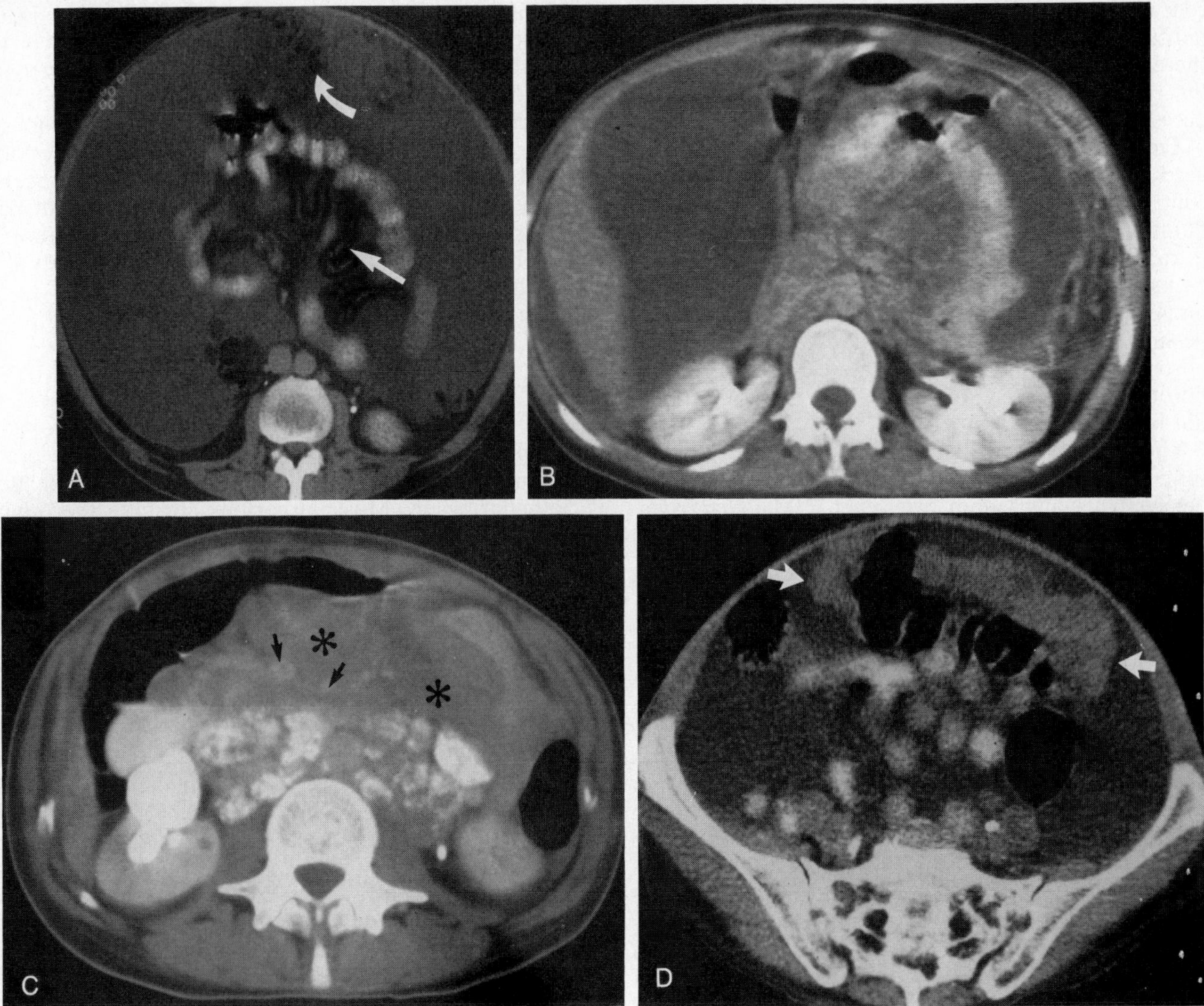

Figure 102–2. Computerized tomographic scan of mesentery and omentum. *A*, Normal omentum and mesentery in a patient with cirrhosis and massive ascites. The mesenteric vessels are well outlined by surrounding mesenteric fat. The mesentery and small bowel loops form a fan-like structure *(straight arrow)*. Omental fat floats freely beneath the anterior abdominal wall *(curved arrow)*. *B*, Tuberculous peritonitis with mesenteric involvement. The mesenteric fat is infiltrated, leading to poor definition of the vessels and mesenteric thickening. There is associated loculated ascites and peritoneal enhancement. *C*, Non-Hodgkin's lymphoma with mesenteric adenopathy. A large confluent mass of lymphomatous nodes *(asterisk)* "sandwiches" the mesenteric vessels *(arrows)*. Bowel loops are displaced. *D*, Ovarian carcinoma with omental metastases. Massive omental metastases form an omental "cake" between the anterior abdominal wall and the transverse colon (*between arrows*). (Courtesy of Faye Laing, M.D., and Michael Federle, M.D., Department of Radiology, San Francisco General Hospital.)

Some patients with mesenteric panniculitis apparently progress to a chronic process, which is probably identical with that described as retractile mesenteritis. These patients with chronic mesenteritis, either from panniculitis or due to retractile mesenteritis, have continual abdominal pain, fever, and weight loss and in addition may develop small bowel obstruction, mesenteric thrombosis, and intestinal lymphatic obstruction, with resultant ascites, steatorrhea, and protein-losing enteropathy.[383, 384] Indeed, protein-losing gastroenteropathy in this setting makes one think of retractile mesenteritis.

Pathology. At laparotomy, patients with mesenteric panniculitis are found to have a thickened mesentery, most often in the mesenteric root, and almost always limited to the small bowel mesentery. A single discrete mass is found in 32 per cent, multiple masses in 26 per cent, and diffuse mesenteric thickening in 42 per cent. Histologic examination of the affected mesentery reveals infiltration of fat by macrophages with abundant foamy cytoplasm, focal lymphocytic infiltration, fat necrosis, fibrosis, and calcification.[380, 385, 386]

In retractile mesenteritis, the mesentery is thickened, fibrotic, and retracted, with opalescent pale gray plaques. There is a dense collagen and fibrous tissue proliferation; less fat necrosis and inflammation are evident than in the earlier panniculitis stage. Rarely, the colonic mesentery and peritoneum may be involved with a similar fibrotic process.[385, 387, 388] The retroperitoneum is involved in retractile mesenteritis in 5 per cent of cases, and the mesentery is involved in retroperitoneal fibrosis in 2 to 3 per cent.[380, 385, 389] However, there is little epidemiologic or pathologic evidence that the two lesions are etiologically related despite their occasional concomitant occurrence.[390]

Treatment and Prognosis. Corticosteroids have been used in symptomatic treatment of mesenteric panniculitis, but it is not clear whether they shorten the duration of the disease or slow the progression to retractile mesenteritis.[380, 385] However, occasional patients may respond dramatically to prednisone or immunosuppresive agents.[391, 392] Surgical treatment should be limited to exploration and biopsy, with bypass of obstructed intestine when indicated. Resection of the fibrotic mass is often not possible and generally should not be attempted.

The prognosis is usually excellent; pain disappears in 75 per cent of patients and the mass regresses in 66 per cent, usually within two years.[380] Malignant lymphomas have developed in 15 per cent of patients, but the basis for this association is unknown.

Mesenteric Fibromatosis (Desmoid Tumors)

Mesenteric fibromatosis, or desmoid, is a benign, noninflammatory fibrous proliferation of the mesentery. It occurs in two forms: an isolated form and a form associated with familial polyposis. About 3 per cent of patients with familial polyposis of the colon may develop the lesion, which usually appears one to three years after abdominal surgery. About one half of those who develop it have other lesions of Gardner's syndrome, such as desmoid, epidermoid, or sebaceous cysts, osteomas, lipomas, or subcutaneous fibromas. Patients with Gardner's syndrome may have a higher incidence, for 14 per cent of one kindred developed mesenteric fibromatosis (see pp. 1504–1507).[393–395]

About 8 per cent of all desmoid tumors are mesenteric, with the rest occurring in the subcutaneous tissue of the abdominal wall (49 per cent) or extra-abdominal tissues (43 per cent). In most cases trauma precipitates the lesion; in other cases estrogens or prostaglandins are factors that have been linked to the pathogenesis of the growths.[396]

Ultrasonography reveals a well-demarcated solid mass with some internal echoes, which on CT shows a nonenhancing mass with soft-tissue density.[397, 398] However, these findings are nonspecific, and surgery is often necessary to define the nature and extent of the lesion.

Mesenteric fibromatosis is usually asymptomatic, and its major importance is that it can be mistaken for metastatic adenocarcinoma in a patient with familial polyposis. However, the fibrous proliferation may be quite aggressive and infiltrative and occasionally causes intestinal perforation or involves mesenteric vessels.[399]

Asymptomatic patients should have only biopsy without excision. The management of other patients may be difficult. With widespread areas of fibromatosis, full excision may be difficult and may lead to further morbidity or need for surgery. It has been suggested that resection should be avoided in favor of intestinal bypass, but wide local excision is recommended by others.[395, 400] Recurrence is common.

Because of the evidence that estrogenic hormones or prostaglandins have a role in growth of the lesion, prostaglandin inhibitors (sulindac) and antiestrogens (tamoxifen) have been used in small numbers of patients with some apparent success.[401, 402] Two recent reports are divided on the efficacy of these agents.[402a, 402b] Radiotherapy and chemotherapy probably have little role in treatment.

Mesenteric and Omental Cysts

Etiology and Pathogenesis. Most mesenteric cysts are mainly chylous lymphatic cysts; some are of mesothelial origin. Most authorities attribute the origin of mesenteric cysts to sequestrations of the lymphatic system, with continued growth of congenitally malformed or malpositioned lymphatics.[403, 404] They may not be closed structures, because they can wax and wane in size and they rarely rupture. Distended lymphaticovenous shunts have been demonstrated, and it is postulated that there may be congenital deficiencies in the formation or persistence of these shunts in the fine lymphaticovenous networks.[405]

Cysts may also be classified as traumatic, neoplastic, infective, or degenerative, but probably few cysts arise as a result of these causes. The frequency of origin from various tissues is unclear. Histologic criteria separate mesenteric cysts (71 per cent of patients) from cystic lymphangiomas, (29 per cent of patients).[406] Mesenteric cysts have cuboidal mesothelial lining cells and lack lymphatic and smooth muscle elements. Cystic lymphangiomas have an endothelial lining, a wall containing small lymphatic spaces, lymphoid tissue, and smooth muscle. Electron microscopy can further differentiate the mesothelial origin of mesenteric cysts and the endothelial nature of cystic lymphangiomas.[137, 406, 407]

Cysts contain fluid which may be serous, chylous, hemorrhagic, or purulent. The presence of chyle depends on proximity to intestinal lacteals, and cysts of any origin may bleed or become infected. Neoplastic cysts are rare and are found in only 3 per cent of patients.[408]

Clinical Features. Mesenteric cysts are five times more common than omental cysts, and both types are more common in females. Mesenteric cysts become symptomatic after 10 years of age in about 75 per cent of cases. Omental cysts are more common in childhood.

Mesenteric cysts may be an asymptomatic, incidental finding in 50 per cent; the other one half of patients present with chronic or acute abdominal pain.[404, 406] Symptoms are usually related to changes in size and position. Patients without symptoms usually have a painless, slow-growing mass, often found incidentally on examination or at the time of surgery. Many patients have chronic pain which is diffuse, nonlocalized, and related to traction on the root of the mesentery. Acute symptoms are present in 20 to 30 per cent of adult patients and 60 per cent of pediatric patients, and are secondary to some complications, including rupture, hemorrhage, volvulus, infection, or intestinal obstruction.

On physical examination a round, smooth, mobile mass may be found which is usually nontender. Omental cysts are usually freely movable in all directions, whereas mesenteric cysts have limited movement longitudinally. Large cysts may simulate ascites with shifting dullness and fluid waves.

There are no definitive diagnostic tests. Contrast studies show displacement of organs or extrinsic compression, and ultrasonography and CT show a uniloculated or multiloculated cystic mass without connection to other normal structures. Cysts are located in the small bowel mesentery in 60 per cent, in the large bowel mesentery in 24 per cent, and in the retroperitoneum in 16 per cent of patients.[408]

Enucleation is the treatment of choice, but resection is occasionally necessary if the cyst is too close to bowel. External marsupialization, aspiration, or internal drainage is not recommended.[403, 408]

Mesenteric and Omental Tumors

Mesenteric tumors are rare and may arise from any of the cellular elements of the mesentery. Fibromas account for about 25 per cent; myomas 15 per cent; lipomatous tumors 15 per cent; histiocytic tumors (xanthogranulomas) 15 per cent; hemangiopericytomas 10 per cent; neurofibromas 5 per cent; and mesenchymomas 5 per cent.[409] The symptoms of mesenteric tumors are nonspecific and include weight loss, abdominal pain, abdominal mass, and the effects of compression of adjacent structures. Most of the connective tissue tumors are well-differentiated, low-grade fibrosarcomas that are locally invasive and may be cured by excision. Many of these tumors may be benign fibromatoses (desmoid tumors) similar to those of Gardner's syndrome. They need not be excised. Indeed, they may even regress or resolve (see discussion above).[410, 411] On the other hand, approximately 50 per cent of the lipomatous, histiocytic, or leiomyomatous tumors are malignant and may metastasize, with a 20 per cent five-year survival.[412, 412a]

Lymphoid tumors of the mesentery have also been described and may be locally infiltrative. Of interest are benign lymphoid tumors (angiofollicular lymph node hyperplasia, or Castleman's disease), which may be present with systemic manifestations such as fever, leukocytosis, hyperglobulinemia, and associated hypochromic microcytic anemia with absence of bone marrow iron. These patients have no evidence of blood loss but do have hypoferremia or resistance to iron therapy; the syndrome is completely reversed by removal of the tumor. It is not clear whether these lesions represent giant lymph node hyperplasia secondary to an inflammatory, immunologic, or infectious process, or whether they are hamartomas or actual lymphoid neoplasms.[413, 414]

Metastatic tumors of the mesentery are more common than primary mesenteric tumors and are usually the result of enlarged lymphomatous or carcinomatous lymph nodes. In one series, mesenteric involvement was present in 30 per cent of non-Hodgkin's lymphoma, 2 per cent of Hodgkin's disease, 38 per cent of ovarian carcinoma, 24 per cent of pancreatic carcinoma, and 12 per cent of colon carcinoma.[371] CT scan shows several patterns: rounded masses, ill-defined masses, and "cakelike" masses (Fig. 102–2). In addition, a stellate mesentery representing thickening and rigidity of the mesentery may be present.[371, 372]

Omental tumors, in contrast to mesenteric tumors, are derived from muscle in 60 per cent of cases (leiomyomas, leiomyosarcomas, or hemangiopericytomas).[415] Abdominal pain, an abdominal mass, and weight loss are seen in patients with large symptomatic tumors (65 per cent), and ascites is more common than in mesenteric tumors. CT scans show several patterns including omental caking (replacement by large masses), small nodules with infiltration, cystic masses, or multiple discrete nodules (Fig. 102–2). Ultrasound defines omental involvement less well.[373] About 40 per cent of omental tumors are malignant; they also tend to produce local invasion and peritoneal implants rather than distant metastases.

Mesenteric Hernias

Various forms of herniation of the mesentery result from anomalous intestinal rotation, with fusion of the mesentery and parietal peritoneum during embryonic development. Mesenteric (internal) hernias account for 1 to 2 per cent of cases of acute intestinal obstruction. They present with chronic, intermittent small intestinal obstruction or acute obstruction. A palpable mass may be present in the upper abdomen in a small number of patients (see p. 1017).

Small bowel mesenteric defects account for 70 per cent of cases (half of which are ileocecal); 28 per cent are mesocolic. The small bowel herniates in 87 per cent, the colon herniates in only 9 per cent, and the stomach herniates in 4 per cent. Most of the defects are single and are 2 to 3 cm in diameter.[416]

Preoperative diagnosis is difficult, but mesenteric hernia should be considered in any patient with intermittent episodes of pain or obstruction. Mesenteric hernias may be missed at operation and should be sought carefully. In addition, if a mesenteric defect is discovered during laparotomy for an unrelated problem, it should be repaired at that time to prevent future herniation and obstruction.

Mesenteric Arteriovenous Fistula

Mesenteric-portal fistulas are sequelae of penetrating wounds or surgical trauma. Patients have cramping abdominal pain, diarrhea, and an abdominal bruit, but a mass is rarely palpable. The major complication is portal hypertension. The diagnosis of mesenteric fistula is easily made with angiography.[417]

Mesenteric Hematoma

Bleeding into the mesentery without associated trauma is usually caused by chronic anticoagulant therapy. Patients present with crampy abdominal pain, and may have an abdominal mass. Contrast studies show nonspecific separation and displacement of bowel loops and may also show signs of submucosal hemmorhage. Ultrasonography shows a complex mass with internal echoes and septation. The diagnosis may be strongly suspected on CT scan, which shows a homogeneous hyperdense mass early in the course of hematoma formation. If the diagnosis is delayed, however, the clot may be isodense or hypodense and mimic a solid or cystic lesion.[418]

Omental Torsion and Infarction

Torsion of the omentum is an acute surgical condition that usually mimics acute appendicitis or acute cholecystitis. The underlying cause of omental torsion is not clear. Predisposing factors that have been suggested are malformation of the omental pedicle, variable amounts and dispositions of omental fat, increased mobility of the right omentum, venous redundancy with omental kinking, or nonspecific inflammatory foci in the omentum.[419] Omental torsion occurs mainly in the fourth and fifth decades, with a male-to-female ratio of 2 to 1. It is rare in children, occurring once in 800 cases of appendicitis.[420] Abdominal pain is the major symptom, localizing in the right lower quadrant in 80 per cent and in the right upper quadrant in about 10 per cent of patients. Nausea, fever, vomiting, abdominal mass, and leukocytosis are each present in about one half of the patients. Nonspecific tenderness, guarding, and ileus are usually present, but the diagnosis may be suspected if a mobile tender mass is palpable in the right abdomen.[421] At laparotomy, vascular engorgement, torsion, and gangrene of the omentum are found. Omentectomy is indicated.

Idiopathic primary omental infarction presents a similar picture of acute right-sided abdominal pain, localized peritoneal signs, fever, and leukocytosis. Because of the acute nature of the clinical picture, radiologic studies are usually not done. If the symptoms are less acute, ultrasonography may show a complex mass and a mixture of solid material and hypoechoic zones, located between the stomach and transverse colon.[422]

A heavy omentum with infarction of the right margin is found at laparotomy and is cured by omentectomy.[423] Various theories have been proposed to explain the segmental nature of the infarction: anomalous venous drainage, rupture of vessels in a heavy omentum, stretching of vessels with subsequent endothelial damage and thrombosis, or disproportionate fat growth with relative ischemia.[424] The finding of tenuous connections between the right omentum and the rest of the omentum has suggested that omental infarction may result from an embryologic variant. The areas of infarction are in those portions of the omentum that have arisen from the ventral mesogastrium, and these have weak bands of fusion and a tenuous blood supply. When this anatomic variant is stressed by congestion or increased intra-abdominal pressure, thrombosis may result.[425]

DISEASES OF THE DIAPHRAGM

General Clinical Features

Patients with diaphragmatic disease usually present with pulmonary symptoms, but they may have only abdominal symptoms if abdominal organs herniate through areas of congenital weakness, defects, or rupture of the diaphragm. In addition, intradiaphragmatic masses may refer pain to the abdomen and simulate abdominal disease.

Diaphragmatic problems are often easily diagnosed or suspected on plain chest films. Ultrasonography and CT scans add the ability to visualize the diaphragm and its attachments, juxtadiaphragmatic masses or fluid collections, and the contents of herniations.[426, 427]

Eventration

Eventration of the diaphragm is a congenital abnormality in which there is a weakness of the central portion of either the right or the left leaf of the diaphragm, owing to absence of muscular tissue in that area; the peripheral musculature and phrenic innervation are intact. Eventration is often an incidental, asymptomatic radiographic finding. Most symptomatic patients present in the fourth or fifth decade of life with nonspecific dyspepsia, epigastric discomfort or burning, and eructation.[428] Occasionally, gastric outlet obstruction may result from volvulus at the cardia or pylorus. Respiratory distress is uncommon in adults, although pulmonary function may be compromised on testing.

The diagnosis may be suggested by dullness to percussion, absent breath sounds, and the presence of bowel sounds over the affected hemidiaphragm. The trachea and heart may be pushed to the contralateral side. If the physical signs are confusing, chest X-ray with fluoroscopy or CT scanning may establish the diagnosis. Symptomatic eventration responds well to surgical repair, which involves resection of the central diaphragm and closure using pericardium or synthetic mesh.

Herniation

Diaphragmatic hernias are due to congenital abnormalities in the formation of the diaphragm. The diaphragm is derived from four embryonic structures: the septum transversum ventrally, the pleuroperitoneal membrane and body wall laterally, and the mesoesophagus mediodorsally. Most commonly, the left pleuroperitoneal membrane fails to fuse with the septum transversum, causing a left posterolateral defect without a hernia sac. If fusion is complete but there is a failure of muscularization posterolaterally, a hernia with a sac is formed. This posterolateral wedge-shaped defect is called the foramen of Bochdalek. Lateral chest films show a single smooth focal bulge centered 4 to 5 cm anterior to either posterior diaphragmatic insertion. Although previous studies reported a left-sided prevalence in 90 per cent, recent CT studies found left-sided hernias were only twice as common as right-sided hernias. In addition, Bochdalek hernias may be more common than was previously thought, since careful retrospective review of 900 CT scans in asymptomatic adults revealed a prevalence of 6 per cent[429] (see p. 597 for information on hiatal hernias).

Bochdalek hernias are asymptomatic in one fourth of patients, but one half have vague, intermittent abdominal pain, and one fourth have chest pain, cardiovascular symptoms, and dyspnea.[430, 431] Incarceration of intestine leads to acute, sharp, substernal pain radiating to the left upper quadrant or back, along with the typical symptoms of intestinal obstruction. The hernia may also contain omentum, stomach, spleen, liver, pancreas, or retroperitoneal fat.

The diagnosis can usually be made on lateral chest film, which reveals a blunted cardiophrenic angle, a small effusion, and a gas-filled intestinal loop. Intestinal contrast studies or pneumoperitoneum may be necessary for small hernias. In addition, if visceral herniation is intermittent, radiologic studies may appear normal if not obtained during acute episodes of pain.[432] CT scanning may demonstrate small, partial diaphragmatic hernias, showing the diaphragmatic defect and adjacent subdiaphragmatic retroperitoneal fat extending into the chest.[429, 431] Because of the danger of strangulation, surgery is always indicated in those patients with incarceration or obstruction.

Congenital defects also occur in the retrocostoxiphoid region, usually on the right, possibly because the pericardial attachment to the diaphragm is more extensive than on the left. These foramen of Morgagni hernias nearly always have a hernial sac. Morgagni hernias are rarely symptomatic but may present with epigastric discomfort, dyspepsia, or bloating. Acute symptoms are almost always due to large bowel obstruction, unlike Bochdalek hernias, although omentum and stomach may also be incarcerated.[433] Lateral chest films are usually diagnostic and may be confirmed with barium enema or CT scanning.[434, 435] Surgical repair is necessary to prevent incarceration and strangulation.

Rupture

Blunt injury to the abdomen may cause diaphragmatic rupture, which has been reported in about 5 per cent of all patients undergoing surgery for trauma.[436] Because the early clinical course may be dominated by accompanying injuries, signs of visceral herniation are often delayed. Patients may present many years later with postprandial fullness, cramps, nausea, vomiting, chest pain, dyspnea, or obvious bowel obstruction or strangulation. Pleuroperitoneal pressure gradients during normal inspiration explain the development of chronic or late diaphragmatic hernias.[437–439]

Diaphragmatic rupture is considered more common on the left side because of an embryologic point of weakness and because of the presence of the liver on the right. Recently, however, several reports have shown an increased incidence of right-sided injury ranging from 20 to 40 per cent.[436, 440, 441] The stomach, colon, omentum, spleen, and small bowel most frequently herniate. The diagnosis may be suspected on physical examination by finding an elevated diaphragm, dullness from effusion, or bowel sounds in the chest. It can be confirmed with chest X-ray, barium studies, or X-ray after pneumoperitoneum. Newer diagnostic modalities may increase the diagnostic yield. Liver scanning demonstrates an abnormally elevated liver and a linear lucency where the liver is wedged through the laceration.[442] Ultrasound and CT scan may demonstrate the tear itself.[443, 444]

Diaphragmatic laceration should be repaired surgically because of the high frequency of later visceral herniation. Diaphragmatic rupture should be suspected in any patient with vague abdominal symptoms and a history of blunt abdominal trauma.

Tumors

Diaphragmatic neoplasms usually cause pleuritic chest pain, but pain may be referred to the epigastrium and simulate intra-abdominal disease. Chest X-rays reveal irregularity of the diaphragm or an enlarged mass that abuts on the diaphragm.[445] Any histologic component of the diaphragm may give rise to benign neoplasms, but the majority of primary malignant neoplasms arise from fibrous tissue.

Excessive subdiaphragmatic fat may separate the superior margin of the liver from the right hemidiaphragm, suggesting tumor, ascites, abscess, or pneumoperitoneum. CT scan clarifies the diagnosis by showing the fatty character of the tissue.[446]

Pseudotumors are another diagnostic pitfall; invaginations of the muscular fibers of the diaphragm into the upper abdomen may appear as nodules of soft tissue density in deep inspiration, and may mimic small tumors by indenting the adjacent stomach, transverse colon, or retroperitoneal fat.[447] Similarly, an *inverted diaphragm* associated with large pleural effusions may cause a left upper quadrant soft tissue density and displacement of abdominal organs.[448]

Diaphragmatic cysts may also cause upper abdominal pain; when located on the right, they suggest possible hepatic or subphrenic abnormalities. These cysts are bronchogenic, mesothelial, or fibrous and may be acquired or congenital.[449]

Intradiaphragmatic abscesses, contained within the leaves of the diaphragm, are rare but may occur following surgery or procedures near the diaphragm. They may be mistaken for subphrenic abscesses, and therefore routine surgical exploration may fail to localize the abscess.[450, 451]

Hiccups

The hiccup is an abrupt inspiratory muscle contraction, the onset of which is followed within 35 ms by closure of the glottis.[452] Because the glottis remains closed until the inspiratory muscle contraction has ceased, there is little or no direct ventilatory effect in adults, although in infants clinically significant changes in ventilation may result.[452, 453] Hiccups result from stimulation of one or more limbs of the reflex arc of the glottis; the afferent limb is composed of the vagus and phrenic nerves and the thoracic sympathetic chain, with the "hiccup center" being located in the spinal cord between C3 and C5. The efferent limb is primarily the phrenic nerve, with efferents to the glottis and accessory respiratory muscles. The hiccup is generated by a supraspinal center, distinct from that which governs respiration. Hiccups may involve one or both diaphragms. It is interesting that they seem to be more frequent in men than in women. Hiccups are usually brief, self-limited episodes, but may be persistent, or rarely, intractable.

Hiccups are caused by or associated with a wide variety of conditions.[454, 455] Self-limited causes are usually gastric distention, sudden temperature changes, alcohol ingestion, excess smoking, or sudden excitement or stress. Causes of persistent hiccups may be considered clinically as arising from the abdomen, neck and thorax, or the central nervous system, the latter including toxic, metabolic, and pharmacologic etiologies. Intra-abdominal processes include subdiaphragmatic abscess or other diaphragmatic irritation, inflammatory and neoplastic processes, gastric distention, and gastrointestinal bleeding. Thoracic and neck disorders include diaphragmatic tumors, pneumonia, phrenic nerve compression, esophageal disease, and myocardial infarction. Central nervous system disorders include intracranial infections and tumors, cerebral ischemia or infarction, the effects of azotemia, hyponatremia, and chemical irritants. Hiccups may also occur in association with general anesthesia.

Persistent hiccups may not be benign and may result in inability to eat, weight loss, exhaustion, insomnia, arrhythmias, and severe reflux esophagitis.[454, 456]

Management of intractable hiccups should include attempts to identify an underlying cause, which should be treated appropriately. For suppression of hiccups, a large number of remedies and drugs have been employed, with variable success. A sequential protocol may be followed, beginning with simple physical maneuvers such as breath holding, sudden fright or pain, breathing into a paper bag, sneezing, pulling on the tongue, swallowing dry granulated sugar, or sipping ice water. If hiccups continue, manual stimulation of the nasopharynx with a finger or catheter or lifting the uvula with a spoon may be tried. Hiccups that remain refractory to these measures will often require the use of pharmacologic agents, such as chlorpromazine, 25 to 50 mg intravenously every six hours; metoclopramide, 10 mg intravenously every four hours; quinidine, 200 mg four times daily; diphenylhydantoin, 100 mg intravenously followed by 100 mg four times daily by mouth; or valproic acid, 15 mg per kg orally. For hiccups unresponsive to these measures, phrenic nerve block or crush can be considered, but even this has failed.[454, 455, 457, 458] Because hiccups may diminish in frequency over hours to days in response to medical treatment or the passage of time, approaches to the phrenic nerve should be reserved for only the most severe and intractable cases.

References

1. Meyers, M. A. Dynamic Radiology of the Abdomen; Normal and Pathologic Anatomy. New York, Springer Verlag, 1976.

1a. Meyers, M. A., Oliphant, M., Berne A. S., et al. The peritoneal ligaments and mesenteries: pathways of intraabdominal spread of disease. Radiology *163*:593, 1987.

2. Sampson, R., and Pasternack, B. M. Current status of surgery of the omentum. Surg. Gynecol. Obstet. *149*:437, 1979.
3. Northover, J. M. A., Williams, E. D. F., and Terblanche, J. Investigation of small vessel anatomy by scanning electron micoscropy of resin casts. J. Anat. *130*:43, 1980.
4. Whittaker, D., Papadimitriou, J. M., and Walters, M. N. The mesothelium and its reactions: a review. C.R.C. Crit. Rev. Toxicol. *10*:81, 1982.
5. Feriani, M., Biasioli, S., Chiaramonte, S., et al. Anatomical bases of peritoneal permeability: a reappraisal. Int. J. Artificial Organs *5*:345, 1982.
6. Gotloib, L., Diginis, G. E., Rabinovich, S., et al. Ultrastructure of normal rabbit mesentery. Nephron *34*:248, 1983.
7. Aune, S. Transperitoneal exchange. Scand. J. Gastroenterol. *5*:85, 99, 161, 241, 253, 1970.
8. Kraft, A., Tompkins, R., and Joseph, J. Peritoneal electrolyte absorption: analysis of portal, systemic venous and lymphatic transport. Surgery *64*:148, 1968.
9. Leak, L. V., and Rahil, K. Permeability of the diaphragmatic mesothelium; the ultrastructural basis for "stomata." Am. J. Anat. *151*:557, 1978.
10. Bettendorf, U. Lymph flow mechanism of the subperitoneal diaphragmatic lymphatics. Lymphology *11*:111, 1978.
11. Raybuck, H., Allen, L., and Haims, W. Absorption of serum from the peritoneal cavity. Am. J. Physiol. *199*:1021, 1960.
12. Lill, S. R., Parsons, R. H., and Buhac, I. Permeability of the diaphragm and fluid resorption from the peritoneal cavity in the rat. Gastroenterology *76*:997, 1979.
13. Shear, L., Swartz, C., Shinaberger, J., et al. Kinetics of peritoneal fluid absorption in man. N. Engl. J. Med. *272*:123, 1965.
14. Shear, L., Castellot, J., Shinaberger, J., et al. Enhancement of peritoneal fluid absorption by dehydration, mercaptomerin, and vasopressin. J. Pharmacol. Exp. Ther. *154*:289, 1966.
15. Zink, J., and Greenway, C. V. Control of ascites absorption in anesthesized cats: effects of intraperitoneal pressure, protein, and furosemide diuresis. Gastroenterology *73*:119, 1977.
16. McKay, T., Zink, J., and Greenway, C. V. Relative rates of

absorption of fluid and protein from the peritoneal cavity of cats. Lymphology *11*:106, 1978.
17. Koninckx, P. R., Ranier, M., and Brosens, I. A. Origin of peritoneal fluid in women—an ovarian exudation product. Br. J. Obstet. Gynecol. *87*:177, 1980.
18. Michel, J., Bercovici, B., and Sachs, T. Comparative studies on the antimicrobial activity of peritoneal and ascitic fluids in human beings. Surg. Gynecol. Obstet. *151*:55, 1980.
19. Simberkoff, M. S., Moldover, N. H., and Weiss, G. Bacterial and opsonic activity of cirrhotic ascites and nonascitic peritoneal fluid. J. Lab. Clin. Med. *91*:831, 1978.
20. Matzner, Y., and Brzezinsky, A. A C5a inhibitor in peritoneal fluid. J. Lab. Clin. Med. *103*:227, 1984.
21. Bercovici, B., and Gallily, R. The cytology of the human peritoneal fluid. Acta Cytol. *22*:124, 1978.
22. Abe, K., Houma, S., and Ito, T. Peritoneal cells in mice: quantitative and qualitative cell morphology. Am. J. Anat. *156*:37, 1979.
23. Cantazaro, P., and Graham, R. Normal peritoneal lymphocytes. Am. J. Pathol. *77*:23, 1974.
24. Van der Berg, W. B., Maarsseveen, A. C. M., Mullen, K. H., et al. Accumulation of T-cells and local anti-PPD antibody production in lymphokine mediated chronic peritoneal inflammation in the guinea pig. J. Pathol. *132*:23, 1980.
25. Mironov, V. A., Gusev, S. A., and Baradi, A. F. Mesothelial stomata overlying omental milky spots: scanning electron microscopic study. Cell Tiss. Res. *201*:328, 1979.
25a. Yoffey, J. M. Peritoneal lymphoid cells. Lymphology *19*:96, 1986.
26. Raftery, A. T. Regeneration of parietal and visceral peritoneum. Br. J. Surg. *60*:293, 1973.
27. Ryan, G. B., Grobety, J., and Majno, G. Mesothelial injury and recovery. Am. J. Pathol. *71*:93, 1973.
28. Raftery, A. T. Regeneration of peritoneum: a fibrinolytic study. J. Anat. *129*:659, 1979.
29. Hau, T., Ahrenholz, D. H., and Simmons, R. L. Secondary bacterial peritonitis: the biologic basis of treatment. Curr. Probl. Surg. *16*:1, 1979.
30. Stangel, J. J., Nisbet, J. D., and Settles, H. Formation and prevention of postoperative abdominal adhesions. J. Reprod. Med. *29*:143, 1984.
31. Teplick, J. C., Haskin, M. E., and Alavi, A. Calcified intraperitoneal metastases from ovarian carcinoma. Am. J. Roentgenol. *127*:1003, 1976.
32. Berliner, L., and Redmond, P. Calcified papillary tumor of the peritoneum. Br. J. Radiol. *53*:1200, 1980.
33. Meyers, M. Peritoneography. Am. J. Roentgenol. *117*:353, 1973.
34. Yeh, H. C. Ultrasonography of peritoneal tumors. Radiology *133*:419, 1979.
35. Jeffrey, R. B. CT demonstration of peritoneal implants. Am. J. Roentgenol. *135*:323, 1980.
36. Roab, L. W., Drayer, B. P., Orr, D. P., et al. Computed tomographic positive contrast peritoneography. Radiology *131*:699, 1979.
37. LaManna, M. M., Saluk, P. H., Zekavat, P. P., et al. Gallium localization in peritonitis. Clin. Nucl. Med. *9*:25, 1984.
38. Crawford, E., and Ellis, H. Generalized peritonitis—the changing spectrum: a report of 100 consecutive cases. Br. J. Clin. Pract. *39*:177, 1985.
39. Stephen, M., and Loewenthal, J. Generalized infective peritonitis. Surg. Gynecol. Obstet. *147*:233, 1978.
40. Lobbato, V., Cioroiu, M., LaRaja, R. D., et al. Peritoneal lavage as an aid to diagnosis of peritonitis in debilitated and elderly patients. Am. Surg. *51*:508, 1985.
41. Richardson, J. D., Flint, L. M., and Polk, H. C. Peritoneal lavage: a useful diagnostic adjunct for peritonitis. Surgery *94*:826, 1983.
42. Vincent, J. L., Puri, V. K., Carlson, R. W., et al. Acute respiratory failure in patients with generalized peritonitis. Resuscitation *10*:283, 1983.
43. Vincent, J. L., Weill, M. H., Puri, V., et al. Circulatory shock associated with purulent peritonitis. Am. J. Surg. *142*:262, 1981.
44. Stewart, D. J. Generalized peritonitis. J. R. Coll. Surg. (Edinburgh) *25*:80, 1980.
45. Dipiro, J. T., Mansburger, J. A., and Davis, J. B. Current concepts in clinical therapeutics: Intraabdominal infections. Clin. Pharmacol. *5*:34, 1986.
46. Solomkin, J. S., Meakins, J. L., Aloo, M. D., et al. Antibiotic trials in intraabdominal infections: a critical evaluation of study design and outcome reporting. Ann. Surg. *200*:29, 1984.
47. Dougherty, S. H. Role of enterococcus in intraabdominal sepsis. Am. J. Surg. *148*:308, 1984.
48. Stephen, M., and Loewenthal, J. Continuing peritoneal lavage in high risk peritonitis. Surgery *85*:603, 1979.
49. Hudspeth, A. S. Radical surgical debridement in the treatment of advanced generalized bacterial peritonitis. Arch. Surg. *110*:1233, 1975.
50. Polk, H. C., and Fry, D. E. Radical peritoneal debridement for established peritonitis: the result of a prospective randomized clinical trial. Ann. Surg. *192*:350, 1980.
51. Roth, R. M., Gleckman, R. A., Gantz, N. M., et al. Antibiotic irrigations: a plea for controlled clinical trials. Pharmacotherapy *5*:222, 1985.
52. Bohnen, J., Boulanger, M., Meakins, J. L., et al. Prognosis in generalized peritonitis: relation to cause and risk factors. Arch. Surg. *118*:285, 1983.
53. Gauntner, W. C., Feldman, H. A., and Puschett, J. B. Peritonitis in chronic peritoneal dialysis patients. Clin. Nephrol. *13*:255, 1980.
54. Mader, J. T., and Reinarz, J. A. Peritonitis during peritoneal dialysis. J. Chron. Dis. *31*:635, 1978.
55. Steinberg, S. M., Kutler, S. J., Nolph, K. D., et al. A comprehensive report on the experience of patients on continuous ambulatory peritoneal dialysis for the treatment of end-stage renal disease. Am. J. Kidney Dis. *6*:233, 1984.
56. Swartz, R. D. Chronic peritoneal dialysis: mechanical and infectious complications. Nephron *40*:29, 1985.
57. Lack, C., Senekjian, H. O., Knight, T. F., et al. Twelve months experience with continuous ambulatory and intermittent peritoneal dialysis. Arch. Intern. Med. *141*:197, 1981.
58. Verbrugh, H. A., Keane, W. F., Hoidal, J. R., et al. Peritoneal macrophages and opsonins: antibacterial defense in patients undergoing chronic peritoneal dialysis. J. Infect. Dis. *147*:1018, 1983.
59. Keane, W. F., Comty, C. M., Verbrugh, H. A., et al. Opsonic deficiency of peritoneal dialysis effluent in continuous ambulatory peritoneal dialysis. Kidney Internat. *25*:539, 1984.
60. Rubin, J., Rogers, W. A., Taylor, H. M., et al. Peritonitis during chronic ambulatory peritoneal dialysis. Ann. Intern. Med. *92*:7, 1980.
61. Prowant, B., Nolph, K., Ryan, L., et al. Peritonitis in continuous ambulatory peritoneal dialysis: analysis of an 8-year experience. Nephron *43*:105, 1986.
62. Arfania, D., Everett, E. D., Nolph, K. D., et al. Uncommon causes of peritonitis in patients undergoing peritoneal dialysis. Arch. Intern. Med. *141*:61, 1981.
63. Gokal, R., Francis, D. M. A., Goodship, T. H. J., et al. Peritonitis in continuous ambulatory peritoneal dialysis. Lancet *2*:1388, 1982.
64. Ghandi, V. C., Kamadana, M. R., Ing, T. S., et al. Aseptic peritonitis in patients on maintenance peritoneal dialysis. Nephron *24*:257, 1979.
65. Spinowitz, B. S., Golden, R. A., Rascoff, J. H., et al. Eosinophilic peritonitis. Clin. Exp. Dialysis Apheresis *6*:187, 1982.
66. Hurley, R. M., Muogbo, D., Wilson, G. W., et al. Cellular composition of peritoneal effluent: response to bacterial peritonitis. Can. Med. Assoc. J. *117*:1061, 1977.
67. Kolmos, H. J. Antibiotic treatment of infectious peritonitis in chronic peritoneal dialysis. Scand. J. Infec. Dis. *17*:219, 1985.
68. Golper, T. A., and Hartstein, A. I. Analysis of the causative pathogens in uncomplicated CAPD-associated peritonitis: duration of therapy, relapses, and prognosis. Am. J. Kidney Dis. *7*:141, 1986.
68a. Report of a working party of the British Society for Antimicrobial Chemotherapy. Diagnosis and management of peritonitis in continuous ambulatory peritoneal dialysis. Lancet *1*:845, 1987.
69. Spence, P. A., Mathews, R. E., Khanna, R., et al. Indications for operation when peritonitis occurs in patients on chronic

ambulatory peritoneal dialysis. Surg. Gynecol. Obstet. *161*:450, 1985.

70. Schulack, J. A., Flannigan, M. J., Nghiem, D. D., et al. Ambulatory peritoneal dialysis: exploratory laparotomy for peritonitis. Arch. Surg. *119*:1400, 1984.
71. Harken, A., and Schochat, S. Gram positive peritonitis in children. Am. J. Surg. *125*:769, 1973.
72. Krensky, A. M., Ingelfinger, J. R., and Groupe, W. E. Peritonitis in childhood nephrotic syndrome: 1970–1980. Am. J. Dis. Child. *136*:732, 1982.
73. Freig, B. J., Votteler, T. P., and McCrackin, G. H. Primary peritonitis in previously healthy children. Am. J. Dis. Child. *138*:1058, 1984.
74. Clark, J. H., Fitzgerald, J. F., and Kleiman, M. D. Spontaneous bacterial peritonitis. J. Pediatr. *104*:495, 1984.
75. Send, S., Lalitha, M. K., Fenn, A. S., et al. Primary peritonitis in children. Ann. Tropic. Pediatr. *3*:53, 1983.
76. McDougal, W., Izant, R., and Zollinger, R. Primary peritonitis in infancy and childhood. Ann. Surg. *181*:310, 1975.
77. Speck, W., Dresdale, S., and McMillan, R. Primary peritonitis in the nephrotic syndrome. Am. J. Surg. *127*:267, 1974.
78. Hoffmann, S. Spontaneous bacterial peritonitis in patients without nephrotic ascites or alcoholic cirrhotic ascites. Danish Med. Bull. *30*:265, 1983.
79. Aklin, H. E., Fisher, K. A., Laleli, Y., et al. Bactericidal activity of ascitic fluid in patients with nephrotic syndrome. Eur. J. Clin. Invest. *15*:138, 1985.
80. Lipsky, P. E., Harden, J. A., Shour, L., et al. Spontaneous peritonitis in systemic lupus erythematosus. JAMA *232*:929, 1975.
81. Isner, J., McDonald, J. S., and Schein, P. S. Spontaneous streptococcus pneumonia peritonitis in a patient with metastatic gastric carcinoma. Cancer *39*:2306, 1977.
82. Kurtz, R. C., and Bronzo, R. L. Does spontaneous bacterial peritonitis occur in malignant ascites? Am. J. Gastroenterol. *77*:146, 1982.
83. Runyon, B. A., Morrissey, R. L., Hoefs, J. C., et al. Opsonic activity of human ascitic fluid: a potentially important protective mechanism against spontaneous bacterial peritonitis. Hepatology *5*:634, 1985.
84. Hau, T., Van Hook, E. J., Simmons, R. L., et al. Prognostic factors of peritoneal infections in transplant patients. Surgery *84*:403, 1978.
85. Alvarez, S., and McCabe, W. R. Extrapulmonary tuberculosis revisted: a review of experience at Boston City and other hospitals. Medicine *63*:25, 1984.
86. Sohocky, S. Tuberculous peritonitis. Am. Rev. Resp. Dis. *95*:398, 1967.
87. Vyravanathan, S., and Jeyarajah, R. Tuberculous peritonitis: a review of 35 cases. Postgrad. Med. J. *56*:649, 1980.
88. Singh, M., Bhargava, A., and Jain, K. Tuberculous peritonitis. N. Engl. J. Med. *281*:1091, 1969.
89. Slavin, R. E., Walsh, T. J., and Pollack, A. D. Late generalized tuberculosis. Medicine *59*:352, 1980.
90. Arafoth, R., Morse, R., Edwards, L. D., et al. Tuberculous peritonitis after laparotomy. Scand. J. Infect. Dis. *4*:139, 1972.
91. Burack, W., and Hollister, R. Tuberculous peritonitis. Am. J. Med. *28*:510, 1960.
92. Karney, W. W., O'Donahue, J. M., Ostrow, J. H., et al. The spectrum of tuberculous peritonitis. Chest *72*:310, 1977.
93. Sunderam, G., McDonald, R. J., Maniatis, T., et al. Tuberculosis as a manifestation of the acquired immune deficiency syndrome. JAMA *256*:362, 1986.
94. Barnes, P., Leedom, J. M., Radin, D. R., et al. An unusual case of tuberculous peritonitis in a man with AIDS. West. J. Med. *144*:467, 1986.
95. Bastani, B., Shariatzadeh, M. R., and Dehdashti, F. Tuberculous peritonitis—report of 30 cases and review of the literature. Q. J. Med. *56*:549, 1985.
96. McKerrow, K. J., and Neale, T. J. Tuberculous peritonitis in chronic renal failure managed by continuous ambulatory peritoneal dialysis. Austral. N. Z. J. Med. *13*:343, 1983.
97. Markman, M. Tuberculous peritonitis developing in a case of documented peritoneal carcinomatosis. West. J. Med. *143*:103, 1985.
98. Sherman, S., Rohwedder, J. J., Ravikrishnan, K. P., et al. Tuberculous enteritis and peritonitis: report of 36 general hospital cases. Arch. Intern. Med. *140*:506, 1980.
99. Hulnick, D. H., Megibow, A. J., Naidich, D. P., et al. Abdominal tuberculosis: CT evaluation. Radiology *157*:199, 1985.
100. Pulliam, J. P., Vernon, D. D., Alexander, S. R., et al. Nontuberculous mycobacterial peritonitis associated with continuous ambulatory peritoneal dialysis. Am. J. Kidney Dis. *2*:610, 1983.
101. Kurnick, P. B., Padmanab, H. U., Bonatsos, C., et al. Mycobacterium gordonae as a human hepato-peritoneal pathogen, with a review of the literature. Am. J. Med. Sci. *285*:45, 1983.
102. Geake, T. M. S., Spitaels, J. M., Moshal, M. G., et al. Peritoneoscopy in the diagnosis of tuberculous peritonitis. Gastrointest. Endosc. *27*:66, 1981.
103. Jorge, A. D. Peritoneal tuberculosis. Endoscopy *16*:10, 1984.
104. Gonnella, J., and Hudson, E. Clinical patterns of tuberculous peritonitis. Arch. Intern. Med. *117*:164, 1966.
105. Borhanmanesh, F., Hekmat, K., Vaezzadeh, K., et al. Tuberculous peritonitis: prospective study of 32 cases in Iran. Ann. Intern. Med. *76*:567, 1972.
106. Dineen, P., Homan, W. P., and Grafe, W. R. Tuberculous peritonitis: 43 years experience in diagnosis and treatment. Ann. Surg. *184*:717, 1976.
107. Khoury, G. A., Payne, C. R., and Harvey, D. R. Tuberculosis of the peritoneal cavity. Br. J. Surg. *65*:808, 1978.
108. Dutt, A. K., Moers, D., and Stead, W. W. Short course chemotherapy for extra-pulmonary tuberculosis: 9 years experience. Ann. Intern. Med. *104*:7, 1986.
109. Palmer, K. R., Patil, D. H., Basran, G. S., et al. Abdominal tuberculosis in urban Britain—a common disease. Gut *26*:1296, 1985.
110. National Consensus Conference on Chemotherapy for Tuberculosis. Standard therapy for tuberculosis, 1985. Chest *87*(suppl.):117, 1985.
111. Wormser, G. P., Leber, G., Tatz, J., et al. Peritonitis in patients with liver disease and ascites: use of Candida albicans as a microbiological clue in differential diagnosis. Am. J. Gastroenterol. *73*:305, 1980.
112. Bayer, A. S., Blumenkrantz, M. J., Montgomerie, J. Z., et al. Candida peritonitis Am. J. Med. *61*:832, 1976.
113. Johnson, R. J., Ramsey, P. G., Gallager, N., et al. Fungal peritonitis in patients on peritoneal dialysis: incidence, clinical features, and prognosis. Am. J. Nephrol. *5*:169, 1985.
114. Eisenberg, E. S., Leviton, I., and Soeiro, R. Fungal peritonitis in patients receiving peritoneal dialysis: experience with 11 patients and review of the literature. Rev. Infect. Dis. *8*:309, 1986.
115. Peterson, P. K., Lee, D., Suh, H. J., et al. Intracellular survival of Candida albicans in peritoneal macrophages from chronic peritoneal dialysis patients. Am. J. Kidney Dis. *7*:146, 1986.
116. Kerr, C. M., Perfect, J. R., Craven, P. C., et al. Fungal peritonitis in patients on continuous ambulatory peritoneal dialysis. Ann. Intern. Med. *99*:334, 1983.
117. Rault, R. Candida peritonitis complicating chronic peritoneal dialysis: a report of 5 cases and review of the literature. Am. J. Kidney Dis. *2*:544, 1983.
118. Solomkin, J. S., Flohr, A. B., Quie, P. G., et al. The role of Candida in intraperitoneal infections. Surgery *88*:524, 1980.

118a. Rutledge, R., Mandel, S. R., and Wild, R. E. Candida species: insignificant contaminant or pathogenic species? Am. Surg. *52*:299, 1986.

119. Reddy, P., Gorelick, D. F., Brasher, C. A., et al. Progressive disseminated histoplasmosis as seen in adults. Am. J. Med. *48*:629, 1970.
120. Saw, E., Shields, S. J., Comer, T. P., et al. Granulomatous peritonitis due to Coccidioides immitis. Arch. Surg. *108*:369, 1974.
121. Chen, K. T. K. Coccidioidal peritonitis. Am. J. Clin. Pathol. *80*:514, 1983.
122. Watson, N., and Johnson, A. Cryptococcal peritonitis. Southern Med. J. *66*:387, 1973.
123. Clift, S. A., Bradsher, R. W., and Chan, C. H. Peritonitis as

an indicator of disseminated cryptococcal infection. Am. J. Gastroenterol. *77*:922, 1982.

124. Blumberg, H., Srinivasan, K., and Parnes, I. Peritoneal schistosomiasis simulating carcinoma. N.Y. State J. Med. *66*:758, 1966.
125. Pearson, R. D., Irons, R. P., Sr., and Irons, R. P., Jr. Chronic pelvic peritonitis due to the pinworm Enterobias vermicularis. JAMA *245*:1340, 1981.
126. Reddy, C., Rao, D., Sarma, E. N. B., et al. Granulomatous peritonitis due to Ascaris lumbricoides and its ova. J. Trop. Med. Hyg. *78*:146, 1975.
127. Lintermans, J. Fatal peritonitis, an unusual complication of Strongyloides stercoralis infestation. Clin. Pediatr. *14*:974, 1975.
128. Kapor, O., Nathwani, B., and Joshi, V. Amebic peritonitis. J. Trop. Med. Hyg. *75*:11, 1972.
129. Rosai, J., and Dehner, L. Nodular mesothelial hyperplasia in hernia sacs. Cancer *35*:165, 1975.
130. Quagilia, A. C. Mesothelial proliferation: a questionable boundary with malignancy. Pathologica *76*:387, 1984.
131. McCaughey, W. T. E. Papillary peritoneal neoplasms in females. Pathol. Ann. *20*:387, 1985.
132. Blaustein, A. Peritoneal mesothelium and ovarian surface cells—shared characteristics. Int. J. Gynecol. Pathol. *3*:361, 1984.
133. Craig, J. R., and Hart, W. R. Extragenital adenomatoid tumor: evidence for the mesothelial theory of origin. Cancer *43*:1678, 1979.
134. Schneider, J. A., and Zelnick, E. J. Benign cystic peritoneal mesothelioma. J. Clin. Ultrasound *13*:190, 1985.
135. Katsube, Y., Mukai, K., and Silverberg, S. G. Cystic mesothelioma of the peritoneum: a report of 5 cases and review of the literature. Cancer *50*:1615, 1982.
136. Miles, J. M., Hart, W. R., and McMahon, J. T. Cystic mesothelioma of the peritoneum: report of a case with multiple recurrences and review of the literature. Cleveland Clin. Q. *53*:109, 1986.
137. Carpenter, H. A., Lancaster, J. R., and Lee, R. A. Multilocular cysts of the peritoneum. Mayo Clin. Proc. *57*:634, 1982.
138. Hansen, R. M., Caya, J. G., Clowry, L. G., Jr., et al. Benign mesothelial proliferation with effusion: clinicopathological entity that may mimic malignancy. Am. J. Med. *77*:887, 1984.
139. Goepel, J. R. Benign papillary mesothelioma of peritoneum: a histologic, histochemical, and ultrastructural study of 6 cases. Histopathology *5*:21, 1981.
140. Genadry, R., Poliakoff, S., Rotmensch, J., et al. Primary papillary peritoneal neoplasia. Obstet. Gynecol. *58*:730, 1981.
141. Dumke, K., Schnoy, N., Specht, G., et al. Comparative light and electron microscopic studies of cystic and papillary tumors of the peritoneum. Virchows Arch. Pathol. Anat. *399*:25, 1983.
142. Lindeque, B. G., Chronje, H. S., and Deale, C. J. C. Prevalence of primary papillary peritoneal neoplasia in patients with ovarian carcinoma. S. Afr. Med. J. *67*:1005, 1985.
143. Riddel, R. H., Goodman, M. J., and Moossa, A. R. Peritoneal malignant mesothelioma in a patient with recurrent peritonitis. Cancer *48*:134, 1981.
144. Stout, A. P. Solitary fibrous mesothelioma of the peritoneum. Cancer *3*:820, 1950.
145. Dervan, P. A., Tobin, B., and O'Connor, M. Solitary (localized) fibrous mesothelioma: evidence against mesothelial cell origin. Histopathology *10*:867, 1986.
146. Antman, K. H. Clinical presentation and natural history of benign and malignant mesothelioma. Semin. Oncol. *8*:313, 1981.
147. Kannerstein, M., Churg, J., and McCaughey, W. T. E. Asbestos in mesothelioma: a review. Pathol. Annu. *1*:81, 1978.
148. McDonald, A. D., and McDonald, J. C. Malignant mesothelioma in North America. Cancer *46*:1650, 1980.
149. Antman, K. H. Current concepts: Malignant mesothelioma. N. Engl. J. Med. *303*:200, 1980.
150. Newhouse, M. Epidemiology of asbestos related tumors. Semin. Oncol. *8*:250, 1981.
151. Gloag, D. Asbestos—can it be used safely? Br. Med. J. *282*:551, 1981.
152. Pooley, F. D. Minerology of asbestos: the physical and chemical properties of the dust they form. Semin. Oncol. *8*:243, 1981.
153. Craighead, J. E., and Mossman, B. T. The pathogenesis of asbestos-related diseases. N. Engl. J. Med. *306*:1446, 1982.
154. Walker, A. M., Laughlin, J. E., Friedlander, E. R., et al. Projections of asbestos related disease, 1980 to 2009. J. Occup. Med. *25*:409, 1983.
155. Gloag, D. Asbestos fibers in the environment. Br. Med. J. *282*:623, 1981.
156. Churg, A., and Warnock, M. L. Asbestos fibers in the general population. Am. Rev. Resp. Dis. *122*:669, 1980.
157. Churg, A., and Warnock, M. L. Asbestos and other ferruginous bodies: their formation and clinical significance. Am. J. Pathol. *102*:447, 1981.
158. Workshop on ingested asbestos. Environ. Health Prospec. *53*:1, 1983.
159. Gardner, M. J., Jones, R. D., Pippard, E. C., et al. Mesothelioma of the peritoneum during 1967–82 in England and Wales. Br. J. Cancer *51*:121, 1985.
160. Selikoff, I. J., Hammond, E. C., and Seidman, H. Latency of asbestos disease among insulation workers in the United States and Canada. Cancer *46*:2736, 1980.
161. Chahinian, A. P., Pajak, T. F., Holland, J. F., et al. Diffuse malignant mesothelioma: prospective evaluation of 69 patients. Ann. Intern. Med. *96*:746, 1982.
162. Levine, D. S. Does asbestos exposure cause gastrointestinal cancer? Dig. Dis. Sci. *30*:1189, 1985.
163. Morgan, R. W., Foliart, D. E., and Wong, O. Asbestos and gastrointestinal cancer: a review of the literature. West. J. Med. *143*:60, 1985.
164. Hourihane, D. A biopsy series of mesotheliomata, and attempts to identify asbestos within some of the tumors. Ann. N.Y. Acad. Sci. *132*:647, 1965.
165. Haderstein, M., Churg, J., Elliot, W. T., et al. Pathogenic effects of asbestos. Arch. Pathol. Lab. Med. *101*:623, 1977.
166. Browne, K., and Smither, W. J. Asbestos related mesothelioma: factors discriminating between pleural and peritoneal sites. Br. J. Indust. Med. *40*:145, 1983.
167. Peterson, J. T., Jr., Greenberg, S. D., and Buffler, P. A. Nonasbestos related malignant mesothelioma: a review. Cancer *54*:951, 1984.
168. Wagner, J. C. Mesothelioma and mineral fibers. Cancer *57*:1905, 1986.
169. Antman, K. H., Corson, J. M., Li, F. P., et al. Malignant mesothelioma following radiation exposure. J. Clin. Oncol. *1*:695, 1983.
170. Risberg, B., Nickels, J., and Wagermark, J. Familial clustering of malignant mesothelioma. Cancer *45*:2422, 1980.
171. Vianna, N. J., and Polan, A. K. Nonoccupational exposure to asbestos and malignant mesothelioma in females. Lancet *1*:1061, 1978.
172. Li, F. P., Lokich, J., Lapey, J., et al. Familial mesothelioma after intense asbestos exposure at home. JAMA *240*:467, 1978.
173. Darke, C., Wagner, M. M. F., and McMillan, G. H. G. HLA-A and B antigen frequencies in an asbestos exposed population with normal and abnormal chest radiographs. Tissue Antigens *13*:228, 1979.
174. Kannerstein, M., and Churg, J. Peritoneal mesothelioma. Human Pathol. *8*:83, 1977.
175. Talerman, A., Montero, J. R., Chilcote, R. R., et al. Diffuse malignant peritoneal mesothelioma in a 13 year old girl: report of a case and review of the literature. Am. J. Surg. Pathol. *9*:73, 1985.
176. Hirsch, A., Brochard, P., DeCremoux, H., et al. Features of asbestos-exposed and unexposed mesothelioma. Am. J. Indust. Med. *3*:413, 1982.
177. Elms, P., and Simpson, P. The clinical aspects of mesothelioma. Q. J. Med. *45*:427, 1976.
178. Brenner, J., Sordillo, P. P., Magill, G. B., et al. Malignant peritoneal mesothelioma. Am. J. Gastroenterol. *75*:311, 1981.
179. Banner, M. T., and Gohel, V. K. Peritoneal mesothelioma. Radiology *129*:637, 1978.
180. Yeh, H. C., and Chahinian, A. P. Ultrasonography and computed tomography of peritoneal mesothelioma. Radiology *135*:705, 1980.

181. Raptopoulos, V. Peritoneal mesothelioma. C.R.C. Crit. Rev. Diagnostic Imaging *24*:293, 1985.
182. Whitley, N. O., Brenner, D. E., Antman, K. H., et al. CT of peritoneal mesothelioma: analysis of 8 cases. Am. J. Roentgenol. *138*:531, 1982.
183. Reuter, K., Raptopoulos, V., Reale, F., et al. Diagnosis of peritoneal mesothelioma: computed tomography, sonography, and fine needle aspiration biopsy. Am. J. Roentgenol. *140*:1189, 1983.
184. Roboz, J., Greaves, J., Silides, D., et al. Hyaluronic acid content of effusions as a diagnostic aid for malignant mesothelioma. Cancer Res. *45*:1850, 1985.
185. Tao, L. C. Cytopathology of mesothelioma. Acta Cytol. *23*:209, 1979.
186. McCallum, R. W., Maceri, D. R., Jensen, D., et al. Laparoscopic diagnosis of peritoneal mesothelioma. Dig. Dis. Sci. *24*:170, 1979.
187. Suzuki, Y. Pathology of human malignant mesothelioma. Semin. Oncol. *8*:268, 1981.
188. Burns, D. R., Greenberg, S. D., Mace, M. L., et al. Ultrastructural diagnosis of epithelial malignant mesothelioma. Cancer *56*:2036, 1985.
189. Colby, T. V., Clayton, F., and Hammond, E. Electron microscopy of body fluids. Clin. Lab. Med. *5*:223, 1985.
190. Singh, G., Whiteside, T. L., and Dekker, A. Immunodiagnosis of mesothelioma. Cancer *43*:2288, 1979.
191. Kjeldsberg, C. R., and Marty, J. Use of immunologic tumor markers in body fluid analysis. Clin. Lab. Med. *5*:233, 1985.
192. Churg, A. Immunohistochemical staining for vimentin and keratin in malignant mesothelioma. Am. J. Surg. Pathol. *9*:360, 1985.
193. Marshal, R. J., Herbert, A., Braye, S. G., et al. Use of antibodies to carcinoembryonic antigen and human milk fat globule to distinguish carcinoma, mesothelioma, and reactive mesothelium. J. Clin. Pathol. *37*:1215, 1984.
194. Waxler, B., Eisenstein, R., and Battifora, H. Electrophoresis of tissue glycosaminoglycans as an aid in the diagnosis of mesotheliomas. Cancer *44*:221, 1979.
195. Antman, K. H., Pomfert, E. A., Aisner, J., et al. Peritoneal mesothelioma: natural history and response to chemotherapy. J. Clin. Oncol. *1*:386, 1983.
196. Antman, K. H., Blum, R. H., and Greenberger, J. S. Multimodality therapy for malignant mesothelioma based on a study of natural history. Am. J. Med. *68*:356, 1980.
197. Gordon, W., Jr., Edmond, K. H., Greenberger, J. S., et al. Radiation therapy in the management of patients with mesothelioma. Int. J. Radiat. Oncol. Biol. Phys. *8*:19, 1982.
198. Rogoff, E., Hailaris, B., and Huvos, A. Long term survival in patients with malignant peritoneal mesothelioma treated with irradiation. Cancer *32*:656, 1973.
199. Aisner, J., and Wiernick, P. H. Chemotherapy in the treatment of malignant mesothelioma. Semin. Oncol. *8*:335, 1981.
200. Vogelzang, N. J., Schultz, S. M., Iannucci, A. M., et al. Malignant mesothelioma: the University of Minnesota experience. Cancer *53*:377, 1984.
201. Lerner, H. J., Schoenfeld, D. A., Martin, A., et al. Malignant mesothelioma: the eastern cooperative oncology groups experience. Cancer *52*:1981, 1983.
202. Markman, M., Cleary, S., Pfeifle, C., et al. Cisplatin administered by the intracavitary route as treatment for malignant mesothelioma. Cancer *58*:18, 1986.
202a. Lederman, G. S., Recht, A., Herman, T., et al. Long-term survival in peritoneal mesothelioma: the role of radiotherapy and combined modality treatment. Cancer *59*:1882, 1987.
203. Antman, K. H., Klegar, K. L., Pomfret, E. A., et al. Early peritoneal mesothelioma: a treatable malignancy. Lancet *2*:977, 1985.
204. Walsch, D., and Williams, G. Surgical biopsy studies of omental and peritoneal nodules. Br. J. Surg. *58*:428, 1971.
205. Garrison, R. N., Kaelin, L. D., and Heuser, L. S. Malignant ascites: clinical and experimental observations. Ann. Surg. *203*:644, 1986.
206. Prolla, J., and Kirsner, J. The gastrointestinal lesions and complications of leukemias. Ann. Intern. Med. *61*:1084, 1964.
207. Ehrlich, A., Stalder, G., Geller, W., et al. Gastrointestinal manifestations of malignant lymphoma. Gastroenterology *54*:1115, 1968.
208. Lewin, K. J., Ranchod, M., and Dorfman, R. F. Lymphomas of the gastrointestinal tract. Cancer *42*:693, 1978.
209. Greer, J. P., Pinson, R. D., Russell, W. G., et al. Malignant plasmacytic ascites: report of 2 cases and a review of the literature. Cancer *56*:2001, 1985.
210. Silverman, J. F. Extramedullary hematoipoetic ascitic fluid cytology in myelofibrosis. Am. J. Clin. Pathol. *84*:125, 1985.
211. Fastaia, J., and Dumont, A. Pathogenesis of ascites in mice with peritoneal carcinomatosis. J. Natl. Cancer Inst. *56*:547, 1976.
211a. Garrison, R. N., Galloway, R. H., and Heuser, L. S. Mechanisms of malignant ascites production. J. Surg. Res. *42*:126, 1987.
212. Feldman, G. Lymphatic obstruction in carcinomatous ascites. Cancer Res. *35*:325, 1975.
213. Bloomer, W. D., and Adelstein, S. J. Mediastinal lymphoscintigraphy reflects cell kinetics of developing malignant ascites. Br. J. Radiol. *52*:756, 1979.
214. Greenbaum, L. Pepstatin, an inhibitor of acid kininogenases and ascites retardant in neoplastic disease. Fed. Proc. *38*:2788, 1979.
215. Domagala, W., Emesin, E. E., and Koss, L. G. Distribution of T-lymphocytes and B-lymphocytes in peripheral blood and effusions of patients with cancer. J. Natl. Cancer Inst. *61*:295, 1978.
216. Tamura, K., Shibata, Y., Matsuda, Y., et al. Isolation and characterization of an immunosuppressive ascitic protein from ascitic fluids of cancer patients. Cancer Res. *41*:3244, 1981.
217. Onsrud, M. Immunosuppressive effects of peritoneal fluids from ovarian cancer patients. Gynecol. Oncol. *23*:316, 1986.
218. Meyers, M. Distribution of intraabdominal malignant seeding. Am. J. Roentgenol. *119*:198, 1973.
219. Epstein, R. J., Oliver, B., McIntosh, P. K., et al. Computed tomography of intraperitoneal malignancy. Austral. N. Z. J. Med. *14*:13, 1984.
220. Brenner, D. E., Shaff, M. I., Jones, H. W., et al. Abdominopelvic computed tomography: evaluation in patients undergoing second look laparotomy for ovarian carcinoma. Obstet. Gynecol. *65*:715, 1985.
221. Clark-Peterson, D. L., Bandy, L. C., Dudzinski, M., et al. Computer tomography in evaluation of patients with ovarian carcinoma in complete clinical remission: correlation with surgical-pathologic findings. JAMA *255*:627, 1986.
222. Martin, J. K., Jr., and Goellner, J. R. Abdominal fluid cytology in patients with gastrointestinal malignant lesions. Mayo Clin. Proc. *61*:467, 1986.
223. Bousfield, L. R., Greenberg, M. L., and Pacey, F. Cytogenetic diagnosis of cancer from body fluids. Acta Cytol. *29*:768, 1985.
224. Ghosh, A. K., Mason, D. Y., and Sprigs, A. I. Immunocytochemical staining with monoclonal antibodies in cytologically "negative" serous effusions from patients with malignant disease. J. Clin. Pathol. *36*:1150, 1983.
225. Pinkus, G. S., and Kurtin, P. J. Epithelial membrane antigen—a diagnostic discriminate in surgical pathology. Human Pathol. *16*:929, 1985.
225a. Weissman, G. S., McKinley, M. J., Budman, D. R., et al. Flow cytometry: a new technique in the diagnosis of malignant ascites. J. Clin. Gastroenterol. *9*:599, 1987.
226. Yamada, S., Tetsutar, T., and Matsumoto, K. Prognostic analysis of malignant pleural and peritoneal effusions. Cancer *51*:136, 1983.
227. Flombaum, C., Issacs, M., Scheiner, E., et al. Management of fluid retention in patients with advanced cancer. JAMA *245*:611, 1981.
228. Greenway, B., Johnson, P. J., and Williams, R. Control of malignant ascites with spironolactone. Br. J. Surg. *69*:441, 1982.
229. Halpin, T. F., and McCann, T. O. Dynamics of body fluids following the rapid removal of large volume of ascites. Am. J. Obstet. Gynecol. *110*:103, 1971.
230. Lifshitz, S., and Buchsbaum, H. J. The effect of paracentesis on serum proteins. Gynecol. Oncol. *4*:347, 1976.
231. Dollinger, M., Krakoff, I., and Karnovsky, D. Quinicrine in

the treatment of neoplastic effusions. Ann. Intern. Med. *66*:249, 1967.
232. Memon, A., and Zawadzki, Z. A. Malignant effusions: diagnostic evaluation and therapeutic strategy. Curr. Probl. Cancer 5:1, 1981.
233. Kefford, R. F., Woods, R. L., Fox, R. M., et al. Intracavitary adriamycin, nitrogen mustard, and tetracycline in the control of malignant effusions. Med. J. Austral. *2*:447, 1980.
234. Ostrowski, M. J. An assessment of the long term results of controlling the re-accumulation of malignant effusions using intracavitary bleomycin. Cancer *57*:721, 1986.
235. Markman, M. Intracavitary chemotherapy. Curr. Probl. Cancer *10*:404, 1986.
236. Brenner, D. E. Intraperitoneal chemotherapy: A review. J. Clin. Oncol. *4*:1135, 1986.
237. Gastrointestinal Tumor Study Group Intraperitoneal Therapy Workshop. Semin. Oncol. *12*(Supplement 4):1, 1985.
238. Kaplan, R. A., Markman, M., Lucas, W. E., et al. Infectious peritonitis in patients receiving intraperitoneal chemotherapy. Am. J. Med. *78*:49, 1985.
239. Markman, M., Cleary, S., Howell, S. B., et al. Complications of extensive adhesion formation after intraperitoneal chemotherapy. Surg. Gynecol. Obstet. *162*:445, 1986.
239a. Howell, S. B., Zimm, S., Markmen, M., et al. Long-term survival of advanced refractory ovarian carcinoma patients with small-volume disease treated with intraperitoneal chemotherapy. J. Clin. Oncol. *5*:1607, 1987.
240. Croll, M. N., and Brady, L. W. Intracavitary uses of colloids. Semin. Nucl. Med. *9*:108, 1979.
241. Kaplan, W. D., Zimmerman, R. E., Bloomer, W. D., et al. Therapeutic intraperitoneal P32: A clinical assessment of the dynamics of distribution. Radiology *138*:683, 1981.
242. Pezner, R. D., Stevens, K. R., Tong, D., et al. Limited epithelial carcinoma of the ovary treated with curative intent by the intraperitoneal instillation of radiocolloids. Cancer *42*:2563, 1978.
243. Regelson, W., and Parker, G. The routinization of intraperitoneal (intracavitary) chemotherapy and immunotherapy. Cancer Invest. *4*:29, 1986.
244. Torisu, M., Katano, M., Kimura, Y., et al. New approach to management of malignant ascites with a streptococcal preparation, OK-432. 1. Improvement of host's immunity and prolongation of survival. Surgery *93*:357, 1983.
245. Berek, J. S., Hacker, N. F., Lichtenstein, A., et al. Intraperitoneal recombinant alfa interferon for "salvage" immunotherapy in stage III epithelial ovarian cancer: A gynecologic oncology group study. Cancer Res. *45*:4447, 1985.
246. Bast, R. C., Jr., Berek, J. S., Obrist, R., et al. Intraperitoneal immunotherapy of human ovarian carcinoma with Corynebacterium parvum. Cancer Res. *43*:1395, 1983.
247. Glass, R., and LaDue, R. Small intestinal obstruction from peritoneal carcinomatosis. Am. J. Surg. *125*:316, 1973.
248. Helzberg, J. H., and Greenberger, N. J. Peritoneovenous shunts in malignant ascites. Dig. Dis. Sci. *30*:1104, 1985.
249. Costroff, K. M., Ross, D. W., and Davis, J. N. Peritoneovenous shunting for cirrhotic vs. malignant ascites. Surgery *161*:204, 1985.
250. Souter, R. G., Wells, C., Tarin, D., et al. Surgical and pathological complications associated with peritoneovenous shunts in management of malignant ascites. Cancer *55*:1973, 1985.
251. Russel, J. G. J., Kroon, B. B. R., and Hart, G. A. M. The Denver type for peritoneovenous shunting of malignant ascites. Surg. Gynecol. Obstet. *162*:235, 1986.
252. Souter, R. G., Tarin, D., and Kettlewell, M. G. W. Peritoneovenous shunts in the management of malignant ascites. Br. J. Surg. *70*:478, 1983.
253. Fernandez, R. N., and Daly, J. M. Pseudomyxoma peritonei. Arch. Surg. *115*:409, 1980.
254. Sanderberg, H. A., and Woodruff, J. D. Histogenesis of pseudomyxoma peritonei. Obstet. Gynecol. *49*:339, 1977.
255. Chejfec, G., Rieker, W. J., Jablokow, V. R., et al. Pseudomyxoma peritonei associated with colloid carcinoma of the pancreas. Gastroenterology *90*:202, 1986.
256. Douds, H. M., and Pitt, M. J. Calcified rims: characteristic but uncommon radiologic finding in pseudomyxoma peritonei. Gastrointest. Radiol. *5*:263, 1980.
257. Yeh, H. C., Shafir, M. K., Slater, G., et al. Ultrasonography and computer tomography in pseudomyxoma peritonei. Radiology *153*:507, 1984.
258. Dachman, A. H., Lichtenstein, J. E., and Friedman, A. C. Mucocele of the appendix and pseudomyxoma peritonei. Am. J. Radiol. *144*:923, 1985.
259. Parsons, J., Grey, J., and Thorbjarnarson, B. Pseudomyxoma peritonei. Arch. Surg. *101*:545, 1970.
260. Hellsten, S. Mucocele and carcinoma of the appendix. Acta Pathol. Microbiol. Scand. *60*:473, 1964.
261. Wackym, P. A., and Grey, G. F., Jr. Tumors of the appendix: I. Neoplastic and nonneoplastic mucoceles. Southern Med. J. *77*:283, 1984.
262. Higa, E., Rosai, J., Pizzimbono, C. A., et al. Mucosal hyperplasia, mucinous cystadenoma, and mucinous cystadenocarcinoma of the appendix. Cancer *32*:1525, 1973.
263. Lember, G., King, R., and Silverberg, S. Pseudomyxoma peritonei. Ann. Surg. *178*:587, 1973.
264. Campbell, J. S., Lou, P., and Ferguson, J. P. Pseudomyxoma peritonei et ovarii with occult neoplasms of appendix. Obstet. Gynecol. *42*:897, 1973.
265. Long, R., Spratt, J., and Dowling, E. Pseudomyxoma peritonei. Am. J. Surg. *117*:162, 1969.
266. Byron, R., Yonemoto, R. H., King, R. M., et al. The management of pseudomyxoma peritonei secondary to ruptured mucocele of the appendix. Surg. Gynecol. Obstet. *122*:509, 1966.
267. Rosato, R., and Seltzer, M. Pseudomyxoma peritonei, case report including in vitro mucolysis. Surgery *68*:301, 1970.
268. Jones, C. M., III, and Homesley, H. D. Successful treatment of pseudomyxoma peritonei of ovarian origin with cisplatinum, doxorubicin, and cyclophosphamide. Gynecol. Oncol. *22*:257, 1985.
269. Sader, A. M., Bahadon, M., and Sattari, M. Granulomatous peritonitis due to *sofia* (sisymbum sophia). Internat. Surg. *62*:364, 1977.
270. Davies, J. D., and Ansell, I. D. Food-starch granulomatous peritonitis. J. Clin. Pathol. *36*:435, 1983.
271. Chen, K. T. K., Kostich, N. D., and Rosai, J. Peritoneal foreign body granulomas to keratin in uterine adenoacanthoma. Arch. Pathol. Lab. Med. *102*:174, 1978.
272. Bokhari, S. I., Desser, K. B., Mouer, J. R. et al. Maternal meconium granulomatous peritonitis. Arch. Intern. Med. *141*:658, 1981.
273. Schwartz, I. S., Bello, G. V., Feigin, G., et al. Maternal vernix caseosa peritonitis following premature rupture of fetal membranes. JAMA *254*:948, 1985.
274. Chen, K. T. K., and Brittini, G. Peritoneal dissemination of pancreatic carcinoma with granulomatous reaction. Arch. Pathol. Lab. Med. *104*:163, 1980.
275. Wong, M., and Rosen, S. Ascites and sarcoidosis due to peritoneal involvement. Ann. Intern. Med. *57*:277, 1962.
276. Daum, F., Boley, S., and Cohen, M. Miliary Crohn's disease. Gastroenterology *67*:527, 1974.
277. Holmes, E., and Eggleston, J. Starch granulomatous peritonitis. Surgery *71*:85, 1972.
278. Tolbert, T. W., and Brown, J. O. Surface powders in surgical gloves. Arch. Surg. *115*:729, 1980.
279. Liebowitz, D., and Valentino, L. A. Exogenous peritonitis. J. Clin. Gastroenterol. *6*:45, 1984.
280. Janoff, K., Wayne, R., Huntwork, B., et al. Foreign body reactions secondary to cellulose lint fibers. Am. J. Surg. *147*:598, 1984.
281. Sternlieb, J. J., McIlrath, D. C., and Van Heerden, J. A. Starch peritonitis and its prevention. Arch. Surg. *112*:458, 1977.
282. Ignatius, J., and Hartmann, W. The glove starch peritonitis syndrome. Ann. Surg. *175*:338, 1972.
283. Warshaw, A. Management of starch peritonitis without the unnecessary secondary operation. Surgery *73*:681, 1973.
284. Cooke, S. A. R., and Hamilton, D. G. The significance of starch powder contamination in the etiology of peritoneal adhesions. Br. J. Surg. *64*:410, 1977.
285. Tinker, M. A., Teicher, I., and Burdman, D. Cellulose gran-

ulomas and their relationship to intestinal obstruction. Am. J. Surg. *133*:134, 1977.
286. Nissim, F., Ashkenazy, M., Borenstein, R., et al. Tuberculoid cornstarch granulomas with caseous necrosis. Arch. Pathol. Lab. Med. *105*:86, 1981.
287. Goodacre, R., Clancy, R. L., Davidson, R. A., et al. Cell mediated immunity to cornstarch in starch induced granulomatous peritonitis. Gut *17*:202, 1976.
288. Grant, J. B. F., Davies, J. D., and Jones, J. V. Allergic starch peritonitis in the guinea pig. Br. J. Surg. *63*:867, 1976.
289. Seaman, W. B., and Wells, J. Complications of barium enema. Gastroenterology *48*:725, 1965.
290. Westfall, R. H., Nelson, R. H., and Musselman, M. M. Barium peritonitis. Am. J. Surg. *112*:760, 1966.
291. Grobmyer, A. J., III, Kerlan, R. A., Peterson, C. M., et al. Barium peritonitis. Am. Surg. *50*:116, 1984.
291a. Gertz, M. A., Pettitt, R. M., Perrault, J., et al. Autosomal dominant familial Mediterranean fever–like syndrome with amyloidosis. Mayo Clin. Proc. *62*:1095, 1987.
292. Meyerhoff, J. Familial Mediterranean fever: report of large family, review of the literature and discussion of the frequency of amyloidosis. Medicine *59*:66, 1980.
293. Ilfeld, D., Weil, S., and Kuperman, O. Immunoregulatory abnormalities in familial Mediterranean fever. Clin. Immunol. Immunopathol. *18*:261, 1981.
294. Levy, M., Ehrenfeld, M., Levo, Y., et al. Circulating immune complexes in recurrent polyserositis. J. Rheumatol. *7*:886, 1980.
295. Bar-Eli, M., Ehrenfeld, M., Levy, M., et al. Leukocyte chemotaxis and recurrent polyserositis. Am. J. Med. Sci. *281*:15, 1981.
296. Melamed, I., Shemer, Y., Zakuth, V., et al. The immune system in familial Mediterranean fever. Clin. Exp. Immunol. *53*:659, 1983.
297. Matzner, Y., and Brzezinkski, A. C5a-inhibitor deficiency in peritoneal fluids from patients with familial Mediterranean fever. N. Engl. J. Med. *311*:287, 1984.
298. Sohar, E., Gafni, J., Pras, M., et al. Familial Mediterranean fever: a survey of 470 cases and review of the literature. Am. J. Med. *43*:227, 1967.
299. Siegal, S. Familial paroxysmal peritonitis: analysis of 50 cases. Am. J. Med. *36*:893, 1964.
300. Lehman, T. J. A., Hanson, V., and Kornreich, H. HLA-B27-negative sacroileitis: a manifestation of familial Mediterranean fever in childhood. Pediatrics *61*:423, 1978.
301. Schwabe, A., and Peters, R. Familial Mediterranean fever in Armenians: an analysis of 100 cases. Medicine *53*:453, 1974.
302. Barakat, M. H., Karnik, A. M., Majeed, H. W. A., et al. Familial Mediterranean fever (recurrent hereditary polyserositis) in Arabs—a study of 175 patients and review of the literature. Q. J. Med. *60*:837, 1986.
303. Voss, M., Gafni, J., Jacob, E. T., et al. Recent advances in familial Mediterranean fever. Adv. Nephrol. *13*:261, 1984.
304. Barakat, M. H., Gumaa, K. A., El-Khawad, A. O., et al. Metaraminol provocative test: a specific diagnostic test for familial Mediterranean fever. Lancet *1*:656, 1984.
305. Tal, Y., Burger, A., Abrahamson, J., et al. Intestinal obstruction caused by primary adhesions due to familial Mediterranean fever. J. Pediatr. Surg. *15*:186, 1980.
306. Zemer, D., Revach, M., Pras, M., et al. A controlled trial of colchicine in preventing attacks of familial Mediterranean fever. N. Engl. J. Med. *291*:932, 1974.
307. Dinarello, C., Wolff, S., and Goldfinger, S. Colchicine therapy for familial Mediterranean fever. N. Engl. J. Med. *291*:934, 1974.
308. Levy, M., and Eliakim, M. Long-term colchicine prophylaxis in familial Mediterranean fever. Br. Med. J. *2*:808, 1977.
309. Peters, R. S., Lehman, T. J. A., and Schwabe, A. D. Colchicine use for familial Mediterranean fever: observations associated with long term treatment. West. J. Med. *138*:43, 1983.
310. Zemer, D., Pras, M., Sohar, E., et al. Colchicine in the prevention and treatment of the amyloidosis of familial Mediterranean fever. N. Engl. J. Med. *314*:1001, 1986.
311. Wright, D. G., Wolf, S. M., Fauci, A. S., et al. Efficacy of intermittent colchicine therapy in familial Mediterranean fever. Ann. Intern. Med. *86*:162, 1977.
312. Halkin, H., Dany, S., Greenwald, M., et al. Colchicine kinetics in patients with familial Mediterranean fever. Clin. Pharmacol. Ther. *28*:82, 1980.
313. Schlesinger, M., Ilfeld, D., Handzel, Z. T., et al. Effect of colchicine on immunoregulatory abnormalities in familial Mediterranean fever. Clin. Exp. Immunol. *54*:73, 1983.
314. Reuben, A., Hirsch, M., and Berlyne, G. M. Renal vein thrombosis as the major cause of renal failure in familial Mediterranean fever. Q. J. Med. *46*:243, 1977.
315. Matolo, N., and Albo, D. Gastrointestinal complications of collagen vascular disease. Am. J. Surg. *122*:678, 1971.
316. Nolph, K., Stoltz, M., and Maher, J. Altered peritoneal permeability in patients with systemic vasculitis. Ann. Intern. Med. *75*:753, 1971.
317. Metzger, A., Coine, M., Lee, S., et al. In vivo LE cell formation in peritonitis due to SLE. J. Rheumatol. *1*:131, 1974.
318. Schochet, A. L., Lain, D., and Kohler, P. F. Immune complex vasculitis as a cause of ascites and pleural effusion in SLE. J. Rheumatol. *5*:33, 1978.
319. Jones, P. E., Rawcliff, E. P., White, N., et al. Painless ascites in SLE. Br. Med. J. *1*:1513, 1977.
320. Wilkins, K. W., Jr., and Hoffman, G. S. Massive ascites in systemic lupus erythematosus. J. Rheumatol. *12*:571, 1985.
321. Efstratapolous, A., and Stourgi, J. Ascites due to allergic purpura. Lancet *2*:168, 1971.
322. Degos, R. Malignant atrophic papulosis. Br. J. Dermatol. *100*:21, 1979.
323. Freund, U., French, W., Carlson, R. W., et al. Hemodynamic and metabolic studies of a case of toxemia of pregnancy. Am. J. Obstet. Gynecol. *127*:206, 1977.
324. Marshall, A. J., Baddeley, H., Barrett, D. W., et al. Practolol peritonitis. Q. J. Med. *46*:135, 1977.
325. Ahmad, S. Sclerosing peritonitis and propranolol. Chest *79*:361, 1981.
326. Castelli, M. J., Armin, A. R., Husain, A., et al. Fibrosing peritonitis in a drug abuser. Arch. Pathol. Lab. Med. *109*:767, 1985.
326a. Marichal, J. F., Faller, B., Brignon, P., et al. Progressive calcifying peritonitis: a new complication of CAPD? Nephron *45*:229, 1987.
327. Ing, T. S., Daugirdas, J. T., and Gandhi, V. C. Peritoneal sclerosis in peritoneal dialysis patients. Am. J. Nephrol. *4*:173, 1984.
328. Slingemeyer, A., Mion, C., Mourad, G., et al. Progressive sclerosing peritonitis: a late and severe complication of maintenance peritoneal dialysis. Trans. Am. Soc. Artificial Int. Organs *29*:633, 1983.
329. Hauglustaine, D., Meerbeek, J. V., Monballyu, J., et al. Sclerosing peritonitis with mural bowel fibrosis in a patient on long term CAPD. Clin. Nephrol. *22*:158, 1984.
330. Shaldon, S., Koch, K. M., Quellhorst, E., et al. Pathogenesis of sclerosing peritonitis in CAPD. Trans. Am. Soc. Artificial Int. Organs *30*:193, 1984.
331. Chejfec, G., Stanley, M. M., Greenlee, H. B., et al. Diffuse peritoneal fibromatosis and cirrhosis following LeVeen peritoneovenous shunt insertion. Gastroenterology *77*:A7, 1979.
332. Smadja, C., and Franco, D. The LeVeen shunt in the elective treatment of intractable ascites in cirrhosis. Ann. Surg. *201*:488, 1985.
333. Cambria, R. P., and Shamberger, R. C. Small bowel obstruction caused by the abdominal cocoon syndrome: possible association with the LeVeen shunt. Surgery *95*:501, 1984.
334. LaFerla, G., McColl, K. E. L., and Crean, G. P. CSF-induced sclerosing peritonitis: a new entity? Br. J. Surg. *73*:7, 1986.
335. Foo, K. T., Eng, K. C., Rauff, A., et al. Unusual small intestinal obstruction in adolescent girls: the abdominal cocoon. Br. J. Surg. *65*:427, 1978.
336. Sieck, J. O., Cowgill, R., and Larkworthy, W. Peritoneal encapsulation and abdominal cocoon: case reports and review of the literature. Gastroenterology *84*:1597, 1983.
336a. Leport, J., DuMayne, J. F. D., Hay, J. M., et al. Chylous ascites and encapsulating peritonitis: unusual complications of

spontaneous bacterial peritonitis. Am. J. Gastroenterol. *82*:463, 1987.
337. McNabb, B. C., Fleming, C. R., Higgins, J. A., et al. Transmural eosinophilic gastroenteritis with ascites. Mayo Clin. Proc. *54*:119, 1979.
338. Adams, H. W., and Mainz, D. L. Eosinophilic ascites. Am. J. Dig. Dis. *22*:40, 1977.
339. Rowland, M., Brown, R. B., and Goldman, M. Eosinophilic peritonitis; an unusual manifestation of spontaneous bacterial peritonitis. J. Clin. Gastroenterol. *7*:369, 1985.
340. Eisenberg, J., Gilbert, S., and Pitcher, J. Ascites with peritoneal involvement in Whipple's disease. Gastroenterology *60*:305, 1971.
341. Iwasaka, T., Yoshinari, O., Yoshimura, T., et al. Endometriosis associated with ascites. Obstet. Gynecol. *66*:72S, 1985.
342. Hulme-Moir, I., and Ross, M. A case of early postpartum abdominal pain due to a hemorrhagic deciduosis peritonei. J. Obstet. Gynecol. Br. Commonwealth *76*:746, 1969.
343. Truong, L. D., Jurco, S., III., and McGavran, M. H. Gliomatosis peritonei: report of 2 cases and review of the literature. Am. J. Surg. Pathol. *6*:443, 1982.
344. Williams, L. J., and Pavlich, F. J. Leiomyomatosis peritonealis disseminata. Cancer *45*:1726, 1980.
345. Brumback, R. A., Brown, B. S., Sobie, P., et al. Leiomyomatosis peritonealis disseminata. Surgery *97*:707, 1983.
346. Rubin, S. C., Wheeler, J. E., and Mikuta, J. J. Malignant leiomyomatosis peritonealis disseminata. Obstet. Gynecol. *68*:126, 1986.
347. Quer, E., Dockerty, M., and Mayo, C. Ruptured dermoid cyst of the ovary simulating abdominal carcinomatosis. Proc. Mayo Clin. *26*:489, 1951.
348. Esensten, M. L., Shaw, S. L., Pak, H. Y., et al. CT demonstration of multiple intraperitoneal teratomatous implants. J. Comp. Asst. Tomog. *7*:1117, 1983.
349. Lee, D., and Pontifex, A. Melanosis peritonei. Am. J. Obstet. Gynecol. *122*:526, 1975.
350. Rose, G., Morrison, E. A., Kirkham, N., et al. Malakoplakia of the pelvic peritoneum in pregnancy: case report. Br. J. Obstet. Gynecol. *92*:170, 1985.
351. Lopez-Zeno, J. A., Keith, L. G., and Berger, G. S. Fitz-Hugh–Curtis syndrome revisited: changing perspectives after half a century. J. Reproduct. Med. *30*:567, 1985.
352. Wolner-Hanssen, P., Westrom, L., and Mardh, P. A. Chlamydial perihepatitis. Scand. J. Infect. Dis. *32*(suppl.):77, 1982.
353. Winkler, W. P., Kotler, D. P., and Saleh, J. Fitz-Hugh–Curtis syndrome in a homosexual man with impaired cell mediated immunity. Gastrointest. Endosc. *31*:28, 1985.
354. Marbet, U. A., Stalder, G. A., Vogtlin, J., et al. Diffuse peritonitis and chronic ascites due to infection with chlamydia trachomatis in patients without liver disease: new presentation of the Fitz-Hugh–Curtis syndrome. Br. Med. J. *293*:5, 1986.
355. Punnonen, R., Terho, P., and Klemi, P. J. Chlamydial pelvic inflammatory disease with ascites. Fertil. Steril. *37*:270, 1982.
356. Wilson, R. O., and Sueldo, C. E. Exudative ascites produced by pelvic inflammatory disease. Obstet. Gynecol. *61*:54S, 1983.
357. Hidvegi, D., Hidvegi, I., and Barrett, J. Douche induced pelvic peritoneal starch granuloma. Obstet. Gynecol. *52*:155, 1978.
358. Fleming, C., Dixon, E., and Harrison, E. Splenosis: autotransplantation of splenic tissue. Am. J. Med. *61*:414, 1976.
359. Leker, J. G., Yonehero, L. O., and Davis, W. C. Traumatic rupture of splenosis. J. Trauma *25*:560, 1985.
360. Pearson, H. A., Johnston, D., Smith, K. A., et al. The born-again spleen: return of splenic function after splenectomy for trauma. N. Engl. J. Med. *298*:1389, 1978.
361. Mazur, E. M., Field, W. W., Cahow, C. E., et al. ITP occurring in a subject previously splenectomized for traumatic splenic rupture. Am. J. Med. *65*:843, 1978.
362. Negus, D., Whimster, I., and Wiernick, G. Peritoneal lymphangiectasis. Br. J. Surg. *53*:740, 1966.
363. Parry, S., Schuhmacher, J., and Llewellyn, R. Abdominal pseudocysts and ascites formation after ventriculoperitoneal shunt procedures. J. Neurosurg. *43*:476, 1975.
364. Yount, R. A., Glazier, M. C., Mealey, J., Jr., et al. Cerebrospinal fluid ascites complicating ventriculoperitoneal shunting. J. Neurosurg. *61*:180, 1984.
365. Nofray, J. F., Henry, H. M., Givens, J. D., et al. Abdominal complications from peritoneal shunts. Gastroenterology *77*:337, 1979.
366. Lees, R. F., Feldman, P. S., Brenbridge, A. N. A., et al. Inflammatory cysts of the pelvic peritoneum. Am. J. Roentgenol. *131*:633, 1978.
367. Berek, J. S., and Darnley, P. D. Massive exudative ascites produced from a tubal pseudocyst in chronic pelvic inflammatory disease. Obstet. Gynecol. *54*:490, 1979.
368. Lewin, K., and McCarthy, L. Peritoneal encapsulation of the small intestine. Gastroenterology *59*:270, 1970.
369. Fataar, S., Morton, P. C. G., Schulman, A., et al. Radiological diagnosis of primary greater omental mass lesions. Clin. Radiol. *32*:325, 1981.
370. Diamond, A., Meng, C., and Golden, R. Arteriography of unusual mass lesions of the mesentery. Radiology *110*:547, 1974.
371. Whitley, N. O., Bohlman, M. E., and Baker, L. P. CT patterns of mesenteric disease. J. Comput. Asst. Tomogr. *6*:490, 1982.
372. Levitt, R. G., Koehler, R. E., and Sagel, S. S. Metastatic disease of the mesentery and omentum. Radiol. Clin. North Am. *20*:501, 1982.
373. Cooper, C., Jeffrey, R. B., Silverman, P. M., et al. Computed tomography of omental pathology. J. Comput. Asst. Tomogr. *10*:62, 1986.
374. Silverman, P. M., Baker, M. E., Cooper, C., et al. CT appearance of diffuse mesenteric edema. J. Comput. Asst. Tomogr. *10*:67, 1986.
375. Shin, M. S., Ferrucci, J. T., Jr., and Wittenberg, J. Computed tomographic diagnosis of pseudoascites (floating viscera syndrome). J. Comput. Asst. Tomogr. *2*:594, 1978.
376. Lewis, V. L., Shaffer, H. A., Jr., and Williamson, B. R. J. Pseudotumoral lipomatosis of the abdomen. J. Comput. Asst. Tomogr. *6*:79, 1982.
377. Siskind, B. N., Weiner, F. R., Frank, M., et al. Steroid induced mesenteric lipomatosis. Comp. Radiol. *8*:175, 1984.
378. Friedman, A. C., Hartman, D. S., Sherman, J., et al. Computed tomography of abdominal fatty masses. Radiology *139*:415, 1981.
379. Reske, M., and Namiki, H. Sclerosing mesenteritis. Am. J. Clin. Pathol. *64*:661, 1975.
380. Kipfer, R., Moertel, C., and Dahlend, D. Mesenteric lipodystrophy. Ann. Intern. Med. *80*:582, 1974.
381. Shah, A. N., and You, C. H. Mesenteric lipodystrophy presenting as an acute abdomen. Southern Med. J. *75*:1025, 1982.
382. Katz, M. E., Heiken, J. P., Glazer, H. S., et al. Intraabdominal panniculitis: clinical, radiographic, and CT features. Am. J. Roentgenol. *145*:293, 1985.
383. Soergel, K., and Hensley, G. Fatal mesenteric panniculitis. Gastroenterology *51*:529, 1966.
384. Aach, R., Kalin, L., and Frick, R. Obstruction of the small intestine due to retractile mesenteritis. Gastroenterology *54*:594, 1968.
385. Durst, A. L., Freund, H., Rosenmann, E., et al. Mesenteric panniculitis: review of the literature and presentation of cases. Surgery *81*:203, 1977.
386. Hartz, R., Stryker, S., Sparberg, M., et al. Mesenteric tumefactions. Am. Surg. *46*:525, 1980.
387. Williams, R. G., and Nelson, J. A. Retractile mesenteritis: Initial presentation as colonic obstruction. Radiology *126*:35, 1978.
388. Han, S. Y., Koehler, R. E., Keller, F. S., et al. Retractile mesenteritis involving the colon; pathologic and radiologic correlation. Am. J. Roentgenol. *147*:268, 1986.
389. Binder, S., Deterling, R., Mahoney, S., et al. Systemic idiopathic fibrosis. Am. J. Surg. *124*:422, 1972.
390. Mitchinson, M. The pathology of idiopathic retroperitoneal fibrosis. J. Clin. Pathol. *23*:681, 1970.
391. Tytgat, G. N., Roozendaal, K., and Winter, W. Successful treatment of a patient with retractile mesenteritis with prednisone and azathioprine. Gastroenterology *79*:352, 1980.

392. Bush, R. W., Hammar, S. P., Jr., and Rudoph, R. H. Sclerosing mesenteritis: response to cyclophosphamide. Arch. Intern. Med. *146*:503, 1986.
393. Simpson, R., Harrison, E., and Mayo, C. Mesenteric fibromatosis in familial polyposis: a variant of Gardner's syndrome. Cancer *17*:525, 1964.
394. Naylor, E. W., Gardner, E. J., and Richards, R. C. Desmoid tumors and mesenteric fibromatosis in Gardner's syndrome: report of kindred 109. Arch. Surg. *114*:1181, 1979.
395. Suarez, V., and Hall, C. Mesenteric fibromatosis. Br. J. Surg. *72*:976, 1985.
396. Reitamo, J. J., Pekka, H., Nykyrie, et al. The desmoid tumor. Am. J. Clin. Pathol. *77*:665, 1982.
397. Barron, R. L., and Lee, J. K. T. Mesenteric desmoid tumors: sonographic and computed tomographic appearance. Radiology *140*:777, 1981.
398. Sampliner, J. E., Paruleker, S., Jain, B., et al. Intraabdominal mesenteric desmoid tumors. Am. Surg. *48*:316, 1982.
399. Shous, A., Estrin, J., and Najarian, J. Gardner's syndrome and fibromatosis. Dis. Colon Rectum *18*:128, 1975.
400. Harvey, J. C., Quan, S. H. Q., and Fortner, J. G. Gardner's syndrome complicated by mesenteric desmoid tumors. Surgery *85*:475, 1979.
401. Belliveau, P., and Graham, A. M. Mesenteric desmoid tumor in Gardner's syndrome treated by sulindac. Dis. Colon Rectum *27*:53, 1984.
402. Waddell, W. R., Gerner, R. E., and Reich, M. P. Nonsteroid anti-inflammatory drugs and tamoxifen for desmoid tumors and carcinoma of the colon. J. Surg. Oncol. *22*:197, 1983.
402b. Klein, W. A., Miller, H., Anderson, M., et al. The use of indomethacin, sulindac, and tamoxifen for the treatment of desmoid tumors associated with familial polyposis. Cancer *60*:2863, 1987.
402b. Jones, I. T., Jozelman, D. G., Fazio, V. W., et al. Desmoid tumors in familial polyposis coli. Ann. Surg. *204*:94, 1986.
403. Walker, A., and Putnam, T. Omental, mesenteric and retroperitoneal cysts. Ann. Surg. *178*:13, 1973.
404. Vanek, V. W., and Phillips, A. K. Retroperitoneal, mesenteric, and omental cysts. Arch. Surg. *119*:838, 1984.
405. Elliott, G., Kliman, M., and Elliott, K. Persistence of lymphaticovenous shunts at the level of the microcirculation: their relationship to lymphangioma of the mesentery. Ann. Surg. *172*:131, 1970.
406. Takiff, H., Calabria, R., Yin, L., et al. Mesenteric cysts and intraabdominal cystic lymphangiomas. Arch. Surg. *120*:1266, 1985.
407. Axiotis, C. A., Zeman, R. K., Chuong, J. H., et al. Intraabdominal lymphangiectatic cysts: an uncommon abdominal lesion in children and young adults. J. Clin. Gastroenterol. *5*:541, 1983.
408. Kurtz, R. J., Heimann, T. M., Beck, A. R., et al. Mesenteric and retroperitoneal cysts. Ann. Surg. *203*:109, 1986.
409. Yannopoulous, K., and Stout, A. P. Primary solid tumors of the mesentery. Cancer *16*:914, 1963.
410. Sturzaker, H. G., Berry, C. L., and McCall, I. Spontaneous resolution of a mesenteric fibromatosis. J. R. Coll. Surg. Edinburgh *22*:395, 1977.
411. Weinberger, H. A., and Ahmed, M. S. Mesenchymal solid tumors of the omentum and mesentery: report of 4 cases. Surgery *82*:754, 1977.
412. Hashimoto, H., Tsuneyoshi, M., and Enjoji, M. Malignant smooth muscle tumors of the retroperitoneum and mesentery: a clinicopathologic analysis of 44 cases. J. Surg. Oncol. *28*:177, 1985.
412a. Moyana, T. N. Primary mesenteric liposarcoma. Am. J. Gastroenterol. *83*:99, 1988.
413. Keller, A., Hochholzer, L., and Castleman, B. Hyaline-vascular and plasma cell types of giant lymph node hyperplasia of the mediastinum and other locations. Cancer *29*:670, 1972.
414. Frizzera, G. Castleman's disease: more questions than answers. Human Pathol. *16*:202, 1985.
415. Stout, A. P., Hendry, J., and Purdie, F. Primary solid tumors of the great omentum. Cancer *16*:231, 1963.
416. Janin, Y., Stone, A. M., and Wise, L. Mesenteric hernia. Surg. Gynecol. Obstet. *150*:747, 1980.
417. Anderson, R., Liebeskind, A., and Lowman, R. Arteriovenous fistula of the mesentery. Am. J. Gastroenterol. *57*:453, 1972.
418. Raghavendra, B. N., Grieco, A. J., Balthazar, E. J., et al. Diagnostic utility of sonography and computed tomography in spontaneous mesenteric hematoma. Am. J. Gastroenterol. *77*:570, 1982.
419. Bradey, S., and Klimon, M. Torsion of the greater omentum or appendices epiploicae. Can. J. Med. *22*:79, 1979.
420. Rich, R. H., and Filler, R. M. Segmental infarction of the greater omentum: a cause of acute abdomen in childhood. Can. J. Surg. *26*:241, 1983.
421. Adams, J. Primary torsion of the omentum. Am. J. Surg. *126*:102, 1973.
422. Naraynsingh, V., Barrow, R., Raju, G. C., et al. Segmental infarction of the omentum: diagnosis by ultrasound. Postgrad. Med. J. *61*:651, 1985.
423. Crowfoot, D. D. Spontaneous segmental infarction of the greater omentum. Am. J. Surg. *139*:262, 1980.
424. DeLaurentis, D., Kim, D., and Hartshorn, J. Idiopathic segmental infarction of the greater omentum. Arch. Surg. *102*:474, 1971.
425. Epstein, L., and Lempke, R. Primary idiopathic segmental infarction of the greater omentum. Ann. Surg. *167*:437, 1968.
426. Naidich, D. P., Megibow, A. J., Ross, C. R., et al. Computed tomography of the diaphragm: normal anatomy and variants. J. Comput. Asst. Tomogr. *7*:633, 1983.
427. Khan, A. N., and Gould, D. A. The primary role of ultrasound in evaluating right sided diaphragmatic humps and juxtadiaphragmatic masses: a review of 22 cases. Clin. Radiol. *35*:413, 1984.
428. Thomas, T. Nonparalytic eventration of the diaphragm. J. Thoracic Cardiovasc. Surg. *55*:586, 1968.
429. Gale, M. E. Bochdalek hernia: prevalence and CT characteristics. Radiology *156*:449, 1985.
430. Ahrend, T., and Thompson, B. Hernia of the foramen of Bochdalek in the adult. Am. J. Surg. *122*:612, 1971.
431. Cope, R. Congenital diaphragmatic hernia: presentations and problems in the adult. Gastrointest. Radiol. *6*:157, 1981.
432. Hight, D. W., Hixson, S. D., Reed, J. O., et al. Intermittent diaphragmatic hernia of Bochdalek: report of a case and literature review. Pediatrics *69*:601, 1982.
433. Comer, T., and Clagett, O. Surgical treatment of hernia of the foramen of Morgagni. J. Thoracic Cardiovasc. Surg. *52*:461, 1966.
434. Fagelman, D., and Caridi, J. G. CT diagnosis of hernia of Morgagni. Gastrointest. Radiol. *9*:153, 1984.
435. Tarver, R. D., Godwin, J. D., and Putnam, C. E. The diaphragm. Radiol. Clin. North Am. *22*:615, 1984.
436. Ward, R. E., Flynn, T. C., and Clark, W. P. Diaphragmatic disruption secondary to blunt abdominal trauma. J. Trauma *21*:35, 1981.
437. Hood, R. Traumatic diaphragmatic hernia. Ann. Thoracic Surg. *12*:311, 1971.
438. Hegarty, M. M., Bryer, J. V., Angorn, I. B., et al. Delayed presentation of traumatic diaphragmatic hernia. Ann. Surg. *188*:229, 1978.
439. McElwee, T. B., Meyers, R. T., and Pennell, T. C. Diaphragmatic rupture from blunt trauma. Am. Surg. *50*:143, 1984.
440. Waldschmidt, M. L., and Laws, H. L. Injuries of the diaphragm. J. Trauma *20*:587, 1980.
441. Esrera, A. S., Landay, M. J., and McClelland, R. N. Blunt traumatic rupture of the right hemidiaphragm: experience in 12 patients. Ann. Thoracic Surg. *39*:525, 1985.
442. Soloman, N. W., and Zukoski, C. F. Isolated rupture of the right hemidiaphragm with eventration of the liver. JAMA *241*:1929, 1979.
443. Ammann, A. M., Brewer, W. H., and Maull, K. I. Traumatic rupture of the diaphragm: real time sonographic diagnosis. Am. J. Roentgenol. *140*:915, 1983.
444. Heiberg, E., Wolverson, M. K., Jagannadharao, B., et al. CT recognition of traumatic rupture of the diaphragm. Am. J. Roentgenol. *135*:369, 1980.
445. Anderson, L., and Forrest, J. Tumors of the diaphragm. Am. J. Roentgenol. *119*:259, 1973.

446. Rao, K. G., and Woodlief, R. M. Excessive right subdiaphragmatic fat: a potential diagnostic pitfall. Radiology *138*:15, 1981.
447. Rosen, A., Auh, Y. H., Rubenstein, W. A., et al. CT appearance of diaphragmatic pseudotumors. J. Comput. Asst. Tomogr. *7*:995, 1983.
448. Dallemand, S., Twersky, J., and Gordon, D. H. Pseudomass of the left upper quadrant from inversion of the left hemidiaphragm: CT diagnosis. Gastrointest. Radiol. *7*:57, 1982.
449. Greenberg, M., Maden, V., Ataii, E., et al. Intradiaphragmatic cyst: a diagnostic challenge. JAMA *230*:1176, 1974.
450. Farquharson, S. M. Intradiaphragmatic abscess. J. R. Coll. Surg. Edinburgh *29*:117, 1984.
451. Mercer, C. D., and Hill, L. D. Intradiaphragmatic abscess: an extremely rare complication of pneumatic dilatation of the esophagus. Dig. Dis. Sci. *30*:891, 1985.
452. Davis, J. N. An experimental study of hiccup. Brain *93*:851, 1970.
453. Brouillette, R. T., Thach, B. T., Abu-Osba, Y. K., et al. Hiccups in infants: characteristics and effects on ventilation. J. Pediatr. *96*:219, 1980.
454. Lewis, J. H. Hiccups: causes and cures. J. Clin. Gastroenterol. *7*:539, 1985.
455. Nathan, M. D., Leshner, R. T., and Keller, A. P. Intractable hiccups (singultus). Laryngoscope *90*:1612, 1980.
456. Shay, S. S., Myers, R. L., and Johnson, L. F. Hiccups associated with reflux esophagitis. Gastroenterology *87*:204, 1984.
457. Williamson, B. W. A., and McIntyre, I. M. C. Management of intractable hiccup. Br. Med. J. *2*:501, 1977.
458. Stromberg, B. V. The hiccup. ENT J. *58*:51, 1979.

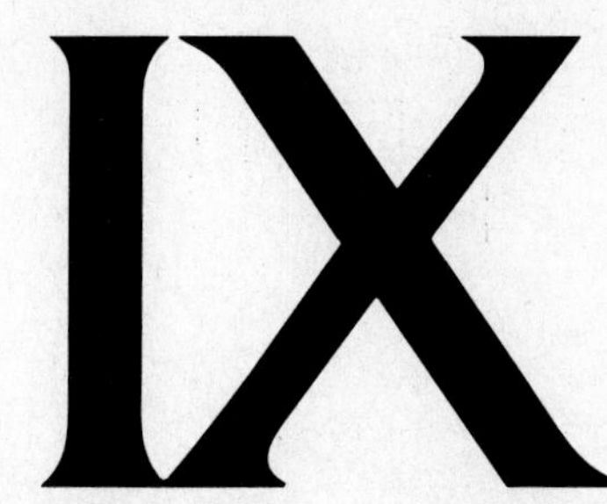

NUTRITIONAL MANAGEMENT

103

Eating Behavior and Nutrient Requirements

DAVID H. ALPERS
IRWIN H. ROSENBERG

The student of gastrointestinal physiology and gastrointestinal disease has always been, to a considerable extent, a student of nutrition as well, because the alimentary canal plays such a critical role in normal nutrition. As much as the practitioner who cares for patients with gastrointestinal disease is concerned with the impact of diet on symptoms and manifestations of disease, so must he or she be concerned with the consequences of altered gastrointestinal function on the nutritional status of the patient. In the constant effort to maximize health, maintenance of good nutrition is a central concern. The physician is asked increasingly to provide nutritional guidance beyond the more familiar functions of diagnosis and therapy. Whatever one's assessment of the conflicting evidence regarding the power of dietary modification to influence susceptibility to certain diseases of the gastrointestinal tract such as cancer, gallstones, diverticulosis, and so forth, there is agreement that many of the other debilitating complications of gastrointestinal disease can be prevented or modified by attention to nutritional status and prevention of nutritional deficits. The most effective management of the patient with gastrointestinal disease therefore requires detailed evaluation of diet and nutritional status and a projection of the continuing interaction of diet and altered gastrointestinal function on the nutritional status of the patient. Proper goals and techniques of nutritional management can then be selected.

Our purpose in this chapter is to present some of the basic considerations that underlie our capacity to assess nutritional status, determine needs, and set goals for treatment. Eating behavior, approaches to dietary assessment, and concepts underlying techniques for evaluation of macronutrient requirements will be discussed.

A determination of the nutritional needs of the individual patient must be carried out in the context of a comprehensive understanding of the nutritional impairments induced by disease (see pp. 1983–1994). A detailed discussion of the normal physiology of the major vitamins and minerals is presented on pages 1045 to 1062. Since this information is important in understanding requirements and replacement doses of these micronutrients, the reader is encouraged to review this chapter. The dietary and other therapeutic options available to the clinician and the principles of decision making that must guide their use are discussed on pages 1994 to 2027.

EATING BEHAVIOR AND NUTRITION

Eating behavior is by nature intermittent. Yet energy needs are continuous. This fundamental challenge of mammalian nutrition has resulted in the evolution of an elaborate set of metabolic controls. These processes must deal with the ebb and flow of nutrients during feeding and in the postabsorptive periods and, in addition, must provide for the maintenance of near-normal function during periods of fasting or when food is unavailable.

From a nutritional perspective, the mechanisms that control appetite and eating behavior are directed to maintaining an energy intake adequate for the needs of the healthy adult, or for the extra needs of growth in the developing child, or for the additional requirements of pregnancy or lactation. Under conditions of disease or trauma, the increased requirements must be met through appropriate modifications in eating behavior or by supplementation if energy balance is to be maintained. Ideally, in addition to calories to meet energy needs, the appropriate intake of proteins, vitamins, and minerals accompanies the intake of a variety of foods that contain these essential nutrients.

In order for the remarkable stability of body weight and body composition to be maintained, there must be neurophysiologic recognition that total calorie intake has met requirements. The precise nature of the internal cues that signal the central nervous system that caloric intake has been appropriate during the preceding day or so is not known. Thus, such signals do not adjust eating behavior on a meal-to-meal time scale. At the time of an individual meal, volume- and chemoreceptors in the stomach and small bowel initiate neural and hormonal responses that contribute to satiety.[1, 2] The nutrient density of the food eaten, in terms of the protein or calorie content per unit volume, is not sensitively perceived, and therefore total calorie or protein intake can fluctuate substantially over the short run.[3] Present evidence indicates that the neurophysiologic mechanisms that control eating behavior recognize calorie deficiencies in humans on roughly a 24- to 48-hour time scale and make compensatory changes in the volume of food eaten over periods of one to two days.[4] That these controls work remarkably well is attested to by the stability of body weight and general nutritional health of the vast majority of the population with access to an adequate food intake. That aberrations in the interplay of these control factors can produce serious and even life-threatening imbalance is represented in the substantial numbers of the population with obesity and with syndromes of anorexia related to manifest disease.

FOOD INTAKE AND BODY WEIGHT CONTROL

Any consideration of body weight begins with the assumption that body weight *is* regulated. The evidence for tight regulation in experimental animals is quite good, but in humans it is much less compelling.[5] The short-term regulation of energy intake is balanced to energy output over 4 to 14 days in humans, as opposed to a 24-hour period in the rat. Because a human being has sufficient fat stored for about one month, there is no need for immediate adjustments. Moreover, hunger and appetite are not reliably linked to energy intake in humans.

Long-term regulation of body weight in humans has been even more difficult to document. However, there is remarkable stability of the body weight in population cohorts studied over many years.[6] On the other hand, although body weight remains stable, body composition may change with age, as the fraction of weight as fat increases.

Assuming that body weight is regulated, it is clear that it is highly variable, according to age, sex, social or genetic background, individual metabolic rates, and other factors. The regulation of food or energy intake is complex, and the complexity begins with the variety of terms used to express the phenomenon. "Food intake" refers to the amount of food ingested, and is useful as a physiologic concept. It is altered by many physiologic, psychologic, and social factors. *Appetite* and *hunger* refer to the desire to eat or the craving for food. These psychologic phenomena trigger food intake, as modified by the time of day, appropriate social setting, and palatability of the food. *Satiety* refers to the feeling when appetite is gratified to excess, and may be triggered after eating by a series of signals from the upper gastrointestinal tract (see below). However, satiety may also refer to the feeling that results from preabsorptive signals (e.g., absence of food sight or smells, unpleasant surroundings). Much that we understand about regulation of food intake depends upon the way in which the problem is studied. The experimentalist usually determines psychologic hunger or appetite for food or the onset of satiety. These end points may have nothing to do with the physiologic need for food. Satiety is easier to assess than long-term control of food intake, the prevalent pattern in humans.[7] Thus, humans cannot easily regulate their energy intake when pregastric stimuli (taste, volume, texture, smell of food) remain the same but energy content is varied. Moreover, even short-term food intake is difficult to study in humans. The physiologic state of the individual also can affect food intake. The best accepted example of taste preference involves lean and obese subjects. Lean subjects tend to prefer high carbohydrate diets, while obese subjects generally prefer food with a higher fat content.

Theories of Food Intake Regulation

The *set point* theory predicts a closed-loop feedback system, in which a sensor accurately monitors energy intake and adjusts it to a fixed reference point.[9] Thus, regulation would be similar to the better understood systems regulating body temperature or plasma osmolarity. Many aspects of body weight regulation follow such a concept, as animals tend to return to their original weight, after they are over- or underfed.[9] However, no such mechanism has been identified that would allow the type of control required of this system.

The *buffer* theory is a simpler concept and requires no such feedback loop. It would require only that change in original equilibrium or rapid fluctuations in food intake or body weight are opposed, but by less finely regulated gradations as with the set point theory. The buffer concept is supported by observations that the set point, if present, is easily disturbed.[10] Such observations include the persistence of decreased weight if short-term starvation occurs in growing rats, the production of persistent obesity by a high-fat diet, the rapid weight gain before hibernation, and the increase in body weight before pregnancy.

Advocates of the set point theory have searched for a physiologic sensor system to support their concept, but none of the proposed systems can explain all the phenomena needed to regulate food intake.[11] These theories are referred to as *appetostats,* and include as their physiologic stimulus glucose (glucostat), fatty acid release (lipostat), amino acids (aminostat), heat generated by body fluids (thermostat), and purines (purinostat).[5] Although each of these proposed nutrient controls has attractive features, none has achieved enough experimental support to gain wide acceptance. The mechanism by which these factors may act may be peripheral (on the gastrointestinal tract and metabolic organs) or central (on the central nervous system). The data available suggest that food intake seems to be regulated by a number of overlapping systems which are complex but seem to work in a coordinated fashion. These factors lead to regulation of both short-term control of food intake (satiety) and long-term control (body weight), although the former level of control is easier to document.

Gastrointestinal Factors Affecting Food Intake

Satiety can occur before much absorption of nutrients takes place. Thus, signals from the gastrointestinal tract must play an important role in the onset of satiety. The oropharynx, stomach, and upper small intestine provide sufficient signals to curtail eating, but other GI organs are probably also involved.[12] Gastric distention is probably one important cue to the onset of satiety, and the level of distention attained is determined in part by the rate of gastric emptying. Rate of gastric emptying, in turn, is related to the composition and concentration of nutrients in the ingesta.[5] As nutrients contact the absorptive surfaces of the duodenum, neural and hormonal signals are sent to the stomach and regulate the rate at which it empties.[13] Thus, it is not any one particular function of the upper GI tract which can be associated with satiety, but rather, it is the coordinated control of gastric and intestinal functions interacting with orosensory factors to determine meal size.

Because their release is triggered by nutrients in the GI tract, a variety of gastric and intestinal peptides have been studied as potential satiety factors. There is considerable evidence, from animal and human studies as well, for a role for cholecystokinin (CCK) in satiety.[12] CCK, which is released from the upper small intestine as a result of nutrient stimulation, has a variety of effects on GI organs. Although not conclusive, there is evidence that its satiety effect is related to its inhibitory effect on gastric emptying rate. Vagotomy has been shown to block CCK's satiety effect, however, implicating a gut-brain circuit. Recent evidence suggests that CCK of intestinal origin, acting via the vagus, stimulates the release of CCK in hypothalamic areas known to be involved in the control of food intake; thus CCK's involvement in satiety is apparently more complex than originally thought.[12]

Many other GI peptides have been shown to affect food intake under experimental conditions, but the evidence for their physiologic role in hunger or satiety is weak. Bombesin has been studied in some detail because of its potent satiety effect upon either peripheral or central administration in rats. Unlike CCK, bombesin's satiety effect is retained after vagotomy, thus suggesting a different mechanism of action for this peptide.

Both insulin and glucagon have also been implicated in mechanisms involved in the control of food intake, primarily via their effects on glucose metabolism. Although exogenous administration of these hormones can stimulate and inhibit eating, respectively, under physiologic conditions they probably play a more indirect role in feeding behavior by acting through the body energy-balance regulator.[5]

Most nutrients are digested, absorbed, and metabolized after the onset of satiety and the termination of eating. Signals that result from postabsorptive events are primarily inhibitory, thus acting as brakes on a centrally mediated tonic drive to eat. As nutrients are utilized or stored, inhibition abates, hunger returns, and eating is initiated once again.

CNS Control of Food Intake

Neurotransmitters

Neurohumoral receptor mechanisms have been postulated for the stimulation of feeding.[11] Catecholamines and β-adrenergic receptor agonists have been extensively implicated. Noradrenergic and dopaminergic fibers have been demonstrated to be involved in the initiation of feeding via the lateral hypothalamic area. Dopamine and serotonin are the monoamines that have been strongly associated with the termination of feeding (satiety). Serotonin may interact with the noradrenergic system as a secondary satiety system. Dopamine levels may increase after eating, perhaps simply the result of the diet itself.[5] These effects of diet stress the care which is needed to evaluate the effects of neurotransmitters on food intake. It seems clear, however, that brain monoamines play an important role in modifying food intake, but they also interact with a variety of other central neurotransmitters and peripheral stimuli.

In addition to the monoamine neurotransmitters, other compounds may play a role in the regulation of food intake. The receptor for endogenous opioids that has been implicated is the kappa receptor; its putative endogenous ligand is dynorphin, which contains leucine-enkephalin at its amino terminus. Leu-enkephalin, however, has effects on feeding intake opposite to dynorphin. Naloxone inhibits feeding in certain experimental models, and exogenous agents that act on the kappa and mu receptors (e.g., butorphenol) stimulate feeding.[11] Blood glucose may alter responsiveness of the mu receptor, as hyperglycemia makes animals more sensitive to opiate blockade. Gamma aminobutyric acid (GABA) and benzodiazepines, which act in conjunction with GABA, can induce feeding and inhibit the serotoninergic satiety system. Norepinephrine-induced feeding may act via GABA release. However, oral GABA decreases feeding in rodents. In sum, the data for GABA are somewhat contradictory.[5]

As discussed above, CCK of intestinal origin has been shown to influence feeding, but there is also good evidence that CCK in the CNS is involved in the control of food intake, and that peripheral and central CCK systems are linked.[14] Of the many postulated peptide mediators of physiologic satiety, CCK is probably the strongest candidate in mammals. Insulin in repeated doses injected into the CNS will induce food intake; the effect is antagonized by glucose injections in the hypothalamus.[5] These types of studies support a central role for insulin in regulating food intake. However, insulin crosses the blood-brain barrier poorly, whereas CCK and other brain-gut peptides are produced in the CNS. Glucocorticoids also may increase food intake, possibly by interacting with central catecholamines.

CNS Centers Regulating Food Intake

Destructive lesions in the ventromedial hypothalamus (VMH) and stimulation of the lateral hypothalamus (LH) lead to hyperphagia and weight gain. This dual theory of satiety (ventromedial) and feeding (lateral hypothalamus) centers has been the focus for experiments in this field for years. This concept is now viewed as an oversimplification. Lesions of the VMH are associated with hyperinsulinemia, decreased growth hormone, vagal hyperactivity, and other abnormalities that contribute to the hyperphagia. Moreover, the VMH communicates with serotoninergic and adrenergic pathways that may modify satiety. Rats with lesions in both LH and VMH can still regulate their body weight but at different set points. In addition, it is not clear that all the effects of LH and VMH lesions are mediated at the site of the lesion. It is uncertain whether it is fibers passing through the LH (e.g., ascending nigro-striatal), rather than LH neurons themselves, that are responsible for the hunger and feeding seen after LH stimulation.[5] Lesions in other areas of the hypothalamus and CNS also affect food intake. In summary, the concept of dual hypothalamic centers regulating feeding is still valid in part, but is not sufficient to explain the central control of food intake.

Abnormalities of Food Intake

Associated with Increased Body Weight

A great deal of evidence suggests that there is a defect in the regulation of body weight and food intake in exogenous obesity. In humans it has been very difficult to separate the physiologic and psychologic drives to eat. Moreover, no consistent defect in metabolic regulation has been shown in obese humans. Because weight seems to remain at a given level for each individual regardless of attempts to alter weight, a case for regulation of body weight at a higher "set point" has been made. These issues are discussed on pages 173 to 199.

Miscellaneous CNS disorders have been associated with obesity (endogenous obesity).[15] These disorders include involvement of the hypothalamus by tumor (especially craniopharyngioma), meningitis, and cysts. However, the incidence of obesity in patients with hypothalamic tumors was the same as in the general population.[15] It appears that obesity occurs only when accompanied by pathologic hyperphagia and is not due to endocrine defects. *Prader-Willi syndrome* is characterized by hyperphagia, obesity, hypogonadism, and mental deficiency. Naloxone has been used to attempt to control the hyperphagia in these patients, although it is not clear that the modest results obtained were due to drowsiness or to a central effect in which opioid mediators play a crucial role.[16] In *Laurence-Moon-Biedl syndrome* retinal degeneration and polydactyly are associated with obesity. Hyperostosis frontalis interna and benign intracranial hypertension have been associated with obesity.[5]

Associated with Decreased Body Weight

Anorexia nervosa is associated with features of decreased sympathetic nervous system activity (bradycardia, hypotension, hypothermia) in keeping with findings in fasted subjects. Low thyroxine, T_3, LH-FSH, and spinal fluid neuropeptides and neurotransmitter levels have been reported, but it is uncertain if these changes are primary in explaining the altered food intake or are secondary to fasting.[17] Anorexia nervosa is discussed in detail elsewhere (see pp. 185–194). Diencephalic tumors have been associated with anorexia as well as hyperphagia, although less frequently.[5] Anorexia is a symptom with multiple causes, ranging from malignancy to the ingestion of medications. The action of drugs can be explained often by interference with one of the initiators of feeding (e.g., dopamine antagonists) or by direct action on the CNS, especially the hypothalamus. Other drugs (or disorders) might produce inhibiting signals from peripheral gastrointestinal organs (e.g., aspirin-induced gastritis, iron-containing medications). Many of the same disorders and drugs that produce anorexia also lead to nausea. It is often difficult to separate the effect of these symptoms, as both lead to decreased body weight.

METABOLIC RESPONSES TO CALORIC INTAKE

When dietary or energy intake is inadequate, critical metabolic responses occur to maintain body function. A primary priority of these metabolic responses is the maintenance of a steady fuel supply to the brain. Because the brain uses glucose for its energy under the usual conditions of feeding at a rate of about 5 gm per hour, it is essential that such a supply be available in both the fasted and the fed states. The brain is also capable of utilizing ketone bodies as an energy source and will do so in preference to glucose if the ketone bodies are presented in sufficiently high concentration.[18] In contrast to certain other tissues, such as skeletal muscle, the brain uses energy at a fairly constant rate, whether waking, sleeping, thinking, or dreaming.

During the influx of nutrients into blood after feeding and absorption, the energy and amino acid needs of the body are readily met from the supply entering from the gastrointestinal tract. When this flow of nutrients has subsided, however, the body's needs then will be met by release of energy from stores (Table 103–1). The generation and maintenance of these stores are

Table 103–1. ENERGY STORES IN NORMAL HUMANS

	Kg	Energy Value (kcal)
Tissues		
Fat	15	141,000
Protein	6	24,000
Carbohydrate		
Muscle glycogen	0.150	600
Liver glycogen	0.075	300
Subtotal		165,900
Circulating Fuels		
Glucose	0.020	80
Free fatty acids	0.0003	3
Triglycerides	0.003	30
Subtotal		113
Total 166,013 kcal		

major metabolic activities in the period immediately after feeding, under the hormonal control of insulin in particular. The excess amino acids, fatty acids, and glucose not required immediately for energy are deposited in the form of proteins, triglycerides, and glycogen. An additional value of this storage process is to modulate the massive extracellular osmotic shifts that might occur between the fed and the fasting states by removing excess nutrients into intracellular storage depots.

The metabolic changes that occur during feeding and fasting can be analyzed by division into four distinct periods defined in relation to the last feeding. They are: (1) the fed state, 0 to 4 hours after eating; (2) the postabsorptive state, 4 to 18 hours after eating; (3) intermediate fasting, 18 hours to three weeks after feeding, and (4) prolonged fasting, beyond three weeks. The metabolic characteristics of these different states are quite distinct, but the transition between them is complex and gradual, representing the interaction of overlapping events.

The *fed state* can be described as the period immediately following the ingestion of a standard carbohydrate-containing meal in a well-nourished individual. Glucose is freely available from absorption in the gastrointestinal tract, supplying the brain with its needed energy. Since that energy requirement is small, much of the absorbed glucose is stored as hepatic and muscle glycogen. Beyond that there is some glucose conversion to fatty acids for storage as triglycerides, largely in adipose tissue.

As the glucose flow subsides in the *postabsorptive state*, the first line of defense against a fall in blood glucose, which would affect the functioning of the brain, is the glycogen stored in the liver. This supply is never more than approximately 75 gm (Table 103–1); therefore, given the 5 to 6 gm hourly requirement for brain function, the hepatic glycogen stores represent only about a 15-hour supply of glucose precursor.[18] The amount of carbohydrate stored in muscle is much larger but is not available as a glucose precursor. Muscle glycogen must be degraded to pyruvate and lactate before these carbon sources can be returned to the circulation.

Intermediate fasting may be total or partial; in the clinical setting, insufficient calorie intake or partial starvation is more common. Certain metabolic responses compensate for energy needs that are not being met by diet.[19] The obvious source of energy when intake is insufficient is *fatty acid*, stored in the adipose tissue in the form of triglyceride (Table 103–1). The initial driving force for long-chain fatty acid oxidation derives from the accelerated release of free fatty acids from adipose tissue as fasting progresses. This process parallels the decline of the postabsorptive rise of circulating insulin and the increase of circulating glucagon, the so-called hormone of fasting. The circulating levels of free fatty acids rise, in part also the result of the action of other hormones, particularly epinephrine.

In peripheral tissues, these free fatty acids are oxidized to carbon dioxide and water in preference to glucose at a rate that is roughly proportional to their circulating level. The liver is capable of either re-esterifying fatty acids into triglycerides or transferring the long-chain fatty acid residues across the mitochondrial membrane, where the oxidative machinery exists.

The end result of fatty acid oxidation is acetate or acetyl coenzyme A. In the presence of rapidly increasing amounts of acetyl units from the β-oxidation of fatty acids and in the absence of the usual activity of the citric acid cycle, which operates at a very slow rate during carbohydrate deprivation, the complete oxidation of acetyl units to CO_2 and water is impaired. However, there is an intact mechanism for condensation into acetone, acetoacetate, and β-hydroxybutyrate (ketone bodies). Since they are water-soluble, these ketone bodies leave the liver in free solution, where they are oxidized in proportion to their circulating levels, often in preference to glucose; thus, they represent an increasingly important energy source during continued calorie deprivation.

The absolute rate of ketogenesis in liver rises rapidly during the first few days of intermediate fasting and then reaches a plateau. Although the level of free fatty acids remains almost constant thereafter, the level of circulating ketone bodies continues to rise. The concentration of ketone bodies in the blood increases from less than 0.1 mEq per liter in the fed state to 6 mEq per liter (β-hydroxybutyrate) after persistent fasting.[20] At this higher level, ketone bodies represent a major energy source for brain metabolism. The decrease in the dependence of brain upon glucose for its energy during *prolonged fasting* or starvation serves to reduce the conversion of body protein reserves to glucose by gluconeogenesis and thus to spare lean body mass from accelerated depletion.

Gluconeogenesis, the creation of glucose from other metabolic precursors, begins in the postabsorptive state as soon as the glucose content of the blood begins to fall. This production of new glucose for maintenance of blood glucose and brain function occurs largely in the liver. Major substrates are 3-carbon nonglucose precursors, including pyruvate and glycerol, and amino acids, particularly alanine from skeletal muscle.[21]

Transhepatic balance studies have revealed that in the usual intermediate period about 50 per cent of the total carbons used in new glucose formation comes from pyruvate, about 20 per cent from amino acids, and 10 per cent from glycerol. About one half of all carbons leaving the liver as glucose are recycled back from the periphery as lactate and pyruvate, the remainder being oxidized to CO_2 and water. The source of the remaining 20 per cent of glucose carbons is not entirely accounted for at present. This proportion of unidentified glucose precursor increases substantially in the accelerated fasting state that occurs when a person is under severe stress.

The quantitative aspects of these processes can be summarized as follows: During a short fast of one to three days, the rate at which body protein is broken down amounts to about 70 gm per day. At this rate, the total body protein content of approximately 6000 gm in an adult man, mostly in skeletal muscle, would be depleted by one third after only three weeks of complete fasting, a circumstance that would lead to severe debility and muscle weakness even in healthy subjects. Because of the increasing availability of ketone bodies during starvation, the brain eventually derives 50 to 70 per cent of its energy supply from ketones. The total glucose production required from hepatic and renal gluconeogenesis drops from about 120 gm at three days of fasting to 90 gm at three weeks, with half of the glucose recycled as lactate. The net negative protein balance falls from 70 gm down to about 20 gm per day. Thus, ketosis clearly must be looked upon as a normal, indeed, as a major component of adaptation to calorie deprivation, particularly to carbohydrate deprivation.

Alcohol and Its Effect on Macronutrient Intake and Metabolism

Alcohol (ethanol) in excess has the potential to affect every organ system in the body. Any discussion of the acute or chronic effects of alcohol use in humans should separate those due to alcohol per se from those due to alcohol-mediated chronic disease. There are data which quantify the amount of alcohol needed to produce nutritional effects in humans.[22] This section discusses the effects on food and calorie intake. Effects on organ function and on vitamin and mineral uptake are covered on pages 1986 to 1987.

Alcohol has a regular effect on the hypothalamic-pituitary axis reflected in an alteration of hormones produced in that region. The better-described effects include diuresis due to inhibition of vasopressin release. Less well characterized are impaired release of thyrotropin releasing hormone and somatostatin. The depression of both hormones is thought to play a role in the symptoms of alcohol withdrawal, as well as in appetite regulation. The more global action of alcohol on the brain resembles a narcotic drug. Alcohol-induced damping of frontal lobe inhibitory controls may affect food intake. Moreover, as alcohol is a calorie source, supplying 7 kcal per gram, it can act as an appetite suppressant. Twelve ounces of beer, 8 ounces of wine, or 2 ounces of distilled liquor each provide about 150 to 180 kcal. The end result of direct caloric effects or indirect CNS effects is to alter the intake of other nutrients. As alcohol intake increases, intake of food decreases. It is not clear if this change is due to altered satiety due to depressive effects of alcohol, to anorexia, either central or peripheral changes (e.g., gastritis), or to biosocial alterations such as disrupted family life or loss of job.

Ingestion of alcohol also alters the body's metabolism of energy sources. This is especially true of a high rate of alcohol consumption, usually found among alcohol abusers (about 50 per cent or more of total caloric intake).[23] Unlike other energy sources, alcohol cannot be stored and must be metabolized by oxidation to acetate. Moreover, its rate of oxidation is relatively constant, without feedback control, so that excessive ingestion leads to larger and larger effects on intermediary metabolism. Most of these effects are manifested in the liver, where over 90 per cent of the alcohol is oxidized. However, fasting or low protein intake can decrease the rate of alcohol metabolism by reducing the amount of hepatic alcohol dehydrogenase. This effect is opposed by the stimulation of the dehydrogenase that is associated with chronic alcohol use in the absence of liver disease.[24]

Among the significant metabolic effects of alcohol oxidation are the impairment of gluconeogenesis (sometimes leading to hypoglycemia), increased lactic acid production, increased ketone body production, decreased uric acid excretion, decreased fatty acid oxidation, and increased fatty acid synthesis.[22] These changes are mediated by the altered redox state, associated with an increased NADH/NAD ratio which results when alcohol is oxidized. The overall changes from normal fasting metabolism (see prior section) include early depletion of glycogen stores, decreased availability of glucose, acidosis from increased ketone production, augmented release of fatty acids from adipose stores, and fatty liver. Because protein and calorie malnutrition is very common in alcohol abusers, as is fatty liver, it is often not possible in any individual to separate the effects of malnutrition from those of alcohol ingestion.[25]

NUTRITIONAL REQUIREMENTS

We have described elaborate metabolic controls directed at meeting basic energy requirements. To formulate an overall plan for nutritional management, one must consider more broadly the nutritional requirements of the patient and the impact of his condition on these requirements. For the individual patient, energy balance in simplest terms means a caloric intake that maintains a steady body weight. Calorie insufficiency, conversely, is reflected in weight loss and calorie overabundance in weight gain. See pages 1983 to 1994 for further discussion of how the physiologic status of the patient influences nutrient requirements importantly. Examples of conditions that can substantially modify nutritional requirements include the stress of infection; trauma, including surgery; alcohol abuse; and malabsorption.

Estimation of Energy Requirement

The components of energy requirements in humans can be summarized as follows: *Total daily energy requirement* = *basal metabolic rate* (BMR) + *energy of activity* + *specific dynamic action of food (SDA).* BMR (or resting energy expenditure, REE) is a measure of the amount of energy expended in order to maintain a living state while at rest and without food; energy of activity is a measure of the energy expended to support a variety of physical activities; and SDA, also referred to as thermic effect of food (TEF) and diet-induced thermogenesis (DIT), is an estimate of the number of calories produced as heat during the ingestion and metabolism of food. Basal metabolic rate accounts for about two thirds of the total energy requirements and is affected by body size (height and weight), age, and sex. Not surprisingly, the BMR values using different individual parameters will not be identical for each method in the same individual.

There are many methods available for estimating these three components. In the following sections only the methods that produce approximations of the energy expenditure will be discussed. A more detailed discussion of available methods for clinical use is available.[26]

Estimation of Resting Energy Expenditure (REE)

Most methods are based on calorimetry, or a measurement of oxygen consumption under carefully controlled conditions, e.g., during fasting, in the morning, and for one hour. A more meaningful metabolic rate would reflect the rate at which energy is consumed in a normal life situation at rest and while eating food. The actual measurements of basal energy requirement only approximate this situation. The clinically useful estimates of REE discussed below are approximations of the actual measurements. Nonetheless, some estimate is to be strongly preferred to none at all.

A method of estimation (devised by Harris and Benedict) based on data from indirect calorimetry has been recommended for general use.[27] These equations have been used with good accuracy to estimate BMR. The formulas for calculating REE (or BMR), using the four variables of age, height, weight, and sex are as follows:

$$BMR_{women} = 655 + (9.5 \times W) + (1.8 \times H) - 4.7 \times A)$$
$$BMR_{men} = 66 + (13.7 \times W) + (5 \times H) - (6.8 \times A)$$

where W is actual or usual weight (kg), H is height (cm), and A is age (years).

The new equations for REE are simpler than those of Harris and Benedict and are based on more comprehensive data.[28] Because people of the same weight but different heights were found to have similar REEs, the formulas derived can be based only on body weight, age, and sex. The new WHO/FAO equations are shown in Table 103–2. The values derived differ from earlier formulas mostly for females, in whom there was an overestimation of weight above 40 kg, which reached nearly 18 per cent by a weight of 80 kg. One should remember that predicted REE (or BMR) may over- or underestimate the measured values (by respirometry) by 20 or even 30 per cent for any individual.

Table 103–2. ESTIMATION OF RESTING ENERGY EXPENDITURE

Age (Years)	Male REE*	Female REE*
<3	0.249 wt − 0.127	0.244 wt − 0.13
3–10	0.095 wt + 2.110	0.085 wt + 2.033
10–18	0.074 wt + 2.754	0.056 wt + 2.898
18–30	0.063 wt + 2.896	0.062 wt + 2.036
30–60	0.048 wt + 4.653	0.034 wt + 3.538
>60	0.049 wt + 2.459	0.038 wt + 2.755

*REE is expressed as millijoules (MJ) per 24 hours, weight in kg. To convert REE to kcal, multiply by 239.2.

Modified from Schofield, W. N. Hum. Nutr. (Clin. Nutr.) *39*(Suppl. 1):5, 1985.

Table 103–3. ESTIMATION OF ADDITIONAL ENERGY EXPENDITURE BY ACTIVITY

Type of Work	Calories Added to BMR (kcal/day)
Sedentary	400–800
Light: office, professional and clerical	800–1200
Moderate: walking, lifting	1200–1800
Heavy: construction, athletic	1800–4500

Modified from Wilmore, D. W. The Metabolic Management of the Critically Ill. New York, Plenum Press, 1977.

Estimates of Energy of Activity

The energy of activity accounts for about one third of total energy expenditures under most conditions. It can vary from 1.5 to 8.5 kcal per kg per hour. This factor is obviously more important in calculating energy requirements for active, ambulatory patients. It should be kept in mind that some types of work (e.g., gardening) can fatigue certain muscle groups without using a large number of calories. Usually, any exercise that results in lifting the body from the ground (e.g., running) uses the most calories. Although precise measurements by calorimetry are available for a wide range of activities, it is easiest to use an approximation when estimating energy needs. Then the total daily range of activity that suits the patient best can be chosen (Table 103–3).

Diet-Induced Thermogenesis (DIT)

Heat or energy production in excess of basal metabolism is caused by the ingestion of nutrients in food. Protein increases heat production by 12 per cent, carbohydrate by 6 per cent, and fat by 2 per cent. A mixed diet will yield approximately a 6 per cent increase in heat, but because of normal variability, 10 per cent is the customary figure used.[26] The calorigenic effect on food seems to be closely related to the energy required for ATP formation, in which protein (via amino acid breakdown and urea synthesis) is the oxidative substrate. Most of the effect is generated in the muscle and liver and is present even after the intravenous administration of nutrients. In hypermetabolic patients, the DIT is lower than normal because heat production is already increased. In calculating additional energy requirements for these patients, the DIT should be estimated at no more than 5 per cent of energy requirements.

Additional Energy Requirements of Illness

Heat production increases with inflammation. However, as oxygen consumption increases owing to fever and new white blood cell production, DIT decreases owing to decreased calorie intake and the energy of activity decreases owing to immobility. For this reason, the daily calorie requirement in ill persons rarely exceeds by very much the requirement of the healthy ones. Thus, the total energy requirement for most patients, even during severe illness, rarely exceeds 3000 kcal per day. In fact, the earlier estimates of massively increased calorie requirements in sepsis have not been substantiated by oxygen consumption studies.[29] Reliable activity estimates for hospitalized patients with different activity levels support adding 20 per cent for a patient confined to bed, and 30 per cent for one who is ambulatory.[30] Severity of illness requires an additional calorie need, provided by measurements made from infected patients or those with thermal injuries.[31] A rough estimate of additional calorie need based on severity of illness would add 10 per cent of estimated resting BMR for mild illness, 25 per cent for moderate illness, and 50 per cent for severe illness. Those without high fever or widespread tissue damage will probably not have such high illness-related requirements. In most cases we tend to overestimate calorie requirements of patients.

Malabsorption is a special case of increased energy requirement. The most accurate but impractical way to assess calorie loss would be calorimetry of the feces. However, one can determine daily fat excretion with a 72-hour fecal fat study. Fat excretion (gm per day) × 9 kcal per gm equals the kcal loss due to fat malabsorption. The fecal calorie loss from fat multiplied by 2.5 approximates the total kilocalorie intake on a Western type of diet. This estimate assumes roughly equivalent malabsorption of carbohydrate and protein.

Example of Estimation of Daily Energy Requirement

The information presented above can be utilized as in the following example: A 40-year-old, 70-kg male office worker presents with Crohn's disease of mild severity. Calorie intake is good, but recent activity has been limited. Malabsorption is not present.

Resting energy expenditure (based on weight and sex)	=	1800 kcal
Activity-related expenditure	=	400
Illness-related expenditure (10 per cent of 1800 kcal)	=	180 kalc
		2380
Diet-induced thermogenesis (10 per cent of 2380 kcal)	=	238
Total	=	2618 kcal

Estimation of Protein Requirement

Protein balance, like energy balance, is an expression of intake relative to utilization and loss. Normally, nitrogen derived from amino acids, the catabolic product of proteins, is excreted in urine and feces and lost from the skin. Unlike the energy that is retained and stored in triglycerides and glycogen, proteins (or amino acids) are not stored in the body for utilization in times of need. Every protein has a function; there is no protein that serves as a storage supply. When excess protein is ingested, only the extra calories are retained and stored while the excess nitrogen is excreted. Extra amino acids are transaminated, making the non-nitrogenous portion of the molecule available as a calorie source.

Obligatory Nitrogen Losses

Urea accounts for over 80 per cent of urinary nitrogen. The remaining nitrogen is accounted for by creatinine, porphyrins, and other nitrogen-containing compounds. Thus, urine loss of nitrogen = urine nitrogen (mg/dl) × daily volume (dl) ÷ 0.8. Urine nitrogen excretion is related to the basal metabolic rate. The larger the body muscle mass, the more transamination of amino acids occurs to fulfill its energy needs. Each kcal needed for basal metabolism leads to the excretion of 1 to 1.3 mg of urinary nitrogen. For the same reason, nitrogen excretion increases during exercise and heavy work.

Fecal and skin losses account for a large proportion of nitrogen loss from the body (about 40 per cent) in normal circumstances, but these vary widely in disease states. Thus, measurement of urinary nitrogen loss alone may provide a predictable assessment of daily nitrogen requirement when it is often needed, i.e., during illness.

Minimal nitrogen loss from a 70-kg person (gm per day) has been estimated as 1.9 to 3.1 in urine, 0.7 to 2.5 in stool, and 0.3 from skin. The total of these figures is a mean loss of nitrogen of 4.4 gm per day. Equivalent protein loss can be calculated by multiplying nitrogen loss by 6.25. Thus, total loss by metabolism of protein is 4.4 × 6.25 or 27.5 gm per day, or 0.39 gm per kg for a 70-kg person. The recommended protein allowance for adults varies from 0.5 to 0.8 gm per kg to allow for a margin of safety and for an inefficiency of utilization of ingested proteins.[32]

Additional Protein Requirements During Growth

Protein requirements are highest during the major growth spurts of infancy and adolescence. During infancy, total body protein is lowest and obligatory losses are greatest. Thus, protein deficiency is most common in infancy. Obligatory protein losses and protein requirements both fall from infancy into childhood. The requirements rise again during adolescence. Minimal requirements for these stages of life are about 1.5 gm per kg per day. The recommended allowance (2 gm per kg per day) exceeds this figure to allow a margin of safety for children who have increased needs or who ingest proteins of low biologic value. These proteins include certain vegetable proteins that do not support growth so well as protein from milk, eggs, or meat. The difference seems largely due to the higher content of essential amino acids in the high-quality animal proteins.

There are increased protein (and calorie) requirements during pregnancy and lactation,[32] but discussion of these is beyond the scope of this book.

Protein Requirements and Gastrointestinal Function

Obligatory loss of protein from the body is a small fraction of total protein synthesized each day. The gastrointestinal tract accounts for a large fraction of this protein turnover. The normal catabolism of proteins by the intestine is shown in Figure 103–1. Between 36 and 50 gm of protein are lost daily owing to shedding of mucosal cells.[33] Pancreatic, gastric, salivary, and biliary proteins provide about 8, 5, 3, and 1 gm per day, respectively, for a total of 17 gm daily. These secreted proteins are digested along with dietary proteins, and about 93 per cent is absorbed. Under normal conditions, the nitrogen derived from about 10 to 15 gm of protein is lost in the stool each day.

Excessive nitrogen losses can occur from organs with a large surface area of epithelial cells. These organs include the intestine, skin, lungs, and kidneys. *Nephrotic syndrome, burns,* and *pneumonia* can lead to a many-fold excessive loss of protein. Only in the case of urinary losses can the amount be easily assessed. Intestinal losses are greatest in those disorders that lead either to decreased digestion or absorption of protein or to increased loss of protein into the lumen.

Nitrogen losses cannot usually be measured in clinical situations. With the exception of major fractures and burns, losses of nitrogen rarely exceed 100 per cent over the basal nitrogen requirement of 4 to 6 gm per day (25 to 40 gm protein) for a 70-kg person.[34] For a hospitalized adult, adequately nourished, receiving high-quality protein intravenously, basal protein requirements can be as low as 0.5 to 0.6 gm per kg of body weight. For an ambulatory patient eating a standard diet of mixed-quality protein, basal requirements should be estimated at 0.7 to 0.8 gm per kg. When estimates of protein requirement during illness are needed, 130 per cent of basal requirements are estimated for mild disease, 160 per cent for moderate disease, and 200 per cent for severe disease. It is unusual for a hospitalized patient with intestinal disease to have a protein requirement in excess of 1.5 gm per kg per day. It is important to recognize an upper limit of protein requirement, since caloric needs for utilizing protein are increased and must be met when protein intake is increased. The rough estimates used are based on limited measurements, and are almost certainly in excess of need.

Caloric Requirement for Protein Utilization

Nitrogen as amino acids ingested without other energy sources will not be efficiently incorporated into protein because of the energy consumed in heat loss during this metabolism. Moreover, incorporation of each amino acid molecule into peptides requires three high-energy phosphate bonds. Any excess of dietary energy over basal needs improves the efficiency of nitrogen utilization. During the period of intense growth in children, about 76 kcal of nonprotein energy are required for each gram of protein.[35] Estimates of energy needed in ambulatory adults are lower, about 50 kcal from nonprotein sources per gram of protein.[32] This high ratio is usually not available with parenteral feeding, since calorie intake is limited by the volume

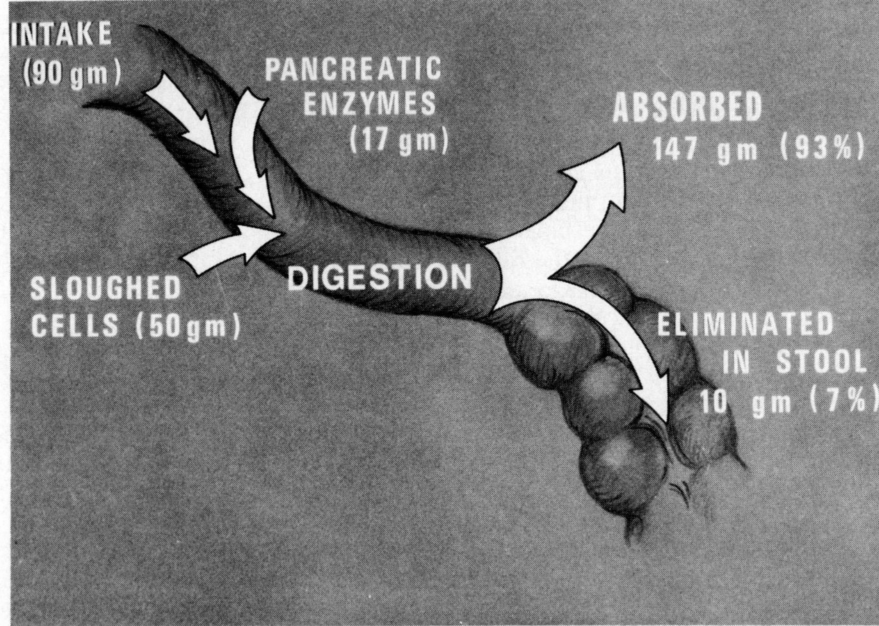

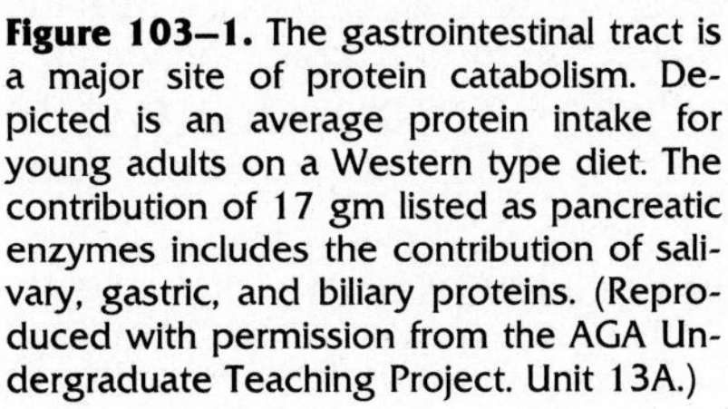
Figure 103–1. The gastrointestinal tract is a major site of protein catabolism. Depicted is an average protein intake for young adults on a Western type diet. The contribution of 17 gm listed as pancreatic enzymes includes the contribution of salivary, gastric, and biliary proteins. (Reproduced with permission from the AGA Undergraduate Teaching Project. Unit 13A.)

needed to be infused. Acceptable figures for parenteral nutrition are about 25 to 30 kcal from nonprotein sources per gram of protein, or 150 to 180 kcal per gram of nitrogen.[36]

Assessment of Caloric Balance

A skillful dietary history that is sufficiently quantitative to be converted into an estimation of total daily nutrient intake for comparison with estimated requirement is a most important aspect of patient assessment. What is the schedule and frequency of eating? Does the patient have a good appetite? Is the appetite satisfied by intake similar to that of others in the family? Does the patient lack appetite or even experience nausea at the consideration of food intake? Does the patient experience early satiety that prevents the completion of a meal? Is food intake followed by exacerbation of symptoms such as abdominal pain or diarrhea? Is there difficulty or pain on swallowing?

Either the physician or the dietitian/nutritionist can arrive at a quantitative estimate of intake by asking the patient to recall dietary intake as accurately as possible. If that intake was reasonably representative of the usual diet, it is possible to approximate total intake of calories, protein, minerals, and vitamins, even fiber, by a calculation using standard tables of food composition.[37] Computer programs based upon these standard sources, which can assist in this task, are becoming increasingly available in many hospitals. Such data can be important in subsequent nutritional management decisions. The physician should be adept at preliminary assessment, as not all problems can be referred to a trained dietitian.

Assessing Energy Intake

The best method that is practicable is a dietary history based on 24-hour recall. Reliability of this method is uncertain, since it depends upon the patient's ability to estimate and remember amounts of food eaten.[38] However, it is usually the only technique available for assessing intake. Food records may be kept by the patient, but these also require accurate estimation of amounts. Calorie counts are useful for hospitalized patients, but the diet assessed is a hospital one, not a home diet. In estimating intake it is helpful to use a reference in which the caloric content is listed according to common package units.[37]

In the assessment of calorie intake, alcohol must be remembered. Since there are 82.9 kcal per ounce of 100-proof alcohol, a convenient formula to estimate calorie intake from alcohol is the following: kcal = 0.8 × proof of beverage × number of ounces. Food preparation often adds many calories to the number listed in calorie charts. The most common and concentrated extra source of calories in food preparation is cooking oil. Since the specific gravity of cooking oil is 0.9, the calories added = number ml × 0.9 × 9 (kcal per gm).

After estimating intake, one must remember that not all sources of nutrients are utilized equally well. Egg protein, for example, the standard against which other protein sources are often compared, is utilized for growth in animals with 85 to 90 per cent efficiency. Plant proteins are utilized for growth only 50 to 80 per cent as well as egg proteins, because they are less completely hydrolyzed by pancreatic enzymes and because their essential amino acid content is lower. An average Western diet provides proteins with an overall efficiency for growth of 80 per cent, since it contains a large proportion of egg, milk, and meat proteins.

Prospective Estimation of Energy Balance

Energy balance in kilocalories per day equals calories obtained minus calories expended. Calories obtained refers to an estimate of dietary intake and/or to a calculation of calories fed enterally or parenterally. Calories expended includes the energy expended through basal or activity-related muscle contraction or that expended owing to disease. Weight gain or loss will occur when energy intake or expenditure predominates. The amount of weight to be gained (or lost) can be estimated using the calculations obtained for energy intake and expenditure. The weekly caloric change (intake-expenditure) × 7 can be divided by 3400 kcal, the caloric equivalent of 1 pound of body weight.[39] Since basal metabolic rates are not linearly related to body weight, this estimation of prospective weight gain or loss is most useful when dealing with a weight change of 10 to 15 per cent.

The various sources of energy should be considered carefully when therapy is planned. Long-chain fatty acids are the most concentrated source of calories (9 kcal per gm). In addition, polyunsaturated fats provide the precursor linoleic acid for arachidonic acid, the major essential fatty acid. However, long-chain fatty acids are ingested as triglycerides and require the most complex metabolism for digestion and absorption. When the intestine is diseased, caloric sources are often limited. Medium-chain triglycerides provide nearly as many calories (8.3 kcal per gm) as long-chain fat, but their use is limited by osmotic diarrhea to providing only a few hundred calories per day. Carbohydrate and protein are energy sources often well tolerated by the diseased intestine, but they provide only 4 kcal per gm. The volume of intake becomes a major problem when these sources provide most of the calories.

Clinical Assessment of Caloric Status

Body weight is the most commonly used measure of caloric status. This is often compared with the usual premorbid weight or the ideal body weight. Those tables that provide averages rather than ideal weight reveal variations with age and are better suited for such comparisons in patients.[26] However, data from either set of standards may be misleading in evaluating patients with recent weight loss related to illness.

Comparison with ideal or average weights in the initial assessment of caloric (or protein) status will only accurately reflect depletion in those patients who were initially at their ideal or average weight. Thus, it is better to compare with the patient's own premorbid weight. Rates of recent weight loss of 2 to 6 per cent per month have been used to predict significant caloric-protein malnutrition.[40]

Although body weight is a simple and reasonably accurate measure, some caveats should be remembered concerning its use. The accuracy of this assessment must be tempered in early weeks of caloric deficit by the fact that fluid loss represents a proportionately greater amount of the body weight decline in this period. Moreover, in the absence of a recorded premorbid weight, the patient is often unable to accurately recall the correct figure.[41] Finally, too much emphasis is often placed on the need for demonstrated weight gain in malnourished hospitalized patients once the nutritional plan is instituted. Increments greater than 2 or 3 lb per week usually suggest fluid overload.

Assessment of Protein Balance

Assessment of Nitrogen or Protein Intake. The usual method relies upon the 24-hour dietary recall and the calculation of protein content of the ingested food, using the tables that are adjusted to usual food portions.[37] When intravenous amino acids or protein are provided, the estimate becomes much easier and more precise.

Estimation of Nitrogen Balance. Determining the severity of the negative balance will allow the physician to estimate the amount of supplement needed for treatment[40] and to discover whether decreased intake or increased losses are the major causative factor. In many cases the results of this assessment will seem obvious and need not be pursued in detail. Criteria for estimating the severity of negative caloric or protein balance have been published.[40]

Nitrogen balance can be readily calculated by measurement of urinary nitrogen losses and the protein content of other draining body fluids. In patients receiving no parenteral or enteral nitrogen intake, 24-hour urinary urea nitrogen (UUN) excretion can be used to estimate the degree of catabolic stress. Assuming steady-state blood urea nitrogen concentration, the UUN will reflect the degree of endogenous protein catabolism and also the increase in metabolic energy demands.[42] The severity of protein catabolism can be correlated with UUN in the following way: A urinary urea nitrogen of less than 8 gm per 24 hours is normal; from 8 to 12 gm per 24 hours is moderate catabolism; from 12 to 16 gm per 24 hours is severe catabolism; and over 16 gm per 2 hours correlates with very severe protein catabolism and metabolic stress.

However, the dependence of the UUN measurement alone can result in the erroneous underestimation of the severity of negative nitrogen balance if major protein losses are occurring from other body sites, particularly the gastrointestinal tract.[31] In such situations it is better to calculate nitrogen balance by measuring all possible nitrogen losses (protein in urine and gastric fluid, draining wounds, and so forth). The total sum of the 24-hour UUN, 20 per cent of the UUN for nonurea urinary nitrogen losses, other measured nitrogen losses, and 2 gm for estimated daily fecal and skin nitrogen losses, is subtracted from the calculated nitrogen intake to estimate nitrogen balance.[31] When the major source of nitrogen loss is in the stool, fecal loss must be measured, not estimated, if nitrogen balance is to be accurately assessed. Such an accurate appraisal of nitrogen balance is only occasionally needed to determine the etiology of protein malnutrition.

Clinical Assessment of Protein Status. Protein status is more difficult to assess than caloric status. Visceral protein can be assessed roughly by the serum albumin value, if the limitations of that measurement are considered. The serum value depends on the state of hydration of the patient and upon alterations in degradation as well as synthesis, both of which are affected by factors other than nutritional status. Moreover, since its half-life is 14 to 21 days, serum albumin records protein deficiency or repletion with a lag period. Serum transferrin is preferred by some because its half-life is shorter and levels fall more rapidly, but interpretation of its values suffer the same problems as with serum albumin. Even when serum albumin provides some index of visceral protein status, it tells nothing about the etiology of deficiency. When protein-losing enteropathy is a cause of protein deficiency, serum albumin and other proteins are also affected (see pp. 283–290).

Somatic protein is measured by factors that reflect muscle mass—i.e., body weight (see above), midarm circumference, or urinary creatinine excretion. Further information on assessment of protein and calorie nutritional status in more severe nutritional deficiency is given on pages 1983 to 1994.

Recommended Dietary Allowances of Protein and Micronutrients

The interpretative collection of current information on nutritional requirements in health is best represented in the reports, updated at four- to five-year intervals, of the Food and Nutrition Board of the U.S. National Academy of Sciences.[32] These recommended dietary allowances, broken down by age group and sex and modified for such conditions as pregnancy and lactation, are designed to cover the requirements of virtually all healthy individuals. With the exception of energy, the allowances are not average requirements but rather a recommended intake sufficient to meet the needs of essentially all healthy individuals.

The recommended dietary allowances for protein (nitrogen), iron, and calcium are based upon balance experiments in which normal requirement is defined as the intake required to achieve zero balance between intake versus output, usually in urine, feces, and skin.

Table 103–4. RECOMMENDED NUTRIENT INTAKES FOR HEALTHY ADULTS*

	Range of Adult Dietary Allowance
Protein, gm	44–56
Vitamin A, μg retinol equivalent	800–1000
Vitamin D, μg	5.0–7.5
Vitamin E, mg α-tocopherol equivalents	8–10
Vitamin C, mg	60
Thiamine, mg	1.0–1.5
Riboflavin, mg	1.2–1.7
Niacin, mg niacin equivalent	13–19
Vitamin B_6, mg	2.0–2.2
Folacin, μg	400
Vitamin B_{12}, μg	3.0
Calcium, mg	800
Phosphorus, mg	800
Magnesium, mg	300–350
Iron, mg	10–18
Zinc, mg	15
Iodine, μg	150
Copper, mg*	2.0–3.0
Manganese, mg*	2.5–5.0
Fluoride, mg*	1.5–4.0
Chromium, mg*	0.05–0.2
Selenium, mg*	0.05–0.2
Molybdenum, mg*	0.15–0.5

*Estimated safe and adequate daily dietary intakes.

From the National Research Council. Recommended Dietary Allowances. Washington, D.C., National Academy of Sciences, 1980.

For most vitamins the recommended allowance is the daily intake required to prevent the appearance of deficiency. Most values assume normal digestion and absorption and normal metabolism. In some cases, estimates of daily turnover by radioisotope or stable isotope tracer techniques are used to determine the amount of nutrient required to maintain body stores. It follows, therefore, that diseases that influence efficiency of absorption or that change the metabolism or nutritional requirements will cause a modification in the safe allowance for that individual (see also pp. 1983 to 1994). It further follows that the recommended *dietary* allowances are at best a rough guide for requirements for enteral nutrient intake by any individual. Such allowances may be an overestimation of parenteral requirements, particularly in the case of micronutrients, since in that case no allowance need be made for the inefficiency of extraction from food and absorption. A listing of these essential nutrients and an estimation of the ranges of required intake of healthy adults are presented in Table 103–4.

References

1. Novin, D., Wyricka, W., and Bray, G. A. Hunger, Basic Mechanisms and Clinical Implications. New York, Raven Press, 1976.
2. Sharma, K. N. Receptor mechanisms in the alimentary tract: Their excitation and functions. *In* Code, C. F. (ed.). Handbook of Physiology. Sec. 6, Vol. 1, Alimentary Canal. Washington, D.C., American Physiological Society, 1967, pp. 225–237.
3. Campbell, R. G., Haskin, S. A., and Van Itallie, T. B. Studies on food-intake regulations in man. Responses to variations in nutritive density in lean and obese subjects. N. Engl. J. Med. *285*:1402, 1971.
4. Van Itallie, T. B., Smith, N. S., and Quatermain, D. Short-term and long-term components in the regulation of food intake. Evidence for a modulatory role of carbohydrate status. Am. J. Clin. Nutr. *30*:742, 1977.
5. Levin, B. E. Neurological regulation of body weight. CRC Crit. Rev. Clin. Neurobiol. *2*:1, 1987.
6. Garrow, J. S. Energy Balance and Obesity in Man. Amsterdam, North-Holland, 1974.
7. Kissileff, H. R., and Van Itallie, T. B. Physiology of the control of food intake. Ann. Rev. Nutr. *2*:271, 1982.
8. Bray, G. A. Obesity—a desire of nutrient or energy balance? Nutr. Rev. *45*:33, 1987.
9. Mrosovsky, N., and Powley, T. L. Set points for body weight and fat. Behav. Biol. *20*:205, 1977.
10. Wirtshafter, D., and Davis, J. D. Set points, setting points and the control of body weight. Physiol. Behav. *19*:75, 1977.
11. Morley, J. E., and Levine, A. S. The central control of appetite. Lancet *1*:398, 1983.
12. Smith, G. P. The peripheral control of appetite. Lancet *2*:88, 1983.
13. Liebowitz, S. F. Neurochemical systems of the hypothalamus in control of feeding and drinking behavior and water-electrolyte excretion. *In* Morgana, P. J., and Parksepp, J. (eds.): Handbook of the Hypothalamus. New York, Marcel Dekker, 1980.
14. Baile, C. A., McLaughlin, C. L., and Della-ferra, M. A. Role of cholecystokinin and opioid peptides in control of food intake. Physiol. Rev. *66*:172, 1986.
15. Bray, G. A., and Gallagher, T. F. Manifestations of hypothalamic obesity in man: a comprehensive investigation of eight patients and a review of the literature. Medicine *54*:301, 1975.
16. Kyriakides, M., et al. Effect of naloxone on hyperphagia in Prader-Willi syndrome. Lancet *1*:876, 1980.
17. Schwabe, A. D. Anorexia nervosa. Ann. Intern. Med. *94*:371–381, 1981.
18. Havel, R. J. Caloric homeostasis and disorders of fuel transport. N. Engl. J. Med. *187*:1186, 1972.
19. Cahill, G. Starvation in man. N. Engl. J. Med. *282*:668, 1970.
20. McGarry, J. D., and Foster, D. W. Regulation of ketogenesis and clinical aspects of the ketogenic state. Metabolism *21*:471, 1972.
21. Felig, P. The glucose-alanine cycle. Metabolism *22*:179, 1973.
22. Turner, T., Mezey, E., and Kimbal, A. Measurement of alcohol-related effects in man: chronic effects in relation to levels of alcohol consumption. Johns Hopkins Med. J. *141*:235, 273, 1977.
23. DeCarli, L., and Lieber, C. Fatty liver in the rat after prolonged intake of ethanol with a nutritionally adequate new liquid diet. J. Nutr. *91*:331, 1967.
24. Kater, R., Crilli, N., and Iber, F. Differences in the rate of ethanol metabolism in recently drinking alcoholic and non-alcoholic subjects. Am. J. Clin. Nutr. *22*:1608, 1969.
25. Mendenhall, C. L., et al. Protein-calorie malnutrition associated with alcoholic hepatitis. Am. J. Med. *76*:211, 1984.
26. Alpers, D. H., Clouse, R. E., and Stenson, W. F. Manual of Nutritional Therapeutics. 2nd ed. Boston, Little, Brown, 1987, Chap. 3.
27. Michel, L., Serrano, A., and Malt, R. A. Nutritional support of hospitalized patients. N. Engl. J. Med. *304*:1147, 1981.
28. Schofield, W. N. Predicting basal metabolic rate, new standards and review of previous work. Human Nutr. Clin. Nutr. *39C*(suppl. 1):5, 1985.
29. Baker, J. P., et al. Randomized trial of total parenteral nutrition of critically ill patients: metabolic effect of varying glucose-lipid ratios as the energy source. Gastroenterology *87*:53, 1984.
30. Kinney, J. M., et al. Tissue compositions of weight loss on surgical patients. Ann. Surg. *168*:459, 1968.
31. Wilmore, D. W. The Metabolic Management of the Critically Ill. New York, Plenum Press, 1977.
32. Recommended Dietary Allowances. The National Research Council. Washington, D.C., National Research Council. Washington, D.C., National Academy of Sciences, 1980.
33. Crosby, W. H. A concept of the pathogenesis of anemia applied to disorders of the intestinal mucosa. Am. J. Dig. Dis. *6*:492, 1961.

34. Munro, H. W., and Allison, J. B. (eds.). Mammalian Protein Metabolism. Vol. II, New York, Academic Press, 1964.
35. Waterlow, J. C., and Payne, P. R. The protein gap. Nature *258*:113, 1975.
36. Hartley, T. F., and Lee, H. A. Investigations into the optimum nitrogen and caloric requirements and comparative nutritive value of three intravenous amino acid solutions in the postoperative period. Nutr. Metab. *19*:201, 1975.
37. Nutritive Value of American Foods in Common Units. Agriculture Handbook No. 456. Washington, D.C., U.S. Department of Agriculture, 1975.
38. Committee on Food Consumption Patterns, National Research Council. Assessing Changing Food Consumption Patterns. Washington, D.C., National Academy Press, 1981.
39. Van Itallie, T. B., and Yang, M. U. Diet and weight loss. N. Engl. J. Med. *297*:1158, 1977.
40. Blackburn, G. N., Bistrian, B. R., Maini, B. S., Schlamm, H. T., and Smith, M. F. Nutritional and metabolic assessment of the hospitalized patient. J. Parent. Ent. Nutr. *5*:11, 1977.
41. Morgan, D. B., et al. The assessment of weight loss from a single measurement of body weight: the problems and limitations. Am. J. Clin. Nutr. *33*:2101–2105, 1980.

Nutritional Deficiency in Gastrointestinal Disease

IRWIN H. ROSENBERG
DAVID H. ALPERS

PATHOGENESIS OF NUTRITIONAL DEFICIENCY IN GASTROINTESTINAL DISEASE

The gastrointestinal tract performs critical functions in the maintenance of adequate nutrition. These functions include ingestion, digestion, absorption, and preliminary metabolism of food. In addition, there is a continuous and large exchange of fluid and electrolytes. Bile salts, secreted by the liver as products of cholesterol metabolism, are required for normal fat absorption. Proteins in the form of enzymes and cells are secreted, digested, and reabsorbed. Nutritional deficiencies can occur whenever disease impairs these functions.

The mechanisms that cause nutritional deficiencies in gastrointestinal diseases are reviewed in Table 104–1.

Inadequate Food Intake

Nutritional deficiency, particularly calorie insufficiency, most often reflects inadequate dietary intake. Patients will often restrict food intake because of anorexia, to prevent symptoms associated with eating, or to avoid foods. Table 104–2 lists those micronutrient deficiencies that result commonly from decreased intake.

Food intake is obviously restricted by nausea; protracted vomiting not only interferes with food ingestion but also commonly results in fluid and electrolyte depletion. Patients who experience pain on swallowing or after eating and those who experience the characteristic worsening of diarrhea after a meal will restrict dietary intake as if by conditioned response. Thus, patients who have diseases that cause narrowing or obstruction of the lumen of any of the gastrointestinal organs and those with inflammatory conditions such as peptic ulcer, Crohn's disease, and biliary tract disease are prone to inadequate dietary intake. Liver disease, particularly hepatitis, is likely to result in anorexia. Radiation-induced nausea, the appetite-suppressing effect of cancer chemotherapy, and digitalis or many other drugs in toxic doses are examples of anorexia associated with therapy. Anorexia dominates the presentation of many cancers, including those of the gastrointestinal tract.

Depression is a frequently overlooked cause of decreased appetite, often misinterpreted as nausea. Associated symptoms of fatigue, alterations in sleep patterns, or emotional lability can assist the physician in distinguishing this disorder as an important factor in inadequate dietary intake.

Some dietary restrictions are justified for their symptomatic benefits, such as the restriction of lactose-rich foods in the diet of the lactose-intolerant individual, the diminution of fat in the patient with steatorrhea and diarrhea, and the reduced intake of high-residue food in some patients (see p. 2005). However, as is emphasized in the discussion of nutritional therapy on page 1971, such restrictions must sometimes be accom-

Table 104–1. PATHOGENESIS OF NUTRITIONAL DEFICIENCIES IN GASTROINTESTINAL DISEASE

Mechanism	Contributing Factors	Example
Decreased oral intake	Anorexia, nausea, vomiting, dysphagia, pain, obstruction, depression	All nutrients
	Iatrogenic: restrictive unbalanced diets	Folate, calcium
	Alcohol	
Malabsorption	Intestinal disease	All nutrients, especially folate and calcium
	Pancreatic disease	Protein
	Intestinal resection or bypass (short bowel)	Calcium, magnesium
	Postgastrectomy	Iron, cobalamin
	Bile salt deficiency	Fat-soluble vitamins
Increased losses	Diarrhea	Sodium, potassium
	Bleeding	Iron
	Protein-losing enteropathy	Albumin
	Fistula drainage	Sodium
	Urinary losses	Folate (in alcoholics)
Increased requirements	Inflammation	Calories
	Fever	Calories
	Cell proliferation	Folate, cobalamin
	Pregnancy	Folate, calcium, iron
	Hemolysis	Folate
Drugs	Anorexia, nausea (many drugs)	All nutrients
	Interference with absorption or metabolism of nutrients	Folate and calcium
	Mucosal toxicity (esp. chemotherapeutic agents)	Sodium, potassium

panied by other alterations in diet in order to prevent or correct nutritional inadequacy. Diets based upon restrictions alone, whether self-imposed or physician-recommended, can lead to nutritional insufficiency.

Although the mechanism for growth retardation in inflammatory bowel disease is not certain, decreased intake of nutrients is one possible cause.[1, 28] Endocrine abnormalities have not been implicated, as thyroid, adrenal, and hypothalamic function appear normal. Severe reduction in caloric intake is a major factor, but enteric protein losses and chronic daily steroid use play a role. The evidence supporting a primary role of decreased nutrient intake includes the dramatic response to aggressive oral or parenteral alimentation.[2–4]

Malabsorption

A second major element in the pathogenesis of nutritional deficiency in patients with gastrointestinal disease is malabsorption, which commonly complicates diseases of the gastrointestinal tract. For a detailed discussion of malabsorption, see pages 263 to 282. Since fat is such an important contributor to total calorie intake, any condition that produces a substantial degree of fat malabsorption places the patient at risk of calorie insufficiency. Diseases affecting the mucosa or the total absorptive surface area of the small intestine, such as celiac sprue or short bowel syndrome after intestinal resection, are most likely to produce combined macro- and micronutrient deficiencies.

Malabsorption is associated with acute and chronic infections involving the gastrointestinal tract. Many infections, whether they involve the gastrointestinal tract directly or not, result in diarrhea. Diarrhea, whether due to enhanced secretion or decreased absorption, contributes to a disturbance of the intestinal

Table 104–2. COMMON CAUSES OF VITAMIN AND MINERAL DEFICIENCIES

Micronutrient Involved	Common Etiologies	Mechanisms
Thiamine, riboflavin pyridoxine, niacin	Alcoholism, anorexia	Inadequate dietary intake
Folic acid	Alcoholism	Inadequate intake, increased urinary loss
	Pregnancy, hemolysis	Increased requirement
	Drugs (esp. sulfasalazine, anticonvulsants)	Decreased absorption
	Intestinal disease	Malabsorption, interrupted EHC of folate
Cobalamin	Ileal disease (esp. Crohn's)	Malabsorption, interrupted EHC of cobalamin
	Postgastrectomy	Lack of intrinsic factor
	Stagnant loop syndrome	Increased utilization by bacteria
Vitamin C	Alcoholism	Inadequate intake
Vitamin A	Alcoholism	Inadequate intake
Vitamins A, D, E	Ileal disease (esp. Crohn's)	Malabsorption
	Obstructive liver or biliary tract disease	Interrupted EHC of bile salts
Vitamin D	Lack of sunlight	Decreased endogenous production
	Drugs, esp. anticonvulsants, cholestyramine	Decreased absorption
Vitamin K	Chronic or acute liver disease	Decreased end organ response
Sodium, potassium	Vomiting, diarrhea	Loss of body stores
Iron	GI bleeding	Loss of body stores (250 mg per unit of blood)
	Pregnancy, infancy	Increased requirement
Calcium	Lactose intolerance	Decreased intake
	Short bowel syndrome	Decreased absorption
Magnesium	Alcoholism	Increased urinary loss
	Short bowel syndrome	Decreased absorption
Phosphate, zinc	Diarrhea	Malabsorption

EHC = enterohepatic circulation.

absorption of multiple nutrients. These losses may result in deficits of protein and vitamins (e.g., folate) that affect the digestive organs secondarily and produce, in turn, further deterioration of the efficiency of digestion and absorption. Several drugs contribute to malabsorption by interfering with absorption of specific nutrients. Examples of such drug-nutrient interactions include corticosteroid inhibition of calcium absorption, interference with folic acid absorption by antacids, cimetidine, sulfasalazine, anticonvulsants, or cholestyramine, and inhibition of fat-soluble vitamin absorption by cholestyramine (see Table 104–2).

Increased Secretion of Protein and Minerals

Closely related to, and sometimes indistinguishable from, conditions that produce nutritional deficits because of malabsorption are conditions that cause increased secretion into the lumen of the small or large intestine and losses of nutrients in the stool. Because the small intestine has the largest surface area and highest normal rate of protein loss of the enteric organs, diseases of the small intestine have the potential for the greatest rate of protein loss. The rates of protein nitrogen loss observed in some intestinal diseases are listed in Table 104–3. Protein-losing enteropathy is common in patients with Crohn's disease and correlates as well as any functional measurement with disease extent and activity.[5]

Increased loss is a problem that is most important in the genesis of certain mineral deficiencies. The most important divalent ions (calcium, magnesium, zinc) are secreted into the bowel via intestinal, pancreatic, and biliary juices. These secreted ions usually are combined with the ingested minerals and compose about 10 to 20 per cent of the luminal minerals requiring absorption.[6,7] All these ions are inefficiently absorbed (less than 40 per cent). One of the reasons is that insoluble salts are formed in the usual alkaline pH of the upper bowel. Magnesium and zinc deficiencies in patients with inflammatory bowel disease, particularly those who have a significant degree of short bowel and chronic diarrhea, reflect this loss of endogenously secreted cation.

The major monovalent cations (Na, K) are also secreted by digestive juices, but they are efficiently absorbed. Nonetheless, their concentration is so high in these juices that deficiency can occur through large losses of diarrheal fluid.

Table 104–3. EXCESS DAILY FECAL NITROGEN LOSS DURING DISEASE*

	Fecal Loss (gm N/day)
Normal	1.7 (0.2–2.5)
Ulcerative colitis	6 (3–9.3)
Total pancreatectomy	6 (4–8)
Pancreatic cancer	3.4 (2.1–5.7)
Extensive small bowel resection	6.8 (2.6–10)
Sprue	3.4 (2.3–4.3)
Cancer of colon	1.8 (1.7–2.0)

*Values refer to means and ranges of observations, reported by Munro, H. N.[8] To convert gm N to gm protein, multiply values by 6.25.

Increased Utilization of Nutrients

Increased nutritional requirements may relate to overutilization of nutrients because of disease. Fever due to inflammation increases basal calorie requirements. Sweating contributes to dermal losses of nitrogen, electrolytes, and trace minerals. Faster enterocyte turnover in celiac disease and in inflammatory bowel disease probably exerts an increased demand on micronutrient stores as well as increasing utilization of protein precursors (see Table 104–1).

The increased requirements of infections or sepsis are best documented.[9] All infections, mild or severe, whether viral, bacterial, or parasitic, result in aberrations of nutrient metabolism with most notable effects on protein balance. These nutritional imbalances result from several mechanisms. First, a period of decreased food intake of variable duration is followed by a period of markedly increased protein requirement to compensate for the losses during acute illness and to rebuild lost lean body tissue. Decreased food intake may result from loss of appetite associated with the infectious disease, but it is also commonly related to the ordered withdrawal of solid food from the infected individual, particularly when the infectious process results in diarrhea. Second, urinary excretion of nutrients, particularly nitrogen and some vitamins, is increased. Third, the metabolic responses to systemic infection demand more nutrients. Not only does the infectious agent augment utilization of nutrients by the host to an abnormal degree, but it also initiates a series of nutritionally costly metabolic responses by the host to the infection. These responses include the synthesis of phagocytes and leukocytes, the production of immunoglobulins, and the synthesis of a variety of nonspecific proteins associated with the reaction to infection.

Thus, there are both increased losses of, and increased requirements for, certain nutrients (particularly protein) during the acute phase of infection. Often a profound negative nitrogen balance can be documented. A third demand for increased nutrients is for the phase of rebuilding, the so-called anabolic phase during recovery. This phase is often several times as long as the catabolic or degradative phase, and, accordingly, the nutritional cost may be very high.

Some of the requirements for nutrients during infections or after trauma have been quantitated. Much of the research has focused on protein utilization and energy requirements in the setting of total parenteral nutrition (see pp. 2007–2027). Earlier estimations of massively increased calorie requirements in surgical sepsis have not been substantiated by oxygen consumption studies.[10] In septic or injured patients, the measured resting energy expenditure exceeded by only 14 per cent the amount predicted by the Harris-

Benedict equation for normal subjects (see Table 103–2). In sepsis complicating surgery or trauma, increases in urinary nitrogen losses as high as 30 per cent per day have been observed. Protein synthesis and metabolism also increase significantly, the former presumably reflecting the efforts by the body to mount hormonal and cellular responses to infection.[11]

Hormonal responses to sepsis or trauma include increases in release of adrenocortical hormones and norepinephrine. Resistance to insulin increases markedly, resulting in continued fat oxidation even when much carbohydrate is given intravenously.[10]

Nutritional Consequences of Conditions Commonly Leading to Vitamin and Mineral Deficiency (Table 104–2)

The causes of deficiency of water and fat-soluble vitamins are not identical to those affecting macronutrients. The difference is explicable by differences in requirements and metabolism. Decreased intake is most important for the water-soluble vitamins, the daily requirement of which is usually a large percentage of the body stores. Cobalamin is the major exception to this generality. The ratio of intake to body stores for folic acid and vitamin C is especially high, and deficiency can rapidly follow diminished intake. Decreased intake of fat-soluble vitamins, on the other hand, is an uncommon cause of deficiency, first, because vitamins D and K are produced endogenously and, second, because the body stores of fat-soluble vitamins in the adult are so large relative to daily intake and requirements. The adipose tissue and liver, in particular, provide very large storage depots for these vitamins.

Dietary deficiency is uncommon for vitamins that are produced endogenously, except for vitamin D. In the case of vitamin D, endogenous synthesis from skin barely provides enough for daily needs (100 to 400 IU). The amount of previtamin converted to vitamin D_3 is limited to 15 to 20 per cent per day, regardless of the amount of light. This limitation is due to photoconversion to other inactive compounds. Therefore, endogenous synthesis alone may not protect against deficiency. The daily production of biotin and vitamin K by intestinal bacteria is considered adequate to meet needs if absorption is satisfactory. Dietary deficiencies of vitamin B_6 and pantothenic acid are rare, and some contribution from intestinal flora is assumed. Vitamin K is absorbed in the colon[12] as well as in the terminal ileum. However, when bile acids are deficient, vitamin K cannot be solubilized and hence is not absorbed.

Malabsorption is a major potential cause of vitamin deficiency. Vitamin A (in the form of retinoic acid), folic acid, and cobalamin undergo enterohepatic circulation; thus, excessive losses are common with malabsorption due to small bowel disease or resection (see pp. 1046–1052). It has been suggested that the loss of bile salts alters hepatic metabolism of vitamin D and leads to the short half-life of the vitamin seen in malabsorption. Decreased hepatic stores of vitamin A and cobalamin are frequent with cirrhosis, since the number of hepatocytes is diminished. This reduction may shorten the time of the onset of deficiency.

All vitamins are needed in larger amounts during pregnancy and growth; folic acid is especially important because of its small body stores. Drug effects can be particularly important in the genesis of vitamin deficiency. Cholestyramine and neomycin may induce bile salt deficiency interfering with fat-soluble vitamin absorption, and cholestyramine may bind vitamin D directly in the gut lumen. Colchicine interferes with release of fat-soluble vitamins from the enterocyte into the circulation. A good example of the interference of drugs with absorption is the effect of the drug sulfasalazine on folic acid metabolism. Sulfasalazine interferes with the absorption and utilization of folate by competitive inhibition in the intestine and other tissues.[13] This can be a contributing factor to malabsorption and malutilization of the vitamin, which leads to subsequent deficiency. Patients with inflammatory bowel disease taking sulfasalazine will often have low serum folate levels. It seems reasonable to treat these patients with 1 mg folic acid daily to prevent folic acid deficiency, even though most patients will not develop folate-responsive anemia.

Alcohol

Because multiple nutritional deficiencies are common in those who use alcohol to excess, some special consideration of the pathogenesis of the nutritional deficiency in alcoholics is deserved. In this analysis, the effects of alcohol itself can be distinguished from the effects of alcohol-induced injury to liver, pancreas, and heart and the secondary effects of these organ impairments on nutritional status.

The schema presented in Table 104–1 on the pathogenetic mechanisms resulting in nutritional deficiency in patients with gastrointestinal disease is entirely applicable to analysis of the effects of excessive alcohol use. As described on page 1976, alcohol, which contains 7 calories per gram, is a potent calorie source, and, in significant doses, is capable of depressing appetite for other foods. In addition, the excessive use of alcohol with or without withdrawal can produce anorexia, nausea, vomiting, and even gastritis. All these factors could contribute to a decreased intake of nutrient containing food, leading eventually to nutrient depletion and deficiency. In high enough doses, alcohol can be shown to interfere with the intestinal absorption of some nutrients. Certainly, chronic alcoholism with attendant malnutrition can result in intestinal abnormalities and malabsorption. Further, when alcoholism leads to disease of the liver or pancreas, maldigestion and malabsorption are common complications which may themselves lead to nutritional deficiency.[14]

Alcohol has many and varied effects on the intestine.[15] It can increase motility, a factor that may be important in the diarrhea of chronic alcoholics. Direct toxic effects on the small intestinal mucosa have been reported. In humans, alcohol may acutely produce hemorrhagic lesions and, after more chronic ingestion, causes ultrastructural abnormalities, especially affecting mitochondria. Alcohol produces major alterations in the brush border membrane, leading to increases in permeability for macromolecules (protein), but decreased uptake of actively transported nutrients, especially glucose and amino acids.[15] Self-limited nonbloody diarrhea is commonly seen in chronic alcoholics after prolonged binges, probably related to rapid intestinal transit. The mild steatorrhea of alcoholics usually is not due to mucosal lesions, but rather to impaired pancreatic function. Fluid and electrolyte absorption is impaired by alcohol in animals, but this has been less well documented in humans. All these effects on nutrient absorption may be worsened by the presence of folate deficiency, which itself leads to structural changes in the enterocyte and mild malabsorption.

The most prevalent vitamin deficiency in alcohol abusers without liver disease is folic acid. Other commonly involved vitamins include B_6, B_1, and B_{12}.[15] The incidence of reduced serum levels is even higher in alcoholics with cirrhosis.

Folate deficiency is the best studied example of vitamin lack in alcoholics. The major causes implicated include (1) decreased intake, (2) decreased absorption, (3) altered tissue utilization, and (4) increased urinary losses.[16, 17] Although many of these same factors may be important in vitamin B_6 deficiency, an additional factor is that cirrhotics metabolize pyridoxal phosphate more rapidly than do normal subjects.[18] Thiamine deficiency in alcoholics is also multifactorial. In addition to decreased intake, impaired active transport of thiamine has been demonstrated.[19] The folate deficiency often found in alcoholics may worsen the malabsorption of thiamine by its direct effect on the enterocyte. When liver disease is present, there is a defect in hepatic thiamine storage and conversion to thiamine pyrophosphate. Severe thiamine deficiency in the presence of acute alcoholism is often overlooked as a cause of lactic acidosis, and rarely, the administration of thiamine can be lifesaving.[20]

The impact of alcohol on nutrient absorption is variable, but in the setting of severely decreased intake of nutrients, serious nutritional deficiency can occur. In fact, chronic alcoholism is among the most common clinical settings for protein-calorie malnutrition and water-soluble vitamin deficiency. Fat-soluble vitamin deficiencies are not so common, with the exception of vitamin A, which requires the liver for its storage and delivery to the peripheral tissues (see pp. 1051–1052). Judging by the incidence of abnormal dark adaptation, subclinical vitamin A deficiency is probably underestimated in alcoholics.[21] Zinc deficiency has been incriminated in this night blindness as well. Subclinical osteopenia is also noted in chronic alcoholics, but the roles of vitamin D or calcium deficiency in this process are not established.[22] It seems likely that hepatic (or pancreatic) abnormalities may be more important than a direct alteration in absorption of these nutrients.

Alcohol use also leads to increased losses of nutrients via both the intestines and the kidneys. Diarrhea and electrolyte losses are commonly associated with chronic alcoholism, bleeding and protein loss are reported, and excessive urinary losses of minerals (especially zinc and magnesium) are well described.

As a depressant drug, alcohol can influence not only alertness, mood, and food intake, but alcohol can also interfere directly with the utilization of nutrients, such as folate in liver and bone marrow. Finally, induction of drug-metabolizing enzyme systems in the liver may result in altered nutrient metabolism including the formation of inactive, inhibitory, or even toxic metabolites.[14]

Cirrhosis

Malabsorption in chronic liver disease is limited to the results of steatorrhea. The steatorrhea is, in turn, due to decreased secretion of bile salts, producing an intraluminal concentration of bile salts that is often below the critical micellar concentration.[23] Reduced micelle formation then leads to decreased lipid absorption. The size of the bile salt pool is also decreased, so that diminished synthesis of bile salts is probably the major cause for reduced secretion. In cholestatic liver disease, obstruction to bile flow may supervene; the most striking malabsorption of lipids occurs in these conditions. Vitamin E deficiency is uncommon, but occurs most often in severe cholestatic disease in children. The progressive neurologic condition presents with areflexia, gait disturbance, decreased proprioceptive and vibratory sensation, and paralysis of gaze. Total serum vitamin E levels may be normal, but the vitamin E total lipid ratio is always low.[24]

Vitamin A and vitamin D deficiencies are seen in chronic liver disease. In some patients with metabolic bone disease and primary biliary cirrhosis, treatment with vitamin D and calcium is not sufficient, despite the expected presence of osteomalacia (see below). Many abnormalities of vitamin D metabolism have been reported in chronic liver disease, including impaired hydroxylation in alcoholics and increased urinary excretion of metabolites in primary biliary cirrhosis.[25, 39]

Postgastrectomy

Weight loss is commonly due to decreased intake, which, in turn, is caused by early satiety or avoidance of symptoms of "dumping" or postprandial diarrhea. Steatorrhea, when it occurs, is usually mild. Sometimes the altered emptying pattern unmasks a subclinical intestinal syndrome, such as lactose intolerance or celiac sprue. The metabolic consequences are quite common and troublesome. Anemia is due to iron deficiency at the earliest times, in part from blood loss, and in part from iron malabsorption. The malabsorption may be related to reduced liberation of food-bound iron, decreased reduction of (nonheme) Fe^{3+} to Fe^{2+}, and bypass of the proximal duodenum, the site of most active iron absorption (see pp. 972–974).

Folate deficiency may occur from inadequate intake. Cobalamin deficiency is uncommon, unless the entire parietal cell region (body) of the stomach has been removed. Metabolic bone disease occurs late (10 to 20 years) after surgery and seems to be due to avoidance of mild products as a source of calcium and vitamin D, bypass of the duodenum as a site of calcium absorption, and rapid intestinal transit.[26]

RECOGNITION OF NUTRITIONAL DEFICIENCY

While taking the patient's history and performing the physical examination, the physician must be aware of the manifestations of the various nutritional disorders for which the patient with disease is at risk. A detailed discussion of the syndromes associated with macronutrient and micronutrient deficiencies is beyond the scope of this text. A summary of malnutrition syndromes is presented in Table 104–4. Because of their clinical importance, or the special challenges they present in management, we will discuss certain nutritional complications of gastrointestinal disease in more detail.

Table 104–4. MALNUTRITION SYNDROMES

Nutrient	Deficiency Syndrome
Calories (energy)	Weight loss, loss of subcutaneous fat, muscle wasting, growth retardation
Protein	Muscle wasting, edema, skin and hair changes, dyspigmentation, hepatomegaly
Essential fatty acid	Scaly, eczematoid skin rash on face and extremities, hepatomegaly
Calcium	Tetany, convulsions, growth failure
Phosphorus	Weakness, osteomalacia
Magnesium	Weakness, tremor, tetany
Iron	Pallor, anemia, weakness, lingual atrophy, koilonychia
Zinc	Hypogeusia, acrodermatitis, slow wound healing, growth failure, hypogonadism—delayed puberty
Copper	Bone marrow suppression
Chromium	Glucose intolerance
Thiamine	Beriberi, muscle weakness, hypesthesia, tachycardia, heart failure
Riboflavin	Angular stomatitis, cheilosis, corneal vascularization, dermatoses
Niacin	Pellagra, glossitis, dermatosis, dementia, diarrhea
Vitamin B_6	Nasolabial seborrhea, peripheral neuropathy
Biotin	Organic aciduria
Folic acid	Macrocytosis, megaloblastic anemia, glossitis
Vitamin B_{12}	Megoblastic anemia, paresthesias, mental changes, combined system degeneration
Vitamin A	Xerophthalmia, hyperkeratosis of skin, night blindness
Vitamin D	Rickets and growth failure in children, osteomalacia in adults
Vitamin K	Bleeding, ecchymoses
Vitamin E	Cerebellar ataxia, areflexia

From Alpers, D. H., Clouse, R. E., and Stenson, W. F. Manual of Clinical Therapeutics. 2nd ed. Boston, Little, Brown and Co., in press, 1987. Used by permission.

Protein-Energy Malnutrition

One of the most common presenting complaints of patients with gastrointestinal disorders is weight loss. Loss of body weight reflects a negative energy balance in which expenditure exceeds intake. Rarely, however, one sees pure energy malnutrition in the clinical setting. Whenever energy intake is inadequate to meet body needs, the metabolic responses described on pages 1974 to 1976 result in a loss of both body protein and stored fat. The term *protein-energy malnutrition* or *protein-calorie malnutrition* refers to those conditions in which energy and protein imbalance have been present long enough to result in structural and functional changes in the patient. When the stress of acute disease is superimposed on more chronic undernutrition, overt clinical manifestations can be anticipated.

The clinical features depend upon the age of onset and the severity of the deficiency. The classic syndromes of kwashiorkor and marasmus are seen in infancy up to the first two to three years of life. Growth retardation is the most prominent clinical manifestation of protein-energy deficiencies in childhood.[27, 28] Mild to moderate deficiencies in children decrease physical and mental activity, appetite, and resistance to common infections and cause diarrhea. In adults, in whom protein requirements for growth are not present, the findings reflect calorie insufficiency—loss of adipose tissue, decrease in skin turgor, weakness, and fatigue. Clinically, reduction of 10 to 20 per cent of ideal or usual body weight usually indicates mild protein-energy malnutrition. Reduction of 20 to 30 per cent of ideal body weight indicates moderate protein-energy malnutrition, and a 30 per cent or greater reduction suggests severe protein-energy malnutrition. In cases of moderate malnutrition there may be evident loss of lean body (skeletal) mass. In severe protein depletion there may be peripheral edema; changes in color and texture of hair, skin, and nails; and fatty liver, which may be reflected by hepatomegaly and elevations of liver enzymes.

Severe protein-calorie malnutrition can result in suppression of immune-responsiveness.[29] The reactions to skin tests of delayed hypersensitivity in the severely debilitated patient are often uniformly negative, indicating anergy; however, the usefulness of these tests in detecting or quantifying protein-calorie malnutrition is quite limited. (The use of anthropometric and laboratory tests to diagnose and identify the severity of calorie-protein malnutrition is discussed on pages 2009 to 2010.)

Vitamin and Mineral Deficiency

Clinical manifestations of micronutrient deficiency are late consequences (Table 104–5). Blood levels of water-soluble vitamins fall relatively early in the course of this deficiency because a major fraction of the body stores is in the blood. With the exception of iron, for

Table 104–5. STAGES OF WATER-SOLUBLE VITAMIN DEFICIENCY

Subclinical Deficiency
1. Lowered plasma levels
2. Lowered cell content
3. Decreased apoenzyme activity
   a. Responsive to coenzyme addition
   b. Altered response to challenge

Clinical Deficiency
4. Functional impairment
   a. On challenge
   b. Spontaneous
5. Tissue organ changes
   a. Reversible
   b. Irreversible

which blood also constitutes a major storage compartment, the correlation between blood levels and body stores is poor for fat-soluble vitamins and the other minerals. Vitamins A and D are carried in the blood by specific binding proteins, and vitamin E is carried in lipoprotein particles. Alterations in levels of these binding proteins could also lead to an erroneous estimate of plasma levels. For the minerals calcium, phosphorus, magnesium, and fluoride, the bone is the major site of body stores, and this site is not in rapid equilibrium with the blood. For some minerals (sodium, potassium, calcium), many compensatory mechanisms exist to maintain blood levels within the normal range. These mechanisms are not, however, designed to regulate body stores but, rather, to regulate extracellular fluid concentrations. Therefore, the use of blood levels to assess deficiency of most minerals is inaccurate.

Another important distinction should be made between tests that correlate with recent dietary intake and those that correlate with body stores. The first group provides information about recent events, while the latter is better for determining the chronic status of any micronutrient. A discussion of these tests follows.

Vitamins

Some tests for assessing intake or absorption and body stores of vitamins commonly deficient in gastrointestinal diseases are listed in Table 104–6.[30–35] Although serum folate levels are widely used to determine folic acid deficiency, this measurement is most sensitive to changes in dietary folate intake. A low serum level can reflect only low recent intake and may not reflect decreased tissue stores. Frequently, low levels reflecting decreased recent intake are further depressed when body stores are depleted. Thus, the red blood cell folate is a more accurate indication of tissue stores than is the serum level, being less variable and reflecting the folate present in the system at the time of red blood cell formation.[30]

No reliable method measures intake of cobalamin, but the Schilling test accurately reflects absorption. The use of simultaneous isotope administration allows the test to be performed in one 24-hour period (see pp. 275–276). The problems with the test involve the collection of urine and the intertest variability. The latter can be as great as 30 to 50 per cent, although the use of ratios with two isotopes (free ^{57}Co-B_{12} and ^{58}Co-B_{12} bound to intrinsic factor) diminishes it somewhat. Because of unexplained variability in results of the double labeled test, the one-stage test is still recommended.[37] It is a mistake to attach too much importance to an arbitrary normal lower limit of 8 per cent excretion. Serum vitamin B_{12} levels usually correlate with body stores, but the latter may not reflect the metabolic state of cobalamin, since up to 75 per cent of strict vegetarians have low serum cobalamin levels without evidence of deficiency.[36] It is likely, however, that these patients will develop deficiency with continued inadequate intake. One third of patients with folate deficiency have low serum vitamin B_{12} levels, although the reasons are not clear. Finally, since some serum vitamin B_{12} radioimmunoassays detect cobalamin analogs as well as cobalamin, a normal vitamin B_{12} level may not rule out true deficiency.[37]

Table 104–6. TESTS FOR COMMON VITAMIN DEFICIENCIES IN GASTROINTESTINAL DISEASE

Vitamin	Test	Values Reflecting Decreased Absorption or Recent Intake	Test	Values Reflecting Decreased Body Stores	Reference
Folic acid	Serum folate	3–5.9 ng/ml	Serum folate	<3 ng/ml	30
	Red blood cell folate	140–160 ng/ml	Red blood cell folate	<140 ng/ml	
			Bone marrow	Megaloblasts	
			Peripheral blood smear	Multilobed polymorphonuclear cells	
Cobalamin	24-hour urinary excretion of ^{57}Co B_{12} (Schilling test)	<8%			31
	Double-labeled Schilling test (^{57}Co, ^{58}Co-IF)	ratio of ^{58}Co/^{57}Co <1.7	Serum B_{12}	<20 pg/ml	32
	Serum B_{12}	120–200 pg/ml	Bone marrow	Megaloblasts	
Vitamin A	Plasma vitamin A	10–19 gm/dl	Plasma vitamin A	<10 gm/dl	33
Vitamin D	Plasma 25 (OH) D	<15 ng/ml	Plasma 25 (OH) D	<10 ng/ml	34
			24-hour urinary calcium	<100 mg/day	
Vitamin K			Prothrombin time	Sample/control ratio <0.88 or >1.12	

Carotene is not stored in the body. Thus, persons with only preformed vitamin A in the diet will have vitamin A in their serum without much carotene. Both carotene and vitamin A intakes are reflected in their serum levels. However, since vitamin A is stored in the liver in large amounts, the serum level is replenished endogenously. Nonetheless, with chronic low intake, the vitamin A level falls, reflecting both low intake and marginal body stores. With continued low intake, levels fall further and reflect decreased body stores. Low carotene levels are meaningful only if carotene is being ingested in the diet, i.e., low levels do not distinguish low intake from poor absorption. Samples should be obtained while the patient is fasting to avoid the fluctuations following meals. Low vitamin A levels can be unrelated to decreased intake or absorption, as in chronic infection and chronic liver disease, owing to decreases in retinol binding protein (see pp. 1051–1052).

Since vitamin K stimulates production of clotting Factors II, VII, IX, and X in the liver, the one-stage prothrombin time is used to assess its presence indirectly. Under the usual conditions of the test, all the clotting factors tested except for Factor V are responsive to vitamin K (II, VII, X). The level of Factor VII is the usual rate-limiting factor. Factor V has a longer half-life than the vitamin K-dependent proteins and is not usually rate-limiting in the reaction. The prothrombin time is not specific for vitamin K deficiency. Prothrombin time may also be prolonged in liver disease, including severe passive congestion of the liver, and in the presence of intravascular coagulation. If parenteral administration of vitamin K (5 to 10 mg) restores the prothrombin time to normal, deficiency of vitamin K becomes evident. Recently, a more sensitive assay of vitamin K status has been proposed based upon measurement of incompletely carboxylated prothrombin reflecting subnormal vitamin K effect.[38]

Vitamin D Deficiency and Metabolic Bone Disease

Osteoporosis and *osteomalacia* are both forms of metabolic bone disease that may complicate gastrointestinal or hepatobiliary disorders.[39]

Osteoporosis, defined histologically as a diminution in trabecular bone mass, is a condition of uncertain etiology in which nutritional, hormonal, and metabolic factors play a contributory role. Osteoporosis may be the result of long-standing negative calcium balance related to deficient calcium absorption or intake, or to factors that increase calcium excretion in the urine. The state of knowledge is not adequate at present to clearly define methods of prevention or to reverse osteoporosis dependably. Osteomalacia, characterized by defective mineralization of bone matrix, is more clearly a nutritional defect. It is related most commonly to inadequate intake, absorption, or utilization of vitamin D, calcium, phosphate, or some combination of these nutrients. Our attention here will be directed to osteomalacia as a form of metabolic bone disease that is both preventable and treatable.

The conditions in which vitamin D deficiency and osteomalacia have been reported and the major elements in the pathogenesis of vitamin D deficiency are listed in Table 104–7. Newer insights into the activation of vitamin D in the liver and then in the kidney to the active dihydroxy forms are described on pages 1052 to 1053. Such knowledge has led to a better understanding of the pathogenesis of vitamin D deficiency as well as to development of new pharmaceutical forms of vitamin D for treatment (see pp. 2002–2003). Gastrointestinal and hepatobiliary disorders could obviously alter the sequence of vitamin D metabolism at several steps: inadequate dietary intake of vitamin D caused by anorexia, early satiety, or other factors; malabsorption of vitamin D secondary to intestinal disease or intraluminal bile salt deficiency; impaired 25-hydroxylase activity in hepatic disorders; hepatic metabolism to inactive metabolites of vitamin D; increased degradation of active forms; or end-organ unresponsiveness, such as failure of severely diseased small intestine in celiac sprue to respond to the appropriate concentrations of 1,25-dihydroxy vitamin D.

How can the clinician diagnose vitamin D deficiency and osteomalacia? Some patients will have clinical osteomalacia manifested by bone pain and a pattern of depressed calcium and phosphorus and elevated alkaline phosphatase. Classic clinical osteomalacia occurs in only a minority of patients with histologic evidence of disease. Standard radiologic techniques require a 50 per cent loss of bone mineral before abnormalities can be detected and, unless specific findings such as Looser's zones are noted, do not identify the cause of the osteopenia. What methods are available for further investigation of patients with clinically silent osteomalacia? More sophisticated measurements of skeletal mineralization, such as computed tomography and dual photon absorptiometry are sensitive and increasingly available but contribute little to etiologic evaluation of osteopenia.[40] These techniques are good predictors of vertebral fracture and can be useful for screening patients at risk for vitamin

Table 104–7. OSTEOMALACIA IN GASTROINTESTINAL DISEASE

Disease	Probable Causes of Deficiency
Postgastrectomy	↓ Intake, malabsorption of vitamin D
Cholestatic liver disease (primary biliary cirrhosis biliary atresia, sclerosing cholangitis)	Malabsorption of vitamin D, cholestyramine binding of vitamin D, diminished hepatic hydroxylation, and increased urinary loss of vitamin D
Cirrhosis	Malabsorption, diminished hydroxylation, increased urinary excretion of vitamin D
Pancreatic insufficiency	Steatorrhea and vitamin D and calcium malabsorption
Celiac sprue	Malabsorption of vitamin D, Ca
Short bowel or ileal resection or bypass (e.g., Crohn's)	Malabsorption of vitamin D and Ca, ? phosphate depletion
Long-term total parenteral nutrition	? ↓ phosphate provision (<600 mg/day)

D deficiency. Their value in screening postmenopausal women for osteoporosis is much less clear.[41] Competitive binding assays for measurement of serum 25-hydroxy vitamin D [25(OH)D] give reproducible results, but correlation with the degree of histologic osteomalacia is uncertain.

Production of 25(OH)D is not closely regulated; that is, the plasma level tends to rise or fall as its precursor is made available. The 25(OH)D in plasma is bound to a binding protein that binds all metabolites, that is only 5 per cent saturated, and that has a plasma half-life of 15 to 30 days. Thus, some vitamin D entering the body is converted to 25(OH)D even if body stores or recent intake are high. The plasma capacity for excess 25(OH)D is very great, and levels rise as intake increases. Moreover, levels remain elevated for some time. Therefore, 25(OH)D levels reflect vitamin D intake or production only in a general way and do not correlate with body stores until these are quite deficient. Levels rise in summer and fall in winter. Pregnancy and use of oral contraceptives increase the vitamin D-binding protein levels. Despite these problems, the 25(OH)D level is the best available test for determining vitamin D status.[27] A low level is almost always found when deficiency is present. The urinary excretion of calcium is a functional assay for vitamin D, but it is not specific and is itself subject to many factors that confuse the interpretation of the test (see pp. 1052–1053.). Nonetheless, the combination of a low 25(OH)D level and decreased urinary calcium is good evidence for vitamin D deficiency.

A definitive diagnosis of osteomalacia can be made only by histologic examination of bone.[42] Bone biopsy can be performed as a simple outpatient procedure under local anesthesia by use of a Bordier needle. Quantitative histometric analysis of undecalcified sections, after special staining and tetracycline labeling of the calcification front, allows accurate distinction of osteomalacia from other bone diseases, such as steroid-induced osteoporosis.[42] Practitioners who suspect osteomalacia in patients with digestive disorders may consider obtaining the benefit of these newer techniques at one of an increasing number of centers where they are available.

Therapy for Osteomalacia. Oral vitamin D maintains vitamin D status less well than endogenous vitamin from skin, which maintains a more constant release and a lower rate of metabolism. Nonetheless, sometimes the most logical approach to therapy is administration of vitamin D to maintain normal serum 25(OH)D levels. The amount of vitamin D required varies greatly from patient to patient. Most patients will respond to oral doses of between 4000 and 12,000 IU, although a rare individual who requires intramuscular administration may be encountered. Therapy with 25(OH)D in an oral dose of 20 to 50 μg per day or $1,25(OH)_2$ vitamin D(0.25 to 0.5 μg per day) shows promise for correction of osteomalacia in hepatic disease, whether malabsorption of or conversion to 25(OH)D, or both, are impaired. Both hydroxylated forms are absorbed in preference to vitamin D in the presence of bile salt depletion. During vitamin D therapy, serum and urinary calcium levels should be monitored regularly to avoid toxic effects of this vitamin, although such toxicity rarely occurs when malabsorption is the underlying illness.

Minerals

The best available tests for assessing intake or absorption and body stores of minerals commonly deficient in gastrointestinal diseases are listed in Table 104–8.[6, 42–49] Serum iron is largely bound to transferrin. At any given time there is 4 to 6 mg of transferrin-bound iron in plasma. However, 25 mg of iron passes each day from the reticuloendothelial cells to the plasma, where it is turned over at a rate of 50 per cent in one hour. Therefore, the measurement of serum iron is inherently unstable. A diurnal variation is seen with higher morning values. Transferrin levels are

Table 104–8. TESTS FOR COMMON MINERAL DEFICIENCIES IN GASTROINTESTINAL DISEASE

Mineral	Test	Values Reflecting Decreased Recent Intake or Absorption	Values Refecting Decreased Body Stores		Reference
Iron	Serum iron		<50 g/dl		42
	Serum iron-binding capacity		<15%		
	Hemoglobin		<14 gm/dl M <12 gm/dl F		
	Serum ferritin		<15 ng/ml M <10 ng/ml F		43
	Marrow iron staining		Decreased		44
Calcium	24-hour urinary excretion	<2 mg/kg/day or <150 mg/day			7
	Ionized serum calcium		<4 mg/dl		45
	Dual-photon absorptiometry		<1 gm/cm²	for vertebral fracture	46
	Quantitative CT scanning		<110 mg/cm³	for vertebral fracture	47
Magnesium	Serum magnesium	<1.5 mEq/L	<1.5 mEq/L		48
	24-hr urinary excretion	<1.3 mM/24h			49
Zinc	Plasma zinc		<100 gm/dl		6
	Hair and nail zinc	<70 ppm			

increased in iron deficiency and in pregnancy even in the absence of iron deficiency. However, transferrin levels are decreased by chronic disease, protein deficiency, or hepatic impairment. Therefore, interpretation of iron-binding capacity is often inconclusive. Serum ferritin levels are proportional to marrow iron. Levels of less than 15 ng/ml for males and 10 ng/ml for females are associated with iron deficiency and decreased stores in adults. Acute liver damage or endogenous ferritin from tumors will raise ferritin levels without changing body stores. Cell damage from inflammatory diseases will also give a falsely high value. Marrow staining is qualitative but separates iron deficiency from other conditions in which serum measurements can be complicated by the presence of chronic disease or increased release of iron from the tissues. However, variation among observers is high, and the visual assessment of stained iron is better for increased stores than for decreased ones. Unfortunately, the absence of visible staining is not always equated with depleted stores, the question for which the test is most commonly performed.

Urinary calcium may correspond to absorption when the intake is constant and subjects are in perfect balance. However, with high protein intake, bone resorption, or renal leak, urinary calcium can vary independently of absorption. It is important to assess urinary excretion only after three or four days on a constant intake after withholding drugs that alter urinary calcium (e.g., thiazides). However, when malabsorption or low intake is present, the urinary excretion does not correlate precisely with the degree of malabsorption. Urinary excretion is maintained to some extent by mobilization of calcium from bone. At levels of absorption and excretion exceeding 2 mg per kg of body weight, urinary calcium equals absorption. However, there is overlap in the low range of normal, so that low values should not be interpreted too rigorously. Plasma ionized calcium may be low when deficiency is severe, but this is a late occurrence. In early or moderate deficiency the normal compensatory mechanisms (parathormone, vitamin D) serve to maintain serum calcium levels in a normal range. Although not a sensitive indicator of calcium deficiency alone, bone densitometry can detect a decrease in bone mass of greater than 10 per cent. Measurement of low density defines low mass but does not identify its cause. Moreover, altered bone mass may be patchy and can be missed unless the appropriate bone is tested. Vertebral fractures are most often seen with osteopenia accompanying gastrointestinal disease, and for these bones the fracture limits have been reasonably well defined.[46, 47] However, density below a certain level identifies the group at risk, but it does not predict the inevitability of fracture or its timing if it occurs.

Serum magnesium values do not correlate linearly with body stores, but a level below 1.5 mEq/L often means that the body stores are reduced. Low values can mean malabsorption, reduced intake, or reduced renal tubular reabsorption or can reflect low serum albumin, to which most magnesium is bound. Moreover, a normal value does not rule out magnesium deficiency, since serum magnesium values are probably dependent upon the action of parathormone and calcitonin. The urinary excretion of magnesium depends upon the intake, absorption, and body stores. When magnesium balance is in equilibrium, and stores are normal, urinary magnesium reflects net absorption, as in the case of calcium.[49] When magnesium stores are depleted, low urine magnesium results from compensatory renal conservation.

Zinc Deficiency

During the past decade, zinc deficiency has been recognized in a number of conditions affecting the gastrointestinal tract.[6, 50] Given the essential role of this trace metal in cell division, protein synthesis, wound healing, lymphocyte function, and testicular and prostatic function as well as a putative role for olfaction and taste, it is not surprising that severe deficiency may give rise to a spectrum of clinical manifestations. Because zinc is present in meats and fish in a highly available form and in most vegetables in a somewhat less absorbable form, dietary deficiency in healthy individuals is uncommon. When deficiency occurs, it is usually a reflection of inadequate absorption or, more commonly, excessive excretion.

When chronic zinc depletion occurs before puberty, particularly in association with multiple nutritional deficiencies including protein and iron malnutrition, a syndrome of growth retardation and hypogonadism is responsive to zinc therapy.[51]

In adults, zinc deficiency may present as a defect in taste or smell, as impaired healing of wounds, and, when more advanced, with characteristic skin lesions. Skin lesions are best characterized in a disorder called acrodermatitis enteropathica, which is related to a genetic defect in zinc absorption. The dermatitis is characterized by epidermal thickening with ulcerations around the body orifices and by thickening and increased pigmentation at the joint creases of the hands and feet. Pustules and vesicular, bullous, seborrheic, or acneiform rashes have been reported. Alopecia, confusion, apathy, and depression have been documented.[52] Similar lesions have been observed in patients treated with total parenteral nutrition without zinc. Patients with Crohn's disease can show low plasma zinc levels,[53] or increased zinc loss in diarrheal fluid,[54] particularly in patients with short bowel syndrome. Diarrheal fluid can contain more than 10 mg of zinc per liter. Thus, the severity of diarrhea can be a good indicator of the risk of zinc depletion in patients with Crohn's disease and other gastrointestinal problems.

At present, zinc deficiency is reliably documented best by symptomatic response to zinc treatment, because the plasma zinc level frequently is misleading. About 80 per cent of zinc in blood is in red blood cells. Thus, minor degrees of hemolysis alter plasma zinc. Hypo- or hyperproteinemia, regardless of cause, affects plasma zinc levels. Drugs may alter zinc binding to plasma proteins. Although normal plasma levels do not rule out deficiency, low levels may indicate deficiency when unaccompanied by hypoproteinemia, acute stress, or polypharmacy.

Documentation of decreased hair zinc may be present in deficiency even before skin lesions occur. However, the problem of external contamination of samples is sufficiently great that this test cannot be used routinely. Other clinical effects of zinc deficiency are negative nitrogen balance in the presence of adequate replacement,[54] a decrease in chemotaxis and leukocytes, diminished lymphocyte function resulting in defective cell-mediated immunity, and abnormalities in wound healing.

Mild and moderate zinc deficiency can be treated by the oral administration of zinc sulfate in doses of 30 to 60 mg of elemental zinc. Severe zinc deficiency with acrodermatitis, diminished response to infection, or poor wound healing, particularly in the face of continuing increased losses in diarrheal fluid or fistula drainage, will usually require intravenous repletion. Although 3 mg of zinc intravenously per day appears to be adequate for maintenance, as much as three to four times that amount may be required to maintain zinc balance in the presence of very rapid losses.

References

1. Kelts, D. G., Grand, R. O., Sher, G., et al. Nutritional basis of growth failure in children and adolescents with Crohn's disease. Gastroenterology *76*:720, 1979.
2. Clark, M. C. Role of nutrition in inflammatory bowel disease: an overview. Gut *27*:51, 72, 1985.
3. Sanderson, I. R., and Walker-Smith, J. A. Crohn's disease in childhood. Br. J. Surg. *72*:587, 1985.
4. Levi, A. J. Diet in the management of Crohn's disease. Gut *26*:985, 1985.
5. Beeken, W., Busch, H. J., and Sylvester, D. L. Intestinal protein loss in Crohn's disease. Digestion *16*:87, 1977.
6. Karcioglu, Z. A., and Sarper, R. M. (eds.). Zinc and Copper in Medicine. Springfield, Illinois, Charles C Thomas, Publisher, 1980.
7. Nordin, B. E. C. (ed.). Calcium, Phosphate, and Magnesium Metabolism. Edinburgh, Churchill Livingstone, 1976.
8. Munro, H. N. A general survey of pathological changes in protein metabolism. *In* Munro, H. N., and Allison, J. B. (eds.). Mammalian Protein Metabolism. New York, Academic Press, 1964, p. 267.
9. Beisel, W. R., Sawyer, W. D., Ryall, E. D., and Crozier, D. Metabolic effects of intracellular infections in man. Ann. Intern. Med. *67*:744, 1967.
10. Askanazi, J., Carpentier, Y. A., Elwyn, D. H., et al. Influence of total parenteral nutrition on fuel utilization in injury and sepsis. Ann. Surg. *191*:40, 1980.
11. Jeejeebhoy, K. N. Protein nutrition in clinical practice. Br. Med. Bull. *37*:11, 1981.
12. Hollander, D. Intestinal absorption of vitamin A, E, D, and K. J. Lab. Clin. Med. *97*:449, 1981.
13. Franklin, J. L., and Rosenberg, I. H. Impaired folic acid absorption in inflammatory bowel disease: effects of salicylazosulfapyridine (Azulfidine). Gastroenterology *64*:517, 1973.
14. Lieber, C. S. Medical disorders of alcoholism: pathogenesis and treatment. Major Probl. Intern. Med. *22*:381, 1982.
15. Wilson, F. A., and Hoyumpa, A. M. Ethanol and small intestinal transport. Gastroenterology *76*:388, 1979.
16. Russell, R. M., Rosenberg, I. H., Wilson, P. D., et al. Increased urinary excretion and diminished turnover of folic acid due to ethanol ingestion. Am. J. Clin. Nutr. *38*:64–70, 1983.
17. Weir, D. G., McGing, P. G., and Scott, J. M. Folate metabolism, the enterohepatic circulation, and alcohol. Biochem. Pharm. *34*:1, 1985.
18. Henderson, J. M., Codner, M. A., Holleris, B., et al. The fasting B_6 vitamin profile and response to a pyridoxine load in normal and cirrhotic subjects. Hepatology *6*:464, 1986.
19. Hoyumpa, A. M., Nichols, S. G., and Schenker, S. Intestinal thiamin transport: effect of chronic ethanol in rats. Am. J. Nutr. *31*:938, 1978.
20. Campbell, C. H. The severe lactic acidosis of thiamin deficiency: acute pernicious or fulminating beriberi. Lancet *2*:446, 1984.
21. Russell, R. M. Vitamin A and zinc metabolism in alcoholism. Am. J. Nutr. *33*:2741, 1980.
22. Bikle, D. D., Genant, H. K., Cann, C., et al. Bone disease in alcohol abuse. Ann. Intern. Med. *103*:42, 1985.
23. Lanspa, S. J., Cahn, A. T. V., Bell, J. S., III, et al. Pathogenesis of steatorrhea in primary biliary cirrhosis. Hepatology *5*:837, 1985.
24. Sokol, R. J., Heubi, J. E., Iannaccone, S. T., et al. Vitamin E deficiency with normal serum vitamin E concentrations in children with chronic cholestasis. N. Engl. J. Med. *310*:1209, 1984.
25. Mawer, E. B., Klass, H. J., Warnes, T. W., and Berry, J. L. Metabolism of vitamin D in patients with primary biliary cirrhosis and alcoholic liver disease. Clin. Sci. *69*:561, 1985.
26. Editorial. Osteomalacia after gastrectomy. Lancet *1*:77, 1986.
27. Alpers, D. H., Clouse, R. E., and Stenson, W. F. Manual of Nutritional Therapeutics. 2nd Ed. Boston, Little, Brown and Co., 1988.
28. Kirschner, B. S., Voinchet, O., and Rosenberg, I. H. Growth retardation in inflammatory bowel disease. Gastroenterology *75*:504, 1978.
29. Dowd, T. S., and Heatley, R. V. The influence of undernutrition on immunity. Clin. Sci. *66*:241, 1984.
30. Davis, R. E. Clinical chemistry of folic acid. Adv. Clin. Chem. *25*:235, 1986.
31. Fairbanks, V. F., Wahner, H. W., and Phyliky, R. C. Tests for pernicious anemia: the "Schilling test." Mayo Clin. Proc. *58*:541, 1983.
32. Lee, D. S. C., and Griffiths, B. W. Human serum vitamin B_{12} assay methods—a review. Clin. Biochem. *18*:261, 1985.
33. Sauberlich, H. E., Skala, J. H., and Dowdy, R. P. Laboratory Tests for the Assessment of Nutritional Status. Cleveland, CRC Press, 1974.
34. Horst, R. L. Recent advances in the quantitation of vitamin D and vitamin D metabolites. *In* R. Kumar, R. (ed.): Vitamin D: Bone and Clinical Aspects. Boston, Martinus Nijhoff, 1984. pp. 423–478.
35. Russell, R. M., Krasinski, S. D., and Dawson-Hughes B. Indices of fat soluble vitamin states. Clin. Nutr. *3*:161, 1984.
36. Chanarin, I. The Megaloblastic Anemias. Oxford, Blackwell, 1968.
37. Kolhouse, J. F., Kondo, H., Allen, N. C., et al. Cobalamin analogues are present in human plasma and can mask cobalamin deficiency because current radioisotope dilution assays are not specific for true cobalamin. N. Engl. J. Med. *299*:785, 1978.
38. Krasinski, S. D., Russell, R. M., Furie, B. C., et al. The prevalence of vitamin K deficiency in chronic gastrointestinal disorders. Am. J. Clin. Nutr. *41*:639, 1985.
39. Meredith, S. C., and Rosenberg, I. H. Gastrointestinal-hepatic disorders and osteomalacia. Clin. Endocrinol. Metab. *9*:131, 1980.
40. Health and Public Policy Committee, American College of Physicians. Radiologic methods to evaluate bone mineral content. Ann. Intern. Med. *100*:908, 1984.
41. Cummings, S. R., and Black, D. Should perimenopausal women be screened for osteoporosis? Ann. Intern. Med. *104*:817, 1986.
42. Teitelbaum, S. L. Osteoporosis and bone biopsy. *In* Avioli, L. V. (ed.): The Osteoporotic Syndrome: Detection, Prevention, and Treatment. New York, Grune & Stratton, 1983, pp. 115–122.
43. Cook, J. D. (ed.). Iron Deficiency. Edinburgh, Churchill Livingstone, 1980.
43. Worwood, M. Serum ferritin. *In* Jacobs, A., and Worwood, M. (eds.): Iron in Biochemistry and Medicine. New York, Academic Press, 1980, pp. 203–244.

44. Carill, J., Jacobs, A., and Worwood, M. Diagnostic methods for iron status. Ann. Clin. Biochem. *23*:168, 1986.
45. Vanstapel, F. H. J., and Lissens, W. D. Free ionized calcium—a critical survey. Ann. Clin. Biochem. *21*:339, 1984.
46. Riggs, B. L., Wahner, H. W., Seeman, E., et al. Changes in bone mineral density of the proximal femur and spine with aging: differences between the postmenopausal and senile osteoporosis syndromes. J. Clin. Invest. *70*:716, 1982.
47. Cann, C. E., Genant, H. K., Kolb, F. O., and Ettinger, B. Quantitative computed tomography for prediction of vertebral fracture risk. Bone *6*:1, 1985.
48. Wacker, W. E. C. Magnesium and Man. Cambridge, Harvard University Press, 1980.
49. Hassov, I., Hasselblad, C., Fastn, S., et al. Magnesium deficiency after ileal resection for Crohn's disease. Scand. J. Gastroenterol. *18*:643, 1983.
50. Underwood, E. J. (ed.). Trace Elements in Human and Animal Nutrition. Ed. 4. New York, Academic Press, 1977.
51. Prasad, A. S., Mirale, A., Jr., Farid, Z., et al. Zinc metabolism in patients with the syndrome of iron deficiency anemia, hepatosplenomegaly, dwarfism and hypogonadism. J. Lab. Clin. Med. *61*:923, 1963.
52. Prasad, A. S. Clinical manifestations of zinc deficiency. Ann. Rev. Nutr. *5*:341, 1985.
53. Solomons, N. W., Rosenberg, I. H., Sandstead, H. H., and Vokhactu, K. P. Zinc deficiency in Crohn's disease. Digestion *16*:87, 1977.
54. Wolman, S. L., Anderson, G. H., Marliss, E. B., and Jeejeebhoy, K. N. Zinc in total parenteral nutrition. Requirements and metabolic effects. Gastroenterology *76*:458, 1979.

105 Dietary Management and Vitamin-Mineral Replacement Therapy

DAVID H. ALPERS

Many diets useful in the treatment of intestinal diseases involve *restriction* of a particular element, for example, fat or lactose. In those cases, care must be taken to ensure that the diet offered is balanced for all major required macro- and micronutrients and meets the estimated caloric and protein needs of the patient. Sometimes supplements must be added to a restrictive diet (e.g., calcium to a low-lactose diet). Other diets alter either the *consistency* of the diet or the *content* of indigestible residue or fiber. These diets do not change the availability of required nutrients in a major way but do have a useful role as treatment of certain intestinal disorders. Useful source books containing specific information on diets are available.[1–4]

Treatment of nutritional deficiencies in most gastrointestinal disorders depends upon the underlying mechanism of the disease. Although some diseases are characterized by increased caloric utilization (e.g., inflammatory bowel disease), most gastrointestinal disorders are characterized either by decreased nutrient intake or by decreased absorption. The problems presented by fat, carbohydrate, or protein malabsorption differ somewhat and are discussed separately. Various disorders associated with altered passage of nutrients through the intestine (e.g., partial obstruction, bypass) lead to problems with intake or absorption of food that can be managed in part by diet. Gastrointestinal disorders commonly lead to deficiency in only certain of the vitamins and minerals. Recognition of these common patterns is useful in dealing with patients who have these chronic disorders. Finally, the role of dietary fiber in the management of intestinal disorders will be discussed.

DISORDERS CHARACTERIZED BY MALABSORPTION OF FAT

Symptomatic Therapy

Low-Fat Diet

Steatorrhea from any cause will diminish when the triglyceride intake is decreased. Diarrhea will also abate, since part of the pathogenesis of diarrhea with steatorrhea is the formation of hydroxy fatty acids in the colon. If fewer fatty acids reach the colon, diarrhea will diminish, and colonic absorption of products of bacterial fermentation will increase. The low-fat (triglyceride) diet is richer in the other caloric sources, especially carbohydrate. The high carbohydrate intake may, however, exacerbate diarrhea if the patient is also unable to absorb carbohydrates.

Many patients complain that fatty foods cause a variety of intestinal symptoms. It is usually sufficient to have these patients avoid fried foods and very fatty meals. Since ingestion of fat is usually not specifically related to the symptoms of cholecystitis, ulcer, irritable bowel syndrome, and so forth, a low-fat diet is usually not indicated. Fat is not unique in stimulating motility; ingestion of protein itself is a potent stimulus for intestinal and gastric motility. Hence, fat need not be singled out for restriction in patients with nonspecific symptoms.

The presence of lipid (and possibly protein as well) in the ileum appears to activate a mechanism that delays transit of a meal through the stomach and small intestine and produces satiety and diminished food intake.[5] Although it is possible that the decreased food intake seen after jejunoileal bypass[6] may be related to this mechanism, fat restriction is indicated in this clinical setting for steatorrhea. The clinical importance of this ileal "brake" is not clear.

Low-fat diets are used to control symptoms and not to reverse abnormal physiology. The best approach is first to determine the usual fat intake of the patient. If this exceeds 100 gm per day, a fat intake that is about 50 per cent of the usual amount should be used. If intake is less than 100 gm but more than 75 gm, 40 to 50 gm of triglyceride can be prescribed to see if symptoms will improve. Restriction to less than 40 gm per day is severe and difficult to maintain. If symptoms are not improved, there is little need to continue this degree of restriction.

The low-fat diet is the best example in gastroenterology of the value of taking a detailed dietary history. Despite the fact that it is difficult to obtain a reliable dietary history with precise accuracy, some of the available methods are reliable.[7] Both the standard food history and a more formal 24-hour recall are easy to use, but depend upon memory and are unreliable. Nonetheless, they can detect major patterns of fat (or of any nutrient) intake, and major defection from the prescribed diet. Food records, preferably with amounts eaten, are much more accurate and can be used easily in an outpatient setting.

Restricting fat is not easy to achieve with Western diets. Most attractive foods high in protein are also rich in fat, which gives good taste, particularly to meats and fish. Triglycerides, the type of fat considered to be an important cause of symptoms, are found in large amounts in many foods. Each cup of milk or ounce of cheese contains 8 gm of triglycerides, and an ounce of lean meat, fish, or poultry, 5 gm; there are negligible amounts in cereals and grains, fruits, and vegetables. A complete list of the fat content of foods is available.[8] The preparation of a low-fat diet is difficult, since the addition of small amounts of some substances increases total fat content significantly. The following formula may be used to calculate the grams of fat in cooking oils, butter, or margarine: grams = number of milliliters × specific gravity (0.91); e.g., 2 tablespoons of olive oil = 30 × 0.9 = 27 grams of triglycerides. Thus, it is apparent that a small volume of cooking fat provides a large portion of dietary fat. Therefore, on a low-fat diet, all foods must be broiled, boiled, or baked.

Chicken and turkey contain less fat than does red meat or fish, especially if the skin is removed. These meats form the staple of the low-fat diet. Red meat trimmed of all fat may also be used. The flat fish (sole, flounder), which contain less fat, are usually served with a sauce when fat intake is not restricted.

Dairy products made with whole or 2 per cent milk contain triglycerides in large amounts. Skim milk should be used. Most cakes, cookies, pies, pastry, candy, and cream sauces or gravies should be avoided. A general list of foods allowed on a restricted-fat diet is presented in Table 105–1.

Essential fatty acids are widespread in animal and especially vegetable fats. Since fat intake is restricted, but not eliminated, essential fatty acid deficiency does not develop on fat restricted diets, and no supplements are needed. When fat is eliminated from the diet, as during total parenteral nutrition, supplements containing essential fatty acids are needed (see pp. 2015–2019).

Medium-Chain Triglycerides

Medium-chain triglyceride (MCT) is theoretically useful in steatorrhea because it is hydrolyzed more rapidly by pancreatic enzymes, because it does not require bile acid micelles for absorption of the products of hydrolysis, and because the products are not absorbed into the lymphatics but directly into the portal circulation. In bile salt deficiency a large fraction of MCTs can be absorbed as triacylglycerols, but long-chain triglycerides are unabsorbed. In the enterocytes these MCTs can be hydrolyzed. Therefore, it is useful in controlling many of the causes of steatorrhea (see pp. 263–282). However, there are a number of problems with the use of MCT. They provide only 8.3 kcal per gm, not 9 kcal gm as do long-chain triglycerides, and they undergo omega oxidation in the body; that is, a second carboxyl group is formed on the first carbon. The resulting dicarboxylic acids cannot be utilized and are excreted.[9] Only a small amount of ingested MCTs are metabolized in this way. Medium-chain fatty acids (MCFAs) do not require carnitine for mitochondrial beta-oxidation and are rapidly oxidized.[10] The large amount of acetyl-CoA produced will be used for synthesis of ketone bodies. Moreover,

Table 105–1. GENERAL OUTLINE OF A LOW-FAT DIET

Fat Intake (gm/day)	Foods Allowed
40	Vegetables, most fruits, bread, cereals with skim milk, two 3-oz servings of lean meat, one egg, 1 tsp margarine
60	*In addition to the above foods:* 2 cups of 2% milk, *or* one more ounce of meat with each serving, *or* one egg, *or* 4 tsp of margarine or oil
75	*In addition to foods allowed on a 60-gm fat diet:* Whole milk instead of 2%, *or* 2 slices of bacon, *or* 4 oz of ice cream, *or* 2 servings of lean meat, 6 oz each

elongation of MCFAs increases when MCTs are used in the diet. The overall response of the liver to MCFAs, however, is to oxidize them rapidly. Thus, they are an available and good source of calories in undernourished patients.

Although the effective caloric content of 1 tablespoon of MCT oil is less than 115 kcal, MCTs are clearly helpful in cases of fat malabsorption. They have been tried with some success as a component of the ketogenic diet for childhood epilepsy and as a component of intravenous lipid emulsion.[10] In general, they are better tolerated by children than by adults.[11] They cannot be used alone, but must be added to other dietary fats. They do produce some side effects. MCTs are ketogenic in normal subjects and even more so in diabetic patients, and should not be given to patients with ketosis or acidosis. In cirrhosis, hepatic metabolism is impaired and MCFAs accumulate in the cerebrospinal fluid, possibly altering energy metabolism but not affecting clinical parameters of encephalopathy. Finally, MCTs in large amounts cause diarrhea, owing to the osmotic effect of medium-chain fatty acids. Nevertheless, MCTs can deliver a small, but perhaps important, addition of calories to a marginal diet. Moreover, since MCTs are also detergent-like, they can help to solubilize fat-soluble vitamins and enhance their absorption. MCTs are best delivered as the oil in a dose up to 15 ml orally, four times a day. This provides about 460 effective calories per day. The oil is most easily ingested plain as a medication, but can be mixed with fruit juice, especially tomato or grape, to obscure the taste. MCTs are also available in complex preparations with proteins, sugars, and other nutrients. When MCTs are used for cooking, they should not be heated above 150 to 160° C. Above this temperature MCTs are oxidized, altering their palatability.

Low-Fat Caloric Supplements

When table foods must be severely restricted to control fat intake, low-fat dietary supplements may be needed to deliver adequate calories. A representative sampling of these is listed in Table 106–1. All of these preparations can be used as complete nutritional supplements, since they contain adequate protein, vitamins, and minerals. Unfortunately, their long-term palatability is not good when they are used alone; they are more useful as supplements, especially if chilled. Some preparations contain mostly digested nutrients and are especially appropriate for use in patients with pancreatic insufficiency, in whom a low-fat, high-protein diet and enzyme replacement are not adequate.

Low Oxalate Diet: The Problem of Hyperoxaluria. The degree of oxaluria is inversely correlated with the degree of fat absorption.[12] Urinary oxalate excretion should be measured for 24 hours in all patients with excessive fat malabsorption, especially those with short bowel syndrome or ileal bypass. The excess of free fatty acids in the lumen in patients with steatorrhea binds calcium, making it unavailable to form an insoluble salt with oxalic acid. Consequently, sodium oxalate is formed, which is much more soluble than the calcium salt. In the presence of bile acid malabsorption, bile acids alter colonic permeability and the sodium oxalate is absorbed by the colon. The major drawback of a low-oxalate diet is that it is often ineffective, since only about 10 per cent of body oxalate is derived from the diet. Therefore, urinary oxalate should be measured again after initiation of the diet to assess its effectiveness. Foods high in oxalate are listed in Table 105–2.

Addition of calcium supplements, which are often required in patients with malabsorption of many causes, is particularly helpful in ileal disease or resection in precipitating oxalate as the calcium oxalate salt in the lumen and in decreasing hyperoxaluria. Such therapy fortunately is useful even if a low-oxalate diet is not prescribed, since such a diet when combined with low fat intake is often too restrictive. Therefore, calcium supplements in the range of 600 to 1000 mg per day of elemental calcium are often used alone for hyperoxaluria.

Specific Therapy: Replacement, Dietary, and Antibiotic

Pancreatic Enzymes

The use of pancreatic enzymes in pancreatic insufficiency is to provide relief of symptoms (diarrhea) and to help patients gain weight. Fat malabsorption does not become significant until lipase output is less than 10 per cent of normal secretion (see pp. 1817–1848). Steatorrhea and creatorrhea result from inadequate secretion of lipase and proteases, respectively, but the severity of symptoms is due largely to steatorrhea. Management is directed toward relief of symptoms and restriction of nutritional status, not toward producing a normal efficiency of fat absorption. Thus, the key feature in choosing a preparation for enzyme replacement is that it contain high levels of lipase and proteases. Tablets, capsules, and enteric-coated or microencapsulated preparations all will be effective in reducing steatorrhea, if adequate amounts of enzyme are ingested. Approximately 30,000 IU of lipase must be taken with each meal to abolish steatorrhea completely. Even then, treatment will be completely successful only if gastric acid does not neutralize lipase

Table 105–2. OXALATE CONTENT OF FOODS

Very High	Moderately High	
Spinach	Parsley	Potatoes
Rhubarb	Green beans	Raw nuts
Cocoa	Collard	Strawberries
Chocolate	Kale	Figs
Tea	Turnip greens	Oranges
Ovaltine	Beets	Some instant coffees
	Brussels sprouts	Cola beverages
	Breads	

activity. Table 105–3 outlines the enzyme activities in various high lipase preparations. Taking all the tablets with a meal is as effective as any other regimen.[13] Because gastric acid inactivates lipase, H_2 blocking agents, taken before meals, will enhance the efficiency of ingested enzymes.[14] However, the use of H_2 blockers is often not necessary. With control of symptoms and re-establishment of positive caloric balance as the goal, three to six tablets with each meal and one or two with snacks is a reasonable dosage schedule for the preparations listed in Table 105–3.

Gluten-Free Diet

This diet is used for treatment of celiac sprue.[1, 15] It is not really effective as nonspecific therapy. The use and details of this diet are discussed on pages 1147 to 1149.

Antibiotics

Effective therapy is available for some illnesses associated with steatorrhea, but it may or may not be specific. A low-fat diet used in conjunction with a specific agent, such as an antibiotic, will often help alleviate symptoms. The pathophysiologic processes of diseases for which antibiotics are successfully used (Whipple's disease or stagnant loop syndrome) are suppressed. Although the therapy is specific, the disease is not cured, since therapy usually must be continued. Steatorrhea in the stagnant or blind loop syndrome is related to the growth of microorganisms that deconjugate bile acids and have a direct toxic effect on the mucosa (see pp. 1289–1297). Theoretically, the constant use of antibiotics could lead to overgrowth of other bacteria that could also produce symptoms. For this reason, the antibiotics are often used in cyclic fashion, either on a two-week pattern (12 days on, 2 days off, treatment) or on a longer cycle (4 to 6 weeks on, 1 week off, treatment). The most frequently used antibiotics in ambulatory patients are tetracycline and erythromycin 250 mg four times a day. These antibiotics are effective against the spectrum of organisms that overgrow the small intestine.[16] Giardiasis can cause steatorrhea, but in this case treatment with antibiotics is usually curative—that is, one course of drug often suffices, and nonspecific therapy is used only during the acute phase of illness.

DISORDERS CHARACTERIZED BY MALABSORPTION OF CARBOHYDRATES

Lactose Intolerance and Low-Lactose Diet

Lactose intolerance defines the syndrome of diarrhea, bloating, and gas following ingestion of lactose.[17] It can be the result of lactase deficiency or of decreased time of exposure to mucosa with a normal or low enzyme level. The latter situation is seen with short bowel syndrome, acute gastroenteritis, or dumping syndrome. Sometimes lactose intolerance and irritable bowel syndrome are present in the same patient. Thus, a low-lactose diet may be used in conjunction with other treatment for irritable bowel (see pp. 263–282 and 1402–1418).

The low-lactose diet is indicated for patients with symptoms of lactose intolerance, as demonstrated by history and/or a positive lactose tolerance test, that is, a blood sugar rise of $\leq$ 20 mg per dl after a lactose load of 50 gm per m^2 in children or 50 gm in adults, accompanied by characteristic symptoms. The hydrogen breath test is more precise, and because of the fact that blood need not be sampled, it is better designed for population studies. It is more sensitive and can detect malabsorption of as little as 2 gm of lactose. Thus, a lower test dose (12.5 gm) can be used, equal to the lactose content of one glass of milk. A rise of more than 20 parts per million is consistent with lactose intolerance. Interpretation of the hydrogen breath test has pitfalls.[17] A small percentage of normal individuals do not produce hydrogen gas; oral antibiotics can suppress bacteria that produce hydrogen; and smoking increases breath H_2 concentration unrelated to carbohydrate intake (see p. 1295). It is not always necessary to employ a test demonstrating lactose intolerance. If the history of intolerance is clear, as it is in about 50 per cent of cases, a trial of a low-lactose diet for five to seven days is indicated. If the diagnosis is in doubt, or if response to lactose withdrawal is uncertain, either the tolerance test or the breath test can be performed.

Low lactose intake is also an integral part of a low available carbohydrate diet (see below). Sometimes a low-lactose diet is used during the acute phase of diarrheal illnesses in which intestinal transit is rapid or lactase deficiency is transient. These illnesses can include acute gastroenteritis, ulcerative colitis, or

Table 105–3. *IN VITRO* ENZYME ACTIVITIES IN SELECTED PANCREATIC ENZYME PREPARATIONS

Preparation	Type	Enzyme Activity (IU/unit)			
		Lipase	*Trypsin*	*Proteolytic*	*Amylase*
Ilozyme	Tablet	3600	3444	6640	329,600
Ku-Zyme HP	Capsule	2330	3082	6090	594,048
Festal	Enteric-coated	2073	488	1800	219,200
Cotazym	Capsule	2014	2797	5840	499,200
Viokase	Tablet	1636	1828	4440	277,333
Pancrease	Microencapsulated	>4000*		>25,000*	

Modified from Graham, D. N. Engl. J. Med. *296*:1314, 1977.
*Manufacturer's estimates. All other determinations made independently.

Crohn's disease. However, it is not necessary to restrict lactose intake in all such cases; the decision is based on empirical grounds. In celiac sprue patients, however, the lactase activity unquestionably is decreased by the disease, and a low-lactose diet is helpful in the initial phase of therapy until the enzyme level is restored some months later (see pp. 1134–1152).

The major indication for very severe restriction of lactose is in the treatment of galactosemia. Small amounts of lactose (up to 3 gm per day) can be well handled by almost all other lactose-intolerant patients.

Treatment for lactose intolerance is usually a low-lactose diet (Table 105–4). Yogurt is the one lactose-containing food that is well tolerated by many lactose-intolerant persons, because the fermentation of lactose continues in the intestinal lumen.[18] Also, lactose content is often lower than equivalent amounts in milk, 7 to 8 gm versus 12 gm per cup. However, tolerance to yogurt must be individualized. Individual susceptibility varies greatly, so that the average patient becomes symptomatic after ingestion of 12 gm of lactose. A few patients, however, become symptomatic after ingestion of 3 gm, and their diets must be more restricted. When lactose intolerance is due to dumping syndrome or short bowel syndrome, however, diarrhea and bloating may be due to other causes, and more strict lactose restriction is not usually helpful.

Lactose is usually added to skim milks to increase their calorie content. Buttermilk, even when naturally fermented, still contains large amounts of lactose. Commercial yogurt contains about 1.5 gm per oz, since milk or cream is added to reduce the fermented taste. Ice creams are made from concentrated milk solids and so are rich in lactose. Sherbets contain fewer milk solids, but ice milks contain much lactose, since it is their only caloric source. Most cheeses contain only 0.5 to 1 gm of lactose per ounce. Since most patients with lactose intolerance can ingest 3 gm of lactose with no ill effects, a few ounces of cheese are allowed on most low-lactose diets. All desserts and sauces made with milk, cream, cheese, or milk chocolate are also avoided in a low-lactose diet. Sorbets, ices, and oleomargarines are not made from milk products and contain no lactose.

A low-lactose diet will be limited in dairy products. Thus, it will be low in calcium, since dairy products constitute the most available source of dietary calcium. Calcium supplements may be necessary, especially in postmenopausal women. Patients on this diet should learn to read all food labels, avoiding all packaged foods with the following words on the label: *milk products, milk solids, whey, lactose, milk sugar, curd, casein, galactose*, or *skim milk powder*. Each individual will discover the amount of lactose that can be tolerated. The physician should not be too rigid in the restriction, since the therapeutic goal is to alleviate symptoms. However, trial-and-error is often needed, since packaged foods frequently do not list the amount of lactose on the label. A few chemically defined products that simulate milk are now available. Corn syrup solids and sodium caseinate as sources for carbohydrates and protein can be used as milk substitutes if they are palatable. The brand available in each area of the country is likely to differ. These products can also be used in treating allergy to milk (see pp. 1113–1123).

Table 105–4. LACTOSE CONTENT OF SELECTED MILK PRODUCTS

Product	Unit	Lactose Content (gm/unit)
Milk		
Whole	1 cup	12
2%	1 cup	9–13
Skim	1 cup	11–14
Chocolate	1 cup	10–12
Sweetened condensed	1 cup	35
Reconstituted dry	1 cup	48
Buttermilk	1 cup	9–11
Cream		
Light	1 tbsp	0.6
Half and Half	1 tbsp	0.6
Whipped	1 tbsp	0.4
Solid Confections		
Ice cream	1 cup	9
Sherbet	1 cup	4
Ice milk	1 cup	10
Yogurt (low fat)	1 cup	7–11
Cheeses		
Hard (e.g., Parmesan)	1 oz	0.6–0.8
Semihard (e.g., Cheddar)	1 oz	0.4–0.6
Soft (e.g., Brie)	1 oz	0.1–0.2
Spreads	1 oz	0.8–1.7
Cottage	1 oz	5–6
Cottage, low fat	1 oz	7–8
Butter	1 tbsp	0.15

Adapted from Welsh, J. D. Am. J. Clin. Nutr. *31*:592, 1978.

Enzyme Replacement for Lactose Intolerance

Milk can be prepared by hydrolysis of the lactose by a yeast enzyme preparation (Lact-Aid, Sugarlo Company, Atlantic City, New Jersey). Mixture of a packet of the preparation (containing lactase from the yeast *Kluyveromyces lactis*) with milk at 4° C results in 70 per cent hydrolysis of the lactose in one day and 90 per cent hydrolysis in two or three days. Prehydrolyzed milk using this yeast preparation is available in many stores. Patients with limited tolerance to lactose can use this milk, which is well accepted, in cooking or on cereal. Of course, nonliquid dairy products cannot be treated in this way, but one to three lactase-containing tablets (Lactaid, Lactrase) may be swallowed with meals to improve lactose tolerance.

Sucrase-Isomaltase Deficiency

This deficiency is rarely encountered in the United States but occurs in about 10 per cent of Eskimos. Diagnosis is made as for lactose intolerance except that the sugar fed during the tolerance test is sucrose rather than lactose. The principles of dietary management are similar to those for lactose intolerance, except that different foods are involved. Sucrose is contained in many unprocessed fruits and, most important, in sugar cane. Thus, table sugar and foods cooked with it are eliminated. A detailed list of foods and their sucrose content has been published.[19] Isomaltose residues are found in limit dextrans after amylase digestion of starch. These dextrans will not be digested in sucrase deficiency but form a small part of the total sucrose-isomaltose intake of a normal diet. Thus, restriction of starch is not usually necessary.

DISORDERS CHARACTERIZED BY PROTEIN LOSS AND/OR MALABSORPTION

Virtually every intestinal disease can be associated with increased protein loss, because protein is normally secreted or lost into the intestine each day (see pp. 283–290 and 1978–1980). Thus, disorders characterized by increased loss of cells or secretions, or decreased efficiency of digestion or absorption, will have increased protein losses ranging from 4 to 40 gm per day (pp. 263–282).

Treatment of protein loss due to an enteropathy or malabsorption differs greatly from that for fat or carbohydrate malabsorption. Significant losses of these latter substances do not cause deficiencies of essential nutrients (except for the small need for essential fatty acids); they do, however, cause symptoms. Protein must be ingested in large quantities each day (0.5 to 1.5 gm per kg) to provide enough essential amino acids for growth and maintenance of tissues. No protein is stored in the body, since all proteins are used for some function. Unlike fat and carbohydrate, then, there is no storage compartment in the body to call on when dietary intake is inadequate without some sacrifice of function. Therefore, when protein is malabsorbed or lost, it must be ingested in excess to allow for the decreased efficiency of absorption.

Dietary Treatment of Protein Loss with Table Foods

While sound in principle, offering table food to compensate for protein loss is difficult. Table foods rich in protein usually contain large amounts of triglycerides.[8] For patients who are absorbing fat as well as protein normally, regular dietary sources of protein may be used, but fat malabsorption is part of most diseases of protein malabsorption or loss, and dietary fat will aggravate both the symptoms and the protein loss. Even in disorders with severe protein loss, such as severe congestive heart failure or intestinal lymphangiectasia, increased dietary fat enhances lymph flow and results in increased secretion of protein into the intestine. Thus, available dietary protein sources in meeting protein loss and malabsorption are often limited.

In general, protein content of table foods may be estimated as follows: milk or milk products, 1 gm per oz; meat, fish, or peanut butter, 7 gm per oz; egg, 7 gm per egg; cooked legumes, 2 gm per oz; cooked rice, cooked pasta, or bread 4 gm per cup; fruits and other vegetables, negligible. Some foods are rich in protein and poor in triglycerides, so that they can be used when steatorrhea is present. Skim milk is a good source but cannot be used when lactose intolerance is present. Shellfish contain many sterols but almost no triglycerides. However, a low-fat dressing must be used if steatorrhea is present. Chicken or turkey without skin is a good source of protein with minimal fat, as is tuna packed in water. Finally, legumes are a relatively rich source of vegetable protein, but they are not rich in protein compared with meats. Moreover, they contain large amounts of nonabsorbable carbohydrates (e.g., raffinose), which can cause bloating and gas. The protein content of common foods is listed in Table 105–5.

Protein Supplements

In order to supply adequate protein in the diet, supplements must often be used. Total protein ingested must often exceed 0.8 gm per kg per day to produce positive protein balance. Unfortunately, it is not always possible to determine when positive balance is achieved, but the assessment of protein requirement can be judged as described on pages 1981 and 2009.

Table 105–5. SUPPLEMENTAL PROTEIN SOURCES IN COMMON FOODS

Food	Serving Size	Approximate Protein Content (gm)	Comment
Whole milk	1 cup	8.5	All milk products contain lactose. Commercially available lactase (Lact-Aid) can be added to milk to hydrolyze over 90 per cent of the disaccharide. Skim milk and nonfat dry milk contain < 1 gm fat per cup. The other milk products contain 4–5 gm fat or more per serving.
Skim milk	1 cup	9	
Nonfat dry milk	1 cup	43	
Ice cream	1 cup	6	
Ice milk	1 cup	6	
Cottage cheese	1 cup	30	
Yogurt (low-fat)	1 cup	8	
Cheese slice	1 oz	6–8	Harder cheeses contain the least lactose. All cheeses are high in fat content.
Egg	1 large	7	
Eggnog	1 cup	12	
Peanut butter	1 tbsp	4	50 per cent of weight is fat (8 gm per tbsp)
Lean beef	1 oz	7	
Fresh fish	1 oz	7	Flat fish have lowest fat content
Tuna	1 oz	8	
Chicken/turkey (without skin)		8	

Any of the low-fat supplements listed in Table 106–1 may be used as sources of protein and carbohydrates. It is important to remember that when protein is ingested, enough additional calories must be provided so that the protein is used as a source of amino acids and is not converted into a source of energy. Usually this protective effect requires a nonprotein calorie per gram protein ratio of 25 to 35.

It is sometimes better to provide protein as a nonfood supplement, along with nonprotein calories in the form of carbohydrate. Such supplements include Casec and PVM powders, providing 4 gm of protein per tbsp and 8.5 gm of protein per scoop, respectively. These are mixed with water and/or flavoring with added table sugar or corn solids (e.g., Polycose) to make a reasonably palatable drink. Often it is best to use both food and nonfood supplements to avoid taste fatigue.

DISORDERS CHARACTERIZED BY MALABSORPTION OF VITAMINS AND MINERALS

Although malabsorption due to diffuse mucosal disease or loss of mucosal surface area can produce deficiency of any vitamin or mineral, certain deficiencies associated with intestinal disorders are seen more commonly than others. This common association may be due to many factors: (1) disease or bypass of an organ uniquely involved in absorption (ileum for cobalamin, duodenum for iron); (2) high requirements for certain nutrients (e.g., folic acid), so that clinical deficiency occurs frequently despite normal body stores; (3) loss of an essential mechanism for absorption (e.g., bile salt absorption for fat-soluble vitamins); (4) inability of the body to compensate for intestinal losses (e.g., iron or zinc loss in stool); (5) inefficient absorption under normal conditions (e.g., calcium, magnesium, iron); and (6) loss of more than one mechanism for absorption (e.g., vitamin D and calcium malabsorption produce calcium deficiency). Tables 105–6 and 105–7 outline the major disorders leading to deficiency of those vitamins and minerals commonly seen with intestinal diseases, as well as representative treatment schedules. These tables are not meant to be comprehensive for all possible deficiency states or for all possible replacement requirements. The reader is referred to more detailed sources for a more extensive discussion of vitamins and mineral deficiency.[20] As the function of the proximal and distal intestine differ, the deficiency states characterizing disorders involving these different anatomic regions also differ. Thus, it is helpful to consider the problems unique to disorders of the proximal and distal small bowel.

Bypass of Proximal Small Intestine

The usual cause of duodenal bypass is gastric surgery for peptic ulcer or obesity. Whereas Billroth I anastomosis or a gastroplasty procedure still leaves the duodenum in its normal anatomic relationship with the stomach, a Billroth II or a gastric bypass diverts the flow of food from the stomach into the jejunum. Patients with a partial gastrectomy and gastroduode-

Table 105–6. REPLACEMENT THERAPY WITH VITAMINS IN GASTROINTESTINAL DISEASE

Vitamin	Condition Commonly Producing Deficiency	Preparation Used	Dose
Folic acid	Gluten-sensitive enteropathy, tropical sprue, medications (e.g., sulfasalazine), alcoholism	Pteroylglutamic acid	1 mg/day p.o.
Cobalamin	Ileal disease or resection, subtotal or total gastrectomy, stagnant loop syndrome	Cyanocobalamin	1000 μg/month I.M.
Other water soluble	Decreased food intake, alcoholism	Multivitamin	1/day p.o.
A	Short bowel syndrome, ileal disease	Retinol	5,000–10,000 IU/day p.o.
D	Short bowel syndrome, ileal disease or resection, biliary obstruction	Vitamin D	50,000 IU 2–3 times/week p.o.
E	Biliary obstruction, short bowel syndrome, abetalipoproteinemia	D-α-tocopherol	100–200 IU/kg/day p.o.
K	Ileal disease or resection, chronic antibiotic therapy biliary obstruction	Vitamin K_3	5–10 mg/day p.o.

Table 105–7. REPLACEMENT THERAPY WITH MINERALS IN GASTROINTESTINAL DISEASE

Mineral	Conditions Commonly Producing Deficiency	Preparation Used	Dose (Elemental)
Iron	Blood loss, Billroth II gastrojejunostomy	Inorganic iron (e.g., sulfate)	60 mg 3 times/day with meals p.o.
Calcium	Short bowel syndrome, ileal disease, steatorrhea of any cause	Calcium carbonate, glubionate	500 mg 1–3 times/day p.o.
Magnesium	Short bowel syndrome, alcoholism	Magnesium oxide	130–360 mg 1–3 times/day p.o.
Zinc	Severe diarrhea (e.g., Crohn's disease), cirrhosis	Zinc sulfate	50 mg 1–3 times/day p.o.

nostomy (Billroth I) have better iron absorption and less iron deficiency than patients with a gastrojejunostomy.[21] Since the major nutrient absorbed primarily by the bypassed duodenum is iron, oral iron preparations are prescribed to prevent iron deficiency. Iron is included in many multivitamin and mineral preparations, the amount of inorganic iron in such products varying greatly, from 10 to 143 mg per tablet. Nearly all the preparations contain vitamin C, 25 to 50 mg, a useful reducing agent in patients with hypo- or achlorhydria after gastric surgery, when insufficient H^+ ions are present to ensure the conversion of ferric ion to soluble ferrous ion complexes. Vitamin C should be prescribed with iron for patients with gastric bypass in whom the acid-producing portion of the stomach is excluded (see pp. 972–974).

Normal daily iron requirements are about 1.2 mg for men and 2.5 mg for women. If 10 per cent is absorbed normally, about 12 to 25 mg of oral inorganic iron daily should be sufficient. The RDA for iron is 10 mg for adult males and 18 mg for females to allow for differences in absorption and for the fact that food iron, especially in vegetables, is less available than heme or inorganic iron. Iron used for oral therapy is usually inorganic, but the elemental iron content varies according to the compound. The approximate content of elemental iron as a percentage of the iron salt is 20 for the sulfate, 30 for the fumarate, and 10 for the gluconate salt. Oral iron preparations should be ingested with meals to avoid the epigastric symptoms caused by direct chemical action on the gastric mucosa.

Some patients are intolerant to oral iron and will not take the pills because of epigastric discomfort or diarrhea. Intravenous iron is preferable to intramuscular iron because larger amounts can be given less frequently and because there is no discomfort associated with the injection. Allergic responses, including anaphylaxis, to intravenous iron are rare, and these can usually be avoided by precautionary steps. All patients should be *previously tested* for sensitivity with 0.5 ml of colloidal iron intravenously. If no reaction is elicited, later that day or on the next day the iron to be injected is *diluted* in 250 to 500 ml of normal saline and *injected slowly* intravenously over a two-hour period. Up to 2 ml of iron (100 mg) can be given intravenously in this fashion. Injection of larger amounts can produce a serum sickness type illness that can last up to 72 hours after the injection.

Bypass of the proximal intestine does not commonly produce vitamin or mineral deficiencies other than iron. The active transport region for calcium absorption is duodenal, but in man the bulk of calcium is absorbed in the jejunum and ileum (see pp. 1057–1058). Folic acid and most other water-soluble vitamins are absorbed largely in the proximal bowel, but only because they are efficiently absorbed by the first segment of bowel to which they are exposed. However, folic acid (26 per cent) and vitamin B_{12} deficiency (20 per cent) are common after ulcer surgery, although less frequent than iron deficiency (48 per cent)[21] (see pp. 971–974). Thus, duodenal bypass produces increased absorption in the jejunum. When there is mucosal disease, however, so that absorption is impaired throughout much or all of the intestine, deficiency of folic acid and other water-soluble vitamins can be seen more regularly. Support for this concept has been provided by the results in patients who have undergone gastric bypass operations for obesity.

Gastric Bypass for Obesity

Despite earlier expectations, gastric exclusion surgery for obesity results in anemia and iron, folate, and vitamin B_{12} deficiencies rather commonly. Anemia has occurred in 18 per cent[22] to 36 per cent[23] of patients. Anemia develops rapidly, with a mean time of 20 months after bypass surgery. In contrast, postgastrectomy deficiencies usually take years to develop.[21] The reasons for the rapid development of anemia are not clear, but it appears that factors other than malabsorption, maldigestion, and altered intake must be operative. Normal Schilling tests have been found in most patients with low serum vitamin B_{12} levels.[23] Perhaps the proteolysis of food-bound cobalamin is impaired after gastric bypass, although this defect has not been demonstrated in these patients, as it has been in postgastrectomy patients.[24] The other micronutrient deficiencies reported in gastric exclusion operations are probably of little clinical importance. A number of cases of Wernicke-Korsakoff syndrome have been reported following recurrent and profuse vomiting. Although thiamine deficiency has been suspected, only one report shows a response to thiamine replacement.[25]

Bypass or Resection of Distal Small Intestine

The clinical disorders that present with this abnormality include Crohn's disease, recurrent adhesions with bowel resection, bowel infarction with resection, and ileal bypass of hypercholesterolemia or obesity (see p. 1106). Treatment consists of a low-fat diet and fat-soluble vitamins, since bile acids are absorbed in the most distal portion of the small intestine. Treatment will vary depending upon whether fatty acid diarrhea or bile acid diarrhea is the predominant syndrome. Bile acid diarrhea classically presents with no or slight steatorrhea, and an abnormal bile acid breath test, in a patient with less than 100 cm of involved or resected ileum. Fatty acid diarrhea is always accompanied by obvious steatorrhea and frequently by an abnormal Schilling test for cobalamin absorption. The length of involved ileum usually exceeds 100 cm. For fatty acid diarrhea, a low-fat diet and fat-soluble vitamins (see above) are used. A low-oxalate diet may or may not be indicated. Cholestyramine is used only when bile acid loss without much steatorrhea is a predominant feature. Cobalamin and divalent cations must often be replaced. Bile acid diarrhea is much less common and may be managed by the use of cholestyramine alone. A low-fat diet may be added if cholestyramine therapy produces steatorrhea. Nutritional management of these syndromes consists of the following measures in addition to a low-fat diet.

Cobalamin (Vitamin B_{12}) Therapy. When vitamin B_{12} therapy is required for ileal disease or resection, the Schilling test will become abnormal long before the serum vitamin B_{12} level falls. The body contains sufficient stores of vitamin B_{12} for one to two years. However, treatment should be started when malabsorption is discovered, not when deficiency becomes evident. Since the enterohepatic circulation accounts for about 10 μg per day, total malabsorption would require 300 μg per month for replacement. Although malabsorption of cobalamin to this extent is uncommon, 500 to 1000 μg per month intramuscularly is recommended as replacement.

Divalent Cations: Calcium, Magnesium, and Zinc Replacement. Low-lactose diets are often used for short bowel syndrome. This removes the most available source of calcium from the diet. For this reason, calcium supplements are almost routine treatment for short bowel syndrome. Additional calcium is needed because at intakes of less than 300 to 400 mg per day, calcium balance is negative owing to loss from the intestinal tract.[26] Calcium supplements are needed, therefore, to prevent negative calcium balance. If calcium absorption normally is 33 per cent efficient and calcium requirement is about 300 to 400 mg per day, the daily allowance for a normal intake is about 1000 mg. If malabsorption decreases calcium retention by 50 per cent, intake should be increased to 2000 mg per day. Ingestion of more calcium each day is usually not helpful in increasing the amount absorbed. Vitamin D replacement frequently is required if the serum 25-OH vitamin D level falls below 10 ng/dl. There is limited information on the relative absorption of calcium salts. Any of the preparations are probably effective, although some patients seem to respond better to the more water-soluble salts (e.g., gluconate, glubionate).

With short bowel syndrome and possible excessive loss of magnesium, oral magnesium supplementation is advisable despite apparent mildness of magnesium deficiency. Magnesium oxide and sulfate are the usual salts prescribed, but both are very insoluble and often cause diarrhea. When magnesium deficiency is severe, parenteral therapy is needed. A reasonable schedule involves the use of magnesium sulfate, 1 gm (8.13 mEq), every four to six hours for five days. Most patients can be maintained with a normal serum magnesium with the use of 32 to 48 mEq of magnesium per day.[27]

The factors that control zinc balance in the human are not well understood. However, the major losses occur through the intestinal tract. Urinary excretion varies rather little no matter what the state of overall zinc balance. Therefore, zinc absorption and balance are regulated by zinc intake. One to 2 mg per day are absorbed from an average intake of 15 mg. Estimations for zinc supplementation in the presence of diarrhea have been made.[28] In addition to normal replacement of 15 mg of elemental zinc per day, one should add about 17 mg per kg per day for stool when diarrhea is present or 12 mg per kg per day for gastric or duodenal fluid loss through vomiting or nasogastric tube.

Fat-Soluble Vitamin Therapy. When steatorrhea is present in short bowel syndrome (especially any cause of diarrhea due to bile salt deficiency), fat-soluble vitamins need to be replaced. These are often offered as water-miscible forms, that is, with detergent added. When the vitamins enter the intestinal tract, they still require bile acid micelles for absorption; hence, if a major cause of steatorrhea is bile acid depletion (e.g., short bowel syndrome), large doses of these vitamins will be needed to achieve some absorption. The exception is vitamin K_3, which is a water-soluble form. When bile acid absorption is intact, fat-soluble vitamin requirements are lower and often can be managed by the use of preparations that offer fat-soluble vitamins in combination with other vitamins and minerals.

The large doses of fat-soluble vitamins needed to treat malabsorption are available only as the individual vitamins and are not contained in a multivitamin preparation. (Vitamin K is not present in *any* multivitamin preparation.) Vitamin E replacement is difficult, because the vitamin is completely water-insoluble. Thus, steatorrhea and fat malabsorption lead to increased fecal loss in the lipid phase. Vitamin E is carried on lipoproteins in serum, not on a specific binding protein, and levels of lipoproteins will be decreased when fat malabsorption is present. In such cases the capacity for carrying vitamin E in serum will be low. Thus, low circulating vitamin E levels are due to both malabsorption and decreased binding capacity. The detection of decreased vitamin E stores is enhanced by measuring the ratio of vitamin E to total serum lipids.[29] Some replacement can be achieved with large oral doses of vitamin E (Table 105–6), but the response is unpredictable. Free tocopherol may be better than the ester, but neither the free vitamin nor any parenteral preparation of vitamin E is yet readily available.

Many available preparations offer fat-soluble vitamins in great excess of the recommended dietary allowance (RDA) and even of the true requirement. Since the requirement in malabsorption is unknown, therapeutic dosage must exceed the RDA. The patient must be watched for toxicity, especially of vitamins A and D. Toxicity is uncommon, however, if steatorrhea is marked, as absorption of the vitamins is limited in this circumstance. The standard vitamin D capsule contains a huge dose of vitamin D (50,000 IU), but cholecalciferol (D_3) is available in liquid form solubilized with polysorbate 80 or polyethylene glycol, at a concentration of 8000 IU per ml. Vitamin A should be administered with care. The RDA assumes an intake of foods in which half of the vitamin is present as retinol and half as beta-carotene, which is biologically less active. However, the therapeutic preparations of 5000 units contain only retinol. Therefore, these preparations offer more activity than is present in 5000 IU available from foods as a mixture of retinol and beta-carotene. The RDA of vitamin A in terms of retinol alone is equivalent to 1000 μg (units). The preparations that contain 5000 units of retinol as the only source of vitamin A offer vitamin A activity that exceeds the RDA by five fold. Thus, toxicity can be seen with the chronic daily use of the more concentrated doses (25,000 to 50,000 units).[30]

Vitamin D is now available in many forms. However, the dose required to treat patients with malabsorption is not known. To avoid toxicity, especially if one uses the more potent preparations, urinary calcium should be measured serially. Although the hydroxylated forms are slightly more water-soluble than the parent vitamin, it is not clear whether they will offer any striking advantage for treatment in fat malabsorption. Bile acid micelles are required for efficient solubilization of 25-OH vitamin D. The more water-soluble form 1, 25-$(OH)_2$ vitamin D has not yet been shown to be advantageous over larger doses of the parent compound for treatment of malabsorption.[31]

Jejunoileal Bypass Surgery for Obesity

Although jejunoileal bypass surgery is rarely performed at present, a large number of patients retain iatrogenic malabsorption from having undergone this operation in the past. The major features of the malabsorption are steatorrhea, anemia, hyperoxaluria with renal stones, hypoxalemia, and hypocalcemia.[32] Although vitamin D is not absorbed well, development of metabolic bone disease is uncommon,[33] presumably because of intestinal adaptation to the bypass. The major reasons for discontinuing this procedure relate to the development of hepatic failure, renal failure due to stones, profound weight loss and weakness, and severe diarrhea.[34] If the patient does not develop one of these serious complications, the symptoms due to malabsorption and nutrient deficiencies can continue to be managed as are the symptoms of short bowel syndrome (see above).

DISORDERS CHARACTERIZED BY ALTERED GASTRIC EMPTYING

Delayed Emptying

The major causes for delayed emptying are mechanical (peptic disease or neoplasm), neurologic (diabetes mellitus and vagotomy), and infectious.

Mechanical Obstruction. Mechanical obstruction is almost always managed by surgical intervention. Even when gastric tumor is metastatic, reestablishment of a patent intestinal tract is important as palliative therapy. If obstruction is incomplete, premixed low-residue enteral feedings can be utilized in preparation for surgery (see pp. 2015–2018). If feeding produces unacceptable symptoms by stimulating motility, enteral feeding should be discontinued and parenteral feeding used preoperatively.

The bland diet is often used in the treatment of ulcer disease. There is no evidence for the value of such a diet, which restricts spices, coarse foods, and spicy foods. Some dietary maneuvers are helpful in ulcer disease. These include the use of frequent, small feedings and the avoidance of nighttime snacks to minimize acid secretion, and the elimination of alcohol, smoking, and caffeine to control symptoms[1] (see pp. 814–909).

Neurologic Causes. Delayed gastric emptying occurs occasionally with diabetes of long duration, especially when peripheral neuropathy is also present. Diarrhea, often an associated symptom, makes nutritional management even more difficult since therapy is often not very effective (see pp. 675–713). The use of small, frequent feedings is often the best approach. Gastric emptying improves with parenteral or oral metoclopramide (10 mg every six hours), but this may not be useful as outpatient therapy,[35] since absorption of medications as well as calories is delayed by the physiologic abnormality. Cisapride, a new prokinetic agent, is a substituted benzamide without extra-gastrointestinal effects. It uniquely induces phase III–like activity. It has been reported to be effective in stimulating liquid and solid gastric emptying in insulin-dependent diabetics, in both acute and chronic administration.[36]

Delayed emptying after vagotomy takes two forms—postoperative ileus and delayed emptying of solid foods. After gastric surgery that includes vagotomy, ileus occasionally is prolonged for one to two weeks. Parenteral delivery of calories is the procedure of choice in this setting. Very rarely the ileus lasts for many weeks, especially if dense adhesions from prior surgery are present. After vagotomy, especially that associated with gastric resection, solid foods empty slowly. The coordinated peristaltic motion of the antrum is impaired after vagotomy, but liquids empty rapidly (see below), whereas solid food resides longer in the stomach (see p. 943). In extreme cases a residual food ball (or *bezoar*) is formed (see p. 743). Usually no special treatment is required because the physiologic defect does not cause symptoms, and bezoar formation is rare. However, patients should be cautioned not to eat excessive amounts of citrus fruits, which most commonly form the core of a gastric food bezoar. Enzymatic treatment to digest phytobezoars has never been demonstrated to be effective, particularly because the bezoar usually resolves with cessation of oral intake for a few days.

Infectious Disorders. Delayed gastric emptying commonly occurs with viral gastroenteritis. The rate of gastric emptying is most rapid when isosmolar foods are ingested (see pp. 675–712). Rarely are the osmotic contents of food or gastric contents known. In the few instances in which the osmolarity is known, the liquids are of low caloric content. For acute illness, however, isosmolar liquids can be used for short periods. The osmolarity of some foods is listed in Table 105–8.[1] To achieve isosmolarity, most liquids must be diluted at least twofold. The presence of fat in food also delays gastric emptying and is better avoided during acute gastroenteritis. Commercial preparations used for

Table 105–8. OSMOLARITY OF SELECTED FOODS

Food	mOsm/Liter
Gatorade	280
Ginger ale	510
Gelatin dessert	535
Tomato juice	595
7-Up	640
Coca-Cola	680
Eggnog	695
Apple juice	870
Orange juice	935
Malted milk	940
Ice cream	1150
Grape juice	1170
Sherbet	1225

treatment of diarrhea are isosmotic and contain sufficient sodium and potassium to replace mild to moderate losses. These oral rehydration solutions are also useful in the management of acute infectious gastroenteritis.

Motor Disorders of the Stomach

Disturbances in normal gastric electric activity have been reported as isolated case reports.[37] The role of gastric dysrhythmia, either tachygastria or bradygastria, has yet to be assessed properly. Table 105–9 lists the clinical conditions that have been associated with gastric dysrhythmias. The patterns of dysrhythmia induced by drugs are similar to those that occur spontaneously.[37] Clinically, these disorders are characterized by severe gastric retention, nausea, vomiting, and weight loss. The symptoms are unrelieved by conventional medical or surgical management and require subtotal gastrectomy for relief. The significance of dysrhythmias is not certain, since they are found in patients with diabetic gastroparesis, a condition in which extrinsic innervation is abnormal, and surgical correction usually is unsuccessful. Moreover, abnormal rhythm is found in stomachs of normal subjects[38] and transiently in the postoperative period. Thus, it is not clear whether gastric dysrhythmias are directly responsible for abnormal motor function or whether they are an epiphenomenon. However, one should consider the disorders listed in Table 105–9 when more usual causes of delayed gastric emptying have been eliminated. Most importantly, the use of mediators with anticholinergic side effects or with opioid action should be minimized or eliminated in patients with delayed gastric emptying.

Rapid Emptying

Rapid emptying of liquids after vagotomy produces a series of symptoms known as the *dumping syndrome* (see p. 944). The symptoms in the first half hour after eating are related to distention of the small bowel with release of vasoactive peptides, including bradykinin. More delayed symptoms are related to reactive hypoglycemia. Symptoms can be controlled by dietary measures and by medication.

The *low available carbohydrate diet* is used in an attempt to decrease the osmolarity of the ingested food. Since most meals are hypertonic and since the intestinal fluid reaches isosmolarity within a few centimeters of the pylorus, ingestion of hypertonic food leads to an increase in intraluminal volume and distention of the bowel. This distention leads to release of active peptides. Although the diet is helpful, any foodstuff, especially carbohydrate or protein, includes large molecular weight substrates that can be hydrolyzed to small osmotically active substances, with subsequent side effects. Therefore, all foods have the potential to cause dumping, and the diet *per se* is only one part of the total therapeutic program, which includes: (1) a low available carbohydrate diet that is low in lactose (see above) as well as dextrose and sucrose; the sugar content of many foods has been characterized; (2) small, frequent feedings to control symptoms; (3) liquids ingested at different times from solids to limit the total fluid load; and (4) anticholinergics to delay gastric emptying (e.g., tincture of belladonna, 10 to 15 drops, 30 minutes before meals). Since the purpose of such a program is to limit symptoms, the degree to which the entire program is followed will depend upon the severity of symptoms.

DISORDERS CHARACTERIZED BY ALTERED GASTROINTESTINAL TRANSIT TIME

Esophageal Stricture

The stricture should be dilated or its cause removed, depending upon the etiology. If obstruction is incomplete, mechanical soft foods or full liquids may be used, depending upon the degree of obstruction. Certain characteristics of these diets must be kept in mind for their successful long-term use: (1) foods need not be bland; (2) milk-based foods form an important part of the diet; (3) flavoring is helpful for some liquids, but vanilla is best tolerated for long periods; (4) medication should be given in liquid form, if possible;

Table 105–9. CLINICAL CONDITIONS ASSOCIATED WITH GASTRIC DYSRHYTHMIAS

Idiopathic gastroparesis	Effect of drugs and hormones
Secondary gastroparesis	Anticholinergics
Diabetes mellitus	Opiates
Anorexia nervosa	Met-enkephalin
Gastric disease	Beta-endorphin
Ulcer	Hormones
Adenocarcinoma	Epinephrine
Asymptomatic state	Glucagon
Postoperative period	Prostaglandin E_2
	Secretin
	Insulin

Modified from Kim, C. H., and Malagelada, J. R. Mayo Clin. Proc. *61*:205, 1986.

and (5) caloric intake must be maintained near the estimated requirement.

The full liquid diet does not usually contain fruits or vegetables. It is easily made adequate in calories, proteins, and essential fatty acids but not in certain vitamins, notably ascorbic acid and thiamine, unless fruit juices and cereals are routinely included.[1–4]

Irritable Bowel Syndrome and Colonic Diverticula (High-Fiber Diet)

The term *dietary fiber* refers to those complex polysaccharides and other polymers that escape digestion in the small intestine. These substances include cellulose, hemicelluloses, gums, mucilages, pectins, and lignins. It is clear that dietary fiber contains many components, and within each fiber class there is much variation. Measurement of fiber involves complicated methods, most of which have not yet been widely available.[39, 40]

Further complicating the understanding and use of fiber content of foods is that analysis of unprocessed food does not always provide an accurate indication of the fiber content of food that is consumed. Freezing and drying, freezing alone, grinding, washing, and so forth alter fiber content. Thus, different preparations of the same food contain different amounts of fiber. These variables (measurement and preparation) lead to the widely divergent statements about the foods allowed or not allowed in high- or low-fiber diets.

The two known functions of fiber include an increase in stool weight and a shortening of bowel transit time.[41, 42] Fiber may decrease intraluminal pressure and its absorbent properties may play a role in human nutrition, but these functions are incompletely understood.

The high-fiber diet is used for treatment of irritable bowel syndrome and diverticulitis[42] (see pp. 1402–1434). Although it is not clear whether total dietary fiber intake in the United States is low, supplemental fiber is helpful in these disorders. This fiber can be supplied either in the diet or as psyllium seed or bran in a dose of 1 teaspoon two or three times a day. Psyllium seed provides a preparation rich in hemicellulose. Most commercial preparations provide 3 to 4 gm of dietary fiber per dose (tsp, wafer, biscuit). Bran provides both cellulose and hemicellulose. Foods grouped according to their crude fiber content are listed in Table 105–10. A high-fiber diet should aim to add the equivalent of about 10 gm of crude fiber to the diet. This increment can be achieved by adding the appropriate distribution of fiber-containing foods or by using bran or psyllium seed.

A high-fiber diet will emphasize whole-grain breads and cereals, fresh fruits, and fresh vegetables. The end result with either approach should be production of a regular pattern of defecation with formed stools. Too much dietary fiber can cause diarrhea. This diet should not be used routinely for chronic constipation alone, as it will often lead only to distention and more obstipation.

Table 105–10. FIBER CONTENT OF COMMONLY USED FOODS

Approximate Content of Dietary Fiber (*gm/serving*)	Representative Foods
5	Bran-containing cereals, stewed prunes, grapes, baked beans, raspberries
4	Peas, broccoli, pear, apple, potato skins, canned fruit, fruit pies
2	Citrus fruits, root vegetables, peanut butter, strawberries, cherries, wheat and corn cereals
1	Melons, white bread, salad vegetables, popcorn, rice cereals
<0.2	Milk, egg, meat, sugar, fats, strained juices

Intestinal Obstruction, Acute Diarrhea, and Bowel Preparation (Low-Fiber Diet)

The low-fiber diet can be fashioned from foods containing little fiber (see Table 105–10). The major indication for this diet is acute diarrhea. Preparation for air-contrast barium enema or colonoscopy and intestinal surgery require a very low fiber intake, approaching a clear liquid diet. These indications require a low-fiber diet only for a few days.

Sometimes a partial low-fiber diet, which does not result in such a severe restriction of fiber, is indicated. Gastric phytobezoars can be treated initially with a full low-fiber diet, but to prevent recurrences, removal of pulpy fruits (citrus, pears) from the diet is often sufficient. With a very narrow ileal segment due to Crohn's disease, only the most indigestible of the fiber sources need to be eliminated (bran buds, corn, nuts), while the other fiber-rich foods can be used in moderation. When the low-fiber diet is used for more chronic problems, content of grains, fruits, and vegetables is reduced. Fat intake and protein are diminished, because about 5 per cent of these macronutrients escape absorption and provide substrates for colonic flora. Even when fat intake is normal, dietary fat enters the colon and helps to maintain a large colonic bacterial population and, thus, stool bulk. However, the commonly applied exclusion of *all* fats from the diet is unnecessary, and some fat intake may be permitted, especially if the diet is to be used chronically. The major problem with the low-fiber diet is that it is often calorically inadequate. This is a disadvantage when nutrition is marginal, especially if the patient is lactose-intolerant. In these circumstances, the diet can be supplemented by one of a variety of preparations designed for enteral feedings (see pp. 2014–2018).

References

1. American Dietetic Association. Handbook of Clinical Dietetics. New Haven, Yale University Press, 1981.
2. Walser, M., Imbembo, A. C., Margolis, S., and Elfert, G. A. Nutritional Management: The Johns Hopkins Handbook. Philadelphia, W. B. Saunders Co., 1984.
3. Pemberton, C., and Gastineau, C. (eds.). Mayo Clinic Diet Manual. Philadelphia, W. B. Saunders Co., 1981.

4. Massachusetts General Hospital, Diet Reference Manual. Boston, Little, Brown, 1984.
5. Welch, I., Saunders, K., and Read, N. W. Effect of ileal and intravenous infusions of fat emulsion on feeding and satiety in human volunteers. Gastroenterology *89*:1293, 1985.
6. Condon, S. C., James, N. J., Wise, L., and Alpers, D. H. Role of caloric intake in the weight loss after jejunoileal bypass in obesity. Gastroenterology *74*:345, 1978.
7. National Research Council. Assessing Changing Food Consumption Patterns. Washington, National Academy Press, 1981.
8. Nutrition Value of American Foods in Common Units. Agriculture Handbook No. 456. Washington, U. S. Department of Agriculture, 1975.
9. Kupfer, D. Endogenous substrates of monooxygenases: fatty acid and prostaglandins. Pharmacol. Ther. *11*:469, 1980.
10. Bach, A. C., and Babayan, V. K. Medium-chain triglycerides: an update. Am. J. Clin. Nutr., *36*:950, 1982.
11. Kaunitz, N. Clinical uses of medium-chain triglycerides. Drug Therapy *8*:91, 1978.
12. Earnest, D. L. Enteric hyperoxaluria. Adv. Intern. Med. *24*:407, 1979.
13. Graham, D. Y. Enzyme replacement therapy of exocrine pancreatic insufficiency in man. N. Engl. J. Med. *296*:1314, 1977.
14. Regan, P. T., Malagelada, J. R., DiMagno, E. P., Glanzman, S. L., and Go, V. L. Comparative effects of antacid, cimetidine, and enteric coating and the therapeutic response to oral enzymes in severe pancreatic insufficiency. N. Engl. J. Med. *297*:854, 1977.
15. Stewart, J. S. Clinical and morphologic response to gluten withdrawal. Clin. Gastroenterol. *3*:109, 1974.
16. Banwell, J. G. Small intestinal bacterial overgrowth syndrome. Gastroenterology *80*:834, 1981.
17. Paige, D. M., and Bayless, T. M. (eds.). Lactose Digestion: Clinical and Nutritional Consequences. Baltimore, Johns Hopkins University Press, 1981.
18. Kolars, J. C., Levitt, M. D., Aoiyi, M., and Sevaino, D. A. Yogurt—an autodigesting source of lactase. N. Engl. J. Med. *310*:1, 1984.
19. Hardinge, M. R., Swarner, J. B., and Crooks, H. Carbohydrates in foods. J. Am. Diet. Assoc. *46*:197, 1965.
20. Alpers, D. H., Clouse, R. E., and Stenson, W. F. Manual of Nutritional Therapeutics. 2nd ed. Boston, Little, Brown, 1987.
21. Hines, J. D., Hoffbrand, A. V., and Mollin, D. L. The hematologic complications following partial gastrectomy: a study of 292 patients. Am. J. Med. *43*:555, 1967.
22. Halverson, J. D. Micronutrient deficiencies after gastric bypass for morbid obesity. Am. Surg. *52*:594, 1986.
23. Amaral, D. F., Thompson, W. R., Caldwell, M. D., et al. Prospective hematologic evaluation of gastric exclusion surgery for morbid obesity. Ann. Surg. *201*:186, 1985.
24. Doscherholmen, A., McMahon, J., and Ripley, D. Impaired absorption of egg vitamin B_{12} in post gastrectomy and achlorhydric patients. J. Lab. Clin. Med. *78*:839, 1971.
25. Fiet, H., Glasberg, M., Ireton, C., et al. Peripheral neuropathy and starvation after gastric partitioning for morbid obesity. Ann. Intern. Med. *96*:453, 1982.
26. Nordin, B. E. C. (ed.). Calcium, Phosphate, and Magnesium Metabolism. Edinburgh, Churchill Livingstone, 1976.
27. Rude, R. K., and Singer, S. F. Magnesium deficiency and excess. Ann. Rev. Med. *32*:245, 1981.
28. Wolman, S. L., Anderson, G., Marliss, E. B., and Jeejeebhoy, K. N. Zinc in total parenteral nutrition: requirements and metabolic effects. Gastroenterology *76*:458, 1979.
29. Sokol, R. J., Heubi, J. E., Iannaccone, S. T., et al. Vitamin E deficiency with normal serum vitamin E concentrations in children with chronic cholestasis. N. Engl. J. Med. *30*:1209, 1984.
30. Oversen, L. Vitamin therapy in the absence of obvious deficiency. What is the evidence? Drugs *27*:148, 1985.
31. Bikle, D. D. Calcium absorption and vitamin D metabolism. Clin. Gastroenterol. *12*:379, 1983.
32. Hocking, M. P., Duerson, M. C., O'Leary, P., and Woodward, E. R. Jejunoileal bypass for morbid obesity: late follow up in 100 cases. N. Engl. J. Med. *308*:995, 1983.
33. Sellin, J. H., Meredith, S. C., Kelly, S., Schrew, H., and Rosenberg, I. H. Prospective evaluation of metabolic bone disease following jejunoileal bypass. Gastroenterology *87*:123, 1984.
34. Halverson, J. D., Scheff, R. J., Gentry, K., and Alpers, D. H. Long term follow-up of jejunoileal bypass patients. Am. J. Clin. Nutr. *33*:472, 1980.
35. Pinker, B. M., Brogdin, R. N., Sawyer, R. P., et al. Metoclopramide: a review of the pharmacological properties and clinical use. Drugs. *12*:81, 1976.
36. Horowitz, M, Maddox, A, Harding, P. E., et al. Effect of cisapride on gastric and esophageal emptying in insulin-dependent diabetes mellitus. Gastroenterology *92*:1899, 1987.
37. Kim, C. H., and Malagelada, J. R. Electrical activity of the stomach: clinical implications. Mayo Clin. Proc. *61*:205, 1986.
38. Stoddard, C. J., Smallwood, R. H., and Duthie, H. L. Electrical arrhythmia in the human stomach. Gut *22*:705, 1981.
39. Spiller, F. B. and Amin, R. J. Dietary fiber in human nutrition. CRC Crit. Rev. Food Sci. Nutr. *7*:39, 1979.
40. Southgate, D. A. T., Bailey, B., Collesin, E., and Waller, A. A guide to calculating intakes of dietary fiber. J. Human Nutr. *30*:303, 1976.
41. Kelsey, J. L. A review of research on the effects of fiber intake in man. Am. J. Clin. Nutr. *31*:142, 1978.
42. Trowell, H., Burkett, D., and Heaton, K. (eds.). Dietary Fiber, Fiber Depleted Foods, and Disease. London, Academic Press, 1985.

106

Intensive Nutritional Support

RAY E. CLOUSE
IRWIN H. ROSENBERG

The high prevalence of malnutrition among hospitalized patients and the impact of malnutrition on prognosis are well recognized.[1–5] Malnourished patients are far sicker in general than are those with better nutritional status. To establish that correction of malnutrition actually decreases morbidity in similar situations is much more difficult,[6] but such evidence is beginning to appear.[7]

Most problems relating to nutritional support arise from the difficulty in meeting calorie and protein requirements. Vitamins and minerals, because of their smaller requirements, are more easily supplemented. Recognized deficiencies of these nutrients usually can be corrected with parenteral or oral supplements. Calorie and nitrogen sources, on the other hand, require larger volumes just to meet daily requirements, let alone to restore normal nutritional status. Therefore, emphasis in this discussion is placed on choosing the most convenient yet effective means of providing these macronutrients.

For nutritional therapy to be effective, reasonable goals must be established. Protein and calorie replacement will not result in rapid restoration of normal nutritional status. The physician, confused by the plethora of commercial products for enteral and parenteral nutrition therapy, must be patient in observing the benefits of his endeavors. Consultation with clinical dietitians and physicians who maintain an updated interest in clinical nutrition will result in the most effective use of nutritional therapy.

OPTIONS AVAILABLE FOR PROTEIN-CALORIE THERAPY

Supplementation With Normal Foods[8]

Ideally, protein and calorie requirements are met and deficiencies are corrected by eating normal foods. This is the most appealing and economical method of nutritional therapy, but it requires that the patient have a satisfactory appetite and an adequate intestinal tract. Dietary management of gastrointestinal disorders is covered more thoroughly on pages 1994 to 2006.

Use of Commercially Available Supplements

Protein and calorie content of the patient's usual diet can be bolstered by the use of commercially available supplements. Calorie supplements can be largely nonprotein (carbohydrates or fats) or protein, or both.[9] What ordinarily are supplements should not be used as the sole dietary constituent unless they are nutritionally complete—that is, the regimen meets daily requirements for vitamins and minerals as well. Many of the supplements have features that make them especially useful in certain gastroenterologic disorders; for example, lactose-free products contain less than 1 gm of the disaccharide per 1000 kcal and are useful for those who do not tolerate this disaccharide. The carbohydrate sources are usually sucrose, glucose oligosaccharides, and corn syrup solids. A few supplements are blenderized formulas containing some fibrous animal or vegetable products. However, most commercially available supplements are devoid of indigestible fiber and are consequently low in residue. Supplements that are also low in fat content provide a substrate that is least conducive to colonic bacterial growth. Low-residue supplements are particularly useful for hospitalized patients in whom decreased ileal effluent is desired (e.g., because of bowel disease, or while undergoing preparation for radiologic or endoscopic procedures). Commercial supplements with increased fiber content have recently become available and may be advantageous for some patients requiring long-term use of liquid products.[10, 11] The features of several commonly used nutritional supplements are summarized in Table 106–1.

Medium-chain triglyceride (MCT) oil is a distilled derivative of coconut oil and can be an important calorie supplement in specific situations. Triglycerides with fatty acid moieties of eight and ten carbons compose over 95 per cent of the oil. They are absorbed even in the presence of minimal amounts of pancreatic enzymes and in the absence of bile salts, and the medium-chain fatty acids appear directly in the portal blood (see pp. 1995–1996).[12, 13] Although this oil can act as a valuable calorie supplement in patients with fat malabsorption of any etiology, only ~400 calories (60 ml) can be effectively used per day.[14]

Partial or Supplemental Parenteral Nutrition Therapy

Protein and calorie requirements can be partially met with intravenous solutions, with a resultant reduction in the degree of negative nitrogen balance from which these patients suffer. Dextrose alone delivered

Table 106–1. CHARACTERISTICS OF A VARIETY OF COMMERCIALLY AVAILABLE ORAL PROTEIN AND/OR CALORIE SUPPLEMENTS

Major Nutrient Provided	Characteristics				Examples
	Low Lactose	*Low Residue*	*Low Fat*	*Nutritionally Complete*	
Protein	√	√	√		Case Powder, Pro Mix, PVM Powder
Calories	√	√	√		Polycose, Cal Powder, Hy-Cal
	√	√			MCT oil,* Controlyte
Protein and calories	√	√	√	√	Precision LR or HN, Vivonex, Flexical Citrotein†
	√	√		√	Ensure, Isocal, Magnacal, Travasorb
	√			√	Enrich

*Medium-chain triglycerides can be a suitable supplement for patients with diseases producing fat malabsorption.
†Vitamin and mineral–supplemented but not recommended as a sole dietary constituent.

in a hypocaloric 5 per cent concentration (170 kcal/liter) reduces urinary nitrogen loss, possibly because of a decrease in protein catabolism from the resultant hyperinsulinemia.[15] Considerable reductions in the nitrogen losses associated with simple starvation occur when as little as 100 to 150 gm of glucose is provided daily. Although urinary urea nitrogen losses (representing protein turnover) can be reduced by more than 50 per cent in this way, fat stores and protein compartments are gradually depleted. Amino acid infusions without additional non-nitrogen calorie sources can also improve negative nitrogen balance.[16–20] Adult postoperative patients given 70 to 100 gm of crystalline amino acids intravenously per day show progressive improvement toward zero in nitrogen balance.[21] Although reduced insulin secretion, allowing an increase in circulation of nonprotein energy sources, might be partially responsible for the "protein-sparing" effect, the mechanism is more complex.[22] The beneficial reduction in negative nitrogen balance is altered little by the coadministration of moderate dextrose, and *positive* nitrogen balance can eventually be achieved in normal subjects only when calorie requirements are also met using such nonprotein calorie sources. Interestingly, nutritional depletion appears to predispose patients to attain positive balance, even when calorie intake is inadequate.[22] Increasing amino acid intake to 2 gm/kg body weight in depleted patients has been shown to produce positive nitrogen balance.[23] Lack of adequate body fat limits the use of this approach, since endogenous energy sources must be utilized to meet all of the daily caloric requirements. Partial parenteral protein and calorie nutrition therapy will reduce negative nitrogen balance at the expense of endogenous fat stores but alone will generally not provide satisfactory support to completely meet daily requirements for calories and proteins or correct established deficiencies.

Intensive Nutritional Support With Tube Feeding or Total Parenteral Nutrition

Oral supplementation with normal foods or with commercially available products is the safest and the most desirable way to meet nutritional requirements and replete diminished stores. Such methods are often ineffective in hospitalized patients who are severely ill and cannot eat, who are anorectic, or who have serious gastrointestinal disorders. More aggressive protein-calorie nutritional therapy, using tube feeding techniques or total parenteral nutrition (TPN), has been successfully employed in the treatment of many hospitalized patients. Requirements of all the essential nutrients can be met with either technique.

SELECTING PATIENTS FOR INTENSIVE NUTRITIONAL THERAPY

A rational approach to the selection of patients for these forms of nutritional therapy is required. Current practice is based largely upon individual experience or retrospective studies that do not compare one option with another. Such controlled studies are clearly needed. The clinician should answer the following questions in considering patients for intensive nutritional support.

Is There a Primary Indication for the Use of TPN with Total Bowel Rest?

There is consensus among practitioners that total bowel rest, rigidly excluding anything by mouth, has an important place in the management of certain gastrointestinal diseases. The logic of minimizing trauma and irritation of inflamed, denuded bowel by decreasing the digestive and absorptive functions of the damaged mucosa to allow for healing and regeneration appears sound. However, the interdigestive period is by no means quiet. Cyclic bursts of vigorous motor activity sweep from the distal stomach to the terminal ileum at intervals of 80 to 120 minutes in normal adults.[24] While passing through the stomach and duodenum, these migrating motor complexes are accompanied by increased gastric and pancreatic secretion.[25] The periodic fasting motor activity is not interrupted by prolonged parenteral nutrition in the dog.[26]

Still, most experience supports the prediction that avoidance of regular oral intake will improve diarrhea and abdominal pain in patients with bowel disorders. Standard peripheral intravenous therapy during total bowel rest therapy can, at best, maintain adequate fluid and electrolyte balance and perhaps ensure maintenance of positive vitamin and some trace mineral balances, but the nutritional deficiencies that are prominent in many patients will only worsen with conventional intravenous management.

"Total" bowel rest and nutritional maintenance or restitution are feasible only when total parenteral alimentation, usually by central venous line, is carried out. The primary indications for bowel rest are discussed in the section on TPN. Some patients with inflammatory bowel disease and patients with severe and protracted gastrointestinal symptoms from other causes are often candidates. This form of therapy has also been used in the management of intestinal fistulas.

What Is the Current Protein-Calorie Nutritional Status of the Patient?

This is a key question in formulating a nutrition support plan. Unfortunately, there is no simple way confidently to establish its answer. Body composition analysis[27] at one point in time has limited value in determining the changes in body composition that result from malnutrition. The body cell mass is particularly affected by malnutrition, and its maintenance or repletion is the goal of nutritional support. Several techniques, including direct[28] and indirect[29] measurement of total body potassium, have been used to calculate the body cell mass, the living, energy-exchanging, oxygen-consuming component of the body.[30] The body cell mass in combination with the extracellular mass (supporting structures) composes the lean body mass. Analysis of body composition by *in vivo* neutron activation techniques has also been used to assess the absolute quantities of various elements (including nitrogen) in the body.[31, 32] This analysis is also more sensitive than routine clinical parameters in detecting deviations of body composition that are associated with malnutrition.[33] Although these techniques are established research tools, they are not practical as screening tests for malnutrition, nor are they as yet feasible for routine clinical application in malnourished individuals.

In the clinical setting, one can estimate fat stores and the degree of depletion of body proteins by combining anthropometry with laboratory blood and urine tests. Not all patients require extensive protein-calorie nutritional assessment. A rapid, "eyeball" assessment using routine clinical information can accurately stratify patients in three fourths of the cases.[34] Some elements in the medical history, such as recent complicated or repeated surgery, protracted medical illness, or 10 per cent weight loss in the past six months, should lead the physician to perform a more careful assessment of nutritional status if deficiencies are not readily apparent. The following tests for depletion of fat stores and protein compartments are readily available to the clinician and may be used to better estimate protein-calorie nutritional status.

Body Weight. A comparison of actual weight (AW) to ideal body weight (IBW) or to usual body weight (UBW) has been used to estimate the severity of protein-calorie malnutrition. Weight and weight change measurements are simple and useful parameters in assessing nutritional status. Acute weight loss of 10 per cent of body mass will result in measurable deterioration of muscle performance, whereas a loss of approximately 40 per cent of body mass in laboratory animals is fatal.[35, 36] A progressive weight loss of no more than 10 per cent in a six-month period is a reasonably safe guideline. The pitfalls of relying solely on weight change as an indication of nutritional states are obvious. Edema fluid, ascites, or rapid swings in hydration will make this measurement very inaccurate.

Triceps Skinfold Thickness. A measure of the triceps skinfold at the midarm level can be compared with anthropometric standards to estimate body adipose tissue stores[37] (Table 106–2). During starvation, body fat is lost proportionately from the subcutaneous tis-

Table 106–2. ANTHROPOMETRIC NORMS FOR TRICEPS SKINFOLD THICKNESS AND MIDARM MUSCLE AREA IN THE ASSESSMENT OF NUTRITIONAL STATUS

		Population Percentiles				
	Age (yr)	***10th***	***25th***	***50th***	***75th***	***90th***
TRICEPS SKINFOLD THICKNESS (mm)						
Male	30	5.5	8.0	12.0	16.0	21.5
	50	6.0	8.0	11.0	15.0	20.0
	70	5.5	8.0	11.0	15.0	19.0
Female	30	12.0	16.0	21.0	26.5	33.5
	50	15.0	20.0	25.0	30.0	36.0
	70	14.0	18.0	23.0	28.0	33.0
MIDARM MUSCLE AREA (sq cm)						
Male	30	50.8	55.9	62.6	71.9	79.9
	50	49.5	55.9	62.6	70.9	79.0
	70	44.7	50.9	57.5	64.6	71.3
Female	30	28.3	32.0	36.3	41.6	49.3
	50	30.1	34.0	39.4	46.8	56.5
	70	30.3	34.5	40.3	47.6	55.7

Adapted from Bishop, C. W., Bowen, P. E., and Ritchey, S. J. Am. J. Clin. Nutr. *34*:2530, 1981.

sues, a depot that contains approximately half of the total body fat; comparison with normative indicators of subcutaneous fat may reflect overall fat losses. Measurement of the subcutaneous fat at more than one site can improve the accuracy of this anthropometric technique.[38] It should be emphasized, however, that comparison of a measurement taken at one point in time to population norms can be misleading when one is trying to determine the degree of malnutrition of an individual patient. For example, a patient initially overweight may have a normal triceps skinfold thickness (and a satisfactory AW:IBW ratio) even after significant weight loss has occurred. This situation is well exemplified by those who become protein-malnourished after intestinal bypass surgery yet are still overweight. Likewise, very lean, athletic subjects may normally carry a percentage of body fat that is low by population norms. For this reason the AW:UBW ratio can be a better predictor of the degree of associated protein depletion than a single measurement of the triceps skinfold.

Efforts must be made to minimize technical errors in all anthropometric measurements. Variance in determination of the triceps skinfold is considerable.[39] Errors may be related to measurement technique (differing locations on the arm, variation in pinch pressure of the calipers) as well as to the undependability of the measurement (from changes in hydration of the adipose tissue, muscle tone).[40] In addition, the skinfold is not a completely accurate measure of body fat; it provides only a correlated value.[41] For these reasons, anthropometric data have limited accuracy in the assessment of nutritional status and should be combined with other assessment parameters in estimating the degree of protein and calorie malnutrition.

Midarm Muscle Measurements. The largest amount of body protein is present in the skeletal muscles. During starvation and metabolic stress (periods of negative nitrogen balance), protein from the skeletal muscle compartment is metabolized along with other body proteins. Weakness of skeletal muscle can be demonstrated when as little as 10 per cent of the lean body mass is acutely lost. The skeletal muscle mass can be estimated by measuring midarm muscle circumference and comparing this measurement with population norms. Midarm muscle area (MMA) is calculated from the circumference of the arm midway between the olecranon process and the acromion while the patient is in a sitting position.[37] The thickness of the skinfold is subtracted from the calculated arm diameter to give the estimated diameter of the muscle compartment. Area of the muscle compartment can then be calculated. Age- and sex-specific reference values for the MMA have been derived from recently published norms for upper arm anthropometry[42] (Table 106–2). Difficulties in using anthropometric data for nutritional assessment are many.[43]

Creatinine-Height Index. The creatinine-height index (CHI)[44] is a more accurate way of estimating total body muscle mass but depends on accurate urinary collections. Creatinine is an end product of muscle metabolism, and steady-state creatinine excretion in a 24-hour period can be used to estimate the somatic protein compartment.[45] The CHI is the ratio of the actual creatinine excreted to the predicted normal excretion for the height of the subject. Ideal urinary creatinine values for men and women are given in Table 106–3. Unfortunately, measures of somatic protein compartment size do not predictably reflect functional capabilities of muscles. Reduction in strength of important muscles, such as the diaphragm, precede measurable reductions in muscle mass as determined by the CHI or MMA.

Circulating Proteins. Suspicion of protein depletion most frequently arises from the observation of abnormally low serum protein levels. Measurable proteins include albumin, transport proteins, and immunoglobulins. Total protein and albumin levels are both nonspecific and insensitive as measures of protein status, although a distinct correlation to body cell mass does exist.[46] When combined with other measurements of protein-calorie nutritional status, serum albumin levels have some predictive value in estimating risk from nutritional depletion.[47] However, albumin levels inconsistently reflect changes in nutritional status as defined by body composition during therapy. Serum transferrin can be directly measured or estimated from the total iron-binding capacity (TIBC) by a linear relation. Although the conversion formula, serum transferrin (mg/dl) = (TIBC × 0.8) − 43, has been suggested,[48] the constants appear to vary considerably depending upon the laboratory. This protein has a smaller body pool and a half-life of eight to ten days and may be a better indicator than is albumin of recent changes in body protein status. Thyroxin-binding prealbumin and retinol-binding protein have even shorter half-lives and possibly more accurately reflect acute changes in the visceral protein compartment. However, measurement

Table 106–3. IDEAL 24-HOUR URINARY CREATININE EXCRETION FOR MEN AND WOMEN IN RELATION TO HEIGHT

Men		Women	
Height (in)	*Ideal Creatinine Excretion (mg/24 hr)*	*Height (in)*	*Ideal Creatine Excretion (mg/24 hr)*
62	1288	58	830
63	1325	59	851
64	1359	60	875
65	1386	61	900
66	1426	62	925
67	1467	63	949
68	1513	64	977
69	1555	65	1006
70	1596	66	1044
71	1642	67	1076
72	1691	68	1109
73	1739	69	1141
74	1785	70	1174
75	1831	71	1206
76	1891	72	1240

Adapted from Blackburn, G. L., Bistrian, B. R., Maini, B. S., et al. JPEN *1*:11, 1979.

of these proteins is currently not widely used in estimation of a patient's protein status. It is clear that no single biochemical marker currently available will consistently reflect protein or calorie nutritional status with the accuracy expected in modern medicine.

Tests of Immune Function. Immunologic competence is impaired in malnutrition. Abnormalities include depressed serum complement levels,[49,50] a decrease in the total number of circulating lymphocytes,[51,52] and depressed reactivity to skin test antigens.[52–54] None of these abnormalities is specific for malnutrition, nor is immunologic incompetence always indicative of protein depletion, but all have been corrected in some patients with intensive total nutritional replacement.[55–57] Demonstration of anergy to a battery of skin test antigens when estimating the severity of protein and calorie malnutrition has been well correlated with in-hospital morbidity,[5,47,58,59] although a causal relationship between immunologic dysfunction and morbidity has not been established.

The overall severity of protein and calorie malnutrition can be estimated from the assessments described. Emphasis should *not* be placed on an individual parameter that does not seem to be in line with the rest of the measurements. Values for the individual measurements to assist in grading severity of nutritional depletion are listed in Table 106–4. Since grading of the severity of malnutrition using these parameters is arbitrary, the abnormal values listed in the table are a composite of various authors' opinions.[9,43,48,60] Patients who are most deceiving in initial evaluation are those who appear to have normal body weight yet are depleted in somatic and visceral proteins. This situation is exemplified by the initially overweight patient who experiences persistent negative nitrogen balance. Anthropometry of the adipose stores will not reveal a deficiency if the patient is still at or above population norms. Likewise, the AW:IBW ratio will be in the normal range. Systematic examination of even the routine laboratory data obtained on most hospitalized patients, such as the serum albumin, TIBC, and peripheral lymphocyte count, especially when there is a history of recent surgery, a protracted medical illness, or 10 per cent weight loss, will keep the clinician from overlooking this group of malnourished patients.

The presence of severe protein or protein and calorie malnutrition on initial evaluation indicates the need to prevent any further deterioration in nutritional status. Since severe depletion represents protracted inadequate nutrition, repletion may be slow when conventional nutritional supplements are given. Many of these patients are candidates for intensive nutritional therapy from the outset.

Patients with mild to moderate protein or protein and calorie malnutrition do not necessarily require intensive nutritional therapy. Other questions must be addressed when selecting such patients for these therapeutic techniques.

How Severe Is the Current Negative Nitrogen and Calorie Balance?

The assessment of protein and calorie balance is covered on pages 1978 to 1981. It is unlikely that a deficit exceeding 1000 kcal/day could be corrected with oral nutritional supplements alone. However, if the daily caloric deficit is small, aggressive forms of nutritional calorie support are generally unnecessary. Urinary urea nitrogen excretion exceeding 10 gm/day is seen in disorders associated with severe catabolism (sepsis, multiple trauma, significant burns).[48] Consequently, persistent negative nitrogen balance of 10 to 12 gm/day or worse should suggest severe calorie-protein imbalance.

What is the Anticipated Duration of Negative Balance?

Although it is difficult to predict the length of time that a patient will be unable to meet calorie and protein demands, the anticipation of the end of persistent negative balance is helpful in choosing patients for intensive nutritional therapy. If it is anticipated that positive nitrogen and calorie balance will be re-estab-

Table 106–4. ASSESSMENT OF PROTEIN AND CALORIE NUTRITIONAL STATUS FROM ANTHROPOMETRIC AND LABORATORY DATA

Measurement of Index	Compartment Best Reflected by the Measurement	Estimated Degree of Malnourishment		
		Mild	*Moderate*	*Severe*
Actual weight/ideal body weight (%)	Somatic protein and fat reserves	80–90%	70–80%	< 70%
Actual weight/usual body weight (%)	Prediction of protein malnourishment	85–95%	75–85%	< 75%
Triceps skinfold thickness (population percentile)	Fat reserves	35–40th	25–35th	< 25th
Midarm muscle area (population percentile)	Skeletal muscle mass	35–40th	25–35th	< 25th
Creatinine-height index (actual Cr excretion/ideal for a given height)	Skeletal muscle mass	0.8–1.0	0.6–0.8	< 0.6
Serum albumin (gm/dl)	Visceral proteins	2.8–3.5	2.1–2.8	< 2.1
Serum transferrin (mg/dl)	Visceral proteins	150–200	100–150	< 100
Total peripheral lymphocyte count (cells/mm³)	Nonspecific	1200–2000	800–1200	< 800
Reactivity to skin test antigens	Nonspecific	+	+	– (anergy)

lished within seven to ten days by using normal foods and nutritional oral supplements, then intensive enteral or parenteral therapy is seldom indicated. If surgery will correct obstruction or eating disability and permit nutritional restitution by mouth, intensive therapy need be used only in those individuals with severe depletion. However, if there is uncertainty about recovery from the illness, and in particular if the patient is severely malnourished, then intensive therapy should be initiated at the outset.

Is the Intestinal Tract Available and Adequate?

Serious gastrointestinal disorders prohibit the use of the intestinal tract because of the further production of symptoms with feeding. Intestinal obstruction, pseudo-obstruction, or ileus will generally prohibit use of the intestinal tract. Although the presence of one of these disorders is not an absolute contraindication to attempted use of enteral therapy, feeding or the infusion of products into the proximal intestinal tract may only exacerbate symptoms of the underlying disorder. Patients with postoperative ileus have been fed in the postoperative period through intraoperatively placed jejunostomy tubes, with rapid establishment of positive nitrogen balance. Colon dysfunction exceeds small bowel dysfunction in postoperative ileus and may explain the success of this technique.[61] In other cases of ileus, especially if low grade without spontaneous abdominal pain, enteral feeding could also be attempted.

It may be difficult to meet daily protein and calorie requirements with foods and supplements in patients with severe malabsorption, whatever the cause. However, malabsorption can usually be overcome and positive calorie and nitrogen balance established by oral feeding if the patient has not previously had intestinal resection. Patients with short bowel syndrome secondary to massive or repeated intestinal resection can significantly benefit from parenteral nutrition. Not only will positive fluid and electrolyte balance be established, but decay in nutritional status will also be prevented. Parenteral nutrition can also be used to ease the transition to oral feeding and to maintain patients over long periods of time at home.[62, 63]

Other situations in which use of the intestinal tract may exacerbate symptoms of the underlying disease include: (1) severe diarrheal illnesses of any etiology, (2) inflammatory disease of the small or large intestine (e.g., Crohn's disease, ulcerative jejunitis, radiation enteritis, diverticulitis), (3) enteric fistulas, and (4) inflammatory disorders of the pancreas and biliary tree. Total parenteral nutrition is not mandatory in these illnesses. However, if recovery of bowel function is not expected within seven to ten days and, in particular, if the degree of metabolic stress is large, parenteral nutrition should be initiated to avoid serious deterioration in nutritional status.

What Is the Safest and Most Cost-Effective Approach to Therapy?

Both forced enteral feeding and total parenteral nutrition are associated with complications that limit the usefulness of the techniques. Gastrointestinal side effects, including bloating, cramping, diarrhea, and vomiting, occur in 10 to 20 per cent of patients treated with nasally placed duodenal feeding tubes.[64] These side effects interfere with treatment but do not result in lasting morbidity. Pulmonary aspiration of stomach contents and esophageal erosion are more serious complications but occur in fewer than 1 per cent of patients treated with small-bore duodenal feeding tubes if precautions are taken to ensure proper placement of the tube.

Total parenteral nutrition is more frequently associated with mechanical, infectious, and metabolic complications (see p. 2018). Septic complications were once reported in up to one third of patients treated with central venous parenteral nutrition, but careful attention to pharmacy preparation techniques and to aseptic catheter care has reduced this incidence considerably. Institutions active in parenteral therapy report septic complication rates not exceeding 5 per cent.[65–67] Other metabolic and catheter-related complications raise the serious morbidity to 5 to 10 per cent. Because of the considerable variability in morbidity from hospital to hospital, local statistics should be considered in deciding whether to use this form of nutrition therapy.

While the theoretical advantages of enteral nutrition therapy are apparent, the practical advantages are remarkable. It is for these reasons that forced enteral nutrition has rapidly established itself as an important form of nutritional therapy today. Technologic advancements in the formulas for tube feeding have allowed tube diameters to be reduced to 3 mm or less. Traumatic complications previously encountered with large nasogastric tubes for gavage feeding now are infrequent. Even in relatively inexperienced hands, successful nutritional support can be offered with a low morbidity. This contrasts with the notable serious morbidity of parenteral nutrition that can be reduced only with concentrated efforts by knowledgeable physicians and paramedical personnel. Cost considerations now have a greater impact on medical decisions, especially for hospitalized patients. The cost comparison of the two forms of forced feeding is striking. The daily inpatient cost of total parenteral nutrition is several hundred dollars above the regular hospital cost.[68] The cost of a standard commercial tube feeding diet is less than one tenth of this. These comparative comments are not meant to denigrate parenteral nutrition. However, they emphasize the desirability of forced enteral nutrition considering the equal utilization of macronutrients when provided by the parenteral or enteral route.[69]

After answering the foregoing questions the clinician should be able to arrive at a satisfactory way of managing the protein and calorie nutritional problems of most patients. There are obviously multiple ways to reach the same end. At times, flow diagrams are helpful in organizing thoughts; a flow diagram useful in selecting patients for intensive nutritional support is presented in Figure 106–1.

Three short case histories illustrate factors in decision-making regarding intensive nutrition support and the points of emphasis in Figure 106–1.

Patient No. 1

A 27-year-old male with known Crohn's disease of the colon is admitted for worsening diarrhea and cramping lower abdominal pain unresponsive to increase in corticosteroid medication. The patient is 90 per cent of ideal body weight and 95 per cent of usual body weight. Triceps skinfold and midarm muscle area are in the fiftieth percentile, serum albumin is 2.9, and lymphocyte count is normal. Radiographic and endoscopic evaluation of the colon is anticipated. There is no history of small bowel disease or other gastrointestinal disease.

Comment. This patient represents a picture of Crohn's colitis in exacerbation. Indications for a nothing-by-mouth regimen or total bowel rest are not absolute. Nutritional assessment reveals a pattern of mild to moderate calorie-protein undernutrition. With further studies planned and the patient unable to tolerate a regular diet that meets calorie needs, continued negative balance can be expected for more than a week. The proximal gastrointestinal tract can be expected to be functional for nutrient absorption. The patient is offered the option of a minimal-residue liquid formula diet to accomplish partial colonic bowel rest with nutritional restitution but chooses to have the formula administered by nasoenteral tube.

Patient No. 2

A 54-year-old woman with extensive radiation enteritis following aggressive radiotherapy for a pelvic tumor 15 years previously enters the hospital with worsening symptoms of postprandial vomiting, inability to eat, and a loss of 15 per cent of usual body weight over the past three months. The admission abdominal film shows multiple air-fluid levels and is consistent with high-grade small bowel obstruction. A decompressing nasoenteral tube is placed; the surgeons are unwilling to operate in face of known multiple strictures complicating radiation enteritis.

Comment. This patient presents a prima facie indication for a nothing-by-mouth regimen or total bowel rest. She requires parenteral nutritional support to prevent worsening of nutritional status while decisions are made regarding subsequent management. Some patients with Crohn's disease in exacerbation who present with worsening symptoms of obstruction with pain and evidence of increased inflammation who are not candidates for surgery are considered in a similar category.

Patient No. 3

A 36-year-old male with a strong alcoholic history enters the hospital for severe epigastric pain and vomiting. Physical

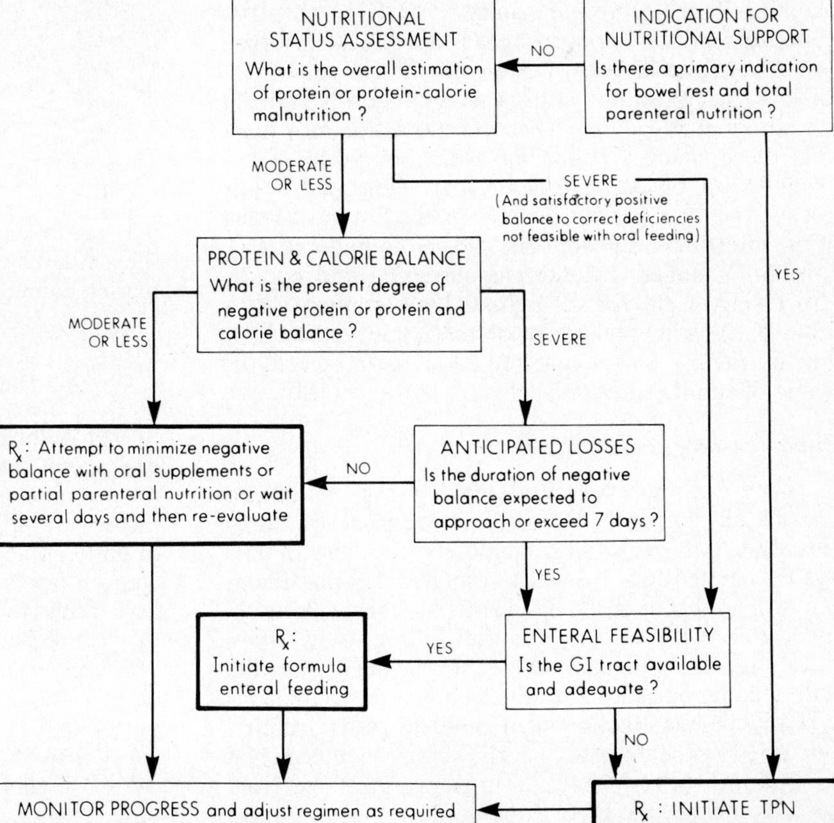

Figure 106–1. A flow diagram useful in selecting candidates for intensive protein and calorie nutritional therapy.

examination, initial X-rays, and serum amylase level are consistent with acute pancreatitis. The patient is treated with nasogastric suction and intravenous fluids. On nutrition assessment after rehydration he is found to have body weight that is 80 per cent of ideal and 80 per cent of his usual weight. Skinfold and muscle area measurements are consistent with moderate protein malnutrition. The serum albumin value is 3.0; the lymphocyte count is normal. His abdominal pain has responded promptly to cessation of oral intake and to nasogastric suction.

Comment. This patient with acute pancreatitis presents with evidence of moderate undernutrition with an acute episode interfering with nutritional intake. It is anticipated that a nothing-by-mouth, nasogastric suction regimen will be required for less than a week, after which time he should be able to be started on feeding and nutritional rehabilitation. Neither forced enteral feeding nor total parenteral nutrition is required for the successful management of this patient.

INTENSIVE ENTERAL NUTRITION THERAPY

Patients with functioning gastrointestinal tracts are candidates for enteral feeding by tube. Tube feeding concepts are not new. However, the introduction of small-caliber feeding tubes and highly dispersed commercial feeding formulas in combination with a generally heightened interest in nutrition has dramatically stimulated applications of this form of intensive nutrition therapy.

Utilization of the intestinal tract when possible has more than aesthetic appeal. Lack of intraluminal nutrient supply eventually results in intestinal mucosal thinning in the laboratory animal.[70, 71] Even with parenteral nutrition support there is a decrease in brush border enzyme activity, DNA content, and total mass of the rat intestine with prolonged deprivation of intraluminal nutrients.[72] There is little reason to suspect that these changes might not eventually occur in humans. Easy reversion to usual oral diets in patients recovering from serious illness would seem most likely if the intestinal tract were not allowed to undergo such atrophic changes. In addition, intestinal and hepatic processing of nutrients is bypassed in parenteral nutrition. The detrimental effects of this, if any, are unclear, but nutrient value of ingested foods may exceed the value of similar nutrients delivered intravenously.

Tube Feeding Techniques

Tubes for forced enteral feeding can be placed transnasally or directly into the stomach or small intestine. Soft tubes with diameters of 3 mm or less are well suited for prolonged nasoduodenal placement and will not produce the nasal and pharyngeal irritation associated with larger or stiffer tubes. It is often advantageous to place the tube into the small intestine with feeding ports distal to the ligament of Treitz. This will reduce the likelihood of duodenogastric reflux[73] but does not eliminate the risk of tracheobronchial aspiration.[74] Several bedside maneuvers can be tried for advancing the tube through the pylorus before resorting to more costly fluoroscopic or endoscopic methods if the tube fails to leave the stomach.[75, 76] Likewise, the tube can be used for nasogastric feeding in many patients if it does not pass spontaneously into the small intestine.[77]

Feeding tubes can also be placed directly into the gastrointestinal tract by several methods. Traditional surgical techniques are being supplanted in many instances by endoscopic, radiologic, or bedside methods that are cost-beneficial and appear to be attended by very low morbidity. This contrasts with rates of significant complications ranging from 10 to 35 per cent for surgical gastrostomy[78] and similar or even higher rates for jejunostomy.[79, 80] For patients who are undergoing anesthesia or an abdominal operation for other reasons, and for those who are not candidates for the simpler procedures, the variety of surgically placed feeding tubes remain as important options.[81] Currently in practice is a recently described technique of *percutaneous gastrostomy*,[82, 83] a method that uses the endoscope to localize an appropriate site and to assist in placement of the feeding tube (Fig. 106–2). This simplified, less expensive approach for obtaining direct access to the gastrointestinal tract may be the preferred method in suitable candidates.[84, 85] Indications for its use are still being developed.

The originally described technique with some modification is still the most commonly utilized method of endoscopic gastrostomy tube placement,[82–84] although alternative methods have appeared.[86] Regardless of technique and despite the serious nature of the underlying illnesses in most patients, complications from endoscopic gastrostomy are relatively uncommon.[84–89] Overall morbidity ranges from 7 to 17 per cent. Abdominal wall infections were initially more frequent until the pioneers of the method began routine use of a single dosage of a cephalosporin shortly before the procedure.[84] Although this use of antibiotics is controversial,[89] the reported rates of wound infection are generally low (2 to 5 per cent). Pneumoperitoneum may be obvious if a large amount of air escapes around the catheter used to puncture the stomach, but this finding immediately after the procedure is not generally of clinical significance.[90] Tube dislodgment, leakage of gastric contents, and fistula development are also rare, each occurring in less than 2 to 4 per cent of cases. Despite the fact that considerable sedation is used for this procedure and that the majority if not all of the endoscopic component is performed with the patient in a supine position, complications related to these factors are apparently unlikely. Death directly related to endoscopic gastrostomy is very uncommon,[89, 91] and laparotomy is rarely needed. These overall complication rates look favorable compared with those of surgical techniques for placement of feeding tubes.

Simplified percutaneous placement of feeding tubes using radiologic guidance has also recently been reported.[92–94] In general, the stomach is inflated using a nasogastric tube and a puncture site is determined using a combination of fluoroscopy and ultrasonography. A guidewire is advanced through the pylorus and

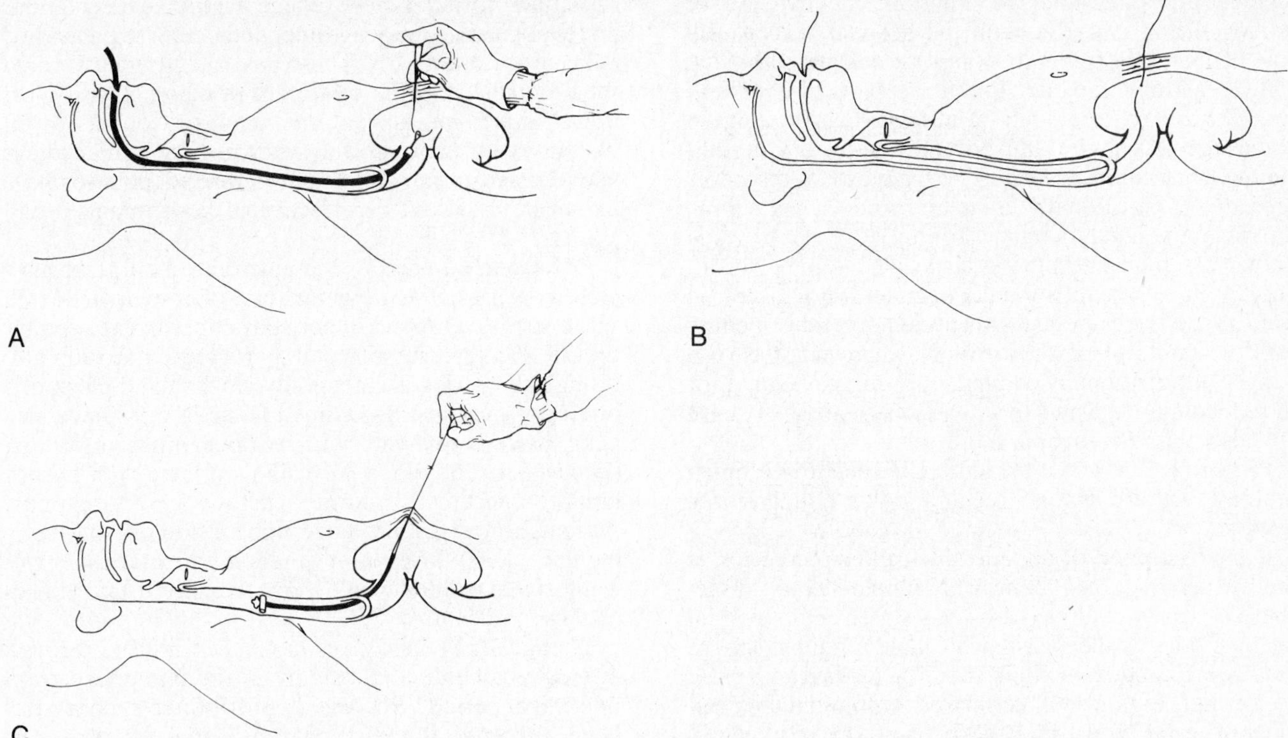

Figure 106–2. Steps in the placement of a percutaneous gastrostomy according to the technique of Ponsky and associates.[82–84] *A,* A needle catheter is used to pierce the abdominal wall and stomach after endoscopic localization of the preferred site. A thread passed through the catheter is grasped with an endoscopic snare. *B,* The endoscope is withdrawn pulling the thread out through the mouth. *C,* The proximal end of the thread is attached to the gastrostomy tube. The thread and tapered tip of the gastrostomy tube are then pulled through the puncture site, firmly anchoring the crosspiece and mushroom tip to the stomach lining. A similar crosspiece is placed externally to ensure good apposition of the gastric and abdominal walls.

into the small bowel. The feeding tube is placed once a satisfactory tract is established with the necessary dilators. Morbidity of this technique may be somewhat higher than that of the endoscopic technique, as determined from the small series that have been reported.[89] Percutaneous transhepatic biliary catheters that have internal drainage access have also been modified as feeding tubes for some patients.[95] A simplified method for establishing a pharyngostomy using a needle puncture technique has also recently been reported.[96] The trend toward development of less expensive techniques for long-term feeding tube access that are attended by low complication rates is readily evident.

Intermittent bolus feeding through a nasogastric or gastrostomy tube is most suitable for the ambulatory patient who does not wish to be confined by a continuous infusion. This is particularly true for patients with neurologic disorders involving the oropharynx and upper esophagus or those with other esophageal disorders. Feeding schedules with incremental increases in bolus volume ultimately can be established such that feedings of 400 ml at three- to four-hour intervals are tolerated. Three to four daytime feedings will meet basal requirements of unstressed patients. Osmolality characteristics of the feeding solution are less important than in direct small bowel intubation if regulatory mechanisms of gastric emptying are intact.

Constant, rather than bolus, infusion of the formula is necessary through feeding tubes placed into the small bowel and is also successful through tubes left in the stomach.[77] This feeding method is often used in hospitalized patients but has no metabolic advantage over bolus feeding techniques.[97] Small bowel infusion bypasses all mechanisms that regulate nutrient delivery to the small bowel from a normally functioning stomach, and, consequently, symptoms similar to those of the dumping syndrome are common. Osmolality of the formulas is an important consideration during small bowel infusion. Dilution of isosmotic formulas to one half or less the original strength is usually recommended during the initiation of feeding. It may be that much of the diarrhea attributed to the high osmolality of feeding solutions is more correctly associated with concomitant antibiotic administration.[98] Slow starter regimens may unnecessarily delay reversal of negative nitrogen balance in many cases.[99] Even with a properly placed small bowel tube, the patient's head should be elevated at least 30 degrees from the horizontal during the infusion to avoid the complication of pulmonary aspiration.

Tube Feeding Diets

Commercial products have replaced hospital-prepared tube feeding diets in most cases. The products are highly dispersed, making the use of small-bore feeding tubes feasible. In addition, the expense of homogenizing table foods in the hospital exceeds the cost of many nutritionally complete commercial diets. The ideal tube feeding diet for a particular patient should meet requirements of all essential nutrients in a reasonable volume and have the necessary modifications to accommodate the gastrointestinal disorders present. A nutritionally complete product will supply the recommended dietary allowance of each of the known essential nutrients in a specified volume. Products that are not nutritionally complete should not be used as the sole dietary constituent for tube feeding over a significant period of time. Characteristics of a variety of nutritionally complete products available for tube feeding are listed in Table 106–5. Most of these are also suitable as oral supplements for the patient with satisfactory appetite, although palatability limits oral use. All are lactose-free and low in nondigestible residue.

Diets composed of oligopeptides and amino acids as the nitrogen sources along with simple sugars, disaccharides, or partially hydrolyzed starch and minimal fat have been called *elemental diets*. Originally these diets were unique in their chemical definition of the major nutrients when compared with homogenized diets of usual foods, and they earned special recognition as chemically defined or defined formula diets. However, the majority of commercial products used today contain specified constituents as the protein, carbohydrate, and fat sources, and consequently the older terminology is nearly obsolete. Diets with amino acids and oligosaccharides as the major calorie source (the original elemental diets) have been specifically studied to determine their usefulness in various gastrointestinal diseases, whereas less information is available comparing these results with those of diets having less-hydrolyzed constituents.

Defined-formula diets reduce gastric acid secretion, increase gastric emptying time, and decrease pancreatic enzyme secretion.[100, 101] These physiologic effects would seem beneficial in the treatment of patients with short bowel syndrome or enteric fistulas. Conversion of patients with short bowel syndrome to oral feedings with defined-formula diets during the adaptation phase has been shown to be effective in both infants[102] and adults.[103]

Fistulas in all parts of the gastrointestinal tract have closed during defined-formula diet therapy with overall success rates of about 70 per cent, a percentage similar to the success rate of total parenteral nutrition, although the series are generally small[104] and closure is often not permanent. Defined-formula diets have also been used in patients with various other disorders, such as anorexia nervosa, Crohn's disease with growth failure, cancer, or routine postoperative situations. Although most studies have utilized the original "elemental" diets, infusion of other, more complex chemically defined diets would seem equally useful for all of these indications.[105]

Chemically defined diets have been infused through a needle-catheter jejunostomy in the immediate postoperative period. Successful nutritional support has been reported in most patients, and complications related to the jejunostomy itself have been infrequent in some series.[106–108] A recent retrospective review of 73 patients undergoing jejunostomy for tube feeding indicates that the morbidity of the procedure may be greater than had been appreciated.[109] Death of seven patients was directly related to the feeding tube. Intolerance to the tube feeding formula may also limit the effectiveness of the technique in a large percentage of patients,[110] particularly when elemental diets are utilized. The chemically defined nonelemental diets appear to be as nutritionally effective as elemental

Table 106–5. CHARACTERISTICS OF REPRESENTATIVE NUTRITIONALLY COMPLETE FORMULAS FOR TUBE FEEDING

Product	kcal*/ 1000 ml	gm protein/ 1000 ml	Approximate Mineral Content† Na mg/L	K mg/L	Cl mg/L	Ca mg/L	P mg/L	Mg mg/L	Osmolality mOsm/kg Water	Comments
Ensure	1060	37	740	1270	1060	530	530	210	450	
Isocal	1040	34	530	1320	1060	630	530	210	300	Low sodium content: 1–1.5 gm/day for most patients (Isocal, Osmolite)
Osmolite	1060	37	540	1060	800	500	540	200	300	
Precision Isotonic	960	29	800	960	1000	640	640	260	300	
Precision LR	1110	26	700	810	1100	580	580	230	525	
Travasorb STD (unflavored)	1000	30	920	1170	1500	500	500	200	450	"Elemental" diets; see text (Travasorb STD through High Nitrogen Vivonex)
Travasorb HN	1000	45	920	1170	1350	500	500	200	450	
Standard Vivonex (unflavored)	1000	21	470	1170	720	560	560	220	550	
High Nitrogen Vivonex (unflavored)	1000	44	530	1170	820	330	330	130	810	
Meritene Powder in Milk	1065	69	1000	3000	2400	2300	1900	385	690	Milk based
Compleat B	1000	40	1200	1300	810	630	1250	250	390	Blenderized food formulas; higher residue; not recommended for small-caliber tube infusion (Compleat B, Formula 2)
Formula 2	1000	38	600	1760	1900	720	560	100	435–510	

*When prepared in standard dilution.
†Refer to manufacturer's literature for content of other minerals and vitamins.

diets and may eliminate much of this intolerance.[105] This technique appears to be an alternative to total parenteral nutrition in severely malnourished patients in whom immediate postoperative nutritional support is desired. The advantage in cost-effectiveness as compared with total parenteral nutrition is considerable, but complications limit enthusiasm for the technique.[111]

Specific disadvantages of the elemental diets reduce their usefulness compared with other formula diets for tube feeding. Lower fat content forces higher carbohydrate content to achieve a satisfactory caloric density. This results in higher osmolality of the diet (Table 106–5). High osmolality is probably in part responsible for the delay in gastric emptying, since gastric emptying rate of liquid varies inversely with osmolality.[112] Direct small bowel infusion overrides this control mechanism; diarrhea is a common problem with any high osmolality diet infusion. In addition, elemental diets are considerably more expensive than many products without amino acids or hydrolyzed peptides as the nitrogen source. Studies comparing the various diets have rarely established any specific benefits of elemental diets over more complex liquid diets.

Differences in the metabolism of the various calorie sources used in enteral diets have been of recent interest, particularly in relation to patients with pulmonary disease. When carbohydrates are completely metabolized in the presence of oxygen to CO_2 and H_2O, one molecule of CO_2 is produced for each molecule of oxygen consumed, and the resultant respiratory quotient (RQ) is 1.0. The RQ for fats is 0.7, less CO_2 being produced in relation to oxygen consumed. Taking into account the different caloric values of fats and carbohydrates, these ratios indicate that isocaloric provision of a diet with higher fat content would be accompanied by less CO_2 production and might be advantageous to patients with severe pulmonary disease.[113, 114] Precipitation of respiratory failure and difficulties with weaning patients from ventilatory support have been attributed to high-carbohydrate parenteral feeding.[115–117] It is possible that the CO_2 production accompanying overfeeding in general has been a major factor in some of these cases. Nevertheless, it is clinically apparent that differing energy sources will affect CO_2 production and minute ventilation and certainly could have detrimental effects. Comparisons of the calculated RQ of various commercially available products indicate that the traditional elemental diets have higher values than other chemically defined diets, reflecting the higher carbohydrate content of the elemental feedings.[118] Products are being designed that contain more fat and have lower RQ values than standard formulations (e.g., Pulmocare, 0.80, versus Ensure Plus, 0.87.[118] These may be useful in selected patients with impaired pulmonary function.

Modified defined formula diets are available for patients with renal failure and liver disease. Renal formulas contain essential amino acids and histidine as the nitrogen sources. In principle, the nonessential amino acids will be formed endogenously, possibly by utilizing retained nitrogen. As a nutritional supplement to a low-protein diet, essential amino acids will reduce the BUN:creatinine ratio and can assist in prolonging the predialysis period without endangering the life expectancy of the patients.[119]

Formulas for liver failure contain a high proportion of branched-chain amino acids (valine, leucine, and isoleucine) and arginine and lesser amounts of aromatic amino acids and methionine. This modification was developed from the observation of a relative increase in plasma concentrations of certain aromatic amino acids and methionine in patients with liver insufficiency and portosystemic encephalopathy.[120–122] Modest improvement in objective and subjective parameters of encephalopathy has been demonstrated with the use of branched-chain amino acids themselves or as alpha-keto analogs in supplemental form to a protein-restricted diet.[121, 123, 124]

These specialized formulas may contain no vitamins and minimal electrolytes; depending on the clinical situation, supplementation will be necessary if no other diet is used. The full extent of the clinical application of these diets and similar commercial products awaits further study.

Tube Feeding at Home

Long-term enteral feeding is accomplished either through a transnasal feeding tube or through a gastrostomy or jejunostomy.[125–128] The simplified methods of gastrostomy described above may become frequently utilized even for patients with relatively short courses of planned nutritional support, such as during radiation therapy or following radical head and neck surgery. However, use of a transnasal feeding tube is certainly more cost-efficient if the patient can tolerate the appearance and other psychological and technical aspects of this approach. It is feasible to continue forced enteral feeding in a patient's home,[125, 126] and the technique is one-tenth to one-twentieth the cost of comparable support with parenteral nutrition.[126] In addition, significant complications are much less frequent with the enteral technique.[125, 126] Patients have been followed systematically for months without detrimental changes in laboratory profile,[127, 128] but gradual development of zinc deficiency has been reported and eventual occurrence of other micronutrient deficiencies is considered possible.[129]

Complications of Tube Feeding

Complications of the nasogastric and nasoenteral tube feeding techniques are infrequent.[64] Nasal passage and oropharyngeal irritation are less common with small-caliber nasogastric or nasoduodenal tubes made of various materials that do not stiffen or become brittle with time. Gastrointestinal distress is more frequent with small bowel infusion than with intragastric feeding and can usually be improved by reducing the infusion rate or temporarily diluting the formula. Diarrhea can result from too-rapid infusion, infusion of hyperosmolar solutions, concomitant antibiotic use, or malabsorption of fats in the formula if underlying gastrointestinal disease is present. Many commercial products available do not contain lactose, so this is no longer a problem. Appropriate modification of the feeding protocol will usually result in a decrease in stool output; occasionally codeine sulfate is necessary. Rare complications mentioned have included inadvertent intravenous administration of the diet[130] and precipitation of pseudo-obstruction syndrome of the colon.[131] Perforation of a bronchus or penetration into the lung parenchyma with passage of the feeding tube into the pleural space can occur if a stylet is used to place a transnasal feeding tube.[132]

Tracheobronchial aspiration and aspiration pneumonia are serious complications of forced enteral feeding. Passage of the tube into the distal duodenum, preferably beyond the ligament of Treitz, should reduce this likelihood. However, even establishment of a feeding jejunostomy may not eliminate tracheobronchial aspiration in those with a prior history of aspiration pneumonia.[109] Patients receiving continuous enteral infusions should have their heads elevated 30 degrees from the horizontal at all times, and those receiving intermittent bolus feeding should remain in a tilted or upright position for at least two hours after each feeding.

Forced feeding with defined diets can result in significant electrolyte abnormalities. Careful monitoring in the first one to two weeks of therapy, similar to protocols for monitoring total parenteral nutrition therapy, is suggested. A syndrome of *hyperosmotic nonketotic dehydration* has occurred as a result of inadequate free water supplementation.[133] Patients with this syndrome appear lethargic, dehydrated, and occasionally febrile and respond to rehydration with hypotonic fluids. In such cases, additional water should be added to the daily regimen.

PARENTERAL NUTRITION

The general indications for parenteral nutrition in gastrointestinal disease are (1) to correct severe nutritional depletion in patients unable to maintain adequate oral intake, and (2) to meet nutritional needs during periods of absolute bowel rest without any enteral intake. Considering the frequency with which nothing-by-mouth regimens or nasogastric suction are used in the management of severe gastrointestinal disorders and the likelihood that such patients suffer from nutritional depletion on presentation, it is not surprising that patients with gastrointestinal disorders have been among those most commonly treated with total parenteral nutrition. The gastrointestinal conditions in which total parenteral nutrition has been an important addition to management are listed in Table 106–6. It should be emphasized that not all, or even the majority, of patients in each diagnostic category need to be treated with total parenteral alimentation. An approach to the selection of patients for intensive nutritional support is found earlier in this chapter.

Table 106–6. EXAMPLES OF GASTROINTESTINAL CONDITIONS FOR WHICH TPN HAS BEEN EMPLOYED

For Nutritional Support in Patients Unable to Eat or Absorb Adequately
Short bowel syndrome
Radiation enteritis
Gastrointestinal cancer
Intestinal pseudo-obstruction
Growth retardation in Crohn's disease
Intractable sprue
For Bowel Rest and Nutritional Restitution
Crohn's disease
Ulcerative colitis
Enterocutaneous fistulas
Pancreatitis

Techniques in Parenteral Nutrition

Parenteral nutrition refers to the intravenous administration of carbohydrates, proteins (as amino acids), and fats, in amounts capable of maintaining or restoring protein and energy needs. The term *total parenteral nutrition* (TPN) deserves some qualification. Many patients selected for protein-calorie therapy may require total support without any other calorie or protein intake. However, in the absence of clinical indications for complete bowel rest or nasogastric or nasoenteric suction, it is possible to use parenteral nutrition therapy to *supplement* an oral intake that by itself cannot meet nutritional goals. Such partial or supplemental nutritional support is often administered by peripheral vein, since the contribution of intravenous nutrition to total calorie requirement is low enough to permit the use of less hypertonic solutions, which can be safely infused into peripheral veins. Central intravenous lines can be used for both partial and total intravenous support. If one establishes nutritional goals for each patient, as described earlier in this chapter, one can select the therapeutic technique best suited to meet these goals. Combined calorie and protein support is generally required in patients who need intensive nutrition support by vein. "Protein-sparing" therapy, which employs intravenous amino acids in hypocaloric regimens, has little specific application in the management of patients with gastrointestinal disease.

Total nutritional support can be performed in some patients via peripheral vein for limited periods of time if one limits the hypertonicity of the solutions. Carbohydrate as dextrose solutions in concentrations of up to 25 to 30 per cent can be used when the administration is into a large central vein. Concentrations above 10 per cent dextrose are considerably hypertonic (> 500 mOsm/liter) and corrosive for use in smaller peripheral veins. Lipid emulsions in concentrations of 10 to 20 per cent by volume have the advantage of delivering a highly concentrated calorie source in an isotonic solution. With the use of such emulsions, it is possible to administer close to 2000 kcal per day by peripheral vein, employing 2.5 liters of 10 per cent dextrose with appropriate amino acids and 1000 ml of a 10 per cent lipid emulsion. By providing more lipid calories, intakes above 2500 kcal/day can be accomplished, but lipid sources should not supply more than 60 to 70 per cent of the daily nonprotein calories. Peripheral vein nutritional support is most attractive in younger patients whose peripheral veins can offer a continuing reliable conduit when calorie requirements can be met within the limitations of peripheral intravenous therapy. Such therapy is usually employed for shorter periods of time, less than two weeks. Peripheral nutrition support therapy also has attractions when the patient is continuing to eat and total caloric requirement can be met by a combination of ingested food or formula plus intravenous nutrition.

Parenteral nutrition by central vein is normally performed through a catheter into the subclavian vein and then into the superior vena cava. To keep complications to a minimum and to maximize therapeutic effectiveness, this technically demanding approach is best executed by an experienced group consisting of a physician or surgeon trained in nutritional decision-making and management in addition to catheter placement, a nurse trained in catheter care and patient monitoring, and a pharmacist responsible for preparation and monitoring of the intravenous solutions. It is helpful also to include a clinical nutritionist to aid in establishing initial goals and to help monitor signs of nutritional progress. Institutions may prefer to have individuals from the aforementioned clinical departments designated as supervisors in parenteral nutrition techniques rather than naming a clinical team. Regardless of the approach, all participants must be well trained in their roles in the parenteral effort.

Principles of TPN Use

A detailed description of catheter insertion and care, preparation of parenteral nutrition solutions, and details of patient monitoring is beyond the scope of this text. Many publications offer detailed guidance on these matters.[9, 134–136] Certain principles in the formulation of a prescription for intravenous nutritional therapy can, nevertheless, be presented.

Setting Nutritional Goals. First, calorie and protein goals must be set, utilizing sound nutritional principles described in this and earlier chapters. In some centers the calorie goals are based on achieving or maintaining ideal body weight based on insurance company actuarial statistics.[137] Weights listed in such tables are those associated with lowest mortality. In some patients the usual body weight may be a more useful basis for judging calorie requirement, particularly when that weight has been the patient's standard for long periods of good health. The daily requirement for most patients with no more than moderate metabolic stress is 30 to 35 kcal/kg for maintenance; for weight gain at a modest rate, 40 kcal/kg may be required.

One gm of protein per kg of ideal body weight or usual body weight per day is usually ample to maintain or promote positive nitrogen balance. Patients with active disease resulting in loss of protein into the gastrointestinal tract or through fistulas often require as much as 1.5 gm of protein/kg/day.

Choosing Calorie Sources. Two sources of nonprotein calories are commercially available: dextrose solutions and lipid emulsions. Both can provide energy through oxidation, and either or both are capable of sparing body protein by providing calories that inhibit protein breakdown for gluconeogenesis. Wolfe demonstrated that maximal suppression of gluconeogenesis was observed with infusion of about 400 gm of glucose, or about 1600 kcal, per day. There appears to be a limit to the capacity to derive energy from infused glucose. The limits of nitrogen-sparing effects of glucose infusion are observed at about 35 kcal/kg/day.[138] Above this dose, one can expect increased fat synthesis from glucose and deposition of fat in the liver. Before widespread use of lipid emulsions, hepatomegaly, right upper quadrant pain, and liver function abnormalities were common complications of intensive nutrition support with hypertonic dextrose and amino acids solutions. Lipid emulsions not only provide a high-energy calorie source of 9 kcal/gm of fat but also provide a source of essential fatty acids, thus preventing essential fatty acid deficiency. Intravenous lipid emulsions are a suitable source of nonprotein calories that contribute to conservation of body protein. Recent clinical studies have confirmed that the most effective approach to providing energy is the combination of carbohydrate and fat. A regimen in which the calorie source is glucose alone compared with the one in which calories were derived nearly equally from fat and glucose resulted in similar weight gain, but protein repletion was achieved only in the combined regimen.[139] Thus, a regimen in which calories are supplied by both dextrose solutions and lipid emulsions, with fat providing 30 per cent or more of total calories, appears to be most effective.

Patients who have difficulty clearing these intravenous lipid particles, which are metabolized almost identically with chylomicrons, are an exception. In such patients, lipid must be given with great care to avoid persistent chylomicronemia and complications such as pancreatitis.

Protein Source. Infusion of a commercial mixture of essential and nonessential amino acids, in a ratio of about 1:4, in the presence of adequate calories can meet needs for protein balance. The optimal calorie to nitrogen ratio appears to be about 160:1 calories per gram.[140] At ratios of 100:1, weight loss and negative nitrogen balance have been observed.

Fluids. The 70-kg adult normally requires about 30 ml of water per kg of body weight or about 1 ml of fluid per kcal per day. The increased requirements of patients with fever, diarrhea, short bowel syndrome, or extensive fistula drainage must be taken into account along with the need for additional electrolytes. In patients with limitations of fluid intake imposed by cardiac status or cirrhosis, total volume will be an important factor in selecting solutions and infusion speed.

Vitamins, Minerals, and Trace Elements. Vitamins and trace minerals are provided in parenteral alimentation solutions in amounts designed to meet daily requirements of patients with disease (Table 106–7). In some cases these doses are several times the recommended dietary dose and therefore may be slightly higher than needed. Research on intravenous vitamin requirements is needed. Still, the usual values appear to have served well in view of the successful support of patients on home total parenteral nutrition for more than ten years. Experience with home total parenteral nutrition has reemphasized the necessity for certain vitamins and trace elements in human nutrition. Deficiency syndromes of biotin,[141] selenium,[142] zinc,[143] or copper[143] have been reported when any of these materials has been excluded from parenteral solutions, underlining the need to include all essential nutrients in parenteral solutions, particularly when prolonged intravenous therapy is planned.

Special problems exist in meeting iron requirements. Iron salts are generally incompatible with the usual intravenous solutions, and iron needs are therefore met by intermittent parenteral infusions or injections.

In the absence of a need to absorb dietary calcium from the gut, the intravenous requirements for vitamin D are uncertain. About 150 to 200 mEq of chloride and 90 to 120 mEq of sodium are required per day. Patients with fistulas in the gastrointestinal tract or those with gastroduodenal drainage may require up to twice that amount.

Many patients with gastrointestinal diseases require large amounts of potassium and magnesium to replace excessive losses in diarrhea. Along with phosphate these electrolytes are incorporated into tissue cells during nutritional repletion. Calcium intake is designed to meet or exceed calcium excretion in urine and stool as predicted from calcium balance studies. Adequate zinc is required for nutritional restitution and for positive nitrogen balance and wound healing. The requirements of zinc may be two or three times normal in patients with diarrhea and gastrointestinal fistulas.

Experience with Parenteral Nutrition in Various Gastrointestinal Disorders

While total parenteral nutrition has added significantly to our capacity to manage severe gastrointestinal disorders, its specific role in therapeutics continues to evolve. Controlled studies are badly needed. A review of reported experience to date, however, provides a helpful perspective.

Ulcerative Colitis. The decision to use total parenteral nutrition in the management of ulcerative colitis is usually based on the goal of maintaining adequate nutritional status in the face of a total bowel rest, nothing-by-mouth regimen in a patient who is losing large amounts of protein as well as blood in the gastrointestinal tract. Such patients are sometimes febrile and hypercatabolic. Parenteral nutrition and bowel rest are commonly viewed as an effort to achieve a clinical remission and avoid total proctocolectomy. Unfortunately, the reported experience does not appear to support the effectiveness of this approach in most instances.[145–150] From this experience one could predict an early clinical remission for one third to one half of the patients, with less than half of the patients actually avoiding surgery. The two controlled studies in this group found no difference between the control group on corticosteroids and diet and the total parenteral nutrition group in the avoidance of total colectomy.[148, 149] For those patients with severe acute colitis who fail to respond to corticosteroids, hospitalization with TPN may achieve nutritional maintenance, while a bowel rest regimen is employed as a final resort prior to surgery. Avoidance of nutritional deterioration rather than avoidance of surgery is probably the best

Table 106–7. TYPICAL DAILY TPN PRESCRIPTION FOR ADULT PATIENTS WITH GASTROINTESTINAL DISORDERS

Calories: about 40 kcal/kg of IBW*		Lipid: ⅓ nonprotein calories	
Protein: 1.0–1.5 gm/kg of IBW		Dextrose: ⅔ nonprotein calories	
Electrolytes and minerals (mEq)		Vitamins	
Sodium	90–120	A (IU)	3300
Potassium	90–150	C (mg)	100
Calcium	12–16	D (IU)	200
Magnesium	150–200	E (IU)	10
Chloride	12–16	K (mg)‡	—
Acetate	20–30	Thiamine, B_1 (mg)	3
Phosphorus	20–40 mmoles	Riboflavin, B_2 (mg)	3.6
Sulfate	12–16	Pyridoxine, B_6 (mg)	4
Trace elements		Niacinamide (mg)	40
Zinc (mg)	3–9	B_{12} (μg)	5
Copper (mg)	1–1.6	Pantothenate (mg)	15
Manganese (mg)	0.5	d-Biotin (μg)	60
Chromium (μg)	10–15	Folic acid (μg)	400
Selenium (μg)	120		
Molybdenum (μg)	20		
Iron†	—		

*IBW, ideal body weight (see reference 137).
†Iron administered as needed IM or by IV piggyback.
‡Vitamin K is administered intramuscularly, 5 mg/week.

justification for this strategy. Prolonged TPN and delay of inevitable surgery is not warranted (see pp. 1435–1477).

Crohn's Disease. From the results of many studies of patients with severe and symptomatic Crohn's disease, reasonable expectations of total parenteral nutrition with bowel rest include (1) weight gain and positive nitrogen balance in almost all patients when sufficient calories and protein are given, and (2) at least temporary remission of symptoms in 40 to 90 per cent of patients with Crohn's disease, with 56 per cent discharged in remission. Active disease of varying severity continues in the remainder (see pp. 1327–1358).

The observations in all the large series detailing remission rates and follow-up have been summarized in Table 106–8.[145–147, 151–155] Although parenteral nutrition and bowel rest are considered the core of therapy, most of these patients received simultaneous corticosteroid therapy. The initial in-hospital remission rate varied from 38 to 90 per cent, averaging 60 per cent. A long-term remission rate on the order of 56 per cent would tend to favor bowel rest and parenteral nutrition, even if, at two years, 10 to 30 per cent of patients require readmission for surgery. Some studies provide a breakdown of results as a function of disease site. For Crohn's colitis alone, Bos and coworkers[152] report remission in 18 out of 44 patients (41 per cent). In the study by McIntyre et al., none of the Crohn's colitis patients on TPN required surgery.[149] In Crohn's disease involving only small bowel, the data suggest a surprisingly good outcome. In a recent study from Toronto, excellent response to TPN was reported in Crohn's patients irrespective of disease location.[154]

Crohn's Disease with Fistulas. Reports that total parenteral nutrition was effective in the management of postoperative gastrointestinal fistulas[156] gave hope that total parenteral nutrition would be helpful also in this difficult and frustrating complication of Crohn's disease. In analyzing the reported experience, one must distinguish fistulas in Crohn's disease from postsurgical or posttraumatic fistulas. In the study of Elson and coworkers,[147] only one of five patients with Crohn's disease and fistulas had lasting benefit from total parenteral nutrition, and that patient had a postoperative enterocutaneous fistula that may not have been directly related to active Crohn's disease. Eisenberg and colleagues[157] had a similar experience: Only 2 of 18 Crohn's disease patients with fistulas treated with total parenteral nutrition avoided surgery. In contrast, Mullen and coworkers[146] evaluated their experience with total parenteral nutrition in the treatment of Crohn's fistulas. Their series included 37 fistulas in 20 patients studied. Fistula closure occurred in 32 per cent. The spontaneous closure rate of small bowel fistulas was twice that observed in large bowel disease. Greenberg and coworkers[151] found spontaneous closure of Crohn's fistulas in six of seven patients receiving total parenteral nutrition and prednisone but observed only one closure in seven patients receiving total parenteral nutrition alone. In Bos's series, only 3 of 12 enterocutaneous fistulas healed (see p. 1338).[152]

Table 106–8. PUBLISHED SERIES DESCRIBING THE USE OF TPN IN CROHN'S DISEASE

Investigator	Year	No. of Patients	Clinical Remission (in hospital) %	Reference
Reilly	1976	21	67	145
Mullen	1978	50	38	146
Elson*	1980	16	75	147
Greenberg*	1981	29	90	151
Bos	1981	59	47	152
Houcke	1980	36	75	153
Ostro	1985	100	77	154
Lerebours	1986	20	95	155

*Prospective studies.

Thus, bowel rest and total parenteral nutrition will lessen fistula drainage and maintain nutritional status. However, the remarkable improvement achieved in the TPN era in healing of noninflammatory fistulas of the gastrointestinal tract[158] cannot be expected in patients with Crohn's disease or radiation enteritis.

Growth Retardation. Growth retardation, variably defined, is reported in about 20 per cent of children and adolescents with Crohn's disease. Since total parenteral nutrition was shown in early studies to reverse growth arrest in all four patients so treated,[159] nutritional restitution, whether by oral or intravenous route, has been increasingly recognized as the principal determinant of restored growth.[160] Usually, oral restitution with supplemental formula diets as needed should be used to sustain adequate calorie and protein intakes and re-establish growth.[161] When symptoms are effectively controlled on drug regimens that avoid high-dose daily steroids, food intake may improve so that nutritional needs for growth are met. In some cases, dietary formula supplements are given by mouth or by tube[162] to achieve caloric and nutritional adequacy. Only rarely is intravenous therapy in the hospital or at home[163] required.

Pancreatic Disease. In patients with acute and, at times, fulminating pancreatic inflammation, a central therapeutic goal is to place the gland "at rest" and decrease the stimulus for production and release of proteolytic enzymes. Therefore, some patients are given parenteral nutritional support to prevent further deterioration during nasogastric suction while oral food intake is completely eliminated.

Two retrospective studies involving 44 and 73 patients with severe acute pancreatitis demonstrate that total parenteral nutrition is feasible in the management of patients with prolonged gastrointestinal tract dysfunction.[164, 165] Although during the first few weeks of therapy the incidence of catheter-associated sepsis was relatively high, the frequency of other total parenteral nutrition–related technical and metabolic complications was not excessive in these severely ill patients, nor was there evidence of unusual intolerance to fat emulsions. Total parenteral nutrition, however, did not significantly alter the mortality or the incidence and severity of non-nutritional complications associated with acute or chronic pancreatitis (see pp. 1814–1872).[165]

Short Bowel Syndrome. Parenteral nutrition has become an important means of managing patients with severe small bowel disease or following resection, both for relatively short periods to allow gut adaptation to occur and for long-term use at home in patients whose functioning small bowel remains inadequate for oral nutritional maintenance. In some patients, particularly those with extensive resections of colon and small bowel, home parenteral nutrition is indicated for greater fluid and electrolyte control as well as for calorie-protein support.

Home Total Parenteral Nutrition

The development of techniques for home total parenteral nutrition has revolutionized the management of patients whose nutritional disability is permanent or of long duration. Such regimens require intensive training of the patient and family and vigorously organized follow-up. Financial savings are substantial compared with TPN in hospital, and home total parenteral nutrition with infusion overnight permits return to a reasonably normal daytime routine and aids in social adjustment. The details of management differ somewhat, but the principles are unchanged. With experience now spanning more than fifteen years, total parenteral nutrition at home is increasingly used, progressively safer, and capable of achieving both nutritional and social rehabilitation in a majority of patients so treated.

The patients in whom total parenteral nutrition has been employed at home represent a difficult challenge for any therapy. Increased survival after massive intestinal resection is directly related to this mode of support. Home total parenteral nutrition has transformed the outcome of severe radiation enteritis and pseudo-obstruction, and some promising results have been reported in the subacute treatment of patients with Crohn's disease at home rather than in the hospital.[166]

Jeejeebhoy[167] first reported his experience with home parenteral nutrition in 12 patients, giving detailed metabolic studies and recommending a nutrient program. The high benefit-to-risk ratio was also reported by Fleming[168] in a series of 19 adult patients treated for a total duration of 485 patient-months. Social rehabilitation was accomplished in 12 of 18 surviving patients, nutritional rehabilitation was achieved in all, and complications were restricted to four catheter-related infections. In pediatric patients, the experience is growing,[163] confirming temporary improvement in growth patterns with nutritional support in those patients with inflammatory bowel disease and growth retardation.

Complications of TPN

Total parenteral nutrition is not an innocuous treatment. The large number of reported complications listed in Table 106–9 emphasizes the importance of carrying out this technique in the setting of an experienced multidisciplinary team or its equivalent.[169]

The most common complications are those related to catheter placement and management.[65] Septic complications can be minimized by maintaining strict and reproducible techniques performed by physicians or surgeons experienced in line insertion and by nurses trained in their management.

As experience with total parenteral nutrition for prolonged periods is extended, some clinical complications have emerged that are not yet clearly understood or predictably prevented. Earlier regimens utilizing excessive carbohydrate calories (actual "hyperalimentation") frequently caused hepatic tenderness and enzyme elevations reflecting hepatic steatosis. Abnormalities of hepatic function, most prominently serum aminotransferase elevations, are observed in over half of patients on TPN, even when calorie sources are balanced between carbohydrates and fat emulsions. The course is benign and abnormalities often disappear spontaneously even when TPN is continued;[170] in others, enzyme abnormalities resolve with decrease or cessation of TPN.

An unusual form of metabolic bone disease is re-

Table 106–9. COMPLICATIONS OF TOTAL PARENTERAL NUTRITION

Complication	Possible Preventive Measure
Catheter Placement	
Subclavian artery puncture, venous thrombosis, hemomediastinum, air embolism, catheter embolism, cardiac arrhythmia, myocardial perforation	Catheter placement by experienced operator; confirmation of catheter site by X-ray
Infection	
Catheter or line contamination, septic thrombophlebitis, bacteremia, fungal septicemia	Meticulous catheter care; exclusive use of catheter for TPN; specially trained nurses
Metabolic Complications	
Hyperglycemia, hyperosmolar coma, ketoacidosis, hypoglycemia, electrolyte or mineral imbalance	Careful monitoring and regular adjustment of prescription; careful control of rate of infusion
Hepatic Complications	
Hepatomegaly, fatty liver, enzyme elevations, cholestasis	Avoidance of carbohydrate overload
Nutritional Deficiencies	
Essential fatty acid, trace minerals (Zn, Cu, Cr, Se, Mn) vitamins (folate, K, B_{12}, biotin, and so forth)	Use of appropriate fat emulsions; trace minerals and all vitamins in intravenous prescription
Other Clinical Complications	Avoid excessive protein, ensure adequate phosphorus
Metabolic bone disease, hypercalciuria, gallstones	

ported in home total parenteral nutrition patients complaining of periarticular bone pain.[144, 171, 172] Bone biopsy changes in some are similar to those in osteomalacia. In others osteoporosis predominates. Both low and high 1,25 (OH) vitamin D levels have been reported. The relationship of this condition to observed hypercalciuria or to vitamin D status in such patients is uncertain. Recent studies have emphasized the role of other nutrients in worsening or ameliorating hypercalciuria and negative calcium balance, which must occur at the expense of the skeleton. Protein/amino acid infusions at doses above 1 gm/kg/day are associated with greater calciuria. The addition of acetate to offset protein-induced urinary acid loads or phosphate to enhance renal calcium retention may reduce urinary calcium losses and thereby restore positive calcium balance.[173]

Pancreatitis has been reported with hypercalcemia in patients on total parenteral nutrition.[174] Another potential cause of pancreatitis is hyperlipemia with inadequate clearing of intravenous lipid emulsion. Increased evidence of cholecystitis and cholelithiasis in patients on long-term total parenteral nutrition probably reflects gallbladder stasis. The increased cholesterol concentration in bile that occurs during fasting is also incriminated. Most of the metabolic abnormalities can be avoided or corrected by careful and regular monitoring of appropriate serum levels.

Summary

Whenever possible, the gastrointestinal tract should be used to correct nutritional deficiencies or prevent further deterioration. However, when total bowel rest is required for symptomatic control, techniques of parenteral nutrition offer opportunities that greatly expand therapeutic options. Total parenteral nutrition can be used to achieve nutritional repletion in the severely malnourished patient, to prevent nutritional deterioration in the patient on bowel rest, and to prepare the severely depleted patient for surgery. For the patient with short bowel syndrome following major intestinal resection, total parenteral nutrition can be used in the immediate postoperative period or for prolonged nutritional support at home until adaptive responses in the intestine permit oral nutritional maintenance. The published experience clearly emphasizes the need for a solid multidisciplinary approach to such therapy if appropriate degrees of safety and effectiveness are to be achieved.

References

1. Bistrian, B. R., Blackburn, G. L., Vitale, J., and Cochran, D. Prevalence of malnutrition in general medical patients. JAMA *235*:1567, 1976.
2. Bistrian, B. R., Blackburn, G. L., Hollowell, E., and Hedsle, R. Protein status of general surgical patients. JAMA *230*:858, 1974.
3. Bollet, A. J., and Owens, S. Evaluation of nutritional status of selected patients. Am. J. Clin. Nutr. *26*:931, 1973.
4. Willgutts, H. D. Nutritional assessment of 1,000 surgical patients in an affluent suburban community hospital. JPEN *1*:25, 1977.
5. Mullen, J. L., Gertner, M. N., Buzby, G. P., Goodhart, G. L., and Rosato, E. F. Implications of malnutrition in the surgical patient. Arch. Surg. *114*:121, 1979.
7. Bastow, M. D., Rawlings, J., and Allison, S. P. Benefits of supplementary tube feedings after fractured neck of femur: a randomized controlled trial. Lancet *287*:1589, 1983.
8. Pennington, J. A. T., and Church, H. N. Bowes and Church's Food Values of Portions Commonly Used. 14th ed. New York, Harper and Row, 1985.
9. Alpers, D. H., Clouse, R. E., and Stenson, W. F. Manual of Nutritional Therapeutics. Boston, Little, Brown and Co., 1983.
10. Bowen, P. E., McCallister, M., Thye, F. W., Taper, L. J., Sherry-Scaman, P. A., and Hecker, A. L. Bowel function and macronutrient absorption using fiber-augmented liquid formula diets. JPEN *6*:588, 1982.
11. Fisher, M., Adkins, W., Hall, L., Scaman, P., Hsi, S., and Marlett, J. The effects of dietary fiber in a liquid diet on bowel function of mentally retarded individuals. J. Ment. Defic. Res. Dec. *29*:(part 4):373, 1985.
12. Greenberger, N. J., Rodgers, J. B., and Isselbacher, K. J. Absorption of medium and long chain triglycerides: factors influencing their hydrolysis and transport. J. Clin. Invest. *45*:217, 1966.
13. Playoust, M. R., and Isselbacher, K. J. Studies on the intestinal absorption and intramucosal lipolysis of a medium chain triglyceride. J. Clin. Invest. *43*:878, 1964.
14. Bockus, H. L., Sarett, H. P., Hashim, S. A., Anderson, C. M., Isselbacher, K. J., and Jeffries, G. H. Practical problems in usage of medium chain triglycerides. *In* Senior, J. R. (ed.). Medium Chain Triglycerides. Philadelphia, University of Pennsylvania Press, 1968.
15. O'Connell, R. C., Morgan, A. P., Aoki, T. T., Ball, M. R., and Moore, F. S. Nitrogen conservation in starvation: graded response to intravenous glucose. J. Clin. Endocrinol. Metab. *39*:555, 1974.
16. Blackburn, G. L., Flatt, J. P., Clowes, G. H. A., and O'Donnell, T. E. Peripheral intravenous feeding with isotonic amino acid solutions. Am. J. Surg. *125*:447, 1973.
17. Schulte, W. J., Condon, R. E., and Kraus, M. A. Positive nitrogen balance using isotonic crystalline amino acid solution. Arch. Surg. *110*:914, 1975.
18. Hoover, H. C., Jr., Grant, J. P., Gorschboth, C., and Ketcham, S. Nitrogen-sparing intravenous fluids in postoperative patients. N. Engl. J. Med. *293*:172, 1975.
19. Freeman, J. B., Stegink, L. D., Fry, L. K., Sherman, B. M., and Denbesten, L. Evaluation of amino acid infusions as protein-sparing agents in normal adult subjects. Am. J. Clin. Nutr. *28*:477, 1975.
20. Greenberg, G. R., and Jeejeebhoy, K. N. Intravenous protein-sparing therapy in patients with gastrointestinal disease. JPEN *3*:427, 1979.
21. Blackburn, G. L. Factors influencing preservation of body cell mass using hypocaloric feeding of isotonic amino acid. Clinical Nutrition Update: Amino Acids. Chicago, AMA Symposium, 1977.
22. Edens, N. K., Gil, K. M., and Elwyn, D. H. The effects of varying energy and nitrogen intake on nitrogen balance, body composition, and metabolic rate. Clin. Chest Med. *7*:3, 1986.
23. Greenberg, G. R., Jeejeebhoy, K. N. Intravenous protein-sparing therapy in patients with gastrointestinal disease. JPEN *3*:427, 1979.
24. Wingate, D. L. Backwards and forwards with the migrating complex. Dig. Dis. Sci. *26*:641, 1981.
25. Vantrappen, G. R., Peeters, T. L., and Janssens, J. The secretory component of the interdigestive migrating motor complex in man. Scand. J. Gastroenterol. *13*:663, 1979.
26. Weisbrodt, N. W., Copeland, E. M., Thor, P. J., and Dudrick, S. J. The myoelectric activity of the small intestine of the dog during total parenteral nutrition. Proc. Soc. Exp. Biol. Med. *153*:121, 1976.
27. Torosian, M. H., Mullen, J. L. Nutritional assessment. *In*: Kaminsky, M. V., Jr. (ed.). Hyperalimentation: A Guide for Clinicians. New York, Marcel Dekker, 1985.
28. Alleyne, G. A. O., Viteri, F., and Alvarado, J. Indices of body composition in infantile malnutrition: total body potassium and urinary creatine. Am. J. Clin. Nutr. *23*:875, 1970.

29. Shizgal, H. M., Spanier, A. H., Humes, J., and Word, C. D. Indirect measurement of total exchangeable potassium. Am. J. Physiol. *233*:F253, 1977.
30. Moore, F. D., Olesen, K. H., McMurray, J. D., Parker, V. H., Ball, M. R., and Boyden, M. C. The body cell mass and its supporting environment. *In* Body Composition in Health and Disease. Philadelphia, W. B. Saunders Co., 1963.
31. Hill, G. L., McCarthy, I. D., Collins, J. P., and Smith, A. H. A new method for the rapid measurement of body composition in critically ill surgical patients. Br. J. Surg. *65*:732, 1978.
32. McNeill, K. G., Mernagh, J. R., Jeejeebhoy, K. N., Wolman, S. L., and Harrison, J. E. In vivo measurements of body protein based on the determination of nitrogen by prompt gamma analysis. Am. J. Clin. Nutr. *32*:1955, 1979.
33. Beddoe, A. H., and Hill, G. L. Clinical measurement of body composition using in vivo neutron activation analysis. JPEN *9*:504, 1985.
34. Baker, J. P., Detsky, A. S., Wesson, D. E., et al. Nutritional assessment: a comparison of clinical judgment and objective measurements. N. Engl. J. Med. *306*:969, 1982.
35. Keys, A., Brozek, J., Henschel, A., Mickelsen, D., Longstree, T., and Taylor, H. The Biology of Human Starvation, Vol. 1. Minneapolis, University of Minnesota Press, 1950, pp. 714–746.
36. Rixon, R. H., and Stevenson, J. A. Factors influencing survival of rats in fasting: metabolic rate and body weight loss. Am. J. Physiol. *188*:332, 1957.
37. Jensen, T. G., Englert, D. M., and Dudrick, S. J. Nutritional Assessment: A Manual for Practitioners. Norwalk, CT, Appleton-Century-Crofts, 1983.
38. Noppa, H., Anderson, M., Bengtsson, C., Bruce, A., and Isaksson, B. Body composition in middle-aged women with special references to the correlation between body fat mass and anthropometric data. Am. J. Clin. Nutr. *32*:1388, 1979.
39. Hall, J. C., O'Quigley, J., Giles, G. R., Appleton, N., and Stocks, H. Upper limb anthropometry: the value of measurement variance studies. Am. J. Clin. Nutr. *33*:1846, 1980.
40. Haas, J. D., and Flegal, K. M. Anthropometric measurements. *In* Newel G. R., and Ellison, N. M. (eds.). Nutrition and Cancer: Etiology and Treatment. New York, Raven Press, 1981.
41. Heymsfield, S. B., McManus, C. B., III, Seitz, S. B., Nixon, D. W., and Andrews, J. S. Anthropometric assessment of adult protein-energy malnutrition. *In* Wright, R. A., and Heymsfield, S. (eds.). Nutritional Assessment. Boston, Blackwell Scientific, 1984.
42. Bishop, C. W., Bowen, P. E., and Ritchey, S. J. Norms for nutritional assessment of American adults by upper arm anthropometry. Am. J. Clin. Nutr. *34*:2530, 1981.
43. Grant, J. P., Custer, P. B., and Thurlow, J. Current techniques of nutritional assessment. Surg. Clin. North Am. *61*:437, 1981.
44. Viteri, F. E., and Alvarado, J. The creatinine height index: its use in the degree of protein depletion and repletion in protein calorie malnourished children. Pediatrics *46*:696, 1970.
45. Forbes, G. B., and Bruining, G. J. Urinary creatinine excretion and lean body mass. Am. J. Clin. Nutr. *29*:1359, 1976.
46. Forse, R. A., and Shizgal, H. M. Serum albumin and nutritional status. JPEN *4*:450, 1980.
47. Buzby, G. P., Mullen, J. L., Matthews, D. C., Hobbs, C. L., and Rosato, E. F. Prognostic nutritional index in gastrointestinal surgery. Am. J. Surg. *139*:160, 1980.
48. Blackburn, G. L., Bistrian, B. R., Maini, B. S., Schlamm, H. T., and Smith, M. F. Nutritional and metabolic assessment of the hospitalized patient. JPEN *1*:11, 1977.
49. Sirisinha, S. R., Suskind, R., Edelman, C., Charupatana, C., and Olson, R. E. Complement and C_3 proactivator levels in children with protein-calorie malnutrition and effect of dietary treatment. Lancet *1*:1016, 1973.
50. Chandra, R. K. Serum complement and immunoconglutinin in malnutrition. Arch. Dis. Child. *50*:225, 1975.
51. Chandra, R. K. Rosette-forming T lymphocytes and cell-mediated immunity in malnutrition. Br. Med. J. *3*:608, 1974.
52. Smythe, P. M., Brereton-Stiles, G. G., Grace, H. J., Mafoyane, A., Schonland, M., Coovadia, M. H., Leoning, W. E. K., Parent, M. A., and Vos, G. H. Thymolymphatic deficiency and depression of cell-mediated immunity in protein-calorie malnutrition. Lancet *2*:939, 1971.
53. Neumann, G. J., Lawlor, C. G., Steihm, E. R., Swendseid, M. E., Newton, C., Herbert, J., Ammann, A. J., and Jacob, M. Immunological response in malnourished children. Am. J. Clin. Nutr. *28*:89, 1975.
54. Bistrian, B. R., Blackburn, G. L., Scrimshaw, N. W., and Flatt, J. P. Cellular immunity in semi-starved states in hospitalized adults. Am. J. Clin. Nutr. *28*:1148, 1975.
55. Law, D. K., Dudrick, S. J., and Abdon, N. I. Immunocompetence of patients with protein-calorie malnutrition. The effects of nutritional repletion. Ann. Intern. Med. *79*:545, 1973.
56. Dionigi, R., Zonta, A., Dominioni, L., Gnes, F., and Ballabio, A. The effects of total parenteral nutrition on immunodepression due to malnutrition. Ann. Surg. *185*:467, 1977.
57. Koster, F., Gaffer, A., and Jackson, T. M. Recovery of cellular immune competence during treatment of protein-calorie malnutrition. Am. J. Clin. Nutr. *34*:887, 1981.
58. Dionigi, P., Dionigi, R., Nazari, S., Bonoldi, A. P., Grizotti, A., Pavesi, F., Tibaldeschi, C., Cividini, F., and Grattoni, I. Nutritional and immunological evaluations in cancer patients. Relationship to surgical infections. JPEN *4*:351, 1980.
59. Kaminski, M. V., Jr., Fitzgerald, M. J., and Murphy, R. J. Correlation of mortality with serum transferrin and anergy. JPEN *1*:27, 1977.
60. Paige, D. M. Manual of Clinical Nutrition. Pleasantville, NJ, Nutrition Publications, 1983.
61. Woods, J. H., Drickson, L. W., Condon, R. E., Schulte, J. H., and Sillin, L. F. Postoperative ileus: a colonic problem. Surgery *84*:527, 1978.
62. Broviac, J. W., and Scribner, B. H. Prolonged parenteral nutrition in the home. Surg. Gynecol. Obstet. *139*:24, 1974.
63. Riella, M. C., and Scribner, B. H. Five years' experience with a right atrial catheter for prolonged parenteral nutrition at home. Surg. Gynecol. Obstet. *143*:205, 1976.
64. Heymsfield, S. B., Bethel, R. A., Ansley, J. D., Nixon, D. W., and Rudman, D. Enteral hyperalimentation: an alternative to central venous hyperalimentation. Ann. Intern. Med. *90*:63, 1979.
65. Padberg, F., Ruggerio, B. S., Blackburn, G. L., and Bistrian, B. R. Central venous catheterization for parenteral nutrition. Ann. Surg. *193*:264, 1981.
66. Sanderson, I., and Deitil, M. Intravenous hyperalimentation without sepsis. Surg. Gynecol. Obstet. *136*:577, 1973.
67. Grant, J. P. Handbook of Total Parenteral Nutrition. Philadelphia, W. B. Saunders Co., 1980, pp. 125–128.
68. Watesko, L. P., Sattler, L. L., and Steiger, E. Cost of a home parenteral nutrition program. JAMA *244*:2303, 1980.
69. Bennegard, K., Kindmark, L., Wickstrom, I., Schersten, T., and Lundholm, K. A comparative study of the efficiency of intragastric and parenteral nutrition in man. Am. J. Clin. Nutr. *40*:752, 1984.
70. Eastwood, G. L. Small bowel morphology and epithelial proliferation in intravenously alimented rabbits. Surgery *32*:613, 1977.
71. Johnson, L. R., Copeland, E. M., Dudrick, S. J., Lichtenberger, L. M., and Castro, A. G. Structural and hormonal alteration in the gastrointestinal tract of parenterally fed rats. Gastroenterology *68*:1177, 1975.
72. Levine, G. M., Deren, J. J., Steiger, E., and Zinno, R. Role of oral intake in maintenance of gut mass and disaccharidase activity. Gastroenterology *67*:975, 1974.
73. Gustke, R. F., Varma, R. R., and Soergel, K. H. Gastric reflux during perfusion of the small bowel. Gastroenterology *59*:890, 1970.
74. Boscoe, M. J., and Rosin, M. D. Fine bore enteral feeding and pulmonary aspiration. Br. Med. J. *289*:1421, 1984.
75. Ramos, S. M., and Lindine, P. Inexpensive, safe and simple nasoenteral intubation—an alternative for the cost conscious. JPEN *10*:78, 1986.
76. Thurlow, P. M. Bedside enteral feeding tube placement into duodenum and jejunum. JPEN *10*:104, 1986.
77. Bethel, R. A., Jansen, R. D., Heymsfield, S. B., Ansler, J. D., Hersh, T., and Rudman, D. Nasogastric hyperalimentation

through a polyethylene catheter: an alternative to central venous hyperalimentation. Am. J. Clin. Nutr. *32*:1112, 1979.

78. Engel, S. Gastrostomy. Surg. Clin. North Am. *49*:1289, 1969.
79. Wasiljew, B. K., Ujiki, G. T., and Beal, J. M. Feeding gastrostomy: complications and mortality. Am. J. Surg. *143*:194, 1982.
80. Adams, M. B., Seabrook, G. R., Quebbeman, E. A., and Condon, R. E. Jejunostomy: a rarely indicated procedure. Arch. Surg. *121*:236, 1986.
81. Rombeau, J. L., Barot, L. R., Low, D. W., and Twomey, P. L. Feeding by tube enterostomy. *In* Rombeau, J. L., and Caldwell, M. D. (eds.). Clinical Nutrition. Vol. 1, Enteral and Tube Feeding. Philadelphia, W. B. Saunders Co., 1984.
82. Gauderer, M. W. L., Ponsky, J. L., and Izant, R. J. Gastrostomy without laparotomy: a percutaneous endoscopic technique. J. Pediatr. Surg. *15*:872, 1980.
83. Ponsky, J. L., and Gauderer, M. W. L. Percutaneous endoscopic gastrostomy: a non-operative technique for feeding gastrostomy. Gastrointest Endosc. *27*:9, 1981.
84. Ponsky, J. L., Gauderer, M. W. L., and Stellato, T. A. Percutaneous endoscopic gastrostomy: review of 150 cases. Arch. Surg. *118*:913, 1983.
85. Larson, D. E., Fleming, C. R., Ott, B. J., Schroeder, K. W. Percutaneous endoscopic gastrostomy: simplified access for enteral nutrition. Mayo Clin. Proc. *58*:103, 1983.
86. Russel, T. R., Brothman, M., and Norris, F. Percutaneous gastrostomy: a new simplified and cost-effective technique. Am. J. Surg. *148*:132, 1984.
87. Strodel, W. E., Eckhauser, F. E., and Lemmer, J. H. Endoscopic percutaneous gastrostomy. Contemp. Surg. *23*:17, 1983.
88. Plumeri, P. A., Wesner, N. N., and Cohen, N. N. Percutaneous endoscopic gastrostomy. Pa. Med. May:57, 1983.
89. Kirby, D. F., Craig, R. M., Tsang, T., and Plotnick, B. H. Percutaneous endoscopic gastrostomies: a prospective evaluation and review of the literature. JPEN *10*:155, 1986.
90. Stasser, W. N., McCullough, A. J., and Marshall, J. B. Percutaneous endoscopic gastrostomy: another cause of "benign" pneumoperitoneum. Gastrointest. Endosc. *30*:296, 1984.
91. Ponsky, J. L. Evolving trends in enteral alimentation. Surg. Ann. *18*:327, 1986.
92. Ho, C-S., Gray, R. R., Goldfinger, M., Rosen, I. E., and McPherson, R. Percutaneous gastrostomy for enteral feeding. Radiology *156*:349, 1985.
93. Tao, H. H., and Gillies, R. R. Percutaneous gastrostomy. AJR *141*:793, 1983.
94. Dills, J. S., and Oglesby, J. Percutaneous gastrostomy. Radiology *149*:449, 1983.
95. Train, J. S., Dan, S. J., and Mitty, H. A. Percutaneous transhepatic hyperalimentation for patients with biliary drainage catheters. AJR *144*:255, 1985.
96. Bucklin, D. L., and Gilsdorf, R. B. Percutaneous needle pharyngostomy. JPEN *9*:68, 1985.
97. Campbell, I. T., Morton, R. P., Cole, J. A., Raine, C. H., Shapiro, L. M., and Still, P. M. A comparison of the effects of intermittent and continuous nasogastric feeding on the oxygen consumption and nitrogen balance of patients after major head and neck surgery. Am. J. Clin. Nutr. *38*:870, 1983.
98. Keohane, P. P., Attrill, H., Love, M., Frost, P., and Silk, D. B. Relation between osmolality of diet and gastrointestinal side effects in enteral nutrition. Br. Med. J. *288*:678, 1984.
99. Rees, R. G., Keohane, P. P., Grimble, G. K., Frost, P. G., Attrill, H., and Silk, D. B. Tolerance of elemental diet administered without starter regimens. Br. Med. J. *290*:1869, 1985.
100. Perrault, J., Devroede, G., and Bounous, G. Effects of an elemental diet in healthy volunteers. Gastroenterology *64*:569, 1973.
101. Bury, K. D., and Jambunathan, G. Effects of elemental diets on gastric emptying and gastric secretion in man. Am. J. Surg. *127*:59, 1974.
102. Christie, D. L., and Ament, M. E. Dilute elemental diet and continuous infusion techniques for management of short bowel syndrome. J. Pediatr. *87*:705, 1975.
103. Voitk, A., Echave, V., Brown, R., and Gurd, F. N. Use of an elemental diet during the adaptive stage of short gut syndrome. Gastroenterology *65*:419, 1973.
104. Bury, K. D. Elemental diets. *In* Fischer, J. E. (ed.). Total Parenteral Nutrition. Boston, Little, Brown and Co., 1976, pp. 395–411.
105. Hinsdale, J. G., Lipkowitz, G. S., Pollock, T. W., Hoover, E. L., and Jaffe, B. M. Prolonged enteral nutrition in malnourished patients with nonelemental feeding. Reappraisal of surgical technique, safety, and costs. Am. J. Surg. *149*:334, 1985.
106. Yeung, C. K., Yound, G. A., Haekett, A. F., and Hill, G. L. Fine needle catheter jejunostomy—an assessment of a new method of nutritional support after major gastrointestinal surgery. Br. J. Surg. *66*:727, 1979.
107. Delany, H. M., Carnevale, N., Garvey, J. W., and Moss, C. M. Post-operative nutritional support using needle catheter feeding jejunostomy. Ann Surg. *186*:165, 1977.
108. Hoover, H. C., Jr., Ryan, J. A., Anderson, E. J., and Fischer, J. E. Nutritional benefits of immediate postoperative jejunal feeding of an elemental diet. Am. J. Surg. *139*:153, 1980.
109. Adams, M. B., Seabrook, G. R., Quebbeman, E. A., and Condon, R. E. Jejunostomy: a rarely indicated procedure. Arch. Surg. *121*:236, 1986.
110. Hayashi, J. T., Wolfe, B. M., and Calvert, C. C. Limited efficacy of early postoperative jejunal feeding. Am. J. Surg. *150*:52, 1985.
111. Smith, R. C., Hartemink, R. J., Hollinshead, J. W., and Gillett, D. J. Fine bore jejunostomy feeding following major abdominal surgery: a controlled randomized clinical trial. Br. J. Surg. *72*:458, 1985.
112. Hinder, R. A., and Kelly, K. A. Canine gastric emptying of solids and liquids. Am. J. Physiol. *233*:E335, 1977.
113. Silberman, H., Silberman, A. W. Parenteral nutrition, biochemistry and respiratory gas exchange. JPEN *10*:151, 1986.
114. Askanazi, J., Weissman, C., Rosenbaum, S. H., Hyman, A. J., Milic-Emili, J., and Kinney, J. M. Nutrition and the respiratory system. Crit. Care Med. *10*:163, 1982.
115. Askanazi, J., Elwyn, D. H., Silverberg, P. A., Rosenbaum, S. H., and Kinney, J. M. Respiratory distress secondary to a high carbohydrate load: a case report. Surgery *87*:596, 1980.
116. Covelli, H. D., Black, J. W., Olsen, M. S., and Beekman, J. F. Respiratory failure precipitated by high carbohydrate loads. Ann. Intern. Med. *95*:570, 1981.
117. Bartlett, R. H., Deckert, R. E., Mault, J. R., and Clark, S. F. Metabolic studies in chest trauma. J. Thorac. Cardiovasc. Surg. *87*:503, 1984.
118. Heymsfield, S. B., Erbland, M., Casper, K., Grossman, G., Roongpisuthipong, C., Hoff, J., and Head, C. A. Enteral nutrition support: metabolic, cardiovascular, and pulmonary interrelations. Clin. Chest Med. *7*:41, 1986.
119. Alvestrand, A., Ahlberg, M., Furst, P., and Bergstrom, J. Clinical experience with amino acid and keto acid diets. Am. J. Clin. Nutr. *33*:1654, 1980.
120. Fischer, J. E., Yoshimura, N., Aguirre, A. L., James, J. H., Cummings, M. G., Abel, R. M., and Deindoerfer, F. Plasma amino acids in patients with hepatic encephalopathy: effects of amino acid infusions. Am. J. Surg. *127*:40, 1973.
121. Maddrey, W. C., Weber, F. L., Coulter, A. W., Chura, C. M., Chapanis, N. P., and Walser, M. Effects of ketoanalogues of essential amino acids in portal-systemic encephalopathy. Gastroenterology *71*:190, 1976.
122. Cascino, A., Cangiano, C., Calcaterra, U., Rossi-Fanelli, F., and Capocaccia, L. Plasma amino acids imbalance in patients with liver disease. Am. J. Dig. Dis. *23*:591, 1978.
123. Fischer, J. E., Rosen, H. M., James, J. H., Ebeid, A. M., James, H. J., Keane, J. M., and Soeters, P. B. The effect of normalization of plasma amino acid on hepatic encephalopathy in man. Surgery *80*:77, 1976.
124. Herlong, H. F., Maddrey, W. C., and Walser, M. The use of ornithine salts of branched-chain ketoacids in portal-systemic encephalopathy. Ann. Intern. Med. *93*:545, 1980.
125. Newmark, S. R., Simpson, S., Beskitt, P., Black, J., and Sublett, D. Home tube feeding for long-term nutritional support. JPEN *5*:76, 1981.
126. Chrysomilides, S. A., and Kaminski, M. V., Jr. Home enteral and parenteral nutrition support. Am. J. Clin. Nutr. *34*:2271, 1981.
127. Woolfson, A. M. J., Ricketts, C. R., Hardy, S. M., Saour, J.

N., Pollard, B. J., and Allison, S. P. Prolonged nasogastric tube feeding in critically ill and surgical patients. Postgrad. Med. J. *52*:678, 1976.

128. O'Hara, I. G., Kennedy, S., and Lizewski, W. Effects of long-term elemental nasogastric feeding on elderly debilitated patients. Can. Med. Assoc. J. *108*:977, 1973.
129. Jhangiani, S., Prince, L., Holmes, R., and Agarwal, N. Clinical zinc deficiency during long-term total enteral nutrition. J Am. Geriatr. Soc. *34*:385, 1986.
130. Stellato, T. A., Danziger, L. H., Nearman, H. S., and Creger, R. J. Inadvertent intravenous administration of enteral diet. JPEN *8*:453, 1984.
131. Kaminski, M. V., Jr. Enteral hyperalimentation. Surg. Gynecol. Obstet. *143*:12, 1976.
132. Miller, K. S., Tomlinson, J. R., and Sahn, S. A. Pleuropulmonary complications of enteral tube feedings. Two reports, review of the literature, and recommendations. Chest *88*:230, 1985.
133. Walike, J. W. Tube feeding syndrome in head and neck surgery. Arch. Otolaryngol. *29*:533, 1969.
134. Dudrick, S. J., Wilmore, D. W., Vars, H. M., and Rhoads, J. E. Long-term total parenteral nutrition with growth, development and positive nitrogen balance. Surgery *64*:134, 1968.
135. White, P. L., and Nagy, M. E. (eds.). Total Parenteral Nutrition. Acton, Mass. Publishing Sciences Group, Inc. 1974.
136. Fischer, J. E. Total Parenteral Nutrition. Boston, Little Brown and Co., 1976.
137. 1979 Build Study. Society of Actuaries and Association of Life Insurance Medical Directors of America, 1980.
138. Wolfe, P. R., O'Donnell, T. F., Stone, M. D., Richmand, D. A., and Burke, J. F. Investigation of factors determining the optimal glucose infusion rate in total parenteral nutrition. Metabolism *29*:892, 1980.
139. MacFis, J., Smith, R. C., and Hill, G. L. Glucose or fat as a non-protein energy source? A controlled clinical trial in patients requiring intravenous nutrition. Gastroenterology *80*:103, 1981.
140. Peters, C., and Fischer, J. E. Studies on calorie to nitrogen ratio for total parenteral nutrition. Surg. Gynecol. Obstet. *151*:1, 1980.
141. Mock, D. M., Delorimer, A. A., Liebman, W. M., Sweetman, L., and Baker, H. Biotin deficiency. Unusual complication of parenteral alimentation. N. Engl. J. Med. *304*:820, 1981.
142. Johnson, R. A., Baker, S. S., Fallon, J. T., Maynard, E. P., Ruskin, J. N., Wen, Z., Ge, K., and Cohen, H. J. An accidental case of cardiomyopathy and selenium deficiency. N. Engl. J. Med. *304*:1210, 1981.
143. Solomons, N. W., Layden, T. J., and Rosenberg, I. R. Plasma trace metals during total parenteral alimentation. Gastroenterology *70*:1022, 1976.
144. Klein, G. L., Horst, R. L., Norman, A. W., Ament, M. E., Slatopolsky, E., and Coburn, J. W. Reduced serum levels of 1,25-dihydroxyvitamin D during long-term total parenteral nutrition. Ann. Intern. Med. *94*:638, 1981.
145. Reilly, J., Ryan, J. A., Strole, W., and Fischer, J. E. Hyperalimentation in inflammatory bowel disease. Am. J. Surg. *131*:192, 1976.
146. Mullen, J. L., Hargrove, W. C., Dudrick, S. J., Fitts, W. T., Jr., and Rosato, E. F. Ten years experience with intravenous hyperalimentation and inflammatory bowel disease. Ann. Surg. *187*:523, 1978.
147. Elson, C. O., Layden, T. J., Nemchausky, B. A., Rosenberg, J., and Rosenberg, I. H. An evaluation of total parenteral nutrition in the management of inflammatory bowel disease. Dig. Dis. Sci. *25*:42, 1980.
148. Dickinson, R. J., Ashton, M. G., Axon, A. T. R., Smith, R. C., Yeung, C. K., and Hill, G. L. Controlled trial of intravenous hyperalimentation and total bowel rest as an adjunct to the routine therapy of acute colitis. Gastroenterology *79*:1199, 1980.
149. McIntyre, P. B., Powell-Tuck, J., Wood, S. R., Lennard-Jones, J. E., Lerebours, E., Hecketsweiler, P., Galmiche, J. P., and Colin, R. Controlled trial of bowel rest in the treatment of severe acute colitis. Gut *27*:481, 1986.
150. Jarnerot, G., Rolny, P., and Sandberg-Gertzen, H. Intensive intravenous treatment of ulcerative colitis. Gastroenterology *89*:1005, 1985.
151. Greenberg, G. R., and Jeejeebhoy, K. N. Total parenteral nutrition in the primary management of Crohn's disease. *In* Perie, A. S. (ed.). Recent Advances in Crohn's Disease. The Hague, Martinus Nijhoff, 1981, pp. 492–498.
152. Bos, L. P., Nube, M., and Weterman, I. T. Total parenteral nutrition in Crohn's disease: A clinical evaluation. *In* Perie A. S. (ed.). Recent Advances in Crohn's Disease. The Hague, Martinus Nijhoff, 1981, pp. 499–506.
153. Houcke, P., Roger, J., Blais, J., Gallot, P., Brunnetaud, J. M., and Paris, J. C. Exclusive parenteral nutrition. Results in 45 acute exacerbations of Crohn's disease. Nouv. Presse Med. *9*:1361, 1980.
154. Ostro, M. J., Greenberg, G. R., Jeejeebhoy, K. N. Total parenteral nutrition and complete bowel rest in the management of Crohn's disease. JPEN *9*:280, 1985.
155. Lerebours, E., Messing, B., Chevalier, B., Bories, C., Colin, R., and Bernier, J. J. An evaluation of total parenteral nutrition in the management of steroid-dependent and steroid-resistant patients with Crohn's disease. JPEN *10*:274, 1986.
156. Soerters, P. B., Ebeid, A. M., and Fischer, J. E. Review of 404 patients with gastrointestinal fistulas. Ann. Surg. *190*:189, 1979.
157. Eisenberg, H. W., Turnbull, R. B., Jr., and Weakley, F. F. Hyperalimentation as preparation for surgery in transmural colitis. Dis. Colon Rectum *17*:469, 1974.
158. Rose, D., Yarborough, M. F., Canizaro, P. C., and Lowry, S. F. One hundred and fourteen fistulas of the gastrointestinal tract treated with total parenteral nutrition. Surg. Gynecol. Obstet. *163*:347, 1986.
159. Layden, T., Rosenberg, J., Nemchausky, B., Elson, C., and Rosenberg, I. Reversal of growth arrest in adolescents with Crohn's disease after parenteral alimentation. Gastroenterology *70*:1017, 1976.
160. Kelts, D. G., Grand, R. J., Shen, G., Watkins, J. B., Werlin, S. L., and Boehme, C. Nutritional basis of growth failure in children and adolescents with Crohn's disease. Gastroenterology *76*:720, 1979.
161. Kirschner, B. S., Klich, J. R., Kalman, S. S., DeFavaro, M. V., and Rosenberg, I. H. Reversal of growth retardation in Crohn's disease with therapy emphasing oral nutritional restitution. Gastroenterology *80*:10, 1981.
162. Morin, C. L., Roulet, M., Roy, C. C., and Weber, A. Continuous elemental enteral alimentation in children with Crohn's disease and growth failure. Gastroenterology *79*:1205, 1980.
163. Strobel, C. T., Byrne, W. J., and Ament, M. E. Home parenteral nutrition in children with Crohn's disease: an effective management alternative. Gastroenterology *77*:272, 1979.
164. Goodgame, J. T., and Fischer, J. E. Parenteral nutrition in the treatment of acute pancreatitis. Ann. Surg. 186:651, 1977.
165. Grant, J. P., James, S., Grabowski, V., Trexler, K. M. Total parenteral nutrition in pancreatic disease. Ann. Surg. *200*:627, 1984.
166. Kushner, R. F., Shapir, J., and Sitrin, M. D. Endoscopic, radiographic and clinical response to prolonged bowel rest and home parenteral nutrition in Crohn's disease. JPEN *10*:568, 1986.
167. Jeejeebhoy, K. N., Langer, B., Tsallas, G., Chu, R. C., Kuksis, A., and Anderson, G. H. Total parenteral nutrition at home: Studies in patients surviving 4 months to 5 years. Gastroenterology *71*:943, 1976.
168. Fleming, C. R., Beart, R. W., Beckner, S., McGill, D. B., and Gaffron, R. Home parenteral nutrition for management of the severely malnourished adult patient. Gastroenterology *79*:11, 1980.
169. Nehme, A. Nutritional support of the hospitalized patient, the team concept. JAMA *243*:1906, 1980.
170. Baker, A. L., and Rosenberg, I. H. Complications of total parenteral nutrition. Am. J. Med. *82*:489, 1987.
171. Klein, G. L., Targoff, C. M., Ament, M. E., Sherrard, D. J.,

Bluestone, R., Young, J. H., Normann, A. W., and Coburn, J. W. Bone disease associated with total parenteral nutrition. Lancet *2*:1041, 1980.

172. Shike, M., Sturtridge, W. C., Tam, C. S., Harrison, J. E., Jones, G., Murray, T. M., Hudson, H., Whitwell, J., Wilson, D. R., and Jeejeebhoy, K. N. A possible role of vitamin D in the group of parenteral nutrition—induced metabolic bone disease. Ann. Intern. Med. *95*:560, 1981.

173. Wood, R. J., Sitrin, M. D., Cusson, G. J., et al. Reduction of total parenteral nutrition-induced urinary calcium loss by increasing the phosphorus in the total parenteral nutrition prescription. JPEN *10*:188, 1986.

174. Izsak, E. M., Shike, M., Roulet, M., and Jeejeebhoy, K. N. Pancreatitis in association with hypercalcemia in patients receiving total parenteral nutrition. Gastroenterology *79*:555, 1980.

INDEX

Note: Page numbers in *italics* refer to illustrations;
Roman numerals refer to illustrations in color section;
page numbers followed by (t) refer to tables.